Dietary Reference Intakes (DRIs): Recommended Dietary Allowances and Adequate Intakes, Vitamins*

Food and Nutrition Board, Institute of Medicine, National Academies

Life Stage Group	Vitamin A (mcg/d)[a]	Vitamin C (mg/d)	Vitamin D (IU/d)[b,c]	Vitamin E (mg/d)[d]	Vitamin K (mcg/d)	Thiamin (mg/d)	Riboflavin (mg/d)	Niacin (mg/d)[e]	Vitamin B6 (mg/d)	Folate (mcg/d)[f]	Vitamin B12 (mcg/d)	Pantothenic Acid (mg/d)	Biotin (mcg/d)	Choline (mg/d)[g]
Infants														
Birth to 6 mo	400*	40*	400[h]	4*	2.0*	0.2*	0.3*	2*	0.1*	65*	0.4*	1.7*	5*	125*
6 to 12 mo	500*	50*	400[h]	5*	2.5*	0.3*	0.4*	4*	0.3*	80*	0.5*	1.8*	6*	150*
Children														
1-3 yr	300	15	600	6	30*	0.5	0.5	6	0.5	150	0.9	2*	8*	200*
4-8 yr	400	25	600	7	55*	0.6	0.6	8	0.6	200	1.2	3*	12*	250*
Males														
9-13 yr	600	45	600	11	60*	0.9	0.9	12	1.0	300	1.8	4*	20*	375*
14-18 yr	900	75	600	15	75*	1.2	1.3	16	1.3	400	2.4	5*	25*	550*
19-30 yr	900	90	600	15	120*	1.2	1.3	16	1.3	400	2.4	5*	30*	550*
31-50 yr	900	90	600	15	120*	1.2	1.3	16	1.3	400	2.4	5*	30*	550*
51-70 yr	900	90	600	15	120*	1.2	1.3	16	1.7	400	2.4[i]	5*	30*	550*
>70 yr	900	90	800	15	120*	1.2	1.3	16	1.7	400	2.4[i]	5*	30*	550*
Females														
9-13 yr	600	45	600	11	60*	0.9	0.9	12	1.0	300	1.8	4*	20*	375*
14-18 yr	700	65	600	15	75*	1.0	1.0	14	1.2	400[i]	2.4	5*	25*	400*
19-30 yr	700	75	600	15	90*	1.1	1.1	14	1.3	400[i]	2.4	5*	30*	425*
31-50 yr	700	75	600	15	90*	1.1	1.1	14	1.3	400[i]	2.4	5*	30*	425*
51-70 yr	700	75	600	15	90*	1.1	1.1	14	1.5	400	2.4[i]	5*	30*	425*
>70 yr	700	75	600	15	90*	1.1	1.1	14	1.5	400	2.4[i]	5*	30*	425*
Pregnancy														
14-18 yr	750	80	600	15	75*	1.4	1.4	18	1.9	600[k]	2.6	6*	30*	450*
19-30 yr	770	85	600	15	90*	1.4	1.4	18	1.9	600[k]	2.6	6*	30*	450*
31-50 yr	770	85	600	15	90*	1.4	1.4	18	1.9	600[k]	2.6	6*	30*	450*
Lactation														
14-18 yr	1200	115	600	19	75*	1.4	1.6	17	2.0	500	2.8	7*	35*	550*
19-30 yr	1300	120	600	19	90*	1.4	1.6	17	2.0	500	2.8	7*	35*	550*
31-50 yr	1300	120	600	19	90*	1.4	1.6	17	2.0	500	2.8	7*	35*	550*

Sources: *Dietary Reference Intakes for Calcium, Phosphorus, Magnesium, Vitamin D, and Fluoride* (1997); *Dietary Reference Intakes for Thiamin, Riboflavin, Niacin, Vitamin B6, Folate, Vitamin B12, Pantothenic Acid, Biotin, and Choline* (1998); *Dietary Reference Intakes for Vitamin C, Vitamin E, Selenium, and Carotenoids* (2000); *Dietary Reference Intakes for Vitamin A, Vitamin K, Arsenic, Boron, Chromium, Copper, Iodine, Iron, Manganese, Molybdenum, Nickel, Silicon, Vanadium, and Zinc* (2001); *Dietary Reference Intakes for Water, Potassium, Sodium, Chloride, and Sulfate* (2005); and *Dietary Reference Intakes for Calcium and Vitamin D* (2011). These reports may be accessed via www.nap.edu.

*NOTE: This table (taken from the DRI reports, see www.nap.edu) presents Recommended Dietary Allowances (RDAs) in **boldface** type and Adequate Intakes (AIs) in lightface type followed by an asterisk (*). An RDA is the average daily dietary intake level; sufficient to meet the nutrient requirements of nearly all (97-98%) healthy individuals in a group. It is calculated from an Estimated Average Requirement (EAR). If sufficient scientific evidence is not available to establish an EAR, and thus calculate an RDA, an AI is usually developed. For healthy breastfed infants, an AI is the mean intake. The AI for other life stage and gender groups is believed to cover the needs of all healthy individuals in the groups, but lack of data or uncertainty in the data prevent being able to specify with confidence the percentage of individuals covered by this intake.

[a] As retinol activity equivalents (RAEs). 1 RAE = 1 mcg of retinol, 12 mcg of β-carotene, 24 mcg of α-carotene, or 24 mcg of β-cryptoxanthin. The RAE for dietary provitamin A carotenoids is twofold greater than retinol equivalents (REs), whereas the RAE for preformed vitamin A is the same as the RE for vitamin A.

[b] As cholecalciferol. 1 mcg of cholecalciferol = 40 IU of vitamin D.

[c] Under the assumption of minimal sunlight.

[d] As α-tocopherol. α-Tocopherol includes RRR-α-tocopherol, the only form of α-tocopherol that occurs naturally in foods, and the 2R-stereoisomeric forms of α-tocopherol (RRR-, RSR-, RRS-, and RSS-α-tocopherol) that occur in fortified foods and supplements. It does not include the 2S-stereoisomeric forms of α-tocopherol (SRR-, SSR-, SRS-, and SSS-α-tocopherol), also found in fortified foods and supplements.

[e] As niacin equivalents (NEs). 1 mg of niacin = 60 mg of tryptophan; 0-6 months = preformed niacin (not NE).

[f] As dietary folate equivalents (DFEs). 1 DFE = 1 mcg of food folate = 0.6 mcg of folic acid from fortified food or as a supplement consumed with food = 0.5 mcg of a supplement taken on an empty stomach.

[g] Although AIs have been established for choline, there are few data to assess whether a dietary supply of choline is needed at all stages of the life cycle, and it may be that the choline requirement can be met by endogenous synthesis at some of these stages.

[h] Life-stage groups for infants were 0-5.9 and 6-11.9 months.

[i] Because 10% to 30% of older people may malabsorb food-bound B12, it is advisable for those older than 50 years to meet their RDA mainly by consuming foods fortified with B12 or a supplement containing B12.

[j] In view of evidence linking folate intake with neural tube defects in the fetus, it is recommended that all women capable of becoming pregnant consume 400 mcg from supplements or fortified foods in addition to intake of food from a varied diet.

[k] It is assumed that women will continue consuming 400 mcg from supplements or fortified food until their pregnancy is confirmed and they enter prenatal care, which ordinarily occurs after the end of the periconceptional period—critical time for formation of the neural tube.

Dietary Reference Intakes (DRIs): Recommended Dietary Allowances and Adequate Intakes, Elements

Food and Nutrition Board, Institute of Medicine, National Academies

Life Stage Group	Calcium (mg/d)	Chromium (mcg/d)	Copper (mcg/d)	Fluoride (mg/d)	Iodine (mcg/d)	Iron (mg/d)	Magnesium (mg/d)	Manganese (mg/d)	Molybdenum (mcg/d)	Phosphorus (mg/d)	Selenium (mcg/d)	Zinc (mg/d)	Potassium (mg/d)	Sodium (mg/d)	Chloride (g/d)
Infants															
Birth to 6 mo	200*a	0.2*	200*	0.01*	110*	0.27*	30*	0.003*	2*	100*	15*	2*	400*	110*	0.18*
6 to 12 mo	260*a	5.5*	220*	0.5*	130*	11	75*	0.6*	3*	275*	20*	3	860*	370*	0.57*
Children															
1-3 yr	700	11*	340	0.7*	90	7	80	1.2*	17	460	20	3	2000*	800*	1.5*
4-8 yr	1000	15*	440	1*	90	10	130	1.5*	22	500	30	5	2300*	1000*	1.9*
Males															
9-13 yr	1300	25*	700	2*	120	8	240	1.9*	34	1250	40	8	2500*	1200*	2.3*
14-18 yr	1300	35*	890	3*	150	11	410	2.2*	43	1250	55	11	3000*	1500*	2.3*
19-30 yr	1000	35*	900	4*	150	8	400	2.3*	45	700	55	11	3400*	1500*	2.3*
31-50 yr	1000	35*	900	4*	150	8	420	2.3*	45	700	55	11	3400*	1500*	2.3*
51-70 yr	1000	30*	900	4*	150	8	420	2.3*	45	700	55	11	3400*	1500*	2.0*
>70 yr	1200	30*	900	4*	150	8	420	2.3*	45	700	55	11	3400*	1500*	1.8*
Females															
9-13 yr	1300	21*	700	2*	120	8	240	1.6*	34	1250	40	8	2300*	1200*	2.3*
14-18 yr	1300	24*	890	3*	150	15	360	1.6*	43	1250	55	9	2300*	1500*	2.3*
19-30 yr	1000	25*	900	3*	150	18	310	1.8*	45	700	55	8	2600*	1500*	2.3*
31-50 yr	1000	25*	900	3*	150	18	320	1.8*	45	700	55	8	2600*	1500*	2.3*
51-70 yr	1200	20*	900	3*	150	8	320	1.8*	45	700	55	8	2600*	1500*	2.0*
>70 yr	1200	20*	900	3*	150	8	320	1.8*	45	700	55	8	2600*	1500*	1.8*
Pregnancy															
14-18 yr	1300	29*	1000	3*	220	27	400	2.0*	50	1250	60	12	2600*	1500*	2.3*
19-30 yr	1000	30*	1000	3*	220	27	350	2.0*	50	700	60	11	2900*	1500*	2.3*
31-50 yr	1000	30*	1000	3*	220	27	360	2.0*	50	700	60	11	2900*	1500*	2.3*
Lactation															
14-18 yr	1300	44*	1300	3*	290	10	360	2.6*	50	1250	70	13	2500*	1500*	2.3*
19-30 yr	1000	45*	1300	3*	290	9	310	2.6*	50	700	70	12	2800*	1500*	2.3*
31-50 yr	1000	45*	1300	3*	290	9	320	2.6*	50	700	70	12	2800*	1500*	2.3*

Sources: Dietary Reference Intakes for Calcium, Phosphorus, Magnesium, Vitamin D, and Fluoride (1997); Dietary Reference Intakes for Thiamin, Riboflavin, Niacin, Vitamin B6, Folate, Vitamin B12, Pantothenic Acid, Biotin, and Choline (1998); Dietary Reference Intakes for Vitamin C, Vitamin E, Selenium, and Carotenoids (2000); and Dietary Reference Intakes for Vitamin A, Vitamin K, Arsenic, Boron, Chromium, Copper, Iodine, Iron, Manganese, Molybdenum, Nickel, Silicon, Vanadium, and Zinc (2001); Dietary Reference Intakes for Water, Potassium, Sodium, Chloride, and Sulfate (2005); and Dietary Reference Intakes for Calcium and Vitamin D (2011). These reports may be accessed via www.nap.edu.

Note: This table (taken from the DRI reports, see www.nap.edu) presents Recommended Dietary Allowances (RDAs) in **boldface** type and Adequate Intakes (AIs) in lightface type followed by an asterisk (*). An RDA is the average daily dietary intake level sufficient to meet the nutrient requirements of nearly all (97–98 percent) healthy individuals in a group. It is calculated from an Estimated Average Requirement (EAR). If sufficient scientific evidence is not available to establish an EAR, and thus calculate an RDA, an AI is usually developed. For healthy breastfed infants, an AI is the mean intake. The AI for other life-stage and gender groups is believed to cover the needs of all healthy individuals in the groups, but lack of data or uncertainty in the data prevent being able to specify with confidence the percentage of individuals covered by this intake.

aLife-stage groups for infants were 0–5.9 and 6–11.9 months.

Dietary Reference Intakes of Energy and Protein From Birth to 18 Years of Age per Day*

	Age	Estimated Energy Requirement	Protein (g)
Infants	0 to 3 months	(89 ×Weight [kg] − 100) + 175 kcal	9.1
	4 to 6 months	(89 × Weight [kg] − 100) + 56 kcal	9.1
	7 to 12 months	(89 × Weight [kg] − 100) + 22 kcal	11
	13 to 36 months	(89 × Weight [kg] − 100) + 20 kcal	13
Boys	3 to 8 years	88.5 − (61.9 × Age [yr] + PA × (26.7 × Weight [kg] + 903 × Height [m]) + 20 kcal	19
	9 to 18 years	88.5 − (61.9 × Age [yrl] + PA × (26.7 × Weight [kg] + 903 × Height [m]) + 25 kcal	34 to 52
Girls	3 to 8 years	135.3 − (30.8 × Age [yr] + PA× (10.0 × Weight [kg] + 934 × Height [m]) + 20 kcal	19
	9 to 18 years	135.3 − (30.8 × Age [yrl] + PA × (10.0 × Weight [kg] + 934 × Height [m]) + 25 kcal	34 to 46

*PA, Physical activity level. Data from the Food and Nutrition Board, Institute of Medicine. *Dietary reference intakes for energy, carbohydrate, fiber, fat, fatty acids, cholesterol, protein, and amino acids (macronutrients).* Washington, DC: National Academies Press; 2002.

Dietary Reference Intakes (DRIs): Recommended Dietary Allowances and Adequate Intakes, Total Water and Macronutrients*

Food and Nutrition Board, Institute of Medicine, National Academies

Life Stage Group	Total Water[a] (L/d)	Total Fiber (g/d)	Linoleic Acid (g/d)	α-Linolenic Acid (g/d)	Protein[b] (g/d)
Infants					
Birth to 6 mo	0.7*	ND	4.4*	0.5*	9.1*
6-12 mo	0.8*	ND	4.6*	0.5*	**11.0**
Children					
1-3 yr	1.3*	19*	7*	0.7*	**13**
4-8 yr	1.7*	25*	10*	0.9*	**19**
Males					
9-13 yr	2.4*	31*	12*	1.2*	**34**
14-18 yr	3.3*	38*	16*	1.6*	**52**
19-30 yr	3.7*	38*	17*	1.6*	**56**
31-50 yr	3.7*	38*	17*	1.6*	**56**
51-70 yr	3.7*	30*	14*	1.6*	**56**
>70 yr	3.7*	30*	14*	1.6*	**56**
Females					
9-13 yr	2.1*	26*	10*	1.0*	**34**
14-18 yr	2.3*	26*	11*	1.1*	**46**
19-30 yr	2.7*	25*	12*	1.1*	**46**
31-50 yr	2.7*	25*	12*	1.1*	**46**
51-70 yr	2.7*	21*	11*	1.1*	**46**
>70 yr	2.7*	21*	11*	1.1*	**46**
Pregnancy					
14-18 yr	3.0*	28*	13*	1.4*	**71**
19-30 yr	3.0*	28*	13*	1.4*	**71**
31-50 yr	3.0*	28*	13*	1.4*	**71**
Lactation					
14-18 yr	3.8*	29*	13*	1.3*	**71**
19-30 yr	3.8*	29*	13*	1.3*	**71**
31-50 yr	3.8*	29*	13*	1.3*	**71**

Source: *Dietary Reference Intakes for Energy, Carbohydrate, Fiber, Fat, Fatty Acids, Cholesterol, Protein, and Amino Acids* (2002/2005) and *Dietary Reference Intakes for Water, Potassium, Sodium, Chloride, and Sulfate* (2005). The report may be accessed via www.n

***Note:** This table (taken from the DRI reports, see www.nap.edu) presents Recommended Dietary Allowances (RDA) in **boldface** type and Adequate Intakes (AIs) in ordinary type followed by an asterisk (*). An RDA is the average daily dietary intake level; sufficient to meet the nutrient requirements of nearly all (97-98%) healthy individuals in a group. It is calculated from an Estimated Average Requirement (EAR).

If sufficient scientific evidence is not available to establish an EAR, and thus calculate an RDA, an AI is usually developed. For healthy breastfed infants, an AI is the mean intake. The AI for other life stage and gender groups is believed to cover the needs of all healthy individuals in the groups, but lack of data or uncertainty in the data prevent being able to specify with confidence the percentage of individuals covered by this intake.

[a]Total water includes all water contained in food, beverages, and drinking water.

[b]Based on grams of protein per kilogram of body weight for the reference body weight (e.g., for adults 0.8 g/kg body weight for the reference body weight).

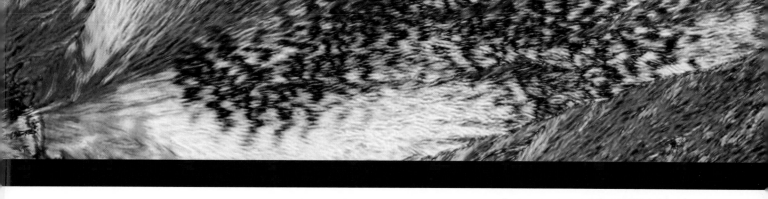

KRAUSE AND MAHAN'S
FOOD & THE NUTRITION CARE PROCESS

15TH EDITION

JANICE L. RAYMOND, MS, RDN, CSG
Clinical Nutrition Director
Thomas Cuisine Management at Providence Mount St. Vincent
Seattle, Washington
Affiliate Faculty
Department of Nutrition and Exercise Science
Bastyr University
Kenmore, Washington

KELLY MORROW, MS, RDN, FAND
Associate Professor
Nutrition Clinic Coordinator
Department of Nutrition and Exercise Science
Bastyr University
Kenmore, Washington

ELSEVIER

Elsevier
3251 Riverport Lane
St. Louis, Missouri 63043

KRAUSE AND MAHAN'S FOOD & THE NUTRITION CARE PROCESS,
FIFTEENTH EDITION

978-0-323-63655-1

Previous editions copyrighted 2017, 2012, 2008, 2004, 2000, 1996, 1992, 1984, 1979, 1972, 1966, 1961, 1957, 1952.

Library of Congress Control Number: 2019956656

Senior Content Strategist: Sandra Clark
Senior Content Development Manager: Lisa Newton
Senior Content Development Specialist: Danielle M. Frazier
Publishing Services Manager: Julie Eddy
Senior Project Manager: Tracey Schriefer
Senior Book Designer: Amy Buxton

Printed in Canada

Last digit is the print number: 9 8 7 6 5 4 3 2 1

Working together
to grow libraries in
developing countries

www.elsevier.com • www.bookaid.org

*This 15th edition is dedicated to the students, professors,
and practitioners who use this text.
We are also incredibly grateful to our authors for sharing their wisdom, experience,
and insight and for their dedication to the field of nutrition and dietetics.*

—The Authors, 15th Edition

*To the residents and patients at Providence Mount St. Vincent who remind
me every day why I chose to work in a health care field devoted to older people.
To my grandparents who helped raise me and taught me the value of listening
to and learning from our elders. Thank you to my husband, Greg, who has
become an enthusiastic chef and did most of the cooking while I was busy
editing. And to Kathy Mahan, who is the reason this book has existed for over
60 years and has always been cutting edge. Thank you for the inspiration.*

—Janice

*To my students at Bastyr University. You continuously inspire me with your
energy and enthusiasm. To my husband Gregg, son Ian, sister Wendy, the chair
of the Nutrition Department at Bastyr, Debra Boutin, and my friends and
colleagues. Thank you for believing in me and providing unending support
and encouragement. To Kathy Mahan: I am honored and grateful that you
have entrusted us to continue your work.*

—Kelly

Diane M. Anderson, PhD, RDN, FADA
Associate Professor
Pediatrics
Baylor College of Medicine
Houston, Texas

Christine Avgeris, RDN, CD
Clinical Dietitian
Nutrition
Seattle Children's Hospital
Seattle, Washington

Cynthia Bartok, PhD, RDN, CD
Associate Professor
Nutrition and Exercise Science
Bastyr University
Kenmore, Washington

Britta Brown, MS, RDN, LD, CNSC
Clinical Dietitian
Nutrition Services
Hennepin Healthcare
Minneapolis, Minnesota

Lindsey Callihan, MS, RDN, CSG
CVS/Coram
Boise, Idaho

Karen Chapman-Novakofski, PhD, RDN, LDN
Food Science and Human Nutrition
University of Illinois
Urbana, Illinois

Ashley Contreras-France, MA, MS, CCC-SLP
Director of Rehabilitation Therapy
Covenant Living at the Shores
Mercer Island, Washington

Mandy L. Corrigan, MPH, RDN, CNSC, FAND, FASPEN
Clinical Manager, Home Nutrition Support
    and Center for Gut Rehabilitation and
    Transplantation
Center for Human Nutrition
Digestive Disease and Surgery Institute
Cleveland, Ohio

Sarah Couch, PhD, RDN
Professor
Rehabilitation, Exercise, and Nutrition
    Sciences
University of Cincinnati
Cincinnati, Ohio

Jean T. Cox, MS, RDN, LN
Patient Educator
Maternity and Family Planning Program
University of New Mexico Hospital;
Volunteer Faculty
Department of OB/GYN
University of New Mexico
Albuquerque, New Mexico

Sheila Dean, DSc, RDN, LDN, CCN, IFMCP
Adjunct Professor
Health Sciences and Human Performance
University of Tampa
Tampa, Florida; Co-Founder
Integrative and Functional Nutrition
    Academy
Palm Harbor, Florida

Ruth DeBusk, PhD, RDN
Family Medicine Residency Program
Tallahassee Memorial HealthCare
Tallahassee, Florida

Judith L. Dodd, MS, RDN, LDN, FAND
Assistant Professor
Sports Medicine and Nutrition
University of Pittsburgh – SHRS
Pittsburgh, Pennsylvania

Lisa Dorfman, MS, RDN, CSSD, CCMS, LMHC, FAND
CEO/Director
Sports Nutrition & Performance
Food Fitness International, Inc
Miami, Florida

Lorena Drago, MS, RDN, CDN, CDE
Diabetes Education
Hispanic Foodways LLC
Forest Hills, New York

L. Karina Díaz Rios, PhD, RDN
Cooperative Extension Specialist in Nutrition
Division of Agriculture & Natural Resources
University of California, Merced
Merced, California

Sharon A. Feucht, MA, RDN, CD
Nutritionist LEND Program (Retired)
Center on Human Development and
    Disability
University of Washington
Seattle, Washington;
Nutritionist
Holly Ridge Early Intervention Center
Bremerton, Washington

Laith Ghazala, MD, FRCP
Fellow
Respiratory Institute
Cleveland Clinic Foundation
Cleveland, Ohio

F. Enrique Gómez, MSc, PhD
Researcher
Nutritional Physiology
National Institute of Medical Sciences and
    Nutrition, Salvador, Zubiran
Mexico City
Mexico

Michael Hahn, BA
Health Science Policy Analyst
All of Us Research Program
National Institutes of Health
Bethesda, Maryland

Jeanette M. Hasse, PhD, RDN, LD, CNSC, FADA
Transplant Nutrition Manager
Simmons Transplant Institute
Baylor University Medical Center
Dallas, Texas

Ginger Hultin, MS, RDN, CSO
Registered Dietitian
Nutrition
Bastyr University
Seattle, Washington

A. Christine Hummell, MS, RDN, LD, CNSC
Clinical Dietitian
Advanced Practitioner I
Center of Human Nutrition
Cleveland Clinic
Cleveland, Ohio

Carol S. Ireton-Jones, PhD, RDN, LD, CNSC, FASPEN, FAND
Nutrition Therapy Specialist
Good Nutrition for Good Living
Dallas, Texas

Jessica Jones, MS, RDN, CDE
Founder
Private Practice
Jessica Jones Nutrition
Richmond, California

Veena Juneja, MSc, RDN
Senior Renal Dietitian
Nutrition
St. Joseph's Healthcare
Hamilton, Ontario
Canada

Martha Kaufer-Horwitz, MSc, DSc, NC, FTOS
Researcher in Medical Sciences
Obesity and Eating Disorders Clinic
National Institute of Medical Sciences and
    Nutrition, Salvador, Zubiran
Mexico City
Mexico

Rachel E. Kay, MS, RDN, CD, CNSC
Clinical Dietitian
Gastroenterology
Seattle Children's Hospital
Seattle, Washington

Bette Klein, MS, RDN, CSP, LD
Advanced Practice II Pediatric Dietitian
Pediatric Gastroenterology
Cleveland Clinic Children's
Cleveland, Ohio

Lauren Kruse, MS, RDN, CNSC
Dietitian
Home Nutrition Support, Center for Human
    Nutrition
Digestive Disease Institute, Cleveland Clinic
Cleveland, Ohio

Glenn Kuz, BSP, PharmD
Clinical Pharmacist
Harborview Medical Center
University of Washington Medical Center
Seattle, Washington

Camille Lyn Lanier, RDN, CD
Pediatric Dietitian
Nutrition
Seattle Children's Hospital
Seattle, Washington

Nicole Larson, PhD, MPH, RDN, LD
Senior Research Associate
Division of Epidemiology and Community
    Health
University of Minnesota
Minneapolis, Minnesota

Tashara M. Leak, PhD, RDN
Lois & Mel Tukman Assistant Professor
Division of Nutritional Sciences
Cornell University
Ithaca, New York;
Assistant Professor of Nutrition Research in
    Medicine
Division of General Internal Medicine
Weill Cornell Medicine
New York, New York

Maureen Lilly, MS, RDN
Registered Dietitian Nutritionist
Nutrition
Chicken Soup Brigade
Seattle, Washington

Mary Demarest Litchford, PhD, RDN, LDN
President
Executive
CASE Software & Books
Greensboro, North Carolina

Michelle Loy, MPH, MS, RDN
Associate Professor
Nutrition and Foods
Fullerton College
Fullerton, California

Lucinda K. Lysen, RDN, RN, BSN
Nutrition Consultant in Private Practice
Orland Park, Illinois

L. Kathleen Mahan, MS, RDN, CD
Functional Nutrition Counselor
Nutrition by Design;
Clinical Associate
Department of Pediatrics
School of Medicine
University of Washington
Seattle, Washington

Gabriela E. Mancera-Chávez, MSc, NC
Professor
College of Sciences and Humanities
Autonomous University of Mexico City;
Independent Consultant
Mexico City
Mexico

Laura E. Matarese, PhD, RDN, LDN, CNSC, FADA, FASPEN, FAND
Professor
Brody School of Medicine and Department
    of Nutrition Science
East Carolina University
Greenville, North Carolina

Mari O. Mazon, MS, RDN, CD
Nutritionist
Center on Human Development and
    Disability
University of Washington
Seattle, Washington

Kelly N. McKean, MS, RDN, CSP, CD
Clinical Pediatric Dietitian
Nutrition
Seattle Children's
Seattle, Washington

Maggie Moon, MS, RDN
Author
The MIND Diet
Nutrition Communications
Los Angeles, California

Kelly Morrow, MS, RDN, FAND
Associate Professor
Nutrition and Exercise Science
Bastyr University
Kenmore, Washington

Diana Noland, MPH, RDN, CCN, IFMCP, LD
Owner
Integrative & Functional Medical Nutrition
    Therapy
FoodFAX
Burbank, California

Patricia Novak, MPH, RDN
Nutrition Consultant
Feeding and Nutrition
Professional Child Development Associates
    (PCDA)
Pasadena, California

Kim Nowak-Cooperman, MS, RDN, CD
Registered Dietitian Nutritionist
Clinical Nutrition
Seattle Children's Hospital
Seattle, Washington

Beth Ogata, MS, RDN, CD, CSP
Lecturer
Department of Pediatrics
University of Washington
Seattle, Washington

Constantina Papoutsakis, PhD, RDN
Senior Director
Nutrition and Dietetics Data Science Center,
    Research International Scientific Affairs
Academy of Nutrition and Dietetics
Chicago, Illinois

Mary H. Purdy, PhD
Professor
Communication Disorders
Southern Connecticut State University
New Haven, Connecticut

Janice L. Raymond, MS, RDN, CSG
Clinical Nutrition Director
Thomas Cuisine Management
Providence Mt. St Vincent
Seattle, Washington;
Affiliate Faculty
Nutrition
Bastyr University
Kenmore, Washington

Rickelle Richards, PhD, MPH, RDN
Associate Professor
Nutrition, Dietetics & Food Science
Brigham Young University
Provo, Utah

Dorene Robinson, RDN, CDN
Editor
website
beyonddiets.com
Seattle, Washington

Justine Roth, MS, CEDRD
Clinical Nutrition Director
Columbia Psychiatry
New York State Psychiatric Institute
New York, New York

Rebecca Rudel, MPH, RDN, CNSC
Graduate Teaching Fellow
DrPH Program
Boston University School of Public Health
Boston, Massachusetts

Mary Russell, MS, RDN, LDN, FAND
Medical Science Liaison II
Medical Affairs
Baxter Healthcare Corporation
Deerfield, Illinois;
Lecturer
Nutrition
Chicago Medical School
North Chicago, Illinois

Janet E. Schebendach, PhD, RDN
Assistant Professor
Psychiatry
Columbia University Medical Center
New York, New York

Elizabeth Shanaman, RDN
Lead Dietitian
Nutrition
Northwest Kidney Centers
Seattle, Washington

Lisa I. Shkoda, RDN, CSO, CSP, CNSC, FAND
Owner
Nutrition for Health RDN Consulting, LLC
Charlottesville, Virginia
Corporate Regional Dietitian
Medical Facilities of America;
Founding Dietitian
Ketogenic Diet Therapy Program
University of Virginia Health System
Charlottesville, Virginia

Jamie S. Stang, PhD, MPH, RDN
Director, Leadership, Education and
    Training Program in Maternal and Child
    Nutrition
Director, Center for Leadership in Maternal
    and Child Public Health
Associate Professor
Division of Epidemiology and Community
    Health
University of Minnesota
School of Public Health
Minneapolis, Minnesota

Catherine S. Sullivan, MPH, RDN, LDN, IBCLC, RLC, FAND
Director, Assistant Professor
Maternal and Child Health-Carolina Global
    Breastfeeding Institute
University of North Carolina at Chapel Hill
Chapel Hill, North Carolina

Kathie Madonna Swift, MS, RDN, LDN, FAND
Co-Founder
www.IFNAcademy.com
Palm Harbor, Massachusetts

Kelly A. Tappenden, PhD, RDN, FASPEN
Professor and Head
Kinesiology and Nutrition
University of Illinois at Chicago
Chicago, Illinois

Christina Troutner, MS, RDN
Research Dietitian
Nutritional Genomics & Digital Health
GB HealthWatch
San Diego, California

Solenne Vanne, MS, RDN
Nutrition
Chicken Soup Brigade
Seattle, Washington

DeeAnna Wales VanReken, MS, RDN, CD, IFNCP
Clinical Nutrition Specialist -
    Gastroenterology
Nutrition Services
Swedish Medical Center
Seattle, Washington

Katy G. Wilkens, MS, RDN
Manager
Nutrition and Fitness Services
Northwest Kidney Centers
Seattle, Washington

Martin M. Yadrick, MBI, MS, RDN, FAND
Director of Nutrition Informatics
Sales & Marketing
Computrition, Inc.
West Hills, California

REVIEWERS

Michael Hahn, BA
Health Science Policy Analyst
All of Us Research Program
National Institutes of Health
Bethesda, Maryland

Cristen L. Harris, PhD, RDN, CSSD, CD, CEP, FAND
Senior Lecturer, Core Faculty
School of Public Health, Nutritional Sciences
    Program
University of Washington
Seattle, Washington

Marion F. Winkler, PhD, RDN, LDN, CNSC, FASPEN
Associate Professor of Surgery and Surgical
    Nutrition Specialist
Brown University School of Medicine and
    Rhode Island Hospital
Providence, Rhode Island

When I was first asked to revise this text in 1975, I said no. Why would I want to take on this herculean task? Times were good. We were wearing miniskirts, bell bottoms, and platform shoes; the Vietnam war was over, and a new Environmental Protection Agency (EPA) had just been established. The Women, Infants, and Children (WIC) program for maternal and child nutrition was beginning, and total parenteral nutrition (TPN), the new "wow" therapy, had just entered the scene. TPN was a powerful tool, and nutritionists knew it. Now we had a way to feed patients with nonfunctioning guts so that they could heal and survive. Feeding a very sick person could be targeted, scientific, and aggressive. TPN enabled premature infants to survive as I would learn with my own preemie a decade later. It was an exciting time for a young dietitian. And then to be able to take over the authorship of this already reputable text—well, wow! It couldn't have been a better entry into a career. I said yes.

Marie Krause first penned this text in 1952, revised it for several editions and then handed it over to me for the 6th edition. Since that time other co-editors (Arlin, Escott-Stump, and Raymond) and I, along with many, many contributors, now considered family, have sought to keep this text in the forefront of nutrition and dietetic education. We have navigated it through the waters of expanding nutrition science and changing clinical care, aiming to offer it as a beacon of learning for students and a reliable reference for clinicians and practitioners. Our goal has been to dispel myths and illuminate the truth. Over the 45 years that my team has been writing and editing this text, we have been honored to hear it referred to as the "nutrition bible." Many of our contributors are nationally acclaimed specialists in their fields and have gone on to write their own books as well as lead major professional nutrition organizations. This tome has become the students' link to these leaders in nutrition.

During its almost 70 years, this textbook has changed considerably. It has been streamlined; content that can more efficiently be found in other texts was omitted. More importantly, new content reflecting current science was added: chapters covering medical nutrition therapy (MNT) for HIV and AIDS and nutrition for sports and performance appeared with the 8th edition (1992), a chapter on nutrigenomics and integrative medicine and herbal therapy in the 10th edition (2000), a chapter on MNT in psychiatric disease in the 12th edition (2008), and one on inflammation and chronic disease in the 14th edition (2017), just to name a few.

This edition has a new name—*Krause and Mahan's Food and the Nutrition Care Process*—and I leave as senior editor and author. My feelings are mixed. I am sad to say goodbye to such a fulfilling and rewarding occupation after four and a half decades, and yet thrilled to leave it in the capable hands of Janice Raymond and Kelly Morrow. Janice has been co-editor and author for the previous two editions. She is experienced in ensuring the information is evidenced-based and logical, and because she continues to work as a clinical dietitian, she ensures it remains relevant. Kelly, who has been a Krause author, will now add her influence as a leader in integrative and functional nutrition in her role as editor.

Using an integrative and functional approach to nutritional care means considering nutrition status as a reflection of not only the nutrient intake of the individual but also the environmental influence on that nutrient intake. For example, what is the influence of the microbiome in the gut on nutrient absorption? Where is the individual's food grown? How is it grown and how does this affect its nutrient content? During processing, are chemicals added to the food, either with or without intent? What is the effect of lifestyle or culture on the individual's food choices? It is exciting and intriguing to think about adding this content to the text.

We plan that the Krause and Mahan text will continue to be the go-to resource for professors and students to learn not only the science of nutrition but also the art of nutrition care. We envision that new learners will turn to it to gain the skills of dietetic/nutrition practice—relating to the individual by asking the right questions, learning the person's story, assessing nutritional needs, and providing nutrition care and learning in a way that the individual and the family can respond to and use.

I hope the writers of future editions will include content with a consciousness toward sustainability and planet renewal as we deal with nourishing an ever-growing population on our limited planet. How will we, the human global population, do that? How and when will we stop contaminating the water and air that provides for life? What changes will need to be made in our food systems to ensure they are sustainable? How will we continue as a species without causing the extinction of other species? Going forward I hope these questions and hopefully many of the answers will be kept in mind as Krause and Mahan is written and revised. It is important work, and I would like to see this text at the center of its progress.

It has been an honor to work with all our wonderful, committed authors and editors as well as the students and teachers who use the book. I am blessed, and it couldn't have happened without you. Thank you from the bottom of my heart. You certainly made it a great ride!

L. Kathleen Mahan
January 6, 2020

PREFACE

Over its 15 editions, this classic text has continued to change in response to the ever-dynamic field of nutrition. And because it remains the most comprehensive nutrition textbook available, it is the reference students take into their internships and careers.

AUDIENCE

Scientific knowledge and clinical information is presented in a form that is useful to students in dietetics, nursing, and other allied health professions in an interdisciplinary setting. It is valuable as a reference for other disciplines such as medicine, dentistry, child development, physical and occupational therapy, health education, and lifestyle counseling. Nutrient and assessment appendices, tables, illustrations, and clinical insight boxes provide practical hands-on procedures and clinical tools for students and practitioners alike.

This textbook accompanies the graduating student into clinical practice as a treasured shelf reference. The popular features remain: having basic information on nutrition in the life cycle all the way through to protocols for clinical nutrition practice in one place, clinical management algorithms, focus boxes that give detailed insight on emerging topics, sample nutrition diagnoses for clinical scenarios, useful websites, and extensive appendices for patient education. All material reflects current evidence-based practice as contributed by authors who are experts in their fields. This text is the first choice in the field of dietetics for students, interns, educators, and clinicians.

ORGANIZATION

This edition follows the Conceptual Framework for Steps of the Nutrition Care Process. All nutritional care process components are addressed to enhance or improve the nutritional well-being of individuals, their families, or populations. The chapters flow according to the steps of assessment, nutrition diagnosis, intervention, monitoring, and evaluation with the separation of the pediatric medical nutrition therapy (MNT) chapters into their own section to assist with that specialty practice.

Part 1, Nutrition Assessment, organizes content for an effective assessment. Chapters here provide an overview of the digestive system, as well as calculation of energy requirements and expenditure, macronutrient and micronutrient needs, nutritional genomics, and food intake. A thorough review of biochemical tests, acid–base balance issues, and medications promote the necessary insight for provision of excellent care. A chapter titled "Inflammation and the Pathophysiology of Chronic Disease" addresses the latest knowledge about inflammation as a cause of chronic disease and the necessity of assessing for it. The final chapter in this section addresses the behavioral aspects of an individual's food choices within the community, a safe food supply, and available resources for sufficient food access.

Part 2, Nutrition Diagnosis and Intervention, describes the critical thinking process from assessment to selection of relevant, timely, and measurable nutrition diagnoses. These nutrition diagnoses can be resolved by the registered dietitian nutritionist (RDN) or trained health professional. The process is generally used for individuals but can be applied when helping families, teaching groups, or evaluating the nutritional needs of a multicultural community or population. A nutrition diagnosis requires an intervention, and interventions relate to food and nutrient delivery (including nutrition support), use of

bioactive substances and integrative medical nutrition, education, counseling, and referral when needed.

Part 3, Nutrition in the Life Cycle, presents in-depth information on nutrition for life stages for conception, pregnancy, and lactation. Chapters on infancy, childhood, and adolescence highlight the importance of nutrition through critical periods of growth. A chapter on adult nutrition highlights risk factors for chronic diseases that usually start appearing in adulthood. Finally, nutrition for the aging adult is discussed in detail because of the growing need for nutrition services in this rapidly expanding population.

Part 4, Nutrition for Weight Management, provides a review of nutrition concepts for the achievement and maintenance of health and prevention of disease. Topics include weight management, disordered eating, dental health, bone health, and sports nutrition.

Part 5, Medical Nutrition Therapy, reflects evidence-based knowledge and current trends in nutrition therapies including integrative approaches. All of the chapters are written and reviewed by experts in their field who present MNT for conditions such as cardiovascular disorders; cancer; diabetes; liver and digestive diseases; renal disease; pulmonary disease; HIV; endocrine disorders (including thyroid disease); and rheumatologic, neurologic, and psychiatric disorders.

Part 6, Pediatric Specialties, describes the role of nutrition therapies in childhood. Chapters provide details for low-birthweight, neonatal intensive-care conditions, genetic metabolic disorders, and developmental disabilities.

NEW TO THIS EDITION

The chapter on food–drug interaction was eliminated this edition. Input from our educators and readers indicated that this chapter was not as useful as in the past due to the rapid changes that occur in the pharmaceutical industry and because computer applications are now in widespread use. We have, however, continued to include a food–drug appendix.

- New appendices on choline, biotin, the Mediterranean diet, and the International Dysphagia Diet Standardisation Initiative (IDDSI).
- Updated and expanded integrative nutrition approaches.
- Expanded section on pregnancy and lactation.
- The chapter titled "Planning the Diet with Cultural Competence" has a new co-author and expanded international nutrition guidelines.
- All chapters were updated with an emphasis on cultural diversity.
- Many new authors have provided new insights to chapters on cancer; GI; HIV; neurology; weight management; analysis of the diet; anemia; nutritional genomics; pulmonary, psychiatric, and cognitive disorders; critical care; and intellectual and developmental disabilities.
- New content highlight boxes on CRISPR, the Indigenous food movement, hearing assessment, Health At Every Size, health disparities, and a tribute to Dr. George Blackburn.

PEDAGOGY

- Unique pathophysiology algorithms and flow charts present the cause, pathophysiology, and the medical nutrition management for a variety of disorders and conditions. They equip the reader with an understanding of the illness as background for providing optimal nutritional care in a variety of healthcare settings.

- *Clinical Insight* boxes expand on clinical information in the text and highlight areas that may go unnoticed. These boxes contain information on studies and clinical resources for the student and practitioner.
- *New Directions* boxes suggest areas for further research by spotlighting emerging areas of interest within the field.
- *Focus On* boxes provide thought-provoking information on key concepts for well-rounded study and the promotion of further discussion within the classroom.
- Useful websites direct the reader to online resources that relate to the chapter topics; however, links are no longer included as they can outdate quickly.
- *Sample Nutrition Diagnosis* boxes present a problem, its etiology, and its signs and symptoms, before concluding with a sample nutrition diagnosis, providing both students and practitioners with "real-life" scenarios they may encounter in practice.
- Key terms are listed at the beginning of each chapter and bolded within the text where they are discussed in more detail.
- Chapter references are current and extensive, with the purpose of giving the student and instructor lots of opportunity for further reading and understanding.

ANCILLARIES

Accompanying this edition is the Evolve website, which includes updated and invaluable resources for instructors and students. These materials can be accessed by going to http://evolve.elsevier.com/Mahan/nutrition/.

INSTRUCTOR RESOURCES

- PowerPoint presentations: More than 900 slides to help guide classroom lectures.
- Image Collection: Approximately 200 images from the text are included in the PowerPoint presentations, as well as more illustrations that can be downloaded and used to develop other teaching resources.
- Audience Response System Questions (for use with iClicker and other systems): Three to five questions per chapter help aid incorporation of this new technology into the classroom.
- Test Bank: Each chapter includes NCLEX-formatted questions with page references specific to that chapter's content to bring you more than 900 multiple-choice questions.
- Animations: Animations have been developed to visually complement the text and the processes described.
- NEW! Case Studies with Answers: Ten detailed clinical case studies using the nutrition care process.

STUDENT RESOURCES

- Study Exercises with Answers: With more than 600 questions, these exercises give instant feedback on questions related to the chapter's content.
- NEW! Case Studies: Ten detailed clinical case studies using the nutrition care process.

Janice L. Raymond, MS, RDN, CD, CSG
Kelly Morrow, MS, RDN, FAND

ACKNOWLEDGMENTS

We sincerely thank the reviewers and especially contributors for this edition who have devoted hours and hours of time and commitment to researching the book's content for accuracy, reliability, and practicality. We are greatly in debt to them and realize that we could not continue to produce this book without them. In particular, we would like to acknowledge Ronona Crowder-Woods for her help with the Diabetes chapter, Hillary Nason on the Mediterranean Diet appendix, Amanda Fredrickson on the Diabetes Exchange List appendix, Linden Hale on the Biotin appendix and Maya DiTraglia on the Choline appendix. Thank you!

We also wish to acknowledge the hard work of Sandra Clark, Senior Content Strategist, who keeps the vision, and Danielle Frazier, Senior Content Developmental Specialist, who can get the "hot off the press" items we'd like included, and Tracey Schriefer, Senior Project Manager, who amazingly keeps the manuscript moving forward as she juggles between us and all others. Thank you!

CONTENTS

PART I: Nutrition Assessment

1 **Intake: Gastrointestinal Digestion, Absorption, and Excretion of Nutrients,** 2
Kelly A. Tappenden, PhD, RDN, FASPEN
The Gastrointestinal Tract, 2
Brief Overview of Digestive and Absorptive Processes, 3
The Small Intestine: Primary Site of Nutrient Absorption, 9
The Large Intestine, 9
Summary, 15

2 **Intake: Energy,** 17
Carol S. Ireton-Jones, PhD, RDN, LD, CNSC, FASPEN, FAND
Energy Requirements, 17
Components of Energy Expenditure, 17
Estimating Energy Requirements, 21
Physical Activity in Children, 25
Calculating Food Energy, 25

3 **Clinical: Water, Electrolytes, and Acid–Base Balance,** 28
Mandy L. Corrigan, MPH, RDN, CNSC, FAND, FASPEN
Lauren Kruse, MS, RDN, CNSC
Body Water, 28
Electrolytes, 33
Acid–Base Balance, 37
Acid Generation, 38
Acid–Base Disorders, 38

4 **Intake: Assessment of Food- and Nutrition-Related History,** 41
Cynthia Bartok, PhD, RDN, CD
L. Kathleen Mahan, RDN, MS, CD
Nutritional Status, 41
Nutrition Screening, 41
Nutrition Assessment, 43
Nutrition-Related History, 44
Food and Nutrient Intake, 46
Food and Nutrient Administration, 53
Nutrition Knowledge, Beliefs, and Attitudes, 54
Nutrition Behaviors, 54
Medication and Complementary or Alternative Medicines, 54
Nutrition Access, 55
Physical Activity and Physical Function, 55
Nutrition Quality of Life, 55

5 **Clinical: Biochemical, Physical, and Functional Assessment,** 57
Mary Demarest Litchford, PhD, RDN, LDN
Biochemical Assessment of Nutrition Status, 57
Nutrition Interpretation of Routine Medical Laboratory Tests, 59
Assessment of Hydration Status, 61
Assessment for Nutritional Anemias, 65
Fat-Soluble Vitamins, 66
Water-Soluble Vitamins and Trace Minerals, 67
Chronic Disease Risk Assessment, 68
Physical Assessments, 70
Nutrition-Focused Physical Examination, 74

6 **Nutritional Genomics,** 81
Ruth DeBusk, PhD, RDN
Michael Hahn, BA
Genetic and Genomic Fundamentals, 82
Modes of Inheritance, 87
Genetic Variation, Inheritance, and Disease, 90
Nutritional Genomics and Chronic Disease, 94
Summary, 101

7 **Inflammation and the Pathophysiology of Chronic Disease,** 104
Diana Noland, MPH, RDN, CCN, IFMNCP, LD
Epidemic of Chronic Disease, 104
Concepts of Chronic Disease Pathophysiology, 105
Inflammation: Common Denominator of Chronic Disease, 106
Nutrient Modulators of Inflammation, 113
Reducing Inflammation in the Body, 118
Summary, 122

8 **Behavioral-Environmental: The Individual in the Community,** 127
Judith L. Dodd, MS, RDN, LDN, FAND
Social Determinants of Health, 128
Nutrition Practice in the Community, 128
Needs Assessment for Community-Based Nutrition Services, 129
National Nutrition Surveys, 130
National Nutrition Guidelines and Goals, 131
Food Assistance and Nutrition Programs, 133
Foodborne Illness, 133
Food and Water Safety, 139
Disaster Planning, 142
Healthy Food and Water Systems and Sustainability, 142
Summary: A Work in Progress, 143

PART II: Nutrition Diagnosis and Intervention

9 **Overview of Nutrition Diagnosis and Intervention,** 146
Constantina Papoutsakis, PhD, RDN
The Nutrition Care Process, 146
Documentation in the Nutrition Care Record, 151
Influences on Nutrition and Health Care, 154
Nutrition Interventions, 158
Nutrition for the Terminally Ill or Hospice Client, 160

10 **Food-Nutrient Delivery: Planning the Diet With Cultural Competence,** 162
Lorena Drago, MS, RDN, CDN, CDE
Martin M. Yadrick, MBI, MS, RDN, FAND
Determining Nutrient Needs, 162
Worldwide Guidelines, 162
Nutritional Status of Americans, 174
National Guidelines for Diet Planning, 176
Food and Nutrient Labeling, 176
Dietary Patterns and Counseling Tips, 180
Cultural Aspects of Dietary Planning, 180

11 **Food and Nutrient Delivery: Bioactive Substances and Integrative Care,** 187
Kelly Morrow, MS, RDN, FAND
    Complementary and Integrative Medicine, 187
    Use of Complementary and Integrative Therapies, 187
    Dietary Supplementation, 191
    Dietary Supplement Regulation, 193
    Assessment of Dietary Supplement Use in Patients, 196

12 **Food and Nutrient Delivery: Nutrition Support Methods,** 208
Carol S. Ireton-Jones, PhD, RDN, LD, CNSC, FASPEN, FAND
Mary Russell, MS, RDN, LDN, FAND
    Rationale and Criteria for Appropriate Nutrition Support, 208
    Enteral Nutrition, 209
    Enteral Nutrition Access, 209
    Parenteral Nutrition, 216
    Complications, 220
    Refeeding Syndrome, 220
    Transitional Feeding, 221
    Nutrition Support in Long-Term and Home Care, 222

13 **Education and Counseling: Behavioral Change,** 226
Karen Chapman-Novakofski, PhD, RDN, LDN
L. Karina Díaz Rios, PhD, RDN
    Behavior Change, 226
    Models for Behavior Change, 227
    Models for Counseling Strategies, 228
    Models for Educational Program Development, 229
    Skills and Attributes of the Nutrition Educator or Counselor, 229
    Assessment Results: Choosing Focus Areas, 232
    Counseling Approaches After the Assessment, 232
    Evaluation of Effectiveness, 235
    Summary, 236

PART III: Nutrition in the Life Cycle

14 **Nutrition in Pregnancy and Lactation,** 240
Jean T. Cox, MS, RDN, LN
Catherine S. Sullivan, MPH, RDN, LDN, IBCLC, RLC, FAND
    Preconception and Fertility, 240
    Conception, 245
    Pregnancy, 250
    Postpartum Period = Preconceptual Period, 286
    Lactation, 286

15 **Nutrition in Infancy,** 310
Kelly N. McKean, MS, RDN, CSP, CD
Mari O. Mazon, MS, RDN, CD
    Physiologic Development, 310
    Nutrient Requirements, 311
    Milk, 314
    Food, 317
    Feeding, 318

16 **Nutrition in Childhood,** 324
Beth Ogata, MS, RDN, CD, CSP
Sharon A. Feucht, MA, RDN, CD
    Growth and Development, 324
    Nutrient Requirements, 326
    Providing an Adequate Diet, 328
    Nutritional Concerns, 335
    Preventing Chronic Disease, 337

17 **Nutrition in Adolescence,** 341
Nicole Larson, PhD, MPH, RDN, LD
Tashara M. Leak, PhD, RDN
Jamie S. Stang, PhD, MPH, RDN
    Growth and Development, 341
    Nutrient Requirements, 344
    Food Habits and Eating Behaviors, 348
    Nutrition Screening, Assessment, and Counseling, 351
    Special Topics, 351

18 **Nutrition in the Adult Years,** 362
Judith L. Dodd, MS, RDN, LDN, FAND
    Setting the Stage: Nutrition in the Adult Years, 362
    Setting the Stage: Messages, 362
    Information Sources, 364
    Lifestyle and Health Risk Factors, 366
    Health Disparities and Global Health, 367
    Nutritional Factors Affecting Adult Women and Men, 367
    Interventions, Nutrition, and Prevention, 368
    Food Trends and Patterns, 369
    Nutritional Supplementation, 369
    Functional Foods, 369
    Adult Health Next Steps, 370

19 **Nutrition in Aging,** 373
Janice L. Raymond, MS, RDN, CSG
Lindsey Callihan, MS, RDN, CSG
    The Older Population, 373
    Gerontology, Geriatrics, and the Spectrum of Aging, 374
    Nutrition in Health Promotion and Disease Prevention, 374
    Theories on Aging, 374
    Physiologic Changes, 375
    Quality of Life, 379
    Nutrition Screening and Assessment, 382
    Nutrition Needs, 382
    Medicare Benefits, 384
    Nutrition Support Services, 384
    Community and Residential Facilities for Older Adults, 385

PART IV: Nutrition for Weight Management

20 **Nutrition in Weight Management,** 392
Lucinda K. Lysen, RDN, RN, BSN
Dorene Robinson, RDN, CDN
Rebecca Rudel, MPH, RDN, CNSC
    Weight Management and Obesity: Its Foundation in Nutritional Medicine, 392
    Body Weight Components, 394
    Regulation of Body Weight, 395
    Overweight and Obesity, 397
    Elements of Energy Balance Dysregulation, 397
    Management of Obesity in Adults, 403
    Weight Management in Children and Adolescents, 415
    Excessive Leanness or Unintentional Weight Loss, 415

21 Nutrition in Eating Disorders, 421
Janet E. Schebendach, PhD, RDN
Justine Roth, MS, CEDRD
   Clinical Characteristics and Medical
      Complications, 424
   Treatment Approach, 425
   Psychologic Management, 426
   Nutrition Management, 427
   Medical Nutrition Therapy and Counseling, 431
   Summary, 437

22 Nutrition in Exercise and Sports Performance, 441
Lisa Dorfman, MS, RDN, CSSD, CCMS, LMHC, FAND
   Bioenergetics of Physical Activity, 441
   Fuels for Contracting Muscles, 442
   An Integrative Approach to Working
      With Athletes, 444
   Nutritional Requirements of Exercise, 444
   Weight Management, 445
   Weight Management and Aesthetics, 446
   Macronutrients, 447
   Carbohydrate, 448
   Protein, 451
   Fat, 452
   Fluid, 453
   Vitamins and Minerals, 456
   Minerals, 459
   Ergogenic Aids, 461
   Popular Ergogenic Aids, 463
   Performance Enhancement Substances and Drugs:
      Doping in Sport, 464

23 Nutrition and Bone Health, 471
Karen Chapman-Novakofski, PhD, RDN, LDN
Rickelle Richards, PhD, MPH, RDN
   Introduction, 471
   Bone Structure and Bone Physiology, 471
   Osteopenia and Osteoporosis, 473
   Nutrition and Bone, 476
   Treatment of Osteoporosis, 478

24 Nutrition for Oral and Dental Health, 482
Janice L. Raymond, MS, RDN, CSG
   Nutrition for Tooth Development, 482
   Dental Caries, 482
   Early Childhood Caries, 487
   Caries Prevention, 487
   Tooth Loss and Dentures, 488
   Other Oral Disorders, 488
   Periodontal Disease, 488
   Oral Manifestations of Systemic Disease, 489

PART V: Medical Nutrition Therapy

25 Medical Nutrition Therapy for Adverse Reactions to Food: Allergies and Intolerances, 494
L. Kathleen Mahan, MS, RDN, CD
Kathie Madonna Swift, MS, RDN, LDN, FAND
   Definitions, 494
   Prevalence, 497
   Etiology, 498
   Pathophysiology of Food Allergy, 498
   Immune System Basics, 498

   Food-Dependent, Exercise-Induced Anaphylaxis
      (FDEIA), 501
   Food Intolerances, 511
   Medical Nutrition Therapy, 514
   Diagnosis, 514
   Intervention, 516
   Monitoring and Evaluation, 517
   Prevention of Food Allergies, 519

26 Medical Nutrition Therapy for Upper Gastrointestinal Tract Disorders, 525
DeeAnna Wales VanReken, MS, RDN, CD, IFNCP
   The Esophagus, 525
   The Stomach, 532
   Gastroparesis, 540

27 Medical Nutrition Therapy for Lower Gastrointestinal Tract Disorders, 544
DeeAnna Wales VanReken, MS, RDN, CD, IFNCP
Rachel E. Kay, MS, RDN, CD, CNSC
Carol S. Ireton-Jones, PhD, RDN, LD, CNSC, FASPEN, FAND
   Common Intestinal Problems, 544
   Diseases of the Small Intestine, 553
   Intestinal Brush-Border Enzyme Deficiencies, 559
   Inflammatory Bowel Disease, 561
   Nutritional Consequences of Intestinal Surgery, 569

28 Medical Nutrition Therapy for Hepatobiliary and Pancreatic Disorders, 579
Jeanette M. Hasse, PhD, RDN, LD, CNSC, FADA
Laura E. Matarese, PhD, RDN, LDN, CNSC, FADA, FASPEN, FAND
   Physiology and Functions of the Liver, 579
   Diseases of the Liver, 581
   Complications of ESLD: Cause and Nutrition
      Treatment, 587
   Nutrition Issues Related to End-Stage Liver
      Disease, 589
   Nutrient Requirements for Cirrhosis, 592
   Herbal and Dietary Supplements and Liver
      Disease, 593
   Liver Resection and Transplantation, 594
   Physiology and Functions of the Gallbladder, 595
   Diseases of the Gallbladder, 595
   Complementary and Integrative Medicine for
      Gallstones, 599
   Physiology and Functions of the Exocrine
      Pancreas, 599
   Diseases of the Exocrine Pancreas, 599
   Complementary and Integrative Medicine for
      Pancreatic Disorders, 602
   Pancreatic Surgery, 602

29 Medical Nutrition Therapy for Diabetes Mellitus and Hypoglycemia of Nondiabetic Origin, 606
Jessica Jones, MS, RDN, CDE
   Incidence and Prevalence, 606
   Categories of Glucose Intolerance, 607
   Screening and Diagnostic Criteria, 611
   Management of Prediabetes, 612
   Management of Diabetes, 613
   Implementing the Nutrition Care Process, 625
   Acute Complications, 633
   Long-Term Complications, 634
   Hypoglycemia of Nondiabetic Origin, 636

30 Medical Nutrition Therapy for Thyroid, Adrenal, and Other Endocrine Disorders, 641

Sheila Dean, DSc, RDN, LDN, CCN, IFMCP

Thyroid Physiology, 641

Assessment in Thyroid Disorders, 643

Hypothyroidism, 644

Polycystic Ovary Syndrome, 648

Hyperthyroidism, 649

Managing Imbalances of the Hypothalamus-Pituitary-Thyroid Axis, 650

Adrenal Disorders, 651

31 Medical Nutrition Therapy for Anemia, 655

Michelle Loy, MPH, MS, RDN

Iron-Related Blood Disorders, 655

Iron Overload, 660

Megaloblastic Anemias, 661

Other Nutritional Anemias, 666

Nonnutritional Anemias, 667

32 Medical Nutrition Therapy for Cardiovascular Disease, 670

Janice L. Raymond, MS, RDN, CSG

Sarah C. Couch, PhD, RDN

Atherosclerosis and Coronary Heart Disease, 670

Genetic Hyperlipidemias, 674

Hypertension, 683

Heart Failure, 693

Cardiac Transplantation, 700

33 Medical Nutrition Therapy for Pulmonary Disease, 705

Laith Ghazala, MD, FRCP

A. Christine Hummell, MS, RDN, LD, CNSC

Bette Klein, MS, RDN, CSP, LD

The Pulmonary System, 705

Chronic Pulmonary Disease, 707

Asthma, 711

Chronic Obstructive Pulmonary Disease, 713

Pulmonary Hypertension, 716

Diffuse Parenchymal Lung Disease, 716

Tuberculosis, 717

Lung Cancer, 718

Obesity Hypoventilation Syndrome, 719

Pleural Effusion, 720

Chylothorax, 720

Acute Respiratory Distress Syndrome, 720

Pneumonia, 721

Lung Transplantation, 722

Bronchopulmonary Dysplasia, 722

34 Medical Therapy for Renal Disorders, 727

Katy G. Wilkens, MS, RDN

Veena Juneja, MSc, RDN

Elizabeth Shanaman, RDN

Physiology and Function of the Kidneys, 727

Renal Diseases, 728

Education, Adherence, and Compliance, 736

Acute Kidney Injury (Acute Renal Failure), 736

Chronic Kidney Disease, 737

End-Stage Renal Disease, 740

35 Medical Nutrition Therapy for Cancer Prevention, Treatment, and Survivorship, 756

Ginger Hultin, MS, RDN, CSO

Pathophysiology, 758

Nutrition and Carcinogenesis, 758

Chemoprevention, 762

Medical Diagnosis and Staging of Cancer, 765

Medical Treatment, 766

Medical Nutrition Therapy, 768

Integrative, Complementary, and Functional Oncology, 773

Nutritional Impact of Cancer Treatments, 774

Nutrition Monitoring and Evaluation, 781

Pediatric Cancer, 781

Nutrition Recommendations for Cancer Survivors, 782

36 Medical Nutrition Therapy for HIV and AIDS, 787

Maureen Lilly, MS, RDN

Solenne Vanne, MS, RDN

The Changing Face of HIV in the United States, 787

Epidemiology and Trends, 788

Pathophysiology and Classification, 788

Medical Management, 790

Medical Nutrition Therapy, 793

HIV in Women, 802

HIV in Children, 803

Integrative and Functional Nutrition (IFN), 803

37 Medical Nutrition Therapy in Critical Care, 807

Britta Brown, MS, RDN, LD, CNSC

Katherine Hall, RDN, LD, CNSC

Metabolic Response to Stress, 807

Hormonal and Cell-Mediated Response, 807

Starvation Versus Stress, 809

Systemic Inflammatory Response Syndrome, Sepsis, and Organ Dysfunction or Failure, 809

Malnutrition: The Etiology-Based Definition, 810

Trauma and the Open Abdomen, 816

Major Burns, 816

Surgery, 819

38 Medical Nutrition Therapy for Rheumatic and Musculoskeletal Disease, 823

F. Enrique Gómez, MSc, PhD

Gabriela E. Mancera-Chávez, MSc, NC

Martha Kaufer-Horwitz, MSc, DSc, NC, FTOS

Etiology, 824

Pathophysiology and Inflammation, 824

Medical Diagnosis and Treatment, 825

Pharmacotherapy, 825

Antiinflammatory Diet, 828

Complementary and Integrative Health Approaches, 828

Microbiota and Arthritis, 829

Osteoarthritis, 829

Rheumatoid Arthritis, 832

Sjögren's Syndrome, 837

Temporomandibular Disorders, 837

Gout, 838

Scleroderma (Systemic Sclerosis or SSc), 840

Systemic Lupus Erythematosus, 841

Spondylarthritides, 842

39 Medical Nutrition Therapy for Neurologic Disorders, 846

Maggie Moon, MS, RDN

Ashley Contreras-France, MA, MS, CCC-SLP

The Nervous System, 846

Dysphagia, 852

Neurologic Diseases of Nutritional Origin, 857

Neurologic Disorders From Trauma, 857

Head Trauma or Neurotrauma, 860

Spine Trauma and Spinal Cord Injury, 864

Neurologic Diseases, 864

40 Medical Nutrition Therapy in Psychiatric and Cognitive Disorders, 882
Christina Troutner, MS, RDN
    The Enteric Nervous System, 883
    Blood Glucose Regulation, 884
    The Role of Nutrients in Mental Function, 884
    Addiction and Substance Abuse, 892
    Anxiety, 894
    Bipolar Disorder, 895
    Dementia and Alzheimer's Disease, 896
    Depression, 901
    Fatigue, Chronic Fatigue Syndrome (CFS), and Fibromyalgia Syndrome (FMS), 903
    Schizophrenia, 905

PART VI: Pediatric Specialties

41 Medical Nutrition Therapy for Low-Birthweight Infants, 912
Diane M. Anderson, PhD, RDN, FADA
    Infant Mortality and Statistics, 912
    Physiologic Development, 912
    Nutrition Requirements: Parenteral Feeding, 914
    Transition From Parenteral to Enteral Feeding, 919
    Nutrition Requirements: Enteral Feeding, 919
    Feeding Methods, 922
    Selection of Enteral Feeding, 923
    Nutrition Assessment and Growth, 926
    Discharge Care, 927
    Neurodevelopmental Outcome, 930

42 Medical Nutrition Therapy for Genetic Metabolic Disorders, 935
Beth N. Ogata, MS, RDN, CD, CSP
Cristine M. Trahms, MS, RDN, FADA
    Newborn Screening, 935
    Disorders of Amino Acid Metabolism, 935
    Phenylketonuria, 939
    Disorders of Organic Acid Metabolism, 947
    Disorders of Urea Cycle Metabolism, 947
    Disorders of Carbohydrate Metabolism, 949
    Disorders of Fatty Acid Oxidation, 950
    Role of the Nutritionist in Genetic Metabolic Disorders, 951

43 Medical Nutrition Therapy for Intellectual and Developmental Disabilities, 954
Kim Nowak-Cooperman, MS, RDN, CD
Patricia Novak, MPH, RDN
Cam Lanier, RDN, CD
Christine Avgeris, RDN, CD
    Medical Nutrition Therapy, 954
    Chromosomal Abnormalities, 960
    Neurologic Disorders, 964
    Fetal Alcohol Syndrome, 973
    Community Resources, 975

Appendices

1 Milliequivalents and Milligrams of Electrolytes, 979
2 Equivalents, Conversions, and Portion (Scoop) Sizes, 980

3 Growth Charts, 981
4 Tanner Stages of Adolescent Development for Girls and Boys, 990
5 Direct Methods for Measuring Height and Weight and Indirect Methods for Measuring Height, 991
6 Determination of Frame Size, 993
7 Adjustment of Desirable Body Weight for Amputees, 994
8 Body Mass Index Table, 995
9 Percentage of Body Fat Based on Four Skinfold Measurements, 996
10 Physical Activity and Calories Expended per Hour, 997
11 Nutrition-Focused Physical Assessment, 1000
12 Laboratory Values for Nutritional Assessment and Monitoring, 1009
13 Nutritional Implications of Selected Drugs, 1031
14 Nutritional Facts on Fluid and Hydration, 1043
15 Enteral (Tube Feeding) Formulas for Adults Marketed in the United States, 1045
16 Sample Stepwise Method to Calculate a Parenteral Nutrition (PN) Formula, 1046
17 Dietary Approaches to Stop Hypertension (DASH) Diet, 1047
18 Exchange Lists and Carbohydrate Counting for Meal Planning, 1049
19 The Ketogenic Diet, 1062
20 The International Dysphagia Diet Standardisation Initiative (IDDSI), 1068
21 Renal Diet for Dialysis, 1073
22 The Antiinflammatory Diet, 1078
23 The Mediterranean Diet, 1082
24 Nutritional Facts on Alcoholic Beverages, 1084
25 Nutritional Facts on Caffeine-Containing Products, 1086
26 Nutritional Facts on Essential (Omega) Fatty Acids, 1087
27 Nutritional Facts on a High-Fiber Diet, 1090
28 Glycemic Index (GI) and Glycemic Load (GL) of Selected Foods, 1092
29 Nutritional Facts on a High-Protein Diet, 1094
30 Nutritional Facts on Vegetarian Eating, 1095
31 Nutritional Facts on Folic Acid, Vitamin B$_6$, and Vitamin B$_{12}$, 1098
32 Nutritional Facts on Choline, 1102
33 Nutritional Facts on Biotin, 1104
34 Nutritional Facts on Vitamin A and Carotenoids, 1105
35 Nutritional Facts on Vitamin C, 1108
36 Nutritional Facts on Vitamin E, 1110
37 Nutritional Facts on Vitamin K, 1112
38 Nutritional Facts on Vitamin D, 1114
39 Nutritional Facts on Calcium, 1116
40 Nutritional Facts on Chromium, 1119
41 Nutritional Facts on Iodine, 1120
42 Nutritional Facts on Iron, 1122
43 Nutritional Facts on Magnesium, 1124
44 Nutritional Facts on Potassium, 1126
45 Nutritional Facts on Selenium, 1127
46 Sodium in Food, 1128
47 Nutritional Facts on Zinc, 1130

PART I

Nutrition Assessment

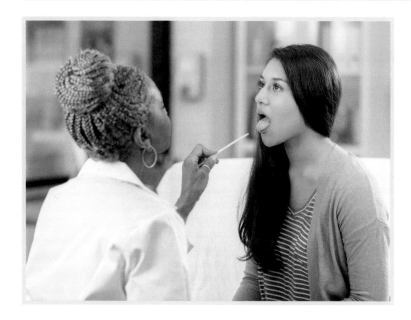

Food provides energy and building materials for countless substances that are essential for the growth and survival of every human being. This section opens with a brief overview of the digestion, absorption, transportation, and excretion of nutrients. These remarkable processes convert complex molecules in food into individual nutrients ready to be used in metabolism. Macronutrients (proteins, fats, and carbohydrates) each contribute to the total energy pool, but ultimately the energy they yield is available for the work of the muscles and organs of the body. The way nutrients become integral parts of the body and contribute to proper functioning depends heavily on the physiologic and biochemical processes that govern their actions. It is now known that these metabolic processes are altered in the presence of acute and chronic inflammation. Understanding the biomarkers and other indicators of inflammation is a critical component of nutrition assessment.

For the health provider, nutrition assessment is the first step in the nutrition care process. To implement a successful nutrition plan, the assessment must include key elements of the patient's clinical, medical, and social history, anthropometric measurements, biochemical and laboratory values, information on medication and herbal supplement use for potential food–drug interactions, plus a thorough food and nutrition intake history. Genetic research is rapidly clarifying how genes and nutrition are interrelated. Nutrigenomics is the study of the effects of foods and nutrients on gene expression and thus nutritional requirements. Thus the chapters in Part I provide an organized way to develop the skills needed to make an assessment in the nutrition care process.

Intake: Gastrointestinal Digestion, Absorption, and Excretion of Nutrients

Kelly A. Tappenden, PhD, RDN, FASPEN

KEY TERMS

amylase, pancreatic
amylase, salivary
brush border membrane
chelation
cholecystokinin (CCK)
chyme
colonic salvage
crypts
diffusion, facilitated
diffusion, passive
dysbiosis
enterocytes
enterohepatic circulation
enterokinase
enzymatic hydrolysis
epithelial cells
gastrin

ghrelin
glucagon-like peptide 2 (GLP-2)
gut–brain axis
isomaltase
lactase
lipase, gastric
lipase, pancreatic
lipase, salivary
lipolytic enzymes
maltase
micelle
microbiome
microbiota
microvilli
motilin
mucosa
parietal cells

pepsin
peristalsis
prebiotic
probiotic
proteolytic enzymes
secretin
segmentation
somatostatin
sucrase
synbiotic
transport, active
transport, passive
trypsin
trypsinogen
unstirred water layer (UWL)
villi

One of the primary considerations for a complete nutrition assessment is to consider the three-step model of "ingestion, digestion, and utilization." In this model, consideration is given to each step to identify all areas of inadequacy or excess. If there is any reason why a step is altered from physical, biochemical, or behavioral-environmental causes, the nutrition provider must select an appropriate nutrition diagnosis for which intervention is required. Intake and assimilation of nutrients should lead to nutritional and overall health.

THE GASTROINTESTINAL TRACT

The GIT is one of the largest organs in the body, has the greatest surface area, has the largest number of immune cells, and is one of the most metabolically active tissues in the body. The unique structure of the GIT enables ample nutrient-processing capacity in healthy humans. The human GIT is about 9 meters long, extending from the mouth to the anus and including the oropharyngeal structures, esophagus, stomach, liver and gallbladder, pancreas, and small and large intestine (Fig. 1.1).

Sections of the chapter were written by Peter L. Beyer, MS, RDN for previous editions of this text.

The GIT is designed to (1) digest the macronutrients protein, carbohydrates, and lipids from ingested foods and beverages; (2) absorb fluids, digested macronutrients, micronutrients, and trace elements; (3) provide a physical and immunologic barrier to pathogens, foreign material, and potential antigens consumed with food or formed during the passage of food through the GIT; (4) coordinate a response to microbes and antigens with the systemic immune system, resulting in controlled levels of tolerance or inflammation; and (5) provide regulatory and biochemical signaling to the nervous system, often involving the intestinal microbiota, via a pathway known as the gut–brain axis.

The human GIT is well suited for digesting and absorbing nutrients from a tremendous variety of foods, including meats, dairy products, fruits, vegetables, grains, complex starches, sugars, fats, and oils. Depending on the nature of the diet consumed, 90% to 97% of food is digested and absorbed; most of the unabsorbed material is of plant origin. Compared with ruminants and animals with a very large cecum, humans are considerably less efficient at extracting energy from grasses, stems, seeds, and other coarse fibrous materials. Humans lack the enzymes to hydrolyze the chemical bonds that link the molecules of sugars that make up plant fibers. However, fibrous foods and any undigested carbohydrates are fermented to varying degrees by bacteria in the human colon; this process can contribute 5% to 10% of the energy needed by humans.

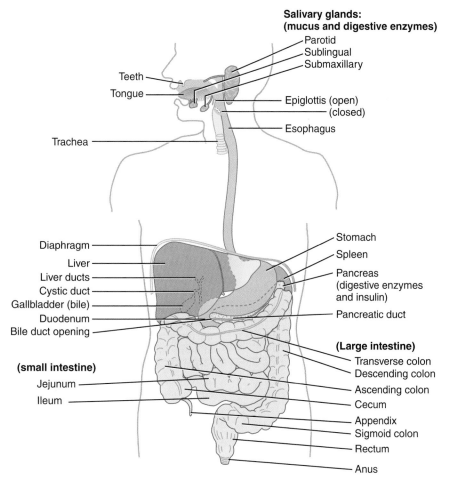

Salivary glands:
(mucus and digestive enzymes)
Parotid
Sublingual
Submaxillary

Teeth
Tongue

Epiglottis (open)
(closed)

Esophagus

Trachea

Diaphragm
Liver
Liver ducts
Cystic duct
Gallbladder (bile)
Duodenum
Bile duct opening

Stomach
Spleen
Pancreas
(digestive enzymes
and insulin)
Pancreatic duct

(Large intestine)
Transverse colon
Descending colon
Ascending colon
Cecum
Appendix
Sigmoid colon
Rectum
Anus

(small intestine)
Jejunum
Ileum

Fig. 1.1 The digestive system.

The structure of the small intestine is carefully designed to allow for a very large surface area that permits the adequate digestion and absorption of the nutrients from food. The lining of this hollow tube, called the mucosa, is configured in a pattern of folds that contains invaginations called crypts and fingerlike projections called villi (Fig. 1.2). These crypt-villus units are lined with a single layer of epithelial cells, many of which are enterocytes that contain even smaller cylindrical extensions called microvilli. The epithelial cells lining the intestinal tract have a life span of approximately 3 to 5 days, and then they are sloughed into the lumen and "recycled," adding to the pool of available nutrients. As the cells migrate from the crypt along the villus, they mature and develop greater digestive and absorptive function.

The health of the body depends on a healthy, functional GIT. Because of the unusually high turnover rate and metabolic requirements of the epithelial cells, gastrointestinal functions are particularly susceptible to impairment due to micronutrient deficiencies, protein-energy malnutrition, and damage resulting from toxins, drugs, irradiation, food allergy reactions, or interruption of its blood supply. Approximately 45% of the energy requirement of the small intestine and 70% of the energy requirement of cells lining the colon are supplied by nutrients passing through its lumen. After only a few days of starvation or intravenous feeding (parenteral nutrition), the intestinal mucosa atrophies (i.e., the surface area decreases and secretions, synthetic functions, blood flow, and absorptive capacity are all reduced). Resumption of food intake stimulates epithelial cell proliferation and return of normal GI function after only a few days. This knowledge justifies the clinical practice of feeding an individual orally and/or enterally (via tube), as opposed to intravenously (or parenterally), when adequate GIT function is present (see Chapter 12).

BRIEF OVERVIEW OF DIGESTIVE AND ABSORPTIVE PROCESSES

The sight, smell, taste, and even thought of food starts the secretions and movements of the GIT. In the mouth, chewing reduces the size of food particles, which are mixed with salivary secretions that prepare them for swallowing. A small amount of starch is degraded by salivary amylase, but digestion in the mouth is minimal. The esophagus transports food and liquid from the oral cavity and pharynx to the stomach. In the stomach, food is mixed with acidic fluid that contains proteolytic and lipolytic enzymes. Small amounts of lipid digestion take place; some proteins change in structure due to denaturation and partial digestion. When food reaches the appropriate consistency and concentration, it is now called chyme and passes from the stomach into the small intestine, where most digestion takes place.

The first 100 cm of the small intestine is highly active, resulting in the digestion and absorption of most ingested food (Fig. 1.3). Here the presence of food stimulates the release of hormones that stimulate the

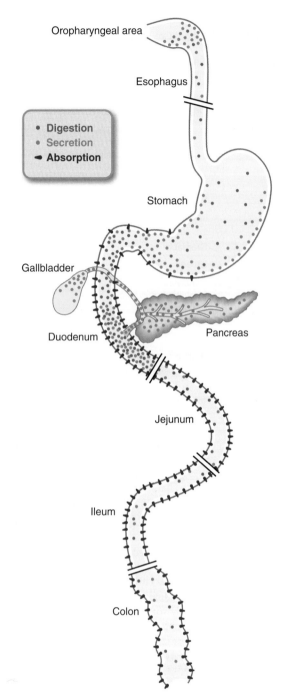

Fig. 1.2 Structure of the human intestine showing crypt-villus architecture and blood and lymph vessels.

Labels on figure:
- Oropharyngeal area
- Esophagus
- Stomach
- Gallbladder
- Duodenum
- Pancreas
- Jejunum
- Ileum
- Colon
- Digestion
- Secretion
- Absorption

production and release of powerful enzymes from the pancreas and bile from the gallbladder. Starches and proteins are reduced to small-molecular-weight carbohydrates and small to medium-size peptides. Dietary fats are reduced from visible globules of fat to microscopic droplets of triglycerides, then to free fatty acids and monoglycerides. Enzymes located on the brush border membrane of the enterocytes further reduce the remaining carbohydrates to monosaccharides and the remaining peptides to single amino acids, dipeptides, and tripeptides.

Large volumes of fluid are used to digest and absorb nutrients. Together with salivary and gastric secretions, secretions from the pancreas, small intestine, and gallbladder secrete 7 L of fluid into the GIT lumen each day—far more than the 2 L ingested through dietary intake each day. All but 100 mL of the total fluid entering the lumen is reabsorbed: about 7 L in the small intestine and about 2 L in the large intestine.

Along the remaining length of the small intestine, almost all the macronutrients, minerals, vitamins, trace elements, and fluid are absorbed before reaching the colon. The colon and rectum absorb most of the remaining fluid delivered from the small intestine. The colon absorbs electrolytes and only a small amount of remaining nutrients. The movement of ingested and secreted material in the GIT is regulated primarily by hormones, nerves, and enteric muscles.

Most nutrients absorbed from the GIT enter the portal vein for transport to the liver where they may be stored, transformed into other substances, or released into circulation. However, end products of most dietary fats are transported into the bloodstream via the lymphatic circulation because they are not water soluble prior to lipoprotein metabolism in the liver (see Chapter 28).

Nutrients reaching the distal small intestine and large intestine, most notably fermentable dietary fiber and resistant starches, are fermented by the microbiota located within the lumen of these intestinal segments. Fermentation produces short-chain fatty acids (SCFAs) and gas. SCFAs provide a preferred fuel source for cells of the intestine, stimulate intestinal cell renewal and function, enhance immune function, and regulate gene expression. In addition, some carbohydrates have "prebiotic" functions that induce the growth and activity of beneficial microbes within the intestinal microbiota. The large intestine also provides temporary storage for waste products. The distal colon, rectum, and anus control defecation.

Enzymes in Digestion

Humans digest food using the chemical process called enzymatic hydrolysis. Cofactors such as hydrochloric acid, bile, and sodium bicarbonate facilitate these processes. Digestive enzymes synthesized in specialized cells of the mouth, stomach, and pancreas are released into the GIT lumen, whereas digestive enzymes synthesized in enterocytes of the small intestine remain embedded within the brush border membrane. Except for fiber and resistant carbohydrates, digestion and absorption of food is completed essentially in the small intestine. Table 1.1 summarizes key enzymes involved in human digestion.

Regulators of Gastrointestinal Activity: Neural and Hormonal Mechanisms

Multiple layers of smooth muscle contract in coordinated patterns to optimize nutrient digestion along the GIT. These smooth muscle movements are regulated by the enteric nervous system and enteroendocrine hormones and facilitate mixing of chyme and digestive secretions (segmentation) or propulsion of luminal contents along the length of the GIT (peristalsis). To enable such coordinated actions, the enteric nervous system is integrated throughout the lining of the GIT and responds to mucosal receptors that sense the composition of chyme and distention of the lumen (i.e., fullness) and send impulses that coordinate the processes of digestion, secretion, absorption, and immunity.

Neurotransmitters from the central nervous system interface with the enteric nervous system to coordinate gastrointestinal functions such as motility, secretion, and blood flow. The GIT then largely regulates its own motility and secretory activity. However, signals from the central nervous system can override the enteric system and affect GIT function. Hormones, neuropeptides, and neurotransmitters in the GIT not only affect intestinal function but also have an effect on other nerves and tissues in many parts of the body. Some examples

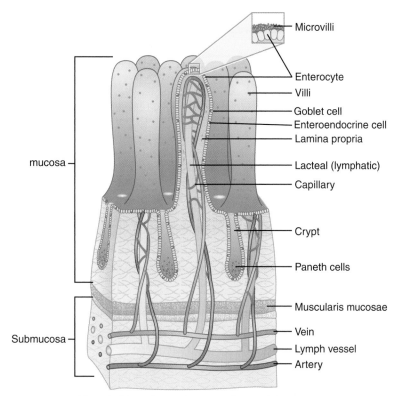

- Microvilli
- Enterocyte
- Villi
- Goblet cell
- Enteroendocrine cell
- Lamina propria
- Lacteal (lymphatic)
- Capillary
- Crypt
- Paneth cells
- Muscularis mucosae
- Vein
- Lymph vessel
- Artery

mucosa

Submucosa

Fig. 1.3 Sites of secretion, digestion, and absorption.

of neurotransmitters released from enteric nerve endings are listed in Table 1.2. In people with gastrointestinal disease (e.g., infections, inflammatory bowel disease, irritable bowel syndrome), the enteric nervous system may be overstimulated, resulting in abnormal secretion, altered blood flow, increased permeability, and altered immune function.

Autonomic innervation is supplied by the sympathetic fibers that run along blood vessels and by the parasympathetic fibers in the vagal and pelvic nerves. In general, sympathetic neurons, which are activated by fear, anger, and stress, tend to slow transit of intestinal contents by inhibiting neurons affecting muscle contraction and inhibiting secretions. The parasympathetic nerves innervate specific areas of the alimentary tract and contribute to certain functions. For example, the sight or smell of food stimulates vagal activity and subsequent secretion of acid from parietal cells within the stomach. The enteric nervous system also sends signals to the central nervous system that are perceived as pain, nausea, urgency or gastric fullness, or gastric emptiness by way of the vagal and spinal nerves. Inflammation, dysmotility, and various types of intestinal damage may intensify these perceptions.

Gastrointestinal Hormones

Regulation of the GIT involves numerous hormones that are secreted by enteroendocrine cells located within the epithelium lining of the GIT. These hormones can regulate function of the cell from which they were secreted (autocrine), on neighboring cells (paracrine), or distant cells by traveling through the blood to their target organs (endocrine).

More than 100 peptide hormones and hormone-like growth factors have been identified. Their actions are often complex and extend well beyond the GIT. Some of the hormones (e.g., of the cholecystokinin [CCK] and somatostatin family) also serve as neurotransmitters between neurons. The GIT secretes more than 30 hormone families,

making it the largest hormone-producing organ in the body (Rehfeld, 2014). Gastrointestinal hormones are involved in initiating and terminating feeding, signaling hunger and satiety, pacing movements of the GIT, governing gastric emptying, regulating blood flow and permeability, priming immune functions, and stimulating the growth of cells (within and beyond the GIT). Ghrelin, a neuropeptide secreted from the stomach, and motilin, a related hormone secreted from the duodenum, send a "hungry" message to the brain. Once food has been ingested, hormones PYY 3-36, CCK, glucagon-like peptide-1 (GLP-1), oxyntomodulin, pancreatic polypeptide, and gastrin-releasing polypeptide (bombesin) send signals to decrease hunger and increase satiety (Rui, 2013). Some of the GI hormones, including some of those that affect satiety, also tend to slow gastric emptying and decrease secretions (e.g., somatostatin). Other GI hormones (e.g., motilin) increase motility.

The signaling agents of the GIT also are involved in several metabolic functions. Glucose-dependent insulinotropic polypeptide (GIP) and GLP-1 are called incretin hormones because they help lower blood sugar by facilitating insulin secretion, decreasing gastric emptying, and increasing satiety. Several of these hormones and analogs are used in management of obesity, inflammatory bowel disease, diarrhea, diabetes, GI malignancies, and other conditions. This area of research is critically important.

Some functions of the hormones that affect gastrointestinal cell growth, deoxyribonucleic acid (DNA) synthesis, inflammation, proliferation, secretion, movement, or metabolism have not been fully identified. Knowledge of major hormone functions becomes especially important when the sites of their secretion or action are diseased or removed in surgical procedures, or when hormones and their analogs are used to suppress or enhance some aspect of gastrointestinal function. Glucagon-like peptide-2 (GLP-2) is an example of a hormone secreted from the distal GIT that increases intestinal surface area and enhances nutrient processing capacity. An analog of GLP-2, named

TABLE 1.1 Summary of Enzymatic Digestion and Absorption

Secretion and Source	Enzymes	Substrate	Action and Resulting Products	Final Products Absorbed
Saliva from salivary glands in mouth	α-amylase	Starch (α-linked polysaccharides)	Hydrolysis to form dextrins and maltose	—
	Lingual lipase	Triglyceride	Hydrolysis to form diglyceride and free fatty acids	—
Gastric secretion from gastric glands in stomach mucosa	Pepsin (activated from pepsinogen in the presence of hydrochloric acid)	Protein	Hydrolysis of peptide bonds to form peptides and amino acids	—
	Gastric lipase	Triglyceride	Hydrolysis to form diglyceride and free fatty acids	—
Exocrine secretions from pancreatic acinar cells, acting in duodenum	Lipase	Fat (in the presence of bile salts)	Hydrolysis to form monoglycerides and fatty acids; incorporated into micelles	Fatty acids into mucosal cells; reesterified as triglycerides
	Cholesterol esterase	Sterols (such as cholesterol)	Hydrolysis to form esters of cholesterol and fatty acids; incorporated into micelles	Cholesterol into mucosal cells; transferred to chylomicrons
	α-Amylase	Starch and dextrins	Hydrolysis to form dextrins and maltose	—
	Trypsin (activated trypsinogen)	Proteins and polypeptides	Hydrolysis of interior peptide bonds to form polypeptides	—
	Chymotrypsin (activated chymotrypsinogen)	Proteins and peptides	Hydrolysis of interior peptide bonds to form polypeptides	—
	Carboxypeptidase (activated procarboxypeptidase)	Polypeptides	Hydrolysis of terminal peptide bonds (carboxyl end) to form amino acids	Amino acids
	Ribonuclease and deoxyribonuclease	Ribonucleic acids (RNA) and deoxyribonucleic acids (DNA)	Hydrolysis to form mononucleotides	Mononucleotides
	Elastase	Fibrous protein (elastin)	Hydrolysis to form peptides and amino acids	—
Small intestine enzymes (embedded in the brush border membrane)	Enterokinase	Trypsinogen	Activates trypsin	Dipeptides and tripeptides
	Aminopeptidase and dipeptidase (also located within the enterocyte cytosol)	Polypeptides	Cleavage of amino acids from the amino terminus of protein (N-terminus) or peptide substrates	Amino acids
	Sucrase	Sucrose	Hydrolysis to form glucose and fructose	Glucose and fructose
	α-Dextrinase (isomaltase)	Dextrin (isomaltose)	Hydrolysis to form glucose	Glucose
	Maltase	Maltose	Hydrolysis to form glucose	Glucose
	Lactase	Lactose	Hydrolysis to form glucose and galactose	Glucose and galactose
	Nucleotidases	Nucleic acids	Hydrolysis to form nucleotides and phosphates	Nucleotides
	Nucleosidase and phosphorylase	Nucleosides	Hydrolysis to form purines, pyrimidines, and pentose phosphate	Purine and pyrimidine bases

TABLE 1.2 Examples of Neurotransmitters and Their Actions

Neurotransmitter	Site of Release	Primary Action
GABA	Central nervous system	Relaxes lower esophageal sphincter
Norepinephrine	Central nervous system, spinal cord, sympathetic nerves	Decreases motility, increases contraction of sphincters, inhibits secretions
Acetylcholine	Central nervous system, autonomic system, other tissues	Increases motility, relaxes sphincters, stimulates secretion
Neurotensin	GI tract, central nervous system	Inhibits release of gastric emptying and acid secretion
Serotonin (5-HT)	GI tract, spinal cord	Facilitates secretion and peristalsis
Nitric oxide	Central nervous system, GI tract	Regulates blood flow, maintains muscle tone, maintains gastric motor activity
Substance P	Gut, central nervous system, skin	Increases sensory awareness (mainly pain), and peristalsis

5-HT, 5-hydroxytryptamine; GABA, α-aminobutyric acid; GI, gastrointestinal.

TABLE 1.3 Functions of Major Gastrointestinal Hormones

Hormone	Site of Release	Stimulants for Release	Organ Affected	Effect on Target Organ
Gastrin	G cells of gastric mucosa and duodenum	Peptides, amino acids, caffeine	Stomach, esophagus, GIT in general	Stimulates secretion of HCl and pepsinogen
		Distention of the antrum		Increases gastric antral motility
		Some alcoholic beverages, vagus nerve		Increases lower esophageal sphincter tone
			Gallbladder	Weakly stimulates contraction of gallbladder
			Pancreas	Weakly stimulates pancreatic secretion of bicarbonate
Secretin	S cells of duodenum	Acid in small intestine	Pancreas	Increases output of H_2O and bicarbonate; increases enzyme secretion from the pancreas and insulin release
			Duodenum	Decreases motility
				Increases mucus output
CCK	I cells of duodenum	Peptides, amino acids, fats, HCl	Pancreas	Stimulates secretion of pancreatic enzymes
			Gallbladder	Causes contraction of gallbladder
			Stomach	Slows gastric emptying
			Colon	Increases motility
				May mediate feeding behavior
GIP	K cells of duodenum and jejunum	Glucose, fat	Stomach	Reduced intestinal motility
Motilin	M cells of duodenum and jejunum	Interdigestive periods, alkaline pH in duodenum	Stomach, small bowel, colon	Promotes gastric emptying and GI motility
GLP-1	L cells of small intestine and colon (density increases in distal GIT)	Glucose, fat, short-chain fatty acids	Stomach	Prolongs gastric emptying
			Pancreas	Inhibits glucagon release; Stimulates insulin release
GLP-2	L cells of small intestine and colon (density increases in distal GIT)	Glucose, fat, short-chain fatty acids	Small intestine, colon	Stimulates intestinal growth and nutrient digestion and absorption

CCK, Cholecystokinin; *GI*, gastrointestinal; *GIP*, glucose-dependent insulinotropic polypeptide; *GIT*, gastrointestinal tract; *GLP-1*, glucagon-like peptide-1; *GLP-2*, glucagon-like peptide-2; *H₂O*, water; *HCl*, hydrochloric acid.

teduglutide, recently has become available for treatment of patients with short bowel syndrome who are dependent on parenteral nutrition to meet their nutrient and fluid requirements (Seidner et al, 2013; see Chapter 27). The key GIT hormones are summarized in Table 1.3.

Gastrin, a hormone that stimulates gastric secretions and motility, is secreted primarily from endocrine "G" cells in the antral mucosa of the stomach. Secretion is initiated by (1) impulses from the vagus nerve, such as those triggered by the smell or sight of food; (2) distention of the antrum after a meal; and (3) the presence of secretagogues in the antrum, such as partially digested proteins, fermented alcoholic beverages, caffeine, or food extracts (e.g., bouillon). When the lumen gets more acidic, feedback involving other hormones inhibits gastrin release (Chu and Schubert, 2013). Gastrin binds to receptors on parietal cells and histamine-releasing cells to stimulate gastric acid, to receptors on chief cells to release pepsinogen, and to receptors on smooth muscle to increase gastric motility.

Secretin, the first hormone to be named, is released from "S" cells in the wall of the proximal small intestine into the bloodstream. It is secreted in response to gastric acid and digestive end products in the duodenum, wherein it stimulates the secretion of pancreatic juice and inhibits gastric acid secretion and emptying (the opposite of gastrin). Neutralized acidity protects the duodenal mucosa from prolonged exposure to acid and provides the appropriate environment

for intestinal and pancreatic enzyme activity. The human receptor is found in the stomach and ductal and acinar cells of the pancreas. In different species, other organs may express secretin, including the liver, colon, heart, kidney, and brain (Chey and Chang, 2014).

Small bowel mucosal "I" cells secrete CCK, an important multifunctional hormone released in response to the presence of protein and fat. Receptors for CCK are in pancreatic acinar cells, pancreatic islet cells, gastric somatostatin-releasing D cells, smooth muscle cells of the GIT, and the central nervous system. Major functions of CCK are to (1) stimulate the pancreas to secrete enzymes, bicarbonate, and water; (2) stimulate gallbladder contraction; (3) increase colonic and rectal motility; (4) slow gastric emptying; and (5) increase satiety. CCK is also widely distributed in the brain and plays a role in neuronal functioning.

Motilin is released by endocrine cells in the duodenal mucosa during fasting to stimulate gastric emptying and intestinal migrating contractions. Erythromycin, an antibiotic, has been shown to bind to motilin receptors; thus analogs of erythromycin and motilin have been used as therapeutic agents to treat delayed gastric emptying (Wijeratne et al, 2016).

Somatostatin, released by "D" cells in the antrum and pylorus, is a hormone with far-reaching actions. Its primary roles are inhibitory and antisecretory. It decreases motility of the stomach and intestine and inhibits or regulates the release of several gastrointestinal hormones. Somatostatin and its analog, octreotide, are being used to treat certain malignant diseases, as well as numerous gastrointestinal disorders such as diarrhea, short bowel syndrome, pancreatitis, dumping syndrome, and gastric hypersecretion (Van Op den Bosch et al, 2009; see Chapters 26 and 27).

Digestion in the Mouth

In the mouth, the teeth grind and crush food into small particles. The food mass is simultaneously moistened and lubricated by saliva. Three pairs of salivary glands—the parotid, submaxillary, and sublingual glands—produce approximately 1.5 L of saliva daily. Enzymatic digestion of starch and lipid is initiated in the mouth due to the presence of amylase and salivary lipase, respectively, in saliva. This digestion is minimal, and the salivary amylase becomes inactive when it reaches the acidic contents of the stomach. Saliva also contains mucus, a protein that causes particles of food to stick together and lubricates the mass for swallowing.

The masticated food mass, or bolus, is passed back to the pharynx under voluntary control, but throughout the esophagus, the process of swallowing (deglutition) is involuntary. Peristalsis then moves the food rapidly into the stomach (see Chapter 39 for a detailed discussion of swallowing).

Digestion in the Stomach

Food particles are propelled forward and mixed with gastric secretions by wavelike contractions that progress forward from the upper portion of the stomach (fundus), to the midportion (corpus), and then to the antrum and pylorus. In the stomach, gastric secretions mix with food and beverages producing a semiliquid slurry called chyme, which is 50% water. An average of 2000 to 2500 mL of fluid is secreted daily in the stomach. These gastric secretions contain hydrochloric acid (secreted by the parietal cells), pepsinogen, gastric lipase, mucus, intrinsic factor (a glycoprotein that facilitates vitamin B_{12} absorption in the ileum), and gastrin. The protease, pepsin, is secreted in an inactive form, pepsinogen, which is converted by hydrochloric acid to its active form. Pepsin is active only in the acidic environment of the stomach and acts to begin the process of protein digestion.

An acid-stable lipase is secreted into the stomach by chief cells. Although this lipase is considerably less active than pancreatic lipase, it contributes to the overall processing of dietary triglycerides. Gastric lipase is more specific for triglycerides composed of medium- and short-chain fatty acids, but the usual diet contains few of these fats. Lipases secreted in the upper portions of the GIT may have a relatively important role in the liquid diet of infants; however, when pancreatic insufficiency occurs, it becomes apparent that lingual and gastric lipases are not sufficient to adequately digest fat from food and prevent lipid malabsorption.

When food is consumed, significant numbers of microorganisms are also consumed. The stomach pH is low, ranging from about 1 to 4. The combined actions of hydrochloric acid and proteolytic enzymes result in a significant reduction in the concentration of viable microorganisms. Some microbes may escape and enter the intestine if consumed in sufficient concentrations or if achlorhydria, gastrectomy, gastrointestinal dysfunction or disease, poor nutrition, or drugs that suppress acid secretions are present. This may increase the risk of pathogenic infection in the intestine.

The lower esophageal sphincter (LES), which lies above the entrance to the stomach, prevents reflux of gastric contents into the esophagus. The pyloric sphincter in the distal portion of the stomach helps regulate the exit of gastric contents, preventing backflow of chyme from the duodenum ntuto the stomach. Obesity, certain food, gastrointestinal regulators, and irritation from nearby ulcers may alter

the performance of sphincters. Certain foods and beverages may alter LES pressure, permitting reflux of stomach contents back into the esophagus (see Chapter 26).

The stomach continuously mixes and churns food and normally releases the mixture in small quantities into the small intestine through the pyloric sphincter. The amount emptied with each contraction of the antrum and pylorus varies with the volume and type of food consumed, but only a few milliliters are released at a time. The presence of acid and nutrients in the duodenum stimulate the regulatory hormone, GIP, to slow gastric emptying.

Most of a liquid meal empties from the stomach within 1 to 2 hours, and most of a solid meal empties within 2 to 3 hours. When eaten alone, carbohydrates leave the stomach the most rapidly, followed by protein, fat, and fibrous food. In a meal with mixed types of foods, emptying of the stomach depends on the overall volume and characteristics of the foods. Liquids empty more rapidly than solids, large particles empty more slowly than small particles, and energy-dense foods empty more slowly than those containing less energy. These factors are important considerations for practitioners who counsel patients with nausea, vomiting, diabetic gastroparesis, or weight management concerns (see Chapters 26 and 20).

Digestion in the Small Intestine

The small intestine is the primary site for digestion of foods and nutrients. The small intestine is divided into the duodenum, the jejunum, and the ileum (see Fig. 1.2). The duodenum is approximately 0.5 m long, the jejunum is 2 to 3 m, and the ileum is 3 to 4 m. Most of the digestive process is completed in the duodenum and upper jejunum, and the absorption of most nutrients is largely complete by the time the material reaches the middle of the jejunum. The acidic chyme from the stomach enters the duodenum, where it is mixed with secretions from the pancreas, gallbladder, and duodenal epithelium. The sodium bicarbonate contained within these secretions neutralizes the acidic chyme and allows the digestive enzymes to work more effectively at this location.

The entry of partially digested foods, primarily fats and protein, stimulates the release of CCK, secretin, and GIP, which, in turn, stimulate the secretion of enzymes and fluids and affect gastrointestinal motility and satiety. Bile, which is predominantly a mixture of water, bile salts, and small amounts of pigments and cholesterol, is secreted from the liver and gallbladder. Through their surfactant properties, the bile salts facilitate the digestion and absorption of lipids, cholesterol, and fat-soluble vitamins. Bile acids are also regulatory molecules; they activate the vitamin D receptor and cell-signaling pathways in the liver and GIT that alter gene expression of enzymes involved in the regulation of energy metabolism (Hylemon et al, 2009). Furthermore, bile acids play an important role in hunger and satiety.

The pancreas secretes potent enzymes capable of digesting all of the major nutrients, and enzymes from the small intestine help complete the process. The primary lipid-digesting enzymes secreted by the pancreas are pancreatic lipase and colipase. Proteolytic enzymes include trypsin and chymotrypsin, carboxypeptidase, aminopeptidase, ribonuclease, and deoxyribonuclease. Trypsin and chymotrypsin are secreted in their inactive forms and are activated by enterokinase (also known as enteropeptidase), which is bound within the brush border membrane of enterocytes within the small intestine. Pancreatic amylase eventually hydrolyzes large starch molecules into units of approximately two to six sugars. Disaccharidase enzymes bound in the enterocyte brush border membrane further break down the carbohydrate molecules into monosaccharides before absorption. Varying amounts of resistant starches and most ingested dietary fiber escape digestion in the small intestine and may add to fibrous material available for fermentation by colonic microbes.

Intestinal contents move along the small intestine at a rate of approximately 1 cm per minute, taking from 3 to 8 hours to travel through the entire intestine to the ileocecal valve; along the way, remaining substrates continue to be digested and absorbed. The ileocecal valve, like the pyloric sphincter, paces the entry of chyme into the colon and limits the amount of material passed back and forth between the small intestine and the colon. A damaged or nonfunctional ileocecal valve results in the entry of significant amounts of fluid and substrate into the colon and increases the chance for microbial overgrowth in the small intestine (see Chapter 26).

THE SMALL INTESTINE: PRIMARY SITE OF NUTRIENT ABSORPTION

The primary organ of nutrient and water absorption is the small intestine, which has an expansive absorptive area. The surface area is attributable to its extensive length, as well as to the organization of the mucosal lining, wherein there are characteristic folds in its mucosal surface that are covered with fingerlike projections called villi and invaginations called crypts (see Fig. 1.2). Enterocytes, a cell type that does much of the digestion and absorption are covered by microvilli, or the brush border membrane, which increases the surface area even further. The combination of folds, the crypt-villus axis, and the brush border membrane creates an enormous absorptive surface of approximately 200 to 300 m^2—a surface area equivalent to a tennis court. The villi rest on a supporting structure called the lamina propria. Within the lamina propria is connective tissue, immune cells, and the blood and lymph vessels that receive the nutrients produced during digestion.

Each day, on average, the small intestine absorbs 150 to 300 g of monosaccharides, 60 to 100 g of fatty acids, 60 to 120 g of amino acids and peptides, and 50 to 100 g of ions. The capacity for absorption in the healthy individual far exceeds the normal macronutrient and energy requirements. Approximately 95% of the bile salts secreted from the liver and gallbladder are reabsorbed as bile acids in the distal ileum. Without recycling bile acids from the GIT (enterohepatic circulation), synthesis of new bile acids in the liver would not keep pace with needs for adequate digestion. Bile salt insufficiency becomes clinically important in patients who have resections of the distal small bowel and diseases affecting the small intestine, such as Crohn's disease, radiation enteritis, and cystic fibrosis. The distal ileum is also the site for vitamin B$_{12}$ (with intrinsic factor) absorption.

Absorptive and Transport Mechanisms

Absorption is a complex process involving many distinct pathways for specific nutrients and/or ions. However, the two basic transport mechanisms used are passive and active transport. The primary differences between the two are whether (1) the nutrient being transported is moving with a concentration gradient or (2) energy in the form of ATP is required because the nutrient being transported is moving against a concentration gradient.

Passive transport does not require energy, and nutrients move from a location of high concentration to low concentration. With passive transport a transport protein may or may not be involved. If the nutrient moves through the brush border membrane without a transport protein, this is termed passive diffusion, or simple passive transport. However, in cases in which a transport protein assists the passage of the nutrient across the brush border membrane, this process is termed facilitated diffusion (Fig. 1.4).

Active transport is the movement of molecules across cell membranes in the direction against their concentration gradient and therefore requires a transporter protein and energy in the form of ATP. Some nutrients may share the same transporter and thus compete for absorption. Transport or carrier systems also can become saturated, slowing the absorption of the nutrient. A notable example of such a carrier is intrinsic factor, which is responsible for the absorption of vitamin B$_{12}$ (see Chapter 26).

THE LARGE INTESTINE

The large intestine is approximately 1.5 m long and consists of the cecum, colon, rectum, and anal tract. Mucus secreted by the mucosa of the large intestine protects the intestinal wall from excoriation and bacterial activity and provides the medium for binding the feces together. Approximately 2 L of fluids are taken from food and beverages during the day, and 7 L of fluid is secreted along the GIT. Under normal circumstances, most of that fluid is absorbed in the small intestine, and approximately 2 L of fluid enters the large intestine. All but 100 to 150 mL of this fluid is absorbed; the remainder is excreted in the feces.

The large intestine is also the site of bacterial fermentation of remaining carbohydrates and amino acids, synthesis of a small amount of vitamins (particularly vitamin K), storage, and excretion of fecal residues. Colonic contents move forward slowly at a rate of 5 cm/h, and some remaining nutrients may be absorbed.

Defecation, or expulsion of feces through the rectum and anus, occurs with varying frequency, ranging from three times daily to once

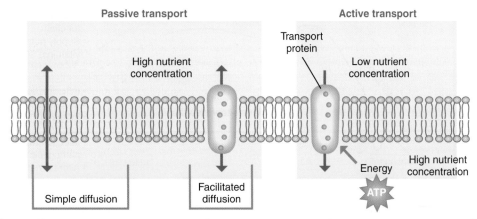

Fig. 1.4 Transport pathways through the cell membrane, as well as basic transport mechanisms. *ATP,* Adenosine triphosphate.

every 3 or more days. Average stool weight ranges from 100 to 200 g, and mouth-to-anus transit time may vary from 18 to 72 hours. The feces generally consist of 75% water and 25% solids, but the proportions vary greatly. Approximately two-thirds of the contents of the wet weight of the stool is bacteria, with the remainder coming from gastrointestinal secretions, mucus, sloughed cells, microbiota, and undigested foods. A diet that includes abundant fruits, vegetables, legumes, and whole grains typically results in a shorter overall GIT transit time, more frequent defecation, and larger and softer stools.

Intestinal Microbiota: The Microbiome

The intestinal microbiota, also called the microbiome, is a dynamic mixture of essential microbes that develops under key influences of genetics, environment, diet, and disease. Bacterial population profiles differ along the gastrointestinal tract, from the lumen to the mucosa, and among individuals. The total microbiota population outnumbers the cells in the human body by a factor of 10 and accounts for 35% to 50% of the volume of the colonic content. Key physiologic functions of the commensal microbiota include (1) protective effects exerted directly by specific bacterial species, (2) control of epithelial cell proliferation and differentiation, (3) production of essential mucosal nutrients, such as short-chain fatty acids and amino acids, (4) prevention of overgrowth of pathogenic organisms, (5) stimulation of intestinal immunity, and (6) development of the gut-brain axis (Kostic et al, 2014; see Chapter 40). Reduced abundance or changes in the relative proportions of these beneficial bacteria, a state called dysbiosis, is associated with various diseases in both children and adults (Buccigrossi et al, 2013; Fig. 1.5).

Normally, relatively few bacteria remain in the stomach and proximal small intestine after meals because bile, hydrochloric acid, and pepsin work as germicides. However, decreased gastric secretions can increase the risk of inflammation of the gastric mucosa (gastritis), increase the risk of bacterial overgrowth in the small intestine, or increase the numbers of microbes reaching the colon. An acid-tolerant bacterium is known to infect the stomach (Helicobacter pylori) and may cause gastritis and ulceration in the host (see Chapter 26).

Bacterial abundance is the greatest and action is most intense in the distal small intestine and the large intestine. After a meal, dietary fiber, resistant starches, remaining parts of amino acids, and mucus sloughed from the intestine are fermented by the microbes present. This process of fermentation produces gases (e.g., hydrogen, carbon dioxide, nitrogen, and, in some individuals, methane) and SCFAs (e.g., acetic, propionic, butyric, and some lactic acids). During the process, several nutrients are formed by bacterial synthesis, such as vitamin K, vitamin B_{12}, thiamin, and riboflavin.

Strategies to stabilize and fortify the beneficial microbes within the microbiota in an attempt to maintain or improve health include the consumption of prebiotics, probiotics, and synbiotics.

Probiotics are live microorganisms, which, when administered in adequate amounts, provide a health benefit to the host. Probiotics can be found within fermented food products (such as yogurt, miso, or sauerkraut) or as a nutritional supplement (Hill et al, 2014). Knowledge of their role in preventing and treating a host of gastrointestinal and systemic disorders has expanded tremendously in recent years (Floch, 2018). However, when recommending a probiotic, practitioners must ensure that the specific microbial species has been shown in properly controlled studies to provide benefits to health (see Chapter 11).

Prebiotics are nondigestible food ingredients that act as a substrate that is selectively utilized by host microorganisms conferring a health benefit. Prebiotics typically require the following three attributes to benefit "beneficial" microbes, such as *Lactobacilli* and *Bifidobacteria* spp.: (1) be able to escape digestion in the upper GIT, (2) be able to be fermented by the microbiota to SCFA(s), and (3) be able to increase the abundance and/or relative proportion of bacteria known to contribute to human health. Good dietary sources of prebiotic carbohydrates include vegetables (including onions, garlic, and asparagus), fruits (especially bananas, apples, stone fruits, and mangos), grains, legumes, chicory, Jerusalem artichokes, soybeans, and wheat bran. Strong evidence exists that consumption of specific prebiotics benefits the GIT including inhibition of pathogens and immune stimulation, cardiometabolic support (e.g., reduction in blood lipid levels, effects upon insulin resistance), mental health benefits (e.g., metabolites that influence brain function, energy, and cognition) and bone health (e.g., mineral bioavailability) (Gibson et al, 2017).

Synbiotics are a synergistic combination of both probiotics and prebiotics in the same food or supplement.

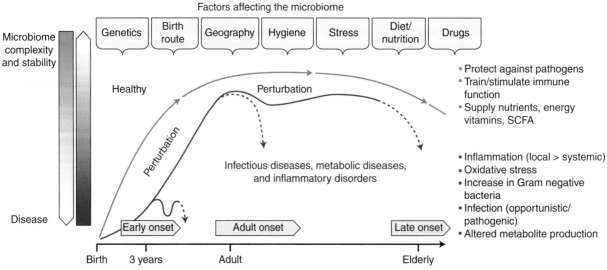

Fig. 1.5 Factors affecting stability and complexity of intestinal microbiota in health and disease. (Redrawn from Kostic AD et al: The microbiome in inflammatory bowel disease: current status and the future ahead, *Gastroenterology* 146:1489, 2014.)

Colonic Salvage of Malabsorbed Energy Sources and Short-chain Fatty Acids

Normally, varying amounts of some small-molecular-weight carbohydrates and amino acids remain in the chyme after leaving the small intestine. Accumulation of these small molecules could become osmotically important were it not for the action of bacteria in the colon. The disposal of residual substrates through production of SCFAs is called colonic salvage. SCFAs produced in fermentation are rapidly absorbed and take water with them. They also serve as fuel for the colonocytes and the microbiota, stimulate colonocyte proliferation and differentiation, enhance the absorption of electrolytes and water, and reduce the osmotic load of malabsorbed sugars. SCFAs also may help slow the movement of GI contents and participate in several other regulatory functions.

The ability to salvage carbohydrates is limited in humans. Colonic fermentation normally disposes of 20 to 25 g of carbohydrates over 24 hours. Excess amounts of carbohydrates and fermentable fiber in the colon can cause increased gas production, abdominal distention, bloating, pain, flatulence, decreased colonic pH, and diarrhea. Over time, adaptation occurs in individuals consuming diets high in fiber. Current recommendations are for the consumption of approximately 14 g of dietary fiber per 1000 kcal consumed each day. This recommendation can be met by consuming ample fruits, vegetables, legumes, seeds, and whole grains and is aimed to (1) support cardiovascular health, (2) maintain the health of the colonic epithelium, (3) prevent constipation, and (4) support stable, health-promoting microbiota.

Digestion and Absorption of Specific Types of Nutrients
Carbohydrates and Fiber

Most dietary carbohydrates are consumed in the form of starches, disaccharides, and monosaccharides. Starches, or polysaccharides, usually make up the greatest proportion of carbohydrates. Starches are large molecules composed of straight or branched chains of sugar molecules that are joined together, primarily in alpha 1-4 or

1-6 linkages. Most of the dietary starches are *amylopectins*, the branching polysaccharides, and amylose, the straight chain–type polymers.

Dietary fiber also is made largely of chains and branches of sugar molecules, but in this case the hydrogens are positioned on the beta (opposite) side of the oxygen in the link instead of the alpha side. Humans have significant ability to digest starch but not most fiber; this exemplifies the "stereospecificity" of enzymes.

In the mouth, the enzyme salivary amylase operates at a neutral or slightly alkaline pH and starts the digestive action by hydrolyzing a small amount of the starch molecules into smaller fragments (Fig. 1.6). Amylase deactivates after contact with hydrochloric acid. If digestible carbohydrates remained in the stomach long enough, acid hydrolysis could eventually reduce most of them into monosaccharides. However, the stomach usually empties before significant digestion can take place. By far, most carbohydrate digestion occurs in the proximal small intestine.

Pancreatic amylase breaks the large starch molecules at the 1-4 linkages to create maltose, maltotriose, and "alpha-limit" dextrins remaining from the amylopectin branches. Enzymes from the brush border of the enterocytes further break the disaccharides and oligosaccharides into monosaccharides. For example, maltase located at the enterocyte brush border membrane breaks down the disaccharide maltose into two molecules of glucose. The brush border membrane also contains the enzymes sucrase, lactase, and isomaltase, which act on sucrose, lactose, and isomaltose, respectively (Fig. 1.7).

The resultant monosaccharides (i.e., glucose, galactose, and fructose) pass through the enterocytes and into the bloodstream via the capillaries of the villi, where they are carried by the portal vein to the liver. At low concentrations, glucose and galactose are absorbed by active transport, primarily by a sodium-dependent active transporter called the sodium-glucose cotransporter (SGLT1). At higher luminal concentrations of glucose, the facilitative transporter GLUT2 becomes a primary route for transport of glucose from the lumen into the enterocyte. Fructose is absorbed from the intestinal lumen across the brush border membrane using the facilitative transporter, GLUT5. All three monosaccharides—glucose, galactose, and fructose—exit the

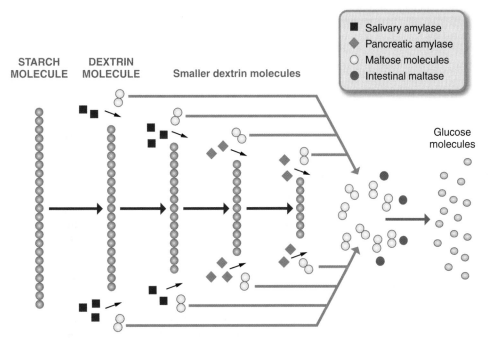

Fig. 1.6 The gradual breakdown of large starch molecules into glucose by digestion enzymes.

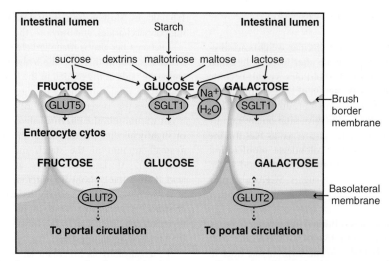

Fig. 1.7 Starch, sucrose, maltotriose, and galactose are digested to their constituent sugars. Glucose and galactose are transported through the apical brush border membrane of the enterocyte by a sodium-dependent transporter, glucose (galactose) cotransporter; fructose is transported by glucose transporter 5 (GLUT5). Glucose, fructose, and galactose are transported across the serosal membrane by the sodium-independent transporter, GLUT2.

basolateral membrane of the enterocyte into portal circulation using the facilitative transporter, GLUT2.

The active transporter, SGLT1, is key to the ability of the small intestine to absorb 7 L of fluid each day and provides the basis for why oral rehydration solutions, rather than water or sugary drinks, should be used to treat dehydration. In addition to transporting sodium and glucose, SGLT1 functions as a molecular water pump. For each molecule of glucose absorbed by SGLT1, two molecules of sodium and 210 molecules of water also are absorbed. Given that this is a major pathway for water absorption in the small intestine, to facilitate water absorption, sodium and glucose also must be present in the right amounts. This explains why the most effective oral rehydration solutions often include both sugar and salt, in addition to water.

Some forms of carbohydrates (i.e., cellulose, hemicellulose, pectin, gum, and other forms of fiber) cannot be digested by humans because neither salivary nor pancreatic amylase has the ability to split the linkages connecting the constituent sugars. These carbohydrates pass relatively unchanged into the colon, where they are partially fermented by bacteria in the colon. However, unlike humans, cows and other ruminants can subsist on high-fiber food because of the bacterial digestion of these carbohydrates that takes place in the rumen. Other resistant starches and sugars are also less well digested or absorbed by humans; thus their consumption may result in significant amounts of starch and sugar in the colon. These resistant starches and some types of dietary fiber are fermented into SCFAs and gases. Starches resistant to digestion tend to include plant foods with a high protein and fiber content such as those from legumes and whole grains.

Proteins

Protein intake in the Western world ranges from approximately 50 to 100 g daily, and a good deal of the protein consumed is from animal sources. Additional protein is added all along the GIT from gastrointestinal secretions and sloughed epithelial cells. The GIT is one of the most active synthetic tissues in the body, and the life span of enterocytes migrating from the crypts of the villi until they are shed is only 3 to 5 days. The number of cells shed daily is in the range of 10 to 20 billion. The latter accounts for an additional 50 to 60 g of protein that is digested and "recycled" and contributes to the daily

supply. In general, animal proteins are more efficiently digested than plant proteins, but human physiology allows for very effective digestion and absorption of large amounts of ingested protein sources.

Protein digestion begins in the stomach, where some of the proteins are split into proteoses, peptones, and large polypeptides. Inactive pepsinogen is converted into the enzyme pepsin when it contacts hydrochloric acid and other pepsin molecules. Unlike any of the other proteolytic enzymes, pepsin digests collagen, the major protein of connective tissue. Most protein digestion takes place in the upper portion of the small intestine, but it continues throughout the GIT. Any residual protein fractions are fermented by colonic microbes.

Contact between chyme and the intestinal mucosa allows for the action of the brush border–bound enterokinase, an enzyme that transforms inactive pancreatic trypsinogen into active trypsin, the major pancreatic protein-digesting enzyme. Trypsin, in turn, activates the other pancreatic proteolytic enzymes. Pancreatic trypsin, chymotrypsin, and carboxypeptidase break down intact protein and continue the breakdown started in the stomach until small polypeptides and amino acids are formed.

Proteolytic peptidases located on the brush border also act on polypeptides, breaking them down into amino acids, dipeptides, and tripeptides. The final phase of protein digestion takes place in the brush border, where some of the dipeptides and tripeptides are hydrolyzed into their constituent amino acids by peptide hydrolases.

End products of protein digestion are absorbed as both amino acids and small peptides. Several transport molecules are required for the different amino acids, probably because of the wide differences in the size, polarity, and configuration of the different amino acids. Some of the transporters are sodium or chloride dependent, and some are not. Considerable amounts of dipeptides and tripeptides also are absorbed into intestinal cells using a peptide transporter, a form of active transport (Wuensch et al, 2013). Absorbed peptides and amino acids are transported to the liver via the portal vein for metabolism by the liver and are released into the general circulation.

The presence of antibodies to many food proteins in the circulation of healthy individuals indicates that immunologically significant amounts of large intact peptides escape hydrolysis and can enter the portal circulation. The exact mechanisms that cause a food to become an allergen are not entirely clear, but these foods tend to be high in protein, to be relatively resistant to complete digestion, and to produce an immunoglobulin response (see Chapter 25). With new technology, it is possible to map and characterize allergenic peptides; this eventually will lead to better diagnosis and development of safe immunotherapy treatments (Melioli et al, 2014).

Almost all protein is absorbed by the time it reaches the end of the jejunum, and only 1% of ingested protein is found in the feces. Small amounts of amino acids may remain in the epithelial cells and are used for synthesis of new proteins, including intestinal enzymes and new cells.

Lipids

Approximately 97% of dietary lipids are in the form of triglycerides, and the rest are found as phospholipids and cholesterol. Only small amounts of fat are digested in the mouth by lingual lipase and in the stomach from the action of gastric lipase. Gastric lipase hydrolyzes some triglycerides, especially short-chain triglycerides (such as those found in butter), into fatty acids and glycerol. However, most fat digestion takes place in the small intestine as a result of the emulsifying action of bile salts and hydrolysis by pancreatic lipase. As in the case of carbohydrates and protein, the capacity for digestion and absorption of dietary fat is in excess of ordinary needs.

Entrance of fat and protein into the small intestine stimulates the release of CCK, secretin, and GIP, which inhibit gastric secretions and motility, thus slowing the delivery of lipids. As a result, a portion of a large, fatty meal may remain in the stomach for 4 hours or longer. In addition to its many other functions, CCK stimulates biliary and pancreatic secretions. The combination of the peristaltic action of the small intestine and the surfactant and emulsification action of bile reduces the fat globules into tiny droplets, thus making them more accessible to digestion by the most potent lipid-digesting enzyme, pancreatic lipase.

Bile is a liver secretion composed of bile acids (primarily conjugates of cholic and chenodeoxycholic acids with glycine or taurine), bile pigments (which color the feces), inorganic salts, some protein, cholesterol, lecithin, and many compounds such as detoxified drugs that are metabolized and secreted by the liver. From its storage organ, the gallbladder, approximately 1 L of bile is secreted daily in response to the stimulus of food in the duodenum and stomach.

Emulsification of fats in the small intestine is followed by their digestion, primarily by pancreatic lipase, into free fatty acids and monoglycerides. Pancreatic lipase typically cleaves the first and third fatty acids, leaving a single fatty acid esterified to the middle glycerol carbon. When the concentration of bile salts reaches a certain level, they form micelles (small aggregates of fatty acids, monoglycerides, cholesterol, bile salts, and other lipids), which are organized with the polar ends of the molecules oriented toward the watery lumen of the intestine. The products of lipid digestion are solubilized rapidly in the central portion of the micelles and carried to the intestinal brush border (Fig. 1.8).

At the surface of the unstirred water layer (UWL), the slightly acidic and watery plate that forms a boundary between the intestinal lumen and the brush border membranes, the lipids detach from the micelles. Remnants of the micelles return to the lumen for further transport. The monoglycerides and fatty acids thus are left to make their way across the lipophobic UWL to the more lipid-friendly membrane cells of the brush border. Upon release of the lipid components, luminal bile salts are reabsorbed actively in the terminal ileum and returned to the liver to reenter the gut in bile secretions. This efficient recycling process is known as the enterohepatic circulation. The pool

of bile acids may circulate from 3 to 15 times per day, depending on the amount of food ingested.

The cellular mechanism(s) whereby fatty acids traverse the brush border membrane include both passive diffusion (a form of transport that does not require energy), and active transport processes. Traditionally, the absorption of lipid was thought to be passive, wherein lipid molecules would solubilize through the brush border membrane in a manner driven by diffusion down the concentration gradient into the enterocyte. The inwardly directed concentration gradient was thought to be maintained in the fed state by the high concentration of fatty acids within the intestinal lumen and the rapid scavenging of free fatty acids for triglyceride reformation once inside the enterocyte. Current theories indicate that both passive diffusion and carrier-mediated mechanisms contribute to lipid absorption. At low fatty acid concentrations, carrier-mediated mechanisms take precedence with little passive diffusion occurring. However, when free fatty acid concentration in the intestinal lumen is high, absorption of fatty acids via passive diffusion becomes quantitatively important.

In the enterocyte, the fatty acids and monoglycerides are reassembled into new triglycerides. Others are further digested into free fatty acids and glycerol and then reassembled to form triglycerides. These triglycerides, along with cholesterol, fat-soluble vitamins, and phospholipids, are surrounded by a lipoprotein coat, forming chylomicrons (see Fig. 1.8). The lipoprotein globules pass into the lymphatic system instead of entering portal blood and are transported to the thoracic duct and emptied into the systemic circulation at the junction of the left internal jugular and left subclavian veins. The chylomicrons then are carried through the bloodstream to several tissues, including liver, adipose tissue, and muscle. In the liver, triglycerides from the chylomicrons are repackaged into very-low-density lipoproteins and transported primarily to the adipose tissue for metabolism and storage.

Under normal conditions approximately 95% to 97% of ingested fat is absorbed into lymph vessels. Because of their shorter length and thus increased solubility, fatty acids of 8 to 12 carbons (i.e., medium-chain fatty acids) can be absorbed directly into colonic mucosal cells without the presence of bile and micelle formation. After entering mucosal cells, they are able to go directly without esterification into the portal vein, which carries them to the liver.

Increased motility, intestinal mucosal changes, pancreatic insufficiency, or the absence of bile can decrease the absorption of fat. When undigested fat appears in the feces, the condition is known as steatorrhea (see Chapter 27). Medium-chain triglycerides (MCTs) have fatty acids 8 to 12 carbons long; MCTs are clinically valuable for individuals who lack necessary bile salts for long-chain fatty acid metabolism and transport. Supplements for clinical use normally are provided in the form of oil or a dietary beverage with other macronutrients and micronutrients.

Vitamins and Minerals

Vitamins and minerals from foods are made available as macronutrients and are digested and absorbed across the mucosal layer, primarily in the small intestine (Fig. 1.9). Besides adequate passive and transporter mechanisms, various factors affect the bioavailability of vitamins and minerals, including the presence or absence of other specific nutrients, acid or alkali, phytates, and oxalates. The liters of fluid that are secreted each day from the GIT serve as a solvent, a vehicle for chemical reactions, and a medium for transfer of several nutrients.

At least some vitamins and water pass unchanged from the small intestine into the blood by passive diffusion, but several different mechanisms may be used to transport individual vitamins across the

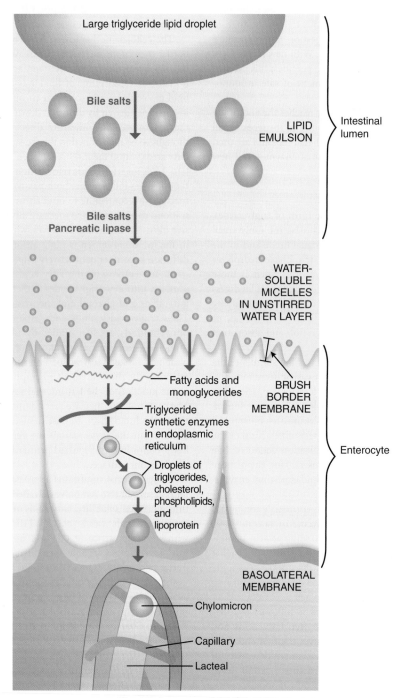

Fig. 1.8 Summary of fat absorption.

mucosa. Drugs are absorbed by a number of mechanisms but often by passive diffusion. Thus drugs may share or compete with mechanisms for the absorption nutrients into intestinal cells.

Mineral absorption is more complex, especially the absorption of the cation minerals. These cations, such as selenium, are made available for absorption by the process of chelation, in which a mineral is bound to a ligand—usually an acid, an organic acid, or an amino acid—so that it is in a form absorbable by intestinal cells (see Chapter 11).

Iron and zinc absorption share several characteristics in that the efficiency of absorption partly depends on the needs of the host. They also use at least one transport protein, and each has mechanisms to increase absorption when stores are inadequate. Because phytates

and oxalates from plants impair the absorption of iron and zinc, absorption is generally better when animal sources are consumed. Fermenting, soaking, sprouting and pretreatment with phytase enzymes improves the bioavailability of iron and zinc from plant based foods such as grains, legumes, nuts and seeds (Gupta et al, 2015). The absorption of zinc is impaired with disproportionately increased amounts of magnesium, calcium, and iron. Calcium absorption into the enterocyte occurs through channels in the brush border membrane, where it is bound to a specific protein carrier for transportation across the basolateral membrane. The process is regulated by the presence of vitamin D. Phosphorus is absorbed by a sodium phosphorus cotransporter, which also is regulated by vitamin D or low phosphate intake.

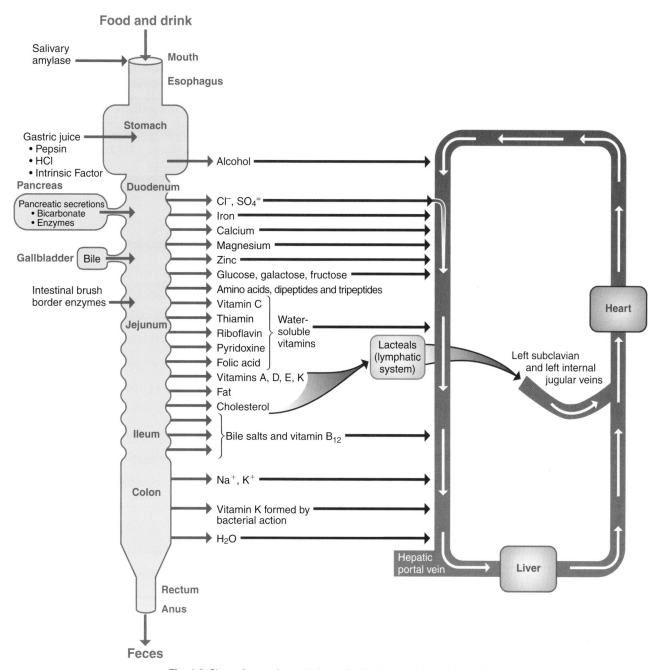

Fig. 1.9 Sites of secretion and absorption in the gastrointestinal tract.

The GIT is the site of important interactions among minerals. Supplementation with large amounts of iron or zinc may decrease the absorption of copper. In turn, the presence of copper may lower iron and molybdenum absorption. Cobalt absorption is increased in patients with iron deficiency, but cobalt and iron compete and inhibit one another's absorption. These interactions are probably the result of an overlap of mineral absorption mechanisms.

Minerals are transported in blood bound to protein carriers. The protein binding is either specific (e.g., transferrin, which binds with iron, or ceruloplasmin, which binds with copper) or general (e.g., albumin, which binds with a variety of minerals). A fraction of each mineral also is carried in the serum as amino acid or peptide complexes. Specific protein carriers are usually not completely saturated; the reserve capacity may serve as a buffer against excessive exposure. Toxicity from minerals usually results only after this buffering capacity is exceeded.

SUMMARY

Assessment of the function of the gastrointestinal tract (GIT) is essential to the nutrition care process. Several nutrition diagnoses can be identified when assessing GIT function. Common or possible nutrition diagnoses related to digestion or metabolism include:

Altered GI function (NC-1.4)

Imbalance of nutrients (NI-5.4)

Increased nutrient needs (NI-5.1)

Altered nutrition related laboratory values (NC-2.2)

Inadequate or excessive fluid intake (NI-3.1 and NI-3.2)

Food–medication interaction (NC-2.3)

USEFUL WEBSITES

American Gastroenterological Association (AGA)
NIH Digestive Diseases
NIH Human Microbiome Project

REFERENCES

Buccigrossi V, Nicastro E, Guarino A: Functions of intestinal microflora in children, *Curr Opin Gastroenterol* 29:31, 2013.

Chey WY, Chang TM: Secretin: historical perspective and current status, *Pancreas* 43:162, 2014.

Chu S, Schubert ML: Gastric secretion, *Curr Opin Gastroenterol* 29:636, 2013.

Floch MH: The role of prebiotics and probiotics in gastrointestinal disease, *Gastroenterol Clin North Am* 47:179, 2018.

Gibson GR, Hutkins R, Sanders ME, et al: The International Scientific Association for Probiotics and Prebiotics (ISAPP) consensus statement on the definition and scope of prebiotics, *Nat Rev Gastroenterol Hepatol* 14:491, 2017.

Gupta RK, Gangoliya SS, Singh NK. Reduction of phytic acid and enhancement of bioavailable micronutrients in food grains, *J Food Sci Technol* 52(2):676–684, 2015.

Hill C, Guarner F, Reid G, et al: Expert consensus document. The International Scientific Association for Probiotics and Prebiotics consensus statement on the scope and appropriate use of the term probiotic, *Nat Rev Gastroenterol Hepatol* 11:506, 2014.

Hylemon PB, Zhou H, Pandak WM, et al: Bile acids as regulatory molecules, *J Lipid Res* 50:1509, 2009.

Kostic AD, Xavier RJ, Gevers D: The microbiome in inflammatory bowel disease: current status and the future ahead, *Gastroenterology* 146:1489, 2014.

Melioli G, Passalacqua G, Canonica GW: Novel in silico technology in combination with microarrays: a state-of-the-art technology for allergy diagnosis and management? *Expert Rev Clin Immunol* 10:1559, 2014.

Rehfeld JF: Gastrointestinal hormones and their targets, *Adv Exp Med Biol* 817:157, 2014.

Rui L: Brain regulation of energy balance and body weight, *Rev Endocr Metab Disord* 14:387, 2013.

Seidner DL, Schwartz LK, Winkler MF, et al: Increased intestinal absorption in the era of teduglutide and its impact on management strategies in patients with short bowel syndrome-associated intestinal failure, *JPEN J Parenter Enteral Nutr* 37:201, 2013.

Van Op den Bosch J, Adriaensen D, Van Nassauw L, et al: The role(s) of somatostatin, structurally related peptides and somatostatin receptors in the gastrointestinal tract: a review, *Regul Pept* 156:1, 2009.

Wijeratne T, Patel AM, Jowhari F, et al: Erythromycin and related macrolides for gastroparesis, *Cochrane Database Syst Rev* 4, 2016

Wuensch T, Schulz S, Ullrich S, et al: The peptide transporter PEPT1 is expressed in distal colon in rodents and humans and contributes to water absorption, *Am J Physiol Gastrointest Liver Physiol* 305:G66, 2013.

Intake: Energy

Carol S. Ireton-Jones, PhD, RDN, LD, CNSC, FASPEN, FAND

KEY TERMS

activity thermogenesis (AT)
basal energy expenditure (BEE)
basal metabolic rate (BMR)
calorie
direct calorimetry
estimated energy requirement (EER)
excess post-exercise oxygen consumption (EPOC)

facultative thermogenesis
fat-free mass (FFM)
high-metabolic-rate organ (HMRO)
indirect calorimetry (IC)
kilocalorie (kcal)
lean body mass (LBM)
metabolic equivalents (METs)
nonexercise activity thermogenesis (NEAT)

obligatory thermogenesis
physical activity level (PAL)
respiratory quotient (RQ)
resting energy expenditure (REE)
resting metabolic rate (RMR)
thermic effect of food (TEF)
total energy expenditure (TEE)

Energy may be defined as "the capacity to do work." The ultimate source of all energy in living organisms is the sun. Through the process of photosynthesis, green plants intercept a portion of the sunlight reaching their leaves and capture it within the chemical bonds of glucose. Proteins, fats, and other carbohydrates are synthesized from this basic carbohydrate to meet the needs of the plant. Animals and humans obtain these nutrients and the energy they contain by consuming plants and the flesh of other animals.

The body makes use of the energy from dietary carbohydrates, proteins, fats, and alcohol; this energy is locked in chemical bonds within food and is released through metabolism. Energy must be supplied regularly to meet the needs for the body's survival. Although all energy eventually takes the form of heat, which dissipates into the atmosphere, unique cellular processes first make possible its use for all the tasks required for life. These processes involve chemical reactions that maintain body tissues, electrical conduction of the nerves, mechanical work of the muscles, and heat production to maintain body temperature.

ENERGY REQUIREMENTS

Energy requirements are defined as the dietary energy intake that is required for growth or maintenance in a person of a defined age, gender, weight, height, and level of physical activity. In children and pregnant or lactating women, energy requirements include the needs associated with the deposition of tissues or the secretion of milk at rates consistent with good health. In ill or injured people, the stressors have an effect by increasing or decreasing energy expenditure.

Body weight is one indicator of energy adequacy or inadequacy. The body has the unique ability to shift the fuel mixture of carbohydrates, proteins, and fats to accommodate energy needs. However, consuming too much or too little energy over time results in body weight changes. Thus body weight reflects adequacy of energy intake, but it is not a reliable indicator of macronutrient or micronutrient adequacy. In addition, because body weight is affected by body composition, a person with a higher lean mass to body fat mass or body fat mass to lean mass may require different energy intakes compared with the norm or "average" person. Obese individuals have higher energy needs because of an increase in body fat mass and lean body mass (Kee et al, 2012).

COMPONENTS OF ENERGY EXPENDITURE

Energy is expended by the human body in the form of basal energy expenditure (BEE), thermic effect of food (TEF), and activity thermogenesis (AT). These three components make up a person's daily total energy expenditure (TEE).

Basal and Resting Energy Expenditure

BEE, or basal metabolic rate (BMR), is the minimum amount of energy expended that is compatible with life. An individual's BEE reflects the amount of energy used for 24 hours while physically and mentally at rest in a thermoneutral environment that prevents the activation of heat-generating processes, such as shivering. Measurements of BEE should be done before an individual has engaged in any physical activity (preferably on awakening from sleep) and 10 to 12 hours after the ingestion of any food, drink, or nicotine. The BEE remains remarkably constant on a daily basis.

Resting energy expenditure (REE), or resting metabolic rate (RMR), is the energy expended in the activities necessary to sustain normal body functions and homeostasis. These activities include respiration and circulation, the synthesis of organic compounds, and the pumping of ions across membranes. REE, or RMR, includes the energy required by the central nervous system and for the maintenance of body temperature. It does not include thermogenesis, activity, or other energy expenditure and is higher than the BEE by 10% to 20%

(Ireton-Jones, 2010). The terms *REE* and *RMR* and *BEE* and *BMR* can be used interchangeably, but *REE* and *BEE* are used in this chapter.

Factors Affecting Resting Energy Expenditure

Numerous factors cause the REE to vary among individuals, but body size and composition have the greatest effect. See Chapter 5 for discussion of methods used to determine body composition.

Age. Because REE is highly affected by the proportion of lean body mass (LBM), it is highest during periods of rapid growth, especially the first and second years of life. Growing infants may store as much as 12% to 15% of the energy value of their food in the form of new tissue. As a child becomes older, the energy requirement for growth is reduced to approximately 1% of TEE. After early adulthood there is a decline in REE of 1% to 2% per kilogram of fat-free mass (FFM) per decade (Keys et al, 1973). Fortunately, exercise can help maintain a higher LBM and a higher REE. Decreases in REE with increasing age may be partly related to age-associated changes in the relative size of LBM components (Cooper et al, 2013).

Body composition. FFM, or LBM, makes up most of the metabolically active tissue in the body and is the primary predictor of REE. FFM contributes to approximately 80% of the variations in REE (Wang et al, 2010). Because of their greater FFM, athletes with greater muscular development have an approximately 5% higher REE than nonathletic individuals. Organs in the body contribute to heat production (Fig. 2.1). Approximately 60% of REE can be accounted for by the heat produced by high-metabolic-rate organs (HMROs): the liver, brain, heart, spleen, intestines, and kidneys). Indeed, differences in FFM between ethnic groups may be related to the total mass of these as well as musculature and presence of obesity (Wang et al, 2012). Relatively small individual variation in the mass of the liver, brain, heart, spleen, and kidneys, collectively or individually, can significantly affect REE (Javed et al, 2010). As a result, estimating the percentage of energy expenditure that appendages (arms and legs) account for in overall daily energy expenditure is difficult, although it is presumably a small amount.

Body size. Larger people generally have higher metabolic rates than smaller people, but tall, thin people have higher metabolic rates than short, stocky people. For example, if two people weigh the same but one person is taller, the taller person has a larger body surface area and a higher metabolic rate. Obesity is a major confounder in the determination of energy needs. Determination of body fat percentage may be helpful in increasing the preciseness of an equation,

but methodology related to measurement of body fat may cause inaccuracies in body fat and REE (Wang et al, 2012).

Climate. The REE is affected by extremes in environmental temperature. People living in tropical climates usually have REEs that are 5% to 20% higher than those living in temperate areas. Exercise in temperatures greater than 86°F imposes a small additional metabolic load of approximately 5% from increased sweat gland activity. The extent to which energy metabolism increases in extremely cold environments depends on the insulation available from body fat and protective clothing.

Gender. Gender differences in metabolic rates are attributable primarily to differences in body size and composition. Women, who generally have more fat in proportion to muscle than men, have metabolic rates that are approximately 5% to 10% lower than men of the same weight and height. However, with aging, this difference becomes less pronounced (Cooper et al, 2013).

Hormonal status. Hormones affect metabolic rate. Endocrine disorders, such as hyperthyroidism and hypothyroidism, increase or decrease energy expenditure, respectively (see Chapter 30). Stimulation of the sympathetic nervous system during periods of emotional excitement or stress causes the release of epinephrine, which promotes glycogenolysis and increased cellular activity. Ghrelin and peptide YY are gut hormones involved in appetite regulation and energy homeostasis (Larson-Meyer et al, 2010). The metabolic rate of women fluctuates with the menstrual cycle. During the luteal phase (i.e., the time between ovulation and the onset of menstruation), metabolic rate increases slightly (Ferraro et al, 1992). During pregnancy, growth in uterine, placental, and fetal tissues, along with the mother's increased cardiac workload, contributes to gradual increases in BEE of around 15% (Chapter 14).

Temperature. Fevers increase REE by approximately 7% for each degree of increase in body temperature above 98.6°F or 13% for each degree more than 37°C, as noted by classic studies (Hardy and DuBois, 1937).

Other factors. Caffeine, nicotine, and alcohol stimulate metabolic rate. Caffeine intakes of 200 to 350 mg in men or 240 mg in women may increase mean REE by 7% to 11% and 8% to 15%, respectively (Compher et al, 2006). Nicotine use increases REE by approximately 3% to 4% in men and by 6% in women; alcohol consumption increases REE in women by 9% (Compher et al, 2006). Under conditions of stress and disease, energy expenditure may increase or decrease, based on the clinical situation. Energy expenditure may be higher in people who are obese (Wang et al, 2012). Energy expenditure may be depressed during starvation and chronic dieting (Volp et al, 2011). A case study demonstrated decreased energy expenditure in people with bulimia that was improved when intake increased consistently (Sedlet and Ireton-Jones, 1989).

Thermic Effect of Food

The thermic effect of food (TEF) is the increase in energy expenditure associated with the consumption, digestion, and absorption of food. The TEF accounts for approximately 10% of TEE (Ireton-Jones, 2010). The TEF may also be called diet-induced thermogenesis, specific dynamic action, or the specific effect of food. TEF can be separated into obligatory and facultative (or adaptive) subcomponents. Obligatory thermogenesis is the energy required to digest, absorb, and metabolize nutrients, including the synthesis and storage of protein, fat, and carbohydrate. Adaptive or facultative thermogenesis is the "excess" energy expended in addition to the obligatory thermogenesis and is thought to be attributable to the metabolic inefficiency of the system stimulated by sympathetic nervous activity.

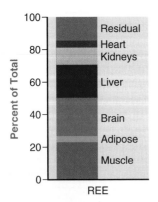

Fig. 2.1 Proportional contribution of organs and tissues to calculated resting energy expenditure. (Modified and used with permission from Gallagher D et al: Organ-tissue mass measurement allows modeling of REE and metabolically active tissue mass, *Am J Physiol Endocrinol Metab* 275:E249, 1998. Copyright American Physiological Society.)

The TEF varies with the composition of the diet, with energy expenditure increasing directly after food intake, particularly after consumption of a meal higher in protein compared with a meal higher in fat (Tentolouris et al, 2008). Fat is metabolized efficiently, with only 4% waste, compared with 25% waste when carbohydrate is converted to fat for storage. The macronutrient oxidation rate is not different in lean and obese individuals (Tentolouris et al, 2008). Although the extent of TEF depends on the size and macronutrient content of the meal, TEF decreases after ingestion over 30 to 90 minutes, so effects on TEE are small. For practical purposes, TEF is calculated as no more than an additional 10% of the REE. Spicy foods enhance and prolong the effect of the TEF. Caffeine, capsaicin, and different teas such as green, white, and oolong tea also may increase energy expenditure and fat oxidation and suppress hunger (Hursel and Westerterp-Plantenga, 2010; Reinbach et al, 2009). The role of TEF in weight management is discussed in Chapter 20.

Enteral nutrition (tube feeding) as well as parenteral nutrition exert a thermic effect on energy expenditure, which should be considered in patients receiving nutrition support. Leuck and colleagues found that energy expenditure of patients receiving enteral nutrition intermittently vs. continuously was increased at night and increased in association with each intermittent feeding (Leuck et al, 2013). A case study of a long-term home parenteral nutrition patient showed an increase in energy expenditure when the intravenous nutrition was being infused (Ireton-Jones, 2010). These are important considerations when predicting overall energy needs for patients receiving enteral or parenteral nutrition (see Chapter 12).

Activity Thermogenesis

Beyond REE and TEF, energy is expended in physical activity, either exercise-related or as part of daily work and movement. This is referred to as activity thermogenesis. Activity thermogenesis (AT) includes nonexercise activity thermogenesis (NEAT), the energy expended during activities of daily living, and the energy expended during sports or fitness exercise.

The contribution of physical activity is the most variable component of TEE, which may be as low as 100 kcal/day in sedentary people or as high as 3000 kcal/day in athletes. NEAT represents the energy expended during the workday and during leisure-type activities (e.g., shopping, fidgeting, even gum chewing), which may account for vast differences in energy costs among people (see Appendix 10). TEE reflects REE, TEF, and energy expended for exercise, as depicted in Fig. 2.2.

Individual AT varies considerably, depending on body size and the efficiency of individual habits of motion. The level of fitness also affects the energy expenditure of voluntary activity because of variations

in muscle mass. AT tends to decrease with age, a trend that is associated with a decline in FFM and an increase in fat mass. In general, men have greater skeletal muscle than women, which may account for their higher AT. The measurement of physical activity is very difficult whether related to children, adolescents, or adults (Mindell et al, 2014). However, this remains an important component of the overall energy intake recommendation suggesting that low-cost quantitative assessment methods are needed (e.g., heart rate monitoring) along with the typical questionnaire and estimate.

Additional Considerations in Energy Expenditure

Excess post-exercise oxygen consumption (EPOC) is influenced by the duration and magnitude of physical activity. In a study of high-intensity intermittent exercise, there was an increase in energy expenditure during activity, although the effect on metabolic rate post-activity was minor (Kelly et al, 2013). Habitual exercise does not cause a significantly prolonged increase in metabolic rate unless FM is decreased and FFM is increased, and then this increase in energy expenditure is mostly during the activity itself.

Amputations resulting from trauma, wounds, or disease processes affect body size; presumably then, they would affect activity energy expenditure. However, a study of energy expenditure related to level of amputation (partial foot to transfemoral) at various speeds of walking was done in unilateral amputees, and no differences in energy expenditure were found between levels of amputation or speed when walking (Göktepe et al, 2010).

Measurement of Energy Expenditure

The standard unit for measuring energy is the calorie, which is the amount of heat energy required to raise the temperature of 1 mL of water at 15°C by 1°C. Because the amount of energy involved in the metabolism of food is fairly large, the kilocalorie (kcal), 1000 calories, is used to measure it. A popular convention is to designate kilocalorie by Calorie (with a capital C). In this text, however, kilocalorie is abbreviated kcal. The *joule* (J) measures energy in terms of mechanical work and is the amount of energy required to accelerate with a force of 1 Newton (N) for a distance of 1 m; this measurement is widely used in countries other than the United States. One kcal is equivalent to 4.184 kilojoules (kJ).

Because various methods are available to measure human energy expenditure, it is important to gain an understanding of the differences in these methods and how they can be applied in practical and research settings.

Direct Calorimetry

Direct calorimetry is possible only with specialized and expensive equipment. An individual is monitored in a room-type structure (a whole-room calorimeter) that permits a moderate amount of activity. It includes equipment that monitors the amount of heat produced by the individual inside the chamber or room. Direct calorimetry provides a measure of energy expended in the form of heat but provides no information on the kind of fuel being oxidized. The method also is limited by the confined nature of the testing conditions. Therefore the measurement of TEE using this method is not representative of a free-living (i.e., engaged in normal daily activities) individual in a normal environment, because physical activity within the chamber is limited. High cost, complex engineering, and scarcity of appropriate facilities around the world also limit the use of this method.

Indirect Calorimetry

Indirect calorimetry (IC) is a more commonly used method for measuring energy expenditure. An individual's oxygen consumption and

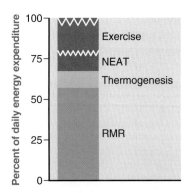

Fig. 2.2 The components of total energy expenditure: activity, thermic effect of food (TEF), and basal or resting metabolic rate.

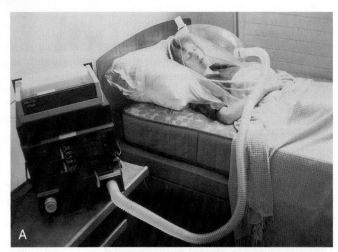
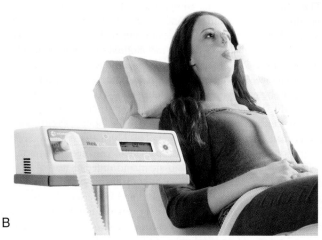

Fig. 2.3 A, Measuring resting energy expenditure using a ventilated hood system. (Courtesy MRC Mitochondrial Biology Unit, Cambridge, England.). **B,** Measuring resting energy expenditure using a handheld system. (Courtesy Korr.)

carbon dioxide production are quantified over a given period. The Weir equation (1949) and a constant respiratory quotient value of 0.85 are used to convert oxygen consumption to REE. The equipment varies but usually involves an individual breathing into a mouthpiece (with nose clips), a mask that covers the nose and mouth, or a ventilated hood that captures all expired carbon dioxide (Fig. 2.3). Ventilated hoods are useful for short- and long-term measurements.

IC measurements are achieved using equipment called a *metabolic measurement cart* or an *indirect calorimeter*. There are various types of metabolic measurement carts, varying from larger equipment that measures oxygen consumption and carbon dioxide production only, to equipment that also has the capability of providing pulmonary function and exercise testing parameters. These larger carts are more expensive because of the expanded capabilities, including measurement interface for IC measurements of hospitalized patients who are ventilator dependent. Metabolic carts often are used at hospitals to assess energy requirements and are found most typically in the intensive care unit (Ireton-Jones, 2010). Individuals and patients who are breathing spontaneously may have their energy expenditure measured with smaller "handheld" indirect calorimeters designed specifically for measuring oxygen consumption while using a static value for carbon dioxide production. These have easy mobility and are relatively low cost (Hipskind et al, 2011).

A strict protocol should be followed before performing IC measurement. For healthy people, a minimum of a 4-hour fast after meals and snacks is recommended. Caffeine should be avoided for at least 4 hours, and alcohol and smoking for at least 2 hours. Testing should occur no sooner than 2 hours after moderate exercise; after vigorous resistance exercise, a 14-hour period is advised (Compher et al, 2006). To achieve a steady-state measurement, there should be a rest period of 10 to 20 minutes before the measurement is taken. An IC measurement duration of 10 minutes, with the first 5 minutes deleted and the remaining 5 minutes having a coefficient of variation less than 10%, indicates a steady-state measurement (Compher et al, 2006). When the measurement conditions listed here are met and a steady state is achieved, energy expenditure can be measured at any time during the day. A suggested protocol for REE measurements is found in Table 2.1.

Energy expenditure can be measured for ill or injured individuals as well (Cooney and Frankenfield, 2012). Equipment used for the patient who is ventilator dependent may be different from that used for the ambulatory individual; however, a protocol specifying the

TABLE 2.1   REE Measurement Protocol (Adults)
REE Measurement Preparation
• Food – fast for 7 hours or 4 hours if < 300 kcal intake
• Caffeine – none for 4 hours
• Nicotine – none for 2.5 hours
• Exercise – none for 4 hours
Simplify: Rule of 4's – no food, caffeine, nicotine, exercise for 4 hours before the REE measurement
REE Measurement Conditions
• Rest period pre-REE: healthy adult 20-30 mins
• Gas collection device:
• Ventilated hood/canopy, mouthpiece & nose clip, facemask
• Ambient room temp 72-77°F
• Quiet and dim light
• Continue for 10 mins or as per individual protocol

Used with Permission: Ireton-Jones, C. Good Nutrition Good Living (Adapted)

conditions of measurement should be used for these patients as well (Ireton-Jones, 2010). When these conditions are met, IC can be applied for measuring the energy expenditure of acute or critically ill inpatients, outpatients, or healthy individuals.

Respiratory Quotient

When oxygen consumption and carbon dioxide production are measured, the respiratory quotient (RQ) may be calculated as noted in the following equation. The RQ indicates the fuel mixture being metabolized. The RQ for carbohydrate is 1 because the number of carbon dioxide molecules produced is equal to the number of oxygen molecules consumed.

RQ = volume of CO_2 expired/volume of O_2 consumed (VCO_2 /VO_2)

RQ values:

    1 = carbohydrate
    0.85 = mixed diet
    0.82 = protein
    0.7 = fat
    ≤0.65 = ketone production

RQs greater than 1 are associated with net fat synthesis, carbohydrate (glucose) intake, or total caloric intake that is excessive, whereas a very low RQ may be seen under conditions of inadequate nutrient intake (McClave et al, 2003). Although RQ has been used to determine the efficacy of nutrition support regimens for hospitalized patients, McClave found that changes in RQ failed to correlate to percent calories provided or required, indicating low sensitivity and specificity that limits the efficacy of RQ as an indicator of overfeeding or underfeeding. However, use of RQ is appropriate as a marker of test validity (to confirm measured RQ values are in physiologic range) and a marker for respiratory tolerance of the nutrition support regimen.

Other Methods of Measuring Energy Expenditure

Alternative methods of measuring energy expenditure remain in the research setting because of the need for specialized equipment and expertise.

Doubly labeled water. The doubly labeled water (DLW) technique for measuring TEE is considered the gold standard for determining energy requirements and energy balance in humans. The DLW method is based on the principle that carbon dioxide production can be estimated from the difference in the elimination rates of body hydrogen and oxygen. After an oral loading dose of water labeled with deuterium oxide (^2H_2O) and oxygen-18 ($H_2^{18}O$)—hence the term *doubly labeled water*—is administered, the ^2H_2O is eliminated from the body as water, and the $H_2^{18}O$ is eliminated as water and carbon dioxide. The elimination rates of the two isotopes are measured for 10 to 14 days by periodic sampling of body water from urine, saliva, or plasma. The difference between the two elimination rates is a measure of carbon dioxide production. Carbon dioxide production then can be equated to TEE using standard IC techniques for the calculation of energy expenditure.

The caloric value of AT can be estimated by using the DLW method in conjunction with IC and can be used to determine adherence to recommended intake and body composition longitudinally (Wong et al, 2014). The DLW technique is most applicable as a research tool; the stable isotopes are expensive, and expertise is required to operate the highly sophisticated and costly mass spectrometer for the analysis of the isotope enrichments. These disadvantages make the DLW technique impractical for daily use by clinicians.

Measuring Activity-Related Energy Expenditure

Triaxial monitors. A triaxial monitor has also been used to measure energy related to activity. It more efficiently measures multidirectional movement by employing three uniaxial monitors. In a review of numerous articles, Plasqui and Westerterp (2007) found that a triaxial monitor correlated with energy expenditure measured using DLW technique. Application of an easily accessible and useable monitor allows determination of real activity levels, thereby reducing errors related to overreporting or underreporting of actual energy expenditure for weight management.

Physical Activity Questionnaire

Physical activity questionnaires (PAQs) are the simplest and least expensive tools for gaining information about an individual's activity level. Reporting errors are common among PAQs, which can lead to discrepancies between calculated energy expenditure and that determined by DLW (Neilson et al, 2008). For healthy individuals, this may account for slowed weight loss or gain and, as such, a need to modify caloric intake.

ESTIMATING ENERGY REQUIREMENTS

Equations for Estimating Resting Energy Expenditure

Over the years several equations have been developed to estimate the REE. Equations are available that allow the estimation of REE as derived from measurement using IC in adults. Until recently, the Harris-Benedict equations were some of the most widely used equations to estimate REE in normal and ill or injured individuals (Harris and Benedict, 1919). The Harris-Benedict equations have been found to overestimate REE in normal-weight and obese individuals by 7% to 27% (Frankenfield et al, 2003). A study comparing measured REE with estimated REE using the Mifflin-St. Jeor equations, Owen equations, and Harris-Benedict equations for males and females found that the Mifflin-St. Jeor equations were most accurate in estimating REE in both normal weight and obese people (Frankenfield et al, 2003). The Mifflin-St Jeor equations were developed from measured REE using IC in 251 males and 247 females; 47% of these individuals had a body mass index (BMI) between 30 and 42 kg/m^2 (Mifflin et al, 1990). Mifflin-St. Jeor equations are used today to estimate energy expenditure of healthy individuals and in some patients and are as follows:

$$\text{Males kcal/:day} = 10\,(\text{wt}) + 6.25\,(\text{ht}) - 5\,(\text{age}) + 5$$
$$\text{Females: kcal/day} = 10\,(\text{wt}) + 6.25\,(\text{ht}) - 5\,(\text{age}) - 161$$
$$\text{Weight} = \text{actual body weight in kilograms}$$
$$\text{Height} = \text{centimeters; age} = \text{years}$$

Although the Harris-Benedict equations have been applied to ill and injured people, these equations, as well as those of Mifflin, were developed for use in healthy individuals, and their application to any other population is questionable. In addition, the database from which the Harris-Benedict equations were developed no longer reflects the population, and therefore use of these equations is not recommended.

Magnetic resonance imaging (MRI), computer tomography (CT), and dual-energy x-ray absorptiometry (DEXA) have been investigated as methods to evaluate REE from determination of LBM and fat mass in humans (Gallagher et al, 1998). While body weight, age, height, and gender may be similar among individuals or groups, body cell mass differs, and this creates the variations in REE that may confound weight loss, gain, or maintenance when predicting REE. Although REE is usually estimated from statistical equations, using imaging techniques to estimate the REE from organ-tissue mass components allows for distinct individuality of REE (Heymsfield et al, 2018). This will provide greater accuracy in determining REE by assessing energy expenditure in relation to body cell mass and body composition.

Energy expenditure of ill or injured patients also can be estimated or measured using IC. Energy expenditure may be affected by illness or injury; however, several studies have shown this increase to be variable from a significant increase to little to none over "normal" energy expenditure. Stable dialysis patients have not been shown to have an increase in REE compared with healthy adults (Dombrowski and Heuberger, 2018). In patients receiving home parenteral nutrition, measured REEs were related to energy expenditures predicted using 20 kcal/kg or the Ireton-Jones equations (Ławiński et al, 2015). Therefore assumptions of REE are often inaccurate—measurement of REE is best even in nonacute patient care. For energy requirements for critically ill patients, see Chapter 37.

Determining TEE

The equations for estimating or measuring energy expenditure begin with REE. Additional factors for TEF and activity must be added. As stated previously, the TEF may be considered as an overall additive factor within activity thermogenesis in calculations of TEE. A simplified way of predicting physical activity additions to REE is through the use of estimates of the level of physical activity, which are then multiplied by the measured or predicted REE. To estimate TEE for minimal activity, increase REE by 10% to 20%; for moderate activity, increase REE by 25% to 40%; for strenuous activity, increase REE by 45% to 60%. These levels are ranges used in practice and can be considered "expert opinion" rather than evidence based at this time.

Estimating Energy Requirements From Energy Intake

Traditionally, recommendations for energy requirements were based on self-recorded estimates (e.g., diet records) or self-reported estimates (e.g., 24-hour recalls) of food intake. However, these methods do not provide accurate or unbiased estimates of an individual's energy intake. The percentage of people who underestimate or underreport their food intake ranges from 10% to 45%, depending on the person's age, gender, and body composition. This occurs in the compromised patient population as well (Ribeiro et al, 2014) (see Chapter 4).

Many online programs are available in which an individual can enter the food and quantity consumed into a program that estimates the macronutrient and micronutrient content. These programs allow users to enter data and receive a summary report, often with a detailed report provided to the health professional as well. Widely available programs include Food Prodigy and the MyPlate Tracker from the U.S. Department of Agriculture (see Chapter 4).

Other Prediction Equations

The National Academy of Sciences, Institute of Medicine (IOM), and Food and Nutrition Board, in partnership with Health Canada, developed the estimated energy requirements for men, women, children, and infants and for pregnant and lactating women (IOM, 2005). The estimated energy requirement (EER) is the average dietary energy intake predicted to maintain energy balance in a healthy adult of a defined age, gender, weight, height, and level of physical activity consistent with good health. In children and pregnant and lactating women, the EER is taken to include the energy needs associated with the deposition of tissues or the secretion of milk at rates consistent with good health. Table 2.2 lists average dietary reference intake (DRI) values for energy in healthy, active people of reference height, weight, and age for each life-stage group (IOM, 2002; 2005).

Supported by DLW studies, prediction equations have been developed to estimate energy requirements for people according to their life-stage group. Box 2.1 lists the EER prediction equations for people of normal weight. TEE prediction equations also are listed for various overweight and obese groups, as well as for weight maintenance in obese girls and boys. All equations have been developed to maintain current body weight (and promote growth when appropriate) and current levels of physical activity for all subsets of the population; they are not intended to promote weight loss (IOM, 2002; 2005).

The EER incorporates age, weight, height, gender, and level of physical activity for people ages 3 years and older. Although variables such as age, gender, and feeding type (i.e., breast milk, formula) can affect TEE among infants and young children, weight has been determined as the sole predictor of TEE needs (IOM, 2002; 2005). Beyond TEE requirements, additional calories are required for infants, young children, and children ages 3 through 18 to support the deposition of tissues needed for growth, nurd for pregnant and lactating women. Thus the EER among these subsets of the population is the sum of TEE plus the caloric requirements for energy deposition.

TABLE 2.2 Dietary Reference Intake Values for Energy for Active Individuals*

Life-Stage Group	Criterion	ACTIVE PAL EER (kcal/day) Male	ACTIVE PAL EER (kcal/day) Female
Infants			
0-6 mo	Energy expenditure + Energy deposition	570	520 (3 mo)
7-12 mo	Energy expenditure + Energy deposition	743	676 (9 mo)
Children			
1-2 yr	Energy expenditure + Energy deposition	1046	992 (24 mo)
3-8 yr	Energy expenditure + Energy deposition	1742	1642 (6 yr)
9-13 yr	Energy expenditure + Energy deposition	2279	2071 (11 yr)
14-18 yr	Energy expenditure + Energy deposition	3152	2368 (16 yr)
Adults			
>18 yr	Energy expenditure	3067†	2403† (19 yr)
Pregnant Women			
14-18 yr	Adolescent female EER + Change in TEE + Pregnancy energy deposition		
First trimester			2368 (16 yr)
Second trimester			2708 (16 yr)
Third trimester			2820 (16 yr)
19-50 yr	Adult female EER + Change in TEE + Pregnancy energy deposition		
First trimester			2403† (19 yr)
Second trimester			2743† (19 yr)
Third trimester			2855† (19 yr)
Lactating Women			
14-18 yr	Adolescent female EER + Milk energy output − Weight loss		
First 6 mo			2698 (16 yr)
Second 6 mo			2768 (16 yr)
19-50 yr	Adult female EER + Milk energy output − Weight loss		
First 6 mo			2733† (19 yr)
Second 6 mo			2803† (19 yr)

*For healthy active Americans and Canadians at the reference height and weight.

†Subtract 10 kcal/day for men and 7 kcal/day for women for each year of age above 19 years.

EER, Estimated energy requirement; *PAL,* physical activity level; *TEE,* total energy expenditure.

From Institute of Medicine of The National Academies: *Dietary reference intakes for energy, carbohydrate, fiber, fat, fatty acids, cholesterol, protein, and amino acids*, Washington, DC, 2002/2005, The National Academies Press.

BOX 2.1 Estimated Energy Expenditure Prediction Equations at Four Physical Activity Levels

EER for Infants and Young Children 0-2 Years (Within the 3rd to 97th Percentile for Weight-for-Height)

EER = TEE + Energy deposition

0-3 months (89 × Weight of infant [kg] − 100) + 175 (kcal for energy deposition)

4-6 months (89 × Weight of infant [kg] − 100) + 56 (kcal for energy deposition)

7-12 months (89 × Weight of infant [kg] −100) + 22 (kcal for energy deposition)

13-35 months (89 × Weight of child [kg] − 100) + 20 (kcal for energy deposition)

EER for Boys 3-8 Years (Within the 5th to 85th Percentile for BMI)§

EER = TEE Energy deposition

EER = 88.5 − 61.9 × Age (yr) + PA × (26.7 × Weight [kg] + 903 × Height [m]) + 20 (kcal for energy deposition)

EER for Boys 9-18 Years (Within the 5th to 85th Percentile for BMI)

EER = TEE + Energy deposition

EER = 88.5 − 61.9 × Age (yr) + PA × (26.7 × Weight [kg] + 903 × Height [m]) + 25 (kcal for energy deposition)

in which

PA = Physical activity coefficient for boys 3-18 years:

PA = 1 if PAL is estimated to be ≥ 1 < 1.4 (Sedentary)

PA = 1.13 if PAL is estimated to be ≥ 1.4 < 1.6 (Low active)

PA = 1.26 if PAL is estimated to be ≥ 1.6 < 1.9 (Active)

PA = 1.42 if PAL is estimated to be ≥ 1.9 < 2.5 (Very active)

EER for Girls 3-8 Years (Within the 5th to 85th Percentile for BMI)

EER = TEE + Energy deposition

EER = 135.3 − 30.8 × Age (yr) + PA × (10 × Weight [kg] + 934 × Height [m]) + 20 (kcal for energy deposition)

EER for Girls 9-18 Years (Within the 5th to 85th Percentile for BMI)

EER = TEE + Energy deposition

EER = 135.3 − 30.8 × Age (yr) + PA × (10 × Weight [kg] + 934 × Height [m]) + 25 (kcal for energy deposition)

in which

PA = Physical activity coefficient for girls 3-18 years:

PA = 1 (Sedentary)

PA = 1.16 (Low active)

PA = 1.31 (Active)

PA = 1.56 (Very active)

EER for Men 19 Years and Older (BMI 18.5-25 kg/m²)

EER = TEE

EER = 662 − 9.53 × Age (yr) + PA × (15.91 × Weight [kg] + 539.6 × Height [m])

in which

PA = Physical activity coefficient:

PA = 1 (Sedentary)

PA = 1.11 (Low active)

PA = 1.25 (Active)

PA = 1.48 (Very active)

EER for Women 19 Years and Older (BMI 18.5-25 kg/m²)

EER = TEE

EER = 354 − 6.91 × Age (yr) + PA × (9.36 × Weight [kg] + 726 × Height [m])

in which

PA = Physical activity coefficient:

PA = 1 (Sedentary)

PA = 1.12 (Low active)

PA = 1.27 (Active)

PA = 1.45 (Very active)

EER for Pregnant Women

14-18 years: EER = Adolescent EER + Pregnancy energy deposition

First trimester = Adolescent EER + 0 (Pregnancy energy deposition)

Second trimester = Adolescent EER + 160 kcal (8 kcal/wk 1 × 20 wk) + 180 kcal

Third trimester = Adolescent EER + 272 kcal (8 kcal/wk × 34 wk) + 180 kcal

19-50 years: = Adult EER + Pregnancy energy deposition

First trimester = Adult EER + 0 (Pregnancy energy deposition)

Second trimester = Adult EER + 160 kcal (8 kcal/wk × 20 wk) + 180 kcal

Third trimester = Adult EER + 272 kcal (8 kcal/wk × 34 wk) + 180 kcal

EER for Lactating Women

14-18 years: EER = Adolescent EER + Milk energy output − Weight loss

First 6 months = Adolescent EER + 500 − 170 (Milk energy output − Weight loss)

Second 6 months = Adolescent EER + 400 − 0 (Milk energy output − Weight loss)

19-50 years: EAR = Adult EER + Milk energy output − Weight loss

First 6 months = Adult EER + 500 − 70 (Milk energy output − Weight loss)

Second 6 months = Adult EER + 400 − 0 (Milk energy output − Weight loss)

Weight Maintenance TEE for Overweight and At-Risk for Overweight Boys 3-18 Years (BMI >85th Percentile for Overweight)

TEE = 114 − 50.9 × Age (yr) + PA × (19.5 × Weight [kg] + 1161.4 × Height [m])

in which

PA = Physical activity coefficient:

PA = 1 if PAL is estimated to be ≥ 1.0 < 1.4 (Sedentary)

PA = 1.12 if PAL is estimated to be ≥ 1.4 < 1.6 (Low active)

PA = 1.24 if PAL is estimated to be ≥ 1.6 < 1.9 (Active)

PA = 1.45 if PAL is estimated to be ≥ 1.9 < 2.5 (Very active)

Weight Maintenance TEE for Overweight and At-Risk for Overweight Girls 3-18 Years (BMI >85th Percentile for Overweight)

TEE = 389 − 41.2 × Age (yr) + PA × (15 × Weight [kg] + 701.6 × Height [m])

in which

PA = Physical activity coefficient:

PA = 1 if PAL is estimated to be ≥ 1 < 1.4 (Sedentary)

PA = 1.18 if PAL is estimated to be ≥ 1.4 < 1.6 (Low active)

PA = 1.35 if PAL is estimated to be ≥ 1.6 < 1.9 (Active)

PA = 1.60 if PAL is estimated to be ≥ 1.9 < 2.5 (Very active)

Overweight and Obese Men 19 Years and Older (BMI ≥ 25 kg/m²)

TEE = 1086 − 10.1 × Age (yr) + PA × (13.7 × Weight [kg] + 416 × Height [m])

in which

PA = Physical activity coefficient:

PA = 1 if PAL is estimated to be ≥ 1 < 1.4 (Sedentary)

PA = 1.12 if PAL is estimated to be ≥ 1.4 < 1.6 (Low active)

PA = 1.29 if PAL is estimated to be ≥ 1.6 < 1.9 (Active)

PA = 1.59 if PAL is estimated to be ≥ 1.9 < 2.5 (Very active)

Overweight and Obese Women 19 Years and Older (BMI ≥ 25 kg/m²)

TEE = 448 − 7.95 × Age (yr) + PA × (11.4 × Weight [kg] + 619 × Height [m])

where

PA = Physical activity coefficient:

PA = 1 if PAL is estimated to be ≥ 1 < 1.4 (Sedentary)

Continued

BOX 2.1   Estimated Energy Expenditure Prediction Equations at Four Physical Activity Levels—cont'd

PA = 1.16 if PAL is estimated to be ≥ 1.4 < 1.6 (Low active)
PA = 1.27 if PAL is estimated to be ≥ 1.6 < 1.9 (Active)
PA = 1.44 if PAL is estimated to be ≥ 1.9 < 2.5 (Very active)

Normal and Overweight or Obese Men 19 Years and Older (BMI ≥ 18.5 kg/m²)

TEE = 864 − 9.72 × Age (yr) + PA × (14.2 × Weight [kg] + 503 × Height [m])
in which
PA = Physical activity coefficient:
PA = 1 if PAL is estimated to be ≥ 1 < 1.4 (Sedentary)
PA = 1.12 if PAL is estimated to be ≥ 1.4 < 1.6 (Low active)
PA = 1.27 if PAL is estimated to be ≥ 1.6 < 1.9 (Active)

PA = 1.54 if PAL is estimated to be ≥ 1.9 < 2.5 (Very active)

Normal and Overweight or Obese Women 19 Years and Older (BMI ≥ 18.5 kg/m²)

TEE = 387 − 7.31 × Age (yr) + PA × (10.9 × Weight [kg] + 660.7 × Height [m])
in which
PA = Physical activity coefficient:
PA = 1 if PAL is estimated to be ≥ 1 < 1.4 (Sedentary)
PA = 1.14 if PAL is estimated to be ≥ 1.4 < 1.6 (Low active)
PA = 1.27 if PAL is estimated to be ≥ 1.6 < 1.9 (Active)
PA = 1.45 if PAL is estimated to be ≥ 1.9 < 2.5 (Very active)

*EER is the average dietary energy intake that is predicted to maintain energy balance in a healthy adult of a defined age, gender, weight, height, and level of physical activity consistent with good health. In children and pregnant and lactating women, the EER includes the needs associated with the deposition of tissues or the secretion of milk at rates consistent with good health.
†PAL is the physical activity level that is the ratio of the total energy expenditure to the basal energy expenditure.
‡TEE is the sum of the resting energy expenditure, energy expended in physical activity, and the thermic effect of food.
§BMI is determined by dividing the weight (in kilograms) by the square of the height (in meters).
BMI, Body mass index; *EER*, estimated energy requirement; *PA*, physical activity; *PAL*, physical activity level; *TEE*, total energy expenditure.
From Institute of Medicine, Food and Nutrition Board: *Dietary reference intakes for energy, carbohydrate, fiber, fat, fatty acids, cholesterol, protein, and amino acids,* Washington, DC, 2002, The National Academies Press, www.nap.edu.

The prediction equations include a physical activity (PA) coefficient for all groups except infants and young children (see Box 2-1). PA coefficients correspond to four physical activity level (PAL) lifestyle categories: sedentary, low active, active, and very active. Because PAL is the ratio of TEE to BEE, the energy spent during activities of daily living, the sedentary lifestyle category has a PAL range of 1 to 1.39. PAL categories beyond sedentary are determined according to the energy spent by an adult walking at a set pace (Table 2.3). The walking equivalents that correspond to each PAL category for an average-weight adult walking at 3 to 4 mph are 2, 7, and 17 miles per day, for low active, active, and very active (IOM, 2002; 2005). All equations are only estimates and individual variations may be wide and unexpected (O'Riordan et al, 2010).

TABLE 2.3   Physical Activity Level Categories and Walking Equivalence*

PAL Category	PAL Values	Walking Equivalence (Miles/Day at 3-4 mph)
Sedentary	1-1.39	
Low active	1.4-1.59	1.5, 2.2, 2.9 for PAL = 1.5
Active	1.6-1.89	3, 4.4, 5.8 for PAL = 1.6
		5.3, 7.3, 9.9 for PAL = 1.75
Very active	1.9-2.5	7.5, 10.3, 14 for PAL = 1.9
		12.3, 16.7, 22.5 for PAL = 2.2
		17, 23, 31 for PAL = 2.5

*In addition to energy spent for the generally unscheduled activities that are part of a normal daily life. The low, middle, and high miles/day values apply to relatively heavyweight (120-kg), midweight (70-kg), and lightweight (44-kg) individuals, respectively.
PAL, Physical activity level.
From Institute of Medicine, The National Academies: *Dietary reference intakes for energy, carbohydrate, fiber, fat, fatty acids, cholesterol, protein, and amino acids,* Washington, DC, 2002/2005, The National Academies Press.

Estimated Energy Expended in Physical Activity

Energy expenditure in physical activity can be estimated using either the method shown in Appendix 10, which represents energy spent during common activities and incorporates body weight and the duration of time for each activity as variables, or using information in Fig. 2.3, which represents energy spent by adults during various intensities of physical activity—energy that is expressed as metabolic equivalents (METs) (IOM, 2002; 2005).

Estimating Energy Expenditure of Selected Activities Using Metabolic Equivalents

METs are units of measure that correspond with a person's metabolic rate during selected physical activities of varying intensities and are expressed as multiples of REE. A MET value of 1 is the oxygen metabolized at rest (3.5 mL of oxygen per kilogram of body weight per minute in adults) and can be expressed as 1 kcal/kg of body weight per hour. Thus the energy expenditure of adults can be estimated using MET values (1 MET = 1 kcal/kg/hr). For example, an adult who weighs 65 kg and is walking moderately at a pace of 4 mph (which is a MET value of 4.5) would expend 293 calories in 1 hour (4.5 kcal × 65 kg × 1 = 293) (Table 2.4).

Estimating a person's energy requirements using the IOM's EER equations requires identifying a PAL value for that person. A person's PAL value can be affected by various activities performed throughout the day and is referred to as the change in physical activity level (Δ PAL). To determine Δ PAL, take the sum of the Δ PALs for each activity performed for 1 day from the DRI tables (IOM, 2002; 2005). To calculate the PAL value for 1 day, take the sum of activities and add the BEE (1) plus 10% to account for the TEF (1 + 0.1 = 1.1). For example, to calculate an adult woman's PAL value, take the sum of the Δ PAL values for activities of daily living, such as walking the dog (0.11) and vacuuming (0.14) for 1 hour each, sitting for 4 hours doing light activity (0.12), and then performing moderate to vigorous activities such as walking for 1 hour at 4 mph (0.20) and ice skating for 30 minutes (0.13) for a total of 0.7. To that value add the BEE adjusted for the 10% TEF (1.1) for the final calculation:

$$0.7 + 1.1 = 1.8$$

TABLE 2.4 Intensity and Effect of Various Activities on Physical Activity Level in Adults*

Physical Activity	METs[†]	Δ PAL/10 min[‡]	Δ PAL/hr[‡]
Daily Activities			
Lying quietly	1	0	0
Riding in a car	1	0	0
Light activity while sitting	1.5	0.005	0.03
Vacuuming	3.5	0.024	0.14
Doing household tasks (moderate effort)	3.5	0.024	0.14
Gardening (no lifting)	4.4	0.032	0.19
Mowing lawn (power mower)	4.5	0.033	0.20
Leisure Activities: Mild			
Walking (2 mph)	2.5	0.014	0.09
Paddling (leisurely)	2.5	0.014	0.09
Golfing (with cart)	2.5	0.014	0.09
Dancing	2.9	0.018	0.11
Leisure Activities: Moderate			
Walking (3 mph)	3.3	0.022	0.13
Cycling (leisurely)	3.5	0.024	0.14
Walking (4 mph)	4.5	0.033	0.20
Leisure Activities: Vigorous			
Chopping wood	4.9	0.037	0.22
Playing tennis (doubles)	5	0.038	0.23
Ice skating	5.5	0.043	0.26
Cycling (moderate)	5.7	0.045	0.27
Skiing (downhill or water)	6.8	0.055	0.33
Swimming	7	0.057	0.34
Climbing hills (5-kg load)	7.4	0.061	0.37
Walking (5 mph)	8	0.067	0.40
Jogging (10-min mile)	10.2	0.088	0.53
Skipping rope	12	0.105	0.63

*PAL is the physical activity level that is the ratio of the total energy expenditure to the basal energy expenditure.
†METs are multiples of an individual's resting oxygen uptakes, defined as the rate of oxygen (O_2) consumption of 3.5 mL of O_2/min/kg body weight in adults.
‡The Δ PAL is the allowance made to include the delayed effect of physical activity in causing excess post exercise oxygen consumption and the dissipation of some of the food energy consumed through the thermic effect of food.
MET, Metabolic equivalent; *PAL*, physical activity level.
Modified from Institute of Medicine of The National Academies: *Dietary reference intakes for energy, carbohydrate, fiber, fat, fatty acids, protein, and amino acids*, Washington, DC, 2002, The National Academies Press.

For this woman, the PAL value (1.8) falls within an active range. The PA coefficient that correlates with an active lifestyle for this woman is 1.27.

To calculate the EER for this adult woman, age 30, use the EER equation for women 19 years and older (BMI 18.5-25 kg/m²); see Box 2.1. The following calculation estimates the EER for a 30-year-old active woman who weighs 65 kg, is 1.77 m tall, with a PA coefficient (1.27):

$$EER = 354 - 6.91 \times Age\ (yr) + PA \times (9.36 \times Weight\ [kg] + 726 \times Height\ [m])$$

$$EER = 354 - (6.91 \times 30) + 1.27 \times ([9.36 \times 65] + [726 \times 1.77])$$

$$EER = 2551\ kcal$$

PHYSICAL ACTIVITY IN CHILDREN

Energy spent during various activities and the intensity and impact of selected activities also can be determined for children and teens (see Box 2.1).

CALCULATING FOOD ENERGY

The total energy available from a food is measured with a bomb calorimeter. This device consists of a closed container in which a weighed food sample, ignited with an electric spark, is burned in an oxygenated atmosphere. The container is immersed in a known volume of water, and the rise in the temperature of the water after igniting the food is used to calculate the heat energy generated.

Not all of the energy in foods and alcohol is available to the body's cells, because the processes of digestion and absorption are not completely efficient. In addition, the nitrogenous portion of amino acids is not oxidized but is excreted in the form of urea. Therefore the biologically available energy from foods and alcohol is expressed in values rounded off slightly below those obtained using the calorimeter. These values for protein, fat, carbohydrate, and alcohol (Fig. 2.4) are 4, 9, 4, and 7 kcal/g, respectively. Fiber is an "unavailable carbohydrate" that resists digestion and absorption; its energy contribution is minimal.

Although the energy value of each nutrient is known precisely, only a few foods, such as oils and sugars, are made up of a single nutrient. More commonly, foods contain a mixture of protein, fat, and carbohydrate. For example, the energy value of one medium (50 g) egg calculated in terms of weight is derived from protein (13%), fat (12%), and carbohydrate (1%) as follows:

$$Protein:\ 13\% \times 50\ g = 6.5\ g \times 4\ kcal/g = 26\ kcal$$

$$Fat:\ 12\% \times 50\ g = 6\ g \times 9\ kcal/g = 54\ kcal$$

$$Carbohydrate:\ 1\% \times 50\ g = 0.05g \times 4\ kcal/g = 2\ kcal$$

$$Total\ =\ 82\ kcal$$

The energy value of alcoholic beverages can be determined using the following equation:

$$Alcohol\ kcal = amount\ of\ beverage\ (oz) \times proof \times 0.8\ kcal/proof/oz.$$

Proof is a description used for alcoholic beverages. It is the proportion of alcohol to water or other liquids in an alcoholic beverage. The standard in the United States defines 100-proof as equal to 50% of ethyl alcohol by volume. To determine the percentage of ethyl alcohol in a beverage, divide the proof value by 2. For example, 86-proof whiskey contains 43% ethyl alcohol. The latter part of the equation—0.8 kcal/proof/1 oz—is the factor that accounts for the caloric density of alcohol (7 kcal/g) and the fact that not all of the alcohol in liquor is available for energy. For example, the number of kilocalories in 1½ oz of 86-proof whiskey would be determined as follows:

$$1\frac{1}{2}\ oz \times 86\%\ proof \times 0.8\ kcal/proof/1\ oz = 103\ kcal$$

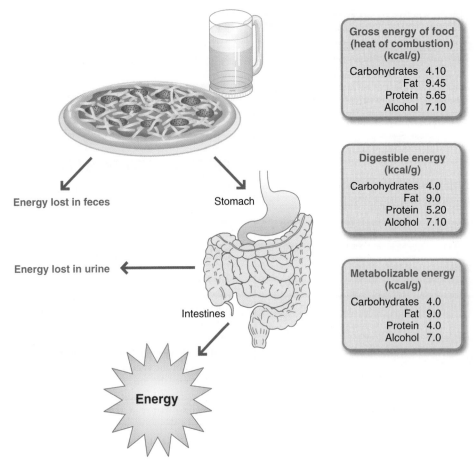

Gross energy of food (heat of combustion) (kcal/g)

Carbohydrates	4.10
Fat	9.45
Protein	5.65
Alcohol	7.10

Digestible energy (kcal/g)

Carbohydrates	4.0
Fat	9.0
Protein	5.20
Alcohol	7.10

Metabolizable energy (kcal/g)

Carbohydrates	4.0
Fat	9.0
Protein	4.0
Alcohol	7.0

Energy lost in feces

Stomach

Energy lost in urine

Intestines

Energy

Fig. 2.4 Energy value of food.

See Appendix 24 for the caloric content of alcoholic beverages.

Energy values of foods based on chemical analyses may be obtained from the U.S. Department of Agriculture (USDA) Nutrient Data Laboratory website or from *Bowes and Church's Food Values of Portions Commonly Used* (Pennington and Spungen, 2009).

Many computer software programs that use the USDA nutrient database as the standard reference are also available and many online websites can be used (see Chapter 4).

Recommendations for macronutrient percentages vary based on the goal of the client and any underlying or overriding disease process. This is discussed in other chapters.

USEFUL WEBSITES/APPS

The Academy of Nutrition and Dietetics: Evidence Analysis Library
American Society for Parenteral and Enteral Nutrition
Food Prodigy
myfitnesspal
MyPlate Tracker
National Academy Press—Publisher of Institute of Medicine DRIs for Energy
U.S. Department of Agriculture Food Composition Tables

REFERENCES

Compher C, Frankenfield D, Keim N, et al: Best practice methods to apply to measurement of resting metabolic rate in adults: a systematic review, *J Am Diet Assoc* 106:881–903, 2006.

Cooney RN, Frankenfield DC: Determining energy needs in critically ill patients: equations or indirect calorimeters, *Curr Opin Crit Care* 18:174–177, 2012.

Cooper JA, Manini TM, Paton CM, et al: Longitudinal change in energy expenditure and effects on energy requirements of the elderly, *Nutr J* 12(1):73, 2013.

Dombrowski A, Heuberger R: Patients receiving dialysis do not have increased energy needs compared with healthy adults, *J Ren Care* 2018. doi:1111/jorc.12248.

Ferraro R, Lillioja S, Fontvieille AM, et al: Lower sedentary metabolic rate in women compared with men, *J Clin Invest* 90:780–784, 1992.

Frankenfield DC, Rowe WA, Smith JS, et al: Validation of several established equations for resting metabolic rate in obese and nonobese people, *J Am Diet Assoc* 103:1152–1159, 2003.

Gallagher D, Belmonte D, Deurenberg P, et al: Organ-tissue mass measurement allows modeling of REE and metabolically active tissue mass. *Am J Physiol* 275:E249–E258, 1998.

Göktepe AS, Cakir B, Yilmaz B, et al: Energy expenditure of walking with prostheses: comparison of three amputation levels, *Prosthet Orthot Int* 34(1):31–36, 2010.

Hardy JD, DuBois EF: Regulation of heat loss from the human body, *Proc Natl Acad Sci U S A* 23:624–631, 1937.

Harris JA, Benedict FG: *A biometric study of basal metabolism in man, Pub no. 279*, Washington, DC, 1919, Carnegie Institute of Washington.

Heymsfield SB, Peterson CM, Bourgeois B, et al. Human energy expenditure: advances in organ-tissue prediction models. *Obes Rev* 19(9):1177–1188, 2018.

Hipskind P, Glass C, Charlton D, et al: Do handheld calorimeters have a role in assessment of nutrition needs in hospitalized patients? A systematic review of literature, *Nutr Clin Pract* 26:426–433, 2011.

Hursel R, Westerterp-Plantenga MS: Thermogenic ingredients and body weight regulation, *Int J Obes (Lond)* 34:659–669, 2010.

Institute of Medicine, Food and Nutrition Board: *Dietary reference intakes for energy, carbohydrate, fiber, fat, fatty acids, cholesterol, protein, and amino acids*, Washington, DC, 2002, National Academies Press.

Institute of Medicine of the National Academies, Food and Nutrition Board: *Dietary reference intakes for energy, carbohydrate, fiber, fat, fatty acids, cholesterol, protein, and amino acids*, Washington, DC, 2005, National Academies Press.

Ireton-Jones C: Indirect calorimetry. In Skipper A, editor: *The dietitian's handbook of enteral and parenteral nutrition*, ed 3, Sudbury, MA, 2010, Jones and Bartlett.

Javed F, He Q, Davidson LE, et al: Brain and high metabolic rate organ mass: contributions to resting energy expenditure beyond fat-free mass, *Am J Clin Nutr* 91:907–912, 2010.

Kee AL, Isenring E, Hickman I, et al: Resting energy expenditure of morbidly obese patients using indirect calorimetry: a systematic review, *Obes Rev* 13:753–765, 2012.

Kelly B, King JA, Goerlach J, et al: The impact of high-intensity intermittent exercise on resting metabolic rate in healthy males, *Eur J Appl Physiol* 113:3039–3047, 2013.

Keys A, Taylor HL, Grande F: Basal metabolism and age of adult man, *Metabolism* 22:579–587, 1973.

Larson-Meyer DE, Ravussin E, Heilbronn L, et al: Ghrelin and peptide YY in postpartum lactating and nonlactating women, *Am J Clin Nutr* 91: 366–372, 2010.

Ławiński M, Singer P, Gradowski Ł, et al: Predicted vs measured energy expenditure in patients receiving home nutrition support, *Nutrition* 31(11-12): 1328–1332, 2015.

Leuck M, Levandovski R, Harb A, et al: Circadian rhythm of energy expenditure and oxygen consumption, *J Parenter Enteral Nutr* 38:263–268, 2013.

McClave SA, Lowen CC, Kleber MJ, et al: Clinical use of the respiratory quotient obtained from indirect calorimetry, *J Parenter Enteral Nutr* 27:21–26, 2003.

Mifflin MD, St. Jeor ST, Hill LA, et al: A new predictive equation for resting energy expenditure in healthy individuals, *Am J Clin Nutr* 51:241–247, 1990.

Mindell JS, Coombs N, Stamatakis E: Measuring physical activity in children and adolescents for dietary surveys: practicalities, problems and pitfalls, *Proc Nutr Soc* 73(2):218–225, 2014.

Neilson HK, Robson PJ, Friedenreich CM, et al: Estimating activity energy expenditure: how valid are physical activity questionnaires? *Am J Clin Nutr* 87:279–291, 2008.

O'Riordan CF, Metcalf BS, Perkins JM, et al: Reliability of energy expenditure prediction equations in the weight management clinic, *J Hum Nutr Diet* 23:169–175, 2010.

Pennington JA, Spungen JS: *Bowes and Church's food values of portions commonly used*, ed 19, Philadelphia, PA, 2009, Lippincott Williams & Wilkins.

Plasqui G, Westerterp KR: Physical activity assessment with accelerometers: an evaluation against doubly labeled water, *Obesity* 15:2371–2379, 2007.

Reinbach HC, Smeets A, Martinussen T, et al: Effects of capsaicin, green tea and CH-19 sweet pepper on appetite and energy intake in humans in negative and positive energy balance, *Clin Nutr* 28:260–265, 2009.

Ribeiro HS, Anastácio LR, Ferreira LG, et al: Energy expenditure and balance among long-term liver recipients, *Clin Nutr* 33:1147–1152, 2014.

Sedlet KL, Ireton-Jones CS: Energy expenditure and the abnormal eating pattern of a bulimic: a case study, *J Am Diet Assoc* 89:74–77, 1989.

Tentolouris N, Pavlatos S, Kokkinos A, et al: Diet induced thermogenesis and substrate oxidation are not different between lean and obese women after two different isocaloric meals, one rich in protein and one rich in fat, *Metabolism* 57:313–320, 2008.

Volp ACP, Esteves de Oliveira FC, Duarte Moreira Alves R, et al: Energy expenditure: components and evaluation methods, *Nutr Hosp* 26(3):430–440, 2011.

Wang Z, Ying Z, Zhang J, et al: Evaluation of specific metabolic rates of major organs and tissues: comparison between nonobese and obese women, *Obesity (Silver Spring)* 20(1):95–100, 2012.

Wang Z, Ying Z, Zhang J, et al: Specific metabolic rates of major organs and tissues across adulthood: evaluation by mechanistic model of resting energy expenditure, *Am J Clin Nutr* 92(6):1369–1377, 2010.

Wong WW, Roberts SB, Racette SB, et al: The doubly labeled water method produces highly reproducible longitudinal results in nutrition studies, *J Nutr* 144:777–783, 2014.

Clinical: Water, Electrolytes, and Acid–Base Balance

Mandy L. Corrigan, MPH, RDN, CNSC, FAND, FASPEN
Lauren Kruse, MS, RDN, CNSC

KEY TERMS

acid–base balance
acidemia
alkalemia
anion gap
antidiuretic hormone
buffer
contraction alkalosis
corrected calcium
dehydration
edema
electrolytes
extracellular fluid (ECF)

hydrostatic pressure
hypervolemia
hyponatremia
insensible water loss
interstitial fluid
intracellular fluid (ICF)
lymph edema
metabolic acidosis
metabolic alkalosis
metabolic water
Na/K-ATPase pump
oncotic pressure (colloidal osmotic pressure)

osmolality
osmolarity
osmotic pressure
renin-angiotensin system
respiratory acidosis
respiratory alkalosis
sensible water loss
"third space" fluid
Total Body Water (TBW)
vasopressin

Fluid, electrolyte, and acid–base management is complex and requires an understanding of the functions and homeostatic mechanisms the body uses to maintain an optimal environment for cell function. Alterations in fluid, electrolyte, and acid–base balance are commonly seen in hospitalized patients and can affect homeostasis both acutely and chronically. Understanding the function and regulation of fluid and electrolytes lends the ability to prevent and treat these imbalances in patients across any disease state.

The volume, composition, and distribution of body fluids have profound effects on cell function. A stable internal environment is maintained through a sophisticated network of homeostatic mechanisms, which are focused on ensuring that water intake and water loss are balanced. Disease, trauma, and surgery can disrupt fluid, electrolyte, and **acid–base balance** and alter the composition, distribution, or amount of body fluids. Even small changes in pH, electrolyte concentrations, and fluid status can adversely impact cell function. If these alterations are not corrected, severe consequences or death can ensue.

BODY WATER

Water is the largest single component of the body. At birth, water is at the highest proportion that it will be throughout the entire human life span and accounts for 75% to 85% of total body weight; this proportion decreases with age and adiposity. Water accounts for 60% to 70% of total body weight in the lean adult but only 45% to 55% in the obese adult. Metabolically active cells of the muscle and viscera have the highest concentration of water; calcified tissue cells have the lowest. Total body water is higher in athletes than in nonathletes, decreases with age, and decreases with diminished muscle mass. Although the

proportion of body weight accounted for by water varies with gender, age, and body fat, there is little day-to-day variation in an individual.

Functions

Water makes solutes available for cellular reactions, regulates body temperature, maintains blood volume, transports nutrients, and is involved with digestion, absorption, and excretion. Loss of 20% of body water (dehydration) may cause death; loss of only 10% may lead to damage to essential body systems. Even mild dehydration (loss of 1% to 2%) can lead to loss of cognitive function and alertness, an increase in heart rate, and a decrease in exercise performance (Murray, 2007). Healthy adults can live up to 10 days without water, and children can live up to 5 days, whereas a person can survive for several weeks without food.

Distribution

Total body water (TBW) is mainly distributed in the intracellular fluid (ICF) and extracellular fluid (ECF). The transcellular fluid is comprised of 3% of TBW and is the small amount of fluid making up cerebral spinal, pericardial, and pleural fluids as well as fluid surrounding the eye. ICF is contained within cells and accounts for two-thirds of total body water. ECF accounts for the remaining one-third of total body water. ECF is the water and dissolved substances in the plasma and lymph, and also includes interstitial fluid (the fluid around the cells in tissues). While the distribution of body water varies under different circumstances, the total amount in the body remains relatively constant. Water intake of foods and beverages is balanced by water lost through urination, perspiration, feces, and respiration. Edema is the abnormal accumulation of fluid in the "third space," including intercellular tissue spaces or body cavities. Fluid in the "third space" is isolated and therefore does not contribute to the functional duties of body water within the body.

CLINICAL INSIGHT

Edema

Edema is the abnormal accumulation of interstitial fluid volume in the "third space," including intercellular tissue spaces or body cavities, that leads to a palpable and/or visible swelling. Fluid in the "third space" is isolated and therefore does not contribute to the functional duties of body water within the body.

The causes of edema can be multifactorial and have four main causes that impact fluid balance (Fig. 3.1).

1. Decrease in **oncotic pressure** (the pressure at the capillary membrane): Circulating plasma proteins decrease in states like protein losing enteropathy, nephrotic syndrome, or liver disease. Circulating proteins normally draw water into the vascular space, but with less circulating proteins there is a decrease in colloid pressure (albumin is the largest contributor to oncotic pressure).

2. Increase in the permeability of the capillaries: Allows protein leaks into the interstitial space, thereby attracting more water out of the vascular space. This can be seen in acute respiratory distress syndrome, trauma, burns, or inflammation.

3. Increase in **hydrostatic pressure**: The force from the increased pressure or blood volume pushes fluid into the interstitial space as seen in disease states such as cirrhosis, congestive heart failure, renal failure, or venous thrombosis.

4. Lymphatic dysfunction: **Lymph edema** is usually localized to specific areas of the body when there is an obstruction of the lymphatic vessels. It occurs when fluid and protein cannot return to circulation, and the trapped protein-rich lymph fluid attracts water. Lymph edema can be seen in cancer patients who have had surgery for lymph node dissection.

Edema is graded based on severity (grades 1, 2, 3, 4+) and can be classified as pitting or nonpitting. If pressure is applied by a finger or thumb to an area with edema, it is classified as pitting edema when an impression or "pit" remains after the finger is removed (Fig. 3.2).

Edema is typically referred to by the location it is present (e.g., pedal edema when present in the feet or peripheral edema when found in the extremities). Edema can also be further categorized as dependent, independent, or generalized. Dependent edema is characterized by the accumulation of fluid in inferior areas. For example, a patient on bed rest with peripheral edema and elevated legs/feet may experience dependent edema in the sacrum and hips with the fluid shifting to an inferior area of the body. Generalized edema is not confined to one area rather fluid accumulates all throughout the body. In contrast, independent edema is isolated to one area of the body (Ratliff, 2015).

When conducting nutrition focused physical examination as part of the nutrition assessment, it's important to evaluate both sides of the body, left and right, for the presence or absence of edema since edema can be unilateral or bilateral.

Water Balance

Water movement is dictated by hydrostatic pressure, diffusion, osmosis, and active transport. Water moves in and out of the ICF and ECF based on the **osmolarity** (ability for osmotic pressure to move fluid between compartments) to obtain equilibrium. Osmotic pressure is directly proportional to the number of particles in the solution and usually refers to the pressure at the cell membrane. The sodium-potassium adenosine triphosphatase pump (**Na/K-ATPase pump**) plays a key role in regulating water balance. In simple terms, osmotic pressure of the ICF is a function of its potassium content because potassium is the predominant intracellular cation. The osmotic pressure of ECF is relative to the sodium content because

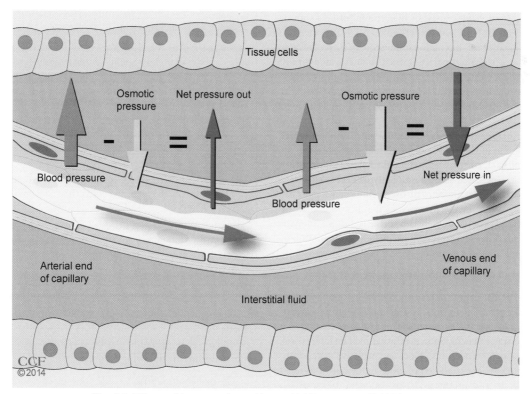

Fig. 3.1 Effects of Intravascular and Interstitial Pressure on Fluid Movement

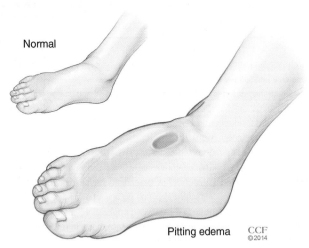

Normal

Pitting edema

CCF
©2014

Fig. 3.2 Pitting Edema

TABLE 3.1	Content of Common Intravenous Fluids			
Fluid	Dextrose (g/L)	Sodium (mEq/L)	Chloride (mEq/L)	Additional Components (mEq/L)
0.45% NaCl	0	77	77	n/a
0.9% NaCl	0	154	154	n/a
3% Saline	0	513	513	n/a
5% Dextrose in water	50	0	0	n/a
$D_5$0.45% NaCl	50	77	77	n/a
$D_5$0.9% NaCl	50	154	154	n/a
10% Dextrose	100	0	0	n/a
Lactated Ringer's (LR)	0	130	109	Potassium 4 Calcium 3 Lactate 28
D_5LR	50	130	109	Potassium 4 Calcium 3 Lactate 28

sodium is the major extracellular cation. Although variations in the distribution of sodium and potassium ions are the principal causes of water shifts between the various fluid compartments, chloride and phosphate also are involved with water balance (see the electrolyte section later in this chapter).

Osmolality is a measure of the osmotically active particles per kilogram of the solvent in which the particles are dispersed. The average sum of the concentration of all the cations in serum is approximately 150 mEq/L. The cation concentration is balanced by 150 mEq/L of anions, yielding a total serum osmolality of approximately 300 mOsm/L. Osmolality or tonicity are words used interchangeably in clinical practice. Normal osmolality or tonicity is 280 to 300 mOsms and values above or below this range are termed hypotonic (typically a sign of water excess) or hypertonic (often a sign of water deficit).

Shifts in water balance can have adverse consequences. Body water is regulated by the gastrointestinal (GI) tract, kidneys, and brain, which keeps body water content fairly constant. Skin, the body's largest organ, also plays a role in regulating temperature and body water. In general, the amount of water intake is approximately equivalent to output each day.

Mechanisms to maintain water equilibrium come from a number of hormones including antidiuretic hormone (aka vasopressin), aldosterone, angiotensin II, cortisone, norepinephrine, and epinephrine (Canada et al, 2015). Increased serum osmolality or decreased blood volume leads to the release of antidiuretic hormone which signals the kidneys to conserve water. In the presence of low ECF volume, the kidneys release renin to produce angiotensin II (the renin-angiotensin system). Angiotensin II has several functions, including stimulation of vasoconstriction and the thirst centers.

Water Intake

Thirst is regulated by the hypothalamus and controls water intake in healthy individuals. Sensitivity to thirst is decreased in older individuals, chronically or acutely ill patients, infants, and athletes leading to a higher potential for water deficits. Sources of water include fluids (oral, enteral tube feeding, parenteral fluids), food, and oxidative metabolism (Tables 3.1, 3.2, and 3.3). The oxidation of foods in the body produces metabolic water as an end product. The oxidation of 100 g of fat, carbohydrate, or protein yields 107, 55, or 41 g of water, respectively,

TABLE 3.2	Percentage of Water in Common Foods		
Food	Percentage	Food	Percentage
Lettuce, iceberg	96	Eggs	75
Celery	95	Bananas	74
Cucumbers	95	Fish, haddock, baked	74
Cabbage, raw	92	Chicken, roasted, white meat	70
Watermelon	92		
Broccoli, boiled	91	Corn, boiled	65
Milk, nonfat	91	Beef, sirloin	59
Spinach	91	Cheese, Swiss	38
Green beans, boiled	89	Bread, white	37
Carrots, raw	88	Cake, angel food	34
Oranges	87	Butter	16
Cereals, cooked	85		
Apples, raw, without skin	84	Almonds, blanched	5
		Saltines	3
Grapes	81	Sugar, white	1
Potatoes, boiled	77	Oils	0

From U.S. Department of Agriculture (USDA), Agricultural Research Service (ARS): Nutrient database for standard reference. http://ndb.nal.usda.gov.

for a total of approximately 200 to 300 mL/day (Whitmire, 2008; Canada, 2015).

Tonicity of body fluids can be measured (serum osmolality) or estimated from the following formula:

$$\text{Osmolality (mOsms)} = (2 \times \text{Serum sodium mEq/L}) + (\text{BUN mg/dL}) + (\text{Blood glucose mg/dL})$$

TABLE 3.3   Water Content of Enteral Nutrition Formulations

Enteral Formula Concentration	Percentage of Free Water
1.0 kcal/mL	84%
1.2 kcal/mL	81%
1.5 kcal/mL	76%
2.0 kcal/mL	69%

CLINICAL INSIGHT

Osmotic Forces

Osmotic pressure is directly proportional to the number of particles in solution and usually refers to the pressure at the cell membrane. Osmotic pressure of intracellular fluid is a function of its potassium content because potassium is the predominant cation there. In contrast, the osmotic pressure of extracellular fluid (ECF) may be considered relative to its sodium content because sodium is the major cation present in ECF. Although variations in the distribution of sodium and potassium ions are the principal causes of water shifts between the various fluid compartments, chloride and phosphate also influence water balance. Proteins cannot diffuse because of their size and thus also play a key role in maintaining osmotic equilibrium. Oncotic pressure, or colloidal osmotic pressure, is the pressure at the capillary membrane. It is maintained by dissolved proteins in the plasma and interstitial fluids. Oncotic pressure helps retain water within blood vessels, preventing its leakage from plasma into the interstitial spaces. In patients with an exceptionally low plasma protein content, such as those who are under physiologic stress or have certain diseases, water leaks into the interstitial spaces, causing edema or third spacing; thus the fluid is called "third space" fluid.

Osmoles and Milliosmoles

Concentrations of individual ionic constituents of extracellular or intracellular fluids are expressed in terms of milliosmoles per liter (mOsm/L). One mole equals the gram molecular weight of a substance; when dissolved in 1 L of water, it becomes 1 osmole (Osm). One milliosmole (mOsm) equals 1/1000th of an osmole.

Osmolality is a measure of the osmotically active particles per kilogram of the solvent in which the particles are dispersed. It is expressed as milliosmoles of solute per kilogram of solvent (mOsm/kg). Osmolarity is the term formerly used to describe concentration—milliosmoles per liter of the entire solution—but osmolality is now the measurement for most clinical work. However, in reference to certain conditions such as hyperlipidemia, it makes a difference whether osmolality is stated as milliosmoles per kilogram of solvent or per liter of solution.

The average sum of the concentration of all the cations in serum is about 150 mEq/L. The cation concentration is balanced by 150 mEq/L of anions, yielding a total serum osmolality of about 300 mOsm/L. An osmolar imbalance is caused by a gain or loss of water relative to a solute. An osmolality of less than 285 mOsm/L generally indicates a water excess; an osmolality of greater than 300 mOsm/L indicates a water deficit.

Water Intoxication and Fluid Overload

Water intoxication occurs as a result of water intake in excess of the body's ability to excrete water. The increased ICF volume is accompanied by osmolar dilution. The increased volume of ICF causes the cells, particularly the brain cells, to swell, leading to headache, nausea, vomiting, muscle twitching, blindness, and convulsions with impending stupor. If left untreated, water intoxication can be fatal. Water intoxication is not commonly seen in normal, healthy individuals. It may be seen in endurance athletes who consume large amounts of electrolyte-free beverages during events, individuals with psychiatric illness, or as a result of water drinking contests (Adetoki et al, 2013).

Fluid overload, or hypervolemia, occurs when excess fluid accumulation is present within the body, leading to excess in circulating blood volume. This may occur as a result of excess fluid intake (via oral, enteral, or parenteral route), injury or illness causing stress to the body, or diagnoses such as kidney, heart, or liver disease. Symptoms of fluid overload may often include generalized or localized swelling, sudden weight gain, dyspnea, orthopnea, pulmonary congestion, or modifications in arterial pressures. Treatment for fluid overload is often dictated by the inherent cause; options may include reduction in fluid intake, diuretic therapy, and sodium restriction.

Water Elimination

Water loss normally occurs through the kidneys as urine and through the GI tract in the feces (measurable, sensible water loss), as well as through air expired from the lungs and water vapor lost through the skin (nonmeasurable, insensible water loss). The kidney is the primary regulator of sensible water loss. Under normal conditions the kidneys have the ability to adjust to changes in body water composition by either decreasing or increasing water loss in the urine. Natural diuretics are substances in the diet that increase urinary excretion, such as alcohol and caffeine.

Insensible water loss is continuous and usually unconscious. High altitude, low humidity, and high temperatures can increase insensible fluid loss through the lungs and through sweat. Athletes can lose 6% to 10% of body weight in sweat loss and fluids need to be replaced. Dehydration leads to an increase in core body temperature, which rises 0.15 to 0.20° C for every 1% of body weight lost due to sweating (Casa et al, 2000). In high-risk conditions, it is suggested athletes evaluate pre- and post-activity fluid loss and consume 1 to 1.25 L of fluid for each 1 kg of body water lost during exercise (Binkley, 2002).

The GI tract can be a major source of water loss (Fig. 3.3). Under normal conditions the water contained in the 7 to 9 L of digestive juices and other ECFs secreted daily into the GI tract is reabsorbed almost entirely in the ileum and colon, except for about 100 mL that is excreted in the feces. Because this volume of reabsorbed fluid is about twice that of the blood plasma, excessive GI fluid losses through diarrhea may have serious consequences, particularly for very young and very old individuals.

Choleric diarrhea, acute diarrhea caused by contaminated food or water containing the bacteria *vibrio cholera*, is responsible for the loss of many lives in developing countries and hydration can be corrected without intravenous fluids. Oral rehydration solution, an isotonic fluid, is a simple mixture of water, sugar, and salt and is highly effective in improving hydration status (Parrish and DiBaise, 2015). Other abnormal fluid losses may occur as a result of emesis, hemorrhage, fistula drainage, burn and wound exudates, gastric and surgical tube drainage, and the use of diuretics.

When water intake is insufficient or water loss is excessive, healthy kidneys compensate by conserving water and excreting more concentrated urine. The renal tubules increase water reabsorption in response to the hormonal action of vasopressin. However, the concentration of the urine made by the kidneys has a limit: approximately 1400 mOsm/L. Once this limit has been reached, the body loses its ability to excrete solutes. The ability of the kidneys to concentrate urine may be compromised in older individuals or in young infants, resulting in increased risk of developing dehydration or hypernatremia, especially during illness.

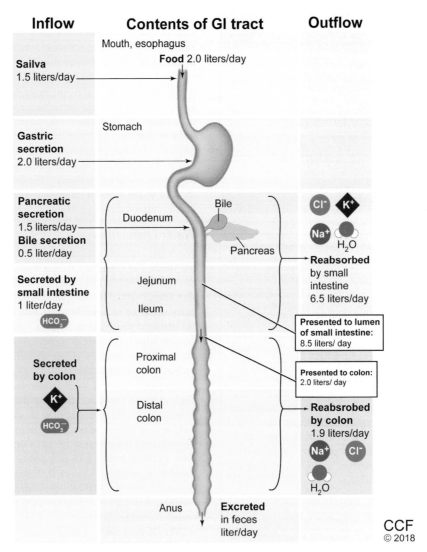

Inflow

Contents of GI tract

Outflow

Mouth, esophagus
Food 2.0 liters/day

Sailva
1.5 liters/day

Stomach

Gastric secretion
2.0 liters/day

Pancreatic secretion
1.5 liters/day
Bile secretion
0.5 liter/day

Duodenum

Bile

Pancreas

Cl⁻ K⁺

Na⁺ H₂O

Reabsorbed
by small intestine
6.5 liters/day

Secreted by small intestine
1 liter/day
HCO₃⁻

Jejunum

Ileum

Presented to lumen of small intestine: 8.5 liters/ day

Presented to colon: 2.0 liters/ day

Secreted by colon
K⁺
HCO₃⁻

Proximal colon

Distal colon

Reabsrobed by colon
1.9 liters/day
Na⁺ Cl⁻

H₂O

Anus

Excreted in feces
liter/day

CCF
© 2018

Fig. 3.3 Content of Gastrointestinal Secretions

Signs of dehydration include headache, fatigue, decreased appetite, lightheadedness, poor skin turgor (although this may be present in well-hydrated older persons), skin tenting on the forearm, concentrated urine, decreased urine output, sunken eyes, dry mucous membranes of the mouth and nose, orthostatic blood pressure changes, and tachycardia. In a dehydrated person the specific gravity, a measure of the dissolved solutes in urine, increases above the normal levels, and the urine becomes remarkably darker.

High ambient temperature and dehydration adversely affect exercise performance. Fluids of appropriate composition in appropriate amounts are essential (see *Clinical Insight*: Water Requirements: When Eight Is Not Enough).

Clinical Assessment of Fluid Status

A variety of methods to estimate fluid requirements are based on age, caloric intake, and weight. Obesity has led to challenges with using weight-based calculations for fluid requirements, as water accounts for only 45% to 55% of body weight for patients with lower proportions of lean body mass. In clinical practice, fluid estimations should be individualized to each patient, especially those with cardiac, liver, or renal failure, and in the presence of ongoing high-volume GI losses.

In most cases a suitable daily water intake (fluids and including foods) is approximately 3.7 L (15.5 cups) for adult males and 2.7 L (11+ cups) for adult females, depending on body size (Institute of Medicine of the National Academies, 2005). Because solid food provides 19% of total daily fluid intake, this equals 750 mL of water or approximately 3 cups daily. When this is added to the 200 to 300 mL (about 1 cup) of water contributed by oxidative metabolism, men should consume about 11.5 cups and women need 7 cups of fluids daily. Total fluid intake comes from drinking water, other liquids, and food; the adequate intake (AI) for water is for total daily water intake and includes all dietary water sources.

Unfortunately there is no gold standard to assess hydration status. Clinicians must carefully assess data from a variety of sources, including physical examination by the medical team, nutrition-focused physical examinations, imaging reports (e.g., identifying abnormal fluid collections within the lungs, ascites), laboratory studies (i.e., serum sodium), subjective report of symptoms from patients, sudden weight changes, medications, and vital signs. In clinical settings it is important to acknowledge all sources of fluid delivery (oral, enteral feeding tube, intravenous fluids, parenteral nutrition, and intravenous fluids given with medications) and all sources of fluid losses including

CLINICAL INSIGHT

Water Requirements: When Eight Is Not Enough

There is no storage form of water, and therefore fluid requirements and fluid losses must be maintained at equilibrium. Often clinicians quickly estimate fluid requirements based on energy requirements (1 mL/kcal for adults and 1.5 mL/kcal for infants) or approximately 35 mL/kg of usual body weight in nonobese adults, 50 to 60 mL/kg in children, and 150 mL/kg in infants.

At certain points within the lifecycle, the body will naturally require more fluid. Infants need more water because of the limited capacity of the kidneys to handle a large renal solute load, higher percentage of body water, and large surface area per unit of body weight. A lactating woman's need for water also increases, approximately 2 ½ to 3 cups per day for milk production.

Knowledge of disease states also helps in determining when higher fluid requirements may occur. Fluid intake should exceed the excretion of sensible and insensible losses in order to prevent dehydration. In patients with Short Bowel Syndrome (SBS), inadequate absorption of fluid can lead to dehydration. SBS patients with an enterostomy (or colon not connected to the small bowel) often have increased fluid requirements and are at an increased risk of dehydration if too much stool is lost due to malabsorption. Like children with infectious diarrhea in developing countries, SBS patients benefit from the use of oral rehydration solutions by mouth, in order to utilize the active co-transport of sodium and glucose molecules at the intestinal brush border, which helps maintain hydration (Matarese, 2005). Use of oral rehydration solution sipped throughout the day and separating fluids from meals can be helpful strategies for helping SBS patients maintain their hydration status. When oral intake alone is not sufficient to prevent dehydration, parenteral fluids may be needed. Use of parental fluids can be temporary (e.g., due to an acute event such as a urinary tract infection in an elderly adult) or chronic for certain disease states (e.g., SBS or gastrointestinal fistula).

Fluid needs of hospitalized patients should be individualized and adequacy of fluid intake assessed from physical examination by the medical team, nutrition-focused physical examinations, imaging reports, laboratory studies (Na, BUN, Cr, Hgb/Hct, albumin, etc.), subjective report of symptoms from patients, sudden weight changes, medications, and vital signs.

TABLE 3.4 Electrolyte Classification

Electrolyte	Location
Cations	
Sodium	Extracellular cation
Potassium	Intracellular cation
Calcium	Extracellular cation
Magnesium	Intracellular cation
Anions	
Chloride	Extracellular Anion
CO2	Extracellular Anion
Phosphorus (inorganic)	Intracellular Anion

fluids, are distributed throughout all body fluids. Electrolytes are responsible for maintenance of physiologic body functions, cellular metabolism, neuromuscular function, and osmotic equilibrium. Although oral intake varies, homeostatic mechanisms regulate the concentrations of electrolytes throughout the body.

Changes in either intracellular or extracellular electrolyte concentrations can have a major impact on bodily functions. The Na/K-ATPase pump closely regulates cellular electrolyte contents by actively pumping sodium out of cells in exchange for potassium. Other electrolytes follow ion gradients (gradient of electrical potential for movement across a membrane).

Calcium

Although approximately 99% of the body's calcium (Ca^{++}) is stored in the skeleton (bones and teeth), the remaining 1% has important physiologic functions. Ionized Ca^{++} within the vascular compartment is a cation with a positive charge. Approximately half of the Ca^{++} found in the intravascular compartment is bound to the serum protein albumin. Thus, when serum albumin levels are low, total Ca^{++} levels decrease because of hypoalbuminemia.

The binding ability of Ca^{++} and its ionized content in blood have implications for normal homeostatic mechanisms. Blood tests for Ca^{++} levels often measure total and ionized Ca^{++} levels. Ionized (or free, unbound) Ca^{++} is the active form of Ca^{++} and is not impacted by hypoalbuminemia. In healthy adults, normal levels for serum total Ca^{++} are about 8.5 to 10.5 mg/dL, whereas normal levels for ionized Ca^{++} are 4.5 to 5.5 mEq/L (refer to the reference ranges for each reporting laboratory).

Functions

Ca^{++} is an extracellular cation necessary for blood clotting; Ca^{++} regulates nerve transmission, muscle contraction, bone metabolism, and blood pressure regulation. Ca^{++} is regulated by parathyroid hormone (PTH), calcitonin, vitamin D, and phosphorus. Through a complex system of regulation among multiple organs, including the kidney, GI tract, and bone, Ca^{++} absorption can be enhanced to increase Ca^{++} reabsorption to maintain homeostasis. When serum Ca^{++} levels are low, PTH causes release of Ca^{++} from the bones and stimulates increased absorption from the GI tract. Calcitonin works in the opposite direction, shutting off the release of Ca^{++} from the bone and decreasing GI absorption. Vitamin D stimulates while phosphorus inhibits Ca^{++} absorption in the GI tract.

In the setting of hypoalbuminemia, serum Ca^{++} levels are not accurate because nearly 50% of Ca^{++} is protein bound. An ionized Ca^{++} level is the most accurate assay for Ca^{++} because it is the active form and is not affected by protein levels. In healthy adults, normal levels for serum total Ca^{++} are approximately 8.5 to 10.5 mg/dL, whereas normal

urine, diuretic medications, and GI secretions (e.g., emesis, gastric secretions, surgical drains, stool, fistulas) (Popkin et al, 2010).

Of note, thirst is not an effective signal to consume fluids in infants, heavily exercising athletes (Casa, 2015), individuals in extreme heat, sick individuals, and older adults who may have a diminished thirst sensation. Hospitalized patients, regardless of the diagnosis, are at risk for water and electrolyte imbalance. Older adults are particularly susceptible because of factors such as impaired renal concentrating ability, fever, diarrhea, vomiting, and a decreased ability to care for themselves.

ELECTROLYTES

Electrolytes are minerals with electric charges that dissociate in a solution into positive or negatively charged ions. Electrolytes can be simple inorganic salts of sodium, potassium, or magnesium, or complex organic molecules; they play a key role in a host of normal metabolic functions (Table 3.4). One milliequivalent (mEq) of any substance has the capacity to combine chemically with 1 mEq of a substance with an opposite charge. For univalent ions (e.g., Na^+), 1 millimole (mmol) equals 1 mEq; for divalent ions (e.g., Ca^{++}), 1 mmol equals 2 mEq (see Appendix 1 for conversion guidelines).

The major extracellular electrolytes are sodium, calcium, chloride, and bicarbonate. Potassium, magnesium, and phosphate are the major intracellular electrolytes. These elements, which exist as ions in body levels for ionized Ca^{++} are 4.5 to 5.5 mEq/L (refer to the reference ranges for each reporting laboratory). When ionized Ca^{++} levels are not available, a simple formula may be used. The corrected calcium formula accounts for a 0.8 mg/dL decrease in Ca^{++} for each 1 g/dL decrease in serum albumin below 4 g/dL. The corrected calcium formula is

$$([4 - \text{Serum albumin (g/dL)}] \times 0.8) + \text{Measured calcium (mg/dL)}$$

Ionized Ca^{++} levels are altered inversely by changes in acid–base balance; as serum pH rises, Ca^{++} binds with protein, leading to decreased ionized Ca^{++} levels. As pH is lowered, the opposite occurs. Because Ca^{++} has an important role in cardiac, nervous system, and skeletal muscle function, hypocalcemia and hypercalcemia can become life threatening.

Common causes of hypercalcemia are cancer with the presence of bone metastases or hyperparathyroidism, when there is a large amount of Ca^{++} moved into the ECF. Symptoms of hypercalcemia include lethargy, nausea, vomiting, muscle weakness, and depression. Treatment usually is directed at treating the underlying cause of the problem, discontinuing Ca^{++}-containing medications, and increasing the excretion of Ca^{++} though the kidneys (by delivery of intravenous fluids followed by diuretic medications).

Hypocalcemia often is marked with numbness or tingling, hyperactive reflexes, tetany, lethargy, muscle weakness, confusion, and seizures. Causes of hypocalcemia include low serum phosphorus or magnesium levels, medications that cause Ca^{++} losses, hypoalbuminemia, vitamin D deficiency, or hypoparathyroidism. Oral Ca^{++} supplements are most often the first-line therapy in the absence of symptoms. Because other hormones, electrolytes, and vitamins are involved in Ca^{++} regulation, these are assessed in the setting of true hypocalcemia. Low phosphorus and magnesium levels must be replete before Ca^{++} levels can be corrected (Rhoda et al, 2011).

Absorption and Excretion

Approximately 20% to 60% of dietary Ca^{++} is absorbed and is tightly regulated because of the need to maintain steady serum Ca^{++} levels in the face of fluctuating intake. The ileum is the most important site of Ca^{++} absorption. Ca^{++} is absorbed via passive transport and through a vitamin D–regulated transport system.

The kidney is the main site of Ca^{++} excretion. The majority of serum Ca^{++} is bound to proteins and not filtered by the kidneys; only about 100 to 200 mg/day is excreted in the urine in normal adults. Ca^{++} is also excreted through sweat and feces.

Sources

Dairy products are the main source of Ca^{++} in the American diet, with some green vegetables, nuts, legumes, canned fish including bones, and Ca^{++}-enriched tofu having moderate amounts of Ca^{++}. Food manufacturers fortify many foods with additional Ca^{++}, such as orange juice that may have some bioavailability (see Appendix 39).

Recommended Intakes

In adults, recommended intakes of Ca^{++} range from 1000 to 1300 mg/day, depending on age and gender. An upper limit for Ca^{++} intake has been estimated to be approximately 2500 to 3000 mg/day (see inside cover). Excessive intake of Ca^{++} may lead to kidney stones and gastrointestinal side effects like constipation.

Sodium

Sodium (Na^+) is the major cation of ECF with a normal range of 135 to 145 mEq/L (refer to the reference ranges for each reporting laboratory). Secretions such as bile and pancreatic juice contain substantial amounts of Na^+. Gastric secretions and diarrhea also contain Na^+, but contrary to common belief, sweat is hypotonic and contains a relatively small amount of Na^+. Approximately 35% to 40% of the total body Na^+ is in the skeleton and the remainder is in body fluids.

Functions

As the predominant ion of the ECF, Na^+ thus regulates extracellular and plasma volume. Na^+ is also important in neuromuscular function and maintenance of acid–base balance. Maintenance of serum Na^+ levels is vital, because severe hyponatremia can lead to seizures, coma, and death.

Extracellular Na^+ concentrations are much higher than intracellular levels (normal serum Na^+ is around 135 mEq/L, whereas intracellular levels are around 10 mEq/L). The sodium-potassium ATP pump is an active transport system that works to keep Na^+ outside the cell through exchange with potassium. The Na/K-ATPase pump requires carriers for Na^+ and potassium along with energy for proper function. Exportation of Na^+ from the cell is the driving force for facilitated transporters, which import glucose, amino acids, and other nutrients into the cells.

Hyponatremia. Assessing hyponatremia or hypernatremia takes into consideration the role of Na^+ in regulating fluid balance and requires evaluation of overall hydration status. Hyponatremia is one of the most common electrolyte disorders among hospitalized patients and occurs in 25% of inpatients. When hyponatremia is below 125 mEq/L, symptoms generally become apparent. Patients may display signs of headache, lethargy, restlessness, decreased reflexes, seizures, or coma in extreme cases. There are three basic causes for hyponatremia. Hypertonic hyponatremia is due to excess delivery of mannitol or hyperglycemia, which causes serum Na^+ to increase by 1.6 mEq for every 100 mg/dL rise in serum glucose. Mannitol is sometimes used for the treatment of cerebral edema or kidney failure. It increases serum osmolality, which leads to dilutional hyponatremia from water movement out of the cells. Isotonic hyponatremia occurs in the presence of hyperlipidemia or hyperproteinemia, because the aqueous component that Na^+ is dissolved and results in a falsely low value (this is mainly a laboratory artifact and is not often seen in clinical practice). The final type is hypotonic hyponatremia. Evaluation depends on fluid status to evaluate the three subtypes.

Isovolemic hyponatremia can be caused by malignancies, adrenal insufficiency, or the syndrome of inappropriate antidiuretic hormone secretion (SIADH). SIADH (see Chapter 30) can result from central nervous system disorders, pulmonary disorders, tumors, and certain medications. The treatment is usually water restriction. Hypervolemic hypotonic hyponatremia is characterized by excess TBW and Na^+ (overall higher excess water than Na^+) because of reduced excretion of water or excess free water administration. Cardiac, renal, or hepatic failure are the most common causes, and patients have edema or ascites on physical examination. The treatment is fluid restriction or diuretics to aid in decreasing TBW, and oral Na^+ restriction also may be beneficial. The final type is hypovolemic hypotonic hyponatremia, characterized by a deficit in TBW and Na^+ that requires treatment with fluid replacement. Often fluid losses leading to hypovolemia hyponatremia include excessive vomiting, excessive sweating (marathon athletes), diarrhea, wound drainage/burns, high-volume gastrointestinal secretions, or excessive diuretic use. Equations to calculate fluid deficits can be used to replace half of the fluid deficit in the first 24 hours. Correcting Na^+ levels must be done slowly (max of 8 to 12 mEq in 24 hours) to prevent osmotic demyelinating syndrome that is seen with rapid correction (Rhoda et al, 2011).

Hypernatremia. A serum Na^+ level greater than 145 mEq/L is classified as hypernatremia, and there are various types. Hypovolemic hypernatremia is caused by a loss of Na^+ and TBW when water losses exceed Na^+ losses. It is important to identify the cause of the fluid losses so that they can be corrected and prevented in the future. The treatment is to slowly replace fluid volume with a hypotonic fluid solution. Hypervolemic hypernatremia is caused by excessive intake of Na^+

resulting in higher Na+ gain than water gains. The treatment is to restrict Na+ (especially in intravenous fluids) and possibly the use of diuretics. Isovolemic hypernatremia is seen with disease states such as diabetes insipidus. Signs of hypernatremia include lethargy, thirst, hyperreflexia, seizures, coma, or death. Formulas for calculating a water deficit are helpful to guide fluid replacement. Free water deficit is calculated as follows (Kingley, 2005):

$$[0.6 \times \text{Weight (kg)}] \times 1 - [140 / \text{Na (mEq/L)}]$$

Absorption and Excretion

Na+ is absorbed readily from the intestine and carried to the kidneys, where it is filtered and returned to the blood to maintain appropriate levels. The amount absorbed is proportional to the intake in healthy adults.

About 90% to 95% of normal body Na+ loss is through the urine; the rest is lost in feces and sweat. Normally the quantity of Na+ excreted daily is equal to the amount ingested. Na+ excretion is maintained by a mechanism involving the glomerular filtration rate, the cells of the juxtaglomerular apparatus of the kidneys, the renin-angiotensin-aldosterone system, the sympathetic nervous system, circulating catecholamines, and blood pressure.

Na+ balance is regulated in part by aldosterone, a mineralocorticoid secreted by the adrenal cortex. When blood Na+ levels rise, the thirst receptors in the hypothalamus stimulate the thirst sensation. Ingestion of fluids returns Na+ levels to normal. Under certain circumstances Na+ and fluid regulation can be disrupted, resulting in abnormal blood Na+ levels. SIADH is characterized by concentrated, low-volume urine and dilutional hyponatremia as water is retained. SIADH can result from central nervous system disorders, pulmonary disorders, tumors, and certain medications. Common drug classes/medications include antidepressants, anticonvulsants, antipsychotic agents, cytotoxic agents, and pain medication are the common medications (Shepshelovich et al, 2017).

Estrogen, which is slightly similar to aldosterone, also causes Na+ and water retention. Changes in water and Na+ balance during the menstrual cycle, during pregnancy, and while taking oral contraceptives are attributable partially to changes in progesterone and estrogen levels.

Dietary Reference Intake

The dietary reference intakes (DRIs) give an upper limit of 2.3 g of Na+ per day (or 5.8 g sodium chloride per day). The mean daily salt intake in the United States is approximately 6 to 12 g/day (Institute of Medicine of the National Academies, 2005), which exceeds the adequate intake (AI) for Na+ of 1.2 to 1.3 g per day for adult males and females (see Table 3.4).

Healthy kidneys are usually able to excrete excess Na+ intake; however, persistent excessive Na+ intake has been implicated in development of hypertension. In addition to its role in hypertension, excessive salt intake has been associated with increased urinary Ca++ excretion, kidney stones, and some cases of osteoporosis. Higher Na+ consumption has been associated with higher weight status, and a positive relationship has been observed between Na+ intake and obesity independent of energy intake (Song et al, 2013; Yoon, 2013; Zhu et al, 2014). In addition, a positive association has been identified between Na+ intake and increased circulation of leptin (secreted by fat cells and influences inflammatory response and Na+ excretion) and tumor necrosis factor alpha (plays a role in inflammation) (Zhu et al, 2014).

Sources

The major source of Na+ is sodium chloride, or common table salt, of which Na+ constitutes 40% by weight. Protein foods generally contain more naturally existing Na+ than do vegetables and grains, whereas fruits contain little or none. The addition of table salt, flavored salts, flavor enhancers, and preservatives during food processing accounts for the high Na+ content of most convenience and fast-food products.

Magnesium

Magnesium is the second most prevalent intracellular cation. Approximately half of the body's magnesium is located in bone, whereas another 45% resides in soft tissue; only 1% of the body's magnesium content is in the ECF. Normal serum magnesium levels are about 1.6 to 2.5 mEq/L; however, about 70% of serum magnesium is free or ionized. The remainder is bound to proteins and is not active.

Function

Magnesium (Mg^{2+}) is an important cofactor in many enzymatic reactions in the body, bone metabolism, central nervous system, and cardiovascular function. Many of the enzyme systems regulated by Mg^{2+} are involved in nutrient metabolism and nucleic acid synthesis, leading to the body's need to carefully regulate Mg^{2+} status.

As with Ca++, severe hypo- or hypermagnesemia can have life-threatening consequences. Physical symptoms of Mg^{2+} abnormalities are similar to those observed with other electrolyte deficiencies, and the challenges with serum measurements discussed earlier make assessment of Mg^{2+} status difficult. Symptoms of hypomagnesemia include muscle weakness, tetany, ataxia, nystagmus, and, in severe cases, ventricular arrhythmia. Frequent causes of hypomagnesemia include excessive stool losses (as seen in short bowel syndrome or malabsorption), inadequate Mg^{2+} in the diet (oral, enteral, or parenteral nutrition), intracellular shifts during refeeding syndrome (Box 3.1; see Chapter 12), acute pancreatitis, burns, alcoholism, diabetic ketoacidosis, and medications causing increased Mg^{2+} losses via the urine. Long-term use of proton pump inhibitors also may be a rare cause (Toh et al, 2015).

Often hypomagnesemia is treated with oral supplementation if no physical symptoms are noted. However, dietitians should monitor cautiously for diarrhea with oral Mg^{2+} supplements if they are not given in divided doses (such as magnesium oxide), which often can increase

---

BOX 3.1   Refeeding Syndrome

Refeeding syndrome is a metabolic response that can be seen upon reintroduction of nutrients to the body in patients that have been without adequate nutrition. Refeeding syndrome can impact patients with malnutrition or those previously well nourished with metabolic stress in the presence of significant illness.

During starvation, the body's metabolism shifts from using glucose to using fat as the main fuel source. When nutrients are provided to the body, there is a metabolic shift. An increase of insulin leads to this intracellular shift, and thus concentrations of electrolytes in the serum fall. Low levels of phosphorus, magnesium, and potassium can be seen, and there are significant risks of cardiac arrhythmia, neurological consequences (seizures, delirium, neuropathy), and respiratory failure. Fluid retention and thiamin deficiency can also occur.

Prevention of Refeeding Syndrome:

1. Patient screening for risk of refeeding syndrome
2. Slow reintroduction and advancement of calories provided from enteral or parenteral nutrition to patients
3. Clinical monitoring (for cardiac, neuro, respiratory, fluid status, etc.)
4. Laboratory monitoring of serum electrolytes and treatment of abnormalities

From Canada T, Tajchman SK, Tucker AM, et al, editors: *ASPEN Fluids, electrolytes and acid base disorders handbook*, Silver Spring, MD, 2015, ASPEN, pp 1–397; Skipper A: Refeeding syndrome or refeeding hypophosphatemia: a systematic review of cases, *Nutr Clin Pract* 27:34–40, 2012; Rhoda KM, Porter MJ, Quintini C: Fluid and electrolyte management: putting a plan in motion, *JPEN J Parenter Enteral Nutr* 35: 675–685, 2011; Kraft MD, Btaiche IF, Sacks GS: Review of the refeeding syndrome, *Nutr Clin Pract* 20:625–633, 2005.

Mg^{2+} losses through the stool. Increased losses through the stool is avoided with supplementation from salts such as magnesium gluconate, magnesium citrate, or magnesium lactate. Intravenous repletion with Mg^{2+} is required with symptomatic signs of deficiency or if serum levels are below 1 mg/dL.

Hypermagnesemia, a serum value greater than 2.5 mg/dL, can be due to excess supplementation or Mg^{2+}-containing medications, severe acidosis, or dehydration. Treatment options include omission of Mg^{2+}-containing medications and correction of the fluid imbalance.

Absorption/Excretion

Approximately 30% to 50% of Mg^{2+} ingested from the diet is absorbed (within the jejunum and ileum though passive and active transport mechanisms). Mg^{2+} is regulated by the intestine, kidney, and bone. Mg^{2+} absorption is regulated to maintain serum levels; if levels drop, more is absorbed and if levels increase, less is absorbed. The kidney is the major regulator of Mg^{2+} excretion, but some Mg^{2+} is also lost via the stool. As magnesium is a cofactor for the Na-K ATPase pump, low magnesium levels should be evaluated and corrected especially when hypokalemia is refractory to repletion (unable to regain a normal level despite delivery of appropriate repletion doses). The kidneys increase potassium excretion in response to hypomagnesemia.

Sources

Mg^{2+} is found in a variety of foods, making an isolated Mg^{2+} deficiency unlikely in otherwise healthy individuals. Highly processed foods tend to have lower Mg^{2+} content, whereas green leafy vegetables, nuts, seeds, legumes, and whole grains are good sources (see Appendix 43).

Dietary Reference Intakes

The recommended intake of Mg^{2+} in adults ranges from 310 to 420 mg/day, depending on age and gender (see inside cover).

Phosphorus

Phosphorus is the primary intracellular anion, and its role in adenosine triphosphate (ATP) is vital in energy metabolism. In addition, phosphorus is important in bone metabolism. About 80% of the body's phosphorus is found in bones. Normal levels for serum phosphorus are between 2.4 and 4.6 mg/dL (refer to the reference ranges for each reporting laboratory).

Functions

Large amounts of free energy are released when the phosphate bonds in ATP are split. In addition to this role, phosphorus is vital for cellular function in phosphorylation and dephosphorylation reactions, as a buffer in acid–base balance, and in cellular structure as part of the phospholipid membrane. Because of the vital role that phosphorus plays in energy production, severe hypophosphatemia can be a life-threatening event. This is seen most often clinically in refeeding syndrome and occurs with the increased use of phosphorus for the phosphorylation of glucose (Skipper, 2012; Rhoda et al, 2011; Kraft et al, 2005). In addition to intracellular shifts, hypophosphatemia can be medication related (insulin, epinephrine, dopamine, erythropoietin, phosphorus-binding medications). Severe and symptomatic hypophosphatemia (<1 mg/dL) can be critical and includes impaired cardiac function, reduced contractions of the diaphragm leading to a weakened respiratory state, confusion, reduced oxygen delivery to tissues, coma, and even death.

Absorption and Excretion

Phosphorus absorption is dependent on serum levels and vitamin D status. Around 80% of phosphorus intake is absorbed in the small bowel when hypophosphatemia is present. The kidney is the major site of phosphorus excretion and regulates phosphorus absorption based on PTH and acid–base status. Phosphorus absorption decreases when vitamin D deficiency occurs or with certain medications that bind phosphorus (e.g., antacids or phosphate binders used in patients with chronic kidney disease).

Sources

Phosphorus is found mainly in animal products, including meats and milk; dried beans, soda, processed foods, baked goods, and seafood or meats soaked in phosphate solutions are common dietary sources in the American diet.

Dietary Reference Intakes

The recommended intake of phosphorus is approximately 700 mg/day, depending on age and gender, with an upper limit of 3500 to 4000 mg (see inside cover).

Potassium

With approximately 98% of potassium (K^+) in the intracellular space, K^+ is the major cation of ICF. The normal serum K^+ concentration is typically 3.5 to 5 mEq/L (refer to the reference ranges for each reporting laboratory).

Functions

With Na^+, K^+ is involved in maintaining a normal water balance, osmotic equilibrium, and acid–base balance. In addition to Ca^{++}, K^+ is important in the regulation of neuromuscular activity. Concentrations of Na^+ and K^+ determine membrane potentials in nerves and muscle. K^+ also promotes cellular growth. The K^+ content of muscle is related to muscle mass and glycogen storage; therefore if muscle is being formed, an adequate supply of K^+ is essential. K^+ has an integral role in the Na/K-ATPase pump.

Hypokalemia and hyperkalemia can have devastating cardiac implications. When hypokalemia is less than 3 mEq/L, symptoms are more apparent and critical. Symptoms of hypokalemia include muscle weakness, cramping in the extremities, vomiting, and weakness. Clinically, hypokalemia occurs with large volume losses of gastrointestinal fluids that contain K^+, insulin delivery, excessive losses through the urine caused by certain medications (diuretics), and diabetic ketoacidosis. Guidelines exist for the treatment of hypokalemia (oral or intravenous medications) and are adjusted in renal impairment because K^+ is excreted by the kidneys.

Hyperkalemia can be critical, especially when levels exceed 6.5 mEq/L and are accompanied by symptoms of muscle weakness, paralysis, respiratory failure, and arrhythmias/ECG changes. Causes of hyperkalemia in a clinical setting include hemolysis causing falsely elevated laboratory results, kidney disease impairing K^+ excretion, medications such as K^+-sparing diuretics, gastrointestinal hemorrhage, rhabdomyolysis, catabolism, metabolic acidosis, or overzealous K^+ supplementation.

Absorption and Excretion

K^+ is absorbed readily from the small intestine. Approximately 80% to 90% of ingested K^+ is excreted in the urine; the remainder is lost in the feces. The kidneys maintain normal serum levels through their ability to filter, reabsorb, and excrete K^+ under the influence of aldosterone. In the setting of hypokalemia, aldosterone secretions are lower, and the kidneys shift to reabsorb K^+ and excrete Na^+.

Sources

K^+-rich food sources include fruits, vegetables, legumes, fresh meat, and dairy products. Salt substitutes commonly contain K^+. Box 3.2

BOX 3.2 Classification of Select Foods by Potassium Content

Low (0-100 mg/serving)*	Medium (100-200 mg/serving)*	High (200-300 mg/serving)*	Very High (>300 mg/serving)*
Fruits	Fruits	Fruits	Fruits
Applesauce	Apple, 1 small	Apricots, canned	Avocados, ¼ small
Blueberries	Apple juice	Grapefruit juice	Banana, 1 small
Cranberries	Apricot nectar	Kiwi, ½ medium	Cantaloupe, ¼ small
Lemon, ½ medium	Blackberries	Nectarine, 1 small	Dried fruit, ¼ cup
Lime, ½ medium	Cherries, 12 small	Orange, 1 small	Honeydew melon, ⅛ small
Pears, canned	Fruit cocktail	Orange juice	Mango, 1 medium
Pear nectar	Grape juice	Peach, fresh, 1 medium	Papaya, ½ medium
Peach nectar	Grapefruit, ½ small	Pear, fresh, 1 medium	Prune juice
Vegetables	Grapes, 12 small	Vegetables	Vegetables
Cabbage, raw	Mandarin oranges	Asparagus, fresh, cooked, 4 spears	Artichoke, 1 medium
Cucumber slices	Peaches, canned	Beets, fresh, cooked	Bamboo shoots, fresh
Green beans, frozen	Pineapple, canned	Brussels sprouts	Beet greens, ¼ cup
Leeks	Plum, 1 small	Kohlrabi	Corn on the cob, 1 ear
Lettuce, iceberg, 1 cup	Raspberries	Mushrooms, cooked	Chinese cabbage, cooked
Water chestnuts, canned	Rhubarb	Okra	Dried beans
Bamboo shoots canned	Strawberries	Parsnips	Potatoes, baked, ½ medium
	Tangerine, 1 small	Potatoes, boiled or mashed	Potatoes, French fries, 1 oz
	Watermelon, 1 cup	Pumpkin	Spinach
	Vegetables	Rutabagas	Sweet potatoes, yams
	Asparagus, frozen	Miscellaneous	Swiss chard, ¼ cup
	Beets, canned	Granola	Tomato, fresh, sauce, or juice; tomato paste, 2 tbsp
	Broccoli, frozen	Nuts and seeds, 1 oz	Winter squash
	Cabbage, cooked	Peanut butter, 2 tbsp	Miscellaneous
	Carrots	Chocolate, 1.5-oz bar	Bouillon, low sodium, 1 cup
	Cauliflower, frozen		Cappuccino, 1 cup
	Celery, 1 stalk		Chili, 4 oz
	Corn, frozen		Coconut, 1 cup
	Eggplant		Lasagna, 8 oz
	Green beans, fresh, raw		Milk, chocolate milk, 1 cup
	Mushrooms, fresh, raw		Milkshakes, 1 cup
	Onions		Molasses, 1 tbsp
	Peas		Pizza, 2 slices
	Radishes		Salt substitutes, ¼ tsp
	Turnips		Soy milk, 1 cup
	Zucchini, summer squash		Spaghetti, 1 cup
			Yogurt, 6 oz

*One serving equals ½ cup unless otherwise specified

categorizes select foods according to their K^+ content. When evaluating K^+ sources and losses, clinicians must consider other nonfood sources of K^+, such as intravenous fluids with added K^+, certain medications containing K^+, and medications that may cause the body to excrete K^+.

Dietary Reference Intakes

The adequate intake level for K^+ for adults is 4700 mg/day. No upper limit has been set. K^+ intake is inadequate in a large number of Americans, as many as 50% of adults. The reason for the poor K^+ intake is simply inadequate consumption of fruits and vegetables. Insufficient K^+ intake has been linked to hypertension and cardiac arrhythmia.

ACID–BASE BALANCE

An acid is any substance that tends to release hydrogen ions in solution, whereas a base is any substance that tends to accept hydrogen ions in solution. The hydrogen ion concentration (H^+) determines acidity.

Because the magnitude of H^+ is small compared with that of other serum electrolytes, acidity is expressed more readily in terms of pH units. A low blood pH indicates a higher H^+ and greater acidity, whereas a high pH value indicates a lower H^+ and greater alkalinity.

Acid–base balance is the dynamic equilibrium state of H^+. Maintaining the arterial blood pH level within the normal range of 7.35 to 7.45 is crucial for many physiologic functions and biochemical reactions. Regulatory mechanisms of the kidneys, lungs, and buffering systems enable the body to maintain the blood pH level despite the enormous acid load from food consumption and tissue metabolism. A disruption of the acid–base balance occurs when acid or base losses or gains exceed the body's regulatory capabilities or when normal regulatory mechanisms become ineffective. These regulatory disturbances may develop in association with certain diseases, toxin ingestion, shifts in fluid status, and certain medical and surgical treatments (Table 3.5). If a disrupted acid–base balance is left untreated, multiple detrimental effects ranging from electrolyte abnormalities to death can ensue.

TABLE 3.5 Four Major Acid–Base Imbalances

Acid-base Imbalance	pH	Primary Disturbance	Compensation	Possible Causes
Respiratory				
Respiratory acidosis	Low	Increased pCO_2	Increased renal net acid excretion with resulting increase in serum bicarbonate	Emphysema; COPD; neuromuscular disease where respiratory function is impaired; excessive retention of CO_2
Respiratory alkalosis	High	Decreased pCO_2	Decreased renal net acid excretion with resulting decrease in serum bicarbonate	Heart failure, pregnancy, sepsis, meningitis, anxiety, pain, excessive expiration of CO_2
Metabolic				
Metabolic acidosis	Low	Decreased HCO_3^-	Hyperventilation with resulting low pCO_2	Diarrhea; uremia; ketoacidosis from uncontrolled diabetes mellitus; starvation; high-fat, low-carbohydrate diet; drugs, alcoholism, kidney disease
Metabolic alkalosis	High	Increased HCO_3^-	Hypoventilation with resulting increase in pCO_2	Diuretics use; increased ingestion of alkali; loss of chloride; vomiting/nasogastric tube suction

ACID GENERATION

The body produces a large amount of acids daily though routine processes such as metabolism and oxidation of food, endogenous production of acid from tissue metabolism, and ingestion of acid precursors. The main acid is carbon dioxide (CO_2), termed a volatile acid, which is produced from the oxidation of carbohydrates, amino acids, and fat. Nonvolatile or fixed acids, including phosphoric and sulfuric acids, are produced from the metabolism of phosphate-containing compounds to form phosphates and phosphoric acid and sulfur-containing amino acids (such as the metabolism of methionine and cysteine). Organic acids, such as lactic, uric, and keto acids, come from the incomplete metabolism of carbohydrates and fats. These organic acids typically accumulate only during exercise, acute illness, or fasting. Under normal conditions, the body is able to maintain normal acid–base status through a wide range of acid intake from foods.

Regulation

Various regulatory mechanisms maintain the pH level within very narrow physiologic limits. At the cellular level, buffer systems composed of weak acids or bases and their corresponding salts minimize the effect on pH of the addition of a strong acid or base. The buffering effect involves formation of a weaker acid or base in an amount equivalent to the strong acid or base that has been added to the system (see Fig. 3.3).

Proteins and phosphates are the primary intracellular buffers, whereas the bicarbonate and H_2CO_3 system is the primary extracellular buffer. The acid–base balance also is maintained by the kidneys and lungs. The kidneys regulate hydrogen ion (H^+) secretion and bicarbonate resorption. The kidneys regulate the pH of the urine by excreting H^+ or HCO_3^- and can make bicarbonate. The kidneys are the slowest-responding mechanism to maintain acid–base balance. The lungs control H^+ through the amount of CO_2 that is exhaled. When more CO_2 is exhaled, it reduces the H^+ concentration in the body. The respiratory system responds quickly to alter either the depth or rate of air movement in the lungs.

ACID–BASE DISORDERS

Acid–base disorders can be differentiated based on whether they have metabolic or respiratory causes. The evaluation of acid–base staus requires analysis of serum electrolytes and arterial blood gas (ABG) values (Table 3.6). There are four main acid–base

TABLE 3.6 Common Arterial Blood Gas Values*

Clinical Test	ABG Value
pH	7.35-7.45
pCO_2	35-45 mm Hg
pO_2	80-100 mm Hg
HCO_3^- (bicarbonate)	22-26 mEq/L
O_2 saturation	>95%

*Check exact reference range at laboratory when interpreting patient results
ABG, Arterial blood gas.

abnormalities: metabolic acidosis, metabolic alkalosis, respiratory acidosis, and respiratory alkalosis. It is important to characterize the type of acid–base disorder because this will dictate the treatment and response or "compensation" mechanism enacted by the body. Metabolic acid–base imbalances result in changes in bicarbonate (i.e., base) levels, which are reflected in the total carbon dioxide (TCO_2) portion of the electrolyte profile. TCO_2 includes bicarbonate (HCO_3^-), carbonic acid (H_2CO_3) and dissolved carbon dioxide; however, all but 1 to 3 mEq/L are in the form of HCO_3^-. Thus, for ease of interpretation, TCO_2 should be equated with HCO_3^-. Respiratory acid–base imbalances result in changes in the partial pressure of dissolved carbon dioxide (pCO_2). This is reported in the ABG values in addition to the pH, which reflect the overall acid–base status.

Metabolic Acidosis

Metabolic acidosis results from increased production or accumulation of acids or loss of base (i.e., HCO_3^-) in the extracellular fluids. Simple, acute metabolic acidosis results in a low blood pH (or acidemia), low HCO_3^-, and normal pCO_2. Examples of metabolic acidosis include diabetic ketoacidosis, lactic acidosis, toxin ingestion, uremia, and excessive HCO_3^- loss via the kidneys or intestinal tract. Multiple deaths previously have been attributed to lactic acidosis caused by administration of parenteral nutrition devoid of thiamin. In patients with metabolic acidosis, the anion gap is calculated to help determine cause and appropriate treatment. An anion gap is the measurement of the interval between the sum of "routinely measured" cations minus the sum of the "routinely measured" anions in the blood. The anion gap is

$$(Na^+ + K^+) - (Cl^- + HCO_3^-)$$

where Na^+ is sodium, K^+ is potassium, Cl^- is chloride, and HCO_3^- is bicarbonate. Normal is 12 to 14 mEq/L (refer to the reference ranges for each reporting laboratory).

Anion gap metabolic acidosis occurs when a decrease in HCO_3^- concentration is balanced by increased acid anions other than chloride. This causes the calculated anion gap to exceed the normal range of 12 to 14 mEq/L. This normochloremic metabolic acidosis may develop in association with diabetic ketoacidosis, lactic acidosis, uremia, ingestion (e.g., methanol, paraldehyde, ethylene glycol, alcohol), or be iatrogenic (Wilson, 2003). Nongap metabolic acidosis occurs when a decrease in HCO_3^- concentration is balanced by an increase in chloride concentration, resulting in a normal anion gap. This hyperchloremic metabolic acidosis may develop in association small bowel fistulae, excess chloride ingestion (from medications or parenteral sources), diarrhea, pancreatic fistulae, renal tubular acidosis, ureterosigmoidostomy, or adrenal insufficiency (Canada et al, 2015).

Metabolic Alkalosis

Metabolic alkalosis results from the administration or accumulation of HCO_3^- (i.e., base) or its precursors, excessive loss of acid (e.g., during gastric suctioning), or loss of ECF containing more chloride than HCO_3^- (e.g., from villous adenoma or diuretic use). Simple, acute metabolic alkalosis results in a high blood pH, or alkalemia. Metabolic alkalosis also may result from volume depletion; decreased blood flow to the kidneys stimulates reabsorption of Na^+ and water, increasing HCO_3^- reabsorption. This condition is known as contraction alkalosis. Alkalosis also can result from severe hypokalemia (serum K^+ concentration <2 mEq/L). As K^+ moves from the intracellular to the extracellular fluid, hydrogen ions move from the extracellular to the intracellular fluid to maintain electroneutrality. This process produces intracellular acidosis, which increases hydrogen ion excretion and HCO_3^- reabsorption by the kidneys.

Respiratory Acidosis

Respiratory acidosis is caused by decreased ventilation and consequent CO_2 retention. Simple, acute respiratory acidosis results in a low pH, normal HCO_3^- and elevated pCO_2. Acute respiratory acidosis can occur as a result of sleep apnea, asthma, aspiration of a foreign object, or acute respiratory distress syndrome (ARDS). Chronic respiratory acidosis is associated with obesity hypoventilation syndrome, chronic obstructive pulmonary disease (COPD) or emphysema, certain neuromuscular diseases, and starvation cachexia. Prevention of overfeeding is prudent as it can worsen acidosis (Ayers and Dixon, 2012).

Respiratory Alkalosis

Respiratory alkalosis results from increased ventilation and elimination of CO_2. The condition may be mediated centrally (e.g., from head injury, pain, anxiety, cerebrovascular accident, or tumors) or by peripheral stimulation (e.g., from pneumonia, hypoxemia, high altitudes, pulmonary embolism, congestive heart failure, or interstitial lung disease). Simple, acute respiratory alkalosis results in a high pH, (or alkalemia), normal HCO_3^-, and decreased pCO_2.

Compensation

When an acid–base imbalance occurs, the body attempts to restore the normal pH by developing an opposite acid–base imbalance to offset the effects of the primary disorder, a response known as compensation. For example, the kidneys of a patient with a primary respiratory acidosis (decreased pH) compensate by increasing HCO_3^- reabsorption, thereby creating a metabolic alkalosis. This response helps increase the pH. Similarly, in response to a primary metabolic acidosis (decreased pH), the lungs compensate by increasing ventilation and CO_2 elimination, thereby creating a respiratory alkalosis. This compensatory respiratory alkalosis helps increase pH.

Respiratory compensation for metabolic acid–base disturbances occurs quickly—within minutes. In contrast, renal compensation for respiratory acid–base imbalances may take 3 to 5 days to be maximally effective (Ayers et al, 2015). Compensation does not always occur, and when it does, it is not completely successful (i.e., does not result in a pH of 7.4). The pH level still reflects the underlying primary disorder. Clinicians must distinguish between primary disturbances and compensatory responses because treatment always is directed toward the primary acid–base disturbance and its underlying cause. As the primary disturbance is treated, the compensatory response corrects itself. Predictive values for compensatory responses are available to differentiate between primary acid–base imbalances and compensatory responses. Clinicians also may use tools such as clinical algorithms.

Acid–Base Balance: Guidelines and Applications to Dietetics Practice

Acid–base balance is a complicated topic that requires a high-level understanding of many complex processes. Table 3.5 displays the anticipated ABG alterations and compensation mechanisms. A few rules of thumb may be helpful to understanding this topic. In uncompensated and simple acid–base disorders, pH and pCO_2 move in opposite directions in respiratory disorders. In uncompensated and simple acid–base disorders, pH and HCO_3^- move in the same direction. When mixed acid–base disorders occur, pCO_2 and HCO_3^- generally move in opposite directions. Regardless of the disorder, the medical team directs the treatment at the underlying cause and uses supporting information from the medical history, current clinical condition, medications, laboratory values, intake and output records, and physical examination to determine the cause. Dietetics professionals play an important role in understanding the physiologic process and how it relates to regulation of electrolyte and fluid balance. Adjustments to the nutrition care plan related to acid–base balance can include shifting chloride and acetate salts in parenteral nutrition, manipulating macronutrients to prevent overfeeding, or adjusting fluid and electrolytes.

REFERENCES

Adetoki A, Evans R, Cassidy G: Polydipsia with water intoxication in treatment resistant schizophrenia, *Prog Neurol Psychiatry* 3:20, 2013.

Ayers P, Dixon C: Simple acid-base tutorial, *JPEN J Parenter Enteral Nutr* 36(1):18–23, 2012.

Ayers P, Dixon C, Mays A: Acid-base disorders: learning the basics, *Nutr Clin Pract* 30:14–20, 2015.

Canada T, Tajchman SK, Tucker AM, et al, editors: *ASPEN Fluids, electrolytes and acid base disorders handbook*, Silver Spring, MD, 2015, ASPEN, pp 1–397.

Casa DJ, DeMartini JK, Bergeron MF, et al: National athletic trainers' association position statement: exertional heat illness, *J Athl Train* 50(9):986–1000, 2015.

Casa DJ, Armstrong LE, Hillman SK, et al: National athletic trainers' association position statement: fluid replacement for athletes, *J Athl Train* 35(2):212–224, 2000.

Institute of Medicine of the National Academies: *Dietary reference intakes for water, potassium, sodium, chloride, and sulfate*, Washington, DC, 2005,

The National Academies Press. Available at: https://www.nap.edu/read/10925/chapter/1.

Kingley J: Fluid and electrolyte management in parenteral nutrition, *Support Line* 27:13, 2005.

Kraft MD, Btaiche IF, Sacks GS: Review of the refeeding syndrome, *Nutr Clin Pract* 20:625–633, 2005.

Murray B: Hydration and physical performance, *J Am Coll Nutr* 26:542S–548S, 2007.

Parrish CR, DiBaise JK: Short bowel syndrome in adults—part 3 Hydrating the adult patient with short bowel syndrome, *Pract Gastroenterol* (138):10–18, 2015. Available at: https://med.virginia.edu/ginutrition/wp-content/uploads/sites/199/2014/06/Parrish_Feb_15.pdf.

Popkin BM, D'Anci KE, Rosenberg IH: Water hydration, and health, *Nutr Rev* 68:439–458, 2010.

Ratliff A: Assessment of fluid accumulation, *Support Line* 37(5):5–10, 2015.

Rhoda KM, Porter MJ, Quintini C: Fluid and electrolyte management: putting a plan in motion, *JPEN J Parenter Enteral Nutr* 35:675–685, 2011.

Shepshelovich D, Schechter A, Calvarysky B, et al: Medication induced SIADH: distribution and characterization according to medication class, *Br J Clin Pharmacol* 83(8):1801–1807, 2017.

Skipper A: Refeeding syndrome or refeeding hypophosphatemia: a systematic review of cases, *Nutr Clin Pract* 27:34–40, 2012.

Song HJ, Cho YG, Lee HJ: Dietary sodium intake and prevalence of overweight in adults, *Metabolism* 62:703–708, 2013.

Toh JW, Ong E, Wilson R: Hypomagnesaemia associated with long-term use of proton pump inhibitors. *Gastroenterol Rep (Oxf)* 3(3):243–253, 2015. doi:10.1093/gastro/gou054.

Whitmire SJ: Nutrition-focused evaluation and management of dysnatremias, *Nutr Clin Pract* 23:108–121, 2008.

Wilson RF: Acid-base problems. In Tintinalli JE, et al, editors: *Emergency medicine: a comprehensive study guide*, ed 6, New York, 2003, McGraw-Hill.

Yoon YS, Oh SW: Sodium density and obesity; the Korea national health and nutrition examination survey 2007–2010, *Eur J Clin Nutr* 67(2):141–146, 2013.

Zhu H, Pollock NK, Kotak I, et al: Dietary sodium, adiposity, and inflammation in healthy adolescents, *Pediatrics* 133:e635–e642, 2014.

4

Intake: Assessment of Food- and Nutrition-Related History

Cynthia Bartok, PhD, RDN, CD
L. Kathleen Mahan, RDN, MS, CD

KEY TERMS

24-hour recall
acceptable intake (AI)
acceptable macronutrient distribution
    range (AMDR)
bioactive compound
calorie count
dietary intake data
dietary reference intakes (DRIs)

food diary
food frequency questionnaire (FFQ)
food record
nutrition assessment
nutrition care indicators
nutrition care process (NCP)
nutrition screening
nutritional status

problem, etiology, signs and symptoms
    (PES) statement
quantitative food patterns
recommended dietary allowance
    (RDA)
tolerable upper level (UL)

NUTRITIONAL STATUS

Nutritional status is the physiologic state or condition of an individual based on the balance between the individual's intake and unique requirement for nutrients (Fig. 4.1). Nutrient intake represents the amount of a nutrient that is absorbed into the body from foods, beverages, medications, and supplements consumed. Thus nutrient intake depends on:

- the amount of a nutrient contained in the diet,
- the bioavailability of a nutrient based on its source, and
- the body's capacity to digest and absorb nutrients within the gastrointestinal system.

Nutrition professionals such as registered dietitian nutritionists (RDNs) and nutrition and dietetic technicians, registered (NDTRs) serve as food and nutrition experts on health care teams. They are in a key position to evaluate the nutrient quantity, quality, and bioavailability of a client's diet. In addition, because many acute and chronic medical conditions impact the body's ability to digest and absorb nutrients from dietary sources, nutrition professionals often evaluate gastrointestinal function when assessing nutritional status.

A nutrient requirement represents the need for a nutrient based on an individual's unique physiologic profile. Adjunctive data such as age, gender, physical activity level, and life cycle stage assist in estimating an individual's nutrient needs in relation to known standards such as the dietary reference intakes (DRIs). In addition, disease status (e.g., nutrient deficiencies), genetics, and medical conditions (e.g., liver disease, inborn errors of metabolism) that further impact nutrient requirements must be carefully considered when estimating nutritional requirements.

Assessment of nutritional status is the foundation of nutrition care and the primary role of the nutrition professional on the research or health care team. Nutritional status assessment can detect a nutrient insufficiency or excess in the early stages, allowing dietary intake and lifestyle to be improved through nutrition intervention before a more significant deficiency or toxicity develops. In the management of acute and chronic diseases, nutritional status assessment provides an important opportunity for the nutrition professional to identify patients who

need medical nutrition therapy (MNT), which ultimately links clients to interventions that support improved health and well-being, and reduce medical care costs (Parkhurst et al, 2013).

As illustrated in Fig. 4.2, imbalances in nutritional status develop over time when intake is higher or lower than an individual can physiologically adapt to. In minor or early nutritional deficits such as stage 1 iron deficiency, the body adapts by increasing absorption of dietary iron to regain balance (see Chapter 31). If the iron deficiency is detected in the early stages through detailed assessment of a food and nutrition history and a ferritin test, the impact may be limited to depletion of stores. If the deficit is substantial or if the requirement for iron is substantially higher than normal, the body's ability to adapt can be exceeded, and a deficiency will ensue. Over time, the imbalance will lead to changes in the biochemistry, anatomy, and physiology of the body, such as overt anemia and chronic fatigue.

While it is theoretically possible to obtain a reasonable estimate of an individual's intake of calories, micronutrients, and macronutrients, nutrition professionals are unlikely to be able to estimate an individual's actual nutrient requirements under most conditions. Thus to accurately assess nutritional status (i.e., a deficiency or excess), the assessment of nutrient intake is combined with additional data in order to support a conclusion that a client's estimated intake is too high or too low to support optimal health (see Fig. 4.2). In a "prototypical" nutritional deficiency, the five domains of assessment data in the nutrition care process (NCP) shown in Box 4.1 can provide the supportive data needed to establish and reveal the severity of a nutritional imbalance. Box 4.2 shows examples of problem, etiology, signs and symptoms (PES) statements created during the NCP that demonstrate how different assessment domain data can be used to describe different types of nutritional status concerns.

NUTRITION SCREENING

Only a portion of individuals or groups ("clients") that present in health care, community, or research settings requires the attention and

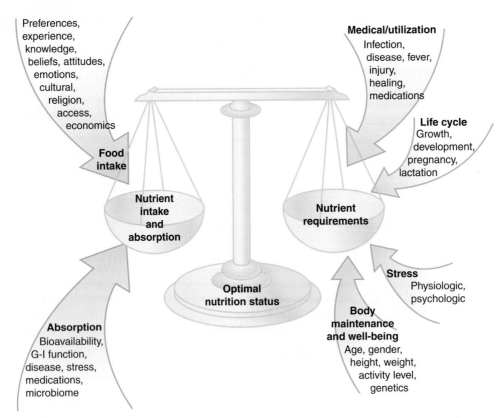

Fig. 4.1 Optimal nutrition status: a balance between nutrient intake and nutrient requirements.

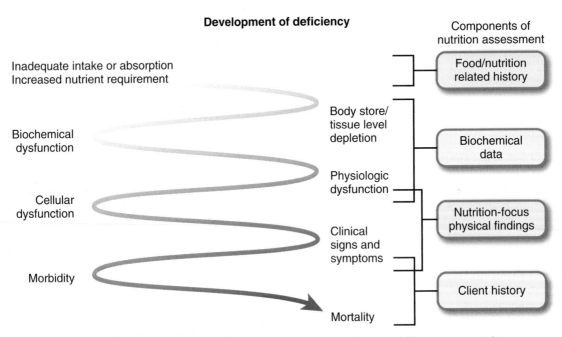

Fig. 4.2 Development of clinical nutritional deficiency and detection by nutrition assessment data.

BOX 4.2   Example Nutrition Diagnosis (PES) Statements for Nutritional Status Problems

Concept: Nutrient Deficiencies Can Be Due to Low Dietary Intake

Inadequate mineral intake (Iron, NI-5.10.1.3) related to knowledge deficit regarding foods high in iron as evidenced by consumption of 30% of the RDA for iron and low ferritin, Hct, and MCHC values.

Concept: Nutrient Deficiencies Can Be Due to Poor Absorption of Nutrients

Altered gastrointestinal (GI) function (NC-1.4) related to *Helicobacter pylori* infection-induced gastritis as evidenced by refractory iron deficiency anemia despite 6 weeks of oral iron therapy.

Concept: Nutrient Deficiencies Can Be Due to High Nutrient Requirements

Increased nutrient needs (Iron, NI-5.1) related to heavy menstrual blood losses as evidenced by iron deficiency anemia (low ferritin, Hct, and MCHC values) despite adequate intake of highly bioavailable heme iron (120% RDA).

services of nutrition professionals. To provide cost-effective nutrition services, the first step is to complete a nutrition screening test or examination to identify clients who currently have or are at risk for nutrition problems. During screening, clients who are determined to be at risk enter into the NCP (Fig. 4.3), and then receive services and care from nutrition professionals. More specifically, clients are screened into the NCP when they have an identifiable nutrition problem (diagnosis) that can be addressed or ameliorated with nutrition intervention(s) delivered by a nutrition professional (AND, 2018a). Thus screening is technically considered to be outside of the NCP.

An ethical aspect of screening is that it connects clients who need specialized care with the services of a nutrition professional, allowing that patient to receive the medical care that is needed to regain health and wellness. A legal aspect of screening is that it legally transfers a portion of the care to the nutrition professional. Medical care facilities identify the timeframe in which every client should be screened and, if needed, the timeframe in which the client should be assessed by an RDN.

Box 4.3 shows the characteristics of optimal screening tools. When available, health care practitioners should utilize population-specific, validated screening tools such as the Nutritional Risk Screening (NRS 2002), the Simple Two-Part Tool, the Malnutrition Screening Tool (MST), the Mini Nutritional Assessment (MNA), and the Malnutrition Universal Screening Tool (MUST). The most recent Evidence Analysis Library (EAL) review from the Academy of Nutrition and Dietetics regarding the performance of screening tools for adults hospitalized in acute care and ambulatory settings suggests that the screening tools listed above have high sensitivity (>90%) and specificity (>90%); but only the MST had both the validity and reliability data to earn a Grade I (good evidence) rating (AND, 2018b). An example screening form developed for subacute and ambulatory elderly populations, the MNA Short Form is shown in Fig. 4.4.

For many settings and patient populations, there are no published screening tools or, if tools do exist, the research supporting their validity and reliability is lacking. In these situations, RDNs often develop a custom-made screening tool for each location (e.g., hospital unit, clinic) or patient population under their care. Examples of potential screening data that could be incorporated into a custom-made screening tool for either pediatric or adult patient groups are shown in Box 4.4.

NUTRITION ASSESSMENT

As shown in Fig. 4.3, clients who are identified as at risk for nutritional problems during the nutritional screening stage formally enter step one of the NCP, nutrition assessment. Nutrition assessment is a "systematic method for obtaining, verifying, and interpreting data needed to identify nutrition-related problems, their causes, and significance" (AND, 2018a). The purpose of completing a nutrition assessment is to determine whether a client has one or more nutrition-related problems (diagnoses). In the NCP, the nutrition diagnoses are documented in step two of the NCP in PES statement format (see Box 4.2 and Chapter 9). After identification of the nutrition diagnoses, the RDN can intervene (NCP step three) to address the nutrition problem and then evaluate and monitor progress (NCP step four) to determine whether the interventions have been effective in achieving key outcomes for the client (see Chapter 9).

Nutrition assessment is a comprehensive evaluation that often includes data from the five NCP domains and a variety of sources (see Box 4.1). On an initial assessment (first visit), the nutrition professional collects data within these five domains in an "ongoing, dynamic process" to determine whether the patterns of the data match the defining characteristics of particular nutrition diagnoses (AND, 2018a). On subsequent visits, the nutrition professional may limit assessment data to nutrition care indicators, which are specific assessment data points that quantify changes associated with the interventions, the nutrition diagnosis, the cause and etiology of the diagnosis, and other health care outcomes defined by evidence-based medicine or regulatory

THE NUTRITION CARE PROCESS MODEL

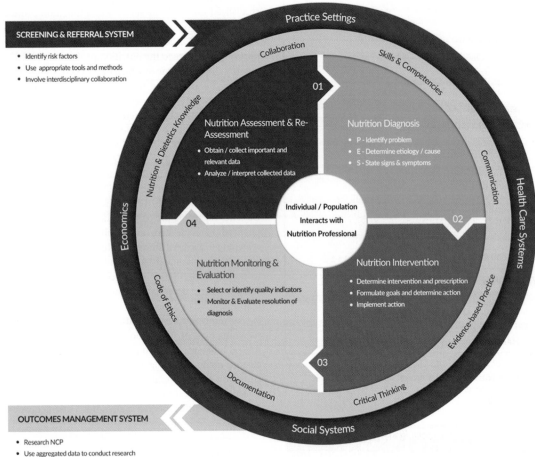

Fig. 4.3 The nutrition care process. (Copyright 2018 Academy of Nutrition and Dietetics. Reprinted with permission.)

BOX 4.3   Characteristics of an Ideal Nutrition Screening Tool

Simple, quick, and easy to use by a variety of health care providers
Utilizes data that are readily available (medical chart, patient report, survey data)
Cost-effective to administer
Reliability:
- Interrater: produces the same screening result when administered by different users
- Intrarater: produces the same screening result when administered by the same user on different occasions

Validity:
- Sensitivity: percentage of clients with nutrition diagnoses identified as "at risk"
- Specificity: percentage of clients without nutrition diagnoses identified as not at risk

Adapted from NSCR: Definitions and Criteria (2009). Academy of Nutrition and Dietetics (AND). https://www.andeal.org/topic.cfm?menu=3584&cat=3958.

---

bodies. Or, the nutrition professional may assess a broader spectrum of data to determine whether other nutrition diagnoses may apply to the client. Critical thinking is important in the process of gathering existing data, using valid and reliable methods to generate new data, interpreting discrepancies in the data, and finding patterns in the data that are consistent with nutritional diagnoses. Any novel data generated by the nutrition professional should be collected, interpreted, and entered into the medical record with integrity, expertise, and validity (AND, 2018a).

NUTRITION-RELATED HISTORY

Part 1 of this text, including Chapters 1 through 10, focuses on the knowledge and skills needed to complete a comprehensive nutrition assessment involving the five domains of assessment data. This chapter will focus on assessment of the domain Food- and Nutrition-Related History, a broad and varied category of data that includes the subdomains and data scope shown in Table 4.1 (AND, 2018a). In brief, Food- and Nutrition-Related History includes assessments of the type

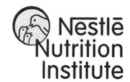
Nestlé Nutrition Institute

Mini Nutritional Assessment
MNA®

Last name:		First name:		
Sex:	Age:	Weight, kg:	Height, cm:	Date:

Complete the screen by filling in the boxes with the appropriate numbers. Total the numbers for the final screening score.

Screening

A Has food intake declined over the past 3 months due to loss of appetite, digestive problems, chewing or swallowing difficulties?
0 = severe decrease in food intake
1 = moderate decrease in food intake
2 = no decrease in food intake ☐

B Weight loss during the last 3 months
0 = weight loss greater than 3 kg (6.6 lbs)
1 = does not know
2 = weight loss between 1 and 3 kg (2.2 and 6.6 lbs)
3 = no weight loss ☐

C Mobility
0 = bed or chair bound
1 = able to get out of bed / chair but does not go out
2 = goes out ☐

D Has suffered psychological stress or acute disease in the past 3 months?
0 = yes   2 = no ☐

E Neuropsychological problems
0 = severe dementia or depression
1 = mild dementia
2 = no psychological problems ☐

F1 Body Mass Index (BMI) (weight in kg) / (height in m²)
0 = BMI less than 19
1 = BMI 19 to less than 21
2 = BMI 21 to less than 23
3 = BMI 23 or greater ☐

IF BMI IS NOT AVAILABLE, REPLACE QUESTION F1 WITH QUESTION F2.
DO NOT ANSWER QUESTION F2 IF QUESTION F1 IS ALREADY COMPLETED.

F2 Calf circumference (CC) in cm
0 = CC less than 31
3 = CC 31 or greater ☐

Screening score ☐☐
(max. 14 points)

12-14 points: Normal nutritional status
8-11 points: At risk of malnutrition
0-7 points: Malnourished

For a more in-depth assessment, complete the full MNA® which is available at **www.mna-elderly.com**

Ref.   Vellas B, Villars H, Abellan G, et al. *Overview of the MNA® - Its History and Challenges*. J Nutr Health Aging 2006;10:456-465.
Rubenstein LZ, Harker JO, Salva A, Guigoz Y, Vellas B. *Screening for Undernutrition in Geriatric Practice: Developing the Short-Form Mini Nutritional Assessment (MNA-SF)*. J. Geront 2001;56A: M366-377.
Guigoz Y. *The Mini-Nutritional Assessment (MNA®) Review of the Literature - What does it tell us?* J Nutr Health Aging 2006; 10:466-487.
® Société des Produits Nestlé, S.A., Vevey, Switzerland, Trademark Owners
© Nestlé, 1994, Revision 2009. N67200 12/99 10M
For more information: www.mna-elderly.com

Fig. 4.4 Mini Nutritional Assessment short form. (Permission by Nestlé Healthcare Nutrition.)

BOX 4.4 Nutritional Risk Factors

Food- and Nutrition-Related History

- Calorie, food group, breastmilk, formula, enteral, or parenteral intake below estimated needs
- Macro- or micronutrient intake below estimated needs
- Diet quality or variety below standards
- Excessive alcohol or drug use
- Poor eating environment
- Medications: polypharmacy, food-drug interactions
- Supplements: excessive intake, food-supplement interactions
- Food beliefs, attitudes, behaviors, knowledge: pica, disordered eating, restrictive eating, picky eating, inability or unwillingness to consume food, knowledge deficit
- Access: limited availability of safe and nutritious foods/beverages, limited access to food preparation facilities or supplies, limited access to resources and programs
- Cognitive or physical impairment that affects eating and food preparation
- Excessive or inadequate physical activity

Anthropometric Measurements

- Weight status: significant weight loss or gain, low or high BMI, inadequate or excessive growth measures
- Body composition: fat or muscle wasting, high waist circumference or waist-to-hip ratio

Biochemical Data, Medical Tests and Procedures

- Abnormal laboratory values: anemia, lipid profile, liver profile, GI profile, kidney function, circulating proteins
- Medical tests: GI function, swallow study, biopsies, ultrasound, endoscopy results

Nutrition-Focus Physical Findings

- Global: muscle or fat wasting, underweight, overweight, edema
- Digestive: poor appetite, nausea, vomiting, diarrhea, constipation, poor dentition, denture problems
- Skin: pressure ulcers, poor wound healing, signs of deficiency/excess
- Other: visual impairment, immobility, cognitive or neurologic impairment

Client History

- Personal: high-risk age (infancy, elderly), literacy, education, tobacco use
- Medical: diagnosis of chronic disease (renal, liver, cardiac, diabetes, gastrointestinal, cancer, AIDS), acute injury (trauma, sepsis, burn), or life cycle stage with high requirements (infancy, childhood, adolescence, pregnancy, lactation)
- Social: socioeconomic limitations, unstable housing, lack of social support, crisis, high stress levels

TABLE 4.1 Nutrition Care Process: Food- and Nutrition-Related History Data

Subdomain	Scope
Food and Nutrient Intake	Total amount, timing, and patterns of intake of foods, beverages, nutrients, and food components
Food and Nutrient Administration	Overall dietary practices, food restrictions, fasting, or food modifications; eating environment; route of administration (oral, enteral, parenteral)
Medication and Complementary/ Alternative Medicine Use	Current and historical use of prescription drugs, over-the-counter drugs, herbs, and other complementary/alternative medicine products
Knowledge/Beliefs/ Attitudes	Knowledge, skills, beliefs, emotions, and attitudes related to food, nutrition, dietary practices, or behavior change
Behavior	Behaviors that impact ability to achieve nutrition-related goals
Factors Affecting Access to Food and Food/Nutrition-Related Supplies	Factors that limit or assist client in obtaining adequate amounts of safe and healthful foods, beverages, and nutrients
Physical Activity and Function	Physical activity level and indicators of physical functioning of the body related to nutritional status
Nutrition-Related Patient/Client-Centered Measures	Client's perception of the nutrition intervention and its impact on quality of life

Adapted from Academy of Nutrition and Dietetics. Nutrition Terminology Reference Manual (eNCPT): Dietetics Language for Nutrition Care. https://www.ncpro.org/pubs/idnt-en/?.

of diet currently and historically consumed by the client, how the diet is consumed, client characteristics that affect dietary needs, and important factors that determine underlying dietary choices and potential responses to future dietary changes.

FOOD AND NUTRIENT INTAKE

The Food and Nutrient Intake subdomain of Food- and Nutrition-Related History includes both assessment of the quantity and quality of foods and beverages in the diet as well as the timing and patterns of food and beverage intake (see Table 4.1). Dietary intake data may be assessed either by asking clients what they have consumed in the past (retrospective intake data) or by having clients record what they are consuming in real time (prospective intake data). Once information

is gathered about the client's diet, the nutrition professional can evaluate whether calorie, macronutrient, micronutrient, and other components of the diet are within health-promoting ranges and patterns.

A food record, or food diary, is the most comprehensive dietary intake tool available for assessing the quantity, quality, and timing of foods and beverages consumed by a client. After the provision of detailed instructions in its use by the nutrition professional, the client (or a trusted support person) prospectively records the foods and beverages consumed over a period of several days or weeks. A food diary form is shown in Fig. 4.5. Analysis of the food diary (discussed below) can provide detailed information on the quantity and quality of foods, beverages, nutrients, and food components consumed, timing and patterns of intake, and bioavailability of nutrients based on food sources (Table 4.2). In addition, the food diary form can be customized to include information that is most needed for client and clinician feedback, such as hunger and fullness scales, emotional responses to eating, location of eating, or physical symptoms (e.g., nausea or diarrhea) that occur after eating. Given that the forms are time consuming to fill out and that they must be filled out during (not after) each eating occasion for optimal validity, the nutrition professional can reduce the client burden by requiring the minimum number of days of records and the minimum data points or details needed to monitor key nutritional outcomes. Studies show that to characterize typical intake patterns, the optimal balance of client burden and data accuracy is obtained with 3 to 4 complete days of data collection with

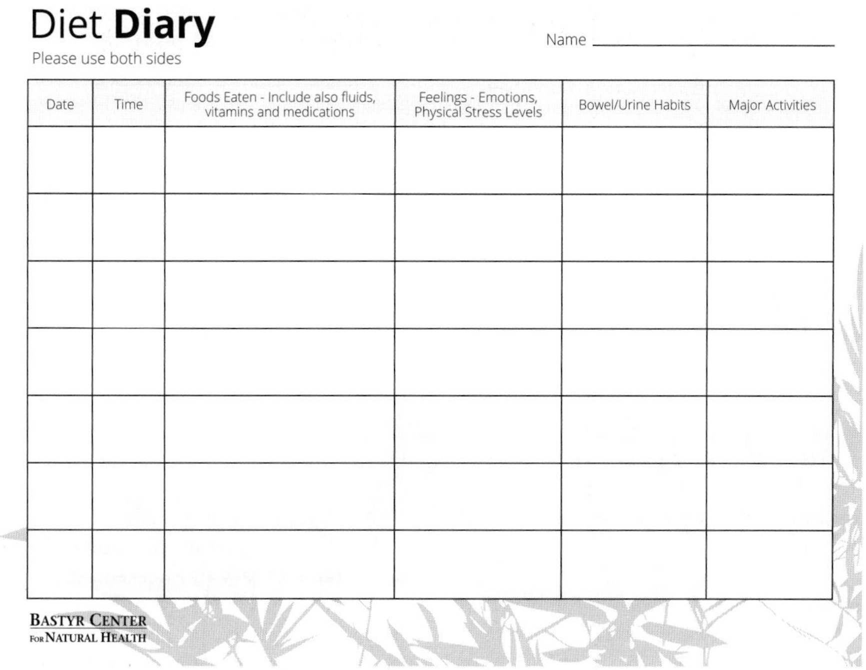

Diet **Diary**

Please use both sides

Name _____

Date	Time	Foods Eaten - Include also fluids, vitamins and medications	Feelings - Emotions, Physical Stress Levels	Bowel/Urine Habits	Major Activities

BASTYR CENTER
FOR NATURAL HEALTH

Fig. 4.5 Food diary. (Permission by Bastyr University.)

TABLE 4.2 **Comparison of Food and Nutrient Intake Assessment Methods**

Method	Advantages	Disadvantages	Best Uses
Food Record (Food Diary)	• Quantitative and qualitative data on foods and beverages consumed • Can provide data on food preparation methods, timing, setting, source, etc. • If items weighed/measured, can provide more accurate portion size data • Real-time recording/less reliance on memory • Modest time and effort for nutrition professional to review	• Client training needed for accuracy • Multiple days needed to characterize diet variety • High client burden • May not capture episodically consumed items • Potential for reactivity (clients change eating patterns in response to recording) • Time consuming for nutrition professional to analyze with software	• Short-term view of the current diet • Motivated and literate client • Analysis of calories, macronutrients, micronutrients, and components of the diet • Analysis of food preparation methods, food quality, ingredients • Data linking food intake with other data (e.g., blood sugar, eating location, distractions, emotions, allergy symptoms)
Food Frequency Questionnaire	• Qualitative data on foods and beverages consumed • Data on diet variety • Less client burden than multiple food records • Low client reactivity • Client can complete in home in paper or online formats • Modest time and effort for nutrition professional to review	• Limited quantitative data possible • Limited data on food preparation methods; no data on settings or timing of intake • Incomplete—not all possible foods listed • Intensive cognitive and memory skills required • Time consuming or costly to analyze with software	• Long-term, holistic view of types of foods consumed in past • Many tools available to assess total diet or certain food groups/types • Motivated and literate client
24-Hour Recall	• Quantitative and qualitative data on foods and beverages consumed • Can provide data on food preparation methods, timing, setting, source, etc. • Quick (20 minutes) and easy to complete in office setting • Low time and effort for nutrition professional to review • Low client reactivity • Low client burden	• Multiple days needed to characterize diet variety • May not capture episodically consumed items • Requires nutrition professional skill and expertise • Time consuming for nutrition professional to analyze with software • Relies on client memory, honesty, skill in reporting food types and portions	• Short-term view of the current diet • Client with limited motivation, skills, or literacy • Analysis of calories, macronutrients, micronutrients, and components of the diet • Analysis of food preparation methods, food quality, ingredients

Continued

TABLE 4.2	Comparison of Food and Nutrient Intake Assessment Methods—cont'd		
Method	**Advantages**	**Disadvantages**	**Best Uses**
Calorie Count	• Actual observation of food intake • Quick (20 minutes) and easy to complete in office setting • Low time and effort for nutrition professional to review • Low client reactivity and burden	• May not represent typical intake patterns or food preferences • Time consuming for nutrition professional to analyze with software	• Short-term view of the current diet • Analysis calorie and macronutrient intake in relation to patient health status • Client with limited motivation, skills, or literacy

Adapted from Thompson FE, Byers T. Dietary Assessment Resource Manual. *J Nutr.* 1994 Nov;124(11 Suppl):2245S-2317S. doi: 10.1093/jn/124. suppl_11.2245s and Dietary Assessment Primer. National Institutes of Health, National Cancer Institute. https://dietassessmentprimer.cancer.gov.

at least 2 weekdays and 1 weekend day (Thompson and Byers, 1994; National Institutes of Health [NIH], 2018a). For some purposes, such as monitoring of food allergy or intolerance symptoms in response to food intake, clients may need to record data for several weeks (see Chapter 25 and Fig. 25.5).

A food frequency questionnaire (FFQ) is a survey completed by the client to retrospectively assess the types of foods and beverages consumed over a specified interval of time (e.g., past 1 month, 6 months, 12 months). In a traditional FFQ, clients indicate the frequency with which they consume various food items of interest—ranging from "never" to multiple times per day (Fig. 4.6). This method is ideal for providing information on typical foods consumed, quality of foods consumed, and diet variety over a prior period of time (see Table 4.2). Semiquantitative FFQs also include assessments of portion sizes or amounts consumed (Fig. 4.7), but questions remain about the validity of quantitative dietary intake data resulting from FFQs (Thompson and Byers, 1994; NIH, 2018a).

Nutrition professionals can select from a wide variety of validated FFQs that are broad or narrow in scope, or potentially adapt an existing FFQ to collect information on just the foods, beverages, or nutrients that are most relevant, important, and vital to the client's clinical situation. For optimal validity, the foods that are listed and the literacy and numeracy skills required to complete the tool should match the client or group that is being assessed.

In a 24-hour recall, the nutrition professional leads the client through a structured interview process to capture information on the quantity and quality of foods and beverages consumed in the previous 24 hours, including details on the timing, amounts, preparation methods, and brands (Thompson and Byers, 1994; NIH, 2018a). In a multiple pass-style of 24-hour recall, the nutrition professional first generates a basic outline of the foods and beverages consumed during the previous 24 hours divided into the meals and snacks the client has defined. On a second pass, the nutrition professional gathers details about foods and beverages consumed, including preparation method, brand name, portion size, key food attributes (whole grain, fortified, enriched, low sodium, etc.), and anchoring activities (while driving, at work, watching TV, etc.).

To improve validity, the nutrition professional can use prompts to help the client remember all foods consumed and ask questions in a neutral and unbiased way ("What was the first time you ate or drank anything after you woke up?" versus "What did you eat for breakfast?"). Carefully collected 24-hour recalls can yield dietary intake data similar to a food record but may miss data on diet variability unless multiple 24-hour recalls are taken over a period of time (see Table 4.2). Advances in technology now include software-directed structured interview formats and automated self-administered tools, such as the National Cancer Institute's Automated Self-Administered 24-Hour

Dietary Assessment Tool (ASA24) for both adults and children (NIH, 2018a; NIH, 2018b).

A calorie count is a method primarily used in inpatient settings such as hospitals and nursing homes (see Table 4.2). Over the course of several weekdays and weekend days, a health care practitioner reviews the client's food trays before and after each eating occasion and estimates the percentage of each food and beverage consumed. Using facility software, which includes information on the portion size and nutritional content of all foods and beverages served in the facility, and the percentage of each item consumed, the nutrition professional can estimate the food and nutrient intake of the client. Often the goal is to determine whether low food and beverage intakes are contributing to an emerging pattern of weight loss and malnutrition so early intervention can occur.

Each of the traditional retrospective and prospective methods currently used in clinical and research settings has specific purposes, strengths, and weaknesses (see Table 4.2). In all methods except the calorie count, intentional under- and overreporting of foods and beverages so the diet appears "healthier" is a concern (Thompson and Byers, 1994; NIH, 2018a). Through setting a comfortable environment with patients, asking neutral questions, and refraining from comments that may be perceived by the client as "judgmental," the nutrition professional may reduce the likelihood of clients consciously or unconsciously altering their intake or misreporting intake data to impress the nutrition professional. The ultimate goal is to select a method that leads to accurate diagnosis of nutrition problems or monitoring of key nutrition care criteria related to interventions.

As these traditional dietary assessment methods are often time and labor-intensive and subject to a variety of sources of error, there has been increasing interest in the use of technology to provide information about dietary intake. New methods include photographic or video imaging of both the preparation and consumption of foods and beverages. In active capture methods an individual takes images of food before and after eating and can supplement the photos with text or voice recordings. In passive capture methods, images or recordings are made continuously throughout the day. Both types of technologies can be used to capture a primary record of the foods and beverages consumed or to enhance other dietary assessment methods such as 24-hour recall or food record.

A review of published studies suggests that photographic or video methods for dietary assessment are effective as a supplement to other self-report measures by revealing unreported and misreported food items (Gemming et al, 2015). When used as the sole method for dietary assessment, if images are of a sufficient quality, reasonable estimates of nutrient intake are possible. These methods often utilize nutrition professionals to evaluate the images of food consumed, but several utilize software to automate this step of the analysis. In addition to

BASTYR CENTER   *the teaching clinic*

FOR NATURAL HEALTH   *of Bastyr University*

Patient name _____ Date of Birth _____/_____/_____

Please check all of the following statements, being careful to use the appropriate box related to the frequency of your personal habits.

Daily	3-5 per week	1-2 per week	1-2 per month	Less than monthly	Never	
						Cook meals at home
						Eat with others
						Eat at restaurants
						Eat at fast food restaurants
						Pastries, cookies, candies, ice cream, other sweets
						Add sugar to coffee, tea, cereals or other foods
						White bread or white flour products
						Colas or other soft drinks
						Artificial sweeteners (saccharin, Nutrasweet, Splenda...)
						Canned foods
						Cold breakfast cereals; list brands :
						Caffeine drinks (coffee, tea, cola, chocolate)
						Deep fried foods (chips, chicken nuggets, fish fillets, French fries)
						Margarine of any type
						Red meat (beef, pork, lamb)
						Processed meat (bologna, bacon, sausages, salami, etc.)
						Chicken or turkey
						Fish
						Shellfish
						Milk: Type (circle) Cow Goat Soy Nut Coconut Rice Flax Other: Fat level (circle) Whole/full fat 2% 1% Non-fat
						Yogurt: Type (circle) Cow Goat Soy Coconut Greek Plain Flavored Fat level (circle) Whole/full fat 2% 1% Non-fat
						Cheese
						Eggs
						Nuts and seeds (almonds, walnuts, cashews...)
						Whole grain hot cereals (oatmeal, Wheatena, etc.)
						Fruit: Type (circle) Fresh Raw Cooked Canned Frozen
						Vegetables: Type (circle) Fresh Raw Cooked Canned Frozen
						Green Leafy: Type (circle) Fresh Raw Cooked Canned Frozen
						100% whole grains or whole grain breads
						Beans and legumes (lentil, kidney, chickpea, etc.)
						Herbs, fresh and dried, or spices
						Water: Type (circle) Tap Filtered Bottled Amount consumed per day: _____ cups/ounces (circle unit)
						Alcohol
						Organic foods

Last Revised October 2016

Fig. 4.6 Simplified food frequency questionnaire. (Permission by Bastyr Center for Natural Health.)

estimating dietary intake, photography and videography can be used to evaluate other aspects of a nutrition assessment including the eating environment, mealtime interactions between caregivers and children, the ability to use eating utensils, feeding difficulties, and methods of food preparation.

Some of these technological advances have trickled down to clients in the form of cellular phone applications (apps), creating an opportunity to collect and analyze food intake and physical activity information for both client and clinician use (Moore, 2018). Originally created for the public to use in self-monitoring health behaviors, several apps also provide options to share tracking data with nutrition professionals and generate useful reports of food and nutrient intake as well as physical activity behaviors (Box 4.5). These apps share many of the same benefits and drawbacks as typical food and physical activity diaries.

Beverage Questionnaire (BEVQ-15)

Instructions:
In the past month, please indicate your response for each beverage type by marking an "X" in the bubble for "how often" and "how much each time".

1. Indicate how often you drank the following beverages, for example, if you drank 5 glasses of water per week, mark 4-6 times per week.

2. Indicate the approximate amount of beverage you drank each time, for example, if you drank 1 cup of water each time, mark 1 cup under "how much each time".

3. Do not count beverages used in cooking or other preparations, such as milk in cereal.

4. Count milk added to tea and coffee in the *tea/coffee with cream beverage category* **NOT** in the milk categories.

Participant ID _____

Date _____

Type of Beverage	Never or less than 1 time per week (go to next beverage)	1 time per week	2-3 times per week	4-6 times per week	1 time per day	2+ times per day	3+ times per day	Less than 6 fl oz (3/4 cup)	8 fl oz (1 cup)	12 fl oz (1 1/2 cups)	16 fl oz (2 cups)	More than 20 fl oz (2 1/2 cups)
	HOW OFTEN (MARK ONE)							**HOW MUCH EACH TIME (MARK ONE)**				
Water	o	o	o	o	o	o	o	o	o	o	o	o
100% Fruit Juice	o	o	o	o	o	o	o	o	o	o	o	o
Sweetened Juice Beverage/Drink (fruit ades, lemonade, punch, Sunny Delight)	o	o	o	o	o	o	o	o	o	o	o	o
Whole Milk	o	o	o	o	o	o	o	o	o	o	o	o
Reduced Fat Milk (2%)	o	o	o	o	o	o	o	o	o	o	o	o
Low Fat/Fat Free Milk (Skim, 1%, Buttermilk, Soymilk)	o	o	o	o	o	o	o	o	o	o	o	o
Soft Drinks, Regular	o	o	o	o	o	o	o	o	o	o	o	o
Diet Soft Drinks/Artificially Sweetened Drinks (Crystal Light)	o	o	o	o	o	o	o	o	o	o	o	o
Sweetened Tea	o	o	o	o	o	o	o	o	o	o	o	o
Tea or Coffee, with cream and/or sugar (includes non-dairy creamer)	o	o	o	o	o	o	o	o	o	o	o	o
Tea or Coffee, black, with/without artificial sweetener (no cream or sugar)	o	o	o	o	o	o	o	o	o	o	o	o
Beer, Ales, Wine Coolers, Non-alcoholic or Light Beer	o	o	o	o	o	o	o	o	o	o	o	o
Hard Liquor (shots, rum, tequila, etc.)	o	o	o	o	o	o	o	o	o	o	o	o
Wine (red or white)	o	o	o	o	o	o	o	o	o	o	o	o
Energy & Sports Drinks (Red Bull, Rockstar, Gatorade, Powerade, etc.)	o	o	o	o	o	o	o	o	o	o	o	o
Other (list):	o	o	o	o	o	o	o	o	o	o	o	o

Virginia Polytechnic Institute and State University, 2010.

Fig. 4.7 BEVQ-15 beverage frequency questionnaire. (Copyright 2012 Academy of Nutrition and Dietetics. Reprinted with permission.) Reference: Hedrick VE, Savla J, Comber DL, et al. Development of a Brief Questionnaire to Assess Habitual Beverage Intake (BEVQ-15): Sugar-Sweetened Beverages and Total Beverage Energy Intake. *J Acad Nutr Diet.* 2012 Jun;112(6):840-9. doi: 10.1016/j.jand.2012.01.023.

BOX 4.5 Apps for Tracking Nutritional Intake and Physical Activity

YouFood Photo Food Journal	Clients can photograph food and beverages consumed, journal about and rate intake, and obtain advice and ideas from community members
	Best for: people who desire nondieting approach, easy ways to monitor intake, and peer support
Recovery Record	Clients record meals and behaviors for eating disorder treatment, clinicians can review results and send feedback
	Best for: people who want to use technology to record data and interact with health care team
Calio	Voice technology allows people to speak data input for food, nutrition, and activity tracker and make requests for analysis of data and advice
	Best for: individuals who desire voice-interface
MyFitnessPal	Food and nutrition tracker with large food database and ability to scan bar codes of processed food items to speed up data entry
	Best for: individuals who desire calorie and weight-loss approach
Calorie Mama & Bitesnap	Provides dietary analysis based only on photos of foods and beverages
	Best for: rough estimates of intake, photo journaling intake
eaTracker	Food and Physical Activity tracker from Dietitians of Canada
	Best for: Canadian foods, research-based foods database
MakeMe	Track and share health goals and data within a team of individuals
	Best for: health challenges at work, fitness centers, and group classes

However, as the app completes the analysis for the clinician, these tools can potentially save clinicians time. The clinician should investigate the app fully before its use to ensure that the data for nutrition and physical activity are accurate and to understand the limits on the app's reliability and validity (Moore, 2018).

Assessment and Interpretation of Energy Intake

A starting point for nearly all dietary analysis work is to assess and evaluate the energy balance of the diet. Adequate calories are needed to sustain the body's structure and function as well as to support health and well-being (physical activity, healing). In addition, the needs for many nutrients (e.g., macronutrients) and food group allowances are established based on calorie intake or needs. Assessment and evaluation of calorie balance requires a thorough and complete dietary assessment tool that captures both the quantity and quality of foods and beverages consumed. Typically, this includes either a multiday food record or multiple 24-hour recalls. Information on foods consumed can then be entered into dietary analysis programs to obtain an estimate of caloric intake (Moore, 2018; Fig. 4.8). The caloric intake value can then be compared with measurements of energy expenditure such as by direct calorimetry, or to estimates of energy requirements from indirect calorimetry or equations based on client characteristics such as age, height, weight, activity level, and injuries (see Chapter 2).

Assessment and Interpretation of Food Group Quantity and Balance

As foods and beverages typically provide the foundation of the diet, analysis of the balance of the foods consumed in the diet is an important role of the nutrition professional. In facilities that have access to software to analyze food records or 24-hour recalls, the software often can provide analysis of the food balance of the diet (Fig. 4.9). In facilities and settings that lack the software, the nutrition professional can develop the skill and experience to quickly translate foods and beverages consumed into standard food group portions or equivalents, adding little time to a 24-hour recall or review of food records, making this an efficient and effective start to nutrition assessment. In settings where clinicians are provided very limited time for dietary analysis, quick estimates of food group quantity and balance may be the only realistic dietary assessment method available.

Quantitative food patterns can also be used as standards by which to evaluate the balance of foods and beverages consumed. Quantitative food patterns show the average amount of food from each food group that should be consumed to meet both calorie and nutrient targets at a variety of calorie levels. Examples of quantitative food patterns that can be used as standards for food group quantity and balance analysis include:

- USDA Food Pattern
- USDA Vegetarian Food Pattern
- USDA Mediterranean Food Pattern
- DASH Diet Pattern
- Diabetes Exchange Meal Pattern

Multi Column: Jane Doe| All Days

Multi-Column

Nutrients	Value	Rcmd	% Rcmd	Nutrients	Value	Rcmd	% Rcmd
Basic Components				Biotin (mcg)	18.09	30.00	60.32%
Gram Weight (g)	4200.55			Vitamin C (mg)	83.51	75.00	111.35%
Calories (kcal)	2078.88	2141.80	97.06%	Vitamin D - IU (IU)	305.80		
Calories from Fat (kcal)	787.22	599.70	131.27%	Vitamin D - mcg (mcg)	7.61	15.00	50.73%
Calories from SatFat (kcal)	239.28	192.76	124.13%	Vitamin E - Alpha-Toco (mg)	4.13	15.00	27.55%
Protein (g)	71.10	47.17	150.72%	Folate (mcg)	183.23	400.00	45.81%
Carbohydrates (g)	277.47	294.50	94.22%	Folate, DFE (mcg)	144.82	400.00	36.21%
Dietary Fiber (g)	25.76	29.99	85.90%	Vitamin K (mcg)	33.27	90.00	36.96%
Soluble Fiber (g)	2.00			Pantothenic Acid (mg)	5.34	5.00	106.85%
Total Sugars (g)	126.51			**Minerals**			
Monosaccharides (g)	22.63			Calcium (mg)	1644.89	1000.00	164.49%
Disaccharides (g)	57.20			Chromium (mcg)	2.93	25.00	11.71%
Other Carbs (g)	125.21			Copper (mg)	0.89	0.90	99.39%
Fat (g)	87.71	66.63	131.63%	Fluoride (mg)	2.15	3.00	71.66%
Saturated Fat (g)	26.59	21.42	124.13%	Iodine (mcg)	114.70	150.00	76.47%
Mono Fat (g)	24.84	23.80	104.39%	Iron (mg)	9.03	18.00	50.18%
Poly Fat (g)	5.57	21.42	26.01%	Magnesium (mg)	265.88	310.00	85.77%
Trans Fatty Acid (g)	0.51			Manganese (mg)	2.16	1.80	119.87%
Cholesterol (mg)	113.05	300.00	37.68%	Molybdenum (mcg)	12.96	45.00	28.80%
Water (g)	3569.45	2700.00	132.20%	Phosphorus (mg)	1238.33	700.00	176.90%
Vitamins				Potassium (mg)	2763.48	4700.00	58.80%
Vitamin A - IU (IU)	24217.06			Selenium (mcg)	45.41	55.00	82.56%
Vitamin A - RAE (RAE)	1464.24	700.00	209.18%	Sodium (mg)	2050.67	2300.00	89.16%
Carotenoid RE (RE)	2232.18			Zinc (mg)	6.45	8.00	80.63%
Retinol RE (RE)	348.15			**Poly Fats**			
Beta-Carotene (mcg)	11625.08			Omega 3 Fatty Acid (g)	0.49	2.14	22.90%
Vitamin B1 (mg)	0.91	1.10	82.94%	Omega 6 Fatty Acid (g)	4.89	19.04	25.66%
Vitamin B2 (mg)	2.30	1.10	209.37%	**Other Nutrients**			
Vitamin B3 (mg)	8.85	14.00	63.19%	Alcohol (g)	0		
Vitamin B3 - Niacin Equiv (mg)	18.33	14.00	130.90%	Caffeine (mg)	145.83		
Vitamin B6 (mg)	0.92	1.30	71.04%	Choline (mg)	173.72	425.00	40.87%
Vitamin B12 (mcg)	2.87	2.40	119.75%				

Fig. 4.8 Nutrient analysis report. (Nutritional analysis from The Food Processor® Nutrition and Fitness Software by ESHA Research, Inc., version 11.0.124, ©2015.)

Strict observance of the defined methods is very important—foods and beverages must be correctly classified into groups, quality standards for food should be met (e.g., caloric and nutrient density), and portion sizes must be correctly converted to obtain accurate food group quantity and balance information in relation to a standard.

Assessment and Interpretation of Food Quality

Research continues to highlight the importance of food and dietary quality in the prevention of chronic disease, which has led to an increased interest in measurement of dietary quality in both research and clinical settings (Gil et al, 2015). After collection of dietary intake data from food diaries, multiple 24-hour recalls, or an FFQ, a clinician can utilize dietary assessment software or other computer analysis programs to evaluate dietary quality using tools such as the Health Eating Index (HEI), the Diet Quality Index (DQI), the Healthy Diet

Indicator (HDI), or the Mediterranean Diet Score (MDS) (Gil et al, 2015). These diet quality methods often not only assess whether a diet achieves sufficient intake of food groups such as fruit, vegetables, beans or pulses, whole grains, and dairy foods but also whether the diet is consistent with nutrient and component standards such as sodium, added sugars, alcohol, and saturated fat. As most clinicians will not have the time or resources to analyze dietary intake data using these methods, an alternative approach is to review food diaries and 24-hour recalls with specific food quality standards in mind, such as the 2015–2020 Dietary Guidelines for Americans.

Assessment and Interpretation of Beverages (Water, Alcohol, and Caffeine)

Assessment of beverage intake can include examination of typical intake patterns of water, milk, fruit juice, fruit drinks, soft drinks, sports

MyPlate: Jane Doe | All Days

MyPlate

Jane Doe | All Days
Female   Age: 28 Yrs.   Height: 5 ft. 6 in.   Weight: 130.00 lb.   Lightly Active   BMI: 20.98

My Plate - Intake vs Recommendation
2200 Calories Pattern

Group	Percent of Rec.	Comparison	Amount (Daily)
Grain Total Intake	101 %		7.09 oz equivalent
Grain Total Recommended			7 oz equivalent
Vegetable Total Intake	26 %		0.78 cup equivalent
Vegetable Total Recommended			3 cup equivalent
Fruit Intake	118 %		2.36 cup equivalent
Fruit Recommended			2 cup equivalent
Dairy Intake	101 %		3.03 cup equivalent
Dairy Recommended			3 cup equivalent
Protein Total Intake	50 %		2.97 oz equivalent
Protein Total Recommended			6 oz equivalent

Make at least half your grains whole grains.

Vary the vegetables that you eat:
   Dark Green Vegetables = 3.00 cups weekly
   Red & Orange Vegetables = 2.00 cups weekly
   Beans and Peas = 3.00 cups weekly
   Starchy Vegetables = 6.00 cups weekly
   Other Vegetables = 7.00 cups weekly

Fig. 4.9 Food analysis report. (Nutritional analysis from The Food Processor® Nutrition and Fitness Software by ESHA Research, Inc., version 11.0.124, ©2015.)

or energy drinks, coffee, tea, and alcoholic beverages. Information from beverage intake, either with or without additional food data, can be used to estimate intake of water, alcohol, and caffeine. In addition, because beverages contain food components with health implications (e.g., calories, water, sugar, alcohol, caffeine, calcium, vitamin D, potassium,) the type and amount of beverages that a person consumes can have health implications for conditions such as obesity and weight gain, bone health, kidney disease, and cardiovascular disease. In a recent nationally representative sample of adults, researchers found that:

- Beverages constitute about 75% to 85% of total daily water intake
- Water (tap and bottled) is the main contributor (30% to 37%) to total dietary water intake
- Beverages contribute 14% to 22% of total energy intake
- Alcohol, soda, and soft drinks are substantial contributors (2% to 6%) to total energy intake, but have little nutritional value (Drewnowski et al, 2013).

If the nutrition professional needs information about total intake of water, alcohol, and caffeine from both foods and beverages, multiple days of food diaries or 24-hour recalls analyzed with commercial dietary assessment software is necessary (see Fig. 4.8). If the nutrition professional simply wants to assess the quantity or quality of beverages in the diet, a simplified FFQ such as the Beverage Intake Questionnaire (BEVQ-15) may be sufficient (Hedrick et al, 2018; see Fig. 4.7). Total water intake can be compared with a variety of methods of estimating water needs to evaluate adequacy (see Chapter 3 and Appendix 14). Caffeine and alcohol intake can be compared with suggested limits in the US Dietary Guidelines or other medical condition-specific guidelines (see Chapter 10).

Assessment and Interpretation of Macronutrients

The fat, protein, carbohydrate, fiber, and water content of the diet can be assessed by analyzing multiple days of food records or 24-hour recalls with commercially available dietary assessment software (see Fig. 4.8). This software also may provide information about specific types of macronutrients such as sugar, soluble fiber, saturated fats, and trans fatty acids. Alternatively, the skilled nutrition professional can assess the calorie containing macronutrients (fat, protein, carbohydrate) in the diet using the diabetic exchange system (Appendix 18).

The DRIs can serve as standards for evaluating the intake of macronutrients in most healthy individuals across the life cycle (see inside cover). **Acceptable intake (AI)** values are set when the research basis for a particular nutrient is limited. The AI represents the daily average intake of a nutrient that appears to be consistent with overall health and nutrient balance in observational studies. AI values for total fiber, linoleic acid, linolenic acid, and water exist and, given the limited research base, they should be used with caution. **Recommended dietary allowance (RDA)** values are set for nutrients with a research base substantial enough to characterize the distribution of nutrient needs of a population subgroup. The RDA represents the daily average intake of a nutrient that would meet the needs of 97% to 98% of a specific population subgroup. RDA values exist for carbohydrates and protein. These RDA values are considered the lower boundary of intake needed to meet needs (i.e., prevent deficiency), rather than the amount needed to promote optimal health and wellness. **Acceptable macronutrient distribution ranges (AMDRs)** are ranges of intake (expressed as a percentage of total calories) for carbohydrates, proteins, and fats that not only meet the needs for essential nutrients but also minimize the risk of chronic diseases. AMDR values exist for carbohydrates, fat, linoleic acid, linolenic acid, and protein. AMDR ranges were developed with intended uses for nutrition assessment and prescription.

Critical thinking of the nutrition professional involves careful consideration of the strengths and weaknesses of the DRIs. Each person's requirements for nutrients is unique; thus, comparison of an individual's intake to a reference such as the RDA should be viewed as an attempt to establish a "likelihood" or "probability" that a particular level of intake is inadequate, adequate, or excessive. In addition, the research base for the DRIs includes only studies of presumably healthy adults. The DRI values are not intended to represent the needs of individuals with known health conditions, trauma, surgery, malnutrition, or any condition that alters nutrient needs. Whenever possible, the nutrition professional should search for standards that are specific to the client's health status or write a nutrition prescription in the chart to specify customized ideal levels of macronutrient intake and timing using evidence-informed practice that will be used as the standard for assessment and intervention.

Particular recommendations exist for added sugars, solid fats, and trans fatty acids from a variety of government and health associations. For example, the following limits have been proposed:
- Saturated fat: <10% of total calories (U.S. Dietary Guidelines); <5-6% total calories (American Heart Association)
- Trans fatty acids: "as low as possible" (American Heart Association, DRIs)
- Sugars: <25 g/d females, <38 g/d males (American Heart Association) or <10% of kcal (U.S. Dietary Guidelines)
- Total solid fats and added sugars (SOFAS): Based on calorie level of the diet, but typically ranges from 160 to 330 kcal/day for most adults (USDA Food Patterns)

Beyond these general recommendations for healthy individuals, standard therapeutic diets such as the Dietary Approaches to Stop Hypertension (DASH) diet include specific recommendations for a variety of dietary components such as saturated fat, cholesterol, and fiber (see Chapter 32 and Appendix 17).

Assessment and Interpretation of Micronutrients

The micronutrient content of the diet can be assessed by analyzing multiple days of food records or 24-hour recalls with the assistance of commercially available dietary assessment software (see Fig. 4.8). If the nutrition professional is interested in micronutrients, careful assessment of foods and beverages that are enriched, fortified, or contain added vitamins and minerals is vital. The dietary assessment software may provide information about specific forms of vitamins in the diet, such as folate versus folic acid, if the foods in the database include such distinctions. However, as the software database is largely from chemical analysis of foods, the nutrition professional will need to consider the food sources of the nutrients in order to factor in the bioavailability of the nutrient levels listed in the report.

As described above, the RDA and AI values provided by the Institute of Medicine can serve as a starting point for establishing a "likelihood" or "probability" that a particular level of intake is inadequate, adequate, or excessive. However, the intake of many micronutrients varies on a day-to-day basis much more than macronutrients. Thus the uncertainty around judgments of intake adequacy involve uncertainty around a person's actual requirement and uncertainty around the typical intake of a micronutrient. For healthy individuals, intake above the RDA is likely adequate but intake below the RDA is not necessarily inadequate. If intake is below the RDA, more data will be needed to interpret nutritional status, such as laboratory values or nutrition-focused physical examination findings (see Appendices 12 and 13). As discussed above, for patients with medical conditions, it is ideal to identify micronutrient recommendations particularly related to that condition (e.g., DASH diet) or write a nutrition prescription in the chart to specify customized ideal levels of specific micronutrients that are evidence-informed and therapeutic for the client.

The **tolerable upper level (UL)** is a DRI value that identifies the highest average daily intake that does not cause adverse effects. In combination with dietary assessment software analysis, the UL value can assist with determining the safety of consuming foods that are enriched, fortified, or otherwise supplemented with nutrients. In addition, the UL value can provide information about the potential risks of nutrient supplementation in healthy individuals. The UL is not intended to apply to individuals who are consuming micronutrient supplements to address nutrient deficiencies, or other medical conditions that have specific micronutrient needs; these situations also require research-based or individual recommendations specific to the client.

Assessment and Interpretation of Other Bioactive Dietary Components

Bioactive compounds include compounds that have "the capability and the ability to interact with one or more component(s) of the living tissue by presenting a wide range of probable effects" (Guaadaoui et al, 2014). According to this framework, natural or synthetic, potentially helpful or harmful, food or nonfood sourced compounds of plant or animal origin would qualify as potentially biologically active in the human body. In this rapidly developing field of study, nutrition professionals are likely to see an ever-expanding list of possible bioactive components and their role in human health and disease. Table 4.3 presents the more common dietary components that nutrition professionals may attempt to assess, interpret, or intervene related to clients.

Assessment of the diet is likely to be limited to qualitative evaluation of the frequency of foods consumed that contain the component of interest. Limited data exist for beneficial bioactive components outside of the typical micronutrients found in foods (e.g. carotenoids). About 800 harmful and beneficial dietary components are monitored in the Total Diet Study, but only in a few hundred foods in the food supply (Total Diet Study, 2019). Few standards exist for interpreting whether intake is within safe, optimal, or health-promoting levels. Nutrition professionals can consult evidence-based MNT guidelines to generate a specific nutrition prescription for a client or refer the client for evaluation by a nutrition professional trained in integrative and functional medicine (refer online to the Academy of Nutrition and Dietetics Practice Group Dietitians in Integrative and Functional Medicine / Find a Practitioner).

FOOD AND NUTRIENT ADMINISTRATION

The subdomain "Food and Nutrient Administration" of Food- and Nutrition-Related History includes details about the client's current and historical approaches to eating, including the current diet order, diets selected or followed in the past, food restrictions and fasting, prior education regarding therapeutic diets, and the eating environment (see Table 4.1). Often this information is obtained through chart review (diet order, prior nutrition education), patient interview, and intake forms. Examples of data points from this section of the Food- and Nutrition-Related History include therapeutic diets implemented on past hospitalizations, prior education on a therapeutic diet, the

TABLE 4.3 Dietary Components and Bioactive Compounds of Interest

Beneficial Component	Potential Food Sources	Potential Implications
Curcumin	Turmeric	Antioxidant, antiinflammatory, anticancer, and neuroprotective properties
Flavonoids	Fruit, vegetables, chocolate, wine, tea	Antiinflammatory, antithrombogenic, antidiabetic, anticancer, and neuroprotective properties
Isothiocyanates	Cruciferous vegetables	Metabolism and elimination of xenobiotics (e.g., carcinogens) from the body, antioxidant and antiinflammatory properties
Phytosterols	Legumes, unrefined vegetable oils, whole grains, nuts, seeds, enriched foods	Reduction in LDL cholesterol
Soy Isoflavones	Soy beans/products	Reduction in breast cancer, improved vascular function
Viscous (soluble) Fiber	Legumes, whole grains and cereals, vegetables, fruits, nuts, and seeds	Reduction in total and LDL cholesterol, lower postprandial insulin and blood glucose levels
Harmful Component	**Potential Food Sources**	**Potential Implications**
Lead	Tap water—leaches in from metal pipes	Neurotoxin, widespread organ damage
Mercury	Seafood, including canned albacore tuna, swordfish	Damage to brain, kidneys, liver, heart, nervous system, developing fetus
Arsenic	Water, rice (whole grain, refined, milks, syrups), fruit juices	Skin, bladder, and lung cancers
Bisphenol A (BPA)	Packaged foods—leaches in from food and beverage containers, linings of food and beverage cans	Organ damage, lowered IQ, miscarriage, hormone disruption

Adapted from Phytochemicals. Linus Pauling Institute, Micronutrient Information Center: https://lpi.oregonstate.edu/mic/dietary-factors/phytochemicals; and Metals. U.S. Food and Drug Administration: https://www.fda.gov/food/chemicals-metals-pesticides-food/metals.

types of weight loss diets attempted in the past and their benefits and drawbacks, foods that should not be served or recommended to the patient with food allergies, access points for enteral or parenteral nutrition, frequency and duration of fasts for religious or health reasons, or whether the client needs or has access to assistance when eating meals. This data is crucial when working with a variety of patients across the life cycle, whether in a facility or home-based setting.

NUTRITION KNOWLEDGE, BELIEFS, AND ATTITUDES

This subdomain includes assessment of the nutrition knowledge and skills as well as important beliefs and attitudes that can enhance or detract from adoption of current or future nutrition interventions (see Table 4.1). This information can be obtained through chart review, patient interview, or intake forms. For example, this type of information can contribute value to the nutrition assessment by showing whether a patient:

- is familiar with foods that contain key therapeutic nutrients
- has the cooking skills needed to implement a therapeutic dietary change
- is likely or unlikely to follow through with a particular nutrition intervention due to religious, cultural, or personal values
- is struggling with emotional eating, negative self-talk, or disordered eating
- is willing to make a dietary change and feels confident in the ability to do so

Clients who have the ability (knowledge and skills) to implement a nutrition intervention are more likely to be successful (see Chapter 13). Similarly, clients whose beliefs and attitudes are consistent with a nutrition intervention are more likely to be willing to implement the intervention. Conversely, nutrition interventions are unlikely to be successful if the client lacks skills or knowledge to implement them, if they conflict with prior nutrition education, or if the client is opposed to carrying out the intervention due to religious, personal, cultural, moral, or ethical values and beliefs.

NUTRITION BEHAVIORS

The Nutrition Behaviors subdomain includes the patient's behaviors, activities, and actions that impact the success of prior, current, and future nutrition interventions (see Table 4.1). For new clients, the RDN can assess behaviors that are likely to be significant barriers to achievement of future dietary change such as restrictive eating, binging, purging, refusal to eat, and unwillingness to try new foods or alter the diet. For returning clients, additional assessments of adherence to the overall nutrition plan can include attendance at scheduled visits and adherence to interventions or self-monitoring activities that were collaboratively developed at previous visits. Clients that present with significant barriers to dietary change or who return multiple times with low adherence may benefit from additional social support, referral to outside agencies, or referral to counselors or psychologists for evaluation.

MEDICATION AND COMPLEMENTARY OR ALTERNATIVE MEDICINES

As foods, beverages, medications, and dietary supplements can interact with each other, careful assessment of these possible interactions is part of the Food- and Nutrition-Related History domain (see Table 4.1). A list of prescription medications, over-the-counter medications, complementary medications, and therapeutic nutritional supplements can be generated from a combination of chart review, patient interview, and intake forms. Based on current scientific knowledge of food–drug interactions, the RDN can assess whether supplements, foods, or beverages (types, patterns, timing) may alter the bioavailability or biological action of drugs, or whether the types of drugs or supplements taken by the patient could alter nutrient absorption, metabolism, excretion, or gastrointestinal (GI) function (taste, smell, appetite) enough to compromise nutritional status (see Appendix 13).

NUTRITION ACCESS

The Nutrition Access subdomain includes assessment of factors that impact the ability to obtain a safe and nutritious diet (see Table 4.1). Some examples include:

- Access to safe and nutritious foods and beverages
- Availability of grocery shopping facilities
- Availability of meal preparation supplies and facilities
- Presence of assistive food preparation and eating devices
- Eligibility for and participation in government and community programs related to food and nutrition

Research has consistently shown that health disparities and health inequities are a result of the social determinants of health or the social and economic conditions under which people live (Centers for Disease Control [CDC], 2018). Addressing these major health inequities is not about providing more health care, but rather about ensuring equal access to the resources needed to make healthier choices and avoid exposures that are harmful to health (CDC, 2018). Successful strategies include linking clients and communities to community and government programs that improve access to safe and nutritious food, clean air and water, recreation opportunities, and preventive health care as well as engaging in public policy and advocacy work (see Chapter 8).

PHYSICAL ACTIVITY AND PHYSICAL FUNCTION

This subdomain includes assessment of indicators of the body's functioning in relation to nutritional status (see Table 4.1). The most common variable assessed is physical activity patterns, which are a key determinant of overall health and energy expenditure and needs. Detailed assessment and interpretation of the dimensions of fitness, such as muscle strength, muscle endurance, cardiovascular endurance, flexibility, and coordination, require additional training or referral to an exercise physiologist. RDNs can complete training for the *Physical Activity Toolkit for Registered Dietitians: Utilizing Resources of Exercise is Medicine*, developed by the Weight Management and Sports, Cardiovascular, and Wellness Nutrition dietetic practice groups in collaboration with the American College of Sports Medicine. This toolkit contains information and resources needed to assess and evaluate the frequency and duration of basic cardiovascular and strength activities (Raynor and Champagne, 2016).

Other indicators of physical functioning in this subdomain include the ability to eat independently or feed others (breastfeed). Information on how to evaluate a child's or adult's physical or cognitive abilities to prepare food or eat independently can be found in Chapters 43 and 19, respectively. Chapter 14 provides a review of potential goals for breastfeeding initiation, duration, and exclusivity as well as methods to assess basic breastfeeding behaviors. Assessment and interpretation of adequacy of breastmilk production (parental) or intake (child) often requires the expertise of an International Board-Certified Lactation Consultant (IBCLC) and access to professional grade breast pumps and infant scales.

NUTRITION QUALITY OF LIFE

The Nutrition Quality of Life subdomain relates to the client's sense of well-being in response to the health challenges that they are experiencing and the nutrition interventions recommended by the nutrition professional (see Table 4.1). Nearly all interventions proposed by the health care team will require resources of the client, which could include money, time, effort, and loss of freedom of choices in health behaviors. Sensitivity toward the impact of an intervention on the client's lifestyle can help establish rapport with the client and create a safe space for the client to discuss real and perceived barriers to implementation of nutrition recommendations. After assessment of the potential impact of nutrition interventions on quality of life, the clinician can make recommendations that are more likely to be adopted by the client.

CLINICAL CASE STUDY

Jessup identifies as a 75-year-old white male of English and French ancestry. He is referred to your private practice for assessment of potential malnutrition. The referral letter from the doctor's visit 2 weeks ago provides you with these pieces of assessment data:

Food- and Nutrition-Related History: Client reported a "moderate" decrease in food intake over the past 2 months.

Anthropometric Data: Current height = 68 inches, current weight = 145 lb, prior weight (3 months ago) = 149 lb.

Biochemical Data, Medical Tests, and Procedures: Low hemoglobin, hematocrit.

Nutrition-Focus Physical Findings: Client reports poor appetite, constipation, and loosening of the dentures.

Client History: Depression and iron deficiency anemia (diagnosed in past 2 weeks), history of hypertension (controlled by medications), loss of wife 7 weeks ago after a prolonged illness, still socially connected (family, friends, church, volunteering).

Nutrition Care Questions

1. Aomplete the Mini Nutritional Assessment Form (see Fig. 4.4) for Jessup. What is his numerical score? What is the interpretation of that score?
2. Which nutritional diagnoses may apply to his situation?
3. During his visit, which key nutritional risk factors (see Box 4.4) and Food- and Nutrition-Related History (see Table 4.1) will you prioritize in your assessment? Which data points will support your ability to narrow down the list of potential nutrition diagnoses you listed in Question 2?
4. Which type of dietary assessment tool found in Table 4.2 do you think is best suited for this client and this situation? Which tool is most likely to give you the dietary intake data you listed in Question 3?
5. What novel data can you provide to the medical team through your assessment? Which methods for collecting food and nutrient intake data could provide the necessary data? Which are most reliable and valid for this client and this setting?

REFERENCES

Academy of Nutrition and Dietetics: *Nutrition terminology reference manual (eNCPT): dietetics language for nutrition care.* Available at: https://www.ncpro.org/pubs/idnt-en/?.

Academy of Nutrition and Dietetics (AND): *NSCR: definitions and criteria (2009).* Available at: https://www.andeal.org/topic.cfm?menu= 3584&cat=3958.

Centers for Disease Control and Prevention: *CDC health disparities & inequalities report (CHDIR),* 2018. Available at: http://www.cdc.gov/minority-health/CHDIReport.html.

Drewnowski A, Rehm CD, Constant F: Water and beverage consumption among adults in the United States: cross-sectional study using data from

NHANES 2005-2010, *BMC Public Health* 13:1068, 2013. doi:10.1186/1471-2458-13-1068.

Gemming L, Utter J, Ni Mhurchu C: Image-assisted dietary assessment: a systematic review of the evidence, *J Acad Nutr Diet* 115(1):64–77, 2015. doi:10.1016/j.jand.2014.09.015.

Gil Á, Martinez de Victoria E, Olza J: Indicators for the evaluation of diet quality, *Nutr Hosp* 31(Suppl 3):128–144, 2015. doi:10.3305/nh.2015.31.sup3.8761.

Guaadaoui A, Benaicha S, Elmajdoub N, et al: What is a bioactive compound? A combined definition for a preliminary consensus, *Int J Nutr Food Sci* 3(3):174–179, 2014.

Hedrick VE, Myers EA, Zoellner JM, et al: Validation of a rapid method to assess habitual beverage intake patterns, *Nutrients* 10(1):E83, 2018. doi:10.3390/nu10010083.

Hedrick VE, Savla J, Comber DL, et al: Development of a Brief Questionnaire to Assess Habitual Beverage Intake (BEVQ-15): sugar-sweetened beverages and total beverage energy intake, *J Acad Nutr Diet* 112(6):840–849, 2012. doi:10.1016/j.jand.2012.01.023.

Metals. U.S. Food and Drug Administration. Available at: https://www.fda.gov/food/chemicals-metals-pesticides-food/metals.

Moore M: *So long, super tracker*, Food and Nutrition Magazine. (July/August):17-18, 2018.

NIH: *Dietary assessment primer*, National Institutes of Health, National Cancer Institute. Available at: https://dietassessmentprimer.cancer.gov.

National Institutes of Health: *ASA24 automated self-administered 24-hour dietary assessment tool*, National Institutes of Health, National Cancer Institute. Available at: https://epi.grants.cancer.gov/asa24/.

Parkhurst L, Quatrara B, Tappenden KA, et al: Critical role of nutrition in improving quality of care: an interdisciplinary call to action to address adult hospital malnutrition, *J Acad Nutr Diet* 113(9):1219–1237, 2013. doi:10.1016/j.jand.2013.05.015.

Phytochemicals. Linus pauling institute, micronutrient information center. Available at: https://lpi.oregonstate.edu/mic/dietary-factors/phytochemicals.

Raynor HA, Champagne CM: Position of the Academy of Nutrition and Dietetics: interventions for the treatment of overweight and obesity in adults, *J Acad Nutr Diet* 116(1):129–147, 2016. doi:10.1016/j.jand.2015.10.031.

Thompson FE, Byers T: Dietary assessment resource manual, *J Nutr* 124 (Suppl 11):2245S–2317S, 1994. doi:10.1093/jn/124.suppl_11.2245s.

Total Diet Study. Food and Drug Administration, 2019. Available at: https://www.fda.gov/food/science-research-food/total-diet-study.

5

Clinical: Biochemical, Physical, and Functional Assessment

Mary Demarest Litchford, PhD, RDN, LDN

KEY TERMS

25 hydroxy vitamin D (25[OH]D₃)
air displacement plethysmogram (ADP)
albumin
analyte
anemia of chronic and inflammatory disease (ACD)
anthropometry
basic metabolic panel (BMP)
bioelectrical impedance analysis (BIA)
body composition
body mass index (BMI)
complete blood count (CBC)
comprehensive metabolic panel (CMP)
C-reactive protein (CRP)
creatinine
dehydration
differential count
dual-energy x-ray absorptiometry (DXA)
edema

erythrocyte sedimentation rate (ESR)
ferritin
functional medicine
Functional Nutrition Assessment
head circumference
height-for-age
hematocrit (Hct)
hemoglobin (Hgb)
hemoglobin A1C (Hgb A1C)
high-sensitivity CRP (hs-CRP)
homocysteine
ideal body weight (IBW)
inflammation
length-for-age
macrocytic anemia
methylmalonic acid (MMA)
microcytic anemia
midarm circumference (MAC)
negative acute-phase reactants

osteocalcin
positive acute-phase reactants
prealbumin (PAB)
Quetelet index (W/H²)
retinol
retinol-binding protein (RBP)
serum iron
statiometer
total iron-binding capacity (TIBC)
transferrin
transthyretin (TTHY)
triceps skin fold (TSF)
urinalysis
usual body weight (UBW)
waist circumference (WC)
waist-to-height ratio (WHtR)
waist-to-hip ratio (WHR)
weight-for-age
weight-for-length

Nutrition assessment may be completed within the context of a traditional medical model or a functional integrative medical model. Clinicians must demonstrate critical thinking skills to observe, interpret, analyze, and infer data to detect new nutrition diagnoses or determine that nutrition-related issues have resolved (Charney and Peterson, 2013). The three sources of information—biochemical data, physical attributes, and functional changes—are viewed in the context of each other, and the trends of data over time are useful to identify patterns consistent with nutrition and medical diagnoses (Fig. 5.1).

Health care reforms are changing the practice of dietetics specific to nutrition assessment in several ways. First, the practice of ordering diets is changing to allow registered dietitian nutritionists (RDNs) the privilege of writing diet orders within the parameters set by the governing body of the health care organization. Second, the practice of ordering routine laboratory tests has changed, and health care providers must justify the need for each laboratory test ordered. Many RDNs have the authority to order laboratory tests with a clinical indicator or International Classification of Diseases (ICD) code to justify the request. RDNs must be proactive to request the authority to write diet orders and order laboratory tests and embrace the responsibilities associated with these privileges. Third, the use of evidence-based

medical guidelines is reshaping the types and frequency of biochemical testing, physical assessments, and functional tests ordered. These changes augment the value of physical and functional assessment as pivotal components of nutrition assessment. Practitioners should assess patients from a global perspective, requesting necessary tests, and not be limited by the history of reimbursement for testing. Also, many consumers are seeking health care services that are not covered currently by traditional insurance and government-funded health care programs. The nutrition professional can determine the validity and usefulness of these requests for testing. Before recommending a biochemical test to be performed, the dietitian should consider: "How will the test results change my intervention?"

BIOCHEMICAL ASSESSMENT OF NUTRITION STATUS

Laboratory tests are ordered to diagnose diseases, support nutrition diagnoses, monitor effectiveness of nutrition preventions, evaluate medication effectiveness, and evaluate nutrition care process (NCP) interventions or medical nutrition therapy (MNT). Acute illness, surgery, or injury can trigger dramatic changes in laboratory test results,

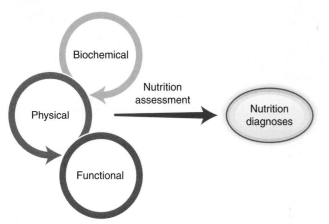

Fig. 5.1 Interrelationship of biochemical data, physical attributes, and functional status.

including rapidly deteriorating nutrition status. However, chronic diseases that develop slowly over time also influence these results, making them useful in preventive care.

Definitions and Applications of Laboratory Test Results

Laboratory assessment is a stringently controlled process. It involves comparing control samples with predetermined substance or chemical constituent (analyte) concentrations with every patient specimen. The results obtained must compare favorably with predetermined acceptable values before the patient data can be considered valid. Laboratory data are the only *objective data* used in nutrition assessment that are "controlled"—that is, the validity of the method of its measurement is checked each time a specimen is assayed by also assaying a sample with a known value.

Laboratory-based nutrition testing, used to estimate nutrient concentration in biologic fluids and tissues, is critical for assessment of clinical and subclinical nutrient deficiencies. As shown in Fig. 5.2, the size of a nutrient pool can vary continuously from a frank deficit to insufficiency to adequate to toxic. Most of these states can be assessed in the laboratory so that nutritional intervention can occur before a clinical or anthropometric change or a frank deficiency occurs (Litchford, 2017). Single test results must be evaluated in light of the patient's current medical condition, nutrition-focused physical examination findings, medications, lifestyle choices, age, hydration status, fasting status at the time of specimen collection, and reference

standards used by the clinical laboratory. Single test results may be useful for screening or to confirm an assessment based on changing clinical, anthropometric, and dietary status. Comparison of current test results to historic baseline test results from the same laboratory is desirable when available. It is vital to monitor trends in test results and patterns of results in the context of genetic and environmental factors. Changes in laboratory test results that occur over time are often an objective measure of nutrition or pharmacologic interventions and modified lifestyle choices.

Specimen Types

Ideally, the specimen to be tested reflects the total body content of the nutrient to be assessed. However, the best specimen may not be readily available. The most common specimens for analysis of nutrients and nutrient-related substances include the following:

- Whole blood: Collected with an anticoagulant if entire content of the blood is to be evaluated; none of the elements are removed; contains red blood cells (RBCs), white blood cells (WBCs), and platelets suspended in plasma
- Serum: The fluid obtained from blood after the blood has been clotted and then centrifuged to remove the clot and blood cells
- Plasma: The transparent (slightly straw-colored) liquid component of blood, composed of water, blood proteins, inorganic electrolytes, and clotting factors
- Blood cells: Separated from anticoagulated whole blood for measurement of cellular analyte content
- Erythrocytes: RBCs
- Leukocytes: WBCs and leukocyte fractions
- Blood spots: Dried whole blood from finger or heel prick that is placed on paper and can be used for selected hormone tests and other tests such as infant phenylketonuria screening
- Other tissues: Obtained from scrapings (i.e., buccal swabs, or biopsy samples)
- Urine (from random samples or timed collections): Contains a concentrate of excreted metabolites
- Feces (from random samples or timed collections): Important in nutritional analyses when nutrients are not absorbed and therefore are present in fecal material or to determine composition of gut flora or microbiota

Less commonly used specimens include the following:

- Breath tests: Noninvasive tool to evaluate nutrient metabolism and malabsorption, particularly of sugars. Emerging breath test technologies are being used to evaluate protein requirements,

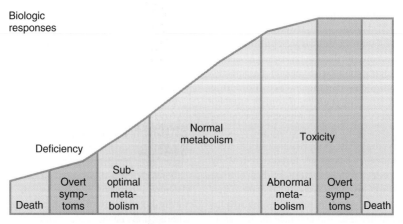

Fig. 5.2 The size of a nutrient pool can vary continuously from frankly deficient, to adequate, to toxic.

inflammatory stress, fructose malabsorption, and bacterial overgrowth in the intestine

- Hair and nails: Easy-to-collect tissue for determining exposure to selected toxic metals
- Saliva: Noninvasive medium with a fast turnover; currently is used to evaluate functional adrenal and other hormone levels
- Sweat: Electrolyte test used to detect sweat chloride levels to determine presence of cystic fibrosis
- Hair and nails specimens have significant drawbacks, including lack of standardized procedures for processing, assay, and quality control and there is potential environmental contamination. Nutrient levels or indices may be less than the amounts that can be measured accurately. Hair can be used for deoxyribonucleic acid (DNA) testing and may be useful in the future as a noninvasive methodology to predict genetic predisposition to disease and effectiveness of MNT (see Chapter 6). Considerable research is being done to improve the usefulness of noninvasive and easy-to-collect specimens that are not routinely ordered.

NUTRITION INTERPRETATION OF ROUTINE MEDICAL LABORATORY TESTS

Clinical Chemistry Panels

Historically the majority of laboratory tests were ordered as panels or groupings; however, the current practice is that the professional ordering of the test must justify the medical need for each test ordered. The bundling or grouping of laboratory tests is changing as health care reforms reshape medical practices to be more cost effective. The most commonly ordered groups of tests are the basic metabolic panel (BMP) and the comprehensive metabolic panel (CMP) that include groups of laboratory tests defined by the Centers for Medicare and Medicaid Services for reimbursement purposes. The BMP and CMP require the patient to fast for 10 to 12 hours before testing. The BMP includes eight tests used for screening blood glucose level, electrolyte and fluid balance, and kidney function. The CMP includes all the tests in the BMP and six additional tests to evaluate liver function. Table 5.1 explains these tests (see Appendix 12).

Complete Blood Count

The complete blood count (CBC) provides a count of the cells in the blood and description of the RBCs. A hemogram is a CBC with a white blood cell differential count (often called a *differential* or *diff*). Table 5.2 provides a list of the basic elements of the CBC and differential, with reference ranges and explanatory comments.

Stool Testing

Mucosal changes in the gastrointestinal (GI) tract are indicated by problems such as diarrhea and bloody or black stool. Tests may be done on a stool sample and can reveal excessive amounts of fat (an indication of malabsorption), the status of the GI flora, and the amounts and types of bacteria present in the gut. Fecal samples may be tested for the presence of blood, pathogens, and gut flora. The fecal occult blood test is ordered routinely for adults older than

TABLE 5.1	Constituents of the Basic Metabolic Panel and Comprehensive Metabolic Panel		
Analytes	Reference Range*	Purpose	Significance
Basic Metabolic Panel (BMP) (All Tests Reflect Fasting State)			
Glucose	70-99 mg/dL; 3.9-5.5 mmol/L (fasting)	Used to screen for diabetes and to monitor patients with diabetes. Individuals experiencing severe stress from injuries or surgery have hyperglycemia related to catecholamine release	Fasting glucose >125 mg/dL indicates DM (oral glucose tolerance tests are not needed for diagnosis); fasting glucose >100 mg/dL is indicator of insulin resistance Monitor levels along with triglycerides in those receiving parenteral nutrition for glucose intolerance
Total calcium	8.5-10.5 mg/dL; 2.15-2.57 mmol/L Normal dependent on albumin level	Reflects the calcium levels in the body that are not stored in bones. Used to evaluate parathyroid hormone function, calcium metabolism and monitor patients with renal failure, renal transplant, and some cancers	Hypercalcemia associated with endocrine disorders, malignancy, and hypervitaminosis D Hypocalcemia associated with vitamin D deficiency and inadequate hepatic or renal activation of vitamin D, hypoparathyroidism, magnesium deficiency, renal failure, and nephrotic syndrome When serum albumin is low, ionized calcium is measured
Na^+	135-145 mEq/L; 135-145 mm/L	Reflects the relationship between total body sodium and extracellular fluid volume as well as the balance between dietary intake and renal excretory function	Used in monitoring various patients, such as those receiving parenteral nutrition or who have renal conditions, uncontrolled DM, various endocrine disorders, ascitic and edematous symptoms, or acidotic or alkalotic conditions; water dysregulation, and diuretics. Increased with dehydration and decreased with overhydration
K^+	3.6-5 mEq/L; 3.6-5 mmol/L	Levels often change with sodium levels. As sodium increases, potassium decreases and vice versa. Reflects kidney function, changes in blood pH, and adrenal gland function	Used in monitoring various patients, such as those receiving parenteral nutrition or who have renal conditions, uncontrolled DM, various endocrine disorders, ascitic and edematous symptoms, or acidotic or alkalotic conditions; decreased K^+ associated with diarrhea, vomiting, or nasogastric aspiration, water dysregulation, some drugs, licorice ingestion, and diuretics; increased K+ associated with renal diseases, crush injuries, infection, and hemolyzed blood specimens.

Continued

TABLE 5.1   Constituents of the Basic Metabolic Panel and Comprehensive Metabolic Panel—cont'd

Analytes	Reference Range*	Purpose	Significance
Basic Metabolic Panel (BMP) (All Tests Reflect Fasting State)			
Cl⁻	101-111 mEq/L; 101-111 mmol/L	Reflects acid–base balance, water balance, and osmolality	Used in monitoring various patients, such as those receiving parenteral nutrition or who have renal conditions, chronic obstructive pulmonary disease, diabetes insipidus, acidotic or alkalotic conditions; increased with dehydration and decreased with overhydration
HCO_3^- (or total CO_2)	21-31 mEq/L; 21-31 mmol/L	Used to assess acid–base balance and electrolyte status	Used in monitoring various patients, such as those receiving parenteral nutrition or who have renal conditions, chronic obstructive pulmonary disease, uncontrolled DM, various endocrine disorders, ascitic and edematous symptoms, or acidotic or alkalotic conditions
BUN or urea	5-20 mg urea nitrogen/dL; 1.8-7 mmol/L	Used to assess excretory function of kidney and metabolic function of liver	Increased in those with renal disease and excessive protein catabolism and overhydration; decreased in those with liver failure and negative nitrogen balance and in females who are pregnant
Creatinine	0.6-1.2 mg/dL; 53-106 μmol/L (males) 0.5-1.1 mg/dL; 44-97 μmol/L (females)	Used to assess excretory function of kidney	Increased in those with renal disease and after trauma or surgery; and decreased in those with malnutrition (i.e., BUN/creatinine ratio >15:1)
Comprehensive Metabolic Panel (CMP) (All Tests Reflect Fasting State and Includes All of the Tests in the BMP and Six Additional Tests)			
Albumin	3.5-5 mg/dL; 30-50 g/L	Reflects severity of illness, inflammatory stress and serves as marker for mortality	Decreased in those with liver disease or acute inflammatory disease and overhydration. Increases with dehydration. It is not a biomarker of protein status
Total protein	6.4-8.3 g/dL; 64-83 g/L	Reflects albumin and globulin in blood	Not a useful measure of nutrition or protein status
ALP	30-120 units/L; 0.5-2 μKat/L	Reflects function of liver; may be used to screen for bone abnormalities	Increased in those with any of a variety of malignant, muscle, bone, intestinal, and liver diseases or injuries
ALT	4-36 units/L at 37° C; 4-36 units/L	Reflects function of liver	Used in monitoring liver function in those receiving parenteral nutrition
AST	0-35 IU/L; 0-0.58 μKat/L	Reflects function of liver; may be used to screen for cardiac abnormalities	Used in monitoring liver function in those receiving parenteral nutrition
Bilirubin	Total bilirubin 0.3-1 mg/dL; 5.1-17 μmol/L Indirect bilirubin 0.2-0.8 mg/dL; 3.4-12 μmol/L Direct bilirubin 0.1-0.3 mg/dL; 1.7-5.1 μmol/L	Reflects function of liver; also used to evaluate blood disorders, and biliary tract blockage	Increased in association with drugs, gallstones, and other biliary duct diseases; intravascular hemolysis and hepatic immaturity; decreased with some anemias
Phosphorous (phosphate)	3-4.5 mg/dL; 0.97-1.45 mmol/L		Hyperphosphatemia associated with hypoparathyroidism and hypocalcemia; hypophosphatemia associated with hyperparathyroidism, chronic antacid ingestion, and renal failure
Total cholesterol	<200 mg/dL; 5.20 mmol/L		Decreased in those with malnutrition, malabsorption, liver diseases, and hyperthyroidism
Triglycerides	<100 mg/dL; <1.13 mmol/L (age and gender dependent)		Increased in those with glucose intolerance (e.g., in those receiving parenteral nutrition who have combined hyperlipidemia) or in those who are not fasting

*Reference ranges may vary slightly among laboratories.

ALP, Alkaline phosphate; *ALT*, alanine aminotransferase; *AST*, aspartate aminotransferase; *BUN*, blood urea nitrogen; *Cl⁻*, chlorine; *CO_2*, carbon dioxide; *DM*, diabetes mellitus; *HCO_3^-*, bicarbonate; *K^+*, potassium; *Na^+*, sodium; *PEM*, protein-energy malnutrition.

age 50 and younger adults with unexplained anemia. Stool culture testing may be ordered in patients with prolonged diarrhea, especially if foodborne illness is suspected. If pathogenic bacteria are isolated in stool culture, appropriate pharmacologic interventions are initiated. Patients with chronic GI symptoms such as maldigestion or unexplained weight loss or gain may benefit from gut flora testing to identify pathologic flora or an imbalance of physiologic flora. In addition, stool tests may be helpful to evaluate the gut microbiota and the effectiveness of probiotic, prebiotic, and synbiotic use.

TABLE 5.2 Constituents of the Hemogram: Complete Blood Count and Differential

Analytes	Reference Range*	Significance
Red blood cells	$4.7\text{-}6.1 \times 10^6/\mu l$ (males); $4.7\text{-}6.1 \ 10^{12}/L$ $4.2\text{-}5.4 \times 10^6/\mu l$ (females); $4.2\text{-}5.4 \ 10^{12}/L$	In addition to nutritional deficits, may be decreased in those with hemorrhage, hemolysis, genetic aberrations, marrow failure, or renal disease or who are taking certain drugs; not sensitive for iron, vitamin B_{12}, or folate deficiencies
Hemoglobin concentration	14-18 g/dL; 8.7-11.2 mmol/L (males) 12-16 g/dL; 7.4-9.9 mmol/L (females) >11 g/dL; >6.8 mmol/L (pregnant females) 14-24 g/dL; 8.7-14.9 mmol/L (newborns)	In addition to nutritional deficits, may be decreased in those with hemorrhage, hemolysis, genetic aberrations, marrow failure, or renal disease or who are taking certain drugs
Hematocrit	42%-52% (males) 35%-47% (females) 33% (pregnant females) 44%-64% (newborns)	In addition to nutritional deficits, may be decreased in those with hemorrhage, hemolysis, genetic aberrations, marrow failure, or renal disease or who are taking certain drugs Somewhat affected by hydration status
MCV	80-99 fl 96-108 fl (newborns)	Decreased (microcytic) in presence of iron deficiency, thalassemia trait and chronic renal failure; normal or decreased in anemia of chronic disease; increased (macrocytic) in presence of vitamin B_{12} or folate deficiency and genetic defects in DNA synthesis; neither microcytosis nor macrocytosis sensitive to marginal nutrient deficiencies
MCH	27-31 pg/cell 23-34 pg/cell (newborns)	Causes of abnormal values similar to those for MCV
MCHC	32-36 g/dL; 32-36% 32-33 g/dL; 32-33% (newborns)	Decreased in those with iron deficiency and thalassemia trait; not sensitive to marginal nutrient deficiencies
WBC	$5\text{-}10 \times 10^9/L$; 5,000-10,000/mm³ (2 yr-adult) $6\text{-}17 \times 10^9/L$; 6,000-17,000/mm³ (<2 yr) $9\text{-}30 \times 10^9$; 9,000-30,000/mm³ (newborns)	Increased (leukocytosis) in those with infection, neoplasia; stress decreased (leucopenia) in those with malnutrition, autoimmune diseases, or overwhelming infections or who are receiving chemotherapy or radiation therapy
Differential	55%-70% neutrophils 20-40% lymphocytes 2-8% monocytes 1%-4% eosinophils 0.5%-1% basophils	*Neutrophilia*: Ketoacidosis, trauma, stress, pus-forming infections, leukemia *Neutropenia*: malnutrition, aplastic anemia, chemotherapy, overwhelming infection *Lymphocytosis*: Infection, leukemia, myeloma, mononucleosis *Lymphocytopenia*: Leukemia, chemotherapy, sepsis, AIDS *Eosinophilia*: Parasitic infestation, allergy, eczema, leukemia, autoimmune disease *Eosinopenia*: Increased steroid production *Basophilia*: Leukemia *Basopenia*: Allergy

*Reference ranges may vary slightly among laboratories.
AIDS, Acquired immune deficiency syndrome; *DNA*, deoxyribonucleic acid; *MCH*, mean corpuscular hemoglobin; *MCHC*, mean corpuscular hemoglobin concentration; *MCV*, mean corpuscular volume.

Urinalysis

The urinalysis test is used as a screening or diagnostic tool to detect substances or cellular material in the urine associated with different metabolic and kidney disorders. Some urinalysis data have broader medical and nutritional significance (e.g., glycosuria suggests abnormal carbohydrate metabolism and possibly diabetes). The full urinalysis includes a record of (1) the appearance of the urine, (2) the results of basic tests done with chemically impregnated reagent strips (often called dipsticks) that can be read visually or by an automated reader, and (3) the microscopic examination of urine sediment. Table 5.3 provides a list of the chemical tests performed in a urinalysis and their significance.

ASSESSMENT OF HYDRATION STATUS

Assessment of hydration status is vital because water dysregulation can be associated with other imbalances such as electrolyte imbalance. Types of water dysregulation include volume depletion or extracellular fluid contraction, dehydration or sodium intoxication, and overhydration or excessive fluid shift into interstitial-lymph fluid compartment. Dehydration often is due to excessive loss of water and electrolytes from vomiting; diarrhea; excessive laxative abuse; diuretics; fistulas; GI suction; polyuria; fever; excessive sweating; or decreased intake caused by anorexia, nausea, depression, or limited access to fluids. Characteristics include rapid weight loss, decreased skin turgor, dry mucous membranes, dry and furrowed tongue, postural hypotension, a weak and rapid pulse, slow capillary refill, a decrease in body temperature (95° to 98° F), decreased urine output, cold extremities, or disorientation (see Chapter 3).

Volume depletion is a state of vascular instability resulting from blood loss, GI bleeding, burns, vomiting, and diarrhea. Volume depletion may occur with low serum sodium (hyponatremia), high blood sodium (hypernatremia), or normal serum sodium levels.

Edema (overhydration), occurs when there is an increase in the extracellular fluid volume. The fluid shifts from the extracellular compartment to the interstitial fluid compartment (see Fig. 3.2 in Chapter 3). Overhydration is caused by an increase in capillary hydrostatic pressure or capillary permeability, or a decrease in colloid osmotic pressure. It often is associated with renal failure, chronic heart failure, cirrhosis of the liver, Cushing's syndrome, excess use of sodium-containing intravenous fluids, and excessive intake of sodium-containing food or medications. Characteristics include rapid weight gain, peripheral edema, distended neck veins, slow emptying of peripheral veins, a bounding and full pulse, rales in the

TABLE 5.3 Chemical Tests in a Urinalysis

Analyte	Expected Value	Significance
Specific gravity	1.010-1.025	Can be used to test and monitor the concentrating and diluting abilities of the kidney and hydration status; low in those with diabetes insipidus, glomerulonephritis, or pyelonephritis; high in those with vomiting, diarrhea, sweating, fever, adrenal insufficiency, hepatic diseases, or heart failure
pH	4.6-8 (normal diet)	Acidic in those with a high-protein diet or acidosis (e.g., uncontrolled DM or starvation), during administration of some drugs, and in association with uric acid, cystine, and calcium oxalate kidney stones; alkaline in individuals consuming diets rich in vegetables or dairy products and in those with a urinary tract infection, immediately after meals, with some drugs, and in those with phosphate and calcium carbonate kidney stones
Protein	2-8 mg/dL	Marked proteinuria in those with nephrotic syndrome, severe glomerulonephritis, or congestive heart failure; moderate in those with most renal diseases, preeclampsia, or urinary tract inflammation; minimal in those with certain renal diseases or lower urinary tract disorders
Glucose	Not detected (2-10 g/dL in DM)	Positive in those with DM; rarely in benign conditions
Ketones	Negative	Positive in those with uncontrolled DM (usually type 1); also positive in those with a fever, anorexia, certain GI disturbances, persistent vomiting, or cachexia or who are fasting or starving
Blood	Negative	Indicates urinary tract infection, neoplasm, or trauma; also positive in those with traumatic muscle injuries or hemolytic anemia
Bilirubin	Not detected	Index of unconjugated bilirubin; increase in those with certain liver diseases (e.g., gallstones)
Urobilinogen	0.1-1 units/dL	Index of conjugated bilirubin; increased in those with hemolytic conditions; used to distinguish among hepatic diseases
Nitrite	Negative	Index of bacteriuria
Leukocyte esterase	Negative	Indirect test of bacteriuria; detects leukocytes

DM, Diabetes mellitus; *GI*, gastrointestinal.

lungs, polyuria, ascites, and pleural effusion. Pulmonary edema may occur in severe cases.

Laboratory measures of hydration status include serum sodium, blood urea nitrogen (elevated out of proportion to serum creatinine), serum osmolality, and urine-specific gravity. Although the laboratory tests are important, decisions regarding hydration should only be made only in conjunction with other information from physical examination, nutrition-focused physical examination, and the clinical condition of the patient. In addition, many other laboratories may be affected by overhydration or dehydration, and accurate interpretation of laboratory results is critical in assessing patients (see Table 5.1).

Inflammation and Biochemical Assessment

Inflammation is a protective response by the immune system to infection, acute illness, trauma, toxins, many chronic diseases, and physical stress. Biochemical indices are affected by inflammation primarily by redirection to synthesis of acute phase reactants. Inflammatory conditions trigger the immune response to release eicosanoids and cytokines, which mobilize nutrients required to synthesize positive acute-phase reactants (which increase in response to inflammation) and leukocytes. Cytokines (interleukin-1beta [IL-1β], tumor necrosis factor alpha [TNF-α], interleukin-6 [IL-6]), and eicosanoids (prostaglandin E2 [PGE2]) influence whole-body metabolism, body composition, and nutritional status. Cytokines reorient hepatic synthesis of plasma proteins and increase the breakdown of muscle protein to meet the demand for protein and energy during the inflammatory response. Moreover, there is a redistribution of albumin to the interstitial compartment, resulting in edema. Declining values of the negative acute-phase reactants (i.e., serum albumin, prealbumin, and transferrin) also reflect the inflammatory processes and severity of tissue injury. In the acute inflammatory state, negative acute phase

reactant values do not reflect current dietary intake or protein status (White et al, 2012).

Cytokines impair the production of erythrocytes and reorient iron stores from hemoglobin and serum iron to ferritin. During infection IL-1β inhibits the production and release of transferrin while stimulating the synthesis of ferritin. Therefore laboratory test results used to predict the risk of nutritional anemias (see Chapter 31) are not useful in assessing the patient with an inflammatory response. Refer to Chapter 7 for more information on the effects of cytokines on organ systems.

As the body responds to acute inflammation, TNF-α, IL-1β, IL-6, and PGE2 increase to a set threshold, then IL-6 and PGE2 inhibit TNF-α synthesis and IL-1β secretion, creating a negative feedback cycle. Hepatic synthesis of positive acute-phase reactants diminishes, and synthesis of negative acute-phase reactants increases. Albumin shifts from the interstitial compartment to the extravascular space where it can be measured as serum albumin. Albumin in the interstitial space cannot be measured, therefore albumin is not a reliable marker for protein status. Iron stores shift from ferritin to transferrin and hemoglobin.

Markers of Inflammation

Biochemical markers of inflammation include positive acute phase reactants and negative acute phase reactants. In the presence of inflammation, the hepatic synthesis of positive acute-phase reactants is *increased* while the synthesis of the negative acute-phase reactants is *depressed*. See Table 5.4 for acute phase reactants. Additional markers of oxidative stress and inflammation can be found in Table 5.5.

Positive Acute Phase Reactants

C-Reactive Protein

C-reactive protein (CRP) is a nonspecific marker of inflammation that may help estimate and monitor the severity of illness.

TABLE 5.4 Acute Phase Reactants

Positive Acute-Phase Reactants	Negative Acute-Phase Proteins
C-reactive protein	Albumin
a_1 antichymotrypsin	Transferrin
a_1-antitrypsin	Prealbumin (transthyretin)
Haptoglobins	Retinol-binding protein
Ceruloplasmin	
Serum amyloid A	
Fibrinogen	
Ferritin	
Complement and components C3 and C4	
Orosomucoid	

High-sensitivity CRP (hs-CRP) is a more sensitive measure of chronic inflammation seen in patients with atherosclerosis and other chronic diseases (Wang et al, 2017). Although the exact function of CRP is unclear, it increases in the initial stages of acute stress—usually within 4 to 6 hours of surgery or other trauma. Furthermore, its level can increase as much as 1000-fold, depending on the intensity of the stress response. When the CRP level begins to decrease, the patient has entered the anabolic period of the inflammatory response and the beginning of recovery when more intensive nutrition therapy may be beneficial. Ongoing assessment and follow-up are required to address changes in nutrition status.

Ferritin

Ferritin is a positive acute-phase protein, meaning that synthesis of ferritin increases in the presence of inflammation. Ferritin is not a reliable indicator of iron stores in patients with acute inflammation, uremia, metastatic cancer, or alcoholic-related liver diseases. Cytokines

TABLE 5.5 Advantages and Disadvantages of Various Biomarkers of Oxidative Stress

Biomarker	Advantages	Disadvantages	Comments
IsoPs (isoprostanes)	Can be detected in various samples (serum, urine) and has been shown to be elevated in the presence of a range of CV risk factors	Current methods of quantification are impractical for large-scale screening.	No evidence linking this biomarker to clinical outcomes yet. F_2-IsoPs show most potential
MDA (mal-ondialdehyde)	Technically easy to quantify spectrophotometrically using the TBARS assay ELISA kits to detect MDA also have good performance. Studies show MDA can predict progression of CAD and carotid atherosclerosis at 3 years	TBARS assay is nonspecific (can detect aldehydes other than MDA) and sample preparation can influence results.	Shows promise as a clinical biomarker; however, does not have a functional impact on the pathophysiology of CVD
Nitrotyrosine (3-NO2-tyr)	Human studies have demonstrated association with CAD independent of traditional risk factors	Circulating levels are not equivalent to tissue levels. Current detection methods are expensive and impractical.	Nitrotyrosine formation on particular cardiovascular proteins has direct effect on function
S-glutathionylation	S-glutathionylation of SERCA, eNOS and Na$^+$–K$^+$ pump demonstrated as biomarkers as well as role in pathogenesis	Detection of S-glutathionylation prone to methodological artifact. Access to tissue (myocardium, vasculature), where modification occurs presents a clinical obstacle	Modified hemoglobin currently being investigated as biomarker
Myeloperoxidase (MPO)	Commercial assays available. An enzyme abundant in granules in inflammatory cells. Strong evidence that MPO correlates with CVD risk	Influenced by sample storage and time to analysis	MPO is a promising biomarker for CVD risk prediction
Oxidized LDL cholesterol (OxLDL)	Forms and occurs in vascular walls as foam cells and stimulates production of proinflammatory cytokines by endothelial cells. Elevated in CAD, increasing OxLDL correlates with increasing clinical severity. Also is predictive of future CAD in healthy population. Good reproducibility from frozen samples	Reduction in OxLDL by antioxidant pharmacotherapy has not been matched by reduction in CVD severity.	ELISAs for OxLDL detection readily available
ROS-induced changes to gene expression	The expression of several genes involved in regulating oxidative stress may be measured simultaneously using microarray technology, potentially increasing the power of this biomarker	Microarray technology can be manually and computationally expensive	It is unclear if expression profiles of cells in biologic samples reflect that in cardiovascular tissues
Serum antioxidant capacity	Activity of antioxidant enzymes such as glutathione peroxidase 1 (GPX-1) and superoxide dismutase (SOD) are demonstrated to be inversely proportional to CAD. Commercial kits available to measure antioxidant capacity. Reproducibly quantified despite frozen sample storage	Antioxidant activity in serum may not reflect that of the cells that are important to the pathogenesis of CVD	Clinical relevance of antioxidant quantification to CVD risk needs further investigation

CAD, Coronary artery disease; CV, cardiovascular; CVD, cardiovascular disease; ELISA, enzyme-linked immunosorbent assay; TBARS, thiobarbituric acid (TBA) reacting substances; eNOS, endothelial nitric oxide synthase; GPX-1, glutathione peroxidase-1, ROS, reactive oxygen species; SERCA, sarcoplasmic reticulum Ca^{2+} -ATPase , SOD, superoxide dismutase.

Adapted from Ho E et al: Biological markers of oxidative stress: applications to cardiovascular research and practice, Redox Biology 1:483, 2013.

and other inflammatory mediators can increase ferritin synthesis, ferritin leakage from cells, or both. Elevations in ferritin occur 1 to 2 days after the onset of the acute illness and peak at 3 to 5 days. If iron deficiency also exists, it may not be diagnosed because the level of ferritin would be falsely elevated.

Erythrocyte Sedimentation Rate

Erythrocyte sedimentation rate (ESR) reflects the rate at which RBCs settle into columns or stacks in a saline or plasma within a given time period. Inflammatory processes lead to increased weight of the RBC and more likely to settle rapidly unlike normal erythrocytes. ESR is useful in differentiating disease entities and is also used to monitor disease therapy (i.e., as ESR increases, the disease state worsens) (Litchford, 2017).

Negative Acute Phase Reactants
Albumin

Albumin is responsible for the transport of major blood constituents, hormones, enzymes, medications, minerals, ions, fatty acids, amino acids, and metabolites. A major role of albumin is to maintain colloidal osmotic pressure, providing approximately 80% of colloidal osmotic pressure of the plasma. When serum albumin levels decrease, the water in the plasma moves into the interstitial compartment and edema results. This loss of plasma fluid results in hypovolemia, which triggers renal retention of water and sodium.

Albumin has a half-life of 18 to 21 days. Levels of albumin remain nearly normal during uncomplicated starvation as redistribution from the interstitium to the plasma occurs. Levels of albumin fall precipitously in inflammatory stress and often do not improve with aggressive nutrition support. Serum levels reflect the severity of illness but do not reflect current protein status or the effects of nutrient-dense supplemental nutrition. For these reasons, a well-nourished but stressed patient may have low levels of albumin and the hepatic transport proteins, whereas a patient who has had significant weight loss and undernutrition may have normal or close to normal levels. Albumin is very sensitive to hydration status, and the practitioner must be aware and document the true cause of an elevated or depressed albumin level.

Albumin is synthesized in the liver and is a measure of liver function. When disease affects the liver, the synthesis of albumin, by the hepatocytes, is impaired. Because of the half-life of albumin, significant changes in liver function are not immediately apparent.

Prealbumin (Transthyretin)

Prealbumin (PAB), officially transthyretin (TTHY), is a hepatic protein transported in the serum as a complex of retinol-binding protein and vitamin A. It transports the thyroid hormones triiodothyronine and thyroxine (T_4), along with T_4-binding globulin. It has a short half-life ($t\frac{1}{2} = 2$ days), and currently it is considered a marker of inflammation. Levels of PAB plummet in inflammatory stress and are not sensitive measures to evaluate the effectiveness of aggressive nutrition support. Moreover, serum levels decrease with malignancy and protein-wasting diseases of the intestines or kidneys. Serum levels do not reflect protein status or the effects of refeeding in the individual with depleted protein reserves. Serum levels also decrease in the presence of a zinc deficiency because zinc is required for hepatic synthesis and secretion of PAB. Consider zinc status from dietary intake and medical history, in addition to inflammation, when interpreting low plasma PAB levels.

PAB levels are often normal in starvation-related malnutrition but decreased in well-nourished individuals who have undergone recent stress or trauma. During pregnancy, the changed estrogen levels stimulate PAB synthesis and serum levels may increase. In nephrotic syndrome, PAB levels also may be increased. Proteinuria and hypoproteinemia are common in nephrotic syndrome, and because PAB is synthesized rapidly, a disproportionate percentage of PAB can exist in the blood, whereas other proteins take longer to produce (Litchford, 2017).

Retinol-Binding Protein

The hepatic protein with the shortest half-life ($t\frac{1}{2} = 12$ hr) is retinol-binding protein (RBP), a small plasma protein that does not pass through the renal glomerulus because it circulates in a complex with PAB. As implied by its name, RBP binds retinol, and transport of this vitamin A metabolite seems to be its exclusive function. RBP is synthesized in the liver and released with retinol. After RBP releases retinol in peripheral tissue, its affinity for PAB decreases, leading to dissociation of the PAB-RBP complex and filtration of apoprotein (apo)-RBP by the glomerulus.

The plasma RBP concentration has been shown to decrease in starvation-related malnutrition. However, RBP levels also fall in the presence of inflammatory stress and may not improve with refeeding. RBP may not reflect protein status in acutely stressed patients. It may even be elevated with renal failure because the RBP is not being catabolized by the renal tubule.

RBP4 is an adipocyte-derived peptide of RBP that influences glucose homeostasis and lipoprotein metabolism. Human clinical trials have demonstrated increased RBP4 levels in obesity, insulin resistance, gestational diabetes, proliferative diabetic retinopathy, and nondiabetic stage 5 chronic kidney disease, ischemic stroke, suggesting a possible relationship between these conditions. Larger clinical trials are needed to define this relationship (Xun et al, 2018; Perduca et al, 2018; Klisić et al, 2017; Zhou et al, 2017).

Transferrin

Transferrin is a globulin protein that transports iron to the bone marrow for production of hemoglobin (Hgb). The plasma transferrin level is controlled by the size of the iron storage pool. When iron stores are depleted, transferrin synthesis increases. It has a shorter half-life ($t\frac{1}{2} = 8$ days) than albumin. Levels diminish with acute inflammatory reactions, malignancies, collagen vascular diseases, and liver diseases. Transferrin levels reflect inflammation and are not useful as a measure of protein status.

Immunocompetence

Inflammation-related malnutrition is associated with impaired immunocompetence, including depressed cell-mediated immunity, phagocyte dysfunction, decreased levels of complement components, reduced mucosal secretory antibody responses, and lower antibody affinity. Assessing immunocompetence (i.e., eosinophils) is also useful in the patient who is being treated for allergies (see Chapter 25).

There is no single marker for immunocompetence except for the clinical outcome of infection or allergic response. Laboratory markers with a high degree of sensitivity include vaccine-specific serum antibody production, delayed-type hypersensitivity response, vaccine-specific or total secretory immunoglobulin A in saliva, and the response to attenuated pathogens. Less sensitive markers include natural killer cell cytotoxicity, oxidative burst of phagocytes, lymphocyte proliferation, and the cytokine pattern produced by activated immune cells. Using a combination of markers is currently the best approach to measuring immunocompetence.

ASSESSMENT FOR NUTRITIONAL ANEMIAS

Anemia is a condition characterized by a reduction in the number of erythrocytes per unit of blood volume or a decrease in the Hgb of the blood to below the level of usual physiologic need. By convention, anemia is defined as Hgb concentration below the 95th percentile for healthy reference populations of men, women, or age-grouped children. Anemia is not a disease but a symptom of various conditions, including extensive blood loss, excessive blood cell destruction, or decreased blood cell formation. It is observed in many hospitalized patients and is often a symptom of a disease process; its cause should be investigated. Clinical nutritionists must distinguish between anemia caused by nutritional inadequacies and that caused by other factors (i.e., dehydration masking falsely low blood values). See Chapter 31 for discussion of the management of anemias.

Classification of Anemia

Nutritional deficits are a major cause of decreased Hgb and erythrocyte production. The initial descriptive classification of anemia is derived from the hematocrit (Hct) value or CBC as explained in Table 5.2. Anemias associated with a mean RBC volume of less than 80 fl (femtoliters) are microcytic; those with values of 80 to 99 fl are normocytic; those associated with values of 100 fl or more are macrocytic (see Chapter 32). Data from the CBC are helpful in identifying nutritional causes of anemia. Microcytic anemia is associated most often with iron deficiency, whereas macrocytic anemia generally is caused by either folate- or vitamin B_{12}–deficient erythropoiesis. However, because of the low specificity of these indexes, additional data are needed to distinguish between the various nutritional causes and nonnutritional causes, such as thalassemia trait and chronic renal insufficiency. Normocytic anemia is associated with the anemia of chronic and inflammatory disease (ACD). This type of anemia is associated with autoimmune diseases, rheumatic diseases, chronic heart failure, chronic infection, Hodgkin's disease and other types of cancer, inflammatory bowel disease, kidney disease and other chronic inflammatory conditions, severe tissue injury, and multiple fractures. ACD does not respond to iron supplementation.

Other information from the CBC that helps differentiate the nonnutritional causes of anemia includes leukocyte, reticulocyte, and platelet counts. When level of leukocytes, reticulocytes, and platelet counts are low, the pattern of results suggests marrow failure. Elevated levels of leukocytes, reticulocytes, and platelet counts are associated with anemia and likely caused by leukemia or infection. ESR testing is ordered when symptoms are nonspecific and if inflammatory autoimmune diseases are suspected. Reticulocytes are large, nucleated, immature RBCs that are released in small numbers with mature cells. When RBC production rates increase, reticulocyte counts also increase. Any time anemia is accompanied by a high reticulocyte count, elevated erythropoietic activity in response to bleeding should be considered. In such cases, stool specimens can be tested for occult blood to rule out chronic GI blood loss. Other causes of a high reticulocyte count include intravascular hemolysis syndromes and an erythropoietic response to therapy for iron, vitamin B_{12}, or folate deficiencies.

Normocytic or microcytic anemia may be caused by chronic or acute blood loss, such as from recent surgery, injury, or from the GI tract as indicated by a positive occult stool test. Note that in those with hemolytic anemias and early iron deficiency anemia, the RBC size may still be normal. Macrocytic anemias include folate deficiency and vitamin B_{12} deficiency. The presence of macrocytic RBCs requires evaluation of folate and vitamin B_{12} status. DNA synthesis is affected negatively by deficiencies of folic acid and vitamin B_{12}, resulting in impaired RBC synthesis and maturation of RBCs. These changes cause large, nucleated cells to be released into the circulation. Although vitamin B_{12}–related anemia is categorized as a macrocytic normochromic anemia, approximately 40% of the cases are normocytic.

Markers of Iron Deficiency Anemias

Hematocrit or Packed Cell Volume and Hemoglobin

Hct and Hgb are part of a routine CBC and are used together to evaluate iron status. Hct is the measure of the percentage of RBCs in total blood volume. Usually the Hct percentage is three times the Hgb concentration in grams per deciliter. The Hct value is affected by an extremely high WBC count and hydration status. Individuals living in high altitudes often have increased values. It is common for individuals older than age 50 to have slightly lower levels than younger adults.

The Hgb concentration is a measure of the total amount of Hgb in the peripheral blood. It is a more direct measure of iron deficiency than Hct because it quantifies total Hgb in RBCs rather than a percentage of total blood volume. Hgb and Hct are below normal in the four types of nutritional anemias and always should be evaluated in light of other laboratory values and recent medical history (see Chapter 31).

Serum Ferritin

Ferritin is the storage protein that sequesters the iron normally gathered in the liver (reticuloendothelial system), spleen, and marrow. As the iron supply increases, the intracellular level of ferritin increases to accommodate iron storage. A small amount of this ferritin leaks into the circulation. This ferritin can be measured by assays that are available in most clinical laboratories. In individuals with normal iron storage, 1 ng/mL of serum ferritin is about 8 mg of stored iron. In healthy adults, the measurement of ferritin that has leaked into the serum is an excellent indicator of the size of the body's iron storage pool.

ACD is the primary condition in which ferritin fails to correlate with iron stores. ACD, a common form of anemia in hospitalized patients, occurs in those with cancer or inflammatory or infectious disorders. It occurs during inflammation because red cell production decreases as the result of inadequate mobilization of iron from its storage sites. In those with chronic inflammatory conditions (i.e., arthritis) depletion of stored iron develops partly because of reduced absorption of iron from the gut due to release of hepcidin. Also the regular use of nonsteroidal antiinflammatory drugs can cause occult GI blood loss. ACD has many forms and must be distinguished from iron deficiency anemia so that inappropriate iron supplementation is not initiated.

Serum Iron

Serum iron measures the amount of circulating iron that is bound to transferrin. However, it is a relatively poor index of iron status because of large day-to-day changes, even in healthy individuals. Diurnal variations also occur, with the highest concentrations occurring midmorning (from 6 am to 10 am), and a nadir, averaging 30% less than the morning level, occurring midafternoon. Serum iron should be evaluated in light of other laboratory values and recent medical history to assess iron status.

Total Iron-Binding Capacity and Transferrin Saturation

Total iron-binding capacity (TIBC) is a direct measure of all proteins available to bind mobile iron and depends on the number of free binding sites on the plasma iron-transport protein transferrin. Intracellular iron availability regulates the synthesis and secretion of transferrin (i.e., transferrin concentration increases in those with iron deficiency).

Transferrin saturation reflects iron availability to tissues (bone marrow erythropoiesis). It is determined by the following equation:

$$\% \text{ Transferrin saturation} = (\text{Serum Fe} / \text{TIBC}) \times 100$$

In addition, when the amount of stored iron available for release to transferrin decreases and dietary iron intake is low, saturation of transferrin decreases.

There are exceptions to the general rule that transferrin saturation decreases and TIBC increases in patients with iron deficiency. For example, TIBC increases in those with hepatitis. It also increases in people with hypoxia, women who are pregnant, or those taking oral contraceptives or receiving estrogen replacement therapy. On the other hand, TIBC decreases in those with malignant disease, nephritis, and hemolytic anemias. Furthermore, the plasma level of transferrin may be decreased in those with malnutrition, fluid overload, and liver disease. Thus although TIBC and transferrin saturation are more specific than Hct or Hgb values, they are not perfect indicators of iron status.

An additional concern about the use of serum iron, TIBC, and transferrin saturation values is that normal values persist until frank deficiency actually develops. Thus these tests cannot detect decreasing iron stores and iron insufficiencies.

Tests for Macrocytic Anemias From B Vitamin Deficiencies

Macrocytic anemias include folate deficiency and vitamin B_{12} deficiency. The nutritional causes of macrocytic anemia are related to the availability of folate and vitamin B_{12} in the bone marrow and require evaluation of both nutrient levels and methyl malonic acid, an intermediate metabolites of vitamin B_{12} metabolism. Both nutrients decrease DNA synthesis by preventing the formation of thymidine monophosphate. Folate and vitamin B_{12} are used at different steps of the synthetic pathway. Impaired RBC synthesis occurs and large, nucleated RBCs then are released into the circulation (see Chapter 31).

Assessing Folate and Vitamin B_{12} Status

Evaluation for macrocytic anemia includes static measurement of folate and vitamin B_{12} deficiency in blood. They can be assayed using tests of the ability of the patient's blood specimen to support the growth of microbes that require either folate or vitamin B_{12}, or radiobinding assays, or immunoassays.

Serum homocysteine. Folate and vitamin B_{12} are required for the synthesis of S-adenosylmethionine (SAM), the biochemical precursor involved in the transfer of one-carbon (methyl) groups during many biochemical syntheses. SAM is synthesized from the amino acid methionine by a reaction that includes the addition of a methyl group and the purine base adenine (from adenosine triphosphate, or ATP). For example, when SAM donates a methyl group for the synthesis of thymidine, choline, creatine, epinephrine, and protein and DNA methylation, it is converted to S-adenosylhomocysteine. After losing the adenosyl group, the remaining homocysteine can be converted either to cysteine by the vitamin B_6–dependent transsulfuration pathway or back to methionine in a reaction that depends on adequate folate and vitamin B_{12}.

When either folate or vitamin B_{12} is lacking, the homocysteine-to-methionine reaction is blocked, causing homocysteine to build up in the affected tissue and spill into the circulation. The vitamin B_6–dependent transsulfuration pathway can metabolize excess homocysteine. Homocysteine has been shown to be sensitive to folate and vitamin B_{12} deficiency.

Therefore an elevated homocysteine level indicates either genetic defects involved in the enzymes that catalyze these reactions, or a deficiency in folate, vitamin B_{12}, or vitamin B_6. Research indicates that several folate gene polymorphisms affecting the methylation of folate and B_{12} contribute risk for several chronic cardiovascular and neurologic disorders (Kagawa et al, 2017; see Chapters 6 and 42).

Folate assessment. Folate most often is measured simultaneously in whole blood with its combined amount from plasma and blood cells, and in the serum alone. The difference between whole-blood folate and serum folate levels then is used to calculate total RBC folate concentration. RBC folate concentration is a better indicator of folate status than serum folate, because folate is much more concentrated in RBCs than in the serum. RBC folate measurement more closely reflects tissue stores and is considered the most reliable indicator of folate status. Folate is absorbed in the jejunum, and its malabsorption has several causes, but a specific test for folate absorption is not available. The presence and extent of deficiency should be assessed in patients with celiac disease, those who have had malabsorptive bariatric surgery, those with a history of long-term use of medications such as anticonvulsants and sulfasalazine, those with chronic alcohol consumption, those with methyltetrahydrofolate reductase (MTHFR) genetic polymorphisms, and those with rheumatoid arthritis taking methotrexate (see Chapters 5 and 8).

Vitamin B_{12} assessment. Vitamin B_{12} is measured in the serum, and all indications are that the serum level gives as much information about vitamin B_{12} status as does the RBC level. If vitamin B_{12} status is compromised, intrinsic factor antibodies (IFAB) and parietal cell antibodies are measured; the presence of antibodies suggests the main cause of macrocytic anemia. Historically the Schilling test was used to detect defects in vitamin B_{12} absorption; it rarely is used today because the test requires that the patient be given radioactive vitamin B_{12} (see Chapter 32). Methylmalonic acid (MMA) levels in serum or urine are more useful to assess B_{12} status.

Vitamin B_{12} and methylmalonic acid. Once a genetic or autoimmune cause is ruled out, the most straightforward biochemical method for differentiating between folate and vitamin B_{12} deficiencies is by measuring the serum or urinary MMA level. MMA is formed during the degradation of the amino acid valine and odd-chain fatty acids. MMA is the side product in this metabolic pathway that increases when the conversion of methylmalonic coenzyme A (CoA) to succinyl CoA is blocked by lack of vitamin B_{12}, a coenzyme for this reaction. Therefore deficiency leads to an increase in the MMA pool, which is reflected by the serum or urinary MMA level. The urinary MMA test is more sensitive than the serum B_{12} test because it indicates true tissue B_{12} deficiency. The serum MMA test may give falsely high values in renal insufficiency and intravascular volume depletion. The urinary MMA test is the only B_{12} deficiency assay that has been validated as a screening tool. Homocysteine and MMA tend to detect impending vitamin deficiencies better than the static assays. This is especially important when assessing the status of certain patients such as vegans or older adults, who could have vitamin B_{12} deficiency associated with central nervous system impairment.

FAT-SOLUBLE VITAMINS

Fat malabsorption often results in impaired absorption of vitamins A, E, D, and K. Factors including low luminal pH, bile salts below the critical micellar concentration, and inadequate triglyceride hydrolysis can interfere with normal bile salt micelle formation, causing impaired absorption of fat-soluble vitamins. Individuals with fat malabsorptive disorders, including those who have had bariatric surgery, are at greatest risk of deficiencies of fat-soluble vitamins. See Appendix 12 for further discussion of tests for assessing specific vitamin adequacy.

Vitamin A

Vitamin A status can be estimated using serum retinol, and the normal level in adults is 30 to 80 mcg/dL. A primary deficiency of vitamin A can result from inadequate intake, fat malabsorption, or liver disorders. A secondary deficiency of vitamin A may be due to decreased bioavailability of provitamin A carotenoids or interference with vitamin A absorption, storage, or transport (e.g., celiac disease, cystic fibrosis, pancreatic insufficiency, malabsorptive weight loss surgery, or bile duct obstruction). Vitamin A deficiency is common in prolonged malnutrition and reported a year or longer after gastric bypass surgery and biliopancreatic weight loss surgery (Parrott et al, 2017). The oxidative stress associated with major surgeries, including gastric bypass surgery, also may interfere with vitamin A absorption and use. Because of shared absorptive mechanisms with vitamin D, serum retinol always should be assessed in the presence of vitamin D supplementation.

Acute or chronic vitamin A toxicity is defined as retinol levels greater than 100 mcg/dL. Hypervitaminosis A has been reported in almost 50% of patients taking 150% of the RDA for vitamin A, in the form of retinol, between 6 to 12 months after laparoscopic sleeve gastrectomy (Aarts et al, 2011). Chronic vitamin A toxicities are associated with loss of hair; dry mucous membranes; dry, rough skin; and even cortical bone loss and fractures (see Appendix 12).

Vitamin D

Individual vitamin D status can be estimated by measuring plasma 25 hydroxy vitamin D (25[OH]D$_3$) levels. Current clinical practice reference ranges have been updated by the Institute of Medicine (IOM, 2011). Traditional levels defining vitamin D sufficiency have been based on the lowest threshold value for plasma 25(OH)D$_3$ (approximately 80 nmol/L or 32 ng/mL) that prevents secondary hyperparathyroidism, increased bone turnover, bone mineral loss, or seasonal variations in plasma parathyroid hormone. The IOM review concluded that individuals are at risk of deficiency at serum 25(OH)D$_3$ levels below 30 nmol or 12 ng/mL and that practically all persons have sufficient serum levels at 50 nmol or 20 ng/mL. The American Geriatric Society (AGS) published a new consensus statement on vitamin D and calcium supplementation for reduction of falls and fractures in adults 65 years and older and for high-risk populations with malabsorption syndromes, those using medications that accelerate vitamin D metabolism, the obese, and those with minimal sun exposure (AGS, 2014).

Vitamin D sufficiency is defined as 25(OH)D$_3$ at 75 nmol/L, or 30 ng/mL (AGS, 2014). Serum levels even higher at 90 to 100 nmol/L (36 to 40 ng/mL) are recommended by some (Bischoff-Ferrari, 2014). The U.S. Preventive Services Task Force (USPSTF) found adequate evidence that daily supplementation with 400 IU or less of vitamin D and 1000 mg or less of calcium—or greater than 400 IU vitamin D or greater than 1000 mg calcium—had no benefit for the primary prevention of fractures in community-dwelling, postmenopausal women without a history of osteoporotic fractures, increased risk for falls, or a diagnosis of osteoporosis (USPSTF, 2018). Optimal levels of 25(OH) D$_3$ have not been defined, and the measurement of serum levels lacks standardization and calibration.

A vitamin D deficiency may be due to inadequate dietary intake, inadequate exposure to sunlight, or malabsorption. Deficiency of vitamin D also can lead to secondary malabsorption of calcium. Calcium malabsorption occurs in chronic renal failure because renal hydroxylation is required to activate vitamin D, which promotes synthesis of a calcium-binding protein in intestinal absorptive cells (see Chapter 34).Vitamin D toxicity is rare, but it has been reported in a few patients taking megadoses of vitamin D. Reported adverse effects include hypercalcemia, hyperphosphatemia, suppressed parathyroid-hormone levels, and hypercalciuria (Taylor and Davies, 2018).

Vitamin E

Vitamin E status can be estimated by measuring serum alpha-tocopherol or the ratio of serum alpha-tocopherol to total serum lipids. A low ratio suggests vitamin E deficiency. Deficiencies are uncommon in the developed world except in individuals with fat malabsorption syndromes. The main symptoms of a vitamin E deficiency include mild hemolytic anemia and nonspecific neurologic effects. In adults, alpha-tocopherol levels less than 5 μg/mL (<11.6 μmol/L) are associated with a deficiency. In adults with hyperlipidemia, a low ratio of serum alpha-tocopherol to lipids (<0.8 mg/g total lipid) is the most accurate indicator.

Vitamin E toxicity is uncommon, but intakes of vitamin E greater than 1000 mg/d may result in a significant bleeding risk, especially if the individual is taking anticoagulation medications. A meta-analysis of the relationship between supplemental vitamin E and all-cause mortality demonstrated that supplementation with vitamin E appears to have no effect on all-cause mortality at doses up to 5500 IU/d (Abner et al, 2011).

Vitamin K

Vitamin K status can be estimated using prothrombin time (PT). PT is used to evaluate the common pathway of blood clotting. The synthesis of clotting factors II, VII, IX, and X are vitamin K dependent. Osteocalcin or bone G1a protein (BGP), a bone turnover marker, may also be used to assess vitamin K status. The production of BGP is stimulated by 1,25 dihydroxy vitamin D (1,25[OH]$_2$D$_3$) and depends on vitamin K. Vitamin K increases the carboxylation of osteocalcin or BGP, but it does not increase its overall rate of synthesis. A reduced vitamin K status is associated with reduced BGP or serum osteocalcin levels. This relationship may explain the pathophysiologic findings of vitamin K–deficiency osteoporosis. The function of osteocalcin is unclear; however, it may exist as a deposition site for hydroxyapatite crystals or it also may affect energy metabolism via the production and action of insulin (Hammami, 2014).

WATER-SOLUBLE VITAMINS AND TRACE MINERALS

Ascorbic Acid

Ascorbic acid or vitamin C is a water-soluble vitamin and also an antioxidant. Vitamin C status can be determined by measuring blood ascorbic acid levels. Values less than 6 mg/dL (<34 micromol/L) suggest insufficiency and values less than 2 mg/dL (<11 micromol/L) suggest a deficiency. Deficiencies are rare in developed countries unless self-imposed dietary intake is highly restrictive. Symptoms of a deficiency include bleeding gums, loose teeth, poor wound healing, and perifollicular hemorrhages. Toxicities have been reported in individuals taking more than 2 g/d for an extended period of time. Individuals consuming more than 1000 mg of ascorbic acid daily may increase their risk of kidney stones. Rebound scurvy may occur in individuals who abruptly stop taking megadoses of ascorbic acid (Ferraro et al, 2016).

B-Vitamins

Vitamin B$_{12}$ and folate are the most common water-soluble vitamin deficiencies reported in adults. Frank deficiencies of other water-soluble vitamins and trace minerals are uncommon in populations that consume a variety of whole foods and fortified foods. Thiamin deficiency has been reported in individuals who chronically consume high levels of alcohol with inadequate thiamin intake, in those with persistent vomiting, in those on high doses of diuretics with poor intake, in those with impaired absorption because of disease or surgery, as well as individuals on long-term parenteral nutrition (PN) without adequate vitamin added. To assess thiamin status, thiamin diphosphate in whole blood is measured because plasma and serum levels reflect recent dietary changes and may be misleading. A deficiency of thiamin results in either wet beriberi, dry beriberi, or Wernicke encephalopathy (WE). Symptoms of wet beriberi include heart failure, tachycardia, and lactic acidosis. Symptoms of dry beriberi are primarily neurologic findings (i.e. peripheral neuropathy, impairment of sensory, motor, and reflex functions). Symptoms of WE include abnormal eye movement, cerebellar dysfunction, and confusion.

Subclinical deficiencies of water-soluble vitamins and other trace minerals may be present in some individuals. However, the current methodologies for evaluating nutritional status of these components are expensive and controversial. See Appendix 12 for further discussion of tests for assessing specific vitamin and trace mineral adequacy.

Markers of Body Composition
Creatinine

Creatinine is formed from creatine, found almost exclusively in muscle tissue. Serum creatinine is used along with blood urea nitrogen (BUN) to assess kidney function (see Chapter 34). Urinary creatinine has been used to assess somatic (muscle) protein status. Creatine is synthesized from the amino acids glycine and arginine with addition of a methyl group from the folate- and cobalamin-dependent methionine–SAM–homocysteine cycle. Creatine phosphate is a high-energy phosphate buffer that provides a constant supply of ATP for muscle contraction. When creatine is dephosphorylated, some of it is converted spontaneously to creatinine by an irreversible, nonenzymatic reaction. Creatinine has no specific biologic function; it is released continuously from the muscle cells and excreted by the kidneys with little reabsorption.

The use of urinary creatinine to assess somatic protein status is confounded by omnivorous diets. Because creatine is stored in muscle, muscle meats are rich sources. The creatinine formed from dietary creatine cannot be distinguished from endogenously produced creatinine. When a person follows a meat-restricted diet, the size of the somatic (muscle) protein pool is directly proportional to the amount of creatinine excreted. Therefore men generally have higher serum levels and excrete larger amounts of creatinine than women, and individuals with greater muscular development have higher serum levels and excrete larger amounts than those who are less muscular. Total body weight is not proportional to creatinine excretion, but muscle mass is. Creatinine excretion rate is related to muscle mass and is expressed as a percentage of a standard value as shown by the following equation for creatinine-height index (CHI):

$$CHI = \text{24-hr urine creatinine (mg)} \times 100 \div$$
$$\text{Expected 24-hr urine creatinine/cm height}$$

Calculated CHI greater than 80% is normal, 60% to 80% suggests mild skeletal muscle depletion, 40% to 60% suggests moderate depletion, and less than 40% suggests severe depletion (Blackburn et al, 1977).

Daily creatinine excretion varies significantly within individuals, probably because of losses in sweat. In addition, the test is based on 24-hour urine collections, which are difficult to obtain. Because of these limitations, urinary creatinine concentration as a marker of muscle mass has limited use in health care settings and is used typically only in research (Table 5.6).

TABLE 5.6 Expected Urinary Creatinine Excretions for Adults Based on Height

ADULT MALES*		ADULT FEMALES†	
Height (cm)	Creatinine (mg)	Height (cm)	Creatinine (mg)
157.5	1288	147.3	830
160.0	1325	149.9	851
162.6	1359	152.9	875
165.1	1386	154.9	900
167.6	1426	157.5	925
170.2	1467	160.0	949
172.7	1513	162.6	977
175.3	1555	165.1	1006
177.8	1596	167.6	1044
180.3	1642	170.2	1076
182.9	1691	172.7	1109
185.4	1739	175.3	1141
188.0	1785	177.8	1174
190.5	1831	180.3	1206
193.0	1891	182.9	1240

*Creatinine coefficient males 23 mg/kg "ideal" body weight.
†Creatinine coefficient females 18 mg/kg "ideal" body weight.

Nitrogen Balance

Nitrogen balance studies are used primarily in research studies to estimate the balance between exogenous nitrogen intake (orally, enterally, or parenterally) and removal of nitrogen-containing compounds (urinary, fecal, wound), and other nitrogen sources. These studies are not a measure of protein anabolism and catabolism because true protein turnover studies require consumption of labeled (stable isotope) protein to track protein use. Even if useful, nitrogen balance studies are difficult because valid 24-hour urine collections are tedious unless the patient has a catheter. In addition, changes in renal function are common in patients with inflammatory metabolism, making standard nitrogen balance calculations inaccurate without calculation of nitrogen retention (Dickerson, 2016). Clinicians using nitrogen balance to estimate protein flux in critically ill patients must remember the limitations of these studies and that positive nitrogen balance may not mean that protein catabolism has decreased, particularly in inflammatory (disease and trauma) conditions.

CHRONIC DISEASE RISK ASSESSMENT

Lipid Indices of Cardiovascular Risk

The American College of Cardiology (ACC) and American Heart Association (AHA) released practice guidelines for the assessment of cardiovascular risk (Stone et al, 2014). These guidelines are referred to as the Adult Treatment Panel 4 (ATP 4) and replace the Adult Treatment Panel 3 (ATP 3). Four high-risk groups are identified:
- Adults with atherosclerotic cardiovascular disease (ASCVD)
- Adults with diabetes, aged 40 to 75 years, with low-density lipoprotein (LDL) levels 70 to 189 mg/dL
- Adults with LDL cholesterol levels of at least 190 mg/dL
- Adults aged 40 to 75 years who have LDL levels 70 to 189 mg/dL and at least 7.5% 10-year risk of atherosclerotic cardiovascular disease

Ten-year risk of atherosclerotic cardiovascular disease is determined using the Framingham 10-year general cardiovascular disease risk equations. Risk factors include age, gender, total cholesterol, high-density lipoprotein (HDL) cholesterol, smoking status, systolic blood pressure, and current treatment for high blood pressure (Box 5.1). The ACC/AHA Guidelines deemphasize use of any markers other than LDL cholesterol and HDL cholesterol. Emerging risk markers for atherosclerotic cardiovascular disease (ACVD) that are not recommended in ATP 4 include differentiating subparticles of LDL by size and grouping by pattern, apolipoprotein B (apoB), and apolipoprotein E (apoE) phenotype. The Cholesterol Expert Panel determined that these markers are not independent markers for risk and do not add to prediction equations. Other researchers propose mathematical models that predict the risk of plaque formation for combined levels of LDL and HDL (Hao and Friedman, 2014). However, the Systematic Review for the 2018 AHA, ACC, and numerous professional organizations and societies published *Guideline on the Management of Blood Cholesterol*. These Guidelines proposed the use of nonstatin lipid modifying medications to reduce the risk of ASCVD. PCSK9 inhibitors and ezetimibe were identified as beneficial, but niacin and cholesterol-ester protein inhibitors were not effective in reducing ASCVD risk (Grundy et al, 2018).

See Chapter 32 for further discussion of the lipid profile and cardiovascular risk.

BOX 5.1 Lipid And Lipoprotein Atherosclerotic Cardiovascular Risk Factors

Laboratory test cutpoints used to calculate 10-year risk of ACVD

Total cholesterol: >200 mg/dL

HDL: <40 mg/dL

LDL: >131 mg/dL

In selected high-risk individuals, these laboratory test cutpoints may be considered:

hs-CRP cutpoints used to assign risk

- <1.0 mg/L = low risk
- 1.1-3.0 mg/L = average risk
- 3.1-9.9 mg/L = high risk
- ≥10 mg/L = very high risk
- If initial value is >3.0 but <10 mg/L, repeat in 2 weeks

Lipoprotein-associated phospholipase A₂ (Lp-PLA₂): used in conjunction with hs-CRP with intermediate or high risk

Apolipoprotein A-1: May be used in addition to LDL-C monitoring as a non-HDL-C marker in patients with serum triglycerides ≥200 mg/dL; decreased level is atherogenic

Apolipoprotein B/A ratio: May be used in addition to LDL-C monitoring as a non-HDL-C marker in patients with serum triglycerides ≥200 mg/dL

Other laboratory test results associated with cardiovascular risk, but not recommended in ATP 4

VLDL density: Remnants are atherogenic

Lp(a): Elevated levels are atherogenic

Serum homocysteine: Increased = greater risk

RBP4: Elevated levels may identify early insulin resistance and associated cardiovascular risk factors

HDL, High-density lipoprotein; *hs-CRP,* high-sensitivity C-reactive protein; *LDL,* low-density lipoprotein; *Lp(a),* lipoprotein little a; *RBP4,* retinol-binding protein 4; *VLDL,* very low-density lipoprotein. Adapted from Stone NJ et al: 2013 ACC/AHA guideline on the treatment of blood cholesterol to reduce atherosclerotic cardiovascular risk in adults: a report of the American College of Cardiology/American Heart Association Task Force on practice guidelines, *Circulation* 129(25 Suppl 2):S1, 2014.

The National Lipid Association (NLA) Expert Panel presents somewhat different treatment goals from the ATP 4. The NLA includes treatment goals for non–HDL cholesterol, LDL cholesterol, and apoB (Jacobson et al, 2014; see Chapter 32).

Patients undergoing lipid assessments should be fasting for 12 hours at the time of blood sampling. Fasting is necessary primarily because triglyceride levels rise and fall dramatically in the postprandial state, and LDL cholesterol values are calculated from measured total serum cholesterol and HDL cholesterol concentrations. This calculation, based on the Friedewald equation, is most accurate when triglyceride concentrations are less than 400 mg/dL.

$$\text{LDL} = \text{Total Cholesterol} - (\text{Triglyceride}/5) - \text{HDL}.$$

The Friedewald equation gives an estimate of fasting LDL cholesterol levels that is generally within 4 mg/dL of the true value when triglyceride concentrations are less than 400 mg/dL (Friedewald, 1972).

Diabetes

In adults with normal glucose control, approximately 4% to 6% of the total Hgb is glycosylated. The percent of this glycohemoglobin or hemoglobin A1C (Hgb A1C) in the blood is related directly to the average blood glucose levels for the preceding 2 to 3 months and does not reflect more recent changes in glucose levels. It is useful in differentiating between short-term hyperglycemia in individuals under stress or who have had an acute myocardial infarction and those with diabetes. Hgb A1C has been added as a diagnostic criterion for diagnosis of diabetes mellitus once the initial value is confirmed by a repeat Hgb A1C above 6.5%, or plasma glucose above 200 mg/dL (11 mmol/L). Historically, Hgb A1C was not used as a diagnostic criterion for gestational diabetes because of changes in red cell turnover (American Diabetes Association [ADA], 2018). Other researchers suggest that combined Hgb A1C and oral glucose tolerance test (OGTT) may be useful in diagnosing gestational diabetes (Renz et al, 2015).

Hgb A1C can be correlated with daily mean plasma glucose (Box 5.2). Each 1% change in Hgb A1C represents approximately 35 mg/dL change in mean plasma glucose. Test results are useful to provide feedback to patients about changes they have made in their nutritional intakes (ADA, 2011). See Chapter 29 for further discussion of Hgb A1C and diabetes management.

Insulin test results reflect both endogenous and exogenous insulin. It may also be used in differentiate type 1 and type 2 diabetes, to diagnose type 2 diabetes in which there is an increased production of insulin with a concurrent increase in blood glucose. Insulin testing is used to identify the etiology of hypoglycemia (plasma glucose < 55 mg/dL) especially if there is a shortage of glucose to the brain due to hypoglycemia and the patient is unconscious due to hypoglycemia. Conditions associated with elevated insulin levels are metabolic syndrome (cluster of conditions associated with the development of type 2 diabetes and cardiovascular disease), obesity, steroid use, acromegaly (abnormal

BOX 5.2 Correlation Between A1C and Mean Plasma Glucose (MPG)

A1C	Approximate MPG (mg/dL)
4	65
5	100
6	135
7	170
8	205

growth of hand hands, feet, and face caused by overproduction of growth hormone by the pituitary gland), Cushing's syndrome (complex hormonal condition manifest with thinning skin, weakness, weight gain, bruising, hypertension, diabetes, osteopetrosis, facial puffiness), type 2 diabetes, insulinoma (tumor of pancreas that produces an excess amount of insulin). Conditions associated with decreased insulin excretion include severe liver disease, type 1 diabetes, and severe heart failure (Buppajarntham, 2014).

C-Peptide

C-peptide is an insulin precursor that is released from the pancreatic beta-cells during cleavage of insulin from proinsulin. It is excreted by the kidney and has a half-life 3 to 4 times longer than that of insulin. C-peptide levels are elevated with insulinomas, sulfonylurea intoxication, insulin resistance, and chronic kidney disease. It is suppressed in type 1 diabetes, and insulin-independent hypoglycemia. C-peptide should be measured in combination with insulin and proinsulin to differentiate between insulin-dependent hypoglycemia and insulin-independent hypoglycemia.

PHYSICAL ASSESSMENTS

Anthropometry

Anthropometry involves obtaining physical measurements of an individual, comparing them to standards that reflect the growth and development of that individual, and using them for evaluating overnutrition, undernutrition, or the effects of nutrition preventions over a period of time. Accurate and consistent measurements require training in the proper techniques using calibrated instruments. Measurements of accuracy can be established by several clinicians taking the same measurement and comparing results. Valuable anthropometric measurements include height, weight, and girth measurements. Skinfold thicknesses and circumference measurements are used in some settings but are associated with a higher rate of inconsistency. Head circumference and length are used in pediatric populations. Birth weight and ethnic, familial, and environmental factors affect these parameters and should be considered when anthropometric measures are evaluated.

Interpretation of Height and Weight in Children and Teens

Currently, reference standards are based on a statistical sample of the U.S. population. The World Health Organization (WHO) international growth standards are based on data from multiple countries and ethnic populations and have been adopted for use in numerous countries. In the United States the expert review panel of WHO and Centers for Disease Control and Prevention (CDC) growth charts recommend the WHO growth standards for children aged less than 24 months and the CDC growth charts for children aged 24 months to 18 years.

Height and weight measurements of children are recorded as percentiles, which reflect the percentage of the total population of children of the same sex who are at or below the same height or weight at a certain age. Children's growth at every age can be monitored by mapping data on growth curves, known as height-for-age, length-for-age, weight-for-age, and weight-for-length curves. Appendix 4 provides pediatric growth charts and percentile interpretations.

Length and Height

The methodology used for determining the length or height of children is determined by the age of the child. Recumbent length measurements are used for infants and children younger than 2 or 3 years of age. Ideally these young children should be measured using a length board as shown in Fig. 5.3. Recumbent lengths in children ages 2 and younger

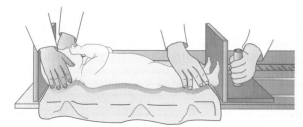

Fig. 5.3 Measurement of the length of an infant.

should be recorded on the birth to 24-month growth grids. Standing height is determined in children using a measuring rod, or statiometer, and should be recorded on the 2- to 20-year growth grids, as in Appendix 4. Sitting heights may be measured in children who cannot stand (see Fig. 43.1). Recording on the proper growth grids provides a record of a child's gain in height over time and compares the child's height with that of other children of the same age. The rate of length or height gain reflects long-term nutritional adequacy.

Weight

Weight in children and teens is a more sensitive measure of nutritional adequacy than height, because it reflects more recent nutritional intake and provides a rough estimate of overall fat and muscle reserves. For children with larger bodies or in those with edema, weight alone makes it difficult to assess overall nutritional status. Weight should be recorded on the age- and gender-appropriate growth grid.

Body weight is interpreted using various methods, including body mass index (BMI), usual weight, and actual weight. BMI is used as a screening tool to identify children and teens who are at risk for overweight or underweight. BMI does not distinguish between excess fat, muscle, and bone mass or fat distribution and should be considered in the context of other growth assessment measurements. Although the calculation of BMI is the same for adults and children, the interpretation of BMI is different in children and teens. BMI is plotted on the CDC BMI-for-age growth charts from which a percentile ranking can be determined. These percentiles are the most commonly used indicator to assess the size and growth patterns of children and teens aged 2 to 20 years in the United States (see Appendix 4). Consistent plotting within a growth channel between the 5% to 85% is considered normal growth although healthy outliers do exist. BMI-for-age weight status categories are noted in Box 5.3.

Interpretation of Height and Weight in Adults

In adults, height and weight measurements are also useful for evaluating nutrition status. Both should be measured because the tendency is to overestimate height and underestimate weight, resulting in an underestimation of the relative weight or BMI. In addition, many adults are losing height as a result of osteoporosis, joint deterioration, and poor posture, and this should be documented.

Measurements of height can be obtained using a direct or an indirect approach. The direct method involves a stadiometer, and the

BOX 5.3 Interpretation of BMI-for-Age Percentiles in Children and Teens	
Percentile Range	**Interpretation**
Less than 5th percentile	Underweight
5th percentile to less than 85th percentile	Healthy weight
85th percentile to less than the 95th percentile	Overweight
Equal to or greater than the 95th percentile	Obese

adult must be able to stand straight or recline flat. Indirect methods, including knee-height measurements, arm span, or recumbent length using a tape measure, may be options for those who cannot stand or stand straight, such as individuals with scoliosis, kyphosis (curvature of the spine), cerebral palsy, muscular dystrophy, contractures, paralysis, or those who are bedridden (see Appendix 6). Recumbent height measurements made with a tape measure while the person is in bed may be appropriate for individuals in institutions who are comatose, critically ill, or unable to be moved. However, this method can be used only with patients who do not have musculoskeletal deformities or contractures (see Box 5.4).

Ideal weight for height reference standards such as the Metropolitan Life Insurance Tables from 1959 and 1983 or the National Health and Nutrition Examination Survey percentiles are no longer used. A commonly used method of determining ideal body weight is the Hamwi Equation (Hamwi et al, 1964). It does not adjust for age, race, or frame size and its validity is questionable. Nonetheless, it is in widespread use by clinicians as a quick method for estimation of ideal weight:

Men: 106 lb for first 5 feet of height and 6 lb per inch over 5 feet; or 6 lb subtracted for each inch under 5 feet

Women: 100 lb for first 5 feet of height and 5 lb per inch over 5 feet; or 5 lb subtracted for each inch under 5 feet

Using the Hamwi method a female who is 5 feet 5 inches tall would have an ideal weight of 125 lb.

Actual body weight is the weight measurement obtained at the time of examination. This measurement may be influenced by changes in the individual's fluid status. Weight loss can reflect dehydration but also can reflect a pattern of suboptimal food intake. The percentage of weight loss is highly indicative of the extent and severity of an individual's illness. The Characteristics of Malnutrition defined by the Academy of Nutrition and Dietetics (AND) and the American Society for Parenteral and Enteral Nutrition (ASPEN) serve as a benchmark for evaluating weight loss (White et al, 2012):

- Significant weight loss: 5% loss in a month, 7.5% loss in 3 months, 10% loss in 6 months
- Severe weight loss: >5% weight loss in a month, >7.5% weight loss in 3 months, >10% weight loss in 6 months

Percentage weight loss = Usual wt − Actual wt/ Usual wt × 100

- For example, if a person's usual weight is 200 lb and he now weighs 180 lb, that is a weight loss of 20 lb.

200 to 180 = 20lb/200lb = 0.10 or 10%

- If this person has lost this 10% in 2 months, that would be more than 7.5% in 3 months and considered SEVERE weight loss.

Another method for evaluating the percentage of weight loss is to calculate an individual's current weight as a percentage of usual weight. Usual body weight (UBW) is a more useful parameter than ideal body weight (IBW) for those who are experiencing involuntary weight loss. However, one problem with using UBW is that it may depend on the patient's memory.

BOX 5.4 Using Height and Weight to Assess a Hospitalized Patient's Nutritional Status

- Measure. Do not just ask a person's height.
- Measure weight (at admission at admission and current).
- Determine percentage of weight change over time (weight pattern).
- Determine percentage above or below usual or ideal body weight.

Body Mass Index

The Quetelet index (W/H^2) or the body mass index (BMI) is used to determine whether an adult's weight is appropriate for height and can indicate overnutrition or undernutrition. BMI accounts for differences in body composition by defining the level of adiposity and relating it to height, thus eliminating dependence on frame size (Stensland and Margolis, 1990). Numerous research studies have demonstrated that individuals with a higher BMI are more likely to experience obesity-related health issues (Flegal et al, 2013), however there is no single body fat measure that clearly differentiates between health from disease or risk of disease. BMI is calculated as follows:

Metric: BMI = Weight (kg) ÷ Height (m)^2

English: BMI = Weight (lb) ÷ Height (in)^2 × 703

Nomograms are also available to calculate BMI, as are various charts (see Appendix 8). The Clinical Insight box: *Calculating BMI and Determining Appropriate Body Weight* gives an example of the BMI calculation.

CLINICAL INSIGHT

Calculating BMI and Determining Appropriate Body Weight

Example: Woman who is 5′8″ (68 in) tall and weighs 185 pounds (lb)
Step 1: Calculate current BMI:
Formula: (Metric)   Weight (kg) 84 kg ÷ Height (m²) (1.72 m) × (1.72 m)
= 84 ÷ 2.96 m² = BMI = 28.4 = overweight
Step 2: Appropriate weight range to have a BMI that falls between 18.5 and 24.9
18.5   (18.5) × (2.96) = 54.8 kg = 121 lb
24.9   (24.9) × (2.96) = 73.8 kg = 162 lb
Appropriate weight range = 121 − 162 lb or 54.8 − 73.8 kg

Formula (English) Weight (lb) ÷ (Height [in] × Height [in]) × 703 = BMI
BMI, Body mass index.

Standards classify a BMI of less than 18.5 for an adult as underweight, a BMI between 25 and 29.9 as overweight, and a BMI greater than 30 as obese. A healthy BMI for adults is considered between 18.5 and 24.9 (CDC, 2018). There are some clinical limitations to the use of BMI as a measure of body fatness. Age, sex, ethnicity, and muscle mass can influence the relationship between BMI and body fat. BMI does not distinguish between excess fat, muscle, and bone mass or fat distribution. BMI is correlated with weight more than fat (CDC, 2018). BMI values tend to increase with age and thereby increasing risk for obesity-related health issues. However, for older adults with chronic conditions, there is increasing evidence that an obesity paradox exists in which an elevated BMI is associated with lower all-cause and cardiovascular mortality compared with patients with lower weight (Winter et al, 2014; Hainer and Aldhoon-Hainerová, 2013; see Chapter 19).

Body Composition

Body composition is a critical component of nutrition assessment and medical status. It is used concurrently with other assessment factors to differentiate the estimated proportions of fat mass, soft tissue body mass, and bone mass. For example, muscular people and athletes may be wrongly classified as overweight because of excess muscle mass contributing to increased weight rather than excessive adipose tissue. Older adults tend to have lower bone density and reduced lean body mass and therefore may weigh less than younger adults of the same height and yet have greater adiposity. Variation in body composition exists among different population groups as well as within the same group. The majority of body composition studies that were performed on whites may not be valid for other ethnic groups. There are differences and similarities between blacks and whites relative to fat-free body mass, fat patterning, and body dimensions and proportions; blacks have greater bone mineral density and body protein compared with whites (Wagner and Heyward, 2000). In addition, optimal BMIs for Asian populations must be in the lower ranges of "normal" for optimal health to reflect their higher risk for cardiovascular disease and diabetes (Araneta et al, 2015). These factors must be considered to avoid inaccurate estimation of body fat and interpretation of risk.

Imaging techniques such as dual-energy x-ray absorptiometry (DXA) and magnetic resonance imaging (MRI) are used in research and clinical settings to assess body composition. The focus of the research on different imaging methodologies is to quantify characteristics of lean soft tissue (LST) that predicts clinical risk and nutrition status. Areas of greatest research are to assess for sarcopenia, sarcopenic obesity (individuals with obesity, low muscle mass, low muscle strength, and low physical performance), and osteosarcopenic obesity (individuals with obesity, bone loss, low muscle mass, low muscle strength, and low physical performance) (Prado and Heymsfield, 2014).

Subcutaneous Fat in Skinfold Thickness

In research studies and selected health care settings, fat-fold or skinfold thickness measurements may be used to estimate body fat in an individual. Skinfold measurement assumes that 50% of body fat is subcutaneous. Because of limitations with accuracy and reproducibility, these measurements are not used routinely in clinical settings.

Circumference Measurements

Circumference measurements may be useful in health care settings in which these measurements are recorded periodically (e.g., monthly or quarterly) and tracked over time to identify trends and potential risk factors for chronic conditions. However, in acutely ill individuals with daily fluid shifts measures of arm circumference and triceps skinfold (TSF) measurements usually are not performed. Use of neck circumference (NC) has been proposed as a marker of overweight, obesity, and associated disease risk in children and adults. Its measurement is a novel, noninvasive screening tool that is easy to do without the privacy concerns associated with waist and hip circumference measurements. NC is measured on bare skin between the midcervical spine and midanterior neck just below the laryngeal prominence (the Adam's apple) with the head in the Frankfurt plane (looking straight ahead). The tape should be as close to horizontal as anatomically feasible (i.e., the tape line in the front of the neck will be at the same height as the tape line in the back of the neck) (Coelho et al, 2016).

Studies of adults and elderly report that NC is associated highly with waist circumference, weight, BMI, and percent body fat. Large NC (> 40.5 cm in males; > 35.7 cm in females) was associated with hypertension and type 2 diabetes (Coelho et al, 2016). Findings from study of a predominantly African American cohort include significant correlations between serum insulin, triglycerides, LDL cholesterol levels, and NC (Arnold et al, 2014).

NC can be used as a reliable tool to identify adolescents with high BMIs (Kelishadi et al, 2016; Androutsos, 2012). The Canadian Health Measures Survey has published reference data for interpretation of NC measurements in Canadian children (Katz et al, 2014).

Bioelectrical Impedance Analysis (BIA)

Bioelectrical Impedance Analysis (BIA) estimates body composition and cellular activity by measuring the bulk of the electrical impedance in the body. The body composition analysis technique is based on the principle that, relative to water, lean tissue has a higher electrical conductivity and lower impedance than fatty tissue because of its electrolyte content. The testing involves application of electrical conductors to the patient's hand and foot, sending a low voltage electrical current through the body. Each body tissue type has a different electrical conductivity property. An algorithm derived from statistical analysis of BIA measurements is used to calculate the parameters measured by this technology. Parameters include total body water, intracellular and extracellular body water (i.e., third spacing of body fluids), fat-free mass, percent body fat, phase angle, and cellular metabolism. The evaluation of cellular metabolism is based on the phase angle. The phase angle measures the relationship between reactance, resistance, and impedance to predict the integrity of cell membranes. High phase angles show that a cell is strong enough to hold water and is a good marker for overall health. Low phase angle show that the cell membrane is weak and may not be able to hold water. BIA can be used to assess for third spacing of fluids even on a subclinical basis.

The BIA method is safe, noninvasive, portable, and rapid. For accurate results the patient should be well hydrated; have not exercised in the previous 4 to 6 hours; and have not consumed alcohol, caffeine, or diuretics in the previous 24 hours. If the person is dehydrated, a higher percentage of body fat than really exists is measured. Fever, electrolyte imbalance, and extreme obesity also may affect the reliability of measurements (Sergi et al, 2017). Presently there are no universally accepted reference norms for interpretation of data. There is limited research using BIA in critical care patients. Monitoring trends in data may be helpful. BIA is contraindicated for individuals who are pregnant, due to ethical concerns, or who have an implanted pacemaker or defibrillator (Buch et al, 2012; Lee and Gallagher, 2008). Fig. 5.4 illustrates a BIA test.

Circumference Measurements in Children

Head circumference measurements are useful in children younger than 3 years of age, primarily as an indicator of nonnutritional abnormalities (i.e., congenital microcephaly, hydrocephalus). Undernutrition must be very severe to affect head circumference; see Box 5.5 and Chapter 15.

Measuring Circumference

Midarm circumference (MAC) is measured in centimeters halfway between the acromion process of the scapula and the olecranon process at the tip of the elbow. MAC should be measured when assessing for nutritional status of children and compared with the standards

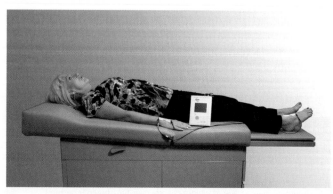

Fig. 5.4 Bioelectrical impedance analysis. (Image reproduced with permission of ImpediMed Limited.)

BOX 5.5 Measuring Head Circumference

Indications
- Head circumference is a standard measurement for serial assessment of growth in children from birth to 36 months and in any child whose head size is in question.

Equipment
- Paper or metal tape measure (cloth can stretch) marked in tenths of a centimeter because growth charts are listed in 0.5-cm increments

Technique
- The head is measured at its greatest circumference.
- The greatest circumference is usually above the eyebrows and pinna of the ears and around the occipital prominence at the back of the skull.
- More than one measurement may be necessary because the shape of the head can affect the location of the maximum circumference.
- Compare the measurement with the National Center for Health Statistics standard curves for head circumference (see Appendices 5 and 9).

Data from Hockenberry MJ, Wilson D: *Wong's nursing care of infants and children*, ed 9, St Louis, 2015, Mosby.

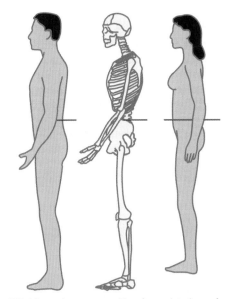

Fig. 5.5 Measuring tape position for waist circumference.

developed by WHO for children aged 6 to 59 months of age (de Onis et al, 1997). It is an independent anthropometric assessment tool in determining malnutrition in children.

Circumference Measurements in Adults

MAC is measured the same way in adults as in children. Combining MAC with triceps skin fold (TSF) measurements allows indirect determination of the arm muscle area (AMA) and arm fat area which can be tracked against a standard and used as an assessment of malnutrition. Because of limitations with accuracy and reproducibility, these measurements are rarely used to assess adult nutrition status.

Waist and Hip Circumference, Waist-to-Hip Ratio, and Waist-to-Height Ratio

Selected circumference measurements may be useful in determining estimated risk for chronic diseases and assessing changes in body composition. Waist circumference (WC) is obtained by measuring the distance around the narrowest area of the waist between the lowest rib and iliac crest and above the umbilicus using a nonstretchable tape measure (Fig. 5.5). Hip circumference is measured at the widest area of the hips at the greatest protuberance of the buttocks. Because fat distribution is an indicator of risk, circumferential or girth measurements may be used. The presence of excess body fat around the abdomen out of proportion to total body fat is a risk factor for chronic diseases associated with obesity and the metabolic syndrome. A WC of greater than 40 inches (102 cm) for men and greater than 35 inches (88 cm) for women is an independent risk factor for metabolic disease (CDC, 2014; Stone et al, 2013). These measurements may not be as useful for those less than 60 inches tall or with a BMI of 35 or greater (CDC, 2014). WC is considered to be a more valid predictor of metabolic risk than BMI, except when BMI is greater than or equal to 35 (CDC, 2018).

To determine the waist-to-hip ratio (WHR), divide the waist measurement by the hip measurement. The WHO defines the ratios of greater than 9.0 in men and greater than 8.5 in women as one of the decisive benchmarks for metabolic syndrome and is consistent with findings of research predicting all cause and cardiovascular disease mortality (Srikanthan et al, 2009; Welborn and Dhaliwal, 2007).

Fig. 5.5 shows the proper location to measure waist (abdominal) circumference.

The waist-to-height ratio (WHtR) is defined as the waist circumference divided by the measured height. WHtR is a measure of the distribution of adipose tissue. Generally speaking, the higher the values of WHtR, the greater the risk of metabolic syndrome and obesity-related atherosclerotic cardiovascular diseases (Schneider et al, 2010). Desirable ratios are less than 0.5 in adults 40 years and younger, between 0.5 and 0.6 in adults aged 40 to 50 years, and 0.6 or less in adults over 50. These targets apply to both males and females and a variety of ethnic groups. For example, a BMI of 25 is equivalent to a WHtR of 0.51. Table 5.7 provides a guide to interpreting WHtR by gender.

A systematic review of evidence on use of WHtR on elderly populations showed evidence that WHtR is associated with obesity and is a predictor of risk factors associated with cardiovascular disease, metabolic syndrome, and diabetes (Corrêa et al, 2016; Ashwell and Gibson, 2016). However, WHtR is not identified as a risk marker in the ACC/AHA ATP 4.

TABLE 5.7 Interpretation of Waist-to-Height Ratio by Gender

Females	Males	
WHtR	WHtR	Interpretation
< 0.35	< 0.35	Underweight; no increased risk
0.35-0.42	0.35-0.43	Slim; no increase risk
0.42-0.49	0.43-0.53	Healthy; no increased risk
0.49-0.54	0.53-0.58	Overweight; increased/high risk
0.54-0.58	0.58-0.63	Obese; increased/high risk
> 0.58	> 0.63	Very obese; very high risk

WHtR, Weight-to-height ratio.
Adapted from Ashwell, M & Gibson, S. Waist-to-height ratio as an indicator of 'early health risk': simpler and more predictive than using a 'matrix' based on BMI and waist circumference. *BMJ Open* 2016; 6:e010159. doi: 10.1136/bmjopen-2015-010159.

Other Methods of Measuring Body Composition
Dual-Energy X-Ray Absorptiometry

Dual-energy x-ray absorptiometry (DXA) measures fat, bone mineral, and fat-free soft tissue. The energy source in DXA is an x-ray tube that contains an energy beam. The amount of energy loss depends on the type of tissue through which the beam passes; the result can be used to measure mineral, fat, and lean tissue compartments. DXA is easy to use, emits low levels of radiation, and is available in the hospital setting, making it a useful tool. Generally, it is found to be a reliable measurement of percentage body fat; however, the patient must remain still for more than a few minutes, which may be difficult for older adults and those in chronic pain. Measurements are influenced by the thickness of tissues and hydration status (Prado and Heymsfield, 2014). Fig. 5.6 illustrates a DXA scan.

Air Displacement Plethysmogram

Air displacement plethysmogram (ADP) relies on measurements of body density to estimate body fat and fat-free masses. Performing an ADP with the BOD-POD device is a densitometry technique found to be an accurate method to measure body composition. ADP appears to be a reliable instrument in body composition assessment for athletes and obese individuals. ADP does not rely on body water content to determine body density and body composition, which makes it potentially useful in those adults with end-stage renal disease (Flakoll et al, 2004; Fig. 5.7).

Indirect calorimetry

Indirect calorimetry is the most accurate method for estimating energy expenditure by measuring inspired and expired oxygen and carbon dioxide. Total energy requirements (TEE) are calculated from the resting energy expenditure (REE) measured for a short period of time using metabolic carts or handheld devices. Studies in healthy populations comparing the data generated from the handheld devices to the data from the traditional indirect calorimetry are both accurate and reliable. However, in studies validating the handheld device in patients with disease or injury the results have not yielded a high degree of clinical accuracy (Zhao et al, 2014). More research is needed to fine-tune the accuracy and reliability of the handheld devices.

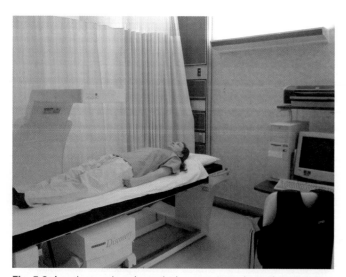

Fig. 5.6 A patient undergoing a dual-energy x-ray absorptiometry scan. (Courtesy the Division of Nutrition, University of Utah.)

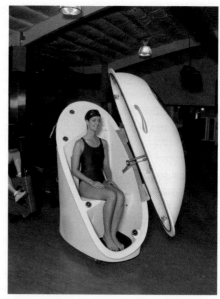

Fig. 5.7 The BOD-POD measures body fat and fat-free mass. (Courtesy COSMED USA, Inc., Concord, CA.)

NUTRITION-FOCUSED PHYSICAL EXAMINATION

Nutrition-focused physical examination (NFPE) is one of the components of nutrition assessment in the NCP model. Data gathered in the NFPE are used in conjunction with food and nutrition history, laboratory and diagnostic test results, physical measurements, and client history to accurately make one or more nutrition diagnoses. The *International Dietetics & Nutrition Terminology Reference Manual* (IDNT) (AND, 2018) defines nutrition-focused physical examination as "findings from an evaluation of body systems, muscle and subcutaneous fat wasting, oral health, suck, swallow/breathe ability, appetite and affect." Unlike a comprehensive clinical examination that reviews all body systems, NFPE is a focused assessment that addresses specific signs and symptoms by reviewing selected body systems.

Approach

A systems approach is used when performing the NFPE, which should be conducted in an organized, logical way to ensure efficiency and thoroughness (Litchford, 2013). Body systems include the following:

- General appearance
- Vital signs
- Skin
- Nails
- Hair
- Head
- Eyes
- Nose
- Mouth
- Neck/chest
- Abdomen
- Musculoskeletal

Equipment

The extent of the NFPE dictates the necessary equipment. Any or all of the following may be used: examination gloves, a stethoscope, a penlight or flashlight, a tongue depressor, scales, calipers, a tape measure, a blood pressure cuff, a watch with a second hand, and dynamometer to measure hand grip strength.

TABLE 5.8   Physical Examination Techniques

Technique	Description
Inspection	General observation that progresses to a more focused observation using the senses of sight, smell, and hearing; note appearance, mood, behavior, movement, facial expressions; most frequently used technique
Palpation	Gentle tactile examination to feel pulsations and vibrations; assessment of body structures, including texture, size, temperature, tenderness, and mobility
Percussion	Assessment of sounds to determine body organ borders, shape, and position; not always used in a NFPE
Auscultation	Use of the naked ear or bell or diaphragm of stethoscope to listen to body sounds (e.g., heart and lung sounds, bowel sounds, blood vessels); not always used in NFPE

Adapted from Litchford MD: *Nutrition focused physical assessment: making clinical connections*, Greensboro, NC, 2013, CASE Software & Books.

Examination Techniques and Findings

Four basic physical examination techniques are used during the NFPE. These techniques include inspection, palpation, percussion, and auscultation (Table 5.8). Appendix 11 discusses NFPE in more detail.

Interpretation of data collected in each component of an NFPE requires critical thinking skills and the following steps in clinical reasoning:

- Identify abnormal findings or symptoms.
- Localize the findings anatomically.
- Interpret findings in terms of probable process.
- Make a hypothesis about the nature of the patient's problem.
- Test the hypothesis by collaborating with other medical professionals and establish a working nutrition diagnosis.
- Develop a plan agreeable to the patient following all the steps of the NCP model (Bickley, 2017) (see Chapter 9).

Guidelines for Assessing Malnutrition in Children

Definitions and guidelines to identify malnutrition in children are evolving. Pediatric malnutrition is defined as an imbalance between nutrient requirements and dietary intake that results in deficits of energy, protein, and micronutrients stores, resulting in impaired growth and development. Pediatric malnutrition is either related to an illness or injury or caused by an environmental circumstance or behavioral factor (Mehta et al, 2013). Specific parameters for determining pediatric undernutrition and malnutrition are being standardized (Becker et al, 2015).

Guidelines for Assessing Malnutrition in Adults

The Academy and the ASPEN Consensus Statement: Characteristics Recommended for the Identification and Documentation of Adult Malnutrition provides a standardized and measurable set of criteria for all health professionals to use to identify malnutrition (White et al, 2012). It uses a cause-based nomenclature that reflects the current understanding of the role of inflammatory response on the incidence, progression, and resolution of adult malnutrition. Moreover, malnutrition syndromes are defined by patient settings, including acute illness or surgery, chronic disease, and environmental or social circumstances. In addition, the presence and degree of inflammation further differentiates types of malnutrition as nonsevere and severe. Nonsevere does not mean not urgent; it means mild to moderate malnutrition or undernutrition (Fig. 5.8).

No single parameter defines malnutrition. The Consensus guidelines identify six characteristics of malnutrition. From these, the clinician must identify a minimum of two characteristics that relate to the context of the concurrent medical condition for a nutrition diagnosis of malnutrition. The characteristics of nonsevere and severe malnutrition are noted in Table 5.9.

Measures of Functionality

Loss of functionality and mobility has a ripple effect on achieving activities of daily living (ADLs) and nutrition-related ADLs. An emerging component of nutrition-focused examination is assessment for muscle strength and functionality. Clinicians may work collaboratively with rehabilitation therapists to assess this and identify strategies to improve physical strength and mobility using diet and exercise.

Physical Activity Assessment

Inclusion of a physical activity assessment is part of a comprehensive nutrition assessment because lifestyle and behavioral factors play a role in the cause and prevention of chronic diseases. Electronic tracking of physical activity through smartphones and other wearable fitness and health tracking devices are useful in collecting, compiling, and preparing summary reports useful to clinicians and patients. Box 5.6 provides a series of questions that can be asked to identify the current levels and interest in future activity levels for ambulatory patients and clients.

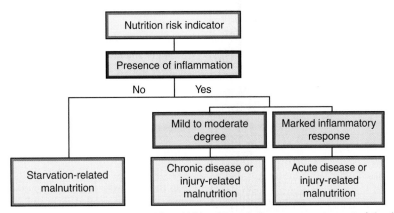

Fig. 5.8 Cause-based malnutrition. (Adapted from White JV et al: Consensus statement of the Academy of Nutrition and Dietetics/American Society for Parenteral and Enteral Nutrition: characteristics recommended for the identification and documentation of adult malnutrition (undernutrition), *J Acad Nutr Diet* 112(5):730, 2012.)

TABLE 5.9   Characteristics of Adult Malnutrition

ACUTE ILLNESS OR INJURY		CHRONIC ILLNESS		SOCIAL OR ENVIRONMENTAL CIRCUMSTANCES	
Nonsevere	Severe	Nonsevere	Severe	Nonsevere	Severe
Interpretation of Weight Loss for Malnutrition by Cause					
1-2% in 1 wk	>2% in 1 wk	5% in 1 wk	>5% in 1 wk	>5% in 1 wk	>5% in 1 wk
5% in 1 mo	>5% in 1 mo	7.5% in 3 mo	>7.5% in 3 mo	>7.5% in 3 mo	>7.5% in 3 mo
7.5% in 3 mo	>7.5% in 3 mo	10% in 6 mo	>10% in 6 mo	>10% in 6 mo	>10% in 6 mo
		20% in 1 yr	>20% in 1 yr	>20% in 1 yr	>20% in 1 yr
Interpretation of Reduced Energy Intake for Malnutrition by Cause					
For >7 days	For > or = to 5 days	For > or = to 1 mo	For > or = to 1 mo	For > or = to 3 mo	For > or = to 1 mo
< 75% of estimated energy needs	< or = to 50% of estimated energy needs	<75% of estimated energy needs	< or = to 75% of estimated energy needs	<75% of estimated energy needs	< or = to 50% of estimated energy needs
Loss of Body Fat					
Mild	Moderate	Mild	Severe	Mild	Severe
Loss of Muscle					
Mild	Moderate	Mild	Severe	Mild	Severe
Fluid Accumulation					
Mild	Moderate to severe	Mild	Severe	Mild	Severe
Reduced Grip Strength					
N/A	Measurably reduced	N/A	Measurably reduced	N/A	Measurably reduced

Adapted from White JV et al: Consensus statement of the Academy of Nutrition and Dietetics/American Society for Parenteral and Enteral Nutrition: characteristics recommended for the identification and documentation of adult malnutrition (undernutrition), *J Acad Nutr Diet* 112(5):730, 2012.

BOX 5.6   Physical Activity Assessment Questionnaire

To be considered physically active, you must get at least:
- 30 minutes of moderate physical activity on 5 or more days a week, OR
- 20 minutes of vigorous physical activity on 3 or more days a week

How physically active do you plan to be over the next 6 months? *(Choose the best answer.)*

_____ I am not currently active and do not plan to become physically active in the next 6 months.

_____ I am thinking about becoming more physically active.

_____ I intend to become more physically active in the next 6 months.

_____ I have been trying to get more physical activity.

_____ I am currently physically active and have been for the last 1-5 months.

_____ I have been regularly physically active for the past 6 months or more.

Compared with how physically active you have been over the last 3 months, how would you describe the last 7 days: *(Check one)*

_____ More active_____ Less active_____ About the same

Recall your participation in activities or in sedentary behaviors, over the past 24 hours:
- Reading, watching TV, or computer time _____ minutes/day
- Fast walking _____ minutes/day
- Physical activity (swimming, tennis, racquetball, similar) _____ minutes/day
- Other physical activity (describe _____) _____ minutes/day

What are the 3 most important reasons why you would consider increasing your physical activity?

☐ Improve my health ☐ Control my weight ☐ Lower my stress

Measures of Strength

With aging, the balanced cycle of muscle synthesis and degradation shifts toward more breakdown than synthesis of muscle tissue (see Chapter 19). The consequence is atrophy of muscle mass and loss of strength and power. Handgrip dynamometry can provide a baseline nutritional assessment of muscle function by measuring grip strength and endurance and is useful in serial measurements. Measurements of handgrip dynamometry are compared with reference standards provided by the manufacturer. Decreased grip strength is an important sign of frailty and is one of the characteristics of severe malnutrition (White et al, 2012). Low grip strength is associated consistently with a greater likelihood of premature mortality, the development of disability, and an increased risk of complications or prolonged length of stay after hospitalization or surgery in middle-aged and older adults (McLean et al, 2014).

Rehabilitation therapists use a number of evidence-based measures of upper and lower extremity physical function and performance that include muscle resistance testing, walking tests, stair climbing, rising from a chair, and balance. A score is determined for each test and summed for interpretation. Working collaboratively with rehabilitation therapists allows for a better understanding of functional measures of performance and how they relate to nutritional status.

Functional Medicine

Functional medicine is an evolving, evidence-based discipline that sees the body with its mutually interactive systems as a whole, rather than as a set of isolated signs and symptoms. The Institute of Functional Medicine (IFM) promotes an evaluation process that recognizes the biochemical, genetic, and environmental individuality of each person. The focus is patient centered, not just disease centered.

TABLE 5.10 Selected Components of Functional Nutrition Assessment

Ingestion	Digestion	Utilization—Cellular and Molecular Functional Relationships
Food, fiber, water, supplements, medication	Adequate microflora	Antioxidants: water-soluble vitamin C, phytonutrients
Intake patterns affected by emotional or disordered eating	Allergies	Methylation and acetylation: dependence on adequate B complex vitamins and minerals
Toxins entering the body via food, skin, inhalants, water, environment (including pesticides and chemicals)	Genetic enzyme deficits	Oils and fatty acids: prostaglandin balance, cell membrane function, vitamin E function
	Hydration	Protein metabolism: connective tissue, enzymes, immune function, etc.
	Infection/inflammatory response	Vitamin D in concert with functional metabolic partner nutrients vitamins A and K
	Lifestyle: sleep, exercise, stressors	

Lifestyle and health-promoting factors include nutrition, exercise, adequate sleep, healthy relationships, and a positive sense of self.

The Functional Nutrition Assessment acknowledges the web-like interconnectedness of internal physiologic factors and identifies root causes of chronic disease by integrating traditional dietetic practice with nutritional genomics (see Chapter 6), the restoration of gastrointestinal function, the quelling of chronic inflammation (see Chapter 7), and the interpretation of nutritional biomarkers. The functional nutrition practitioner organizes the data collected from a detailed intake that includes exploration of core areas of imbalance: dietary, hormonal, oxidative stress, environmental exposures, immune function, and psychological and spiritual health. This leads a unique and personalized assessment of disease for each individual within the framework of the NCP (see Table 5.10, Fig. 5.9, and Chapter 11).

CLINICAL CASE STUDY

Gia, a 58-year-old F, is admitted to City Hospital following a work-related accident. She has a history of hypertension, obesity, and unsuccessful weight loss attempts using restrictive diets. She loves fried foods, soft drinks, and sweets. Her medical profile today is:

Age	58 years old	
Height	59 in	
Weight	200 lb	
	Normal Value	Gia's Values
Glucose	70-99 mg/dL;4.1-5.9 mmol/L	142 mg/dL; 7.8 mmol/L
Calcium	9.0-10.5 mg/dL; 2.25-2.62 mmol/L	9.1 mg/dL; 2.27 mmol/L
Sodium	136-145 mEq/L; 136-145 mmol/L	145 mEq/L; 145 mmol/L
Potassium	3.5-5.0 mEq/L; 3.5-5.0 mmol/L	3.6 mEq/L; 3.6mmol/L
CO_2	23-30 mEq/L/ 23-30 mmol/L	25 mEq/L/ 25 mmol/L
Chloride	98-106 mEq/L; 98-106 mmol/L	98 mEq/L; 98 mmol/L
BUN	10-20 mg/dL; 3.6-7.1 mmol/L	30 mg/dL; 10.7 mmol/L
Creatinine	F 0.5-1.1 mg/dL; 44-97 μmol/L	0.9 mg/dL; 79.6 μmol/L
	M 0.6-1.2 mg/dL; 53-106 μmol/L	
Albumin	3.5-5.0 g/dL; 35-50 g/L	3.8 g/dL; 38 g/L
Total protein	6.4-8.3 g/dL; 64-83 g/L	8.0 g/dL; 80 g/L
ALP	30-120 U/L; 0.5-2.0 μkat/L	35 U/L; 0.5 μkat/L
ALT	4-36 units/L; 4-36 units/L	28 units/L; 28 units/L
AST	0-35 units/L; 0-0.58 μkat/L	23 units/L; 0.38 μkat/L
Bilirubin, total	0.3-1.0 mg/dL; 5.1-17μmol/L	1.5 mg/dL; 25.65 μmol/L
RBC	F 4.2-5.4 × 10^6 mL; 4.2-5.4 × 10^{12} L	5.1 × 10^6 mL; 5.1 × 10^{12} L
	M 4.7-6.1 × 10^6 mL; 4.7-6.1 × 10^{12} L	
Hgb	F 12-16 g/dL; 7.4-9.9 mmol/L	11 g/dL; 7 mmol/L
	M 14-18 g/dL; 8.7-11.2 mmol/L	
Hct	F 37-47%; 0.37-0.47	30%; 0.30
	M 42-52%; 0.42-0.52	

MCV	80-95 mm³; 80-95 fL	108 mm³; 108 fL
MCH	27-31 pg	33 pg
MCHC	32-36 g/dL;32%-36%	40 g/dL; 40%
WBC	5000-10000/mm³ ;5-10 x 10^9	8 × 10^9
Total cholesterol	< 200 mg/dL; <5.2 mmol/L	245 mg/dL
LDL	<130 mg/dL	145 mg/dL
HDL	F > 55 mg/dL	30 mg/dL
	M > 45 mg/dL	
Triglycerides	F 35-135 mg/dL; 0.4-1.52 mmol/L	
	F 40-160 mg/dL; 0.45-1.81 mmol/L	210 mg/dL

Gia is referred for medical nutrition therapy. NFPE indicates a prefrail female, with excessive abdominal fat stores, low muscular development, and no fluid accumulation. Assess her nutrition status using the data provided.

Nutrition Diagnostic Statement

- Altered laboratory values related to chronic restrictive dieting as well as overeating highly processed foods as evidenced by signs of nutritional anemia and dyslipidemia.

Nutrition Care Questions

1. Considering Gia's medical history, what does her laboratory report for hemoglobin, hematocrit, and mean corpuscular volume suggest?
2. What does her laboratory report for total cholesterol, LDL, HDL, and triglycerides values suggest?
3. What does her laboratory report for sodium, blood urea nitrogen suggest?
4. What additional laboratory tests would be helpful for a comprehensive nutrition assessment?

ALP, Alkaline phosphate; *ALT,* alanine aminotransferase; *AST,* aspartate aminotransferase; *BUN,* blood urea nitrogen; *CO₂,* carbon dioxide; *Hct,* hematocrit; *Hgb,* hemoglobin; *MCH,* mean corpuscular hemoglobin; *MCHC,* mean corpuscular hemoglobin concentration; *MCV,* mean corpuscular volume; *RBC,* red blood cell; *WBC,* white blood cell.

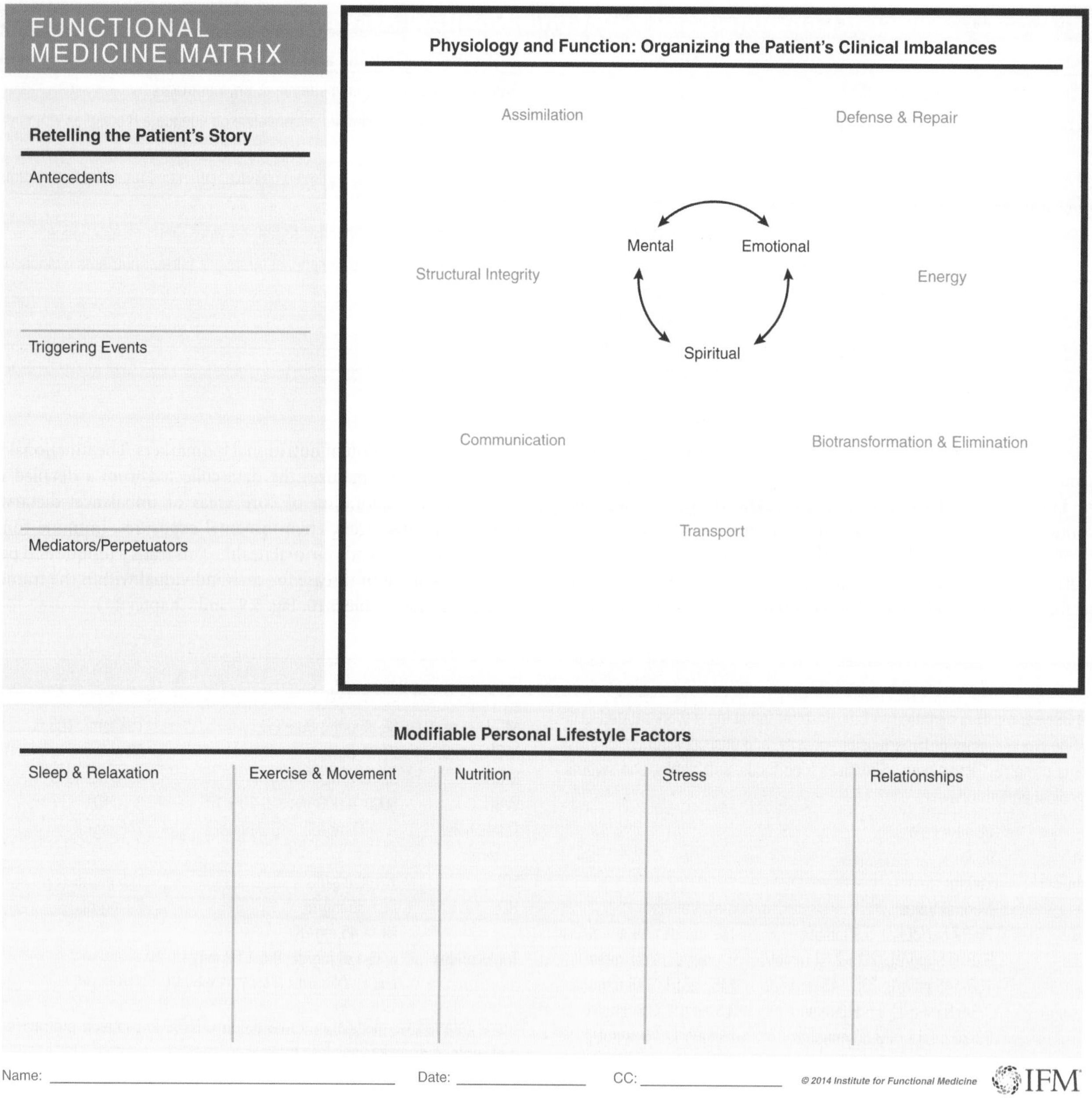

FUNCTIONAL MEDICINE MATRIX

Retelling the Patient's Story

Antecedents

Triggering Events

Mediators/Perpetuators

Physiology and Function: Organizing the Patient's Clinical Imbalances

Assimilation   Defense & Repair

Mental   Emotional

Structural Integrity   Energy

Spiritual

Communication   Biotransformation & Elimination

Transport

Modifiable Personal Lifestyle Factors

Sleep & Relaxation	Exercise & Movement	Nutrition	Stress	Relationships

Name: _____   Date: _____   CC: _____   © 2014 Institute for Functional Medicine   IFM

Fig. 5.9 Functional Medicine Matrix Model.

USEFUL WEBSITES

Academy of Nutrition and Dietetics, Evidence Analysis Library
Assessment Tools for Weight-Related Health Risks
Body Mass Index Assessment Tool
Centers for Disease Control and Prevention—Growth Charts
Centers for Disease Control and Prevention—Weight Assessment
Dietitians in Integrative and Functional Medicine

REFERENCES

Aarts EO, Janssen IM, Berends FJ: The gastric sleeve: losing weight as fast as micronutrients? *Obes Surg* 21:207–211, 2011.

Abner EL, Schmitt FA, Mendiondo MS, et al: Vitamin E and all-cause mortality: a meta-analysis, *Curr Aging Sci* 4(2):158–170, 2011.

American Diabetes Association (ADA): Diagnosis and classification of diabetes mellitus, *Diabetes Care* 343:62, 2011.

American Diabetes Association: Classification and diagnosis of diabetes: standards of medical care in diabetes—2019, *Diabetes Care* 41(Suppl 1): S13–S27, 2018. doi:10.2337/dc18-S002.

American Geriatric Society Workgroup on vitamin D supplementation for older adults: Consensus statement: vitamin D for prevention of falls and the consequences in older adults, *J Am Geriatr Soc* 62:147–152, 2014.

Androutsos O, Grammatikaki E, Moschonis G, et al: Neck circumference: a useful screening tool of cardiovascular risk in children, *Pediatr Obes* 7:187–195, 2012.

Araneta MR, Kanaya AM, Hsu WC, et al: Optimum BMI cut points to screen Asian Americans for type 2 diabetes, *Diabetes Care* 38(5):814–820, 2015.

Arnold TJ, Schweitzer A, Hoffman HJ, et al: Neck and waist circumference biomarkers of cardiovascular risk in a cohort of predominantly African-American college students: a preliminary study, *J Acad Nutr Diet* 114(1):107–116, 2014.

Ashwell M, Gibson S: Waist-to-height ratio as an indicator of 'early health risk': simpler and more predictive than using a 'matrix' based on BMI and waist circumference, *BMJ Open* 6:e010159, 2016.

Becker P, Carney LN, Corkins MR, et al: Consensus statement of the Academy of Nutrition and Dietetics/American Society for Parenteral and Enteral Nutrition: indicators recommended for the identification and documentation of pediatric malnutrition (undernutrition), *Nutr Clin Prac* 30: 147–161, 2015.

Bickley LS: *Bates guide to physical assessment*, Philadelphia, PA, 2017, Wolters Kluwer.

Bischoff-Ferrari HA: Optimal serum 25-hydroxyvitamin D levels for multiple health outcomes, *Adv Exp Med Biol* 810:500–525, 2014.

Blackburn GL, Bistrian BR, Maini BS, et al: Nutritional and metabolic assessment of the hospitalized patient, *JPEN J Parenter Enteral Nutr* 1:11–22, 1977.

Buch E, Bradfield J, Larson T, et al: Effect of body composition analysis on function of implanted cardiac devices, *Pacing Clin Electrophysiol* 35(6):681–684, 2012.

Buppajarntham S, Staros EB: *Insulin*, February 14, 2014. Available at: https://emedicine.medscape.com/article/2089224-overview#a2.

Centers for Disease Control and Prevention (CDC): *Overweight and obesity*. Available at: http://www.cdc.gov/obesity/.

Charney P, Peterson SJ: Critical thinking skills in nutrition assessment and diagnosis, *J Acad Nutr Diet* 113:1545, 2013.

Coelho HJ, Sampaio RA, Gonçalvez IO, et al. Cutoffs and cardiovascular risk factors associated with neck circumference among community-dwelling elderly adults: a cross-sectional study, *Sao Paulo Med J* 134(6):519–527, 2016.

Corrêa MM, Thumé E, De Oliveira ER, et al: Performance of the waist-to-height ratio in identifying obesity and predicting non-communicable diseases in the elderly population: a systematic literature review, *Arch Gerontol Geriatr* 65:174–182, 2016.

Dickerson RN: Nitrogen balance and protein requirements for critically Ill older patients, *Nutrients* 8:226, 2016.

Ferraro PM, Curhan GC, Gambaro G, et al: Total, dietary, and supplemental vitamin c intake and risk of incident kidney stones, *Am J Kidney Dis* 67(3):400–407, 2016.

Flakoll PJ, Kent P, Neyra R, et al: Bioelectrical impedance vs air displacement plethysmography and dual-energy X-ray absorptiometry to determine body composition in patients with end-stage renal disease, *JPEN J Parenter Enteral Nutr* 28:13–21, 2004.

Flegal K, Kit BK, Orpana H, et al: Association of all-cause mortality with overweight and obesity using standard body mass index categories a systematic review and meta-analysis, JAMA 309(1):71–82, 2013.

Friedewald WT, Levy RI, Fredrickson DS: Estimation of the concentration of low-density lipoprotein cholesterol in plasma, without use of the preparative ultracentrifuge, *Clin Chem* 18:499–502, 1972.

Grundy SM, Stone NJ, Bailey AL, et al: Systematic Review for the 2018 AHA/ACC/AACVPR/AAPA/ABC/ACPM/ADA/AGS/APhA/ASPC/NLA/PCNA Guideline on the Management of Blood Cholesterol, *Circulation* 2018. Available at: https://www.ahajournals.org/doi/10.1161/CIR.0000000000000625. (Published online ahead of print).

Hainer V, Aldhoon-Hainerová I: Obesity paradox does exist, *Diabetes Care* 36(Suppl 2):S276–S281, 2013

Hammami MB: *Serum osteocalcin*, 2014. Available at: http://emedicine.msedscape.com/article/2093955-overview.

Hamwi GJ, Fajans SS, Sussman KE, et al: *Diabetes mellitus, diagnosis and treatment*, New York, NY, 1964, American Diabetes Association.

Hao W, Friedman A: The LDL-HDL profile determines the risk of atherosclerosis: a mathematical model, *PLoS One* 9:e90497, 2014.

Jacobson TA, Ito MK, Maki KC, et al: National Lipid Association recommendations for patient-center management of dyslipidemia, *J Clin Lipidol* 8:473–488, 2014.

Kagawa Y, Hiraoka M, Kageyama M, et al: Medical cost savings in Sakado City and worldwide achieved by preventing disease by folic acid fortification, *Congenit Anom (Kyoto)* 57(5):157–165, 2017.

Katz SL, Vaccani JP, Clarke J, et al: Creation of a reference dataset of neck sizes in children: standardizing a potential new tool for prediction of obesity-associated diseases? *BMC Pediatr* 14:159, 2014.

Kelishadi R, Djalalinia S, Motlagh ME, et al: Association of neck circumference with general and abdominal obesity in children and adolescents: the weight disorders survey of the CASPIAN-IV study, *BMJ Open* 6(9):e011794, 2016. Available at: https://bmjopen.bmj.com/content/6/9/e011794#block-system-main.

Klisić A, Kavarić N, Bjelaković B, et al: The association between retinol-binding protein 4 and cardiovascular risk score is mediated by waist circumference in overweight/obese adolescent girls, *Acta Clin Croat* 56(1):92–98, 2017.

Lee SY, Gallagher D: Assessment methods in human body composition, *Curr Opin Clin Nutr Metab Care* 11:566–572, 2008.

Litchford MD: *Laboratory assessment of nutritional status: bridging theory & practice*, Greensboro, NC, 2017, CASE Software & Books.

Litchford MD: *Nutriton-focused physical assessment: making clinical connections*, Greensboro, NC, 2013, Case Software and Books.

McLean RR, Shardell MD, Alley DE, et al: Criteria for clinically relevant weakness and low lean mass and their longitudinal association with incident mobility impairment and mortality: the foundation for the National Institutes of Health (FNIH) sarcopenia project, *J Gerontol A Biol Sci Med Sci* 69:576–583, 2014.

Mehta NM, Corkins MR, Lyman B, et al: Defining pediatric malnutrition: a paradigm shift toward etiology-related definitions, *J Parenter Enteral Nutr* 37:460–481, 2013.

Parrott J, Frank L, Rabena R, et al: American society for metabolic and bariatric surgery integrated health nutritional guidelines for the surgical weight loss patient 2016 update: micronutrients, *Surg Obes Relat Dis* 13(5): 727–741, 2017.

Perduca M, Nicolis S, Mannucci B, et al: Human plasma retinol-binding protein (RBP4) is also a fatty acid-binding protein, *Biochim Biophys Acta Mol Cell Biol Lipids* 1863(4):458–466, 2018.

Prado CM, Heymsfield SB: Lean tissue imaging: a new era for nutritional assessment and intervention, *J Parenter Enteral Nutr* 38:940–953, 2014.

Renz PB, Cavagnolli G, Weinert LS, et al: HbA1c test as a tool in the diagnosis of gestational diabetes mellitus, *PLoS One* 10(8):e0135989, 2015 doi:10.1371/journal.pone.0135989.

Schneider HJ, Friedrich N, Klotsche J, et al: The predictive value of different measures of obesity for incident cardiovascular events and mortality, *J Clin Endocrinol Metab* 95:1777–1785, 2010.

Sergi G, De Rui M, Stubbs B, et al: Measurement of lean body mass using bioelectrical impedance analysis: a consideration of the pros and cons, *Aging-Clin Exp Res* 29(4):591–597, 2017.

Srikanthan P, Seeman TE, Karlamangla AS, et al: Waist-hip-ratio as a predictor of all-cause mortality in high-functioning older adults, *Ann Epidemiol* 19:724–731, 2009.

Stensland SH, Margolis S: Simplifying the calculation of body mass index for quick reference, *J Am Diet Assoc* 90:856, 1990.

Stone NJ, Robinson JG, Lichtenstein AH, et al: 2013 ACC/AHA guideline on the treatment of blood cholesterol to reduce atherosclerotic cardiovascular risk in adults: a report of the American College of Cardiology/American Heart Association Task Force on Practice Guidelines, *J Am Coll Cardiol* 63(25 Pt B):2889–2934, 2014.

Taylor PN, Davies JS: A review of the growing risk of vitamin D toxicity from inappropriate practice, *Br J Clin Pharmacol* 84:1121–1127, 2018.

US Preventive services Task Force, Grossman DC, Curry SJ, et al: Vitamin D, calcium, or combined supplementation for the primary prevention of fractures in community-dwelling adults US Preventive Services Task Force Recommendation Statement, *JAMA* 319(15):1592–1599, 2018.

Wagner DR, Heyward VH: Measures of body composition in blacks and whites: a comparative review, *Am J Clin Nutr* 71:1392–1402, 2000.

Wang A, Lui J, Li C, et al: Cumulative exposure to high sensitivity C-reactive protein predicts risk of cardiovascular disease, *J Am Heart Assoc* 6(10):e005610, 2017.

Welborn TA, Dhaliwal SS: Preferred clinical measures of central obesity for predicting mortality, *Eur J Clin Nutr* 61:1373–1379, 2007.

White JV, Guenter P, Jensen G, et al: Consensus statement of the Academy of Nutrition and Dietetics/American Society for Parenteral and Enteral Nutrition: characteristics recommended for the identification and documentation of adult malnutrition (undernutrition), *J Acad Nutr Diet* 112: 730–738, 2012.

Winter JE, MacInnis RJ, Wattanapenpaiboon N, et al: BMI and all-cause mortality in older adults: a meta-analysis, *Am J Clin Nutr* 99:875–890, 2014.

Xun C, Zhao Y, Wang W, et al: Circulating RBP4 increase and its diagnosis of chronic kidney disease, *Ann Clin Lab Sci* 48(2):205–207, 2018.

Zhao D, Xian X, Terrera M, et al: A pocket-sized metabolic analyzer for assessment of resting energy expenditure, *Clin Nutr* 33(2):341–347, 2014.

Zhou Z, Chen H, Ju H, et al: Circulating retinol binding protein 4 levels in nonalcoholic fatty liver disease: a systematic review and meta-analysis, *Lipids Health Dis* 16:180, 2017.

6

Nutritional Genomics

Ruth DeBusk, PhD, RDN
Michael Hahn, BA

KEY TERMS

autosome
bioactive food components
candidate gene approach
chromosome
coding region
codon
deoxyribonucleic acid (DNA)
dominant
ELSI
epigenetics
epigenetic inheritance
epigenetic marks/tags
epigenome, epigenomics
expression genome-wide association
   studies (eGWAS)
exon
gene, genetics
gene variant/genetic variation
Genetic Information Nondiscrimination
   Act (GINA)
genome, genomics

genome-wide association study (GWAS)
genomic imprinting
genotype
heterozygous
histone
homozygous
intervening sequences
intron
karyotype
ligand
mendelian inheritance
messenger RNA (mRNA)
metabolome, metabolomics
microbiome, microbiomics
mitochondrial DNA (mtDNA)
mitochondrial (maternal) inheritance
mutation
nucleotide
nutrigenetics
nutrigenomics
nutritional genomics

obesogen
penetrance
pharmacogenomics
phenotype
polymorphism
posttranslational modification
precision (personalized) health
promoter region
proteomics
recessive
regulatory region
response elements
rs number
sex chromosome
signal transduction
single nucleotide polymorphism (SNP)
somatic
transcription
transcription factors
transcriptomics
translation

Imagine meeting with clients and having an assessment of their genetic capabilities and disease susceptibilities. Add to that information their laboratory reports as well as insight into their lifestyle choices: the foods they eat, their exercise habits, how well they manage their thoughts and emotions, how supportive their relationships are, the quantity and quality of their sleep, and their degree of toxic exposures. Further, as a well-trained nutrition professional, you understand the complex interconnections among their genetic profile, lifestyle choices, and chronic disease. It's routine for you to assess the molecular, biochemical, and physiologic mechanisms contributing to the client's current health status and to translate this information into effective therapeutic interventions that can restore health or prevent disease, as needed. Such a scenario is what's envisioned for the era of precision (personalized) health where therapy is tailored to each individual so that nutrition professionals can help clients optimize their health and describe the promise that nutritional genomics brings to the field of nutrition and dietetics.

Nutrition research is focused increasingly on the mechanisms that underlie these interactions and on projecting how this understanding can be translated into clinical interventions for more effective chronic disease management and prevention. Health is a continuum that spans wellness at one end and illness at the other. Genes are an important component in determining at which end of this continuum we find ourselves; they determine our unique signature of susceptibility to being well or ill. However, research into chronic disease is teaching us that environmental factors such as diet and other lifestyle choices made on a daily basis strongly influence who among the susceptible will actually develop dysfunction and disease. Food choices, physical activity habits, sleep patterns, thoughts and emotions, and systems of meaning—relationships with self and others and one's sense of purpose in life—affect cellular function at the molecular, biochemical, and physiologic levels. The influence of these environmental factors is modifiable through daily choices and, when appropriate to the genetic makeup, has the potential for changing the health trajectory from a poor quality of life filled with disease and disability to one of thriving and flourishing.

This understanding of the key role of choices regarding these modifiable lifestyle factors is enabling clinicians to assess to the root cause of chronic disease, to identify the molecular and biochemical mechanisms that underlie symptoms, and to tailor therapy to the individual's uniqueness. As a result, the promise of the molecular era is not only to manage chronic disease more effectively but also to restore health and, ultimately, to prevent chronic disease from developing. The interactions among genes, diet and other lifestyle factors, and their influence on health and disease are the focus of nutritional genomics.

GENETIC AND GENOMIC FUNDAMENTALS

Genetics is the science of heredity. It is the study of individual genes and their variations, how they give rise to measurable traits and the mechanisms by which traits (genes) are inherited from one generation to the next. Genomics focuses on the full set of an organism's genes, its genome, and how genes interact with each other and with the environment. Genetic research focuses on identifying genes in an organism, their location, the function of the proteins they encode, and how genes are associated with various traits, some health-promoting, some disease-promoting. Genomic research looks at the structure and functions of the whole genome, including interactions between different groups of genes or other elements. Whereas genetics was initially concerned with diseases that arise from a change in a single gene, genomics has broadened the focus to include the complex interaction of multiple genes, variations in these genes, and environmental factors that influence their expression. This focus positions genomic-related research and clinical applications primarily on addressing chronic disease, which involves the interaction among genes and environmental factors. The Human Genome Project was a multinational collaboration formed to identify each of the approximately 3 billion nucleotide building blocks of the human genome. See Box 6.1 for background information on the importance of this project to the progress of understanding the interconnections among genes, environment, and health.

The basic unit of heredity is the gene, which is made up of DNA (deoxyribonucleic acid). The nucleotide sequence of a gene encodes the instructions for making a protein or a peptide component of a protein. Changes in the nucleotide sequence of the DNA are translated into the amino acid sequence of the protein and can potentially change the ability of that protein to perform its role. These changes are passed from parent to child and are the basis for inheritance of traits. In higher organisms the DNA is housed within the nucleus of cells (Fig. 6.1). The DNA molecule is a double helix consisting of two strands of nucleotide subunits held together by hydrogen bonds. Each nucleotide contains the sugar deoxyribose, the mineral phosphorus, and one of four nitrogen-containing bases: adenine (A), thymine (T), guanine (G), or cytosine (C). Any base can sit next to one another, but across strands of the helix, these bases pair specifically: A pairs with T, G pairs with C (Fig. 6.2). The nucleotides are arranged in a linear order, and this order determines the particular information encoded in a stretch of DNA that results in the synthesis of a protein. The nucleotide sequence of DNA is unique to the individual and is called its genotype.

To be useful to the cells, information in the DNA first must be decoded and translated into proteins, which perform the work of the organism's "operating system." A sequence of DNA nucleotides that encodes the information for synthesizing a protein is called a gene. Human DNA contains approximately 20,000 genes. Each gene has a location or "address" at a specific site on a particular chromosome. Long stretches of nucleotides often are found between genes along the chromosome. Such sequences are called intervening sequences and compose the majority of the DNA in humans. These sequences do not code for proteins, but they are not "junk DNA" as originally thought. Instead, they perform structural and regulatory functions, such as controlling when, where, and how much of a protein is produced.

The large amount of genetic material in the nucleus is distributed among multiple chromosomes, which are formed by wrapping DNA tightly around specific proteins called histones. Human beings have 23 pairs of chromosomes, 22 autosomes, and 2 sex chromosomes. One copy of each member of a pair comes from the mother and the other from the father. Females have two X chromosomes; males have one X and one Y chromosome. The nucleus of each human cell contains all 46 chromosomes.

BOX 6.1 The Human Genome Project

The Human Genome Project (HGP) has been the impetus for a fundamental shift to integrating genetic principles into health care. This ambitious project was a $15 billion international effort that began in 1990, headquartered within the U.S. by the Department of Energy and the National Institutes of Health. The initial goal was to identify each of the 3 billion nucleotides in human DNA, the genetic material (genome). Subsequent goals would include (1) cataloging each gene in the human genome, (2) identifying each gene and its protein product, (3) detecting changes in genes and their association with disease susceptibility, and (4) shedding light on how environmental triggers influence genes and disease susceptibility. Additionally, the genomes of other organisms would be sequenced to enable their use as model systems in the laboratory in order to explore key mechanisms, from retrieving encoded information from DNA to understanding gene-environment interactions.

The HGP completed the sequencing phase in 2003, much earlier than expected. However, identifying the human sequence did not automatically provide answers to all the key questions that were needed to develop clinical applications that could be used to restore health and prevent disease, particularly for the chronic diseases whose prevalence was significant worldwide. A number of disciplines emerged corresponding to the various steps in the processes, from retrieving information to translating that information into proteins to regulating gene expression. This latter process includes epigenetics, which has been a bit of a "missing link" in understanding how genes give rise to chronic diseases, which is essential for developing effective clinical applications and for disease prevention. See Box 6.2 for information about the primary "omic" disciplines that have emerged. Each of these disciplines has continued developing as a primary research focus and is contributing valuable insight into the gene/environment/health and disease connections.

Another major accomplishment of the initial HGP work has been the advances that have occurred in genetic technologies, without which this work would not have been able to move forward so quickly. Advances include the ability to move from studying single genes and their variations to high-throughput whole genome sequencing that has greatly increased the speed with which the work can be conducted and decreased the cost of sequencing. Additionally, the genomes of numerous other organisms have been sequenced. Some of these organisms, such as the laboratory mouse, have served a valuable role as model systems for understanding human processes. The genetics and environmental conditions of model systems can be manipulated and the molecular, biochemical, and physiologic outcomes studied as well as the heritability of any changes noted. The HGP also emphasized educating genetic scientists and clinicians, integrating the results of genetic research into clinical practice, and developing sophisticated computer technology (bioinformatics) in order to make sense of the large volume of data that would be generated. As a result of this collaborative effort on a global scale, the era of precision health, only dreamed about in 1990, is now a viable goal for health care. For a history of the Human Genome Project, see the National Human Genome Research Institute's website.

DNA, The Molecule of Life

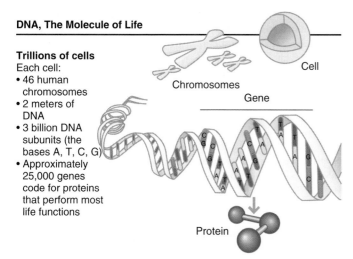

Trillions of cells

Each cell:
- 46 human chromosomes
- 2 meters of DNA
- 3 billion DNA subunits (the bases A, T, C, G)
- Approximately 25,000 genes code for proteins that perform most life functions

Fig. 6.1 DNA, the Molecule of Life. Cells are the fundamental working units of every living system. All the instructions needed to direct their activities are contained within the chemical deoxyribonucleic acid. (From U.S. Department of Energy, Human Genome Program: www.ornl.gov/hgmis.)

DNA Replication Prior to Cell Division

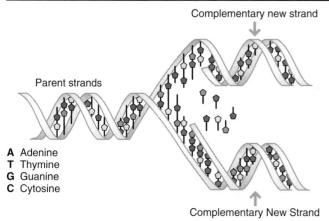

A Adenine
T Thymine
G Guanine
C Cytosine

Fig. 6.2 DNA Replication Prior to Cell Division. Each time a cell divides into two daughter cells, its full genome is duplicated; for humans and other complex organisms, this duplication occurs in the nucleus. During cell division the deoxyribonucleic acid (DNA) molecule unwinds, and the weak bonds between the base pairs break, allowing the strands to separate. Each strand directs the synthesis of a complementary new strand, with free nucleotides matching up with their complementary bases on each of the separated strands. Strict base-pairing rules are adhered to (i.e., adenine pairs only with thymine [an A-T pair] and cytosine with guanine [a C-G pair]). Each daughter cell receives one old and one new DNA strand. The cells' adherence to these base-pairing rules ensures that the new strand is an exact copy of the old one. This minimizes the incidence of errors (mutations) that may greatly affect the resulting organism or its offspring. (From U.S. Department of Energy, Human Genome Program: www.ornl.gov/hgmis.)

Gene Expression: Transcription and Translation

To initiate the process of decoding the DNA, the condensed chromosomes housing the genes first must open (decondense) to allow access to the information in the DNA nucleotide sequence. A common mechanism employed is the covalent attachment of acetyl groups to the histone proteins associated with the chromosomes. This action

relaxes the DNA and makes it accessible to the enzymes involved in transcription (the decoding process). Information decoding involves transcription by ribonucleic acid (RNA) polymerase into pre-messenger RNA (pre-mRNA) and subsequent translation of mRNA into the amino acid sequence of the protein according to a universal genetic code. The architecture of a gene typically includes a promoter region, where the RNA polymerase attaches and a coding region (also called a "structural region") that contains the encoded information for synthesizing that gene's protein. Within the coding region are sequences of nucleotides called exons that correspond to the order of the amino acids in the gene's protein product. The coding region also contains introns (sequences that are interspersed between exons and do not code for amino acids needed for synthesizing proteins).

Upstream from the promoter region is the regulatory region that controls the ability of the polymerase to attach to the promoter, thereby influencing whether transcription occurs. Within this region are response elements, DNA sequences that serve as binding sites for regulatory proteins such as transcription factors and their bound ligands. The binding of transcription factors triggers the recruitment of additional proteins to form a protein complex that in turn changes the expression of that gene by changing the conformation of the promoter region, increasing or decreasing the ability of RNA polymerase to attach and transcribe (express) the gene. The array of response elements within the promoter region can be complex, allowing for the binding of multiple transcription factors that in turn fine-tune the control of gene expression. It is through the binding of transcription factors to response elements that environmental factors such as the bioactive components in food essentially "talk" to a gene, conveying information that more or less of its protein product is needed.

Once transcribed, the pre-mRNA must be processed (posttranscriptional processing) to form mature messenger RNA (mRNA) from which the introns have been removed and the nucleotide sequence of the mRNA is ready to be translated into the amino acid sequence of the encoded protein. The protein synthesis process is called translation. Each set of three nucleotides makes up a codon, which in turn specifies a particular amino acid and its position within the protein (Figs. 6.3 and 6.4).

DNA Genetic Code Dictates Amino Acid Identity and Order

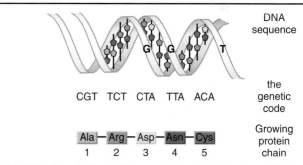

Fig. 6.3 DNA Genetic Code Dictates Amino Acid Identity and Order. All living organisms are composed largely of proteins. Proteins are large, complex molecules made up of long chains of subunits called amino acids. Twenty different kinds of amino acids are usually found in proteins. Within the gene, each specific sequence of three deoxyribonucleic acid bases (codons) directs the cells protein-synthesizing machinery to add specific amino acids. For example, the base sequence ATG codes for the amino acid methionine. Because three bases code for one amino acid, the protein coded by an average-sized gene (3000 bp) contains 1000 amino acids. The genetic code is thus a series of codons that specify which amino acids are required to make up specific proteins. *A*, adenine; *bp*, base pairs; *C*, cytosine; *G*, guanine; *T*, thymine. (From U.S. Department of Energy, Human Genome Program: www.ornl.gov/hgmis.)

BOX 6.2 Genomics and Other "Omic" Disciplines

Several new disciplines, technologies, and tools applicable to health care have developed from the Human Genome Project. The major disciplines have been genomics, proteomics, metabolomics, and microbiomics. **Genomics** is the study of organisms and their genetic material (the genome): composition, organization, and function.

The genome (total DNA sequence) is transcribed into coding and noncoding RNA transcripts. **Transcriptomics** is the study of the transcripts produced: the types of transcripts genome-wide and the amount produced. The coding RNA contains information needed to synthesize proteins and was originally thought to be the only functional type of RNA. Transcriptomics research has revealed that the majority of the genome is transcribed but that noncoding RNA comprises most of the transcripts produced. Although their physiologic roles are only beginning to be understood, some of these transcripts are being found to be associated with disease.

Proteomics focuses in part on identifying the protein encoded by each gene, the protein's function, and the effect of a mutation in a gene on the structure and function of the encoded protein. Research in proteomics also includes identifying the posttranslational modifications of proteins, such as enzymatic cleavage to generate an active protein or the addition of chemical groups such as in glycosylation and phosphorylation.

Metabolomics is the study of the substrates and products of metabolism (the metabolites). The goal is to identify each metabolite and its role in the metabolic processes carried out in cells, biofluids, tissues, and organs.

Microbiomics concerns the microbial ecology of body cavities, such as the digestive tract and the oral cavity, another important body cavity in nutrition practice. Beneficial and pathogenic microbes colonize these cavities and influence health. The Human Microbiome Project (https://hmpdacc.org) has been instrumental in identifying which microbes are present in health and disease and sequencing the genomes of each.

Pharmacogenomics, which is conceptually similar to nutritional genomics, involves using genomics to analyze the genetic variations in the genes that encode the drug-metabolizing enzymes and using this information to predict a patient's response to a drug. Genetic variability can lead to differing function in these enzymes, which explains why a drug may have the intended effects for one person, be ineffective for another, and be harmful to a third. In addition to identifying individuals for whom the drug therapy will be beneficial, it's possible to calculate the appropriate starting dosage and minimize adverse events. The common blood-thinning medication warfarin provides an example of pharmacogenomics and its clinical applications (see Box 6.14).

Many genetic technologies and tools have been developed for the various "omics" disciplines. Basic DNA sequencing technology applied to microbiomics has significantly shortened the time needed to identify pathogenic microorganisms, which allows antimicrobial therapy to be initiated much sooner than previously possible. Next-generation sequencing technology enables research and clinical laboratories to generate complete genomic profiles in a fraction of the time and cost of earlier technology. The vast amount of data generated by these disciplines has led to rapid growth in the field of bioinformatics. The ability of sophisticated computers to organize, store, and retrieve massive amounts of data has been integral to the rapid advances of the genomics era.

Following translation, most proteins need further processing (**posttranslational modification**) before they are active. This occurs with proenzyme and prohormones that must be enzymatically processed before becoming active or other proteins that are phosphorylated or glycosylated prior to being functional.

Investigation of these downstream steps in the gene expression process has created new fields, often called the "omics" (Hasin et al, 2017). These disciplines correlate with the major steps in the process of genetic information retrieval and translation: transcriptomics, posttranscriptional and posttranslational processing, proteomics, metabolomics, and epigenomics (see Box 6.2).

Genomic Regulation of Gene Expression

In higher organisms such as human beings, the expression of the information encoded within the genes is regulated at the chromosome level and at the DNA level. In both cases the strategy is the same: physically block or allow access to the genes in order to prevent or allow the expression of genes. As described earlier, the large amount of DNA in the genome is condensed and not available for transcription. The region of the chromosome to be transcribed must first be opened (relaxed) before RNA polymerase can access the promoter of the gene of interest. The attachment of acetyl or other chemical groups to the histone proteins relaxes the chromosome and permits access to the DNA. In the absence of the attachment of these chemical groups, the chromosome stays condensed, the promoter is not accessible, and the gene is not expressed (Fig. 6.5).

A similar process is used at the DNA level for promoting or inhibiting transcription once the chromosome has relaxed except that the chemical group is frequently a methyl group. Recall the architecture of a typical gene as having a regulatory region, a promoter region, and a coding region. When methyl groups are attached to the DNA in the promoter region, the RNA polymerase is physically blocked from attaching and initiating transcription. For transcription to occur in higher organisms, methyl groups must be removed, and specialized proteins called transcription factors must bind to the DNA in the regulatory region.

Health or Disease?

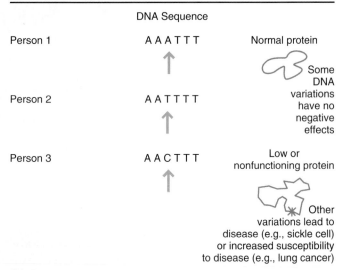

Fig. 6.4 DNA Sequence Variation in Genes Can Change the Protein Produced. Human beings differ from each other in only an estimated 0.1% of the total sequence of nucleotides that compose deoxyribonucleic acid. These variations in genetic information are thought to be the basis for the physical and functional differences between individuals. Some variations in a person's genetic code will have no effect on the protein that is produced; others can lead to disease or an increased susceptibility to a disease. (From U.S. Department of Energy, Human Genome Program: www.ornl.gov/hgmis.)

Transcription factors have a DNA binding site and a ligand binding site. This latter site can bind a small molecular weight "sensor" molecule (a **ligand**) that changes the conformation of the transcription factor and changes its ability to bind to DNA. In higher organisms binding may involve multiple transcription factors, each binding its specific ligand. Depending on the gene, multiple transcription factors may connect with

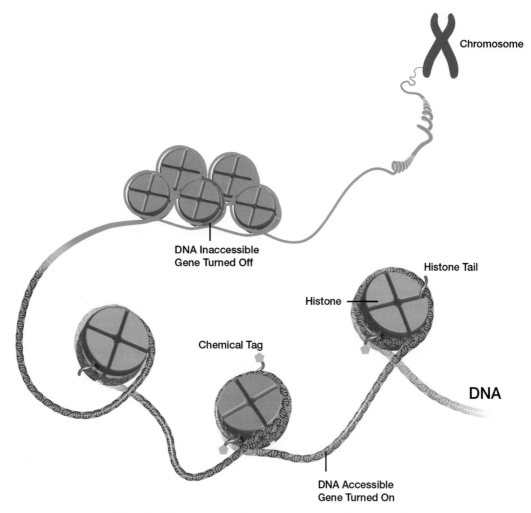

Fig. 6.5 Epigenetic regulation of gene expression through histone modification and DNA methylation. (Image credit: Darryl Leja, National Human Genome Research Institute, NIH.)

DNA individually or form a complex that then allows attachment to the DNA. The expression of some genes is activated by the complex and for others transcription is silenced.

Food plays key roles in the regulation of gene expression. The acetyl and methyl groups originate from food and many of the ligands that bind to transcription factors are derived from food. Food is an important source of information for all organisms to "sense" and respond to their environment. In lower organisms the interaction with DNA is direct. Food molecules placed into the growth medium surrounding the organisms, such as bacteria, can turn on or off genes. The classic examples of regulation of gene expression in lower organisms by food can be seen with the sugar lactose and the amino acid histidine. The disaccharide lactose is not typically in the bacterium's growth medium. The genes coding for the proteins needed to move lactose into the cell and to cleave the sugar into its glucose and galactose components are silenced until lactose is detected. In contrast, the presence of the nutrient histidine in the growth medium silences the genes needed for its biosynthesis. Since histidine is an essential amino acid, these genes are normally expressed constitutively (always "on"). In this way the organism conserves its energy by sensing the environment, detecting histidine, silencing biosynthesis, and making use of the histidine in the environment.

In both the lactose and histidine examples, there is communication between the environment and the DNA to silence or activate genes, as appropriate to the health of the organism. The process of sensing and responding to the external and internal environments differs in complexity among organisms but the basic motif is the same. Genes that encode routinely needed proteins are constitutively expressed and silenced by a feedback mechanism when the quantity of the end product is sufficient. As the end product level falls, gene expression resumes. Genes whose protein products are not routinely needed are silenced until needed, at which point gene expression is activated until the environmental trigger (such as lactose) is exhausted and expression is silenced.

Human beings have similar but more complex processes for sensing their environment and some of these aspects can be inherited. The process in higher organisms is called signal transduction and there are more steps and more players involved in the process. Food contains numerous bioactive molecules from plants and animals that play important roles in regulating gene expression by serving as "sensors" of the external environment. Among these bioactives are familiar compounds such as isoflavones from soybeans, curcumin from the spice turmeric, glucosinolates from cruciferous vegetables, and epigallocatechin-3-gallate from green tea. For additional information on food molecules as sensors, examples of common bioactive food molecules, and examples of the intricate system of transducing these environmental signals to silence or activate genes, see Boxes 6.3 and 6.4.

BOX 6.3 How Food and Genes Communicate

Transcription factors are specialized proteins that bind DNA in one region of the protein and bind a small molecular weight ligand in another region. The complex then binds to DNA and influences gene expression. In this way, food-derived molecules (often referred to as **bioactive food components**) and nonfood molecules such as toxic environmental chemicals communicate with genes and influence which ones are switched on or off, as needed.

These ligands may regulate transcription of genes needed for their metabolism. Alternatively, they may communicate a broader message, such as the presence of chronic inflammation and the need to dampen the expression of genes that produce proinflammatory cytokines. Examples of bioactive food components include the omega-3 fatty acids involved in silencing transcription of proinflammatory genes, derivatives of vitamin A and vitamin D, and numerous plant-derived small molecular weight ligands (phytonutrients). See Box 6.4 for further discussion of phytonutrients.

In human beings this process of sensing the environment and communicating with DNA is a more complex version of the ability of lower organisms to sense nutrients in the growth medium and turn on or off the expression of genes needed for nutrient metabolism. In higher organisms there are more steps and more players involved in the process but the basic theme is the same: to protect the organism by responding appropriately to the state of the ever-changing environment. If the molecule that triggers the switching on (or off) of a gene is fat-soluble (hydrophobic) and of small molecular weight, it typically can pass through the cellular and nuclear membranes and bind to DNA through DNA-binding transcription factors. Examples include the steroid hormones, vitamin A, vitamin D, and thyroid hormones. If the molecule is large or water-soluble (hydrophilic), it will not readily pass through membranes. Instead it will dock with receptors on the outer cell membrane. Docking sets off the process of **signal transduction**, a multistep cascade that amplifies the initial signal and ultimately results in an activator molecule binding to a transcription factor that in turn binds to DNA and activates or inhibits expression of the target gene. Numerous food-derived molecules are involved in signal transduction.

The nuclear factor-κB (NF-κB) family of transcription factors provides an example of such a signal transduction model of gene regulation in higher organisms. These transcription factors regulate numerous genes involved with inflammation, immunity, cell proliferation and differentiation, and apoptosis (programmed cell death). The NF-κB factors reside in the cytoplasm and are kept inactive by the binding of inhibitors. When a signal molecule from the environment connects to receptors on the cell surface, a stepwise cascade is initiated that activates the NF-κB transcription factors. The active factors then translocate to the nucleus to bind to genes whose expression is under their regulation.

Activators of this family of transcription factors are molecules that sound the alarm that the organism is under attack, such as tissue necrosis factor alpha (TNFα), interleukin-1 (IL-1), and reactive oxygen species (free radicals). In contrast, several food phytonutrients have been shown to help maintain the inactive state of NF-κB and protect against inflammation. These molecules have been found in the cruciferous vegetables (indole-3-carbinol, 3,3′-diindolylmethane), in soybeans (genistein and other isoflavones), and in curcumin, from the spice turmeric.

BOX 6.4 Bioactive Food Components: Phytonutrients

Food contains many thousands of biologically active molecules (referred to as "bioactive food components") that are being investigated for their health benefits. Bioactives derived from plants are called "phytonutrients" ("phyto" in Greek meaning "plants"). The original term for these bioactives was "phytochemicals" but was changed to phytonutrients because expressed discomfort with the term "chemicals." Although not technically nutrients, phytonutrients are emerging as important metabolic components.

From a dietary standpoint, the most commonly studied phytonutrients have been those from fruits, vegetables, legumes, cereal grains, nuts, seeds, teas, olive oil, wine, herbs, spices, and dark chocolate (Upadhyay and Dixit, 2015; Andreesu et al, 2018). Phytonutrients regulate numerous cellular and molecular pathways, such as preventing cell proliferation and aggregation, protecting against inflammation and oxidative stress, potentiating signals from the environment, and regulating gene expression in response to environmental triggers. The benefits of these compounds are being investigated in many prevalent chronic disorders, such as cancer, vascular disease (hypertension, dyslipidemia, smooth muscle proliferation leading to intimal thickening), diabetes (glucose intolerance, insulin resistance), and neurodegeneration.

Polyphenols are the largest category of phytonutrients and include simple phenolic acids, stilbenes, curcuminoids, chalcones, lignans, flavonoids, and isoflavones. Common food sources of polyphenols include genistein and daidzein (soy), resveratrol (purple grape skins, red wine), quercetin (onions), catechins and epicatechins (beans, green tea, black tea, apricots, chocolate), proanthocyanidins (apples, cocoa, berries), and curcumin (turmeric, mustard, curries). Curcumin is also antiinflammatory and, as such, is potentially helpful in virtually all of the chronic disorders since low-grade chronic inflammation is an underlying mechanism. Glucosinolates are sulfur-rich compounds that occur in cruciferous vegetables, such as broccoli, cauliflower, Brussels sprouts, and kale. Metabolism of glucosinolates yields isothiocyanates (e.g., sulforaphane) and indoles (e.g., indole-3-carbinol), which have been found to have anticarcinogenic properties (Lampe and Peterson, 2002; Peterson et al, 2002). The cruciferous vegetables and their glucosinolate components also play an important role in biotransformation, which is a key mechanism for protecting the body against cancer.

Of the polyphenols, isoflavones, curcumin, glucosinolates, resveratrol, and epigallocatechin-3-gallate (EGCG) from green tea have been of particular interest because they are known to influence gene expression through epigenetic mechanisms (Vanden Berghe, 2012). Isoflavones, curcumin, and EGCG are important inhibitors of the proinflammatory NF-κB signaling cascade. Resveratrol and curcumin are examples of polyphenols that can activate SIRT1, a histone deacetylase involved in inflammatory pathways, including NF-κB. There are numerous cell signaling mechanisms involved in epigenetic regulation of gene expression; NF-κB is an important example because it regulates several proinflammatory processes that contribute to chronic inflammation that underlies chronic disorders. Scientific research continues to support the recommendation for a mostly plant-based diet that includes a wide variety of foods as essential to long-term health. Several overviews of phytonutrients, their health benefits, and their mechanisms can be found in Rescigno et al, 2018; Lee et al, 2018; Rescigno et al, 2017; Upadhyay and Dixit, 2015; and Gupta and Prakash, 2014.

In addition to these mechanisms, noncoding RNAs are also involved in regulating gene expression. These RNAs are produced during transcription but are not mRNA and therefore do not direct protein synthesis. There are long noncoding RNAs (lncRNA) and short noncoding RNAs (sncRNA), which include microRNAs (miRNA) and small nucleotide RNAs (snRNA). The finding that these RNAs are not simply extra nucleotides that were removed during maturation of pre-mRNA into mRNA is fairly recent. The roles of these various RNAs are being investigated and include gene silencing as a major target (Mattick, 2018). Several thousand early-stage studies in mouse models and human tissues have been reported. Both long and short RNAs have been linked to various metabolic disorders: diabetes, obesity, cardiovascular disease, cardiometabolic syndrome, neurologic disorders, nonalcoholic fatty liver disease, and various cancers.

Epigenomics and Gene Expression

The regulation of gene expression occurs at two levels: genomic and epigenomic. "Epi" in Greek means "above," as in "above" the genetic code. Genomic control takes place within the regulatory region of genes, upstream from the promoters. Epigenetics and epigenomics relate to processes that alter gene expression through modification of histone proteins or DNA without changing the sequence of the DNA, thereby keeping the information in DNA intact. This point is important since DNA encodes the information for making RNAs and proteins, which are critical for the translation of this information into an operating system that generates human function. Epigenetics is concerned with the processes involved in regulating gene expression, how genes are turned on or off and the mechanisms involved. These processes are particularly critical during the various stages of normal human growth and development. Epigenomics, in contrast, is the collective set of epigenetic tags in a genome. Although the DNA sequence is the same from cell to cell, the pattern of gene expression is different among different cell types and these patterns can be inherited. The pattern of epigenetic marks (or "tags") that are characteristic of each cell type determines the gene expression pattern (i.e., which genes are active or silent at any given point). Epigenetic marks represent an additional set of instructions beyond the DNA genetic code that governs the process of decoding DNA into RNA and protein. Epigenomic research focuses on understanding which epigenetic marks are within a genome, how changes arise, the influence of epigenetic patterns on physiologic function, and how the marks are inherited.

Epigenetic gene regulation is achieved through the addition or deletion of chemical groups to histone proteins or methyl groups to DNA. To date, the more common tags are acetyl groups added to histone proteins and methyl groups to DNA but phosphorylation, ubiquitylation, and sumoylation (attachment of SUMO groups—small ubiquitin-like modifiers) are also used. During development of the fertilized embryo most of the epigenetic marks are erased (genomic reprogramming) but some remain and are passed from parent to child. In this way the child inherits some of the parents' life experiences that led to the epigenetic patterns in the egg and sperm. Research and advances in technology will likely expand the library of potential epigenetic tags as well as our understanding of epigenetic inheritance.

Identical (monozygotic) twins are a natural example of the influence of epigenetics in human beings. The twins are not identical phenotypically despite having identical genotypes. Epigenetic regulation of gene expression contributes to this phenomenon, which is called monozygotic discordance (also epigenetic drift). See Box 6.5 for a further exploration of the role of epigenetics in the differences in anthropomorphic features and disease susceptibility as monozygotic twins age.

Epigenetic marks provide the instructions for the development and differentiation of each cell type and for directing their aggregation into tissues and organs. With the exception of red blood cells, which have no nucleus, each of the cells in higher organisms contains the full set of DNA in the nucleus. During development, these cells differentiate into the various types of cells needed to operate the organism, such as eye cells, bone cells, liver cells, heart cells, and so on. Each cell type is specialized for particular tasks, which requires that certain of its genes be transcribed and others be silenced. The importance of nutrition during the prenatal and postnatal developmental periods cannot be

---

BOX 6.5 Epigenetics and Identical Twins

Have you ever wondered why most identical twins and other monozygotic multiples have increasingly obvious phenotypic differences as they age in spite of having the same DNA? Commonly encountered differences include physical features, disease susceptibility, and personality. Twins reared apart tend to exhibit greater observable differences. However, not all monozygotic twins exhibit this pattern. The basis for these differences lies, at least in part, with different epigenetic signatures, which leads to differential regulation of gene expression and the phenomenon of "monozygotic discordance," also called "epigenetic drift." Early investigations by Fraga and colleagues (Fraga et al, 2005; Poulsen et al, 2007) found that monozygotic (MZ) twins were identical in their epigenetic patterns early in life but that the epigenetic patterns of DNA methylation and histone acetylation in older MZ twins was considerably different. These studies were significant in explaining how different phenotypes could arise from apparently identical genotypes.

Recently the situation has grown even more complex. Waterland and colleagues discovered that the timing of the restoration of the epigenetic marks in monozygotic twins determines how similar the marks are between the twins (Van Baak et al, 2018). These marks are erased during fertilization and restored during very early embryonic development. Monozygotic siblings form when the very early embryo splits in two and each embryo develops into a separate individual. If the epigenetic marks are reset before the embryo splits, the epigenetic pattern will be the same for both twins, called "epigenetic supersimilarity". If the marks are reset after the embryo splits, there will be differences in epigenetic patterns between the twins. In both cases the DNA sequence is identical, but the epigenetic pattern is identical or different depending on the timing of resetting the epigenetic marks.

Two findings from this study are intriguing and under further study. One is the link between the genes involved in epigenetic supersimilarity and the development of cancer. The other is a rethinking of the use of monozygotic twins as a model system for estimating the risk of disease contributed by genes vs. environment. The lack of stratification of the twins in such studies based on their epigenetic pattern at birth may have led to an overestimation of genetic contribution to disease.

---

overemphasized because the diet is the source not only of the nutrients needed for growth but for the epigenetic marks that direct growth, development, and differentiation. Research suggests that many other stressors in addition to food insufficiency have an epigenetic effect, such as poverty, stress, and toxic exposure. A new discipline, social epigenomics, has arisen that focuses on social experiences throughout the lifespan and investigation of the key environmental triggers and their epigenetic effects. See Box 6.6 for additional information.

MODES OF INHERITANCE

Three processes influence how traits are transmitted from one generation to the next: mendelian inheritance, mitochondrial inheritance, and epigenetic inheritance.

Mendelian Inheritance

Each cell's nucleus contains a complete set of genetic material (genome), divided among 22 pairs of chromosomes (autosomes) and 2 sex chromosomes for a total of 46 chromosomes. During cell division (mitosis), all 46 chromosomes are duplicated and distributed to each new cell. During meiosis, one member of each of the autosome and sex chromosome pairs is distributed to an egg or sperm. Upon fertilization, the full set of 46 chromosomes is restored.

Because genes are carried on chromosomes, the rules governing the distribution of chromosomes during mitosis and meiosis

BOX 6.6   Social Epigenomics

Social epigenomics is concerned with the negative and positive influences of social experiences throughout the lifespan. These experiences do not alter the DNA sequence, only the epigenetic marks attached to the DNA and histone proteins. The epigenetic pattern (epigenome), in turn, alters gene expression. This feature is important because genes that might normally protect against a disease (such as cancer tumor-suppressor genes) may be turned off and genes that promote disease (such as cancer oncogenes) may be turned on.

The focus of research in this area is to investigate the key environmental drivers for altering the epigenetic pattern and their influences on function. Numerous factors are being found to cause changes in the epigenetic pattern, from food to stress to toxic chemicals to aging. The encouraging aspect of this work is that these influencers on epigenetic patterns are potentially modifiable. Research is identifying what the environmental triggers are and the mechanisms by which they influence gene expression.

Since 2008 the National Institutes on Minority Health and Health Disparities has established a program for funding research highlighting social epigenomics, particularly as it includes the health of minorities and health disparities in the U.S. population, especially as a result of racism and discrimination. The expectation is that, by identifying epigenetic modifications, it may be possible to detect disease susceptibilities early and tailor interventions that can prevent chronic conditions from manifesting. See the National Institutes of Health website on research on social epigenomics to address health disparities for information on the types of research studies that are being conducted.

govern the distribution of genes and any changes (mutations, gene variants) they may contain. These rules describe the mendelian inheritance of a gene, named after Gregor Mendel, who first deduced that the inheritance of traits was governed by a predictable set of rules. It is possible to track a mutation through multiple generations by knowing these rules of inheritance. This transmission is depicted typically as a pedigree and can be used to predict the probability of a genetic change being inherited by a particular family member. When the change causes a disease, a pedigree can be helpful in predicting the probability that another family member will inherit the disease. The Family History Initiative through the CDC offers helpful online tools for organizing information about your family history.

Mendelian transmission can be autosomal or sex-linked, dominant or recessive. There are five classic modes of mendelian inheritance: autosomal dominant, autosomal recessive, X-linked dominant, X-linked recessive, and Y-linked. An individual's genotype obeys the laws of inheritance, but the phenotype (the observable/measurable expression of the genotype) may not. Each gene in an individual is present in two copies (alleles), one on each chromosome (with the exception of traits carried on the male X or Y chromosome). When the alleles are the same (either both are the common or usual version or both are the mutant or variant form), the individual is said to be homozygous. If the alleles are different, the individual is heterozygous (also called a carrier).

Whether a gene is dominant or recessive refers to whether a trait is expressed (can be measured, observed) in a heterozygous individual who has one common allele and one variant allele. If a trait is expressed when only a single copy of a variant allele is present, the allele is said to be dominant (i.e., the variant allele determines the phenotype). Alleles that do not dominate the genotype when only a single copy is present are called recessive. The variant allele is present in the genome, but the trait is not expressed unless two copies of this allele are expressed. Further confounding the nomenclature is the

concept of penetrance. Even when a pedigree suggests that a gene is present that should lead to the individual displaying a certain phenotype, the phenotype (often a disease) may not be evident. Such a gene is said to have reduced penetrance, meaning that not everyone who has the gene expresses it in a form that is readily measurable. "Measurable form" much depends on what is able to be measured with current technology. Many alleles thought to be recessive 50 years ago can be detected today as the result of new and more sensitive technologies. Penetrance is of interest to nutrition professionals because it can also reflect the inability of a genetic variation to impair function and cause disease unless the individual is exposed to specific environmental triggers, such as diet and lifestyle factors. Modifying these factors potentially can improve outcomes for those with such variants. Expect the terminology to continue to be updated as knowledge advances about the associations among genes, lifestyle, and functional outcomes.

Mitochondrial Inheritance

Mitochondria are subcellular organelles that are essential for energy production and are thought to have originated from bacteria (therefore no chromosomes). In addition to genetic material in the nucleus, the mitochondria in each cell also contain DNA. Human mitochondrial DNA (mtDNA) codes for 14 proteins essential to oxidative phosphorylation and energy production and 2 ribosomal RNAs and 22 transfer RNAs needed for mitochondrial protein synthesis. The remainder of the proteins are coded for by nuclear DNA. In contrast to nuclear DNA, mtDNA is small (16,569 base pairs), circular, and exists in multiple copies within each mitochondrion, the number varying among cell types. As with nuclear DNA, changes in mtDNA can lead to disease.

Traits resulting from mitochondrial genes have a characteristic inheritance pattern; they are nonmendelian because mitochondria and their genetic material typically pass from mother to child, called mitochondrial or maternal inheritance. This biologic principle has become the basis for anthropological studies that trace lineage and population migration patterns through the centuries. It also has provided a way to trace familial diseases caused by changes in mtDNA.

Epigenetic Inheritance

Epigenetic inheritance illustrates another mechanism by which genetic information is passed between generations. Inheritance occurs by the genome being passed by parents through germline (egg and sperm) cells to their offspring. Somatic (body) cells also pass on their epigenetic marks each time they divide, which is essential for cells to maintain their specialization (as heart cells, kidney cells, etc.).

An important point here is that epigenetic marks appear not to be permanent (lifelong) at the time of fertilization. Lifestyle choices throughout the lifespan can alter these marks (the epigenome) as a result of the organism responding to information communicated from the ever-changing environment. The triggers may be traditional nutrients, phytonutrients, exercise, stress, sleep sufficiency, cytokines, toxins, hormones, and drugs. The fact that epigenetic marks are passed on to daughter cells, whether gametes or somatic cells, means that any changes in the marks can be inherited and can influence gene expression in subsequent generations. The quality of our lifestyle choices, and their appropriateness for our particular genetic makeup, matters.

Epigenetics is increasingly considered to be one important factor in sorting out why the presence, in the genome, of single nucleotide polymorphisms (SNPs) that appear to be strongly associated with a particular chronic disorder are typically not sufficient to lead to chronic disease. The presence of these gene variants, a change in a nucleotide in a genetic sequence, can cause an aberration in coding of proteins and can increase the susceptibility for developing a chronic disease—but this is not a guarantee. Food and other lifestyle choices appear to be essential triggers for activating the susceptibility for chronic disease and epigenetic marks. With their ability to regulate gene expression, food and lifestyle choices appear to be at least some of the underlying mechanisms.

Groundbreaking research demonstrating the influence of diet on physiologic outcomes and the connection to epigenetics was conducted by Waterland and Jirtle (2003), showing the effect of specific nutrients on phenotype. See Box 6.7 for more information on these experiments. Applicability of these types of findings to human beings can be found in studies such as the Dutch Hunger Winter Families Study (Roseboom et al, 2006; Rooji et al, 2010; Bygren, 2013). The Dutch Hunger Winter study is a retrospective cohort study that supports the possibility of transgenerational epigenetic inheritance in human beings as well as the importance of prenatal nutrition. This study investigated the offspring of mothers who were pregnant during the Dutch Hunger Winter famine that followed World War II. Undernutrition during fetal development could be traced to health consequences for these children during later life. See Box 6.8 for details.

BOX 6.7 Epigenetic Inheritance: Influence of Nutrition

Researching the underlying genetic and metabolic basis for a trait or disease requires the ability to control a number of the variables, such as mating, diet, and other lifestyle choices.

For this reason, model systems have evolved in which researchers can get an understanding of the genetic, biochemical, and physiological mechanisms prior to designing human studies. The laboratory mouse has been of particular value because it has a sufficiently similar operating system to that of human beings. This feature has allowed researchers to predict from mouse studies what is likely occurring in human beings. It was through the use of mice whose coat color could be controlled through genetic and dietary manipulation that Waterland and Jirtle (2003) were able to provide insight into the complexity of epigenetics and its heritability.

The researchers selected a strain of mice with a mutation in the *Asip* gene, more commonly referred to as the *agouti* ("a-goo-tee") gene. The mutation involved the insertion of a DNA fragment into the promoter region of the agouti gene. The mutation is designated A^{vy} (agouti viable yellow allele) and it is dominant. Genetically identical A^{vy}/A^{vy} mice with yellow coats were bred with *a/a* wild-type ("normal") mice with dark brown coats and fed the standard laboratory mouse chow. The offspring (F1 generation) were genetically A^{vy}/a. Since the A^{vy} allele is dominant, all the offspring were expected to have yellow coats. Instead, there was a range of coat colors varying from yellow to yellow-brown ("mottled") to brown and these colors persisted into adulthood. The insightful hypothesis of Waterland and Jirtle was that epigenetics was responsible for the coat color results, potentially caused by methylation of the A^{vy} allele, and that this effect could be inherited.

The researchers then tested whether methylation was involved. They designed a study in which dark-coated *a/a* females were bred to A^{vy}/A^{vy} yellow males. The females were divided into two groups. Both groups received the standard laboratory chow, but half the mothers received a supplement of folate, vitamin B_{12}, choline, and betaine, which provided a methyl donor-rich diet. The supplement was begun 2 weeks before mating and continued during pregnancy and lactation. All the offspring were A^{vy}/a. The unsupplemented mothers had offspring with yellow or yellow-brown coats, as expected. Most of the offspring from the mothers on the methyl-rich diet, however, had a mottled coat with a mix of brown and yellow (called *pseudoagouti*). Clearly, the mother's diet affected the coat color of the offspring and these effects persisted into adulthood. An investigation into what may be causing the difference in phenotype among genotypically identical siblings detected a correlation between mottled coat and degree of methylation of the *agouti* gene, which suggested that the methyl-rich diet led to epigenetic silencing of the A^{vy} allele.

Furthermore, this effect of diet was clearly heritable. In subsequent experiments (Cropley et al, 2006) found that feeding the females of the "grandmother" generation a methyl-rich diet but not enriching the daughter offspring's diet still produced a number of second-generation offspring with mottled brown coats, which suggested that the effect the diet had on coat color could be transmitted to succeeding generations. These studies laid the groundwork for research investigating diet and other lifestyle factors for potential transgenerational effects.

BOX 6.8 Epigenetic Inheritance: The Dutch Famine Study

A retrospective cohort study suggests that the existence of transgenerational epigenetic inheritance that was seen in the mouse studies (see Box 6.7) also occurred in humans. The Dutch Hunger Winter Families Study investigated over 2414 offspring of mothers who were pregnant during the extreme famine in the Netherlands during the harsh winter of 1944 to 1945. The de Rooij et al study (2010) provides an overview of the history of the famine, which resulted from the coalescence of the food embargo during World War II and a particularly severe winter that decimated food crops. All social classes were affected. Daily caloric intake at the peak of the famine was extremely low for the adult population (estimated at 400 to 800 calories/day). Although pregnant women were allotted extra food, there was insufficient food to meet the need. The famine period was followed by plentiful food as these children grew to adulthood. Studies of adult offspring from these mothers found elevated rates of cardiovascular disease and accompanying altered lipid profiles, obesity, type 2 diabetes, and age-associated cognitive decline (Roseboom et al, 2006; de Rooij et al, 2010; Bygren, 2013).

As regrettable in terms of human suffering as the famine was, it has generated valuable understanding of the developmental origins of health and disease and has increased awareness of the critical nature of diet and lifestyle during the prenatal period. Further, researchers have been able to correlate starvation during stages of gestation with effects of the famine on offspring (de Rooij et al, 2010). Children exposed to the famine in the latter third of pregnancy were small at birth and remained small throughout life. Impaired renal function was correlated with those exposed to starvation during midpregnancy (Roseboom et al, 2006). Those exposed in the early stages of pregnancy tended to have the elevated rates of cardiovascular disease, obesity, and cognitive decline in adulthood (de Rooij et al, 2010). More recently, Franke et al (2018) have used neuroimaging of these offspring compared with healthy individuals of the same age and found that undernutrition during early gestation resulted in distinct differences in brain structure as well as premature brain aging.

Changes in epigenetic marks are suspected of contributing to the health outcomes seen with undernutrition in prenatal life. Researchers are examining prenatal and adult epigenetic signatures in human beings and animal model systems to gain a better understanding of the influence of various types of stress during the prenatal period. A recent review by Cao-Lei et al (2017) summarizes the current understanding of this association.

At this time, epigenetic inheritance is the least understood of the mechanisms of inheritance but is under active study globally by numerous laboratories. At least three mechanisms are involved: histone modification, DNA modification, and noncoding RNAs. As discussed earlier, epigenetic marks resulting from histone and DNA modifications can be passed down through the generations. Just how far the reach extends is not yet known, but there is a clear pattern at least from grandparents to children to grandchildren. The importance here to nutrition professionals is that food and other lifestyle choices matter—what grandparents ate has the potential to influence subsequent generations. The details of these processes are beyond the scope of this chapter, but readers should be aware that diet and other lifestyle factors are powerful levers for changing one's health trajectory. As such, they are powerful tools for improving clients' health.

Expect that, in time, understanding epigenetic mechanisms will be essential for the development of effective nutrition therapy. Current reviews explore epigenetic inheritance in mammals as well as other animals and plants and in neurodevelopmental disorders, including current applications to autism (Radford, 2018; Dall'Aglio et al, 2018).

Genomic Imprinting

Typically, the human genome contains two working copies of each gene, one copy from each parent. For some genes, however, only one copy is switched on and transcribed. The other copy is epigenetically silenced through the addition of chemical groups. In other words, genes are silenced in a parent-of-origin specific manner. Epigenetic marks, typically methyl groups, are added in order to silence particular genes in the egg and other genes in the sperm. This process is called genomic imprinting.

The nucleotide sequences of the same gene in the father and the mother are much the same but not identical due to variations occurring over time. One parent may have a sequence that produces a functional protein from that gene. The other parent may have a change in their DNA, producing an altered protein that leads to impaired function. If the father's (paternal) copy of the gene is the one with the mutation and the mother's (maternal) copy is normal, the normal gene can usually compensate for the influence of the mutated gene (and vice versa if the maternal copy is mutated and the paternal copy is normal). However, if the gene involved is one that is epigenetically marked and it's the normal copy that's silenced, there will be insufficient normal protein to compensate and typically dysfunction and disease result. What's critical is which copy, paternal or maternal, is activated and which is silenced.

Imprinted genes are particularly important in the control of normal growth and development, including prenatal development, brain development, and postnatal metabolism (Girardot et al, 2013; Perez et al, 2016; Nilsson et al, 2018). Only a small number of genomic imprinting abnormalities have been reported to date. The reason is likely that the basis for such abnormalities can be difficult to detect and confirm. See Box 6.9 for examples of two well-known human disorders involving genomic imprinting and the importance of maternal and paternal genetic contributions. For additional examples of genomic imprinting and human disease, Kalish et al (2014) explores the role of imprinting in Beckwith-Wiedemann and Russell-Silver syndromes. Fifty percent of individuals with Beckwith-Wiedemann are estimated to have methylation defects, which suggests a role for nutrition therapy in addressing folate status (Dagar et al, 2018).

Current research efforts are now wide-ranging beyond chromosomal disorders. The potential role of genomic imprinting is being investigated in numerous diseases affecting growth, development, and differentiation. A few examples include cancer, autism spectrum disorders, the development of the brain and brain disorders, food allergy, and assisted reproductive technology (Liu et al, 2018).

BOX 6.9   Genomic Imprinting: Angelman and Prader-Willi Syndromes

Two examples of known developmental disorders arising from genomic imprinting abnormalities are Angelman's and Prader-Willi's syndromes. Both involve a microdeletion of chromosome 15. However, because of the phenomenon of genomic imprinting, which of the two syndromes develops is due to whether the deletion is passed from the father to the child or from the mother to the child.

Angelman's syndrome is a neurologic disorder with developmental disabilities; speech impediments; jerky gait; and a smiling, laughing demeanor. In this syndrome the genomically imprinted gene *UBE3A* associated with the ubiquitin pathway is involved. In Angelman's syndrome the paternal copy of this gene is silenced and the maternal copy is expressed.

If the maternal copy has a mutation in the imprinted gene or, as in the case of the microdeletion, the gene is lost, the gene is not present and cannot produce the normal protein needed. Angelman's syndrome develops.

Similarly, the *SNRPN* gene (which plays a role in mRNA splicing) is in the same region of the chromosome 15 microdeletion as the *UBE3A* gene but is associated with a different developmental disability, Prader-Willi's syndrome. In this case the maternal copy of the gene is silenced and the paternal copy is expressed. When the microdeletion is on the paternal contribution, the *SNRPN* gene is lost to deletion and the maternal gene is not expressed.

Prader-Willi's syndrome is also characterized by developmental disabilities, decreased muscle tone, and an extreme drive for food (see Chapter 43).

It is quite possible that these two examples are only the tip of the iceberg in terms of the developmental disabilities that likely involve genomic imprinting.

X-Inactivation

Another epigenetic example is X-inactivation, which may appear to be an example of genomic imprinting but is not. Imprinting involves the inactivation of working genes; X-inactivation involves inactivating an entire chromosome. Further, the two mechanisms are quite different. The need for X-inactivation stems from human males typically having one X chromosome and females having two X chromosomes. The assumption is that having twice the amount of gene expression from the X chromosome would be information overload due to the large number of genes (over 1000). Instead, one of the X chromosomes in females is inactivated early in development through a combination of epigenetic marks: hypermethylation of the DNA and condensation of the chromosome. The choice of whether the mother's or the father's X chromosome is inactivated appears to be random and varies from cell to cell. The selection occurs during early fetal development and continues through the numerous cell divisions required. Females therefore are mosaics. If the active X chromosome carries one or more genes associated with a disease and there are sufficient numbers of cells expressing this gene, symptoms characteristic of that disease may be observed. See Balaton et al (2018) for a review of the process of X-inactivation.

GENETIC VARIATION, INHERITANCE, AND DISEASE

Historically, human genetic research focused on identifying the mechanisms by which traits were passed from parent to child, such as physical traits or certain rare diseases that appeared within extended families. Genetic diseases were considered to be a separate category of disease, limited to those rare heritable disorders that resulted either from changes to a single gene or alterations at the chromosomal level. Either type of change can have a devastating effect on the metabolic and functional ability of the individual.

Today it is recognized that most diseases are genetic in origin, either from errors in the DNA nucleotide sequence and the information it encodes or from alteration in the expression of this information and its conversion into our functional abilities. Changes to the genetic material, whether to the chromosomal DNA, mtDNA, or even a single nucleotide, have the potential to alter one or more proteins that may be critical to the operation of the cells, tissues, and organs of the body. Changes to the genetic material at each of these levels can have important consequences to our metabolic and functional abilities.

Although DNA is physically quite stable, changes in the nucleotide sequence occur. Each time a cell divides or an egg or sperm cell forms, there's the potential for errors to occur in duplicating the DNA or distributing the chromosomes into the egg or sperm. Environmental exposures such as ultraviolet light and toxic chemicals can cause breaks in the DNA and changes may be introduced during repair. Changes to the DNA are commonly referred to as mutations but they're also called genetic variations, gene variants, or just "variants." They may involve a single nucleotide, a segment of a chromosome, or a whole chromosome. Although a change may be harmful to the organism, it may also be neutral or beneficial in effect. Mutation is the basis for evolution. When a change occurs that provides a survival benefit to the organism, that organism is able to grow to maturity and reproduce, and its descendants will continue to reproduce and contribute the mutation to the gene pool that characterizes that population.

The order of nucleotides within the DNA sequence determines the amino acid sequence of the protein that's produced. Which amino acid is altered determines the physical conformation (shape) of the protein, which influences how functional the protein is (Fig. 6.5). Whereas particular changes (mutations) in some genes have a devastating effect on function and lead to a disease, changes in other genes may have a much less drastic functional impact or no apparent effect at all. Some changes actually improve function, and many silent mutations have no effect. Where on the continuum the individual's functional ability falls depends on (1) how critical a gene is to the overall function of the organism, (2) whether a gene is expressed at the level needed and at the point in time needed, and (3) where in the gene the change occurs.

A change in the DNA sequence can affect the production or the function of the encoded protein and influence that protein's ability to fulfill its physiologic role. Either outcome can influence the extent of dysfunction that occurs. A classic example is the HBB gene, which encodes the beta-subunit of hemoglobin. A change in this gene involving a single nucleotide causes the debilitating disease sickle cell anemia. The variant beta-hemoglobin molecule is impaired in its ability to bind and deliver oxygen to cells. Additionally, under conditions of low oxygen, the hemoglobin-carrying red blood cells assume a rigid sickle shape, which can cause blockage of small blood vessels, most commonly leading to severe pain crises but sometimes organ damage, stroke, and even death. As knowledge and technology related to the connections among genes, mutation, and disease has progressed, it has become clear that there is a spectrum of disease severity, depending on the location of the altered nucleotide within the HBB gene.

Clinically, this type of knowledge has been helpful in explaining why individuals with a mutation in the same gene can have quite different symptoms. As an example, over a thousand mutations have been identified in the DNA sequence of the cystic fibrosis transmembrane conductance regulator gene (CFTR). What is observed clinically (the phenotype) is a spectrum of functional outcomes ranging from severe cystic fibrosis to much milder disease (see Chapter 33). Clinicians will need to look more fully into the genetic makeup of an individual to determine where on the functional spectrum the mutations fall. Of particular interest are the functional consequences of changes in the structure of proteins coded for by genes that provide the metabolic machinery for the cells, such as enzymes, receptors, transporters, antibodies, hormones, neurotransmitters, and communicators.

Thus a gene can exist in slightly different forms as a result of a seemingly minor change, such as one nucleotide replacing another. The term for the different forms of a gene is allele (or polymorphism if multiple alleles have been detected for a gene). As a result, genes have protein products with differing amino acid sequences (isoforms) and often different functions. Polymorphism is an important concept because it explains why human beings, although 99.9% alike genetically, are distinctly different. The 0.1% difference is sufficient to explain the obvious physical variations among humans. It is also the basis for more subtle differences that may not be readily observable, such as in the functional ability of a key metabolic enzyme to catalyze its reaction. Such variations likely underlie many of the inconsistencies observed in therapeutic outcomes and in nutritional intervention research. Researchers around the world are working to make the connections among gene variants, health and disease outcomes, and effective therapeutic interventions with the goal of improving health outcomes. Directly editing the genome is one strategy to improve health. See Box 6.10 to see how this technology is being applied in research and medicine.

BOX 6.10 Genome Editing: CRISPR

Genome editing has been a staple of science fiction for many years. In reality, gene editing has been a tool of scientists to introduce changes in the DNA of model organisms from bacteria to fruit flies and even large mammals so that the health effects of mutations (variants) can be studied. Genome editing has also been done to a variety of foods including corn, soybeans, zucchini, and sugar beets. The methods for introducing these mutations have been slow, expensive, and imprecise, sometimes creating random variants (such as with radiation) or requiring multiple generations to achieve the desired outcome.

A new technology called CRISPR (which stands for clusters of regularly interspaced short palindromic repeats) has given scientists a way to quickly, accurately, and inexpensively edit the genome. Adapted from the natural antiviral defense system in bacteria, CRISPR allows specific areas of the genome to be added, removed, or changed. The system uses small pieces of RNA to bind to a specific location in the target DNA, which then allows a CRISPR-associated protein (Cas) to cut the DNA. Cas9 is most often used, but other enzymes can also be combined with CRISPR such as Cas11 and Cpf1. The cell's DNA repair mechanism then repairs the break, introducing changes also encoded on the guide RNA.

Since CRISPR is much more accurate and efficient than previous genome editing technologies, researchers are exploring the possibility of using it to correct genetic diseases in humans. Single-gene disorders such as sickle cell anemia, cystic fibrosis, and other mendelian disorders are likely first candidates for this treatment. However, reports of changes in nontargeted parts of the genome (called off-target effects) raise the possibility of unintended consequences such as cancer or other diseases. The early failures of gene therapy and the availability of current disease-managing therapies have led health researchers to proceed with caution. The applicability of this technology to complex diseases and the line between fighting disease and unnecessary enhancement also remain provocative topics.

The technology also opens debate about responsible ways to edit human genomes. Editing a person's own cells, known as somatic editing, affects only the individual; editing germline cells (sperm and eggs) or those of embryos has the potential to affect future generations. Unregulated experiments on human embryos have already occurred, spurring the need for researchers, policymakers, and the public to discuss the ethics, limits, and potential of this powerful technology.

BOX 6.11   Detecting Gene Variants: Candidate Gene vs. GWAS

For a gene variant to be clinically useful, it must be well-characterized in terms of its association with a disease state, occur frequently in the population being studied (and, preferably, in multiple populations), and have a well-documented effective therapeutic intervention. There have been two main approaches to identifying gene variants that are associated with increased risk of developing common diseases: candidate gene studies and genome-wide association studies (GWAS). The **candidate gene approach** was the original tool. It focuses on functional variants and positional variants. Functional variants result from mutations in genes whose products are known to be involved in the mechanisms underlying the disease of interest. The positional approach is similar but searches for variants that are physically close to genes known to be involved in the underlying mechanisms. Candidate gene studies have the limitation that they're dependent on knowledge of the mechanisms underlying the disease of interest. If the mechanisms have not been thoroughly defined, it is likely that novel genes will not be detected. Further, a large cohort is often needed in order to include sufficient subjects homozygous for the risk allele. Candidate genes have been most successful for single gene disorders.

Lifestyle-related chronic diseases, however, tend to be complex traits and the complexity is further compounded by the epigenetic component. Development of these diseases typically requires the interaction of a genetic susceptibility created by a gene variant with environmental factors. These factors are typically modifiable and involve lifestyle choices such as the food we eat, whether we exercise regularly, how well we manage our thoughts and emotions, the quality of relationships and systems of meaning, the quality and quantity of our sleep, and our exposure to toxins such as tobacco smoke and other air pollution, food-borne toxic chemicals, and alcohol.

With the rapid advances in genetic technology it has been possible and economically feasible to scan the entire genome in search of common genetic variations. For example, a GWAS scan might involve a set of individuals with the same diagnosis and search for common genetic variations among these individuals or between populations. There are no predetermined target genes and thousands of variants and thousands of individuals can be investigated, which has greatly increased the speed at which gene variants have been detected. The *Catalog of Published Genome-Wide Association Studies* can be searched by diseases of interest to learn which gene variants have been identified to date. The large amounts of data generated by either approach, but particularly by the GWAS approach, greatly benefits from the development of bioinformatics and its high-capacity computer organization and analysis.

The rate of progress of applying genomics in clinical applications is associated strongly with progress in identifying associations between diseases and **single nucleotide polymorphisms** (SNPs, pronounced "snips"). Once a strong association has been determined, diagnostic tests and appropriate diet and lifestyle interventions can be developed and tested for efficacy. As the name for this genetic variation suggests, the change involves a single nucleotide. The initial molecular approach to associating mutations with susceptibility to disease was to look for SNPs (changes) in genes that encoded important metabolic proteins. This approach has been somewhat successful but not sufficiently successful in understanding the genetic and environmental complexity of chronic disorders. As a result, more recently the speed of whole genome sequencing has increased substantially and the cost has decreased, which have allowed a shift to **genome-wide association studies (GWAS)** as the preferred genomic tool for detecting SNPs. GWAS allows the detection of patterns of multiple SNPs associated with a disease and is particularly useful for complex disorders. See Box 6.11 for additional information.

In addition to SNPs, other types of variations also may play an important role in the genotypic and phenotypic variation among humans. Loss or gain of more than one nucleotide (deletions and insertions, respectively), duplication of nucleotide sequences, copy number variants, and restructuring of regions within a chromosome (inversions and translocations) also have important consequences to function. The most recent cataloging of human genetic variation has been the 1000 Genomes Project (www.internationalgenome.org) (Box 6.12). The earlier SNP cataloging was predominantly of individuals of European descent with some African American and Asian representation and is now undergoing expansion to multiple ethnic groups.

Disease at the Chromosomal Level

Change in the number of chromosomes, or the arrangement of DNA within a chromosome, is almost always detrimental and often fatal to the individual. Chromosomal disorders are detected by means of a **karyotype**, a visualization of all the chromosomes in picture form. Mutations that involve a change in the number or structure of a chromosome are often lethal events because chromosomes contain multiple genes and the ensuing chaos of having too little or too much

BOX 6.12   The 1000 Genomes Project

Like the Human Genome Project, the 1000 Genomes Project is a significant step forward in the goal of personalizing therapy. Advances in DNA technology and the subsequent cost-savings allowed researchers to expand the number of genomes and populations represented in the human genome database beyond the original Euro-centric data set. The genomes of 2504 individuals from 26 populations representing 5 continental regions were sequenced. The populations include a diverse sampling of the human population: African, American (north, central, and south American, including Native American), East Asian, European, and South Asian.

The goal of the project was to identify genetic variations that occurred in 1% or greater of the populations studied. Over 84.7 million single nucleotide polymorphisms (SNPs), 3.6 million short insertion/deletion structural variants, and 60,000 other structural variants were detected in these individuals, many clustered in haplotypes. The researchers estimate that >99% of the SNPs projected to be in the human genome at 1% or greater in frequency have been identified. This project is a major step forward for personalized health care. Future research will likely focus on detecting strong associations between specific genetic regions and particular diseases and then on developing effective therapeutic approaches. Bioinformatics has played a significant role in analyzing the extremely large data sets that were generated and will continue to be essential for subsequent research. The steady progress in knowledge, technology, and trained manpower focusing on genetic variation is revolutionizing the way clinicians think about the clinical aspects of medicine, pharmacology, and nutrition. Given the magnitude of variation among individuals, clinical approaches will increasingly accommodate the shift from one-size-fits-all to personalized approaches (1000 Genomes Project Consortium, 2015).

---

information, or information being expressed at the wrong time, is detrimental to the organism. However, it is possible that parts of chromosomes will break away and attach to another chromosome or that a region of a chromosome will be duplicated. Such events are not always lethal but do typically cause abnormal symptoms. There are numerous chromosomal aberrations that have been defined, many of which have nutritional implications such as assistance with feeding. Descriptions of the changes and their consequences can be found in clinical genetics textbooks as well as online in resources such as the

Genetic and Rare Diseases Information Center and the Mendelian Inheritance in Man compendium.

An example of a nonfatal chromosomal abnormality is trisomy 21 (Down's syndrome). Typically seen is an extra copy of the whole chromosome resulting from an error in distributing the chromosomes during sperm or egg formation. However, the characteristics of Down's syndrome are due to a small region of chromosome 21, so that even if only that tiny piece of DNA is present in triplicate, the syndrome results. Other developmental syndromes are caused by the loss of a portion of a chromosome (a partial deletion). In Beckwith-Wiedemann's syndrome (a chromosome 11 deletion), changes are characterized by organ overgrowth, including an oversized tongue, which leads to feeding difficulties and undernutrition.

Nutrition professionals play an important role in the therapy of those with chromosomal disorders, because these individuals often have oral-motor problems that affect their nutritional status and cause growth problems in early life. Later in development, body weight may become an issue, and nutrition therapy is helpful in controlling weight, diabetes, and cardiovascular complications. Varying degrees of mental insufficiency often complicate therapy. Nutrition professionals can help mitigate the detrimental effects of these disorders on nutritional status (see Chapter 43).

Disease at the Mitochondrial Level

Due to the major role that mitochondria play in energy production, alterations in mtDNA are frequently degenerative and have varied clinical manifestations because of the multiple copies of mtDNA, not all of which may contain the genetic change. Mutations in mtDNA can manifest at any age and include neurologic diseases, cardiomyopathies, and skeletal myopathies. An increasing number of diseases are being linked to mutations in mtDNA. One of the earliest disorders to be traced to mtDNA is Wolfram's syndrome, a form of diabetes with associated deafness. Subsequently, gene variants have been found that relate to each of the components of the oxidative phosphorylation pathway. The physiologic consequences of these mutations typically involve organs that have a high demand for energy, such as the heart, kidneys, brain, and muscles. See the National Institutes of Health Genetics Home Reference website for information on mtDNA-based disorders and MITOMAP, a human mitochondrial genome database, for specifics on human mtDNA variants.

Disease at the Molecular Level

The majority of disease conditions associated with genomics involve changes at the molecular level. Changes to the DNA typically involve a single nucleotide change or several nucleotides within a single gene through substitutions, additions, or deletions in the regulatory, promoter, or coding regions. Alterations in the regulatory or promoter region may increase or decrease the quantity of protein produced or alter the ability of the gene to respond to environmental signals. Alterations in the coding region may affect the amino acid sequence of the protein, which in turn can affect the conformation and function of the protein and thereby the functioning of the organism. Because the majority of human genes reside on chromosomes, gene variations are transmitted according to mendelian inheritance and are subject to modification from epigenetic markings.

Autosomal dominant single-gene disorders that have nutritional implications include several that may result in developmental disabilities, oral-motor problems, susceptibility to weight gain, and difficulties with constipation. Examples include Albright hereditary osteodystrophy, which commonly results in dental problems, obesity, hypocalcemia, and hyperphosphatemia; chondrodysplasias, which often result in oral-motor problems and obesity; and Marfan syndrome, which involves cardiac disease, excessive growth, and increased nutritional needs. Familial hypercholesterolemia (type 2 familial dyslipidemia) results from a defective low-density lipoprotein receptor (LDLR gene), transmitted as an autosomal dominant trait. Symptoms include elevated levels of total cholesterol, elevated levels of LDL cholesterol, and increased risk of atherosclerosis.

Autosomal recessive disorders are more common. They were traditionally detected because the mutation had a detrimental effect on the newborn infant that led to serious developmental consequences or death. Sickle cell anemia is an example of an autosomal recessive disease, caused by inheriting two copies of the variant HBB gene. Metabolic disorders of amino acid, carbohydrate, and lipid metabolism, designated as inborn errors of metabolism (IEM), are similarly heritable and associated with a particular mutation. IEM disorders are the earliest known examples of nutritional genomics, and dietary modification remains the primary treatment (see Chapter 42). A brief overview of IEM from a genetic perspective is included here to emphasize the important role of the nutrition professional in restoring health to these individuals and to contrast IEM with chronic disorders, which result from the same type of genetic change but affect function less severely. A classic example of an IEM of amino acid metabolism is phenylketonuria (PKU), which is an autosomal recessive disorder. PKU results from a mutation in the gene coding for the enzyme phenylalanine hydroxylase, leading to an inability to convert phenylalanine to tyrosine. Lifelong dietary restriction of phenylalanine enables individuals with PKU to live into adulthood and enjoy a quality life.

Hereditary fructose intolerance (HFI) is another example of an autosomal recessive IEM of carbohydrate metabolism. A mutation in the ALDOB gene encoding aldolase B (fructose-1,6-biphosphate aldolase) impairs the catalytic activity of the enzyme and prevents fructose from being converted to glucose. Breast-fed infants are typically asymptomatic until fruit is added to the diet. Nutrition therapy involves the elimination of fructose, sorbitol, and the fructose-containing disaccharide sucrose. In the absence of understanding the presence of this genetic lesion and the need to eliminate these sweeteners from the diet, the individual typically proceeds to develop hypoglycemia, vomiting, and ultimately kidney failure, leading to death.

These disorders highlight the power of understanding the underlying genetic mutation when developing nutrition therapeutic approaches. First, the family history may give a hint that a genetic mutation is present. Although the genetic mutation (genotype) is permanent, the phenotype is not. In spite of an individual having mutations that predispose to disease, eliminating specific foods and food ingredients essentially keeps the disease susceptibility silent, and the infant will enjoy normal development. Nutrition professionals are invaluable for being able to detect the problem and recommend the appropriate therapy sufficiently early to prevent disease symptoms from manifesting and causing serious developmental issues.

The X-linked dominant fragile X syndrome also affects nutritional status. Fragile X syndrome is characterized by developmental delays, mental impairment, and behavioral problems. The lesion occurs within the FMR1 gene on the X chromosome in which a cytosine-guanine-guanine trinucleotide segment is repeated more times than the usual number for human beings. The multiple repeats of this trinucleotide make the X chromosome susceptible to breakage. Another X-linked dominant disorder is a form of hypophosphatemic rickets. This disorder is found in males and females, is resistant to vitamin D therapy, and is characterized by bone anomalies, which include dental malformations and resultant feeding challenges.

X-linked recessive conditions include nephrogenic diabetes insipidus, adrenoleukodystrophy, and Duchenne muscular dystrophy (DMD) disorders. Individuals with X-linked recessive nephrogenic diabetes insipidus are unable to concentrate urine and exhibit polyuria and polydipsia. This disorder usually is detected in infancy and can manifest as dehydration, poor feeding, vomiting, and failure to thrive. X-linked recessive adrenoleukodystrophy results from a defect in the enzyme that degrades long-chain fatty acids. These fats accumulate and lead to brain and adrenal dysfunction and ultimately motor dysfunction. X-linked recessive DMD is characterized by fatty infiltration of muscles and extreme muscle wasting. Children typically are confined to a wheelchair by the time they reach their teens and need assistance with feeding.

Y-linked inheritance disorders primarily involve male sex determination. At this time no nutrition-related disorders have been assigned conclusively to the Y chromosome.

In summary, any gene potentially can undergo mutation, which can affect the function of its protein and the health of the individual. Its location within the nuclear DNA or mtDNA determines its mode of inheritance. See Chapter 42 for more information about genetic and metabolic disorders.

Disease at the Epigenetic Level

Although epigenetic mechanisms are major contributors to chronic disease through the gene-environment interactions, much remains to be discovered regarding the usual epigenomic patterns of each gene involved and the mechanisms by which that pattern is altered in response to environmental triggers. Details must await the outcomes of the many studies currently underway. Instead, let's take a moment to acknowledge the valuable contributions of nutrition pioneers who alerted the field to the importance of nutrition-related epigenetics to health. Ornish demonstrated the power of nutrition and lifestyle therapy to change cardiovascular disease and prostate cancer outcomes and linked the latter work to regulation of prostate gene expression (Ornish et al, 2008). Kallio et al (2007) demonstrated that changing the carbohydrate composition of the diet affects gene expression, which includes genes that regulate insulin signaling. Stover has long studied the basis for individual differences in diet-related disease from an epigenetic standpoint and sounded an early alarm on the need to use care in the concentration of folate used in enriching flour products, dietary supplements, and medication because of folate's role as the primary source of methyl groups used to silence gene expression (Stover et al, 2018). Their insight has contributed substantially to the understanding that nutrition is critically important at the molecular level as well as the biochemical, metabolic, and physiologic levels.

NUTRITIONAL GENOMICS AND CHRONIC DISEASE

Health care providers are gradually incorporating the various "omic" disciplines into assessment, diagnosis, intervention, and monitoring/evaluation. To do so requires a deep foundation of knowledge that connects genetic and epigenetic signatures to particular disease states so that an appropriate target for therapy is identified. Additionally, assessment and diagnosis must be followed by interventions known to restore health to those with existing disease or to prevent future disease in those susceptible who do not yet manifest symptoms. This overall approach is well underway for the single gene disorders for which gene variants have been identified and connected to the biochemical and physiologic consequences, and for which effective interventions have been developed, tested, and applied.

In contrast, the majority of clinic visits are for patients with one or more complex chronic diseases. Restoring health or preventing disease in the case of chronic disorders is an ambitious undertaking that will likely require decades of basic and clinical research before the potential is fully realized. Even when there are not yet well-defined nutritional genomics protocols for particular disorders, diet-and-lifestyle therapy can often be helpful.

Of particular interest to nutrition professionals is the emerging discipline of nutritional genomics and its role in precision/personalized nutrition. Nutritional genomics is a field of study focused on the interaction between genes, diet, lifestyle factors, and human health. Included within nutritional genomics are nutrigenetics, nutrigenomics, and nutrition-related aspects of epigenetics and epigenomics, which provide insight into how environmental factors regulate gene expression. Nutritional genomics and its subdisciplines encompass numerous other disciplines: molecular biology, biochemistry, intermediary metabolism, transcriptomics, proteomics, metabolomics, the microbiome, neuroscience, and behavioral change. See the Academy of Nutrition and Dietetics review on nutritional genomics for an overview of current progress in the field (Rozga and Handu, 2018). As these disciplines evolve, practitioners will increasingly be able to tailor diet and lifestyle choices to the genetic makeup of each client.

Nutrigenetics concerns the effect of genetic variation on the response to nutrients and other dietary input. For example, an often-cited illustration of nutrigenetics involves a variant in the 5,10-methylenetetrahydrofolate reductase (*MTHFR*) gene. Mutations in this gene can result in a substantial decrease in enzyme activity which is responsible for converting dietary folate or folic acid into 5-methyl folate, the active form. Individuals with such a mutation would need additional folate in the diet for optimal health.

Nutritional genomics is being advanced for clinical applications to common chronic disorders such as cancer, type 2 diabetes, obesity, and vascular disease, as well as important physiologic processes such as inflammation and biotransformation. At this time human clinical studies are limited, and the field is focused on developing the research foundation to be able to make the connections among gene variants, disease, functional impact, and effective interventions. Early adopters are developing nutrigenetic test panels intended to guide practitioners and their clients in identifying susceptibilities and offering recommendations for health promotion. Clients are bringing their test results to nutrition professionals for help with implementing these recommendations. Where there are variants common across nutrigenetic panels, these will be briefly discussed in order to make readers aware of what they may encounter in practice. Expect considerably more variants to be identified and increasingly targeted interventions to be developed in the years ahead.

Genetic Testing and Nutrition Care Process

The long-term promise of nutritional genomics is the ability to identify diet-gene interactions and translate this information into diet-and-lifestyle approaches personalized to the individual. In the shorter term, the expectation is that the information can be used to move away from one-size-fits-all to identifying categories of individuals with chronic disease who would benefit from a similar therapeutic approach based on their genetic makeup and modified for their specific environmental challenges. Genomics will be fundamental in this effort since gene variants will be the basis for identifying susceptibility. Epigenetics will be similarly important because it is the key to gene expression patterns in response to lifestyle choices.

The first step in nutrigenetic testing is assessment. Genome sequencing is used to query the client's genome to identify genetic variants present. Epigenomics will potentially be added in the not-too-distant future to identify epigenetic signatures and their influence on gene expression. Genomic analysis is accomplished either by genetic technology that detects specific variants (typically referred to as microarray chips), through sequencing of the gene-related parts of the genome (whole exome sequencing), or through whole genome sequencing. The evolution of DNA sequencing technology to the present next-generation sequencing has greatly decreased the cost and the time needed for sequencing and is rapidly becoming the preferred technology for chronic disease research. Once the sequence is obtained, there are numerous computer algorithms that can detect particular gene variants of interest. Some filters are readily available; others are proprietary to companies in the business of converting the presence of gene variants into recommendations for improving health and decreasing disease susceptibility.

The following points should be considered before taking a nutrigenetic test or when assisting your clients in understanding the test results that they or their providers have ordered.

- Evaluate the credentials of the company/laboratory that will be doing the testing. Is testing being conducted in an appropriately credentialed laboratory (at least CLIA-certified)?
- How will the client's privacy be protected?
- What is the cost of the test?
- To whom will the test results be sent?
- How long before the results will be available?
- Is the DNA sample destroyed following analysis? If saved, how will it be used in the future? The consumer will need to provide written consent to have their sample retained and used for future analyses.
- What will be included in the report of the test results?
- Which variants will be examined and are rs numbers reported along with the SNP?
- What is the association of each variant with a disease? Does the company make the studies available that link the variants (SNPs) with diseases?
- Which lifestyle choices are particularly important in promoting disease when this variant is present?

Several prominent nutritional genomics researchers have proposed guidelines for evaluating the validity of nutrigenetic testing and its use for dietary advice (Grimaldi et al, 2017). Additionally, the Academy of Nutrition and Dietetics' 2014 nutritional genomics position paper describes the various governmental agencies that have at least some oversight of nutritional genomics, particularly direct-to-consumer testing (Camp and Trujillo, 2014).

The information that is generated by genetic tests can provide insight into an individual's present health status and future disease susceptibilities to a much greater degree than has been possible to date. Clients will want to know that their information will be held private like any other health care data and that it cannot be used to discriminate against them in obtaining employment or insurance. Unintended consequences of genetic testing are often causes of concern for clients, and the increase in genetic testing across health care makes understanding those consequences especially important for nutrition professionals. See Box 6.13 for more on this topic.

Working with nutrigenetic test reports requires familiarity with the nomenclature used. Variants are named by the gene they represent, typically as three to five letters and written in italics. For the vast number of genes, human beings have two copies. Therefore when describing the gene and nucleotides present (whether wild-type/usual or variant/mutant) certain conventions are used. If the two nucleotides are wild-type, the individual is described as being homozygous wild-type. If one wild-type and one variant are present, the individual is heterozygous, also called a "carrier." If both nucleotides are the variant nucleotide, the individual is homozygous variant. Wild-type and variant states may be referred to as the wild-type allele and the variant or risk allele, which simply refers to the fact that either the wild-type sequence is present or the variant sequence is present or, in the case of a carrier, one of each is present.

The *MTHFR* gene is a now classic example of a nutrigenetic biomarker. A variant of this gene, *MTHFR* C677T (also written as 677C>T) involves the normal nucleotide C (for cytidine) being replaced by a T (thymidine) nucleotide at position 677 in the *MTHFR* gene sequence. Individuals homozygous wild-type have a C at this position in both copies of this gene. Heterozygotes have 1 C and 1 T and those homozygous for the variant have a T at this position in both copies of the gene.

Additionally, each variant is assigned an "**rs number**" (reference SNP cluster ID). The above *MTHFR* variant is rs1801133. A different variant within this same gene is the *MTHFR* A1298C and is labeled rs1801131). The rs number is critical because it denotes a specific location within the DNA and different mutations often create different functional outcomes. The lack of rs numbers in the earlier genomic literature has often made it difficult to discern which mutation is being analyzed for its gene-environment interactions. Both researchers and

BOX 6.13 ELSI: Ethical, Legal, and Social Implications of Genomics

For the various "omic" technologies to be helpful in the clinic, clients must be comfortable with their use. Of particular concern to clients has been whether genetic information in the hands of insurers or employers could lead to discrimination against applicants. These and other issues are the subject of debate and research into the ethical, legal, and social implications (ELSI) of genetic research and technologies.

From the beginning of the Human Genome Project, scientists, policymakers, and the public have worked to address **ELSI** issues in genetic research and technologies to inform and protect the public. Some of the potential harms have been addressed by legislation. Genetic-related information is defined as Protected Health Information by the passage of the Health Insurance Portability and Accountability Act (HIPAA). The passage of the **Genetic Information Nondiscrimination Act (GINA)** in 2008 is another important milestone in ensuring that genetic information will not be used to discriminate against Americans with respect to employment or health insurance. This legislation specifically prohibits the use of genetic information by health insurers to deny healthy individuals coverage or to charge higher than usual premiums because that individual may develop a disease in the future. It also bars employers from making hiring, firing, promotion, or job placement decisions based on genetic information.

However, as the popularity of direct-to-consumer genetic testing has increased, the issue of privacy and nondiscrimination continues to be of concern to consumers and to various governmental agencies. The Federal Trade Commission has begun taking a careful look at how companies supplying these tests protect the consumer's privacy. The nutrition professional should be aware of this concern and be ready to educate clients who are considering genetic testing.

Research into ELSI topics is ongoing and is emerging as a research field in its own right. The National Human Genome Research Institute's ELSI research program, established in 1990, continues to conduct research into ELSI issues. A list of the types of research being conducted can be found on the National Human Genome Research Institute website under ELSI. The European Union's Horizon 2020 research and innovation program is developing another asset, the ELSI Knowledge Desk which is also available on their website. Databases are also available that can be helpful to researchers and consumers, such as the ELSI Helpdesk and ELSI Knowledge Database online funded by the European Union's Horizon 2020 research and innovation program.

commercial companies typically now give the rs number along with the variant's gene and mutation. SNPs, such as *MTHFR,* are the most common type of mutation encountered in nutrigenetic testing but be aware that other types of mutations are possible, such as deletions, insertions, and copy number variants and that each variant has an rs number.

The next step is to take the variants identified and make predictions as to which variants increase one's susceptibility to particular diseases and then to select appropriate health-promoting interventions for these susceptibilities. Many genomics researchers and health care professionals question the reliability of the testing and its present clinical utility. The weakness would seem not to be the technology itself, which has been in place for decades and is a mainstay in research laboratories and, more recently, in clinical laboratories. The weakness is the link between a particular variant and the strength of its association with promoting disease and in the efficacy of the recommended therapeutic intervention. Be aware that the research into which variants are strongly associated with which diseases is early-stage. Many, many variants have been identified but few exhibit both a strong association and prevalence within multiple populations. In most cases, multiple genes variants, not a single SNP, as well as specific environmental exposures are needed for a disease to develop. The nutrition professional will need to be able to translate the implications of the variants in the nutrigenetic test report and the potential disease susceptibilities and link them to a therapeutic plan that can reasonably be expected to improve the client's health. The report accompanying the test results should be helpful in this regard, coupled with the nutrition professional's knowledge of appropriate nutritional approaches and of the lifestyle changes that will be needed for health restoration and sustained health promotion.

Inflammation

Chronic inflammation is an underlying mechanism for virtually all chronic diseases. Diet-and-lifestyle interventions are typically antiinflammatory in nature across the board for each of the primary lifestyle recommendations: nutrition, physical activity, managing thoughts and emotions, developing supportive relationships, obtaining sufficient quantity and quality of sleep, and minimizing toxin exposure. Interventions focus on preventing inflammation and on antiinflammatory approaches to existing inflammation. See Chapter 7 for a comprehensive discussion of inflammation, biomarkers, and antiinflammatory therapy.

Commonly used gene variants considered to increase susceptibility to an inflammatory state are those associated with inflammatory biomarkers: C-reactive protein (*CRP*), interleukin-1beta (*IL1ß*), interleukin-6 (*IL6*), and tumor necrosis factor alpha (*TNF*). *CRP* is produced by the liver in response to inflammation. Interleukin-1 and interleukin-6 proteins are cytokines produced as part of the inflammatory process. These proteins function as cell signaling molecules that activate the immune system, which involves inflammatory processes. Inflammation is typically self-limiting and abates when the infection or injury is under control. In the case of chronic disease, however, the inflammatory response is essentially stuck in the "on" position.

Biotransformation (Detoxification)

A parallel between pharmacogenomics and nutritional genomics can be seen with the phase I and phase II biotransformation/detoxification pathways that are active in the digestive tract and liver. In a two-phase process, this metabolic system converts drugs and other potentially toxic molecules into chemical forms that can be excreted. Phase I activates the toxic molecule to form a reactive oxygen species (free radical) through the activity of various cytochrome P450 enzymes (CYPs). Subsequently, in Phase II glutathione-S-transferases (GSTs) and other enzymes add chemical groups to the activated molecule to render it more soluble and less toxic. Knowing the genomic status of the genes that code for these various enzymes would be helpful for predicting which nutritional approaches would be beneficial to support the biotransformation process and when specific medications are used (see Box 6.14).

The gene variants commonly found in genetic test panels that include biotransformation are from the family of *CYP* genes, the *GST* genes, and two super oxide dismutase (*SOD*) genes. One or more of the *CYP* genes typically include: *CYP2D6, CYP2C19, CYP3A4, CYP1A2, CYP29, CYP2B6,* and *CYP2E1.* There are three common *GST* variants: GSTM, GSTP1, and GSTT1. The SOD genes represented are *SOD1* (copper-zinc SOD) and *SOD2* (manganese-dependent SOD) that

---

BOX 6.14 Application of Pharmacogenomics: Warfarin

One of the earliest clinical applications of the "omic" disciplines has been in pharmacogenomics, which is similar in concept to nutritional genomics. Pharmacogenomics involves using genomics to analyze the genetic variations in the genes that encode the drug-metabolizing enzymes and predict the outcomes when variants interact with specific drugs. Genetic variability can lead to differing function in these enzymes, which explains why a drug may have the intended effects for one person, be ineffective for another, and be harmful to a third. By identifying known mutations in biochemical pathways involved in the drug's metabolism, it becomes possible to identify individuals for whom the drug therapy will be beneficial but also to assist with calculating the appropriate dose from the outset of therapy. For drugs with narrow therapeutic windows of efficacy, prescribing the correct dosage from the outset of therapy improves efficacy and reduces the potential for adverse events. Several drugs have now been associated with gene variants and genetic testing is available before beginning therapy.

The blood-thinning medication warfarin has a narrow therapeutic window and is widely used. Associated with frequent adverse events, warfarin was one of the earliest drugs to which pharmacogenomics was applied. Variation in the *CYP2C9, VKORC1,* or *CYP4F2* genes influence its safe use. The most recent comprehensive trial to test the clinical utility of warfarin pharmacogenetics is the Clarification of Optimal Anticoagulation Through Genetics (COAG) trial

(Gage et al, 2017). The data demonstrated that genotype-guided dosing of warfarin was superior to standard management in two ways: (1) efficacy, in increasing the amount of drug in the therapeutic range over the period of the trial and (2) safety, for reducing adverse events up to 30 days following the end of the trial.

An interesting aspect of this trial points out a major limitation of genomics to date: the database of gene variants has been developed primarily from individuals of European descent. Gene pools vary among different ancestral populations and, to be effective, recommendations must be based on the gene variants appropriate to each population. The COAG trial did not test for the *CYP2C9*8* variant that is an important predictor of warfarin dose in African Americans (Nagai et al, 2015). These individuals spent less time within the therapeutic window and did not receive the full effect of the drug. Because the study population was 91% white, the overall effectiveness of the drug for the genotyped arm was not affected. However, genotyping for warfarin will likely not be recommended for African Americans until further research clarifies the set of gene variants that best provides safety and efficacy for this population. This limitation in the gene variant database is well recognized by researchers and a global effort is underway to expand the database. See Box 6.12 for additional information. This project is expanding the populations included and helping identify common mutations associated with specific ethnic groups. Additionally, various countries are establishing databases that represent their specific populations.

protect against free radicals generated during biotransformation. Gene variants in any of the proteins involved in biotransformation can potentially alter the effectiveness of the process.

Cancer

"Omic" clinical research and applications are currently the most advanced for cancer compared with other chronic diseases. The influence of epigenetic marks on gene expression is directly associated with the development of cancer and its characteristic unregulated growth. The expression of oncogenes (tumor-promoting genes) and tumor suppressor genes must be carefully orchestrated to maintain normal growth and development. Oncogenes are typically silenced epigenetically and tumor suppressor genes are activated. If either of these systems malfunction, the risk for cancer could be increased. An example would be a methyl group attaching to a tumor suppressor gene by mistake and turning off its expression. Or, if someone lacked sufficient folate in the diet, an oncogene may not be sufficiently turned off.

Although total personalization of cancer therapy, or any other medical therapy, for an individual is in the forefront of discovery, a number of early steps using "omic" technologies have already been successful in helping tailor therapy and for early detection of treatment failure. Cytotoxic chemotherapy has been the prevailing cancer therapy to date. Although successful in many respects, this approach is relatively nonspecific in that it targets both cancerous and noncancerous cells. One of the goals of precision health is to harness the "omic" disciplines into personalized therapy appropriate for individuals and their particular type of cancer. This approach requires knowledge of the molecular landscape in which the cancer exists (i.e., the person's genomic and epigenomic makeup and the molecular characteristics of the cancer itself). Molecular defects in the individual's genome and epigenome, and in the cancer itself, can provide valuable information about potential therapeutic targets. See Luoh and Flaherty (2018) for an overview of the types of cancers being studied and treated using this approach.

Gene Variants and Cancer

Well-known examples of applying genomics to cancer include detection of BRCA1 and BRCA2 genes in diagnosing breast cancer and the hMLH1 and hMSH2 genes in diagnosing hereditary nonpolyposis colorectal cancer (HNPCC). Genetic testing is also available for detecting susceptibility to these types of cancer. Genomic testing is also being used to distinguish specific tumor characteristics to help differentiate one cancer from another. Genetic diagnostics help determine which therapeutic approach will likely be successful and, during therapy, help detect early treatment failure. As options for early detection and prevention emerge, tailorerd diet-and-lifestyle options will become common in treatment of cancer.

Epigenetics and Cancer

Dietary nutrients and bioactive food components can affect epigenetic processes in multiple ways, from providing nutrients needed to protect against cancer to suppressing gene expression of key components in the signal cascades that lead to cancer promotion (or the enzymes needed for DNA methylation or histone acetylation) to changing the availability of substrates needed for the various enzymatic reactions involved. The nutritional genomics/epigenomics-oriented research being conducted focuses on dietary nutrients and bioactive food components that change gene expression through epigenetic mechanisms (Andreescu et al, 2018).

With traditional nutrients, a main focus is on one-carbon metabolism, which supplies the methyl groups for DNA methylation and histone acetylation, in addition to numerous other important processes such as DNA repair. These nutrients include folate and folic acid, riboflavin, pyridoxine, vitamin B_{12}, choline, and methionine. Other common dietary components being studied for their cancer-protective properties include dietary fiber, vitamin C, vitamin E, and selenium. In addition to serving as ligands for transcription factors, polyunsaturated fats are essential for downregulating the expression of those transcription factors involved in switching on proinflammatory genes. Examples include transcription factors used for hepatic metabolism of carbohydrates, lipids, and bile acids (Jump et al, 2013).

For the bioactive food components, identification of bioactives from plants is a particularly active area of research because a substantial number of health benefits have been reported for these compounds. The polyphenol and glucosinolate categories of phytonutrients are the most studied for cancer treatment and prevention. Epigenetic changes to tumor suppressor genes can silence these genes and lead to increased risk of tumor development.

Type 2 Diabetes

Type 2 diabetes mellitus (T2DM) is a chronic disorder that accounts for the vast majority of individuals with diabetes (see Chapter 29). T2DM is complex and results from gene variants interacting with bioactive food components and other lifestyle triggers that result in epigenetic modifications to the genome. The hallmarks of this type of diabetes are insulin resistance and failure of the insulin-producing beta cells of the pancreas. Numerous studies have reported the efficacy of diet-and-lifestyle approaches for managing and preventing T2DM. Nutritional genomics will add to the understanding of this complex disease by identifying gene variants that significantly increase the risk of developing T2DM. Additionally, nutritional genomics research will identify gene–diet/lifestyle interactions and mechanisms by which these interactions epigenetically influence gene expression, which will help in developing new and effective interventions.

Gene Variants and T2DM

A few rare mutations have been found that predispose to T2DM, but they do not explain the high prevalence of the disease. Rather than resulting from a single gene mutation, T2DM appears to be due to the contributions of a number of variants interacting with diet-and-lifestyle triggers. Some of the variants are in genes that have obvious connections to glucose homeostasis, but many are not. The following variants are among the more promising in terms of the strength of their association with risk of developing type 2 diabetes: Transcription factor 7-like 2 (TCF7L2), solute carrier family 30 member 8 (SLC30A8), peroxisome proliferator activated receptor gamma (PPARG), adiponectin (ADIPOQ), fat mass and obesity protein/alpha-ketoglutarate dependent dioxygenase (FTO), clock circadian regulator (CLOCK), and melanocortin 4 receptor (MC4R). SLC30A8 is a zinc transporter that is required for insulin synthesis and secretion. The ADIPOQ, CLOCK, FTO, and MC4R variants are associated with obesity and increased risk for developing T2DM. PPARG is a transcription factor involved with lipid metabolism and adipocyte differentiation that regulates the expression of multiple genes. It has been implicated in diabetes, obesity, cancer, and atherosclerosis. For further depth into any of these variants, visit the Gene website from the National Center for Biotechnology Information or the Genetics Home Reference website from the National Institutes of Health.

TCF7L2 is involved with insulin secretion and exhibits the strongest association by far with susceptibility to T2DM. The TCF7L2 gene encodes a transcription factor that plays a key role in the WNT signal transduction pathway. Further, TCF7L2 has been detected in multiple populations. In studies with Indian (Chandak et al, 2007), Chinese Han (Dou et al, 2013), Japanese (Horikoshi et al, 2007), Mexican

American (Lehman et al, 2007), African (Yako et al, 2016), and white European (Groves et al, 2006) populations, the variant occurred frequently and increased the risk of T2DM by 30% to 50%. *TCF7L2* has also been found to predispose individuals with metabolic syndrome to developing T2DM (Katsoulis et al, 2018).

Epigenetics and T2DM

Studies have long suggested that T2DM is strongly associated with diet-and-lifestyle choices, most notably food choices (especially dietary fat) and exercise habits. T2DM has been assumed to be genetic in origin but, with the exception of *TCF7L2*, the large number of gene variants that have been identified appear to weakly contribute to T2DM susceptibility. The answers appear to be (1) there are multiple genes involved and (2) epigenetic mechanisms involving diet-and-lifestyle triggers are important contributors. Research to detect epigenetic changes in response to nutrients and bioactive food components is in progress.

A nutrient-sufficient antiinflammatory diet in which carbohydrate and fat consumption is controlled for quantity and quality continues to be a cornerstone of T2DM care. Increasingly, a focus is being placed on the incorporation of a variety of phytonutrients into the diet. Results from the Nurses' Health Study (NHS) and its follow-up (NHS II) (Sun et al, 2015), as well as the Health Professionals Follow-Up Study (Wedick et al, 2012), suggest that regular consumption of phytonutrient-rich plant foods helped lower the risk of developing T2DM.

In addition to diet and exercise, other daily lifestyle choices influence the physiologic imbalances that lead to chronic inflammation and must be incorporated into lifestyle change programs if the positive changes are to be sustained long term. Examples include chronic psychological and physiological stress and exposure to chemicals and toxins. Hopefully, health care will move toward approaches for T2DM and for chronic disease in general that target the underlying chronic inflammation along with contemporary neuroscience-based behavioral change programs that enable those at risk to address their barriers to making healthy lifestyle choices.

For more in-depth information about the genomic and epigenetic aspects of T2DM, see recent reviews by Silveira et al (2019), Xue et al (2018), and Ortega et al (2017).

Obesity

Obesity is usually indicated by body mass index (BMI), which is measured in kg/m^2. It is important to assess each person individually, including weight history, waist circumference, and body composition as people with larger body sizes can be metabolically healthy in some cases. Different countries use somewhat different BMI scores to define obesity, but a common global standard is that set by the World Health Organization (WHO), which classifies a BMI of ≥ 25 kg/m^2 in adults as overweight/preobese, a BMI ≥ 30 kg/m^2 as obese, and a BMI ≥ 40 kg/m^2 as extremely obese. WHO has also set BMI standards for children up to 5 years old and 5 to 19 years old. The prevalence of obesity is steadily rising. In the United States the 2015 to 2016 National Health and Nutrition Examination Survey found 39.8% of adults and 18.5% of youth to be obese (Hales et al, 2017).

In addition to being a storage organ ready to provide for future energy needs, adipose tissue is an active metabolic tissue that is important in whole body energy balance. Adipose tissue secretes adipokines, which are cell signaling proteins. Adipokine examples include leptin, adiponectin, and proinflammatory adipokines, such as the interleukins and tumor necrosis alpha cytokines discussed in the type 2 diabetes section. When leptin (*LEP*) binds to leptin receptors (*LEPR*) in the hypothalamus, binding sends the signal of satiety, followed by a reduction in the desire to eat and a stimulated thermogenesis. The

foundational work was done in mouse model systems and subsequently found to be operative in human beings (Ghilardi et al, 1996; Dulloo et al, 2002). Adiponectin is a protein hormone adipokine encoded by the *ADIPOQ* gene and produced by adipocytes. It appears to be important for metabolic balance, particularly in reference to the insulin resistance, oxidative stress, and chronic inflammation characteristic of the metabolic syndrome (Achari and Jain, 2017). In particular the balance between adiponectin and leptin has been correlated with the obesity component of metabolic syndrome. A decrease in the adiponectin/leptin ratio increases the risk of obesity, inflammation, and development of the metabolic syndrome (Frühbeck et al, 2017).

ADIPOQ is a gene of interest because of its association with obesity but also potentially for type 2 diabetes and metabolic syndrome. One of the SNPs in this gene (-11391G>A, rs17300539) appears to link increased levels of adiponectin with decreased risk of obesity. In white Americans, those with one or more copies of the variant allele (A) had elevated adiponectin levels and decreased weight, waist and hip circumference, and BMI (Warodomwichit et al, 2009). These researchers further detected a gene-diet interaction between the variant allele (A) and monounsaturated fat (MUFA). When MUFA intake was equal to or greater than 13% of total energy, those with one or more copies of the A allele (AA or AG genotype) had a lower BMI compared with individuals with the GG genotype (2 copies of the non-variant G allele). No effect of the A allele was seen for waist circumference, insulin resistance or for saturated fat or polyunsaturated fats. Other researchers have reported increased risk of obesity in the presence of SNPs in *ADIPOQ* in the North Indian Punjabi population (Kaur et al., 2018) and in the Tunisian population (Zayani et al, 2018). These interesting findings with *ADIPOQ* will likely continue to be studied in multiple populations and under varying dietary conditions.

As with leptin, much of the initial work with adiponectin has been carried out using mouse model systems, with research in human beings following more recently. Given the apparent importance of these genes in energy metabolism, the lack of consistency is likely due to a large volume of research but very few polymorphisms are linked to increased risk of developing obesity across multiple populations. Additionally, the complexity of obesity and the multitude of molecules involved has made it challenging to untangle the multiple interactions that increase or decrease risk of developing obesity (Jagannadham et al, 2016). A recent review by Unamuno et al (2018) provides insight into the complexity of dysfunctional adipose tissue and the ensuing dysregulation of adipokine secretion, which leads to chronic inflammation and increased risk of chronic disorders such as insulin resistance, type 2 diabetes, atherosclerosis, cancer, and, most likely, obesity.

The focus of the various research studies is highly varied, from identifying genes that increase risk of obesity, to identifying the environmental cues that trigger overeating and epigenetic changes in the brain, adipose tissue, and liver; from factoring in the composition of the food supply with its increased toxin load and abundance of high-calorie processed foods, to understanding the complex behavioral aspects of why we make the food choices we do. The epigenetic mechanisms that link obesity to increased risk of T2DM and cardiovascular disease add yet more complexity. Clearly, why and how humans become obese is multifaceted and multiple disciplines will be involved in defining the mechanisms and finding effective solutions. The addition of contemporary neuroscience and behavioral research to the search for answers as to why and how we become obese is expanding our insight into this challenging dilemma (see Chapter 20).

The sections that follow highlight genes and gene variants that are among those with a stronger association with obesity than most variants, along with a discussion of the role of epigenetics in obesity. The fact that environmental factors play a major role in triggering the development of obesity reminds us of the difficulties of identifying even the primary factors within today's obesogenic environment. It also provides encouragement that attention to the behavioral aspects of making health-promoting choices day-by-day throughout the lifespan can have a positive influence on shifting one's health trajectory from disease susceptibility to health and vitality.

Gene Variants and Obesity

In terms of its genetic basis, obesity has been categorized as both monogenic and polygenic. Monogenic (single gene) obesity has historically referred to those genes that, when mutated, lead to severe obesity. Examples of well-studied gene variants associated with monogenic obesity include mutations in *MC4R* (melanocortin-4 receptor), *LEP*, and *LEPR*. In contrast, polygenic (multigene) obesity has been referred to as "common obesity" where multiple genes and environmental triggers are involved. This basis for obesity occurs frequently. In common obesity, mutation in a single gene contributes only a small degree of risk; development of the susceptibility to becoming obese is strongly dependent on the interaction with environmental triggers. However, the recent finding by Fairbrother et al (2018) that mutations in *MC4R* are found frequently in obese individuals in the general population makes this type of all or nothing categorization questionable. This revelation is not surprising given that most, if not all, gene-function-disease associations are being found to constitute a continuum of phenotypes ranging from silent to mild to severe effects on function. However, be aware that this type of classification is in the literature and can cause confusion. In this section the focus will be on what has, to date, been termed common obesity involving multiple genes and multiple environmental triggers.

Also not surprising is the large number of genes identified as contributors to the predisposition for obesity, particularly since GWAS studies have come to be used routinely in the search for genes of interest and their polymorphisms. One gene that has for several years been found to have a strong association with common obesity and to occur frequently in multiple populations is *FTO* (Loos and Yeo, 2014). This gene encodes the fat mass and obesity protein (an alpha-ketoglutarate dependent dioxygenase). Its mechanism of action appears to be related to the regulation of adipose tissue development, which suggests body composition is affected (Yang et al, 2017). Variations in the *FTO* gene have been found in multiple populations. Its effect is greater in European descendants than in African or Asian populations (Loos and Yeo, 2014; Merritt et al, 2018).

Gene-diet interactions have been reported for SNPs in the *FTO* gene. Data from a cross-sectional study found that those with the A allele of *FTO* gene who reported high levels of dietary fat and low levels of physical activity had higher BMI values than those with the A allele who reported a lower-fat diet (Sonestedt et al, 2009). A low-carbohydrate diet appeared to attenuate the effect of the high-fat diet in those with the risk allele. Lappalainen and colleagues (2012) investigated the effect of this same SNP on BMI in subjects in the Finnish Diabetes Prevention Study. This group also found elevated BMI values in those consuming a high-fat diet. More recently Vimaleswaran et al (2016) reported a gene-diet interaction in a second *FTO* SNP in an Asian Indian population. Individuals with the SNP who also consumed a high-carbohydrate diet had increased risk of being obese. Physical inactivity seemed to also influence obesity risk in these individuals.

Two other genes that influence not only obesity but also insulin sensitivity/resistance are the suppressor of cytokine signaling 3 (*SOCS3*) gene and the peroxisome proliferator-activated receptor gamma (*PPARG2*) gene. *SOCS3* inhibits cytokine signal transduction (part of the inflammatory response) through the Janus kinase/signal transducer and activator of transcription (JAK/STAT) signaling pathway. *SOCS3* is frequently overexpressed in obesity and diabetes (Galic et al, 2014). In an expression genome-wide association study (eGWAS), Xu et al (2018) found that the *SOCS3* promoter was hypomethylated in obese individuals. Within this low-methylated *SOCS3* group, those who had had five or more majorly stressful life events were at increased risk of obesity.

The *PPARG* gene is a nuclear receptor that functions as a transcription factor and is a key contributor to fat cell formation. It is frequently referred to as the "master regulator" of adipogenesis and differentiation (Mukherjee et al, 1997). Gene-diet interactions for the PPARG gene have been reported, originally by Memisoglu et al (2003) and more recently by Rodrigues and colleagues (2017). In a subgroup of the Nurses' Health Study, Memisoglu and colleagues investigated the interaction between the *PPARG2* Pro12Ala SNP (the Pro allele is the wild-type allele and the Ala allele the variant allele) and dietary fat intake. Those with the Pro/Pro genotype who also had the highest dietary fat intake had significantly higher BMI values than those who had the lowest dietary fat intake. There did not appear to be a gene-diet interaction with the Ala allele with respect to BMI. Rodrigues et al (2018) reported on severely obese individuals and found that those with one or more copies of the Ala allele had higher BMI values and higher polyunsaturated fat intake. It is not unusual to encounter these types of inconsistencies as researchers attempt to identify SNPs that influence physiologic processes in response to lifestyle choices. Typically the pattern will become clearer as the volume of studies increases.

Because of the large number of variants that have been reported since GWAS became the primary tool for identifying obesity-related variants and the need to screen multiple populations to detect variants that occur frequently in several populations, expect the research to be ongoing.

Additionally, the variants will need to be strongly associated with particular environmental triggers. Obesogenic environments are highly variable among individuals even within the same population, which further compounds the amount of work ahead to clearly link variants with effective clinical interventions.

Epigenetics and Obesity

Beyond the methylation, acetylation, and miRNA studies being conducted with the various gene variants, environmental triggers that promote epigenetic modifications are being studied to gain insight into how these triggers promote the transformation of obesity susceptibility into overt disease. Today's environment is frequently referred to as obesogenic. Two aspects of the environment that are under study are environmental pollutants and their role in promoting obesity and the composition of the gut microbiota. The term "obesogen" refers to environmental pollutants that promote obesity but the term has expanded over time as it has become apparent that a wide variety of pollutants lead to oxidative stress and inflammation, which promote not only obesity but diabetes, vascular disease, cancer, and various other inflammatory disorders (Grün and Blumberg, 2006). Categories of common pollutants include persistent organic pollutants (POPs), heavy metals, and air pollution. POPs include polychlorinated biphenyls (PCBs), organochloride pesticides, and endocrine disruptors, hormone-like compounds that mimic natural hormones and disrupt the normal functioning of the endocrine system, which includes altering normal gene expression patterns. See reviews by Muscogiuri et al (2017) and by Darbre (2017) for additional information.

The gut microbiota refers to the community of different microorganisms (bacteria, yeast, viruses) that live within the digestive tract. The gut "microbiome" that is often spoken of technically refers to the genomes of these various microbes but is often used synonymously with the organisms themselves (the "microbiota"). These organisms can be beneficial or pathogenic. The benefits include maintenance of the integrity of the digestive tract, which promotes digestive functions and the integrity of the barrier function of a healthy gut mucosa. The microbiota also contribute nutritionally by synthesizing folate, biotin, and vitamin K and digesting insoluble fiber to generate short-chain fatty acids that serve as fuel for enterocytes. Earlier in this chapter it was noted that genomic technology has been successfully applied to identifying the microbes, which has been helpful for research purposes but also for laboratory testing so that pathogenic microbes can be rapidly identified and antimicrobial therapy begun.

The presence of pathogens in the microbiota can cause mild to severe digestive tract imbalances and can lead to infection and erosion of the gut barrier, chronic activation of the immune system, and chronic inflammation. One of the side effects of the presence of gram-negative bacteria is that, as they die, they release lipopolysaccharide (LPS) molecules from their cell walls. LPS is a potent activator of the innate immune system as well as a number of proinflammatory systems, which further promotes and sustains chronic inflammation.

The microbiota composition also appears to be important in weight management. When the gut microbiota of lower weight and obese human beings are compared, the overweight/obese individuals have lower fecal bacterial diversity, impaired glucose regulation, dyslipidemia, and greater low-grade inflammation (Le Chatelier et al, 2013; Mathur & Barlow, 2015). Studies suggest that one of the potentially important differences in obesity is that the *Firmicutes:Bacteroidetes* ratio changes substantially and that a Western-style diet high in refined carbohydrates and fat influences the quantity and composition of the microbiota associated with weight gain (Ley et al, 2005; Jumpertz et al, 2011). See reviews by Duranti et al (2017), Selber-Hnatiw et al (2017), Davis (2016), and Castaner et al (2018) for details on the role of the microbiota in health and disease.

Nutrition can exacerbate or protect against the effects of environmental toxins and the gut microbiota (Hoffman et al, 2017). Dietary fats such as saturated fats can enhance the proinflammatory effects of pollutants whereas omega-3s can interfere with the signaling process and downregulate inflammation. Diets rich in bioactive components that serve as antioxidants or antiinflammatory agents can diminish the negative impact of obesogens (see Box 6.4). Similarly, nutrition can alter the microbiota and promote health or disease.

Finally, identifying the mechanisms by which environmental cues lead to alterations in gene expression is a major research focus. One of the epigenetic associations that's been identified relates to the distinction between inflammation induced by obesity compared with inflammation induced by infection or tissue trauma. Obesity-induced inflammation is systemic rather than localized and is a low-intensity but chronic reaction whereas the classic inflammatory process is self-limiting. The toll-like receptor (TLR) signaling pathway involves a family of proteins. TLR4 is a major component of obesity-induced inflammation. Activation of this signaling system promotes gene expression of inflammatory cytokines and NF-κB regulated proinflammatory genes (Rocha et al, 2016; Rogero and Calder, 2018).

Activation of the TLR4 pathway occurs through the presence of environmental triggers, such as saturated fatty acids (supplied by the diet or from triglycerides stored in adipose tissue) and LPS (produced by bacteria that populate the microbiome). Rocha et al (2018) suggest that saturated fatty acids alter the microbial ecology of the gut and result in increased bacterial production of LPS, which is a known activator of the TLR4 signaling pathway. Further, this increase in LPS leads to oxidative stress that in turn triggers the production of atherogenic lipids such as oxidized LDL and oxidized phospholipids that are also known triggers of the TLR4 system. The elevated levels of saturated fatty acids further exacerbate the situation by contributing additional LDL-cholesterol in the presence of oxidative stress that increases the amount of oxidized LDL, which further promotes atherogenesis. The TLR4 signaling pathway is also connected to the activation of transcription factors such as NF-κB (see Box 6.3), which regulates expression of a number of proinflammatory genes that produce cytokines and other inflammatory mediators. It's easy to see how the obesity-induced inflammatory response, once initiated, would self-perpetuate in the presence of such environmental conditions. The omega-3 polyunsaturated fatty acids eicosapentaenoic acid (EPA) and docosahexaenoic acid (DHA) supplied through food or dietary supplements are able to interfere with signaling cascades and have an antiinflammatory effect by preventing activation by either the saturated fats or LPS. Reviews by Lopomo et al (2016) and Hoffman and Hennig (2017) examine various topics relating to how epigenetic modifications are related to obesity, including the transgenerational effects of these changes and what that means for future generations.

Vascular Disease

The complexity of vascular disease provides numerous opportunities for genomic analysis to help distinguish among the various subtypes as well as to apply pharmacogenomic testing. Two applications already in use concern medications relating to blood clotting (warfarin) and platelet aggregation (clopidogrel). Box 6.14 gives an overview of the clinical utility of this type of testing.

A large proportion of the vascular disorders commonly seen in clinic are those with strong associations to diet and lifestyle: hypertension and dyslipidemia (cardiovascular, cerebrovascular, and peripheral vascular diseases; elevated LDL-cholesterol, decreased HDL-cholesterol, and hypertriglyceridemia). Each of these chronic disorders decreases quality of life, increases medical costs, and elevates risk of premature death. As with other chronic disorders, low-grade inflammation and oxidative stress are assumed to play an important role in converting disease susceptibility to development of disease. Fortunately, the major environmental triggers that promote vascular disease are lifestyle choices: diet, exercise, and smoking, each of which is modifiable.

Gene Variants and Vascular Disease

The earliest gene variants incorporated into assessment testing are candidate genes that encode proteins known to be associated with vascular disease: those that suggested predisposition to chronic inflammation and oxidative stress, formation of blood clots, predisposition to high blood pressure, or development of dyslipidemia (Curti et al, 2011). The proinflammatory variants include *CRP, IL1ß, IL6,* and *TNF* discussed in the Inflammation section of this chapter. Oxidative stress predisposition has been associated with the glutathione-S-transferase genes *GSTM1, GSTP1, GSTT1,* and the superoxide dismutase enzymes *SOD2* and *SOD3*. For blood clot formation and susceptibility to venous thrombosis, the most commonly included variant is Factor V Leiden (*F5*). The hypertension variant has been *ACE,* the gene that encodes angiotensinogen-converting enzyme. Dyslipidemia variants are those that code for the proteins involved in the various lipoproteins, such as *APOA1, APOA2, APOA5,* and *APOE*.

Considering the multiple aspects of both cardiovascular and cerebrovascular disease, there will likely be many more variants identified before a comprehensive vascular genetic panel is constructed. That said, information from the presently available variants can provide insight into potential susceptibilities to developing vascular disease but expect stronger associations to be identified as research continues. In addition to the goal of screening multiple populations to find variants that occur frequently and have a strong association with vascular disease, there is also a need to identify variants that predict susceptibility among the specific populations. For example, venous thromboembolism (VTE) is more prevalent in African Americans than in other populations but frequently missed by gene panels that derive from European populations. One promising lead has come from a GWAS study that found three variants in the thrombomodulin gene (THBD) that decreases expression and increases the risk of VTEs in African Americans (Hernandez et al, 2016).

At this point a combination of candidate gene and GWAS studies has identified over 400 variants that influence hypertension susceptibility alone. Similar to challenges with categorizing cancer as a single disease, the complexity of vascular disease makes it challenging to identify gene variants that have a strong association with a specific aspect of susceptibility to developing vascular disorders. As a result, each aspect of this complex disease will continue to be investigated to find variants that have a strong association with distinct subcategories of vascular disease.

Epigenetics and Vascular Disease

As it has become obvious that numerous environmental factors increase susceptibility to developing vascular disorders, epigenetic mechanisms have become an additional focus of nutritional genomic research into vascular disease. Epigenetic research will help define the mechanisms by which lifestyle choices influence gene expression. It also provides insight into lifestyle-oriented therapeutic options for managing existing disease and preventing future disease.

Given the complexity of vascular disease and the large number of associated candidate gene and GWAS loci found to have an association with these disorders, the most effective health-promoting approach for nutrition professionals is to address the modifiable lifestyle choices available to clients. With the escalating global prevalence of vascular disease, as well as obesity and T2DM that increase vascular susceptibility, expanding the therapeutic approach to include modifiable lifestyle factors beyond food choices will be needed. These behavioral changes entail eliminating smoking, curbing alcohol intake, avoiding food- and air-borne toxins, adopting an antiinflammatory diet, exercising, managing stress, developing supportive relationships, and getting sufficient quantity and quality of sleep. The epigenetic component of chronic disease development appears to be strong, which suggests that all of us have at least some level of susceptibility that, if continually challenged with inappropriate lifestyle choices, will lead to manifestation of any number of inflammation-based chronic disorders.

The nutrition practice of the future will incorporate aspects of not only genomics and epigenomics but contemporary neuroscience and behavioral change as well. Nutrition professionals are ideally suited to deliver this information but also to counsel clients as they address the often-challenging behavioral changes that are needed to restore their health from vascular and other chronic diseases and prevent disease susceptibility from becoming an inevitability.

SUMMARY

Genomics, epigenetics, and the various "omic" disciplines that have emerged are adding a new dimension to nutrition science and medical nutrition therapy. It has opened up a new way of thinking about how food influences gene expression and, ultimately, our disease susceptibility and health. As nutrition moves into an era of precision health, the molecular and biochemical aspects of nutrition will become increasingly important tools for nutrition professionals. As a human being, each client will be generally like other members of our species yet have sufficient genetic heterogeneity to give each distinctive differences. The vision for the era ahead is to get ever closer to being able to assess, diagnose, intervene, monitor, and evaluate each client's unique situation. This depth of information will be helpful in developing interventions that will more effectively manage existing disease

and restore health, as well as identify early genetic susceptibilities and prevent them from developing into disease.

During the past 50 years the focus for health care has been on treating disease, and physicians have had increasingly sophisticated drugs, surgery, and technologies available to meet this challenge. However, with the understanding that chronic disease is genetically based but environmentally influenced, the focus is now on targeted intervention and prevention. Although the first applications of this changed focus in health care involve the medical and pharmaceutical aspects of acute care, nutrition therapy is expected to figure prominently as a cornerstone of care in preventing and managing chronic, diet-and-lifestyle-related diseases.

Although our genetic makeup sets the stage, environmental factors such as nutrition and other lifestyle choices determine who among the susceptible actually develops chronic disease (Henning et al, 2018). In addition to our food choices, other lifestyle choices also epigenetically influence function and are as central as food if our clients are to enjoy robust health. A comprehensive overview by Abdul et al (2018) on the influence of lifestyle choices on epigenetic mechanisms and health suggests that the role of the nutrition professionals will be expanding in the years ahead. Similarly, social epigenomics is a developing field that will appeal to nutrition professionals given our history of concern for the health of the underserved individuals in our society. Nutrition professionals are well-positioned to play a major role in this new era of personalized health care. You can prepare to meet this challenge by developing a solid foundation in the various sciences needed for effective lifestyle therapy, from molecular nutrition to nutritional genomics/epigenetic-related disciplines to neuroscience and contemporary behavioral change programs.

CLINICAL CASE STUDY

Amalia is a 32-year-old Hispanic female who was diagnosed with depression 3 years ago by her primary care physician and referred to the clinic's psychologist. Multiple family members suffer from depression in Amalia's family. Amalia has been faithfully attending her monthly counseling sessions since that time and, although her affect has improved somewhat, she feels like she's not getting better. In fact, has recently been getting worse. Her chief complaint is exhaustion, to the extent that she has lost interest in her church work and social activities that in the past have brought her pleasure. Increasingly she feels too tired to manage self-care such as cooking. She has been eating fast-food take out and snacking on ready-to-eat processed foods. Her physician prescribed an antidepressant, but she stopped taking it some time ago because she says she does not want to take medication to feel better. Her comprehensive metabolic panel is unremarkable; however, a genetic panel reveals she has a homozygous mutation in the *MTHFR* C677T gene. The psychologist has referred her for nutrition and genetic counseling.

Nutrition Diagnostic Statements

- Undesirable food choices related to fatigue and depression as evidenced by consumption of highly processed, nutrient-poor fast foods.
- Altered nutrition-related laboratory value related to personal genetic variation as evidenced by a mutation in the *MTHFR* C677T and potential increased need for B vitamins, especially folate.

Nutrition Care Questions

1. What is the difference between a heterozygous and a homozygous mutation in a gene?
2. What are your thoughts about what might be causing Amalia's symptoms of depression and fatigue?
3. What is the significance of having a MTHFR C677T mutation?
4. What foods may help improve Amalia's nutrition status, especially foods that would support her genetic aberration?

USEFUL WEBSITES

CDC Genomics (educational materials, blogs, weekly literature updates)

The ELSI Knowledge Desk

Epigenetics and Epigenomics, the Future of Nutritional Science

Epigenomics. National Institutes of Health

Family History Initiative

Gene (National Center for Biotechnology Information)

Genetic and Rare Diseases Information Center

Genetic Information and Nondiscrimination Act of 2008

Genetics Home Reference

Human Genome Project

The International Genome Sample Resource

National Center for Advancing Translational Sciences (National Institutes of Health)

National Human Genome Research Institute (educational materials, including ELSI-related)

National Institutes of Health dbSNP (extensive information about each single nucleotide polymorphism)

NIMHD Social Epigenomics Research

Scitable by Nature Education

REFERENCES

Abdul QA, Yu BP, Chung HY, et al: Epigenetic modifications of gene expression by lifestyle and environment, *Arch Pharm Res* 40:1219–1237, 2018.

Achari AE, Jain SK: Adiponectin, a therapeutic target for obesity, diabetes, and endothelial dysfunction, *Int J Mol Sci* 18:E1321, 2017.

Andreescu N, Puiu M, Niculescu M: Effects of dietary nutrients on epigenetic changes in cancer, *Methods Mol Biol* 1856:121–139, 2018.

Balaton BP, Dixon-McDougall T, Peeters SB, et al: The eXceptional nature of the X chromosome, *Hum Mol Genet* 27(R2):R242–R249, 2018.

Bygren LO: Intergenerational health responses to adverse and enriched environments, *Annu Rev Public Health* 34:49–60, 2013.

Camp KM, Trujillo E: Position of the academy of nutrition and dietetics: nutritional genomics, *J Acad Nutr Diet* 114(2):299–312, 2014.

Cao-Lei L, de Rooij SR, King S, et al: Prenatal stress and epigenetics, *Neurosci Biobehav Rev* S0149-7634(16)30726-6, 2017.

Castaner O, Goday A, Park YM, et al: The gut microbiome profile in obesity: a systematic review, *Int J Endocrinol* 2018:4095789, 2018.

Chandak GR, Janipalli CS, Bhaskar S, et al: Common variants in the TCF7L2 gene are strongly associated with type 2 diabetes mellitus in the Indian population, *Diabetologia* 50:63–67, 2007.

Cropley JE, Suter CM, Beckman KB, et al: Germ-line epigenetic modification of the murine A^vy allele by nutritional supplementation, *Proc Natl Acad Sci USA* 103:17308–17312, 2006.

Curti ML, Jacob P, Borges MC, et al: Studies of gene variants related to inflammation, oxidative stress, dyslipidemia, and obesity: implications for a nutrigenetic approach, *J Obes* 2011:497401, 2011.

Dagar V, Hutchison W, Muscat A, et al: Genetic variation affecting DNA methylation and the human imprinting Beckwith-Wiedemann syndrome, *Clin Epigenetics* 10:114, 2018.

Dall'Aglio L, Muka T, Cecil CAM, et al: The role of epigenetic modifications in neurodevelopmental disorders: a systematic review, *Neurosci Biobehav Rev* 94:17–30, 2018.

Darbre PD: Endocrine disruptors and obesity, *Curr Obes Rep* 6:18–27, 2017.

Davis CD: The gut microbiome and its role in obesity, *Nutr Today* 51:167–174, 2016.

de Rooij SR, Wouters H, Yonker JE, et al: Prenatal undernutrition and cognitive function in late adulthood, *Proc Natl Acad Sci U S A* 107:16881–16886, 2010.

Dou H, Ma E, Yin L, et al: The association between gene polymorphism of TCF7L2 and type 2 diabetes in Chinese Han population: a meta-analysis, *PLOS One* 8:e59495, 2013.

Dulloo AG, Stock MJ, Solinas G, et al: Leptin directly stimulates thermogenesis in skeletal muscle, *FEBS Lett* 515:109–113, 2002.

Duranti S, Ferrario C, van Sinderen D, et al: Obesity and microbiota: an example of an intricate relationship, *Genes Nutr* 12:18, 2017.

Fairbrother U, Kidd E, Malagamuwa T, et al: Genetics of severe obesity, *Curr Diab Rep* 18:85, 2018.

Fraga MF, Ballestar E, Paz MF, et al: Epigenetic differences arise during the lifetime of monozygotic twins, *Proc Natl Acad Sci U S A* 102:10604–10609, 2005.

Franke K, Gaser C, Roseboom TJ, et al: Premature brain aging in humans exposed to maternal nutrient restriction during early gestation, *Neuroimage* 173:460–471, 2018.

Frühbeck G, Catalán V, Rodríguez A, et al: Involvement of the leptin-adiponectin axis in inflammation and oxidative stress in the metabolic syndrome, *Sci Rep* 7:6619, 2017.

Gage BF, Bass AR, Lin H, et al: Effect of genotype-guided warfarin dosing on clinical events and anticoagulation control among patients undergoing hip or knee arthroplasty: The GIFT randomized clinical trial, *JAMA* 318:1115, 2017. (Erratum in: *JAMA* 319, 1281, 2018.)

Galic S, Sachithanandan N, Kay TW, et al: Suppressor of cytokine signaling (SOCS) proteins as guardians of inflammatory responses critical for regulating insulin sensitivity, *Biochem J* 461:177–188, 2014.

Ghilardi N, Ziegler S, Wiestner A, et al: Defective STAT signaling by the leptin receptor in diabetic mice, *Proc Natl Acad Sci U S A* 93:6231–6235, 1996.

Girardot M, Feil R, Llères D: Epigenetic deregulation of genomic imprinting in humans: causal mechanisms and clinical implication, *Epigenomics* 5:715–728, 2013.

Grimaldi KA, van Ommen B, Ordovas JM, et al: Proposed guidelines to evaluate scientific validity and evidence for genotype-based dietary advice, *Genes Nutr* 12:35, 2017.

Grün F, Blumberg B: Environmental obesogens: organotins and endocrine disruption via nuclear receptor signaling, *Endocrinology* 147:S50–S55, 2006.

Gupta C, Prakash D: Phytonutrients as therapeutic agents, *J Complement Integr Med* 11:151–169, 2014.

Hales CM, Carroll MD, Fryar CD, et al: *Prevalence of obesity among adults and youth: United States, 2015-2016*. NCHS Data Brief No. 288, October 2017, U.S. Department of Health and Human Services, Centers for Disease Control and Prevention, National Center for Health Statistics.

Hasin Y, Seldin M, Lusis A: Multi-omics approaches to disease, *Genome Biol* 18:83, 2017.

Hennig B, Petriello MC, Gamble MV, et al: The role of nutrition in influencing mechanisms involved in environmentally mediated diseases, *Rev Environ Health* 33:87–97, 2018.

Hernandez W, Gamazon ER, Smithberger E, et al: Novel genetic predictors of venous thromboembolism risk in African Americans, *Blood* 127:1923–1929, 2016.

Hoffman JB, Petriello MC, Hennig B: Impact of nutrition on pollutant toxicity: an update with new insights into epigenetic regulation, *Rev Environ Health* 32:65–72, 2017.

Horikoshi M, Hara K, Ito C, et al: A genetic variation of the transcription factor 7-like 2 gene is associated with risk of type 2 diabetes in the Japanese population, *Diabetologia* 50:747–751, 2007.

Jagannadham J, Jaiswal HK, Agrawal S, et al: Comprehensive map of molecules implicated in obesity, *PLoS One* 11:e0146759, 2016.

Jump DB, Tripathy S, Depner CM: Fatty acid-regulated transcription factors in the liver, *Annu Rev Nutr* 33:249–269, 2013.

Jumpertz R, Le DS, Turnbaugh PJ, et al: Energy-balance studies reveal associations between gut microbes, caloric load, and nutrient absorption in humans, *Am J Clin Nutr* 94:58–65, 2011.

Kallio P, Kolehmainen M, Laaksonen DE, et al: Dietary carbohydrate modification induces alterations in gene expression in abdominal subcutaneous adipose tissue in persons with the metabolic syndrome: the FUNGENUT study, *Am J Clin Nutr* 85:1417–1427, 2007.

Kalliomäki M, Collado MC, Salminen S, et al: Early differences in fecal microbiota composition in children may predict overweight, *Am J Clin Nutr* 87:534–538, 2008.

Kalish JM, Jiang C, Bartolomei MS: Epigenetics and imprinting in human disease, *Int J Dev Biol* 58:291–298, 2014.

Katsoulis K, Paschou SA, Hatzi E, et al: TCF7L2 gene variants predispose to the development of type 2 diabetes mellitus among individuals with metabolic syndrome, *Hormones (Athens)* 17:359–365, 2018.

Kaur H, Badaruddoza B, Bains V, et al: Genetic association of ADIPOQ gene variants (-3971A>G and +276G>T) with obesity and metabolic syndrome in North Indian Punjabi population, *PLoS One* 13:e0204502, 2018.

Lampe JW, Peterson S: Brassica, biotransformation and cancer risk: genetic polymorphisms alter the preventive effects of cruciferous vegetables, *J Nutr* 132:2991–2994, 2002.

Lappalainen T, Lindström J, Paananen J, et al: Association of the fat mass and obesity-associated (FTO) gene variant (rs9939609) with dietary intake in the Finnish Diabetes Prevention Study, *Br J Nutr* 108:1859–1865, 2012.

Le Chatelier E, Nielsen T, Qin J, et al: Richness of human gut microbiome correlates with metabolic markers, *Nature* 500:541–546, 2013.

Lee YH, Song NY, Suh J, et al: Curcumin suppresses oncogenicity of human colon cancer cells by covalently modifying the cysteine 67 residue of SIRT1, *Cancer Lett* 431:219–229, 2018.

Lehman DM, Hunt KJ, Leach RJ, et al: Haplotypes of transcription factor 7-like 2 (TCF7L2) gene and its upstream region are associated with type 2 diabetes and age of onset in Mexican Americans, *Diabetes* 56:389–393, 2007.

Ley RE, Bäckhed F, Turnbaugh P, et al: Obesity alters gut microbial ecology, *Proc Natl Acad Sci USA* 102:11070–11075, 2005.

Loos RJ, Yeo GS: The bigger picture of FTO: the first GWAS-identified obesity gene, *Endocrinology* 10:51–61, 2014.

Lopomo A, Burgio E, Migliore L, et al: Epigenetics of obesity, *Mol Biol Transl Sci* 140:151–184, 2016.

Luoh SW, Flaherty KT: When tissue is no longer the issue: tissue-agnostic cancer therapy comes of age, *Ann Intern Med* 169:233–239, 2018.

Mattick JS: The state of long non-coding RNA biology, *Noncoding RNA* 4:E17, 2018.

Mathur R, Barlow GM: Obesity and the microbiome, *Expert Rev Gastroenterol Hepatol* 9:1087–1099, 2015.

Memisoglu A, Hu FB, Hankinson SE, et al: Interaction between a peroxisome proliferator-activated receptor gamma gene polymorphism and dietary fat intake in relation to body mass, *Hum Mol Gene* 12:2923–2929, 2003.

Merritt DC, Jamnik J, El-Sohemy A: FTO genotype, dietary protein intake, and body weight in a multiethnic population of young adults: a cross-sectional study, *Genes Nutr* 13:4, 2018.

Mutch DM, Zulyniak MA, Rudkowska I, et al: Lifestyle genomics: addressing the multifactorial nature of personalized health, *Lifestyle Genom* 11(1):1–8, 2018.

Mukherjee R, Jow L, Croston GE, et al: Identification, characterization, and tissue distribution of human peroxisome proliferator-activated receptor (PPAR) isoforms PPARgamma2 versus PPARgamma1 and activation with retinoid X receptor agonists and antagonists, *J Biol Chem* 272:8071–8076, 1997.

Muscogiuri G, Barrea L, Laudisio D, et al: Obesogenic endocrine disruptors and obesity: myths and truths, *Arch Toxicol* 91:3469–3475, 2017.

Nagai R, Ohara M, Cavallari LH, et al: Factors influencing pharmacokinetics of warfarin in African-Americans: implications for pharmacogenetic dosing algorithms, *Pharmacogenomics* 16, 217–225, 2015.

Naj AC, Schellenberg GD, Alzheimer's Disease Genetics Consortium: Genomic variants, genes, and pathways of Alzheimer's disease: an overview, *Am J Med Genet B Neuropsychiatr Genet* 174(1):5–26, 2017.

Nilsson EE, Sadler-Riggleman I, Skinner MK: Environmentally induced epigenetic transgenerational inheritance of disease, *Environ Epigenet* 4:dvy016, 2018.

Ornish D, Magbanua MJ, Weidner G, et al: Changes in prostate gene expression in men undergoing an intensive nutrition and lifestyle intervention, *Proc Natl Acad Sci U S A* 105:8369–8374, 2008.

Ortega Á, Berná G, Rojas A, et al: Gene-diet interactions in type 2 diabetes: the chicken and egg debate, *Int J Mol Sci* 18:E1188, 2017.

Perez JD, Rubinstein ND, Dulac C: New perspectives on genomic imprinting, an essential and multifaceted mode of epigenetic control in the developing and adult brain, *Annu Rev Neurosci* 39:347–384, 2016.

Peterson S, Schwarz Y, Li SS, et al: CYP1A2, GSTM1, and GSTT1 polymorphisms and diet effects on CYP1A2 activity in a crossover feeding trial, *Cancer Epidemiol Biomarkers Prev* 18:3118–3125, 2009.

Poulsen P, Esteller M, Vaag A, et al: The epigenetic basis of twin discordance in age-related diseases, *Pediatr Res* 61:38R–42R, 2007.

Radford EJ: Exploring the extent and scope of epigenetic inheritance, *Nat Rev Endocrinol* 14:345–355, 2018.

Rescigno T, Micolucci L, Tecce MF, et al: Bioactive nutrients and nutrigenomics in age-related diseases, *Molecules* 22:E105, 2017.

Rescigno T, Tecce MF, Capasso A: Protective and restorative effects of nutrients and phytochemicals, *Open Biochem J* 12:46–64, 2018.

Rocha DM, Caldas AP, Oliveira LL, et al: Saturated fatty acids trigger TLR4-mediated inflammatory response, *Atherosclerosis* 244:211–215, 2016.

Rodrigues APDS, Rosa LPS, da Silva HD, et al: The single nucleotide polymorphism PPARG2 Pro12Ala affects body mass index, fat mass, and blood pressure in severely obese patients, *J Obes* 12:2743081, 2018.

Rogero MM, Calder PC: Obesity, inflammation, toll-like receptor 4 and fatty acids, *Nutrients* 10:E432, 2018.

Roseboom T, de Rooij S, Painter R: The Dutch famine and its long-term consequences for adult health, *Early Hum Dev* 82:485–491, 2006.

Rozga M, Handu D: Nutritional genomics in precision nutrition: an evidence analysis library scoping review, *J Acad Nutr Diet* S2212–2672(18):30744, 2018. [Epub ahead of print]

Selber-Hnatiw S, Rukundo B, Ahmadi M, et al: Human gut microbiota: toward an ecology of disease, *Front Microbiol* 8:1265, 2017.

Silveira AC, Dias JP, Santos VM, et al: The action of polyphenols in diabetes mellitus and Alzheimer's disease: a common agent for overlapping pathologies, *Curr Neuropharmacol* 17(7):590–613, 2019.

Sonestedt E, Roos C, Gullberg B, et al: Fat nd carbohydrate intake modify the association between genetic variation in the FTO genotype and obesity, *Am J Clin Nutr* 90:1418–1425, 2009.

Stover PJ, James WPT, Krook A, et al: Emerging concepts on the role of epigenetics in the relationships between nutrition and health, *J Intern Med* 284:37–39, 2018.

Sun Q, Wedick NM, Tworoger SS, et al: Urinary excretion of select dietary polyphenol metabolites is associated with lower risk of type 2 diabetes in proximate but not remote follow-up in a prospective investigation in 2 cohorts of US women, *J Nutr* 145:1280–1288, 2015.

Unamuno X, Gómez-Ambrosi J, Rodríguez A, et al: Adipokine dysregulation and adipose tissue inflammation in human obesity, *Eur J Clin Invest* 48:e12997, 2018.

Upadhyay S, Dixit M: Role of polyphenols and other phytochemicals on molecular signaling, *Oxid Med Cell Longev* 2015:504253, 2015.

Van Baak TE, Coarfa C, Dugué PA, et al: Epigenetic supersimilarity of monozygotic twin pairs, *Genome Biol* 19:2, 2018.

Vanden Berghe W: Epigenetic impact of dietary polyphenols in cancer chemoprevention: lifelong remodeling of our epigenomes, *Pharmacol Res* 65:565–576, 2012.

Vimaleswaran KS, Bodhini D, Lakshmipriya N, et al: Interaction between FTO gene variants and lifestyle factors on metabolic traits in an Asian Indian population, *Nutr Metab (Lond)* 13:39, 2016.

Warodomwichit D, Shen J, Arnett DK, et al: ADIPOQ polymorphisms, monounsaturated fatty acids, and obesity risk: the GOLDN study, *Obesity (Silver Spring)* 17:510–517, 2009.

Waterland RA, Jirtle RL: Transposable elements: targets for early nutritional effects on epigenetic gene regulation, *Mol Cell Biol* 23:5293–5300, 2003.

Wedick NM, Pan A, Cassidy A, et al: Dietary flavonoid intakes and risk of type 2 diabetes in US men and women, *Am J Clin Nutr* 95:925–933, 2012.

Xue A, Wu Y, Zhu Z, et al: Genome-wide association analyses identify 143 risk variants and putative regulatory mechanisms for type 2 diabetes, *Nat Commun* 9:2941, 2018.

Yako YY, Guewo-Fokeng M, Balti EV, et al: Genetic risk of type 2 diabetes in populations of the African continent: a systematic review and meta-analyses, *Diabetes Res Clin Pract* 114:136–150, 2016.

Yang Q, Xiao T, Guo J, et al: Complex relationship between obesity and the fat mass and obesity locus, *Int J Biol Sci* 13:615–629, 2017.

Zayani N, Hamdouni H, Boumaiza I, et al: Association of ADIPOQ, leptin, LEPR, and resistin polymorphisms with obesity parameters in Hammam Sousse Sahloul Heart Study, *J Clin Lab Anal* 32:e22227, 2018.

1000 Genomes Project Consortium, Auton A, Brooks LD, et al: A global reference for human genetic variation, *Nature* 526(7571):68–74, 2015.

Inflammation and the Pathophysiology of Chronic Disease

Diana Noland, MPH, RDN, CCN, IFMCP, LD

KEY TERMS

adipokines
allostasis
antecedents
autoimmune
autophagy
biochemical individuality
body fluid viscosity
C-reactive protein–high sensitivity
   (CRP-hs)
coenzyme Q_{10}
conditionally essential
curcumin
cyclooxygenases (COX)
cytochrome P450 enzymes
cytokines
delta-6-desaturase
eicosanoid cascade
enteroimmunology

genesis of disease
glutathione
health continuum
hyperinsulinemia
inflammation
interleukin-6 (IL-6)
leukotrienes
lipoic acid
lipoxins
lipoxygenases (LOX)
long-latency nutrient insufficiencies
maresins
mediators
metabolic syndrome
"new-to-nature" molecules
nutrient-partner principle
nutrition transition
prolonged inflammation

prostaglandins
protectins
reactive oxygen species (ROS)
resolvins
quercetin
sarcopenia
sarcopenic obesity
sedimentation rate
specialized proresolving mediators (SPM)
systems biology
total inflammatory load
triage theory
triggers
tumor necrosis factor alpha (TNF-α)
vagal nerve
visceral adipose tissue (VAT)
xenobiotics

EPIDEMIC OF CHRONIC DISEASE

Chronic disease in the twenty-first century is a recent phenomenon in the history of the human race. Its recognition began after World War II at the same time the very significant nutrition transition began to occur, first in industrialized countries, then globally (see Chapter 10 *Focus On*: Nutrition Transition). The nutrition transition includes technology that enables synthesis of "new-to-nature" molecules (Bland, 2007), rapid increases in environmental toxin exposure, and decreased physical activity. New behavior patterns have promoted a decrease in home cooking along with increases in convenience food consumption and eating out. All of these changes are accompanied by the increased use of processed, less nutrient-dense food; decreased intake of whole fruits and vegetables; and increased consumption of sugar and high-sugar–containing foods. These components of the nutrition transition do not appear to have been beneficial to the human race, because the effects are rapidly and globally increasing the risk of being overweight and obese, along with producing epidemic levels of chronic diseases at earlier ages (Hruby and Hu, 2015) (see *Clinical Insight*: Is Chronic Disease an Epidemic?).

Despite the fact that the United States spends more money on health care than any other country, according to a report by the Centers for Disease Control and Prevention (CDC), 90% of the health care dollars in the United States are spent on chronic disease management (CDC, 2018). As people are living longer, the number of years spent living with disability has increased. The fact of the growing

CLINICAL INSIGHT

Is Chronic Disease an Epidemic?

- According to the Centers for Disease Control (CDC, 2018) and the World Health Organization (WHO, 2018):
- 1 out of 3 U.S. adults will have diabetes by 2050.
- 70% of U.S. deaths will be from chronic disease.
- Global cancer rates could increase by 70% 2015 to 2035.
- Two of three U.S. adults will be overweight or obese.
- One-third of cancer deaths will be due to the five leading behavioral and dietary risks (high BMI, low fruit and vegetable intake, lack of physical activity, smoking, and alcohol use).
- Younger Americans will likely face a greater risk of mortality throughout life than previous generations (related to obesity).
- The three most preventable risk factors are unhealthy diet, smoking, and physical inactivity.

incidence of chronic disease has driven the global civilian and governmental health care systems to seek new answers to this nearly universal challenge.

The global effort to improve understanding of this chronic disease phenomenon is bringing the realization that these chronic diseases have long incubation periods (years to decades), thus they may not be observable during their early stages and may be present in an otherwise healthy-looking person. Focusing on preventive care with earlier detection of signs, symptoms, and biomarkers that were previously thought insignificant allows for a chance to reverse the disease process before it becomes a serious affliction. The new phenotype of "fat, fatigued, and in pain" in combination with associated conditions is descriptive of many chronic disease states considered to be preventable "lifestyle" diseases. The genotype, or genetic makeup, of a person may increase the propensity toward a chronic disease, but lifestyle—what one eats and thinks and where one lives—may be the most powerful cause of these "lifestyle" chronic diseases (CDC, 2018; Elwood et al, 2013).

CONCEPTS OF CHRONIC DISEASE PATHOPHYSIOLOGY

An understanding of the following basic concepts is essential when addressing the newly identified characteristics of chronic disease pathophysiology: systems biology, allostasis, autophagy, the health continuum, genesis of disease, long-latency nutrient insufficiencies, and nutrient-partner principle.

Systems Biology

The emerging new paradigm of systems biology is the basis for a broader understanding of chronic disease. Systems biology is based on the understanding that all body systems work together interdependently. It is an interdisciplinary field that focuses on complex interactions within biological systems and includes the intersection of biology, informatics, computer science, physics, and engineering. Using this collaborative approach, scientists can identify biomarkers and genetic, dietary, and lifestyle influences on health and construct innovative models for prevention and treatment of disease (Trachana et al, 2018).

The global movement in health care toward systems biology and holistic and personalized approach to medicine is expanding. The registered dietitian nutritionist (RDN), as a member of the health care team, has a larger role to improve the nutritional status of each individual with dietary and lifestyle modifications as a foundational component of addressing chronic disease.

Allostasis

This is a condition of metabolic stability with adjustments for environmental influences and stresses through physiologic changes. Allostasis will be established even under inflammatory conditions but not always for optimal function. The maintenance of these changes over a long period of time can lead to wear and tear of the body. Inflammation may be initiated for tissue adaptation and yet may involve collateral damage. Inflammation is particularly relevant to obesity and its associated adverse health conditions, such as type 2 diabetes, cardiovascular disease, autoimmunity, and cancer. The ensuing systemic low-grade inflammation promotes a multitude of pathologic and self-perpetuating events, such as insulin resistance (Mather et al, 2013), endothelial dysfunction, and activation of oncogenic pathways (Baffy and Loscalzo, 2014).

For the nutritionist in clinical practice, the challenge is assessing metabolism and levels of inflammation at the cellular-molecular level available indirectly by using improved laboratory testing technology and scientific discovery of biochemical markers. For example, the biomarker C-reactive protein–high sensitivity (CRP-hs) has been shown to be the strongest univariate predictor of the risk of cardiovascular events. It is a systemic marker of inflammation within the internal milieu related most often to bacterial infection, trauma, and neoplastic activity with acute and chronic expression. Some studies indicate that the omega-3 fat eicosapentaenoic acid (EPA) from fish and fish oil has

an antiinflammatory effect and suppresses CRP-hs. Refer to Chapter 5 for additional information about CRP-hs.

Autophagy

Autophagy, or "self-eating," is a major regulatory cellular mechanism providing the cells an ability to clean up "cellular debris" occurring from normal metabolic activity. It is a survival mechanism required for maintaining cellular homeostasis after infection, mitochondrial damage, or endothelial reticulum stress. Autophagy results in the lysosomal degradation of organelles, unfolded proteins, or foreign extracellular material that provides a microenvironment supportive of healthy tissue. Defects in autophagy have been shown to result in pathologic inflammation influencing health and disease (Abraham and Medzhitov, 2011; Moloudizargari et al, 2017; Prado et al, 2014).

Health Continuum

Health is measured on a continuum from birth to death. "Health is the perfect, continuing adjustment of an organism to its environment" (Wyle, 1970). Chronic disease management for an individual must include considering the entire health continuum history to determine which factors along the way relate to one's current health condition. When collecting the patient's history during the assessment, plotting the person's health milestones as they relate to major life events can be helpful. This is often referred to as a health timeline.

Genesis of Disease

Triggers, antecedents, and mediators are critical terms that are part of the genesis of disease that underlies the patient's signs and symptoms, illness behaviors, and demonstrable pathology. Triggers are the distinct entities or events that provoke disease or its symptoms. They are usually insufficient for disease formation; host response is an essential component. Antecedents are congenital or developmental aspects of the individual that can include gender, family history, and genomics. These act to set the stage for the body's response to the trigger. Mediators are intermediates that are the primary drivers of disease; these are biochemical (Di Gennaro and Haeggström, 2012) but can be influenced by psychosocial factors such as smoking or stress (Avitsur et al, 2015; see Fig. 5.9 in Chapter 5).

Long-Latency Nutrient Insufficiencies

Long-latency nutrient insufficiencies (i.e., subclinical [below-optimum] or deficient nutrient pools resulting from chronic poor intake and genotype) contribute over time to development of chronic disease. New tools have to be included in nutrition practice to expand beyond just detection of overt clinical deficiencies (Heaney, 2012). There must be further identification of biomarkers, usually biochemical and phenotypic, which are indicative of early chronic disease and are evidence based.

The nutrient deficiencies defined in the early 1900s are the end-stage and the result of specific index diseases. An example of this is the discovery that vitamin C deficiency caused scurvy in British sailors. Scurvy produces obvious clinical symptoms and death within months of the absence of vitamin C intake. In contrast, a more recent discovery is that years of subclinical vitamin C deficiency (without classic scurvy symptoms) can cause a less recognizable form of scorbutic progression in the form of periodontal gum disease (periodontitis) (Alagl and Bhat, 2015; Japatti et al, 2013). Many other functions of vitamin C are compromised because of this "subclinical" deficiency. Pioneering biochemist Bruce Ames proposed that there should be two categories of nutrients according to their essentiality for immediate survival and reproduction (survival-nutrients), and nutrients that function in long-term health (longevity-nutrients) (Ames, 2018).

Nutrient-Partner Principle

Nutrient balance is the foundation of nutrition science, and this concept is expanding to appreciate the principle that, in addition to macronutrients requiring balance, there are known partner nutrients involved in an individual's nutrition and inflammatory status. An example of application of the **nutrient-partner principle** is the common recommendation for adults to take calcium supplements along with vitamin D. Another example is calcium and magnesium. For years, no attempt was made to routinely assess an individual's intake of magnesium, even though the National Health and Nutrition Examination Survey (NHANES) studies showed that 70% to 80% of the U.S. population had magnesium intakes below the recommended daily allowance (RDA). With recent recognition of this calcium-magnesium partnership, many calcium supplements now contain magnesium in a 2:1 or 1:1 Ca:Mg ratio, and nutrition guidelines include the consumption of more vegetables and greens containing magnesium and calcium. The principle of nutrients as well as metabolic systems having synergistic relationships are seen in Box 7.1.

Triage Theory

The concept of nutrient **triage theory** states that "during poor dietary supply, nutrients are preferentially utilized for functions that are important for survival." As a consequence, some tissues may be lacking during times of insufficiency. As proposed by the triage theory, a modest deficiency of nutrients/cofactors triggers a built-in rationing mechanism that favors the proteins needed for immediate survival and reproduction (survival proteins) while sacrificing those needed to protect against future damage (longevity proteins). Impairment of the function of longevity proteins results in an insidious acceleration in the risk of diseases associated with aging. This may result in a chronic deficiency in the person with inadequate nutrient intake that occurs for years and often for decades (Ames, 2006; Ames, 2010; McCann and Ames, 2011).

To summarize (Ames, 2018; Maggio et al, 2014):

- Most tissues need most nutrients.
- Inadequate intakes of most nutrients impair the function of most systems.
- The classical deficiency diseases occur at only the extremes of "inadequacy" (see Fig. 5.2 in Chapter 5).

BOX 7.1 Nutrient and System Partner Principles

Nutrient Partners
- Calcium – Zinc – Copper
- Omega 6 GLA/DGLA – Arachidonic Acid – Omega 3 EPA/DHA
- Sodium chloride – potassium – calcium
- B Complex (B1-B2-B3-B5-B6-B9 (folate)-B12-Biotin-Choline)
- Antioxidants – reactive oxygen species (ROS)
- Albumin – globulin

System Partners and Rhythm Cycles:
- Autonomic Nervous System: sympathetic – parasympathetic
- Circadian Rhythm: 24-hour balanced rhythm
- Acid-Base Balance
- Microbiome: oral, nasal, skin, lung, vaginal, gastrointestinal
- Hormones-biochemistry
  - Cortisol – insulin – glucose
  - Estrogen – progesterone – testosterone
  - T4-T3 (total and free forms)
  - HPTA axis – Hippocampus – Pituitary – Thyroid – Adrenal

- The role of nutritional status as a key factor of successful aging is very well recognized (McCann and Ames, 2011).
- "Adequate" adult nutrition can be best conceptualized as preventive maintenance.

INFLAMMATION: COMMON DENOMINATOR OF CHRONIC DISEASE

Inflammation is the natural, reaction of a healthy immune system as it responds to injury or infection, or flight or fright scenarios. See Box 7.2 for a classic description of inflammation.

The immune system's response to physiologic and metabolic stress is to produce proinflammatory molecules such as **adipokines** and **cytokines**. These cell-signaling molecules aid in cell-to-cell communication and stimulate the movement of cells toward sites of inflammation in conditions of infection and injury. Thus the immune system responds and the resulting inflammation is intimately connected.

According to Undurti N Das, MD, in the Molecular Basis of Health and Disease:

Inflammation is the complex biological response of vascular tissue to harmful stimuli such as pathogens, damaged cells or irritants that consists of both vascular and cellular responses. Inflammation is a protective attempt by the organism to remove the injurious stimuli and initiate the healing process and to restore both structure and function. Inflammation may be local or systemic. It may be acute or chronic.

Optimally, the immune system's function is to keep the body healthy, responding appropriately with an inflammatory response to environmental influences, such as short-lived infection and injury, and then returning the body to an alert system of defense. This function depends on the body's ability to recognize "self" and "nonself." When the immune response is successful, the tissue returns to a state of wellness, or metabolic stability described as allostasis. If many areas of the body's defense system, such as the gastrointestinal barrier, stomach acidity, skin, or various orifices (e.g., eye, ear, nose, lung, vagina, uterus), are compromised, there is diminishing recognition of "self" and "nonself" until the body is repaired. The longer the physiologic injury continues, the greater the loss of the ability to recognize "self" and "nonself" (Fasano, 2012; Wu et al, 2014).

If the underlying cause is not resolved, the immune response can get "stuck" in a state of prolonged inflammation. Locked into this state for a while, the immune system loses its ability to recognize "self" and "nonself," a critical survival skill and the core of immunology (Gonzalez et al, 2011; Paul, 2010).

Prolonged Inflammation

Prolonged inflammation, known as chronic inflammation, sustained inflammation, or nonresolving inflammation, leads to a progressive

---

BOX 7.2 The Five Classic Signs of Inflammation, First Described and Documented by Aulus Cornelius Celsus (ca 25 BC-ca 50), a Roman Physician and Encyclopaedist

- **Dolor** - "pain"
- **Calor** - "heat"
- **Rubor** - "redness"
- **Tumor** - "swelling"
- **Functio laesa** - "injured function" or "loss of function."

shift in the type of cells present at the site of inflammation and is characterized by simultaneous destruction and healing of the tissue from the inflammatory process. Multiple studies have suggested that prolonged inflammation plays a primary role in the pathogenesis of chronic diseases (e.g., cardiovascular disease, cancer, diabetes), when the immune response is to increase the ratio of proinflammatory to antiinflammatory cytokines (Bauer et al, 2014; Franceschi and Campisi, 2014).

In the chronology of chronic disease progression, inflammation is at first subclinical, often referred to as "silent inflammation." This insidious inflammation remains below the threshold of clinical diagnosis. Cellular and tissue damage can occur in the body for years before being noticed. It is like a "smoldering" fire with a small whiff of smoke and heat being evident before it finally bursts into a flame. Some refer to early chronic disease as a "smoldering disease" (Noland, 2013). Inflammation in chronic disease is described as:

Low-grade, chronic, systemic inflammation may be defined as a 2- to 3-fold elevation of circulating inflammatory mediators, usually associated with the innate arm of the immune system. It is a state that develops slowly (in contrast to pathologic acute inflammatory responses, to sepsis for example), and its origin cannot be easily identified (in contrast to chronic inflammatory diseases such as rheumatoid arthritis and inflammatory bowel disease, where additional symptoms identify local dysregulated inflammation). This makes it difficult to develop appropriate therapeutic strategies that target both cause and symptom (inflammation) in a concerted fashion (Calçada et al, 2014).

Of concern is the initiation of prolonged inflammation in utero from the maternal inflammatory environment, thereby programming the fetus for a lifetime of chronic disease (European Foundation for the Care of Newborn Infants [EFCNI], 2015; Lane, 2014; Fisher et al, 2012; Fleisch et al, 2012; see Chapter 14).

Inflammation is a very complex condition, and there are many protein biomarkers that are acute phase reactants. Clinical elevations of inflammatory biomarkers, such as CRP-hs (plasma), sedimentation rate, interleukin-6 (IL-6), and tumor necrosis factor alpha (TNF-α), represent systemic markers of inflammation that are exacerbated by insulin resistance (IR) and hyperinsulinemia (Das, 2010, 2011; see Table 7.1). Diseases associated with increased levels of inflammatory markers include heart disease, diabetes, autoimmune diseases, and

TABLE 7.1 Biomarkers of Prolonged Inflammation

Test	Reference	Association
Blood Specimen		
8-hydroxy-2-deoxyguanosine	< 7.6 ng/mL	DNA increased ROS and cell proliferation*
Asymmetric dimethylarginine (ADMA)	<18 years: not established ≥18 years: 63-137 ng/mL	Inhibitor of L-arginine (Arg)-derived nitric oxide (NO)
C-reactive protein sensitivity	≤3.0 mg/L	Systemic inflammation related to bacterial infection, trauma, VAT, neoplastic activity
CA-125	0-35 U/mL	Inflammation in abdomen Ovarian cancer Uterine fibroids
CA 15-3/CA 27-29	<32 U/mL	Breast cancer, advanced
CA-19-9 Carbohydrate Ag 19-9 (screening test)	<55 U/mL Up to 20% of individuals do not express CA 19-9.	Pancreatic cancer Infections in liver, gallbladder, and pancreas.
CEA (other specimens also)	12-100 years: 0-5.0 ng/mL	Cancer
CD4 Lymphocyte CD4%		HIV infections, autoimmune
CD8 Count		Infections Lymphoma
Ceruloplasmin (bound copper/ acute phase reactant)	18-46 mg/dL	Acute phase reactant Cancer (elevated) Wilson's Disease (low) Menkes syndrome (low)
Eosinophils	1%-4%	Elevated inflammatory marker of allergies / sensitivities, helminthic, parasites, autoimmune, neoplasms
Ferritin (storage iron)	Males ≥5 years: 24-150 ng/mL Females ≥5 years: 12-150 ng/mL	Acute Phase Reactant Hemochromatosis (genetic) Iron Toxicity
Fibrinogen / Platelets	150-450 mg/dL / 150-450 billion/L	Disseminated intravascular coagulation (DC) Liver disease
Homocysteine (Hcy)	0-15 μmol/L	Block in homocysteine metabolism to cystathionine relate to B$_6$, B$_{12}$, folate, betaine cofactors

Continued

TABLE 7.1   Biomarkers of Prolonged Inflammation—cont'd

Test	Reference	Association
IgA Total or IgA specific	50-350 mg/dL	Elevated in lymphoproliferative disorders; chronic infections; autoimmune; celiac disease
IgE Total or IgE specific	800-1500 mg/dL	Elevated immediate-response inflammatory allergic disorders; parasitic infections
IgG Total or IgG specific	800-1500 mg/dL	Elevated inflammation marker of delayed sensitivities; chronic infections
Interleukin-1 (IL-1)	<3.9 pg/mL	Bone formation, insulin secretion, appetite regulation, fever reduction, neuronal development
Interleukin 8 (IL-8)	<17.4 pg/mL < or = 5 pg/mL (2014)	Neoplasms / promotes angiogenesis Obesity Oxidative stress
Insulin (Korkmaz, 2014)	2.0-12.0 µIU/mL	Elevated inflammatory insulin resistance
Lipid Peroxides	<2.60 nmol/mL	Inflammatory elevation when risk of oxidative stress / elevated triglycerides
Liver enzyme: ALT	0-35/U/L	Inflammatory elevation in liver disease
Liver enzyme: AST	0-35 U/L	Inflammatory elevation with liver, kidney, muscle infection, or injury
Liver enzymes: Alk Phos	30-120 U/L	Inflammatory elevation related to liver, bone, placenta
Liver enzyme: GGT	0-30 U/L	Elevated inflammatory marker of liver disease, neoplasms, toxicity
Liver enzyme: LDH	50-150 U/L	
Prostate Specific Antigen (PSA)	Total PSA ≤4.0 ng/mL % Free PSA >25 % (calc)	Prostate inflammation Prostate cancer
Rheumatoid Factor (RF)	Less than 40-60 U/mL Less than 1:80 (1-80) titer	Rheumatoid arthritis Sjogren's Autoimmune disease
Sedimentation Rate (ESR) Westergren	Male <50 years old:<15 mm/hr Male >50 years old:<20 mm/hr Female <50years old:<20 mm/hr Female >50 years old:<30 mm/hr	Systemic inflammation marker related to autoimmune; viral infections; rouleaux; carcinoid influence
Total Protein	60-80 g/L (6.0-8.0 g/dL)	Total protein in serum
Albumin	35 - 50 g/L (3.5-5.0 g/dL) (half-life ~ 20 days)	Acute phase reactant
Globulin	2.6-4.6 g/dL	Chronic inflammation, low albumin levels, and other disorders
TH17 Interleukin 17 (IL-17)	0.0-1.9 pg/mL	Fungal, bacterial, viral infections, autoimmune conditions
TNF-α	1.2-15.3 pg/mL	Systemic inflammation Acute phase reactant Alzheimer's, infection, depression, IBD, cancer
Uric Acid	2-7 mg/dL	Antioxidant, elevated in abnormal urate cycle exacerbated by protein in diet, gout, other
VEGF	31-86 pg/mL	Cancer, angiogenesis
White blood cell count	4.5- 11 x 10³/µL	(Elevated) Leukocytosis, bacterial infections, anemia, cigarette smoking (Low) Cancer, radiation, severe infection
Stool Specimen		
Calprotectin	2-9 years 166 µg/g of feces 10-59 years 51 µg/g of feces ≥ 60 years 112 µg/g of feces	Inflammatory bowel disease Intestinal inflammation Neoplasms
Lactoferrin	Negative	Intestinal inflammation
Pancreatic elastase I	> 200 µg/g	Exocrine pancreatic function
Urine		
5-hydroxyindoleacetate (5-HIAA)	1.6-10.9 µg/mL creatinine	Elevated with inflammatory breakdown of serotonin
p-hydroxyphenyllactate (HPLA)	<1.45 µg/mL creatinine	Inverse relationship to depletion of ascorbic acid

*Normal value ranges may vary slightly among different labs

TABLE 7.2 Autoimmune Specific Inflammatory Markers

Biomarker Test	Reference Range	Specimen	Association
Sedimentation Rate (ESR)	Men: 0-15 mm/h Women: 0-20 mm/h	Blood serum	Collagen diseases Inflammatory diseases Infections Toxicity, heavy metals
C-Reactive Protein-hs (CRP-hs)	<1.0 mg/dL	Blood	Systemic inflammation Metabolic Syndrome
Rheumatoid Factor (RF)	0-39 IU/mL nonreactive 40-79 IU/mL weakly reactive >80 reactive	Blood	Rheumatoid arthritis Sjögren's syndrome Joint pain Rheumatoid conditions
Antigliadin Antibody Deamidated Gliadin Antibody, IgA, IgG	0-19 Negative 20-30 Weak Positive >30 Moderate to Strong positive	Blood serum	Celiac disease Dermatitis herpetiforme Non-Celiac gluten sensitivity
Endomysial antibody test (IgA-EMA)	Negative normal individuals Negative Gluten-free diet		Dermatitis herpetiforme, celiac disease
Tissue Transglutaminase IgA/IgG (tTG-IgA)	<4.0 U/mL (negative) 4.0-10.0 U/mL (weak positive) >10.0 U/mL (positive) Reference values apply to all ages.	Blood serum	Celiac disease (indicates Rx biopsy, gene HLA_DQ2/DQ8) Dermatitis herpetiforme Villi Atrophy
SS-A Sjögren's/Ro IgG	<1.0 U (negative) > or = 1.0 U (positive) Reference values apply to all ages.	Blood	Connective tissue disease (Systemic lupus erythematosus, Sjögren's, Rheumatoid arthritis)
SS-B Sjögren's	<1.0 U (negative) > or = 1.0 U (positive) Reference values apply to all ages.	Blood	Connective tissue disease, including Sjögren's syndrome, systemic lupus erythematosus (SLE)
ANA antibody titer	<1:40 normal (or < 1/0 IU) is negative	Blood serum	Multiple autoimmune conditions, systemic lupus erythematosus (SLE)
Anti-dsDNA Test IgG	<30.0 IU/mL (negative) 30.0-75.0 IU/mL (borderline) >75.0 IU/mL (positive) Negative is considered normal. Reference values apply to all ages.	Blood	
Cyclic Citrullinated Peptide Antibody (Anti-CCP)	<20.0 U (negative) 20.0-39.9 U (weak positive) 40.0-59.9 U (positive) > or = 60.0 U (strong positive) Reference values apply to all ages.	Blood	Rheumatoid arthritis Arthritis
Anti-Desmoglein 1/3 IgG antibody Blister biopsy	negative	Blood Skin tissue	Pemphigus vulgaris Pemphigus foliaceus Epidermolysis bullosa acquisita

possibly cancer and Alzheimer's disease (Birch et al, 2014; Luevano-Contreras et al, 2017; Wu, 2013). See Tables 7.2 through 7.4 and Boxes 7.3 and 7.4 for more examples of common disease specific biomarkers.

Other common physiologic changes shared by these inflammatory conditions include changes in nutrient tissue pools, plasma, and red blood cell (RBC) membrane composition of polyunsaturated fatty acids and antioxidants. This multifactorial syndrome (referred to as metabolic syndrome) is related to obesity, and more importantly, insulin resistance and visceral adipose tissue (VAT) as evidenced by central adiposity. (See Chapter 29 for discussion of the metabolic syndrome). However, the expression of prolonged inflammation is individual and doesn't necessarily manifest in all the characteristics described above.

For the nutritionist and dietitian to incorporate the related factors of prolonged inflammation into the nutrition assessment, it is useful to conceptualize an overview of a person's total inflammatory load (Fig. 7.1). It is a compilation of every factor in the patient's history or story that contributes to the inflammation that a person carries.

As various factors are identified within diet, lifestyle, environment, and genetics, the pattern of where the most inflammatory risk is being generated becomes clear and gives a basis of how to intervene with a plan for medical nutrition therapy (MNT).

Antigens

Antigens are a source of inflammation that become amplified with chronic exposure (see Chapter 25). During assessment of the total

TABLE 7.3 Neurologic Specific Inflammatory Markers

Biomarker Test	Reference	Specimen	Association
RBC Fatty Acid Analysis	Mean +/− SD	Blood	Membrane integrity
Lipid Panel	170-200 mg/dL	Blood	CHD risk
Triglycerides	50-80 mg/dL	Blood	Adult: CHD risk
Total Cholesterol	Men: 37-40 mg/dL	Blood	Child: abnormal cholesterol
HDL	Women: 40-85 mg/dL		metabolism
LDL	Adult <130 mg/dL or <3.4 mmol/L		
	Child <110 mg/dL or <2.8 mmol/L		
CREATINE KINASE			
Creatinine	0.76-1.27 mg/dL	Blood	Kidney function
BUN	8-27 mg/dL		
GFR	>60 mL/min/BSA		
Glucose, fasting	65-99 mg/dL	Blood, urine	Glucose status
Insulin, fasting	2.0-19.6 µIU/mL	Blood	Insulin status
HgbA1C	4.8%-6.4%	Blood	Average BS over 120 days
25OH vit D	30-150 ng/mL	Blood, saliva	Vitamin D status

TABLE 7.4 Endocrine (noncancer) Specific Inflammatory Markers

Biomarker Test (Mother)	Reference	Specimen	Association
RBC Fatty Acid Analysis	Mean +/− SD	Blood	Membrane integrity
Lipid Panel	170-200 mg/dL	Blood	CHD
Total Cholesterol	Men: 37-40 mg/dL		Cholesterol/lipid metabolism
HDL-chol	Women: 40-85 mg/dL		Liver stress
LDL-chol	Adult <130 mg/dL or <3.4 mmol/L		CHD risk
Triglycerides	Child <110 mg/dL or <2.8 mmol/L		CHD risk
	<150 mg/dL		Abnormal cholesterol
			Metabolic syndrome
			Carnitine insufficiency
			High simple sugar/alcohol diet
			CHD risk
Celiac Panel	<4 U/mL no antibody detected		Small intestine villi atrophy
tTG IgG/IgA	<20 Units antibody not detected		Gluten sensitivity
Anti-Gliadin antibody			Gluten-free diet
tissue Transglutaminase IgG/IgA			
Antigen (Food IgG/IgE)	Per laboratory		
Insulin, fasting	2.0-19.6 µIU/mL	Blood	Insulin status
HgbA1C	4.8%-6.4%	Blood	Average BS over 120 days
TSH	Adult 0.2-5.4 mU/L blood	Blood	Thyroid function
Vitamin $D_2$5-OH	30-150 ng/mL	Blood, saliva	Vitamin D status

inflammatory load of an individual, the "antigenic load" is important. Antigens usually are thought to come from foods to which one is either allergic or sensitive, but also can be derived from cosmetics, clothing, inhalants, furniture, household building materials, and other substances in the environment. Antigens from food are much more likely to be significant when a person has lost gut barrier integrity and a situation of intestinal permeability, sometimes referred to as "leaky gut" exists (Fasano, 2012). This condition provides access for larger molecules to enter the internal microenvironment, setting off a cascade of immunologic responses (see Chapters 25 and 27).

Genomics

Predictive genomic testing, family history, and personal history are gathered as the practitioner hears the patient's story during an assessment. This information helps paint a picture of biochemical individuality, that each person has genetic and chemical uniqueness, which influences the response to inflammation. Since the completion of the Human Genome Project (2003), the rapid development of genomic testing for clinical application has greatly enhanced the toolbox of the nutrition practitioner. Nutrigenomics, nutrigenetics, and epigenetics are new fields of study about the way the individual metabolically interacts with their environment (Dick, 2015; see Chapter 6).

Body Composition

Chronic diseases are related directly to increased body fat exacerbated by physical inactivity, poor diet, lack of restorative sleep, and immune stress, all of which drive increased inflammation. Of equal importance with increased body fat percentage is the fat distribution. Central adiposity at all ages is the most serious health concern. VAT has been discovered to have endocrine functions with the secretion of several

---

BOX 7.3 Cardiometabolic Specific Inflammatory Markers

- Increased body fat %, most often with elevated BMI and VAT.
  - BMI
  - Waist Circumference
  - Waist/Height Ratio
  - Waist/Hip Ratio
  - Body fat % (bioelectric impedance, air or water displacement plethysmograph, DEXA, calipers)
- Blood Biomarkers of prolonged inflammation in CVD/cardiometabolic syndrome with diabetes
  - Hyperlipidemia/Hypertriglyceridemia
  - Total Cholesterol/HDL Ratio
  - Fasting Glucose/Fasting Insulin
  - HgbA1C
  - C-Reactive Protein-high sensitivity (CRP-hs or CRP-cardio)
  - Homocysteine
- Imaging: Coronary calcium scan
- Myeloperoxidase (blood)
- Other associations for CVD/cardiometabolic syndrome/diabetes:
  - Sympathetic dominant metabolism (metabolic stress)
  - Stress (biochemical, glandular, emotional, environmental, smoking)
  - Poor sleep
  - Apnea

BOX 7.4 Cancer-Specific Inflammatory Markers

- Various metabolic markers measuring inflammatory hallmarks of cancer
  - Adhesion: Fibrinogen and platelets (blood)
  - Metastasis promoters:
  - Copper (Cu): Zinc Ratio 1.0 or less (rate limiting to metastatic enzymes)
  - Ceruloplasmin (contributes to the total Cu load)
  - Angiogenesis promoters (Dai et al, 2014): VEGF, adhesion factors.
- Tumor-promoting inflammation: Specific type of cancer markers (examples: ovarian cancer CA 125, breast cancer CA 15-3, prostate cancer PSA). Various proinflammatory cytokines and chemokines: TNF-α, IL-8, IL-6, etc.
  - Glycolysis (Warburg Effect: sugar is primary fuel of cancer cells)
  - Growth factors
  - Genome instability/mitochondrial DNA
  - Loss of apoptosis/cell immortality

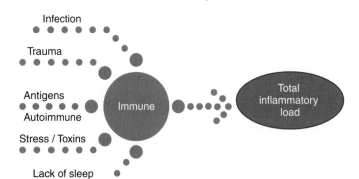

Total Inflammatory Load

Copyright 2013 Diana Noland, MPH RD CCN LD

Fig. 7.1 Total Inflammatory Load.

Body composition can be assessed, and if found to be abnormal based an individual's lean body mass (LBM) and fat mass (FM), it should be considered a primary marker for monitoring prolonged inflammation (Biolo et al, 2015; Juby, 2014).

According to Khan, S et al, (2014):

Obesity today stands at the intersection between inflammation and metabolic disorders causing an aberration of immune activity, and resulting in increased risk for diabetes, atherosclerosis, fatty liver, and pulmonary inflammation to name a few.

Energy Dysregulation

Another underlying physiologic system involved in inflammation is compromised mitochondrial production of adenosine triphosphate (ATP) (Cherry and Piantadosi, 2015). Assessment of mitochondrial function focuses on structure and function by considering conutrients such as coenzyme Q_{10}, and alpha-lipoic acid and gamma(γ)-linolenic acid (GLA) (already produced by the body), and their protective effects against inflammation and oxidative stress. Quelling systemic prolonged inflammation promotes a healthier microenvironment for improved mitochondrial function and energy production.

Mitochondrial disease or dysfunction is an energy production problem. Almost all cells in the body have mitochondria that produce a body's essential energy, ATP. Mitochondrial diseases disturb cellular function and reduce mitochondrial energy output. When that happens, some body systems may be impaired causing muscle weakness, organ dysfunction, hormone imbalance, disrupted cognition, and lowered immunity (Miller et al, 2018). The complaint of fatigue is the most common phenotypic expression of mitochondrial dysfunction (see *Clinical insight*: Inflammaging).

The ratios of carbohydrate, fat, and protein influence mitochondrial function, primarily affecting glucose-insulin regulation. During each assessment, determination of the most favorable macronutrient ratios and individual nutrient requirements provides the foundation for the most effective interventions for restoring mitochondrial health and general wellness. There is an increasing popularity and evidence base for low-carbohydrate, paleo, and ketogenic diets for mitochondrial support for some conditions, such as epilepsy, neurodegenerative diseases, and oncology (Allen et al, 2014). It is worth noting that the nutritional assessment of an individual should include a diet history to evaluate the macronutrients consumed. Because of the common tendency for a high protein intake as part of a low-carbohydrate diet, the excess protein may potentially increase gluconeogenesis, thus thwarting the benefit of low carb by increasing available metabolic glucose. The principle of the ketogenic diet (KD) replaces all but

known inflammatory adipokines, such as resistin, leptin, and adiponectin, and TNF-α—all contributing to the systemic total inflammatory load (Hughes-Austin et al, 2014). **Sarcopenia** results from a wasting of lean body mass and muscle strength from the ongoing inflammatory burden and is exacerbated by decreased physical activity (da Silva et al, 2019). **Sarcopenic obesity** is accompanied by increased body fat percentage, especially the deposit of VAT with increasing waist circumference, but for some individuals the loss of muscle and increased fat mass percentage can exist for any body mass index (BMI) range—underweight, normal weight, or overweight and obesity. This underscores the importance of assessing more detail than only BMI (Gonzalez et al, 2017; Norman and Matthews, 2008). The BMI alone does not adequately characterize the distribution of adipose tissue and recommendations exist for more specific measures with better predictive value (Gonzalez et al, 2017). The nutritionist's tools for assessing sarcopenia vary from using the waist-to-hip ratio, waist-to-height ratio, bioelectric impedance analysis (BIA), handgrip strength (dynamometer), or dual-energy x-ray absorptiometry (DXA), when available (Springstroh et al, 2016) (see Chapter 5 and *Clinical Insight*: Sarcopenic Obesity).

low and nonstarchy vegetable carbohydrates (20 to 100 g cholesterol [CHO]) with low to moderate amounts of proteins (0.8 to 1.0 g protein/kg ideal body weight) and high amounts of short-chain, medium chain and monounsaturated, and polyunsaturated fats, preferably from whole and unprocessed foods (Miller et al, 2018; see Appendix 19).

CLINICAL INSIGHT

Sarcopenic Obesity

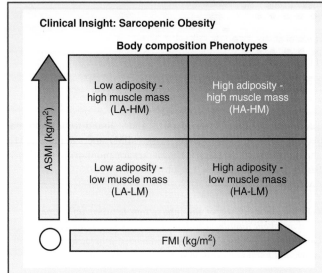

Clinical Insight: Sarcopenic Obesity

Body composition Phenotypes

ASMI (kg/m²) / FMI (kg/m²)

- Low adiposity - high muscle mass (LA-HM)
- High adiposity - high muscle mass (HA-HM)
- Low adiposity - low muscle mass (LA-LM)
- High adiposity - low muscle mass (HA-LM)

In this figure, body composition is depicted by a spectrum of ASMI and FMI (low to high). On the basis of the Baumgartner model (Waters and Baumgartner, 2011), these phenotypes can be depicted as follows:

LA-HM = low adiposity with high muscle mass (individuals with low FMI and high ASMI)

HA-HM = high adiposity with high muscle mass (individuals with high FMI and ASMI)

LA-LM = low adiposity with low muscle mass (individuals with low ASMI and FMI)

HA- LM = high adiposity with low muscle mass (individuals with high FMI and low ASMI).

Those with **LA-HM would be the least healthy.**

Cutoffs were defined according to the following deciles:

LA-HM (ASMI: 50-100; FMI: 0-49.99)

HA-HM (ASMI: 50-100; FMI: 50-100)

LA-LM (ASMI: 0-49.99; FMI: 0-49.99)

HA-LM (ASMI: 0-49.99; FMI: 50-100).

ASMI, Appendicular skeletal muscle mass index; *FMI,* fat mass index. Carla MM Prado et al: A population-based approach to define body-composition phenotypes, *Am J Clin Nutr,* 99:1369, 2014.

CLINICAL INSIGHT

Inflammaging

Aging is a ubiquitous complex phenomenon that results from environmental, genetic, and epigenetic events in different cell types and tissues and their interactions throughout life. A pervasive feature of aging tissues and most, if not all, age-related diseases is chronic inflammation. "Inflammaging" describes the low-grade, chronic, systemic inflammation in aging, in the absence of overt infection ("sterile" inflammation) and is a highly significant risk factor for morbidity and mortality in the elderly (Franceschi and Campisi, 2014).

Microbiome

After the Human Genome Project, the National Institutes of Health (NIH) launched studies for genomic identification and characterization of the microorganisms associated with healthy and diseased humans. The exciting findings focus on five body sites (mouth, skin, vagina, nose/lung, and the gastrointestinal [GI] tract). The total number of genes in the human microbiome is 10 times greater than the human genome. When the delicate microbiome community in and on the body is disturbed and altered from healthy baseline, it becomes a factor in promoting prolonged inflammation and affects the way food is metabolized in the body. The loss of microbiome diversity and the presence of specific undesirable or virulent bacteria appears to be a common finding related to various diseases (Fasano, 2012; Viladomiu et al, 2013).

The cause of these changes in the patterns of microbiota from "healthy" to dysfunctional appears to be influenced by genetics, diet, exposure to environmental toxins, and antibiotic use (National Institutes of Health [NIH], 2014). After a pathology has been determined, the systems biology-based practitioner often uses stool testing to provide more quantitative and specific functional information regarding the condition of the gut environment and microbiology. Laboratory tests for inflammatory markers such as calprotectin, lactoferrin, and pancreatic elastase 1 in the gut, much like sedimentation rate or CRP-hs and immunoglobulin A (IgA) are markers of inflammation in the blood (Gommerman, 2014). Because the GI tract contains about 70% of the immune system, it is important to assess the condition of the GI tract—from the mouth to the anus—as part of the total inflammatory load of an individual (Underwood, 2014). A new field of study regarding diseases that are related to disturbances in the gut environment and the immune system is called enteroimmunology (Lewis, 2014; Tsai, 2018; Fig. 7.2).

Hypercoagulation

With inflammation comes an increasingly unhealthy degree of coagulation within body fluids. At some point, the microenvironment becomes too congested, facilitating the development of chronic diseases such as cancer, cardiovascular disease, autoimmune diseases, and infectious diseases (Karabudak et al, 2008). This increase in body fluid viscosity promotes secretion of more proinflammatory immune cytokines and chemokines that can set the stage for chronic disease. Autophagy is the normal response to raise the level of proteolytic enzymes to "clean up" the cell debris and prepare it for recycling or elimination (Gottlieb and Mentzer, 2010; Gurkar et al, 2013; Rahman and Rhim, 2017; Wallace et al, 2014).

Dietary factors helping maintain healthy fluid viscosity are hydration, plant-based diets, polyunsaturated fatty acids (PUFAs), and monounsaturated fats (MUFAs) (Naghedi-Baghdar et al, 2018). Common biomarkers of increased body fluid viscosity are blood fibrinogen with platelets, and urinalysis measurements of specific gravity and the presence of "cloudiness" or mucus.

Infection

Acute infections are easily recognized and diagnosed because of their blatant signs and symptoms such as fever, leukocytosis, pus, and tachycardia. Subclinical infection processes, on the contrary, may go unnoticed for years or decades while promoting a "smoldering," under-the-radar, inflammatory condition that wears away at the integrity of the body cells and tissues. Good examples are hepatitis C virus (HCV), which begins as an acute infection but persists as a chronic infection in the liver (Vescovo et al, 2014), and human papilloma virus (HPV), which becomes chronic in cervical tissue and may lead to cervical cancer.

All chronic infections raise the level of immune response to produce inflammatory mediators and are exacerbated by nutrient insufficiencies

---

ENTEROIMMUNOLOGY

Enteroimmunology includes underlying pathophysiologies of many, if not all, autoimmune diseases. About 50% of the body's immune cells are housed in the intestine. The intestine secretes the largest amount of inflammatory cytokines in the body. What happens in an inflamed GUT has the potential to exacerbate inflammation throughout the body.

Common nonspecific symptoms in enteroimmune disease

Area Affected	Symptoms
Cognitive	Mental fog, poor concentration, learning difficulties, poor memory, lethargy, apathy, rage, restlessness, hyperactivity
Sensory	Vertigo, lightheadedness, tinnitus
Emotional	Anxiety, moodiness, depression, aggressiveness, irritability
Somatic	Headaches, insomnia, fatigue, joint pain, muscle pain, stiffness, weakness, weight gain, fluid retention, non-ischemic chest pain
Gastrointestinal	Dyspepsia, bloating, belching, constipation, abdominal cramping, nausea, excessive flatulence
Respiratory	Congestion, excessive phlegm and mucous, dyspnea, chronic cough, gagging
Adapted from Lewis (2013)	

Some neurologic diseases associated with enteroimmunopathies

- Autism
- Alzheimer's disease
- Parkinson's disease
- Multiple sclerosis
- Depression
- Bipolar disorder
- Schizophrenia
- Migraine headaches
- Cerebellar ataxia
- Certain seizure disorders

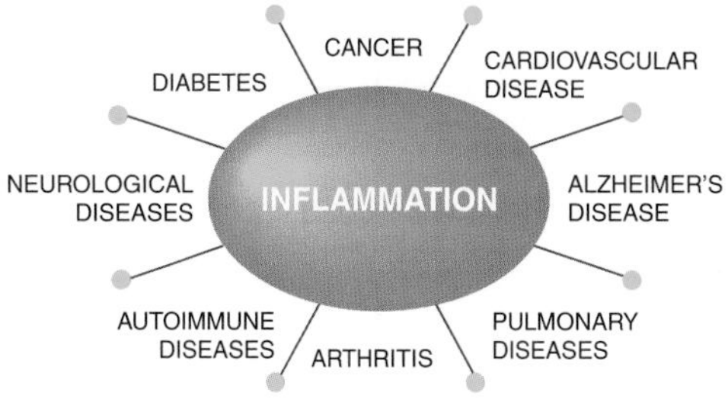

CANCER — CARDIOVASCULAR DISEASE — DIABETES — ALZHEIMER'S DISEASE — NEUROLOGICAL DISEASES — **INFLAMMATION** — AUTOIMMUNE DISEASES — ARTHRITIS — PULMONARY DISEASES

Fig. 7.2 Enteroimmunology.

and deficiencies and imbalances between prooxidant and antioxidant conditions (Cokluk et al, 2015). Other nutrients, when insufficient for optimum function, are involved in permitting chronic infections to persist over decades include vitamin D, vitamin C, and methylation nutrients such as folate, B_{12}, B_6, and B_2, which act as conutrients in inflammation and immune-control mechanisms (Ames, 2010). In addition, the health of the microbiome in the gastrointestinal tract, the skin, and other body orifices plays a critical role in inflammation and immune strength or weakness.

Stress

Stress is proinflammatory. The sources of metabolic stress may include injury, infection, musculoskeletal misalignment, lack of sleep, strong emotions, unhealthy diet, smoking, quality-of-life challenges, or lack or excess of physical activity. Whatever the source, stress can increase nutrient requirements contributing to depletion and the level of oxidative stress risks damage to body cells and tissues.

NUTRIENT MODULATORS OF INFLAMMATION

For the three prostaglandins and their metabolites formed from the eicosanoid cascade, there are vitamin, mineral, and antioxidant nutrients and hormones that act as rate-limiting cofactors for the shared

delta-5 and delta-6 desaturase and the elongase enzymes. These enzymes are required for conversion of the essential fatty acids (EFA) and PUFAs to prostaglandins. These conutrients, listed in Figs. 7.3 and 7.4, have the important ability to modulate the fatty acids and their antiinflammatory products that have key roles in the pathophysiology of chronic disease and systemic inflammation that contributes to its progression.

In addition to nutrient cofactors and hormones (like insulin) influencing the biochemistry of the eicosanoid and fatty acid metabolism of an individual, there is emerging evidence of genotype and epigenetic effects from environmental triggers that affect the genetic expression. The key genes modulating the conversion enzymes are FAD1, FAD2, and ELOVL5 (see Chapter 6). The omega-6 and omega-3 eicosanoids also share the three genes that can influence an individual's activity and efficiency of the desaturase and elongase enzymes used in conversion of the eicosanoid molecules (see Fig. 7.3).

If genomic test data is available for the nutritionist in developing a nutritional intervention, the knowledge of the influence of FAD1, FAD2, and ELOVL5 on the eicosanoid desaturases and elongase enzymes can help guide an intervention (Chisaguano et al, 2013). Chisaguano and colleagues in 2013 described the findings that children who have heterozygous or homozygous single polymorphisms for the FAD2 and ELOVL5 genes are at much higher risk of developing the inflammatory condition of atopic eczema. Upon fatty acid testing

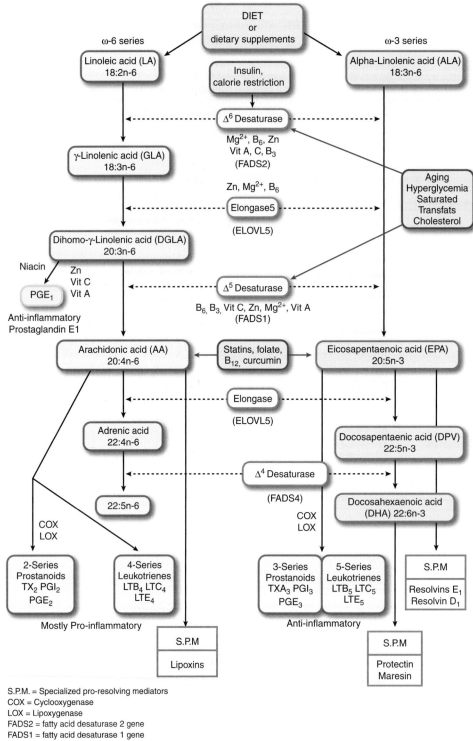

Fig. 7.3 Mechanisms of essential fatty acids and eicosanoid metabolites in modulating inflammation. Inflammatory biological responses are driven by a balance between feedback loops, much like a "toggle" switch, influenced by messages from hormones, lifestyle, and nutrient cofactors (see primary enzyme nutrient-cofactors listed in diagram). The eicosanoid biological cascade responses receive environmental messages from diet, lifestyle, infection, and trauma. From the essential fatty acids (LA, ALA), downstream metabolites are produced dependent on hormonal messages, genotype, and adequate nutrient cofactors of enzymatic conversion activity. Acute inflammatory triggers to initiate a healing response from infection or trauma are then resolved to homeostasis by specialized proresolving mediators (SPM) in healthy subjects. This complex dance of biochemical activity is handicapped by interfering conditions (see activity in RED) noted in the diagram above). Nutrition status from regular intake over the life span of essential fatty acids and nutrient dense whole foods build the foundation for healthy eicosanoid management of acute and prolonged inflammation.

these children were found to have lower omega-6 dihomo-γ-linolenic acid (DGLA) and arachidonic acid (AA) (Chisaguano et al, 2013). Clinical application of this information and thorough assessment of an individual's fatty acid status and dietary intake can be used when developing a nutrition plan to support adequate intake of essential fatty acids (see Figs. 7.3 and 7.4).

Nutrient insufficiencies and imbalances that accompany prolonged inflammation initially can go unrecognized. Along with possible insufficient dietary intake of nutrients, there can potentially be imbalances of the body nutrient reservoirs. Various stressors or genomic single nucleotide polymorphisms (SNPs) (see Chapter 6) can also cause increased nutrient requirements to meet metabolic needs, and those depleted nutrients become "conditionally essential" for an individual. Dr. Robert P. Heaney has provided a simplified conceptual diagram called the sigmoid curve to illustrate the concepts of dynamic varied nutrient needs of the physiologic "nutrient needs spectrum" (Fig. 7.5).

Nutriture is a term that refers to the state of nutrition. Skill in assessing the nutriture of body tissues requires knowledge about nutrient interactions with other molecular compounds (e.g., hormones, nutrients, reactive oxygen species [ROS]). Manipulating biologic function with nutrition must include consideration of the "rate limiting" restrictions on a biochemical system. Like a food recipe, if any ingredient is inadequate or missing, the final product is flawed.

Examples of some critical nutrient-partner balances are omega-6 and omega-3 fatty acids, vitamin D and vitamin A, magnesium and calcium, and folate, B_6, B_2, and B_{12}. In whole or unprocessed foods,

these nutrients naturally exist in balance, such as vitamin A and D in cod liver oil, in liver, and in eggs (see Box 7.1).

The nutrient partners most strongly associated with influencing prolonged inflammation are discussed below.

Omega-6 Linoleic Acid and Omega-3 Alpha-Linolenic Acid (Essential Fatty Acids)

Fish ingestion several times a week has been associated with reduced risk of chronic disease, especially cardiac disease. It is a characteristic of the Mediterranean Diet (Pallauf et al, 2013), the Asian Diet (Kruk, 2014), and the more recently studied Nordic or Viking Diet described in the Systems Biology in Controlled Dietary Interventions and Cohort Studies (SYSDIET) (Kolehmainen et al, 2015; Uusitupa et al, 2013). The human metabolism of oils in fish and their bioactive mediators provide important factors in inflammatory processes. The relationship of diet to inflammatory biochemistry supports a strong position for the nutritionist to develop individualized interventions to ensure adequate balance of the eicosanoid-producing foods that decrease inflammation.

Three main groups of prostaglandin metabolites are formed from the two initial essential fatty acids in the eicosanoid cascade (linoleic acid [LA] and alpha-linolenic acid [ALA]): prostaglandin 1 (PGE1) (omega 6 DGLA-derived antiinflammatory), prostaglandin 2 (PGE2) (omega 6-arachidonic-derived proinflammatory), and prostaglandin 3 (PGE3) (omega 3-derived antiinflammatory). These metabolites are precursors for a wide range of bioactive lipid mediators influencing

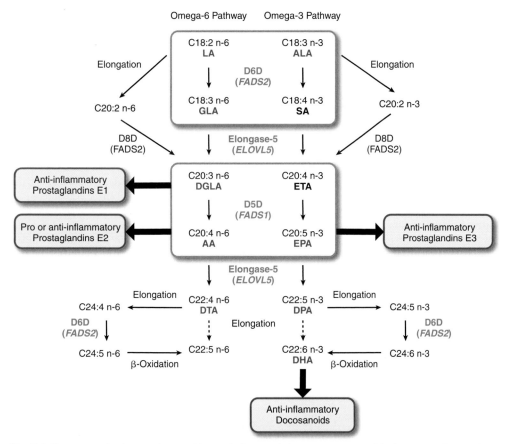

Fig. 7.4 Summary of primary eicosanoid metabolites and the genes responsible for conversion to downstream metabolites. Chisaguano M, Montes R, Pérez Berezo T, et al. Gene expression of desaturase (FADS1 and FADS2) and elongase (ELOVL5) enzymes in peripheral blood: association with polyunsaturated fatty acid levels and atopic eczema in 4-year-old children. *PloS One* 2013; 8, e78245.

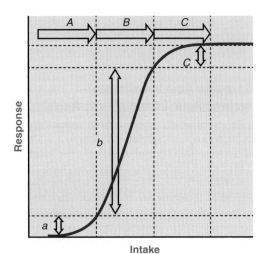

Typical sigmoid curve showing physiological response as a function of nutrient intake. Depicted are the expected responses from *equal* increments in intake, starting from a low basal intake, and moving to progressively higher starting levels. Intake increments A, B, and C produce responses, a, b, and c, respectively. Only intakes in the B region produce responses large enough adequately to test the hypothesis that the nutrient concerned elicits the response in question. (Copyright Robert P. Heaney, MD., 2010. All rights reserved. Used with permission.)

Fig. 7.5 Sigmoid Curve (Heaney, 2010) PERMISSION BY ROBERT HEANEY Heaney RP: The Nutrient Problem, *Nutr Rev* 70:165, 2012.

inflammation. The RDN can assess and then develop an individualized intervention to return the individual's metabolic balance in these three groups of metabolites of the eicosanoid series. The most accurate way to assess fatty acid status is to evaluate dietary fat intake (Table 7.5), absorptive capacity (bile adequacy, pancreatic function), and RBC fatty acids (Kelley et al, 2009). Collecting this nutrition data for an individual during assessment can reveal important underlying physiologic imbalances.

The balance between the two eicosanoid signaling molecule pathways (derived from the essential PUFAs, omega-3 ALA, and omega-6 LA or dietary intake), exerts inflammatory control in response to the metabolic environment (Gil et al, 2015; Patton, 2014; Zreik and Behrman, 2018). Prostaglandins contribute to the regulation of vascular tone, platelet function, and fertility (Ricciotti and FitzGerald, 2011; Stipanuk and Caudill, 2013; Kemiläinen et al, 2016). They also play key roles as inflammatory mediators and modulators of tumor biology and are major regulators of growth and transport in epithelial cells (Varga et al, 2014). The metabolism of these hormone-like molecules is modulated by dietary intake and are of primary importance to the RDN when considering the source of chronic inflammation. The hormone-like prostaglandins formed as downstream metabolites are the primary metabolic control for acute and chronic inflammation. The seminal observation that omega-3 EPA could modulate eicosanoid biosynthesis to suppress arachidonic acid biosynthesis, an omega-6 fatty acid, was first made in 1962 (Machlin) and 1963 (Mohrhauer and Holman) and initiated research on the use of fish and fish oil supplements to reduce inflammation by suppressing the proinflammatory arachidonic acid. Omega-3 DHA (C22) is an interesting molecule formed from the eicosanoid 20-carbon cascade with antiinflammatory effects (Shichiri et al, 2014; Kemiläinen et al, 2016). EPA and docosahexaenoic acid (DHA) are found in fish oil, as well as DHA being found in algae. DHA and EPA are biochemically reversible, meaning they can be

metabolized from one molecule to the other. DHA is a critical component of many body tissues such as the eye and brain, and it contributes to modulation of metabolic inflammation. EPA, DHA, and AA can produce the more newly recognized specialized proresolving mediators (SPMs), including resolvins, protectins, maresins, and lipoxins, that reduce inflammation during events like injury, infection, and antigen exposure. The body has redundant systems to provide essential molecules for metabolism.

The key eicosanoid metabolic intersections in the eicosanoid cascade are omega-6 GLA, DGLA, and AA promoting the antiinflammatory PGE1 and proinflammatory PGE2 series while coexisting with omega-3 EPA and DHA, promoting the antiinflammatory PGE3 series. As the knowledge of the functions of these eicosanoid metabolites has matured over the past 50 years, their synergistic relationships and the need to keep them in homeostatic balance is now appreciated (Das, 2011). The omega-6 and omega-3 eicosanoids share the same desaturase and elongase enzymes, so there is a competition between the two, where production of biologically active EPA and DHA is dependent on the availability of cofactor nutrients (Reed et al, 2014).

It is now known that fatty acid intake can influence and change physiologic responses to inflammation by modification of eicosanoid metabolism to favor synthesis of antiinflammatory prostaglandins and leukotrienes (produced by the oxidation of AA). Assessment of dietary fat intake and tissue status provides more targeted information that can help manage chronic inflammation (Arm et al, 2013; Dahlin and Weiss, 2016). As more randomized controlled trial (RCT) studies are available, it is hoped this will result in an improved model for the study of nutrient synergistic influences on metabolism. Wergeland and colleagues designed a multivariable study of a combination of fatty acid therapies that showed a suppression of inflammation in multiple sclerosis described as a "beneficial disease-modifying effect of increased intake of polyunsaturated fatty acids (PUFAs)" (Wergeland et al, 2012). Even as far back as 1993, Berth-Jones and Graham-Brown hypothesized that "since both ω6 and ω3 essential fatty acids may possess antiinflammatory properties, it is possible that giving both together will have a synergistic effect" (1993). There are a growing number of studies targeting key eicosanoid and downstream lipid mediators with the ability to modulate physiologic processes involving immunity, hormonal balance, inflammatory mediators, and cell membrane integrity including GLA (Horrobin et al, 2002), DGLA (Chisaguano et al, 2013), AA (Carlson et al, 2018; Amézaga et al, 2018), EPA, and DHA (Harris et al, 2017).

Metabolically, the five primary eicosanoids (GLA, DGLA, AA, EPA, DHA) collaborate and compete for shared enzymes in forming the prostaglandin groups: PGE1, PGE2, and PGE3 series (see Figs. 7.3 and 7.4). Each plays a critical role in the control of inflammatory conditions. Until the research interest in the 1990s of the dynamic influence omega-3 EPA has on elevated omega-6 AA, dietary intake of the essential fatty acids was the main determinant of the levels of these fatty acids in tissue composition.

However, as awareness of omega-3 and its function increased, a large portion of the U.S. population is now adding omega-3 fatty acids to their regular nutraceutical intake. In some individuals who take more than 500 mg EPA and/or DHA daily, this may cause AA and GLA biosynthesis to be suppressed with the potential to unbalance the levels of these two molecules (Horrobin et al, 2002). "Nutrient partners" require balance for optimum metabolic function. A nutrition assessment should consider the fatty acid supplements a client is taking and for how long, in addition to the amount in the diet to assess the potential for imbalance of eicosanoid and other lipid cellular components. If laboratory testing of fatty acid parameters is available, a quantitative evaluation of RBC or plasma fatty acids can be added to the nutritional assessment (Djoussé et al, 2012; Guo et al, 2010).

TABLE 7.5 Fat-Oil Dietary Intake Survey

Fats and Oils
Please indicate how many times PER WEEK you eat the following fats/oils.

OMEGA 9 (stabilizer)	__ Almond Oil	__ Olives / Olive Oil
Oleic Fatty Acid	__ Almonds	__ Cashews
~50% of daily fat calories	__ Almond butter	__ Sesame Seeds/Tahini
	__ Avocados	__ Hummus (tahini oil)
	__ Peanuts	__ Macadamia Nuts
	__ Peanut butter (natural/soft)	__ Pine Nuts
OMEGA 6 (controllers)	__ Eggs (whole), organic (AA)	__ Evening Primrose (GLA)
Essential Fatty Acid Family	__ Meats (commercial) (AA)	__ Black Currant Oil (GLA)
~30% of daily fat calories	__ Meats (grass-fed, org) (AA)	__ Borage Oil (GLA)
LA→GLA→DGLA→AA	__ Brazil nuts (raw)	__ Hemp Oil / seeds
	__ Pecan (raw)	__ Grapeseed Oil
	__ Hazelnuts/Filberts (raw)	__ Sunflower Seeds (raw)
	__ Seed oils (cold-press)	__ Pumpkin seeds (raw)
OMEGA (fluidity/communicators)	__ Fish Oil capsule: ↑DHA	__ Flax Oil (cold-press)
Essential Fatty Acid Family	__ Fish Oil capsule: ↑TEPA	__ UDO's DHA Oil
~10% of daily fat calories	__ Fish (salmon/fin-fish)	__ Algae
ALA→EPA→DHA	__ Fish (shellfish)	__ Greens Powder w/algae
	__ Flax seeds/meal	__ Chia seeds
BENEFICIAL SATURATED (structure)	__ Coconut Oil	__ Meats, grass-fed
Short-chain/Medium-chain Triglycerides	__ Butter, organic	__ Wild game
~10% of daily fat calories	__ Ghee (clarified butter)	__ Poultry, organic
	__ Dairy, raw & organic	__ Eggs, whole organic
DAMAGED FATS/OILS (promoting stress to cells & tissues)	__ Margarine	__ Doughnuts (fried)
	__ Reg. vegetable oils (corn, sunflower, canola)	__ Deep-fried foods
Should be <5% (try to avoid)	__ Mayonnaise (Commercial)	__ Chips fried in oil
Trans Fats	__ Hydrogenated Oil (as an ingredient)	__ Regular salad dressing
Acrylamides	__ "Imitation" cheeses	__ Peanut Butter (JIF, etc.)
Odd-Chain Fatty Acids	__ Tempura	__ Roasted nuts / seeds
VLCFA/damaged		__ Products with hydrogenated fats

©2004, Diana Noland MPH, RDN, CCN, IFMCP, LD

Prostaglandin 1 Series (PGE1): Antiinflammatory

PGE1 metabolites are part of the balancing act between prostaglandin groups to manage inflammation, with a primary antiinflammatory effect on the tissue microenvironment. PGE1 is particularly important for the effects of GLA and its conversion to DGLA in managing inflammation. GLA not only attenuates intracellular inflammation by converting to DGLA (Arm et al, 2013) but also reduces inflammation in the extracellular matrix as is present in diabetic nephropathy (Kim et al, 2012). Evidence suggests skin integrity involved with autoimmune and other inflammatory conditions has a "conditionally essential" (DiSilvestro et al, 2017) need for GLA (Chung et al, 2018; Andersson-Hall et al, 2018).

Another physiologic function of the fatty acids is that GLA, DGLA, EPA, and DHA, if kept in balance, can function as inhibitors of tumor cell proliferation and migration in in-vitro and in-vivo conditions (Rahman et al, 2013; Wang et al, 2012; Yao et al, 2014).

Prostaglandin 2 Series (PGE2): Proinflammatory When in Excess

PGE2's ability to increase tissue inflammation when in excess is part of the cause of inflammation with pain, swelling, fever, redness, and constriction of blood vessels that lead to loss of function. AA increases with acute injury to trigger inflammation and increased blood flow for tissue healing, but with the prolonged character of chronic disease, AA can get "stuck" in an elevated state and continue to damage tissue and encourage degeneration. Neoplastic disease can overproduce PGE2 in the tumor environment and has been found to simulate the growth and formation of a substantial number of carcinomas (Goodwin, 2010).

AA can become dangerously elevated, especially when dietary intake is deficient in omega-3 ALA, EPA, and DHA to act as an AA counterbalance. In the United States and most industrialized countries, some populations have high AA levels because of low intake of omega-3 oils and large intakes of highly processed PUFAs and trans fats.

The preponderance of information about AA is that it increases inflammation. It is important to acknowledge that AA in healthy humans can also help stabilize cell membranes and reduce inflammation. AA has essential functions in platelet aggregation and vasoconstriction, for example. Targeted nutrition therapy must have a goal of healthy homeostasis requiring monitoring to ensure omega-3 supplementation does not cause AA levels to fall too low (Khan, S et al, 2014).

Prostaglandin 3 Series (PGE3): Antiinflammatory

Another aspect of antiinflammatory action lies in the PGE3 prostaglandin group and their metabolites, leukotriene-5 series and others, which promote suppression of AA, GLA, and DGLA. They have been most studied in relation to cardiovascular pathologies such as vascular and coagulation health, but often the suppression of GLA goes unnoticed and unappreciated potentially suppressing production of the antiinflammatory PGE1 prostaglandins derived from DGLA.

Lipoxygenases (LOX)

Lipoxygenases (LOX) are AA downstream intermediates that produce inflammatory leukotrienes-4 (PGE2) or antiinflammatory leukotrienes-5 (PGE3). LOX-4 and LOX-5 molecules can modulate inflammation, mostly as mediators of cell signaling and as modifiers of cell membrane structures. Practical examples of structural changes are in red blood cell maturation, modification of lung barrier function to improve bronchial function in asthma conditions, and others. The LOX molecules also act as a substrate in the mobilization of fatty acids in membranes involving beta-oxidation metabolism of fatty acids. The LOX are expressed more intensely under physiologic stress (Allaj et al, 2013).

Cyclooxygenases (COX)

Another group of eicosanoid metabolites, the cyclooxygenase (COX) products, have an important role in reproduction and in the inflammatory response with inflammatory COX (PGE2) molecules and antiinflammatory COX (PGE1 and PGE3).

Specialized Proresolving Mediators (SPM)

More recent recognition of further downstream metabolites of a different class are called SPMs derived from both w3 and w6 PUFA. These SPM lipid molecules are capable of initiating a resolution phase of inflammation to return metabolism to tissue homeostasis. These SPMs are lipoxins, resolvins, protectins, and maresins (see Fig. 7.3). These mediators appear to explain some of the antiinflammatory effects of PGE1, PGE2, and PGE3 metabolites (Chiang and Serhan, 2017).

REDUCING INFLAMMATION IN THE BODY

Modern research of EFAs and their metabolites has been concerned mainly with the therapeutic impact on the inflammatory process. However, as with all systems in the body, there are opposing mediators in the body's regulation of these systems to achieve homeostasis or allostasis to promote survival. Among the primary mediators of inflammation are biogenic amines, such as histamine and serotonin, cytokines, prostaglandins, thromboxanes, and leukotrienes. The PGE1 and PGE3 antiinflammatory action opposes and balances the PGE2 inflammatory systems. Both are required for a healthy metabolism. For instance, derivatives of the omega-6 GLA and DGLA acids regulate the inflammatory process through their opposed activity and synergism with EPA, by directing formation at the crossroads to the antiinflammatory PGE1, or the inflammatory PGE2 molecules. In parallel metabolism, the derivatives of the omega-3 ALA, EPA, DHA, and others form the antiinflammatory PGE3 metabolites, while at the same time inhibiting the transformation of AA to leukotrienes and conversion of DGLA to the PGE1 molecules. This antiinflammatory action of the omega-3 eicosanoids is most researched because of their powerful suppression of AA associated with cardiovascular disease (Tousoulis et al, 2014).

It is important to understand the enzymes responsible for healthy metabolic conversions from the essential fatty acids, LA and ALA, and how to target them with foods and nutrients. These enzymes are illustrated on the eicosanoid cascade (see Fig. 7.3). The desaturase enzymes (delta-5 and delta-6) and the elongase enzymes are shared and are in competition between the omega-6 and omega-3 pathways.

Delta-6-desaturase transforms LA into GLA and ALA to EPA by adding additional double bonds. Of all the endogenous conversion steps in the eicosanoid cascade, the one driven by delta-6-desaturase is the least efficient. It is not biochemically equipped to handle the conversion of high dietary intake of LA found in the standard American diet (Kurotani et al, 2012). The delta-6-desaturase can also be less efficient in the presence of hyperinsulinemia which is associated with obesity and the metabolic syndrome (Simopoulos, 2017). In the competition for the enzyme between the omega-6 and omega-3 metabolites, a preference has been shown toward the omega-3s. However, these enzyme systems are affected by the adequacy of nutrient cofactors such as zinc, vitamin B_6, and magnesium and other physiologic and pathologic factors, such as hyperglycemia, that can lead to GLA deficiency.

The ratio of omega-6 to omega-3 fatty acids in the Western diet is between 10:1 and 21:1, whereas the diet of ancestral humans had a ratio of closer to 1:1; the ratio in the Western diet has been related to chronic disease (Simopoulos, 2016). Poor eicosanoid-related enzyme function is seen often in type 2 diabetes related to the hyperglycemia in the early stages of that disease (Forouhi et al, 2016). GLA supplementation has been shown to bypass the inefficient rate-limiting delta-6-desaturase system in the formation of LA to GLA and then to DGLA, and determines which pathway it will follow—either antiinflammatory PG1 or inflammatory AA-PG2 and their derivatives. EPA has been shown in the omega-3 pathway to bypass the delta-6-desaturase conversion of ALA to EPA (Innis, 2014; see Fig. 7.3). A balance of essential fatty acids is important to quell excessive prolonged inflammation.

A targeted approach using dietary, nutraceutical, and/or enteral and parenteral lipids directs PUFAs to shift the metabolism of eicosanoids toward homeostasis, thereby attributing potent antiinflammatory effects (Triana Junco et al, 2014; Waitzberg and Torrinhas, 2015; see Chapter 12). There are promising research data from Europe where olive oil–based intravenous lipids have been used for a decade, indicating that by using different intravenous appropriate fat sources, inflammation can be reduced.

Short-term and long-term inflammatory stimulation influence COX pathways in shifting them to the "less inflammatory" COX (PGE3 and thromboxane [TX]-3), and the resolvins derived from EPA and DHA polyunsaturated fatty acids (LC PUFAs) through COX-2 enzymatic epoxidation (5-lipoxygenase), thereby offering protection against inflammation (Khan, S et al, 2014; Uddin, 2011).

Dietary therapies to improve balance and promote adequate GLA to DGLA conversion that directs DGLA toward conversion to the PGE1 prostanoids include weight management, improving insulin sensitivity, and adequate nutrient stores of vitamin D, EFA, zinc, magnesium, B_6, and others, as well as increased intake of GLA-rich oils (evening primrose, black currant, borage). Nutraceuticals and food sources studied include GLA-rich plant oils from evening primrose, black currant, and borage (Pickens et al, 2015).

The nutritionist who is skilled in assessing an individual's fatty acid balance, by first performing a dietary intake survey (see Table 7.5), and more specifically by obtaining an RBC fatty acid analysis, can more accurately target interventions to see improved outcomes in managing inflammation. With the information from an RBC fatty acid test, one can calculate an Omega-3 Index, a prognostic indicator of eicosanoid and EFA balance especially related cardiovascular disease (Harris et al, 2012; von Schacky, 2014; Fig. 7.6).

These assessment parameters provide a roadmap that is able to guide individualized lipid interventions. With this information, the levels of lipids in the body can be manipulated toward a healthy composition, restoring a degree of optimum inflammation-immune

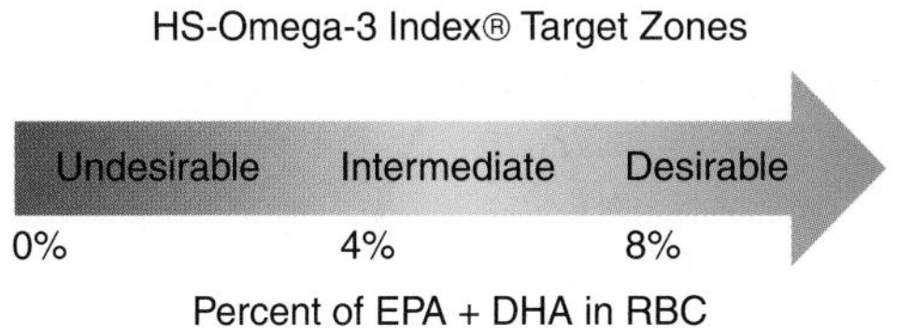

HS-Omega-3 Index® Target Zones

Fig. 7.6 HS-Omega-3 Index® Target Zones.

response in all systems of the body. Targeted nutrient therapy using food, dietary supplements, and functional foods can be mediators of these metabolic enzyme systems and help take advantage of the membrane and tissue malleability affected by dietary and lifestyle changes. These therapies usually require 2 to 12 months of nutrient therapy to achieve successful outcomes.

Cytochrome P450 Enzymes

Cytochrome P450 (CYP450) enzymes are essential for the production of cholesterol, steroids, prostacyclins, and thromboxane A_2. They are also involved in the first-pass hydroxylation of endogenous and exogenous toxic molecules in the biotransformation and transport of toxins for elimination via the feces and bile, urine, and sweat. If the enzyme function is suppressed by poor integrity of the enzyme structure, abnormal pH microenvironment, hepatic inflammation, altered availability of nutrient cofactors, or CYP450 genotypes, then there is a backup of toxins and an increase in an individual's toxic load. These CYP450 enzymes are expressed primarily in the liver, but they also occur in the small intestine, kidneys, lungs, and placenta.

More tools for assessment of all the systems of the body's metabolism are becoming available. Testing for the CYP450 SNP, for instance, allows recognition of a person's metabolic strengths and weaknesses that can influence nutritional interventions (see Chapter 6). Although the science is still evolving and being validated, nutrigenomic testing may be helpful for providers (including dietitians) to personalize food and nutrition recommendations.

Vitamin D

Vitamin D (cholecalciferol) actually functions as a prohormone with multiple roles, including hormone and immune modulation, antiinflammatory and antitumor effects, and apoptosis support (Pfotenhauer and Shubrook, 2017). This suggests that vitamin D is able to physiologically contribute to the regulation of all immune responses, by means of the vitamin D receptor (VDR) expressed in the nucleus of these cells. Epidemiologic, genetic, and basic studies indicate a potential role of vitamin D in the pathogenesis of certain systemic and organ-specific autoimmune diseases (Agmon-Levin et al, 2013).

Vitamin D is activated in the skin upon exposure to UV sunlight or artificial rays (therapeutically used in northern and southern extreme latitudes), as well as obtained by dietary sources (fatty fish, fish eggs or caviar, organ meats, egg yolk, and mushrooms; see Appendix 38). The past decade has spotlighted attention on an apparent global epidemic of low vitamin D status. Many chronic diseases are associated with increased prevalence of lowered vitamin D levels as vitamin D 25-OH vit D levels fall below 30 ng/mL (75 nmol/L) (see Chapter 5). Recommendations to test for 25-OH vit D and supplement vitamin D are common to increase blood levels to a goal of at least 30 ng/mL (75 nmol/L), but some recommend higher. Optimal serum levels of vitamin D have not been defined (see Chapter 5). An estimate is that for each additional 1000 IU/day of vitamin D intake, the serum 25(OH) vit D may increase by 4 to 5 ng/mL (10 to 20 nmol/L) (Stipanuk and Caudill, 2013).

Vitamin D exhibits antiinflammatory effects (Khan, M et al, 2014; Krishnan et al, 2012; Krishnan et al, 2013). Also, as a nutrient partner, vitamin A (retinol/retinyl palmitate) has a relationship with vitamin D in the sharing of the retinoid X receptor (RXR) with the VDR, establishing a synergistic effect between the two. In nature, vitamins A and D are always found together (e.g., liver, egg yolk; see Appendix 38). Because of the close proximity to this RXR nuclear receptor in all cells, there is a synergistic relationship. If one is too high or too low, it can affect the function of the other. For optimal health, it is important to have adequate intake of vitamin A and optimal vitamin D status (Schmutz et al, 2016).

Minerals

Magnesium

Magnesium is involved with more than 300 identified enzyme systems in metabolism and blood levels are inversely correlated with C-reactive protein blood values (Dibaba et al, 2015). NHANES data involving over 14,000 people between 1971 and 2006 revealed 60%-80% of the population had low serum levels (Zhang et al, 2018b). The potential beneficial effect of magnesium intake on chronic disease may be, at least in part, explained by its inhibition of inflammation (Dibaba et al, 2015).

The NHANES 1999 to 2000 study revealed that 60% of the U.S. population consumed inadequate dietary magnesium from low vegetable and whole grain intake. Low dietary magnesium intake has been related to several health outcomes, including those related to metabolic and inflammatory processes such as hypertension, metabolic syndrome (DiNicolantonio et al, 2017), type 2 diabetes (Hruby et al, 2017), cardiovascular diseases (Liu and Chacko, 2013; Stevanovic et al, 2011), osteoporosis, and some cancers (e.g., colon, breast) (Nielsen, 2010).

Magnesium requires the microenvironment of other essential nutrients, especially its nutrient-partners, calcium and zinc. Dietary intake of chlorophyll-rich vegetables, nuts, and seeds and whole grains provides adequate magnesium if digestion and absorption are functioning well (see Appendix 43). Recently López-Alarcón and colleagues, in their study linking low-grade inflammation with obesity in children, looked at several inflammation-related biomarkers and concluded that the most significant determinants of inflammation were a magnesium-deficient diet and central obesity (López-Alarcón et al, 2014).

Zinc

Zinc is a primary cofactor for more than 300 enzymes, many of which are involved in inflammatory processes. See Appendix 47 for food sources of zinc. Intracellular zinc is required for cell signaling within the intestinal tissue triggered by the inflammatory cytokine TNF-α (Ranaldi et al, 2013). Zinc deficiency leads to thymic atrophy and decreased function. The thymus gland is responsible for the production of T-lymphocytes, a critical part of immunity.

Zinc is the nutrient partner to copper, so when assessing zinc status, copper also should be considered. Gibson and colleagues (2008) have described loss of taste (especially in the elderly) with zinc deficiency, and this should be noted when taking a history from an individual. Because alkaline phosphatase (Alk Phos) is a zinc-dependent/zinc sensitive enzyme, a low measurement may suggest further investigation is needed for zinc deficiency. Serum zinc levels only provide information about frank zinc deficiency and are not reliable to assess for marginal status. Currently, assessing for dietary intake is the most efficient way to estimate zinc adequacy.

Methylation

Methylation is universal throughout metabolism, and methyl donors are primary promoters of healthy methylation. The B complex vitamins work synergistically and are critical to the methylation process. Folate, B_6, B_2, and B_{12} have been shown to be the most rate-limiting when insufficient. Although the results are preliminary, there may be metabolic advantages to supplementing with methylated forms of B vitamins. This is true, for example, with the methylation defect SNPs MTHFR 677C or MTHFR 1298C when the 5-MTHF form of folate rather than the synthetic folic acid is used (Bailey et al, 2010; Manshadi et al, 2014; Miller, 2010; Vollset, 2013) (see *Clinical Insight*: Synthetic and Bioactive B-Complex Vitamins).

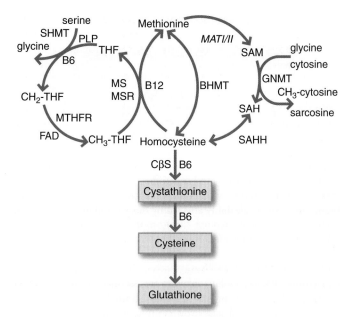

Fig. 7.7 Methylation Mechanism.

CLINICAL INSIGHT

Synthetic and Bioactive B-Complex Vitamins

B-Complex Vitamins	Synthetic Form/ Common Name	Bioactive Natural Form in Foods
B1	Thiamin mononitrate Thiamin hydrochloride	Thiamin (benfotiamine)
B2	Riboflavin	Riboflavin-5-phosphate
B3	Nicotinic acid Niacin (generic term)	Nicotinamide adenine dinucleotide (NAD) NAD phosphate (NADP) Niacinamide
B5	Pantothenic acid D-pantothenate Panthenol	Pantothenate
B6	Pyridoxine-HCl	Pyridoxine-5-phosphate (P5P)
B12	Cyanocobalamin	Methylcobalamin Hydroxycobalamin Adenosylcobalamin
B9	Folic Acid	Folinic Acid 5-Methyltetrahydrofolate 5-Formyltetrahydrofolate
B7	Biotin	Biotin (Biocytin)

To date, the methylation system most associated with inflammation of chronic disease is the methylation of DNA, which is especially sensitive. Chronic diseases related to methylation from epigenetic influences from the environment relate to potential development and promotion of cancer (Ehrlich, 2002), inflammatory bowel disease such as Crohn's disease (Karatzas et al, 2014), cognitive dysfunction, mood disorders (Hing et al, 2014), and cardiovascular disease (Delbridge et al, 2015).

The mechanisms supporting methylation have important implications in inflammation and immune response (Kominsky et al, 2010). These mechanisms rely on B vitamin cofactors and the role they play in homocysteine metabolism as well as the eicosanoid cascade which produces the inflammation reducing prostaglandins (Nazki et al, 2014). These methyl factors are involved in turning on gene expression associated with neurotransmitters, nitric oxide (NO), and methionine metabolism, which are precursors to antiinflammatory compounds that protect against oxidative stress.

The methylation genes are currently the most studied of the SNPs and able to provide data for clinical application. Most national laboratories provide testing for the genes MTHFR C667T, MTHFR 1298C, and COMT. Others are available at specialty labs (see Chapter 6 and Fig. 7.7).

Flavonoids and Antioxidant Nutrients

Flavonoids or bioflavonoids are phytonutrients associated with the varied colors found in fruits and vegetables. These phytonutrients provide antiinflammatory antioxidant functions beneficially messaging the immune system (Islam et al, 2016; Jeena et al, 2013). They provide protection against free radical and reactive oxygen species (ROS) activity that cause inflammation, and they modulate epigenetic effects by interacting with the fatty acid and prostaglandin status of a person.

When the antioxidant and flavonoid status is inadequate to protect cells and tissues, accelerated damage occurs, promoting degeneration, and depleting the health of the individual. The most studied flavonoid compound researched to date is curcumin, a component of the spice turmeric (Agrawal et al, 2015; Tuorkey, 2014). Another example is quercetin, a component of citrus pulp, apples, and onions, which is a yellow flavonoid with antiinflammatory action toward mast cells. Quercetin-rich foods are helpful in quelling allergic or sensitivity reactions (Kim et al, 2014; Lee et al, 2013). Both of these flavonoid compounds, as well as others, are also available in supplemental form for targeted nutritional therapy when indicated (Box 7.5).

Several antioxidant systems are involved in protection against these ROS—especially within the electron transport system in the mitochondria. Among the 80 or more known antioxidants, ascorbate (vitamin C) has been shown to react with other biologic antioxidants referred to as the "antioxidant network." Ascorbate acts as a central reducing agent regenerating other biologic antioxidants (Stipanuk and Caudill, 2013). Ascorbate interacts with the vitamin E complex to provide protection to water- and lipid-soluble surfaces in membranes.

BOX 7.5   Selected Flavonoid Antioxidants

Alpha Lipoic Acid	Glutathione
Astaxanthin	Lutein
Citrus Bioflavonoids	Lycopene
CoQ10	Quercetin
Curcumin	Resveratrol
Epigallocatechin 3 Gallate (EGCG)	Zeaxanthin

Other key members of the antioxidant network are glutathione, another water-soluble antioxidant that is synthesized in all cells and which supports the central role of ascorbate and vitamin E; lipoic acid with its water and lipid molecular components and sometimes considered the "universal antioxidant"; and coenzyme Q_{10} that functions in protecting lipid structures, especially in cardiac muscle and mitochondrial membranes. Antioxidants work synergistically to quell ROS activity. These nutrients are natural metabolites in healthy individuals and can be used as supplements for health-compromised individuals if indicated.

Gut Ecology and the Microbiome

The gastrointestinal tract has many functions in the health of an individual, and one of them is in immune integrity. This is because the largest immune organ is located within the gastrointestinal tract as gut-associated lymphoid tissue (GALT) and mucosa-associated lymphoid tissue (MALT), containing innate and acquired immune systems as well as about 3 pounds of symbiotic microbial organisms. The condition of the gut lymphoid tissue and the microbial ecology has a large influence on the body's inflammatory state (Lewis, 2014). The inverse relationship of gut barrier integrity and ecology with organ specific or systemic inflammation is well documented (Goldman and Schafer, 2012; Hold et al, 2014; Kinnebrew and Pamer, 2012; Pastorelli et al, 2013; Ruth and Field, 2013).

Medical nutrition therapy recommendations to support the microbial ecology include increasing intake of fermented foods and fiber, decreasing highly processed foods, and avoiding inflammatory antigens, especially those that affect the gastrointestinal tract (such as food allergens). Therapeutic use of functional foods (Abuajah, 2015), pre- and probiotics (Isolauri and Salminen, 2015), and fiber supplements can sometimes be used to restore optimum gut function and reduce inflammation (Luoto et al, 2013; see Chapters 25 and 27).

Lifestyle

Lifestyle factors such as poor sleep, physical inactivity, and smoking contribute to inflammation and chronic disease. Toxic environmental exposures, stress, social isolation and poor interpersonal relationships have also been identified as influencing factors (Tay et al, 2013; Umberson and Montez, 2010).

Sleep: Circadian Rhythm

The CDC targets sleep insufficiency as an important public health challenge with 50 to 70 million U.S. adults diagnosed with sleep disorders (CDC, 2018; CDC 2014a). Sleep quality and duration, "feeling refreshed" upon awaking, and having good energy throughout the day until bedtime are the signs of adequate sleep. Good-quality sleep helps reduce blood markers of inflammation including CRP-hs (Irwin et al, 2016). Common habits that disrupt sleep include watching TV or looking at computers and cell phones. Electronic devices produce penetrating light that reduces the body's production of melatonin (the natural sleep hormone responding to darkness). Sleep apnea, snoring, and for some, consumption of caffeinated food and drinks also contribute to poor sleep quality. The cumulative effects of poor sleep affect metabolic activities that may lead to weight gain, mood disorders, and feelings of stress (Heaney, 2012). Sleep problems can contribute to diseases such as hypertension, heart disease, depression, and diabetes.

Clinical Insight

The Role of the Vagus Nerve in Inflammation

The status of a person's vagus nerve is often not considered in assessing chronic inflammation. The vagus nerve the longest cranial nerve connecting the brain to the body, and regulating many systems, especially gastrointestinal function and inflammation. Poor vagal tone inhibits the ability to achieve parasympathetic function influencing optimum digestion (Yuen et al, 2017; Gerritsen et al, 2018). During a physical examination a simple screening for vagal tone is having a patient perform a gag reflex status by using a tongue depressor pushing down on the tongue starting at the tip and incrementally proceeding toward the back of the tongue till sensing a beginning gag response. The healthy vagal tone should produce a gag response within 1 to 2 cm of depressing the tip of the tongue. An important role of the vagal nerve is controlling the promotion of SPM and resolution of inflammation. This would be important if a patient history includes a vagotomy (Mirakaj et al, 2014). Lifestyle interventions can be recommended that have strong evidence to improving vagal tone and function, effecting control of inflammation (e.g., meditation, yoga, laughing, gargling) (Gerritsen et al, 2018; Loizzo, 2016).

Physical Activity

In the medical literature, physical activity is often associated with an improvement in inflammatory markers. Participants in the Multi Ethnic Study of Atherosclerosis (mean age 64) who exercised from a moderate to vigorous level had reduced blood levels of multiple inflammatory markers including IL-6, leptin, and resistin (an adipocyte specific hormone associated with insulin resistance). These results were found in all ethnicities and were not diminished by the presence of obesity or other cardiometabolic risk factors (Vella et al, 2016). Multiple studies have shown an inverse relationship between physical activity and inflammatory markers such as CRP-hs and TNF-α (Woods et al, 2012). In young sedentary adults, 12 weeks of aerobic training improved aerobic capacity but did not reduce inflammatory markers. In some cases, inflammatory markers were increased leading the authors to conclude that the antiinflammatory potential of physical activity may be population and situationally specific (Sloan et al, 2018). Although studies on the effect on inflammation are mixed, the overall health benefit of physical activity in most people cannot be disputed.

Stress of Life

Some health professionals and researchers have theorized that prolonged unresolved stress on the body is one of the primary promoters of early aging and chronic disease. The unresolved state of stress, whether emotional, physical, or perceived, or from infection or injury, triggers the immune system to respond with more inflammatory cytokines. The analogy used to describe unrelenting stress is getting ready for the "fight or flight" response, with nowhere to run. Under the influence of a short-term stressor, the body is able to clear the inflammatory and stress signals. That cannot happen with unrelenting chronic stress (Liu et al, 2017)

Toxin Load

Toxins are endogenous and exogenous xenobiotics, toxic substances within a biologic organism, that damage the metabolism.

In the modern world, since World War II, there have been 80,000 or more synthetic chemicals and many toxic metals released into the environment, increasing the exposure of plant and animal life to an unprecedented level (NRDC, 2019). Although many historical compounds such as smoking are toxic (Adams et al, 2015), many toxic compounds are "new-to-nature" molecules not before present in the environment (Aris and Leblanc, 2011; Bland, 2007). An example is trans fatty acids (Ganguly and Pierce, 2015).

The metabolisms of plants and animals usually have difficulty providing the systems to process and eliminate these toxins when incorporated into the organism. Industrial and food industry pressures have challenged attempts at governmental regulation of these toxic compounds. The result has been increasing tissue levels of some of these toxins when tissue testing is performed. Examples of these increased levels are shown in studies of newborn cord blood, which have found multiple environmental chemicals in a population of urban U.S. newborns (Morello-Frosch et al, 2016).

Another example is studies of toxic cadmium and lead metals in Korean populations residing near abandoned metal mines. A study of more than 5000 Koreans found notably higher toxic metal levels in those residing within a 2-km radius of the mines than in the general population in Korea and other countries (Park et al, 2014). Cadmium and lead are known carcinogens and are related to central nervous system (CNS) disturbances and cardiovascular and renal diseases with accompanying prolonged inflammation.

A study on hermetic (low-level) exposure to cadmium and arsenic related to clinical symptoms found that low dietary protein intake affected enzyme activity such that depressed biologic systems and long-term adaptations were inadequate (Dudka et al, 2014). Lack of dietary vegetable micronutrient and phytonutrient intake has repeatedly been shown to increase the inflammatory effects of toxins such as toxic metals, chemicals, and pesticides (Bakırcı et al, 2014, Jeena et al, 2013). Adequate intake of macro- and micronutrients may provide protection from toxin exposures such as from high intake of vegetables and adequate protein.

Assessment and Reducing Prolonged Inflammation in Chronic Diseases

The Patient's Story

Nutrition assessment includes gathering information about the whole person and begins by hearing the patient's story and forming the therapeutic relationship that is foundational for the most effective outcomes. It is a type of detective work partnering with the client to uncover root causes of underlying physiologic imbalances, including inflammation that frame the intervention.

The patient's story is a term inclusive of the whole of the patient's history and current state of health; it is a collection of all data that potentially can contribute to the individual's health. In the therapeutic encounter the data is collected from the personal interview, study of medical records, family history from multiple generations if possible, clinical observation, and current laboratory records. Most often a pattern suggesting metabolic genotypes can be recognized. Examples like cardiovascular, autoimmune, or neurologic events repeated in family members, especially at young ages or in multiple relatives, should prompt the nutritionist to investigate possible metabolic mechanisms and SNPs. Quantitative laboratory or clinical confirmation of an altered metabolism may be appropriate before planning an intervention.

Personal health history, from gestation through the present, can be obtained via creation of a timeline of major life events and health challenges. This can give insight into patterns that have contributed to a person's current state of health or disease. For example, infants not breastfed are found to have more difficulty in maintaining healthy gut microbiota, and increased incidence of allergies and asthma. These infants may benefit from probiotic supplementation (Prescott and Nowak-Wegrzyn, 2011).

Medical History and Data

Inflammation is a common denominator in nearly every chronic disease. Most evidence of this phenotype among humans, centers around various aspects of the metabolic syndrome described as presenting with a cluster of risk factors including insulin resistance (IR)/hyperinsulinemia, increased VAT (increased body fat percentage and waist circumference), elevated blood triglycerides (TG)/lowered high-density cholesterol (HDL-chol), hypertension, and raised fasting glucose (dysglycemia) (Watson, 2014). An additional biomarker is seen commonly as elevated CRP-hs blood values greater than 1.0. Increased understanding of dysregulation of glucose metabolism and its various causes helps define the complex condition of prolonged inflammation (Patel and Patel, 2015).

Biochemical markers also can be important factors in personalizing an individual's "total inflammatory load." Inflammatory markers such as sedimentation rate (blood) are significant in monitoring the progression of chronic inflammatory processes (see Chapter 5).

Predictive genomic testing has provided new tools for personalizing assessment of individual metabolism. The use of SNP testing is growing at a rapid pace. It is important to appreciate the SNP as a "predictive" value and not as a "diagnostic" tool. An example is the identification of an association between a vitamin D receptor SNP with breast cancer (VDR genes such as CDX2 and BGL) (Khan, M et al, 2014). The VDR gene may influence risks of some cancers and their prognosis. This encourages closer monitoring of vitamin D status in cancer patients (Huss et al, 2019).

Vitamin D is involved in enhancing the management of metabolic inflammation because of its "prohormone" and immune modulating effects. This comprehensive candidate-gene analysis demonstrates that the risk of multiple VDR polymorphisms results in lower VDR mRNA levels. Polymorphisms of the vitamin D receptor gene (VDR) have been shown to be associated with several complex diseases, including osteoporosis. This could affect the vitamin D signaling efficiency and may contribute to the increased fracture risk in some populations (Zhang et al, 2018a).

Gathering the patient's story and combining it with other data like anthropometrics, medical history, and the nutrition focused physical examination (see Appendix 11) allows a pattern to emerge of nutritional and metabolic priorities. This provides the clinician with important information to develop a nutrition intervention to promote optimal health and wellness.

Developmental Inflammatory-Related Conditions

Developmental inflammatory-related conditions bring a focus to the uterine environment, where there is recognition of the importance of preprogramming the fetus. Epigenetic messages to the fetus can impact long-term health and risk of disease. In the infant and toddler years, negative physical and psychosocial exposures, including violence, abuse, bullying and racism, can also influence health into adulthood. If the fetus and young child do not grow in a healthy environment, the inflammatory processes of chronic disease take root and will challenge the individual throughout their life (Claycomb et al, 2015; EFCNI, 2015; Lane, 2014; see Chapters 15 and 16).

SUMMARY

Chronic disease is an epidemic that is affected by diet and lifestyle, and chronic disease pathophysiology is the result of genetics and epigenetic influences. Sustained inflammation is the common denominator in most chronic disease. Nutrition and lifestyle are modulators of sustained inflammation (Box 7.6).

The nutritionist has an important role in the interdisciplinary management of chronic disease. Having the skills to recognize early signs and symptoms of inflammation enable the nutritionist to identify nutritional priorities and individual strategies to reduce inflammation and restore health and well-being.

Whole foods, "functional foods," targeted dietary supplements when indicated, and lifestyle changes can be foundational in achieving wellness. Dietitians with an understanding of the immune and inflammatory response and its relationship to chronic disease will have the capacity for more effective nutrition assessments and interventions.

BOX 7.6 Food, Nutraceuticals, and Lifestyle as Medicine to Manage Inflammation

Food
Whole Foods Diet
Mediterranean Diet
Med-Asian Diet
Nordic Diet
Fruits and vegetables
Beneficial fats
Pure water
Targeted nutrients
Low-antigen foods for the individual
Low toxin–containing foods
Foods and cookware toxin-free
   (aluminum, BPA, perfluorooctanoic
   acid [PFOA]-free)

Nutraceuticals
Quercetin
Rutin
Curcumin
Proteolytic enzymes
Enzyme therapy
Rx nutrition therapy
Guidance for dietary supplements

Lifestyle
Sleep
Physical activity
Beliefs
Community

USEFUL WEBSITES

American Academy of Sleep Medicine
Angiogenesis Foundation
Dietitians in Integrative and Functional Medicine
Inflammation Research Foundation
National Institutes of Health: Tox Town

REFERENCES

Abraham C, Medzhitov R: Interactions between the host innate immune system and microbes in inflammatory bowel disease, *Gastroenterology* 140:1729–1737, 2011.

Abuajah CI: Functional components and medicinal properties of food: a review, *J Food Sci Technol* 52:2522–2522, 2015.

Adams T, Wan E, Wei Y, et al: Secondhand smoking is associated with vascular inflammation, *Chest* 148(1):112–119, 2015.

Agmon-Levin N, Theodor E, Segal RM, et al: Vitamin D in systemic and organ-specific autoimmune diseases, *Clin Rev Allergy Immunol* 45:256–266, 2013.

Agrawal R, Sandhu SK, Sharma I, et al: Development and evaluation of curcumin-loaded elastic vesicles as an effective topical anti-inflammatory formulation, *AAPS PharmSciTech* 16:364–374, 2015.

Alagl AS, Bhat SG: Ascorbic acid: new role of an age-old micronutrient in the management of periodontal disease in older adults, *Geriatr Gerontol Int* 15:241–254, 2015.

Allaj V, Guo C, Nie D: Non-steroid anti-inflammatory drugs, prostaglandins, and cancer, *Cell Biosci* 3:8, 2013.

Allen BG, Bhatia SK, Anderson CM, et al: Ketogenic diets as an adjuvant cancer therapy: history and potential mechanism, *Redox Biol* 2:963–970, 2014.

Ames BN: Low micronutrient intake may accelerate the degenerative diseases of aging through allocation of scarce micronutrients by triage, *Proc Natl Acad Sci U S A* 103(47):17589–17594, 2006.

Ames BN: Prevention of mutation, cancer, and other age-associated diseases by optimizing micronutrient intake, *J Nucleic Acids* 2010:725071, 2010. doi:10.4061/2010/725071.

Ames BN: Prolonging healthy aging: longevity vitamins and proteins, *Proc Natl Acad Sci U S A* 115(43):10836–10844, 2018.

Amézaga J, Arranz S, Urruticoechea A, et al: Altered red blood cell membrane fatty acid profile in cancer patients, *Nutrients* 10(12):E1853, 2018.

Andersson-Hall U, Carlsson NG, Sandberg AS, et al: Circulating linoleic acid is associated with improved glucose tolerance in women after gestational diabetes, *Nutrients* 10(11):E1629, 2018.

Aris A, Leblanc S: Maternal and fetal exposure to pesticides associated to genetically modified foods in Eastern Townships of Quebec, Canada, *Reprod Toxicol* 31:528–533, 2011.

Arm JP, Boyce JA, Wang L, et al: Impact of botanical oils on polyunsaturated fatty acid metabolism and leukotriene generation in mild asthmatics, *Lipids Health Dis* 12:141, 2013.

Avitsur R, Levy S, Goren N, et al: Early adversity, immunity and infectious disease, *Stress* 18(3):289–296, 2015.

Baffy G, Loscalzo J: Complexity and network dynamics in physiological adaptation: an integrated view, *Physiol Behav* 131:49–56, 2014.

Bailey RL, Mills JL, Yetley EA, et al: Unmetabolized serum folic acid and its relation to folic acid intake from diet and supplements in a nationally representative sample of adults aged ≥60 y in the United States, *Am J Clin Nutr* 92:383–389, 2010.

Bakırcı GT, Yaman Acay DB, Bakırcı F, et al: Pesticide residues in fruits and vegetables from the Aegean region, Turkey, *Food Chem* 160:379–392, 2014.

Bauer UE, Briss PA, Goodman RA, et al: The Health of Americans 1 Prevention of chronic disease in the 21st century: elimination of the leading preventable causes of premature death and disability in the USA, *Lancet* 384:45–52, 2014.

Berth-Jones J, Graham-Brown RA: Placebo-controlled trial of essential fatty acid supplementation in atopic dermatitis, *Lancet* 341:1557–1560, 1993.

Biolo G, Di Girolamo FG, Breglia A, et al: Inverse relationship between "a body shape index" (ABSI) and fat-free mass in women and men: insights into mechanisms of sarcopenic obesity, *Clin Nutr* 34:323–327, 2015.

Birch AM, Katsouri L, Sastre M: Modulation of inflammation in transgenic models of Alzheimer's disease, *J Neuroinflammation* 11:25, 2014.

Bland J: The correct therapy for diagnosis: new-to-nature molecules vs natural, *Integr Med* 6:20–23, 2007.

Calçada D, Vianello D, Giampieri E, et al: The role of low-grade inflammation and metabolic flexibility in aging and nutritional modulation thereof: a systems biology approach, *Mech Ageing Dev* 136–137:138–147, 2014.

Carlson SE, Gajewski BJ, Alhayek S, et al: Dose–response relationship between docosahexaenoic acid (DHA) intake and lower rates of early preterm birth, low birth weight and very low birth weight, *Prostaglandins Leukot Essent Fatty Acids* 138:1–5, 2018.

Centers for Disease Control and Prevention: *Chronic disease prevention and health promotion*, 2018. Available at: http://www.cdc.gov/chronicdisease/about/index.htm. Accessed January 5, 2019.

Centers for Disease Control and Prevention: *Insufficient sleep is a public health epidemic*, 2014a. Available at: https://www.cdc.gov/sleep/index.html. Accessed January 30, 2019.

Centers for Disease Control and Prevention: *R2-p: research to practice at NIOSH*, 2018. Available at: http://www.cdc.gov/niosh/r2p/. Accessed January 31, 2019.

Cherry AD, Piantadosi CA: Regulation of mitochondrial biogenesis and its intersection with inflammatory responses, *Antioxid Redox Signal* 22(12):965–976, 2015.

Chiang N, Serhan CN: Structural elucidation and physiologic functions of specialized pro-resolving mediators and their receptors, *Mol Aspects Med* 58:114–129, 2017.

Chisaguano AM, Montes R, Pérez-Berezo T, et al: Gene expression of desaturase (FADS1 and FADS2) and elongase (ELOVL5) enzymes in peripheral blood: association with polyunsaturated fatty acid levels and atopic eczema in 4-year-old children, *PLoS One* 8:e78245, 2013.

Chung BY, Park SY, Jung MJ, et al: Effect of evening primrose oil on Korean patients with mild atopic dermatitis: a randomized, double-blinded, placebo-controlled clinical study, *Ann Dermatol* 30(4):409–416, 2018.

Claycomb KJ, Brissette CA, Ghribi O: Epigenetics of inflammation, maternal infection and nutrition, *J Nutr* 145(5):1109S–1115S, 2015.

Cokluk E, Sekeroglu MR, Aslan M, et al: Determining oxidant and antioxidant status in patients with genital warts, *Redox Rep* 20(5):210–214, 2015.

Dahlin A, Weiss ST: Genetic and epigenetic components of aspirin-exacerbated respiratory disease, *Immunol Allergy Clin North Am* 36(4):765–789, 2016.

Das UN: *Metabolic syndrome pathophysiology: the role of essential fatty acids*, 2010, Wiley-Blackwell.

Dai B, Zhang Y, Zhan Y, et al: A novel tissue model for angiogenesis: evaluation of inhibitors or promoters in tissue level, *Sci Rep* 4:3693, 2014. doi:10.1038/srep03693.

Das UN: *Molecular basis of health and disease*, Netherlands, 2011, Springer.

da Silva JR, Wiegert EVM, Oliveira L, et al: Different methods for diagnosis of sarcopenia and its association with nutritional status and survival in patients with advanced cancer in palliative care, *Nutrition* 60:48–52, 2019.

Delbridge LM, Mellor KM, Wold LE: Epigenetics and cardiovascular disease, *Life Sci* 129:1–2, 2015.

Dibaba DT, Xun P, He K: Dietary magnesium intake is inversely associated with serum C-reactive protein levels: meta-analysis and systematic review, *Eur J Clin Nutr* 69:409, 2015.

Dick DM, Agrawal A, Keller MC, et al: Candidate gene-environment interaction research: reflections and recommendations, *Perspect Psychol Sci* 10:37–59, 2015.

Di Gennaro A, Haeggström JZ: The leukotrienes: immune-modulating lipid mediators of disease, *Adv Immunol* 116:51–92, 2012.

DiNicolantonio JJ, O'Keefe JH, Wilson W: Subclinical magnesium deficiency: a principle driver of cardiovascular disease and a public health crisis, *Open Heart* 5:1–16, 2017.

DiSilvestro RA, Hart S, Marshall T, et al: Enhanced aerobic exercise performance in women by a combination of three mineral Chelates plus two conditionally essential nutrients, *J Int Soc Sports Nutr* 14:42, 2017.

Djoussé L, Matthan NR, Lichtenstein AH, et al: Red blood cell membrane concentration of cis-palmitoleic and cis-vaccenic acids and risk of coronary heart disease, *Am J Cardiol* 110:539–544, 2012.

Dudka I, Kossowska B, Senhadri H, et al: Metabonomic analysis of serum of workers occupationally exposed to arsenic, cadmium and lead for biomarker research: a preliminary study, *Environ Int* 68:71–81, 2014.

Ehrlich M: DNA methylation in cancer: too much, but also too little, *Oncogene* 21:5400–5413, 2002.

Elwood P, Galante J, Pickering J, et al: Healthy lifestyles reduce the incidence of chronic diseases and dementia: evidence from the caerphilly cohort study, *PLoS One* 8:e81877, 2013.

European Foundation for the Care of Newborn Infants: *Healthy pregnancy: fetal programming and chronic diseases in later life*, 2015. Available at: https://www.efcni.org/wp-content/uploads/2018/03/Factsheet_Healthy_pregnancy_Fetal_programming.pdf. Accessed January 30, 2019.

Fasano A: Leaky gut and autoimmune diseases, *Clin Rev Allergy Immunol* 42:71–78, 2012.

Feldman D, Pike JW, Adams J: *Vitamin D*, ed 3, San Diego, CA, 2011, Academic Press.

Fisher RE, Steele M, Karrow NA: Fetal programming of the neuroendocrine-immune system and metabolic disease, *J Pregnancy* 2012:792934, 2012.

Fleisch AF, Wright RO, Baccarelli AA: Environmental epigenetics: a role in endocrine disease, *J Mol Endocrinol* 49:R61–R67, 2012.

Forouhi NG, Imamura F, Sharp SJ, et al: Association of plasma phospholipid n-3 and n-6 polyunsaturated fatty acids with type 2 diabetes: the EPIC-InterAct Case-Cohort Study, *PLoS Med* 13(7):e1002094, 2016.

Franceschi C, Campisi J: Chronic inflammation (inflammaging) and its potential contribution to age-associated diseases, *J Gerontol A Biol Sci Med Sci* 69(Suppl 1):S4–S9, 2014.

Ganguly R, Pierce GN: The toxicity of dietary trans fats, *Food Chem Toxicol* 78:170–176, 2015.

Gerritsen RJS, Band GPH: Breath of life: the respiratory vagal stimulation model of contemplative activity, *Front Hum Neurosci* 12:397, 2018.

Gibson RS, Hess SY, Hotz C, et al: Indicators of zinc status at the population level: a review of the evidence, *Br J Nutr* 99(Suppl 3):S14–S23, 2008.

Gil Á, Martinez de Victoria E, Olza J: Indicators for the evaluation of diet quality, *Nutr Hosp* 31:128–144, 2015.

Goldman L, Schafer A: *Goldman's cecil medicine*, ed 24, Philadelphia, 2012, Elsevier.

Gonzalez S, Gonzalez-Rodriguez AP, Suarez-Alvarez B, et al: Conceptual aspects of self and non self discrimination, *Self Nonself* 2(1):19–25, 2011.

Gommerman JL, Rojas OL, Fritz JH: Re-thinking the functions of IgA(+) plasma cells, *Gut Microbes* 5:652–662, 2014.

Gonzalez MC, Isabel M, Correia TD, Heymsfield SB. A requiem for BMI in the clinical setting, *Curr Opin Clin Nutr Metab Care* 20(5):314–321, 2017.

Goodwin GM: *Prostaglandins: biochemistry, functions, types and roles (cell biology research progress)*, ed 1, 2010, Nova Science Publishers, Inc.

Gottlieb RA, Mentzer RM: Autophagy during cardiac stress: joys and frustrations of autophagy, *Annu Rev Physiol* 72:45–59, 2010.

Guo Z, Miura K, Turin TC, et al: Relationship of the polyunsaturated to saturated fatty acid ratio to cardiovascular risk factors and metabolic syndrome in Japanese: the INTERLIPID study, *J Atheroscler Thromb* 17:777–784, 2010.

Gurkar AU, Chu K, Raj L, et al: Identification of ROCK1 kinase as a critical regulator of Beclin1-mediated autophagy during metabolic stress, *Nat Commun* 4:2189, 2013.

Harris C, Buyken A, Koletzko S, et al: Dietary fatty acids and changes in blood lipids during adolescence: the role of substituting nutrient intakes, *Nutrients* 9(2):E127, 2017.

Harris WS, Pottala JV, Lacey SM, et al: Clinical correlates and heritability of erythrocyte eicosapentaenoic and docosahexaenoic acid content in the Framingham Heart Study, *Atherosclerosis* 225:425–431, 2012.

Heaney RP: The nutrient problem, *Nutr Rev* 70:165–169, 2012.

Hing B, Gardner C, Potash JB: Effects of negative stressors on DNA methylation in the brain: implications for mood and anxiety disorders, *Am J Med Genet B Neuropsychiatr Genet* 165B:541–554, 2014.

Hold GL, Smith M, Grange C, et al: Role of the gut microbiota in inflammatory bowel disease pathogenesis: what have we learnt in the past 10 years, *World J Gastroenterol* 20:1192–1210, 2014.

Horrobin DF, Jenkins K, Bennett CN, et al: Eicosapentaenoic acid and arachidonic acid: collaboration and not antagonism is the key to biological understanding, *Prostaglandins Leukot Essent Fatty Acids* 66(1):83–90, 2002.

Hruby A, Gausch-Ferré M, Bhupathiraju SN, et al: Magnesium intake, quality of carbohydrates, and risk of type 2 diabetes: results from three U.S. cohorts, *diabetes care* 40(12):1695–1702, 2017.

Hruby A, Hu FB: The epidemiology of obesity: a big picture, *Pharmacoeconomics* 33(7):673–689, 2015.

Hughes-Austin JM, Wassel CL, Jiménez J, et al: The relationship between adiposity associated inflammation and coronary artery and abdominal aortic calcium differs by strata of central adiposity: the Multi-Ethnic Study of Atherosclerosis (MESA), *Vasc Med* 19:264–271, 2014.

Huss L, Butt ST, Borgquist S, et al: Vitamin D receptor expression in invasive breast tumors and breast cancer survival, *Breast Cancer Res* 21(1):84, 2019. doi:10.1186/s13058-019-1169-1.

Innis SM: Omega-3 fatty acid biochemistry: perspectives from human nutrition, *Mil Med* 179(Suppl 11):S82–S87, 2014.

Irwin MR, Olmstead R, Carroll JE: Sleep disturbance, sleep duration, and inflammation: a systematic review and meta-analysis of cohort studies and experimental sleep deprivation, *Biol Psychiatry* 80(1):40–52, 2016.

Islam MA, Alam F, Solayman M, et al: Dietary phytochemicals: natural swords combating inflammation and oxidation-mediated degenerative diseases, *Oxid Med Cell Longev* 2016:5137431, 2016.

Isolauri E, Salminen S: The impact of early gut microbiota modulation on the risk of child disease: alert to accuracy in probiotic studies, *Benef Microbes* 6(2):167–171, 2015.

Japatti SR, Bhatsange A, Reddy M, et al: Scurvy-scorbutic siderosis of gingiva: a diagnostic challenge—a rare case report, *Dent Res J* (Isfahan) 10:394–400, 2013.

Jeena K, Liju VB, Kuttan R: Antioxidant, anti-inflammatory and antinociceptive activities of essential oil from ginger, *Indian J Physiol Pharmacol* 57:51–62, 2013.

Juby AG: A healthy body habitus is more than just a normal BMI: implications of sarcopenia and sarcopenic obesity, *Maturitas* 78:243–244, 2014.

Karabudak O, Ulusoy RE, Erikci AA, et al: Inflammation and hypercoagulable state in adult psoriatic men, *Acta Derm Venereol* 88:337–340, 2008.

Karatzas PS, Mantzaris GJ, Safioleas M, et al: DNA methylation profile of genes involved in inflammation and autoimmunity in inflammatory bowel disease, *Medicine (Baltimore)* 93:e309, 2014.

Kelley DS, Siegel D, Fedor DM, et al: DHA supplementation decreases serum C-reactive protein and other markers of inflammation in hypertriglyceridemic men, *J Nutr* 139:495–501, 2009.

Kemiläinen H, Adam M, Mäki-Jouppila J, et al: The hydroxysteroid (17β) dehydrogenase family gene HSD17B12 is involved in the prostaglandin synthesis pathway, the ovarian function, and regulation of fertility, *Endocrinology* 157(10):3719–3730, 2016.

Khan MI, Bielecka ZF, Najm MZ, et al: Vitamin D receptor gene polymorphisms in breast and renal cancer: current state and future approaches (review), *Int J Oncol* 44:349–363, 2014.

Khan SA, Ali A, Khan SA, et al: Unraveling the complex relationship triad between lipids, obesity, and inflammation, *Mediators Inflamm* 2014:502749, 2014a.

Kim B, Choi YE, Kim HS, et al: Eruca sativa and its flavonoid components, quercetin and isorhamnetin, improve skin barrier function by activation of peroxisome proliferator-activated receptor (PPAR)-α and suppression of inflammatory cytokines, *Phytother Res* 28:1359–1366, 2014.

Kim DH, Yoo TH, Lee SH, et al: Gamma linolenic acid exerts anti-inflammatory and anti-fibrotic effects in diabetic nephropathy, *Yonsei Med J* 53: 1165–1175, 2012.

Kinnebrew MA, Pamer EG: Innate immune signaling in defense against intestinal microbes, *Immunol Rev* 245:113–131, 2012.

Kolehmainen M, Ulven SM, Paananen J, et al: Healthy Nordic diet downregulates the expression of genes involved in inflammation in subcutaneous adipose tissue in individuals with features of the metabolic syndrome, *Am J Clin Nutr* 101:228–239, 2015.

Kominsky DJ, Campbell EL, Colgan SP: Metabolic shifts in immunity and inflammation, *J Immunol* 184:4062–4068, 2010.

Krishnan AV, Swami S, Feldman D: Equivalent anticancer activities of dietary vitamin D and calcitriol in an animal model of breast cancer: importance of mammary CYP27B1 for treatment and prevention, *J Steroid Biochem Mol Biol* 136:289–295, 2013.

Krishnan AV, Swami S, Feldman D: The potential therapeutic benefits of vitamin D in the treatment of estrogen receptor positive breast cancer, *Steroids* 77:1107–1112, 2012.

Kruk J: Lifestyle components and primary breast cancer prevention, *Asian Pac J Cancer Prev* 15:10543–10555, 2014.

Kurotani K, Sato M, Ejima Y, et al: High levels of stearic acid, palmitoleic acid, and dihomo-γ-linolenic acid and low levels of linoleic acid in serum cholesterol ester are associated with high insulin resistance, *Nutr Res* 32:669–675, 2012.

Lane RH: Fetal programming, epigenetics, and adult onset disease, *Clin Perinatol* 41(4):815–831, 2014.

Lee CC, Shen SR, Lai YJ, et al: Rutin and quercetin, bioactive compounds from tartary buckwheat, prevent liver inflammatory injury, *Food Funct* 4:794–802, 2013.

Lewis CA: *Enteroimmunology: a guide to the prevention and treatment of chronic inflammatory disease*, ed 3, Carrabelle, FL, 2014, Psy Press.

Liu S, Chacko S: Dietary Mg intake and biomarkers of inflammation and endothelial dysfunction. *Magnesium in human health and disease*, New York, 2013, Humana Press.

Liu YZ, Wang YX, Jiang CL: Inflammation: the common pathway of stress-related diseases, *Front Hum Neurosci* 11:316, 2017.

Loizzo JJ: The subtle body: an interoceptive map of central nervous system function and meditative mind–brain–body integration, *Ann N Y Acad Sci* 1373(1):78–95, 2016.

López-Alarcón M, Perichart-Perera O, Flores-Huerta S, et al: Excessive refined carbohydrates and scarce micronutrients intakes increase inflammatory mediators and insulin resistance in prepubertal and pubertal obese children independently of obesity, *Mediators Inflamm* 2014:849031, 2014.

Luevano-Contreras C, Gomez-Ojeda A, Macias-Cervantes MH, et al. Dietary advanced glycation end products and cardiometabolic risk, *Curr Diab Rep* 17:63, 2017.

Luoto R, Collado MC, Salminen S, et al: Reshaping the gut microbiota at an early age: functional impact on obesity risk, *Ann Nutr Metab* 63 (Suppl 2):17–26, 2013.

Machlin LJ: Effect of dietary linolenate on the proportion of linoleate and arachidonate in liver fat, *Nature* 194:868–869, 1962.

Maggio R, Viscomi C, Andreozzi P, et al: Normocaloric low cholesterol diet modulates Th17/Treg balance in patients with chronic hepatitis C virus infection, *PLoS One* 9(12):e112346, 2014.

Manshadi D, Ishiguro L, Sohn KJ, et al: Folic acid supplementation promotes mammary tumor progression in a rat model, *PLoS ONE* 9:e84635, 2014.

Mather KJ, Steinberg HO, Baron AD: Insulin resistance in the vasculature, *J Clin Invest* 123(3):1003–1004, 2013. doi:10.1172/JCI67166.

McCann JC, Ames BN: Adaptive dysfunction of selenoproteins from the perspective of the triage theory: why modest selenium deficiency may increase risk of diseases of aging, *FASEB J* 25:1793–1814, 2011.

Miller ER, Juraschek S, Pastor-Barriuso R, et al: Meta-analysis of folic acid supplementation trials on risk of cardiovascular disease and risk interaction with baseline homocysteine levels, *Am J Cardiol* 106:517–527, 2010.

Miller VJ, Villamena FA, Volek JS: Nutritional ketosis and mitohormesis: potential implications for mitochondrial function and human health, *J Nutr Metab* 2018:5157645, 2018. doi:10.1155/2018/5157645.

Mirakaj V, Dalli J, Granja T, et al: Vagus nerve controls resolution and pro-resolving mediators of inflammation, *J Exp Med* 211(6):1037–1048, 2014.

Mohrhauer H, Holman RT: The effect of dose level of essential fatty acids upon fatty acid composition of the rat liver, *J Lipid Res* 4:151–159, 1963.

Moloudizargari M, Asghari MH, Ghobadi E, et al: Autophagy, its mechanisms and regulation: implications in neurodegenerative diseases, *Ageing Res Rev* 40:64–74, 2017.

Morello-Frosch R, Cushing LJ, Jesdale BM, et al: Environmental chemicals in an urban population of pregnant women and their newborns from San Francisco, *Environ Sci Technol* 50(22):12464–12472, 2016.

Naghedi-Baghdar H, Nazari Sm, Taghipour A, et al: Effect of diet on blood viscosity in healthy humans: a systematic review, *Electron Physician* 10(3):6563–6570, 2018.

National Institutes of Health: *National human genome research institute*: skin microbiome, 2014. Available at: https://www.genome.gov/27559614/2014-news-feature-the-skin-microbiome-more-than-skin-deep/. Accessed January 30, 2019.

National Resources Defense Council: *Take out toxics*, 2019. Available at: http://www.nrdc.org/health/toxics.asp. Accessed January 30, 2019.

Nazki FH, Sameer AS, Ganaie BA: Folate: metabolism, genes, polymorphisms and the associated diseases, *Gene* 533:11–20, 2014.

Nielsen FH: Magnesium, inflammation, and obesity in chronic disease, *Nutr Rev* 68:333–340, 2010.

Noland D: DN 881 *Introduction to dietetics and integrative medicine*, Kansas City, MO, 2013, University of Kansas Medical Center.

Norman K, Matthews DE: Old tools, new insights' assessment of nutritional and metabolic status, *Curr Opin Clin Nutr Metab Care* 11(6):693–700, 2008.

Pallauf K, Giller K, Huebbe P, et al: Nutrition and healthy ageing: calorie restriction or polyphenol-rich "MediterrAsian" diet, *Oxid Med Cell Longev* 2013:707421, 2013.

Park DU, Kim DS, Yu SD, et al: Blood levels of cadmium and lead in residents near abandoned metal mine areas in Korea, *Environ Monit Assess* 186:5209–5220, 2014.

Pastorelli L, De Salvo C, Mercado JR, et al: Central role of the gut epithelial barrier in the pathogenesis of chronic intestinal inflammation: lessons learned from animal models and human genetics, *Front Immunol* 4:280, 2013.

Patel H, Patel VH: Inflammation and metabolic syndrome—an overview, *Curr Res Nutr Food Sci* 3(3):263–268 , 2015.

Pfotenhauer KM, Shubrook JH: Vitamin D deficiency, its role in health and disease and current supplement recommendations, *J Am Osteopath Assoc* 117:301–305, 2017.

Paul WE: Self/nonself—immune recognition and signaling: a new journal tackles a problem at the center of immunological science, *Self Nonself* 1: 2–3, 2010.

Pickens CA, Sordillo LM, Comstock SS, et al: Plasma phospholipids, non-esterified plasma polyunsaturated fatty acids and oxylipids are associated with BMI, *Prostaglandins Leukot Essent Fatty Acids* 95:31–40, 2015.

Prado CM, Siervo M, Mire E, et al: A population-based approach to define body-composition phenotypes, *Am J Clin Nutr* 99:1369–1377, 2014.

Prescott S, Nowak-Węgrzyn A: Strategies to prevent or reduce allergic disease, *Ann Nutr Metab* 59(Suppl 1):S28–S42, 2011.

Rahman MA, Rhim H: Therapeutic implication of autophagy in neurodegenerative diseases, *BMB Rep* 50(7):345–354, 2017.

Rahman MM, Veigas JM, Williams PJ, et al: DHA is a more potent inhibitor of breast cancer metastasis to bone and related osteolysis than EPA, *Breast Cancer Res Treat* 141:341–352, 2013.

Ranaldi G, Ferruzza S, Canali R, et al: Intracellular zinc is required for intestinal cell survival signals triggered by the inflammatory cytokine TNFα, *J Nutr Biochem* 24:967–976, 2013.

Reed S, Qin X, Ran-Ressler R, et al: Dietary zinc deficiency affects blood linoleic acid: dihomo-γ-linolenic acid (LA:DGLA) ratio; a sensitive physiological marker of zinc status in vivo (Gallus gallus), *Nutrients* 6:1164–1180, 2014.

Ricciotti E, FitzGerald GA: Prostaglandins and inflammation, *Arterioscler Thromb Vasc Biol* 31:986–1000, 2011.

Ruth MR, Field CJ: The immune modifying effects of amino acids on gut-associated lymphoid tissue, *J Anim Sci Biotechnol* 4:27, 2013.

Schmutz EA, Zimmermann MB, Rohrmann S: The inverse association between serum 25-hydroxyvitamin D and mortality may be modified by vitamin A status and use of vitamin A supplements, *Eur J Nutr* 55(1): 393–402, 2016.

Shichiri M, Adkins Y, Ishida N, et al: DHA concentration of red blood cells is inversely associated with markers of lipid peroxidation in men taking DHA supplement, *J Clin Biochem Nutr* 55:196–202, 2014.

Simopoulos AP: An increase in the Omega-6/ Omega-3 fatty acid ratio increases the risk for obesity, *Nutrients* 8(3):128, 2016.

Simopoulos AP, Di Nicolantonio JJ. Mediterranean Diet: W-6 and w-3 fatty acids and diabetes, *Am Jour Clin Nutr* 106(3):953–954, 2017

Sloan RP, Shapiro PA, McKinley PS, et al: Aerobic exercise training and inducible inflammation: results of a randomized controlled trial in healthy, young adults, *J Am Heart Assoc* 4(17):e010201, 2018.

Springstroh KA, Gal NJ, Ford AL, et al: Evaluation of handgrip strength and nutritional risk of congregate nutrition program participants in Florida, *J Nutr Gerontol Geriatr* 35(3):193–208, 2016.

Stevanovic S, Nikolic M, Stankovic A, et al: Dietary magnesium intake and coronary heart disease risk: a study from Serbia, *Med Glas* 8:203–208, 2011.

Stipanuk MH, Caudill MA, editors: *Biochemical, physiological, and molecular aspects of human nutrition,* ed 3, St Louis, MO, 2013, Elsevier.

Tay L, Tan K, Diener E, et al: Social relations, health behaviors, and health outcomes: a survey and synthesis, *Appl Psychol Health Well Being* 5:28–78, 2013.

Tousoulis D, Plastiras A, Siasos G, et al: Omega-3 PUFAs improved endothelial function and arterial stiffness with a parallel antiinflammatory effect in adults with metabolic syndrome, *Atherosclerosis* 232:10–16, 2014.

Trachana K, Bargaje R, Glusman G, et al: Taking systems medicine to heart, *Circ Res* 122(9):1276–1289, 2018.

Triana Junco M, García Vázquez N, Zozaya C, et al: An exclusively based parenteral fish-oil emulsion reverses cholestasis, *Nutr Hosp* 31:514–516, 2014.

Tsai CY, Tang CY, Tan TS, et al: Subgingival microbiota in individuals with severe chronic periodontitis, *J Microbiol Immunol Infect* 51(2):226–234, 2018.

Tuorkey MJ: Curcumin a potent cancer preventive agent: mechanisms of cancer cell killing, *Interv Med Appl Sci* 6:139–146, 2014.

Uddin M, Levy BD: Resolvins: natural agonists for resolution of pulmonary inflammation, *Prog Lipid Res* 50(1):75–88, 2011.

Umberson D, Montez JK: Social relationships and health: a flashpoint for health policy, *J Health Soc Behav* 51:S54–S66, 2010.

Underwood MA: Intestinal dysbiosis: novel mechanisms by which gut microbes trigger and prevent disease, *Prev Med* 65:133–137, 2014.

United Nations General Assembly: *Political declaration of the high-level meeting of the general assembly on the prevention and control of non-communicable diseases,* 2011. Available at: http://www.who.int/entity/nmh/events/un_ncd_summit2011/en/. Accessed January 31, 2019.

Uusitupa M, Hermansen K, Savolainen MJ, et al: Effects of an isocaloric healthy Nordic diet on insulin sensitivity, lipid profile and inflammation markers in metabolic syndrome—a randomized study (SYSDIET), *J Intern Med* 274:52–66, 2013.

Varga J, De Oliveira T, Greten FR: The architect who never sleeps: tumor-induced plasticity, *FEBS Lett* 588:2422–2427, 2014.

Vella CA, Allison MA, Cushman M, et al: Physical activity and adiposity-related inflammation: the MESA, *Med Sci Sports Exerc* 49(5):915–921, 2016.

Vescovo T, Refolo G, Romagnoli A, et al: Autophagy in HCV infection: keeping fat and inflammation at bay, *Biomed Res Int* 2014:265353, 2014.

Viladomiu M, Hontecillas R, Yuan L, et al: Nutritional protective mechanisms against gut inflammation, *J Nutr Biochem* 24:929–393, 2013.

Vollset SE, Clarke R, Lewington S, et al: Effects of folic acid supplementation on overall and site-specific cancer incidence during the randomised trials: meta-analyses of data on 50,000 individuals, *Lancet* 381:1029–1036, 2013.

von Schacky C: Omega-3 index and cardiovascular health, *Nutrients* 6:799–814, 2014.

Waitzberg DL, Torrinhas RS: The complexity of prescribing intravenous lipid emulsions, *World Rev Nutr Diet* 112:150–162, 2015.

Wallace KL, Zheng LB, Kanazawa Y, et al: Immunopathology of inflammatory bowel disease, *World J Gastroenterol* 20:6–21, 2014.

Wang X, Lin H, Gu Y: Multiple roles of dihomo-g-linolenic acid against proliferation diseases, *Lipids Health Dis* 11:25, 2012.

Waters DL, Baumgartner RN: Sarcopenia and obesity, *Clin Geriatr Med* 27(3):401–21, 2011.

Watson RR, editor: *Nutrition in the prevention and treatment of abdominal obesity,* Waltham, MA, 2014, Elsevier.

Wergeland S, Torkildsen Ø, Bø L, et al: Polyunsaturated fatty acids in multiple sclerosis therapy, *Acta Neurol Scand Suppl* 195:70–75, 2012.

Woods JA, Wilund KR, Martin SA, Kistler BM. Exercise, inflammation and aging, *Aging Dis* 3:130–140, 2012.

World Health Organization: *Cancer,* 2018. Available at: http://www.who.int/mediacentre/factsheets/fs297/en/. Accessed January 5, 2019.

Wu C, Li F, Niu G, et al: PET imaging of inflammation biomarkers, *Theranostics* 3:448–466, 2013.

Wu Y, Lach B, Provias JP, et al: Statin-associated autoimmune myopathies: a pathophysiologic spectrum, *Can J Neurol Sci* 41:638–647, 2014.

Wylie CM: The definition and measurement of health and disease, *Public Health Rep* 85:100–104, 1970.

Yao QH, Zhang XC, Fu T, et al: ω-3 polyunsaturated fatty acids inhibit the proliferation of the lung adenocarcinoma cell line A549 in vitro, *Mol Med Rep* 9:401–406, 2014.

Yuen AW, Sander JW: Can natural ways to stimulate the vagus nerve improve seizure control? *Epilepsy Behav* 67:105–110, 2017.

Zhang L, Yin X, Wang J, et al: Associations between VDR gene polymorphisms and osteoporosis risk and bone mineral density in postmenopausal women: a systematic review and meta-analysis, *Sci Rep* 8(1):981, 2018a.

Zhang X, Xia J, Del Gobo LC, et al: Serum magnesium and mortality in the general US population: results from the NHANES I epidemiologic follow-up study, *Circulation* 133:AP146, 2018b.

Zreik T, Behrman H: *Glob. libr. women's med. (ISSN: 1756-2228)* 2008; doi:10.3843/GLOWM.10313 *Under review—Update due 2018.* The Prostaglandins: Basic Chemistry and Action.

8

Behavioral-Environmental: The Individual in the Community

Judith L. Dodd, MS, RDN, LDN, FAND

KEY TERMS

biosecurity
bioterrorism
community needs assessment
Department of Homeland Security (DHS)
Federal Emergency Management Agency (FEMA)
food defense
food desert
Food Safety and Inspection Service (FSIS)
food security
foodborne illness
genetically modified organisms (GMOs)
Hazard Analysis Critical Control Points (HACCP)
Hunger-Free Kids Act

National Food and Nutrition Survey (NFNS)
National Health and Nutrition Examination Survey (NHANES)
National Nutrient Databank (NND)
National Nutrition Monitoring and Related Research (NNMRR) Act
nutrition policy
pandemic
policy development
primary prevention
public health assurance
risk assessment
risk management
secondary prevention

social determinants of health
Special Supplemental Nutrition Program for Women, Infants, and Children (WIC)
Supplemental Nutrition Assistance Program (SNAP; formerly the food stamp program)
Sustainable Development Goals (SDGs)
tertiary prevention
U.S. Department of Health and Human Services (USDHHS)
What We Eat in America

Community nutrition is a constantly evolving and growing area of practice with the broad focus of serving the general population across all cultures, genders, geographic locations, and socioeconomic conditions. Although this practice area encompasses the goals of public health, in the United States the current model has been shaped and expanded by prevention and wellness initiatives that evolved in the 1960s. Because the thrust of community nutrition is to be proactive and responsive to the needs of the community, current emphasis areas include access to a nutritionally adequate and safe food supply along with disaster and pandemic control, food and water safety, and controlling environmental risk factors related to obesity and other health risks. Food safety continues to be in the public health picture. Although traditional safety concerns continue to exist, potential safety issues such as genetic modification of the food supply is a new and growing concern and must be recognized as a part of community nutrition. In addition, the reliance on eating food away from home and previously processed foods adds to the risk for food borne illness.

Historically public health was defined as "the science and art of preventing disease, prolonging life, and promoting health and efficiency through organized community effort." The public health approach, also known as a population-based or epidemiologic approach, differs from the clinical or patient care model generally seen in hospitals and other clinical settings. In the public health model the client

is the community, a geopolitical entity. The focus of the traditional public health approach is primary prevention with health promotion, as opposed to secondary prevention with the goal of risk reduction, or tertiary prevention with rehabilitation efforts. Changes in the health care system, technology, and attitudes of the nutrition consumer have influenced the expanding responsibilities of community nutrition providers. Growing involvement in and access to technology, especially social media, has framed new opportunities and challenges in public health and community nutrition.

In 1988 the Institute of Medicine published a landmark report that promoted the concept that the scope of community nutrition is a work in progress. This report defined a mission and delineated roles and responsibilities that remain the basis for community nutrition practice. The scope of community-based nutrition encompasses efforts to prevent disease and promote positive health and nutritional status for individuals and groups in settings where they live and work. The focus is on well-being and quality of life. "Well-being" goes beyond the usual constraints of physical and mental health and includes other factors that affect the quality of life within the community. Today's terminology promotes "wellness," and like the definition for "well-being," this state goes beyond the absence of illness to a dynamic process. Community members need a safe environment and access to housing, safe and nourishing food, income, employment, and education. The mission of community nutrition is to promote standards and conditions in which all people can be healthy and can achieve a state of wellness.

Portions of this chapter were written by Cynthia Taft Bayerl and Lisa Mays.

SOCIAL DETERMINANTS OF HEALTH

The social determinants of health are the conditions in which people are born, grow, live, work, and age. These circumstances are shaped by the distribution of money, power, and other resources at global, national, and local levels. A summary report of conditions throughout the world, including the United States, by the World Health Organization (WHO) describes how stress, social exclusion, discrimination, working conditions, unemployment, lack of social support, addiction, quality of the food, and access to transportation affect opportunities in life and overall health (WHO, 2011). The report described how people with fewer economic resources suffer from more acute and chronic disease and ultimately have shorter lives than their wealthier counterparts. This disparity drew attention to the remarkable sensitivity of health to the social environment, including psychological and social influences, and how these factors affect physical health and longevity. The report proposed that public policy can shape a social environment, making it more conducive to better health for all. Although such action was described as a challenging task, WHO leadership noted that if policy makers and advocates focused on policy and action for health needs to address the social determinants of health, the stage could be set addressing the causes of ill health before they lead to problems. (WHO, 2011; Wilkinson and Marmot, 2011). In 2015 WHO affiliated countries adopted Sustainable Development Goals (SDGs) meant to provide specific targets to be achieved over 15 years. Since 2005 WHO has continued to publish world health statistics. In 2016 the focus of the series was on monitoring the progress of SDGs. The 2018 series provides information on 36 health-related indicators (WHO, *World Health Statistics 2018: Monitoring Health for the SDGs*, 2018).

Programming and services can be for any segment of the population. The program or service should reflect the diversity of the designated community, such as the politics, geography, culture, ethnicity, ages, genders, socioeconomic issues, and overall health status. Along with primary prevention, community nutrition provides links to programs and services with goals of disease risk reduction and rehabilitation.

In the traditional model, funding sources for public health efforts were monies allocated from official sources (government) at the local, state, or federal level. Currently nutrition programs and services are funded alone or from partnership between a broad range of sources, including public (government), private, and voluntary health sectors. As public source funding has declined, the need for private funding has become more crucial. The potential size and diversity of a designated "community" makes collaboration and partnerships critical, because a single agency may be unable to fund or deliver the full range of services. In addition, it is likely that the funding will be for services or product (in-kind) rather than cash. Creative funding and management skills are crucial for a community nutrition practitioner.

NUTRITION PRACTICE IN THE COMMUNITY

Nutrition professionals recognize that successful delivery of food and nutrition services involves actively engaging people in their own community. The pool of nutrition professionals delivering medical nutrition therapy (MNT) and nutrition education in community-based or public health settings continues to expand. Telemedicine has become a growth area both through private practice and organized health care. In addition, community outreach is evidenced by the presence of registered dietitian nutritionists (RDN), and other health professionals in for-profit or retail settings such as supermarkets, big-box stores, or pharmacies as well as in gyms and fitness-oriented clubs.

The objectives of *Healthy People 2020* offer a framework of measurable public health outcomes that can be used to assess the overall health of a community. Although the settings may vary, there are three core functions in community nutrition practice: (1) community needs assessment, (2) policy development, and (3) public health assurance. These areas are also the components of community nutrition practice, especially community needs assessment as it relates to nutrition. The findings of these needs assessments shape policy development and protect the nutritional health of the public.

Although there is shared responsibility for completion of the core functions of public health, official state health agencies have primary responsibility for this task. Under this model, state public health agencies, community organizations, and leaders have responsibility for assessing the capacity of their state to perform the essential functions and to attain or monitor the goals and objectives of *Healthy People 2020*. Along with monitoring and evaluation, work is continuing on what will be the 2030 edition of Healthy People. This, along with work on the Dietary Guidelines for 2025, provides an opportunity for local involvement as well as shaping the national initiatives.

A Framework for Public Health Action: Friedan's Pyramid

Local health agencies are charged with protecting the health of their population groups by ensuring that effective service delivery systems are in place. In 2010 Dr. Thomas Frieden, MD, at the Centers for Disease Control published an article that described a new way of thinking about community-based health services (Frieden, 2010). In his article "A Framework for Public Health Action: The Health Impact Pyramid," Frieden describes a five-tier pyramid derived from evidence-based research (Fig. 8.1). The Pyramid describes the potential impact of various types of public health interventions and provides a framework to improve health. Each layer describes the spheres that influence the involvement of the community in health services including nutrition. The foundation of this Pyramid (see Fig. 8.1) depicts the largest and broadest involvement of partners and communities, which Frieden describes as more powerful in influencing positive health outcome than the more traditional model of one-to-one intervention (depicted at the top of the figure).

Friedan's Pyramid illustrates, in ascending order, the interventions that could change the context to make an individual's default decisions healthy (Frieden, 2010). In addition, the Pyramid includes clinical interventions that require limited contact but confer long-term protection, ongoing direct clinical care, health education, and counseling. Friedan's point is that interventions focusing on lower levels of the Pyramid tend to be more effective because they reach broader segments of society and require less individual effort. Implementing interventions at each of the levels can achieve the maximum possible sustained public health.

Government's Role in Public Health

The federal government can support the development and dissemination of public health knowledge and provide funding. Box 8.1 provides a list of government agencies related to food and nutrition. Typical settings for community nutrition include public health agencies (state and local), including the Special Supplemental Nutrition Program for Women, Infants, and Children (WIC). WIC is a federal program that allocates funds to states and territories for specific foods, health care referrals, and nutrition education for low-income, nutritionally at-risk pregnant, breastfeeding, and non-breastfeeding postpartum women; infants; and children up to age 5 years. This program is a specific, nutrition-based food package that has evolved over the years to provide for the individual needs of the client and has adapted to changes in society and in health needs. Inclusion of fresh fruits and vegetables, foods that meet the needs of a diverse client base and food intolerances or allergies are examples of how this program is tailored and evolving.

Factors that Affect Health

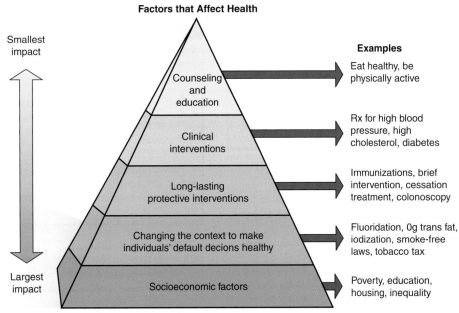

Fig. 8.1 The Health Impact Pyramid.

The expansion of community-based practice beyond the scope of traditional public health has opened new employment and outreach opportunities for nutrition professionals. Nutrition professionals often serve as consultants or may establish community-based practices. Nutrition services are often available in programs for senior adults, in community health centers, in early intervention programs, within health maintenance organizations, at food banks and shelters, in schools (including Head Start), and in physicians' offices or clinics through direct contact and telemedicine models.

Effective practice in the community requires a nutrition professional who understands the effect of economic, social, and political issues on health. Many community-based efforts are funded or guided by legislation resulting in regulations and policies. Community practice requires an understanding of the legislative process and an ability to translate policies into action. In addition, the community-based professional needs a working knowledge of funding sources and resources at the federal, state, regional, and local level in the official, nonprofit, and private sectors.

NEEDS ASSESSMENT FOR COMMUNITY-BASED NUTRITION SERVICES

Nutrition services should be organized to meet the needs of a "community." Once that community has been defined, a community needs assessment is developed to shape the planning, implementation, and evaluation of nutrition services. Evidence-based assessment tools are available to aid in this process. The Centers for Disease Control and Prevention's (CDC) *Community Guide* is a work-in-progress source of tools. This source provides information on various topics related to health risk factors, such as nutrition, obesity, physical activity, tobacco use, and diabetes. Information on policies, programs or services, funding, research, and education are included. Community needs are ever changing and this site provides an opportunity to be updated as new information is shared (CDC, 2018).

Box 8.2 lists other organizations and centers such as involved in healthcare policy. Resources are available to communities for use in health and nutrition policy (course of action adopted by government, community agency or business) that include technical assistance to support communities in the process of developing policies and conducting assessments. Such tools and assistance can result in meaningful strategies and programming.

Community Needs Assessment

A community needs assessment is a current snapshot of a defined community with a goal of identifying the health risks or areas of greatest concern to the community's well-being. To be effective, the needs assessment must be a dynamic document responsive to changes in the community. A plan is only as good as the research used to shape the decisions, so a mechanism for ongoing review and revision should be built into the planning.

A needs assessment is based on objective data, including demographic information and health statistics. Information should represent the community's diversity and be segmented by such factors as age, gender, socioeconomic status, disability, and ethnicity. Examples of information to be gathered include current morbidity and mortality statistics, number of low-birth-weight infants, deaths attributed to chronic diseases with a link to nutrition, and health-risk indicators such as incidence of smoking or obesity. *Healthy People 2020* outlines the leading health indicators that can be used to create target objectives. Ongoing evaluation of progress on these indicators builds on objectives and adds new direction. Subjective information such as input from community members, leaders, and health and nutrition professionals can be useful in supporting the objective data or in emphasizing questions or concerns. The process mirrors what the business world knows as market research.

Another step should be cataloging accessible community resources and services. As an example, consider how environmental, policy, and societal changes have contributed to the rapid rise in obesity over the past few decades. Resources to consider are affordable access to walkable neighborhoods, housing, recreation facilities, and health-promoting foods (CDC, 2014).

In nutrition planning the goal is to determine who and what resources are available to community members when they need food or nutrition-related products or services. For example, what services are available for MNT, nutrition and food education, home care, child care, or job or home-related skills training? Are there safe areas for exercise or recreation? Is there access to affordable transportation? Is there compliance with disability legislation? Are mechanisms in place for emergencies that may affect access to adequate and safe food and water?

At first glance some of the data gathered in this process may not appear to relate directly to nutrition, but an experienced community nutritionist or a community-based advisory group with public health professionals can help connect this information to nutrition- and diet-related issues. Often the nutritional problems identified in a review of nutrition indicators are associated with dietary inadequacies, excesses, or imbalances that can be triggers for disease risk (Box 8.3). Careful attention should be paid to the special needs of adults and children

with disabilities or other lifestyle-limiting conditions. Once evaluated, the information is used to propose needed services, including MNT as discussed in other chapters, as part of the strategy for improving the overall health of the community.

Sources for Assessment Information

Community practitioners must know how to locate relevant resources and evaluate the information for validity and reliability. Knowing the background and intent of any data source and identifying the limitations and the dates when the information was collected are critical points to consider when selecting and using such sources. Census information is a starting point for beginning a needs assessment. Morbidity and mortality and other health data collected by state and local public health agencies, the CDC, and the National Center for Health Statistics (NCHS) are useful. Federal agencies and their state program administration counterparts are data sources; these agencies include the **U.S. Department of Health and Human Services (USDHHS)**, U.S. Department of Agriculture (USDA), and the Administration on Aging. Local providers such as community hospitals and agencies, WIC, child care agencies, health centers, and universities with a public health or nutrition department are additional sources of information. Nonprofit organizations such as the March of Dimes, the American Heart Association (AHA), the American Diabetes Association, and the American Cancer Society (ACS) also maintain population statistics. Health insurers are a source for information related to health care consumers and geographic area. Food banks and related agencies may be able to provide insights into food access and security (see Box 8.3).

NATIONAL NUTRITION SURVEYS

Nutrition and health surveys at the federal and state level provide information on the dietary status of a population, the nutritional adequacy of the food supply, the economics of food consumption, and the effects of food assistance and regulatory programs (Box 8.4). Public guidelines for food selection usually are based on survey data. The data are also used in policy settings; program development; and funding at the national, state, and local levels. Until the late 1960s, the USDA was the primary source of food and nutrient consumption data. Although much of the data collection is still at the federal level, other agencies and states are now generating information that can build a comprehensive picture of the health and nutrition of the public.

National Health and Nutrition Examination Survey

The National Health and Nutrition Examination Survey (NHANES) provides a framework for describing the health status of the nation.

Sampling the noninstitutionalized population, the initial study began in the early 1960s, with subsequent studies on a periodic basis from 1971 to 1994. NHANES has been collected on a continuous basis since 1999. NHANES scientists and technicians travel the country in specialized buses equipped with mobile examination rooms. The process includes interviewing approximately 6000 individuals each year in their homes and following approximately 5000 individuals with a complete health examination. Since its inception, each successive NHANES has included changes or additions that make the survey more responsive as a measurement of the health status of the population. NHANES I to III included medical history, physical measurements, biochemical evaluation, physical signs and symptoms, and diet information using food frequency questionnaires and a 24-hour recall. Design changes added special population studies to increase information on underrepresented groups. NHANES III (1988 to 1994) included a large proportion of persons age 65 years and older. This information enhanced understanding of the growing and changing population of senior adults. Currently, reports are released in 2-year cycles. Sampling methodology is planned to oversample high-risk groups not previously covered adequately (low income, those older than the age of 60, African Americans, and Hispanic Americans). Information on NHANES including currently analyzed materials is cataloged at the CDC website.

Continuing Survey of Food Intake of Individuals: Diet and Health Knowledge Survey

The Continuing Survey of Food Intake of Individuals (CSFII) was a nationwide dietary survey instituted in 1985 by the USDA. In 1990 CSFII became part of the USDA National Nutrition Monitoring System. Information from previous surveys is available from the 1980s and 1990s. The Diet and Health Knowledge Survey (DHKS), a telephone follow-up to CFSII, began in 1989. The DHKS was designed as a personal interview questionnaire that allowed individual attitudes and knowledge about healthy eating to be linked with reported food choices and nutrient intakes. Early studies focused on dietary history and a 24-hour recall of dietary intake from adult men and women ages 19 to 50. The 1989 and 1994 surveys questioned men, women, and children of all ages and included a 24-hour recall (personal interview) and a 2-day food diary. Household data for these studies were determined by calculating the nutrient content of foods reported to be used in the home during the survey. These results were compared with nutrition recommendations for persons matching in age and gender. The information derived from the CSFII and DHKS is still useful for decision makers and researchers in monitoring the nutritional adequacy of American diets, measuring the effect of food fortification on nutrient intakes, tracking trends, and developing dietary guidance and related programs. In 2002 both surveys merged with NHANES to become the National Food and Nutrition Survey (NFNS), or What We Eat in America.

National Food and Nutrition Survey: What We Eat in America

The integrated survey What We Eat in America is collected as part of NHANES. Food-intake data are linked to health status from other NHANES components, allowing for exploration of relationships between dietary indicators and health status. The USDHHS is responsible for sample design and data, whereas the USDA is responsible for the survey's collection and maintenance of the dietary data. Data are released at 2-year intervals and are accessible from the NHANES website (USDA, Agricultural Research Service, 2014).

National Nutrition Monitoring and Related Research Act

In 1990 Congress passed Public Law 101-445, the National Nutrition Monitoring and Related Research (NNMRR) Act. The purpose of this law is to provide organization, consistency, and unification to the survey methods that monitor the food habits and nutrition of the U.S. population and to coordinate the efforts of the 22 federal agencies that implement or review nutrition services or surveys. Data obtained through NNMRR are used to direct research activities, develop programs and services, and make policy decisions regarding nutrition programs such as food labeling, food and nutrition assistance, food safety, and nutrition education. Reports of the various activities are issued approximately every 5 years and provide information on trends, knowledge, attitudes and behavior, food composition, and food supply determinants. They are available from the National Agricultural Library database.

National Nutrient Databank

The National Nutrient Databank (NND), maintained by the USDA, is the United States' primary resource of information from private industry, academic institutions, and government laboratories on the nutrient content of foods. Historically the information was published as the series *Agriculture Handbook 8*. Currently, the databases are available to the public on tapes and on the Internet. The bank, which is updated frequently, is computer based and is currently available online at the USDA website. This databank is a standard source of nutrient information for commercial references and data systems on ingredients, raw and cooked products. When using sources other than the USDA site, clinicians should check the sources and the dates of the updates for evidence that these sources are reliable and current.

The Centers for Disease Control and Prevention

The CDC is a component of the USDHHS. It monitors the nation's health, detects and investigates health problems, and conducts research to enhance prevention. The CDC is also a source of information on health for international travel. Housed at CDC is the NCHS, which is the lead agency for NHANES, morbidity and mortality, BMI, and other health-related measures. Public health threats also are monitored by CDC.

NATIONAL NUTRITION GUIDELINES AND GOALS

Policy development describes the process by which society makes decisions about problems, chooses goals, and prepares the means to reach them. Such policies may include health priorities and dietary guidance.

Early dietary guidance had a specific disease approach. The 1982 National Cancer Institute (NCI) landmark report, *Diet, Nutrition and Cancer*, evolved into *Dietary Guidelines for Cancer Prevention*. These were updated and broadened in 2004, combining recommendations on energy balance, nutrition, and physical activity. The ACS and the American Institute for Cancer Research (AICR) are excellent resources along with materials from the NCI. Another federal agency, the National Heart, Lung, and Blood Institute, provided three sets of landmark guidelines for identifying and treating lipid disorders between 1987 and 2010.

AHA guidelines continue to focus on reducing risks for hypertension and coronary artery disease (see Chapter 32). The guidelines now have a common focus on increasing the intake of fruits, vegetables, legumes, and nuts and recommend a Mediterranean diet pattern (see Appendix 24) or DASH plan (see Appendix 18).

Building on another consumer-friendly, single health guideline (5-a-Day for Better Health), the NCI, the National Institutes of Health (NIH), and the Produce for Better Health Foundation put a focus on fruits and vegetables in all forms (fresh, frozen, canned, dried). This guidance was built around the message that fruits and vegetables are naturally low in fat and good sources of fiber, several vitamins and minerals, and phytonutrients. In keeping with evidence-based messages, five to nine servings of fruits and vegetables a day are recommended to promote good health under the name of "Fruits and Veggies: More Matters" (Produce for Better Health Foundation, 2019). Understanding serving sizes that meets personal needs has become another key message. The *More Matters* banner continues as the branding for health guidelines and is an ongoing message for My Plate and the *Dietary Guidelines for Americans* (DGA) (U.S. Dietary Guidelines for Americans). In addition, this provides further support for incorporating a plant-based focus on health-supporting eating (Produce for Better Health Foundation, 2018).

The release of My Plate after the update on the DGA in 2010 made this a source of a strong and ongoing public health message with materials focusing across the life cycle, professional and consumer updates, and a robust social media presence (see Chapter 10).

Dietary Guidelines for Americans

Senator George McGovern and the Senate Select Committee on Nutrition and Human Needs presented the first *Dietary Goals* for the United States in 1977. In 1980 the goals were modified and issued jointly by the USDHHS and the USDA as the *Dietary Guidelines for Americans* (DGA). The original guidelines were a response to an increasing national concern for the rise in overweight, obesity, and chronic diseases such as diabetes, coronary artery disease, hypertension, and certain cancers. The approach continues to be one of health promotion and disease prevention, with special attention paid to specific and often underserved population groups (see Chapter 10).

The release of the DGA led the way for a synchronized message to the community. The common theme has been a focus on a diet lower in sodium and saturated fat, with emphasis on foods that are sources of fiber, complex carbohydrates, and lean or plant-based proteins. The message is based on food choices for optimal health using appropriate portion sizes and calorie choices related to a person's physiologic needs. Exercise, activity, and food safety guidance are standard parts of this dietary guidance. The current DGA are evidence based. The expert committee report provides scientific documentation that is used widely in health practice. The ongoing work for the next edition is continuing to support the need for evidence-based advice by validated experts. The DGA have become a central theme in community nutrition assessment, program planning, and evaluation; they are incorporated into programs such as the School Meals program and Congregate Meals for seniors. Updated every 5 years, the 2010–2015 revision, released in 2015, is currently undergoing discussions to formulate the next steps. Included are webinars and online meetings open to both professionals and the public to solicit input.

The 2010 DGA created the path for our current food guide, My Plate, and set the stage for programs such as More Matters to evolve. The 2015–2020 DGA are setting the stage for what will be released in 2020. Guidelines are continuing to move toward an emphasis on plant-based choices with a focus on inclusion of omega-3 and monounsaturated fats and on reducing added sugars and sodium (Dietary Guidelines 2015–2020). Since discussions are open to the public, nutrition professionals should monitor and provide input to the shaping of these guidelines. To access the portal for input contact the U.S. Dietary Guidelines website.

Food Guides

In 1916 the USDA initiated the idea of food grouping in the pamphlet *Food for Young Children*. Food grouping systems have changed in shape (wheels, boxes, pyramids, and plates) and numbers of groupings (four, five, and seven groups), but the intent remains consistent: to present an easy guide for healthful eating. In 2005 an Internet-based tool called *MyPyramid.gov: Steps to a Healthier You* was released. In 2011 MyPyramid.gov was replaced with My Plate (chooseMyPlate.gov.) along with a version for children called *chooseMyPlate.gov/kids*. These food guidance systems focus on health promotion and disease prevention and are updated whenever DGA guidance changes. This program has become a leading public education resource. Resources available include downloadable tip sheets and a variety or resources for both the public and the educator.

Healthy People and the Surgeon General's Report on Nutrition and Health

The 1979 report of the Surgeon General, *Promoting Health/Preventing Disease: Objectives for the Nation*, outlined the prevention agenda for the nation with a series of health objectives to be accomplished by 1990. In 1988 *The Surgeon General's Report on Nutrition and Health* further stimulated health promotion and disease prevention by highlighting information on dietary practices and health status. Along with specific health recommendations, documentation of the scientific basis was provided. Because the focus included implications for the individual as well as for future public health policy decisions, this report remains a useful reference and tool. *Healthy People 2000: National Health Promotion and Disease Prevention Objectives* and *Healthy People 2010* were the next generations of these landmark public health efforts. Both reports outlined the progress made on previous objectives and set new objectives for the next decade.

During the evaluation phase for setting the 2010 objectives, it was determined that the United States made progress in reducing the number of deaths from cardiovascular disease, stroke, and certain cancers. Dietary evaluation indicated a slight decrease in total dietary fat intake. However, during the previous decade there has been an increase in the number of persons who are overweight or obese, a risk factor for cardiovascular disease, stroke, and other leading chronic diseases and causes of death.

Objectives for *Healthy People 2020* have specific goals that address nutrition and weight, heart disease and stroke, diabetes, oral health, cancer, and health for seniors. These goals are important for consumers and health care providers. The website for *Healthy People 2020* offers an opportunity to monitor the progress on past objectives as well as on the shaping of future health initiatives.

National School Lunch Program and School Breakfast Program

The National School Lunch Program (NSLP) and School Breakfast Program (SBP) are federal assistance programs that provide free or reduced-cost meals for low-income students in public schools and in nonprofit private residential institutions. These are administered at a state level through the education agencies that generally employ RDNs and registered dietetic technicians. In 1998 the program was expanded to include after-school snacks in schools with after-hours care. This program, along with backpack or weekend and summer programs, has continued to be expanded. Local community groups are often involved in expanding the reach to underserved populations.

Currently the guidelines for calories, percent of calories from fat, percent of saturated fat, and the amount of protein and key vitamins and minerals must meet the DGA, but there is ongoing evaluation and interpretation to stay in line with population needs. Efforts have been made to meet My Plate guidelines for whole grains, more fruits and vegetables, and skim or 1% milk. In addition, the issues of education of recipients to accept these foods and use of local foods and community gardens are evolving processes that are happening in communities.

A requirement for wellness policies in schools that participate in the NSLP and SBP is in place (USDA, Local School Wellness). The *School Nutrition Dietary Assessment Study IV*, a nationally representative study fielded during school year 2009–2010 to evaluate nutritional quality of children's diets, identified that most schools offered and served NSLP lunches and SBP met the School Meal Initiative (SMI) and DGA minimum levels of target nutrients. Progress was made on meeting the SMI standard for reducing fat. However, few schools offered or served meals that met all the SMI standards. Efforts continue on increasing whole grains, fresh fruits, and a greater variety of vegetables as well as reducing the level of fat and added sugars.

On December 14, 2010, the Hunger-Free Kids Act was signed into law. It expanded the after-school meal program, created a process for a universal meal program that allows schools with a high percentage of low-income children to receive meals at no charge, allowed states to increase WIC coverage from 6 months to 1 year, mandated WIC use electronic benefits by 2020, and improved the nutritional quality of foods served in school-based and preschool settings by developing new nutrition standards.

The Recommended Dietary Allowances and Dietary Reference Intakes

The recommended dietary allowances (RDAs) were developed in 1943 by the Food and Nutrition Board of the National Research Council of the National Academy of Sciences. The first tables were developed at a time when the U.S. population was recovering from a major economic depression and World War II; nutrient deficiencies were a concern. The intent was to develop intake guidelines that would promote optimal health and lower the risk of nutrient deficiencies. As the food supply and the nutrition needs of the population changed, the intent of the RDAs was adapted to prevention of nutrition-related disease. Until 1989 the RDAs were revised approximately every 10 years.

The RDAs always have reflected gender, age, and life-phase differences: there have been additions of nutrients and revisions of the age groups. However, recent revisions are a major departure from the single list some professionals still view as the RDAs. Beginning in 1998 an umbrella of nutrient guidelines known as the dietary reference intakes *(DRIs)* was introduced. Included in the DRIs are RDAs, as well as new designations including guidance on safe upper limits (ULs) of certain nutrients. As a group the DRIs are evaluated and revised at intervals, making these tools reflective of current research and population base needs (see Chapter 10).

FOOD ASSISTANCE AND NUTRITION PROGRAMS

Public health assurance addresses the implementation of legislative mandates, maintenance of statutory responsibilities, support of crucial services, regulation of services and products provided in the public and private sector, and maintenance of accountability. This includes providing for food security, which translates into having access to an adequate amount of healthful and safe foods.

Food security, or access by individuals to a readily available supply of nutritionally adequate and safe foods programs, is an ongoing challenge. The Supplemental Nutrition Assistance Program (SNAP), formerly known as food stamps, along with food banks and pantries, home-delivered meals, child nutrition programs, supermarkets, and other food sources have been highlighted to focus on the issues of quality, access, and use. For example, research on neighborhood food access indicates that low availability of health-promoting food in area stores is associated with low-quality diets of area residents (Rose et al, 2010). See Table 8.1 for a list of food and nutrition assistance programs. *Clinical Insight:* The History of the Supplemental Nutrition Assistance Program (SNAP) provides additional information on this program.

There is an ongoing movement to encourage goals emphasized in My Plate, to add more vegetables and fruits, to increase minimally processed foods, and to increase education for SNAP recipients as well as other food and nutrition assistance programs. The presence of food deserts is a concept that has become a focus of research and community planning. Food deserts are described as neighborhoods and rural areas with limited access to fresh, healthy, affordable food. This is a definition that continues to be disputed and updated (USDA Food Dessert Locator). USDA has described it as a neighborhood where the nearest supermarket or grocery store is 1 to 3 miles away for urban residents and 10 miles for rural settings. One of the complicating factors of a description is that convenience stores, gas stations, all-purpose shopping areas and pharmacies, as well as home delivery sites, have included food in their offerings. What is real is the potential for food insecurity and for selections of health-promoting foods to be limited. The Economic Research Service (ERS) of the USDA estimated that in 2016, 12.3% of U.S. households (about 15.6 million households reaching over 41 million people) experienced food insecurity at some time during the year. Food insecurity is when lack of resources limits access to adequate food for all household members. SNAP, WIC, School Meals, Senior Meals were the resource for about 59% food-insecure households in 2016 (Oliveira, 2018). It is critical for the community-based RDN to have accurate and up-to-date knowledge on the specific community they serve.

FOODBORNE ILLNESS

The CDC has estimated that each year at least one in six Americans (or 48 million people) get sick, 128,000 are hospitalized, and 3000 die of foodborne diseases (Table 8.2). The majority of foodborne illness outbreaks reported to the CDC result from bacteria, followed by viral outbreaks, chemical causes, and parasitic causes. Segments of the population are particularly susceptible to foodborne illnesses; vulnerable individuals such as pregnant women and the elderly are more likely to become ill and experience complications. Availability of safe food access, storage, and preparation skills vary in populations and may not be predictable by national or even local guidance.

The 2000 edition of the DGA was the first to include food safety, important for linking the safety of the food and water supply with health promotion and disease prevention. This acknowledges the potential for foodborne illness to cause acute illness and long-term chronic complications. Since 2000 all revisions of the DGA have made food safety a priority. Persons at increased risk for foodborne illnesses include young children; pregnant women; older adults; persons who are immunocompromised because of human immunodeficiency virus or acquired immunodeficiency syndrome, steroid use, chemotherapy, diabetes mellitus, or cancer; alcoholics; persons with liver disease, decreased stomach acidity, autoimmune disorders, or malnutrition; persons who take antibiotics; and persons living in institutionalized settings. The latter includes those living in group home care settings. Costs associated with foodborne illness include those related to investigation of foodborne outbreaks and treatment of victims, employer costs related to lost productivity, and food industry losses related to lower sales and lower stock prices. Table 8.2 describes common foodborne illnesses and their signs and symptoms, timing of onset, duration, causes, and prevention.

All food groups have ingredients associated with food safety concerns. There are concerns about microbial contamination of fruits and vegetables, especially those imported from other countries. An increased incidence of foodborne illness occurs with new methods of food production or distribution and with increased reliance on commercial food sources (AND, 2014). Improperly cooked meats can harbor organisms that trigger a foodborne illness. Even properly cooked meats have the potential to cause foodborne illness if the food handler allows raw meat juices to contaminate other foods during preparation. Sources of a foodborne illness outbreak vary, depending on such factors as the type of organism involved, the point of contamination, and the duration and temperature of food during holding.

Text continued on page 139

TABLE 8.1   U.S. Food Assistance and Nutrition Programs

Program Name	Goal/Purpose	Services Provided	Target Audience	Eligibility	Funding	Level of Prevention*
After-School Snack Program	Provides reimbursement for snacks served to students after school	Provides cash reimbursement to schools for snacks served to students after the school day. Snacks must contain two of four components: fluid milk, meat/meat alternate, vegetable or fruit or full-strength juice, whole-grain or enriched bread.	Children younger than 18 whose school sponsor a structured, supervised after-school enrichment program and provide lunch through the NSLP	School programs located within the boundaries of eligible low-income areas may be reimbursed for snacks served at no charge to students.	USDA	Primary, secondary
Child and Adult Care Food Program	Provides nutritious meals and snacks to infants, young children, and adults receiving day care services, as well as infants and children living in emergency shelters	Provides commodities or cash to help centers serve nutritious meals that meet federal guidelines	Infants, children, and adults receiving day care at childcare centers, family day care homes, and homeless shelters		USDA FNS	Primary, secondary
Commodity Supplemental Food Program	Provides no-cost monthly supplemental food packages composed of commodity foods to populations perceived to be at nutritional risk	Provides food packages; nutrition education services are available often through extension service programs; program referrals provided	Generally children ages 5-6, postpartum non-breastfeeding mothers from 6-12 months' postpartum, seniors	Between 130% and 185% of the poverty guideline	USDA FNS	Primary, secondary
Disaster Feeding Program	Makes commodities available for distribution to disaster relief agencies	Commodities are provided to disaster victims through congregate dining settings and direct distribution to households.	Those experiencing a natural disaster	Those experiencing a natural disaster	USDA FNS	Primary
TEFAP	Commodities are made available to local emergency food providers for preparing meals for the needy or for distribution of food packages.	Surplus commodity foods are provided for distribution.	Low-income households	Low-income households at 150% of the federal poverty income guideline	USDA FNS	Primary
EFSP	Funds are used to purchase food and shelter to supplement and extend local services.	EFSP provides funding for the purchase of food products, operation costs associated with mass feeding and shelter, limited rent or mortgage assistance, providing assistance for first month's rent, limited off-site emergency lodging, and limited utility assistance.	Those in need of emergency services	Primary	FEMA	Primary
Head Start	Provides agencies and schools with support and guidance for half- and full-day child development programs for low-income children	Programs receive reimbursement for nutritious meals and snacks and USDA-donated commodities, support for curriculum, social services, and health screenings.	Low-income children ages 3-5; parents are encouraged to volunteer and be involved.	Same as NSLP	USDA (food) USDHHS (health)	Primary, secondary
National School Breakfast Program	Provides nutritionally balanced, low-cost or free breakfasts to children enrolled in participating schools	Participating schools receiving cash subsidies and USDA-donated commodities in return for offering breakfasts that meet same criteria as school lunch and offering free and reduced-price meals to eligible children.	Children preschool age through grade 12 in schools; children and teens 20 years of age in residential childcare and juvenile correctional institutions	Same as NSLP	USDA FNS	Primary, secondary
NSLP	Provides nutritionally balanced, low-cost or free lunches to children enrolled in participating schools	Participating schools receive cash subsidies and USDA-donated commodities in return for offering lunches that meet dietary guidelines and 1/3 of RDA for protein, iron, calcium, vitamins A and C, and calories and for offering free and reduced-price meals to eligible children	Children preschool age through grade 12 in schools; children and teenagers 20 years of age and younger in residential childcare and juvenile correctional institutions	185% of federal poverty income guideline for reduced-price lunches; 130% for free lunches	USDA FNS	Primary, secondary

Program	Description	Function	Target audience	Income standard	Administering agency	Level of prevention
Nutrition Program for the Elderly/Area Agencies on Aging	Provides commodity and cash assistance to programs providing meal services to older adults	Provides nutritious meals for older adults through congregate dining or home-delivered meals	Older adults	No income standard applied	USDHHS administers through state and local agencies; USDA cash and commodity assistance	Primary
Seniors' Farmers Market Nutrition Program	Provides fresh, nutritious, unprepared, locally grown fruits, vegetables, and herbs from farmers' markets, roadside stands, and community-supported agriculture programs to low-income seniors	Coupons for use at authorized farmers' markets, roadside stands, and community-supported agriculture programs (Foods that are not eligible for purchase with coupons by seniors are dried fruits or vegetables, potted plants and herbs, wild rice, nuts, honey, maple syrup, cider, and molasses.)	Low-income adults older than age 60	Low-income seniors with household incomes not exceeding 195% of the federal poverty income guideline	USDA FNS	Primary
SNAP	Provides benefits to low-income people that they can use to buy food to improve their diets	Provides assistance such as food stamps	Any age	For households in the 48 contiguous states and the District of Columbia. To get SNAP benefits, households must meet certain tests, including resource and income tests.	USDA FNS	Primary, secondary
Special Milk Program	Provides milk to children in participating schools who do not have access to other meal programs	Provides cash reimbursement for milk with vitamins A and D at RDA levels served at low or no cost to children; milk programs must be run on nonprofit basis.	Same target audience as school lunch and school breakfast programs	Eligible children do not have access to other supplemental foods programs.	USDA FNS	Primary, secondary
Summer Food Service Program	Provides healthy meals (per federal guidelines) and snacks to eligible children when school is out, using agriculture commodity foods	Reimburses for up to two or three meals and snacks served daily free to eligible children when school is not in session; cash based on income level of local geographic area or of enrolled children	Infants and children 18 years of age and younger served at variety of feeding sites		USDA FNS	Primary, secondary
WIC	Provides supplemental foods to improve health status of participants	Nutrition education, free nutritious foods (protein, iron, calcium, vitamins A and C), referrals, breastfeeding promotion	Pregnant, breastfeeding, and postpartum women up to 1 year; infants, children up to 5 yrs.	185% of federal poverty income guideline nutritional risk	UDSA FNS, home state support	Primary, secondary, tertiary
WIC FMNP	Provides fresh, unprepared, locally grown fruits and vegetables to WIC recipients, and to expand the awareness, use of and sales at farmers' markets	FMNP food coupons for use at participating farmers' markets stands; nutrition education through arrangements with state agency	Same as WIC recipients	Same as WIC recipients	USDA FNS	Primary

*Level of prevention rationale: Programs that provide food only are regarded as primary; programs that provide food, nutrients at a mandated level of recommended dietary allowances, or an educational component are regarded as secondary; and programs that used health screening measures on enrollment were regarded as tertiary.

EFSP, Emergency Food and Shelter Program; FEMA, Federal Emergency Management Agency; FMNP, Farmers Market Nutrition Program; FNS, Food and Nutrition Service; NSLP, National School Lunch Program; RDA, recommended daily allowance; SNAP, Special Nutrition Assistance Program; USDA, U.S. Department of Agriculture; USDHHS, U.S. Department of Health and Human Services; WIC, Special Supplemental Nutrition Program for Women, Infants, and Children.

TABLE 8.2 Common Foodborne Illnesses

Illness	Signs and Symptoms	Onset and Duration	Causes and Prevention	Comments
Bacillus cereus	Watery diarrhea, abdominal cramping, and vomiting	6-15 hours after consumption of contaminated food; duration 24 hours in most instances	Meats, milk, vegetables, and fish have been associated with the diarrheal type; vomiting-type outbreaks have generally been associated with rice products; potato, pasta, and cheese products; food mixtures such as sauces, puddings, soups, casseroles, pastries, and salads may also be a source.	B. cereus is a gram-positive, aerobic spore former.
Campylobacter jejuni	Diarrhea (often bloody), fever, and abdominal cramping	2-5 days after exposure; duration 2-10 days	Drinking raw milk or eating raw or undercooked meat, shellfish, or poultry; to prevent exposure, avoid raw milk and cook all meats and poultry thoroughly; it is safest to drink only pasteurized milk; the bacteria also may be found in tofu or raw vegetables. Hand-washing is important for prevention; wash hands with soap before handling raw foods of animal origin, after handling raw foods of animal origin, and before touching anything else; prevent cross-contamination in the kitchen; proper refrigeration and sanitation are also essential.	Top source of foodborne illness; some people develop antibodies to it, but others do not. In persons with compromised immune systems, it may spread to the bloodstream and cause sepsis; may lead to arthritis or to GBS; 40% of GBS in the United States is caused by campylobacteriosis and affects the nerves of the body, beginning several weeks after the diarrheal illness; can lead to paralysis that lasts several weeks and usually requires intensive care.
Clostridium botulinum	Muscle paralysis caused by the bacterial toxin: double or blurred vision, drooping eyelids, slurred speech, difficulty swallowing, dry mouth, and muscle weakness; infants with botulism appear lethargic, feed poorly, are constipated, and have a weak cry and poor muscle tone	In foodborne botulism symptoms generally begin 18-36 hours after eating contaminated food; can occur as early as 6 hours or as late as 10 days; duration days or months	Home-canned foods with low acid content such as asparagus, green beans, beets, and corn; outbreaks have occurred from more unusual sources such as chopped garlic in oil, hot peppers, tomatoes, improperly handled baked potatoes wrapped in aluminum foil, and home-canned or fermented fish. Persons who home-can should follow strict hygienic procedures to reduce contamination of foods; oils infused with garlic or herbs should be refrigerated; potatoes that have been baked while wrapped in aluminum foil should be kept hot until served or refrigerated; because high temperatures destroy the botulism toxin, persons who eat home-canned foods should boil the food for 10 minutes before eating.	If untreated, these symptoms may progress to cause paralysis of the arms, legs, trunk, and respiratory muscles; long-term ventilator support may be needed. Throw out bulging, leaking, or dented cans and jars that are leaking; safe home-canning instructions can be obtained from county extension services or from the U.S. Department of Agriculture; honey can contain spores of C. botulinum and has been a source of infection for infants; children younger than 12 months old should not be fed honey.
Clostridium perfringens	Nausea with vomiting, diarrhea, and signs of acute gastroenteritis lasting 1 day	Within 6-24 hours from the ingestion	Ingestion of canned meats or contaminated dried mixes, gravy, stews, refried beans, meat products, and unwashed vegetables. Cook foods thoroughly; leftovers must be reheated properly or discarded.	
Cryptosporidium parvum	Watery stools, diarrhea, nausea, vomiting, slight fever, and stomach cramps	2-10 days after being infected	Contaminated food from poor handling. Hand washing is important.	Protozoa causes diarrhea among immune-compromised patients.
Enterotoxigenic Escherichia coli (ETEC)	Watery diarrhea, abdominal cramps, low-grade fever, nausea, and malaise	With high infective dose, diarrhea can be induced within 24 hours	Contamination of water with human sewage may lead to contamination of foods; infected food handlers may also contaminate foods; dairy products such as semisoft cheeses may cause problems, but this is rare.	More common with travel to other countries; in infants or debilitated elderly persons, electrolyte replacement therapy may be necessary.

TABLE 8.2 Common Foodborne Illnesses—cont'd

Illness	Signs and Symptoms	Onset and Duration	Causes and Prevention	Comments
Escherichia coli O157:H7 Enterohemorrhagic E. coli (EHEC)	Hemorrhagic colitis (painful, bloody diarrhea)	Onset is slow, usually approximately 3-8 days after ingestion; duration 5-10 days	Undercooked ground beef and meats, from unprocessed apple cider, or from unwashed fruits and vegetables; sometimes water sources; alfalfa sprouts, unpasteurized fruit juices, dry-cured salami, lettuce, spinach, game meat, and cheese curds. Cook meats thoroughly, use only pasteurized milk, and wash all produce well.	Antibiotics are not used because they spread the toxin further; the condition may progress to hemolytic anemia, thrombocytopenia, and acute renal failure, requiring dialysis and transfusions; HUS can be fatal, especially in young children; there are several outbreaks each year, particularly from catering operations, church events, and family picnics; E. coli O157:H7 can survive in refrigerated acid foods for weeks
Listeria monocytogenes (LM)	Mild fever, headache, vomiting, and severe illness in pregnancy; sepsis in the immunocompromised patient; meningoencephalitis in infants; and febrile gastroenteritis in adults	Onset 2-30 days; duration variable	Processed, ready-to-eat products such as undercooked hot dogs, deli or lunchmeats, and unpasteurized dairy products; post pasteurization contamination of soft cheeses such as feta or Brie, milk, and commercial coleslaw; cross-contamination between food surfaces has also been a problem. Use pasteurized milk and cheeses; wash produce before use; reheat foods to proper temperatures; wash hands with hot, soapy water after handling these ready-to-eat foods; discard foods by their expiration dates.	May be fatal. Caution must be used by pregnant women, who may pass the infection on to their unborn child.
Norovirus	Gastroenteritis with nausea, vomiting, and/or diarrhea accompanied by abdominal cramps; headache, fever/chills, and muscle aches also may be present.	24-48 hours after ingestion of the virus, but can appear as early as 12 hours after exposure	Foods can be contaminated either by direct contact with contaminated hands or work surfaces that are contaminated with stool or vomit or by tiny droplets from nearby vomit that can travel through air to land on food; although the virus cannot multiply outside of human bodies, once on food or in water, it can cause illness; most cases occur on cruise ships.	Symptoms are usually brief and last only 1 or 2 days; however, during that brief period, people can feel very ill and vomit, often violently and without warning, many times a day; drink liquids to prevent dehydration.
Salmonella	Diarrhea, fever, and abdominal cramps	12-72 hours after infection; duration usually 4-7 days	Ingestion of raw or undercooked meat, poultry, fish, eggs, unpasteurized dairy products; unwashed fruits and raw vegetables (melons and sprouts). Prevent by thorough cooking, proper sanitation, and hygiene.	There are many different kinds of Salmonella bacteria; S. typhimurium and S. enteritidis are the most common in the United States. Most people recover without treatment, but some have diarrhea that is so severe that the patient needs to be hospitalized; this patient must be treated promptly with antibiotics; the elderly, infants, and those with impaired immune systems are more likely to have a severe illness.
Shigellosis	Bloody diarrhea, fever, and stomach cramps	24-48 hours after exposure; duration 4-7 days	Milk and dairy products; cold mixed salads such as egg, tuna, chicken, potato, and meat salads. Proper cooking, reheating, and maintenance of holding temperatures should aid in prevention; careful hand washing is essential.	This is caused by a group of bacteria called Shigella; it may be severe in young children and the elderly; severe infection with high fever may be associated with seizures in children younger than 2 years old.

Continued

TABLE 8.2 Common Foodborne Illnesses—cont'd

Illness	Signs and Symptoms	Onset and Duration	Causes and Prevention	Comments
Staphylococcus aureus	Nausea, vomiting, retching, abdominal cramping, and prostration	Within 1-6 hours; rarely fatal; duration 1-2 days	Meat, pork, eggs, poultry, tuna salad, prepared salads, gravy, stuffing, cream-filled pastries. Cooking does not destroy the toxin; proper handling and hygiene are crucial for prevention.	Refrigerate foods promptly during preparation and after meal service.
Streptococcus pyogenes	Sore and red throat, pain on swallowing; tonsillitis, high fever, headache, nausea, vomiting, malaise, rhinorrhea; occasionally a rash occurs	Onset 1-3 days	Milk, ice cream, eggs, steamed lobster, ground ham, potato salad, egg salad, custard, rice pudding, and shrimp salad; in almost all cases, the foodstuffs were allowed to stand at room temperature for several hours between preparation and consumption.	Entrance into the food is the result of poor hygiene, ill food handlers, or the use of unpasteurized milk. Complications are rare; treated with antibiotics.
Vibrio vulnificus	Vomiting, diarrhea, or both; illness is mild	Gastroenteritis occurs about 16 hours after eating contaminated food; duration about 48 hours	Seafood, especially raw clams and oysters, that has been contaminated with human pathogens; although oysters can only be harvested legally from waters free from fecal contamination, even these can be contaminated with V. vulnificus because the bacterium is naturally present.	This is a bacterium in the same family as those that cause cholera; it yields a Norovirus; it may be fatal in immunocompromised individuals.
Yersinia enterocolitica	Common symptoms in children are fever, abdominal pain, and diarrhea, which is often bloody; in older children and adults, right-sided abdominal pain and fever may be predominant symptom and may be confused with appendicitis.	1-2 days after exposure; duration 1-3 weeks or longer	Contaminated food, especially raw or undercooked pork products; postpasteurization contamination of chocolate milk, reconstituted dry milk, pasteurized milk, and tofu are also high-risk foods; cold storage does not kill the bacteria. Cook meats thoroughly; use only pasteurized milk; proper hand washing is also important.	Infectious disease caused by the bacterium Yersinia; in the United States most human illness is caused by Y. enterocolitica; it most often occurs in young children. In a small proportion of cases, complications such as skin rash, joint pains, or spread of bacteria to the bloodstream can occur.

GBS, Guillain-Barré Syndrome; HUS, hemolytic uremic syndrome.
Adapted with permission from Escott-Stump S: *Nutrition and diagnosis-related care*, ed 7, Baltimore, 2011, Lippincott Williams & Wilkins. Other sources: http://www.cdc.gov/health/diseases.

CLINICAL INSIGHT

The History of the Supplemental Nutrition Assistance Program (SNAP)

In the years after World War II, hunger and extreme malnutrition was a serious and pervasive problem in the United States. By the mid-1960s, one fifth of American households had poor diets. Among low-income households, this rate nearly doubled to 36% (United States Department of Agriculture [USDA] and Agricultural Research Service [ARS], 1969). According to studies at the time, these rates of hunger, especially in low-income areas of the South, had a serious effect on the public at the time because of malnutrition and vitamin deficiency (Wheeler, 1967). Many Americans learned how serious the problem was in their living rooms when CBS News aired a landmark documentary, *Hunger in America*, in 1968. The documentary featured malnourished children with distended bellies and stories from everyday people about how hunger affected their lives—something that other Americans couldn't believe was happening in their backyard (Center on Budget and Policy Priorities, November 2008). A public outcry resulted in the federal government's modern nutrition assistance system that began in the early 1960s as the Food Stamp program. Originally created as a small program during World War II to help bridge the gap between plentiful farm surpluses and urban hunger, it was discontinued in the 1950s because of the prosperous economy. President John F. Kennedy reintroduced it through an executive order in 1961 as a broader pilot program. As part of President Lyndon B. Johnson's War on Poverty initiative, Congress finally made it permanent. It has since been reauthorized and strengthened several times and is today known as the Supplemental Nutrition Assistance Program (SNAP) (USDA Food and Nutrition Service [FNS], 2010). Another important supplemental food program is for Women, Infants, and Children (WIC) and was developed in the 1970s to provide specialized nutrition assistance and support to low-income pregnant women, infants, and children up to age 5 (USDA and Economic Research Service [ERS], 2009).

In 2013 SNAP helped more than 47 million Americans afford a nutritionally adequate diet in a typical month. It also kept about 4.9 million people out of poverty in 2012, including 1.3 million children (Center on Budget and Policy Priorities, 2015). A recent study has shown that after these expansions in the 1960s and 1970s, disadvantaged children with access to nutrition assistance in early childhood and who had mothers that received assistance during pregnancy, had improved health and education outcomes, better growth curves, and fewer diagnoses of heart disease and obesity (Hoynes et al, 2012). Today, state agencies administering SNAP have the option of providing nutrition education to SNAP participants through federal grants and matching fund programs (USDA, 2017).

Erik R. Stegman, MA, JD

Targeted food safety public education campaigns are important. However, the model for food safety has expanded beyond the individual consumer and now includes the government, the food industry, the food growers, and the general public. Several government agencies provide information through websites with links to the CDC, the USDA Food Safety and Inspection Service (FSIS), the Environmental Protection Agency (EPA), the National Institute of Allergy and Infectious Diseases (NIAID), and the Food and Drug Administration (FDA). A leading industry program, ServSafe, provides food safety and training certification and was developed and administered by the National Restaurant Association. Because the U.S. food supply comes from a global market, food safety concerns are worldwide. The 2009 Country of Origin Labeling (COOL) legislation requires that retailers provide customers with the source of foods such as meats, fish, shellfish, fresh and frozen fruits and vegetables, and certain nuts and herbs (USDA, 2013). The USDA Agricultural Marketing Service has responsibility for COOL implementation. Future practice must include awareness of global food safety issues (see *Focus On*: Global Food Safety).

Hazard Analysis Critical Control Points

An integral strategy to reduce foodborne illness is risk assessment and management. Risk assessment entails hazard identification, characterization, and exposure. Risk management covers risk evaluation, option assessment and implementation, and monitoring and review of progress. One formal program, organized in 1996, is the Hazard Analysis Critical Control Points (HACCP), a systematic approach to the identification, evaluation, and control of food safety hazards. HACCP involves identifying any biologic, chemical, or physical agent that is likely to cause illness or injury in the absence of its control. It also involves identifying points at which control can be applied, thus preventing or eliminating the food safety hazard or reducing it to an acceptable level. Restaurants and health care facilities are obligated to use HACCP procedures in their food handling practices.

◎ FOCUS ON

Global Food Safety

The United States imports produce, meat, and seafood from other countries to meet the consumer demands for foods that are not readily available in the country. Global importation creates potential danger to the public. Our current food supply is becoming much harder to trace to a single source. Because of this, safety concerns must be addressed globally, as well as in the United States. Leadership from food growers, producers, distributors, and those involved in food preparation is essential to ensure a safe food supply. Protecting the food supply chain requires several safety management systems such as hazard analysis, critical control points, good manufacturing practice, and good hygiene practice. Food safety also includes attention to issues such as the use of toxins and pesticides in countries where standards and enforcement may be variable, as well as the importance of clean water. Finally, the effect of global warming on food production is an increasing concern.

Those who serve populations at the greatest risk for foodborne illness have a special need to be involved in the network of food safety education and to communicate this information to their clients (Fig. 8.2). Adoption of the HACCP regulations, food quality assurance programs, handling of fresh produce guidelines, technologic advances designed to reduce contamination, increased food supply regulations, and a greater emphasis on food safety education have contributed to a substantial decline in foodborne illness.

FOOD AND WATER SAFETY

Although individual educational efforts are effective in raising awareness of food safety issues, food and water safety must be examined on a national, systems-based level (AND, 2014). Several federal health initiatives include objectives relating to food and water safety, pesticide and allergen exposure, food-handling practices, reducing disease incidence associated with water, and reducing food- and water-related exposure to environmental pollutants. Related agencies can be found in Table 8.3.

Contamination

Controls and precautions concerning limiting potential contaminants in the water supply are of continuing importance. Water contamination with arsenic, lead, copper, pesticides and herbicides, mercury, dioxin, polychlorinated biphenyls (PCBs), chlorine, and *Escherichia coli* continues to be highlighted by the media. Lead has become a major concern in some areas due to old water pipes and plumbing. It was estimated that many public water systems, built using early twentieth-century technology, will need to invest more than $138 billion during the next 20 years to ensure continued safe drinking water (AND, 2014). The aging infrastructure has become an ongoing concern in older urban areas. The effect on the potential safety of food and drinks (including baby formula requiring water to be added) that have contact with these contaminants is an ongoing issue being monitored by advocacy and professional groups and governmental agencies.

Of interest to many is the issue of the potential hazards of ingestion of seafood that has been in contact with methyl mercury present naturally in the environment and released into the air from industrial pollution. Mercury has accumulated in bodies of water (i.e., streams, rivers, lakes, and oceans) and in the flesh of seafood in these waters (USDA and EPA, n.d.). The body of knowledge on issues such as this is being updated constantly, and current recommendations are to restrict the consumption of certain fish such as shark, mackerel, tilefish, tuna, and swordfish by pregnant women (FDA, 2013; Centers for Food Safety and Applied Nutrition et al, 2013). (See Chapter 14 for further discussion.) Other contaminants in fish, such as PCBs and dioxin, are also of concern (California Office of Environmental Health Hazard Assessment [OEHHA], 2014). Disposal of plastic containers and water bottles are another ongoing issue that merits researching the effect to the fishing industry and the consumer and the steps being taken.

Precautions are in place at the federal, state, and local levels that must be addressed by nutrition and dietetics professionals whose roles include advocacy, communication, and education. Members of the public and local health officials must understand the risks and the importance of carrying out measures for food and water safety and protection. The EPA and the Center for Food Safety and Applied Nutrition (CFSAN) provide ongoing monitoring and guidance. In addition, food and water safety and foodborne illness issues are monitored by state and local health departments.

Organic Foods and Pesticide Use

The use of pesticides and contaminants from the water supply affect produce quality. The debate continues about whether organic foods are worth the extra cost. However, the beneficial effects of organic farming also must be considered (see *Focus On*: Is It Really Organic, and Is It Healthier?).

Genetic Modification/Genetic Engineering

An emerging safety issue is that of genetically modified organisms (GMOs). A GMO is a plant or animal in which the genetic material has been altered in a way that does not occur naturally. The process of

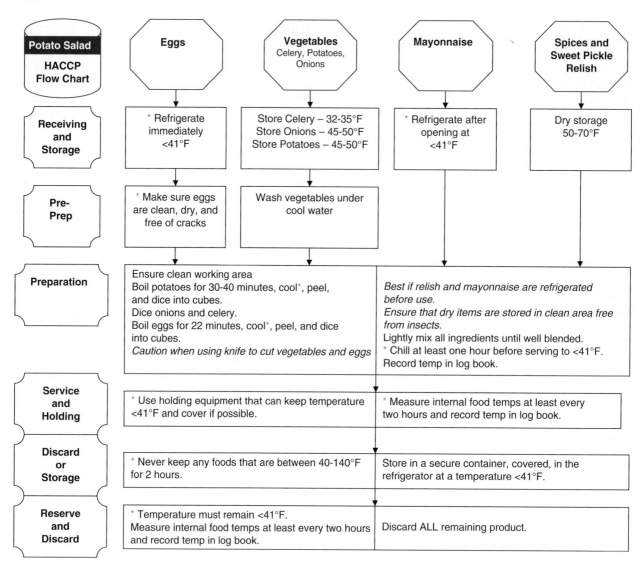

Fig. 8.2 The Six Steps of HACCP and a sample flow chart.

making GMOs is called genetic engineering (GE). The most recent data from the International Service for the Acquisition of Agri-biotech Applications shows that more than 18 million farmers in 26 countries—including 19 developing nations—planted over 185 million hectares (457 million acres) of GMO crops in 2016. This is a 3% increase over 2015. More than 26 countries have total or partial bans on the use of GMO crops and they remain controversial in the United States. Currently labeling of GMO/GE foods is voluntary, but there continues to be public demand to require it be labeled. The FDA is studying the issue. Once again, this is an issue that should be on the monitoring list of nutrition and dietetics professionals to be alert to valid and current research.

Bioterrorism and Food-Water Safety

Bioterrorism is the deliberate use of microorganisms or toxins from living organisms to induce death or disease. Threats to the nation's food and water supplies have made food **biosecurity**, or precautions to minimize risk, an issue when addressing preparedness planning. The CDC has identified seven foodborne pathogens as having the potential to be used by bioterrorists to attack the food supply: tularemia, brucellosis, *Clostridium botulinum* toxin, epsilon toxin of

Clostridium perfringens, *Salmonella*, *Escherichia coli*, and *Shigella*. These pathogens, along with potential water contaminants, such as mycobacteria, *Legionella*, *Giardia*, viruses, arsenic, lead, copper, methyl butyl ether, uranium, and radon, are the targets of federal systems put in place to monitor the safety of the food and water supply. Current surveillance systems are designed to detect foodborne illness outbreaks resulting from food spoilage, poor food handling practices, or other unintentional sources, but they were not designed to identify an intentional attack.

Consequences of a compromised food and water supply are physical, psychological, political, and economic. Compromise could occur with food being the primary agent such as a vector to deliver a biologic or chemical weapon or with food being a secondary target, leaving an inadequate food supply to feed a region or the nation. Intentional use of a foodborne pathogen as the primary agent may be mistaken as a routine outbreak of foodborne illness. Distinguishing normal illness fluctuation from an intentional attack depends on having in place a system for identification, preparedness planning, rapid communication, and central analysis. FDA has organized information for **food defense**, or protecting the food and water supply from deliberate attacks. (FDA, 2018).

TABLE 8.3 Food and Water Safety Resources

Academy of Nutrition and Dietetics	http://www.eatright.org/	Fruits and Veggies: More Matters	http://www.fruitsandveggies morematters.org/
Agricultural Marketing Services, USDA	http://www.ams.usda.gov/AMSv1.0/	National Broiler Council	http://www.eatchicken.com
American Egg Board	http://www.aeb.org	National Cattleman's Beef Association	http://www.beef.org/
North American Meat Institute	https://www.meatinstitute.org/	National Institutes of Health	http://www.nih.gov
CFSAN	http://www.fda.gov/Food/	National Food Safety Database	http://www.foodsafety.gov
CFSCAN—Food and Water Safety— Recalls, Outbreaks & Emergencies	http://www.fda.gov/Food/ RecallsOutbreaksEmergencies/ default.htm	National Restaurant Association Educational Foundation	http://www.nraef.org/
CDC	http://www.cdc.gov	The Partnership for Food Safety Education	http://www.fightbac.org
CDC Disaster	https://emergency.cdc.gov/ bioterrorism/ https://www.cdc.gov/disasters/ index.html	Produce Marketing Association	http://www.pma.com
		PulseNet	http://www.cdc.gov/pulsenet/
		U.S. Department of Agriculture	http://www.usda.gov
FEMA	http://www.fema.gov	U.S. Department of Agriculture Food Safety and Inspection Service	http://www.fsis.usda.gov
Food Chemical News	http://www.foodchemicalnews.com		
Food Marketing Institute-retail	http://www.fmi.org	U.S. Department of Education	http://www.ed.gov
Food Marketing Institute—Food Safety	http://www.fmi.org/docs/facts- figures/foodsafety.pdf?sfvrsn=2	U.S. Department of Health and Human Services	http://www.hhs.gov/
FoodNet	http://www.cdc.gov/foodnet/	U.S. EPA—Office of Ground and Drinking Water	http://www.epa.gov/safewater
Food Safety, Iowa State University	http://www.extension.iastate. edu/foodsafety/	U.S. EPA Seafood Safety	http://www.epa.gov/ost/fish
Grocery Manufacturers of America	http://www.gmabrands.org	U.S. Food and Drug Administration	http://www.fda.gov
International Food Information Council	http://www.foodinsight.org/	U.S. Poultry and Egg Association	http://www.uspoultry.org/

Note: Websites are updated frequently. Go to the home website and use a search to find the desired resources.

◎ FOCUS ON

Is It Really Organic, and Is It Healthier?

There are a variety of reasons why organic foods can be considered as facilitating the creation of a healthful, sustainable food system (McCullum-Gómez and Scott, 2009; Scialabba, 2013). First, some organic fruits, vegetables, and juices may contain more antioxidants and polyphenols compared with their conventionally grown counterparts (Barański et al, 2014), although there is an ongoing debate regarding the potential nutritional advantages of consuming organic versus conventional fruits and vegetables and other plant products (Barański et al, 2014; Smith-Spangler et al, 2012). Other researchers reported that organic soybeans contain significantly more total protein and zinc, and less saturated fat and total omega-6 fatty acids than conventional and genetically engineered soybeans (Bøhn et al, 2014). Second, organically raised meat may reduce the development of human antibiotic resistance and lessen air and water pollution (American Medical Association, 2009). Researchers have found a lower prevalence of antibiotic-resistant *Salmonella* (Sapkota et al, 2014) and antibiotic-resistant Enterococci (Sapkota et al, 2011) on U.S. conventional poultry farms that transitioned to organic practices. Third, a published meta-analysis (Palupi et al, 2012) found that organic dairy products contained significantly higher protein, total omega-3 fatty acids, and conjugated linoleic acid than those of conventional types. Another study reported that individual omega-3 fatty acid concentrations and the concentration of conjugated linoleic acid were higher in organic milk (Benbrook et al, 2013). In an ongoing cohort study, consumption of organic dairy products was associated with a lower risk of eczema during the first 2 years of life. These authors hypothesize that "a high intake of omega-3 fatty acids and/or conjugated linoleic acids from organic dairy products by the child is protective against eczema (independent of atopy) and that . . . the mother's intake of these fatty acids during pregnancy and lactation contributes

to this protection" (Kummeling et al, 2008). More recent research found that cows fed a 100% organic grass- and legume-based diet produce milk with elevated levels of omega-3 fatty acids and conjugated linoleic acid, thus providing a healthier balance of fatty acids (Benbrook et al, 2018).

Fortunately, organic foods are increasing their presence in the marketplace. Organic sales account for over 4% of total U.S. food sales, although organic products account for a much larger share in some food product categories. Certified organic acreage and livestock have been expanding in the U.S., particularly for fruits, vegetables, dairy, and poultry (Greene, 2014). In 2017 organic sales totaled 49.4 billion dollars with fruits and vegetables accounting for 16.5 billion dollars (McNeil, 2018). These foods are produced following practices described in the USDA National Organic Program (NOP), a marketing program with a certification process throughout the production and manufacturing chain, which describes the practices that are required for labeling a product "organic" (USDA, n.d.). Organic foods that are certified through the USDA NOP must also meet the same state and federal food safety requirements as nonorganic foods (Riddle and Markhart, 2010).

In organic farming, raw animal manure must be composted (§205.203), "unless it is: i) applied to land used for a crop not intended for human consumption; ii) incorporated into the soil not less than 120 days before the harvest of a product whose edible portion has direct contact with the soil surface or soil particles; or iii) incorporated into the soil not less than 90 days before the harvest of a product whose edible portion does not have direct contact with the soil surface or soil particles" (Electronic Code of Federal Regulations, Title 7: Agriculture, Part 205 – National Organic Program, 2017).

Organic agriculture offers numerous opportunities to reduce exposure to agricultural pesticides through the community food and water supply, which may

Continued

Is It Really Organic, and Is It Healthier?—cont'd

be detrimental to human health—particularly for high-risk groups including pregnant women, infants, young children, farmers, and farmworkers (American College of Obstetricians and Gynecologists Committee Opinion, 2013; Costa et al, 2014; Misiewicz and Shade, 2018). Long-term/low-dose exposure to pesticides has also been linked to neurodegenerative diseases such as Parkinson's disease and Alzheimer's disease (Baltazar et al, 2014). Studies with children reveal that there are dramatic reductions in organophosphate (OP) pesticide exposure with the consumption of organic food (Lu et al, 2008). Research with adults found that the consumption of an organic diet for 1 week significantly reduced OP pesticide exposure. These authors recommend consumption of organic food as a precautionary approach to reducing pesticide exposure (Oates et al, 2014). More recently, researchers compared French adults who frequently consumed organic foods to those who never consumed organic foods and found a 25% reduction in overall cancer risk. More specifically, eating an organic diet significantly reduces the risk of developing non-Hodgkin lymphoma (86%),

all lymphomas (76%), and postmenopausal breast cancer (34%) (Baudry et al, 2018).

Organically grown foods also promote a more sustainable food system by reducing energy requirements for production, impacting local economic development, reducing soil erosion, rehabilitating poor soils, and sequestering carbon in soil, which may reduce carbon levels in the atmosphere (Gattinger et al, 2012; Jaenicke, 2016; Scialabba, 2013; Williams et al, 2017). In addition, biodiversity is enhanced in organic agricultural systems (Tuck et al, 2014), which makes these farms more resilient to unpredictable weather patterns and pest outbreaks. Organic farming also favors insect-pollinated forb species richness and flower cover, presumably due to the lack of herbicide use (Happe et al, 2018). Finally, public investment in organic agriculture facilitates wider access to organic food for consumers, helps farmers capture high-value markets, and conserves natural resources including soil and water.

by Christine McCullum-Gomez, PhD, RDN

Experience with the series of hurricanes in 2005 emphasized the need to provide access to a safe food and water supply after emergencies and disasters. Access to food and water may be limited, which results in social disruption and self-imposed quarantine. These situations require a response different from the traditional approach to disaster relief, during which it is assumed that hungry people will seek assistance and have confidence in the safety of the food that is offered. In the event of a disaster, dietetics professionals can play a key role by being aware of their environment, knowing available community and state food and nutrition resources, and participating in coordination and delivery of relief to victims of the disaster.

DISASTER PLANNING

Dietetics and health professionals working in food service are expected to plan for the distribution of safe food and water in any emergency situation. This may include creating and choosing food preparation and distribution sites, establishing temporary kitchens, preparing foods with limited resources, and keeping prepared food safe to eat through HACCP procedures. One of the most vulnerable groups is infants. The American Academy of Pediatrics has guidelines for infant feeding during disasters (https://www.aap.org/en-us/advocacy-and-policy/aap-health-initiatives/Breastfeeding/Documents/InfantNutritionDisaster.pdf).

Planning, surveillance, detection, response, and recovery are the key components of public health disaster preparedness. The key agencies are the USDA, the Department of Homeland Security (DHS), the Federal Emergency Management Agency (FEMA), the CDC, and the FDA. In conjunction with DHS, USDA operates Protection of the Food Supply and Agricultural Production (PFSAP). PFSAP handles issues related to food production, processing, storage, and distribution. It addresses threats against the agricultural sector and border surveillance. PFSAP conducts food safety activities concerning meat, poultry, and egg inspection and provides laboratory support, research, and education on outbreaks of foodborne illness.

Ready.gov of the DHS is an education toolkit on how to prepare for a national emergency, including possible terrorist attacks. In addition, the USDA Food Safety and Inspection Service (FSIS) operates the Food Threat Preparedness Network (PrepNet) and the Food Biosecurity Action Team (F-Bat). PrepNet ensures effective coordination of food security efforts, focusing on preventive activities to protect the food supply. F-Bat assesses potential vulnerabilities along the farm-to-table continuum, provides guidelines to industry on food security and increased plant

security, strengthens FSIS's coordination and cooperation with law enforcement agencies, and enhances security features of FSIS laboratories (Bruemmer, 2003).

CDC has three operations relating to food security and disaster planning: PulseNet, FoodNet, and the Centers for Public Health Preparedness. PulseNet is a national network of public health laboratories that performs deoxyribonucleic acid fingerprinting on foodborne bacteria, assists in detecting foodborne illness outbreaks and tracing them back to their source, and provides linkages among sporadic cases. FoodNet is the Foodborne Diseases Active Surveillance Network, which functions as the principle foodborne disease component of the CDC's Emerging Infections Program, providing active laboratory-based surveillance. The Centers for Public Health Preparedness fund academic centers linking schools of public health with state, local, and regional bioterrorism preparedness and public health infrastructure needs.

CFSAN in the FDA is concerned with regulatory issues such as seafood HACCP, safety of food and color additives, safety of foods developed through biotechnology, food labeling, dietary supplements, food industry compliance, and regulatory programs to address health risks associated with foodborne chemical and biologic contaminants. CFSAN also runs cooperative programs with state and local governments.

FEMA, under the DHS, provides emergency support functions after a disaster or emergency. FEMA identifies food and water needs, arranges delivery, and provides assistance with temporary housing and other emergency services. Agencies that assist FEMA include the USDA, the Department of Defense, the USDHHS, the EPA, and the General Services Administration. Major players include nonprofit volunteer agencies such as the American Red Cross, the Salvation Army, and community-based agencies and organizations. Disaster management is evolving as it is tested by manufactured and natural disasters.

HEALTHY FOOD AND WATER SYSTEMS AND SUSTAINABILITY

This chapter began with a note that community nutrition is a constantly evolving and growing area of practice with the broad focus of serving the population at large with a thrust to be proactive and responsive to the needs of the community. Today's communities and community needs differ, but regardless of environmental, social, and geographic variations, a goal of all nutrition and dietetics professionals is to promote and sustain access to safe, affordable, and health-promoting food sources.

In 2014 the Academy of Nutrition and Dietetics issued *Standards of Professional Performance* that addressed building and supporting sustainable, resilient, and healthy food and water systems (AND, 2014). These standards are meant to provide guidance to every RDN beyond the usual safety standards. This paper identifies sustainability as the ability to maintain the system for the long term. Resilience means a system can withstand interruptions that occur. From a community nutrition aspect, a practical example of resilience is that standards are in place for access to health-supporting and safe food and water even after a flood, natural disaster, or funding interruption. The sustainability is rooted in how the system is built, guided, and nourished. Public and private programs and resources are critical components and must meet the tests of resiliency to be sustainable to meet funding requirements.

The safety, adequacy, and quality of the food and water supply along with energy sources are components that build sustainability and resiliency. The nutrition and dietetics professional can be a major player but must have the expertise and competency as well as the initiative to build as well as promote standards and conditions in which people can reach the goal of being healthy.

SUMMARY: A WORK IN PROGRESS

This chapter is a work in progress, a snapshot of the evolving world of community nutrition that is changing even faster with Internet access. Changes are inherent in food, health, food access and safety, and our global environment. The nutrition and dietetics professional is an important player but needs to be current; engaged; and alert to legitimacy, science, and currency of sources. Networking with other community professionals, agencies, schools, universities, and organizations can provide both access and resources. However, as nutrition and dietetics professionals, decisions and actions need to be defensible as meeting both ethical and science-based standards. This means seeking updated and science-based sources and resources.

Below are listed useful websites, many with access to regular updates on problems, issues, and solutions.

USEFUL WEBSITES

Academy of Nutrition and Dietetics
American Heart Association
Centers for Disease Control
Centers for Science in the Public Interest (CSPI)
ChangeLab Solutions
Dietary Guidance and Dietary Guidelines for Americans
Environmental Protection Agency
Federal Emergency Management Agency
Feeding America
Food Safety
Fruits and Vegetables: More Matters
Hazard Analysis Critical Control Points
Head Start
Healthy People 2010 and 2020
Homeland Security
National Academies Press—Dietary Reference Intakes
National Center for Health Statistics
National Health and Nutrition Examination Study
Robert Wood Johnson Foundation
U.S. Department of Agriculture Farm to School Initiative
U.S. Department of Agriculture Food Safety Resources
U.S Department of Agriculture **MyPlate**
U.S. Department of Agriculture Nutrition Assistance Programs
U.S. Department of Agriculture SNAP-Ed Connection
Yale Rudd Center for Food Policy & Obesity

REFERENCES

Academy of Nutrition and Dietetics, Cody MM, Stretch T: Position of the Academy of Nutrition and Dietetics: food and water safety, *J Acad Nutr Diet* 114:1819–1829, 2014.

American College of Obstetricians and Gynecologists, Committee on Health Care for Underserved Women, American Society for Reproductive Medicine Practice Committee, et al: Exposure to toxic environmental agents, *Fertil Steril* 100:931–934, 2013.

American Medical Association. *Report of the Council on Science and Public Health.* (CSAPH). *CSAPH Report 8-A-09.* Sustainable Food AMA House of Delegates Annual Meeting, Chicago, IL, 2009. Available at: https://www.ama-assn.org/sites/ama-assn.org/files/corp/media-browser/public/about-ama/councils/Council%20Reports/council-on-science-public-health/a09-csaph-sustainable-food.pdf.

Baltazar MT, Dinis-Oliveira RJ, de Lourdes Bastos M, et al. Pesticides exposure as etiological factors of Parkinson's disease and other neurodegenerative diseases—a mechanistic approach, *Toxicol Lett* 230(2):85–103, 2014.

Barański M, Srednicka-Tober D, Volakakis N, et al: Higher antioxidant and lower cadmium concentrations and lower incidence of pesticide residues in organically grown crops: a systematic literature review and meta-analyses, *Br J Nutr* 112:794–811, 2014.

Baudry J, Assmann KE, Touvier M, et al. Association of frequency of organic food consumption with cancer risk: findings from the NutriNet-Santé Prospective Cohort Study, *JAMA Intern Med* 178(12):1597–1606, 2018. doi:10.1001/jamainternmed.2018.4357.

Benbrook CM, Butler G, Latif MA, et al: Organic production enhances milk nutritional quality by shifting fatty acid composition: a United States-wide, 18-month study, *PLoS One* 8:e82429, 2013, doi:10.1371/journal.pone.0082429.

Benbrook CM, Davis DR, Heins BJ, et al. Enhancing the fatty acid profile of milk through forage-based rations, with nutrition modeling of diet outcomes, *Food Sci Nutr* 6(3):681–700, 2018. doi:10.1002/fsn3.610.

Bøhn T, Cuhra M, Traavik T, et al. Compositional differences in soybeans on the market: glyphosate accumulates in Roundup Ready GM soybeans, *Food Chem* 153:207–215, 2014.

Bruemmer B: Food biosecurity, *J Am Diet Assoc* 103:687–691, 2003.

California Office of Environmental Health Hazard Assessment: *Chemicals in fish*, 2014. Available at: https://oehha.ca.gov/fish/advisories.

Center for Food Safety and Applied Nutrition, U.S. Department of Health and Human Services, U.S. Food and Drug Administration: *Food*, 2013. Available at: https://www.fda.gov/Food/default.htm.

Center on Budget and Policy Priorities: *Making America stronger: The U.S. Food Stamp Program*, November 3, 2008. Available at: https://www.youtube.com/watch?v=aqOV-hK0sP4; https://www.fns.usda.gov/school-meals/child-nutrition-programs; https://www.fns.usda.gov/tn/local-school-wellness-policy.

Center on Budget and Policy Priorities: *Supplemental Nutrition Assistance Program (SNAP)*, 2015. Available at: http://www.thisissnap.org/.

Centers for Disease Control and Prevention: *Healthy People 2020 and National Center for Health Statistics*, 2014. Available at: https://www.cdc.gov/nchs/healthy_people/hp2020.htm; https://www.cdc.gov/nchs/fastats/default.htm.

Centers for Disease Control and Prevention: *The community guide*, 2018. Available at: http://www.thecommunityguide.org/.

Costa C, García-Lestón J, Costa S, et al: Is organic farming safer to farmers' health? A comparison between organic and traditional farming, *Toxicol Lett* 230(2):166–176, 2014. Available at: http://dx.doi.org/10.1016/j.toxlet.2014.02.011.

Electronic Code of Federal Regulations (e-CRF), Title 7: Agriculture. Part 205 – National Organic Program, January 1, 2017. Available at: https://www.gpo.gov/fdsys/pkg/CFR-2017-title7-vol3/xml/CFR-2017-title7-vol3-part205.xml.

Food and Drug Administration: *Food defense*, 2018. Available at: https://www.fda.gov/Food/FoodDefense/default.htm.

Frieden TR: A framework for public health action: the health impact pyramid, *Am J Public Health* 100:590–595, 2010.

Gattinger A, Muller A, Haeni M, et al: Enhanced top soil carbon stocks under organic farming, *Proc Natl Acad Sci U S A* 109:18226–18231, 2012.

Greene C: *Overview—Organic agriculture.* Washington, DC, April 7, 2014, United States Department of Agriculture, Economic Research Service. Available at: http://www.ers.usda.gov/topics/natural-resources-environment/organic-agriculture.aspx.

Happe AK, Riesch F, Rösch V, et al. Small-scale agricultural landscapes and organic management support wild bee communities of cereal field boundaries, *Agric Ecosyst Environ* 254:92–98, 2018.

Healthy People 2010: *National health promotion and disease prevention objectives,* Washington, DC, 2000, U.S. Department of Health and Human Services.

Healthy People 2020: *National health promotion and disease prevention objectives,* Washington, DC, 2010, U.S. Department of Health and Human Services. Available at: http://www.healthypeople.gov/2020/default.aspx.

Hoynes H, Schanzenbach DW, Almond D: *Long run impacts of childhood access to the safety net* [White paper], 2012. Available at: http://www.nber.org/papers/w18535.

Jaenicke EC: *U.S. organic hotspots and their benefit to local economies. Hotspot identification, formation, impacts, and policy recommendations,* Washington, DC, May 2016, Organic Trade Association. Available at: https://ota.com/sites/default/files/indexed_files/OTA-HotSpotsWhitePaper-OnlineVersion.pdf.

Kummeling I, Thijs C, Huber M, et al: Consumption of organic foods and risk of atopic disease during the first 2 years of life in the Netherlands, *Br J Nutr* 99:598–605, 2008.

Lu C, Barr DB, Pearson MA, et al: Dietary intake and its contribution to longitudinal organophosphorus pesticide exposure in urban/suburban children, *Environ Health Perspect* 116:537–542, 2008.

McCullum-Gómez C, Scott AM: *Hot topic: perspective on the benefits of organic foods,* September 2009. Available at: http://www.hendpg.org/docs/Resources%20-%20public/Hot-Topic-Perspective-Benefits-Organic-Foods-2009.pdf.

McNeil M: *Maturing U.S. organic sector sees steady growth of 6.4 percent in 2017.* Press Release, Washington, DC, May 18, 2018, Organic Trade Association. Available at: https://ota.com/news/press-releases/20236. Accessed October 19, 2018.

Misiewicz T, Shade J: *Organic agriculture: critical issue report: occupational pesticide exposure. Reducing occupational pesticide exposure in farmers and farmworkers,* Boulder, CO, September 2018, The Organic Center. Available at: https://www.organic-center.org/wp-content/uploads/2018/09/Reducing-Occupational-Pesticide-Exposure.pdf.

Oates L, Cohen M, Braun L, et al: Reduction in urinary organophosphate pesticide metabolites in adults after a week-long organic diet, *Environ Res* 132:105–111, 2014.

Oliveira V, United States Department of Agriculture, Economic Research Service: *The food assistance landscape: FY 2017 Annual Report,* 2018. Available at: https://www.ers.usda.gov/webdocs/publications/88074/eib-190_summary.pdf?v=43174.

Palupi E, Jayanegara A, Ploeger A, et al: Comparison of nutritional quality between conventional and organic dairy products: a meta-analysis, *J Sci Food Agric* 92:2774–2781, 2012.

Produce for Better Health Foundation: *Guidelines,* 2018. Available at: https://fruitsandveggies.org/about/

Produce for Better Health Foundation: *Fruit and Veggies More Matters,* 2019. Available at: http://www.fruitsandveggiesmorematters.org.

Riddle J, Markhart B: *What is organic food and why should I care?* Lamberton, MN, 2010, University of Minnesota, Organic Ecology Research and Outreach Program, Southwest Research and Outreach Center. Available at: https://www.scribd.com/document/199266366/University-of-Minnesota-Organic-Food-Report.

Rose D, Bodor JN, Hutchinson PL, et al: The importance of a multi-dimensional approach for studying the links between food access and consumption, *J Nutr* 140:1170–1174, 2010.

Sapkota AR, Hulet RM, Zhang G, et al: Lower prevalence of antibiotic-resistant Enterococci on U.S. conventional poultry farms that transitioned to organic practices, *Environ Health Perspect* 119:1622–1628, 2011.

Sapkota AR, Kinney EL, George A, et al: Lower prevalence of antibiotic-resistant Salmonella on large-scale U.S. conventional poultry farms that transitioned to organic practices, *Sci Total Environ* 476:387–392, 2014.

Scialabba N: Organic agriculture's contribution to sustainability, *Crop Manag* 12, 2013. doi:10.1094/CM-2013-0429-09-PS.

Smith-Spangler C, Brandeau ML, Hunter GE, et al: Are organic foods safer or healthier than conventional alternatives?: a systematic review, *Ann Intern Med* 157:348–366, 2012.

Tuck SL, Winqvist C, Mota F, et al: Land-use intensity and the effects of organic farming on biodiversity: a hierarchical meta-analysis, *J Appl Ecol* 51:746–755, 2014, doi:10.1111/1365-2664.12219.

U.S. Department of Agriculture: *Food desert locator.* Available at: https://www.fns.usda.gov/tags/food-desert-locator.

U.S. Department of Agriculture: *Organic standards,* n.d. Available at: https://www.ams.usda.gov/grades-standards/organic-standards

U.S. Department of Agriculture: *State SNAP-Ed contacts,* 2017. Available at: https://snaped.fns.usda.gov/state-contacts.

U.S. Department of Agriculture, Agricultural Marketing Service: *Country of origin labeling,* 2013. Available at: http://www.ams.usda.gov/AMSv1.0/cool.

U.S. Department of Agriculture, Agricultural Research Service: *Dietary levels of households in the United States, Spring 1965,* 1969. Available at: http://www.ars.usda.gov/SP2UserFiles/Place/80400530/pdf/6566/hfcs6566_rep_6.pdf.

U.S. Department of Agriculture, Agricultural Research Service: *What we eat in America (WWEIA), NHANES,* 2014. Available at: https://www.cdc.gov/nchs/nhanes/wweia.htm.

U.S. Department of Agriculture, Economic Research Service: *The WIC program,* 2009. Available at: https://www.fns.usda.gov/wic/women-infants-and-children-wic.

U.S. Department of Agriculture, Food and Nutrition Service: *From food stamps to the supplemental nutrition assistance program: legislative timeline.* Available at: http://www.fns.usda.gov/sites/default/files/timeline.pdf.

U.S. Department of Health and Human Services: *Dietary guidelines,* 2015. Available at: http://www.health.gov/dietaryguidelines/.

U.S. Dietary Guidelines for Americans. Available at: https://health.gov/DietaryGuidelines/; https://www.usda.gov/media/blog/2018/03/01/2020-2025-dietary-guidelines-americans-we-want-hear-you.

U.S. Food and Drug Administration (SDA) and Environmental Protection Agency (EPA): *Mercury and fish,* n.d. Available at: https://www.epa.gov/mercury/guidelines-eating-fish-contain-mercury.

Wheeler R: Hungry children: special report, *J South Reg Counc* 6:15, 1967.

WHO is in Geneva, Switzerland. That's the only location listed on the site.

Wilkinson RG, Marmot MG, editors: *Social determinants of health: the solid facts,* ed 2, Denmark, 2003, World Health Organization.

Williams DM and Francis CA, et al. Organic farming and soil properties: an assessment after 40 years, Agronomy 109(2), 2017.

World Health Organization: *Closing the gap: policy into practice on social determinants of health,* World Health Organization.

World Health Organization: *World Health Statistics 2018: Monitoring health for the SDGs Sustainable Development Goals,* 2018, World Health Organization.

PART II

Nutrition Diagnosis and Intervention

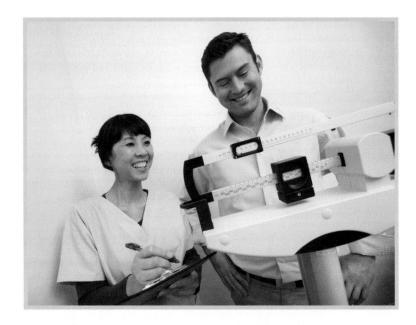

The type of nutrition care provided to an individual or population varies depending on the findings of the assessment process (step one of the nutrition care process). The environment, surgery or trauma, food allergies, inadequate access to safe or sufficient food, stage of growth and development, harmful beliefs, lack of knowledge, and socioeconomic issues can all affect whether an individual or population maintains adequate nutrition status. In the healthy individual or population, omission of a specific food group or intake of high-energy, nutrient-poor foods does not lead to failed nutritional status overnight. It is the prolonged imbalanced intake that leads to chronic disease. Dramatic and acute insufficiency combined with acute disease also leads to undesirable nutritional consequences. Indeed, inadequacy of the types or amounts of macro- or micronutrients, fluid, or even physical activity may cause a decline in health status or immunity and dysfunction and disease.

The establishment of nutrition diagnoses helps define and promote effective care according to specific nutrition problems. Such problems may be found in an individual, a group (such as persons who have diabetes or celiac disease), or even a community (such as sites where local produce is grown in mineral-depleted soil.)

Step two of the nutrition care process involves an analysis of the factors affecting adequacy of the current nutritional intake and overall nutritional status. In most cases, institutions use standards of care, national or disease-specific evidence-based practice guidelines that describe recommended actions in the nutrition care process (NCP). These comparative standards serve as the basis for assessing the quality of care provided.

Step three of the NCP is intervention, which involves planning and implementation. This includes the selection and carrying out of interventions that resolve, lessen, or manage the cause of the nutrition problem. For example, nutrition education is an appropriate intervention for the person who has little knowledge of how to manage a gluten-free diet. And this requires a counseling approach that takes into account the client's level of readiness to change. It may be helpful to refer the individual to available cookbooks, health services, and support groups. Manipulation of dietary components, provision of enteral or parenteral nutrition, or in-depth nutrition counseling may also be needed. Coordination of care between hospital and home and community is important for life long management of nutrition and chronic disease.

The final step of the NCP is specific to the client's (individual or population) monitoring and evaluation, and is focused on the important and relevant signs and symptoms identified in the assessment. The findings of monitoring and evaluation become the basis for reassessment as the NCP cycle repeats with subsequent interactions (encounters or visits) with the client.

9

Overview of Nutrition Diagnosis and Intervention

Constantina Papoutsakis, PhD, RDN

KEY TERMS

advance directives
Affordable Care Act (ACA)
assessment, diagnosis, interventions, monitoring, evaluation (ADIME) format
case management
Centers for Medicare and Medicaid Services (CMS)
Chronic care model (CCM)
comparative standards
critical pathways
discharge planning
disease management
electronic health record (EHR)
electronic medical record (EMR)
etiology

Health Insurance Portability and Accountability Act (HIPAA)
managed-care organizations (MCOs)
national provider identifier (NPI)
nutrition care process (NCP)
nutrition care process model (NCPM)
nutrition care process terminology (NCPT)
nutrition diagnosis
nutrition diagnosis etiology matrix
nutrition prescription
nutrition screening
order-writing privileges (OWPs)
palliative care
Patient Reported Outcome Measures (PROMs)
patient-centered medical home (PCMH)

people-centered care (PCC)
personal health record (PHR)
preferred-provider organizations (PPOs)
problem, etiology, signs and symptoms (PES)
problem-oriented medical records (POMR)
protected health information (PHI)
room service
sentinel events
standards of care
Standards of Professional Performance (SOPPs)
subjective, objective, assessment, plan (SOAP) note format
The Joint Commission (TJC)
utilization management

Nutrition care is a systematic group of professional activities that aim to identify nutritional needs and provide care to address these needs. Nutrition care can occur in a variety of settings and populations, involving members of the multidisciplinary team, as appropriate. For example, nutrition care occurs in schools with children and in collaboration with a school nurse and the education staff as well as in public health departments with a variety of populations and in collaboration with public health officials. Nutrition care also occurs in clinical settings (e.g., skilled nursing facilities, dialysis clinics, and hospital settings), in populations who are acutely or chronically ill, and in collaboration with the medical team (e.g., nurses, physicians, pharmacists, physical therapists). Comprehensive care may involve different health care providers (e.g., the physician, registered dietitian nutritionist [RDN], nurse, pharmacist, physical or occupational therapist, social worker, speech therapist, and case manager) who are integral in achieving desired outcomes, regardless of the care setting. The client is a core member of the team that participates actively in all major decisions throughout the care process, whenever possible. Overall, the nutrition care process model (NCPM) (the graphic representation of the NCP) defines the term client as the individual and/or populations, and this definition encompasses supportive members such as

family, caregivers, and structures including social service agencies and faith-based organizations (Swan et al, 2017). For consistency, the same definition of the term client will be used throughout the present chapter.

A collaborative approach helps ensure that care is coordinated and that team members and the client are aware of all goals and priorities. Team conferences, formal or informal, are useful in all settings: a clinic, a hospital, the home, the community, a long-term care facility, or any other site where nutrition problems may be identified. Coordinating the activities of health care professionals also requires documentation of the process and regular discussions to offer complete nutritional care. Standardization of the care process (the nutrition care process, NCP) improves consistency and quality of care and enables collection and assessment of nutrition related outcome measures.

THE NUTRITION CARE PROCESS

The nutrition care process (NCP) is a standardized framework of professional activities for the provision of nutrition care established by the Academy of Nutrition and Dietetics (AND, known as the Academy, formerly the American Dietetic Association [ADA]). The NCP model has been embraced by nutrition and dietetics professionals across borders. Most importantly, international input has been a salient influence on the model's continuous improvement (Swan et al, 2017). Per the Academy, the NCP is a process for identifying, planning for, and meeting nutritional needs. The nutritional needs referred to in this definition may be of an individual, specific group, or population. Furthermore, the NCP gives the profession a framework for critical thinking and decision making, which

---

Portions of this chapter were written by Pamela Charney, PhD, RDN, CHTS-CP and Alison Steiber, PhD, RDN. Sections of this chapter were written by Sylvia Escott-Stump, MA, RDN, LDN for previous editions of this text.

may assist in defining the roles and responsibilities of registered dietitian nutritionists (RDN) and registered nutrition and dietetic technicians (NDTR) in all practice settings and professional levels (AND, 2018).

The current update of the model highlights the following themes: support for people-centered care (PCC) where the individual or population is at the very center (see Fig. 4.3), use of concise language, and professionals' responsibility for outcomes management (Swan et al, 2017). The NCP includes four steps that are the responsibility of the RDN: (1) nutrition assessment, (2) nutrition diagnosis, (3) nutrition intervention, and (4) monitoring and evaluation (Swan et al, 2017). Nutrition screening and outcomes management are vital to safe, high-quality nutrition care; however, they are not included as separate steps in the NCP because they are not unique to nutrition and dietetics and may be performed by others qualified professionals.

Each step of the NCP has corresponding terminology that allows for standardized documentation. This terminology is called the nutrition care process terminology (NCPT) (previously the international dietetics and nutrition terminology [IDNT]) (Swan et al, 2019). Originally, the terminology was available in print form. Currently, the complete terminology of approximately 1700 terms can only accessed in a web-based format known as the electronic NCPT (eNCPT) for a nominal cost (AND, 2018a). Also, a select subset of the current NCPT is found in print form (AND, 2017). Using standardized terminology within the documentation process is critical. Systematic and accurate collection of outcomes data allows caregivers a process to determine whether interventions are effective in improving or resolving the nutrition diagnosis. To facilitate the collective aggregation of nutrition care data using the NCPT, the Academy has developed a web-based tool, the Academy Nutrition and Dietetics Health Informatics Infrastructure (ANDHII) (Murphy and Steiber, 2015). Also, an evaluation method to check if the NCP is used appropriately has been applied in different settings. This method is known as the NCP Chains (Hakel-Smith et al, 2005; Murphy et al, 2018). This is important methodology for all nutrition and dietetics students, educators, and professionals who have a vested interest in checking the quality of NCP application. If an RDN works in a public health department and has implemented a program for reducing obesity in an inner city population, he or she would have to be able to collect standardized parameters pre- (assessment) and post (monitoring) intervention and compare them for change (evaluation) to determine whether the intervention was effective. Without standardized language and corresponding definitions, different terms are used for the same condition and thus reduce the ability to show effectiveness of interventions. Recently, the eNCPT added a new collection of terms focused on public health interventions. The eNCPT continues to add terminology to meet the evolving needs of the nutrition and dietetics profession using a rigorous terminology submission process (AND, 2018b).

Nutrition Screening

The purpose of nutrition screening is to identify clients who are at nutrition risk and thus should be referred to the RDN for assessment of nutritional status. Nutrition screening can be done in all settings: hospitals, clinics, long-term care facilities, schools, and food banks. When available, population-specific, validated tools should be used for screening (see Chapter 4). Regulatory agencies, including The Joint Commission (TJC), include nutrition screening in their standards. Most health care facilities have developed a multidisciplinary admission screening process that is completed by nursing staff during admission to the facility. Nutrition screening can be incorporated into this admission assessment. Facilities that use an electronic health record (EHR) should build an automatic referral to the RDN when screening criteria are met. The nutrition risk screen should be quick, easy to administer, and cost effective. Table 9.1 lists information that is

TABLE 9.1	**Nutrition Risk Screening**	
Responsible Party	**Action**	**Documentation**
Admitting health care professional	Assess weight status— Has the client lost weight without trying before admission?	Check yes or no on admission screen.
Admitting health care professional	Assess GI symptoms— Has the client had GI symptoms preventing usual intake over the past 2 weeks?	Check yes or no on admission screen.
Admitting health care professional	Determine need to consult RDN.	If either screening criterion is "yes," consult RDN for nutrition assessment.

GI, Gastrointestinal; *RDN*, registered dietitian nutritionist.

included frequently in a nutrition screen. Also see Box 4.3 and Fig. 4.4 in Chapter 4 for additional examples.

When the Academy's Evidence Analysis Library (EAL) team conducted a systematic review of acute care screening tools, they determined that the Malnutrition Screening Tool (MST), the Mini-Nutrition Assessment-short form (MNA), and the Nutrition Risk Screen-2002 (NRS) had acceptable reliability and validity in various hospital settings (AND, 2010). See Chapter 4 for a description of these screening tools. When used in a hospital setting, rescreening should occur at regular intervals during the admission. Policies for nutrition rescreening should take into account the average length of time a client will stay at the facility.

Nutrition Assessment and Reassessment

The purpose of nutrition assessment is to obtain, verify, and interpret data needed to identify nutrition-related problems and their causes, importance, and relevance. Nutrition assessment data that is used to justify the nutrition diagnosis (the step that follows nutrition assessment) is typically recorded as "signs and symptoms" in the nutrition diagnosis statement and is also referred to as "evidence." Nutrition assessment is needed when the screening tool identifies the client to be at nutritional risk (see Chapter 4 through Chapter 7 for detailed discussions of nutrition assessment). The Integrative and Functional Medicine radial in Fig. 9.1 presents a summary of all the aspects of the client's lifestyle that go into a functional assessment as designated in the center with ADIME (assessment, diagnosis, intervention, monitoring and evaluation), and personalized nutrition care. Nutrition assessment parameters have specific corresponding terms, which should be used during documentation. These terms are classified into five domains (food/nutrition related history, anthropometrics, biochemical, nutrition-focused physical examination findings, and client history) (AND, 2017a). The NCPT also provides comparative standards. Comparative standards are criteria, or relevant norms and standards against which nutrition assessment data is compared with to identify nutrition problems (see Chapter 4 and Appendices 12 and 13).

Nutrition Diagnosis

RDNs evaluate all the information from the nutrition assessment to determine a nutrition diagnosis. Accurate diagnosis of nutrition problems is guided by critical evaluation of assessment data combined with good judgment and decision-making skills. The purpose of identifying the presence of a nutrition diagnosis is to identify and describe a

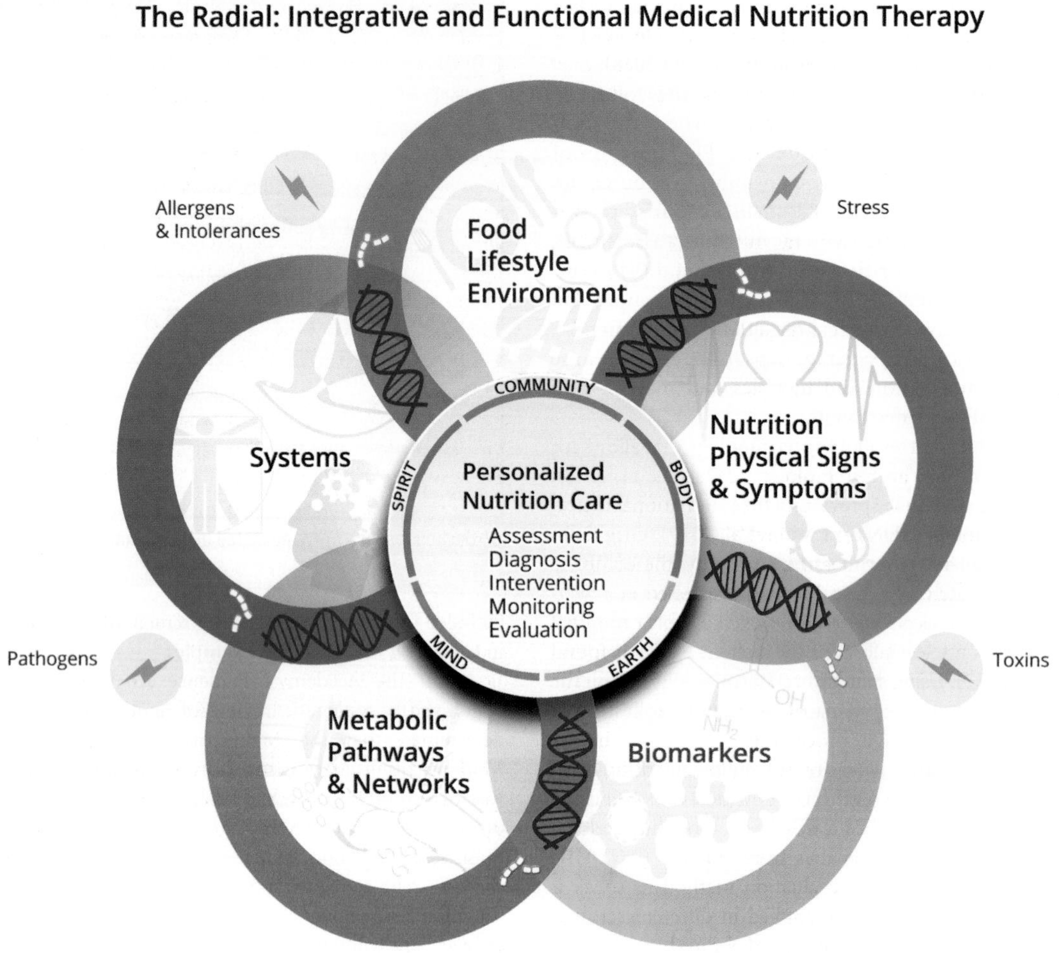

The Radial: Integrative and Functional Medical Nutrition Therapy

Fig. 9.1 The Integrative and Functional Medicine Radial. (Copyright 2010. 2018. KM Swift, D Noland and E. Redmond.)

specific problem or problems that can be resolved or improved through nutrition intervention by a nutrition and dietetics professional (Swan et al, 2017). Clients with nutrition diagnoses may be at higher risk for nutrition-related complications, such as increased morbidity, increased length of hospital stay, and infection with or without complications. Nutrition-related complications can lead to a significant increase in costs associated with hospitalization, lending support to the early diagnosis of nutrition problems followed by prompt intervention (AND, 2015).

The process of aggregating assessment data and using critical thinking to determine important and relevant nutrition diagnoses should also lead to the identification of the "cause" or etiology of the problem. For example, while assessing a client with significant recent weight loss, the RDN may discover that the person is food insecure because of a lack of money or food assistance. Although the RDN can diagnose "unintended weight loss" and begin providing a high calorie diet to the client during a hospital stay, this treatment will not resolve the root cause of the diagnosis (lack of food in the home). Conversely, by provision of nutrition education to the client while in the hospital and enrolling the client into a food assistance program such as Meals on Wheels after he or she gets home, the RDN may prevent the diagnosis from reoccurring. Identification of the etiology is not always possible; however, when it is, it allows for greater understanding of the conditions in which the diagnosis came about and allows for an individualized intervention. Additionally, when the etiology cannot be changed, the focus

of the interventions should be directed at managing or lessening the signs and symptoms of the nutrition problem.

Many facilities use standardized formats to facilitate communication of nutrition diagnoses. The nutrition diagnosis is documented using the problem, etiology, signs, and symptoms (PES) format in a simple, clear statement. A basic rule of the NCPT is that the problem must be a nutrition diagnosis term from the NCPT without deviations (verbatim). Correct application of the NCPT supports standardized documentation and consequent aggregation of related data for research, reporting, and analytics. For example, "inadequate energy intake" (an official NCPT nutrition diagnostic term) will have to be documented and not a similar variation of it such as "lack of sufficient caloric consumption." In some instances there are formally accepted synonyms, and these can be used interchangeably. For example, "food- and nutrition-related knowledge deficit" may be replaced by "limited food and nutrition related knowledge." The etiology component can be either an NCP term or a free-text explanation of the root cause of the problem. When constructing a PES statement, it is advised to use the nutrition diagnosis etiology matrix (available in the NCPT) to identify whether the selected nutrition problem is matched to the selected etiology category (AND, 2017a). The nutrition diagnosis etiology matrix is a table that categorizes all nutrition diagnosis terms by all described etiology categories (there are 10 etiology categories). It is also important to review carefully the reference sheet (a comprehensive profile of an NCP term) of the selected nutrition diagnosis term to understand the definition of that term, the various etiologies listed, and common signs and symptoms associated with the nutrition problem. (AND, 2017a). These are just some of the fundamental benefits of reviewing the reference sheets. Signs and symptoms should be documented in as specific and quantifiable a manner as possible. For example, it is best practice to write that a client has "lost 15 lbs within the last 3 months" rather than write "recent weight loss." Methods used for documenting nutrition care in the health record are determined at the facility level. RDNs in private practice should also develop a systematic method for documenting care provided. Signs and symptoms listed in the PES statement need to be data already documented in the assessment step. Assessment data that are selected as signs and symptoms and justify/support the nutrition problem constitute the "evidence" component when assessing NCP application completeness (Murphy et al, 2018).

Nutrition Intervention

Nutrition interventions are the actions taken to treat nutrition problems by resolving the etiology and/or reducing/managing the related signs and symptoms. Nutrition intervention involves two steps: planning and implementation. Whenever possible, the nutrition intervention should target the etiology identified during the assessment step of NCP. Thus if the nutrition diagnosis is *Excessive Carbohydrate* and the etiology is *lack of knowledge about high-carbohydrate foods*, then the appropriate intervention could be *Nutrition Education, Priority Modifications* (*education focused on which foods are high in carbohydrate*).

As previously stated, intervention directed at the etiology is not always possible. When the RDN cannot treat the etiology of the nutrition diagnosis directly, the treatment should focus on ameliorating and/or managing the signs and symptoms of the diagnosis. For example, a frequent etiology of malnutrition in hospitalized adult clients is inflammation. The RDN may not be able to intervene directly in the inflammatory process; however, inflammation can increase the client's nutritional needs. Therefore although the RDN may not be able to reduce the inflammation, the RDN can increase the amount of nutrients provided to the client through high-calorie foods, nutritional supplements, or other nutrition support therapies.

During the planning phase of the nutrition intervention, the RDN, client, and others as needed collaborate to identify goals that will signify success of the intervention. Whether in an inpatient or outpatient clinical setting, a significant component of the plan may be the nutrition prescription. A nutrition prescription is a detailed description of the nutrient needs of that particular client. Typically, this can include recommended needs for energy, protein, and fluid but also may include nutrients pertinent to the client's condition such as carbohydrate needs in diabetes, potassium needs in renal disease, or sodium needs in hypertension.

Client-centered goals are set first, and then implementation begins. Interventions may include food and nutrition therapies, nutrition education, counseling, or coordination of care such as providing referral for financial or food resources. Because the care process is continuous, the initial plan may change as the condition of the client changes, as new needs are identified, or if the interventions prove to be unsuccessful.

Interventions should be specific; they are the "what, where, when, and how" of the client's care. For example, in a client with "inadequate oral food or beverage intake," a goal may be to increase portion sizes at two meals per day. This could be implemented through provision of portions that are initially 5% larger with a gradual increase to 25% larger portion sizes. Interventions should be communicated to the health care team and discussed with the client to ensure understanding of the intervention and its rationale, whenever possible. Thorough communication by the RDN increases the likelihood of adherence to the intervention. Box 9.1 presents the NCP applied to a sample client, JW.

The nutrition intervention terminology is organized in five categories (domains) within the NCPT: (1) food and/or nutrient delivery, (2) nutrition education, (3) nutrition counseling, (4) coordination of nutrition care by a professional, and (5) population-based nutrition action. Interventions can occur in all settings. For example, a woman with little knowledge of heart-healthy foods may need a group class on cooking or an educational session on changing the type of fats in her diet (nutrition education). An RDN working for the Women Infant and Children (WIC) clinic may counsel a pregnant woman on initiating breastfeeding as an intervention (nutrition counseling). A clinical RDN may write orders for initiation and progression of enteral feeding for a child with cystic fibrosis (food and/or nutrient delivery). The RDN may communicate to the social worker the nutrition needs for a client post discharge to ensure that the client continues to improve (coordination of nutrition care). As an example of a population-based nutrition action, an RDN working at the lobbying level may aim to achieve legislative action to facilitate supportive infrastructure, guidelines, and regulations for farm-to-table initiatives.

All of these are types of interventions that RDNs may plan and implement.

Monitoring and Evaluation of Nutrition Care

The fourth step in the NCP involves monitoring and evaluation of the effect of nutrition interventions. This clarifies the effect that the RDN has in the specific setting, whether health care, education, consulting, food services, or research. During this step, the RDN first determines indicators that should be monitored. These indicators should match the signs and symptoms identified during the assessment process. For example, if excessive sodium intake was identified during the assessment, then an evaluation of sodium intake against criteria (a comparative standard or a mutually agreed goal level) is needed at a designated time for follow-up.

In the clinical setting the objective of nutrition care is to achieve and maintain optimal nutrition status for the client or population being served; thus interventions must be monitored and progress toward goals or criteria must be evaluated frequently. This ensures that unmet goals are addressed, and care is evaluated and modified in a timely manner. Evaluation of the monitored indicators provides objective data to demonstrate effectiveness of nutrition interventions, regardless of the setting or focus. If goals are written in measurable terms, evaluation is relatively easy because a change in the indicator is compared with the status of the indicator before implementation of the nutrition intervention.

An example in clinical practice is the sample case in Box 9.1. Here, monitoring and evaluation include weekly reviews of nutritional intake, including an estimation of energy intake. If intake was less than the goal of 1800 kcal, the evaluation may be: "JW was not able to increase his calorie intake to 1800 kcal because of his inability to cook and prepare meals for himself." This also points to a missed nutrition diagnosis: JW does not have access to tools and supplies needed to cook for himself. A revision in the care plan and implementation at this point may include the following: "JW will be provided a referral to local agencies (Meals on Wheels) that can provide meals at home." The new diagnosis and intervention then are implemented with continued monitoring and evaluation to determine whether the new goal can be met.

When evaluation reveals that goals are not being met or that new needs have arisen, the process begins again with reassessment, identification of new nutrition diagnoses, and formulation of a new NCP cycle. For example, in JW's case, during his hospitalization, high-calorie snacks were provided. However, monitoring reveals that JW's usual eating pattern does not include snacks, and thus he was not consuming them when in the hospital. The evaluation showed these snacks to be an ineffective intervention. JW agrees to a new intervention: the addition of one more food to his meals. Further monitoring and evaluation

BOX 9.1 Applying the Nutrition Care Process for Patient JW

JW is a 70-year-old male who was admitted to the hospital for mitral valve replacement surgery. JW lives alone in his own home. JW is a widower and states that he hasn't been able to prepare meals for the past 6 months. The nutrition risk screen reveals that he has lost weight without trying and has been eating poorly for several weeks before admission, leading to referral to the RDN. Client reports 15 lb weight loss in the last 3 months.

Assessment (Step 1)
Chart review, client interview, and nutrition-focused physical examination reveal the following:

Biomedical Data, Medical Tests and Procedures
Glucose and electrolytes: WNL
Albumin: 3.8 g/dL
Cholesterol/triglycerides: WNL

Anthropometric Measurements
Height: 70"
Admission weight: 130 lb (15 lb weight loss over 3 months)
Usual Body Weight: 145 lb
BMI: 18.3 < 18.5

Food/Nutrition-Related History
Food intake: Client reports indicate estimated intake of 1200 kcal/day, irregular meals, drinks 4-6 cups of coffee per day.

Client History
History of hypertension, thyroid dysfunction, asthma, prostate surgery
Medications: Inderal, Lipitor, and levothyroxine
New widower; reports depression and loneliness without his wife
Has some social support from neighbors and community center but states he doesn't like to ask for help
Comparative standard: 1600 kcal (based on 25-30 kcal/kg current body weight)

Nutrition Diagnosis (Step 2)
Basic critical thinking: JW has been consuming fewer calories than required and has little interest in eating. There is support available in the community but JW doesn't like to "impose" on others.
RDN diagnoses nutrition problems and establishes objectives for his care.

PES Statements
- Unintended weight loss *related to* self-reported depression *as evidenced by* 10% weight loss in 3 months and reported intake of less than 75% of estimated requirements.
- Inadequate oral intake *related to* self-reported depression *as evidenced by* estimated inadequate energy intake, reported intake less than 75% of estimated requirements, weight loss of 15 lbs in 3 months.
- Limited access to food *related to* lack of food planning and purchasing skills *as evidenced by* estimated inadequate energy intake (less than 75% of estimated requirements), weight loss of 15 lbs in 3 months, and current BMI = 18.3.

Method to Progress to Nutrition Intervention
Identification of the nutrition diagnoses allows the RDN to focus the nutrition intervention on treatment of the cause of the problem (in this case the missing meals). As a reminder the nutrition intervention consists of two parts planning and implementation. A nutrition prescription and a collection of supporting goals may comprise the planning portion of the intervention (Step 3). Goal setting to establish short-term and long-term plans are often

needed. In the education process the client and the RDN must jointly establish achievable goals. Goals should be expressed in behavioral terms and stated in terms of what the patient will do or achieve when the goals are met. Goals should reflect the educational level and the economic and social resources available to the client and the family.

Nutrition Intervention (Step #3)
Plan
Nutrition prescription: 1800 kcal regular diet

Overall goals
Provide diet to meet JW's needs during hospitalization
Monitor weight
Refer to social services following discharge

Short-Term Goal
During the hospitalization, JW will maintain his current weight; after discharge he will begin to slowly gain weight up to a target weight of 145 lb.

Implementation:
While in the hospital, JW will include nutrient-dense foods in his diet, especially if his appetite is limited.

Coordination of Nutrition Care by a Nutrition Professional:
Nursing to weigh patient daily.

Nutrition Education – Content: Priority modifications:
Educate patient on importance of adequate energy intake to meet nutrient needs to prevent further weight loss until he is able to return to adequate oral intake.
Verbalize understanding of Nutrition Education—Content: Priority modifications for current course of dietary intake to prevent further weight loss.

Long-Term Goal
JW will modify diet to include adequate calories through the use of nutrient-dense foods to prevent further weight loss and eventually promote weight gain.

Implementation:
After discharge, JW will attend a local senior center for lunch on a daily basis to help improve socialization and caloric intake.

Coordination of Nutrition Care by a Nutrition Professional:
Social worker to coordinate referral to local senior center.

Method to monitor progress and evaluation
Choosing the means for monitoring if the interventions and nutritional care activities have met the goals is important. Evaluation of the monitoring criteria will provide the RDN with information on outcomes, and this should occur over time. Finally, documentation is important for each step of the process to ensure communication between all parties.

For JW, weekly weight measurements and nutrient intake analyses are required while he is in the hospital and biweekly weight measurements are taken at the senior center or clinic when he is back at home. If nutrition status is not improving, which in this case would be evidenced by JW's weight records, and the goals are not being met, it is important to reassess JW and perhaps develop new goals for new implementation approaches.

Monitoring and Evaluation (Step 4)
Indicator: energy intake
Criteria: 1800 kcal/day, will monitor energy intake weekly
Indicator: body weight
Criteria: target weight: 145 lb, will monitor weight weekly during hospital stay

PES, Problem, etiology, and signs and symptoms; *RDN*, registered dietitian nutritionist; *WNL*, within normal limits.

will be needed to ascertain if this new intervention improves his intake. The monitoring and evaluation step may function as the stepping stone for reassessment. In this fashion, the NCP is not static but continues to a next cycle of steps using prior information and relevant, new information that has been identified and informs next NCP steps.

Evidence-Based Guidelines

In health care, providers must use the best available evidence in caring for clients. The Center for Evidence Based Medicine defines evidence-based practice as "the conscientious, explicit and judicious use of current best evidence in making decisions about the care of individual patients." Best evidence includes properly designed and executed prospective, randomized controlled trials (PRCT), systematic reviews of the literature, and meta-analysis to support decisions made in practice (CEBM, 2014; Sackett et al, 1996). Evidence-based guidelines (EBGs) are developed by first conducting a systematic review and then using the conclusion of the systematic review to develop practice-based guidelines. A work group of subject matter experts and specially trained analysts work together to evaluate the research and to develop recommendations for client care. These guidelines give providers a summary of the best available evidence by which to conduct their practice.

Appropriate use of EBGs may lead to improved quality of care. RDNs must be able to evaluate the EBG and determine whether a guideline is appropriate in a given situation for a given client. Many health care professional organizations and practice specialties have developed EBGs. Because of potential significant differences in quality and applicability, RDNs must be able to evaluate these guidelines.

In the 1990s, the Academy began developing nutrition practice guidelines and evaluating how guideline use affected clinical outcomes; diabetes management was among the first clinical situations examined. These evidence-based nutrition practice guidelines (EBNPGs) are disease- and condition-specific recommendations with corresponding toolkits. The EBNPGs include major recommendations, background information, and a reference list. To assist the RDN in implementing the EBNPG into their routine care, the guidelines are organized by the NCP steps as appropriate, and NCPT is used in guidelines and within the toolkits (Papoutsakis et al, 2017).

EBNPGs and associated toolkits assist nutrition and dietetics professionals to provide effective nutrition care, especially for clients with diabetes and early stages of chronic kidney disease (CKD). Medical nutrition therapy (MNT) provided by a Medicare Part B licensed provider can be reimbursed when the EBNPGs are used and all procedural forms are documented properly and coded (Parrott et al, 2014). Benefits of nutrition therapy can be communicated to physicians, insurance companies, administrators, or other health care providers using evidence provided from these guidelines.

To define professional practice by the RDN, the Academy published a Scope of Dietetics Practice Framework, a Code of Ethics, and the Standards of Professional Performance (SOPPs) (AND, 2018). Specialized standards for knowledge, skills, and competencies required to provide care at the generalist, specialist, and advanced practice level for a variety of populations are now complete for many areas of practice.

The Academy's EAL is a credible and current resource to answer questions that arise during provision of nutrition care. Use of the EAL may protect the professional and the public from the consequences of ineffective care. These guidelines are extremely valuable for educating students, staff orientation, competence verification, and training of RDNs.

Accreditation and Surveys

Accreditation by The Joint Commission (TJC) and other accrediting agencies involves review of the systems and processes used to deliver health care along with evaluation of actual care processes. TJC survey teams evaluate health care institutions to determine the level of compliance with established minimum standards. For example, TJC requires that nutrition screening be completed within 24 hours of admission to acute care but does not mandate a method to accomplish screening. However, policies must be applied consistently and must reflect commitment to provision of high-quality, timely nutrition services to all clients.

The "Care of the Patient" section of the TJC Accreditation Manual for Hospitals contains standards that apply specifically to medication use, rehabilitation, anesthesia, operative and other invasive procedures, and special treatments, as well as nutrition care standards. The focus of the nutrition standards of care is provision of appropriate nutrition care in a timely and effective manner using an interdisciplinary approach. Appropriate care requires screening of clients for nutrition needs, assessing and reassessing client needs, developing a nutrition care plan, ordering and communicating the diet order, preparing and distributing the diet order, monitoring the process, and continually reassessing and improving the nutrition care plan. A facility can define who, when, where, and how the process is accomplished, but TJC specifies that a qualified dietitian must be involved in establishing this process. A plan for the delivery of nutrition care may be as simple as providing a regular diet for a client who is not at nutritional risk or as complex as managing enteral feedings in a ventilator-dependent client, which involves the collaboration of multiple disciplines.

RDNs are involved actively in the survey process. Standards set by TJC play a large role in influencing the standards of care delivered to clients in all health care disciplines. For more information, see the TJC website.

Dietitians also are involved with surveys from other regulatory bodies, such as a state or local health department, a department of social services, or licensing organizations. Introduction of diagnostic-related groups (DRG) in the mid-1980s led to decreasing acute care length of stay (LOS). However, some clients who no longer need acute hospital care but are not ready to care for themselves at home are admitted to "subacute" care units (these are often called rehabilitation units) that are regulated by Centers for Medicare and Medicaid Services (CMS). Subacute units also undergo an annual review by CMS. (See Chapter 19 for more information.)

Sentinel events are unanticipated events that involve death, serious physical or psychologic injury, or the risk thereof (TJC, 2017). When there is a sentinel event, the outcomes must be documented in the medical record and there must be clinical and administrative follow-up to document steps taken to prevent recurrence of the event. Regardless of the source of the survey, clinicians must follow all regulations and guidelines at all times and not just when a survey is due.

DOCUMENTATION IN THE NUTRITION CARE RECORD

MNT and other nutrition care provided must be documented in the health or medical record. The health record is a legal document; if interventions are not recorded, it is assumed that they have not occurred. Documentation affords the following advantages:

- It ensures that nutrition care will be relevant, thorough, and effective by providing a record that identifies the problems and sets criteria for evaluating the care.
- It allows the entire health care team to understand the rationale for nutrition care, the means by which it will be provided, and the role each team member must play to reinforce the plan and ensure its success.

The health record serves as a tool for communication among members of the health care team. Most health care facilities are using or in the process of implementing electronic health records (EHRs) to document client care, store and manage laboratory and test results, communicate with other entities, and maintain information related to an individual's health. During the transition to EHRs, those using paper documentation maintain paper charts that typically include sections for physician orders, medical history and physical examinations,

TABLE 9.2 Evaluation of a Note in SOAP Format

	Outstanding 2 Points	Above Expectations 1 Point	Below Expectations 0 Points	Score
DATE & TIME		Present	Not present	
S (SUBJECTIVE) Tolerance of current diet Reports of wt loss or appetite decrease Chewing or swallowing difficulties Previously unreported food allergies Pertinent diet history information	Pertinent components documented Captures essence of pt's perception of medical problem	Accurately summarizes most of the pertinent information	One or more pertinent elements missing	
O (OBJECTIVE) Diet order √ Pt dx Ht, wt, DBW, % DBW √ UBW, % UBW Pertinent laboratory values √ Diet-related meds Estimated nutrient needs (EER & protein)	All necessary elements documented accurately	Necessary elements documented No more than one item missing or irrelevant data documented	One or more pertinent elements omitted and irrelevant data documented	
A (ASSESSMENT) S + O = A Nutritional status assessed Appropriateness of current diet order noted Interpretation of abnormal laboratory values (to assess nutritional status) Comments on diet history (if appropriate) Comments on tolerance of diet (if appropriate) Rationale for suggested changes (if appropriate)	Sophisticated assessment drawn from items documented in S & O Appropriate conclusions drawn	Appropriate, effective assessment, but not based on documentation in S & O	Unacceptable assessment or no assessment Disease pathophysiologic findings documented as assessment of nutritional status	
DATE, SIGNATURE & CREDENTIALS		Present	Not present	

DBW, Desired body weight; *Dx,* diagnosis; *EER,* estimated energy requirements; *F/U,* follow up; *ht,* height; *PO,* by mouth; *PRN,* as necessary; *pt,* patient; *Rx,* prescription; *SOAP,* subjective, objective, assessment, plan; *TF,* tube feeding; *TPN,* total parenteral nutrition; *UBW,* usual body weight; *wt,* weight.
Courtesy Sara Long, PhD, RDN.

laboratory test results, consults, and progress notes. Although the format of the health record varies depending on facility policies and procedures, in most settings all professionals document care in the medical record. The RDN must ensure that all aspects of nutrition care are summarized succinctly in the medical record. The NCPT developed by the Academy is used to document the NCP in several countries around the world including Australia, Canada, China, Denmark, Sweden, New Zealand, Norway, and Taiwan (AND, 2017a).

Medical Record Charting

Problem-oriented medical records (POMR) are used in many facilities. The POMR is organized according to the client's primary problems. Entries into the medical record can be done in many styles. A common form is the subjective, objective, assessment, plan (SOAP) note format (Table 9.2).

The assessment, diagnosis, interventions, monitoring, evaluation (ADIME) format reflects the steps of the NCP (Box 9.2; Table 9.3).

BOX 9.2 Chart Note Using ADIME

Nutrition Assessment
- Pt is 66-year-old woman admitted with heart failure
- Ht: 162 cm; Wt: 56 kg; IBW: 52-58 kg
- Laboratory values within normal limits
- Estimated energy needs: 1570-1680 kcal (28-30 kcal/kg/day)
- Estimated protein needs: 56-73 g protein (1-1.3 g/kg/day)
- Current diet order is "Regular - no added salt" with pt consuming 95% of meals recorded
- Consult for nutrition education received

Nutrition Diagnosis
- Food- and nutrition-related knowledge deficit related to lack of prior nutrition-related education on low sodium diet as evidenced by client reports no prior education provided, new Heart Failure medical diagnosis.

Nutrition Intervention
Plan:
- Nutrition prescription: 1600 kcal/day no added salt (3 g Na) diet

Implementation:
Nutrition education – Content: Priority modifications:
- Provided client with written and verbal instruction on a no added salt diet (3 g) diet.
- Client verbalized understanding of Nutrition Education – Content: Priority Modifications for current salt restriction (3 g Na) to manage heart failure.
- To develop and provide client 1-day menu using dietary restrictions.
Coordination of Nutrition Care by a Nutrition Professional:
- Provided contact information for outpatient clinic.

Monitoring and Evaluation
- Indicator: dietary Na intake
- Criteria: 3 g Na/day via 24 hr dietary recall
J Wilson, MS, RDN 1/2/18

ht, height; *IBW,* ideal body weight; *wt,* weight.

TABLE 9.3 Evaluation of a Note in ADIME Format

	Outstanding 2 Points	Above Expectations 1 Point	Below Expectations 0 Points	Score
DATE & TIME		Present	Not present	
A (ASSESSMENT) Reports of wt loss or appetite decrease Chewing or swallowing difficulties Previously unreported food allergies Pertinent diet history information Estimated nutrient needs (EER & protein) Diet order √ Pt dx Ht, wt, DBW, % DBW √ UBW, % UBW if appropriate Pertinent laboratory values √ Diet-related meds	Pertinent components documented Captures essence of pt's perception of medical problem	Accurately summarizes most of the pertinent information	One or more pertinent elements missing or irrelevant data documented	
D (NUTRITION DIAGNOSIS) Written in PES statement(s) using standardized language for the nutrition care process	Necessary PES statement(s) stated accurately & prioritized	No more than one item missing	Not written in PES statement format or standardized language not used Medical dx listed as nutrition dx	
I (INTERVENTION) Aimed at etiology (cause) of nutr dx; can be directed at reducing effects of signs & symptoms Planning: prioritize nutr dx, jointly establish goals w/ pt, define nutrition Rx, identify specific nutr interventions Implementation: action phase, includes carrying out & communicating plan of care, continuing data collection & revising nutr intervention as warranted based on pt's response	Appropriate & specific plan(s) AND implementation to remedy nutr dx documented	Plans or implementation missing Vague plans or intervention documented	MD's orders documented as intervention, or inappropriate plan or intervention documented.	
M (MONITORING) & E (EVALUATION) Determines progress made by pt & if goals are being met Tracks pt outcomes relevant to nutr dx Can be organized into one or more of following: Nutr-Related Behavioral & Environmental Outcomes Food & Nutrient Intake Outcomes Nutr-Related Physical Sign & Symptom Outcome Nutr-Related Pt-Centered Outcome	Appropriate nutr care outcomes relevant to nutr dx & intervention plans & goals documented. Nutr care outcomes defined, specific indicators (can be measured & compared with established criteria) identified	No more than one item missing	Nutr care outcome not relevant to nutr dx, intervention, or plans/ goals. Nutr care outcomes cannot be measured or compared with established criteria.	
DATE, SIGNATURE & CREDENTIALS		Present	Not present	

ADIME, Assessment, diagnosis, intervention, monitoring, evaluation; *DBW,* desirable body weight; *dx,* diagnosis; *EER,* estimated energy requirement; *ht,* height; *MD,* medical doctor; *meds,* medications; *nutr,* nutrition; *PES,* problem, etiology, signs and symptoms; *pt,* patient; *Rx,* prescription; *UBW,* usual body weight; *w/,* with; *wt,* weight.
Courtesy Sara Long, PhD, RDN.

See Table 9.4 for examples of nutrition diagnostic (PES) statements. However, each client and situation is different, and the NCP should be individualized appropriately.

Documentation must be accurate, clear, and concise and must be able to convey important information to the physician and other health care team members. All entries made by the RDN should address the issues of nutrition status and needs. Those using EHRs must use great caution when using "copy and paste" functions to document care.

Electronic Health Records and Nutrition Informatics

Beginning in the 1990s, costs for computer memory decreased, hardware became more portable, and computer science advanced to make computers and technology a permanent fixture in health care.

Additional impetus to change standard practice came with publication of several Institute of Medicine (IOM) reports that brought to light a high rate of preventable medical errors along with the recommendation to use technology as a tool to improve health care quality and safety (Institute of Medicine, 2000).

Clinical information systems used in health care are known by different names; although some use electronic medical record (EMR), electronic health record (EHR), and personal health record (PHR) interchangeably, there are important differences. An EHR describes information systems that contain all the health information for an individual over time regardless of the care setting. An EMR is a clinical information system used by a health care organization to document client care during one episode of care or admission. EHRs and EMRs are maintained by health care providers or organizations. In contrast, the PHR is a system used by individuals to maintain health information. A PHR can be web or paper based or integrated into a facility's EMR. Information in the PHR is controlled by the person, not the provider or health care organization.

EHRs include all of the information typically found in a paper-based documentation system along with tools such as clinical decision support, electronic medication records, computerized provider order entry, and alert systems that support clinicians in making decisions regarding client care. Current government regulations include requirements to implement and "meaningfully use" EHRs to enter, store, retrieve, and manage information related to client care. Dietitians must have at least a basic understanding of technology and health information management to ensure a smooth transition from paper to EHR and to use effectively the powerful tools provided by a well-designed EHR. Such transitions include development of nutrition screens for client admission, documentation, information sharing, decision support tools, and order entry protocols. Customization capabilities vary depending on vendor contracts and facility requirements. Because it can take several years to implement an EHR, RDNs managing nutrition services must be involved in EHR system decisions from the very beginning. The Academy's EHR toolkit, which is available on the eNCPT website, is an important resource to help RDNs communicate effectively their specific EHR needs (AND, 2017a). Also, there are standards that have been developed to "spell-out" what RDNs need to have included in the EHR in order to apply the NCP. The Academy has developed such a standard by the name of Electronic Nutrition Care Process Record System (ENCPRS) (Health Level Seven International, 2010). In paper and electronic formats, health records and the information contained are vital conduits for communicating client care to others, providing information for quality evaluation and improvement, and serving as a legal document. RDN documentation includes information related to NCPs. Documentation must follow the facility policy and be brief and concise while accurately describing actions taken to those authorized to view the record. Fig. 9.2 shows how a computerized health record may look when using the ADIME method.

Current efforts are focused on ensuring that health information stored in clinical information systems can be exchanged safely and securely between providers and facilities. Systems that are able to share information seamlessly are "interoperable." Although this concept seems simple on the surface, problems with interoperability can be very difficult and expensive to overcome. RDNs in private practice and ambulatory care must ensure that systems they are using have the capability to share health information.

The transition from paper health records to EHRs is facilitated by thorough planning, training, and support. Many health care professionals do not have sufficient experience with health care technology to understand the practice improvement that can be realized with proper implementation and use of technology. Others may resist any change in the workplace that interrupts their current workflow. These clinicians are not resisting change because they are afraid of technology; instead, resistance is based on real or imagined fears that technology will impede their workflow or hinder client care.

INFLUENCES ON NUTRITION AND HEALTH CARE

The health care environment has undergone considerable change related to the provision of care and reimbursement in the last decade. Governmental influences, cost containment issues, changing demographics, and the changing role of the client as a "consumer" have influenced the health care arena. The United States currently spends more on health care than any other nation, yet health care outcomes lag far behind those seen in other developed nations. Exponential increases in health care costs in the United States have been a major impetus for drives to reform how health care is provided and paid for in the United States.

Confidentiality and the Health Insurance Portability and Accountability Act

Privacy and security of personal information are a concern in all health care settings. In 1996 Congress passed the Health Insurance Portability and Accountability Act (HIPAA) (Centers for Medicare and Medicaid Services, 2018). The initial intent of HIPAA was to ensure that health insurance eligibility is maintained when people change or lose jobs. The Administrative Simplification provisions of HIPAA require development of national standards that maintain privacy of electronically transmitted protected health information (PHI). In 2013 the HIPAA Omnibus Rule expanded client rights to their own health information, strengthened rules surrounding privacy and confidentiality of PHI, and increased penalties for unauthorized sharing or loss of PHI (U.S. Department of Health and Human Services, 2015).

HIPAA requires that health care facilities and providers (covered entities) take steps to safeguard PHI. Although HIPAA does not prevent sharing of client data required for care, clients must be notified if their medical information is to be shared outside of the care process, or if protected information (e.g., address, email, income) is to be shared. Violations of HIPAA rules have resulted in large fines, loss of jobs, and criminal prosecution. In an effort to avoid the serious repercussions of HIPAA violations, health care institutions have implemented mandatory annual education on HIPAA for each employee.

Payment Systems

One of the largest influences on health care delivery in the last decade has been changes in health care payment methods. There are several common methods of reimbursement: private insurance, cost-based reimbursement, negotiated bids, and DRGs. DRG codes is a collection of codes that determines how much money Medicare and some health insurance agencies will pay for a patient's hospital stay. Under the DRG system, a facility receives payment for a client's admission based on the principal diagnosis, secondary diagnosis (comorbid conditions), surgical procedure (if appropriate), and the age and gender of the client. Approximately 500 DRGs cover the entire spectrum of medical diagnoses and surgical treatments. Preferred-provider organizations (PPOs) and managed-care organizations (MCOs) also are changing health care. MCOs

TABLE 9.4   Sample PES Statements Based on Medical Diagnosis*

Medical Diagnosis	Nutrition Diagnosis** (Problem)	Etiology (E)	Signs/Symptoms (S)
Obesity	Obesity	Excessive energy intake and physical inactivity	Current weight 175% desired body weight, BMI 38 kg/m², reported overconsumption of energy-dense food and large amounts of computer use and other sedentary activities
	Excessive energy intake	Food and nutrition-related knowledge deficit concerning energy intake	Diet history; intake approximately 150% estimated requirements, and BMI 38 kg/m²
	Physical inactivity	Time constraints	Reports of 8-10 hours of daily screen time (computer and television), BMI > 30
Cancer	Unintended weight loss	Decreased ability to consume sufficient energy	Cancer chemotherapy, reports of nausea and poor intake (<50% of estimated needs), weight loss of 10% usual body weight within 30 days
	Inadequate oral intake	Decreased ability to consume sufficient energy	Nausea from chemotherapy, weight loss of 10% usual body weight within 30 days, reports of insufficient intake of energy from diet (<50% of estimated needs).
Newly diagnosed type 2 diabetes	Food- and nutrition-related knowledge deficit	Lack of prior nutrition-related education	New medical diagnosis of Type 2 Diabetes Mellitus, and measured fasting glucose of 230 mg/dL
Major trauma GI surgery with complications	Altered GI function	Decreased ability to consume sufficient energy	Intubation after GI surgery, NPO × 48 hours.
Anorexia nervosa	Disordered eating pattern	Environmental-related obsessive disorder to be thin	BMI<17.5, estimated energy intake <25% of estimated needs at least 7 days before admission, and anorexia nervosa
Heart failure	Excessive fluid intake	Cardiac dysfunction	Heart Failure, reported estimated fluid intake 150% more than physician-ordered restriction
	Inability to manage self-care	Food- and nutrition-related knowledge deficit concerning self-care	Three admissions for fluid overload in past 2 months, Congestive Heart Failure
Dysphagia	Limited food acceptance	Decreased ability to consume sufficient energy	Reports of inadequate intake (<75% of estimated needs), inability to consume most foods served
	Swallowing difficulty	Cerebrovascular accident	Dysphagia, abnormal swallow study, decreased estimated food intake (<75% of estimated needs).
Referral for social services	Limited access to food	Lack of financial resources	Lack of resources for food, Patient/SWS reports disqualified from SNAP program

*These are only examples. Each client is different; each nutrition problem diagnosed by the RDN has an etiology and signs/symptoms that are unique to that client.
**Each client may have more than one nutrition diagnosis.

finance and deliver care through a contracted network of providers in exchange for a monthly premium, changing reimbursement from a fee-for-service system to one in which fiscal risk is borne by health care organizations and physicians.

The Patient Protection and Affordable Care Act (PPACA) was signed into law by President Obama on March 23, 2010. PPACA is the most significant change to the U.S. health care system since the 1965 passage of legislation that created Medicare and Medicaid. The goal of PPACA or the Affordable Care Act (ACA) is to ensure that affordable health insurance is available to all Americans. ACA uses several methods to improve access to health insurance including subsidies, state insurance exchanges, and assurance of coverage for preexisting conditions (U.S. Government Publishing Office, 2010) (see *Clinical Insight*: The ACA: How Does Nutrition Fit?)

Quality Management

To contain health care costs while providing efficient and effective care that is consistently of high quality, practice guidelines, or standards of care, are used. These sets of recommendations serve as a guide for defining appropriate care for a client with a specific diagnosis or medical problem. They help ensure consistency and quality for providers and clients in a health care system and, as such, are specific to an institution or health care organization. Critical pathways, or care maps, identify essential elements that should occur in the client's care and define a timeframe in which

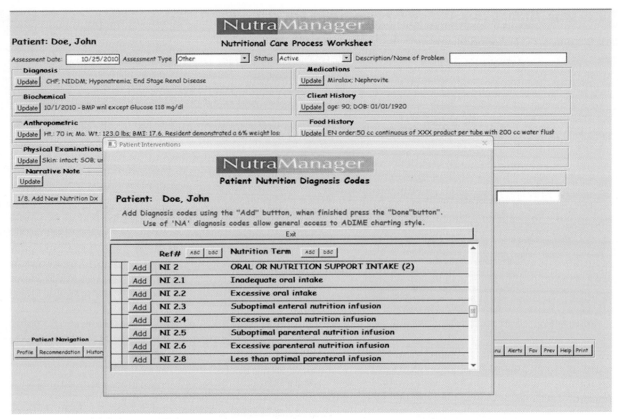

Fig. 9.2 Example of electronic chart note using drop-down boxes on computer. (Courtesy Maggie Gilligan, RDN, owner of NUTRA-MANAGER, 2010.)

each activity should occur to maximize client outcomes. They often use an algorithm or flowchart to indicate the necessary steps required to achieve the desired outcomes. Disease management is designed to prevent a specific disease progression or exacerbation and to reduce the frequency and severity of symptoms and complications. Education and other strategies maximize compliance with disease treatment. Educating a client with type 1 diabetes regarding control of blood glucose levels would be an example of a disease management strategy aimed at decreasing the complications (nephropathy, neuropathy, and retinopathy) and the frequency with which the client needs to access the care provider. Decreasing the number of emergency room visits related to hypoglycemic episodes is a sample goal.

Patient-Centered Care and Case Management

The case management process is aimed at achieving client care goals in a cost-effective, efficient manner. It is an essential component in delivering care that provides a positive experience for the client, ensures optimal clinical outcomes, and uses resources wisely. Case management involves assessing, evaluating, planning, implementing, coordinating, and monitoring care, especially in clients with chronic disease or those who are at high risk. In some areas, dietitians have added skill sets that enable them to serve as case managers. Client-centered care has become a movement in the United States that puts more decision making in the hands of the consumer. It places more emphasis on outcomes, sometimes at the expense of physician autonomy (Bardes, 2012). In long-term care the goal is focused on ensuring dignity as well as choice (see Chapter 19).

Utilization management is a system that strives for cost efficiency by eliminating or reducing unnecessary tests, procedures, and services. Here, a manager usually is assigned to a group of clients and is responsible for ensuring adherence to pre-established criteria.

The patient-centered medical home (PCMH) is a new development that focuses on the relationship between the client and personal physician. The personal physician takes responsibility for coordinating health care for the client and coordinates and communicates with other providers as needed. Other providers such as nurses, dietitian nutritionists, health educators, and allied health professionals may be called on by the client or personal physician for preventive and treatment services. When specialty care is needed, the personal physician becomes responsible for ensuring that care is seamless and that transitions between care sites go smoothly. The RDN should be considered part of the medical home treatment plan.

Regardless of model, the facility must manage client care prudently. Nutrition screening can be important in identifying clients who are at nutrition risk. Early identification of these factors allows for timely intervention and helps prevent the comorbidities often seen with malnutrition, which may cause the LOS and costs to increase. CMS has identified conditions such as heart failure, heart attack, and pneumonia, to name a few, for which no additional reimbursement will be received if a client is readmitted to acute care within 30 days of a prior admission. Although many view this rule as punitive, it does provide an opportunity for RDNs to demonstrate how nutrition services, including client education, can save money through decreased readmissions.

Other recent developments include "never events." Never events are those occurrences that should never happen in a facility that provides

CLINICAL INSIGHT

The ACA: How Does Nutrition Fit?

To get paid for their services of nutritional counseling under the Affordable Care Act (ACA), registered dietitian nutritionists (RDNs) must gain an understanding of the language and steps involved in reimbursement as well as how to become a provider. According to Medicare standards, a medical nutrition therapy (MNT) provider must have completed the educational and clinical experience required of an RDN (AND, 2018). Next, he or she has to obtain the 10-digit **National Provider Identifier (NPI)**, required for billing and credentialing (a term used by insurance companies, the payers, for enrolling service providers). Credentialing is a binding contract of services, conditions, and diseases for which nutritional counseling will be paid, codes to use, and the fee schedule. The diagnosis code (ICD-10) and Common Procedure Terminology (CPT) are required for billing purposes. The ICD-10 describes the person's medical condition, obtained from the physician, and the CPT documents the procedure performed by the RDN. MNT has been designated as 97802 (initial visit), 97803 (follow-up), 97804 (group [2 or more individuals]) procedural codes that are applicable for nutritional counseling for the ACA.

By researching insurance companies, RDNs can find out if MNT is covered, if RDNs are accepted into network, the covered diagnosis and procedure codes, the limits to MNT, and the fee schedules. The fee schedule is the payment per billing unit (blocks of 15 minutes, or per visit). Plans differ, even if they are offered by the same insurance company.

From changes stimulated by the passage of the ACA, it is evident that the chronic care model is replacing the acute care model. A **chronic care model (CCM)** is a multidisciplinary and multifaceted approach for chronic disease management and prevention, whose premise is the development of self-management skills while enhancing the patients' relationships to their care and the team providing that care (Coleman et al, 2009). With this CCM comes development of the Patient-Centered Medical Home (PCMH), Accountable Care Organizations (ACOs) and Comprehensive Primary Care Initiative Projects (CPCI), which combine PCMH and ACOs. A PCMH's focus is on the patient-provider relationship incorporating the team approach (Boyce, 2012).

After the passage of the ACA, ACOs were formed to provide a team approach for coordinating the care provided by doctors, hospitals, and other allied health providers for Medicare patients. Seven states and regions participate in the CPCI, but it is expected to grow, requiring the dietitian-nutritionist to think beyond the traditional MNT model of fee for service, to comprehensive care and new areas of practice, such as primary care settings rather than hospitals (AND, 2018). A survey conducted in 2014 demonstrated that RDNs have inadequate awareness (about 40%) of and poor participation (20%) in the PCMH, which adds to the urgency for RDNs to become educated about the ACA and their activity in its implementation (AND, 2014).

Patricia Davidson DCN, MS, RDN, CDE

Academy of Nutrition and Dietetics: *Payment* (website): https://www.eatrightpro.org/payment.
Academy of Nutrition and Dietetics: *PCMH/ACO Workgroup report, June 2014* (website https://www.eatrightpro.org/-/media/eatrightpro-files/practice/patient-care/pcmhaco_workgroup_report_final.pdf?la=en&hash=3FF564E9CA95ADBEE19293B7F7D2D464C4AA27BD.
Boyce B: Paradigm shift in health care reimbursement: a look at ACOs and bundled service payments, *J Acad Nutr Diet* 112:974, 2012.
Coleman K et al: Evidence on the Chronic Care Model in the new millennium, *Health Aff* 28:75, 2009.

high-quality, safe, people-centered care (PCC). CMS will not reimburse facilities for additional costs of care related to "never events." RDNs must pay attention to new or worsening pressure ulcers and central line infections as potential "never events."

Staffing

Staffing also affects the success of nutrition care. Clinical RDNs may be centralized (all are part of a core nutrition department) or decentralized (individual dietitians are part of a unit or service that provides care to clients), depending on the model adopted by a specific institution. Certain departments such as food service, accounting, and human resources remain centralized in most models because some of the functions for which these departments are responsible are not related directly to client care. Dietitians should be involved in the planning for any redesign of client care (see *Focus On*: Nutrition Standardized Language and Coding Practices). The methods of the *Registered Dietitian Staffing and Productivity Benchmarking Study* is an important resource on how a staffing model could be applied to determine RDN staffing requirements (Hand et al, 2015).

◎ FOCUS ON

Nutrition Standardized Language and Coding Practices

The history of the International Classification of Diseases (ICD) can be traced to the mid-1600s and the London Bills of Mortality. It was not until the late 1800s that ICD codes were introduced in health care. The ICD coding system has been revised and updated several times and is used by most countries. Because ICD initially was developed as a system to track causes of death, its use for coding medical diagnoses has been criticized. The United States has been using ICD-10 since October 2015.

Medical records departments review medical records and assign codes to the medical diagnoses based on specific findings documented by health care providers as well as complicating factors ("comorbidities") to determine reimbursement rates. Commonly, pulmonary, gastrointestinal, endocrine, mental disorders, and cancer can lead to malnutrition as a comorbid factor. Thus coordinated nutrition care and coding for malnutrition are important elements in patient services.

A study by Parrott et al (2014) found that self-employed RDNs are more likely to be reimbursed by private or commercial payers, and RDNs working in clinic settings are more likely to be reimbursed by Medicare. RDNs must know and be accountable for the business and clinical side of their nutrition practices (Parrott et al, 2014).

In private practice, use of correct codes and following payers' claims processing policies and procedures are essential. For example, an NPI is a 10-digit number that is required on claims. To apply for an NPI, RDNs can complete the online application at the NPPES website.

ICD, International Classification of Disease; *NPI*, National Provider Identifier; *NPPES*, National Plan and Provider Enumeration System; *RDN*, registered dietitian nutritionist.

NUTRITION INTERVENTIONS

The RDN is responsible for provision of food and nutrition services that are reliable and highly individualized. RDNs are responsible for using evidence-based practice that is not compromised by market forces.

The evaluation of general and modified diets requires in-depth knowledge of the nutrient content of foods. In particular, it is essential to be aware of the nutrient-dense foods that contribute to dietary adequacy and to be able to recommend how foods can be fortified to increase their nutrition value (see *Focus On*: Food First in Chapter 19.). A knowledge of protein-rich foods required for healing is also essential. As outlined in the later disease-focused chapters, balance and professional judgment are needed. For example, sometimes a person with healing needs also has kidney dysfunction so the amount of protein and type of protein recommended is more complex.

Interventions: Food and Nutrient Delivery

The nutrition prescription, written by the RDN, designates the type, amount, and frequency of nutrition based on the individual's disease process and disease management goals. The prescription may specify a caloric level or other restriction to be implemented. It also may limit or increase various components of the diet, such as carbohydrate, protein, fat, alcohol, fiber, water, specific vitamins or minerals, bioactive substances such as phytonutrients, or probiotics. RDNs write the nutrition prescription after the diagnosis of nutrition problems.

The CMS issued a rule in 2014 that allows RDNs employed in hospitals to enter diet orders independently into a client's health record, without requiring the supervision or approval of a physician or other practitioner (Centers for Medicare and Medicaid Services, 2014). Specifically, RDNs are permitted to become privileged by hospital medical staff to enter independent diet orders (and optionally order laboratory tests to monitor effectiveness of dietary plans and orders) subject to state laws governing licensing and scope-of-practice. The process of obtaining ordering privileges requires medical staff or review board evaluation of each practitioner's qualifications and demonstrated competency to perform these tasks. Recent information shows that providing nutrition-related order-writing privileges (OWPs) to RDNs enhances the quality of client care, improves related outcomes, and controls costs associated with provided care (Phillips and Doley, 2017). In states where licensure laws or other regulations preclude RDNs from ordering diets directly, the nutrition prescription should be conveyed to the responsible licensed health care provider (e.g., physicians, physician assistants, and advanced practice nurses) to approve and enter the appropriate orders for oral diet, oral nutritional supplements, and enteral or parenteral nutrition. The ability to enter orders does not absolve the RDN of the need to communicate and coordinate care with the provider who is ultimately responsible for all aspects of client care.

Therapeutic or modified diets are based on a general, adequate diet that has been altered to provide for individual requirements, such as digestive and absorptive capacity, alleviation or arrest of a disease process, and psychosocial factors. In general, the therapeutic diet should vary as little as possible from the individual's normal diet. Personal eating patterns and food preferences should be recognized, along with socioeconomic conditions, religious practices, and any environmental factors that influence food intake, such as where the meals are eaten and who prepares them (see "Cultural Aspects of Dietary Planning" in Chapter 10).

A nutritious and adequate diet can be planned in many ways. One foundation of such a diet is the chooseMyPlate Food Guidance System described in Chapter 10. This is a basic plan; additional foods or more of the foods listed are included to provide additional energy and increase the intake of required nutrients for the individual. The Dietary Guidelines for Americans also are used in meal planning and to promote wellness. The dietary reference intakes (DRIs) and specific nutrient recommended dietary allowances are formulated for healthy persons, but they also are used as a basis for evaluating the adequacy of therapeutic diets. Nutrient requirements specific to a particular person's genetic makeup, disease state, or disorder always must be taken into account during diet planning.

Modifications of the Normal Diet

Normal nutrition is the foundation on which therapeutic diet modifications are based. Regardless of the type of diet prescribed, the purpose of the diet is to supply needed nutrients to the body in a form that it can handle. Adjustment of the diet may take any of the following forms:

- Change in consistency of foods (liquid diet, pureed diet)
- Increase or decrease in energy value of diet (weight-reduction diet, high-calorie diet)
- Increase or decrease in the type of food or nutrient consumed (sodium-restricted diet, lactose-restricted diet, fiber-enhanced diet, high-potassium diet)
- Elimination of specific foods (MSG-free, gluten-free diet)
- Adjustment in the level, ratio, or balance of protein, fat, and carbohydrate (diet for blood sugar control, ketogenic diet, renal diet, high protein diet)
- Rearrangement of the number and frequency of meals (diet for someone elderly, postgastrectomy diet)
- Change in route of delivery of nutrients (enteral or parenteral nutrition)

Diet Modifications in Hospitalized Clients

Food is an important part of nutrition care. Attempts must be made to honor client preferences during illness and recovery from surgery. This means that the client must be involved in the decision to follow a therapeutic diet. Imagination and ingenuity in menu planning are essential when planning meals acceptable to a varied client population. Attention to color, texture, composition, and temperature of the foods, coupled with a sound knowledge of therapeutic diets, are required for menu planning. However, to the client, good taste and attractive presentation are most important. When possible, client choices of food are most likely to be consumed. The ability to make food selections gives the client an option in an otherwise limiting environment.

Hospitals and long-term care facilities are required to adopt a nutrition care manual that serves as the reference for the diets served in the facility. For this purpose, the Academy has developed online nutrition care manuals (AND, 2018c). All hospitals or health care institutions have basic, routine diets designed for uniformity and convenience of service. These standard diets are based on the foundation of an adequate diet pattern with nutrient levels as derived from the DRIs. Types of standard diets vary but generally can be classified as general or regular or modified in consistency. The diets should be realistic and meet the nutritional requirements of the clients. The most important consideration of the type of diet offered is providing foods that the client is willing and able to eat and that accommodate any required dietary modifications. Shortened lengths of stay in many health care settings result in the need to optimize intake of calories and protein, and this often translates into a liberal approach to therapeutic diets. This is especially true when the therapeutic restrictions may compromise intake and subsequent recovery from surgery, stress, or illness.

Regular or General Diet

"Regular" or "general" diets are used routinely and serve as a foundation for more diversified therapeutic diets. In some institutions a diet that has no restrictions is referred to as the regular or house diet. It is used when the client's medical condition does not warrant any limitations. This is a basic, adequate, general diet of approximately 1600 to 2200 kcal; it usually contains 60 to 80 g of protein, 80 to 100 g of fat, and 180 to 300 g of carbohydrate. Although there are no particular food restrictions, some facilities have instituted regular diets that are low in saturated fat, sugar, and salt to follow the dietary recommendations for the general population. In other facilities the diet focuses on providing foods the client is willing and able to eat, with less focus on restriction of nutrients. Many institutions have a selective menu that allows the client certain choices; the adequacy of the diet varies based on the client's selections. More recent developments in health care food service include use of "room service" similar to the hotel room service model; clients have complete freedom to choose what and when they will eat.

Consistency Modifications

Modifications in consistency may be needed for clients who have limited chewing or swallowing ability. See Chapter 39 and Appendix 20 for more information on consistency modifications and clients with neurologic changes that require these diets.

Clear liquid diets include some electrolytes and small amounts of energy from tea, broth, carbonated beverages, clear fruit juices, and gelatin. Milk and liquids prepared with milk are omitted, as are fruit juices that contain pulp. Fluids and electrolytes often are replaced intravenously until the diet can be advanced to a more nutritionally adequate one.

Little scientific evidence supports the use of clear liquid diets as transition diets after surgery. The average clear liquid diet contains only 500 to 600 kcal, 5 to 10 g of protein, minimum fat, 120 to 130 g of carbohydrate, and small amounts of sodium and potassium. It is inadequate in calories, fiber, and all other essential nutrients and should be used only for short periods. In addition, full liquid diets also are not recommended for a prolonged time. If needed, oral supplements may be used to provide more protein and calories and could be offered as liquids with which to take medications if appropriate.

Food Intake

Food served does not necessarily represent the actual intake of the client. Prevention of malnutrition in the health care setting requires observation and monitoring of the adequacy of client intake. This nutrient intake analysis is described in Chapter 4. If food intake is inadequate, measures should be taken to provide foods or supplements that may be better accepted or tolerated. Regardless of the type of diet prescribed, the food served and the amount actually eaten must be considered to obtain an accurate determination of the client's energy and nutrient intake. Snacks and calorie-containing beverages consumed between meals also are considered in the overall intake. The RDN must maintain communication with nursing and food service personnel to determine adequacy of intake.

Acceptance and Psychologic Factors

Meals and between-meal snacks are often highlights of the day and are anticipated with pleasure by the client. Mealtime should be as positive an experience as possible. In whatever setting the client is eating, it should be comfortable for the client. Food intake is encouraged in a pleasant room with the client in a comfortable eating position in bed or sitting in a chair located away from unpleasant sights or odors. Eating with others often promotes better intake.

Arrangement of the tray should reflect consideration of the client's needs. Dishes and utensils should be in a convenient location. Independence should be encouraged in those who require assistance in eating. The caregiver can accomplish this by asking clients to specify the sequence of foods to be eaten and having them participate in eating. Even visually impaired persons can eat unassisted if they are told where to find foods on the tray. For clients who require eating assistance it is important that food be served when a caregiver is ready to assist so the foods are at an optimal temperature. Occupational therapists are helpful for recommending special utensils (such as weighted spoons) and for developing a plan for eating independence.

Poor acceptance of foods and meals may be caused by unfamiliar foods, a change in eating schedule, improper food temperatures, the client's medical condition, or the effects of medical therapy. Food acceptance is improved when personal selection of menus is encouraged.

Clients should be given the opportunity to share concerns regarding meals, which may improve acceptance and intake. The attitude of the caregiver is important for encouraging acceptance of a therapeutic diet. The nurse who understands that the diet contributes to the restoration of the client's health communicates this conviction by actions, facial expressions, and conversation. Clients who understand that the diet is important to the success of their recovery usually accept it more willingly. When the client must adhere to a therapeutic dietary program indefinitely, a counseling approach helps him or her achieve nutritional goals (see Chapter 13). Because they have frequent contact with clients, nurses and nursing assistants play an important role in a client's acceptance of nutrition care. Ensuring that the nursing staff is aware of the client's nutrition care plan can greatly improve the probability of success.

Interventions: Nutrition Education and Counseling

Nutrition education is an important part of nutrition care provided to individuals and populations. The goal of nutrition education is to help the client acquire the knowledge and skills needed to make changes, including modifying behavior to facilitate sustained change. Nutrition education and dietary changes can result in many benefits, including management of the disease or symptoms, improved health status, enhanced quality of life, and decreased health care costs.

As the average length of hospital stays has decreased, the role of the inpatient dietitian in educating inpatients has changed to providing brief education or "survival skills." This education includes the types of foods to limit, timing of meals, and portion sizes. Many clients now transfer to a rehabilitation facility to complete their recovery to lower the cost of care. RDNs are able to follow them for longer periods of time and are able to continue nutrition counseling started in the hospital. Follow-up outpatient counseling should be encouraged at discharge. See Chapter 12 for managing nutrition support and Chapter 13 for counseling.

Intervention: Coordination of Care

Nutrition care is part of discharge planning. Education, counseling, and mobilization of resources to provide home care and nutrition support are included in discharge procedures. Completing a discharge nutritional summary for the next caregiver is imperative for optimal care. Appropriate discharge documentation includes a summary of nutrition therapies and outcomes; pertinent information such as weights, laboratory values, and dietary intake; relevant drug-nutrient interactions; expected progress or prognosis; and recommendations for follow-up services. Types of therapy attempted and failed can be very useful information. The amount and type of instruction given, the client's comprehension, and the expected degree of adherence to the prescribed diet are included. An effective discharge plan increases the likelihood of a positive outcome for the client.

Regardless of the setting to which the client is discharged, effective coordination of care begins on day 1 of a hospital or nursing home stay and continues throughout the institutionalization. The client should be included in every step of the planning process whenever possible to ensure that decisions made by the health care team reflect the desires of the client.

When needed, the RDN refers the client to other caregivers, agencies, or programs for follow-up care or services. For example, use of the home-delivered meal program of the Older Americans Act Nutrition Program traditionally has served frail, homebound, older adults, yet studies show that older adults who have been discharged recently from the hospital may be at high nutritional risk but not referred to this service (Sahyoun et al, 2010; see Chapter 19). Thus the RDN plays an essential role in making the referral and coordinating the necessary follow-up.

NUTRITION FOR THE TERMINALLY ILL OR HOSPICE CLIENT

Maintenance of comfort and quality of life are most typically the goals of nutrition care for the terminally ill client. Dietary restrictions are rarely appropriate. Nutrition care should be mindful of strategies that facilitate symptom and pain control. Recognition of the various phases of dying—denial, anger, bargaining, depression, and acceptance—will help the health care professional understand the client's response to food and nutrition support.

The decision as to when life support should be terminated often involves the issue of whether to continue enteral or parenteral nutrition. With advance directives, the client can advise family and health care team members of individual preferences with regard to end-of-life issues. Food and hydration issues may be discussed, such as whether tube feeding should be initiated or discontinued, and under what circumstances. Nutrition support should be continued as long as the client is competent to make this choice (or as specified in the client's advance directives).

In advanced dementia, the inability to eat orally can lead to weight loss (see Chapter 19). One clear goal-oriented alternative to tube feeding may be the order for "comfort feeding only" to ensure an individualized eating plan (Palecek et al, 2010). Palliative care encourages the alleviation of physical symptoms, anxiety, and fear while attempting to maintain the client's ability to function independently.

Hospice home care programs allow terminally ill clients to stay at home and delay or avoid hospital admission. Quality of life is the critical component. Indeed, individuals have the right to request or refuse nutrition and hydration as medical treatment. RDN intervention may benefit the client and family as they adjust to issues related to the approaching death. Families who may be accustomed to a modified diet should be reassured if they are uncomfortable about easing dietary restrictions. Ongoing communication and explanations to the family are important and helpful. RDNs should work collaboratively to make recommendations on providing, withdrawing, or withholding nutrition and hydration in individual cases and serve as active members of institutional ethics committees. The RDN, as a member of the health care team, has a responsibility to promote use of advanced directives of the individual client and to identify their nutritional and hydration needs. Quality of life and other Patient Reported Outcome Measures (PROMs) are becoming increasingly important as a concrete approach to monitor PCC.

CLINICAL CASE STUDY

Mr. B, a 47-year-old white male, 6 ft 2 in tall and weighing 200 lb, is admitted to the hospital with chest pain. Three days after admission, at patient care rounds, it is discovered that Mr. B has gained 30 pounds over the last 2 years. Review of the health record reveals the following laboratory data: LDL is 240 mg/dL (desirable 130), HDL is 30 mg/dL (desirable 50), triglyceride is 350 mg/dL (desirable <200). Blood pressure is 120/85. Current medications: multivitamin/mineral daily. Cardiac catheterization is scheduled for tomorrow. Diet history reveals frequent consumption of high-fat foods. 24-hour recall: 3200 kcal and 150 g of fat.

Nutrition Diagnostic Statements
- Altered nutrition-related laboratory values related to undesirable food choices as evidenced by elevated LDL and low HDL, and diet history of frequent consumption of high-fat foods.
- Excessive fat and energy intake related to consumption of high-fat foods at all meals as evidenced by 24-hour recall of 3200 kcal and 150 g of fat.

Nutrition Care Questions
1. What other information do you need to develop a nutrition care plan?
2. Was nutrition screening completed in a timely manner? Discuss the implications of timing of screening versus implementing care.
3. Develop a chart note, using ADIME format, based on this information and the interview you conduct with the client.
4. What nutrition care goals would you develop for this client during his hospital stay?
5. What goals would you develop for this client after discharge? Discuss how the type of health care insurance coverage the client has might influence this plan.

HDL, High-density lipoprotein; *LDL,* low-density lipoprotein.

USEFUL WEBSITES

Academy of Nutrition and Dietetics
Academy of Nutrition and Dietetics Health Informatics Infrastructure
Centers for Medicare and Medicaid Services
electronic Nutrition Care Process Terminology (eNCPT)
Nutrition Care Manual
The Joint Commission

REFERENCES

Academy of Nutrition and Dietetics: *About eNCPT*, 2018a. Available at: www.ncpro.org.

Academy of Nutrition and Dietetics: *Abridged Nutrition Cate Process Terminology* (NCPT), *reference manual,* ed 2017, Chicago, 2017, Academy of Nutrition and Dietetics.

Academy of Nutrition and Dietetics: *Terminology submission instructions,* 2018b. Available at: www.ncpro.org/terminology-submission-process.

Academy of Nutrition and Dietetics, Evidence Analysis Library: NSCR: *adult nutrition screening tool comparison (2009),* 2010. Available at: www.andeal.org/topic.cfm?menu=3584.

Academy of Nutrition and Dietetics, Evidence Analysis Library: *Medical nutrition therapy effectiveness systematic review (2013–15),* 2015. Available at: www.andeal.org/topic.cfm?menu=5284&cat=3676.

Academy of Nutrition and Dietetics: *Nutrition care manual,* 2018c. Available at: www.nutritioncaremanual.org.

Academy of Nutrition and Dietetics Quality Management Committee: Academy of Nutrition and Dietetics: revised 2017 standards of practice in nutrition care and standards of professional performance for registered dietitians, *J Acad Nutr Diet* 118:132–140.e15, 2018.

Bardes CL: Defining "patient-centered medicine", *N Engl J Med* 366:782–783, 2012.

Centers for Medicare and Medicaid Services: *HIPAA general information*, 2018. Available at: www.cms.gov/Regulations-and-Guidance/Administrative-Simplification/HIPAA-ACA/index.html.

Centre for Evidence-Based Medicine: *What is evidence based medicine*, 2014. Available at: http://www.cebm.net/.

Centers for Medicare & Medicaid Services: *Rules and regulations – medicare and medicaid programs; regulatory provisions to promote program efficiency, transparency, and burden reduction; part II – final rule - pages 27105-27157 (FR DOC # 2014-10687)*, 2014. Available at: https://www.gpo.gov/fdsys/pkg/FR-2014-05-12/pdf/2014-10687.pdf.

Hakel-Smith N, Lewis NM, Eskridge KM: Orientation to nutrition care process model standards improves nutrition care documentation by nutrition practitioners, *J Am Diet Assoc* 105:1582–1589, 2005.

Hand RK, Jordan B, DeHoog S, et al: Inpatient staffing needs for registered dietitian nutritionists in 21st century acute care facilities, *J Acad Nutr Diet* 115:985–1000, 2015.

Health Level Seven International: *Electronic Nutrition Care Process Record System (ENCPRS) functional profile*, 2010. Available at: http://www.hl7.org/special/committees/projman/searchableprojectindex.cfm?action=edit&ProjectNumber=706.

Institute of Medicine Committee on Quality of Health Care in America: *To err is human: building a safer health system*, Washington, DC, 2000, National Academies Press.

Joint Commission: *Sentinel event policy and procedures*, 2017. Available at: http://www.jointcommission.org/Sentinel_Event_Policy_and_Procedures/.

Murphy WJ, Steiber AL: A new breed of evidence and the tools to generate it: introducing ANDHII, *J Acad Nutr Diet* 115:19–22, 2015.

Murphy WJ, Yadrick MM, Steiber AL, et al: Academy of Nutrition and Dietetics Health Informatics Infrastructure (ANDHII): a pilot study on the documentation of the nutrition care process and the usability of ANDHII by registered dietitian nutritionists, *J Acad Nutr Diet*, 118: 1966–1974, 2018.

Palecek EJ, Teno JM, Casarett DJ, et al: Comfort feeding only: a proposal to bring clarity to decision-making regarding difficulty with eating for persons with advanced dementia, *J Am Geriatr Soc* 58:580–584, 2010.

Papoutsakis C, Moloney L, Sinley RC, et al: Academy of Nutrition and Dietetics methodology for developing evidence-based nutrition practice guidelines, *J Acad Nutr Diet* 117:794–804, 2017.

Parrott JS, White JV, Schofield M, et al: Current coding practices and patterns of code use of registered dietitian nutritionists: the Academy of Nutrition and Dietetics 2013 coding survey, *J Acad Nutr Diet* 114:1619-1629.e5, 2014.

Phillips W, Doley J: Granting order-writing privileges to registered dietitian nutritionists can decrease costs in acute care hospitals, *J Acad Nutr Diet* 117:840–847, 2017.

Sackett DL, Rosenberg WM, Gray JA, et al: Evidence based medicine: what it is and what it isn't, *BMJ* 312:71–72, 1996.

Sahyoun NR, Anyanwu UO, Sharkey JR, et al: Recently hospital-discharged older adults are vulnerable and may be underserved by the Older Americans Act nutrition program, *J Nutr Elder* 29:227–240, 2010.

Swan WI, Vivanti A, Hakel-Smith NA, et al: Nutrition care process and model update: toward realizing people-centered care and outcomes management, *J Acad Nutr Diet* 117:2003–2014, 2017.

Swan WI, Pertel DG, Hotson B, et al: Nutrition Care Process (NCP) update part 2: developing and using the NCP terminology to demonstrate efficacy of nutrition care and related outcomes, *J Acad Nutr Diet* 119(5):840–855, 2019. doi:10.1016/j.jand.2018.10.025.

U.S. Department of Health and Human Services: *Omnibus HIPAA rulemaking*, 2015. Available at: www.hhs.gov/hipaa/for-professionals/privacy/laws-regulations/combined-regulation-text/omnibus-hipaa-rulemaking/index.html.

U.S. Government Publishing Office: *Public law 111 – 148 - patient protection and affordable care act*, 2010. Available at: www.gpo.gov/fdsys/granule/PLAW-111publ148/PLAW-111publ148/content-detail.html.

10

Food-Nutrient Delivery: Planning the Diet With Cultural Competence

Lorena Drago, MS, RDN, CDN, CDE
Martin M. Yadrick, MBI, MS, RDN, FAND

KEY TERMS

adequate intake (AI)
daily reference value (DRV)
daily value (DV)
Dietary Guidelines for Americans (DGA)
dietary reference intake (DRI)
estimated average requirement (EAR)
flexitarian
food deserts

food insecurity
functional food
health claim
Healthy Eating Index (HEI)
Lactoovovegetarian
Lactovegetarian
MyPlate Food Guidance System
nutrition facts label

phytochemicals
recommended dietary allowance (RDA)
reference daily intake (RDI)
semivegetarian
tolerable upper intake level (UL)
vegan
vegetarian

An appropriate diet is adequate and balanced and considers the individual's characteristics, such as age and stage of development, taste preferences, and food habits. It also reflects the availability of food, storage and preparation facilities, socioeconomic conditions, cultural practices and family traditions, and cooking skills. An adequate and balanced diet meets all the nutritional needs of an individual for maintenance, repair, living processes, growth, and development. It includes energy and all nutrients in proper amounts and in proportion to each other. The presence or absence of one essential nutrient may affect the availability, absorption, metabolism, or dietary need for others. The recognition of nutrient interrelationships provides further support for the principle of maintaining food variety to provide the most complete diet.

Registered dietitian nutritionists (RDNs) and registered nutrition and dietetic technicians (NDTRs) translate food, nutrition, and health information into food choices and diet patterns for groups and individuals. With increasing knowledge of the relationship between diet and incidence of chronic disease among Americans, the importance of an appropriate diet cannot be overemphasized. In this era of vastly expanding scientific knowledge, food intake messages for health promotion and disease prevention change frequently.

DETERMINING NUTRIENT NEEDS

According to the Food and Nutrition Board (FNB) of the National Academies of Sciences, Engineering, and Medicine, choosing a variety of foods should provide adequate amounts of nutrients. A varied diet also may ensure that a person is consuming sufficient amounts of functional food constituents that, although not defined as nutrients, have biologic effects and may influence health and susceptibility to disease. Examples include foods containing dietary fiber and

carotenoids, as well as lesser known phytochemicals (components of plants that have protective or disease-preventive properties) such as isothiocyanates in Brussels sprouts or other cruciferous vegetables and lycopene in tomato products.

WORLDWIDE GUIDELINES

Numerous standards serve as guides for planning and evaluating diets and food supplies for individuals and population groups. The Food and Agriculture Organization (FAO) and the World Health Organization (WHO) of the United Nations have established international standards in many areas of food quality and safety, as well as dietary and nutrient recommendations. In the United States the FNB has led the development of nutrient recommendations since the 1940s. Since the mid-1990s, nutrient recommendations developed by the FNB have been used by the United States and Canada.

The U.S. Departments of Agriculture (USDA) and Health and Human Services (USDHHS) have a shared responsibility for issuing dietary recommendations, collecting and analyzing food composition data, and formulating regulations for nutrition information on food products. Health Canada is the agency responsible for Canadian dietary recommendations, nutritional health and well-being of Canadians, and evidenced-based nutrition policies and standards. Eating Well with Canada's Food Guide aims to improve health, meet nutrient needs, and reduce the risk of nutrient-related conditions and diseases. In South America, several countries such as Argentina, Brazil, Chile, Uruguay, and Venezuela released dietary guidelines in the late 1990s or early 2000s. Among 27 Latin American and Caribbean countries, 24 have established food-based dietary guidelines. In Latin America and the Caribbean, the dietary guidelines and food guides are changing from a focus solely on undernutrition to now include obesity. The

Mexican dietary guidelines were developed by a group of interdisciplinary experts in the fields of nutrition (including dietetics), food security, and public health convened by the National Academy of Medicine and the National Institute of Public Health to prevent the double burden of malnutrition and obesity and other chronic diseases related to food. The Mexican dietary and physical activity guidelines for the general population emphasize the enjoyment of eating in a family setting; eating whole grains; drinking water and *aguas frescas* (cold beverages made by blending fruit with water or by infusing fruits, seeds or grains, or flower petals with water) without sugar; and avoiding highly processed foods, sweetened beverages, and grain-based desserts. In El Salvador, the Nutrition Division of the Ministry of Health develops the Salvadoran Dietary Guidelines. The dietary guidelines recommend consuming a variety of fresh foods, fruits, vegetables, and avoiding fast foods, fried foods, canned foods, desserts, and sweetened beverages.

The Guatemalan Ministry of Public Health and Social Assistance, in coordination with the National Program of Chronic Noncommunicable Diseases of the Ministry of Public Health and Social Assistance with support from the Pan American Health Organization/WHO, the Nutrition Institute of Central America and Panama, and other institutions developed the Guatemalan Dietary Guidelines. The Guidelines promote a "protective diet," which allows the population to make better decisions to avoid malnutrition while preventing obesity and chronic diseases, such as hypertension and diabetes, among others. The daily recommendations include physical activity and consumption of fruits, vegetables, and two tablespoons of beans with each tortilla as these are economical and healthy foods. To combat malnutrition and anemia, consumption of beef, chicken, liver, or fish is recommended at least twice per week. The Honduran Ministry of Health published the Honduran Dietary Guidelines in 2011 and revised them in 2013. Key messages include eating a variety of foods such as fruits and vegetables daily and beef, fish, or offal at least twice a week to promote growth and strengthen the body. The Dominican Republic Ministry of Public Health, with other public health collaborators, developed the dietary guidelines. The objectives of the dietary guidelines are to promote a healthy diet based on seven food groups to prevent diseases due to deficit or excess in the consumption of food; improve the feeding habits of the Dominican population through the promotion of a healthy and balanced diet; and encourage a healthy lifestyle through the routine practice of physical activity and healthy habits. The Colombian Institute of Family Welfare developed the Colombian Dietary Guidelines, emphasizing the consumption of a variety of food sources; daily intake of fruits, vegetables, and dairy; and physical activity. It encourages the consumption of legumes twice a week and eating organ meats once a week to prevent anemia. Sweetened beverages, "junk food," processed and high-sodium foods, and animal sources of food are discouraged. The Bengoa Foundation for Food and Nutrition published the Venezuelan Dietary Guidelines. The core messages focus on eating a variety of foods in adequate amounts in a family setting with good food and good hygiene practices.

In Australia, the guidelines are available through the National Health and Medical Research Council of the Department of Health. In 1996 the WHO and FAO published guidelines for the development and use of food-based dietary guidelines (FAO/WHO, 1996). On the African continent, dietary guidelines have been developed in Benin, Kenya, Namibia, Nigeria, Seychelles, Sierra Leone, and South Africa. Asian countries, including Bangladesh, India, Indonesia, Malaysia, Nepal, Philippines, Singapore, and Thailand released dietary guidelines in the late 1990s and early 2000s.

Several countries have developed food-based dietary guidelines that are illustrated using images including a pyramid, a house, a

staircase, or a palm tree. In the United States the **MyPlate Food Guidance System**, shown in Fig. 10.1, replaced the previous MyPyramid diagram. For comparison, see Eating Well with Canada's Food Guide as shown in *Clinical Insight*: Nutrition Recommendations for Canadians and Fig. 10.2. Mexico's *El Plato del Bien Comer*, with its five plate sections including one for legumes, is shown in Fig. 10.3. The Healthy Colombian Family Plate *Plato Saludable de la Familia Colombiana* (Fig. 10.4) has a six-section plate that includes animal/vegetable protein, fruits and vegetables, grains and starchy vegetables, sweetened foods and fast foods, fats and oil, and dairy. There is an exercise icon to encourage regular physical activity. The Dominican Republic utilizes the mortar, a staple kitchen tool in the Dominican cuisine. Guatemala and Honduras use a pot containing the recommended food groups in proportion to how much they should be consumed. The Australian Guide for Healthy Eating uses a pie-shaped image with the five food groups represented proportionally in terms of recommended intakes (Fig. 10.5). There is a separate Australian Guide to Health Eating for Aboriginal and Torres Strait Islanders (Fig. 10.6). In Japan, the Ministry of Health, Labour and Welfare and the Ministry of Agriculture, Forestry and Fisheries jointly developed their Dietary Guidelines in 2000, and in 2005 published the "Japanese Food Guide Spinning Top" (with revisions in 2010) to encourage a well-balanced diet (Fig. 10.7). The Chinese Nutrition Society released the latest update to its dietary Pagoda in 2016. The 2016 dietary pagoda is a revision of the 2007 Food Pagoda. Compared with the 2007 version, the number of guidelines is reduced from ten to six (Fig. 10.8). Several other countries use images to illustrate their food-based dietary guidelines, including the

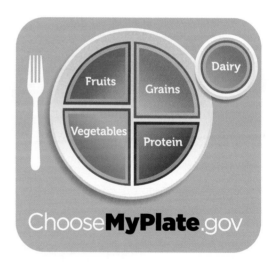

MyPlate Messages

- Find your healthy eating style and maintain it for a lifetime
- Make half your plate fruits and vegetables: vary your veggies, focus on whole fruits
- Make half your grains whole grains
- Move to low-fat or fat-free milk or yogurt
- Vary your protein routine
- Make small changes

Fig. 10.1 MyPlate showing the five essential food groups. (Courtesy the United States Department of Agriculture.) Retrieved from http://www.choosemyplate.gov/.

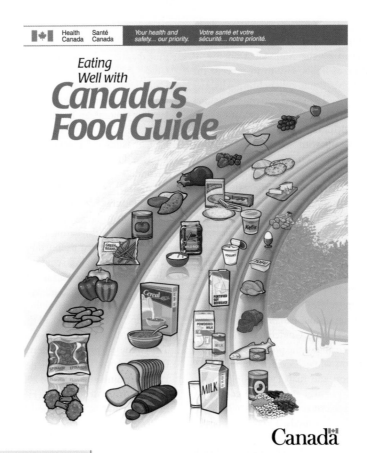

Fig. 10.2 Eating Well with Canada's Food Guide. (Courtesy Health Canada. Data from Health Canada: Eating well with Canada's food guide, Her Majesty the Queen in Right of Canada, represented by the Minister of Health Canada, 2011.) Retrieved from https://www.canada.ca/content/dam/hc-sc/migration/hc-sc/fn-an/alt_formats/hpfb-dgpsa/pdf/food-guide-aliment/view_eatwell_vue_bienmang-eng.pdf.

Make each Food Guide Serving count...
wherever you are – at home, at school, at work or when eating out!

▸ **Eat at least one dark green and one orange vegetable each day.**
- Go for dark green vegetables such as broccoli, romaine lettuce and spinach.
- Go for orange vegetables such as carrots, sweet potatoes and winter squash.

▸ **Choose vegetables and fruit prepared with little or no added fat, sugar or salt.**
- Enjoy vegetables steamed, baked or stir-fried instead of deep-fried.

▸ **Have vegetables and fruit more often than juice.**

▸ **Make at least half of your grain products whole grain each day.**
- Eat a variety of whole grains such as barley, brown rice, oats, quinoa and wild rice.
- Enjoy whole grain breads, oatmeal or whole wheat pasta.

▸ **Choose grain products that are lower in fat, sugar or salt.**
- Compare the Nutrition Facts table on labels to make wise choices.
- Enjoy the true taste of grain products. When adding sauces or spreads, use small amounts.

▸ **Drink skim, 1%, or 2% milk each day.**
- Have 500 mL (2 cups) of milk every day for adequate vitamin D.
- Drink fortified soy beverages if you do not drink milk.

▸ **Select lower fat milk alternatives.**
- Compare the Nutrition Facts table on yogurts or cheeses to make wise choices.

▸ **Have meat alternatives such as beans, lentils and tofu often.**

▸ **Eat at least two Food Guide Servings of fish each week.***
- Choose fish such as char, herring, mackerel, salmon, sardines and trout.

▸ **Select lean meat and alternatives prepared with little or no added fat or salt.**
- Trim the visible fat from meats. Remove the skin on poultry.
- Use cooking methods such as roasting, baking or poaching that require little or no added fat.
- If you eat luncheon meats, sausages or prepackaged meats, choose those lower in salt (sodium) and fat.

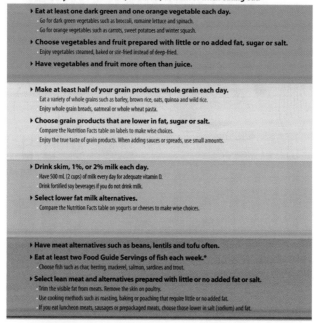

Enjoy a variety of foods from the four food groups.

Satisfy your thirst with water!

Drink water regularly. It's a calorie-free way to quench your thirst. Drink more water in hot weather or when you are very active.

* Health Canada provides advice for limiting exposure to mercury from certain types of fish. Refer to www.healthcanada.gc.ca for the latest information.

Advice for different ages and stages...

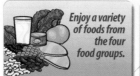

Children

Following *Canada's Food Guide* helps children grow and thrive.

Young children have small appetites and need calories for growth and development.

- Serve small nutritious meals and snacks each day.
- Do not restrict nutritious foods because of their fat content. Offer a variety of foods from the four food groups.
- Most of all... be a good role model.

Women of childbearing age

All women who could become pregnant and those who are pregnant or breastfeeding need a multivitamin containing **folic acid** every day. Pregnant women need to ensure that their multivitamin also contains **iron**. A health care professional can help you find the multivitamin that's right for you.

Pregnant and breastfeeding women need more calories. Include an extra 2 to 3 Food Guide Servings each day.

Here are two examples:
- Have fruit and yogurt for a snack, or
- Have an extra slice of toast at breakfast and an extra glass of milk at supper.

Men and women over 50

The need for **vitamin D** increases after the age of 50.

In addition to following *Canada's Food Guide*, everyone over the age of 50 should take a daily vitamin D supplement of 10 µg (400 IU).

Eat well and be active today and every day!

The benefits of eating well and being active include:
- Better overall health.   - Feeling and looking better.
- Lower risk of disease.   - More energy.
- A healthy body weight.   - Stronger muscles and bones.

Be active

To be active every day is a step towards better health and a healthy body weight.

Canada's Physical Activity Guide recommends building 30 to 60 minutes of moderate physical activity into daily life for adults and at least 90 minutes a day for children and youth. You don't have to do it all at once. Add it up in periods of at least 10 minutes at a time for adults and five minutes at a time for children and youth.

Start slowly and build up.

Eat well

Another important step towards better health and a healthy body weight is to follow *Canada's Food Guide* by:

- Eating the recommended amount and type of food each day.
- Limiting foods and beverages high in calories, fat, sugar or salt (sodium) such as cakes and pastries, chocolate and candies, cookies and granola bars, doughnuts and muffins, ice cream and frozen desserts, french fries, potato chips, nachos and other salty snacks, alcohol, fruit flavoured drinks, soft drinks, sports and energy drinks, and sweetened hot or cold drinks.

Read the label

- Compare the Nutrition Facts table on food labels to choose products that contain less fat, saturated fat, trans fat, sugar and sodium.
- Keep in mind that the calories and nutrients listed are for the amount of food found at the top of the Nutrition Facts table.

Limit trans fat

When a Nutrition Facts table is not available, ask for nutrition information to choose foods lower in trans and saturated fats.

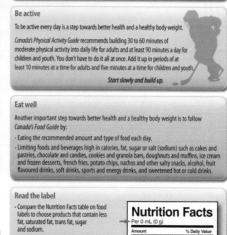

Nutrition Facts		
Per 0 mL (0 g)		
Amount		**% Daily Value**
Calories 0		
Fat 0 g		0 %
Saturates 0 g		0 %
+ Trans 0 g		
Cholesterol 0 mg		
Sodium 0 mg		0 %
Carbohydrate 0 g		0 %
Fibre 0 g		0 %
Sugars 0 g		
Protein 0 g		
Vitamin A 0 %	Vitamin C	0 %
Calcium 0 %	Iron	0 %

Take a step today...

✓ Have breakfast every day. It may help control your hunger later in the day.

✓ Walk wherever you can – get off the bus early, use the stairs.

✓ Benefit from eating vegetables and fruit at all meals and as snacks.

✓ Spend less time being inactive such as watching TV or playing computer games.

✓ Request nutrition information about menu items when eating out to help you make healthier choices.

✓ Enjoy eating with family and friends!

✓ Take time to eat and savour every bite!

For more information, interactive tools, or additional copies visit Canada's Food Guide on-line at:
www.healthcanada.gc.ca/foodguide

or contact:

Publications
Health Canada
Ottawa, Ontario K1A 0K9
E-Mail: publications@hc-sc.gc.ca
Tel.: 1-866-225-0709
Fax: (613) 941-5366
TTY: 1-800-267-1245

Également disponible en français sous le titre :
Bien manger avec le Guide alimentaire canadien

This publication can be made available on request on diskette, large print, audio-cassette and braille.

How do I count Food Guide Servings in a meal?

Here is an example:

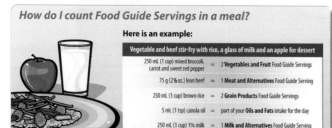

Vegetable and beef stir-fry with rice, a glass of milk and an apple for dessert	
250 mL (1 cup) mixed broccoli, carrot and sweet red pepper	= 2 **Vegetables and Fruit** Food Guide Servings
75 g (2½ oz.) lean beef	= 1 **Meat and Alternatives** Food Guide Serving
250 mL (1 cup) brown rice	= 2 **Grain Products** Food Guide Servings
5 mL (1 tsp) canola oil	= part of your **Oils and Fats** intake for the day
250 mL (1 cup) 1% milk	= 1 **Milk and Alternatives** Food Guide Serving
1 apple	= 1 **Vegetables and Fruit** Food Guide Serving

Fig. 10.2, cont'd

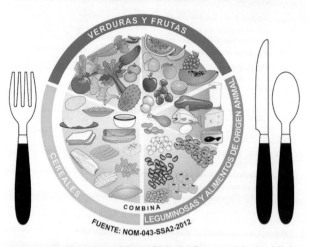

Fig. 10.3 El Plato del Bien Comer (The Plate of Good Eating). (Courtesy Mexico Ministry of Health.) Retrieved from https://www.ciad.mx/notas/item/1409-conozca-el-plato-del-buen-comer.

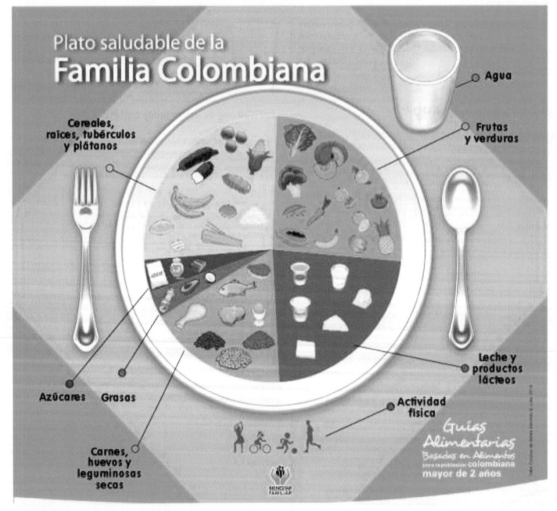

Fig. 10.4 Plato *Saludable de la Familia Colombiana.* Retriebved from https://www.icbf.gov.co/sites/default/files/guias_alimentarias_para_poblacion_colombiana_mayor_de_2_anos_0.pdf.

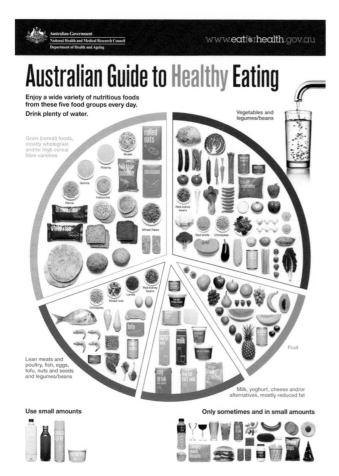

Fig. 10.5 Australian Guide to Healthy Eating. (*Courtesy the Australian Government, National Health and Medical Research Council, Department of Health and Ageing.*) Retrieved from https://www.eatforhealth.gov.au/sites/default/files/content/The%20Guidelines/n55_agthe_large.pdf.

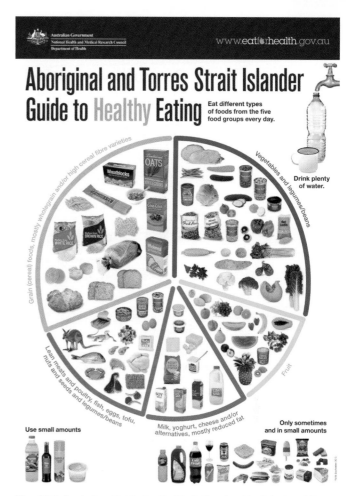

Fig. 10.6 Australian Guide to Health Eating for Aboriginal and Torres Strait Islanders. Retrieved from https://www.eatforhealth.gov.au/sites/default/files/content/The%20Guidelines/final_igthe_a3_poster_-_lr.pdf.

Netherlands (Fig. 10.9), France (Fig. 10.10), Greece (Fig. 10.11), Hungary (Fig. 10.12), Ireland (Fig. 10.13), Saudi Arabia (Fig. 10.14), Slovenia (Fig. 10.15), South Korea (Fig. 10.16), and the United Kingdom (Fig. 10.17). The dietary guidelines from Brazil and Venezuela include mention of the environment in which one eats, the time spent consuming a meal, and the importance of eating in a family setting (Guia alimentar para a população Brasileira, 2015). The Brazilian guidelines also offer advice on choosing fresh or freshly made foods at the grocery store and at restaurants and suggest that the consumer look objectively at food product advertisements.

Dietary Reference Intakes

American standards for nutrient requirements have been the **recommended dietary allowances (RDAs)** established by the FNB of the former Institute of Medicine (IOM), now the National Academy of Medicine.

They were first published in 1941 and most recently revised for certain nutrients in 2019. Each revision incorporates the most recent research findings. In 1993 the FNB developed a framework for the development of nutrient recommendations, called **dietary reference intakes (DRIs)**. Nutrition and health professionals always should use updated food composition databases and tables and inquire whether data used in computerized nutrient analysis programs have been revised to include the most up-to-date information. An interactive DRI

calculator is available at the USDA's website. This can be used to determine an individual's daily nutrient recommendations based on the DRI, including energy, macronutrients, vitamins, and minerals, as well as calculating body mass index (BMI).

DRI Components

The DRI model expands the previous RDA and Canada's Recommended Nutrient Intakes (RNI), which focused only on levels of nutrients for healthy populations to prevent deficiency diseases. To respond to scientific advances in diet and health throughout the life cycle, the DRI model now includes four reference points: **adequate intake (AI)**, estimated average requirement (EAR), RDA, and tolerable upper intake level (UL), as well as acceptable macronutrient distribution ranges (AMDR).

The **AI** is an average daily intake level that is based on observed or experimentally determined approximations of nutrient intake by a group (or groups) of healthy people when sufficient scientific evidence is not available to calculate an RDA. Some key nutrients are expressed as an AI, including potassium (see Chapter 3). The **estimated average requirement (EAR)** is the average daily requirement of a nutrient for healthy individuals based on gender and stage of life. It is the amount of a nutrient with which approximately one-half of individuals would have their needs met and one-half would not. The EAR should be used for assessing the nutrient adequacy of populations but not for individuals.

Text continued on page 175

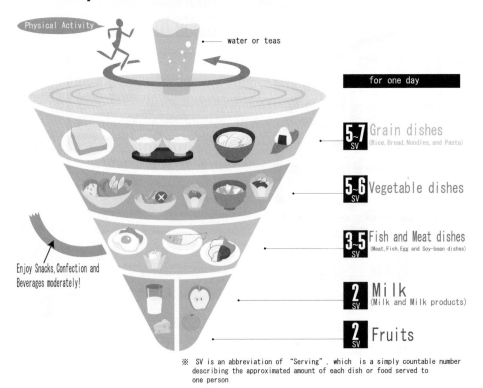

Fig. 10.7 Japanese Food Guide Spinning Top. (Courtesy the Ministry of Health, Labour and Welfare and the Ministry of Agriculture, Forestry and Fisheries.) Retrieved from http://www.mhlw.go.jp/bunya/kenkou/pdf/eiyou-syokuji5.pdf.

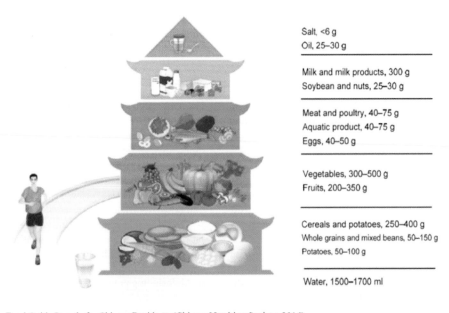

Food Guide Pagoda for Chinese Residents (Chinese Nutrition Society, 2016)

Fig. 10.8 The Food Guide Pagoda for Chinese People Courtesy from the Chinese Nutrition Society. Retrieved from https://www.ncbi.nlm.nih.gov/pmc/articles/PMC5018612/.

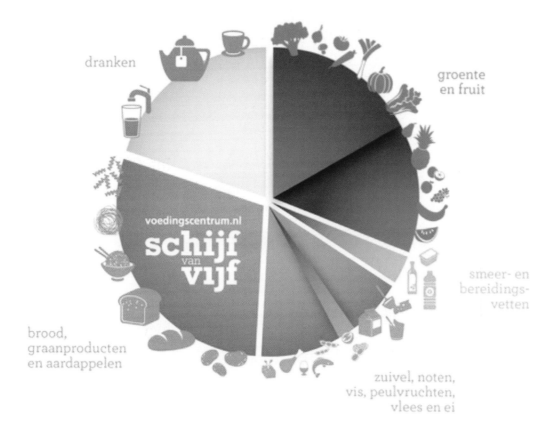

Fig. 10.9 The Wheel of Five (Netherlands). (Courtesy the Netherlands Nutrition Center.) Retrieved from http://www.afvallenkanwel.nl/wp-content/uploads/2010/12/schijfvanvijf.jpg.

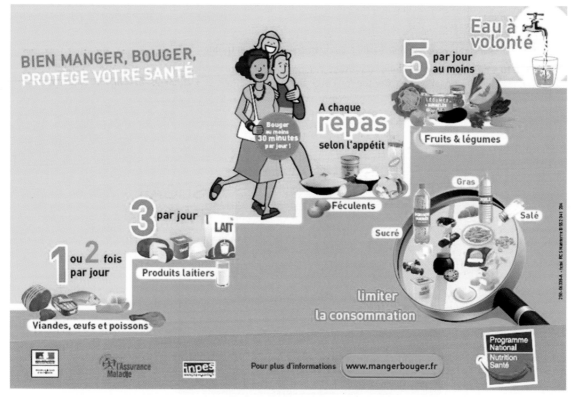

Fig. 10.10 French Stairs. (Courtesy Institut national de prévention et d'éducation pour la santé.) Retrieved from https://www.eufic.org/en/healthy-living/article/food-based-dietary-guidelines-in-europe.

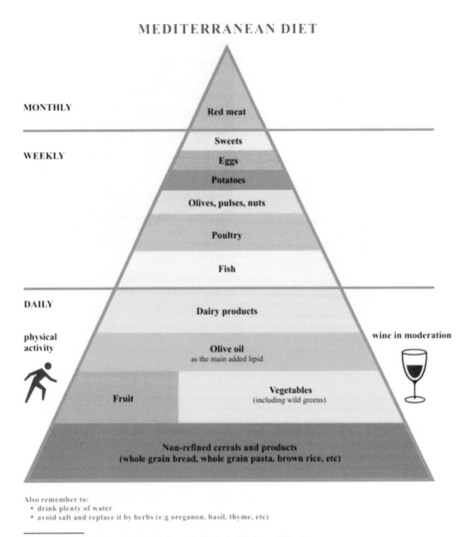

Fig. 10.11 Greek Food Pyramid. (Courtesy National and Kapodistrian University of Athens, School of Medicine-WHO Collaborating Center for Food and Nutrition Policies.) *Archives of Hellenic Medicine*, 1999, 16:516.

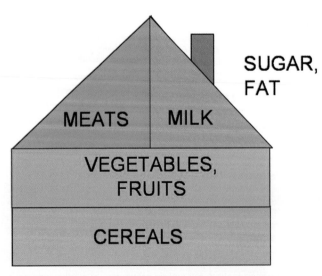

Fig. 10.12 House of Healthy Nutrition—Hungary (Courtesy National Institute for Food and Nutrition Science.) Retrieved from https://www.eufic.org/en/healthy-living/article/food-based-dietary-guidelines-in-europe.

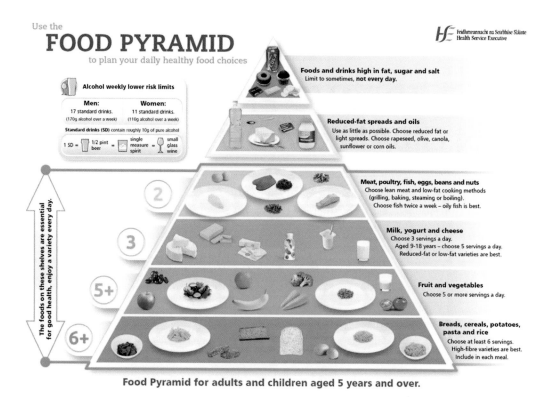

Fig. 10.13 Food Pyramid—Ireland (Courtesy Ireland Department of Health.) Retrieved from https://www.healthpromotion.ie/hp-files/docs/HPM00833.pdf.

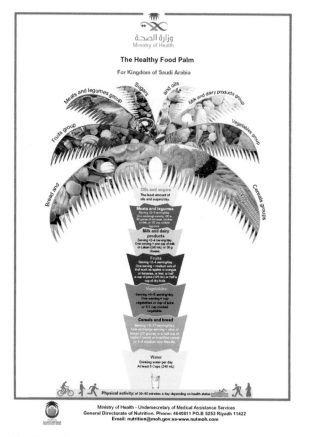

FIG. 10.14 The Healthy Food Palm—For Kingdom of Saudi Arabia. (Courtesy Ministry of Health.) Retrieved from https://www.moh.gov.sa/en/Ministry/MediaCenter/Publications/Documents/.

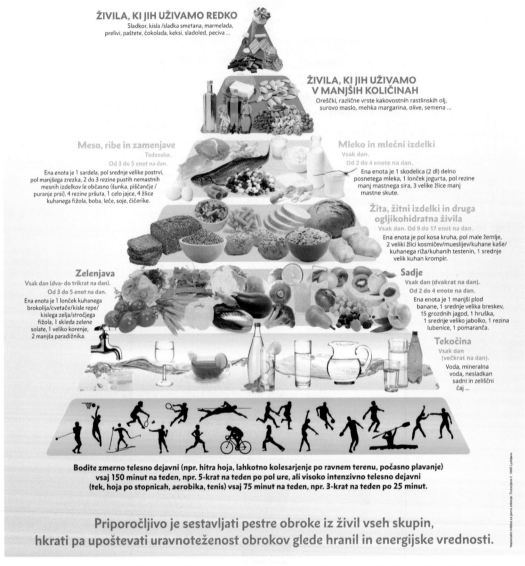

Fig. 10.15 Food Pyramid—Slovenia. (Courtesy National Institute of Public Health. Food Pyramid – Slovenia.) Retrieved from http://www.fao.org/nutrition/education/food-based-dietary-guidelines/regions/countries/slovenia/en/.

Food Balance Wheels

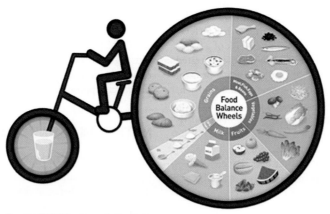

Copyright © 2010 The Korean Nutrition Society.

Fig. 10.16 The Food Balance Wheels—Republic of Korea. (Courtesy Ministry of Health and Welfare, Republic of Korea and the Korean Nutrition Society.) Retrieved from http://www.fao.org/nutrition/education/food-based-dietary-guidelines/regions/countries/republic-of-korea/en/.

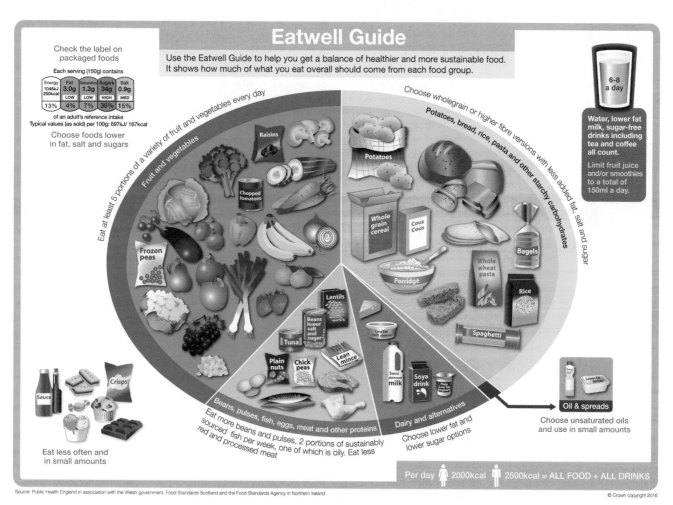

Fig. 10.17 The eatwell guide—United Kingdom. (Courtesy Crown copyright. Public Health England in association with the Welsh government, Food Standards Scotland, and the Food Standards Agency in Northern Ireland.) Retrieved from https://www.nhs.uk/Livewell/Goodfood/Documents/The-Eatwell-Guide-2016.pdf.

The RDA presents the amount of a nutrient needed to meet the requirements of almost all (97% to 98%) of the healthy population of individuals for whom it was developed. An RDA for a nutrient should serve as an intake goal for individuals, not as a benchmark for adequacy of diets of populations. Finally the tolerable upper intake level (UL) was established for many nutrients to reduce the risk of adverse or toxic effects from consumption of nutrients in concentrated forms—either alone or combined with others (not in food)—or from enrichment and fortification. A UL is the highest level of daily nutrient intake that is unlikely to have any adverse health effects on almost all individuals in the general population. The DRIs for the macronutrients, vitamins, and minerals, including the ULs, are presented on the inside covers of this text. The AMDRs are ranges of intakes of macronutrients associated with reduced risk of chronic disease. The AMDRs for fat, carbohydrate, and protein are based on energy intake by age group. See Table 10.1 and the DRI tables on the inside covers of this text.

Target Population

Each of the nutrient recommendation categories in the DRI system is used for specific purposes among individuals or populations. As noted previously, the EAR is used for evaluating the nutrient intake of populations. The AI and RDA can be used for individuals. Nutrient intakes between the RDA and the UL may further define intakes that may promote health or prevent disease in the individual.

Age and Gender Groups

Because nutrient needs are highly individualized depending on age, gender, and the reproductive status of females, the DRI framework has 10 age groupings, including age group categories for children, adolescents, men and women 51 to 70 years of age, and those older than 70 years of age. It separates three age group categories each for pregnancy and lactation—14 to 18 years, 19 to 30 years, and 31 to 50 years of age.

Reference Men and Women

The requirement for many nutrients is based on body weight, according to reference heights and weights that are specific to gender and stage of life. Reference height and weight information used in determining the DRIs was obtained from the Centers for Disease Control and Prevention (CDC)/National Center for Health Statistics (NCHS) growth charts. Although this does not necessarily imply that these weight-for-height values are ideal, at least they make it possible to define recommended allowances appropriate for the greatest number of people.

NUTRITIONAL STATUS OF AMERICANS

Food and Nutrient Intake Data

Information about the diet and nutritional status of Americans and the relationship between diet and health is collected primarily by the CDC via its NCHS and National Health and Nutrition Examination Survey (NHANES).

Unfortunately, gaps still exist between actual consumption and government recommendations in certain population subgroups. Nutrition-related health measurements indicate that overweight and obesity are increasing from lack of physical activity. Data from the combined NHANES and NHANES National Youth Fitness Survey showed that only about 25% of youth ages 12 to 15 engage in moderate to vigorous physical activity for more than 60 minutes daily. In males, this number decreased as weight increased (NHANES, 2012). Hypertension remains a major public health problem in middle-age and older adults and in non-Hispanic blacks in whom it increases the risk of stroke and coronary heart disease (see Chapter 32). Osteoporosis develops more often among non-Hispanic whites than non-Hispanic blacks (see Chapter 23). Concern about preventable conditions, along with an increased emphasis on sustainability, has led to many hospitals taking on the challenge for healthier food intake (see *Focus On*: The "Healthy Food in Health Care" Pledge).

TABLE 10.1 **Acceptable Macronutrient Distribution Ranges**					
NUTRIENT	**AMDR (PERCENTAGE OF DAILY ENERGY INTAKE)**			**AMDR SAMPLE DIET ADULT, 2000-KCAL/DAY DIET**	
	1-3 Years	**4-18 Years**	**>19 Years**	**%Reference***	**g/Day**
Protein[†]	5-20	10.30	10.35	10	50
Carbohydrate	45-65	45-65	45-65	60	300
Fat	30-40	25-35	20-35	30	67
α-Linolenic acid (*omega-3)[‡]	0.6-1.2	0.6-1.2	0.6-1.2	0.8	1.8
Linoleic acid (omega-6)	5-10	5-10	5-10	7	16
Added sugars[§]	≤25% of total calories			500	125

*Suggested maximum.
[†]Higher number in protein AMDR is set to complement AMDRs for carbohydrate and fat, not because it is a recommended upper limit in the range of calories from protein.
[‡]Up to 10% of the AMDR for α-linolenic acid can be consumed as EPA, DHA, or both (0.06%-0.12% of calories).
[§]Reference percentages chosen based on average DRI for protein for adult men and women, then calculated back to percentage of calories. Carbohydrate and fat percentages chosen based on difference from protein and balanced with other federal dietary recommendations.
AMDR, Acceptable macronutrient distribution range; *DHA*, docosahexaenoic acid; *DRI*, dietary reference intakes; *EPA*, eicosapentaenoic acid.
Modified from Food and Nutrition Board, Institute of Medicine: *Dietary reference intakes for energy, carbohydrate, fiber, fat, fatty acids, cholesterol, protein, and amino acids*, Washington, DC, 2002/2005: National Academies Press.

◎ FOCUS ON

The "Healthy Food in Health Care" Pledge

Health care facilities across the nation have recognized that their systems of purchasing, producing, and distributing food may be misaligned with the U.S. dietary guidelines and have joined a movement to change their practices. One organization promoting this plan is called "Health Care Without Harm." In 2009, The American Medical Association (AMA) approved a new policy resolution in support of practices and policies within health care systems that promote and model a healthy and ecologically sustainable food system. The resolution also calls on the AMA to work with health care and public health organizations to educate the health care community and the public about the importance of healthy and ecologically sustainable food systems. Hospitals are using the online pledge form to commit to these nine steps:

1. Work with local farmers, community-based organizations, and food suppliers to increase the availability of locally sourced food.
2. Encourage vendors and/or food management companies to supply food that is, among other attributes, produced without synthetic pesticides and hormones or antibiotics given to animals in the absence of diagnosed disease and food which supports farmer health and welfare and ecologically protective and restorative agriculture.

3. Increase offering of fruit and vegetables, nutritionally dense and minimally processed foods, and unrefined foods and reduce unhealthy (trans and saturated) fats and sweetened foods.
4. Implement a stepwise program to identify and adopt sustainable food procurement. Begin where fewer barriers exist and immediate steps can be taken. For example, the adoption of rBGH-free milk, fair trade coffee, or organic fresh produce in the cafeteria.
5. Communicate to group purchasing organizations an interest in foods that are identified as local and/or third-party certified.
6. Educate patients and community members about nutritious, socially just, and ecological sustainable healthy food practices and procedures.
7. Minimize or beneficially reuse food waste and support the use of food packaging and products which are ecologically protective.
8. Develop a program to promote and source from producers and processors that uphold the dignity of family, farmers, workers, and their communities and support sustainable and humane agriculture systems.
9. Report annually on implementation of this pledge.

Modified from *Health Care without Harm* (website): https://noharm-uscanada.org/content/us-canada/healthy-food-health-care-pledge.

CLINICAL INSIGHT

Nutrition Recommendations for Canadians

The revision to Canada's Food Guide to Healthy Eating, released in 2007, developed age- and gender-specific food intake patterns. These suggested patterns include 4 to 7 servings of vegetables and fruits, 3 to 7 servings of grain products, 2 to 3 servings of milk or milk alternatives, and 1 to 3 servings of meat or meat alternatives. Canada's Eating Well with Canada's Food Guide contains four main food groupings presented in a rainbow shape.

Tips include the following:

- Eat at least one dark green and one orange vegetable each day.
- Make at least half of your grain products whole grain each day.
- Compare the Nutrition Facts table on food labels to choose products that contain less fat, saturated fat, trans fat, sugar, and sodium.

- Drink skim, 1% or 2% milk, or fortified soy beverages each day.
- Include a small amount—30-45 mL (2-3 tbsp)—of unsaturated fat each day.
- Eat at least two Food Guide Servings of fish each week.

It is recommended that adults accumulate at least 2½ hours of moderate to vigorous physical activity each week and that children and youth accumulate at least 60 minutes per day. The Canadian Food Guide recognizes the cultural, spiritual, and physical importance of traditional Aboriginal foods as well as the role of nontraditional foods in contemporary diets, with a First Nations, Inuit, and Métis guide available. The guide is available in 12 languages.

Data from Health Canada: *Eating Well with Canada's Food Guide, Her Majesty the Queen in Right of Canada, represented by the Minister of Health Canada, 2011* (website): from http://www.hc-sc.gc.ca/fn-an/food-guide-aliment/index-eng.php.
Eating Well with Canada's Food Guide – First Nations, Inuit, and Métis: from http://hc-sc.gc.ca/fn-an/pubs/fnim-pnim/index-eng.php.

Finally, in spite of available choices, many Americans experience food insecurity, meaning that they lack access to adequate and safe food for an active, healthy life. More than one in seven American households, including 12 million children, struggle to have enough to eat. In many lower socioeconomic neighborhoods, food deserts exist, where foods like fresh fruits and vegetables are not available at affordable prices. This is often accompanied by poor public transportation options. The Academy of Nutrition and Dietetics published a position paper on food insecurity in the United States in 2017.

Healthy Eating Index

The Center for Nutrition Policy and Promotion of the USDA releases the Healthy Eating Index (HEI) to measure how well people's diets conform to recommended healthy eating patterns. The index provides a picture of foods people are eating, the amount of variety in their diets, and compliance with specific recommendations in the Dietary Guidelines for Americans (DGA) (USDHS, 2015). The HEI is designed to assess and monitor the dietary status of Americans by evaluating 12 components, each representing different aspects of a healthy diet. The HEI was last updated after the release of the 2015–2020 DGA. The dietary components used in HEI-2015 include nine related to adequacy: whole fruits, total fruits, whole grains, dairy, total protein foods, seafood and plant proteins, greens and beans, total vegetables, fatty acids, and four components for which moderation is recommended: refined grains, sodium, saturated fat, and added sugars (Krebs-Smith et al, 2018). One change since HEI-2010 is in the algorithm used to count legumes in the diet, which is now allocated to both the vegetable and the protein components.

NATIONAL GUIDELINES FOR DIET PLANNING

Eating can be one of life's greatest pleasures. People eat for enjoyment and to obtain energy and nutrients. Although many genetic, environmental, behavioral, and cultural factors affect health, diet is equally important for promoting health and preventing disease. Over the past several decades, attention has been focused increasingly on the relationship between nutrition and chronic diseases and conditions. Although this interest derives somewhat from the increasing percentage of older adults in the population as well as their longevity, it also is prompted by the desire to prevent premature deaths from diseases such as coronary heart disease, diabetes mellitus, and cancer. Approximately two-thirds of deaths in the United States are caused by chronic disease.

Current Dietary Guidance

In 1969 President Nixon convened the White House Conference on Nutrition and Health (White House conference on food, nutrition and health, 1969). Increased attention was being given to prevention of hunger and disease. The development of dietary guidelines in the United States is discussed in Chapter 8. Guidelines directed toward prevention of a particular disease, such as those from the National Cancer Institute; the American Diabetes Association; the American Heart Association; and the National Heart, Lung, and Blood Institute's cholesterol education guidelines, contain recommendations unique to particular conditions.

Implementing the Guidelines

The task of planning nutritious meals centers on including the essential nutrients in sufficient amounts as outlined in the most recent DRIs, in addition to appropriate amounts of energy, protein, carbohydrate (including fiber and sugars), fat (especially saturated and trans fats), cholesterol, and sodium. Suggestions are included to help people meet the specifics of the recommendations. When specific numeric recommendations differ, they are presented as ranges.

To help people select an eating pattern that achieves specific health promotion or disease prevention objectives, nutritionists should assist individuals in making food choices (e.g., to reduce saturated fat, to increase fiber). Although numerous federal agencies are involved in the issuance of dietary guidance, the USDA and USDHHS lead the effort. The DGA first were published in 1980 and are revised every 5 years; the 2015–2020 guidelines are included (Box 10.1). The DGA are designed to provide evidence-based nutrition information for people ages 2 and older to help them make healthy choices in their daily diet. The information in the DGA is used by the federal government to create educational materials for consumers and helps guide development of federal food and nutrition education programs (Dietary Guidelines 2015-2020: Introduction https://health.gov/dietaryguidelines/2015/guidelines/introduction/dietary-guidelines-for-americans/).

BOX 10.1 The 2015–2020 Dietary Guidelines for Americans

1. Follow a healthy eating pattern across the lifespan.
2. Focus on variety, nutrient density, and amount.
3. Limit calories from added sugars and saturated fats and reduce sodium intake.
4. Shift to healthier food and beverage choices.
5. Support healthy eating patterns for all.

Retrieved from http://www.health.gov/dietaryguidelines/2015/guidelines/.

FOOD AND NUTRIENT LABELING

To help consumers make choices between similar types of food products that can be incorporated into a healthy diet, the FDA established a voluntary system of providing selected nutrient information on food labels. The regulatory framework for nutrition information on food labels was revised and updated by the USDA (which regulates meat, poultry products, and eggs) and the FDA (which regulates all other foods) with enactment of the Nutrition Labeling and Education Act (NLEA) in 1990. The labels became mandatory in 1994. In 2016 the FDA announced the new nutrition facts label layout, designed to better educate consumers on the relationship between diet and chronic disease. Some of the changes include a larger type size for display of calories including declaration of actual amounts of Vitamin D, calcium, iron, and potassium (in addition to their percent daily value), and a better explanation of the meaning of daily value. The new labels also include a separate line for added sugars because many health experts recommend decreasing intake of sugars in favor of more nutrient-dense foods, as well as to help decrease overall caloric intake (Fig. 10.18). Compliance is currently set for January 1, 2020 for manufacturers with $10 million or more in food sales, and January 1, 2021 for those with less than $10 million in food sales.

Mandatory Nutrition Labeling

As a result of the NLEA, nutrition labels must appear on most foods, except products that provide few nutrients (such as coffee and spices), restaurant foods, and ready-to-eat foods prepared on site, such as supermarket bakery and deli items. Providing nutrition information on many raw foods is voluntary. However, the FDA and USDA have called for a voluntary point-of-purchase program in which nutrition information is available in most supermarkets. Nutrition information is provided through brochures or point-of-purchase posters for the 20 most popular fruits, vegetables, and fresh fish and the 45 major cuts of fresh meat and poultry. Several food

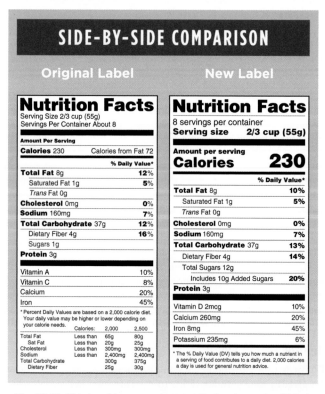

Fig. 10.18 Side-by-side comparison: original and new food label.

processors in the United States and elsewhere have tried implementing front-of-package labeling that employed a score, symbols, or color coding to reflect a product's overall nutrient content. Some of these systems, however, were confusing to consumers and have since been discontinued.

Nutrition information for foods purchased in restaurants is widely available at the point of purchase or from websites. FDA regulations require restaurant chains, retail food establishments, and vending machines with 20 or more locations to disclose calorie information on their menus or menu board (or on a sign or sticker on or adjacent to the vending machine). Additional nutrient information that must be made available upon request includes total calories, total fat, saturated fat, trans fat, cholesterol, sodium, total carbohydrates, fiber, sugars, and protein.

The new regulations also cover ready-to-eat unpackaged foods in delicatessens or supermarkets that meet the requirements above. If a food makes the claim of being organic, it also must meet certain criteria and labeling requirements. Use of the term *organic* is governed by USDA rather than FDA.

Standardized Serving Sizes on Food Labels

Serving sizes of products are set by the United States government based on reference amounts commonly consumed by Americans. For example, a serving of milk is 8 oz, and a serving of salad dressing is 2 tbsp. Standardized serving sizes make it easier for consumers to compare the nutrient contents of similar products (Fig. 10.18).

Nutrition Facts Label

The nutrition facts label on a food product provides information on its per-serving calories and calories from fat. The label must list the amount (in grams) of total fat, saturated fat, trans fat, cholesterol, sodium, total carbohydrate, dietary fiber, sugar, and protein. For most of these nutrients the label also shows the percentage of the daily value (DV) supplied by a serving, showing how a product fits into an overall diet by comparing its nutrient content with recommended intakes of those nutrients (Table 10.2). DVs are not recommended intakes for individuals; they are simply reference points to provide some perspective on daily nutrient needs and are based on a 2000-kcal diet. For example, individuals who consume diets supplying more or fewer calories can still use the DVs as a rough guide to ensure that they are getting adequate amounts of vitamin C, for example, but not too much saturated fat.

The DVs are listed for nutrients for which RDAs already exist (in which case they are known as reference daily intakes [RDIs]) (Table 10.3) and for which no RDAs exist (in which case they are known as daily reference values [DRVs] [Table 10.4]). However, food

TABLE 10.2 Daily Value (Based on 2000 kcal Diet)

Nutrient	Amount
Total Fat	78 grams (g)
Saturated Fat	20 g
Cholesterol	300 milligrams (mg)
Sodium	2300 mg
Potassium	4700 mg
Total Carbohydrate	275 g
Added Sugars	50 g
Dietary Fiber	28 g
Protein	50 g
Vitamin A	900 micrograms (mcg) Retinol Activity Equivalents (RAE)
Vitamin C	90 mg
Calcium	1300 mg
Iron	18 mg
Vitamin D	20 mcg
Vitamin E	15 mg alpha-tocopherol
Vitamin K	120 mcg
Thiamin	1.2 mg
Riboflavin	1.3 mg
Niacin	16 mg Niacin Equivalents (NE)
Vitamin B$_6$	1.7 mg
Folate	400 mcg Dietary Folate Equivalents (DFE)
Vitamin B$_{12}$	2.4 mcg
Biotin	30 mcg
Pantothenic acid	5 mg
Choline	550 mg
Phosphorus	1250 mg
Iodine	150 mcg
Magnesium	420 mg
Zinc	11 mg
Selenium	55 mcg
Copper	0.9 mg
Manganese	2.3 mg
Chromium	35 mcg
Molybdenum	45 mcg
Chloride	2300 mg

From National Institutes of Health *Dietary Supplement Label Database: Labeling Daily Values,* retrieved from https://www.dsld.nlm.nih.gov/dsld/dailyvalue.jsp.

TABLE 10.3 Reference Daily Intakes

Nutrient	Amount
Vitamin A	900 mcg RAE
Vitamin C	90 mg
Thiamin	1.2 mg
Riboflavin	1.3 mg
Niacin	16 mg NE
Calcium	1300 mg
Iron	18 mg
Vitamin D	20 mcg
Vitamin E	15 mg alpha-tocopherol
Vitamin B$_6$	1.7 mg
Folic acid	400 mcg DFE
Vitamin B$_{12}$	400 mcg DFE
Phosphorus	1250 mg
Iodine	150 mcg
Magnesium	420 mg
Zinc	11 mg
Copper	0.9 mg
Biotin	30 mcg
Pantothenic acid	5 mg
Selenium	55 mcg

From Food Labeling: Revision of the Nutrition and Supplement Facts Labels. Retrieved from https://s3.amazonaws.com/public-inspection.federalregister.gov/2016-11867.pdf.

TABLE 10.4 Daily Reference Values

Food Component	DRV	Calculation
Fat	78 g	35% of kcal
Saturated fat	20 g	10% of kcal
Cholesterol	300 mg	Same regardless of kcal
Carbohydrates (total)	275 g	55% of calories
Added Sugars	50 g	
Fiber	28 g	14 g per 1000 kcal
Protein	50 g	10% of kcal
Sodium	2300 mg	Same regardless of kcal
Potassium	3500 mg	Same regardless of kcal

DRV, Daily reference value.
NOTE: The DRVs were established for adults and children over 4 years old. The values for energy yielding nutrients below are based on 2000 calories per day.

labels use only the term *daily value.* RDIs provide a large margin of safety; in general, the RDI for a nutrient is greater than the RDA for a specific age group. As new DRIs are developed in various categories, labeling laws are updated. Box 10.2 provides tips for reading and understanding food labels.

Nutrient Content Claims

Nutrient content terms such as *reduced sodium, fat free, low-calorie,* and *healthy* must meet government definitions that apply to all foods (Box 10.3). For example, *lean* refers to a serving of meat, poultry, seafood, or game meat with less than 10 g of fat, less than 4 g of saturated fat, and less than 95 mg of cholesterol per serving or per 100 g. Extra lean meat or poultry contains less than 5 g of fat, less than 2 g of saturated fat, and the same cholesterol content as lean, per serving, or per 100 g of product.

BOX 10.2 Tips for Reading and Understanding Food Labels

Interpret the percent daily value (%DV).
- Nutrients with %DV of 5 or less are considered low or poor sources.
- Nutrients with %DV of 10 to 19 or less are considered moderate or "good sources."
- Nutrients with %DV of 20 or more are considered high or "rich sources."

Prioritize nutrient needs and compare %DV levels accordingly. For example, if a consumer wishes to lower osteoporosis risk versus limiting sodium, a packaged food containing 25%DV calcium and 15%DV sodium may be considered a sensible food selection.

Note the calories per serving and the servings per container. Consider how the energy value of a specific food fits into the total energy intake "equation." Be conscious of the portion size that is consumed and "do the math" as to how many servings per container that portion would be.

Be aware of specific nutrient content claims. As shown in Box 10.3, there are many nutrient content claims, but only specific ones may relate to personal health priorities. For example, if there is a positive family history for heart disease, the "low fat" nutrient claim of 3 grams or less per serving may serve as a useful guide during food selection.

Review the ingredient list. Ingredients are listed in order of prominence. Pay particular attention to the top five items listed. Ingredients that contain sugar often end in *-ose.* The term *hydrogenated* signals that trans fats may be present. Sodium-containing additives also may be present in multiple forms.

BOX 10.3 Nutrient Content Claims

Free: *Free* means that a product contains no amount of, or only trivial or "physiologically inconsequential" amounts of, one or more of these components: fat, saturated fat, cholesterol, sodium, sugar, or calories. For example, *calorie-free* means the product contains fewer than 5 calories per serving, and *sugar-free* and *fat-free* both mean the product contains less than 0.5 g per serving. Synonyms for *free* include *without, no,* and *zero.* A synonym for fat-free milk is *skim.*

Low: *Low* can be used on foods that can be eaten frequently without exceeding dietary guidelines for one or more of these components: fat, saturated fat, cholesterol, sodium, and calories. Synonyms for low include *little, few, low source of,* and *contains a small amount of.*
- **Low fat:** 3 g or less per serving
- **Low saturated fat:** 1 g or less per serving
- **Low sodium:** 140 mg or less per serving
- **Very low sodium:** 35 mg or less per serving
- **Low cholesterol:** 20 mg or less and 2 g or less of saturated fat per serving
- **Low calorie:** 40 calories or less per serving

Lean and extra lean: *Lean* and *extra lean* can be used to describe the fat content of meat, poultry, seafood, and game meats.
- **Lean:** less than 10 g fat, 4.5 g or less saturated fat, and less than 95 mg cholesterol per serving and per 100 g
- **Extra lean:** less than 5 g fat, less than 2 g saturated fat, and less than 95 mg cholesterol per serving and per 100 g

Reduced: *Reduced* means that a nutritionally altered product contains at least 25% less of a nutrient or of calories than the regular, or reference, product. However, a *reduced* claim cannot be made on a product if its reference food already meets the requirement for a "low" claim.

Less: *Less* means that a food, whether altered or not, contains 25% less of a nutrient or of calories than the reference food. For example, pretzels that have 25% less fat than potato chips could carry a *less* claim. *Fewer* is an acceptable synonym.

Light: *Light* can mean two things:
- First, that a nutritionally altered product contains one-third fewer calories or half the fat of the reference food. If the food derives 50% or more of its calories from fat, the reduction must be 50% of the fat.
- Second, that the sodium content of a low-calorie, low-fat food has been reduced by 50%. In addition, *light in sodium* may be used on food in which the sodium content has been reduced by at least 50%.
- The term *light* still can be used to describe such properties as texture and color, as long as the label explains the intent (e.g., *light brown sugar* and *light and fluffy*).

High: *High* can be used if the food contains 20% or more of the daily value for a particular nutrient in a serving.

Good source: *Good source* means that one serving of a food contains 10% to 19% of the daily value for a particular nutrient.

More: *More* means that a serving of food, whether altered or not, contains a nutrient that is at least 10% of the daily value more than the reference food. The 10% of daily value also applies to *fortified, enriched, added, extra,* and *plus* claims, but in these cases the food must be altered.

Data adapted from Food and Drug Administration. Retrieved from https://www.accessdata.fda.gov/scripts/cdrh/cfdocs/cfcfr/CFR Search.cfm?fr=101.54 and https://www.fda.gov/downloads/food/guidanceregulation/guidancedocumentsregulatoryinformation/ucm535370.pdf.

Health Claims

A **health claim** is allowed only on appropriate food products that meet specified standards. The government requires that health claims be worded in ways that are not misleading (e.g., the claim cannot imply that the food product itself helps prevent disease). Health claims cannot appear on foods that supply more than 20% of the DV for fat, saturated fat, cholesterol, and sodium. The following is an example of a health claim for dietary fiber and cancer: "Low-fat diets rich in fiber-containing grain products, fruits, and vegetables may reduce the risk of some types of cancer, a disease associated with many factors." Box 10.4

lists health claims that manufacturers can use to describe food-disease relationships. In 2013 the FDA added a regulation that defines "gluten-free," to clarify its voluntary use in food labeling and to help consumers with celiac disease to avoid foods containing gluten (see Chapters 25 and 27).

BOX 10.4   Health Claims for Diet–Disease Relationships

Calcium and Osteoporosis

- "Adequate calcium throughout life, as part of a well-balanced diet, may reduce the risk of osteoporosis."

Calcium, Vitamin D, and Osteoporosis

- "Adequate calcium and vitamin D, as part of a well-balanced diet, along with physical activity, may reduce the risk of osteoporosis."

Sodium and Hypertension

- "Diets low in sodium may reduce the risk of high blood pressure, a disease associated with many factors."

Dietary Fat and Cancer

- "Development of cancer depends on many factors. A diet low in total fat may reduce the risk of some cancers."

Dietary Saturated Fat and Cholesterol and Risk of Coronary Heart Disease

- "While many factors affect heart disease, diets low in saturated fat and cholesterol may reduce the risk of this disease."

Fiber-Containing Grain Products, Fruits and Vegetables, and Cancer

- Low-fat diets rich in fiber-containing grain products, fruits, and vegetables may reduce the risk of some types of cancer, a disease associated with many factors."

Fruits, Vegetables, and Grain Products That Contain Fiber, Particularly Soluble Fiber, and Risk of Coronary Heart Disease

- "Diets low in saturated fat and cholesterol and rich in fruits, vegetables, and grain products that contain some types of dietary fiber, particularly soluble fiber, may reduce the risk of heart disease, a disease associated with many factors."

Fruits and Vegetables and Cancer

- "Low-fat diets rich in fruits and vegetables [foods that are low in fat and may contain dietary fiber, vitamin A, or vitamin C] may reduce the risk of some types of cancer, a disease associated with many factors. Broccoli is high in vitamins A and C, and it is a good source of dietary fiber."

Folate and Neural Tube Defects

- "Healthful diets with adequate folate may reduce a woman's risk of having a child with a brain or spinal cord defect."

Dietary Noncariogenic Carbohydrate Sweeteners and Dental Caries

- Full claim: "Frequent between-meal consumption of foods high in sugars and starches promotes tooth decay. The sugar alcohols in [name of food] do not promote tooth decay"; Shortened claim on small packages only: "Does not promote tooth decay."

Soluble Fiber from Certain Foods and Risk of Coronary Heart Disease

- "Soluble fiber from foods such as [name of soluble fiber source, and, if desired, name of food product], as part of a diet low in saturated fat and cholesterol, may reduce the risk of heart disease. A serving of [name of food product] supplies __ grams of the [necessary daily dietary intake for the benefit] soluble fiber from [name of soluble fiber source] necessary per day to have this effect."

Soy Protein and Risk of Coronary Heart Disease

- "25 grams of soy protein a day, as part of a diet low in saturated fat and cholesterol, may reduce the risk of heart disease. A serving of [name of food] supplies __ grams of soy protein."
- "Diets low in saturated fat and cholesterol that include 25 grams of soy protein a day may reduce the risk of heart disease. One serving of [name of food] provides __ grams of soy protein."

Plant Sterol/Stanol Esters and Risk of Coronary Heart Disease

"Foods containing at least 0.65 gram per of vegetable oil sterol esters, eaten twice a day with meals for a daily total intake of least 1.3 grams, as part of a diet low in saturated fat and cholesterol, may reduce the risk of heart disease. A serving of [name of food] supplies __ grams of vegetable oil sterol esters."

"Diets low in saturated fat and cholesterol that include two servings of foods that provide a daily total of at least 3.4 grams of plant stanol esters in two meals may reduce the risk of heart disease. A serving of [name of food] supplies __ grams of plant stanol esters."

FDA Modernization Act Health Claims

Whole Grain Foods and Risk of Heart Disease and Certain Cancers

- "Diets rich in whole grain foods and other plant foods and low in total fat, saturated fat, and cholesterol may reduce the risk of heart disease and some cancers."

Potassium and the Risk of High Blood Pressure and Stroke

- "Diets containing foods that are a good source of potassium and that are low in sodium may reduce the risk of high blood pressure and stroke."

Fluoridated Water and Reduced Risk of Dental Carries

- "Drinking fluoridated water may reduce the risk of [dental caries or tooth decay]."

Saturated Fat, Cholesterol, and Trans Fat, and Reduced Risk of Heart Disease

- "Diets low in saturated fat and cholesterol, and as low as possible in trans fat, may reduce the risk of heart disease."

Substitution of Saturated Fat in the Diet with Unsaturated Fatty Acids and Reduced Risk of Heart Disease

- "Replacing saturated fat with similar amounts of unsaturated fats may reduce the risk of heart disease. To achieve this benefit, total daily calories should not increase."

Data from Food and Drug Administration (website): https://www.fda.gov/downloads/Food/GuidanceRegulation/GuidanceDocuments RegulatoryInformation/UCM265446.pdf.

DIETARY PATTERNS AND COUNSELING TIPS

Vegetarian Diet Patterns

Vegetarian diets are popular. Those who choose them may be motivated by philosophic, religious, or ecologic concerns, or by a desire to have a healthier lifestyle. Considerable evidence attests to the health benefits of a vegetarian diet. For example, studies of Seventh-Day Adventists indicate that the diet helps lower rates of metabolic syndrome and cardiovascular disease (Rizzo et al, 2011).

Of the millions of Americans who call themselves vegetarians, many eliminate "red" meats but eat fish, poultry, and dairy products. A lactovegetarian does not eat meat, fish, poultry, or eggs but does consume milk, cheese, and other dairy products. A lactoovovegetarian also consumes eggs. A vegan does not eat any food of animal origin. The vegan diet is the only vegetarian diet that has any real risk of providing inadequate nutrition, but this risk can be avoided by careful planning (see Appendix 30). A type of semivegetarian is known as a flexitarian. Flexitarians generally adhere to a vegetarian diet for the purpose of good health and do not follow a specific ideology. They view an occasional meat meal as acceptable. A public health awareness campaign called Meatless Monday advocates that Americans have a vegetarian meal at least 1 day per week to help reduce the incidence of preventable chronic health conditions such as diabetes, obesity, and cardiovascular disease.

Vegetarian diets tend to be lower in iron than omnivorous diets, although the nonheme iron in fruits, vegetables, and unrefined cereals usually is accompanied either in the food or in the meal by large amounts of ascorbic acid that aids in iron assimilation. Vegetarians who consume no dairy products may have low calcium intakes, and vitamin D intakes may be inadequate among those in northern latitudes where there is less exposure to sunshine. The calcium in some vegetables is made unavailable for absorption by the presence of oxalates. Although phytates in unrefined cereals also can make calcium unavailable, this is not a problem for Western vegetarians, whose diets tend to be based more on fruits and vegetables than on the unrefined cereals of Middle Eastern cultures.

Long-term vegans may develop megaloblastic anemia because of a deficiency of vitamin B_{12}, found only in foods of animal origin. The high levels of folate in vegan diets may mask the neurologic damage of a vitamin B_{12} deficiency. Vegans should have a reliable source of vitamin B_{12} such as fortified breakfast cereals, fortified soy beverages, or a supplement. Although most vegetarians meet or exceed the requirements for protein, their diets tend to be lower in protein than those of omnivores. Lower protein intake usually results in lower saturated fat intake because many high-protein animal products are also rich in saturated fat (Academy of Nutrition and Dietetics, 2016).

Well-planned vegetarian diets are safe for infants, children, and adolescents and can meet all of their nutritional requirements for growth. They are also adequate for pregnant and lactating females. The key is that the diets be well planned. Vegetarians should pay special attention to ensure that they get adequate calcium, iron, zinc, and vitamins B_{12} and D. Calculated combinations of complementary protein sources is not necessary, especially if protein sources are reasonably varied. Useful information on vegetarian meal planning is available at the Academy of Nutrition and Dietetics website.

CULTURAL ASPECTS OF DIETARY PLANNING

To plan diets for individuals or groups that are appropriate from a health and nutrition perspective, RDNs and health providers must use resources that are targeted to the specific client or group. Numerous population subgroups in the United States and throughout the world have specific cultural, ethnic, or religious beliefs and practices to consider. These groups have their own set of dietary practices, which are important when considering dietary planning (Diabetes Care and Education Dietetic Practice Group, 2010). The IOM report entitled *Unequal Treatment* recommended that all health care professionals receive training in cross-cultural communication to help reduce ethnic and racial disparities in health care. Cultural competence training improves the skills and attitudes of the clinician and can facilitate a dialogue that encourages the client to share more information during a session (Betancourt and Green, 2010).

Attitudes, rituals, and practices surrounding food are part of every culture in the world, and there are so many cultures that it defies enumeration. Many world cultures have influenced American cultures as a result of immigration and intermarriage. This makes planning a menu that embraces cultural diversity and is sensitive to the needs of a specific group of people a major challenge. It is tempting to simplify the role of culture by attempting to categorize dietary patterns by race, ethnicity, or religion. However, this type of generalizing can lead to inappropriate labeling and misunderstanding.

To illustrate this point, consider the case of Native Americans. There are more than 560 different federally recognized tribes in 35 states. The food and customs of the tribes in the Southwest are different from those of the Northwest. With traditional foods among Native Americans, the situation is complicated further by the fact that many tribes were removed from their traditional lands in the nineteenth century by the government and forced to accept the foods provided by the federal government. Another example of the complexity of diet and culture in the United States is that of African Americans. "Soul food" is commonly identified with African Americans from the South. Traditional food choices, likely borne out of hard times, limited choices, and creativity, may include greens such as collards, mustard, and kale prepared with pork; beans; field peas; yams; fried meats; grits; and cornbread. However, this by no means represents the diet of all African Americans. Similarly, the diet of Mexican Americans does not necessarily equal that of immigrants from Central and South America. Mexican cuisine is not homogenous. There are seven regions of Mexican cuisine, each with its distinctive culinary variations. Baby goat is commonly eaten in the Northern region, which also produces a wide variety of cheeses and wheat tortillas. The South Pacific Coast of Mexico includes Oaxaca, Guerrero, and Chiapas. Oaxaca is known for its seven mole varieties, and corn tortillas are the staple of this region.

When faced with planning a diet to meet the needs of an unfamiliar culture, it is important to avoid forming opinions that are based on inaccurate information or stereotyping (see Chapter 13). Some cultural food guides have even been developed for specific populations to help manage disease conditions.

Religion and Food

Dietary practices have been a component of religious practice for all of recorded history. Some religions forbid the eating of certain foods and beverages; others restrict foods and drinks during holy days. Specific dietary rituals may be assigned to members with designated authority or with special spiritual power (e.g., a *shohet*, certified to slaughter animals in accordance with Jewish law). Sometimes dietary rituals or restrictions are observed based on gender. Dietary and food preparation practices (e.g., halal and kosher meat preparation) can be associated with rituals of faith.

TABLE 10.5 Some Religious Dietary Practices

	Buddhist	Hindu	Jewish (Orthodox)	Muslim	Christian Roman Catholic	Christian Eastern Orthodox	Christian Mormon	Christian Seventh-Day Adventist
Beef	A	X						A
Pork	A	A	X	X				X
Meats, all	A	A	R	R	R	R		A
Eggs/dairy	O	O	R			R		O
Fish	A	R	R			R		A
Shellfish	A	R	X			O		X
Alcohol		A		X			X	X
Coffee/tea				A			X	X
Meat/dairy at same meal			X					
Leavened foods			R					
Ritual slaughter of meats			+	+				
Moderation	+			+				+
Fasting*	+	+	+	+	+	+	+	+

*Fasting varies from partial (abstention from certain foods or meals) to complete (no food or drink).
+, Practiced; A, avoided by the most devout; O, permitted, but may be avoided at some observances; R, some restrictions regarding types of foods or when a food may be eaten; X, prohibited or strongly discouraged.
Modified from Kittler PG et al: *Food and culture*, ed 7, Belmont, Calif, 2017, Wadsworth/Cengage Learning; Escott-Stump S: *Nutrition and diagnosis-related care*, ed 8, Baltimore, MD, 2015, Lippincott Williams & Wilkins.

Fasting is practiced by many religions. It has been identified as a mechanism that allows one to improve one's body, to earn approval, or to understand and appreciate the suffering of others. Attention to specific eating behaviors such as overeating, use of alcoholic or stimulant-containing beverages, and vegetarianism also are considered by some religions. Before planning menus for members of any religious group, clinicians must gain an understanding of the traditions or dietary practices (Table 10.5). In all cases, discussing the personal dietary preferences of an individual is imperative (Kittler et al, 2017).

Health Literacy

Health literacy is defined as the degree to which individuals have the capacity to obtain, process, and understand basic health information and services needed to make appropriate health decisions (Healthy People 2010, USDHHS). Approximately 80 million Americans have limited health literacy (Kutner, 2006). Low health literacy is associated with poorer health outcomes and poorer use of health care services. Poor health literacy affects all levels of the health care experience. It obstructs provider–patient communications and affects health outcome and patient self-management. Minority groups, older adults, poor persons, nonnative speakers of English, and those with less than a high school education have high rates of restricted health literacy.

The components of health literacy include (AHRQ):
1. Cultural and conceptual knowledge
   a. Health beliefs, attitudes, and practices and the perceptions of illness, health risks, and benefits.
2. Oral Literacy
   a. Listening and speaking
3. Print literacy
   a. Reading and writing

4. Numeracy
   a. Use of numbers and math skills in everyday activities (Strategies to Enhance Numeracy Skills, 2015).

There is evidence to support the importance of health literacy for the management and treatment of diet-related diseases such as hypertension, diabetes, and cardiovascular disease. Health literacy is associated with glycemic management.

The goal of nutrition education and counseling is to promote healthy eating behaviors and provide individuals with knowledge and skills to make sound decisions conducive to health and well-being. RDNs provide verbal and visual information during the nutrition education and counseling sessions to increase understanding and help clients implement actionable goals. Restricted health literacy is a barrier to health behavior change (Academy of Nutrition and Dietetics).

Cultural Context

People from different cultural backgrounds determine how to define health, recognize illness, seek medical treatment, and relate to health care providers. The explanatory model of illness suggests that individuals develop conceptual models to explain illness. This includes beliefs about why the condition started, how long will it last, and how it should be treated. In a study by Lemley and Spies (2015), Mexican Americans believed that *susto*, a folk illness in which a person experiences an episode of fright, causes diabetes. Aloe vera (*sábila*), and prickly cactus (*nopal*) are some of the herbal remedies used to treat diabetes. Providers play an important role and must develop awareness and utilize available tools to provide cross-cultural counseling.

Models of Cultural Competence

The Campinha-Bacote model (1999) of cultural competence has five constructs that can be utilized by dietetic professionals to leverage their knowledge and acquire cross-cultural communication skills to improve patient satisfaction and improve health outcomes. They are the following:

1. **Awareness:**
   - Examine your own cultural background and your own personal beliefs and practices. How do your own perceptions improve or hinder the relationship with patients/clients?
   - Ask your client: What are some of your food and health beliefs and practices?
2. **Knowledge:**
   - Gain insight on the client's explanatory model of illness and dietary practices. Even when a cultural group shares common cultural traits, no group is homogenous and there are more variations within cultural groups than across cultural groups.
   - **Ask your client:**
     - What do you think caused your health condition? (i.e., diabetes, high blood pressure.)
     - Do you think that diabetes is caused by eating too many processed foods?
3. **Skill:**
   - Collect relevant cultural data to perform an assessment, evaluation, and counseling. Assess the client's therapeutic uses of foods.
     - **Ask your client:**
       - What is your preferred language?
       - Is there anything I should learn about your culture, beliefs, or religious practices that would help me take better care of you?
       - What do you call your illness and what do you think caused it?
       - Do you receive advice from traditional healers or others?
       - What kinds of foods do you eat to keep healthy?
       - What kinds of foods do you avoid when you are ill?
       - Do you avoid any foods for cultural or religious reasons?
       - How do you think you should manage or treat your condition? (i.e., high cholesterol, hypertension, arthritis, fatty liver, etc.)
4. **Encounter:**
   - How many face-to-face encounters have you had with the cultural group? What skills, knowledge, and tools do you need to improve the outcome of this encounter? Acquaint yourself with your clients' traditional foods and dietary practices. Assess the acculturation of dietary practices.
   - **Ask clients:**
     - What are your favorite foods?
     - Which foods do you dislike?
     - What foods do you commonly eat?
     - How often do you eat them?
     - Which foods do you eat on special occasions and holidays?
     - What new foods have you tried?
     - Which traditional foods do you no longer eat or eat infrequently?
5. **Desire:** Dietetic professionals seeking to become culturally competent should know that cultural competency is a continuously evolving process and the ability to effectively work with an individual, family, or community requires lifelong knowledge, adaptation, and flexibility.

Culturally Specific Education Tools

- Develop a food plan that is linguistically and culturally appropriate that incorporates traditional and newly acquired food choices.
- Provide food lists that includes foods from the patient's culture.
- Consider life experience of cultural groups prior to migrating to the United States, where there might have been exposure to other cultures and food influences.
- Consider the client's food insecurity and food availability that may hinder access to recommended nutrition recommendations.
- Translate educational materials into the client's preferred language
  - Translating education materials into the client's preferred language should take into consideration the client's literacy in his or her native language.
  - Consider the client's language variations. For example, Spanish has different variations in Latin America. When developing education materials, the best practice is to test the material to include the target audience dialect.

Oral Literacy

In order to have a successful patient–health care provider encounter, clients need to articulate health concerns, verbalize symptoms, explain medical history, and ask appropriate questions.

Patients need to understand medical diagnosis and treatment directions to be able to make appropriate health decisions. A person who does not fully comprehend diagnosis and treatment may be at risk of adverse events. Patients with limited health literacy are less likely to understand medical terminology and ask questions during a health care visit.

Oral Communication Tools

- Use living-room, nonmedical language. Use words that you would use to explain to non-health care providers. Below are some health and nutrition terms and suggested alternatives.
  - **Medical Conditions**

Cardiac problems	Heart problems
Diabetes	Blood sugar is elevated
Heart failure	Heart is not pumping well
Hyperlipidemia	Blood has too many fats
Hypertension	High blood pressure
Osteoporosis	Soft, breakable bones

  - **Nutrition Concepts**

Calorie	Amount of energy the body gets from food
Carbohydrate	Provides energy/fuel to the body like fuel to a car
Carbohydrate and diabetes	The part of foods that turns into sugar
Protein	Building blocks needed for growth & repair
Fat	Provides the body with energy and helps it use vitamins

- **Use the patient's words**: If the patient says "tummy" or "belly" you may use abdomen and explain that abdomen is another word for tummy or belly.
- **Limit and repeat information**: Stick to three key points and repeat them
- **Use graphics**: Use pictures or food models to demonstrate important concepts
- **Use teach-back**: Confirm client understanding by asking them to tell you or show you. For example, "Tell me, what are you going to do at home?" or "Show me how are you going to use the nutrition facts label." Remember: You are not testing the patient's knowledge; you are testing how well you explained the information.

Print Literacy

Clients' inability to complete nutritional assessments and questionnaires can affect the accuracy of their medical and nutritional history. Dietetic professionals rely on printed materials to educate and reinforce key concepts such as menu planning, nutrition facts labels, nutrient composition of foods, and food lists. A number of studies have shown moderate evidence that patients with low health literacy have difficulty taking medications as prescribed and had poor comprehension and poor interpretation of the nutrition label (Berkman, 2011). Reading food labels is not a good predictor of interpreting the information correctly. In a study that examined the use of the food label, only 60% of participants responded correctly when asked how many carbohydrates were in half a bagel (Rothman, 2006).

Written Communication Tools

Use the following tips when writing nutrition education materials (Goody and Drago, 2009):

- Write the most important information first, as patients with restricted health literacy may only read the first sentences.
- Keep paragraphs and sentences short because readers tend to skip information that appears difficult to read.
- Break complex information into chunks to enhance comprehension and retention.
- Use simple language and define medical terms. For example, an endocrinologist is a doctor who treats people with diabetes, and hemoglobin A1C is an average of blood sugar levels.
- Use definitive language. For example: A food diary *may* help you identify foods that you eat (passive). You *will* benefit from keeping a food diary (active).
- Write actionable content. Indicate what actions must be taken and break them down into steps. For example:
  - Eat whole grains such as whole wheat, brown rice.
    - Select cereals that have whole wheat and brown rice listed as the first ingredients on the food label.
- Provide benefits that the patient will gain when making changes. For example:
  - When you lower your blood sugar you will feel less thirsty and will be able to sleep better without making many trips to the bathroom.
- Provide tips to overcome barriers. For example:
  - Remember, small changes count: Even 10 minutes of activity is better than none. Walk for 10 minutes a day, three times a week during your lunch break.
- Add interactive content to increase retention.
- Have health professionals check for accuracy and have the target audience check for understanding.
- Use white space judiciously.
- Visit https://healthfinder.gov for examples to write and format health and nutrition education materials that are easy to read and understand and are actionable.

Use the following tips when selecting written education materials:

- Select material that is linguistically appropriate for the group that it is intended to reach. Hispanic subgroups speak different versions of Spanish. For example, the word *bocadillo* means "snack" in some Spanish speaking countries, but it means guava paste in Colombia. If you are writing a menu encouraging a snack and use the word *bocadillo*, it can have very different outcomes. Test the materials with the intended audience first.
- Select material that is culturally appropriate. A food exchange list that is translated into the patient's preferred language may lack many traditional foods.
- Ensure that printed materials are easy to understand. There are three commonly used readability formulas: Fry formula, SMOG, and Flesch Reading Ease. Search the Internet for "readability formulas."

- Select materials that are written at a fifth or sixth grade level.
- Select materials that your patients understand: Word choice, organization of information, and formatting affect comprehension. These methods are available to test comprehension:
  - Agency for Healthcare Research and Quality's Patient Education Materials Assessment Tool (PEMAT) used to assess written and audiovisual materials.
  - Use the CDC Clear Communications Index to assess your health communications materials, including behavioral recommendations and risk information (http://www.cdc.gov/ccindex).
  - The Suitability Assessment of Materials (SAM) assesses the cultural appropriateness and how materials stimulate learning.

Include Engaging Content in your Reading Materials

Write or select materials that contain engaging content. Interactive material helps reaffirm information and increase retention. Consider adding interactive tools such as the following:

- Fill in the blanks
- Multiple choice
- True/false questions
- Short quizzes
  Explain the reasons why answers were right or wrong.

Numeracy in Health and Nutrition

Numeracy is "the ability to access, use, interpret, and communicate mathematical information and ideas, to engage in and manage mathematical demands of a range of situations in adult life" (PIAAC, 2009). Numeracy skills are an important component of health literacy. Numeracy-related tasks are ubiquitous in health care and self-care management. Numeracy skills are needed to:

- Interpret test results (not being able to identify blood glucose within normal limits)
- Take medications appropriately and calculate dosages
- Read and interpret the nutrition label

Diabetes self-care involves tasks that require numeracy skills. These are:

Monitoring

- Taking medication including oral and injectables
- Interpreting nutrition food label
  - Using fractions, decimals, percentages, and proportions
- Multistep problem solving
  - Interpreting blood glucose readings
  - Calculating carbohydrate intake
- Approximately 25% of patients could not determine what glucose values were within normal range of 80 to 120 mg/dL.
- Approximately 56% of patients could not count carbohydrates in a prepackaged snacks.
- Approximately 59% of patients could not calculate insulin dose based on blood glucose reading and carbohydrate intake.

Measuring Numeracy Skills

There are several tests to measure numeracy skills that measure arithmetic skills and calculations without a health focus (Rothman, 2008):

- Wide Range Achievement Test (WRAT 3)
- Kauffman Test of Educational Achievement (K-TEA)
- Key Math
- Woodcock Johnson

The Diabetes Numeracy Test (DNT) is a scale to measure diabetes-related numeracy deficits. There are short and long versions.

Numeracy Skills Tools

- Use words and numbers to decrease misinterpretation. For example, instead of solely using words such as "rare" or "common" include numerical terms. For example, this condition is rare—it affects 1 in 10,000 people.

- Do the math for your patients. For example, instead of saying "Losing 5% to 7% of weight has shown to lower blood sugar levels," say "Losing 5% to 7% of weight (about 10 to14 lbs for a person weighing 200 lbs) has shown to lower blood sugar levels."
- Use visuals to explain nutrition concepts that require arithmetic calculations. Provide a conversion chart to help patients calculate basic arithmetic concepts.

- When helping clients use measuring cups:
  - 1 cup = ½ cup + ½ cup
  - 1 cup = 1/3 cup + 1/3 cup + 1/3 cup
  - 1 cup = ¼ cup + ¼ cup + ¼ cup + ¼ cup
- When helping clients interpret nutrition labels:
  - If a serving is ¾ cup, use: ½ cup + ¼ cup
  - If a serving is ½ cup, use: ¼ cup + ¼ cup

◎ FOCUS ON

Nutrition Transition

The term *nutrition transition*, coined in the early 1990s, describes alterations in diet, body composition, and physical activity patterns in people in developing countries undergoing rapid urbanization and demographic, socioeconomic, and acculturative changes (Popkin, 2001; Shetty, 2013). The shifts in traditional ways, value systems, and behaviors experienced in emerging economies such as India, China, the Middle East, North Africa, and Latin America are associated with notable increases in nutrition-related chronic diseases, while infectious and nutrition related deficiency diseases persist. Consequently, these populations face a double burden of disease—the struggles of undernutrition coexist with the maladies of overnutrition within the same individual, family, or community (Schmidhuber and Shetty, 2005).

Rapid advancements in medicine, food production, and agricultural technologies, along with the liberalization of markets leading to changes in food distribution and retail, have proven to be a double-edged sword in these countries. On the one hand, enormous economic developments and health benefits

have accrued; on the other, myriad challenges marked by nutritional imbalances and chronic disease trajectories have risen (World Health Organization/Food and Agriculture Organization, 2013). Inequalities in income and access to quality food and health care exist. Inactive lifestyles and increased toxic burden exposure and processed food consumption at the expense of indigenous foods are important nutrition transition determinants. In addition, there is increased vulnerability of individuals because of epigenetic fetal programming changes (Barker, 2006).

Several holistic, sustainable nutrition intervention approaches using a food-based and community involvement focus are currently underway to address nutrition transition worldwide (Sunguya et al, 2014; Vorster et al, 2011). These initiatives are directed at achieving optimal and balanced nutrition for all using evidence-based interventions and timely policies (Garmendia et al, 2013).

Sudha Raj, PhD, RDN, FAND

✳ THE INDIGENOUS FOOD SOVEREIGNTY MOVEMENT

A new movement to improve health and food access has taken off in indigenous communities across the world: "food sovereignty." This movement is founded on the belief that these communities have the right to define their own food policy systems—including agriculture, labor, fishing, and land—according to their traditional and cultural understandings of their environment and unique needs.

The need to redefine food systems in these communities is serious. American Indian and Alaska Native (AI/AN) communities in the United States suffer from some of the most severe health disparities in the country. Childhood obesity rates in these communities often surpass 50%, and there was a 110% increase in diagnosed diabetes cases from 1990 to 2009 in AI/AN youth ages 15 to 19 years. AI/AN people are also twice as likely as the overall U.S. population to experience some manner of nutrition-related health problem.

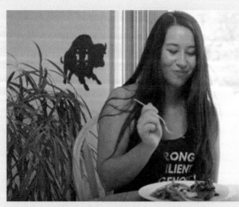

Generations of failed federal food policy, lack of access to healthy food, and the need for better education are all significant contributors to this challenge in tribal communities. Federal programs such as those that distributed surplus commodity foods on reservations aligned with other policies designed to assimilate

AI/AN people and helped make many of these communities reliant on food with very little nutritional value. Food like fry bread have their roots in these programs. Access to markets with fresh foods is another serious challenge. Most reservation areas in the country reside in "food deserts" according to the USDA—meaning they do not have access to a grocery store every 10 miles within the community. The Navajo Nation alone, which spans over 27,000 square miles, only has 10 full time grocery stores.

AI/AN youth leaders, like Mariah Gladstone of the Blackfeet Nation, are leading many of these grassroots movements. Recognizing the need for cooking education, Mariah started *Indigikitchen*, an online cooking show aimed at teaching indigenous cooking methods with traditional ingredients to viewers. Youth leaders are also working in food sovereignty coalitions across the country to advocate for flexibility in federal food programs to invest in indigenous gardens and agriculture, and to promote indigenous cooking knowledge and ingredients in programs like Supplemental Nutrition Assistance Program Education (SNAP-Ed). For more information about *Indigikitchen*, visit https://indigikitchen.com. For more information on the food sovereignty movement and policy recommendations, visit the Indigenous Food and Agriculture Initiative at University of Arkansas School of Law at http://indigenousfoodandag.com.

Erik Stegman, Carry the Kettle First Nation (Nakoda), JD, MA, is the Executive Director of the Center for Native American Youth at the Aspen Institute.

References

Center for Native American Youth: *"Our Identities as Civic Power: The State of Native Youth 2017." State of Native Youth Report,* Washington, DC, 2017, Center for Native American Youth at The Aspen Institute.

Echo Hawk Consulting: *Feeding Ourselves: Food access, health disparities, and the pathways to healthy Native American communities,* Longmont, CO, 2015, Echo Hawk Consulting.

University of Arkansas: *School of law indigenous food and agriculture initiative.* Available at: http://indigenousfoodandag.com/

CLINICAL CASE STUDY

George is a 65-year-old Navajo (Dine) male who lives in a traditional hogan. English is his second language. He lives in a food desert and eats a lot of canned foods and processed foods as well as foods his wife and other family grows and preserves. He does not drink milk but does consume other dairy products. He has a body mass index of 32 and a family history of heart disease. He has come to you for advice on increasing his calcium intake and decreasing his sodium intake because he thinks it will help his blood pressure.

Nutrition Diagnostic Statement

• Food and nutrition related knowledge deficit related to patient needs additional information about the relationship between calcium, sodium and blood pressure as evidenced by typical day intake containing highly processed foods.

Nutrition Care Questions

1. What type of dietary guidance would you offer George?
2. What type of dietary plan is realistic for him?
3. What are the cultural considerations for educating George about his diet?
4. How can food labeling information be used to help George meet his nutrition goals?

USEFUL WEBSITES

Academy of Nutrition and Dietetics
Center for Nutrition Policy and Promotion, U.S. Department of Agriculture
Centers for Disease Control—Health Literacy
Cost of Food at Home
Dietary Guidelines for Americans
Ethnic Food Guides
European Food and Information Council
Food and Drug Administration, Center for Food Safety and Applied Nutrition
Food and Nutrition Information Center, National Agricultural Library, U.S. Department of Agriculture
Health Canada
Healthy Eating Index
International Food Information Council Foundation
MyPlate Food Guidance System
National Academy of Medicine
National Center for Health Statistics—National Health and Nutrition Examination Survey
Nutrition.gov (U.S. government nutrition site)
U.S. Department of Agriculture

REFERENCES

Academy of Nutrition and Dietetics: *How to explain basic nutrition concepts.* Available at: https://www.eatrightpro.org/practice/practice-resources/international-nutrition-pilot-project/how-to-explain-basic-nutrition-concepts.

Academy of Nutrition and Dietetics: Position of the Academy of Nutrition and Dietetics: vegetarian diets, *J Acad Nutr Diet* 116:1970–1980, 2016.

AHRQ: *Health literacy universal precautions toolkit*, ed 2, Available at: https://www.ahrq.gov/sites/default/files/publications/files/healthlittoolkit2_3.pdf.

Barker D: Commentary: birthweight and coronary heart disease in a historical cohort, *Int J Epidemiol* 35:886–887, 2006.

Berkman ND, Sheridan SL, Donahue KE, et al: Low health literacy and health outcomes: an updated systematic review, *Ann Intern Med* 155:97–107, 2011.

Betancourt JR, Green AR: Commentary: linking cultural competence training to improved health outcomes: perspectives from the field, *Acad Med* 85:583–585, 2010.

Campinha-Bacote J: A model and instrument of addressing cultural competence in health care, *J Nurs Educ* 38:203–207, 1999.

Cavanaugh K, Huizinga MM, Wallston KA, et al: Association of numeracy and diabetes control, *Am Intern Medicine* 148:737–746, 2008.

Diabetes Care and Education Dietetic Practice Group, Goody CM, Drago L, editors: *Cultural food practices*, Chicago, 2010, American Dietetic Association.

FAO/WHO: *Preparation and use of Food-Based Dietary Guidelines. Report of a joint FAO/WHO consultation*, Nicosia, Cyprus, 1996, WHO. Available at: www.fao.org/docrep/X0243E/x0243e00.htm.

Garmendia ML, Corvalan C, Uauy R: Addressing malnutrition while avoiding obesity: minding the balance, *Eur J Clin Nutr* 67:513–517, 2013.

Goody CM, Drago L: Using cultural competence constructs to understand food practices and provide diabetes care and education, *Diabetes Spectrum* 22(1):43–47, 2009.

Guia alimentar para a população Brasileira: *Dietary guidelines for Brazilians*, 2015. Available at: http://bvsms.saude.gov.br/bvs/publicacoes/dietary_guidelines_brazilian_population.pdf.

Katz MG, Jacobson TA, Veledar E, et al: Patient literacy and question-asking behavior during the medical encounter: a mixed-methods analysis, *J Gen Intern Med* 22(6):782–786, 2007.

Kittler PG, Sucher KP, Nelms M: *Food and culture*, ed 7, Belmont, CA, 2017, Wadsworth/Cengage Learning.

Krebs-Smith SM, Pannucci TE, Subar AF, et al: Update of the Healthy Eating Index: HEI-2015. *J Acad Nutr Diet* 118(9):1591–1602, 2018.

Kutner MG, Greenberg E, Jin Y, et al: *The health literacy of America's adults: results from the 2003 National Assessment of Adult Literacy (NCES2006-483)*, Washington, DC, 2006, U.S. Department of Education, National Center for Education Statistics.

Lemley M, Spies LA: Traditional beliefs and practices among Mexican American immigrants with type II diabetes: a case study, *J Am Assoc Nurse Pract* 27(4):185–189, 2015.

NHANES: *National youth fitness survey, centers for disease control and prevention*, 2012. Available at: http://www.cdc.gov/nchs/nnyfs.htm.

PIAAC Numeracy Expert Group: *"PIAAC Numeracy: a conceptual framework"*, *OECD Education Working Papers, No. 35*, Paris, France, 2009, OECD Publishing. Available at: https://doi.org/10.1787/220337421165.

Popkin BM: The nutrition transition and obesity in the developing world, *J Nutr* 131:871S–873S, 2001.

Rizzo NS, Sabaté J, Jaceldo-Siegl K, et al: Vegetarian dietary patterns are associated with a lower risk of metabolic syndrome: the adventist health study 2, *Diabetes Care* 34:1225–1227, 2011.

Rothman RL, Montori VM, Cherrington A, et al: Perspective: the role of numeracy in health care, *J Health Commun* 13(6):583–595, 2008.

Rothman, RL, Housam R, Weiss H, et al: Patient understanding of food labels, *Am J Prev Med* 31(5):391–398, 2006.

Schmidhuber J, Shetty P: The nutrition transition to 2030. Why developing countries are likely to bear the major burden, *Acta Agr Scand* 2:150–166, 2005.

Shetty P: Nutrition transition and its health outcomes, *Indian J Pediatr* 80(Suppl 1):S21–S27, 2013.

Strategies to Enhance Numeracy Skills: 2016. Available at: https://nam.edu/wp-content/uploads/2016/05/Strategies-to-Enhance-Numeracy-Skills.pdf.

U.S. Department of Health and Human Services, U.S. Department of Agriculture: *2015 – 2020 Dietary Guidelines for Americans*, ed 8, 2015. Available at: http://health.gov/dietaryguidelines/2015/guidelines/.

Vorster HH, Kruger A, Margetts BM: The nutrition transition in Africa: can it be steered into a more positive direction? *Nutrients* 3:429–441, 2011.

White House conference on food, nutrition and health, *Am J Clin Nutr* 11:1543, 1969.

WHO/FAO: *Diet, nutrition and the prevention of chronic diseases, Report of Joint WHO/FAO Expert Consultation*, Geneva, 2013, World Health Organization.

11

Food and Nutrient Delivery: Bioactive Substances and Integrative Care

Kelly Morrow, MS, RDN, FAND

KEY TERMS

adverse events (AEs)
acupuncture
alternative medicine
American Botanical Council
American Herbalists Guild
Ayurveda
bioactive compound
botanical medicine
chi (qi)
chiropractic medicine
Codex Alimentarius Commission (Codex)
Commission E Monographs
complementary medicine
complementary and alternative medicine (CAM)

complementary and integrative medicine (CIM)
dietary supplement
Dietary Supplement Health and Education Act of 1994 (DSHEA)
Dietary Supplement Label Database
drug nutrient interaction (DNI)
East Asian medicine
excipients
functional medicine
generally recognized as safe (GRAS)
health claim
holistic medicine
homeopathy
integrative medicine

megadose
meridians
moxibustion
naturopathy
National Center for Complementary and Integrative Health (NCCIH)
new dietary ingredient (NDI)
pharmacognosy
phytochemical
phytotherapy
structure function claim
subluxation
third party certification
Tolerable Upper Limit (UL)
vis medicatrix naturae

COMPLEMENTARY AND INTEGRATIVE MEDICINE

Some people may be confused by the multiple names used to describe natural medicine approaches. Holistic medicine, from the Greek word *holos*, means "whole." Holistic therapies are based on the theory that health is a vital dynamic state that is determined by the balance between physical, mental, and spiritual parameters. Vis medicatrix naturae, the healing force of nature, is the underlying precept of holistic medicine. The philosophy states that when a person lives according to the laws of nature, the body has the ability to self-heal or the overall health of the individual will improve. Examples would include the adoption of a whole foods, mostly unrefined diet, maintaining a level of physical activity, use of plant-based (herbal) medicines and dietary supplements, and meditation to reduce stress. This theory is primarily applied to conditions where diet and lifestyle influence health to a large degree such as cardiovascular disease, diabetes, and many inflammatory conditions. Alternative medicine refers to nonmainstream therapies used *in place* of conventional medicine. For example, the use of an herbal preparation instead of a drug. Integrative medicine and complementary medicine refer to holistic therapies used *in combination with* conventional medicine. Most people who use holistic or nonmainstream therapies also use conventional medicine (National Center for Complementary and Integrative Health [NCCIH], 2018; see Tables 11.1 and 11.2).

Functional medicine is another iteration of holistic medicine that has gained esteem in recent years. It shifts the disease-centered focus of conventional medical practice to a more individualized and patient-centered approach (IFM, 2018). The goal is to evaluate the whole person rather than individual symptoms or organs and to consider care in relation to both prevention and treatment of chronic disease. Functional medicine practitioners, including medical doctors, naturopathic doctors, chiropractors, nurse practioners, and dietitians, acknowledge a web-like interconnectedness of internal physiologic factors within the body. Acting within their scope of practice, they use nutrition therapy, dietary supplements, lifestyle modifications, and physical manipulations as the foundation of medical care. Functional medicine providers assess for core imbalances, including dietary intake, hormones and neurotransmitters, markers of oxidative stress, environmental exposures, immune function, and psychological and spiritual health.

The Academy of Nutrition and Dietetics (AND) practice group, Dietitians in Integrative and Functional Medicine (DIFM), has developed a nutrition-oriented functional medicine radial for dietetics practitioners to assess clients using Integrative and Functional Medical Nutrition Therapy (IFMNT) (Noland, 2019). A functional nutrition assessment can overlap with the nutrition care process (NCP) and includes expanded categories in the clinical, biochemical, and physical domains (see Chapter 5 and Fig. 5.9).

USE OF COMPLEMENTARY AND INTEGRATIVE THERAPIES

According to the National Center for Complementary and Integrative Health (NCCIH), almost 53% of adults and 12% of children in the

Portions of this chapter were written by Cynthia A. Thomson, PhD, RDN, for the previous edition of this text.

TABLE 11.1 Common Holistic Therapies According to the National Center for Complementary and Integrative Health (NCCIH)

Complementary and Integrative Medical systems	Naturopathy, traditional Chinese medicine (also known as East Asian medicine), Ayurveda, and homeopathy
Mind/Body therapies	Meditation, prayer, art or music therapy, and cognitive behavior therapy
Biologically based therapies	Herbs, whole-foods diets, and nutrient supplementation
Manipulative therapies	Massage, chiropractic medicine, osteopathy, and yoga
Energy therapies	Qi gong, magnetic therapy, or reiki

National Center for Complementary and Integrative Health (NCCIH). Complementary, Alternative or Integrative Health: What's In a Name? http://nccam.nih.gov/health/whatiscam.

TABLE 11.2 Description of Commonly Used Complementary and Integrative Therapies

Naturopathy (Naturopathic Medicine)	Naturopathy is a form of primary care medicine that uses the healing power of nature, *vis medicatrix naturae*, to restore and maintain optimum health. Guiding principles include the following: *Primum non nocere*—First do no harm *Tolle causam*—Treat the root cause of illness *Docere*—Doctor as teacher Therapeutic methods and substances are used that work in harmony with a person's self-healing process, including diet and nutrient therapy, botanical medicine, psychotherapy, physical and manipulative therapy, minor surgery, prescription medicines, naturopathic obstetrics (natural childbirth), homeopathy, and acupuncture. Licensed in the United States to practice in 23 states and 2 territories. Training includes pathology, microbiology, histology, physical and clinical diagnosis, **pharmacognosy** (clinical training in botanical medicine), hydrotherapy, physiotherapy, therapeutic nutrition, and homeopathy.
Chiropractic	Chiropractic therapy embraces many of the same principles as naturopathy, particularly the belief that the body has the ability to heal itself and that the practitioner's role is to assist in that process. Like naturopathy, chiropractic care focuses on wellness and prevention and favors noninvasive treatments. Chiropractors do not prescribe drugs or perform surgery. The focus is on locating and removing interferences to the body's natural ability to maintain health, called **subluxations** (specifically musculoskeletal problems that lead to interference with the proper function of the nervous and musculoskeletal systems). Therapeutic approach is the manual manipulation of the body, such as spinal adjustment and massage and lifestyle recommendations, including physical exercises and stretching. Two fundamental precepts: (1) The structure and condition of the body influence how well the body functions, and (2) the mind-body relationship is important in maintaining health and in promoting healing. Licensed and regulated in all 50 states and in 30 countries. Must complete a 4-year program from a federally accredited college of chiropractic and, like other licensed practitioners, successfully pass an examination administered by a national certifying body.
Homeopathy	The root words of *homeopathy* are derived from the Greek *homios*, meaning *like* and *pathos*, meaning *suffering*. Homeopathy is a medical theory and practice advanced to counter the conventional medical practices of 200 years ago. It endeavors to help the body heal itself by treating like with like, commonly known as the "law of similars." The law of similars is based on the theory that, if a large amount of a substance causes symptoms in a healthy person, a smaller amount of the same substance can be used to treat an ill person. Samuel Hahnemann, an eighteenth-century German physician, is credited with founding homeopathy. The amounts of the remedies used in homeopathic medicines are extremely diluted. According to homeopathic principles, remedies are potentized and become more powerful through a shaking process called succussion. Homeopathic tinctures are made from a variety of source materials including botanicals, minerals, and animal tissues. Dosages are based on the following dilutions. A remedy becomes stronger the more it is diluted. X: 1 drop tincture in 10 drops water C: 1 drop tincture in 100 drops water M: 1 drop tincture in 1000 drops water The minimum-dose principle means that many homeopathic remedies are so dilute that no actual molecules of the healing substance can be detected by chemical tests. The goal of homeopathy is to select a remedy that will bring about a sense of well-being on all levels—physical, mental, and emotional—and that will alleviate physical symptoms and restore the patient to a state of wellness and creative energy. Although this form of medicine has a long history of use, clinical evidence on the efficacy of homeopathy is highly contradictory. In 2017, the FDA proposed new safety regulations for homeopathic medicines, specifically for those that contain potentially toxic substances or are used for life threatening conditions. This is especially significant for those who are vulnerable (infants and children, the elderly, and immune compromised). Homeopathic treatments are highly individualized using thousands of remedy combinations which makes the practice difficult to study using randomized and blinded trials. This presents a research challenge that will not soon be overcome.

TABLE 11.2	**Description of Commonly Used Complementary and Integrative Therapies—cont'd**
East Asian medicine	Based on the concept that energy, also termed **chi (qi)** or life-force energy, is central to the functioning of the body. Chi is the intangible force that animates life and enlivens all activity. Wellness is a function of the balanced and harmonious flow of chi, whereas illness or disease results from disturbances in its flow. Wellness also requires preserving equilibrium between the contrasting states of yin and yang (the dual nature of all things). The underlying principle is preventive in nature, and the body is viewed as a reflection of the natural world. Four substances—blood, jing (essence, substance of all life), shen (spirit), and fluids (body fluids other than blood)—constitute the fundamentals. The nutritional modality has several components: food as a means of obtaining nutrition, food as a tonic or medicine, and the abstention from food (fasting). Foods are classified according to taste (sour, bitter, sweet, spicy, and salty) and property (cool, cold, warm, hot, and plain) to regulate yin, yang, chi, and blood. The **meridians** are channels that carry chi and blood throughout the body. These are not channels per se, but rather they are invisible networks that act as energy circuits, unifying all parts of the body and connecting the inner and the outer body; organs are not viewed as anatomic concepts but as energetic fields.
Acupuncture	Acupuncture is the use of thin needles, inserted into points on the meridians, to stimulate the body's chi, or vital energy. **Moxibustion**, the application of heat using moxa, dried leaves from mugwort, along meridian acupuncture points for the purpose of affecting chi and blood so as to balance substances and organs, is related to acupuncture. This therapy is used to treat disharmony in the body, which leads to disease. Disharmony, or loss of balance, is caused by a weakening of the yin force in the body, which preserves and nurtures life, or a weakening of the yang force, which generates and activates life. The concept of yin and yang expresses the dual nature of all things, the opposing but complementary forces that are interdependent on each other and must exist in equilibrium. According to the National Certification Commission for Acupuncture and Oriental Medicine (NCCAOM), acupuncturists are licensed to practice in 46 states and the District of Columbia.
Ayurveda	Ayurveda is a 5000-year-old system of natural healing that originated in India. *Ayur* means life and *Veda* means science of knowledge. Assessment and treatment are based on three fundamental forces that govern the internal and external environments and determine an individual's constitution and overall health: Vata (wind): energetic, creative, and adaptable. If out of balance, can be anxious, dry, thin, and have poor concentration. Pitta (fire): intense, driven, and strong. If out of balance, can be compulsive, irritable, inflamed, and have poor digestion. Kapha (earth): nurturing, methodical, and stable. When out of balance, can be sluggish, phlegmatic, and gain weight easily. Mental and physical health are achieved when these forces are in balance. Therapeutic modalities include diet, herbal and lifestyle recommendations, massage, and aromatherapy.
Massage therapy/body work	The philosophy behind massage therapy and body work is that there is a healing that occurs through the action of touching. Massage therapy became a profession in the United States in the 1940s and has grown in use over the last several decades. The key principles of body work are the importance of increasing blood circulation, moving lymphatic tissue to remove waste and release toxins, calming the spirit, enhancing physiologic functions of body systems, and improving musculoskeletal function. This therapy also has been widely used to reduce stress and increase energy.

United States use nonmainstream health care approaches. Worldwide, the prevalence is 12% of the adult population in Canada, 26% in the United Kingdom, 56% in Malaysia, and 76% in Japan (Harris et al, 2012). Preferences in medical care are influenced by economic and sociocultural factors. In poor countries where access to modern medicine is limited, there is a heavy reliance on herbalists and traditional healers. In affluent countries, the decision to use natural therapies usually aligns with personal beliefs and preferences and is used commonly in addition to Western medicine (Harris et al, 2012).

The use of integrative therapies has been evaluated four times in the National Health Interview Survey (NHIS)—in 2002, 2007, 2012, and most recently 2017—with a data set limited to yoga, meditation, and chiropractic manipulation. In U.S. adults, the most popular integrative modalities include the use of nonvitamin, nonmineral supplements such as fish oil, glucosamine, probiotics, and melatonin (52%), chiropractic or osteopathic manipulation (10.3%), yoga (14.3%), and meditation (14.2%) (Peregoy et al, 2014; Falci et al, 2016). The Council for Responsible Nutrition (CRN) conducts an annual survey of over 2000 adults in the United States and reports on the use of dietary supplement use. CRN reports the use of dietary supplements in 76% of the adult population. Discrepancies exist in exact numbers between the NHIS and CRN, however the prevalence

of use is significant (CRN, 2017). In children, the prevalence of use of integrative medicine approaches did not change significantly since 2007 except for an increase in use of yoga and a decrease in the use of nontraditional healers. Nonvitamin, nonmineral dietary supplements, chiropractic and osteopathic manipulations, and yoga were the most common modalities used. The most common reasons cited were for back, neck, and musculoskeletal pain; colds; anxiety; and stress.

Fig. 11.1 highlights the most common forms of integrative medicine used by adults in the United States.

A significant number of Americans use some form of integrative medicine with increases seen in yoga, meditation, homeopathic treatments, acupuncture, and naturopathy. Use has been shown to be greatest among those age 55 and older, living in the West and Northeast of the United States, female gender, and higher socioeconomic status and education level (CRN, 2017). By race or ethnicity, use of integrative approaches varies, with white adults (37.9%) and non–Hispanic other races (37.3%) having the highest use and Hispanic (22%) and black adults (19.3%) reporting lower rates of use (Clark et al, 2015). Among a survey of 5057 registered dietitians in the Academy of Nutrition and Dietetics (AND), the most common use of integrative approaches includes vitamin, mineral, and other dietary supplements

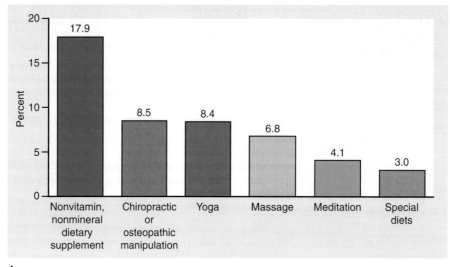

A

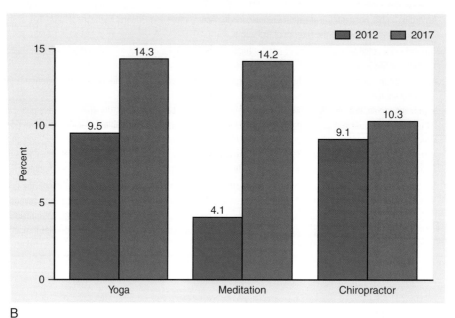

B

Fig. 11.1 A, Percentage of adults who used complementary health approaches in the past 12 months, by type of approach: United States, 2012. (Retrieved from http://www.cdc.gov/nchs/data/databriefs/db146.pdf.) **B,** Percentage increase by adults who used complementary approaches including yoga, meditation, and chiropractic care between 2012 and 2017 in the United States, 2018. (Retrieved from https://www.cdc.gov/nchs/data/databriefs/db325-h.pdf)

(such as probiotics and fatty acids) (55% to 75%), mind-body therapies (32%), herbs (22%), and detoxification (7%) (Augustine et al, 2016).

Integrative therapies are often considered when conventional medicine is not perceived as effective by the patient. Examples include chiropractic medicine for back pain, acupuncture for pain relief, and select dietary supplementation for conditions such as macular degeneration, depression, and digestive complaints. Integrative approaches are also commonly used when they are supported by significant evidence of efficacy. The NHIS survey also suggested that integrative medicine use increased when conventional treatments were too costly.

As a result of the increased interest in integrative therapies, the Office of Alternative Medicine of the National Institutes of Health (NIH) was created in 1992 to evaluate their effectiveness. This office became the twenty-seventh institute or center within the NIH in 1998,

when it was renamed the National Center for Complementary and Alternative Medicine (NCCAM). In 2015 the name was changed again to the National Center for Complementary and Integrative Health (NCCIH) because the use of complementary and integrative medicine in the United States is so common, it no longer warrants the term "alternative." Complementary and alternative medicine (CAM) had been the most common term used to describe the use of holistic medicine, although this term may be falling out of favor and is being replaced by complementary and integrative medicine (CIM). The NCCIH explores complementary and integrative healing practices scientifically using research, training, outreach, and integration (NCCIH, 2018). There continues to be an expansion of training opportunities and medical reimbursement for integrative therapies in the conventional medical system including the U.S. Department of Veterans Affairs (VA), and many nursing and medical curricula include training in integrative medicine.

In 2011 the Bravewell Collaborative, a philanthropic organization that works to improve health care, published results from a national survey on the use of integrative medicine among 29 major integrative medical centers and programs across the United States. Top conditions for which the centers reported the most success in treatment included chronic pain, gastrointestinal disorders, depression, anxiety, and stress. The most common interventions included nutrition, dietary supplements, yoga, meditation, acupuncture, massage, and pharmaceuticals (Horrigan et al, 2012). The Academic Consortium for Integrative Medicine and Health was formed in 1999 with the goal of "transforming the healthcare system and promoting integrative medicine and health for all." Its members include over 70 academic health centers across the United States including Cleveland Clinic, Stanford, Duke, Georgetown, Harvard, Johns Hopkins, Tufts, Yale, UCLA, and a number of state universities. The Consortium provides mentoring and training and disseminates information about integrative approaches based on rigorous scientific research (Academic Consortium for Integrative Medicine and Health, 2018).

DIETARY SUPPLEMENTATION

More than half of all Americans are taking some form of dietary supplement, and many of them may not be well informed about what they are taking (Gahche et al, 2014). Historically, dietetics professionals focused their assessment, care plan, and counseling on diet or food-related recommendations. The demand for information about dietary supplements from dietetics professionals is high. The 2018 Position Paper of the AND on micronutrient supplementation calls on registered dietitian nutritionists and dietetic technicians to be reliable experts with information on nutrient supplementation by keeping up to date on issues associated with regulation, safety, and efficacy of dietary supplements (AND, 2018).

Defining Dietary Supplements

According to the Food and Drug Administration (FDA), a dietary supplement is a substance that is taken orally and is intended to add nutritional value to the diet (Food and Drug Administration, 2015). Dietary supplements can come in many forms, including teas, tablets, capsules, powders, and liquids. A complete description can be found in Box 11.1.

BOX 11.1   FDA Definition of a Dietary Supplement

Intended to be a supplement to the diet

Intended to be taken by mouth; this excludes other routes of administration, such as intranasal, transdermal, and suppository

Contains one or more dietary ingredients, including the following:

  Macronutrients (protein, carbohydrates, fats)

  Vitamins and minerals

  Herbs and botanicals

  "Other" dietary substances that are either grandfathered in or are approved as

New dietary ingredients (NDIs), such as:

  Phytochemicals (such as curcumin from Turmeric)

  Bee pollen

  Probiotics

  Glandulars (products made from dessicated animal glands)

  Some hormones, including melatonin and DHEA

Does not contain any unapproved ingredients, such as:

  Thyroid hormone, cortisol, estrogen, progesterone, or testosterone

  Pathogenic bacteria

  Human tissue

Herbal Medicine

Herbal medicine has been used since the beginning of time and has a written history of more than 5000 years. In many parts of the world, it is the primary source of medicine (AHG, 2019). Herbs and plants provide a large array of phytochemicals and bioactive compounds (plant-based chemicals and compounds) that have biologic activity within the human body. Although some of the phytochemicals have been identified and characterized, many of them have unknown actions and may interact with pharmaceutical drugs (Gurley, 2012). When herbs are used in combination with each other or in concentrated forms (such as in a capsule or tincture), the likelihood for a drug nutrient interaction (DNI) or side effect increases.

Botanical medicines are made up of a variety of plant parts including leaves, flowers, stems, bark, rhizomes, and roots. They are produced in a variety of forms and are used orally and topically, including teas, infusions, decoctions, extracts, and pills as shown in Box 11.2. Topical application of botanicals or nutrients such as salves and aroma therapy are not classified as dietary supplements under the current regulatory definition because they are not ingested. The Commission E Monographs on phytomedicines were developed in Germany in 1998 by an expert commission of scientists and health care professionals as references for practice of phytotherapy, the science of using plant-based medicines in an evidence-based way to prevent or treat illness. Other useful herbal references including the American Botanical Council and the American Herbalists Guild are listed at the end of the chapter.

Trends in the Dietary Supplement Industry

According to the National Health and Nutrition Examination Survey (NHANES) 1999-2010, the most common reasons people use dietary supplements are to improve or maintain health, supplement the diet, support bone health (in women), lower cholesterol, and improve immunity (Bailey et al, 2013; Gahche et al, 2014).

The industry has grown steadily for the past 30 years. Industry sales were more than $43.5 billion in 2017 and sales are expected to continue to increase (Morton, 2018). The most popular supplements according to NHANES and the CRN include multivitamins and minerals (MVM), vitamin D, vitamin C, omega-3 fatty acids, lutein, probiotics, and protein powders. Among children, the most common dietary supplements include multivitamins, immune support supplements like vitamin C, omega-3 fatty acids, antacids, vitamin D, and melatonin (Quato et al, 2018). Herbal supplement sales increased 8.5% in 2017. Herbs that experienced the strongest growth in sales include turmeric (*Curcuma longa*), wheat grass (*Triticum aestivum*), barley grass (*Hordeum vulgare*), elderberry (*Sambucus nigra*), fenugreek (*Trigonella foenum-graecum*), echinacea (*Echinacea spp.*), and cranberry (*Vaccinium macrocarpon*), (Smith et al, 2018).

Multivitamin Efficacy

Most people take an MVM to increase nutrient levels in the diet or fill perceived gaps in nutrition. Dietary surveillance data from the National Center for Health Statistics (NCHS) and NHANES reveal that most adults and children in the United States are not meeting dietary guidelines and are underconsuming dark greens, orange vegetables, legumes, and whole grains (Bowman et al, 2018). Total nutrient intakes for vitamin D, vitamin E, calcium, vitamin A, vitamin C, and magnesium have been found to be significantly below the estimated average requirement (EAR), and less than 3% of the population is meeting the adequate intake (AI) for potassium (Drake and Frei, 2018).

Use of multivitamins and minerals has been shown to improve micronutrient status among adults and children (Bailey et al, 2012;

BOX 11.2 Botanical Formulations

Type	Form
Bulk Herbs	
	Sold loose to be used as teas, in cooking, and in capsules; rapidly lose potency; should be stored in opaque containers, away from heat and light.
Beverages	
Teas	Beverage weak in concentration; fresh or dried herbs are steeped in hot water and strained before drinking.
Infusions	More concentrated than teas; steep fresh or dried herbs for approximately 15 min to allow more of the active ingredients to be extracted than for teas. A cold infusion is made by steeping an herb over time in a cold liquid.
Decoctions	Most concentrated of the beverages, made by simmering the root, rhizome, bark, or berries for 30-60 min to extract the active ingredients.
Extracts	
	Herbs are extracted with an organic solvent to dissolve the active components; forms a concentrated form of the active ingredients. Standardized extracts concentrate a specific constituent(s) of an herb. Removal of the solvent creates a solid extract.
Tinctures	Extract in which the solvent is alcohol, glycerine, honey, or occasionally vinegar. Ratios are listed as herb:quantity of solvent. A 1:1 tincture is equal parts herb and solvent.
Glycerites	Extract in which the solvent is glycerol or a mixture of glycerol and water; more appropriate for children than an alcohol based tincture.
Salve	An infusion of herbs in oil and beeswax that is used topically. This preparation is not considered to be a dietary supplement under DSHEA.
Pill Forms	
	Pills should be taken with at least 8 oz of water to avoid leaving residue in the esophagus.
Capsules	Herbal material is enclosed in a hard shell made from animal-derived gelatin or plant-derived cellulose (vegetarian caps).
Tablets	Herbal material is mixed with filler material (excipients) to form the hard tablet; may be uncoated or coated with starches and polymers.
Lozenges	Also called *troches*; method of preparation allows the active components to be readily released in the mouth when chewed or sucked.
Soft gels	Soft capsule used to encase liquid extracts such as fatty acids or vitamin E.
Essential oils	Fragrant, volatile plant oils; used for aromatherapy, bathing; concentrated form and not to be used internally unless specifically directed (such as enteric-coated peppermint oil capsules).

Blumberg et al, 2017). Unfortunately, increased nutrient intake has not translated into reduced risk of chronic disease in people without overt nutrient deficiencies. Research reviews by the NIH State of Science Panel and the U.S. Preventive Services Task Force have evaluated observational and randomized controlled trials (RCTs) of more than 400,000 people using single or paired vitamins or MVM and have not found evidence that they reduce chronic disease or prevent early death with the exception of some forms of cancer and potentially cardiovascular disease, especially for long-term users of MVMs (Fortmann et al, 2013; Blumberg et al, 2018). Two trials, the Supplementation in Vitamins and Mineral Antioxidants Study (SU.VI.MAX) and the Physicians' Health Study II (PHS-II), found a small reduction in cancer incidence for men only after 12 ½ years (SU.VI.MAX) and 8 years (PHS-II) of supplementation (Fortmann et al, 2013; Gaziano et al, 2012). More recently, analysis of male physicians in the Physicians' Health Study I cohort who reported taking an MVM for more than 20 years showed a lower risk of cardiovascular events. In a nationally representative sample of women from NHANES, those who took an MVM for more than 3 years had lower cardiovascular mortality although the results were deemed nonsignificant when the results were fully adjusted for confounding variables (Rautiainen et al, 2016; Bailey et al, 2015). Trials looking at cognitive decline and all-cause mortality have not shown statistically significant incidence of harm or benefit (Fortmann et al, 2013). Chronic diseases are complex and usually have multifactorial causes. Studying the effect of an MVM on nutrient intake and overall health is a difficult undertaking. Almost all Americans are taking in supplemental forms of nutrients via fortified foods, which complicates efforts to quantify the impact of taking an MVM supplement. In observational trials, people take a variety of MVMs with differing compositions and potencies. People who self-select to take an MVM are usually healthier and have better diets, suggesting that MVMs may not be helpful for most well-nourished people. A few long-term RCTs evaluated the merits of MVMs, and the results have been population or gender specific and not generalizable to the entire U.S. population (Fortmann et al, 2013). MVMs may have efficacy based on assessment of individual needs, especially with the advent of nutrigenomics and personalized nutrition, but are not generally useful for all people. In those who do supplement with MVMs, there is little evidence for harm, however assessment should include a risk for exceeding upper limits on nutrients, especially when multiple supplements are taken at the same time (Blumberg et al, 2018).

Antioxidant Supplements

Oxidative stress is implicated in a variety of disease states, and many Americans take antioxidant supplements. A Cochrane review of 78 RCTs with 296,707 participants found that all-cause mortality was increased slightly with regular antioxidant use. The effect was strongest with beta carotene in smokers, and high-dose vitamin E and vitamin A. Vitamin C and selenium were not found to increase mortality but also did not improve longevity (Bjelakovic et al, 2012). Antioxidant supplements may be beneficial, however, for prevention of age-related macular degeneration (AMD). In the Age-Related Eye Disease Study (AREDS), high-dose vitamin C (500 mg), vitamin E (400 IU), beta carotene (15 mg), and zinc (80 mg) had a significant reduction in the risk of developing AMD after taking the antioxidant supplements for 6.3 years. The effects were still present after a 10-year follow-up (Chew et al, 2013). For the majority of people, it is probably best to get antioxidants and phytonutrients by eating a variety of plant-based foods, including fruits, vegetables, herbs, spices, nuts, seeds, legumes, and whole grains.

Potentially At-Risk Populations

Although dietary supplement use is most common among people who are least likely to have a nutrient deficiency, the AND has identified several populations and life cycle stages that potentially could benefit from dietary supplements (AND, 2018). Table 11.3 outlines potentially at-risk populations. Clinicians should be aware of these at-risk

TABLE 11.3 Populations Potentially at Risk for Nutrient Deficiencies

At-Risk Population or Life Cycle Stage	Nutrients of Concern that Could Potentially Be Corrected by Supplementation
Those living in poverty (especially children)	Iron, calcium, magnesium, folate, vitamins A, B_6, C, D, and E
Those taking oral contraceptives	Zinc, folic acid, B_6, and B_{12}
Adolescent females	Iron and calcium
Pregnancy	Iron and folic acid
Older adults	B_{12} and vitamin D, multiple micronutrients
Those following calorie-restricted weight loss diets	Multiple nutrients
People with dark pigmented skin	Vitamin D
People with malabsorption (inflammatory bowel disease, gastric bypass)	Multiple nutrients
Those who avoid food groups due to allergy or preference including strict vegetarians and vegans	Multiple nutrients, iron, zinc, calcium, B_{12}
Those with genetic predisposition to nutrient deficiencies (i.e., MTHFR or vitamin D receptor mutations)	Folate, B_{12}, vitamin D. Use of nutrigenomic testing is still an emerging science.
Those with advanced macular degeneration (AMD)	Vitamin C, vitamin E, zinc, copper, lutein, and zeaxanthin
Smokers	Vitamin C
Those with alcoholism	Folate and thiamin
People taking medications that deplete nutrients	Multiple nutrients

Adapted from the Academy of Nutrition and Dietetics. Position of the Academy of Nutrition and Dietetics: Micronutrient Supplementation. *J Acad Nut Diet* 118(11):2162-2173, 2018.

subgroups and complete a nutrition assessment to determine the need for supplementation on an individual basis if nutrition status cannot be improved by dietary changes alone.

DIETARY SUPPLEMENT REGULATION

Dietary supplements are regulated by two government agencies, the FDA, which oversees safety concerns, and the Federal Trade Commission (FTC), which oversees advertising, label, and health claims. Before 1994, dietary supplements existed in limbo under the general, but unspecified, regulation of the FDA. The Dietary Supplement Health and Education Act of 1994 (DSHEA) defined dietary supplements under the category of food and explicitly removed them from consideration as drugs or dietary additives. This was seen as a victory to the dietary supplement industry and consumers; they had become accustomed to open access in ability to manufacture and purchase dietary supplements without many restrictions.

Dietary supplement regulation set forth by DSHEA includes the following (NIH, 1994):

- Generally recognized as safe (GRAS) status to all supplements produced before October 15, 1994. This allows manufacturers to continue to sell all of the products that were on the market at the time DSHEA was passed. Any company that introduces a new dietary supplement must send notification and safety information to the FDA 75 days before selling the supplement.
- A supplement facts panel that defines how ingredients must be listed on the label. See Fig. 11.2 for an example of a dietary supplement label.
- Structure function claims vs. health claims: Supplement companies are no longer allowed to list disease states or make specific health claims on a dietary supplement label. A structure function claim allows for a description that includes a structure or function of the body or a stage of life. "Supports strong bones" is an allowable structure function claim; "Prevents osteoporosis" is not. The label must also include the disclaimer, "This statement has not been

Supplement Facts

Serving Size 1 Capsule

Amount Per Capsule	% Daily Value
Calories 20	
Calories from Fat 20	
Total Fat 2 g	3%*
Saturated Fat 0.5 g	3%*
Polyunsaturated Fat 1 g	†
Monounsaturated Fat 0.5 g	†
Vitamin A 4250 IU	85%
Vitamin D 425 IU	106%
Omega-3 fatty acids 0.5 g	†

* Percent Daily Values are based on a 2,000 calorie diet.
† Daily Value not established.

Ingredients: Cod liver oil, gelatin, water, and glycerin.

Fig. 11.2 A dietary supplement facts label per Food and Drug Administration regulation as defined under the Dietary Supplement Health Education Act. (From http://www.fda.gov/ucm/groups/fdagov-public/documents/image/ucm070717.gif.)

evaluated by the Food and Drug Administration. This product is not intended to diagnose, treat, cure, or prevent any disease." Opponents of DSHEA feel that structure function claims are too similar to drug claims and encourage dietary supplements to be used like drugs. By contrast, a health claim can mention a disease state as long as it has met the significant scientific agreement standard of the FDA and can exist on foods and dietary supplements.

For example, "soluble fiber from foods such as oat bran, as part of a diet low in saturated fat and cholesterol, may reduce the risk of heart disease." The FDA has approved only a limited number of health claims.

- Disseminating product literature: Dietary supplement manufacturers and retailers are no longer able to display product information or technical data sheets next to products because they can mislead consumers and make dietary supplements appear to be drugs.
- Because a wide variety of dietary supplements are available, including some hormones and megadose vitamins, it is up to consumers to be educated about the dietary supplement they choose to consume. The NIH founded the Office of Dietary Supplements (ODS) in 1994 to fund research and disseminate credible information on dietary supplements to consumers. On this government website, consumers can find basic consumer information, technical data sheets about dietary supplements and herbs, and FDA warnings.
- Good manufacturing procedures (GMPs) were adopted in 2007 and went into full enforcement in 2010. According to the GMPs, manufacturers of dietary supplements must meet minimum standards for production and are subject to random audits. The GMPs regulate the design and construction of manufacturing plants, maintenance and cleaning procedures, manufacturing procedures, quality control procedures, testing of materials, handling of consumer complaints, and maintaining records (FDA, 2010).

Under DSHEA, dietary supplements are regulated only for safety and not for efficacy. Manufacturers are beholden to follow the regulatory laws governing dietary supplements; however, they do not have to send any premarket notification to the FDA except for structure function claims and safety documentation for new dietary ingredients (NDIs) that were not used before 1994. The FDA randomly inspects more than 300 dietary supplement manufacturers per year. According to the Natural Products Insider via information obtained through the Freedom of Information Act (FOIA), in fiscal year 2018, 75 inspections (~24% of inspections) resulted in GMP violations and companies were cited by the FDA. The most common noncompliance issues were failure to test products for identity, potency, and purity (Long, 2018). The FDA is increasing its auditing program every year. With repeated audits, many of the noncompliant companies will be forced to comply or shut down, which will help ensure increased safety in the industry. For now, health care providers should recommend dietary supplements only from reputable companies. The FDA does not publish data on which companies pass or do not pass inspections. This information can only be obtained via the FOIA or by looking on the FDA warning letters database under the company name.

Ensuring Dietary Supplement Safety

Under DSHEA, the FDA bears the burden of proving a supplement is unsafe. This can be a challenging task once a product is released onto the market. To date, only two dietary supplements have been banned by the FDA over safety issues, *Ephedra sinica* in 2004, and dimethylamylamine (DMAA) in 2013. Both have been linked to cardiovascular toxicity and death. The most common supplements with health and safety concerns are those used for weight loss, performance enhancement (ergogenic aids), and sexual dysfunction (FDA, 2018). These supplements have the highest risk of contamination and adulteration with unapproved dietary ingredients and pharmaceutical drugs, especially when purchased from obscure retailers and on the Internet. Internet sales of dietary supplements is one of the fastest-growing retail markets and is also the hardest to regulate. Consumers can often find banned supplements easily on the Internet. In a 2014 study, researchers found that when products are recalled or banned by the FDA, a significant number of them are still available online. Of 274 supplements

recalled between 2009 and 2012, 85% of the sports supplements, 67% of weight loss, and 20% of sexual enhancement products were still available and still contained the banned ingredient (Cohen et al, 2014).

In December 2006 the Dietary Supplement and Nonprescription Drug Consumer Protection Act was signed into law, requiring mandatory reporting by manufacturers and retailers of known serious adverse events (AEs) related to dietary supplement and over-the-counter (OTC) medications. Serious AEs include a life-threatening event, incapacitation, hospitalization, a birth defect, or death. These must be reported to the FDA MedWatch website and can be filed by an individual, a health care provider, or an industry representative. In addition, supplement manufacturers are required by law to have contact information on supplement bottles. AE reports are forwarded to the Center for Food Safety and Applied Nutrition, where they are further evaluated by qualified reviewers (FDA, 2013). Health care providers and consumers are not mandatory reporters under the law but are strongly encouraged to report AEs.

Between 2008 and 2011 the FDA and poison control centers received almost 13,000 AE reports related to dietary supplements. Of those, 71% were considered serious AEs. During that same time, the FDA logged 2.7 million adverse drug events, of which 63% were considered serious (Government Accountability Office, 2013). The 2013 Annual report of the American Poison Control Centers revealed 1692 deaths due to drugs and zero deaths due to dietary supplements. Less than 1% of Americans experience AEs related to dietary supplements and the majority are classified as minor (Brown, 2017). It is estimated that many AEs from taking supplements are not being reported or are not being reported correctly. Common barriers from consumers include downplaying the significance, not knowing where or how to report, and embarrassment. After nine years of tracking (2004 to 2013), the Centers for Disease Control and Prevention (CDC) released a report indicating that an estimated 23,000 emergency department visits per year could be attributed to dietary supplements. Among young adults ages 20 to 34, the most common supplements causing AEs were for weight loss and energy (ergogenic aids) and the most common symptoms were tachycardia, chest pain, and palpitations. For adults 65 and older, AEs were mostly attributed to choking on micronutrient pills. Twenty percent of dietary supplement related emergency visits were for unsupervised children who ingested dietary supplements (Geller et al, 2015). Health care providers who wish to stay abreast of alerts from the FDA can subscribe to the MedWatch email list on the FDA website. The ODS website is another resource for information about current warnings and recalls as well as consumer tips for buying and taking dietary supplements safely.

Botanical supplements are increasing in popularity, and some have the likelihood for producing AEs, especially when taken in combination products and in concentrated form. Most of the common herbs used in the United States do not pose a great risk for a drug nutrient interaction (DNI). Of the herbs most commonly used, St. John's wort is the most problematic and has been shown to reduce efficacy of many drugs, including antiretrovirals for HIV, antirejection medications for organ transplants, oral contraceptives, cardiac medications, chemotherapy, and cholesterol medications. Two other herbs have been shown to have a high risk for DNI, including goldenseal (*Hydrastis canadensis*) and black pepper (*Piper nigrum*), although black pepper is only a problem in supplemental form and not in amounts commonly found in food (Gurley et al, 2012).

In recent years the ODS has worked collaboratively with several organizations and experts to develop a Dietary Supplement Label Database of dietary supplements used in the United States. Because the database provides specific information on the nutrient, herbal, or other constituents contained in a supplement, it allows clinicians to

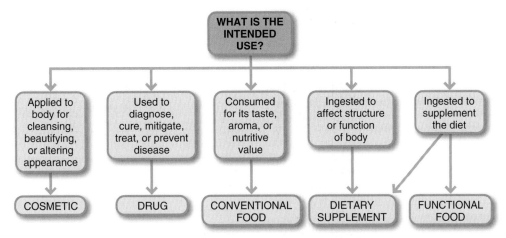

Fig. 11.3 Use of dietary supplementation in clinical practice requires use of a credible resource for evaluation and application. (From Thomson CA, Newton T: Dietary supplements: evaluation and application in clinical practice. *Topics Clin Nutr* 20(1):32, 2005. Reprinted with permission.)

assess more accurately the appropriate use of select supplements by their patients (Fig. 11.3). The database includes dietary supplement label information for more than 76,000 dietary supplement products, including the ingredients, daily values, and structure and function claims. The ODS offers Supplement Fact Sheets containing information about dietary supplements that is linked to PubMed, allowing clinicians and consumers to access to peer-reviewed information on use in human trials, AEs associated with use, and information regarding the mechanism of action. The Natural Medicines Comprehensive Database and Consumer Lab (subscriptions needed) offer similar information.

Third Party Certification

The FDA and FTC have primary jurisdiction for ensuring dietary supplements are safe and do not have misleading advertising. With approximately 85,000 products on the market, this is a daunting task. Because supplement manufacturers are audited randomly, it is not easy for consumers to know whether a company is truly following GMPs and their products are free from adulteration. Several private companies offer third party certification in the supplement industry. Consumer Lab is a well-known and affordable subscription-based company that randomly pulls supplements from store shelves to test them for potency, identity, and purity. Subscribers to the Consumer Lab website are able to access reports that reference specific brands. The U.S. Pharmacopeia (USP), the National Sanitation Foundation (NSF), and the Therapeutic Goods Association (TGA) each certify supplement companies for compliance with federal GMPs. Once verified, companies can display a stamp on their supplement labels that signifies the products have been third party certified. In addition, NSF offers a "Certified for Sport" certification for supplements that are used by competitive athletes to ensure they are not contaminated with illegal substances.

The Codex Alimentarius Commission (Codex) is an agency with international significance. It was created in 1963 by two U.N. organizations, the Food and Agriculture Organization and the World Health Organization, to protect the health of consumers and to ensure fair practices in international food trade. Codex participants work on the development of food standards, codes of practice, and guidelines for products such as dietary supplements. Codex standards and guidelines are developed by committees from 180 member countries, where they voluntarily review and provide comments on standards at several stages in the development process.

Quality Issues in Dietary Supplements

Not all dietary supplements are high quality. As discussed previously, many manufacturers are not in full compliance with DSHEA, which means many substandard and contaminated and adulterated products are on the market. Many of the popular brands in health food stores and major retail outlets are likely safe. Products bought off the Internet and from obscure retailers may be adulterated and/or may not meet label claims. What determines quality in a supplement must go beyond the safety issues to address the quantity, formulations, and quality of all ingredients used.

Quantity of Ingredients

Many MVMs contain megadoses of nutrients, which greatly exceed the RDA and may or may not be appropriate for each individual consumer. Some individuals may benefit from high doses of certain nutrients because of genetic variations in enzyme function or other pharmacologic effects of megadoses. Examples include increased need for folate with an MTHFR gene variant or reduction in triglycerides with megadoses of niacin (Ames et al, 2002; Boden et al, 2014).

It is important to assess for upper limits, especially when patients are taking multiple sources of nutrients. Most water-soluble vitamins do not have overt toxicity at high doses with the exception of niacin (flushing, prickly heat, and liver irritation in some people) and pyridoxine (reversible neuropathy). Fat-soluble vitamins can become toxic more quickly, such as vitamin A (hepatotoxicity and teratogenicity) and vitamin D (nephrolithiasis, calcification of soft tissue). Often vitamin A is listed in its provitamin form, beta carotene, which does not pose the same health risks as retinol at high doses.

Minerals can become toxic more easily than vitamins, so they often are not formulated using megadoses. In some cases, people may take a megadose of a mineral for a limited time, such as zinc for the common cold. To ensure patient safety, it is important to coordinate care with a physician when a patient is taking a megadose of a mineral. Although it is not a megadose, the FDA limits potassium content in dietary supplements to 99 mg because of the prevalence of chronic kidney disease. In patients with end stage kidney disease, high potassium levels can cause cardiac arrhythmia or arrest.

Formulations

Dietary supplements come in many formulations, including capsules, tablets, gels, chewables, liquids, and powders. The form a consumer selects has to do with convenience, preference, and affordability.

Supplement powders can be added easily to foods and beverages, but most have added sugars to increase palatability. Chewable and liquid supplements often are missing multiple nutrients to increase taste appeal, so it is important to assess the label to ensure it meets the patient's needs.

Tablets tend to be more compressed than capsules and require a fewer number of pills to achieve the optimal dosage. Capsules tend to be easier to swallow but less concentrated than tablets. Gelatin capsules may not be suitable for vegetarians. Some companies make vegetarian capsules out of vegetable cellulose to accommodate vegetarian consumers. Other nutrient forms that may not be suitable for vegetarian clients include cholecalciferol (often from fish oil or lambswool) and vitamin A/retinol (also usually from fish oil). Vegetarian formulations usually contain ergocalciferol and beta carotene as alternatives. Some manufacturers produce cholecalciferol from lichen and mushrooms, which are vegetarian sources.

Excipients

Excipients are extra ingredients added to dietary supplements to increase bulk, mask "off flavors," add color, and improve compressibility and flow through machinery. To assess whether a dietary supplement is right for an individual, it is important to consider the quality of the excipients used. Some contain allergens and/or potentially unfavorable ingredients, such as wheat starch, lactose, hydrogenated oils, artificial colors. When choosing a dietary supplement, it is important to read the label for quantity and quality of active ingredients and excipients.

Vitamins

Most vitamins in dietary supplements are similar across brands with the exception of B_6 (pyridoxine), B_{12} (cyanocobalamin), folate (folic acid), and vitamin E. Some formulations contain active, methylated, or phosphorylated forms of these nutrients such as in active B_6: pyridoxal 5′-phosphate, active B_{12}: methylcobalamin or adenosylcobalamin, and active folate: methyltetrahydrofolate. Individuals with genetic polymorphisms, nervous system disorders, increased oxidative stress, or impaired digestion may benefit from the increased bioavailability of these nutrients; however, research is limited on their widespread need and efficacy. In addition, the active forms tend to be more expensive (Head, 2006; Hendren, 2013). A review published in 2015 refutes the necessity of coenzyme forms of cobalamin, finding that all forms,

including cyanocobalamin are equally effective at treating B_{12} deficiency (Obeid et al, 2015).

Vitamin E can be made synthetically or extracted naturally from soybean oil, sunflower oil, or other vegetable oils. Natural vitamin E (d-alpha tocopherol) is more expensive but has a greater bioavailability than synthetic vitamin E (dl-alpha tocopherol) (Landvik, 2004; AND, 2018). High-quality vitamin E products usually contain mixed tocopherols and tocotrienols in addition to the d-alpha tocopherol, which is thought to mimic more closely what one would get from eating a food source of vitamin E. Tocotrienols have been shown to possess potent antioxidant and antiinflammatory qualities, although dietary sources such as nuts, seeds, and plant-based oils may be superior to dietary supplements (Peh et al, 2016).

Minerals

Chelated minerals bound to an amino acid or a Krebs cycle intermediary are considered the most easily absorbed form of a mineral supplement, especially in specific populations such as older adults, preterm infants, people with low stomach acid, and those with compromised digestion including inflammatory bowel disease (IBD) and celiac disease but may not be better than other forms in healthy young people (Chermesh et al, 2006). Examples of chelated minerals include citrate, malate, bisglycinate, succinate, aspartate, and picolinate. Chelated minerals are less concentrated that ionic minerals and therefore more pills will often be needed to obtain the same dose. Chelated minerals can also be more expensive. Ionic mineral preparations such as carbonates and oxides should be taken with food, especially protein, to increase absorption (Straub, 2007).

ASSESSMENT OF DIETARY SUPPLEMENT USE IN PATIENTS

Health care professionals should be aware that patients often do not report their use of botanicals or other dietary supplements. Therefore practitioners must inquire specifically about the use of supplements by their patients. To facilitate disclosure, health care providers, including RDNs should approach patients in an open-minded, nonjudgmental manner. Key questions to ask are summarized in Box 11.3. Ideally,

---

BOX 11.3 Evaluating Dietary Supplement Use: The Patient–Health Care Provider Information Exchange

Ask
- What dietary supplements are you taking (type: vitamin, mineral, botanical, amino acid, fiber, including brand and dose)?
- Why are you taking these dietary supplements? Include review of patient's medical diagnosis and symptoms for reasons why they may be taking supplements (e.g., osteoarthritis, heart disease, high blood pressure, premenstrual syndrome [PMS], fatigue).
- How long have you been taking these dietary supplements?
- What dose or how much are you taking? For each, include supplement form and manufacturer.
- With what frequency are you taking each supplement?
- Where were the supplements purchased (e.g., health food store, Internet, health care provider)?
- Who recommended the supplement (e.g., media, physician, nurse, dietitian, integrative medicine practitioner, friend, family)?

Evaluate
- Dietary intake (including intake of fortified foods and beverages, and nutritional and sports bars)

- Health status and health history—include lifestyle habits (e.g., smoking, alcohol, physical activity level)
- Biochemical profile, laboratory data
- Prescribed and over-the-counter (OTC) medications
- Clinical response to supplements
- Adverse events, symptoms

Educate
- Scientific evidence of benefit and effectiveness
- Potential interaction with foods, nutrients, and medications or other dietary supplements
- Appropriate dose, brand, and chemical form; duration of supplementation; appropriate follow-up
- Quality of products, manufacturers, good manufacturing practices (U.S. Pharmacopeia [USP], Consumer Labs)
- Mechanism of action of the primary active ingredient
- Appropriate storage of the dietary supplement
- Administration instructions: With or without food? Potential food-supplement interactions?

BOX 11.3 Evaluating Dietary Supplement Use: The Patient–Health Care Provider Information Exchange—cont'd

- Awareness and reporting of any side effects or adverse events, symptoms
- Recommend necessary dietary changes to support needs. Food should come first.

Document

- List specific supplements and brand names of each supplement being taken.

- Record batch number from bottle in case of an adverse event.
- Record patient perception and expected level of compliance.
- Monitor efficacy and safety, including health outcomes and adverse effects.
- Record medication-supplement or supplement-supplement interactions.
- Plan for follow-up.

From Practice Paper of the American Dietetic Association: Dietary supplements, *J Am Diet Assoc* 105(3):466, 2005. Reprinted with permission.

BOX 11.4 Dietary Supplements that Affect Blood Clotting and Should Be Discontinued 10 to 14 Days Before Surgery or Certain Medical Tests

Ajoene, birch bark, cayenne, Chinese black tree fungus, cumin, evening primrose oil, feverfew, garlic, ginger, *Ginkgo biloba*, ginseng, grapeseed extract, milk thistle, omega-3 fatty acids, onion extract, St. John's wort, turmeric, vitamins C and E

Reference: American College of Surgeons. College of Education: *Medication and Surgery Before Your Operation* (website): http://www.facs.org/patienteducation/medications.html.

BOX 11.5 International Dietetics and Nutrition Terminology (IDNT) that Applies to the Documentation of Dietary Supplement Use Among Patients

Assessment Terminology: Food and Nutrient Intake, Medication and Complementary and Alternative Medicine Use and Knowledge, Beliefs and Attitudes

Diagnosis Terminology: Inadequate bioactive substance intake (NI-4.1), Excessive bioactive substance intake (NI-4.2), Increased nutrient needs (NI-5.1), Decreased nutrient needs (NI-5.4), Imbalance of nutrients (NI-5.5), Less than optimal intake of types of fats (NI-5.6.3), Less than optimal intake of types of proteins or amino acids (NI-5.7.3), Inadequate fiber intake (NI-5.8.6), Inadequate vitamin intake (specify) (NI-5.9.1), Excessive vitamin intake (specify) (NI-5.9.2)

Inadequate mineral intake (specify) (NI-5.10.1), Excessive mineral intake (specify) (NI-5.10.2), Predicted suboptimal nutrient intake (specify) (NI-5.11.1), Predicted excessive nutrient intake (specify) (NI-5.11.2), Impaired nutrient utilization (NC-2.1), Altered nutrition related laboratory values (specify) (NC-2.2), Food-medication interaction (NC-2.3), Predicted food-medication interaction (NC-2.4), Food and nutrition related knowledge deficit (NB-1.1), Unsupported beliefs and attitudes about food or nutrition related topics (NB-1.2), Limited adherence to nutrition related recommendations (NB-1.6)

Intervention Terminology: Vitamin and mineral supplements (specify) (ND-3.2), Bioactive substance management (specify) (ND-3.3), Nutrition related medication management: Nutrition related complementary/alternative medicine (ND-6.3), Nutrition education (specify) (E-1), Nutrition counseling (specify) (C-1), Collaboration and referral of nutrition care (RC-1)

---

patients should be encouraged to bring all of their dietary supplements and medications into the clinic to be evaluated. In this way the health care provider can review doses (including those above the **tolerable upper limit [UL]**), forms, frequency of use, rationale for use, side effects, and the patient-perceived efficacy of each supplement (AND, 2018). This should be done on a regular basis. It is particularly important that dietary supplement use be reviewed before surgery because some dietary supplements and botanicals alter the rate of blood coagulation. Box 11.4 provides specific recommendations regarding the discontinuation of dietary supplements before surgery to avoid complications associated with prolonged bleeding time. In addition, patients on blood-thinning medications may have to be monitored for a potential interaction with these supplements (American College of Surgeons, 2012).

For assessing patients for dietary supplement use using the NCP, potential diagnosis and intervention codes are shown in Box 11.5.

Recommendation and Sale of Dietary Supplements

Many health care professionals are uncomfortable recommending dietary supplements. Clinical guidelines for recommending and selling dietary supplements have been published previously by the Academy of Nutrition and Dietetics (Thompson et al, 2002). Dietitians and nutritionists who recommend dietary supplements must take the initiative to develop their knowledge, skills, and resources to provide accurate and safe recommendations. The AND has developed *The Academy Scope of Practice Decision Tool: A Self-Assessment Guide* for dietetics providers; it is available through the AND website. It can be used to assess competence and scope of practice as defined by training, place of employment, and state of residence. It is advisable to use this tool before beginning any new practice, including recommending or selling dietary supplements.

When recommending dietary supplements to clients, clinicians should use an evidence- or science-based approach and document thoroughly in the patient's medical chart. Documentation should include the supplement name, dosage, form, duration of use, and a short description of supporting evidence. Each provider is responsible to cross-check for contraindications and potential DNIs and document any risks in the patient's medical chart. See Box 11.6 for guidelines for choosing dietary supplements and botanical products and Box 11.7 for information about usage, dosage, and safety of some of the most commonly used dietary supplements.

Resources for Clinicians

As awareness of dietary supplement use expands within the health care community, the number of evidence-based resources available to clinicians is also growing considerably. Clinicians should have access to online and print resources that are updated at regular intervals. Resources that provide references to the original research are preferable. A list of evidence-based resources can be found at the end of the chapter. In addition, accessing available medical literature is advised, given that there are a growing number of studies being published in peer-reviewed literature.

BOX 11.6 Guidelines for Choosing Dietary Supplements and Botanical Products

- Ensure the supplement is appropriate for the individual patient based on state of health, dietary deficiency, and scientific evidence.
- Consider multiple sources of dietary supplements including fortified foods, bars, cereals, and beverages to ensure patients are not exceeding safe intake limits.
- Check for potential drug-nutrient interactions and be aware of side effects and contraindications. For example, fish oil can reduce blood clotting in high doses and antioxidant supplements can inhibit the effects of some chemotherapy drugs.
- Investigate the quality of the manufacturer to ensure a quality product. Look for companies that have third party certification (National Sanitation Foundation [NSF], U.S. Pharmacopeia [USP]), or well-known companies with a longstanding reputation for quality. Check Consumer Labs or the Food and Drug Administration (FDA) warning letters website for documented problems.

- Use the dietary supplement label to obtain important information, including the following:
  - Product identity (including scientific or botanical names), form, and dosage
  - Allergy information in case the patient has a dietary restriction. Excipients (inactive ingredients) are often the source of allergens or unwanted ingredients.
  - A lot number, which is helpful if problems arise because it allows the product to be tracked through each stage of the manufacturing process.
  - An expiration date
- After determining that a manufacturer and its product meet these standards, compare prices among products of similar quality. Prices can vary widely.

National Institutes of Health, Office of Dietary Supplements. *Dietary Supplements: What You Need to Know.* http://ods.od.nih.gov/HealthInformation/DS_WhatYouNeedToKnow.aspx. Academy of Nutrition and Dietetics. Position of the Academy of Nutrition and Dietetics: Micronutrient Supplementation. *J Acad Nut Diet* 118(11):2162–2173, 2018.

BOX 11.7 Popular Dietary Supplements and Their Efficacy

Supplement	Benefits	Dosage	Potential Contraindications	Quality Considerations
Vitamins				
Vitamin B_6	Effective for hereditary sideroblastic anemia, pyridoxine-dependent seizures; Likely effective for hyperhomocysteinemia, age-related macular degeneration, hypertension, calcium oxalate kidney stones, pregnancy induced nausea and vomiting	Most supplemental doses are 5-50 mg/day. 25 mg every 8 hours for pregnancy induced nausea and vomiting. Doses up to 200 mg/day have been used for carpel tunnel, but close monitoring is recommended.	Doses up to 200 mg/day appear to be tolerated by most people, although high doses can cause hypotension and reversible neuropathy.	Available as pyridoxine and pyridoxal 5'-phosphate (coenzyme form).
Vitamin B_{12}	Effective for pernicious anemia and B_{12} deficiency. Likely effective for hyperhomocysteinemia; possibly effective for age-related macular degeneration	Doses in supplements are often in megadoses due to lack of toxicity. Can be taken orally and injected. Common dosage range is 2.4-1000 mcg/day.	Most risk is associated with intravenous forms, not oral forms. People with pernicious anemia will not benefit from oral dosing.	Available as cyanocobalamin, methylcobalamin and adenosylcobalamin (coenzyme forms). Active form may be beneficial for those with genetic polymorphisms; however all forms of B_{12} have been found effective for correcting B_{12} deficiency.
Vitamin C	Effective for scurvy; likely effective for iron absorption enhancement; possibly effective for age-related macular degeneration, cancer prevention, common cold prevention and treatment, complex regional pain syndrome, hypertension, osteoarthritis, sunburn	Doses vary widely but usually range from 100-2000 mg/day. Use divided doses for enhanced absorption.	Safe at lower doses and in amounts found in foods. Higher doses can cause diarrhea and gastrointestinal cramping. Greater than 500 mg is contraindicated for those who have a history of calcium oxalate kidney stones.	Mineral ascorbates (buffered vitamin C) or Ester C® may be better tolerated (less gastrointestinal [GI] distress) than ascorbic acid for some people.

BOX 11.7 Popular Dietary Supplements and Their Efficacy—cont'd

Supplement	Benefits	Dosage	Potential Contraindications	Quality Considerations
Vitamin D	Effective for familial hypophosphatemia, hypoparathyroidism, osteomalacia, psoriasis, renal osteodystrophy, and rickets. Likely effective for corticosteroid induced osteoporosis, fall prevention in older adults, osteoporosis. Possibly effective for prevention of cancer, dental caries, multiple sclerosis, respiratory tract infections, rheumatoid arthritis, and obesity.	Dose is usually based on individual serum levels and can vary from person to person. Optimal serum level is considered to be 30-50 nmol/L. In research, doses range from 400 IU to 50,000 IU/day. The tolerable upper limit (UL) is 4000 IU (100 mcg)/day.	Exceeding the UL and elevated serum concentrations are associated with calcification of soft tissues (damage to the heart, blood vessels, and kidney), and increased risk for kidney stones. Risk may be increased in postmenopausal women who also take supplemental calcium. Best to coordinate care with primary care provider and monitor blood levels.	Cholecalciferol (D_3) is the most common supplement and is usually sourced from fish or sheep (lanolin), lichen, or mushrooms. Ergocalciferol (D_2) is suitable for vegetarians and vegans.
Vitamin E	Effective for vitamin E deficiency. Possibly effective for slowing cognitive decline in Alzheimer's disease, improving response to erythropoietin in hemodialysis, reducing cisplatin induced neurotoxicity and pain in rheumatoid arthritis, prevention of dementia, dysmenorrhea, premenstrual syndrome (PMS), Parkinson's disease, and radiation induced fibrosis and increasing muscle strength in older adults.	Most supplements are between 50 and 2000 IU. Most common dose is 200-400 IU/day.	Doses above 400 IU/day may increase risk for bleeding, prostate cancer, and have prooxidant effects.	D-alpha tocopherol is the natural form of vitamin E and dl-alpha tocopherol is the synthetic form. Natural forms with mixed tocopherols, specifically gamma tocopherol, may have cardioprotective effects. Supplemental Vitamin E has been linked with prostate cancer in the SELECT trial. This result was not found in other studies (Physicians' Health Study II [PHS II] and Women's Health Study (WHS)).
Folic acid/Folate	Effective for folate deficiency. Likely effective for hyperhomocysteinemia, methotrexate toxicity, and neural tube defects. Possibly effective for age-related macular degeneration, depression, hypertension.	Recommended dietary allowance (RDA) level is recommended in most people, although those with MTHFR variant or chronic conditions may need higher levels (200 mcg-5 mg/day has been used although 800 mcg-1000 mg is most common). Coordinate care with physician for megadose amounts. The Institute of Medicine (IOM) recommends adults limit their intake from supplements and fortification to 1000 mg/d	Excess folic acid (5 mg and above) can cause B_{12} deficiency. Folic acid supplements can also mask B_{12} deficiency. Caution with folic acid supplementation in those at risk for colon cancer.	Supplemental sources have greater bioavailability than folate in food. People with a MTHFR variant may have increased need for folate. The methylated form, methylenetetrahydrofolate is also used.
Minerals Calcium	Effective for dyspepsia, hyperkalemia, and renal failure (as a phosphate binder). Likely effective for osteoporosis, corticosteroid induced osteoporosis, hyperparathyroidism, and premenstrual syndrome. Possibly effective for reducing risk of colorectal cancer, hypercholesterolemia, hypertension, and prevention of weight gain.	500-1000 mg/day is a typical dose. Do not exceed the UL.	High doses can increase risk for kidney stones, cardiovascular disease (CVD), and constipation. CVD risk is greater in postmenopausal women who take supplemental calcium. Caution in patients with hyperparathyroidism.	Chelated forms such as citrate and malate are better absorbed than carbonate unless taken with a meal. Coadministration with vitamin K may be helpful to reduce risk of hypercalcemia except in those taking blood-thinning medications

Continued

BOX 11.7 Popular Dietary Supplements and Their Efficacy—cont'd

Supplement	Benefits	Dosage	Potential Contraindications	Quality Considerations
Chromium	Effective for chromium deficiency. Possibly effective for reducing blood sugar in diabetes, decreasing low-density lipoprotein (LDL) cholesterol, and triglycerides.	Studies have used 150-1000 mcg/day. Adequate intakes are thought to be 25-35 mcg/day for adults. No UL has been established.	Trivalent chromium is found in appropriate dietary supplements. Poor quality brands may contain hexavalent chromium, which is toxic and linked to cancer. Caution in those with diabetes, renal impairment. Higher doses may cause dermatitis and/or gastrointestinal irritation.	Chromium picolinate is the most common form and is thought to be well absorbed.
Iron	Effective for iron deficiency anemia and pregnancy induced anemia. Possibly effective for ACE inhibitor induced cough, cognitive function, restless leg syndrome, and heart failure	RDA is recommended unless blood work indicates increased need. Needs increase in pregnancy. Vegetarians may need higher levels because of decreased bioavailability from plant foods. 4-6 mg/kg/day or 60-120 mg/day for those with anemia. Some research shows intermittent doses (several times a week to weekly) can be effective for prevention of anemia in multiple populations.	Ensure the presence of iron deficiency anemia before supplementing with iron (also check ferritin level). Do not exceed the UL except with coordination of care with a physician. Excessive iron intake can cause nausea, constipation, and black stools and may increase the risk of heart disease.	Chelated iron (citrate, bisglycinate) and Feosol® (carbonyl iron) may be better tolerated and cause fewer gastrointestinal side effects.
Magnesium	Effective for constipation, dyspepsia, preeclampsia, and eclampsia. Possibly effective for asthma prevention, cancer associated neuropathic pain, chronic fatigue syndrome, chronic obstructive pulmonary disease (COPD), cluster headaches, osteoporosis, diabetes (improved blood glucose control), and vasospastic angina. IV forms are effective for cardiac arrhythmia, acute pre term labor and acute asthma attacks. Magnesium is often used in fibromyalgia and migraine headache, but the results are mixed.	Typical dose is 100-500 mg/day. Exceeding the UL from supplements (350 mg/day) is not recommended because of potential for diarrhea.	The most common side effects with high doses are diarrhea, bloating, and reduction in blood pressure. Serious side effects are a risk with IV magnesium, including hypotension, nausea, and ataxia.	Chelated forms such as citrate, bisglycinate, and amino acid chelate may be better absorbed and tolerated (less GI side effects) than oxide form.
Selenium	Possibly effective for autoimmune thyroiditis, dyslipidemia, prevention of HIV virus replication and increased immune cell count, reduced risk of cancer and cancer mortality with good selenium status. Used as an antioxidant supplement as a cofactor for selenocysteine and glutathione production.	Daily recommended intake is 55-70 mcg/day although most supplemental doses are in the 100-200 mcg range. Exceeding the UL of 400 mcg/day is not recommended.	Gastrointestinal symptoms, nausea, and vomiting are most common with high doses. Acute toxicity may impair liver, kidney, and cardiac function.	Brazil nuts are an excellent source of selenium. Selenium and vitamin E have a synergistic effect and are best taken together.

BOX 11.7   Popular Dietary Supplements and Their Efficacy—cont'd

Supplement	Benefits	Dosage	Potential Contraindications	Quality Considerations
Zinc	Likely effective for diarrhea and Wilson's disease. Possibly effective for acne, age-related macular degeneration, anemia, anorexia nervosa, attention deficit hyperactivity disorder, burns, common cold, dandruff, depression, diabetic foot ulcers, diaper rash, halitosis, gingivitis, herpes simplex virus, muscle cramps, radiation mucositis, osteoporosis, peptic ulcers, pressure ulcers, sickle cell disease, vitamin A deficiency, warts	Doses vary depending on condition. 15-45 mg/day range is common. Much higher doses sometimes given for wound healing short term. Coordination of care recommended.	Mostly nontoxic below the UL of 40 mg/day in adults. High zinc intake can deplete copper and can cause nausea, dermatitis, and copper deficient anemia.	Take zinc supplements with copper to prevent depletion of copper. Zinc lozenges have been used to prevent and treat the common cold.

Other Supplements

Supplement	Benefits	Dosage	Potential Contraindications	Quality Considerations
Arginine	Possibly effective for angina, erectile dysfunction, hypertension, necrotizing enterocolitis (NEC), peripheral artery disease, post-surgery recovery, and preeclampsia.	Therapeutic dose range is thought to be from 400-6000 mg/day. There is no tolerable upper limit and higher doses (up to 30 g/day) have been used. Coordination of care recommended	High doses may increase bleeding in those on warfarin, may lower blood sugar and blood pressure. Caution in those with history of myocardial infarction or cancer	No special production or quality control issues with arginine. L- arginine is the active form.
Beta-glucans	Likely effective for hyperlipidemia. Possibly effective for allergic rhinitis (hay fever), cancer survival, and postoperative infection. Beta glucans can stimulate the immune response including upregulating natural killer cells and tumor necrosis factor.	3 g beta-glucan/day (from oats) per the FDA as a cholesterol lowering food. In supplements, 2-16 g/day is common dosing for hyperlipidemia.	Generally well tolerated with few side effects. May cause mild gastrointestinal symptoms in some. Can lower blood pressure and blood sugar	Found widely in plant-based foods, especially oats and mushrooms.
Coenzyme Q$_{10}$ (Ubiquinone)	Possibly effective for mitochondrial encephalomyopathies, age-related macular degeneration, cardiovascular mortality, congestive heart failure, diabetic neuropathy, HIV/AIDS, hypertension, ischemic reperfusion injury, migraine headache, and Parkinson's disease.	Doses vary from 30-600 mg/day. The most common dosing is 100-200 mg/d in divided doses	Very few side effects reported other than mild nausea, headache, and skin itching. May decrease blood pressure. Caution with people on blood-thinning medications	Oil-based preparations may be better absorbed. Ubiquinol is the active form and may be more biologically active, although most people are able to convert ubiquinone to ubiquinol without problems.
Creatine	Possibly effective for athletic performance enhancement (muscle mass and muscle strength) and age-related muscle loss.	Usually taken as a loading dose of 20 grams per day for 4-7 days followed by a maintenance dose of 2-10 grams per day for up to 14 weeks in conjunction with strength training. Doses up to 30 g have been taken safely short term.	Considered safe for healthy people. Increased fluid needs when taking creatine. Caution with kidney disease especially if taking nonsteroidal antiinflammatory drugs (NSAIDs). Increased symptoms of anxiety and depression have been noted.	Usually sold as creatine monohydrate.

Continued

BOX 11.7 Popular Dietary Supplements and Their Efficacy—cont'd

Supplement	Benefits	Dosage	Potential Contraindications	Quality Considerations
DHEA Dehydroepiandrosterone	Possibly effective for aging skin and depression. Mixed results in studies on use in adrenal insufficiency, depression, chronic fatigue syndrome, fibromyalgia, HIV/AIDS, osteoporosis, physical performance, sexual dysfunction, weight loss. Most doctors treat with DHEA based on individual laboratory values.	Dose should be recommended by a physician and based on laboratory results. Doses range from 5-450 mg/day.	May increase estrogen and testosterone and risk for hormone imbalance and cancer. May increase acne, facial hair growth, and cause other hormonal side effects. Avoid with hormone blockers such as tamoxifen. Multiple contraindications.	7 Keto dehydroepiandrosterone (DHEA) is a metabolite of DHEA that is not converted into estrogen or testosterone and is thought to be a safer alternative to DHEA.
Fish oil	Effective for hypertriglyceridemia. Likely effective for cardiovascular disease. Possibly effective prevention of restenosis after angioplasty and coronary artery bypass grafts, attention deficit hyperactivity disorder, bipolar disorder, cachexia, dysmenorrhea, heart failure, hypertension, psoriasis, Raynaud's syndrome, rheumatoid arthritis, stroke. Conflicting evidence for depression, eczema, inflammatory bowel disease, autism.	1-4 g/day of eicosapentaenoic acid (EPA) and docosahexaenoic acid (DHA) combined. Up to 3 g/day is considered generally recognized as safe (GRAS) and the Food and Drug Administration (FDA) recommends not exceeding 2 g/d EPA/DHA from dietary supplements.	More than 3 g/day EPA/DHA may increase risk for bleeding, bruising, and elevation in blood sugar. Caution with people on blood-thinning medications and those with diabetes (may increase blood glucose above 3 grams EPA/DHA).	Molecular distilled fish oil is considered the best quality. For vegetarians, flaxseed oil may also be beneficial. Use cold pressed oil in dark bottles or refrigerate. The International Fish Oil Standards (IFOS) website lists brands that have passed strict international standards for purity.
Glucosamine	Possibly effective for mild to moderate osteoarthritis; conflicting or insufficient evidence to rate effectiveness for interstitial cystitis and temporomandibular (TMJ) disorders and postoperative recovery.	Typical dose for joint conditions is 1500 mg/day taken in 2-3 divided doses. Lower doses of 400-1000 mg/day have been used for other conditions.	Considered to be a safe supplement for most people. Most is sourced from shellfish, so may be an allergen in some. High doses can disrupt blood sugar metabolism in those with diabetes. Caution in those with renal dysfunction or in those taking warfarin.	Most research has been done on glucosamine sulfate form, although glucosamine hydrochloride has also been used with success. Glucosamine is often sold in combination with chondroitin for added benefit.
Glutamine	Possibly effective for use in burn patients, bone marrow transplants, burns, critical illness (trauma), AIDS wasting, and to improve nitrogen balance after surgery. Conflicting evidence for use with diarrhea (especially due to chemotherapy), oral mucositis, inflammatory bowel disease and short bowel syndrome.	5-30 g/day orally is a typical dose. Doses in IV or total parenteral nutrition (TPN) in the critically ill may be higher.	Considered safe. Many drugs deplete body stores of glutamine. Caution with higher doses in those with renal or liver impairment due to nitrogen content.	Take separately from food (especially protein) for maximal absorption.

BOX 11.7   Popular Dietary Supplements and Their Efficacy—cont'd

Supplement	Benefits	Dosage	Potential Contraindications	Quality Considerations
Melatonin	Likely effective for delayed sleep phase syndrome and sleep disorders, especially in the blind. Possibly effective for insomnia, benzodiazepine withdrawal, jet lag. High doses have been used to promote tumor regression in some forms of cancer.	500 mcg-5 mg/day have been used in research. 3-5 mg/day is the most common dose. 10-40 mg has been used for tumor regression—coordination of care with an oncologist is essential.	Generally regarded as safe for use up to 3 months and is even tolerated in neonates. Most common side effects are headache, nausea, and drowsiness. May lower blood pressure and disrupt hormone balance.	Usually taken 30 minutes before bed for sleep disorders.
Probiotics (lactobacillus acidophilus and bifidobacteria)	Likely effective for rotaviral diarrhea. Possibly effective for antibiotic associated diarrhea, atopic dermatitis (eczema), clostridium difficile diarrhea, chemotherapy induced diarrhea, constipation, Helicobacter pylori inflammation, infantile colic, irritable bowel syndrome, pouchitis, respiratory tract infections, travelers diarrhea, ulcerative colitis	Dosage varies and is measured in colony forming units (CFUs). Range is 1-450 billion CFU depending on the disease condition and therapeutic goal.	May be contraindicated in the immune suppressed, those with central line placement (especially saccharomyces boulardii), and in those on hemodialysis due to risk of sepsis. May cause diarrhea in high doses especially if the supplement contains prebiotics like inulin. May be contraindicated in premature infants with risk of bacteremia.	Refrigeration is important to preserve quality in most products; however, some products are shelf stable. Yeast-based probiotics (saccharomyces boulardii) are shelf stable.
Herbs				
Chamomile *Matricaria recutita* (German Chamomile)	Possibly effective for anxiety, colic, diarrhea, dyspepsia, and oral mucositis.	250-1100 mg/day in capsules or 1-4 cups/day as tea.	GRAS. Caution in those with allergy to ragweed or Asteraceae family.	Ensure correct plant is used. German chamomile (not Roman Chamomile) is the most common.
Cinnamon *Cinnamomum cassia*	Possibly effective for reducing fasting glucose in diabetes.	Typical dose is 120 mg-6 g/day in capsules or 1 tsp/day in food.	Generally safe. Caution in people with diabetes or blood sugar dysregulation or in those with impaired liver function. May enhance blood-thinning effects of warfarin.	Cassia cinnamon is more biologically active than Ceylon cinnamon for blood sugar regulation.
Cranberry *Vaccinium macrocarpon*	Possibly effective for urinary tract infection, (prevention and treatment). Preliminary evidence for reducing urinary odor and improving symptoms in benign prostatic hyperplasia (BPH).	As juice: 1 oz cranberry concentrate or 10 oz cranberry cocktail (sweetened). As capsules: 300-500 mg twice/day or 200 mg twice/day with 25% standardization of proanthocyanidins (PAC).	Generally safe. Caution with sugar in juice for diabetics, may increase calcium oxalate kidney stones.	Blueberries have similar constituents and may be similarly beneficial. Many supplements are standardized to contain a specific amount of PAC. This preparation may have a stronger effect.
Echinacea angustifolia, pallida and *purpurea*	Possibly effective for the common cold. Insufficient evidence for influenza, herpes simplex virus, human papilloma virus, and otitis media.	Can be taken as a capsule, tablet, tea, or tincture. Doses vary and are dependent on the variety used and preparation. 5 mL fresh juice or 20 drops in water every 2 hours, 4 mL 10 times per day for the first day of a cold then three times a day for the duration.	Caution in people with allergy to Asteraceae family (daisy, sunflower), and those on immunosuppressive medications.	Sometimes standardized to contain a specific amount of echinacoside or cichoric acid.

Continued

BOX 11.7   Popular Dietary Supplements and Their Efficacy—cont'd

Supplement	Benefits	Dosage	Potential Contraindications	Quality Considerations
Fenugreek *Trigonella foenum-graecum*	Possibly effective for improving blood sugar control in diabetes and dysmenorrhea. Conflicting evidence for promoting lactation, PCOS and hyperlipidemia.	Highly variable. 5-100 grams of ground seeds added to food although 2-5 grams 2-3 times per day is most common.	Long term studies lacking although the seeds are a staple some Asian cuisine. Therapeutic doses in children may be unsafe and not recommended for use during pregnancy (uterine stimulant). Few side effects noted. More than 100 grams may cause hypoglycemia. Avoid use with diabetes medications.	Ensure quality brand. In one case seeds were contaminated with E Coli and caused death. Generally recognized as safe (GRAS) as a food.
Garlic *Allium sativum*	Possibly effective for atherosclerosis, reducing blood sugar in diabetes, reducing blood lipids in hyperlipidemia, hypertension. Conflicting evidence for the common cold and cancer prevention.	2-5 g fresh garlic, 0.4-1.2 g dried powder, 2-5 mg oil, or 300-1000 mg extract to deliver 2-5 mg allicin (active constituent) per day. One clove fresh garlic has also been used.	Generally well tolerated. Higher doses may cause gastric irritation, body odor, and decreased blood pressure. Caution with those who are taking blood thinners and hypoglycemic drugs.	Comes in many forms in supplements. Those that preserve allicin content may be more effective. Aged extracts have shown benefits as well because of the multitude of sulfur compounds present.
Green tea *Camellia sinensis*	Likely effective for hyperlipidemia. Possibly effective for coronary artery disease, hypotension, Parkinson's disease. Conflicting evidence for cancer prevention, cardiovascular disease, and for weight loss.	Epigallocatechin (EGCG) epicate-chin gallate, and epicatechin levels vary when taken as tea. 3 cups daily is a common dosage. Standardized extracts (60%-97% polyphenols) of 200-500 mg/day are common for a variety of conditions. 10% topical cream for skin aging and acne.	Well tolerated in most people. Most side effects come from the caffeine content (nervousness, anxiety, sleeplessness, and increased blood pressure). Use with caution in patients with psychiatric or cardiovascular conditions.	Decaffeinated versions are available to eliminate caffeine side effects.
Kava Kava *Piper methysticum*	Possibly effective for anxiety; insufficient evidence for benzodiazepine withdrawal, stress reduction, insomnia, and menopausal anxiety.	60-400 mg standardized extract per day.	Typical therapeutic doses are tolerated by most. Significant evidence of liver injury. Caution in people with liver disease. Chronic use can cause dry, scaly skin and photosensitivity.	Often standardized to contain 30%-70% kavalactones. May be best to start at lower doses and titrate up.
Milk thistle *Silybum marianum*	Although it is commonly used to reduce inflammation and fibrosis in liver disease, it is possibly effective for lowering fasting glucose in diabetes, and for dyspepsia. There is conflicting and insufficient evidence for alcohol related liver disease, amanita mushroom poisoning, cirrhosis, and hepatitis induced liver damage.	160-1200 mg/day based on condition treated. Take as divided doses. 140 mg standardized extract taken three times per day is a common dose.	Low toxicity risk. Can cause a mild laxative effect if taken in large amounts. Rare risk of allergic reaction. May lower blood sugar. May mildly inhibit CYP 34A, 2C19, and 2D6 cytochrome enzymes.	Often standardized to contain 70%-80% silymarin. Tea preparation is not recommended because of poor water solubility. Whole, ground milk thistle seeds can be added to food.
Red Yeast Rice (RYR) *Monascus purpureus*	Likely effective for hyperlipidemia. Possibly effective for CVD and diabetes and HIV/AIDS related dyslipidemia. Preliminary evidence for use in nonalcoholic fatty liver disease (NAFLD).	The most common dose is 600- 2400 mg/day. It is estimated that average intake of naturally occurring RYR in Asia is 14-55 g/day.	Limited data on adverse events. Side effects appear to be similar to those with low-dose statin medications (headache, gastrointestinal discomfort, and muscle pain). May increase liver enzymes.	Contains naturally occurring lovastatin (Monacolin K). Dosing is difficult because of natural variations in products. It is illegal in the United States to standardize Monacolin K levels in supplements.

BOX 11.7	Popular Dietary Supplements and Their Efficacy—cont'd			
Supplement	**Benefits**	**Dosage**	**Potential Contraindications**	**Quality Considerations**
St. John's Wort *Hypericum perforatum*	Likely effective for mild to moderate depression. Possibly effective for menopausal symptoms, somatization disorder. Conflicting or insufficient evidence for anxiety, obsessive compulsive disorder, premenstrual syndrome, seasonal affective disorder. Can be used topically for wound healing.	Typical dose is 300-450 mg three times per day. Coordination of care with a physician is important.	**Has the most drug nutrient interactions of any common herb.** Inhibits CYP 34A, 2C19, and 2C9 cytochrome enzymes and the P-glycoprotein (P-gp) transporter. Reduces the effectiveness of immunosuppressive, antiretroviral, cardiovascular, and oral contraceptive medications among others. Can cause photosensitity.	Typically standardized at 0.3% hypericin.
Turmeric *Curcuma longa*	Possibly effective for allergic rhinitis, depression, hyperlipidemia, NAFLD, ulcerative colitis, and osteoarthritis. Conflicting evidence for Alzheimer's disease, colorectal cancer, Crohn's disease, irritable bowel syndrome, rheumatoid arthritis, and ulcerative colitis.	500 mg-2 g curcumin per day depending on disease condition. Higher doses taken in divided doses.	Safe in amounts eaten in food. Higher doses can lower blood pressure and blood sugar and increase risk of bleeding. Caution in those with liver and gall bladder diseases and in those taking blood-thinning medications.	May be best absorbed when taken with food, especially a meal that contains fat. Curcumin supplements bound to phosphatidyl choline (Meriva) may be better absorbed.

Natural Medicines Comprehensive Database. https://naturalmedicines.therapeuticresearch.com/.
Linus Pauling Institute. https://lpi.oregonstate.edu/mic.
Consumer Lab. https://www.consumerlab.com/.

CLINICAL CASE STUDY

Ellen is a 60-year-old white female who was referred from her primary care provider for evaluation of her dietary supplements. Medical history includes hypertension, hypercholesterolemia, osteopenia, mild depression, and memory problems. Two years ago, she had angioplasty (PTCA) with a stent placement in her coronary artery. Ellen is a retired school teacher, married, and has two grown children. Her neighbor works in a supplement store and recommended some herbs and supplements to address Ellen's health concerns.

At the initial consult Ellen reports she is taking the following supplements: calcium carbonate 1200 mg/d, garlic (*Allium sativum*) 500 mg/d, *Ginkgo biloba* 240 mg/d, and St. John's wort (*Hypericum perforatum*) 900 mg/d. Her prescription medications include warfarin, simvastatin, sertraline, and atenolol.

Height: 64" Weight: 165 lbs BMI: 28.4
Blood pressure readings: 134/92, 140/95 "This is higher than it usually is" Ellen reports.
Recent labs:
Total cholesterol: 284 mg/dL
High-density lipoprotein (HDL): 36 mg/dL
Low-density lipoprotein (LDL): 140 mg/dL
Prothrombin times (INR) has been inconsistent lately.
Typical dietary intake includes the following:
Breakfast: Total cereal with milk and calcium fortified orange juice

Lunch: Frozen entrée—beef and broccoli with rice and a Diet Coke
Snack: Strawberry yogurt and pretzels, coffee with milk
Dinner: Meatloaf, mashed potatoes with gravy and carrots. Glass of red wine.
Dessert: Chocolate ice cream, coffee with milk

Nutrition Diagnostic Statements

- Predicted food medication interaction (NC-2.4) related to a food and nutrition knowledge deficit about DNI's as evidenced by taking St. John's Wort with sertraline and the potential for serotonin syndrome.
- Altered nutrition related laboratory value (NC-2.2) related to knowledge deficit about DNI's, as evidenced by taking ginkgo and garlic with warfarin and inconsistent INRs

Nutrition Care Questions

1. Using the Office of Dietary Supplements Fact Sheets (ODS website), identify what each dietary supplement Ellen is taking is used for and if it has good evidence to support use.
2. List any potential drug nutrient interactions (DNIs) Ellen may have with her current concomitant use of medications and dietary supplements.
3. Looking at Ellen's lab tests, is there any evidence she may be having a DNI?
4. Does Ellen need to be taking a calcium supplement? Are there any potential risks with taking 1200 mg/day with a positive history of cardiovascular disease (CVD)?

USEFUL WEBSITES

Free Sites

FDA MedWatch
Linus Pauling Micronutrient Information Center
Medscape Drug Interaction Checker
National Center for Complementary and Integrative Health
Natural Products Association
Office of Dietary Supplements
Operation Supplement Safety (U.S. Department of Defense)

Subscription Sites

Cochrane Database Review
Consumer Lab
Dietitians in Integrative and Functional Medicine (DIFM) practice group through the Academy of Nutrition and Dietetics
Institute for Functional Medicine
Natural Medicines Database

Text/Print

Moyad M. *The Supplement Handbook*, New York, 2014, Rodale.

Resources for Herbal Medicine

American Botanical Council (ABC)
American Herbal Products Association (AHPA)
American Herbalists Guild (AHG)
Dr. Duke's Phytochemical and Ethnobotanical Database

REFERENCES

Academic Consortium for Integrative Medicine and Health: *Introduction*, 2018. Available at: https://imconsortium.org/.

Academy of Nutrition and Dietetics: Position of the Academy of Nutrition and Dietetics: micronutrient supplementation, *J Acad Nut Diet* 118(11):2162–2173, 2018.

American College of Surgeons, College of Education: *Medication and surgery before your operation*, 2014. Available at: http://www.facs.org/patienteducation/medications.html.

American Herbalists Guild: *Herbal medicine fundamentals*, 2019. Available at: http://www.americanherbalistsguild.com/herbal-medicine-fundamentals.

Ames BN, Elson-Schwab I, Silver EA: High dose vitamin therapy stimulates variant enzymes with decreased coenzyme binding affinity (increased K(m)): relevance to genetic disease and polymorphisms, *Am J Clin Nutr* 75:616–658, 2002.

Augustine MB, Swift KM, Harris SR, et al: Integrative medicine: Education, Perceived knowledge, attitudes and practice among Academy of Nutrition and Dietetics Members, *J Acad Nutr Diet* 116(2):319–329, 2016.

Bailey RL, Fakhouri TH, Park Y, et al: Multivitamin-mineral use is associated with reduced risk of cardiovascular disease mortality among women in the United States, *J Nutr* 145:572–578, 2015.

Bailey RL, Fulgoni VL III, Keast DR, et al: Do dietary supplements improve micronutrient sufficiency in children and adolescents? *J Pediatr* 161:837–842, 2012.

Bailey RL, Gahche JJ, Miller PE, et al: Why US adults use dietary supplements, *JAMA Intern Med* 173(5):355–361, 2013.

Bjelakovic G, Nikolova D, Gluud LL, et al: Antioxidant supplements for prevention of mortality in healthy participants and patients with various diseases, *Cochrane Database Syst Rev* 3:CD007176, 2012. doi:10.1002/14651858.CD007176.pub2.

Blumberg JB, Bailey RL, Sesso HD, et al: The evolving role of multivitamin/multi-mineral supplement use among adults in the age of personalized nutrition, *Nutrients* 10:E248–E265, 2018.

Blumberg JB, Frei BB, Fulgoni VL, et al: Impact of frequency of multi-vitamin/multi-mineral supplement intake on nutritional adequacy and nutrient deficiencies in U.S. adults, *Nutrients* 9:849–864, 2017.

Boden WE, Sidhu MS, Toth PP: The therapeutic role of niacin in dyslipidemia management, *J Cardiovasc Pharmacol Ther* 19(2):141–158, 2014.

Bowman SA, Clemens JC, Friday JE, et al: *Food patterns equivalents intakes by Americans: what we eat in America, NHANES 2003-2004 and 2015-2016*. Food Surveys Research Group. Dietary Data Brief No. 20, November 2018.

Brown AC: An overview of herb and dietary supplement efficacy, safety and government regulations in the United States with suggested improvements. Part 1 of 5 series, *Food Chem Toxicol* 107:449–471, 2017.

Chermesh I, Tamir A, Suissa A, et al: Ferrus calcium citrate is absorbed better than iron bisglycinate in patients with Crohn's disease, but not in healthy controls, *Dig Dis Sci* 51(5):942–945, 2006.

Chew EY, Clemons TE, Agrón E, et al: Long-term effects of vitamins C and E, β-carotene, and zinc on age-related macular degeneration: AREDS report no. 35, *Ophthalmology* 120(8):1604–1611.e4, 2013.

Cohen PA, Maller G, DeSouza R, et al: Presence of banned drugs and dietary supplements following FDA recalls. *JAMA* 312(16):1691–1693, 2014.

Council for Responsible Nutrition: *2017 CRN Consumer survey on dietary supplements*, 2017. Available at: http://crnusa.org/resources/2017-crn-consumer-survey-dietary-supplements.

Drake VJ and Frei B: *Micronutrient inadequacies in the US population: an overview*, 2018. Available at: https://lpi.oregonstate.edu/mic/micronutrient-inadequacies/overview#references.

Falci L, Shi Z, Greenlee H: Multiple chronic conditions and use of complementary and alternative medicine among US adults: results from the 2012 National Health Interview Survey, *Prev Chronic Dis* 13:E61, 2016.

Food and Drug Administration: *Guidance for industry: current good manufacturing practice in manufacturing, packaging, labeling, or holding operations for dietary supplements; small entity compliance guide*, 2010. Available at: http://www.fda.gov/food/guidanceregulation/guidancedocumentsregulatoryinformation/dietarysupplements/ucm238182.htm.

Food and Drug Administration: *Reports received and reports entered into FAERS by year*, 2012. Available at: http://www.fda.gov/Drugs/GuidanceComplianceRegulatoryInformation/Surveillance/AdverseDrugEffects/ucm070434.htm.

Food and Drug Administration: *Guidance for industry: questions and answers regarding adverse event reporting and recordkeeping for dietary supplements as required by the dietary supplement and Nonprescription Drug Consumer Protection Act*, 2013. Available at: https://www.fda.gov/regulatory-information/search-fda-guidance-documents/guidance-industry-questions-and-answers-regarding-labeling-dietary-supplements-required-dietary.

Food and Drug Administration: *Q and A on dietary supplements: what is a dietary supplement?* 2015. Available at: http://www.fda.gov/Food/DietarySupplements/QADietarySupplements/default.htm#what_is.

Food and Drug Administration: *Tainted products marketed as dietary supplements potentially dangerous*, 2018. Available at: https://www.accessdata.fda.gov/scripts/sda/sdNavigation.cfm?sd=tainted_supplements_cder.

Fortmann SP, Burda BU, Senger CA, et al: *Vitamin, mineral and multivitamin supplements for the primary prevention of cardiovascular disease and cancer: a systematic evidence review for the U.S. preventive services task force*, Report No.: 14-05199-EF-1. Rockville, MD, 2013, Agency for Healthcare Research and Quality.

Gahche J, Bailey R, Burt V, et al: *Centers for disease control and prevention. Dietary supplement use among US adults and children has increased since NHANESIII 2014*. Available at: http://www.cdc.gov/nchs/data/databriefs/db61.pdf.

Geller AI, Shehab N, Weidle NJ, et al: Emergency department visits for adverse events related to dietary supplements, *N Engl J Med* 373(16):1531–1540, 2015.

Gaziano JM, Sesso HD, Christen WG, et al: Multivitamins in the Prevention of Cancer in Men: The Physicians' Health Study II Randomized Controlled Trial. *JAMA* 308(18):1871–1880, 2012.

Government Accountability Office: *Dietary supplements: FDA may have opportunities to expand its use of reported health problems to oversee products*, 2013. Available at: http://www.gao.gov/assets/660/653113.pdf.

Gurley BJ: Pharmacokinetic herb-drug interactions (Part 1): origins, mechanisms, and the impact of botanical dietary supplements, *Planta Med* 78:1478–1489, 2012.

Gurley BJ, Fifer EK, Gardner Z: Pharmacokinetic herb-drug interactions (Part 2): drug interactions involving popular botanical dietary supplements and their clinical relevance, *Planta Med* 78:1490–1514, 2012.

Harris PE, Cooper KL, Relton C, et al: Prevalence of complementary and alternative medicine (CAM) use by the general population: a systematic review, *Int J Clin Prac* 66(10):924–939, 2012.

Head KA: Peripheral neuropathy: pathogenic mechanisms and alternative therapies, *Altern Med Rev* 11(14):294–329, 2006.

Hendren RL: Autism: biomedical complementary treatment approaches, *Child Adolesc Psychiatr Clin N Am* 22:443–456, 2013.

Horrigan B, Lewis S, Abrams D, et al: *Integrative medicine in America. How integrative medicine is being practiced in clinical centers across the United States,* 2012, The Bravewell Collaborative. Available at: http://www.bravewell.org/current_projects/mapping_field/.

Institute for Functional Medicine: *What is functional medicine?* 2018. Available at: http://www.functionalmedicine.org/about/whatisfm.

Landvik S: Vitamin E from supplements has good bioavailability, *Am J Clin Nutr* 80(3):784–785, 2004.

Long J: *FDA still finding same cGMP deficiencies at dietary supplement facilities,* 2018, Natural Products Insider. Available at: https://www.naturalproductsinsider.com/regulatory/fda-still-finding-same-cgmp-deficiencies-dietary-supplement-facilities.

Morton C: *State of the supplements industry. Nutrition business journal (Data brief online),* 2018. Available at: https://www.newhope.com/sites/newhope360.com/files/state-of-the-supplement-industry-2018.pdf.

National Center for Complementary and Integrative Health: *Complementary, alternative, or integrative health: what's in a name?* 2018. Available at: http://nccam.nih.gov/health/whatiscam.

National Institutes of Health: *Dietary supplement Health and Education Act of 1994* Public law 103-417 103rd Congress, 1994. Available at: https://ods.od.nih.gov/About/DSHEA_Wording.aspx.

Noland and Raj: Academy of Nutrition and Dietetics: Revised 2019 Standards of Practice and Standards of Professional Performance for Registered Dietitian Nutritionists (Competent, Proficient, and Expert) in Nutrition in Integrative and Functional Medicine. *Jour of the Acad of Nut and Diet* 119(6):1019–1036.e47, 2019

Obeid R, Fedosov SN, Nexo E, et al: Cobalamin coenzyme forms are not likely to be superior to cyano- and hydroxyl-cobalamin in prevention or treatment of cobalamin deficiency, *Mol Nutr Food Res* 59(7): 1364–1372, 2015.

Peh HY, Tan WS, Liao W, et al: Vitamin E therapy beyond cancer: tocopherol vs. tocotrienol, *Pharmacol Ther* 162:152–169, 2016.

Peregoy JA, Clarke TC, Jones LI, et al: Regional variation in use of complementary health approaches by US adults, *NCHS Data Brief* (146):1–8, 2014.

Quato DM, Alexander GC, Guadamuz JS, et al: Prevalence of dietary supplement use in US children and adolescents, 2003-2014, *JAMA Pediatr* 172(8):780–782, 2018.

Rautiainen S, Rist PM, Glynn R, et al: Multivitamin use and the risk of cardiovascular disease in men, *J Nutr* 146:1235–1240, 2016.

Smith T, Kawa K, Eckl V, et al: Herbal Supplement Sales in US Increased 8.5% in 2017, Topping $8 Billion, *Herbal Gram* 119:62–71, 2018.

Straub DA: Calcium supplementation in clinical practice: a review of forms, doses, and indications, *Nutr Clin Pract* 22(3):286–296, 2007.

Thompson C, Diekman C, Fragakis AS, et al: Guidelines regarding the recommendation and sale of dietary supplements, *J Am Diet Assoc* 102(8):1158–1164, 2002.

Food and Nutrient Delivery: Nutrition Support Methods

Carol S. Ireton-Jones, PhD, RDN, LD, CNSC, FASPEN, FAND
Mary Russell, MS, RDN, LDN, FAND

KEY TERMS

advance directives
bolus enteral feeding
catheter
central parenteral nutrition (CPN)
closed enteral system
computerized provider order entry
   (CPOE)
durable medical equipment (DME)
   provider
enteral nutrition (EN)
essential fatty acid deficiency (EFAD)
French size
gastrointestinal decompression
gastrojejunostomy

gastric residual volume (GRV)
hang time
hemodynamic stability
home enteral nutrition (HEN)
home parenteral nutrition (HPN)
intermittent enteral feeding
intravenous lipid emulsion (ILE)
multiple lumen tube
nasoduodenal tube (NDT)
nasogastric tube (NGT)
nasojejunal tube (NJT)
open enteral system
osmolality
osmolarity

parenteral nutrition (PN)
percutaneous endoscopic gastrostomy
   (PEG)
percutaneous endoscopic jejunostomy
   (PEJ)
peripheral parenteral nutrition (PPN)
peripherally inserted central catheter
   (PICC)
polymeric enteral formula
rebound hypoglycemia
refeeding syndrome
sentinel event
total nutrient admixture (3-in-1)
transitional feeding

Nutrition support is the delivery of formulated enteral or parenteral nutrients for the purpose of maintaining or restoring nutritional status. Enteral nutrition (EN) refers to nutrition provided through the gastrointestinal tract (GIT) via a catheter or a tube or stoma that delivers nutrients distal to the oral cavity. Parenteral nutrition (PN) is the provision of nutrients intravenously.

RATIONALE AND CRITERIA FOR APPROPRIATE NUTRITION SUPPORT

When patients cannot or will not eat enough to support their nutritional needs for more than a few days, nutrition support should be considered as part of the integrated care plan. Using the GIT (EN vs. using PN alone) helps preserve the intestinal mucosal barrier function and integrity. In critically ill patients, feeding the GIT has been shown to attenuate the catabolic response and preserve immunologic function (McClave et al, 2016). Research shows less septic morbidity, fewer infectious complications, and significant cost savings in critically ill adult patients who received EN vs. PN. There is limited evidence that EN vs. PN affects hospital length of stay (LOS), but an impact on mortality has not been demonstrated (Academy of Nutrition and Dietetics [AND] and Evidence Analysis Library [EAL], 2012). A 2014 study

found no significant difference in 30-day mortality in critically ill adults who received nutrition support by the parenteral or the enteral route (Harvey et al, 2014). Another more recent study of ventilated adults with shock noted that early isocaloric EN did not reduce mortality or the risk of secondary infections but was associated with a greater risk of digestive complications compared with early isocaloric PN (Reignier et al, 2018). Conversely, a recent meta-analysis and systematic review noted that EN compared with PN had no overall effect on mortality but resulted in fewer infectious complications and shorter intensive care unit LOS (Elke et al, 2016).

A variety of diseases and conditions may result in the need for nutrition support (Table 12.1). PN should be used in patients who are or will become malnourished and who do not have sufficient gastrointestinal function to be able to restore or maintain optimal nutritional status (McClave et al, 2016). EN should be considered when an individual has a functional GIT and is unable or unwilling to consume sufficient nutrients to meet estimated nutritional needs. Fig. 12.1 presents an algorithm for selecting appropriate routes for EN and PN. Although these guidelines provide ideas, the choice of the most optimal method of nutrition support can be challenging. For example, the small bowel feeding access for EN may not be available in every health care setting. In such a case, PN may be the only realistic option for provision of nutrition support. PN may be used temporarily until adequate gastrointestinal function to support EN or oral intake returns, or PN may be used to supplement EN or oral intake to meet needs effectively for energy, protein, and other key nutrients. "Transitional

Sections of this chapter were written by Janice L. Raymond, MS, RDN, CSG for the previous edition of this text.

TABLE 12.1 Conditions That May Require Nutrition Support

Recommended Route of Feeding	Condition	Typical Disorders
Enteral nutrition	Inability to eat	Neurologic disorders (dysphagia)
		Facial trauma
		Oral or esophageal trauma
		Congenital anomalies
		Respiratory failure (on a ventilator)
		Traumatic brain injury
		Comatose state
		GI surgery (e.g., esophagectomy)
	Inability to eat enough	Hypermetabolic states such as with burns
		Cancer
		Heart failure
		Congenital heart disease
		Impaired intake after orofacial surgery or injury
		Anorexia nervosa
		Failure to thrive
		Cystic fibrosis
	Impaired digestion, absorption, metabolism	Severe gastroparesis
		Inborn errors of metabolism
		Crohn's disease
		Short bowel syndrome with minimum resection
		Pancreatitis
Parenteral nutrition	Gastrointestinal incompetency	Short bowel syndrome—major resection
		Severe acute pancreatitis with intolerance to enteral feeding
		Severe inflammatory bowel disease
		Small bowel ischemia
		Intestinal atresia
		Severe liver failure
		Persistent postoperative ileus
		Intractable vomiting/diarrhea refractory to medical management
		Distal high-output fistulas
		Severe GI bleeding
	Critical illness with poor enteral tolerance or accessibility	Multi-organ system failure
		Major trauma or burns
		Bone marrow transplantation
		Acute respiratory failure with ventilator dependency and gastrointestinal malfunction
		Severe wasting in renal failure with dialysis
		Small bowel transplantation, immediate after surgery

GI, Gastrointestinal.
McClave SA et al: Guidelines for the provision and assessment of nutrition support therapy in the adult critically ill patient, *J Parenter Enteral Nutr; 40*:159-211, 2016.

Feeding," described later in the chapter, refers to the provision of nutrition support via two or more methods, until nutrition adequacy is reached via oral intake alone.

Although specific nutrition support regimens may be standardized for specific disease states or courses of therapy, each patient presents a unique challenge. Nutrition support frequently must be adapted to address unanticipated developments or complications. An optimal treatment plan requires interdisciplinary collaboration that is aligned closely with the comprehensive plan of patient care. In rare cases, nutrition support may be warranted but physically impossible to implement. In other situations, nutrition support may be possible but not warranted because it presents an unacceptable risk or is not indicated because of the prognosis or the patient's right to self-determination.

In all cases, it is important to prevent errors in ordering, delivering, and monitoring of nutrition support to prevent undesirable risks or outcomes (sentinel events) such as an unexpected death, serious physical injury with loss of limb or function, or psychological injury (Joint Commission, 2017). A computerized provider order entry (CPOE) system allows prescribers to enter an order directly into a computer, often aided by decision-support technology to help facilitate accuracy and clinical effectiveness.

ENTERAL NUTRITION

Enteral implies using the GIT, usually via a feeding tube with the tip in the stomach or small bowel. The location of nutrient administration and type of enteral access device are selected after the patient is determined to be a candidate for EN. (The process for determining whether an individual is a candidate for EN is described later.) Enteral access selection depends on the (1) anticipated length of time enteral feeding will be required, (2) degree of risk for aspiration or tube displacement, (3) patient's clinical status, (4) adequacy of digestion and absorption, (5) patient's anatomy (e.g., after previous surgical resection or in extreme obesity), and (6) whether future surgical intervention is planned.

Feeding tubes may be referred to by their French size, which is a measure of the outer tube diameter. One French unit is 0.33 mm. A French size of 5 to 12 typically is considered "small bore," and a French size of more than 14 is considered "large bore."

ENTERAL NUTRITION ACCESS

Short-Term Enteral Nutrition Support

Nasogastric Access

Nasogastric tubes (NGTs) are used most commonly to access the GIT, for gastric decompression (i.e., draining the fluid normally secreted by the stomach when the normal emptying process is slowed), medication delivery, and/or feeding. They are appropriate only for those patients who require short-term (no more than 3 to 4 weeks) EN. Typically, the tube is inserted at the bedside by a nurse or physician (or a registered dietitian with appropriate clinical privileges) and passed through the prognose into the stomach (Fig. 12.2). Polyurethane or silicone tubes of various diameters, lengths, and design features may be used, depending on formula characteristics and feeding requirements. These tubes are soft, flexible, and often well tolerated by patients. Tube placement is verified by aspirating gastric contents in combination with auscultation of air insufflation into the stomach or by radiographic confirmation of the tube tip location. The American Society for Parenteral and Enteral Nutrition (ASPEN) Enteral Nutrition Practice Recommendations offer detailed information on this process (Bankhead et al, 2009).

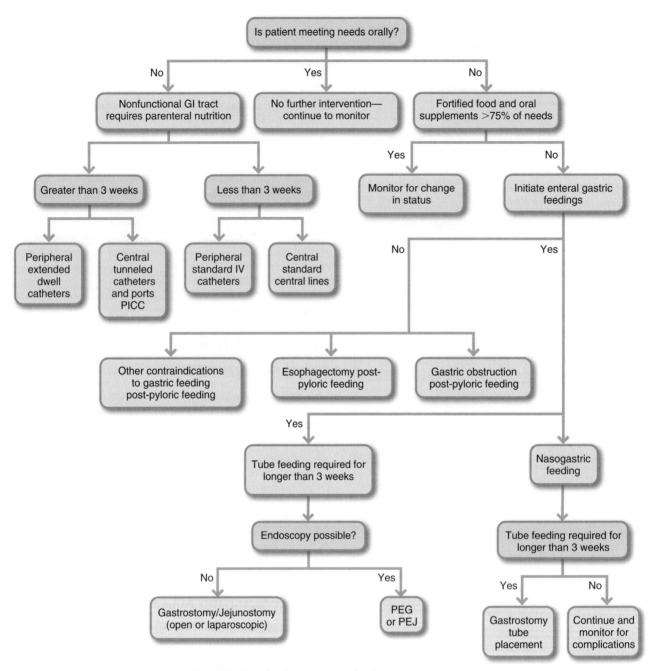

Fig. 12.1 Algorithm for route selection for nutrition support.

NGT feedings are provided by bolus administration or by intermittent or continuous infusions (see *Administration* later in this chapter). Patients with normal gastrointestinal function are often fed via this route, which takes advantage of normal digestive, hormonal, and bactericidal processes in the stomach. Rarely, complications occur (Box 12.1).

Gastric Versus Small-Bowel Access

Placement of a feeding tube into the stomach may be more straightforward and less time consuming than placing a tube into the small bowel. However, ease of access is only one consideration. Critically ill patients, including those who have undergone surgery, or suffered a head injury or major intraabdominal trauma, may not tolerate gastric feeding (see Chapter 37).

Signs and symptoms of intolerance to gastric feeding include, but are not limited to, the following:
- Abdominal distention and discomfort
- Vomiting
- Persistent diarrhea

Some clinicians believe that intragastric feeding increases the risk of aspiration pneumonia; the data on this subject are not totally clear (Bankhead et al, 2009; McClave et al, 2016).

Nasoduodenal or Nasojejunal Access

Patients who do not tolerate gastric feedings and require relatively short-term EN support may benefit from placement of a **nasoduodenal tube (NDT)** or a **nasojejunal tube (NJT)**, described by the point at which the tube tip terminates. These tubes may be placed with

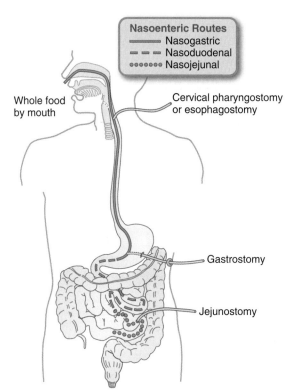

Fig. 12.2 Diagram of enteral tube placement.

BOX 12.1 Potential Complications of Nasoenteric Tubes

Esophageal strictures
Gastroesophageal reflux resulting in aspiration pneumonia
Tracheoesophageal fistula
Incorrect position of the tube leading to pulmonary injury
Mucosal damage at the insertion site
Nasal irritation and erosion
Pharyngeal or vocal cord paralysis
Rhinorrhea, sinusitis, otitis media
Ruptured gastroesophageal varices in hepatic disease
Ulcerations or perforations of the upper gastrointestinal tract and airway

Adapted from McClave SA et al: Guidelines for the provision and assessment of nutrition support therapy in the adult critically ill patient, J Parenter Enteral Nutr 40:159-211, 2016; Cresci G: Enteral access. In Charney P, Malone A: *Pocket guide to enteral nutrition*, ed 2, Chicago, 2013, Academy of Nutrition and Dietetics, p 62.

endoscopic or fluoroscopic guidance (Fig. 12.3, *A*); using a computer guidance system (Fig. 12.3, *B*); or intraoperatively as part of a surgical procedure.

Some practitioners may place a feeding tube intragastrically with the goal of migration into the duodenum by peristalsis; this process is unlikely to result in desired location of the feeding tube tip and inevitably delays initiation of appropriate EN. Spontaneous migration never achieves jejunal tip placement.

Long-Term Enteral Access
Gastrostomy or Jejunostomy

When EN is required for more than 3 to 4 weeks, placement of a surgically or endoscopically guided gastrostomy or jejunostomy feeding

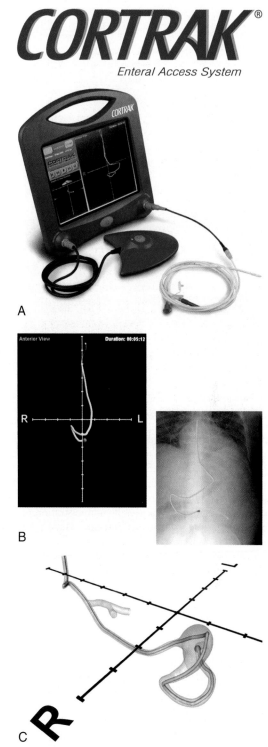

Fig. 12.3 Computerized Cortrak tube feeding placement system. **A**, CORTRAK System; **B**, CORTRAK anterior view compared with abdominal radiograph; **C**, 3-dimensional graphic representation of a CORTRAK feeding tube in post-pyloric position. (Used with permission from COR-PAK MedSystems.)

tube should be considered to maximize patient comfort (Fig. 12.4) and minimize nasal and upper GIT irritation (see Box 12.1). This tube may be placed during a required surgical or endoscopic procedure to maximize efficiency and cost effectiveness.

Percutaneous endoscopic gastrostomy (PEG) or percutaneous endoscopic jejunostomy (PEJ) is a nonsurgical technique for placing

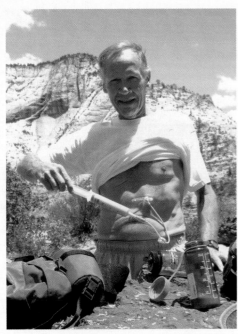

Fig. 12.4 A man with a gastrostomy tube out hiking. (From Oley Foundation, Albany, NY: www.oley.org.)

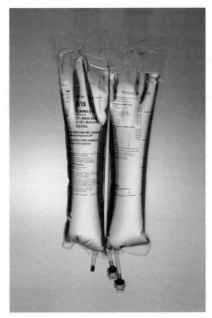

Fig. 12.5 Baxter Clinimix Compounding System. (Image provided by Baxter Healthcare Corporation. CLINIMIX is a trademark of Baxter International Inc.)

a tube directly into the stomach through the abdominal wall, using an endoscope and local anesthesia. The tube is guided from the mouth into the stomach or the jejunum and brought out through the abdominal wall. The short procedure time and limited anesthesia requirements have contributed to making it a very common method for long-term feeding tube placement.

Tubes placed by PEG (note the PEG is the procedure, not the tube, although clinicians commonly refer to "PEGs" as the tube) are generally large bore (French size), facilitating administration of medications and reducing the incidence of clogging. These tubes may be connected to a short piece of tubing used to infuse a bolus feeding or connect to a bag of formula. Some tubes placed by PEG are flush to the skin, or "low profile." These tubes, also known as "buttons," are a good choice for children, and for adults with dementia, both of whom may be likely to pull out a tube that protrudes from the skin. Active individuals, and those who prefer a sleeker profile under clothing, also may opt for this type of tube. Fig. 12.5 shows a component from a skin level balloon G-tube kit, designed to improve patient comfort and increase the length of time the G-tube may remain in place. To prevent the accidental parenteral infusion (into the blood) of enteral formula, a universal connector that is incompatible with IV equipment has been developed. Fig. 12.5 shows a silicone G-tube with a purple connector, which is incompatible with a Luer lock syringe or an IV connection. This innovation, recently made the industry standard, is designed to reduce the risk of accidental connection or infusion.

A tube placed by PEG may be converted to a **gastrojejunostomy** using fluoroscopy or endoscopy by threading a small-bore tube through the larger tube into the jejunum.

Other Minimally Invasive Techniques

High-resolution video cameras have made percutaneous radiologic and laparoscopic gastrostomy and jejunostomy enteral access an option for patients in whom endoscopic procedures are contraindicated. Using fluoroscopy, a radiologic technique, a feeding tube may be guided into the stomach or the jejunum and then brought

through the abdominal wall to provide access for enteral feedings. Laparoscopic or fluoroscopic techniques offer alternative options for enteral access.

Gastrojejunal dual tubes, used for early postoperative feeding, are available for endoscopic or surgical placement. These tubes are designed for patients who may require prolonged **gastrointestinal decompression** (removal of the contents of the stomach through a nasogastric tube). The **multiple lumen tube** includes one lumen for decompression and one for feeding into the small bowel.

Formula Content and Selection

Many enteral formulations, marketed for a wide variety of clinical conditions and indications, are currently available (Escuro and Hummell, 2016):

- Enteral formulas are classified as (1) standard, (2) elemental or semi-elemental, (3) specialty or disease-specific, (4) blenderized, and (5) modular. A variety of formulas are available in each of these categories. Health care organizations, including hospitals and long-term care organizations, typically develop a formulary of products to be used within the facility. Selection of an enteral formula for a specific patient should involve consideration of the patient's nutrient needs, GIT function, and clinical status.

In the past, **osmolality** was considered key to EN tolerance, and belief was widespread that EN formulas should be the same osmolality as body fluids (290 mOsm/kg). However, studies in the mid-1980s showed that patients tolerate feedings across a wide range of osmolality, and clinical experience of many clinicians has reinforced those study results.

Cost of a formula and its availability after discharge from the hospital or other facility may be barriers for clinicians, patients, families, and facility administrators.

Formulas may be classified based on protein or overall macronutrient composition. The nutrition needs of most patients may be met with a standard or **polymeric enteral formula** (McClave et al, 2016). These formulas contain intact macronutrients (1 to 2 kcal/mL), are lactose free, and frequently may be used as an oral supplement and an enteral feeding. The higher nutrient density (1.5 to 2 kcal/mL) formulas are useful when fluid restriction is required (cardiopulmonary, renal, and/or hepatic dysfunction), and for patients with intolerance to a higher feeding volume. Products intended to supplement oral diets may be used for EN in some cases; these products are flavored and may contain simple sugars to enhance palatability (see Appendix 15).

The manufacture and labeling of enteral formulas are regulated by the Food and Drug Administration (FDA), which classifies enteral formulas as medical foods (a subclassification of foods for special dietary use). As such, these products are exempt from specific nutrition labeling requirements in the Code of Federal Regulations. The products must be labeled as "intended to be used under medical supervision" (FDA, 2014).

Manufacturers are not obligated to register enteral products with the FDA or obtain FDA approval before placing them on the market. Many EN formulas lack rigorous scientific evidence to support their specific composition, and their marketing materials are not subject to the rigorous standards used for prescription drugs. Evaluation of the efficacy of EN products and the statements made in marketing materials and by company representatives requires the attention of qualified registered dietitian nutritionists (RDNs). RDNs should evaluate claims of pharmacologic effects and other specific benefits using clinical evidence before choosing a specific product for a formulary or for a specific patient (Box 12.2).

Blenderized (Homemade) Tube Feedings

Tube feedings made from common ingredients such as eggs, sugar, and wine have been used since the 1500s. Blenderized tube feedings (BTFs) were commonly used in the United States throughout the first half of the twentieth century (Vassilyadi et al, 2013). Clinicians often are concerned about nutritional adequacy, food safety, and the additional burden preparation of BTF places on the caregivers. Advantages of BTF may include cost effectiveness (because commercial formulas may not be covered by insurance), health benefits from using whole foods, and ability to tailor the formula exactly to patient needs. The social bond between the caregiver who prepares the feeding (possibly from foods served to the rest of the family) and the patient also is cited as a strong driver for BTF use. Hurt and colleagues found that more than 80% of a small sample of home EN patients at the Mayo Clinic in Rochester, MN, wanted to use BTF (Hurt et al, 2015). In the last several years, several commercially prepared BTF have appeared on the market, such as Liquid Hope™ and Real Food Blends™. Compleat® has been marketed by Nestle for a number of years, and Abbott Nutrition will soon market a BTF.

BOX 12.2 Factors to Consider When Choosing an Enteral Formula

Ability of the formula to meet the patient's nutrient requirements
Caloric and protein density of the formula (i.e., kcal/mL, g protein/mL, mL fluid/L)
Gastrointestinal function
Sodium, potassium, magnesium, and phosphorus content of the formula, especially for patients with cardiopulmonary, renal, or hepatic failure
Form and amount of protein, fat, carbohydrate, and fiber in the formula relative to the patient's digestive and absorptive capacity
Cost effectiveness of formula
Patient compliance
Cost-to-benefit ratio

Homemade BTFs are contraindicated for patients who are immunocompromised and should be hung for no more than 2 hours. All BTF may be contraindicated for infusion through tubes smaller than 10 French, for continuous feeding (unless the recommended formula hang time is followed), if a fluid restriction of less than 900 mL/day is required, in cases of multiple food allergies, and if a jejunostomy tube (JT) is used (Novak et al, 2009). Some state regulations prohibit use of BTF in long-term care facilities (see *New Directions*: Pureed by Gastrostomy Tube—the PBGT Diet).

✳ NEW DIRECTIONS

Pureed by Gastrostomy Tube—the PBGT Diet

The Pureed by Gastrostomy (G) Tube (PBGT) Diet is a specialized, nutritionally balanced blended food feeding given by G-tube. It was originally designed to decrease or eliminate symptoms of retching and gagging which can be a complication of a Nissen Fundoplication surgery. In addition to improving tolerance of bolus feeds for individuals who are volume sensitive, the PBGT diet is also used by families seeking an alternative to commercial formulas. The goals of the PBGT diet are to:

- Decrease frequency of gastrostomy tube feedings and transition from drip feedings
- Meet all nutritional and fluid requirements
- Improve weight gain, growth, and overall nutritional status
- Encourage increased opportunities for oral intake
- Improve and sustain quality of life for individuals and their families

The PBGT diet is different from the usual blended tube feeding in that it is calculated and formulated by a registered dietitian nutritionist (RDN) to provide an individual with complete nutrition through small, calorie-dense gastrostomy tube boluses, thereby eliminating the need and cost for a feeding pump. In addition to the easier preparation of the PBGT, special attention is also given to the variety of foods, nutrient content, cost, and ease of the 5- to 10-minute bolus administration (Pentiuk et al, 2011).

The use of Stage 2 infant foods promotes consistency in the viscosity of the diet, provides availability and affordability, and eliminates the need for an expensive blender. They can be premeasured and individually sealed in containers that can be easily used in formula rooms within hospitals if allowed by hospital policy. Families can be educated on the easy preparation method and proper storage, along with additional fluid and vitamin and mineral supplementation guidelines (O'Flaherty et al, 2011; O'Flaherty, 2015).

Therese O'Flaherty MS, RDN, CSP, LD

Protein

The amount of protein in available commercial enteral formulas varies from 6% to 37% of total kilocalories. The protein typically is derived from casein, whey, or soy protein isolate. Standard formulas provide intact protein; elemental formulas contain di- and tripeptides and amino acids, which are absorbed more easily. Specialized formulas (that are marketed for hepatic or severe renal failure or for cases of multiple, severe allergies) usually include crystalline amino acids.

Specific amino acids may be added to some enteral formulas. Branched chain amino acids have been used in formulas for patients with severe hepatic disease, and arginine has been added to formulas marketed for critically ill patients. Strong evidence to support these additions is not available. (See Chapter 37 for further discussion.)

Carbohydrate

Carbohydrate content in enteral formulas varies from 30% to 85% of kilocalories. Corn syrup solids typically are used in standard formulas.

Sucrose is added to flavored formulas that are meant for oral consumption. Hydrolyzed formulas contain carbohydrate from cornstarch or maltodextrin.

Carbohydrate or fiber that cannot be processed by human digestive enzymes is added frequently to enteral formulas. Fibers are classified as water soluble (pectins and gums) or water insoluble (cellulose or hemicellulose). The effectiveness of different fibers added to enteral formulas in treating GIT symptoms of critically ill patients is controversial. The Adult Critical Illness guidelines, in the Evidence Analysis Library of the Academy of Nutrition and Dietetics (AND and EAL, 2012), suggests that the RDN "consider using soluble fiber to prevent and/or manage diarrhea."

Fructooligosaccharides (FOS), which are prebiotics, have been added to enteral formulas, often in combination with a source of dietary fiber, for more than 15 years. More recently inulin, another fermentable oligosaccharide, has been added to some enteral formulas. Both FOS and inulin are associated with fermentable oligosaccharides, disaccharides, monosaccharides, and polyols (FODMAPs), which are poorly absorbed short-chain carbohydrates (Escuro and Hummell, 2016).

FOS have been shown to stimulate the production of beneficial bifidobacteria, and when combined with dietary fiber may produce beneficial changes in colonic pH, fecal microbiota, and short-chain fatty acid concentrations. Animal models provide evidence that FOS may help to achieve colonization resistance against *Clostridium difficile*. Use of formulas with a high FODMAPs content may exacerbate and play a role in diarrhea, especially in individuals who receive antibiotics that affect the intestinal microbiome (Escuro and Hummell, 2016).

The Society of Critical Care Medicine (SCCM)/ASPEN guidelines suggest that "mixed-fiber formula not be used routinely" in adult critically ill patients "to promote regularity or prevent diarrhea" and also "to consider a fermentable soluble fiber additive (FOS, inulin) for routine use in all stable MICU/SICU patients placed on standard enteral formulations if there is evidence of diarrhea" (McClave et al, 2016).

All commercially available enteral formulas are lactose free, because lactase insufficiency may be encountered in acutely ill patients. (Atkinson and Worthley, 2003).

Lipid

Lipid content of enteral formulas varies from 1.5% to 55% of the total kilocalories. In standard formulas, lipid as (typically) canola, soybean, and/or safflower oil provides between 15% and 30% of the total kilocalories. Elemental formulas contain minimal amounts of fat, typically in the form of medium-chain triglycerides (MCTs) rather than long-chain triglycerides (LCTs).

Most of the lipid in standard enteral formulas is in the form of LCTs and MCTs. Some formulas contain "structured lipids," which are a mix of LCTs and MCTs and contain properties of both. Most of the LCTs found in structured lipids are omega-3 fatty acids (such as eicosapentaenoic acid and docosahexaenoic acid); these omega-3 fatty acids may have antiinflammatory effects (see Chapter 7).

MCTs do not require bile salts or pancreatic lipase for digestion and are absorbed directly into the portal circulation. The percentage of fat as MCT in enteral formulas varies from 0% to 85%. About 2% to 4% of daily energy intake from linoleic and linolenic acid is necessary to prevent essential fatty acid deficiency (EFAD). MCTs do not provide linoleic or linolenic acids; the clinician must ensure that patients who receive high MCT enteral formulas receive linoleic and linolenic acids from other sources.

Vitamins, Minerals, and Electrolytes

Most, but not all, available formulas provide the dietary reference intakes (DRIs) for vitamins and minerals in a volume that may be administered to most patients. Because the DRIs are intended for healthy populations, not specifically for individuals (whether healthy or acutely or chronically ill), it is difficult to know for certain whether the vitamin and mineral provision from these formulas is adequate. Formulas intended for patients with renal or hepatic failure are intentionally low in vitamins A, D, and E; sodium; and potassium. Conversely, disease-specific formulas often are supplemented with antioxidant vitamins and minerals and marketed to suggest that these additions improve immune function or accelerate wound healing. Definitive studies demonstrating these effects are not available.

Electrolyte content of enteral formulas is typically modest compared with the oral diet. Patients who experience large electrolyte losses (e.g., because of diarrhea, fistula, emesis) likely will require electrolyte supplementation. Salt must be added to home-prepared BTFs in order to provide an adequate sodium intake.

Fluid

Adult fluid needs often are estimated at 1 mL of water per kilocalorie consumed, or 30 to 35 mL/kg of usual body weight. Patients fed exclusively by EN, especially if it is a concentrated formula, may receive insufficient fluid (water) to meet their needs. Insufficient fluid intake and administration of a high-fiber product can lead to undesirable consequences, including inadequate urine output, constipation, and formation of a fiber bezoar (a hard ball of fiber that may develop within the human stomach). All sources of fluid, including feeding tube flushes, medications, and intravenous fluids, should be considered when assessing a patient's fluid intake relative to individual needs.

Standard (1 kcal/mL) formulas contain about 85% water by volume; concentrated (2 kcal/mL) formulas contain only about 70% water by volume. Additional water (as flushes and for additional hydration) are often necessary to meet fluid needs and help assure tube patency.

Administration

EN may be administered as a bolus, or as an intermittent or continuous feeding. Administration method selection should accommodate the patient's clinical status, living situation, and quality-of-life considerations. One method may serve as a transition to another method as the patient's status changes.

In a closed enteral system, the container or bag is prefilled with sterile liquid formula by the manufacturer and is "ready to feed" after connecting to the patient's feeding access. In an open enteral system, the contents of formula cans or packages are poured into a separate, empty container or bag and then connected to the feeding access.

Hang time is the length of time an enteral formula hanging at room temperature is considered safe for delivery to the patient. Most facilities allow a 4-hour hang time for a product in an open system and 24 to 48 hours for products in closed system (manufacturer's directions should always be followed).

Bolus

Syringe bolus enteral feedings can be suitable for patients with adequate gastric emptying who are clinically stable (see Fig. 12.4). Administered over 5 to 20 minutes, these feedings are more convenient and less expensive than pump or gravity bolus feedings and should be encouraged when tolerated. A 60-mL syringe may be used to infuse the formula. If bloating or abdominal discomfort develops, the patient should wait 10 to 15 minutes before infusing the remainder of formula allocated for that feeding. Patients with normal gastric function generally tolerate 500 mL or more of formula per feeding; therefore, three or four bolus feedings per day typically provide their daily nutritional requirements. Some individuals, especially if elderly, may not tolerate larger boluses and require smaller, more frequent feedings. Formula at room temperature is better tolerated than cold formula; however, food safety must be the primary consideration. Follow label directions for storing partially used cans of formula.

Intermittent and Cyclic

Quality-of-life issues are often the reason for the initiation of intermittent enteral feedings. Cyclic regimens allow mobile patients an improved quality of life by offering time "off the pump" and more autonomy. They are initiated to allow time for treatments, therapies, and activities. Intermittent feedings can be given by pump or gravity drip. Gravity feeding is accomplished by pouring formula into a feeding bag that is equipped with a roller clamp. The clamp is adjusted to the desired drips per minute. A typical daily feeding schedule is four to six feedings, each administered over 20 to 60 minutes. Formula administration is initiated at 100 to 150 mL per feeding and increased incrementally as tolerated. Patients who most often succeed with this regimen are motivated, organized, alert, and mobile. Cyclic feeding also allows for time away from tube feeding. This feeding regimen is a good choice for patients who are receiving physical therapy or participate in other activities that require mobility. A typical daily feeding schedule is 90 to 150 mL per hour of formula administered over 18 to 20 hours. This regimen, often started at night, can be used to transition to an oral diet.

Continuous

Continuous infusion of EN requires a pump. This method is appropriate for patients who do not tolerate the volume of infusion used with the bolus, cyclical, or intermittent methods. Patients with compromised gastrointestinal function because of disease, surgery, cancer therapy, or other physiologic impediments are candidates for continuous feedings. Patients with a feeding tube tip in the small intestine should be fed only by continuous or cyclic infusion. (Use of bolus or gravity feeding in these patients is strongly discouraged, although anecdotal verbal reports of use of both have been shared by some providers.) The feeding rate goal, in milliliters per hour, is set by dividing the total daily volume by the number of hours per day of administration. Full strength feeding is started at one quarter to one half of the hourly goal rate and advanced every 8 to 12 hours to the final volume. Dilution of formulas is not necessary and can lead to underfeeding. High osmolality formulas may require more time to achieve tolerance and should be advanced conservatively.

One possible drawback to continuous feedings occurs if the patient requires medication that must be administered on an empty stomach. For example, when administering phenytoin (Dilantin) it is recommended that tube feedings be stopped before and after administration. The times vary by situation and medication.

Enteral pumps for home use are small and easy to handle. Many pumps run for up to 8 hours on battery power, with a "plug-in" option, allowing flexibility and mobility for the patient. Pump sets typically include bags and tubing compatible with proper pump operation. Feeding bags should be labeled in accordance with the ASPEN Enteral Nutrition Practice Guidelines and should include the name of the formula and its concentration, the date and time the bag was filled, and the initials of the health care provider who hung the feeding.

Monitoring and Evaluation
Monitoring for Complications

Box 12.3 provides a comprehensive list of complications associated with EN. Many complications can be prevented or managed with careful patient monitoring.

Aspiration, a common concern for patients receiving EN, is a controversial topic. Many experts believe that aspiration of throat contents and saliva is as much as or more important than aspiration of formula. To minimize the risk of aspiration, patients should be positioned with their heads and shoulders above their chests during and immediately after feeding (Bankhead et al, 2009; McClave et al, 2016).

Significant disagreement exists about the value of gastric residual volumes (GRV) as an indicator of EN tolerance. GRV procedures are not standardized and checking GRV does not protect patients from aspiration. GRV does not have to be checked regularly in patients who are stable on a feeding regimen and those who have a long history on tube feedings. In critically ill tube-fed patients the best methods for reducing the risk of aspiration include elevation of the head of the bed,

---

BOX 12.3 Complications of Enteral Nutrition

Access
Leakage from ostomy/stoma site
Pressure necrosis/ulceration/stenosis
Tissue erosion
Tube displacement/migration
Tube obstruction/occlusion

Administration
Microbial contamination
Enteral misconnections or misplacement of tube, causing infection, aspiration pneumonia, peritonitis, pulmonary or venous infusion
Regurgitation
Inadequate delivery for one or more reasons

Gastrointestinal
Constipation
Delayed gastric emptying/elevated gastric residual volume
Diarrhea
   Osmotic diarrhea, especially if sorbitol is present in liquid drug preparations
   Secretory
Distention/bloating/cramping
Formula choice/rate of administration
Intolerance of nutrient components
Maldigestion/malabsorption
Nausea/vomiting

Metabolic
Drug-nutrient interactions
Glucose intolerance/hyperglycemia/hypoglycemia
Dehydration/overhydration
Hypernatremia/hyponatremia
Hyperkalemia/hypokalemia
Hyperphosphatemia/hypophosphatemia
Micronutrient deficiencies (notably thiamin)
Refeeding syndrome

Data from Russell M: Complications of enteral feedings. In Charney P, Malone A (eds): *Pocket guide to enteral nutrition*, ed 2, Chicago, 2013, Academy of Nutrition and Dietetics, p 170.

continuous subglottic suctioning, and oral decontamination (Bankhead et al, 2009; McClave et al, 2016).

In the presence of gastroparesis, doses of a promotility drug (like metoclopramide) may increase gastrointestinal transit, improve EN delivery, and improve feeding tolerance (McClave et al, 2016).

Diarrhea is a common EN complication, often related to the antibiotic therapy, colonic bacterial overgrowth, and gastrointestinal motility disorders associated with acute and critical illness. Hyperosmolar medications such as magnesium-containing antacids, sorbitol-containing elixirs, and electrolyte supplements also contribute to diarrhea. Adjustment of medications or administration methods may reduce or eliminate the diarrhea. FOS, pectin, guar gum, bulking agents, and antidiarrheal medications also can be beneficial. (Use care to avoid clogging the feeding tube when using bulking agents or pectin.) A predigested formula is rarely the best "first line" option, because the formula is typically not the cause of the diarrhea.

Constipation is a concern with EN, particularly among bed-bound patients who receive long-term feedings. Fiber-containing formulas or stool-bulking medication may be helpful; daily provision of adequate fluid is important. Narcotic pain relievers slow GIT activity; iron supplements can cause constipation. Diarrhea may coexist with constipation because liquid stool can pass a fecal impaction.

Monitoring for Tolerance and Nutrient Intake Goals

Monitoring the patient's *actual* (not prescribed) intake and tolerance is necessary to ensure that all nutrition goals are achieved and maintained. Monitoring of metabolic and gastrointestinal tolerance, hydration status, weight, and lean body mass is extremely important (Box 12.4). Practice guidelines, institutional protocols, and standardized ordering procedures should be developed and used to ensure optimal, safe monitoring of EN (McClave et al, 2016).

Time is often lost from the prescribed feeding schedule because of issues such as NPO (nothing by mouth) status for medical procedures, clogged tubes, dislodged or misplaced tubes, and perceived or actual gastrointestinal intolerance. The result of "held" feedings is always inadequate nutrition with the risk of onset, or worsening, of malnutrition. Adjustment in the tube feeding regimen must be made. For example, if tube feedings are being turned off for 2 hours every afternoon for physical therapy, the feeding rate on the feeding should be increased and the feeding time decreased to accommodate the therapy schedule.

PARENTERAL NUTRITION

PN provides nutrients directly into the bloodstream intravenously. PN is indicated when the patient or individual is unable to take adequate nutrients orally or enterally. PN may be used as an adjunct to oral or EN to meet nutrient needs (Mundi et al, 2017; Derenski et al, 2016). Alternatively, PN may be the sole source of nutrition during recovery from illness or injury or may be a life-sustaining therapy for patients who have lost the function of their intestine for nutrient absorption. As any type of nutrition support other than oral is invasive, it is important to evaluate ethical issues if the patient is terminal or has a short life expectancy (Schwartz et al, 2016).

Getting Started with Parenteral Nutrition

After the patient has been deemed to require nutrition support via the parenteral route, the clinician must choose between central and peripheral access. *Central access* refers to catheter tip placement in a large, high-blood-flow vein such as the superior vena cava; this is central parenteral nutrition (CPN). Peripheral parenteral nutrition (PPN) refers to catheter tip placement in a small vein, typically in the hand or forearm.

The osmolarity of the PN solution dictates the location of the catheter; central catheter placement allows for the higher caloric PN formulation and therefore greater osmolarity (Table 12.2). The use of PPN is limited: it is short-term therapy and therefore has a minimum effect on nutritional status because the type and amount of fluids that can be provided peripherally are limited and most often do not fully meet nutrition requirements. Volume-sensitive patients such as those with cardiopulmonary, renal, or hepatic failure are not good candidates for PPN. PPN may be appropriate when used as a supplemental feeding or in transition to enteral or oral feeding, or as a temporary method to begin feeding when central access has not been initiated. Calculation of the osmolarity of a parenteral solution is important to ensure venous tolerance. Osmolarity, or mOsm/mL, is used to calculate IV fluids rather than osmolality, which is used for body fluids.

BOX 12.4 Monitoring the Patient Receiving Enteral Nutrition

Abdominal distention and discomfort
Confirm proper tube placement and maintain head of bed >30 degrees (daily)
Change feeding delivery container and tubing (daily)
Fluid intake and output (daily)
Gastric residual volume if appropriate (not for jejunal tubes)
Signs and symptoms of edema or dehydration (daily)
Stool frequency, volume, and consistency (daily)
Weight (at least three times/wk)
Nutritional intake adequacy (daily)
Clinical status (daily)
Nutrition focused physical exam (daily)
Serum electrolytes, blood urea nitrogen, creatinine, (daily until stable, then two to three times/wk)
Serum glucose, calcium, magnesium, phosphorus (daily until stable, then weekly)

Data from McClave SA et al: Guidelines for the provision and assessment of nutrition support therapy in the adult critically ill patient, *J Parenter Enteral Nutr* 40:159-211, 2016.
Shelton M: Monitoring and evaluation of enteral feedings. In Charney P, Malone A: *Pocket guide to enteral nutrition*, ed 2, Chicago, 2013, AND, p. 153.

TABLE 12.2 Osmolarity of Nutrients in PN Solutions

Nutrient	Osmolarity (mOsm/mL)	Sample Calculations
Dextrose 5%	0.25	500 mL = 125 mOsm
Dextrose 10%	0.505	500 mL = 252 mOsm
Dextrose 50%	2.52	500 mL = 1260 mOsm
Dextrose 70%	3.53	500 mL = 1765 mOsm
Amino acids 8.5%	0.81	1000 mL = 810 mOsm
Amino acids 10%	0.998	1000 mL = 998 mOsm
Lipids 10%	0.6	500 mL = 300 mOsm
Lipids 20%	0.7	500 mL = 350 mOsm
Electrolytes	Varies by additive	
Multitrace elements	0.36	5 mL = 1.8 mOsm
Multivitamin concentrate	4.11	10 mL = 41 mOsm

Data from RxKinetics: *Calculating Osmolarity of an IV Admixture* (website): http://www.rxkinetics.com/iv_osmolarity.html.

Access
Peripheral Access

PPN solutions should be hypoosmolar, that is, not more than 800 to 900 mOsm/kg to allow infusion through a peripheral, midline, or mid-clavicular intravenous catheter. Clear criteria must be identified to determine when it is appropriate to use PPN, as phlebitis is a common complication (Sugrue et al, 2018). Most often PPN is used as a "bridge" to either return to EN or CPN.

Short-Term Central Access

Catheters used for CPN ideally consist of a single lumen. If central access is needed for other reasons, such as hemodynamic monitoring, drawing blood samples, or giving medications, multiple-lumen catheters are available (Derenski et al, 2016). To reduce the risk of infection, the catheter lumen used to infuse CPN should be reserved for that purpose only. Catheters are inserted most commonly into the subclavian vein and advanced until the catheter tip is in the superior vena cava, using strict aseptic technique. Alternatively, an internal or external jugular vein catheter can be used with the same catheter tip placement. However, the motion of the neck makes this site much more difficult for maintaining the sterility of a dressing. Radiologic verification of the tip site is necessary before infusion of nutrients can begin. Strict infection control protocols should be used for catheter placement and maintenance. Fig. 12.6 shows alternative venous access sites for CPN; femoral placement is also possible.

A peripherally inserted central catheter (PICC) may be used for short- or moderate-term infusion in the hospital or in the home. This catheter is inserted into a vein in the antecubital area of the arm and threaded into the subclavian vein with the catheter tip placed in the superior vena cava. Trained nonphysicians can insert a PICC, whereas placement of a tunneled catheter is a surgical procedure. All catheters must have radiologic confirmation of the placement of the catheter tip before initiating any infusion.

Long-Term Central Access

A commonly used long-term catheter is a "tunneled" catheter. This single- or multiple-lumen catheter is placed in the cephalic, subclavian, or internal jugular vein and fed into the superior vena cava (Opilla, 2016). A subcutaneous tunnel is created so that the catheter exits the skin several inches from its venous entry site. This allows the patient to care for the catheter more easily as is necessary for long-term infusion. Another type of long-term catheter is a surgically implanted

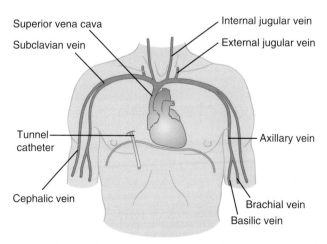

Fig. 12.6 Venous sites from which the superior vena cava may be accessed.

port under the skin where the catheter normally would exit at the end of the subcutaneous tunnel. A special needle must access the entrance port. Ports can be single or double; an individual port is equivalent to a lumen. Both tunneled catheters and PICCs can be used for extended therapy in the hospital or for home infusion therapy. Care of long-term catheters requires specialized handling and extensive patient education.

Parenteral Solutions
Protein

Commercially available standard PN solutions contain all essential amino acids and only some of the nonessential amino acids. Nonessential nitrogen is provided principally by the amino acids alanine and glycine, usually without aspartate, glutamate, cysteine, and taurine. Specialized solutions with adjusted amino acid content that contain taurine are available for infants, for whom taurine is thought to be conditionally essential.

The concentration of amino acids in PN solutions ranges from 3% to 20% by volume. Thus a 10% solution of amino acids supplies 100 g of protein per liter (1000 mL). The percentage of a solution usually is expressed as its final concentration after dilution with other nutrient solutions. The caloric content of amino acid solutions is approximately 4 kcal/g of protein provided. Protein needs are calculated based on the nutrition assessment data related to disease, injury, or clinical/nutrition status and range between 15% and 20% of total energy intake (Mueller et al, 2011).

Carbohydrates

Carbohydrates are supplied as dextrose monohydrate in concentrations ranging from 5% to 70% by volume. The dextrose monohydrate yields 3.4 calories per gram. As with amino acids, a 10% solution yields 100 g of carbohydrates per liter of solution.

Maximum rates of carbohydrate administration should not exceed 5 to 6 mg/kg/min, calculated over a 24-hour infusion period, in critically ill patients. When PN solutions provide 15% to 20% of total calories as protein, 20% to 30% of total calories as lipid, and the balance from carbohydrate (dextrose), infusion of dextrose should not exceed this amount. Excessive administration can lead to hyperglycemia, hepatic abnormalities, or increased ventilatory drive (see Chapter 33).

Lipids

Intravenous lipid emulsions (ILE) provide calories and the essential fatty acids (EFA), linoleic acid (LA) and alpha-linolenic acid (ALA) in PN to avoid EFAD (Derenski et al, 2016; Mundi et al, 2017)

Approximately 2% to 4% of calories from linoleic acid and 0.25% of calories from alpha-linoleic acid are required to prevent EFAD (Derenski et al, 2016; Gramlich et al, 2015). Administration should not exceed 2 g of ILE per kilogram of body weight per day, although recommendations of 1 to 1.5 g/kg are common. Triglyceride levels should be monitored and when triglycerides exceed 400 mg/dL, the ILE should be discontinued. All ILE should be administered through a 1.2-micron filter.

A 10% ILE contains 1.1 kcal/mL, whereas a 20% emulsion contains 2 kcal/mL. Providing 20% to 30% of total calories as lipid emulsion should result in a daily dosage of approximately 1 g of fat per kilogram of body weight. For critically ill patients who receive sedation in an ILE, these calories should be included in the nutrient intake calculations to avoid overfeeding or underfeeding (Drover et al, 2010). Diprivan (propofol) is an example of a sedation/anesthesia agent administered as an injectable infusion in a soybean oil-based ILE providing approximately 1.1 kcal/mL infused. In the hospital, lipid is infused for 24 hours when mixed with the dextrose and amino acids. Alternatively, lipids can be provided separately by infusion via an infusion pump. For adult patients receiving home parenteral nutrition (HPN), the PN most often is infused during 10 to 12 hours per day with the lipid as part of the PN solution. It may be infused as a daily component of the HPN or a few times per week (Kirby et al, 2017).

Selection of ILE should be based on individual patient requirements and ILE lipid content. The ILE currently available in the United States are composed of aqueous suspensions of soybean oil with egg yolk phospholipid as the emulsifier (Intralipid®, Fresenius Kabi [marketed by Baxter Healthcare in the United States], and Nutrilipid® B. Braun), or a mixture of soybean, medium chain, olive, and fish oil (Smoflipid, Fresenius Kabi) or fish oil only (Omegaven, Fresenius Kabi). The ILE containing egg phospholipids should not be used when a patient has an egg allergy.

These ILE contain varying levels of omega-6 polyunsaturated fatty acids, omega-3 fatty acids, and monounsaturated fat. Until 2016, 100% soybean oil-based ILE were available in the United States. A multi-oil ILE, Smoflipid (Fresenius Kabi) has been used in Europe for many years with clinical studies in critical care and long-term HPN patients indicating that it is safe and well tolerated (Antébi et al, 2004; Klek et al, 2013) and is now used in the United States. Because of the multiple lipid types in the emulsion, the plasma fatty acid pattern demonstrated a rise in EPA- and DHA-derived lipid mediators and maintenance of an adequate vitamin E status (Puiggròs et al, 2009; Gramlich et al, 2015).

Omegaven (Fresenius Kabi) is a fish oil–based ILE now available in the United States. Proposed benefits of fish oil lipid emulsion, as well as those that contain MCTs, include decreased inflammatory effects and less immunosuppression (Manzanares et al, 2014; Driscoll, 2017).

Careful attention to the caloric load as well as the adequacy of EFA is important when these are used.

For the clinician, the choice of ILE must include risks and benefits of each formulation. As soybean oil is primarily proinflammatory omega-6 fatty acids, this is a consideration when higher amounts are administered to a patient, especially for a long-term HPN patient or critically ill patient. Additionally, when ILE is limited, as with lipid lowering techniques to prevent intestinal failure associated liver

disease, dextrose must be increased to assure adequate calories are provided. This can cause hyperglycemia. Therefore the use of an ILE with decreased levels of soybean oil and increased levels of fish oil can be advantageous (Gramlich et al, 2015; Klek et al, 2013).

Electrolytes, Vitamins, Trace Elements

General guidelines for daily requirements for electrolytes are given in Table 12.3, for vitamins in Table 12.4, and for trace elements in Table 12.5. Parenteral solutions also represent a significant portion of total daily fluid and electrolyte intake. Once a solution is prescribed and initiated, adjustments for proper fluid and electrolyte balance may be necessary, depending on the stability of the patient. The choice of the salt form of electrolytes (e.g., chloride, acetate) affects acid-base balance (Derenski et al, 2016).

Parenterally administered multivitamin and mineral preparations are designed to meet most patient's needs. These levels may be inadequate in some situations when additional individual supplementation is required (Vanek et al, 2012). Patients receiving PN as their sole source of nutrition should receive added multivitamins and trace

TABLE 12.3 Daily Electrolyte Requirements During Total Parenteral Nutrition—Adults

Electrolyte	Standard Intake/Day
Calcium	10-15 mEq
Magnesium	8-20 mEq
Phosphate	20-40 mmol
Sodium	1-2 mEq/kg + replacement
Potassium	1-2 mEq/kg
Acetate	As needed to maintain acid-base balance
Chloride	As needed to maintain acid-base balance

From McClave SA et al: Guidelines for the provision and assessment of nutrition support therapy in the adult critically ill patient, *J Parenter Enteral Nutr* 33:277, 2009.

TABLE 12.4 Adult Parenteral Multivitamins: Comparison of Guidelines and Products

Vitamin	NAG-AMA Guidelines	FDA Requirements	MVI-12	MVI-13 (Infuvite) Baxter
A (retinol)	3300 units (1 mg)	3300 units (1 mg)	3300 units (1 mg)	3300 units (1 mg)
D (ergocalciferol cholecalciferol)	200 units (5 mcg)	200 units (5 mcg)	200 units (5 mcg)	200 units (5 mcg)
E (mcg-tocopherol)	10 units (10 mg)	10 units (10 mg)	10 units (10 mg)	10 units (10 mg)
B_1 (thiamin)	3 mg	6 mg	3 mg	6 mg
B_2 (riboflavin)	3.6 mg	3.6 mg	3.6 mg	3.6 mg
B_3 (niacinamide)	40 mg	40 mg	40 mg	40 mg
B_5 (dexpanthenol)	15 mg	15 mg	15 mg	15 mg
B_6 (pyridoxine)	4 mg	6 mg	4 mg	6 mg
B_{12} (cyanocobalamin)	5 mcg	5 mcg	5 mcg	5 mcg
C (ascorbic acid)	100 mg	200 mg	100 mg	200 mg
Biotin	60 mcg	60 mcg	60 mcg	60 mcg
Folic acid	400 mcg	600 mcg	400 mcg	600 mcg
K		150 mcg	0	150 mcg

AMA, American Medical Association; *FDA*, U.S. Food and Drug Administration; *MVI-12* and *MVI-13*, multivitamin supplements; *NAG*, National Advisory Group.
Vanek V et al: A.S.P.E.N. position paper: recommendations for changes in commercially available parenteral multivitamin and multi-trace element products, *Nutr Clin Prac* 27:440, 2012.

TABLE 12.5 Daily Trace Element Supplementation for Adult Parenteral Formulations

Trace Element	Intake
Chromium	10-15 mcg
Copper	0.3-0.5 mg
Manganese	60-100 mcg
Zinc	2.5-5.0 mg
Selenium	20-60 mcg

elements daily and be monitored closely, especially those who are critically ill. Patients receiving PN short-term or peripherally should also receive daily multivitamins and trace elements. If PN is provided, there is no reason to leave out these important additives. Monitoring of manganese and chromium status is recommended for patients receiving PN for longer than 6 months (Buchman et al, 2009). In most cases, manganese is not needed as a daily infusion as it is provided in adequate amounts as a contaminant in glass vials. Similarly, chromium is usually not needed daily.

In certain cases, additional multivitamins may be required to treat a specific deficiency such as thiamine infusion in patients with refeeding syndrome or a deficiency due to poor intake. Recognizing the importance of providing specific nutrients may obviate the development of a more complex problem.

Iron is not normally part of parenteral infusions because it is not compatible with lipids and may enhance certain bacterial growth. In addition, care must be taken to ensure that a patient can tolerate the separate iron infusion. When patients receive iron on an outpatient basis, the first dose should be done in a controlled setting (such as an outpatient infusion suite) to observe for any reactions that the patient may experience.

One of the challenges in PN in the last 5 years has been the occurrence of drug shortages that have affected micro- and macronutrients, including ILE, multivitamins, multitrace elements, and electrolytes including phosphorous. Patients in the hospital, at home, and in long-term care receiving not only PN but also other intravenous and injectable therapies have been affected. This problem is expected to be ongoing, and therefore clinicians should be aware of alternative products as well as methods to allocate safely products in short supply.

Fluid

Fluid needs for PN or EN are calculated similarly. Maximum volumes of CPN rarely exceed 3 L, with typical prescriptions of 1.5 to 3 L daily. In critically ill patients, volumes of prescribed CPN should be coordinated closely with their overall care plan (Mundi et al, 2017). The administration of other medical therapies requiring fluid administration, such as intravenous medications and blood products, necessitates careful monitoring. Patients with cardiopulmonary, renal, and hepatic failure are especially sensitive to fluid administration. For HPN, higher volumes may be best provided in separate infusions. For example, if additional fluid is required because of high output by the patient, then a liter bag of intravenous fluid containing minimal electrolytes may be infused during a short time during the day if the PN is infused overnight. See Appendix 16 on calculating PN prescriptions.

Compounding Methods

PN prescriptions historically have required preparation or compounding by competent pharmacy personnel under laminar airflow hoods using aseptic techniques. Hospitals may have their own compounding pharmacy or may purchase PN solutions that have been compounded outside the hospital in a central location and then returned to the hospital for distribution to individual patients. A third method of providing PN solutions is to use multichamber bag technology, whereby solutions are manufactured in a quality-controlled environment using good manufacturing processes. PN solutions of two chamber bags contain amino acids (with or without electrolytes) and dextrose and are available in multiple formulas with varying amounts of dextrose and amino acids, making them suitable for CPN or PPN infusion. Some multichamber bag formulas may contain lipids in a third chamber; however, these are not currently available in the United States but are available in Europe and Canada. They contain conservative amounts of electrolytes or may be electrolyte free. These products have a shelf life of 2 years and do not have to be refrigerated unless the product covering has been opened to reveal the infusion bag. They do not contain vitamins or trace elements that can be added to the solutions; therefore, the clinician must add vitamins/minerals to the patient's treatment plan to avoid any deficiencies. Institutions frequently use standardized solutions, which are compounded in batches, thus saving labor and lowering costs; however, flexibility for individualized compounding should be available when warranted (Ayers et al, 2014).

Prescriptions for PN are compounded in two general ways. One method combines all components except the fat emulsion, which is infused separately. The second method combines the lipid emulsion with the dextrose and amino acid solution and is referred to as a **total nutrient admixture** or **3-in-1** solution. The PN Safe Practices Guidelines provide clinicians with information on many techniques and procedures that enhance safety and prevent mistakes in the preparation of PN (Boullata et al, 2014).

A number of medications, including antibiotics, vasopressors, narcotics, diuretics, and many other commonly administered drugs, can be compounded with PN solutions. In practice this occurs infrequently because it requires specialized knowledge of physical compatibility or incompatibility of the solution contents. The most common drug additives are insulin for persistent hyperglycemia and histamine-2 antagonists to avoid gastroduodenal stress ulceration. One other consideration is that the PN usually is ordered 24 hours before its administration, and patient status may have changed.

Administration

The methods used to administer PN are addressed after the goal infusion rate has been established. For critically ill and hospitalized patients, a 24-hour infusion rate is used. However, for patients transitioning to a long term or lifetime of receiving PN, infusion rate should be decreased to a 10- to 12-hour cycle per day to complete activities of daily living and improve quality of life (Kirby et al, 2017). Nevertheless, general considerations as listed in Box 12.5 can be applied to almost any protocol.

Continuous Infusion

Parenteral solutions usually are initiated below the goal infusion rate via a volumetric pump and then increased incrementally over a 2- or 3-day period to attain the goal infusion rate. Some clinicians start PN based on the amount of dextrose, with initial prescriptions containing 100 to 200 g daily and advancing over a 2- or 3-day period to a final goal. With high dextrose concentrations, abrupt cessation of CPN should be avoided, particularly if the patient's glucose tolerance is abnormal. If CPN is to be stopped, it is prudent to taper the rate of infusion in an unstable patient to prevent **rebound hypoglycemia**, low blood sugar levels resulting from abrupt cessation. For most stable patients this is not necessary.

BOX 12.5   Nutrition Care Process for Enteral and Parenteral Nutrition

Assessment
1. Clinical status, including medications
2. Fluid requirement
3. Route of administration
4. Energy (kcal) requirement
5. Protein requirement
6. Carbohydrate/lipid considerations
7. Micronutrient considerations
8. Formula selection or PN solution considerations
   A. Concentration (osmolarity)
   B. Protein content
   C. Carbohydrate/lipid content
   D. Micronutrient content
   E. Special formula considerations
9. Calculations
   A. Energy: use kcal/mL formula
   B. Protein: use g/1000 mL
   C. Fat and micronutrient considerations: units/1000 mL
   D. Fluid considerations: extra water, IV fluids (including medications)

Nutrition Diagnosis
1. Identify the problems affecting oral nutritional intake.
2. Identify problems related to access or administration of tube feedings.
3. Write PES statements. These may include inadequate or excess infusion of enteral or parenteral nutrition, or other nutrition diagnoses.

Intervention
1. Each problem should have an intervention and a way to evaluate it.
2. Recommend method and how to begin feedings.
3. Recommend how to advance feedings.
4. Determine how fluids will be given in adequate amounts.
5. Calculate final feeding prescription.

Monitoring and Evaluation
1. Describe clinical signs and symptoms to monitor for feeding tolerance.
2. List laboratory values and other measurements to be monitored.
3. Determine how feeding outcomes will be evaluated.

IV, Intravenous; *PES*, problem, etiology, and signs and symptoms; *PN*, parenteral nutrition.

Cyclic Infusion

Individuals who require PN at home benefit from a cyclic infusion; this entails infusion of PN for 8- to 12-hour periods, usually at night. This allows the person to have a free period of 12 to 16 hours each day, which may improve quality of life. The goal cycle for infusion time is established incrementally when a higher rate of infusion or a more concentrated solution is required. Cycled infusions should not be attempted if glucose intolerance or fluid tolerance is a problem. The pumps used for home infusion of PN are small and convenient, allowing mobility during daytime infusions. Administration time may be decreased because of patient ambulation and bathing, tests or other treatments, intravenous administration of medications, or other therapies.

Monitoring and Evaluation

As with enteral feeding, routine monitoring of PN is necessary more frequently for the patient receiving PN in the hospital (Mundi et al, 2017). For patients receiving HPN, initial monitoring is done on a weekly basis or less frequently as the patient becomes more stable on PN. Monitoring is done not only to evaluate response to therapy but also to ensure compliance with the treatment plan (Kirby et al, 2017).

COMPLICATIONS

Infection

The primary complication associated with PN is infection (Box 12.6). Therefore strict adherence to protocols and monitoring for signs of infection such as chills, fever, tachycardia, sudden hyperglycemia, or elevated white blood cell count are necessary. Monitoring of metabolic tolerance is also critical. Electrolytes, acid-base balance, glucose tolerance, renal function, and cardiopulmonary and hemodynamic stability (maintenance of adequate blood pressure) can be affected by PN and should be monitored carefully. Table 12.6 lists parameters that should be monitored routinely.

The CPN catheter site is a potential source for introduction of microorganisms into a major vein. Protocols to prevent infection vary and should follow Centers for Disease Control and Prevention guidelines (O'Grady et al, 2011). Catheter care and prevention of catheter-related bloodstream infections are of utmost importance in the hospital and alternate settings. These infections not only are costly but also may be life-threatening. Catheter care is dictated by the site of the catheter and the setting in which the patient receives care.

REFEEDING SYNDROME

Patients who require enteral or PN therapies may have been eating poorly before initiating therapy because of the disease process and may be moderately to severely malnourished. Aggressive administration of nutrition, particularly via the intravenous route, can precipitate refeeding syndrome with severe, potentially lethal electrolyte fluctuations involving metabolic, hemodynamic, and neuromuscular problems. Refeeding syndrome occurs when energy substrates, particularly carbohydrate, are introduced into the plasma of anabolic patients.

Proliferation of new tissue requires increased amounts of glucose, potassium, phosphorus, magnesium, and other nutrients essential for tissue growth. If intracellular electrolytes are not supplied in sufficient quantity to keep up with tissue growth, low serum levels of potassium, phosphorus, and magnesium develop. Low levels of these electrolytes are the hallmark of refeeding syndrome, especially hypophosphatemia (Skipper, 2012). Carbohydrate metabolism by cells also causes a shift of electrolytes to the intracellular space as glucose moves into cells for oxidation. Rapid infusion of carbohydrate stimulates insulin release, which reduces salt and water excretion and increases the chance of cardiac and pulmonary complications from fluid overload.

Patients starting on PN who have received minimal nutrition for a significant period should be monitored closely for electrolyte fluctuation and fluid overload. A review of baseline laboratory values, including glucose, magnesium, potassium, and phosphorus should be completed and any abnormalities corrected before initiating nutrition support, particularly PN. Conservative amounts of carbohydrate and

BOX 12.6   Parenteral Nutrition Complications

Mechanical Complications
Air embolism
Arteriovenous fistula
Brachial plexus injury
Catheter fragment embolism
Catheter misplacement
Cardiac perforation
Central vein thrombophlebitis
Endocarditis
Hemothorax
Hydromediastinum
Hydrothorax
Pneumothorax or tension pneumothorax
Subcutaneous emphysema
Subclavian artery injury
Subclavian hematoma
Thoracic duct injury

Infection and Sepsis
Catheter entrance site
Catheter seeding from bloodborne or distant infection
Contamination during insertion
Long-term catheter placement
Solution contamination

Metabolic Complications
Dehydration from osmotic diuresis
Electrolyte imbalance
Essential fatty acid deficiency
Hyperosmolar, nonketotic, hyperglycemic coma
Hyperammonemia
Hypercalcemia
Hyperchloremic metabolic acidosis
Hyperlipidemia
Hyperphosphatemia
Hypocalcemia
Hypomagnesemia
Hypophosphatemia
Rebound hypoglycemia on sudden cessation of PN in patient with unstable glucose levels
Uremia
Trace mineral deficiencies

Gastrointestinal Complications
Cholestasis
Gastrointestinal villous atrophy
Hepatic abnormalities

Adapted from McClave SA et al: Guidelines for the provision and assessment of nutrition support therapy in the adult critically ill patient, *J Parenter Enteral Nutr* 33:277, 2009.

TABLE 12.6   Inpatient Parenteral Nutrition Monitoring (Critical/Acute Care)

Variable to be Monitored	SUGGESTED FREQUENCY	
	Initial Period*	Later Period*
Weight	Daily	Weekly
Serum electrolytes	Daily	1-2/wk
Blood urea nitrogen	3/wk	Weekly
Serum total calcium or ionized Ca^+, inorganic phosphorus, magnesium	3/wk	Weekly
Serum glucose	Daily	3/wk
Serum triglycerides	Weekly	Weekly
Liver function enzymes	3/wk	Weekly
Hemoglobin, hematocrit	Weekly	Weekly
Platelets	Weekly	Weekly
WBC count	As indicated	As indicated
Clinical status	Daily	Daily
Catheter site	Daily	Daily
Temperature	Daily	Daily
I&O	Daily	Daily

Initial period is that period in which a full glucose intake is being achieved. *Later period* implies that the patient had achieved a steady metabolic state. In the presence of metabolic instability, the more intensive monitoring outlined under initial period should be followed. *I&O,* Intake and output; *WBC,* white blood cell.
I&O refers to all fluids going into the patient: oral, intravenous, medication; and all fluid coming out: urine, surgical drains, exudates. McClave SA et al: Guidelines for the provision and assessment of nutrition support therapy in the adult critically ill patient, *J Parenter Enteral Nutr* 33:277, 2009.

adequate amounts of intracellular electrolytes should be provided. The initial PN formulation usually should contain 25% to 50% of goal dextrose concentration and be increased slowly to avoid the consequences of hypophosphatemia, hypokalemia, and hypomagnesemia. PN compatibilities must be assessed when very low levels of dextrose are provided with higher levels of amino acids and electrolytes. The syndrome also occurs in enterally fed patients, but less often because of the effects of the digestive process.

In managing the nutrition care process, refeeding syndrome is an undesirable outcome that requires monitoring and evaluation. Most often, the nutrition diagnosis may be "excessive carbohydrate intake" or "excessive infusion from enteral or parenteral nutrition" in the undernourished patient. Thus in the early phase of refeeding, nutrient prescriptions should be moderate in carbohydrate and supplemented with phosphorus, potassium, and magnesium.

TRANSITIONAL FEEDING

All nutrition support care plans strive to use the GIT when possible, either with EN or by a total or partial return to oral intake. Therefore patient care plans frequently involve transitional feeding, moving from one type of feeding to another, with several feeding methods used simultaneously while continuously administering estimated nutrient requirements. This requires careful monitoring of patient tolerance and quantification of intake from parenteral, enteral, and oral routes. Most experts advise that initial oral diets be low in simple carbohydrates and fat, as well as lactose free. These provisions make digestion easier and minimize the possibility of osmotic diarrhea. Attention to individual tolerance and food preferences also helps maximize intake. During the transition stage from HPN to home enteral nutrition (HEN) or an oral diet, careful attention should be paid to assuring multivitamin and mineral adequacy. This may require laboratory assessment of micronutrients if a deficiency is suspected.

Parenteral to Enteral Feeding

To begin the transition from PN to EN, introduce a minimal amount of enteral feeding at a low rate of 30 to 40 mL/hr to establish gastrointestinal tolerance. When there is severe gastrointestinal compromise, predigested formula to initiate enteral feedings may be better tolerated. Once formula has been given during a period of hours, the parenteral rate can be decreased to keep the nutrient levels at the same prescribed amount. As the enteral rate is increased by 25 to 30 mL/hr increments every 8 to 24 hours, the parenteral prescription is reduced accordingly. Once the patient is tolerating about 75% of nutrient needs by the enteral route, the PN solution can be discontinued. This process ideally takes 2 to 3 days; however, it may become more complicated depending on the degree of gastrointestinal function. At times the weaning process may not be practical, and PN can be stopped sooner, depending on overall treatment decisions and likelihood for tolerance of enteral feeding.

Parenteral to Oral Feeding

The transition from parenteral to oral feeding ideally is accomplished by monitoring oral intake and concomitantly decreasing the PN to maintain a stable nutrient intake. Approximately 75% of nutrient needs should be met consistently by oral intake before the PN is discontinued. The process is less predictable than the transition to enteral feeding. Variations include the patient's appetite, motivation, and general well-being. It is important to continue monitoring the patient for adequate oral intake once PN has been stopped and to initiate alternate nutrition support if necessary. Generally, patients are transitioned from clear liquids to a diet that is low in fiber and fat and is lactose free. It takes several days for the GIT to regain function; during that time, the diet should be composed of easily digested foods.

Special nutrient needs can be employed, especially when transitioning a patient with gastrointestinal disorders such as short bowel syndrome. Specialized nutrients, optimized drug therapy, and nutrition counseling should be comprehensive to improve outcome. Some PN patients may not be able to discontinue PN fully but may be able to use PN less than 7 days per week, necessitating careful attention to nutrient intake. A skilled RDN can coordinate diet and PN needs for this type of patient.

Enteral to Oral Feeding

A stepwise decrease also is used to transition from EN to oral feeding. It is effective to move from continuous feeding to a 12- and then an 8-hour formula administration cycle during the night; this reestablishes hunger and satiety cues for oral intake during daytime. In practice, oral diets often are attempted after inadvertent or deliberate removal of a nasoenteric tube. This type of interrupted transition should be monitored closely for adequate oral intake. Patients receiving EN who desire to eat and for whom it is not contraindicated can be encouraged to do so. A transition from liquids to easy-to-digest foods may be necessary during a period of days. Patients who cannot meet their needs by the oral route can be maintained by a combination of EN and oral intake.

Oral Supplements

The most common types of oral supplements are commercial formulas meant primarily to augment the intake of solid foods. They commonly provide 250 to 360 kcal/8 oz or 240-mL portion and approximately 8 to 14 g of intact protein. Some products have 360 or 500 or as much as 575 kcal in a can. There are different types of products for different disease states, but many of these are brought to market with little to no scientific evidence to support their efficacy.

Fat sources are often LCTs, although some supplements contain MCTs. More concentrated and thus more nutrient-dense formulas are also available. A variety of flavors, consistencies, and modifications of nutrients are appropriate for various disease states. Some oral supplements provide a nutritionally complete diet if taken in sufficient volume.

The form of carbohydrate is a key factor to patient acceptance and tolerance. Supplements with appreciable amounts of simple carbohydrate taste sweeter and have higher osmolalities, which may contribute to gastrointestinal intolerance. Individual taste preferences vary widely, and normal taste is altered by certain drug therapies, especially chemotherapy. Concentrated formulas or large volumes can contribute to taste fatigue and early satiety. Thus oral nutrient intake and the intake of prescribed supplements should be monitored.

Oral supplements that contain hydrolyzed protein and free amino acids such as those developed for patients with renal, liver, and malabsorptive diseases tend to be mildly to markedly unpalatable, and acceptance by the patient depends on motivation. Formulas for renal and liver disease may lack sufficient vitamins and minerals and are not nutritionally complete and therefore useful only to the specific population.

Although commercially available modular supplements are used most commonly for convenience, modules of protein, carbohydrate, or fat or commonly available food items can produce highly palatable additions to a diet. As examples, liquid or powdered milk, yogurt, tofu, or protein powders can be used to enrich cereals, casseroles, soups, or milk shakes. Thickening agents are now used to add variety, texture, and esthetics to pureed foods, which are used when swallowing ability is limited (see Chapter 39). Imagination and individual tailoring can increase oral intake, avoiding the necessity for more complex forms of nutrition support.

NUTRITION SUPPORT IN LONG-TERM AND HOME CARE

Long-Term Care

Long-term care (LTC) usually refers to a skilled nursing facility but includes subacute care for rehabilitation. Health care provided in this environment focuses on quality of life, self-determination, and management of acute and chronic disease. Indications for EN and PN are generally the same for older patients as for younger adults and vary according to the age, gender, disease state, and most importantly, the care goals of the individual. PN is often provided to these facilities by offsite pharmacies that specialize in LTC. These providers may employ dietitians and specially trained nurses to assist the facilities with education and training.

Oral supplements have gained widespread use in LTC over the last two decades, again for convenience. However, they appear to have detrimental effects, and real food always should be attempted first. A major goal in LTC is the elimination of canned nutrition supplements because they are seen as a detriment to eating real food. (See Chapter 19 for a discussion of the dining standards for LTC).

Advance directives are legal documents that residents use to state their preferences about aspects of care, including those regarding the use of nutrition support. These directives may be written in any setting, including acute or home care but are especially useful in LTC to guide interventions on behalf of LTC residents when they are no longer able to make decisions (Schwartz et al, 2016)

Differentiation between the effects of advanced age and malnutrition is an assessment challenge for dietitians working in LTC (see Chapter 19). This is an area of active research, as is the influence that nutrition support has on the quality of life among LTC residents. Studies generally show that use of nutrition support in older adults is beneficial only in specific situations and especially when used in conjunction with physical activity. Patients who are actively pursuing physical therapy are good candidates for nutrition support. However, when there is a terminal illness or condition, starting nutrition support may have no advantage and can prolong suffering. Tube feeding has not been shown beneficial in people with dementia who's decreased intake is part of the disease process. Dietitians should be strong patient advocates in end-of-life decisions. RDNs should be involved in writing and implementing the policies in their institutions.

Home Care

Home enteral nutrition (HEN) or home parenteral nutrition (HPN) support usually entails the provision of nutrients or formulas, supplies, equipment, and professional clinical services. Resources and technology for safe and effective management of long-term enteral or parenteral therapy are widely available for the home care setting. Although home nutrition support has been available for more than 30 years, few outcome data have been generated. Because mandatory reporting requirements do not exist in the United States for patients receiving home nutrition support, the exact number of patients receiving this support is unknown.

The elements needed to implement home nutrition successfully include identification of appropriate candidates and a feasible home environment with responsive caregivers, a choice of a suitable nutrition support regimen, training of the patient and family, and a plan for medical and nutritional follow-up by the physician as well as by the home infusion provider (Box 12.7). These objectives are best achieved through the coordinated efforts of an interdisciplinary team (see *Clinical Insight*: Home Tube Feeding—Key Considerations).

Patients receiving HEN may receive supplies only, or formula and supplies with or without clinical oversight by the provider. Many enteral patients receive services from a durable medical equipment (DME) provider that may or may not provide clinical services. A home infusion provider provides intravenous therapies, including home PN, intravenous antibiotics, and other therapies. Home nursing agencies may be associated with a DME company or a home infusion agency to provide nursing services to home EN or PN patients. Often the patient's reimbursement source for home therapy plays a major role in determining the type of home infusion provider. In fact, reimbursement is a key component of a patient's ability to receive home therapy of any kind and should be evaluated early in the care plan so that appropriate decisions can be made before discharge or initiating a therapy.

Companies that provide home infusion services for EN or PN can be private or affiliated with acute care facilities. Criteria for selecting a home care company to provide nutrition support should be based on

CLINICAL INSIGHT
Home Tube Feeding—Key Considerations

What Is the Best Kind of Tube?
In general, nasal tubes should be avoided because they are more difficult to manage, clog easily, are easily dislodged, and over time can cause tissue irritation and even erosion. Percutaneous endoscopic gastrostomy (PEG) tubes are now the most common and preferred method for home tube feedings. They can be either low profile (flat to the abdomen), button-type tubes, or they can have a short piece of tubing attached through the abdomen and into the stomach. The button tubes require some manual dexterity to access and can be difficult to use for patients who are very obese. Percutaneous endoscopic jejunostomy (PEJ) tubes are best for patients who require post-pyloric feedings as a result of intolerance of gastric feeding, but PEJ feedings require a pump, which severely limits mobility of the patient.

What Is the Best Method of Administration?
Bolus feeding is the easiest administration method and generally should be tried first. It should be started slowly at half of an 8-oz can four to six times a day. If bolus feeding is not tolerated, gravity feeding is a second option. It does require a bag and pole but can be accomplished fairly quickly and requires less manual dexterity than bolus feeding.

Pump feeding is sometimes necessary when a patient requires small amounts of formula delivered slowly. Although it is well tolerated, it has major implications for a patient at home because even the simplest pump is often viewed as "high tech." Its use greatly limits mobility, and, like any piece of equipment, it can break and interrupt feeding schedules.

What Is the Best Way to Educate the Patient and Caregiver?
- Directions should be written in common measurements such as cups, tablespoons, and cans rather than milliliters.
- The enteral nutrition regimen should be as simple as possible; use whole cans of formula rather than partial cans.
- Additives to the feedings should be minimized to avoid confusion and clogging of the feeding tubes.
- Provide clear directions for gradually increasing to the goal feeding rate.
- Provide clear directions for water flushing of the tube and for additional water requirements to prevent dehydration.
- Discuss common problems that may come up and provide guidance for resolving them.
- Make sure that the patient or caregiver can demonstrate understanding of the feeding process by either explaining it or by doing it.

the company's ability to provide ongoing monitoring, patient education, and coordination of care. However, in today's world hospital or patient insurance contracts often dictate the PEN provider. When a patient is receiving home EN or PN, it is important to determine whether the provider has an RDN on staff or access to the services of an RDN. The RDN is uniquely qualified not only to provide oversight and monitoring for the patient while receiving EN or PN but also to provide the appropriate nutrition counseling and food suggestions when the patient transitions between therapies.

Ethical Issues

Whether to provide or withhold nutrition support is often a central issue in end-of-life decision making. For patients who are terminally ill or in a persistent vegetative state, nutrition support can extend life to the point that issues of quality of life and the patient's right to self-determination come into play. Often surrogate decision makers are

---

BOX 12.7 Considerations When Deciding on Home Nutrition Support

Sanitation of the home environment to preserve the patient's health and reduce risk of infection

Potential for improvement in quality of life and nutritional status

The financial and time commitment needed by patient or family; potential loss of income outside the home in some cases

Ability to understand the techniques for administration of the product and safe use of all equipment and supplies

Any physical limitations that prevent the implementation of HEN or HPN therapy

Capacity for patient or caregiver to contact medical services when needed

HEN, Home enteral nutrition; *HPN*, home parenteral nutrition.

involved in treatment decisions. The nutrition support clinician has a responsibility to know whether documentation, such as a living will regarding the patient's wishes for nutrition support, is in the medical record and whether counseling and support resources for legal and ethical aspects of patient care are available to patients and their significant others.

CLINICAL CASE STUDY

A 24-year-old has newly diagnosed type 1 diabetes mellitus and Crohn's disease. She recently had surgery for removal of one third of her ileum. She is 75% of her usual weight, which is 125 lb; she is 65 inches tall. She requires specialized nutrition support for several months until her body adapts to the shortened bowel.

Nutrition Diagnostic Statements
- Involuntary weight loss related to poor intake, surgery, and pain during flare-up of Crohn's disease as evidenced by 25% weight loss.
- Inadequate oral food and beverage intake related to recent ileal resection as evidenced by 75% of usual weight and need for artificial nutrition.

Nutrition Care Questions
1. What immediate nutrition support method would be recommended?
2. What long-term nutrition support plan is likely to be designed?
3. What specialty products, if any, may be beneficial?
4. What parameters would you monitor to determine tolerance and response to the nutrition plan?

USEFUL WEBSITES

Academy of Nutrition and Dietetics—Evidence Analysis Library (member/subscription access only)
American Society for Parenteral and Enteral Nutrition
European Society for Parenteral and Enteral Nutrition
Infusion Nurses Society
Medscape—Integrated Med Information
Oley Foundation

REFERENCES

Academy of Nutrition and Dietetics, Evidence Analysis Library: *Critical illness guidelines*, 2012. Available at: http://andevidencelibrary.com/topic.cfm?cat54800.

Antébi H, Mansoor O, Ferrier C, et al: Liver function and plasma antioxidant status in intensive care unit patients requiring total parenteral nutrition: comparison of 2 fat emulsions, *J Parenter Enteral Nutr* 28(3):142–148, 2004.

Atkinson M, Worthley LI: Nutrition in the critically ill patient: part III: Enteral nutrition. *Crit Care Resusc* 5(3):207–215, 2003.

Ayers P, Adams S, Boullata J, et al: A.S.P.E.N. parenteral nutrition safety consensus recommendations, *J Parenter Enteral Nutr* 38:296–333, 2014.

Bankhead R, Boullata J, Brantley S, et al: Enteral nutrition practice recommendations, *J Parenter Enteral Nutr* 33:122–167, 2009.

Boullata JI, Gilbert K, Sacks G, et al: A.S.P.E.N. clinical guidelines: parenteral nutrition ordering, order review, compounding, labeling, and dispensing, *JPEN J Parenter Enteral Nutr* 38:334–377, 2014.

Buchman AL, Howard LJ, Guenter P, et al: Micronutrients in parenteral nutrition: too little or too much? The past, present, and recommendations for the future, *Gastroenterology* 137(Suppl 5):S1–S6, 2009.

Derenski K, Catlin J, Allen L: Parenteral nutrition basics for the clinician caring for the adult patient, *Nutr Clin Prac* 31(5):578–595, 2016.

Driscoll, DF: Pharmaceutical and clinical aspects of lipid injectable emulsions, *J Parenter Enteral Nutr* 41(1):125–134, 2017.

Drover JW, Cahill NE, Kutsogiannis J, et al: Nutrition therapy for the critically ill surgical patient: we need to do better! *J Parenter Enteral Nutr* 34:644–652, 2010.

Elke G, van Zanten AR, Lemieux M, et al: Enteral versus parenteral nutrition in critically ill patients: an updated systematic review and meta-analysis of randomized controlled trials, *Crit Care* 20:117, 2016.

Escuro AA, Hummell AC: Enteral formulas in nutrition support practice: Is there a better choice for your patient? *Nutr Clin Pract* 31:709–722, 2016.

Food and Drug Administration: *Medical foods guidance documents & regulatory information*, 2014. Available at: http://www.fda.gov/Food/GuidanceRegulation/GuidanceDocumentsRegulatoryInformation/MedicalFoods/.

Gramlich L, Meddings L, Alberda C, et al: Essential fatty acid deficiency in 2015: the impact of novel intravenous lipid emulsions, *J Parenter Enteral Nutr* 39(Suppl 1):61S–66S, 2015.

Harvey SE, Parrott F, Harrison DA, et al: Trial of the route of early nutritional support in critically ill adults, *N Engl J Med* 371:1673–1684, 2014.

Hurt RT, Edakkanambeth Varayil J, Epp LM, et al: Blenderized tube feeding use in home enteral nutrition patients: a cross-sectional study, *Nutr Clin Pract* 30:824–829, 2015.

Joint Commission: *Sentinel event policy and procedures*, 2017. Available at: http://www.jointcommission.org/Sentinel_Event_Policy_and_Procedures/.

Kirby DF, Corrigan ML, Hendrickson E, et al: Overview of home parenteral nutrition: an update, *Nutr Clin Prac* 32(6):739–727, 2017.

Klek S, Chambrier C, Singer P, et al: Four-week parenteral nutrition using a third generation lipid emulsion (SMOFlipid) – a double-blind, randomised, multicenter study in adults, *Clinical Nutrition* 32:224–231, 2013.

Manzanares W, Dhaliwal R, Jurewitsch B, et al: Parenteral fish oil lipid emulsion in the critically ill: a systematic review and meta-analysis, *J Parenter Enteral Nutr* 38:20–28, 2014.

McClave SA, Taylor BE, Martindale RG, et al: Guidelines for the provision and assessment of nutrition support therapy in the adult critically ill patient: Society of Critical Care Medicine (SCCM) and American Society for Parenteral and Enteral Nutrition (A.S.P.E.N.), *J Parenter Enteral Nutr* 40:159–211, 2016. Available at: https://www.ncbi.nlm.nih.gov/pubmed/26773077.

Mueller C, Compher C, Ellen DM, et al: A.S.P.E.N. clinical guidelines: nutrition screening, assessment, and intervention in adults, *J Parenter Enteral Nutr* 35:16–24, 2011.

Mundi MS, Nystrom EM, Hurley DL, et al: Management of parenteral nutrition in hospitalized adult patient, *J Parenter Enteral Nutr* 41(4):535–549, 2017.

Novak P, Wilson KE, Ausderau K, et al: The use of blenderized tube feedings, *Infant Child Adolesc Nutr* 1:21–23, 2009.

O'Flaherty T, Santoro K, Pentiuk S: Calculating and preparing a pureed-gastrostomy tube (PBGT) diet for pediatric patients with retching and gagging post-fundoplication, *Infant Child Adolesc Nutr* 3:361–364, 2011.

O'Flaherty T: Use of a pureed by gastrostomy tube diet (PBGT) to promote oral intake: Review and case study, *Support Line* 37:21, 2015.

O'Grady NP, Alexander M, Burns, LA, et al. Guidelines for the prevention of intravascular catheter-related infections. Clin Infect Dis, 52(9):e162-1193, 2011.

Opilla M: Parenteral nutrition access. In Ireton-Jones C, editor: *Out-patient nutrition care and home nutrition support*, Boca Raton, FL, 2016, CRC Press, p 164.

Pentiuk S, O'Flaherty T, Santoro K, et al: Pureed by gastrostomy tube diet improves gagging and retching in children with fundoplication, *JPEN J Parenter Enteral Nutr* 35:375–379, 2011.

Puiggròs C, Sánchez J, Chacón P, et al: Evolution of lipid profile, liver function, and pattern of plasma fatty acids according to the type of lipid emulsion administered in parenteral nutrition in the early postoperative period after digestive surgery, *J Parenter Enteral Nutr* 33:501–512, 2009.

Reignier J, Boisramé-Helms J, Brisard L, et al: Enteral versus parenteral early nutrition in ventilated adults with chock: a randomised, controlled, multi-center, open-label, parallel-group study (NUTRIREA-2), *Lancet* 391: 133–143, 2018.

Schwartz DB, Olfson K, Goldman B, et al: Incorporating palliative care concepts into nutrition practice, *Nutr Clin Prac* 31(3):305–315, 2016.

Skipper A: Refeeding syndrome or refeeding hypophosphatemia: a systematic review of cases, *Nutr Clin Pract* 27(1):33–40, 2012.

Sugrue D, Jarrell AS, Kruer R, et al: Appropriateness of peripheral parenteral nutrition use in adult patients at an academic center, *Clin Nutr ESPEN* 23:117–121, 2018.

Vanek VW, Borum P, Buchman A, et al: A.S.P.E.N. position paper: recommendations for changes in commercially available parenteral multivitamin and multi-trace element products, *Nutr Clin Prac* 27:440–491, 2012.

Vassilyadi F, Panteliadou AK, Panteliadis C: Hallmarks in the history of enteral and parenteral nutrition: from antiquity to the 20th century, *Nutr Clin Prac* 28:209–217, 2013.

13

Education and Counseling: Behavioral Change

Karen Chapman-Novakofski, PhD, RDN, LDN
L. Karina Díaz Rios, PhD, RDN

KEY TERMS

acceptance and commitment therapy
   (ACT)
alignment
behavior change
behavior modification
beneficence
cognitive behavioral therapy (CBT)
cognitive dissonance
cultural competency
discrepancy
deep structure

double-sided reflection
empathy
health belief model (HBM)
health literacy
maleficence
motivational interviewing (MI)
negotiation
normalization
nutrition counseling
nutrition education
peer educator

PRECEDE-PROCEED model
reflective listening
reframing
self-efficacy
self-management
social cognitive theory (SCT)
social-ecological model
stages of change
surface structure
theory of planned behavior (TPB)
transtheoretical model (TTM)

Key factors in changing dietary behaviors are the person's awareness that a change is needed and the motivation to change. Within the nutrition care process, nutrition education and nutrition counseling both provide information and motivation, but they do differ. Nutrition education can be individualized or delivered in a group setting; it is usually more preventive than therapeutic, and there is a transmission of knowledge. Nutrition counseling is most often used during medical nutrition therapy, one-on-one. In the one-on-one setting, the nutritionist sets up a transient support system to prepare the client to handle social and personal demands more effectively while identifying favorable conditions for change. The goal of both nutrition education and nutrition counseling is to help individuals make meaningful changes in their dietary behaviors.

BEHAVIOR CHANGE

Although there are differences between education and counseling as intervention techniques, the distinctions are not as important as the shared and desired outcome—behavior change. Behavior change requires a focus on the broad range of activities and approaches that affect the individual choosing food and beverages in their community and home environment. Behavior modification implies the use of techniques to alter a person's response to environmental cues through positive and negative reinforcement, and reduction of maladaptive behaviors. In the context of nutrition,

both education and counseling can assist the individual in achieving short-term or long-term behavioral goals to improve health outcomes.

Factors Affecting the Ability to Change

Multiple factors affect a person's ability or desire to change, the educator's ability to teach new information and skills, and the counselor's ability to stimulate and support progressive changes.

The Social-Ecological Model (McLeroy et al, 1988; Fig. 13.1) illustrates the different levels of influence that affect change: personal, interpersonal, institutional, community, and policy levels. This multi-level, comprehensive model is often used to guide health promotion and disease prevention programs. The 2015–2020 Dietary Guidelines for Americans support the use of the Social-Ecological Model for pursuing changes in diet and physical activity behaviors (U.S. Department of Health and Human Services and U.S. Department of Agriculture, 2015).

Financial constraints; perceived lack of time; situational expectations; lack of preparation, knowledge, and skills; low motivation; and inadequate family or social support are some of the personal and interpersonal factors that may be barriers for obtaining and maintaining an adequate diet (Munt et al, 2017). With a population that is culturally diverse, it is imperative to appreciate the differences in understanding, beliefs, and values that may influence the ability to change.

Physical and emotional factors may also make it hard to change, especially for some populations. Older adults need education and counseling programs that address their former positive or negative experiences with food and eating behaviors, their financial and food security situations along with their willingness to use food assistance programs, transportation issues, physical changes that affect food access and intake, and social

---

Sections of this chapter were written by Linda Snetselaar, PhD, RDN for the previous edition of this text.

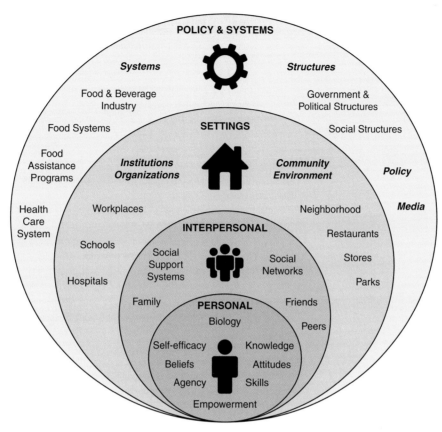

Fig. 13.1 The Social-Ecological Model. Behavior change can be influenced at the personal, interpersonal, institutional, community, and policy levels. (Adapted from: Conducting Effective SNAP-Ed Evaluations: A Step-by-Step Guide. In Contento IR. Nutrition Education: Linking research, theory, and practice [2nd ed.], 2011.)

influences (Oemichen et al, 2016). For families, time restraints, child-parent interplay, sibling dynamics, stressful everyday life, and a low priority for diet within the arena of parental concerns may also hinder changes in food intake (Norman et al, 2015). For children, barriers to sound eating choices include food marketing, taste preferences, food insecurity, and the availability of competing foods of low nutritional quality (Ogle et al, 2017; Nicklas et al, 2013). Across all ages, culture affects not only what foods are eaten and how, but also perceptions about education, counseling, health, and health care.

MODELS FOR BEHAVIOR CHANGE

Changing behavior is the ultimate goal for nutrition counseling and education. Providing a pamphlet or a list of foods can reinforce information, but it usually is not enough to change eating behavior. Behavioral science has provided valuable insight into the many different factors that influence what someone eats and has helped identify several mediators of people's eating behavior on which to intervene. Health professionals, including registered dietitian nutritionists, can support individuals in deciding what and when to change by using a variety of health behavior theories. Some of the theories for behavior change most commonly used are listed in Table 13.1, with examples described in the following paragraphs.

Health Belief Model

The **health belief model (HBM)** focuses on a disease or condition and factors that may influence behavior related to that disease (Rosenstock, 1974; James et al, 2012). These factors include perceived threat and severity

from the disease, as well as cues to action from the environment and perceived benefits, barriers, and self-efficacy related to engaging in preventive or disease management behaviors. The HBM has been used most with behaviors related to diabetes and osteoporosis, focusing on barriers to and benefits of changing behaviors (Babatunde et al, 2011; Plawecki and Chapman-Novakofski, 2013). The clinician may ask what they perceive could be the outcome if they had osteoporosis, as this information may be part of the decisional balance to change an eating behavior.

Social Cognitive Theory

Social cognitive theory (SCT) explains the reciprocal interaction among personal, behavioral, and environmental factors (Bandura, 1977, 1986). This means a person's behavior is modeled by the environment, and conversely, the person has the ability to shape their environment to achieve behavioral goals. Because it is one of the most comprehensive theories, SCT is particularly useful to understand complex behaviors, such as eating. Some of the most relevant SCT concepts to counseling include self-efficacy, self-regulation through goal setting, and relapse prevention by means of positive reinforcement (Matwiejczyk et al, 2018; Vilaro et el, 2016). Behavior modeling is especially important to emphasize when counseling parents with young children (Yee et al, 2017). The nutrition counselor may assess the client's self-efficacy and guide them to set realistic goals and to develop the skills needed to change their eating behavior.

Theory of Planned Behavior

The **theory of planned behavior (TPB)** is an extension of the theory of reasoned action, conceived in the 1960s to describe intentions as

TABLE 13.1	Overview of Behavior Theories Used in Nutrition Education and Counseling
Health Belief Model (HBM)	Perceived susceptibility: Clients beliefs regarding the chance that they may get a condition or disease Perceived severity: An individual's belief of how serious a condition and its consequences are Perceived benefits: An individual's belief in the positive effects of the advised action in reducing the risk or the seriousness of a condition Perceived barriers: An individual's belief about the tangible and psychological costs of the advised action Self-efficacy: Clients believe they are capable of performing the desired action Cues to action: Strategies to activate one's readiness to change a behavior
Social Cognitive Theory (SCT)	Personal factors: Outcome expectations, self-efficacy, reinforcements, impediments, goals and intentions, relapse prevention Behavioral factors: Knowledge and skills, self-regulation and control, and goal setting Environmental factors: Include imposed, selected, and created environments
Theory of Planned Behavior (TPB)	Subjective norms: The people who may influence the patient Attitudes: What the patient thinks about the behavior Perceived control: How much control the patient has to change things that affect the behavior Behavioral intention: Whether the patient plans to perform the behavior
Transtheoretical Model (TTM), or Stages of Change Model	Precontemplation: The individual has not thought about making a change. Contemplation: The individual has thought about making a change but has done no more than think about it. Preparation: The individual has taken some steps to begin to make the desired change. Action: The individual has made the change and continues it for less than 6 months. Maintenance: The individual has continued the behavior for longer than 6 months. Termination: The individual no longer thinks about the change; it has become a habit.

precursors of behavior at a given time and place. The original theory was expanded to account for the ability of people to exert control over their behavior. The theory was intended to explain all behaviors over which people have the ability to exert self-control. (Ajzen, 1991; Fishbein and Ajzen, 2010). Intentions are predicted by attitudes, subjective norms (important others), and perceived control (self-efficacy). This theory is most successful when a discrete behavior is targeted (e.g., vegetable intake), but has also been used for healthy diet consumption (Sheats et al, 2013).

Transtheoretical Model of Change

The transtheoretical model (TTM), or stages of change model, has been used for many years to alter addictive behaviors, and is often described as "tailored education." TTM describes behavior change as a process in which individuals progress through a series of six distinct stages of change, as shown in Fig. 13.2 (Prochaska and Norcross, 2001), whereby they move from experiential to behavioral processes of change. The value of the TTM is in determining the individual's current stage, then using change processes matched to that stage (Mochari-Greenberger et al, 2010).

MODELS FOR COUNSELING STRATEGIES

Cognitive behavioral therapy (CBT) focuses on identifying and changing erroneous perceptions of the self, environment, and behavioral consequences. CBT will often identify behaviors and thoughts that have a negative impact on desired behavioral goals and apply strategies to change those behaviors and thoughts (Beck, 2005). CBT counselors can help clients explore troubling themes, strengthen their coping skills, and focus on their well-being (Dobson and Dobson, 2017).

CBT is often used for obesity interventions, eating disorders, and chronic disease management when depression also exists, such as in heart failure and diabetes. CBT is also used in a range of psychological and psychiatric disorders (Freedland et al, 2015; Tovote et al, 2015).

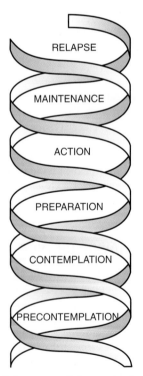

Fig. 13.2 A model of the stages of change. In changing, a person progresses up these steps to maintenance. If relapse occurs, the client gets back on the steps at some point and works up them again.

Acceptance and commitment therapy (ACT) helps to enhance mindfulness by focusing on thoughts and feelings related to valued behavior. Rather than trying to change thoughts or feelings as in CBT, ACT strives to create a new internal network that is flexible, compassionate, accepting, and reflective of one's life values (Hayes et al, 1999). ACT has been used in counseling for overweight and obesity (Järvelä-Reijonen et al, 2018) and self-management of diabetes (Shayeghian, 2016) as well as for programs addressing chronic pain (Graham et al, 2016).

Motivational interviewing (MI) is a counseling style that allows the client to identify behavioral goals by encouraging a conversation about ambivalence to change (Miller and Rollnick, 2012). It has been used in a variety of conditions to guide clients to identify discrepancies between how they would like to behave and how they are behaving, and ultimately to promote their motivation to change toward improving dietary outcomes (Spahn et al, 2010). The following are key principles of MI (Miller and Rollnick, 2012):

Partnership

In MI, information is transmitted from one expert to another. This implies a paradigm shift from traditional counseling where the client is the recipient of information prescribed by an expert. The nutrition counselor practicing MI assumes the role of a learner by actively listening to the client's language about change and allowing them to openly and safely share the beliefs, values, and expectations that affect their ability to change. Acknowledging the client's autonomy and inherent knowledge of themselves are at the center of the MI interpersonal dynamics.

Acceptance

Practicing MI requires unconditional acceptance of the client's humanity. This is achieved by recognizing the client's inherent worth, by conveying empathy and offering affirmation, and by providing autonomy support. The nutrition counselor demonstrates empathy by displaying an understanding of the client's perspective rather than a judgmental attitude, affirms the client's efforts and resources, and supports client's chosen path to change.

> Client: I want to lose weight, but with three children, two jobs, and a degree to finish, I just don't have time.
> Nutrition Counselor: That is a lot to handle. If this is not the best time, I understand. If and when you want my help, I am ready to listen and help as I can.

Compassion

The nutrition counselor practicing MI deliberately focuses on advancing the client's well-being and best interests concerning their dietary choices. This means prioritizing the client's expressed needs and values over the provision of authoritative guidance.

> Client: I need to get a meal out fast for my family or they are out the door.
> Nutrition Counselor: It is hard to get that meal out quickly and have it be healthy. Can we look at some quick meals that are also healthy?

Evocation

Practicing MI means inviting new perspectives without imposing them. Perceptions can be shifted, and the client is the most valuable resource in finding solutions to problems. The role of the nutrition counselor is to help with this process by encouraging the evocation of dietary experiences and the resources developed as a result of those. As the client reviews situations in their lives and barriers to dietary changes, the nutrition counselor will hear ambivalence—on the one hand, the client wants to make changes; on the other hand, the client questions the feasibility or importance of changing. Identifying the advantages and disadvantages of modifying a behavior, or developing discrepancy, is a crucial process in making changes.

> Client: I want to follow the new eating pattern, but I just can't afford it.

> Nutrition Counselor: Let's look at your diet record and find some healthy, low-cost options.

When an atmosphere of acceptance is established, this pondering process represents an opportunity to express empathy and affirm internalized motivation to change. For example, clients who are wary of describing why they are not ready to change may become much more open to change if they perceive openness to their resistive behaviors. When it becomes okay to discuss resistance, the rationale for its original existence may seem less relevant.

> Client: I just feel that my level of enthusiasm for making these changes is low. It all seems like too much effort.
> Nutrition Counselor: I appreciate your concerns. Many people feel frustrated when they try to make dietary changes. Tell me more about your concerns and feelings.

Belief in one's own capability to change, or self-efficacy, is an important motivator. The client is responsible for choosing and carrying out personal change. The nutrition counselor can respect the client's autonomy and support self-efficacy by offering to practice behaviors or activities to develop skills while the counselor is available to help.

> Client: I just don't know what to buy once I get to the grocery store. I end up with hamburgers and potato chips.
> Nutrition Counselor: Let's think of one day's meals right now. Then we can make a grocery list from that.

MODELS FOR EDUCATIONAL PROGRAM DEVELOPMENT

The PRECEDE-PROCEED model is a participatory health program planning model that has been used in a variety of health topics and communities to systematically plan and evaluate behavior change programs. PRECEDE consists of four planning phases represented in its acronym for Predisposing, Reinforcing, Enabling, Constructs in Education/Ecological Diagnosis and Evaluation. This reflects the needs assessment and participatory planning of the educational program. PROCEED's acronym stands for Policy, Regulatory, and Organizational Constructs in Educational and Environmental Development and provides a framework for program implementation and evaluation (Green et al, 1980). This model has been applied to develop a number of nutrition education programs (Walsh et al, 2014; Kattelmann et al, 2014).

The Behavior Change Wheel (BCW) is a new method to develop interventions to change eating behavior that consists of three steps— define the behavior and understand its determinants (i.e., ability, opportunity, and motivation); identify intervention options suitable to address behavioral determinants (e.g., education, persuasion, skill-building, modeling); and devise content and implementation strategy (i.e., educational techniques and mode of delivery). It also considers policy categories to leverage for the program implementation (Atkins and Michie, 2015).

SKILLS AND ATTRIBUTES OF THE NUTRITION EDUCATOR OR COUNSELOR

Cultural Competency

The ability to productively engage clients from different cultural backgrounds is a distinctive mark of effective nutrition educators and counselors (Bruening et al, 2015). Culture it is the framework through which people perceive and interact with the world. Thus, understanding cultural expressions on eating choices is fundamental to providing meaningful guidance. Cultural identity comprises a combination of permanent (e.g., age, ethnicity/race, language, sexual orientation), modifiable (e.g., educational status, socioeconomic status, occupation, religion, geographic residence, food choices), and contextual (e.g., historical, social, political forces) factors. Refer to Chapter 10: Planning the Diet with Cultural Competency.

Educating or counseling with cultural competency requires acknowledging both surface and deep structure factors affecting eating choices. Surface structure refers to attributes that are easily observable, such as food preferences, traditions, and language. Surface structures allow first-hand contact; however, they are often sources of stereotypes and can create communication interference. For instance, language is often the primary surface structure issue that is addressed. Although knowing several languages is an asset, many rely on interpreters. Relying on unofficial interpreters, such as family or friends, is rarely a good choice because of a lack of familiarity with nutrition and health concepts. Using professional interpreters is also not without limitations in that the educator needs to understand not only the client but also the interpreter. The educator should maintain contact with the client and explain the role of the interpreter (Box 13.1). Using common terms, avoiding slang and words with multiple meanings, is a practice recommended when working with clients who have limited language skills. Always speak directly to the client, even when using an interpreter, and watch the client for nonverbal responses during the translation. Movements such as gestures, facial expressions, and postures are often the cause of confusion and misinterpretations in intercultural communication. Rules regarding eye contact are usually complex and vary according to attributes such as gender, physical distance, and social status (see *Clinical Insight:* Body Language and Communication Skills).

Deep structure culture includes psychosocial factors that are not readily apparent, such as beliefs, values, attitudes, norms, and stressors affecting eating choices, as well as the personal and interpersonal context of the intervention. Because culture is complex, shape-shifting, and ultimately inseparable from its social and economic context, it is impossible to consider it as an isolated or static phenomenon. Any understanding of a particular cultural context is always incompletely true, always somewhat out of date and partial (Gregg et al, 2006). The culturally competent nutrition practitioner facilitates the consideration of individual- or group-specific deep structure factors in all steps of the nutrition care process. The following are principles common to the several proposed models of cultural competency:

Cultural Awareness

Culturally competent nutrition practitioners assess their own surface and deep structure cultural makeup to identify personal and professional assumptions, beliefs, and attitudes that may affect their ability to effectively connect with the client (Campinha-Bacote, 2002; Jongen et al, 2018; Wright and Lundy, 2014). Heightening awareness of personal biases and becoming comfortable with cultural differences (see *Clinical Insight:* The Counselor Looks Within) allows the counselor to be more effective in understanding what the client may need to move forward.

BOX 13.1 Federal Regulations for Translation and Interpreting in Medical Settings

As part of the regulations for nondiscrimination administered by the Department of Health and Human Services, additional provisions were added to Section 1557 of the Affordable Care Act in 2016 concerning support for those with limited English proficiency. Reasonable language assistance is required in the form of an interpreter or translator. However, video remote interpreting may be allowed. In addition, acceptance of language assistance from the client is not required.

CLINICAL INSIGHT
The Counselor Looks Within

Before entering a counseling relationship and after reflecting on the session, nutritionists should look inward and consider any factors that affect their own thinking and how they might affect the client. The nutritionist should reflect on ethical issues, such as the autonomy of the client, and beneficence (good) versus maleficence (harm). An example may be when a client decides not to set goals for blood glucose levels and not to learn the amounts of carbohydrates in foods (autonomy). These choices serve as barriers to the benefit the counselor would make in teaching these self-management tools (beneficence) and the need for nonmaleficence (do no harm). Whenever clients decide a behavior change is not right for them, the counselor's role is not to force the issue but to encourage its future consideration.

Client's Perspective

Culturally competent communication considers deep structure issues, such as the role of the individual within a group, and why certain foods are prepared and preferred (Broyles et al, 2011). The culturally competent nutrition practitioner explores how clients perceive their own nutritional status, including their understanding of the causes and consequences; previous use of integrative remedies, care, and information sources; the level of cognitive or emotional attachment to integrative treatments; and the expectations around the impending dietary treatment. It is also important to prompt clients to describe how their nutritional issue affects and is affected by their social environment, as potential barriers or facilitators to change.

Informed Negotiation

Developing a culturally relevant intervention plan is a collaborative effort between the client and the practitioner. It requires summarizing deep structure attributes that influence the client's eating choices, communicating the rationale behind proposed evidence-based nutrition prescriptions, and reaching consensus for a meaningful integration of both. Cognitive dissonance may arise when the client expresses opinions, worldviews, or values different from the ones held by the nutrition educator or counselor. Acknowledging opposing views, instead of debating them, can help maintain open and productive communication. The client may show hesitation or lack of confidence to adopt certain dietary prescriptions or express a desire for retaining traditional or nonevidence-based practices. Allowing the client to actively participate in setting their own nutritional goals can increase ownership and accountability, convey respect for the client's values, and increase the level of trust.

Empathy and Rapport

Cultural awareness and understanding of the client's perspectives about their nutritional status is necessary for the nutrition practitioner to gain empathy and establish rapport with the client. In turn, this can improve the quality of the communication, setting the conditions for the negotiation of a sound action plan (Diaz Rios and Chapman-Novakofski, 2018).

Learning the skills to elicit the client's individual beliefs and interpretations and to negotiate conflicting beliefs is important to proper care, regardless of the social or cultural backgrounds of the client (Constantinou et al, 2018). When developing culturally sensitive interventions, the PRECEDE-PROCEED model can provide the framework to guide appreciation for the target audience's surface and deep cultural structures (Cuy Castellanos et al, 2013; DePue et al, 2010).

CLINICAL INSIGHT

Body Language and Communication Skills

Active listening forms the basis for effective nutrition counseling. There are two aspects to effective listening: nonverbal and verbal. Nonverbal listening skills consist of varied eye contact, attentive body language, a respectful but close space, adequate silence, and encouragers. Eye contact is direct yet varied. Lack of eye contact implies that the counselor is too busy to spend time with the client. When the counselor leans forward slightly and has a relaxed posture and avoids fidgeting and gesturing, the client will be more at ease. Silence can give the client time to think and provide time for the counselor to contemplate what the client has said. Shaking one's head in agreement can be a positive encourager, leading to more conversation. Moving forward slightly toward the client is an encourager that allows for more positive interaction.

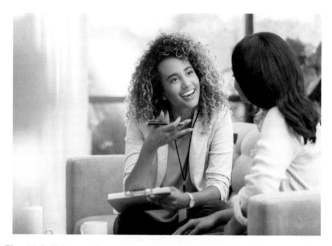

Fig. 13.3 This nutrition counselor is effectively using verbal and nonverbal communication skills, including eye contact and leaning in, to build rapport with a client. From www.istockphoto.com.

Asking Questions

Information gathering is an instrumental quality of effective counselors and educators as they consistently ask open-ended questions that prompt fruitful discussions. Data questions can provide valuable information but rarely lead to effective discussion (e.g., "What did you eat?"), and knowledge questions can sometimes elicit a defensive response depending on the context in which they are asked (e.g., "Can you tell me what you know about sodium?").

Open-ended questions allow the client to express a wider range of ideas, whereas closed questions (e.g., data questions or yes/no questions) can help in targeting concepts and eliminating tangential discussions. For the person who is not ready to change, targeted discussions around difficult topics can help focus the session. The nutritionist asks questions that must be answered by explaining and discussing, not by one-word answers. This is particularly important for someone who is not ready to change because it opens the discussion to discover problem areas that keep the client from being ready. The following statements and questions are examples that create an atmosphere for discussion:

- "We are here to talk about your dietary change experiences to this point. Could you start at the beginning and tell me how it has been for you?"
- "What are some things you would like to discuss about your dietary changes so far? What do you like about them? What don't you like about them?"

Framing the optimal discussion question is not easy and requires the counselor to be self-reflective on which questions were successful. Teaching counseling skills has included simulated patient–counselor scenarios with a standardized patient (Tada et al, 2018); a tool has been developed to evaluate these skills called the Feedback on Counseling Using Simulation (FOCUS) (Henry and Smith, 2010). Verbal and nonverbal communication is important; for the latter, maintaining an appropriate facial expression and using affirmative gestures are important (Collins et al, 2011).

Building Rapport

The ability to build rapport is one of the most useful skills in counseling and education. However, it can also be a challenging skill to develop. A client who appears hostile, unusually quiet, or dismissive may have more success with someone with a similar background or experience. In those cases, working with a peer educator may be most effective. The **peer educator** should ideally share similarities with the target clientele in terms of age or ethnicity, and have primary experience in the nutrition topic (e.g., breastfeeding) (Jain, 2014; Perez-Escamilla et al, 2008). Peer educators are usually community health workers or paraprofessionals. The Expanded Food and Nutrition Education Program (EFNEP) has demonstrated the effectiveness and cost efficiency of peer educators (Baral et al, 2013). In perinatal and Special Supplemental Nutrition Program for Women, Infants, and Children (WIC) clinics, breastfeeding peer counselors are often highly effective in helping new mothers with their questions and concerns (Bartholomew et al, 2017).

Reflective Listening

Nutrition counselors not only listen but also try to tag the feelings that surface as a client is describing difficulties with an eating pattern. Listening is not simply hearing the words spoken by the client and paraphrasing them back. Fig. 13.3 shows a nutrition counselor listening reflectively to a client.

Reflective listening involves a guess at what the person feels and is phrased as a statement, not a question. By stating a feeling, the nutrition counselor communicates understanding. The following are three examples of listening reflectively:

Client: I really do try, but I am retired and my husband always wants to eat out. How can I stay on the right path when that happens?

Nutrition Counselor: You feel frustrated because you want to make dietary changes, but at the same time you want to be spontaneous with your husband. Is this correct? *(reflective listening; TPB, subjective norms; HBM, barriers; SCT, personal factors)*

Client: I feel like I let you down every time I come in to see you. We always discuss plans and I never follow them. I almost hate to come in.

Nutrition Counselor: You are feeling like giving up. You haven't been able to modify your diet, and it is difficult for you to come into our visits when you haven't met the goals we set. Is this how you are feeling? *(reflective listening)* Can you think of a specific time when you feel that you had an opportunity to achieve your plan, but didn't? *(HBM, barriers)*

Client: Some days I just give up. It is on those days that I just eat whatever I want and I can't make good decisions about what to eat.

Nutrition Counselor: You just lose the desire to try to eat well on some days and that is very depressing for you. Do I have that right? *(rephrasing)* Are those days when something in particular has happened?" *(HBM, barriers)*

Affirming

Counselors often understand the idea of supporting a client's efforts to follow a new eating style but do not put those thoughts into words. When the counselor affirms someone, there is alignment and normalization of the client's issues. In **alignment** the counselor expresses understanding about the difficult times. **Normalization** means telling clients they are within reason and that it is normal to have such reactions and feelings. The following statements indicate affirmation:

- "I know that it is hard for you to tell me this. But thank you."
- "You have had amazing competing priorities. I feel that you have done extremely well, given your circumstances."
- "Many people I talk with express the same problems. I can understand why you are having difficulty."

Summarizing

The nutrition counselor periodically summarizes the content of what the client has said by covering all the key points. Simple and straightforward statements are most effective, even if they involve negative feelings. If conflicting ideas arise, the counselor can use the strategy exemplified by the statement, "On the one hand you want to change, but you still feel attached to the way you have been eating." This helps the client recognize the ambivalence in thinking that often prevents behavior change.

ASSESSMENT RESULTS: CHOOSING FOCUS AREAS

Health and Nutrition Literacy

Low **health literacy** is common among older adults, minorities, and those who are medically underserved or have a low socioeconomic status (Health Resources and Services Administration, 2017). Health literacy is the degree to which an individual has the capacity to obtain, communicate, process, and understand basic health information and services needed to make appropriate health decisions (Patient Protection and Affordable Care Act of 2010, Title V). The problem of low health literacy can lead to poor management of chronic health conditions, as well as low adherence to recommendations. Useful resources available from the Agency on Healthcare Research and Quality (AHRQ) are *Rapid Estimate of Adult Health Literacy in Medicine (REALM)* and *Short Assessment of Health Literacy for Spanish Adults (SAHLSA-50)* (AHQR, 2016). Additional nutrition-targeted evaluation measures include the Newest Vital Sign which focuses on a nutrition facts label (Rowlands et al, 2013) and the Nutrition Literacy Assessment Instrument, which evaluates several components including understanding of nutrition and health, macronutrients, household food measurement, food labels and numeracy, and food groups (Gibbs and Chapman-Novakofski, 2013). Although there are some areas of overlap when discussing nutrition literacy and food literacy, specific guidelines or definitions are lacking (Velardo, 2015). Often, relying on the client's educational attainment provides some guidance about capacity to understand directions, information, or skills, but asking the clients to repeat explanations in their own words can also help the nutrition educator evaluate the client's level of understanding.

Assessing Readiness to Change

One purpose of assessment is to identify the client's stage of change and to provide appropriate help in facilitating change. The assessment should be completed in the first visit if possible. If the conversation extends beyond the designated time for the session, the assessment steps should be completed at the next session. The nutritional assessment requires gathering the appropriate anthropometric, biochemical, clinical, dietary, and socioeconomic data relating to the client's condition. The nutritional diagnosis then focuses on any problems related to food or nutrient intake.

Determining present eating habits provides ideas on how to change in the future. A reflective review of the client's eating behavior will identify areas needing change, and help the client create goals that will have the most positive effect on health. For example, if the nutrition diagnoses include excessive fat intake (nutrient intake), inappropriate intake of food fats, excessive energy intake, inadequate potassium intake, food- and nutrition-related knowledge deficit (nutrition behavior), and impaired ability to prepare foods or meals, the counselor may need to focus on the last diagnosis before the others. If all other diagnoses are present except impaired ability to prepare foods or meals, the nutritionist may want to have a discussion about whether excessive fat intake, inappropriate intake of types of food fats, or excessive energy intake are related to knowledge deficit and which of them is more appealing or possible for the client to focus on first.

Once the nutrition diagnosis is selected for intervention, it is important to assess readiness for change. Using a ruler that allows the client to select their level of intention to change is one method of allowing client participation in the discussion. The counselor asks the client, "On a scale of 1 to 10, how ready are you right now to make any new changes to eat less fat? (1 = not ready to change; 10 = very ready to change)." The dietitian nutritionist may use this method with each nutrition diagnosis to help the client decide where to focus first.

Three possibilities for readiness exist: (1) not ready to change; (2) unsure about change; (3) ready to change. These three concepts of readiness have condensed the six distinct stages of change described in this chapter to assist the counselor in determining the level of client readiness. There are many concepts to remember, and readiness to change may fluctuate during the course of the discussion. The counselor must be ready to move back and forth between the phase-specific strategies. If the client seems confused, detached, or resistant during the discussion, the counselor should return and ask about readiness to change. If readiness has lessened, tailoring the intervention is necessary. Not every counseling session has to end with the client's agreement to change; even the decision to think about change can be a useful conclusion.

COUNSELING APPROACHES AFTER THE ASSESSMENT

Not-Ready-To-Change Counseling Sessions

In approaching the "not-ready-to-change" stage of intervention, there are three goals: (1) facilitate the client's ability to consider change, (2) identify and reduce the client's resistance and barriers to change, and (3) identify behavioral steps toward change that are tailored to each client's needs. At this stage, identifying barriers (HBM), the influence of subjective norms and attitudes (TPB), or personal and environmental factors (SCT) that may have negative influences on the intention to change can be helpful. To achieve these goals, several communication skills are important to master: asking open-ended questions, listening reflectively, affirming the patient's statements, summarizing the patient's statements, and eliciting self-motivational statements.

The four communication strategies (asking open-ended questions, listening reflectively, affirming, and summarizing) are important when eliciting self-motivational statements. The goals are for the client to realize that a problem exists, develop concern, and acknowledge the positive steps in the future that can be taken to correct the problem. These realizations set the stage for later efforts at dietary change. Examples of questions to use in eliciting self-motivational feeling statements follow.

Problem Recognition

- "What things make you think that eating out is a problem?"
- "In what ways has following this eating pattern been a problem?"

Concern

- "How do you feel when you can't follow your dietary recommendations?"
- "In what ways does not being able to follow your dietary recommendations concern you?"
- "What do you think will happen if you don't make a change?"

Intention to Change

- "The fact that you're here indicates that at least a part of you thinks it's time to do something. What are the reasons you see for making a change?"
- "If you were 100% successful and things worked out exactly as you would like, what would be different?"
- "What things make you think that you should keep on eating the way you have been?" And in the opposite direction, "What makes you think it is time for a change?"

Optimism

- "What encourages you that you can change if you want to?"
- "What do you think would work for you if you decided to change?"

Clients in this "not-ready-to-change" category have already told the counselor they are not doing well at making changes. Usually if a tentative approach is used that asks permission to discuss the problem, the client will not refuse. One asks permission by saying, "Would you be willing to continue our discussion and talk about the possibility of change?" At this point, it is helpful to discuss thoughts and feelings about the current status of dietary change by asking open-ended questions:

- "Tell me why you picked _____ on the ruler." (Refer to previous discussion on the use of a ruler.)
- "What would have to happen for you to move from a _____ to a _____ (referring to a number on the ruler)? How could I help get you there?"
- "If you did start to think about changing, what would be your main concern?"

To show real understanding about what clients are saying, it is beneficial to summarize the statements about their progress, difficulties, possible reasons for change, and what needs to be different to move forward. This paraphrasing allows clients to rethink their reasoning about readiness to change. The mental processing provides new ideas that can promote actual change.

Ending the Session

Counselors often expect the client to be ready to decide to make changes and set goals. However, it is important in this stage to realize that traditional goal setting will result in feelings of failure on both the part of the client and the nutritionist. If the client is not ready to change, respectful acknowledgment of this decision is important. The counselor might say, "I can understand why making a change right now would be very hard for you. The fact that you are able to indicate this as a problem is very important, and I respect your decision. Our lives do change, and, if you feel differently later on, I will always be available to talk with you. I know that, when the time is right for you to make a change, you will find a way to do it." When the session ends, the counselor will let clients know that the issues will be revisited after they have had time to think. Expression of hope and confidence in the client's ability to make changes in the future, when the time is right, will be beneficial. Arrangements for follow-up contact can be made at this time.

With a client who is not ready to change it is easy to become defensive and authoritarian. At this point, it is important to avoid pushing, persuading, confronting, coaxing, or telling the client what to do. It is

reassuring to a nutritionist to know that change at this level will often occur outside the office. The client is not expected to be ready to do something during the visit.

Unsure-About-Change Counseling Sessions

The only goal in the "unsure-about-change" session is to build readiness to change. This is the point at which changes in eating behavior can escalate. This "unsure" stage is a transition from not being ready to deal with a problem eating behavior to preparing to continue the change. It involves summarizing the client's perceptions of the barriers to a healthy eating style and how they can be eliminated or circumvented to achieve change. Heightened self-efficacy may provide confidence that goals can be achieved. A restatement of the client's self-motivational statements assists in setting the stage for success. The client's ambivalence is discussed, listing the positive and negative aspects of change. The nutritionist can restate any statements that the client has made about intentions or plans to change or to do better in the future.

One crucial aspect of this stage is the process of discussing thoughts and feelings about current status. Use of open-ended questions encourages the client to discuss dietary change progress and difficulties. Change is promoted through discussions focused on possible reasons for change. The counselor might ask the question: "What would need to be different to move forward?"

This stage is characterized by feelings of ambivalence. The counselor encourages the client to explore ambivalence to change by thinking about "pros" and "cons." Some questions to ask are:

- "What are some of the things you like about your current eating habits?"
- "What are some of the good things about making a new or additional change?"
- "What are some of the things that are not so good about making a new or additional change?"

By trying to look into the future, the nutrition counselor can help a client see new and often positive scenarios. As a change facilitator, the counselor helps to tip the balance away from being ambivalent about change toward considering change by guiding the client to talk about what life might be like after a change, anticipating the difficulties as well as the advantages. An example of an opening to generate discussion with the client might be: "I can see why you're unsure about making new or additional changes in your eating habits. Imagine that you decided to change. What would that be like? What would you want to do?" The counselor then summarizes the client's statements about the "pros" and "cons" of making a change and includes any statements about wanting, intending, or planning to change.

The next step is to negotiate a change. There are three parts to the negotiation process. The first is setting goals. Set broad goals at first and hold more specific nutritional goals until later. "How would you like things to be different from the way they are?" and "What is it that you would like to change?"

The second step in negotiation is to consider options. The counselor asks about alternative strategies and options and then asks the client to choose from among them. This is effective because, if the first strategy does not work, the client has other choices. The third step is to arrive at a plan, one that has been devised by the client. The counselor touches on the key points and the problems and then asks the client to write down the plan.

To end the session the counselor asks about the next step, allowing the client to describe what might occur next in the process of change. The following questions provide some ideas that might promote discussion:

- "Where do you think you will go from here?"
- "What do you plan to do between now and the next visit?"

Resistance Behaviors and Strategies to Modify Them

Resistance to change is the most consistent emotion or state when dealing with clients who have difficulty with dietary change. Examples of resistance behaviors on the part of the client include contesting the accuracy, expertise, or integrity of the nutrition counselor; or directly challenging the accuracy of the information provided (e.g., the accuracy of the nutrition content). The nutrition counselor may even be confronted with a hostile client. Resistance may also surface as interrupting, when the client breaks in during a conversation in a defensive manner. In this case the client may speak while the nutrition counselor is still talking without waiting for an appropriate pause or silence. In another, more obvious manner, the client may break in with words intended to cut off the nutrition counselor's discussion.

When clients express an unwillingness to recognize problems, cooperate, accept responsibility, or take advice, they may be denying a problem. Some clients blame other people for their problems (e.g., spouses or partners may blame each other for their inability to make dietary changes). Other clients may disagree with the nutrition counselor when a suggestion is offered, but they frequently provide no constructive alternative. The familiar "Yes, but . . ." explains what is wrong with the suggestion but offers no alternative solution.

Clients try to excuse their behavior. A client may say, "I want to do better, but my life is in a turmoil since my husband died 3 years ago." An excuse that was once acceptable is reused even when it is no longer a factor in the client's life.

Some clients make pessimistic statements about themselves or others. This is done to dismiss an inability to follow an eating pattern by excusing poor compliance as just a given resulting from past behaviors. Examples are "My partner will never help me" or "I have never been good at sticking with a goal. I'm sure I won't do well with it now."

In some cases, clients are reluctant to accept options that may have worked for others in the past. They express reservations about information or advice given. "I just don't think that will work for me." Some clients will express a lack of willingness to change or an intention not to change. They make it very clear that they want to stop the dietary regimen.

Often clients show evidence that they are not following the nutrition counselor's advice. Clues that this is happening include using a response that does not answer the question, providing no response to a question, or changing the direction of the conversation.

These types of behaviors can occur within a counseling session as clients move from one stage to another. They are not necessarily stage-specific, although most are connected with either the "not ready" or "unsure-about-change" stages. A variety of strategies are available to assist the nutrition counselor in dealing with these difficult counseling situations. These strategies include reflecting, double-sided reflection, shifting focus, agreeing with a twist, emphasizing personal choice, and reframing. Each of these options is described in the following paragraphs.

Reflecting. In reflecting, the counselor identifies the client's emotion or feeling and reflects it back. This allows the client to stop and reflect on what was said. An example of this type of counseling is, "You seem to be very frustrated by what your wife says about your food choices."

Double-Sided Reflection. In double-sided reflection, the counselor uses ideas that the client has expressed previously to show the discrepancy between the client's current words and the previous ones. For example:

Client: I am doing the best I can. (Previously this client stated that she sometimes just gives up and doesn't care about making dietary modifications.)

Nutrition Counselor: On the one hand you say you are doing your best, but on the other hand I recall that you said you just felt like giving up and didn't care about making dietary changes. Do you remember that? How was that point in time different than now?

Shifting Focus. Clients may hold onto an idea that they think is getting in the way of their progress. The counselor might question the feasibility of continuing to focus on this barrier to change when other barriers may be more appropriate targets. For example:

Client: I will never be able reduce my saturated fat intake as long as my grandchildren come to my house and want snacks.

Nutrition Counselor: Are you sure that this is really the problem? Is part of the problem that you like those same snacks?

Client: Oh, you are right. I love them.

Nutrition Counselor: Could you compromise? Could you ask your grandchildren which of this long list of low saturated fat snacks they like and then buy them?

Agreeing with a Twist. This strategy involves offering agreement, then moving the discussion in a different direction. The counselor agrees with a piece of what the client says but then offers another perspective on the problem. This allows the opportunity to agree with the statement and the feeling, but then to redirect the conversation onto a key topic. For example:

Client: I really like eating out, but I always eat too much, and my blood sugars go sky high.

Nutrition Counselor: Most people do like eating out. Now that you are retired it is easier to eat out than to cook. I can understand that. What can we do to make you feel great about eating out so that you can still follow your eating plan and keep your blood glucose values in the normal range?

Reframing. With reframing the counselor changes the client's interpretation of the basic data by offering a new perspective. The counselor repeats the basic observation that the client has provided and then offers a new hypothesis for interpreting the data. For example:

Client: I gave up trying to meet my dietary goals because I was having some difficulties when my partner died, and I have decided now that I just cannot meet those strict goals.

Nutrition Counselor: I remember how devastated you were when he died and how just cooking meals was an effort. Do you think that this happened as a kind of immediate response to his death and that you might have just decided that all of the goals were too strict at that time? *(Pause)*

Client: Well, you are probably right.

Nutrition Counselor: Could we look at where you are now and try to find things that will work for you now to help you in following the goals we have set?

These strategies help by offering tools to ensure that nutrition counseling is not ended without appropriate attempts to turn difficult counseling situations in a more positive direction.

Ending the Session. Counselors should emphasize that any future action belongs to the client, that the advice can be taken or disregarded. This emphasis on personal choice (autonomy) helps clients avoid feeling trapped or confined by the discussion. A sense of self-efficacy reflects the belief about being capable of influencing events and choices in life. These beliefs determine how individuals think, feel, and behave. If people doubt their capabilities, they will have weak commitments to their goals. Success breeds success, and failure breeds a sense of failure. Having resilience, positive role models, and effective coaching can make a significant difference.

Ready-To-Change Counseling Sessions

Setting goals. The major goal in the "ready-to-change" session is to collaborate with the client to set goals that include a plan of action. The nutrition counselor provides the client with the tools to use in meeting nutrition goals. This is the stage of change that is most often assumed when a counseling session begins. To erroneously assume this stage means that inappropriate counseling strategies set the stage for failure. Misaligned assumptions often result in lack of adherence on the part of the client and discouragement on the part of the nutritionist. Therefore it is important to discuss the clients thoughts and feelings about where they stand relative to the current change status. Use of open-ended questions helps the client confirm and justify the decision to make a change and in which area. The following questions may elicit information about feelings toward change:

- "Tell me why you picked _____ on the ruler."
- "Why did you pick (nutrition diagnosis 1) instead of (other nutrition diagnoses)?"

In this stage, goal setting is extremely important. Here the counselor helps the client set a realistic and achievable short-term goal: "Let's do things gradually. What is a reasonable first step? What might be your first goal?"

Action Plan. Following goal setting, an action plan is set to assist the client in mapping out the specifics of goal achievement. Identifying a network to support dietary change is important. What can others do to help?

Early identification of barriers to adherence is also important. If barriers are identified, plans can be formed to help eliminate these roadblocks to adherence.

Many clients fail to notice when their plan is working. Clients can be asked to summarize their plans and identify markers of success. The counselor then documents the plan for discussion at future sessions and ensures that the clients also have their plans in writing. The session should be closed with an encouraging statement and reflection about how the client identified this plan personally. Clients are experts about what influences their behavior. Compliment the client on carrying out the plan. Ways to express these ideas to clients are:

- "You are working very hard at this, and it's clear that you're the expert about what is best for you. You can do this!"
- "Keep in mind that change is gradual and takes time. If this plan doesn't work, there will be other plans to try."

The key point for this stage is to avoid telling the client what to do. Clinicians often want to provide advice. However, it is critical that the client express ideas of what will work best: "There are a number of things you could do, but what do you think will work best for you?" The next contact may be in person, online, or by phone.

Following up with clients by phone or a telemedicine portal have become popular counseling methods for many nutritionists. The dietitian nutritionist utilizing telemedicine services in their practice is required to follow certain regulations. The Academy of Nutrition and Dietetics (AND) has developed practice tips for the utilization of these services (AND, 2018). When behavior and counseling theories are combined with phone counseling, the results have been effective in managing weight, type 2 diabetes, and metabolic syndrome (Muñoz Obino et al, 2017). Telephone counseling in itself has been reported to be effective in achieving weight reduction (Schmittdiel et al, 2017), and online programs and telehealth interventions have also been successful (Muñoz Obino et al, 2017; Kelly et al, 2016).

✳ NEW DIRECTIONS

Counseling and Educating Online

More counselors and educators are turning to online connections with their clients and target audiences. Although the basics of counseling and education remain the same, there are additional issues to consider. If clients are recording food intake and physical activity through mobile technology or telemedicine, it is important to to consider how often to monitor and provide feedback. While many best practices in nutrition education include the use of mobile technology, consideration should be given to whether a company will develop the website or app, and will the sites be maintained in a constantly changing technological world.

Telenutrition is defined by the Academy of Nutrition and Dietetics as "the interactive use, by a RDN [registered dietitian nutritionist], of electronic information and telecommunications technologies to implement the Nutrition Care Process . . ." (AND, 2018). A systematic review of apps for lifestyle improvements concluded that in eight of nine included studies, apps were effective for improving lifestyles (Lunde et al, 2018). Barriers to successful app use include the cost of apps, data entry burden, and loss of interest and discontinued use of apps (Sun et al, 2017). Clinicians should be aware of privacy and security aspects of telenutrition. Personal data should be encrypted, and all patient privacy policies upheld (Boulos et al, 2014). While the Food and Drug Administration (FDA) does regulate apps that are intended for use as an accessory to a regulated medical device (Glucometers), it does not regulate apps that function as an electronic or personal health record system (U.S. Department of Health and Human Services [USDHHS] and FDA, 2018).

EVALUATION OF EFFECTIVENESS

Counseling

Clinicians and educators need to evaluate their services. Just completing the process does not mean that outcomes will match the goals. When the AND Evidence Analysis Library Nutrition Counseling Workgroup conducted a review of literature related to behavior change theories and strategies used in nutrition counseling, they found the following (Spahn et al, 2010):

1. Strong evidence supports the use of CBT in facilitating modification of targeted dietary habits, weight, and cardiovascular and diabetes risk factors.
2. MI is a highly effective counseling strategy, particularly when combined with CBT.
3. Few studies have assessed the application of the TTM or SCT on nutrition-related behavior change.
4. Self-monitoring, meal replacements, and structured meal plans are effective; financial reward strategies are not.
5. Goal setting, problem solving, and social support are effective strategies.
6. Research is needed in more diverse populations to determine the most effective counseling techniques and strategies.

A systematic review of nutrition therapy by a registered dietitian nutritionist compared with dietary advice by others concluded that individualized nutrition therapy by a registered dietitian nutritionist led to greater effects on clinical outcomes such as hemoglobin A1C, body weight, and blood lipids (Møller et al, 2017). On the other hand, a systematic review comparing either dietary counseling or high energy supplements' effects on dietary intake found dietary counseling alone less effective. Many other topics and populations can be found in the literature. Looking for systematic reviews and meta-analyses will help to stay current on what is working best.

Educational Programs

LOGIC Models are often used to evaluate a program's effectiveness. The simplest version includes inputs (resources or investments into a program), outputs (activities, services, and events) and outcomes (behavior change of individuals, groups, or communities), although some include multiple levels within these three broad categories (McLaughlin and Jordan, 1999). LOGIC Models have guided evaluation of national nutrition programs (Levine et al, 2012) as well as educational programs at the individual level, such as a video program to improve dietary habits of children (Beasley et al, 2012).

The three evaluation phases in the PRECEDE-PROCEED model are commonly applied to determine (1) program feasibility and whether it was implemented as intended (i.e., process evaluation); (2) program effectiveness at eliciting desired change in target behaviors (i.e., outcome evaluation); and (3) program contribution to changes in ecological and structural determinants of behavior (i.e., impact evaluation).

SUMMARY

Effective nutrition education and counseling requires skill development and practice. It is important to have an understanding of the individual and cultural needs of the client and knowledge of the variety of behavior change theories that can help clarify the client's behavior change process. Monitoring and evaluation of outcomes will ensure effectiveness of the interventions offered.

CLINICAL CASE STUDY

Mrs. Lee is originally from mainland China, and primarily speaks and reads in Mandarin Chinese. She has been living in Chicago for several years with her husband and daughter, and has numerous health problems, including high blood pressure, diabetes, and glaucoma. You have been asked to counsel her about making changes in her diet. Using an interpreter, you discover she is also having difficulty buying and preparing food and depends on her daughter for help. Because her vision is poor, she will not be able to use printed materials that you have in your office that have been translated into Chinese.

Nutrition Diagnostic Statement
- Impaired ability to prepare food and meals (NB-2.4) related to inability to see as evidenced by client report and history of glaucoma.

Nutrition Care Questions
1. What steps should you take to make her comfortable with this session?
2. Should you invite family members to attend the counseling session? Why or why not?
3. What tools might be useful to help Mrs. Lee understand portions or types of food that she should select?
4. Would a supermarket tour be useful? Why or why not?
5. What other types of information will be needed to help Mrs. Lee?

USEFUL WEBSITES

American Counseling Association
Behavioral Health Dietetic Practice Group (DPG) Academy of Nutrition and Dietetics
MINT: Excellence in Motivational Interviewing
Society for Nutrition Education and Behavior
Think Cultural Health
University of Wisconsin LOGIC Model in Program Planning and Evaluation

REFERENCES

Academy of Nutrition and Dietetics: *Practice tips: telehealth challenges and opportunities*, 2018. Available at: https://www.eatrightstore.org/product-type/case-studies-and-practice-tips/practice-tips-telehealth-challenges-and-opportunities.

Agency on Healthcare Research and Quality: *Health literacy measurement tools*, 2016. Available at: https://www.ahrq.gov/topics/health-literacy.html.

Ajzen I: The theory of planned behavior, *Organ Behav Hum Decis Process* 50:179–211, 1991.

Atkins L, Michie S: Designing interventions to change eating behaviours, *Proc Nutr Soc* 74(2):164–170, 2015.

Babatunde OT, Himburg SP, Newman FL, et al: Theory-driven intervention improves calcium intake, osteoporosis knowledge, and self-efficacy in community-dwelling older Black adults, *J Nutr Educ Behav* 43(6): 434–440, 2011.

Bandura A: *Social foundations of thought and action*, Englewood Cliffs, NJ, 1986, Prentice-Hall.

Bandura A: *Social learning theory*, New York, 1977, General Learning Press.

Baral R, Davis GC, Blake S, et al: Using national data to estimate average cost effectiveness of EFNEP outcomes by state/territory, *J Nutr Educ Behav* 45(2):183–187, 2013.

Bartholomew A, Adedze P, Soto V, et al: Historical perspective of the WIC program and its breastfeeding promotion and support efforts, *J Nutr Educ Behav* 49(7):S139–S143.e1, 2017.

Beasley N, Sharma S, Shegog R, et al: The Quest to Lava Mountain: using video games for dietary change in children, *J Acad Nutri Diet* 112(9): 1334–1336, 2012.

Beck AT: The current state of cognitive therapy: a 40-year perspective, *Arch Gen Psychiatry* 62:953–959, 2005.

Boulos MN, Brewer AC, Karimkhani C, et al: Mobile medical and health apps: state of the art, concerns, regulatory control and certification, *Online J Public Health Inform* 5(3):229–229, 2014.

Broyles SL, Brennan JJ, Burke KH, et al: Cultural adaptation of a nutrition education curriculum for Latino families to promote acceptance, *J Nutr Educ Behav* 43(4 Suppl 2):S158–S161, 2011.

Bruening M, Udarbe AZ, Yakes Jimenez E, et al: Standards of Practice and Standards of Professional Performance for Registered Dietitian Nutritionists (Competent, Proficient, and Expert) in Public Health and Community Nutrition, *J Acad Nutr Diet* 115(10):1699–1709.e39, 2015.

Campinha-Bacote J: The process of cultural competence in the delivery of healthcare services: a model of care, *J Transcult Nurs* 13(3):181–184, 2002.

Cuy Castellanos D, Downey L, Graham-Kresge S, et al: Examining the diet of post-migrant Hispanic males using the precede-proceed model: predisposing, reinforcing, and enabling dietary factors, *J Nutr Educ Behav* 45(2):109–118, 2013.

Collins LG, Schrimmer A, Diamond J, et al: Evaluating verbal and non-verbal communication skills, in an ethnogeriatric OSCE, *Patient Educ Couns* 83(2):158–162, 2011.

Constantinou CS, Papageorgiou A, Samoutis G, et al: Acquire, apply, and activate knowledge: a pyramid model for teaching and integrating cultural competence in medical curricula, *Patient Educ Couns* 101(6):1147–1151, 2018.

DePue JD, Rosen RK, Batts-Turner M, et al: Cultural translation of interventions: diabetes care in American Samoa, *Am J Public Health* 100(11):2085–2093, 2010.

Diaz Rios LK, Chapman-Novakofski K: Latino/Hispanic participation in community nutrition research: An interplay of decisional balance, cultural competency, and formative work, *J Acad Nutr Diet* 118(9):1687–1699, 2018.

Dobson D, Dobson K: *Evidence-based practice of cognitive-behavioral therapy*, ed 2, New York, 2017, Guilford Press.

Fishbein M, Ajzen I: *Predicting and changing behavior: the reasoned action approach*, New York, 2010, Psychology Press (Taylor & Francis).

Freedland KE, Carney RM, Rich MW, et al: Cognitive Behavior Therapy for depression and self-care in heart failure patients. A randomized clinical trial, *JAMA Intern Med* 175(11):1773–1782, 2015.

Gibbs H, Chapman-Novakofski K: Establishing content validity for the Nutrition Literacy Assessment Instrument (NLAI), *Prev Chronic Dis* 10:E109, 2013.

Graham CD, Gouick J, Krahé C, et al: A systematic review of the use of Acceptance and Commitment Therapy (ACT) in chronic disease and long-term conditions, Clin Psychol Rev 46:46–58, 2016.

Green LW and Kreuter MW: *Health education planning: a diagnostic approach*, Mountain View, California, 1980, Mayfield.

Gregg J, Saha S: Losing culture on the way to competence: the use and misuse of culture in medical curriculum, *Acad Med* 81:542–547, 2006.

Hayes SC, Strosahl KD, Wilson KG: *Acceptance and commitment therapy: an experiential approach to behavior change*, New York, NY, US, 1999, Guilford Press.

Health Resources and Services Administration, Office of Health Equity: *Health literacy*, 2017. Available at: https://www.hrsa.gov/about/organization/bureaus/ohe/health-literacy/index.html#.

Henry BW, Smith TJ: Evaluation of the FOCUS (Feedback on Counseling Using Simulation) instrument for assessment of client-centered nutrition counseling behaviors, *J Nutr Educ Behav* 42(1): 57–62, 2010.

Jain N: Increasing black, asian and minority ethnic (Bame) patient & community awareness – using the peer educator model, *J Ren Care* 40(Suppl 1): 36–40, 2014.

James DC, Pobee JW, Oxidine D, et al: Using the health belief model to develop culturally appropriate weight-management materials for African-American women, *J Acad Nutr Diet* 112(5):664–670, 2012.

Järvelä-Reijonen E, Karhunen L, Sairanen E, et al: The effects of acceptance and commitment therapy on eating behavior and diet delivered through face-to-face contact and a mobile app: a randomized controlled trial, *Int J Behav Nutr Phys Act* 15:22, 2018.

Jongen C, McCalman J, Bainbridge R: Health workforce cultural competency interventions: a systematic scoping review, *BMC Health Serv Res* 18:232, 2018.

Kattelmann KK, White AA, Greene GW, et al: Development of young adults eating and active for health (YEAH) internet-based intervention via a community-based participatory research model, *J Nutr Educ Behav* 46(2):S10–S25, 2014.

Kelly JT, Reidlinger DP, Hoffmann TC, et al: Telehealth methods to deliver dietary interventions in adults with chronic disease: a systematic review and meta-analysis, *Am J Clin Nutr* 104(6):1693–1702, 2016.

Levine E, Abbatangelo-Gray J, Mobley AR, et al: Evaluating MyPlate: an expanded framework using traditional and nontraditional metrics for assessing health communication campaigns, J Nutr Educ Behav 44(4): S2–S12, 2012.

Lunde P, Nilsson BB, Bergland A, et al: The effectiveness of smartphone apps for lifestyle improvement in noncommunicable diseases: systematic review and meta-analyses, *J Med Internet Res* 20(5):e162, 2018.

Matwiejczyk L, Mehta K, Scott J, et al: Characteristics of effective interventions promoting healthy eating for pre-schoolers in childcare settings: an umbrella review, *Nutrients* 10(3):293, 2018.

McLaughlin JA, Jordan GB: Logic models: a tool for telling your programs performance story, *Eval Program Plann* 22(1):65–72, 1999.

McLeroy KR, Bibeau D, Steckler A, et al: An ecological perspective on health promotion programs, *Health Educ Q* 15(4):351–377, 1988.

Miller WR, Rollnick S: *Motivational interviewing: helping people change*, New York, 2012, Guilford Press.

Mochari-Greenberger H, Terry MB, Mosca L: Does stage of change modify the effectiveness of an educational intervention to improve diet among family members of hospitalized cardiovascular disease patients? *J Am Diet Assoc* 110(7):1027–1035, 2010.

Møller G, Andersen HK, Snorgaard O: A systematic review and meta-analysis of nutrition therapy compared with dietary advice in patients with type 2 diabetes, *Am J Clin Nutr* 106(6):1394–1400, 2017.

Muñoz Obino KF, Aguiar Pereira C, Caron-Lienert RS: Coaching and barriers to weight loss: an integrative review, *Diabetes Metab Syndr Obes* 10:1–11, 2016.

Munt AE, Partridge SR, Allman-Farinelli M: The barriers and enablers of healthy eating among young adults: a missing piece of the obesity puzzle: a scoping review, *Obes Rev* 18:1–17, 2017.

Nicklas TA, Jahns L, Bogle ML, et al: Barriers and facilitators for consumer adherence to the dietary guidelines for Americans: the health study, *J Acad Nutr Diet* 113(10):1317–1331, 2013.

Norman A, Berlin A, Sundblom E, et al: Stuck in a vicious circle of stress. Parental concerns and barriers to changing children's dietary and physical activity habits, *Appetite* 87(1):137–142, 2015.

Oemichen M, Smith C: Investigation of the food choice, promoters and barriers to food access issues, and food insecurity among low-income, free-living Minnesotan seniors, *J Nutr Educ Behav* 48(6): 397–404, 2016.

Ogle AD, Graham DJ, Lucas-Thompson RG, et al: Influence of cartoon media characters on children's attention to and preference for food and beverage products, *J Acad Nutr Diet* 117(2):265–270, 2017.

Pérez-Escamilla R, Hromi-Fiedler A, Vega-López S, et al: Impact of peer nutrition education on dietary behaviors and health outcomes among Latinos: a systematic literature review, *J Nutr Educ Behav* 40: 208–225, 2008.

Plawecki K, Chapman-Novakofski K: Effectiveness of community intervention in improving bone health behaviors in older adults, *J Nutr Gerontol Geriatr* 32(2):145–160, 2013.

Prochaska JO, Norcross JC: Psychotherapy: theory, research, practice, *Training* 38(4):443–448, 2001.

Rosenstock IM: The health belief model and preventive health behavior, *Health Educ Behav* 2(4):354–386, 1974.

Rowlands G, Khazaezadeh N, Oteng-Ntim E, et al: Development and validation of a measure of health literacy in the UK: the newest vital sign, *BMC Pub Health* 13(1):116, 2013.

Schmittdiel JA, Adams SR, Goler N, et al: The impact of telephonic wellness coaching on weight loss: a "Natural Experiments for Translation in Diabetes (NEXT-D)" Study, *Obesity (Silver Spring)* 25(2):352–356, 2017.

Shayeghian Z, Hassanabadi H, Aguilar-Vafaie ME, et al: A randomized controlled trial of acceptance and commitment therapy for type 2 diabetes management: the moderating role of coping styles, *PLoS One* 11(12):e0166599, 2016.

Sheats JL, Middlestadt SE, Ona FF, et al: Understanding African American women's decisions to buy and eat dark green leafy vegetables: an application of the reasoned action approach, *J Nutr Educ Behav* 45(6): 676–682, 2013.

Spahn JM, Reeves RS, Keim KS, et al: State of the evidence regarding behavior change theories and strategies in nutrition counseling to facilitate health and food behavior change, *J Am Diet Assoc* 110: 879–891, 2010.

Sun L, Wang Y, Greene B, et al: Facilitators and barriers to using physical activity smartphone apps among Chinese patients with chronic diseases, *BMC Med Inform Decis Mak* 17:44, 2017.

Tada T, Moritoshi P, Sato K, et al: Effect of simulated patient practice on the self-efficacy of Japanese undergraduate dietitians in Nutrition Care Process Skills, *J Nutr Educ Behav* 50(6):610–619, 2018.

Tovote KA, Schroevers MJ, Snippe E, et al: Long-term effects of individual mindfulness-based cognitive therapy and cognitive behavior therapy for depressive symptoms in patients with diabetes: a randomized trial, *Psychother Psychosom* 84(3):186–187, 2015.

U.S. Department of Health and Human Services, Food and Drug Administration: *Mobile medical applications*, 2018. Available at: https://www.fda.gov/MedicalDevices/DigitalHealth/MobileMedicalApplications/default.htm.

U.S. Department of Health and Human Services and U.S. Department of Agriculture: *2015 – 2020 Dietary Guidelines for Americans*, ed 8, 2015. Available at: https://health.gov/dietaryguidelines/2015/guidelines/.

Velardo S: The nuances of health literacy, nutrition literacy, and food literacy, *J Nutr Educ Behav* 47(4):385–389, 2015.

Vilaro MJ, Staub D, Xu C, et al: Theory-Based Interventions for Long-Term Adherence to improvements in diet quality: an in-depth review, *Am J Lifestyle Med* 10(6):369–376, 2016.

Walsh J, White AA, Kattelmann KK: Using PRECEDE to Develop a weight management program for disadvantaged young adults, *J Nutr Educ Behav* 46(2):S1–S9, 2014.

Weiss BD, Mays MZ, Martz W, et al: Quick assessment of literacy in primary care: the newest vital sign, *Ann Fam Med* 3(6):514–522, 2005.

Wright L, Lundy M: Perspectives of cultural competency from an international service learning project, *J Acad Nutr Diet* 114(7):996–1000, 2014.

Yee AZH, Lwin MO, Ho SS: The influence of parental practices on child promotive and preventive food consumption behaviors: a systematic review and meta-analysis, *Int J Behav Nutr Phys Act* 14:47, 2017.

PART III

Nutrition in the Life Cycle

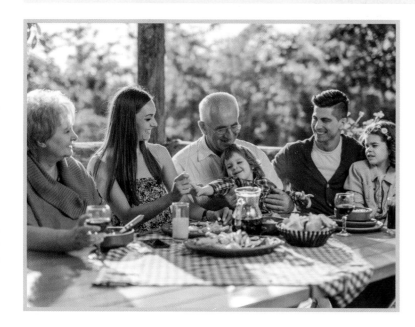

The importance of nutrition throughout the life cycle cannot be refuted. However, the significance of nutrition during specific times of growth, development, and aging is becoming increasingly appreciated.

Health professionals have recognized for quite some time the effects of proper nutrition during pregnancy on the health of the infant and mother, even after her childbearing years. However, looking at "nutrition in the womb" encompasses not only maternal health history and nutrition but also paternal nutrition and the health of sperm before conception. "Fetal origins" have far more lifelong effects on the new life than originally thought.

Establishing good dietary habits during childhood lessens the possibility of inappropriate eating behavior later in life. Although the influence of proper nutrition on morbidity and mortality usually remains unacknowledged until adulthood, dietary practices aimed at preventing the degenerative diseases that develop later in life should be instituted in childhood.

During early adulthood many changes begin that lead to the development of chronic disease, the so-called diseases of aging, years later. Many of these changes can be accelerated or slowed over the years, depending on the genetic makeup of the individual, quality of the nutritional intake, the health of the gut, and the function of the immune system.

With the rapid growth of the population of older adults has evolved a need to expand the limited nutrition data currently available for these individuals. Although it is known that energy needs decrease with aging, little is known about whether requirements for specific nutrients increase or decrease. Identifying the unique nutritional differences among the various stages of aging is becoming even more important.

14

Nutrition in Pregnancy and Lactation

Jean T. Cox, MS, RDN, LN
Catherine S. Sullivan, MPH, RDN, LDN, IBCLC, RLC, FAND

KEY TERMS

amylophagia
assisted reproductive technology (ART)
baby-led weaning
colostrum
conception
congenital anomalies
developmental origins of health
    and disease (DOHaD)
fetal alcohol syndrome (FAS)
fetal origins of disease
foremilk
galactogogue
geophagia
gestational diabetes mellitus (GDM)
gestational hypertension

gravida
HELLP syndrome
hindmilk
hyperemesis gravidarum (HG)
intrauterine fetal demise (IUFD)
intrauterine growth restriction (IUGR)
lactogenesis I
lactogenesis II
large for gestational age (LGA)
let-down
low birth weight (LBW)
macrosomia
mature milk
Montgomery glands
mother-led weaning

nausea and vomiting in pregnancy (NVP)
neural tube defects (NTDs)
oxytocin
pagophagia
perinatal mortality
pica
postpartum depression (PPD)
preeclampsia
prolactin
ptyalism gravidarum
small for gestational age (SGA)
teratogen
transitional milk

Optimal nutrition during pregnancy actually begins preconceptually. The placenta and developing fetus must receive all the necessary nutrients for growth and development from the mother. The old cliché that the "fetus is the perfect parasite" implies fetuses take all they require at the expense of the host. However, at some point nutritional deficiency can result in a preterm delivery. After birth, quality nutrition during lactation continues providing the nutritional building blocks for normal cerebral development and growth of all body organs in the neonate.

This time period—growing a new human being—sets the stage for the health of future generations. The quality and quantity of nourishment to the developing zygote, then fetus, then neonate, then adult emerge as one explanation for diseases that manifest in adulthood. This concept is known as fetal origins of disease or developmental origins of health and disease (DOHaD) (Guéant et al, 2013).

PRECONCEPTION AND FERTILITY

The focus on preconceptual nutrition and health is important for both women and men. Infertility affects 10% to 12% of U.S. couples of reproductive age, and extremes in body mass index (BMI) in either partner may be one cause. Women with a BMI less than 20 have an increased risk of anovulation. Men and women have increased rates of subfertility when overweight or obese, and fat distribution patterns may be important. Obesity appears to negatively affect the sperm (both concentration and motility), oocyte (development, quality, and ovulation), embryo, and the endometrium, including uterine receptivity (Catalano and Shankar, 2017). Elevated BMI negatively affects the fertility of both men and women in a dose-dependent manner. The

potential mechanisms that obesity negatively affects fertility are many and likely include direct effects and comorbidities, but also endocrine, genetic, epigenetic, hormonal, and inflammation factors (Craig et al, 2017; Broughton and Moley, 2017). Elevated serum cholesterol levels in both partners are associated with an increased time to pregnancy (Schisterman et al, 2014). Preconceptual control of diabetes of both parents improves birth outcomes (Kotelchuck and Lu, 2017). Weight loss (by reducing calories from fat and carbohydrates) and increased physical activity may be helpful, but the evidence is stronger for women than for men. However, the benefit of preconception weight loss is not yet established with clinical trials (Stephenson et al, 2018) and treatment results don't always match expectations. Although 5% weight loss often is cited to improve fertility, there is not a clear dose-response relationship, and the degree of weight loss is not a good surrogate for perinatal benefit (Legro, 2017). Conception during active weight loss can be harmful. Refer to the Postbariatric Surgery section later in this chapter. The use of weight loss drugs is not recommended. While weight loss should theoretically be the first line of therapy, eliminating tobacco and alcohol, increasing physical activity, and stress management may be more productive for improved conception (Luke, 2017).

As yet, there is no documented ideal diet for increased fertility but it may include components of heart healthy (Chavarro and Schlaff, 2018) and Mediterranean diet patterns (Broughton and Moley, 2017), as well as the New Nordic diet pattern. Specific dietary changes have been shown to decrease ovulatory disorders and improve fertility and embryonic growth trajectory (Berti et al, 2017). Zinc deficiency negatively affects oocyte development in animal models (Hester et al, 2017). Iodine deficiency has been associated with decreased fertility in women (Pearce, 2018). Vitamin D deficiency in men and women can be associated with infertility (Pludowski et al, 2013). For women, vitamin D deficiency may be associated with insulin resistance and metabolic syndrome in polycystic ovary syndrome (PCOS), as well as follicular development. For men, vitamin D deficiency is associated with lower testosterone levels and lower sperm quality. However, in both cases, neither causality nor ability to treat has yet been demonstrated and there is little evidence that supplementation is beneficial without evidence of deficiency (Chavarro and Schlaff, 2018). Calcium has been shown to be important in males for spermatogenesis, sperm motility, hyperactivation, and acrosome (area of the sperm that contains digestive enzymes to break down the outer layers of the ovum) reactions. Healthier sperm counts are associated with optimal dietary zinc, folic acid, and antioxidants, as well as avoidance of tobacco and alcohol (Gaur et al, 2010). Recommendations for improved male fertility include eating a diet higher in fiber, with a lower glycemic index (including high-fat dairy products and monounsaturated fats but reducing trans fats) and lower in animal protein. They may also see improvements by consuming a multivitamin daily, being moderately physically active, and obtaining iron from plant sources. However, there is also very preliminary evidence of decreased sperm quality among those consuming a self-described vegan diet (Orzylowska et al, 2016). Whether the effect can be attributed to low caloric intake, low intake of vitamin B$_{12}$ or zinc, an increased intake of isoflavones with high soy intake, an increased intake of pesticides, or other unidentified factors is not yet known and intervention trials have not been done. Oxidative stress is associated with impaired spermatogenesis. However, the evidence for taking supplemental antioxidants appears weak and inconsistent. The optimal types and dosages of the specific antioxidants are not yet known, and individuals also may exhibit variable responses (Mora-Esteves and Shin, 2013). On the other hand, supplementation is not likely to be harmful, assuming it is at levels of the recommended dietary allowance (RDA) or less. Whether supplements are as effective as a diet rich in antioxidants is unknown. Although studies exist to the contrary, the American Society for Reproductive Medicine states there is little evidence that herbal supplements improve fertility or affect infant gender (Practice Committee, 2017).

Preconceptual guidance is based on findings that many women enter pregnancy with suboptimal nutritional status, including obesity, and with low intakes of fiber, long-chain polyunsaturated fatty acids (LCPUFA), protein, zinc, iron, phosphorus, potassium, calcium, magnesium, vitamins A and D, folate, riboflavin, and choline (Monk et al, 2013; Rai et al, 2015). Even overweight and obese women can have low nutrient intakes and, in some studies, have been seen to be more nutritionally vulnerable than other pregnant women (Dubois et al, 2018). Although current public health recommendations primarily promote folic acid supplementation, many other nutrients are also important in the periconceptual period. Micronutrient supplementation can improve maternal status but may not improve child health outcomes if started after conception (Stephenson et al, 2018). How much before conception this supplementation is needed is unknown and likely varies by maternal nutrient status. Optimal nutrient intakes are associated with lower risk of growth-restricted babies (low birth weight [LBW] or small for gestational age [SGA]) or preterm births (Table 14.1). Thus a preconceptual multivitamin-multimineral supplement may confer more benefit than single supplements for a pregnant woman, or gravida, especially in the context of low background food intake.

Preconception educational programs for both parents are promoted, but evidence of effectiveness and benefit is inconsistent.

TABLE 14.1 Examples of Nutrients Likely Important in the Periconceptual Period: Preconception Through Organogenesis

System or Function	Nutrients
Brain and nervous system	Iron, zinc, iodine, LCPUFA, vitamins A, B$_6$, B$_{12}$, folic acid, copper, protein, selenium
Placental function and structure	Iron, LCPUFA, vitamins E, C, B$_{12}$, zinc, selenium, copper, omega-3 PUFA, folate
Inflammation and immune function	Vitamins A, D, zinc, fatty acids
Oxidative stress	Vitamins C, E, B$_6$, B$_{12}$, folic acid
Embryogenesis	Vitamins A, B$_6$, B$_{12}$, folic acid, zinc

Adapted from Cetin I et al: Role of micronutrients in the periconceptional period, *Hum Reprod Update* 16:80, 2010; Monk C et al: Research review: maternal prenatal distress and poor nutrition—mutually influencing risk factors affecting infant neurocognitive development, *J Child Psychol Psychiatry* 54:115, 2013; Ramakrishnan U et al: Effect of women's nutrition before and during early pregnancy on maternal and infant outcomes: a systematic review, *Paediatr Perinat Epidemiol* 26:285, 2012. *LCPUFA*, Long-chain polyunsaturated fatty acids; *PUFA*, polyunsaturated fatty acids.

There is also little evidence for which interventions are most effective (Goldstein et al, 2016). However, it appears that nutrition interventions may be more effective in promoting change than those targeting smoking and alcohol cessation (Temel et al, 2014). In addition, these programs are targeted at those planning pregnancies, not the general public, and likely won't resonate with many. Even if these programs could address the parents of the estimated 50% of pregnancies that are unplanned, the issues that can be addressed quickly (smoking, alcohol use, vitamin supplementation, caffeine, etc.) are limited. Because some preconceptual issues, including obesity and harmful dietary patterns, require long-term interventions, there are calls for a more public health or marketing approach to improve the health status of potential parents (Stephenson et al, 2018).

Toxins

Screening women for alcohol, tobacco (including e-cigarettes, vapors), and recreational drug use is critical and also may be important for occupational toxin exposure. Marijuana (*Cannabis sativa*) use is now legalized in some states. It does not appear to affect semen parameters but the prevalence of infertility increases among women reporting marijuana use (Practice Committee, 2017). Animal models have demonstrated an increase in birth defects (Hennessy, 2018) but human studies are confounded with polysubstance abuse and often ignore the timing of exposure (American College of Obstetricians and Gynecologists [ACOG], 2017a). In addition, the potency has increased over time. The chemicals cross the placenta and fetal cannabinoid receptors are active as early as 14 weeks. Marijuana use affects the central nervous system and animal models show it negatively affects fetal brain development. The prevalence of SGA babies and stillbirths both increase among those using marijuana and, if associated with cigarette smoking, may increase the risk of preterm birth (ACOG, 2017a; ACOG, 2018d). In vitro studies, using first trimester placental villous cells from terminated pregnancies transplanted to a nutrient medium, demonstrate poor placental growth and function, including lower taurine transport to the fetus, when the fetus is exposed to high amounts of alcohol in early pregnancy (Lui et al, 2014). Women may be at risk for entering pregnancy with toxic levels of mercury, and the types of fish eaten should be discussed (see *Focus On*: Omega-3 Fatty Acids in Pregnancy and Lactation). The effect of maternal caffeine intake on infertility is often debated. No increased risk of miscarriage has been seen with caffeine consumption less than 200 mg/day, but consumption of more than 500 mg/day is associated with decreased fertility (Practice Committee, 2017). Caffeine is not a teratogen (a substance that causes malformation in an embryo or fetus), and does not affect semen parameters (see Appendix 25).

⊚ FOCUS ON

Omega-3 Fatty Acids in Pregnancy and Lactation

Our ancestors likely consumed a diet with equal amounts of omega-3 and omega-6 fatty acids. American diets currently are estimated to contain much higher levels of omega-6 than omega-3 fatty acids. This dramatic change in the ratio is thought to affect overall disease prevalence as well as pregnancy outcome. However, there is no evidence that the absolute amounts of essential fatty acids (EFA) provided by any culture are inadequate for the placenta, fetus, or infant growth (Lauritzen and Carlson, 2011). Adequacy of EFA intake is highly individual based on dietary intake, food access, and food preferences.

Fatty acids are found in all cell membranes. The fetal brain contains equal amounts of omega-6 (arachidonic acid) and omega-3 (docosahexaenoic acid [DHA]). Arachidonic acid intake is seldom limited. The omega-3s, primarily eicosapentaenoic acid (EPA) and DHA, are important for fetal neurodevelopment, vasodilation, reduced inflammation, and thrombosis inhibition. Although EPA is thought to be beneficial, the separate effects have not yet been tested because purified EPA supplements are only recently available.

DHA is important for the growth and development of the fetal central nervous system and the retina. It may play a beneficial role in the fetal immune function and may help lower the risk of food allergy (Larqué et al, 2012). DHA may also be helpful regarding birth weight, as well as maternal depression. There is some evidence that supplementing all pregnant women with DHA may be a cost-effective way to lower the risk of early preterm delivery (Shireman et al, 2016). A recent Cochrane review found that increased overall intake of the omega-3 long-chain polyunsaturated fatty acids (LCPUFAs) (from food or supplements) reduced the risk of both preterm (< 37 weeks) and early preterm (< 34 weeks) births (Middleton et al, 2018). Cochrane also concluded that more research is needed to determine the long-term effects on mother and child; to determine the metabolic and neurodevelopment pathways; and to determine whether, and how, the outcomes vary by the different types of omega-3 fatty acids, as well as the effects of the timing, dosage, and characteristics of women.

DHA is selectively and preferentially transferred across the placenta (Lauritzen and Carlson, 2011). Fetal DHA accretion is highest in the last half of pregnancy, reaching 30 to 45 mg/day in the last trimester (Koletzko et al, 2007), primarily to the brain and adipose tissue, and in the first few months of life. DHA must be mobilized from maternal stores or the prenatal diet must include adequate amounts of preformed DHA. Transfer rates are highly variable and are lower among women with obesity, preeclampsia, hypertension, and diabetes (type 1, type 2, and gestational diabetes) (Lauritzen and Carlson, 2011). Women who smoke and have growth restricted fetuses also have lower transfer rates. It is thought that short interconceptual periods may cause a mother to enter a subsequent pregnancy depleted. The amount of DHA in the blood that optimizes maternal and infant outcomes, as well as the intake levels to achieve that level, is still unknown. An average daily intake of 200 mg DHA during pregnancy and lactation currently is recommended, but studies are underway testing the benefit of larger amounts (Carlson et al, 2017). Current intakes are often far lower. Intakes of up to 1 g/day of DHA or 2.7 g/day of total omega-3 PUFAs appear safe (Koletzko et al, 2007). The main food source of DHA is fatty, cold-water fish, and a couple of meals per week of low-mercury fish during pregnancy provide adequate amounts of DHA. Those fish that are low in methylmercury but high in DHA include salmon, sardines, trout, herring, anchovies, and mackerel (not King mackerel). Caviar and brains (do not use where prion contamination is of concern) are also particularly high in DHA. Other foods also may be used, depending on local availability and acceptability of safe sources. Check the local food composition tables for options.

Vegetable sources of omega-3 fats (alpha-linolenic acid [ALA]) include flaxseeds and nuts, especially walnuts. The conversion rate to DHA is usually very low but improves during pregnancy (Burdge et al, 2017). However, biomagnification by the placenta doesn't appear to compensate for the absence of preformed EPA or DHA. DHA fortified eggs can be helpful, but other fortified foods contain very little DHA. Foods labeled as fortified with omega-3s likely contain ALA. In dietary supplements, algae source EPA and DHA is another useful vegetarian option.

Any pregnant woman allergic to fish should seek an algal source of supplemental DHA. It is currently unknown if EPA or other components (e.g., other fatty acids, vitamin D, iodine, and selenium) are also important (Oken et al, 2013). Fish oil supplements contain EPA and DHA, although better long-term outcomes are seen with fish consumption than with supplements. Caution is advised, though, with the fish liver oils (such as cod liver oil) because of high preformed vitamin A levels.

The breastfed infant obtains DHA through maternal milk when the mother eats sufficient quantities of foods containing DHA. If the exclusively breastfeeding mother is not consuming fish or DHA supplements, a DHA supplement can be given to the infant. For women who are unable, or choose not to breastfeed, most infant formulas in the United States are fortified with DHA.

There is no dietary reference intake (DRI) for either EPA or DHA in the United States. The benefit of maternal supplementation has not been proven as of yet and there are potential epigenetic effects that must also be considered. Maternal fish consumption is associated with better child neurodevelopment, at least in observational studies subject to confounding. Perhaps supplementation is merited only for those women with very low intakes of LCPUFAs and/or for premature infants who had insufficient time to accumulate enough.

Promoting a variety of safe seafood choices is preferable. Women have consumed less fish since the mercury advisories were issued (McGuire et al, 2016). They must be reassured that fish can be eaten safely as a good protein source as long as care is taken in choosing and preparing the fish (see Box 14.7). If at least some of the high DHA sources are chosen, pregnancy outcomes, as well as infant neurodevelopment and visual acuity, may improve. In addition, if women eat these fish during pregnancy, they are also likely to continue eating them postpartum, improving the maternal repletion and the child's DHA accretion that continues after birth.

Exposure of men and women to environmental chemicals, including pesticides, heavy metals, and organic solvents, is associated with an increased time to pregnancy. However, most studies are plagued with important confounders (age, smoking, alcohol use, parity, use of contraceptives, underlying disease) and causality cannot be determined. It is also unknown whether men and women have different susceptibility to the effects of environmental toxins. The strongest evidence of adverse effect is with pesticide and lead exposure. Pesticide exposure affects semen quality and increases risk of sterility (ACOG, 2013b; Table 14.2).

A father's regular preconceptual smoking is associated with DNA damage to the sperm, but it is unclear whether male fertility is reduced (Practice Committee, 2017). Smoking also increases the risk that his child will have acute lymphoblastic leukemia, but the absolute risk is still very small, raising it from 27 per million births to 34 per million births (Van der Zee et al, 2013). Maternal smoking is associated with an increased rate

TABLE 14.2 Examples of Reproductive Health Effects of Prenatal Exposure to Environmental Contaminants

Chemicals	Exposure Sources and Pathways	Reproductive or Developmental Health Effects
Pesticides	Pesticides are applied in large quantities in agricultural, community, and household settings. In 2001 more than 1.2 billion pounds of pesticides were used in the United States. Pesticides can be ingested, inhaled, and absorbed by the skin. The pathways of pesticide exposure include food, water, air, dust, and soil.	Impaired cognitive development Impaired neurodevelopment Impaired fetal growth Increased susceptibility to testicular cancer Childhood cancer
Solvents	Examples include benzene, toluene, xylene, styrene, 1-bromopropane, 2-bromopropane, perchloroethylene, and trichloroethylene. Solvents include some of the highest production volume chemicals in the United States. They are used in plastics, resins, nylon, synthetic fibers, rubber, lubricants, dyes, detergents, drugs, pesticides, glues, paints, paint thinners, fingernail polish, lacquers, detergents, printing and leather tanning processes, insulation, fiberglass, food containers, carpet backing, and cleaning products. Solvents are a component of cigarette smoke. Exposure is primarily through breathing contaminated air.	Fetal loss Miscarriage
Toluene	Exposure occurs from breathing contaminated air at the workplace, in automobile exhaust, and in some consumer products, paints, paint thinners, fingernail polish, lacquers, and adhesives.	Decreased fetal and birth weight Congenital malformations
Phthalates	Phthalates are synthetically derived. They are used in a variety of consumer goods, such as medical devices, cleaning and building materials, personal care products, cosmetics, pharmaceuticals, food processing, and toys. Exposure occurs through ingestion, inhalation, and dermal absorption.	Reduced masculine play in boys Reduced anogenital distance Shortened gestational age Impaired neurodevelopment in girls
Lead	Occupational exposure occurs in battery manufacturing and recycling, smelting, car repair, welding, soldering, firearm cleaning and shooting, and stained glass ornament and jewelry production. Nonoccupational exposure occurs in older homes where lead-based paints were used, water pipes, imported ceramics and pottery, herbal remedies, traditional cosmetics, hair dyes, contaminated soil, toys, and costume jewelry.	Alterations in genomic methylation Intellectual impairment Increased likelihood of allergies
Mercury	Mercury from coal-fired power plants is the largest man-made source of mercury pollution in the United States. Primary human exposure is by consumption of contaminated seafood.	Reduced cognitive performance Impaired neurodevelopment
Polychlorinated biphenyls	Polychlorinated biphenyls were used as industrial insulators and lubricants. They were banned in the 1970s but are persistent in the aquatic and terrestrial food chains, resulting in exposure by ingestion.	Development of attention-deficit/hyperactivity disorder-associated behavior Increased body mass index Reduced IQ
Air pollutants	Common air pollutants include carbon monoxide, lead, ground-level ozone, particulate matter, nitrogen dioxide, and sulfur dioxide. Air pollution arises from a variety of sources, including motor vehicles, industrial production, energy (coal) production, wood burning, and small local sources such as dry cleaners.	Low birth weight Birth defects
Cigarette smoke	Cigarette smoke exposure includes active smoking, passive smoking, or both.	Miscarriage Intrauterine growth restriction Low birth weight Preterm delivery Decreased semen quality
Perchlorate	Perchlorate is used to produce rocket fuel, fireworks, flares, and explosives and also can be present in bleach and some fertilizers. Sources of exposure are contaminated drinking water, food, and other nonwater beverages. Infants also may be exposed through breastmilk.	Altered thyroid function
Perfluorochemicals	Perfluorochemicals are widely used man-made organofluorine compounds with many diverse industrial and consumer product applications. Examples are perfluorooctane sulfonate and perfluorooctanate, which are used in cookware products with nonstick surfaces and in packaging to provide grease, oil, and water resistance to plates, food containers, bags, and wraps that come into contact with food. They persist in the environment. Occupational exposure and general population exposure occur by inhalation, ingestion, and dermal contact.	Reduced birth weight

Continued

TABLE 14.2   Examples of Reproductive Health Effects of Prenatal Exposure to Environmental Contaminants—cont'd

Chemicals	Exposure Sources and Pathways	Reproductive or Developmental Health Effects
Polybrominated diphenyl ethers	These include flame retardant materials that persist and bioaccumulate in the environment. They are found in furniture, textiles, carpeting, electronics, and plastics that are mixed into but not bound to foam or plastic.	Impaired neurodevelopment Premature delivery Low birth weight Stillbirth
Bisphenol-A	Bisphenol-A is a chemical intermediate for polycarbonate plastic and resins. It is found in food, consumer products, and packaging. Exposure occurs through inhalation, ingestion, and dermal absorption.	Recurrent miscarriage Aggression and hyperactivity in female children
Formaldehyde	Formaldehyde is used in the production of wood adhesives, abrasive materials, and other industrial products and in clinical laboratories and embalming. It is found in some germicides, fungicides, insecticides, and personal care products. Routes of exposure are oral, dermal, and inhaled.	Spontaneous abortion Low birth weight
Antineoplastic drugs	This class of chemotherapy drugs presents an occupational exposure for nurses and other health care professionals.	Spontaneous abortion Low birth weight
Anesthetic gases	Anesthetic gases are administered by inhalation in health care settings and veterinary care. Occupational exposure is a risk for nurses, physicians, dentists, veterinarians, and other health care professionals who work in settings where anesthetic gases are used.	Congenital anomalies Spontaneous abortion
Ethylene oxide	Ethylene oxide is used to sterilize heat-sensitive medical items, surgical instruments, and other objects that come into contact with biologic tissues. Occupational exposure is a risk in some health care settings, particularly sterilization units. Exposure is through inhalation.	Spontaneous abortion and pregnancy loss Preterm and postterm birth

Reprinted with permission from American College of Obstetricians and Gynecologists: Exposure to toxic environmental agents, companion document. Retrieved from https://www.acog.org/-/media/Committee-Opinions/Committee-on-Health-Care-for-Underserved-Women/ExposuretoToxic.pdf, 2013d.

of miscarriage (Practice Committee, 2017). Habitual alcohol consumption may be associated with reduced semen quality and changes in testosterone and sex hormone-binding globulin levels. Although higher intakes are of more concern, even five drinks per week have been associated with a reduced sperm count and concentration, as well as a reduction in the percentage of spermatozoa with normal morphology (Jensen et al, 2014).

Obesity and Endocrine Conditions

Preconceptual obesity raises risk for men and women. In men, elevated BMI is associated with lower success with in vitro fertilization (IVF).

Maternal prepregnant obesity is correlated with lower rates of conception, higher rates of congenital anomalies, and lower live birth rates (Merhi et al, 2013). Obesity affects oocyte development, ovulation, embryo development, endometrial development, implantation, and pregnancy loss. Obesity in pregnancy and postpartum is correlated with lactation failure (Garcia et al, 2016). Those with known diabetes and hypothyroidism, as well as hypertension, should be in good control before conception. Although weight loss improves fertility for women, it has less effect on fertility in men (see *Focus On*: Special Case of Obesity).

◎ **FOCUS ON**

Special Case of Obesity

The rates of obesity have increased dramatically in industrialized and, to a lesser extent, in developing countries (see Chapter 20). Among women with obesity, rates of conception are lower and congenital anomalies (neural tube defects [NTDs], cardiovascular anomalies, oral clefts, anorectal atresia, hydrocephaly, limb reductions, spina bifida) occur more frequently and are detected less often prenatally than in the general population. Rates of NTDs increase with the degree of obesity. For women with severe obesity, rates are more than triple that for women with normal weight. Supplementation with folic acid is not as protective for these women, but the benefit of supplementing with more than 400 mcg folic acid/day has not been studied.

Women with obesity have an exaggerated response to the normal physiologic changes of pregnancy. They have increased risk of cardiac dysfunction, proteinuria, sleep apnea, nonalcoholic liver disease, gestational diabetes, and preeclampsia (American College of Obstetricians and Gynecologists [ACOG], 2015d). Genetic, hormonal, and biochemical environments are altered, influencing fetal growth and

organ development. Women who enter pregnancy with a body mass index (BMI) greater than 30 have a higher risk of spontaneous abortion (SAB, i.e., miscarriage), intrauterine fetal demise (IUFD) or stillbirth, with the risk of many complications increasing linearly (Nelson et al, 2010). These women are more likely to have intrapartum, operative, and postoperative complications, including anemia and postpartum depression. Increased risks of maternal morbidity and mortality are associated with increasing degrees of obesity (Lisonkova et al, 2017). Women with obesity are less likely to initiate breastfeeding and more likely to experience lactation failure.

Normal fetal growth patterns are disrupted. Risk is increased for macrosomia, birth injury (shoulder dystocia, brachial plexus injury, fetal hypoxia), and childhood obesity, but there are also significant rates of growth-restricted babies and preterm deliveries. Infants of women with obesity are more likely to require admission to the neonatal intensive care unit (NICU). There is a linear association between maternal BMI and neonatal death and both neonatal morbidity and maternal complications are significantly higher when maternal BMI is at least 60 (Kim et al, 2017).

Special Case of Obesity—cont'd

Although excessive gestational weight gain is common among women who are overweight or obese, and this weight gain is associated with similar increased risks, the prepregnant BMI is usually thought to be the more important factor. Weight loss before pregnancy is recommended and women who have undergone bariatric surgery are less likely to develop gestational diabetes, hypertension, preeclampsia, or to have a macrosomic infant. Weight loss medications are not recommended because of safety concerns at conception (ACOG, 2015d). The optimal timing and extent of that weight loss is being examined.

How maternal obesity mediates poor maternal and fetal outcomes is not clear (Catalano and Shankar, 2017). There are likely genetic and fetal-maternal interactions. It was thought that exposure to hyperglycemia was the main predictor, but it is now recognized that other factors are also important, including hypertriglyceridemia, insulin and insulin resistance, androgens, leptin, increased blood pressure, inflammation, and oxidative stress. Both placental and fetal functioning are affected. Obesity and inflammation are causally linked to insulin resistance. How maternal inflammation affects developmental programming, leading to increased infant adiposity, is not known but there is some evidence that fetal inflammation exists also. Obesity, with low levels of adiponectin, is associated with increased fetal growth. The normal twofold to threefold increase in serum cholesterol and free fatty acid levels during pregnancy are exaggerated in women with obesity. Placentas of these women have altered elevated inflammation markers and lower steroid hormone levels, possibly in response to maternal hyperinsulinemia. These placentas contain higher lipid levels but modified uptake of the LCPUFAs. Triglycerides do not pass through the placenta easily, but there is increased placental transfer of metabolites and an increase in fetal fat deposits with obesity. Altered placental development or function, leading to altered amino acid transfer, contributes to a fetal hyperinsulinemic state. In addition, obesity is associated with tissue-specific changes in mitochondrial function and elevated oxidative stress. High lipid levels also may cause epigenetic changes in lipid sensing and metabolism genes. Obesity may also alter the regulation of appetite, satiety, and adipocyte maturation of the fetus. Iron status in the context of obesity is understudied (Vricella, 2017). These women may have less plasma volume expansion, resulting in higher hemoglobin values. On the other hand, because of the increased inflammation associated with obesity, they potentially have higher hepcidin levels, lowering hemoglobin levels.

Babies that are exclusively breastfed are less likely to be obese later in life (Uwaezuoke et al, 2017). Both the nutrient and hormonal content of breastmilk is altered with maternal obesity. In addition, the infant microbiome is also altered because of the changes in human milk oligosaccharides. Developmental programming and interactions with the early diet are likely to both be important (Catalano and Shankar, 2017).

Babies born to obese mothers have permanently altered body weight-regulating mechanisms, including the hypothalamic response to leptin, regulation of appetite, and pancreatic beta-cell physiology. There are also changes in the adipose tissue. They are more likely to have obesity, hypertension, and diabetes as adults. In addition, these babies have increased risk of allergy and atopy, possibly through the intestinal dysbiosis and reduced microbial diversity. Maternal obesity also negatively affects maturation and development of the neonate's immune system but the roles of maternal nutrition and exposure to infections and/or their treatments are as yet unclear (Godfrey et al, 2017b). The role of both the maternal and newborn gut microbiome in fetal programming is unknown but may be important (Zhou and Xiao, 2018). Maternal obesity is associated with an increased risk of autism spectrum disorders, developmental delay, and attention-deficit/hyperactive disorder (ACOG, 2015d). Animal research has identified potential mechanisms, including concentrations of fatty acids and glucose, high concentrations of leptin and insulin, and inflammatory mediators interleukins and tumor necrosis factor that cross the placenta and influence neuroendocrine development, neuronal proliferation, and brain development (Godfrey et al, 2017b). Interactions with the environment and epigenetic effects are also likely important. However, the relative impact of maternal obesity, gestational weight gain, and dietary patterns is not yet clear (Catalano and Shankar, 2017).

It appears that both preconception and periconception times are critical. Improving metabolic function preconceptually improves perinatal outcomes. Interpregnancy intervention to lower weight improves placental function and fetal development.

PCOS affects up to 10% of women of reproductive age but prevalence varies widely between populations (Bellver et al, 2018). Whether PCOS affects oocyte quality is unknown. The testosterone-estrogen balance is altered, resulting in insulin resistance and infertility. Some research suggests that 5% to 10% weight loss is preferred to the use of metformin for ovulation induction in patients with PCOS (Usadi and Legro, 2012; see Chapter 30). Both metabolic syndrome and PCOS are associated with lower fertility rates, along with increased pregnancy and neonatal risks, even when controlling for the obesity. These problems are likely the result of multiple mechanisms, including inflammation, some of which may overlap with the two conditions, and some of which have not yet been identified. Obesity is often a comorbidity that may amplify the effects of PCOS but it is not a diagnostic criterion (ACOG, 2018a). Weight loss for both metabolic syndrome and PCOS is recommended as a first course of treatment because obesity is, in itself, associated with decreased fertility. However, in the case of PCOS, weight loss will not address the underlying hyperandrogenemia and likely will not be helpful if the patient is not overweight or obese. Because 50% to 70% of people with PCOS have insulin resistance regardless of BMI, optimizing glucose control may be beneficial (Bellver et al, 2018). A male equivalent of PCOS may also exist but the impact on reproductive function still needs investigation (Cannarella et al, 2018).

Optimal antioxidants appear to be helpful, as well as vitamin D and omega-3 PUFAs from fish, but the relatively importance of supplements vs. diets rich in these components is not clear. Herbal and dietary supplements are promoted for PCOS treatment (see *Focus On: Herbal and Dietary Supplements*).

A healthy diet and exercise program helps parents prepare for an optimal pregnancy outcome, with the goal of achieving normal weight before conception. However, although preconceptual intervention is recommended, it is seldom achieved because half of pregnancies in the United States are unplanned. In addition, advances in assisted reproductive technology (ART) mean that "parents" may be egg or sperm donors or surrogate mothers. The preconceptual health of these "parents" is likely also important but the impact is unknown.

CONCEPTION

Conception involves a complex series of endocrine events in which a healthy sperm fertilizes a healthy ovum (egg) within 24 hours of ovulation. Conception does not guarantee successful pregnancy outcome.

◎ FOCUS ON

Herbal and Dietary Supplements

Some herbal and dietary supplements are promoted for PCOS and/or metabolic syndrome treatment. However, for many, the supporting evidence is insufficiently reliable to rate their effectiveness. For others, there is concern even if the herbal supplements are thought to be effective, because of the potential negative effect on a pregnancy. Specifically, berberine is likely unsafe in pregnancy because it crosses the placenta and may harm the fetus. It may also stimulate uterine contractions. N-acetyl cysteine is also mentioned as useful in treating PCOS. However, it also crosses the placenta. Melatonin may inhibit ovulation but the critical dose is unknown and it is not recommended. Inositol (myo-inositol, D-chiro-inositol) appears to be safe for use in pregnancy. Its use with folic acid appears to lower triglycerides and/or testosterone and improve ovarian function, including ovulation rates in overweight women with PCOS, working as well as metformin (Jellin and Gregory, 2018). A combination of the two forms of inositol may be more effective than a single form. However, a Cochrane systematic review found no differences between inositol and placebo on BMI, waist-hip ratio, the number of people who ovulated, serum testosterone, triglycerides, cholesterol, fasting glucose, or fasting insulin (Monash University, 2018). Data is still limited and inositol use should be considered experimental. Dosage appears critical and there are potential adverse effects among non-obese women, so caution is advised (Noventa et al, 2016).

As in the general population, the use of herbal and dietary supplements for many conditions is common during pregnancy. For many herbs, the supporting evidence is insufficiently reliable to rate their effectiveness or safety, especially in the first trimester. Common local herbs should be investigated carefully for their safety during pregnancy. Even those with the same names can have different effects. For example, German chamomile appears to be of little concern during pregnancy, while Roman chamomile appears to increase the risk for preterm delivery and LBW (Trabace et al, 2015) and may be an abortifacient (Jellin and Gregory, 2018). Many herbs may cause uterine contractions and/or bleeding and are contraindicated in pregnancy, including ingested aloe vera latex, cat's claw, cinnamon volatile oil, oregano tea, avocado leaf tea, rue, sage tea, damiana, and large amounts of parsley or celery seeds (Kennedy et al, 2016; Rivera et al, 2006).

Caution is advised with the use of all herbal and dietary supplements because safety, purity, and effectiveness cannot always be guaranteed due to the way they are regulated by the Food and Drug Administration (FDA). Interactions with prescribed medications can occur, affecting treatment decisions (Kennedy et al, 2016). Even some herbs considered helpful during pregnancy can have unexpected consequences. For example, raspberry leaf and blackberry leaf tea can cause hypoglycemia in patients with gestational diabetes (Cheang et al, 2016). Women should advise their health care provider about any medication use, including dietary and herbal supplements, and the risk vs. benefit should be carefully considered. See Natural Medicines Comprehensive Database for specific detailed information. Also see Chapter 11.

Occult loss rates are estimated to be 41% to 70%, depending on the timing and sensitivity of the pregnancy test (Kwak-Kim et al, 2010). Among clinically recognized pregnancies, the overall early pregnancy loss rate is 10% but varies widely by the age of the mother (ACOG, 2015e).

The Carnegie Stages are a system used to describe predictable embryonic changes and developmental milestones. As noted in Table 14.3, as well as in Table 14.1 and Box 14.1, optimal conditions, including the absence of hostile factors and optimal status of many nutrients, are thought to be critical preconceptually and during fetal organogenesis.

TABLE 14.3 The Carnegie Stages of Human Gestation Through 16 Weeks Postovulation

Carnegie Stage (time postovulation)	Structure Size	Highlighted Developmental Events with Selected Potential Nutrient Implications
Stage 1 Fertilization (1 day)	0.1-0.15 millimeters (mm); smaller than the size of a pencil point	Fertilization begins when the sperm penetrates the oocyte. This requires the sperm, which can survive up to 48 hours, to travel 10 hours up the female reproductive tract. Then the sperm must successfully penetrate the zona pellucida, a tough membrane surrounding the egg, a process that takes approximately 20 minutes. Once the fertilization is successful, the structure now becomes a zygote. This is the end of the fertilization process. **Optimal amounts of folate** are needed for cell division and formation of DNA.
Stage 2 First Cell Division (1.5-3 days)	0.1-0.2 mm	Zygote begins to divide. Division begins to occur approximately every 20 hours. When cell division generates a mass of approximately 16 cells, the zygote now becomes a morula, a mulberry shaped structure. The newly created morula leaves the fallopian tube and enters the uterine cavity 3-4 days after fertilization.
Stage 3 Early Blastocyst (4 days)	0.1-0.2 mm	The morula enters the uterus and cell division continues. A cavity (hole), known as a blastocele, forms in the middle of the morula. Cells are flattening and compacting inside this cavity. The zona pellucida remains the same size as it was after fertilization, with the cavity in the center. The entire structure is now called a blastocyst. Two cell types are forming: embryoblasts, on the inside of the blastocele, and trophoblasts, on the outside portion of the blastocele.
Stage 4 Implantation Begins (5-6 days)	0.1-0.2 mm	Pressure from the blastocele expanding in the middle of the blastocyst against the rigid wall of the zona pellucida creates a "hatching" of the blastocyst from this zona pellucida. Separation of the embryoblasts and trophoblasts is complete. The outer layer of trophoblast cells secretes an enzyme that erodes the epithelial lining of the uterus so the blastocyst can implant. Trophoblast cells also secrete hCG, which stimulates the corpus luteum (the yellow glandular mass in the ovary formed by an ovarian follicle that has matured and discharged its ovum) to continue progesterone production, important in maintaining the blood-rich uterine lining. Progesterone is also later produced by the placenta. Five days is the latest that an IVF embryo would be transferred. **Consider vitamin D.**

TABLE 14.3	**The Carnegie Stages of Human Gestation Through 16 Weeks Postovulation—cont'd**	
Carnegie Stage (time postovulation)	**Structure Size**	**Highlighted Developmental Events with Selected Potential Nutrient Implications**
Stage 5 Implantation Complete (7-12 days)	0.1-0.2 mm	Trophoblast cells continue to destroy cells of the uterine lining, creating blood pools and stimulating new capillaries to grow. This begins the growth of the placenta. The blastocyst inner cell mass differentiates into the epiblast (top layer of cells, becoming the embryo and the amniotic cavity) and the hypoblast (lower layer of cells, becoming the yolk sac). Ectopic pregnancies are those that do not implant in the uterus at this time, eventually becoming a life-threatening problem.
Stage 6 Primitive Streak (13 days)	0.2 mm	Placental formation: Chorionic villi "fingers" form, anchoring the embryo to the uterus. Blood vessels begin appearing. Stalk formation: The embryo is attached to the developing placenta by a stalk, which later becomes part of the umbilical cord. Gastrulation: A narrow line of cells, called the *primitive streak,* appears on the surface of the two-layered embryonic disc. Cells migrate in, with bilateral symmetry, from the outer edges of the disc to the primitive streak and begin to form three layers: the ectoderm (top layer of the embryonic disc that will later form skin, hair, lenses of the eye, lining of the internal and external ear, nose, sinuses, mouth, anus, tooth enamel, pituitary and mammary glands, and all parts of the nervous system), the mesoderm (middle cell layer that will later form muscles, bones, lymphatic tissue, spleen, blood cells, heart, lungs, and reproductive and excretory systems), and the endoderm (inner cell layer that will later form the lining of the lungs, the tongue, the tonsils, the urethra and associated glands, the bladder, and the digestive tract). **Consider vitamins A, E, C, copper, and DHA.**
Stage 7 Neurulation (16 days)	0.4 mm	Gastrulation continues, forming the three-layered embryonic disc. Neural crest cells originate at the top of the neural tube and migrate extensively throughout the embryo, differentiating into many cell types, including neurons, glial cells, pigmented cells of the epidermis, epinephrine-producing cells of the adrenal glands, and various skeletal and connective tissues of the head. Fetal alcohol syndrome results from disruption of the migration of neural crest cells. **Consider vitamins A, E, folic acid, choline, zinc, selenium, DHA, and antioxidants.**
Stage 8 (17-19 days)	1-1.5 mm	The embryonic area is now shaped like a pear, with the head region broader than the tail. The ectoderm has thickened to form the neural plate. The edges rise, forming the concave neural groove. This groove is the precursor of the embryo's nervous system, one of the first organs to develop. Blood cells are already developed and begin to form channels alongside the epithelial cells that are also forming. *Sonic hedgehog (Shh)* is one of three genes that are now secreted from the notochord (rod-shaped body composed of mesoderm cells). These genes encode for signaling molecules involved in patterning processes during embryogenesis, including the development of cerebral neurons, the separation of the single eye field into two bilateral fields, hair growth, and limb development. A repression of Shh by the notochord initiates pancreatic development. **Consider vitamin B_{12}, omega-3 fatty acids, folate, cholesterol, and choline.**
Stage 9 Appearance of Somites (19-21 days)	1.5-2.5 mm	Embryo looks like a peanut with a larger head end compared with the tail end. One to three pairs of somites (mesoderm tissue that looks like "bumps") are now present, with every ridge, bump, and recess indicating cellular differentiation. The head fold rises on either side of the primitive streak. Endocardial (muscle) cells begin to fuse and form into the early embryo's two heart tubes. Secondary blood vessels now appear in the chorion/placenta. Hematopoietic cells (forming blood cells) and endothelial cells (forming blood vessels) appear on the yolk sac simultaneously. **Consider folic acid, copper, and iron.**
Stage 10 (21-23 days)	1.5-3.0 mm	At this time, the embryo looks like an old fashioned key-hole with a big oval top, with an ear of corn in the bottom two thirds of the structure. Rapid cell growth elongates the embryo and expands the yolk sac. By the end of this stage, 4-12 somite pairs can exist. Cells that will become the eyes and ears appear. Neural folds begin to rise and fuse, "zippering" the neural tube closed. Failure of this closure results in a neural tube defect, including anencephaly and spina bifida, which varies in severity depending on location and extent of the area left open. The two endocardial tubes fuse into one. This heart tube takes on an S-shaped form and cardiac muscle contraction begins. **Consider folate, B_6, B_{12}, choline, vitamin A, zinc, copper, and methionine.**

Continued

TABLE 14.3   **The Carnegie Stages of Human Gestation Through 16 Weeks Postovulation—cont'd**

Carnegie Stage (time postovulation)	Structure Size	Highlighted Developmental Events with Selected Potential Nutrient Implications
Stage 11 (23-25 days)	2.5-3.0 mm	Embryo has a modified S-curve shape with a bulb-like tail and a stalk connecting to the developing placenta. Somites increase to 20 pairs, at which point the forebrain is completely closed. The primitive tubal heart is beating and peristalsis begins. **Consider Vitamin A.**
Stage 12 (25-27 days)	3-5 mm	Embryo now has a C-shape. Brain and spinal cord are the largest tissue in the embryo. Face is becoming apparent; eyes and ears are beginning to form. Heart valves and septa may become apparent. Blood system is developing. Blood cells follow the surface of the yolk sac (where they originated), then move along the central nervous system to the chorionic villi, part of the maternal blood system. Liver cells are beginning to form, before the rest of the digestive system. Upper limb buds appear. **Consider vitamin A, folic acid, choline, methionine, and zinc.**
Stage 13 (26-30 days)	4-6 mm; size of the head of a pencil eraser	More than 30 somite pairs are now evident, precursors of multiple organ systems. First thin surface layer of skin appears to cover the embryo. Back muscles and ribs begin to form. The digestive epithelium layer begins to differentiate, eventually developing into the liver, lung, stomach, and pancreas.
Stage 14 (31-35 days)	5-7 mm	Brain and head are growing rapidly, sections of the brain and spinal cord wall are becoming differentiated. The eye is developing and the nasal plate can be detected. The adenohypophyseal pouch, later developing into the anterior pituitary, is defined. The esophagus is forming and lung sacs appear. Ureteric buds and the metanephros, later developing into the kidney, appear. Upper limbs elongate and innervation begins. **Consider LCPUFA (especially DHA and AA), protein, zinc, iron, choline, copper, iodine, vitamin A, and folate.**
Stage 15 (35-38 days)	7-9 mm	Brain is still larger than the trunk. Maxillary and mandibular arches are more prominent. The stomodeum, the depression in the ectoderm that will develop into the mouth and oral cavity, appears. Retinal pigment may appear in the optic cup. Symmetric and separate nasal pits appear as depressions in the nasal disc. Future cerebral hemispheres are distinct. Blood flowing through the atrioventricular canal is now divided into left and right streams. Handplate, forearm, arm, and shoulder may now be discerned in the upper limb bud. Lower limb bud begins to develop and innervation begins.
Stage 16 (37-42 days)	9-11 mm	Hindbrain, responsible for heart regulation, breathing, and muscle movements, begins to develop. Future lower jaw is now visible. Nasal pits rotate to face ventrally as head widens. Cardiac tube begins to develop. Mammary gland tissue begins to mature. Mesentery, the tissue that attaches the intestines to the rear abdominal wall and supplies them with blood, nerves, and lymphatics, is now defined. Hands begin to develop. Thigh, leg, and foot areas can now be distinguished. **Consider vitamin A.**
Stage 17 (42-44 days)	10-13 mm	Jaw and facial muscles are developing. The nasofrontal groove becomes distinct. An olfactory bulb (sense of smell) forms in the brain. Teeth buds (without a clear cell arrangement) begin to form. Heart separates into four distinct chambers. The diaphragm forms and the pituitary gland, trachea, larynx, and bronchi begin to form. Intestines begin to develop within the umbilical cord, later migrating to the abdomen when there is space. Primitive germ cells arrive at the genital area, responding to genetic instructions on whether they develop into female or male genitals. Digital rays are apparent on feet and hands. **Consider vitamin K.**
Stage 18 (44-48 days)	11-14 mm	Body appears more like a cube. Eyelids begin to develop, eyes are pigmented. Nipples appear on the chest. Kidneys begin to produce urine. Ossification of the skeleton begins. **Consider calcium, phosphorus, magnesium, vitamins A, D, and K.** See Chapter 23.
Stage 19 (48-51 days)	13-18 mm	Semicircular canals are forming in the inner ear, enabling a sense of balance and body position. Gonads are forming. Knee and ankle locations are now apparent, joints are more distinct. Toes are nearly completely notched and toenails begin to appear. Bone cartilage begins to form a more solid structure. Muscles develop and strengthen.
Stage 20 (51-53 days)	15-20 mm	Spontaneous movement begins. Nose is fully formed. Anal membrane is perforated. Testes or ovaries, as well as toes, are distinguishable.
Stage 21 (53-54 days)	17-22 mm	Eyes are well developed but have not yet migrated forward from the side of the head. External ears have not yet migrated up. Tongue is developing. Intestines begin to recede into the abdominal cavity. Failure to recede may result in either *gastroschisis* or *omphalocele*.

TABLE 14.3 The Carnegie Stages of Human Gestation Through 16 Weeks Postovulation—cont'd

Carnegie Stage (time postovulation)	Structure Size	Highlighted Developmental Events with Selected Potential Nutrient Implications
Stage 22 (54-56 days)	19-24 mm	Development of multiple organs continues. Upper lip now fully formed. The brain can signal muscle movement. Limbs begin to ossify (replacing cartilage with bone), starting in the upper limbs. **Consider the bone nutrients.** See Chapter 23.
Stage 23 Embryonic Period Ends (56-60 days)	23-26 mm	Head is erect and round. External ear is completely developed. Retina is fully pigmented. Eyelids begin to unite and are half closed. Taste buds begin to form. Bones of the palate begin to fuse. Primary teeth are at cap state (cells are now arranged and look like a cap). Upper and lower limbs are well formed; fingers and toes no longer webbed. Intestines continue to migrate from the umbilical cord into the body cavity. Layers of rather flattened cells (precursors to the surface layer of skin) replace the thin ectoderm. **Consider vitamins A, D, and K, calcium, phosphorus, magnesium, protein, and omega-3 fatty acids.**
(61-68 days, approximately 10 weeks)	31-42 mm	Basic brain structure is complete and the brain mass is rapidly growing. Sockets for all 20 teeth are formed in the gum line. Face has human appearance. Vocal cords form and the fetus can make sounds. Fetus develops reflexes. Digestive tract muscles can function and practice contraction. Nutrient-extracting villi line the folded intestines. The liver begins to secrete bile (thick, brown-green liquid containing bile salts, bile pigments, cholesterol, and inorganic salts), which is stored in the gallbladder. The thyroid and pancreas are fully developed. The pancreas produces insulin. Genitalia are not yet fully formed. Fingernails begin growing. Skin is very sensitive. **Consider folate, omega-3 fatty acids, vitamins D, A, choline, Bs, protein, zinc, iron, copper, magnesium, and iodine.**
(12 weeks)	Length: crown-rump length 61 mm (almost 2.5 inches) Weight: 8-14 g (0.3-0.5 oz)	Fetus begins to move around as muscle and nervous systems continue to develop. Heartbeat can be detected. Sucking muscles develop, salivary glands begin to function. Sweat glands and body hair begin to grow. Scalp hair pattern is discernible. Fetus inhales and exhales amniotic fluid, essential for the development of the air sacs in the lungs. Spleen is fully functional, removing old red blood cells and producing antibodies.
(Approximately 14 Weeks)	Length: 80-104 mm (3.2-4.1 inches) Weight: 25 g (almost 1 oz)	Bones continue to form, muscles strengthen. Eyes face more forward and ears are near their final position. Torso is growing rapidly, increasing its proportion to the head. Limbs are well developed. Toenails begin to grow. Heart pumps 25 quarts of blood/day (by the time of delivery it will be 300 quarts/day). Breathing, swallowing, and sucking are all becoming more developed. **Consider vitamin A, protein, and the bone nutrients.** See Chapter 23.
(16 weeks)	Length: 109-117 mm (4.3-4.6 inches) Weight: 80 g (approximately 2.8 oz)	The placenta is now the size of the fetus. The umbilical cord system grows and thickens, with the blood providing nourishment to the fetus through considerable force. 7.5 oz (250 mL) of amniotic fluid surround the conceptus. Eyes and ears are in correct positions. Fetus can blink, ears stand out from head. Fingerprints and toe prints develop. Circulation is completely functional. Meconium, the product of cell loss, digestive secretions, and swallowed amniotic fluid, begins to accumulate in the intestines. Nerves are being coated with myelin, a fatty substance that speeds nerve cell transmission and insulates them for uninterrupted impulses. **Consider omega-3 fatty acids, iron, vitamin A, and cholesterol.**

Adapted from *The Visible Embryo* (website): http://www.visembryo.com/. *AA*, Arachidonic acid; *DNA*, deoxyribonucleic acid; *hCG*, human chorionic gonadotropin; *LCPUFA*, long-chain polyunsaturated fatty acids, *DHA*, docosahexaenoic acid.

BOX 14.1 Potential Risk Factors for Development of Birth Defects

Assisted reproductive technologies (ART)

Genetic alterations

Gene-environmental interactions, such as maternal smoking

Hypoxia during pregnancy

Infection during pregnancy (bacterial, parasitic, viral)

In utero exposure to toxins or heavy metals (lawn chemicals, formaldehyde, endocrine disruptors, agricultural products, pesticides, carbon monoxide, radiation, mercury, lead)

Maternal medical conditions (diabetes, hypothyroidism, phenylketonuria)

Maternal medication or substance exposure (including but not restricted to isotretinoin, phenytoin, carbamazepine, triamterene, trimethoprim, warfarin, and radioactive iodine), illicit recreational substances, alcohol

Nutrient deficits during early pregnancy (iodine, vitamin B_{12}, vitamin D, vitamin A [also excess], vitamin K, copper, zinc, folic acid, choline)

Obesity

Older mother or father

PREGNANCY

Physiologic Changes of Pregnancy

Blood Volume and Composition

Blood volume expands by nearly 50% by the end of pregnancy, with wide variability among women. This increased blood volume results in decreased levels of hemoglobin, serum albumin, other serum proteins, and water-soluble vitamins, primarily after the end of the first trimester. In contrast, serum concentrations of fat-soluble vitamins and other lipid fractions such as triglycerides, cholesterol, and free fatty acids increase to ensure sufficient transport to the fetus. A compilation of laboratory values by trimester is available, and selected values are listed in Table 14.4. However, wide individual variability makes determination of an inadequate intake or a deficient nutrient state difficult. Normal hematocrit and hemoglobin values change by trimester and cutpoints increase with altitude and smoking status, as shown in Table 14.5.

Cardiovascular and Pulmonary Function

Increased cardiac output accompanies pregnancy, and cardiac size increases by 12%. Blood pressure, primarily diastolic, decreases during the first two trimesters because of peripheral vasodilation but may return to prepregnancy values in the third trimester. Mild lower extremity edema is normal, resulting from the pressure of the expanding uterus on the inferior vena cava.

Maternal oxygen requirements increase and the threshold for carbon dioxide lowers, which can make the pregnant woman feel dyspneic. Compensation results from more efficient pulmonary gas exchange and larger chest diameter. In the third trimester, the diaphragm is pushed upwards by the growing uterus, which may also contribute to maternal dyspnea.

Gastrointestinal Function

During pregnancy the function of the gastrointestinal (GI) tract changes in several ways that affect nutritional status. Gums may bleed more easily because of increased blood flow. In the first trimester nausea and vomiting may occur, followed by a return of appetite that may be ravenous (see Nausea and Vomiting, Hyperemesis Gravidarum, and Ptyalism). Cravings for and aversions to foods are common (see Cravings, Aversions, and Pica). Increased progesterone concentration relaxes the uterine muscle to allow for fetal growth while also decreasing GI motility with increased reabsorption of water. This often results in constipation. However, early hormonal changes can also cause diarrhea (see Constipation, Hemorrhoids, and Diarrhea). A relaxed lower esophageal sphincter and pressure on the stomach from the growing uterus can cause regurgitation and gastric reflux (see Heartburn).

Gallbladder emptying becomes less efficient because of the effect of progesterone on muscle contractility. Constipation, dehydration, and a low-calorie diet are risk factors for gallstone development. During the second and third trimesters, the volume of the gallbladder doubles and its ability to empty efficiently is reduced. Bile composition also changes, becoming more sludge-like, increasing the intrinsic risk of gallstones.

Immune Function

Pregnancy has been thought of as a time of overall immunosuppression but there is little evidence to support that idea. Instead, it appears to be a time of immunotransformation. It is hypothesized that the slow, gradual release of paternal/fetal antigens may somehow induce

TABLE 14.4 Selected Reference Ranges for Nutrient Levels in Nonpregnant and Pregnant Women, by Trimester

Component	Nonpregnant Adult	First Trimester	Second Trimester	Third Trimester
Albumin, g/dL	4.1-5.3	3.1-5.1	2.6-4.5	2.3-4.2
Protein, total, g/dL	6.7-8.6	6.2-7.6	5.7-6.9	5.6-6.7
Cholesterol, total, mg/dL	< 200	141-210	176-299	219-349
Triglycerides, mg/dL	< 150	40-159	75-382	131-453
Vitamin A (retinol), mcg/dL	20-100	32-47	35-44	29-42
Vitamin B_{12}, pg/mL	279-966	118-438	130-656	99-526
Vitamin C, mg/dL	0.4-1.0	Not reported	Not reported	0.9-1.3
Vitamin D, 25 hydroxy, ng/mL	14-80	18-27	10-22	10-18
Vitamin E, mcg/mL	5-18	7-13	10-16	13-23
Folate, red blood cell, ng/mL	150-450	137-589	94-828	109-663
Calcium, total, mg/dL	8.7-10.2	8.8-10.6	8.2-9.0	8.2-9.7
Copper, mcg/dL	70-140	112-199	165-221	130-240
Ferritin, ng/mL	10-150	6-130	2-230	0-116
Hemoglobin, g/dL	12-15.8	11.6-13.9	9.7-14.8	9.5-15.0
Hematocrit, %	35.4-44.4	31.0-41.0	30.0-39.0	28.0-40.0
Magnesium, mg/dL	1.5-2.3	1.6-2.2	1.5-2.2	1.1-2.2
Selenium, mcg/L	63-160	116-146	75-145	71-133
Zinc, mcg/dL	75-120	57-88	51-80	50-77

Adapted from Abbassi-Ghanavati M et al: Pregnancy and laboratory studies: a reference table for clinicians, *Obstet Gynecol* 114:1326, 2009.

TABLE 14.5 Maximum Hemoglobin and Hematocrit Values for Prenatal Anemia Diagnosis

Trimester	Hemoglobin Cutpoints at Sea Level	Hematocrit Cutpoints at Sea Level
First	< 11.0 g/dL	< 33.0%
Second	< 10.5	< 32.0
Third	< 11.0	< 33.0
Altitude adjustments: must be added to the above cutpoints for accurate diagnosis		
3000-3999 feet above sea level 1000 meters	+0.2 g/dL	+0.5%
4000-4999 feet	+0.3	+1.0
5000-5999 feet 1500 meters	+0.5	+1.5
6000-6999 feet 2000 meters	+0.7-+0.8	+2.0
7000-7999 feet	+1.0	+3.0
8000-8999 feet 2500 meters	+1.3	+4.0
9000-9999 feet 3000 meters	+1.6-+1.9	+5.0
10,000-11,000 feet	+2.0	+6.0
3500 meters	+2.7	+8.0
4000 meters	+3.5	+10.5
4500 meters	+4.5	+13.5
Cigarette smoking: may be added to the above cutpoints for accurate diagnosis		
0.5 to < 1.0 pack per day	+0.3 g/dL	+1.0 %
1.0 to < 2.0 packs per day	+0.5	+1.5
≥ 2.0 packs per day	+0.7	+2.0
All smokers	+0.3 g/dL	+1.0 %

Adapted from Centers for Disease Control and Prevention: Recommendations to prevent and control iron deficiency in the United States, *MMWR Recomm Rep* 47:1, 1998; World Health Organization (WHO): *Haemoglobin concentrations for the diagnosis of anaemia and assessment of severity.* Vitamin and Mineral Nutrition Information System. WHO/NMH/NHD/MNM/11.1, 2011. http://www.who.int/vmnis/indicators/haemoglobin.pdf.

tolerance rather than rejection, thus not requiring the same immunosuppression as is necessary for transplant recipients. Some humoral and cell-mediated immunologic functions do appear to be suppressed, likely to aid in the acceptance of the "foreign" fetus. However, other immunologic cells appear to be upregulated. The fetal immune system appears to affect the maternal response (Mor et al, 2011). The placenta is an effective barrier to many pathogens but also produces signals and regulates the immune response at both the implantation site and also systemically (Silasi et al, 2015) and, at least in the murine model, peripheral blood measures of immune function may not be appropriate windows on the maternal-fetal interface (Lewis et al, 2018).

Pregnancy has both proinflammatory and antiinflammatory periods (Mor et al, 2011). It is now known that the first trimester, as well as just

NEW DIRECTIONS
Immune Function and Brain Development

Maternal chronic low-grade inflammation, causing inflammation in the fetus, appears to affect fetal brain structure development, negatively affecting neurodevelopment (Miller and Georgieff, 2017). This inflammation may be caused by over- or undernutrition, but also maternal stress or anxiety. Fetal inflammation is directly toxic to the developing brain but also reduces the availability of nutrients essential for neural migration, neuronal growth, and differentiation.

In addition, it is now thought that immune molecules are important in regulating the development of the brain (Bilbo et al, 2018). Current research has been guided by the working hypothesis that prenatal inflammatory events, including a response to infection but also exposure to environmental toxins, can disrupt the normal expression of immune molecules in the brain called microglia during critical periods of development, increasing the risk of neurodevelopmental disorders, including autism spectrum disorder. Causality has not yet been determined and most of the current research is still with animal models. Whether and how dietary changes would affect this process is also still unknown.

before labor, are proinflammatory. The early proinflammatory response is necessary for optimal endometrial vascularity and is, therefore, associated with a successful pregnancy. The second and most of the third trimester are antiinflammatory states, when the mother and fetus are in relative equilibrium. Exposure to infections, toxins, and environmental pollution, as well as maternal psychological stress, all affect maternal immune function and inflammation in utero (Claycombe et al, 2015). When the inflammatory response is exaggerated, as in the case of obesity, the risk of negative consequences increases, including the risk of both preterm labor and preeclampsia. The exaggerated inflammatory response may also negatively affect fetal brain development (see *New Directions:* Immune Function and Brain Development). There are also likely negative epigenetic effects (Claycombe et al, 2015).

It is still not completely clear how the immune system and pregnancy affect each other but the interaction is critical for the survival of this mother and child and, possibly, for future pregnancies. Although nutrition is likely important in affecting the inflammatory response during pregnancy, the extent of the dietary influence (Vannuccini et al, 2016), the specific dietary patterns and components (Claycombe et al, 2015), and the importance of individual differences (Bjørke-Monsen et al, 2016) are all still unknown but are currently under investigation (see Chapter 7).

Metabolic Responses

The metabolism of macronutrients changes during pregnancy. This response varies between normal weight women and women with obesity (Table 14.6).

Renal Function

The glomerular filtration rate (GFR) increases by 50% during pregnancy, although the volume of urine excreted each day is not increased. Renal plasma flow increases because of the increased GFR with lower serum creatinine and blood urea nitrogen concentrations. Renal tubular resorption is less efficient than in the nonpregnant state, and glucosuria, because of increased GFR, may occur along with increased excretion of water-soluble vitamins and amino acids. Small amounts of glucosuria increase the risk for urinary tract infections.

Placenta and Uterine Environment

The fetus is not provided nutrients and oxygen through the placenta until after blood flow is established to the placenta through

TABLE 14.6 Metabolic Changes During Pregnancy for Women of Normal Weight and Obese

Component	Normal Weight	Obese
Fat deposition with gestational weight gain	Gestational fat gain is primarily accumulated centrally, both subcutaneous and visceral fat. Visceral accumulation may increase as pregnancy progresses.	Locations are similar, amount may be less
Lipid metabolism	50% to 80% increase in basal fat oxidation and in response to glucose, marked hyperlipidemia	Hyperlipidemia is exaggerated
Amino acid metabolism	Protein synthesis increases in the second (15%) and third (25%) trimesters	Unknown, but limited evidence suggests anabolic response may be impaired
Glucose metabolism, insulin resistance	Improved fasting glucose levels, glucose tolerance and insulin sensitivity in early pregnancy, then insulin sensitivity decreases 50% to 70% by third trimester	Early fasting glucose improves less if at all, more insulin resistance, which increases serum levels of all macronutrients

Adapted from Nelson SM et al: Maternal metabolism and obesity: modifiable determinants of pregnancy outcome, *Human Reprod Update* 16:255, 2010.

the uterine spiral arteries, around 10 weeks of gestation. Before that, nourishment is through secretions from both the fallopian tubes and the endometrial glands, also known as uterine glands. The fallopian tube secretions are initially high in simple carbohydrates but become more complex farther down the tubes (Burton, 2018). These secretions are modified in response to the presence of gametes (Avilés et al, 2010) and also after fertilization (Leese et al, 2008). They include many growth factors, cytokines, and antioxidants (Ménézo et al, 2015). Animal studies have shown that many nutrients, including amino acids, potassium, and lactate, are present in concentrations higher than in maternal plasma, while glucose, pyruvate, and total protein concentrations are lower. The nutrients enter the egg through endocytosis and, in both mice and rats, a maternal diet low in protein negatively affects the growth and development of the embryo, including the cardiovascular phenotype (Leese et al, 2008). The contents of the endometrial secretions, called "uterine milk," are also not completely understood but are rich in glucose, lipids, glycoproteins, and growth factors (Burton, 2018). These secretions enter through the intervillous spaces of the placenta, going to the yolk sac and feeding the developing fetus. Whether maternal diet or obesity affects the contents of these secretions is unknown (Burton et al, 2016) but at least glycogen is stored in these glands (Jones et al, 2015). The uterine gland secretions impact uterine receptivity and blastocyst implantation (Kelleher et al, 2016). The growth factors in the secretions that stimulate placental growth may be triggered by the trophoblast itself (Burton, 2018).

Maternal nutritional status affects placental development, growth, nutrient transport, and endocrine capabilities (Burton et al, 2016). Some nutrients, including iron, iodine, zinc, folate, selenium, and vitamin A, are known to be critically important preconceptually. Optimal maternal status improves pregnancy outcomes and reduces the risk of preeclampsia, gestational diabetes mellitus (GDM), and preterm delivery possibly by improving placental functioning by reducing placental oxidative stress and inflammation (Richard et al, 2017). Other nutrients, including magnesium, appear to directly affect placental development. However, very little is known about the effects of nutritional status on the development of the placenta. Maternal BMI (both high and low), body composition, past nutritional status, current diet, fuel reserves, and epigenetics are all likely important (Burton, 2018).

Placental weight is not a useful proxy measure for placental function (Burton et al, 2016). The placenta grows throughout the pregnancy, including exponentially in the third trimester, but the growth appears to be tightly regulated (Myatt and Thornburg, 2018). Small placentas can adapt to increase nutrient transporters. However, when, how, and by how much the placenta adapts is not completely clear, nor is the reserve capacity. When the placental capacity to adapt is limited, or if the placental function is impaired, fetal development may be impaired, affecting long-term health (Burton et al, 2016). For example, the effect of GDM on placental anatomy is not fully understood but sex-specific alterations are evident that may affect nutrient transport (Castillo-Castrejon and Powell, 2017), including docosahexaenoic acid (DHA) (Léveillé et al, 2018). Whether there are independent effects of GDM and obesity is not yet clear. Obesity appears to affect the placental function in a sex-specific way, where males continue to grow and females adapt a more conservative strategy, ensuring survival (Myatt and Thornburg, 2018). High altitude also affects placental development and function (Burton et al, 2016) (Fig. 14.1).

Nutrients pass through the placenta by a variety of mechanisms. Maternal nutrient status would directly affect those transferred through diffusion or endocytosis/exocytosis. However, the transport of other nutrients can be upregulated through facilitated transport, exchange transport, and active transport (Fig. 14.2). Transport mechanisms have not yet been identified for all nutrients. In addition, the placenta can synthesize proteins for transport to the fetus and may also be a source of glucose, choline, and fatty acids (Burton et al, 2016; Nugent and Bale, 2015; Myatt and Thornburg, 2018).

The placenta is very active metabolically, consuming 80% of the oxygen it takes from maternal circulation at midgestation and 40% to 60% in late gestation (Zhang et al, 2015). It plays a dynamic role in optimizing the resource allocation between the mother and the fetus. It responds to maternal nutrient availability but paternal genes also play a role, promoting the growth of placental tissues. It is not clear if obesity alters specific nutrient transporters. The sex of the fetus/placenta is also critical and, in general, placental adaptation is greater with female offspring (Brett et al, 2014). How the mother and fetus signal each other is not yet clear. However, it is known that the fetus is not just a passive recipient of maternal nutrients but, instead, actually directs how much is transferred through the placenta, including trying to match the perceived nutrient availability. For example, there is a down-regulation of protein transfer in the case of intrauterine growth restriction (IUGR). When an abnormal situation is identified and interventions are implemented, it is unknown whether these transport mechanisms adapt to the new environment or, once set, are relatively permanent.

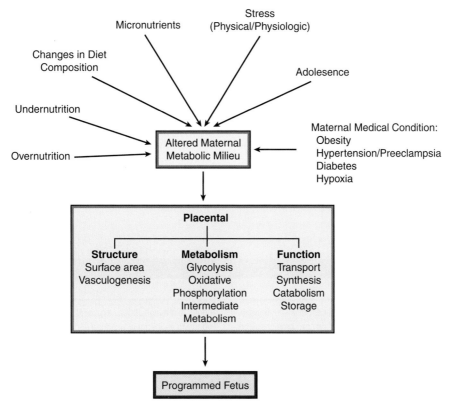

Fig. 14.1 Summary of potential stressors that can alter the placental structure and function, affecting the nutrient availability and therefore the programming of the fetus. (Adapted from Myatt L, Thornburg KL: Effects of Prenatal Nutrition and the Role of the Placenta in Health and Disease, *Methods Mol Biol* 1735: 19, 2018.)

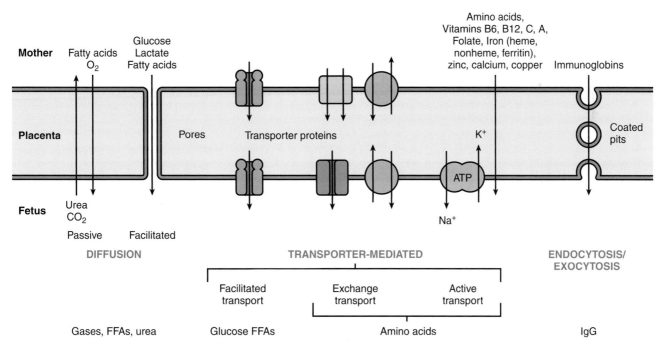

Fig. 14.2 Representation of the known processes by which materials cross the placental membrane. (Adapted from Burton GJ, Fowden AL, Thornburg KL: Placental Origins of Chronic Disease, *Physiol Rev* 96:1509, 2016; Cao C, Fleming MD: The placenta: the forgotten essential organ of iron transport, *Nutr Rev* 74:421, 2016; Grieger JA, Clifton VL: A review of the impact of dietary intakes in human pregnancy on infant birthweight, *Nutrients* 7:153, 2014; Myatt L, Thornburg KL: Effects of Prenatal Nutrition and the Role of the Placenta in Health and Disease, *Methods Mol Biol* 1735: 19, 2018; Nugent BM, Bale TL: The omniscient placenta: Metabolic and epigenetic regulation of fetal programming, *Front Neuroendocrinol* 39:28, 2015; Richard K, Holland O, Landers K et al: Review: Effects of maternal micronutrient supplementation on placental function, *Placenta* 54:38, 2017.)

The placenta produces several hormones responsible for regulating fetal growth and the development of maternal support tissues. It is the conduit for the exchange of nutrients, oxygen, and waste products. The placenta also provides a selective barrier, protecting the fetus from pathogens, teratogens, and other toxins (see Clinical Insight: Consumption of Human Placenta), but its defenses can be overwhelmed. In addition, it is now thought that the placenta may contain a unique microbiome, hypothesized to be important in the development of the fetal immune system, lowering the risk of allergies (Prince et al, 2015). It is also known now that the trophoblast invades the lymphatic system (as well as the spiral arteries and uterine veins) but whether access to the lymph triggers maternal immune tolerance is unknown (Moser et al, 2018).

Placental insults compromise the ability to nourish the fetus, regardless of how well-nourished the mother is. These insults can be the result of poor placentation from early pregnancy or small infarcts associated with preeclampsia and other hypertensive disorders. When the placenta has a reduced functional capacity for whatever reason, the result is often intrauterine growth restriction (IUGR). However, as mentioned before, the placenta also has the ability to respond to a poor environment. For example, women affected by the World War II Dutch famine in their first trimesters had larger placentas, resulting in normal weight infants (Belkacemi et al, 2010).

A less-than-optimal environment in utero can lead to a mismatch between available nutrients and the genetically determined fetal drive for growth. The goal is to support a healthy environment through a proper balance of nutrients and the avoidance of teratogens (see *Clinical Insight*: High-Risk Pregnancies with Nutritional Components).

CLINICAL INSIGHT

Consumption of Human Placenta

In many areas, women are now being offered their placentas after delivery. While some people want to save it for cultural reasons, many are now choosing to eat their placentas for many self-reported benefits. Placentophagy is promoted as a potential way to lower the risk of postpartum depression and improve infant bonding, as well as replace the iron and other nutrients lost during pregnancy and delivery. It is also promoted as a source of energy, a lactation promoter, an immune system booster, and as a way to decrease pain and bleeding after delivery (Farr et al, 2018).

Placentas do contain hormones that may be beneficial but the therapeutic effect has not been demonstrated (Young et al, 2016b; Young et al, 2018a; Young et al, 2018b). The placenta is a significant source of iron but normal consumption amounts are unlikely to make a significant difference in the postpartum iron status (Gryder et al, 2017). The placenta is a source of other nutrients as well, including selenium, protein, and cholesterol (Chang et al, 2017). However, there is wide variability between women (Young et al, 2016a).

The placenta is also a potential source of pathogens, toxins, and heavy metals, depending on prenatal exposure. Theoretically, maternal consumption could trigger alloimmunization, exposing her to genetically different cells or tissues, triggering an immune response and, therefore, harming future pregnancies (Farr et al, 2018). A recent case report cited maternal ingestion of dried placenta as a likely source of Group B strep infection in a newborn, possibly increasing maternal intestinal and skin colonization, facilitating transfer to the infant. Dried placenta powder is not sterile and when stored over 6 months, has been a source of *Paenibacillus macerans*, bacteria that produce histamine in preserved foods, potentially causing foodborne chemical intoxication (Johnson et al, 2018).

The processing is not regulated by the Food and Drug Administration (FDA) and is not standardized. The placenta must be handled carefully, including being refrigerated soon after delivery. The consumption of placenta should be discouraged if the mother or baby has a viral infection (Johnson et al, 2018) or if the mother was exposed to heavy metals during pregnancy. It should not be eaten raw, including in a smoothie. If dried and encapsulated, it should be steamed first to lower the risk of pathogen transmission.

CLINICAL INSIGHT

High-Risk Pregnancies with Nutritional Components

Approximately 10% of all pregnancies are considered "high risk," meaning there is a maternal preexisting complication or a situation that antedates pregnancy or presents in the current gestation that puts the mother or the fetus at risk for a poor outcome. Many of these may include nutritional concerns as well. Women who present with the following issues need increased medical surveillance and nutrition assessment to ensure the most favorable outcomes, controlled medical costs, and the fewest complications.

Anemias: microcytic or macrocytic

Cardiovascular issues: maternal cardiac structural defects, preexisting cardiovascular disease

Endocrine issues: polycystic ovary syndrome, thyroid disease, gestational diabetes, type 1 or 2 diabetes

Functional alterations: deafness, blindness, paralysis, paraplegia, quadriplegia

Gastrointestinal issues: food allergies, celiac disease, Crohn's disease, ulcerative colitis, postbariatric surgery, gallstones

Hyperemesis gravidarum

Hypertension: preexisting, pregnancy-induced, preeclampsia

Infections: HIV and AIDS, malaria, dental disease, intestinal parasites

Maternal genetic diseases or intellectual developmental disability

Medical problems: lupus, myasthenia gravis, cystic fibrosis, pancreatitis, phenylketonuria, cancer, sickle cell disease

Multiple fetuses

Obesity: BMI ≥30

Pica

Psychiatric: eating disorders, depression, bipolar disorders, Munchausen syndrome, suicidal ideation, substance abuse

Respiratory issues: asthma, tuberculosis, adult respiratory distress disorder

Surgeries: cancers, gallbladder, appendectomy, trauma

Young age—teenagers

AIDS, Acquired immune deficiency syndrome; *HIV*, human immunodeficiency virus.

All nutrients are thought to be important, although some are better studied than others. Table 14.1 lists some potential functions. However, more complex interactions involving multiple functions are also likely critical. For example, multiple nutrients are involved in the creation of bone (see Chapter 23) and brain (Table 14.7). When either macro- or micronutrients are lacking, the timing of the deficit is important in predicting the impact of that insult (Monk et al, 2013) When critical periods are missed, the damage will be irreversible, even if the nutrient supply later appears adequate (Georgieff et al, 2015). Nutrients known to have critical or sensitive periods include protein, LCPUFAs, glucose, iron, zinc, copper, iodine, selenium, and vitamins B_6, B_{12}, A, K, folate, and choline. In the case of fetal neurodevelopment, the younger the brain, the more it is able to recover from an insult. However, the brain is not a homogenous organ and does not develop in a single trajectory, so the specific risks depend on the region of the brain as well as the timing, dose, and duration of the perturbation (Georgieff et al, 2015; Georgieff, 2017).

Effects of Nutritional Status on Pregnancy Outcome
Fetal Growth and Development

In the early 1900s U.S. women with poor nutritional status had adverse pregnancy outcomes with hemorrhage at delivery, prolonged labor, and LBW infants, conditions still of concern today in many developing countries. Because of blockades during World War II, previously well-nourished Dutch populations were exposed to severe food restrictions for 6 months, with available rations as low as 500 kcals/day (Lumey et al, 2007). Higher rates of miscarriage (spontaneous abortion [SAB]), stillbirths, neonatal deaths, and congenital malformations were noted in offspring born to women who conceived during the famine. Surviving infants were smaller if exposed to famine late in gestation (Roseboom et al, 2011). Similar findings have been found in other countries as well. In addition, individuals may be at higher risk of undernutrition because of preexisting medical conditions or because of either physical or cultural limitations on food availability.

Even if a mother is not starving, the developing fetus may be unable to obtain optimal nutrients from someone who is compromised nutritionally, resulting in growth restriction. The causes of IUGR are many and include maternal, fetal, and placental factors (Box 14.2). Infants born with LBW (<2500 g), especially those with very LBW (<1500 g), are at higher risk for perinatal mortality (infant death occurring between 28 weeks of gestation and 4 weeks postpartum). Babies who are born with LBW may suffer from necrotizing enterocolitis, respiratory distress syndrome, intraventricular hemorrhage, cerebral palsy, or retinopathy of prematurity (see Chapter 41).

In addition to fetal growth restriction, any adverse maternal condition, including poor nutritional status, puts the fetus at risk for being delivered preterm. Prematurity leads to increased risk of neonatal morbidity and mortality, especially if the baby is also growth restricted. Preterm delivery rates are rising in developed countries and are higher in the United States than in Europe (Bloomfield, 2011). In the United States rates are highest among non-Hispanic black women, and it is unclear if early fetal developmental programming is playing a role. Preterm delivery rates are higher with ART, among both singletons and multiples, possibly explained in part by the underlying medical conditions that also increase infertility (ACOG, 2016a).

Although obesity does not predict optimal nutrition, it is somewhat protective for preterm delivery. However, prepregnant underweight, combined with low weight gain during pregnancy, has an additive effect on preterm delivery and LBW risk. Even for those women of normal weight, low weight gain doubles the risk of preterm delivery, while weight loss triples the risk (Bloomfield, 2011). Short interconceptual periods are associated with increased rates of preterm births. In a recent study, those women who were underweight, with an interconceptual period of less than 6 months, and who had inadequate weight gain had an increased risk of nearly 3.5 times, resulting in over 25% rate of preterm delivery (Lengyel et al, 2017).

TABLE 14.7 Key Nutrients for Fetal and Neonatal Brain Development

Nutrient	Function in Brain Development	Negative Effect of Deficiency
Long-chain polyunsaturated fatty acids, primarily DHA and AA	Cell membrane formation, myelin, synaptosomes, intracellular communication, signal transduction	Neurodevelopment, visual development
Protein	Neuronal and glial structural proteins, synaptic structures and numbers, neurotransmitter peptide production especially in cerebellum, hippocampus, and cerebral cortex	Overall central nervous system growth, neurodevelopment
Zinc	Cofactor in enzymes mediating protein and nucleic biochemistry, growth, gene expression, neurotransmitters, especially affecting cerebellum, limbic system, cerebral cortex, temporal lobe, frontal lobe	Attention, motor development delays, short-term memory, brain growth
Iron	Myelination, dendritogenesis, synaptogenesis, neurotransmission, especially in the hippocampus, striatum, frontal cortex	Global intelligence, general motor development, neurodevelopment, attention, memory, language, auditory recognition
Choline	Methylation, myelin, neurotransmitters, especially affecting hippocampus, septum, striatum, anterior neocortex, midposterior neocortex	Visual spatial and auditory memory in rodents (no information yet available for humans)
Copper	Iron transport, antioxidant activity, neurotransmitter synthesis, neuronal and glial energy metabolism, especially affecting cerebellum	Motor control, cognitive function
Iodine	Thyroid synthesis, neuronal synthesis, myelination	Cognitive function
Vitamin A	Structural development, antioxidant	Visual function
Folate	One-carbon metabolism	Neural tube development

Adapted from Monk C et al: Research review: maternal prenatal distress and poor nutrition—mutually influencing risk factors affecting infant neurocognitive development, *J Child Psychol Psychiatry* 54:115, 2013.

BOX 14.2   Potential Causes of Intrauterine Growth Restriction (IUGR)

Maternal Factors

Medical conditions: chronic hypertension, preeclampsia (early in gestation), diabetes, systemic lupus erythematosus, chronic kidney disease, inflammatory bowel disease, severe lung disease, cancer, hyperemesis gravidarum

Infections: syphilis, toxoplasmosis, cytomegalovirus, rubella, hepatitis B, herpes simplex virus 1 or 2, HIV-1, *Helicobacter pylori*, malaria

Malnutrition: low prepregnant weight; small maternal size; poor weight gain (especially in the last half of pregnancy); obesity (especially if combined with weight loss); nutrient deficiencies, including protein, vitamins A, B's, C, folic acid, zinc, calcium, iron; recent history of pregnancy; high parity; multiple pregnancy; history of IUGR; active eating disorders

Social conditions: very young age; poverty; lack of food because of war, famine, natural disasters (earthquake, tsunami); physical or mental abuse; substance abuse (cigarettes, alcohol, heroin, cocaine); exposure to teratogens; exposure to therapeutic medications (antimetabolites, warfarin, phenytoin)

Fetal Factors

Genetic: race, ethnicity, sex, genetic disorders

Parity: first baby often weighs less than subsequent siblings

Chromosomal anomalies: chromosomal deletions; trisomy 13, 18, 21

Congenital malformations: anencephaly, gastrointestinal atresia, Potter syndrome, pancreatic agenesis

Placental Factors

Placental insufficiency: reduced blood flow, impaired transfer of nutrients

Anatomic problems: multiple infarcts, aberrant cord insertions, umbilical vascular thrombosis and hemangiomas, premature placental separation, small placenta

Adapted from Alisi A et al: Intrauterine growth retardation and nonalcoholic fatty liver disease in children, *Int J Endocrinol* 2011:269853, 2011; Wu G et al: Biological mechanisms for nutritional regulation of maternal health and fetal development, *Paediatr Perinat Epidemiol* 26:4, 2012a.

Oxidative stress, metabolic stress, and inflammation may all be important factors in increasing risk of preterm delivery, and it appears that periconceptual malnutrition is more important than nutrition later in pregnancy. Those women who are still growing or who have eating disorders may have competition for nutrients. Supplementation with macronutrients may be helpful, but there are no preconceptual studies. Supplementation with LCPUFAs, protein, and vitamins E and C are not effective (ACOG, 2012). Although no ideal diet has been identified, one containing fruits, vegetables, whole grains, and fish has been observed to be associated with lower risk of preterm delivery. Probiotics might be helpful (Englund-Ögge et al, 2014) and smoking cessation is helpful (ACOG, 2012). Particular toxins may increase the risk of prematurity. One study found nearly double the risk of preterm delivery if women consumed more than four servings of diet soda per day (Bloomfield, 2011), although that finding has been disputed (La Vecchia, 2013). Licorice (*Glycyrrhiza glabra* root) blocks the enzyme that inactivates cortisol, and the effect on preterm delivery risk is dose-related. Similar results are seen when the mother is exposed to psychological stress (see *Clinical Insight: Stress during Pregnancy*). The role of paternal nutrition in preterm delivery risk is unexplored (Bloomfield, 2011).

The effect of poor maternal nutrition or exposure to toxins may follow the infant for decades. A very preterm, growth-restricted baby may suffer permanent brain damage. Neural tube defects (NTDs) may cause lifelong problems with mobility and bodily functions. Fetal alcohol syndrome (FAS) is a major cause of intellectual developmental disability. However, even those babies who are born with no apparent defects may suffer increased risk of chronic diseases because of a less-than-optimal prenatal environment. See Fig. 14.3 for a summary of the effects of maternal malnutrition.

Epigenetic Effects

Compromises in structural or cognitive potential may not be evident when an infant is born but may manifest later in life. A child with IUGR, often resulting from maternal hypertension or severe malnutrition or anemia, may have permanent mild neurodevelopmental cognitive abnormalities. Babies born preterm or growth restricted are more likely to have a higher risk of obesity, type 2 diabetes, hypertension, and cardiovascular disease (CVD) later in life (Simeoni et al, 2018). Those babies exposed to the Dutch famine early in gestation were at highest risk of CVD and had double the risk for schizophrenia, as well as an increased risk of stress sensitivity and breast cancer. Those

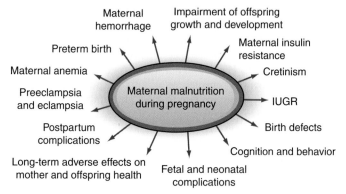

Fig. 14.3 Major negative effects of maternal malnutrition (both under- and overnutrition) on mother and infant.

exposed midpregnancy were three times more likely to develop microalbuminuria and decreased creatinine clearance, as well as having an increased risk for obstructive airway disease; growth restriction was common among those affected in the later trimesters (Roseboom et al, 2011; Matusiak et al, 2014).

Girls born preterm are more likely to deliver preterm with their own pregnancies and more likely to develop anorexia nervosa (Bloomfield, 2011). Immune function, learning ability, mental health, cancer, and aging are likely affected by LBW. Functional neural pathways controlling appetite and satiety likely develop in the third trimester, so preterm infants may experience disruptions in their development.

Those babies born large for gestational age (LGA) or exposed to maternal hyperglycemia or maternal obesity are at increased risk of chronic diseases, likely through multiple mechanisms (see *Focus On: Special Case of Obesity*).

Birth weight may not be the only predictor for the propensity for adult disease. Exposure to high folate during pregnancy is associated with insulin resistance and obesity in later life if combined with low vitamin B_{12} levels, and increased rates of cancer are associated with supraphysiologic intakes of methyl donors (Milagro et al, 2013; see Chapter 6). Maternal and paternal nutritional imbalances are likely to increase the risk of metabolic syndrome (DelCurto et al, 2013).

Exposure to endocrine-disrupting chemicals (substances found in the environment that interfere with the synthesis, metabolism, or action of the body's hormones) may modify gene expression and the effects, including increased risk of obesity, insulin resistance, and type 2 diabetes, may be nonlinear (i.e., low doses may be more harmful than high doses) (Barouki et al, 2012). In one study, mothers who ate an unbalanced high-protein diet (1 pound red meat/day, no carbohydrate) during late pregnancy produced offspring who experienced higher cortisol levels when exposed to stress as adults (Bloomfield, 2011).

This developmental plasticity can be helpful. However, when there is a mismatch between in utero programming and the later environment, the risk of chronic disease rises. A fetus may develop a "thrifty phenotype," adapting to poor nutritional conditions by being more efficient in acquiring and conserving energy. However, when later exposed to an environment with higher availability, this "thrifty" adaptation may predispose the offspring to the diseases of affluence, including obesity and type 2 diabetes. In addition, harm may also be caused by overcompensation later with excessive catch-up growth. Altered organ structure, cell numbers, and metabolic functioning, including premature aging of tissues, all appear important (Burton et al, 2016).

Exposure of the embryo or fetus to specific maternal nutrients, as well as environmental contaminants, can turn the imprinting genes that control growth and development on or off, but the amounts, timing, and effects are still being investigated. Paternal nutrient imbalance and gene-environment interactions are also likely important (Barouki et al, 2012; DelCurto et al, 2013). Although the concept of the DOHaD originally focused on undernutrition, overnutrition also is being studied. Effects of macro- and micronutrients, as well as phytonutrients and hypoxia, are being examined, primarily through animal studies so far, and the ideal maternal and paternal diet for epigenetic effects has not yet been established (Vanhees et al, 2014). It appears that the epigenetic effect of preconceptual obesity is stronger for maternal than paternal obesity (Godfrey et al, 2017b). However, the paternal diet before conception does appear to affect the offspring epigenetically and there is evidence that the sperm epigenome is rapidly remodeled after weight loss following bariatric surgery (Block and El-Osta, 2017). Parental diet, body composition, metabolism, and stress exposure all appear important, but the effects are sex-specific. Mechanisms include epigenetic, cellular, physiologic, and metabolic changes (Fleming et al, 2018).

New research also is focusing on the grandchildren of people affected by the Dutch famine (Roseboom et al, 2011) to document the long-term epigenetic effects (Fig. 14.4). Preliminary results show that under- and overnutrition are important issues, but there are differences in response by sex, and the timing of the insult matters (Vanhees et al, 2014; Preston et al, 2018).

The preconceptual nutritional role in altering the epigenome is still being actively explored. Animal research shows components of a preconceptual diet may resolve toxicant epigenetic changes (Owen et al, 2013). Maternal and paternal weight and nutritional status, as well as that of previous generations, are likely important in affecting, and being affected by, genetic variations. Because of the increased appreciation for the periconceptual effects on the lifetime health of the offspring, there are calls for much better guidance and parental preparation before conception (Fleming et al, 2018) (see Chapter 6).

Nutrient Requirements During Pregnancy

Nutrition during pregnancy often is equated with weight gain because weight is most easily and consistently measured. However, maternal weight gain is not necessarily predictive of health outcomes, especially for heavier women. In general, although the mother needs to eat a little more when she is pregnant or breastfeeding, she needs to eat more carefully because most nutrient requirements increase more during pregnancy and lactation than do the calorie requirements (Fig. 14.5). The U.S. dietary reference intakes (DRIs) are found on the inside cover. Estimated requirements during pregnancy and lactation vary between countries (see additional information on the Evolve website for recommendations from WHO and 16 governments or regions worldwide) but there is a call to improve the consistency in the development of these values across cultures (National Academies of Sciences, Engineering, and Medicine, 2018). For most nutrients, there is little guidance by trimester or for pregnancies with more than one fetus.

Energy

Additional energy is required during pregnancy to support the metabolic demands of pregnancy and fetal growth. Metabolism increases by an average of 15% in the singleton pregnancy, but with wide variability especially in the third trimester. The DRI for energy increases by only 340 kcal/day during the second trimester and by 452 kcal/day in the third trimester. If maternal weight gain is within the desirable limits, the range of acceptable energy intakes varies widely, given large individual differences in energy output and basal metabolic rate. Modifying intakes to achieve recommended weight gain (see Pregnancy Weight Gain Recommendations) is more useful than calculating caloric requirements.

Exercise. Energy expended in voluntary physical activity is the largest variable in overall energy expenditure. Physical activity increases energy expenditure proportional to body weight. However, most pregnant women compensate for increased weight gain by slowing their

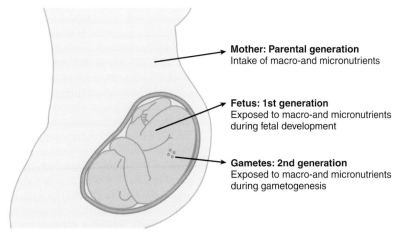

Fig. 14.4 Transgenerational inheritance of epigenetic modifications induced by exposure to macro- and micronutrients. (Adapted from Vanhees K, Vonhögen IG, van Schooten FJ et al: You are what you eat, and so are your children: the impact of micronutrients on the epigenetic programming of offspring, *Cell Mol Life Sci* 71:271, 2014.)

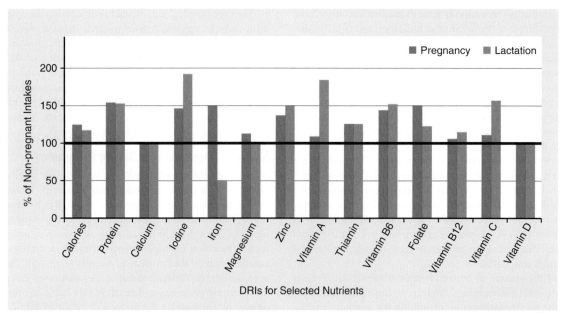

Fig. 14.5 Percent of nonpregnant DRIs for selected nutrients for pregnancy and lactation. Calculations are based on a 25-year-old woman (65 inches, 126 pounds prepregnant weight), pregnant with a singleton in the third trimester and lactation in the first 6 months.

work and movement pace. Therefore total daily energy expenditure may not be substantially greater than before pregnancy.

The ACOG recommends at least 20 to 30 minutes of moderate intensity exercise on most, if not all, days for pregnant women without contraindications (ACOG, 2015a). Short duration strenuous exercise appears unconcerning, but the impact of long duration strenuous exercise on the fetus is unknown (Szymanski and Satin, 2012). Elite athletes may need to modify their exercise routines (Bø et al, 2018). Excessive exercise, combined with inadequate energy intake, may lead to suboptimal maternal weight gain and poor fetal growth. Therefore a pregnant woman should always discuss exercise with her health practitioner. Although there is limited evidence that exercise helps modify gestational weight gain, there is also no evidence of harm and in observational studies exercise has been associated with lower risk of gestational diabetes, pregnancy-induced hypertension, and preeclampsia (Seneviratne et al, 2015). The effect of maternal exercise on offspring susceptibility to chronic diseases is being explored in animal research but results are mixed and the type, timing, intensity, and dose of optimal exercise are all unknowns (Blaize et al, 2015). However, not all epigenetic effects may be positive. There is limited evidence that excessive paternal exercise is associated with an offspring's thrifty phenotype (Dhasarathy et al, 2017).

Protein

Additional protein is required to support the synthesis of maternal and fetal tissues. This demand increases throughout gestation and is maximized during the third trimester. Caution is advised when reading the DRI tables. The baseline protein RDA of 0.8 g/kg current body weight/day for pregnant women is 46 g only for someone with a prepregnant weight of 126 pounds. The protein calculation in the first half of pregnancy is the same as that for nonpregnant women but the required intake increases as weight increases. The RDA calculation increases in the second half of pregnancy to 1.1 gm/kg current body weight/day. This would be 71 g/day only for that same reference woman who is also gaining weight appropriately. For many women, the protein requirement

is higher. For each additional fetus, the Institute of Medicine (IOM) recommends an additional 50 g/day starting in the second trimester (Otten et al, 2006), but because protein is also used as an energy source, the total may be as much as 175 g/day for the normal-weight woman carrying a twin gestation who is consuming 3500 kcal/day (Goodnight and Newman, 2009).

The WHO uses slightly different calculations. They also calculate a baseline requirement using current body weight. However, the estimates of increased needs are presented as standard amounts/day for everyone. The 2007 recommendations are designed to support a total 13.8 kg weight gain. However, some researchers recommend the older (1985) and more conservative guidelines (Millward, 2012) (Table 14.8).

There is concern that nitrogen balance studies may underestimate protein needs, especially when considering that the increased requirements of specific amino acids may be disproportionately higher according to animal research (Elango and Ball, 2016). There is some call to increase protein requirements, including increasing the protein intake earlier in pregnancy. Recent research found optimal intake was 1.2 g/kg/day at 16 weeks and 1.52 g/kg/day at 36 weeks when estimated by indicator amino acid oxidation. However, the method is not universally accepted and further research is necessary. Protein deficiency during pregnancy has adverse consequences, including poor fetal growth. Protein also is involved in the synthesis of hormones and neurotransmitters. Limited intakes of protein and energy usually occur together, making it difficult to separate the effects of energy deficiency from those of protein deficiency. Although most women in the United States likely eat more than enough protein, there are some for whom particular attention must be paid, including those consuming a vegetarian diet, those who are still growing themselves, or those who are pregnant with multiples. The optimal balance of protein to total calories has yet to be determined and recommendations, as well as intakes, vary across cultures (Blumfield and Collins, 2014). Caution is advised when considering very high protein supplements. Intakes at the high end of the acceptable macronutrient distribution ranges (AMDR) (i.e., 30% to 35% of calories from protein) have been associated with an increased risk of poor fetal growth in some

TABLE 14.8 Protein Intake Recommendations

	Prepregnancy	First Trimester	Second Trimester	Third Trimester	Notes
U.S. DRIs	0.8 g/kg current body weight/day	0.8 g/kg current weight/day	1.1 g/kg current weight/day starting in the second half of pregnancy	1.1 g/kg current weight/day	
WHO, 2007	0.83 g/kg current body weight/day	Baseline + 0.7 g/day	Baseline + 9.6 g/day	Baseline + 31.2 g/day	
WHO, 1985	0.83 g/kg current body weight/day	Baseline + 1.2 g/day	Baseline + 6.1 g/day	Baseline + 10.7 g/day	Average increase 6 g/day above baseline requirements

Adapted from Millward DJ: Identifying recommended dietary allowances for protein and amino acids: a critique of the 2007 WHO/FAO/UNU report, *Br J Nutr* 108(Suppl 2):S3, 2012.

studies, although the mechanism is unclear. Current U.S. practice often targets protein intakes at 20% of total calories, possibly higher for multiples. WHO recommends 23% of calories come from protein (Millward, 2012). Supplementation, if necessary, should be done with food rather than with protein supplements. For example, someone consuming 2240 kcal from 6 cups/day of 2% milk, 8 oz of meat, six servings of starch, three vegetable servings, two fruit servings, and six fat servings gets 23% of calories from protein (128 g). If using skim milk, the total is 1970 kcal with 26% from protein.

Carbohydrates

The RDA for carbohydrates increases slightly, helping maintain appropriate blood glucose and prevent ketosis. Intakes may be greater in women consuming more calories, but careful carbohydrate choices are needed to include all the daily nutrients for pregnancy. Priority should be given to complex carbohydrates from whole grains, fruits, and vegetables rather than just simple sugars, including refined liquid sugars, whether natural (juices) or industrially produced (soda).

Fiber

Daily consumption of whole-grain breads and cereals, leafy green and yellow vegetables, and fresh and dried fruits should be encouraged to provide additional minerals, vitamins, and fiber. The DRI for fiber during pregnancy is 14 g/day/1000 kcal and, if met, will help a great deal in managing the constipation that often accompanies pregnancy.

Lipids

As with nonpregnant women, there is no DRI for total lipids during pregnancy. The amount of fat in the diet should depend on energy requirements for proper weight gain. However, recommendations for omega-6 polyunsaturated fatty acid (PUFA) (linoleic acid) and omega-3 PUFA (alpha-linolenic acid) increase slightly. Although not a DRI, the recommended intake of DHA is 200 mg/day and can be met by one to two portions of fish per week (Carlson et al, 2017) (see *Focus On: Omega-3 Fatty Acids in Pregnancy and Lactation*).

Vitamins

All vitamins and minerals are needed for optimal pregnancy outcome. In some instances requirements may be met through diet. For others a supplement, started preconceptually, is often necessary. Many, but not all, vitamin and mineral recommendations increase with pregnancy, but the magnitude of the increase varies by nutrient (see the DRI tables on the inside cover and Fig. 14.5).

Folate. The RDA for dietary folate equivalents increases to support maternal erythropoiesis, DNA synthesis, and fetal and placental growth. Low folate levels are associated with miscarriages, LBW, and preterm birth. Early maternal folate deficiency is associated with an increased incidence of congenital malformations, including NTDs, orofacial clefts, and congenital heart defects (Obeid et al, 2013). Approximately 3000 new cases of NTDs occur in the United States annually and over 300,000 babies are born worldwide with NTDs (CDC, 2018a), but prevalence varies widely, from 6.9/10,000 births in the Western Pacific to 21.9/10,000 births in the Middle East (ACOG, 2017b). Although spina bifida and anencephaly are the most common, other NTDs can also occur (Table 14.9). The neural tube closes by 28 days of gestation, before most women realize they are pregnant. In addition, more than half of all U.S. pregnancies are unplanned. Therefore the CDC recommends that all women of childbearing age, in anticipation of possible pregnancy, increase their intake of folic acid by 400 mcg/day, the synthetic version that is available in supplements and fortified foods, especially some breakfast cereals (CDC, 2018a). The U.S. Preventive Services Task Force (USPSTF) recommends 400 to 800 mcg/day of folic acid preconceptually. Women who have had a previous NTD-affected pregnancy should consume 400 mcg/day when not planning to conceive and those planning pregnancy should consider 4000 mcg/day (4 mg/day) from 3 months before to 3 months after conception (ACOG, 2017b). Other situations that may merit the higher supplementation levels include women who have an NTD themselves, whose partner has an NTD, or whose partner has a previously affected child. These higher doses should be taken as a separate supplement and not as part of a multivitamin supplement to avoid excess intakes of other nutrients in the multivitamin. Although this level is recommended by many medical providers, there are calls to reevaluate these higher recommendations because of evidence that the lower doses may be equally effective in preventing recurrent NTDs (Dolin et al, 2018). Supplementation recommendations vary by country (Moussa et al, 2016) and may take the genetic susceptibility to low folate status into account (Colson et al, 2017) so local guidelines should be followed. Although the 800-mcg dose achieves recommended blood levels in 4 weeks, the 400-mcg dose requires 8 to 12 weeks to reach these levels (Berti et al, 2011). Also available is 5-methyltetrahydrofolate, the primary circulating form of folate. It is proposed to be better used, especially by those with polymorphisms (see Chapter 6), and without the detrimental rise in unmetabolized folic acid. However, its role in preventing NTDs or other birth defects is untested in clinical trials (Obeid et al, 2013). In addition, concern about unmetabolized folic acid may be unwarranted in some cases, as it was found to be undetectable if pregnant women took 400 mcg/day throughout the pregnancy, in addition to consuming 100 mcg/day from fortified grains, even among those with the C677T polymorphism

TABLE 14.9 Neural Tube Defects

Neural Tube Defect	Malformation
Cranial	
Anencephaly	Failure of fusion of cephalic portion of neural folds; absence of all or part of brain, skull, and skin
Encephalocele	Failure of complete skull formation; extrusion of brain tissue into membranous sac
Exencephaly	Failure of scalp and skull formation; exteriorization of abnormally formed brain
Iniencephaly	Defect of cervical and upper thoracic vertebrae; abnormally formed brain tissue and extreme retroflexion of upper spine
Spinal	
Craniorachischisis	Coexisting anencephaly and open neural tube defect, often in the cervical–thoracic region
Holorachischisis	Failure of fusion of vertebral arches; entire spinal cord exposed
Meningocele	Failure of fusion of caudal portion of neural tube; meninges exposed
Myelomeningocele	Failure of fusion of caudal portion of neural tube; meninges and neural tissue exposed
Myeloschisis	Failure of fusion of caudal portion of neural tube; flattened mass of neural tissue exposed
Spina bifida	Failure of fusion of caudal portion of neural tube, usually of 3-5 contiguous vertebrae; spinal cord or meninges, or both, exposed to amniotic fluid

Adapted from American College of Obstetricians and Gynecologists Committee on Practice Bulletins-Obstetrics: Practice Bulletin No. 187: Neural Tube Defects, *Obstet Gynecol* 130:e279, 2017b.

(Pentieva et al, 2016). The impact of higher doses of folic acid causing higher, and concerning, levels of unmetabolized folic acid is not well-established but is being studied (Plumptre et al, 2015).

Red blood cell folate levels exceeding 906 nmol/L (400 ng/mL) have been associated with the fewest NTDs (Obeid et al, 2013), although the mechanism of folic acid is still unknown (ACOG, 2017b). Natural folate is less bioavailable and has not been shown to raise blood levels as well as the synthetic folic acid or to lower the risk of NTDs. Although theoretically natural folate could be effective, 6 to 12 cups of raw spinach (more than 2 cups cooked) daily is the bioequivalent level of natural folate that is found in one bowl of fortified breakfast cereal. Look for 100% of the daily value/serving.

Women who are obese or who smoke, consume alcohol moderately or heavily, or use recreational drugs are at risk for marginal folate status, as are those with malabsorption syndromes or genetic differences related to methylation and the metabolic use of dietary folate, including the estimated 11% of the U.S. population with the MTHFR 677 C to T variation (Caudill, 2010). European prevalence is estimated to be 10% to 22% (Obeid et al, 2013), but not all populations with the C677T polymorphism show higher rates of NTDs (ACOG, 2017b). Other polymorphisms are also being investigated for increased risk for NTDs. Although increased folate intake may be helpful in some situations, added riboflavin also may be beneficial (see Chapters 5 and 6).

Women using antiseizure medications must be monitored closely when starting folic acid because it can reduce their seizure control.

Enriched grain products in the United States are fortified with folic acid and are estimated to provide an average 200 mcg/day, with resulting higher blood folate levels and reduced (19% to 54%) NTD rates (Caudill, 2010). However, with the increased popularity of the low carbohydrate diets, estimated intake has been reduced recently and is associated with increased risk of NTDs (Desrosiers et al, 2018). Because NTD rates remain higher among the Hispanic population in the United States, fortification of corn masa flour is now approved by the FDA but implementation is voluntary and not widespread.

Over 70 countries now fortify grain products but this fortification is not universally practiced because of concerns about exposing the entire population to extra folic acid. Possible adverse effects of increased folic acid intake include masking of vitamin B_{12} deficiency, tumor promotion, epigenetic hypermethylation, interference with antifolate treatments, and an increase in miscarriages and multiple births. Widespread problems have not been seen. However, high intakes of folic acid also have potential epigenetic effects, but data are fragmentary and sometimes conflicting. Caution is advised with the use of pharmacologic doses. For example, although some studies have seen no negative effects on DNA methylation at doses up to 4000 mcg/day (Crider et al, 2011), other studies have found that, in the context of low vitamin B_{12} status, supplementing pregnant women with just 500 mcg/day was associated with an increased risk of diabetes among the women (Paul and Selhub, 2017) and of offspring adiposity and insulin resistance at age 6 (Yajnik et al, 2008).

On the other hand, adequate folic acid in the second trimester may decrease inflammation, and folate status is associated inversely with the severity of bacterial vaginosis, a documented risk factor for preterm delivery (Dunlop et al, 2011). Murine studies have found that the negative effect of maternal exposure to bisphenol-A is effectively neutralized by maternal supplementation with folic acid, betaine, and choline (Guéant et al, 2013). Supplementation with methyl donors, such as folic acid, also may reduce the harmful effects of fumonisin (a mycotoxin produced by *Fusarium* molds that grow on agricultural commodities, especially corn, that has been associated with increased risk of NTDs) contamination. Spermatozoid folate deficiency among men exposed to dioxins may increase the risk of spina bifida in their offspring. Supplementation during early pregnancy (at least 800 mcg/day) may reduce the risk of autism spectrum disorders after prenatal exposure to pesticides (Schmidt et al, 2017).

While folic acid supplementation does not completely eliminate the risk of NTDs, up to 70% of NTDs could be prevented with the periconceptual use of 400 mcg folic acid/day (ACOG, 2017b). Optimal levels of other methyl donors (B_2, B_6, B_{12}, and choline) and inositol may also lower the risk of NTDs and improve birth weight. There is speculation that paternal folate deficiency might also explain part of the residual risk of NTDs (Guéant et al, 2013).

Vitamin B_6. Pyridoxine functions as a cofactor for many decarboxylase and transaminase enzymes, especially those involved in amino acid metabolism. Although this vitamin catalyzes a number of reactions involving neurotransmitter production, it is not known whether this function is involved in the relief of nausea and vomiting. Because meat, fish, and poultry are good dietary sources, deficiency is not common, and routine prenatal vitamins contain sufficient amounts (Hovdenak and Haram, 2012). Regarding nausea and vomiting, standard doses of 10-25 mg three to four times per day (ACOG, 2018b) have questionable efficacy but do not appear to be dangerous.

Vitamin B_{12}. Cobalamin is required for enzyme reactions and for generation of methionine and tetrahydrofolate. It is important in growth and development, including immune function (Wu et al, 2012a).

Vitamin B_{12} is naturally found exclusively in foods of animal origin, so vegetarians, especially vegans, are at risk for dietary vitamin B_{12} deficiency and should consume fortified foods or supplements. Also at risk are those people with malabsorption, including those with Crohn's disease involving the terminal ileum, women who have had gastric bypass surgery, and those using proton pump inhibitor medications (see Chapters 26 and 27). People taking metformin also may be at risk. Deficiencies in folate and vitamin B_{12} have been related to depression in adults. Inadequate amounts of folate and B_{12} may negatively affect infant cognitive and motor development as well as increase the risk of NTDs and inadequate fetal growth.

Choline. Choline is needed for structural integrity of cell membranes, cell signaling, and nerve impulse transmission and is a major source of methyl groups. Choline and folate are metabolically interrelated. Both support fetal brain development and lower risk of NTDs and orofacial clefts (Zeisel, 2013). Animal studies show choline is neuroprotective after prenatal alcohol exposure (Blusztajn et al, 2017). Maternal supplementation during the third trimester was recently seen in a small study to improve the offspring's information processing speed (Caudill et al, 2018). While 480 mg/day was helpful, 930 mg/day produced larger effects. Preliminary animal data shows prenatal supplementation with choline may be helpful in minimizing the harm caused by iron deficiency by helping restore some of the neural plasticity (Georgieff et al, 2015). Choline also appears to be important in placental functioning, including playing a role in the remodeling of the spiral arteries, and may affect maternal and fetal responses to stress. The DRI for choline increases slightly during pregnancy and there are calls for it to be reexamined and possibly raised (Caudill et al, 2018). Genetic variations and concurrent intakes of folate and methionine may affect requirements, and de novo synthesis may not meet fetal and maternal needs (Zeisel, 2013). Choline-rich foods include milk, meat, and egg yolks, and women not eating these foods may need supplementation (see Appendix 32). Many popular prenatal supplements do not contain choline or, if so, contain very little (25 to 50 mg) (Zeisel et al, 2018). Large supplemental doses may cause GI discomfort, but a small study using 750 mg during pregnancy did not identify adverse effects (Zeisel, 2013).

Vitamin C. The DRI for vitamin C increases during pregnancy and may be even higher for those who smoke, abuse alcohol or drugs, or regularly take aspirin. Daily consumption of good food sources should be encouraged. Low plasma levels are associated with preterm labor (Dror and Allen, 2012), possibly because of its antioxidant function or its role in collagen synthesis. However, supplemental vitamin C is not recommended for the prevention of premature rupture of membranes (PROM). Previously supplementation with vitamin C (1000 mg) along with vitamin E (400 IU) was promoted for the possible prevention of preeclampsia. However, it is not currently recommended (ACOG, 2013c) and actually may increase risk of gestational hypertension and PROM. Vitamin C is actively transported across the placenta, so there is also potential for excessive levels in the fetus (Dror and Allen, 2012).

Vitamin A. Vitamin A is critical during periods of rapid growth and important in cellular differentiation, ocular development, immune function, and lung development and maturity as well as gene expression (Wu et al, 2012a). Low vitamin A levels are associated with IUGR and increased risk of maternal and neonatal mortality, possibly due to the protective role of carotenoids against oxidative stress (Zielińska et al, 2017). Malformations are seen in animals exposed to deficiencies, but confirmation of human malformations has not been well-established. However, a recent case report demonstrated that vitamin A deficiency following bariatric surgery resulted in recurrent fetal and neonatal losses, with preterm delivery, pulmonary hypoplasia, and

microphthalmia in the surviving fetuses (Mackie et al, 2018). Among women positive for human immunodeficiency virus (HIV), improved vitamin A status is associated with improved birth weight, possibly by improving immunity (Hovdenak and Haram, 2012).

Excess preformed vitamin A is teratogenic, so high intake is of most concern in the first trimester. Supplementation is usually not necessary and is often limited to 5000 IU/day, although doses up to 10,000 IU/day are not associated with increased risk of malformations (Hovdenak and Haram, 2012). The acne medication isotretinoin is a vitamin A analog, and exposed fetuses are at extremely high risk for fetal anomalies and miscarriages. Women should stop its use for at least 1 month before conception. Other retinoids (etretinate, acitretin) would also be of concern (Harris et al, 2017). Beta-carotene is not associated with birth defects.

Although no cases have been seen, theoretically someone eating liver could consume as much preformed vitamin A as has been associated with fetal anomalies, so large amounts of liver, liver pâté, and liverwurst or braunschweiger are not recommended in the first trimester. Although guidance from some countries recommends avoiding liver throughout pregnancy because of its vitamin A content, ACOG does not. The vitamin A content of the livers from different animals varies considerably. Acute vitamin A poisoning has been documented with the livers from seals, whales, polar bears, and multiple species of saltwater fish, especially from the tropics (Dewailly et al, 2011). All of these livers should be avoided. Fish liver oils (halibut, shark, and cod) are also very high in vitamin A and should be avoided (McLaren and Kraemer, 2012). Livers from sheep and ox contain very high levels, as do all livers of animals fed feedstuffs fortified with vitamin A and all should be avoided (Scotter et al, 1992). Using data from the current U.S. Department of Agriculture (USDA) food composition tables, both veal and moose livers should be avoided. Livers from ringed seal and turkey should be very limited. Livers from other animals generally have lower vitamin A contents. Quantities eaten should be limited. Check your local food composition databases for details on the livers most commonly consumed in your area.

Vitamin D. According to the IOM, vitamin D requirements do not increase during pregnancy and intakes of 600 IU/day (15 mcg/day) are sufficient when considering bone health. The few dietary sources of vitamin D are salmon and other fatty fish, as well as some fortified breakfast cereals and mushrooms exposed to UV light, and seal and whale blubber and polar bear liver (Holick, 2017). Not all dairy products are fortified, but liquid milk is a good source, usually containing 100 IU/8 oz (see Appendix 38).

Vitamin D deficiency is recognized increasingly in dark-skinned and veiled women living in latitudes where sun exposure is low. Women who are at risk of entering pregnancy with low vitamin D levels also include those with BMI more than 30, those with fat malabsorption, and those with high use of sunblock, along with poor dietary intake. Screening for vitamin D status is advised for those women (ACOG, 2011).

Severe vitamin D deficiency is associated with congenital rickets and newborn fractures and also may manifest as seizures, although it is unknown if calcium insufficiency also plays a role (Brannon and Picciano, 2011). There is concern that low maternal vitamin D status may negatively affect fetal bone accrual. However, small studies have shown that although maternal supplementation can increase cord blood levels, there is no effect on fetal calcium, phosphorus, parathyroid hormone (PTH), or skeletal parameters (Kovacs, 2012). A recent study found no association between maternal vitamin D status and her offspring's bone mineral content at ages 9 to 10 years (Lawlor et al, 2013).

Vitamin D metabolism changes in pregnancy, with the conversion of 25(OH)D to 1,25(OH)$_2$D drastically increased (Hollis and Wagner, 2017). 1,25(OH)$_2$D levels are 2 to 3 times nonpregnant levels by 12 weeks of gestation and keep rising throughout the pregnancy, depending on 25(OH)D availability. These levels are not associated with hypercalciuria or hypercalcemia and appear to be driven by the pregnancy itself rather than by increasing vitamin D-binding protein levels. Mechanisms are still unknown but likely include an uncoupling of renal 1-alpha-hydroxylase from feedback control and upregulating it twofold to fivefold for reasons other than calcium homeostasis (Kovacs, 2012). It is assumed that high 1,25(OH)$_2$D values increase delivery of vitamin D to maternal tissues and may modulate innate and adaptive immunity, including possibly an immunomodulatory role in preventing fetal rejection. Vitamin D may be important in regulating gene expression and in promoting successful implantation so preconceptual levels, and therefore supplementation, may be important (Hollis and Wagner, 2017). It also may have a role in preventing preeclampsia, preterm delivery, gestational diabetes, bacterial vaginosis, and the need for cesarean delivery. In addition, it may be involved in the development of the infant's immune function and development of allergy as well as other developmental programming (Brannon and Picciano, 2011), including risk of type 1 diabetes (Kovacs, 2012). However, associations are inconclusive, often contradictory and confounded, and lack causality. Although supplementation raises maternal vitamin D levels, it has not been consistently associated with improved obstetric outcomes (Roth et al, 2017). However, a recent trial found that women who achieved blood concentrations of at least 40 ng/mL had at least a 60% lower risk of preterm delivery and that the risk reduction was 78% among nonwhite women (McDonnell et al, 2017). Optimal serum levels of 25(OH)D during pregnancy are not yet known but must be at least 20 ng/mL (50 nmol/L) for bone health (ACOG, 2011). Other experts suggest serum levels at least 32 ng/mL (80 nmol/L) is better for pregnancy and it has been proposed that optimal levels of 1,25(OH)$_2$D and, therefore, optimal fetal outcomes can be achieved only with blood levels of 40 ng/mL (100 nmol/L) (Hollis and Wagner, 2017). Others propose even higher levels (Heyden and Wimalawansa, 2018). On the other hand, increased risk of growth restriction at levels exceeding 70 nmol/L and child eczema at levels exceeding 75 nmol/L also have been reported (Brannon and Picciano, 2011). Research is active and ongoing and debate is vigorous. Vitamin D supplementation may be needed to reach desired serum concentrations, although there is insufficient evidence to recommend routine supplementation and WHO recommends against it (Roth et al, 2017). A dose of 1000 to 2000 IU/day of vitamin D appears safe (ACOG, 2011). Although some researchers have found no hypercalciuria with 4000 IU/day (the tolerable upper intake level [UL]), caution is advised. In those studies, only spot checks of urine were done, not 24-hour urine collections, and there was no long-term follow-up on kidney stone formation rates (Kovacs, 2012). Very high supplementation (≥1000 mcg = 40,000 IU/day) has been associated with hypercalcemia, and although vitamin D does not appear to be teratogenic in the doses usually given, some animal data suggest the need for concern (Roth, 2011). The potency of vitamin D supplements is variable and many contain less than the labeled amounts (LeBlanc et al, 2013).

Current data is inconsistent, with small, low quality studies. In an attempt to answer critical questions, many trials are planned or are currently ongoing. In addition to determining the optimal serum levels, the optimal timing of supplementation and the effect of different lifestyles, body types, baseline status, the role of the placenta, and genotypes (both maternal and fetal) are all currently unknown (Hollis and Wagner, 2017; Størdal et al, 2017).

Vitamin E. Vitamin E requirements do not increase. Although deficiency is speculated to cause miscarriage, preterm birth, preeclampsia, and IUGR, vitamin E deficiency specifically has not yet been reported in human pregnancy. Vitamin E is an important lipophilic antioxidant, but supplementation of vitamin E (along with vitamin C) is not an effective strategy for preventing preeclampsia nor does it reduce risk of fetal or neonatal loss, SGA, or preterm delivery. Supplementation actually may be proinflammatory, preventing the switch from Th1 cytokines (proinflammatory) to Th2 cytokines (antiinflammatory) that is normal during pregnancy (Hovdenak and Haram, 2012; see Appendix 36 for food sources of vitamin E).

Vitamin K. Although vitamin K requirements do not increase during pregnancy, usual diets often do not provide sufficient vitamin K, as most food sources (e.g., dark leafy green vegetables) are not consumed in recommended amounts. Vitamin K has an important role in bone health as well as in coagulation homeostasis, so adequate amounts during pregnancy are vital (see Chapter 23). Vitamin K deficiency has been reported in women who have had hyperemesis gravidarum, Crohn's disease, or gastric bypass, and a case report describes a deficiency associated with intrahepatic cholestasis of pregnancy (Maldonado et al, 2017). See Appendix 37 for sources of vitamin K.

Minerals

Calcium. Hormonal factors strongly influence calcium metabolism in pregnancy. Human placental lactogen modestly increases the rate of maternal bone turnover. Although estrogen inhibits bone resorption, accretion and resorption increase. Maternal absorption of calcium across the gut doubles during pregnancy (Kovacs, 2016). PTH often drops in North American and European women consuming adequate calcium. In areas with lower calcium diets that are also rich in phytates, PTH levels stay the same or increase and more research is necessary on the limitations of maternal response when intakes are marginal or low (Olausson et al, 2012). These changes maintain maternal serum calcium levels and promote calcium retention to meet progressively increasing fetal skeletal demands for mineralization. Fetal hypercalcemia and subsequent endocrine adjustments ultimately stimulate the mineralization process. The placenta appears to protect the developing fetus unless there is maternal hypocalcemia with severe hypoparathyroidism (Kovacs, 2015).

The net effects of pregnancy and lactation on the maternal skeleton are not yet clear. Bone mineral is mobilized during pregnancy and replenished starting in later lactation. The degree of bone changes varies considerably by site and also between individuals. It appears that genetics, endocrine responses, and nutritional factors are all important. No prospective studies have examined whether there is increased risk of osteoporosis later in life attributed to pregnancy or lactation and retrospective studies are inconsistent. Higher intakes are associated with improved calcium balance when intakes are low, but some evidence suggests that supplementation may temporarily disrupt the process of adaptation to habitually low intakes (Olausson et al, 2012).

Approximately 30 g of calcium is accumulated during pregnancy, primarily in the fetal skeleton (25 g), but there is wide variation. The remainder is stored in the maternal skeleton, held in reserve for the calcium demands of lactation. Most fetal accretion occurs during the last half of pregnancy, increasing from 50 mg/day at 20 weeks of gestation to 330 mg/day at 35 weeks (Olausson et al, 2012). There is conflicting evidence regarding whether maternal calcium intake affects a child's long-term accretion.

In addition to its role in bone formation, low calcium intake is associated with increased risk of IUGR and preeclampsia (Hovdenak and Haram, 2012). Calcium also is involved in many other processes, including blood clotting, intracellular proteolysis, and nitric oxide synthesis, and it has a role in regulating uterine contractions (Wu et al, 2012a).

The requirement for calcium during pregnancy does not increase. However, many women enter pregnancy with low intakes and often need encouragement to increase consumption of calcium-rich foods. Dairy products are the most common sources of dietary calcium.

Milk, including extra dry milk powder, can be incorporated into foods. One-third cup of dried skim milk is equivalent to 1 cup of fluid milk. Small amounts can be added to liquid milk while much more can be added to foods with stronger flavors. Although most of the dry milk sold in the United States is nonfat, powdered whole milk is also available in the ethnic food sections of grocery stores. Yogurt is often well accepted, and using plain nonfat yogurt with fruit and minimal added sugar can maximize nutrients without providing as many extra calories. Greek yogurt, although higher in protein, may contain less calcium than regular yogurt. Although cheese can be used, often the higher calories from fat become a limiting factor. Lactose intolerance can be managed (see Chapter 25).

Soy milks are fortified with calcium, but this often precipitates to the bottom of the container. It is difficult to reincorporate the sludge, with the milk containing only 31% of the labeled amount without shaking, 59% with shaking (Heaney and Rafferty, 2006). The fortificant should be calcium carbonate for best absorption. Other drinks, including enriched rice, coconut, and nut milks, are often low in protein, and caution is advised. Regarding vegetable sources of calcium, the concern is one of quantity and bioavailability (Table 14.10; see also Appendix 39).

Care should be taken when considering the use of calcium supplements. Among nonpregnant adults, bone building is better with dietary calcium than with supplements (Booth and Camacho, 2013). Overconsumption of calcium through food is not common. However, elevated serum calcium levels can result from excess antacid ingestion if the UL is exceeded (see Heartburn).

Copper. Diets of pregnant women are often marginal in copper, and requirements rise slightly in pregnancy. In addition to primary deficiency from genetic mutation (Menkes disease), secondary deficiency (from increased zinc or iron intake, the use of certain drugs, or a history of gastric bypass surgery) is also of concern. Copper deficiency alters embryo development and induced copper deficiency has been shown to be teratogenic. There is decreased activity of cuproenzymes, increased oxidative stress, altered iron metabolism, abnormal protein cross-linking, decreased angiogenesis, and altered cell signaling (Uriu-Adams et al, 2010). Copper interacts with iron, affecting neurocognitive and neurobehavioral development. Although not commonly included in prenatal supplements, it is recommended that copper be supplemented when zinc and iron are given during pregnancy. Good sources of copper include organ meats, seafood, nuts, seeds, and whole grain products. Because of the relatively large amounts consumed, tea, milk, potatoes, and chicken are also important sources (Otten et al, 2006).

Fluoride. The role of fluoride in prenatal development is controversial, and fluoride requirements do not increase during pregnancy. Development of primary dentition begins at 10 to 12 weeks of gestation and the first four permanent molars and eight of the permanent incisors are forming during the final trimester. Thus 32 teeth are developing during gestation. Controversy involves the extent to which fluoride is transported across the placenta and its value in utero in the development of caries-resistant permanent teeth (see Chapter 24).

Most bottled water does not contain fluoride. Fluoride is often added to the municipal water supply in the United States to achieve the intake level recommended by CDC. In other countries, salt and milk are common vehicles for fortification. Fluoride levels exceeding the maximum contamination level of municipal water supplies are problematic for bones and teeth. These elevated levels also appear to be neurotoxic for the developing fetus (Barrett, 2017).

Iodine. Iodine is part of the thyroxine molecule, with a critical role in the metabolism of macronutrients as well as in fetal neuronal myelination and gene expression (Wu et al, 2012a). Because the thyroid hormone synthesis increases 50% during pregnancy, iodine requirements also increase (Stagnaro-Green and Pearce, 2012). Severe iodine deficiency is associated with increased risk of miscarriage, congenital anomalies, fetal goiter, and stillbirth, as well as prematurity, poor fetal growth, and decreased IQ. Infant cretinism, although rare in the United States, is a significant public health problem. Iodine deficiency is the most common cause of preventable intellectual developmental disability in the world (Leung et al, 2013).

TABLE 14.10 Comparison of Absorbable Calcium With 1 Cup Milk

Food	Calcium Content	Fractional Absorption	Estimated Absorbed Calcium	Amount Needed to Equal 1 c Milk
Milk	300 mg/c	32.1%	96.3 mg	1.0 cup
Beans, pinto	44.7 mg/0.5 c*	26.7	11.9	4.05 cups, cooked*
Beans, red	40.5 mg/0.5 c	24.4	9.9	4.85 cups
Beans, white	113 mg/0.5 c	21.8	24.7	1.95 cups
Bok choy	79 mg/0.5 c	53.8	42.5	1.15 cups
Broccoli	35 mg/0.5 c	61.3	21.5	2.25 cups
Cheddar cheese	303 mg/1.5 oz	32.1	97.2	1.5 oz
Chinese mustard greens	212 mg/0.5 c	40.2	85.3	0.55 cup
Chinese spinach	347 mg/0.5 c	8.36	29.0	1.65 cups
Kale	61 mg/0.5 c	49.3	30.1	1.6 cups
Spinach	115 mg/0.5 c	5.1	5.9	8.15 cups
Sweet potatoes	44 mg/0.5 c	22.2	9.8	4.9 cups
Tofu with calcium	258 mg/0.5 c	31.0	80.0	0.6 cup
Yogurt, regular	300 mg/c	32.1	96.3	1.0 cup

*All vegetables are cooked portions.
Adapted from Weaver CM et al: Choices for achieving adequate dietary calcium with a vegetarian diet, *Am J Clin Nutr* 70:543s, 1999.

Worldwide, many people are at risk for iodine deficiency caused by low intake of milk or by consuming produce grown in iodine-deficient soils, especially if eating locally and consuming goitrogens or exposed to perchlorate contamination. Fish and seafood are good sources. Iodine content varies between and within species. It is higher in white fish than oily fish and levels are highest at and just below the skin. Marine fish contain six times the amount found in fresh water fish. Other seafood is also a good source. Cooking losses are much higher with boiling than with frying or grilling (Bouga et al, 2018).

An estimated 70% of the world population has access to iodized salt (Pearce et al, 2013). Salt iodization is voluntary in the United States and Canada. Iodized salt rarely is used in processed foods, the primary source of dietary sodium, and must be labeled if used. Kosher salt and sea salt do not naturally contain iodine. Women should be encouraged to use iodized salt when cooking at home and to limit the intake of processed foods made with uniodized salt.

Median urinary iodine values in the United States have declined, mainly because of the reduction of iodine in dairy and bread products, such that 35% of U.S. women of childbearing age now have urinary iodine values suggesting mild iodine deficiency or insufficiency (Leung et al, 2013). Similar reductions have been seen in women in other developed countries as well (Pearce et al, 2013). A recent study estimated 21% to 44% of U.S. pregnant women in the third trimester may have inadequate iodine levels, using a new quantitative modeling tool (Lumen and George, 2017). Although the effects of severe iodine deficiency on fetal brain development are well established, the effects of milder deficits are not as clear. Results of supplementation studies are mixed regarding thyroid function and the neurodevelopment of children, but children of women with mild to moderate deficiency demonstrate better neurocognitive scores if mothers were supplemented starting very early in pregnancy, that is, by 4 to 6 weeks of gestation (Leung et al, 2013). Current research is studying the effect of iodine supplementation on obstetric outcomes and long-term child development. Because of the concern that a subset of the population may be at risk for mild deficiency, the American Thyroid Association recommends that women receive 150 mcg/day during pregnancy and lactation as potassium iodide, given the variability of iodine content in kelp and seaweed (Leung et al, 2013; ACOG, 2015b). A recent study in the United States found that 61% of prenatal vitamins contain iodine and that those that were available over the counter were more likely to contain it (71%) than those available by prescription (46%) (Lee et al, 2017). Iodine content ranged from 10 to 450 mcg according to product labels, but the majority (89%) contained at least 150 mcg. Another U.S. study found that adult multivitamins were more likely to contain iodine (74.2%) than those labeled prenatal vitamins (57.6%) (Patel et al, 2018). Although the adult multivitamins consistently used potassium iodide, that was only true for 73.5% of those labeled as prenatal vitamins. In addition, the accuracy of labeled content of multivitamins sold in the United States is also of concern.

High iodine levels are also of concern, potentially causing the same symptoms as low levels. There is concern about the safety of iodine supplementation in areas of iodine sufficiency, but the problems appear to be temporary (Pearce et al, 2013). There are individual differences in the ability to handle high iodine intakes but most healthy people adapt within a few days and produce normal levels of thyroid hormones (Hamby et al, 2018). However, the fetus and neonate are particularly sensitive to high iodine levels, especially the preterm infant, because the homeostatic mechanisms do not mature until 36 weeks of gestation (Pearce, 2018).

Problems have been seen with high intakes of seaweeds. The iodine content of seaweeds is variable and depends primarily on the species of seaweed but also the parts of the plant consumed, the growing conditions, and the preparation methods (Roleda et al, 2018). Of most concern are the brown seaweeds, including kombu and kelp, because they are known to be the most efficient accumulators of iodine, followed by red seaweeds (Teas et al, 2004). Frequent consumption of these seaweeds could far exceed the UL (Desideri et al, 2016), even when cooking methods (iodine is water soluble) and bioavailability issues are taken into account (Roleda et al, 2018; Domínguez-González et al, 2017). Congenital hypothyroidism resulting from high prenatal intake of seaweeds has been documented (Nishiyama et al, 2004). Very high breastmilk iodine levels also have been seen among Korean women ingesting the customary brown seaweed soup postpartum, utilized for its nutrient content but also thought to facilitate maternal weight loss and enhance breast milk production (Hamby et al, 2018).

As a reminder, postpartum thyroiditis affects an estimated 5.4% of all women (Stagnaro-Green and Pearce, 2012). Thyroiditis can manifest as either hyper- or hypothyroidism, and both can affect breastmilk production.

Iron. The RDA for iron significantly increases in pregnancy. An estimated 42% of pregnant women worldwide have iron deficiency anemia with wide regional variability. Although prevalence is highest in developing countries, an estimated 33% of low-income pregnant women in the United States are anemic in the third trimester (Murray-Kolb, 2011).

Inadequate iron consumption may lead to poor hemoglobin production, followed by compromised delivery of oxygen, as well as iron, to the uterus, placenta, and developing fetus. The placenta contains multiple iron transporter proteins for both heme and nonheme iron but they are not yet fully described, especially for heme iron (Fisher and Nemeth, 2017). There is some evidence that ferritin can also be transported, as well as preliminary evidence that dietary heme iron is preferentially transported to the fetus (O'Brien and Ru, 2017). Iron transport is regulated, balancing maternal and fetal needs (Cao and Fleming, 2016). The fetus appears to drive placental iron transport, although it is unclear how the placenta senses the fetal demand. Fetal hepcidin, as we currently understand it, usually remains low, allowing high transfer rates of iron from the placenta to the fetus. However, there is speculation that elevated fetal hepcidin levels, as might be found in fetal inflammation, (i.e., chorioamnionitis), may inhibit the transfer of iron from the placenta to the fetus (Fisher and Nemeth, 2017). Supplementation may improve maternal status but doesn't necessarily improve cord levels because fetal transfer can be sustained until maternal anemia becomes too severe (hemoglobin < 9 g/dL or serum ferritin < 13.6 mcg/L) (Georgieff, 2017).

Iron deficiency anemia (IDA) is associated with IUGR (threefold increase in LBW), preterm delivery (twofold increased incidence), increased fetal and neonatal mortality, and if severe (hemoglobin < 9 g/dL), with complications during delivery (Auerbach, 2018). IDA also is associated with increased fetal cortisol production and oxidative damage to fetal erythrocytes (Hovdenak and Haram, 2012). Early iron deficiency affects fetal brain development and the regulation of brain function in multiple ways (see Table 14.7). Because erythropoiesis gets priority over the brain and other organs, fetal brain iron deficiency can occur before maternal IDA is identified and better functional measures are needed (Georgieff, 2017). Neonatal iron deficiency can result if the mother is extremely iron deficient, but maternal hypertension and therefore restricted blood flow, as well as maternal smoking and prematurity, also increase the risk. Infants of mothers with diabetes are also more likely to develop iron deficiency because of increased fetal demands with macrosomia and fetal hyperglycemia/hyperinsulinemia increasing fetal oxygen consumption, but also with hyperglycosylation of the placental transferrin receptors restricting iron transport to the fetus (Rao and Georgieff, 2012), all resulting in a 40% reduction in brain iron concentration. These changes result in long-term neurobehavioral impairments affecting temperament, interactions with others, learning, and memory and also may result in genomic changes.

Maternal effects of IDA include fatigue, dyspnea, light-headedness, and poor exercise tolerance. Prenatal weight gain is likely to be low. The mother is at risk of increased blood loss with uterine atony during delivery, thus increasing her risk of needing a blood transfusion. Wound healing and immune function are impaired. She is more likely to suffer from postpartum depression, poor maternal/infant interaction, and impaired lactation. There is some evidence that negative alterations in cognition, emotions, quality of life, and behavior may occur before overt IDA is reached, but the degree of iron deficiency associated with negative consequences remains unknown. Treatment during pregnancy improves maternal iron status postpartum and also is associated with improved infant development (Murray-Kolb, 2011).

Plasma volume increases 50% from baseline, and normal erythrocyte volume increases by 20% to 30% in pregnancy. This marked increase in the maternal blood supply during pregnancy, as well as fetal needs, greatly increases the demand for iron. The estimated total requirement for pregnancy is 1190 mg, but with the cessation of menses, the average net deficit is 580 mg. Added to her normal requirements, a pregnant woman often needs to absorb 17 mg/day by the third trimester. Normal absorption is often 1 to 2 mg/day from a normal diet, and 3 to 5 mg/day if the diet contains high-iron foods (Lee and Okam, 2011). Absorption of both heme and nonheme iron increases during pregnancy. Hepcidin levels decrease in the second and third trimesters, thus increasing the available iron to the placenta and therefore, the fetus (Fisher and Nemeth, 2017). However, the mechanism that causes this decrease in maternal hepcidin is not yet known and it is also unknown how iron supplementation affects hepcidin levels during pregnancy. While hepcidin certainly affects the availability of nonheme iron, there is also some evidence that it impacts heme iron availability as well. Elevated maternal hepcidin levels, causing lower than optimal transfer of iron to the placenta, would be important in the case of inflammation. However, the normal inflammation of healthy pregnancies does not seem to increase hepcidin. Pregnancies with more intense inflammation may, however, cause hepcidin levels to increase and therefore, iron availability to drop. How important this is in the case of the inflammation associated with maternal obesity or excessive weight gain is currently unclear. The effect of supplementation on intestinal absorption is also unclear, as is the possible increased risk of higher exposure with increased intake (Brannon et al, 2017), as well as the role of unabsorbed iron on the microbiome. Most accretion occurs after the twentieth week of gestation, when maternal and fetal demands are greatest. Those at highest risk of IDA are women with inadequate iron stores, including those with short interconceptual periods, those with poor habitual intakes, those with impaired absorption including a history of bariatric surgery or chronic use of antacids, and those who have experienced red cell destruction from malaria or excessive blood loss from heavy menstrual flow or prior hookworm infections.

A first trimester serum ferritin level may be assessed and if less than 20 mcg/L, supplementation may be necessary (Lee and Okam, 2011). However, checking red blood cell indices on the complete blood count (CBC) (see Chapter 5) is often adequate. Hemoglobin and hematocrit values normally decrease in the second trimester (see Table 14.5). Not decreasing may be a sign of poor blood volume expansion, which is associated with increasing risk of a growth-restricted infant, preterm delivery, and stillbirth (Luke, 2015). Serum values should increase again in the third trimester for best outcomes, but often this rise is not seen and intervention is merited. If anemia does not improve with iron therapy (i.e., an increase of 1 g hemoglobin or 3% in hematocrit by 4 weeks [CDC, 1998]), it is advised to check vitamins B_6, B_{12}, and folate

status, although many other nutrients, including protein, cobalt, magnesium, selenium, zinc, copper, vitamins A and C, lipids, and carbohydrate, also may play a role (Lee and Okam, 2011; Mechanick et al, 2013; Wu et al, 2012a).

High iron status is also associated with poor fetal growth, preterm delivery, preeclampsia, gestational diabetes, and stillbirth. However, the mechanism(s) are unclear but may include the actual iron status (increased viscosity and therefore compromised blood flow and/or poor placental perfusion), relative zinc and copper deficiencies, oxidative stress with supplementation, altered gut microbiome, and/or poor plasma volume expansion itself (Brannon and Taylor, 2017; Fisher and Nemeth, 2017). Serum ferritin may also just be a proxy measure for inflammation, especially in the context of maternal obesity (Vricella, 2017). There are no good functional measures of replete vs. excess iron status (Brannon and Taylor, 2017), nor is there a good way to adjust serum ferritin or hepcidin for inflammation but there is evidence that the obesity-associated inflammation does not override the influence of low iron status on hepcidin signaling (O'Brien and Ru, 2017).

Because many women do not enter pregnancy with sufficient iron stores to cover the physiologic needs of pregnancy, iron supplementation (usually as a ferrous salt) often is prescribed, but the amount of elemental iron contained varies by the preparation (Office of Dietary Supplements [ODS], 2018). The iron in the supplement already is reduced (i.e., ferrous rather than ferric), so taking the supplement with water is effective and consuming it with juice is not necessary. As with all nonheme sources, supplements should not be taken with coffee, tea, or milk to optimize absorption. Iron supplements should be taken separately from the prenatal vitamins to minimize the competition with other minerals. Absorption is best if taken on an empty stomach, but tolerance is often worse. Multiple supplements should be taken separately from each other to maximize absorption, but diminishing absorption is seen with increasing dosage, so tolerance of side effects should be balanced against need. Enteric-coated and delayed-release preparations produce fewer side effects, but because they are not well absorbed they are not recommended. Intravenous iron can be used during pregnancy, even as a first line treatment, in the second and third trimesters (Auerbach, 2018).

Iron supplementation is controversial. CDC and WHO recommend routine early iron supplementation to lower the risk of maternal anemia, LBW, and preterm delivery (WHO, 2016b). The USPSTF states that while supplementation may improve maternal iron status, the evidence supporting routine supplementation to improve either maternal or infant clinical outcomes is inconclusive (Cantor et al, 2015). ACOG recommends screening everyone and supplementing those with documented IDA. However, for those at risk of chronic iron overload, including those with hemochromatosis and beta-thalassemia, iron supplementation may not be recommended. Iron supplements may cause oxidative damage and may exacerbate inflammation. Consequently, overtreatment of IDA is now thought to be associated with preterm delivery, IUGR, and GDM (Hovdenak and Haram, 2012; see Chapter 7 for other examples of oxidative damage). Intermittent supplementation (one to two times per week) may be effective (Kaiser and Campbell, 2014), possibly by minimizing the increase in hepcidin levels (Auerbach, 2018). Nonphysiologic intakes of iron, as would be achieved with supplementation, may increase the risk of infections, especially important for people living in unsanitary settings (Prentice et al, 2017). In areas where bacterial and protozoal infections, especially malaria, are of concern, food fortification providing smaller doses at a time may be safer than supplementation. In addition, iron supplements are extremely dangerous for small children. Doses as little as 36 mg elemental iron/kg body weight have been lethal (ODS, 2018), so mothers must be reminded to keep supplements out of the reach of children.

Because of the concerns with iron supplementation, including compliance, safety, and effectiveness, emphasizing dietary sources of iron is necessary. The best sources of iron are red meats, including wild meats, (see Appendix 43) because of their heme content, and many organ meats may contain even higher levels of iron. It is important to limit the amount of liver and liver products (pâté, liverwurst, braunschweiger) in the first trimester because of their high vitamin A contents.

Vegetable sources, containing only nonheme iron, are less well absorbed, and volume may become the limiting factor, especially late in pregnancy. Absorption can be enhanced by eating them with ascorbic acid or a little meat.

Women who follow vegetarian diets should pay particular attention to iron and try to prevent having their hematocrit drop so far that it cannot recover sufficiently. Followers of Jehovah's Witness also must pay close attention to their iron levels. Because they choose not to receive blood transfusions, these women should receive nutrition counseling on high-iron foods early in pregnancy, with reinforcement as the pregnancy continues.

Magnesium. Magnesium functions as an enzyme cofactor and activator. The full-term fetus accumulates 1 g of magnesium during gestation, and maternal deficiency may interfere with fetal growth and development, including possible teratogenesis (Hovdenak and Haram, 2012). Recommendations for magnesium increase slightly during pregnancy, but its role in preterm labor, preeclampsia, gestational diabetes, and poor fetal growth is not well understood (Dalton et al, 2016). Magnesium sulfate is sometimes used to treat women with preeclampsia, but whether supplementation of magnesium for any of these conditions is helpful when a woman is not deficient in magnesium is unknown. Maternal magnesium deficiency has been speculated to play a part in increased risk for sudden infant death syndrome (SIDS), but prospective supplementation trials have not been done. Moderate magnesium deficiency is associated with subtle renal deficits in offspring (Richard et al, 2017). Optimal magnesium levels may be beneficial in helping prevent leg cramps (see Edema and Leg Cramps). However, too few data are available to give supplementation recommendations (Hovdenak and Haram, 2012). See Appendix 43 for good dietary sources. Prolonged, high doses of magnesium supplements should be avoided (see Heartburn).

Phosphorus. Phosphorus is found in a variety of foods, and deficiency is rare if one is able to eat normally. Requirements do not rise with pregnancy. However, low phosphorus levels, indicative of "refeeding syndrome," have been found in women experiencing severe vomiting or other situations resulting in starvation. Hypophosphatemia can be life threatening because phosphorus is important in energy metabolism as a component of adenosine triphosphate (ATP) and must be replenished promptly (see Chapter 12).

Selenium. Selenium functions as an antioxidant and is important for reproduction. Low selenium status is associated with recurrent miscarriages, preeclampsia, and IUGR. The DRI increases slightly during pregnancy, but there are no evidence-based recommendations for supplementation (Hovdenak and Haram, 2012). Excess selenium intake is also of concern, especially if women eat locally from areas where soil selenium contents are high. There are no known areas in the United States or Canada with recognized cases of selenosis. See Appendix 45.

Sodium. The hormonal milieu of pregnancy affects sodium metabolism. Increased maternal blood volume leads to increased glomerular filtration of sodium. Compensatory mechanisms maintain fluid and electrolyte balance.

Rigorous sodium restriction stresses the renin-angiotensin-aldosterone system. Although moderation in the use of salt and other sodium-rich foods is appropriate for most people, aggressive restriction is usually unwarranted in pregnancy. For pregnant women with edema, the use of diuretics is not recommended but correcting high sodium intakes from the diet is warranted. Normal intakes are often much higher than the DRI, which does not increase during pregnancy. ACOG has previously recommended that sodium intake should not be restricted below 2300 mg/day, which is higher than the current DRI. (ACOG, 2013c). Use of iodized salt should be encouraged, but processed food consumption, the source of more than 75% of dietary sodium in the United States, should be limited because of the noniodized salt content.

Zinc. Zinc is critical for growth and development, and requirements rise during pregnancy. A zinc-deficient diet does not result in effective mobilization of zinc stored in the maternal skeletal muscle and bone. Therefore a compromised zinc status develops rapidly. Zinc is part of 100 enzymes related to the metabolism of macronutrients (Hovdenak and Haram, 2012). It provides a structural function in many tissues, including some proteins involved in gene expression. Deficiency is highly teratogenic, leading to congenital malformations, including anencephaly and possibly oral clefts. Even a mild zinc deficiency may lead to impaired fetal growth and brain development, as well as impaired immune function. Women with untreated low zinc levels associated with acrodermatitis enteropathica have increased risk of miscarriage, fetal growth restriction, hypertension, preeclampsia, preterm delivery, and intrapartum hemorrhage.

Zinc is widely available and good sources include red meat, seafood, whole grains, and some fortified breakfast cereals (see Appendix 47). Supplementation exceeding that found in prenatal vitamins usually is not required but may be necessary for women with GI disorders that affect absorption. Overt deficiency is rare in the United States, but rates are higher where the main staple foods are high in phytates (i.e., the unrefined cereals), and women following a vegetarian diet may experience low zinc bioavailability. High levels of iron supplementation may inhibit zinc absorption if both are taken without food (Kaiser and Campbell, 2014).

Pregnancy Weight Gain Recommendations
General Weight Gain Recommendations

With a singleton gestation, less than half of the total weight gain of a normal-weight pregnant woman resides in the fetus, placenta, and amniotic fluid. The remainder is in maternal reproductive tissues (breast tissues and uterus), interstitial fluid, blood volume, and maternal adipose tissue. Increased subcutaneous fat in the abdomen, back, and upper thigh serves as an energy reserve for pregnancy and lactation. The normal distribution of weight is illustrated in Fig. 14.6.

Recommended weight gains to support a healthy pregnancy vary by prepregnant BMI and are summarized in Table 14.11. Designed for

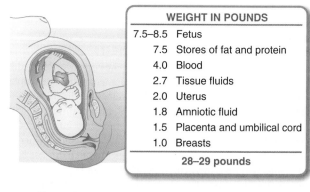

WEIGHT IN POUNDS	
7.5–8.5	Fetus
7.5	Stores of fat and protein
4.0	Blood
2.7	Tissue fluids
2.0	Uterus
1.8	Amniotic fluid
1.5	Placenta and umbilical cord
1.0	Breasts
28–29 pounds	

Fig. 14.6 Distribution of weight gain during pregnancy.

TABLE 14.11 U.S. Institute of Medicine (IOM) Prenatal Weight Gain Goals

Prepregnant Weight Category	Total Singleton Weight Gain	Rates of Gain in 2nd and 3rd Trimesters for Singletons* Mean/week (Range)	Total Twins Weight Gain (Provisional guidelines)
Underweight BMI < 18.5	28-40 lb [12.5-18 kg]	1 lb (1-1.3) [0.51 kg (0.44-0.58)]	Insufficient information available for guideline
Normal weight BMI 18.5-24.9	25-35 lb [11.5-16 kg]	1 lb (0.8-1) [0.42 kg (0.35-0.50)]	37-54 lb [17-25 kg]
Overweight BMI 25.0-29.9	15-25 lb [7-11.5 kg]	0.6 lb (0.5-0.7) [0.28 kg (0.23-0.33)]	31-50 lb [14-23 kg]
Obese BMI ≥ 30.0	11-20 lb [5-9 kg]	0.5 lb (0.4-0.6) [0.22 kg (0.17-0.27)]	25-42 lb [11-19 kg]

*Calculations assume a first trimester gain for singleton pregnancy of 1 to 3 kg (2.2 to 6.6 lb) for women who are underweight, normal weight, or overweight and 0.5 to 2 kg (1.1 to 4.4 lb) for those who are in the obese category.
Adapted from Rasmussen KM et al: Recommendations for weight gain during pregnancy in the context of the obesity epidemic, *Obstet Gynecol* 116:1191, 2010; Rasmussen KM, Yaktine AL: *Weight gain during pregnancy: reexamining the guidelines*, Washington, DC, 2009, IOM, NRC.

women living in healthy environments, the IOM weight gain guidelines balance the risk of adverse birth outcomes with the mother's risk of postpartum weight retention. Insufficient gain, especially if also associated with prepregnant underweight, is associated with increased risk of SGA babies and spontaneous preterm deliveries. Excessive gain often results in LGA babies, with increased risk during delivery. Excessive gain is also the strongest predictor of later maternal obesity. Outcomes are best when women gain within the recommended ranges. However, less than one third of pregnant women do so, and most (especially those who are overweight or obese) gain too much, although a significant proportion of underweight women gain too little (Siega-Riz and Gray, 2013). Women want advice on how much weight they should gain but a recent study found that 26% received no guidance from their health care provider (Deputy et al, 2018). Those that received advice tried to follow it, even if it was inappropriate, resulting in both inadequate and excessive gains among those studied.

Height and, ideally, prepregnant weight should be measured, not asked, to determine prepregnant BMI. Self-reported prepregnancy weight can be used if necessary but it is subject to error and is usually underreported (Headen et al, 2017). If prepregnant weight is unknown or unreliable, use the weight at the first visit, assuming she is early in pregnancy, as a good estimate of prepregnant weight. If she starts prenatal care late and has no idea of her prepregnant weight, estimate that she has had appropriate gain to that point. Later in pregnancy BMI is not a robust estimate of body fat because of the increase in total body water (Catalano and Shankar, 2017).

Women need guidance on target weight gains. One third of women try to keep the same weight or even lose weight during pregnancy (Rasmussen and Yaktine, 2009). Weight gain should be monitored as a way to evaluate progress and to intervene when necessary. The pattern of weight gain is also important. In an observational cohort, excessive first trimester weight gain was a stronger predictor of maternal weight retention, higher waist circumference, and higher blood pressure than was weight gain later in pregnancy (Walter et al, 2015). It is also associated with toddler obesity, in spite of having no effect on birthweight (Karachaliou et al, 2015). Higher rates of weight gain in the second trimester are associated with higher birth weight, especially among women whose prepregnant BMI is less than 26 (Rasmussen and Yaktine, 2009). Maternal weight gain plotted on the appropriate grid is an effective teaching tool. See Appendix 3 for all pregnancy weight gain grids, as well as tables (using pounds/inches and kilograms/centimeters)

to quickly choose the correct grid without needing to calculate the prepregnant BMI.

Weight loss during pregnancy should be discouraged. There are no intervention studies documenting benefit (Furber et al, 2013). As adipose tissue is mobilized, semivolatile organic compounds may be released (see *Clinical Insight:* What's in That Fat When You Lose It in Chapter 20). Because of the accelerated starvation characteristic of pregnancy, women are more likely to develop ketonemia and ketonuria after a 12- to 18-hour fast, with ketone levels higher than in nonpregnant women. Although the fetus has a limited ability to metabolize ketones, these compounds may adversely affect fetal brain development (Rasmussen and Yaktine, 2009). In addition, mobilized protein stores, increased free fatty acids, urinary nitrogen excretion, and lower plasma glucose, insulin, and gluconeogenic amino acids have been seen, resulting in increased risk of IUGR and preterm birth (Furber et al, 2013).

Prenatal weight gain guidelines vary somewhat worldwide (Scott et al, 2014). WHO has discussed, but not implemented, different weight gain guidelines based on ethnic differences in body composition and, therefore, different risks (Ma et al, 2016). The IOM guidelines are based on observational, not interventional, data. Thus some countries do not advocate either a particular weight gain or even routine weighing after determining the prepregnant BMI status. Although there are many small intervention studies, large trials are not yet available. It also must be noted that it is unclear whether maternal weight gain itself is a critical variable or whether it is a marker for nutritional status. Even so, tracking weight gain is useful and when variation from normal patterns is noted, more questions should be asked. While seeing the grid or hearing the actual weight may be stressful for some, many women find the visual tracking of their weight gain against the appropriate grid both effective and also reassuring. Just tracking weight gain without guidance or support is not beneficial.

Obesity Weight Gain Recommendations

Pregravid obesity is described as class I (BMI 30 to 34.9), class II (BMI 35 to 39.9), and class III (BMI at least 40). The IOM's weight gain recommendation of 11 to 20 pounds does not distinguish between these classes (Rasmussen and Yaktine, 2009). Optimal gestational weight gains for these groups are not yet known and research continues, with some evidence that lower gains, or even loss, can be managed successfully as individuals may balance intakes well enough to avoid ketonemia. Overweight, and therefore overnutrition, is not the same as good quality nutrition and, in fact, obesity is associated with lower serum levels of carotenoids; vitamins C, D, B$_6$, K; folate; iron; and selenium (Saltzman and Karl, 2013; see also Chapter 20). Individual guidance and clinical judgment, including optimizing nutrient intakes and encouraging exercise, is necessary, and fetal growth must be monitored. Although weight gain targets may be too high for some women, evidence suggests that the risk of preterm delivery, IUGR, and perinatal mortality all increase if the weight gain is too restrictive. Epigenetic effects also must be considered. Inadequate weight gain and weight loss should not be encouraged (ACOG, 2015d). The United States, Canada, Australia, New Zealand, and Great Britain have similar, but not identical, guidelines regarding the management of obesity in pregnancy but all recommend that a nutrition consultation should be offered to all women who are overweight or obese before pregnancy (Vitner et al, 2019). No study has yet examined the pregnancy outcomes of low weight gain/weight loss resulting from insufficient food intake vs. that resulting from replacing foods containing excessive fats and sweets with those of higher nutrient, but lower caloric contents.

Postbariatric Surgery. The high prevalence of obesity has resulted in an increase in bariatric surgeries. Although prepregnancy weight loss may improve fertility, it has the potential to provide a suboptimal uterine environment for the developing fetus, and adequate nutrient supplementation is essential. Which nutrients are most likely to be deficient will be determined by the type of surgery and the nutritional status since that surgery (see Chapter 20), but commonly include protein, as well as vitamins D, folate, B$_{12}$, B$_1$, and A; iron; calcium; magnesium; copper; and zinc. Other deficiencies, although potentially severe, are more sporadic (Saltzman and Karl, 2013) but may include vitamins C, B$_6$, B$_2$, niacin, E, and K; selenium; and essential fatty acids (with biliopancreatic diversion). If anemia does not respond to treatment, vitamin B$_{12}$, folate, protein, copper, selenium, and zinc should be assessed (Mechanick et al, 2013). ACOG recommends women be evaluated for nutrient deficiencies and supplemented as needed (ACOG, 2015d).

The optimal timing of pregnancy following bariatric surgery is still unclear. Although 1 year has been commonly cited, ACOG now recommends delaying pregnancy for 18 months to avoid the period of rapid weight loss. However, a recent study is more conservative (Parent et al, 2017). They found that if pregnancy occurred within 2 years of surgery, the risk of prematurity increased (14% vs. 8.6%), as did the rates of neonatal intensive care unit (NICU) admission (15.2% vs. 11.3%), SGA prevalence (13% vs. 8.9%), and low APGAR scores (17.5% vs. 14.8%), compared with a matched cohort. They suggest that women should wait at least 3 years to conceive. An individualized approach has also been suggested, delaying pregnancy until the weight has been stable for 2 years and with all nutrient deficiencies treated prior to conception. However, many women don't follow this advice and are likely to be entering pregnancy with less than ideal nutrient status.

An optimum nutrient prescription and caloric requirement for pregnant women after bariatric surgery has not been determined and must be individualized. Protein intake recommendations following surgery are higher than normal (1.0 to 2.1 g/kg ideal body weight) but it is unknown what further increase is needed for pregnancy. Specific vitamin and mineral recommendations are also unknown. These women may have more difficulty eating enough if they have had a restrictive procedure and the gastric band may need to be adjusted. Those with bypass procedures may have malabsorptive problems and many women may develop food intolerances. In addition, women with a history of bariatric surgery may be less willing to gain enough weight after having invested so much in losing it, so guidance with reassurance and support may be necessary (see Chapter 20). Although the weight gain guidelines are based on prepregnant BMI and are the same as for those without surgery, they are difficult to achieve for these women. Focus on high nutrient, low volume foods and minimize the intake of foods that don't help fetal growth or development.

These women need to be monitored carefully during pregnancy and their prenatal care may need to be modified. Practitioners should have a high degree of suspicion when hearing about discomforts. The gastric band can slip, causing an obstruction that can mimic hyperemesis but can result in fetal death (Jacquemyn and Meesters, 2014). This band migration can happen years after surgery, after uneventful pregnancies, and also after delivery. Roux-en-Y surgery has been shown to increase the risk of bowel obstruction. GI hemorrhage, anastomotic leaks, internal or ventral hernias, gastric rupture, peptic ulcers, cholelithiasis, and band erosion have all been seen. Those experiencing dumping syndrome (primarily after Roux-en-Y) may require glucose monitoring rather than trying to use the glucola to diagnose gestational diabetes. Glucose monitoring may also need to be modified. Because these women experience higher, shorter glucose peaks and lower lows, identification of a problem may be missed if the common 2-hour window is used (Bonis et al, 2016; Feichtinger et al, 2017).

Earlier research found little or no difference in pregnancy outcomes after bariatric surgery but studies were small, short term, and had inconsistent results. Newer studies are larger and have matched controls, enabling researchers to better characterize the additional risk for pregnancy after bariatric surgery, taking into account the elevated risk of continued obesity. Women who have had bariatric surgery often have successful pregnancy outcomes, with lower rates of gestational diabetes, hypertension, preeclampsia, macrosomia, and childhood obesity than seen among women with obesity who have not undergone bariatric surgery (Kassir et al, 2016). However, they also have higher risk of fetal growth restriction and preterm births (Kwong et al, 2018), including higher miscarriage and neonatal mortality rates after surgery (Kassir et al, 2016). If women have had Roux-en-Y or biliopancreatic diversion surgery, with or without the duodenal switch, they may also have higher risk of fetal malformations (Pelizzo et al, 2014), but there appears to be no consistent increase in the risk of malformations. Some have found an increased risk of NTDs and case reports describe the consequences of specific nutrient deficiencies, including vitamins K, B$_{12}$, and A.

The estimation of nutritional risk from bariatric surgery has risen over time, as evidenced by the increased number of nutrients being monitored, the testing frequency, and the level of routine supplementation recommended. Current guidelines (Parrott et al, 2017) are not specific to pregnancy (see Chapter 20). Studies regarding pregnancy following bariatric surgery are ongoing (Jans et al, 2016), including examining the effect of bariatric surgery on breastmilk composition, and better guidance is expected in the future. As with other dietary supplements, bariatric multivitamin-multimineral supplements are not standardized and some fit the profile of prenatal nutrient recommendations better than others do.

Multiple Births

The incidence of multiple births in the United States is rising because of the increased use of fertility drugs and ART, age at conception, and obesity rates among pregnant women (ACOG, 2016b). Multifetal gestations cause significant maternal physiologic adaptations beyond the usual pregnancy changes, including increased plasma volume, metabolic rate, and increased insulin resistance (Goodnight and Newman, 2009).

These infants have a greater risk of preterm delivery with accompanying IUGR or LBW than do singletons. Adequate maternal weight gain, especially early in pregnancy (before 20 weeks), has been shown to be particularly important for optimal growth and time in-utero

(Greenan et al, 2017). A common rule of thumb is to target a 24-pound gain by 24 weeks of gestation for twins (Goodnight and Newman, 2009) but intervention should begin in the first trimester. The IOM weight gain guidelines for twins are provisional (see Table 14.11 and Appendix 3) but are supported by more recent research (Hutcheon et al, 2018). The effect of chorionicity on optimal weight gain is unknown. For those pregnant with triplets or other higher-order multiples, there is limited information available, but best practice advice does exist. Target a gain of at least 36 pounds by 24 weeks of gestation for triplets (Stone and Kohari, 2015). Mean gestational weight gain for triplets is 45 to 51 pounds (20.5 to 23 kg) at 32 to 34 weeks. For quadruplets, it is 46 to 68 pounds (20.8 to 31 kg) at 31 to 32 weeks (Rasmussen and Yaktine, 2009) but better outcomes have been seen with higher gains (Luke et al, 2017; Luke, 2015).

The optimal nutrient requirements for twins and higher-order multiples are not yet known but are certainly higher than for singleton pregnancies. There are more fetuses and more placentas needing nourishment. In addition, the increased maternal weight may increase inflammation and therefore negatively affect the nutrient transport (Cao and O'Brien, 2013). It is assumed that at least the milk and meat food groups need to be doubled for twins, increasing as needed for optimal fetal growth, with even higher servings for the higher order multiples (Luke et al, 2017).

A summary of current nutritional plans for twins is summarized in Table 14.12 but may have to include iodine and choline as well; newer evidence cautions against high doses of vitamins C and E (see Hypertension and nutrient sections) (ACOG, 2013c). Because of a greater need for nutritional density in the diet, it is recommended that only 40% of calories come from carbohydrate, with 20% from protein, and 40% from fat (Goodnight and Newman, 2009). A woman pregnant with multiples has increased nutrient needs but decreased space. Counseling should focus on the consumption of very high nutrient foods. She must eat very frequently, possibly every hour, and must focus on foods that aid fetal growth each time she eats. Using fruits and vegetables as desserts rather than snacks often helps, as does suggesting that she eat before drinking liquids. Consumption of any foods that don't help fetal growth and development should be discouraged.

Adolescent Pregnancy

Public health initiatives have helped reduce the incidence of teen pregnancies overall, but it continues as a major problem in the United States among some minority groups (CDC, 2018c). Risk factors for poor outcome in pregnant adolescents are listed in Box 14.3.

Increased rates of LBW and preterm delivery are especially common among those who are very young and underweight, for whom there may be competition for nutrients between the mother and the fetus (see Chapter 17). Poor outcomes are also common in obese teens that become pregnant. Many teens enter pregnancy with suboptimal nutritional status, especially for iron, calcium, and folic acid. In one study, women in the United States who gave birth as teens were more likely to be overweight or obese as adults (Chang et al, 2013).

Improved dietary practices can be one of the most important factors for the pregnant teen. In counseling young mothers, the nutrition professional must be aware of the teen's psychosocial and literacy levels, her economic status and level of independence, as well as her cultural environment, all of which may influence her food choices.

Complications and Nutritional Implications

Many of the following complications follow from the normal hormonal changes during pregnancy. These changes cause the GI transit to slow so that more nutrients are available to the fetus. However, that causes more nausea and vomiting, constipation, and heartburn. Although

TABLE 14.12 Nutrient Recommendations for Women Pregnant with Twins

Nutrient	Twins	Comments
Calories	Underweight: 4000 kcal Normal: 3000-3500 kcal Overweight: 3250 kcal Obese: 2700-3000 kcal	Estimated needs are 40-45 kcal/kg. Monitor weight gain and modify calories to meet target weight goals.
Protein	Underweight: 200 g Normal: 175 g Overweight: 163 g Obese: 150 g	Target 20% of calories from protein. Choose concentrated sources as space becomes limiting.
Carbohydrate	Underweight: 400 g Normal: 350 g Overweight: 325 g Obese: 300 g	Encourage low glycemic choices.
Fat	Underweight: 178 g Normal: 156 g Overweight: 144 g Obese: 133 g	Encourage healthy fats.
Vitamin D	1000 IU/day or more as needed (1000 IU/day raises blood 5 mg/dL)	Assessment of maternal levels should be considered in first and early third trimesters to allow alterations in the supplemental dose, especially important if the mother is on bed rest.
Vitamin C	500-1000 mg/day	This is half of the UL of 1800-2000 mg/day. See more recent cautions.
Vitamin E	400 mg/day	This is half of the UL of 800-1000 mg/day. See more recent cautions.
Zinc	15 mg/day (T1); 30-45 mg/day (T2-3)	Diet alone may not be enough. Supplementation may be required.
Iron	30 mg/day as part of 1 multivitamin/day (T1), 2 multivitamins/day (T2 and T3)	Twin gestation requirement is likely double that of singletons. Higher intakes may be needed for treatment of anemia.
Folic acid	800-1000 mcg/day, 4 mg if with a history of NTD	
Calcium	1500 mg/day (T1); 2500-3000. mg (T2-3)	UL: 2500 mg/day, consider limiting if there is a history of kidney stones.
Magnesium	400 mg/day (T1); 800-1200. mg/day (T2-3)	
DHA + EPA	300-1000 mg/day	

Adapted from Goodnight W, Newman R: Optimal nutrition for improved twin pregnancy outcome, *Obstet Gynecol* 114:1121, 2009; Luke B: Nutrition for multiples, *Clin Obstet Gynecol* 58:585, 2015; Luke B, Eberlein T, Newman R: *When you're expecting twins, triplets, or quads*, ed 4, New York, 2017, Harper. *DHA*, Docosahexaenoic acid; *EPA*, eicosapentaenoic acid; *NTD*, neural tube defect; *T*, trimester; *UL*, tolerable upper limit.

BOX 14.3 Risk Factors for Poor Pregnancy Outcome in Teenagers

- Young maternal age
- Pregnancy less than 2 years after onset of menarche
- Poor nutrition and low prepregnancy weight
- Preexisting anemia
- Inappropriate weight gain (too low and too high)
- Obesity
- Sexually transmitted disease or infection
- Substance abuse: smoking, drinking, and drugs
- Poverty
- Lack of social support
- Low educational level
- Rapid repeat pregnancies
- Lack of access to age-appropriate prenatal care
- Late entry into the health system
- Unmarried status
- Unstable housing, shelter living, homelessness

normal, these complications can be uncomfortable and potentially dangerous but can be managed.

Constipation, Hemorrhoids, and Diarrhea

With the hormonal changes of pregnancy, women become constipated if they fail to consume adequate water and fiber. Women who receive iron supplements often complain of constipation. Those who are treated with ondansetron for nausea and vomiting often experience severe constipation. Compression of the pelvic floor by the fetus, as well as straining during stooling (Valsalva), increases the risk for hemorrhoids. Increased consumption of fluids and fiber-rich foods (see Appendix 27), including dried fruits (especially prunes), usually controls these problems. Some women also may require a bulking type of stool softener but laxatives containing stimulants are not recommended. Adding unprocessed wheat bran to foods is safe and effective.

Diarrhea may also be caused by a change in hormones early in pregnancy. It may also occur when a mother is starting labor. Infectious and other medical causes should be ruled out. See Chapter 27 for treatment options. Prevention of dehydration is important.

Cravings, Aversions, and Pica

Most women change their diets during their pregnancies as a result of medical advice, cultural beliefs, or changes in food preference and appetite. Food intake in pregnancy may be affected, both positively and negatively, by changes in hormone levels. There is limited research on pregnancy's effect on the various hormones related to appetite control. Taste preferences often change during pregnancy, likely due to the pregnancy hormones affecting both the taste buds and the central nervous system (Faas et al, 2010). Food avoidances may not reflect a mother's conscious choice but may include an adverse response to smell caused by an enhanced perception of aromas, a heightened gag response, getting ill while eating or smelling a particular food, or altered gastric comfort.

Cravings and Aversions. Cravings and aversions are powerful urges toward or away from foods, including foods about which women experience no unusual attitudes when not pregnant. In the United States the most commonly craved foods are sweets, fruits, and dairy products, or foods that can be eaten quickly. The most common aversions reported are to alcohol, coffee, meats, and the smell of frying.

However, cravings and aversions are not limited to any particular food or food groups, they often overlap, and cultural differences exist. For examples, see Table 14.13.

Pica. Consumption of nonfood substances or food items in nonphysiologic amounts (pica) during pregnancy most often involves geophagia (consumption of dirt or clay), amylophagia (laundry starch, corn starch, or uncooked rice), or pagophagia (ice). Other substances include paper, burnt matches, stones or gravel, charcoal, rock salt, bleach, cigarette ashes, baby powder, baking soda, soap, tires, and coffee grounds. Although some of the common substances are of little concern, others are dangerous to the mother. The local poison control center can give guidance on which require immediate intervention.

Pica is common in pregnancy, and the incidence of pica in the United States is estimated to be 14% to 44%, with wide variability between groups (Scolari Childress and Myles, 2013). Pica is not limited to any one geographic area, race, culture, or social status, but there are cultural components related to the substances chosen and the acceptability of disclosure. Preferred substances often are imported from home countries, including soil or clay and blocks of magnesium carbonate.

The cause of pica is poorly understood. One theory suggests that pica relieves nausea and vomiting, although pica often appears later in pregnancy when nausea and vomiting are not so prevalent. One hypothesis is that it is due to a deficiency of an essential nutrient, most often iron, but zinc, calcium, and potassium also have been mentioned (Cardwell, 2013). Although it is hypothesized that the craving causes one to eat the nonfood substance that contains the missing nutrients, that is seldom the case. Pica also can be a craving for smell or texture as well as taste. IDA has been associated with the olfactory craving in pica (Hansen et al, 2017) and chewing ice has been shown to improve alertness and response times on a neuropsychological test for people who are anemic but not for others (Hunt et al, 2014). Taste perceptions often change, but whether that is associated with lower zinc levels is not known.

Malnutrition can be a consequence of pica when nonfood substances displace essential nutrients in the diet. Starch in excessive amounts contributes to obesity and can negatively affect glucose control. Large intakes of baking soda can raise blood pressure and extreme doses (1 box/day) have caused rhabdomyolysis and cardiomyopathy (Scolari Childress and Myles, 2013). Excessive intakes of baking powder can mimic preeclampsia. Substances may contain toxic compounds or heavy metals, parasites, or other pathogens. The absorption of iron or other minerals may be disrupted. Excessive geophagia can result in intestinal obstruction or perforation (Young, 2011).

Recommending stopping a pica often fails, either because of the strong physiologic drive or the cultural perception that not complying with the craving will cause harm to the fetus. Rather than insisting on cessation, resulting only in less willingness to admit the pica, a more productive approach is to offer a better alternative. For example, allowing the mother to continue to smell the wet dirt, but trading its consumption for a burned tortilla, toast, or jicama often is successful. Pica often is associated with IDA, but whether the pica is a result, a cause, or a marker of other concurrent deficiencies is unknown. However, treatment with very high iron foods often decreases the cravings and infusions of iron have resulted in a cessation of the pagophagia, as well as restless legs (Auerbach and Adamson, 2016).

Diabetes Mellitus

Gestational diabetes mellitus (GDM), carbohydrate intolerance with onset or recognition during pregnancy, encompasses two distinct groups—those who have unrecognized preexisting diabetes and those for whom the pregnancy precipitates the carbohydrate intolerance.

TABLE 14.13 Reported Cravings and Aversions by at Least 10% of Pregnant Women in Published Studies

Country	Cravings	Aversions
Ethiopia	Meat sauce, cheese, milk	Wheat, coffee, wheat bread, meat sauce
Tanzania	Meat, mangoes, yogurt, oranges	Rice, meat, fish, eggs
Nigeria	Cereals, vegetables, beans, yams, cassava, plantain, nonalcoholic beverages, fruits, meats, milk, fish	Alcohol, plantains, cassava, yams, fish, meat, milk, nonalcoholic beverages, beans, fruits, cereals
South Africa	Fruits, sour foods, sweets, cold drinks	Meat
Iraq	Meat, chicken, milk, eggs, fruits, milk	Melons, onions, leeks, radishes, spices
Saudi Arabia	Salty foods, sour foods, milk	Tea, coffee, cola, meat, spicy foods
Italy	Fruit, pasta	Meat, smoke, perfumes, coffee (taste, smell), white wine
England	Fruit and fruit juices, including citrus, sweets, chocolate, biscuits, ice cream, milk and milk products, vegetables, sweet meats, liquids, meats	Tea, coffee, highly flavored or spicy foods, including curries, meats, fish, eggs, smell of fried or fatty foods, cigarette smoke/tobacco, cocoa, vegetables
Ecuador	Fruit and fruit juices, meat, poultry, fish and seafood, eggs	Meat, poultry, fish, seafood, chicken and quail eggs, vegetables, white rice, wheat noodles, corn, barley
Jamaica	Water, ice, milk and milk drinks, fruit and fruit juices, vegetables, sweet drinks, meats, fish	Meat, rice, wheat dumplings, yams, milk, fruit and fruit juices, sweet drinks, fish
United States	Sweets, chocolate, fruit and fruit juice, citrus, pickles, ice cream, ice milk, pizza, beef, chips, spicy foods, raw vegetables, milk and other dairy, fish, ethnic foods, meat, grains, nuts and nut butters, salty foods, cookies, Italian sauce, breads/cereals	Meat, beef, fish, eggs, vegetables, ethnic foods, greasy foods, coffee, tea, legumes, alcohol, grains, sweets, fruits, cigarettes, Italian sauce, spicy foods

Adapted from. Patil CL, Abrams ET, Steinmetz AR, et al: Appetite sensations and nausea and vomiting in pregnancy: an overview of the explanations, *Ecol Food Nutr* 51:394, 2012.

Women with risk factors for type 2 diabetes (including but not limited to a history of GDM, known impaired glucose metabolism, and BMI ≥30) should be screened early in pregnancy using standard diagnostic criteria (ACOG, 2018c; American Diabetes Association [ADA], 2019; see Chapter 29). According to the ADA, those women identified with diabetes in the first trimester should be given a diagnosis of overt diabetes rather than GDM. Universal screening with a hemoglobin A1C at the first prenatal visit is common and will often identify these people.

Women identified by early screening, as well as those with known preexisting diabetes (either type 1 or 2), should be referred to a Certified Diabetes Educator (CDE) and/or a diabetes management team. Fetuses of mothers with poorly controlled diabetes at conception are at risk for multiple congenital anomalies. See Chapter 29 for management guidelines.

As pregnancy progresses and insulin resistance increases, GDM resulting from the pregnancy may appear. GDM rates in the United States are 5% to 6% of the prenatal population (National Institutes of Health [NIH], 2013), but the prevalence can be much greater in high-risk groups, including women with a high BMI, advanced maternal age, and personal and family history (first-degree relative with diabetes). Rates are higher among African American, Asian, Hispanic, Native American, and Pacific Islander women compared with non-Hispanic white women (ACOG, 2018c).

A diagnosis of GDM is associated with increased risk of gestational hypertension and of preeclampsia, as well as increased risk of type 2 diabetes and CVD later in life. Fetal implications include hyperinsulinemia, macrosomia (often defined as a baby weighing more than 4000 g), and, therefore, increased risk of delivery complications, including shoulder dystocia and cesarean delivery. The neonate is more likely to require admission to NICU and to experience respiratory distress syndrome and metabolic complications, including hyperbilirubinemia and hypoglycemia. Infant iron levels may be lower because of overgrowth and therefore increased demand (Monk et al, 2013). Other nutrients also may be low. Fetal programming, with increased long-term risk of obesity and type 2 diabetes, is also of concern.

Although some practitioners believe that GDM may represent the early stages of type 2 diabetes, others feel that women should not be labeled at all with a GDM diagnosis. However, treatment for GDM is merited because it lowers the risk by 40% for gestational hypertensive disorders, reduces the risk of macrosomia, and therefore reduces the risk of shoulder dystocia from 3.5% to 1.5% (NIH, 2013).

The diagnostic criteria for GDM are controversial. Historically, the United States and other countries have used a two-step process, whereas the WHO has advocated a one-step approach. Table 14.14 summarizes selected current guidelines but other cutoffs and testing protocols also exist (Agarwal, 2015). Recently the International Association of the Diabetes and Pregnancy Study Groups (IADPSG) advocated for a universal one-step approach developed from the Hyperglycemia and Adverse Pregnancy Outcomes (HAPO) trials. All previous protocols were designed to identify women at risk of developing type 2 diabetes later in life while the HAPO study was the first to correlate glucose values with pregnancy outcomes. Because only one elevated value is diagnostic, using the more liberal IADPSG criteria results in a twofold to threefold increase in the number of people defined as having GDM, arriving at a national prevalence of 15% to 20% (NIH, 2013).

Because of the increased cost to the medical system and the patient, increased patient stress with likely increased interventions, combined with concern that treatment may not be as beneficial for those at the lower glucose levels, a NIH consensus committee concluded there is currently insufficient evidence to recommend changing to the IADPSG

TABLE 14.14 **Screening and Diagnosis of Gestational Diabetes Mellitus (GDM) at 24 to 28 Weeks of Gestation: Blood Glucose Thresholds and Testing Protocols**

Approach	Fasting mg/dL	1-hour mg/dL	2-hour mg/dL	3-hour mg/dL	Source
TWO STEP: universal screening; only those ≥ cutoff need diagnostic test					
Screening: (nonfasting) 50 g glucose load, value ≥		130, 135, or 140			
Diagnosis: (fasting) 100 g load, 2 values ≥	95	180	155	140	Carpenter and Coustan
100 g load, 2 values ≥	105	190	165	145	National Diabetes Data Group
ONE STEP: universal testing					
Diagnosis: (fasting) 75 g load, 1 value ≥	92-125*	180	153-199*		World Health Organization (WHO)**
75 g load, 1 value ≥	92	180	153		International Association of the Diabetes and Pregnancy Study Groups

*Values above these cutpoints are considered diagnostic of diabetes mellitus in pregnancy rather than GDM, as is a random plasma value of ≥ 200 mg/dL with diabetes symptoms.
**Considered diagnostic of GDM when found any time during the pregnancy.
Adapted from National Institutes of Health consensus development conference statement: diagnosing gestational diabetes mellitus, March 4-6, 2013, *Obstet Gynecol* 122:358, 2013; World Health Organization: WHO recommendation on the diagnosis of gestational diabetes in pregnancy, March 8, 2018 (website): https://extranet.who.int/rhl/topics/preconception-pregnancy-childbirth-and-postpartum-care/antenatal-care/who-recommendation-diagnosis-gestational-diabetes-pregnancy-0.

approach (NIH, 2013). Those concerns have now been studied and some practices have returned to using the two-step approach after finding no improvement in maternal or neonatal outcomes in spite of increased diagnoses and interventions (Pocobelli et al, 2018).

The ADA and ACOG recommend screening all pregnant women for GDM (unless already identified with diabetes) at 24 to 28 weeks of gestation (ACOG, 2018c; ADA, 2019). Only those with an abnormal result on the 1-hour screen receive the 3-hour diagnostic test. ACOG recommends that the choice of a screening cutpoint and the choice of diagnostic tests (using the Carpenter and Coustan criteria if testing serum or plasma, or the National Diabetes Data Group criteria if testing plasma), be guided by local community GDM prevalence rates (ACOG, 2018c). Although current practice requires two abnormal values for a diagnosis of GDM, further study is recommended to see if those with only one elevated value also benefit from treatment.

As with preexisting diabetes, those women with GDM should be followed carefully during pregnancy and managed by a diabetes team that includes a CDE. See Chapter 29 for diet and exercise recommendations, including target glucose values. Medications may be necessary to manage blood sugars. Insulin and some oral hypoglycemic agents (e.g., metformin and glyburide) can be used. Long-term use of metformin is associated with decreased vitamin B_{12} levels, but its use only in late pregnancy has not been shown to be problematic for maintenance of normal B_{12} levels (Gatford et al, 2013). There is intriguing preliminary evidence that myoinositol may be helpful in preventing or treating GDM and its use appears to be safe (Werner and Froehlich, 2016). However, its use in treating GDM is not endorsed by the Cochrane Review because of the limited data available (Brown et al, 2016). Inositol does not appear to lower the risk of an LGA baby and other clinically meaningful outcomes have not been reported. Optimal dose, frequency, and timing of supplementation are all currently unknown, as are the long-term effects. Its

preconceptual use, along with other micronutrients and probiotics, to help improve insulin sensitivity is currently being studied (Godfrey et al, 2017a).

Women with GDM should be screened for persistent diabetes at 4 to 12 weeks postpartum, usually with fasting and 2-hour (after a 75g glucose load) blood sugars, and at least every 3 years for diabetes or prediabetes, using nonpregnancy diagnostic criteria (ADA, 2019; see Chapter 29).

Eating Disorders

The rates of eating disorders during pregnancy are 1% for anorexia nervosa and slightly more for bulimia, with the prevalence likely underestimated (Cardwell, 2013) because of voluntary nondisclosure or because the medical practitioner is not assessing the risk (Leddy et al, 2009). Anorexia and bulimia are associated with increased risk of miscarriage, birth defects, hyperemesis, IUGR, and micronutrient deficiencies, as well as postpartum depression and impaired infant bonding. For those with binge eating, excessive weight gain, macrosomia, and increased cesarean rates are seen. Those that purge may have caries or fractured teeth severe enough that they cannot chew meat.

The effect of pregnancy on the individual with an eating disorder varies, but 70% may show improvement, especially with purging behaviors (Harris, 2010). However, pregnancy does not cure the eating disorder and symptoms often are exacerbated after delivery. In fact, in some cases the newborn is seen as "too fat," to the point of restricting food, administering suppositories or enemas, or inducing vomiting. A team approach to treating the mom is helpful in those cases.

For the woman with an eating disorder, pregnancy may be particularly frightening because of the loss of control and disturbed body image. Anorexia can be diagnosed during pregnancy. Substance abuse, as well as the use of laxatives or diet pills, may be coping mechanisms. Insulin has been used as a purging mechanism. Women may fear being weighed and may need reassurance that the nausea and vomiting of pregnancy is not necessarily a resurgence of purging. Fatigue, irritability, and depression may be due to starvation. These pregnant women should be treated with particular care, including focusing on healthy eating for optimal fetal growth and development (see Chapter 21).

Edema and Leg Cramps

Mild physiologic edema is usually present in the third trimester and should not be confused with the pathologic, generalized edema associated with preeclampsia. Normal edema in the lower extremities is caused by the pressure of the enlarging uterus on the vena cava, obstructing the return of blood flow to the heart. When a woman reclines on her side, the mechanical effect is removed, and extravascular fluid is mobilized and eventually eliminated by increased urine output. No dietary intervention is required, assuming her protein intake is adequate. If, however, her urine is dark and/or she has swelling in her hands, increased fluid intake is recommended and excessive salt consumption should be reduced.

Increased fluid intake also is recommended for leg cramps. Women should be advised to stretch with their toes pointing back toward their bodies rather than away from them. Massage and heat application may help treat the cramp. Optimal calcium intake may reduce the prevalence of leg cramps. The literature is conflicting about the benefit of magnesium supplementation for prevention or treatment of pregnancy-related leg cramps (Zhou et al, 2015). Caution is advised against large intakes of supplements.

Heartburn

Gastric esophageal reflux is common during the latter part of pregnancy and often occurs at night. The pressure of the enlarged uterus on the intestines and stomach, along with the relaxation of the esophageal sphincter due to hormonal changes, may result in regurgitation of stomach contents into the esophagus. Relief measures may include eating smaller meals, limiting fluids with meals, limiting caffeine, chocolate, mint, carbonated beverages, tomatoes, citrus, fat, and spicy foods, as well as chewing gum, walking, and staying upright for at least 3 hours after a meal, but interventions have not been evaluated for effectiveness (Kaiser and Campbell, 2014). Using more pillows at night also may help (see Chapter 26).

Although heartburn medicines can be used, they are not benign and use should be limited. Taking excessive calcium carbonate can cause life-threatening milk-alkali syndrome (hypercalcemia, renal sufficiency, and metabolic alkalosis). Hypercalcemia-induced pancreatitis has also been documented (Trezevant et al, 2017). The UL of 2500 mg of elemental calcium (food plus supplements) should be observed. If a couple of calcium carbonate tablets (two regular strength Tums contain 400 mg calcium; two ultrastrength tablets provide 800 mg) do not resolve the heartburn, switching to those containing magnesium may be beneficial. However, prolonged use of high-dose magnesium-containing antacids is associated with offspring kidney stones, hypotonia, and respiratory distress (Bustos et al, 2017). Antacids containing bicarbonate may cause maternal and fetal metabolic acidosis, as well as fluid overload and are not recommended in pregnancy. Proton pump inhibitors may reduce the bioavailability of many nutrients, including vitamins C, B_{12}, calcium, magnesium, and nonheme iron. The use of antacids also potentially can increase the risk of food allergies by impeding gastric protein digestion, but whether that translates into a higher risk of food allergy or asthma for the child is unclear. Some herbal medicines, including aloe vera juice, are promoted for treatment of heartburn. However, caution is advised because animal research demonstrates some preparations of aloe contain latex which might induce abortion and/or stimulate menstruation (Zielinski et al, 2015).

Hypertension

Hypertension observed during pregnancy may be preexisting or observed for the first time. Elevated blood pressure that is first diagnosed in pregnancy may be relatively benign. However, a rise in blood pressure, accompanied by other changes listed in this chapter, can be a sign of preeclampsia, a progressive, systemic problem affecting 3% to 8% of pregnancies worldwide and the leading cause of maternal and neonatal morbidity and mortality (Myers, 2017). Although delivery resolves the problem for most, some women develop hypertension after delivery.

Chronic hypertension predates pregnancy and is associated with fetal growth restriction. Avoidance of severe hypertension is a goal, but the optimal blood pressure during pregnancy for someone with preexisting hypertension is unclear (see Chapter 32). Appropriate weight gain, a modified Dietary Approaches to Stop Hypertension (DASH) diet (see Appendix 17), and regular aerobic exercise for those without complications are recommended. Although excessive sodium should be reduced, ACOG has previously recommended that intake should not be less than 2300 mg/day (ACOG, 2013c). Calcium supplementation for those with low calcium intakes may be helpful. Some antihypertensive medications can be used during pregnancy but may need to be modified during breastfeeding.

Gestational hypertension is defined as elevated blood pressure that appears after 20 weeks of gestation, but without proteinuria or other findings. Some women (up to 50%) go on to develop preeclampsia, while others may have no risk except the elevated blood pressure (ACOG, 2019). They are treated the same as those with chronic hypertension and monitored for worsening of symptoms. Gestational hypertension may predict increased risk for future hypertension. Optimal periconceptual nutrition is important, including focus on folate, sodium, calcium, potassium, iron, copper, and zinc intakes (Tande et al, 2013).

Some women who develop hypertension during pregnancy go on to develop preeclampsia. Risk factors include women who are primiparous and obese, but other risk factors include a personal or family history of preeclampsia, chronic hypertension, diabetes (type 1, type 2, or GDM), chronic renal disease, history of thrombophilia, systemic lupus erythematosus, antiphospholipid antibody syndrome, obstructive sleep apnea, multifetal pregnancy, IVF (especially following oocyte donation [Myers, 2017]), and maternal age of at least 35 years (ACOG, 2019). However, the presence of these risk factors doesn't necessarily guarantee that an individual will develop preeclampsia. For example, while women who are obese are twice as likely to develop preeclampsia compared with women with a lower BMI, only one in ten women with obesity develop preeclampsia (Myers, 2017). In addition, most cases of preeclampsia occur in healthy, nulliparous women with no apparent risk factors (ACOG, 2019). Paternal factors also likely play a role. Risk increases with advanced paternal age, paternal obesity, and family history of early-onset CVD. Paternal genes also may be important—increased risk for preeclampsia is seen if the man has fathered a preeclamptic pregnancy or if he was born of a preeclamptic pregnancy (Dekker et al, 2011). Maternal smoking reduces the risk by 35% (ACOG, 2013c), but if preeclampsia occurs, the severity increases (Trogstad et al, 2011). Risk of recurrence in a subsequent pregnancy is 25% (Myers, 2017). Risk of preeclampsia is less likely in subsequent pregnancies with the same partner than when the mother is pregnant with a new partner.

Preeclampsia involves dysfunction of multiple organ systems. It is dynamic, progressive, and once evident, is not reversible. Delivery is needed because it is potentially fatal for mother and baby. Growth restriction is common and babies are often also premature in an effort to avoid the mother progressing to severe preeclampsia, eclampsia (new onset grand mal seizures), or HELLP syndrome (hemolysis, elevated liver enzymes, and low platelets), all of which have high rates of maternal morbidity and mortality (ACOG, 2019). Those women with superimposed preeclampsia onto chronic hypertension (13% to 40% of women) have much worse consequences (ACOG, 2013c). Women with preeclampsia that develops near term have double the risk of CVD later in life, but the risk of CVD is nearly 10-fold for those who must be delivered at less than 34 weeks of gestation because of preeclampsia (Roberts and Bell, 2013).

Preeclampsia has historically been defined by elevated blood pressure and proteinuria, but guidelines now recommend not waiting for the proteinuria to appear. Box 14.4 summarizes diagnostic criteria designed to facilitate earlier diagnosis and therefore earlier treatment.

The causes of preeclampsia are under intense investigation. It appears to be a two-stage process, with a poorly perfused placenta (from failed remodeling of the maternal spiral arteries) being the root cause (ACOG, 2013c). Reduced perfusion and increased velocity of blood perfusing the intervillous spaces alters placental function and leads to maternal disease through oxidative and endoplasmic reticulum stress and inflammation, as well as modified endothelial function and angiogenesis. The second stage, called *maternal syndrome,* is a cascade of events, but what links the hypoxic placenta and the maternal syndrome is unclear and possibly involves oxidative stress. The hypertension and proteinuria are only a small part of the syndrome and reduced perfusion of any organ in the body can lead to hemorrhage and necrosis. Not all women with inadequate placental perfusion develop preeclampsia. A woman's underlying disease (e.g., diabetes, hypertension), lifestyle (e.g., obesity, activity, sleep), genetics, and environmental conditions (e.g., air pollution) may affect the maternal response (Roberts and Bell, 2013). The inflammatory response is accentuated in preeclampsia. Predictive tests are being studied but are not ready for clinical use (ACOG, 2019). It is now thought that preeclampsia is actually a syndrome of many diseases with subsets of pathophysiology and varied contributions of maternal and placental factors (Roberts and Bell, 2013).

Prevention of preeclampsia has not yet been effective, although daily low-dose aspirin may be beneficial (ACOG, 2019). Although previously recommended, vitamin C and E supplements do not prevent occurrence of preeclampsia or adverse outcomes and may be associated with increased risk of gestational hypertension and LBW. Calcium supplementation may help reduce symptom severity if a mother's baseline calcium intake has been less than 600 mg/day (ACOG, 2013c). There is insufficient evidence to demonstrate effectiveness of fish oil, garlic, vitamin D or folic acid supplementation, nor of sodium restriction (ACOG, 2019). Avoiding excessive weight gain and tightly controlling diabetes may help. Protein and calorie restriction for women with obesity does not reduce the risk of either gestational hypertension or preeclampsia and may increase the risk of IUGR. Bed rest does not appear to reduce risk. Diuretics are not recommended. Moderate exercise (30 minutes/day) is recommended as during normal pregnancy, but it is unclear whether it can help reverse the endothelial dysfunction and prevent adverse pregnancy outcomes. Obesity, leptin, insulin, and free fatty acids appear to affect various stages of preeclampsia. Endothelial cell disorder from placental ischemia and hypoxia appear important. An imbalance of angiogenic factors, immune factors, inflammation, endothelin (a protein that constricts blood vessels), nitric oxide, oxidative and endoplasmic reticulum stress, the stress response gene hemeoxygenase and its catalytic product carbon monoxide, and the effect of statins are all being studied.

For those women with a history of preeclampsia, weight loss, increased physical activity, smoking cessation, and optimization of blood glucose levels and nutrient intakes preconceptually are recommended. During pregnancy, helping women maintain a normal rate of weight gain, with optimal calcium intake and fruits and vegetables (antioxidants), may be beneficial. Encourage notifying the medical provider immediately if there is a sudden onset of face or hand swelling, persistent headaches, seeing spots or changes in eyesight, pain in the upper right quadrant or stomach, nausea and vomiting in the second half of pregnancy, rapid weight gain, or difficulty breathing.

Although delivery resolves the preeclampsia for most, a subset of women have a worsening of preeclampsia after delivery and others may first develop preeclampsia postpartum, including HELLP syndrome. Pain medications may have to be modified. Blood pressure may be labile for months but usually normalizes by 1 year postpartum. Postpartum hypertension may predict future chronic hypertension (ACOG, 2013c).

Nausea and Vomiting, Hyperemesis Gravidarum, and Ptyalism

Morning sickness, nausea and vomiting in pregnancy (NVP), affects 50% to 90% of all pregnant women during the first trimester and usually resolves by 20 to 22 weeks of gestation, although up to 10% of women suffer with it until delivery (Bustos et al, 2017). The cause of NVP is unclear but likely includes a genetic predisposition, combined with changes in human chorionic gonadotropin (hCG), estrogen, and progesterone levels. Recently an increase in the half-life of endokinin B,

---

BOX 14.4   Preeclampsia Diagnostic Criteria

Elevated blood pressure
  Confirmed ≥160 or ≥110 for anyone (confirmed over a few minutes) or ≥140 or ≥90 after 20 weeks of gestation (confirmed over 4 hours) if previously normal

AND

Proteinuria
  ≥300 mg/24-hour urine collection, an extrapolated amount from a timed collection, protein/creatinine ratio ≥0.3, or dipstick reading of 2+ if no other quantitative methods are available

OR

Elevated blood pressure
  Confirmed ≥160 or ≥110 for anyone (confirmed over a few minutes) or ≥140 or ≥90 after 20 weeks of gestation (confirmed over 4 hours) if previously normal

AND

New onset of any of the following:
  Thrombocytopenia: platelets <100,000/microliter
  Renal insufficiency: serum creatinine >1.1 mg/dL or doubling of serum creatinine concentration in absence of other renal disease
  Impaired liver function: elevated liver transaminases to twice normal blood concentrations
  Pulmonary edema
  Cerebral or visual symptoms

Adapted from American College of Obstetricians and Gynecologists (ACOG): ACOG Practice Bulletin No. 202: Gestational Hypertension and Preeclampsia, Obstet Gynecol 133:e1, 2019.

a tachykinin produced by the placenta to increase blood flow, has also been proposed as a cause (Lowry and Woods, 2018) because it also stimulates the NK1R receptor in the brain, causing nausea and vomiting in some women. NVP may be mediated through the vestibuloocular reflex pathway and those with a history of motion sickness or migraines are at increased risk. Those pregnant with a female fetus, multiple fetuses, or a molar pregnancy (sperm fertilizes an empty egg, resulting in no embryo but a placenta that develops into an abnormal mass of cells) are more likely to suffer with either NVP or hyperemesis gravidarum, as are those with hyperthyroid disorders, GI disorders, preexisting diabetes, or a psychiatric illness. Maternal age more than 30 years and smoking are protective, but paternal smoking increases risk (Fejzo et al, 2012). NVP is associated with more favorable pregnancy outcomes, including fewer birth defects; reduced risk of miscarriage, preterm delivery, or stillbirth; and greater birth weight.

Treatment for NVP involves managing the symptoms. Motion, specific odors, loud noises, bright or flickering lights, and adverse climate conditions may trigger the nausea. Fortunately, most women with NVP are functional, able to work, do not lose weight, and are helped by simple dietary measures. Many dietary and lifestyle recommendations have not been evaluated in the literature (Kaiser and Campbell, 2014). Although the quality of the evidence is low, it appears that ginger preparations (tablets, syrup, capsules, or ginger biscuits) are more effective than placebos in reducing the severity of symptoms (O'Donnell et al, 2016), possibly by multiple mechanisms (Marx et al, 2017). However, while ginger reduces the nausea, it may not reduce the episodes of emesis and does not work for many people, especially those with hyperemesis (Dean and O'Hara, 2015). Ginger supplements can be offered as a first line therapy (250 mg capsules 4x/day) (ACOG, 2018b) but should not be used for women on anticoagulation therapy because of the increased risk of bleeding with platelet function inhibition (Bustos et al, 2017). Ginger has also been reported to increase symptoms for some, including heartburn and throat burning during vomiting (Dean and O'Hara, 2015). If the symptoms are already severe, ginger is unlikely to be helpful and therefore delays more effective treatment.

Acupressure of the P6 point of the wrist may have limited benefit but neither acupuncture nor electrical nerve stimulation appear to be effective (ACOG, 2018b). Noise reduction and hypnosis also can be helpful. If not tolerated, stopping the prenatal vitamins may help, but women should continue the supplemental folic acid if possible, and often taking the prenatal vitamins before bed or with food during the largest meal of the day is tolerated. Others recommend adding supplemental thiamin (at least 5 mg/day) to lower the risk of Wernicke's encephalopathy (Fejzo et al, 2016). Various antinausea medications are also available, with different modes of action and risk levels. Vitamin B_6, in combination with doxylamine, is often used (ACOG, 2018b). Whether the vitamin B_6 alone is effective as well as what form of the B_6 is best are both unclear but it appears that the metabolites pyridoxine and pyridoxal may function as prodrugs (Matok et al, 2014). Marijuana, while it is promoted by some to help with NVP, is not recommended (ACOG, 2018b). In fact, cannabinoid hyperemesis syndrome, potentially fatal, has been documented (Nourbakhsh et al, 2018).

Small, frequent snacks of carbohydrate foods, including crackers or dry cereal, reduce nausea for some, whereas protein foods may help others (Erick, 2014). Some women crave potato chips. Some do not tolerate odors and are bothered by hot foods, preferring foods that are cold or at room temperature. Smelling lemons may help block noxious odors. Avoiding hunger by eating more frequently often helps, as does separating dry foods from liquids. Avoiding highly spiced foods or bitter foods is helpful for some, but for others taste sensitivity decreases and strong flavors are craved. Women should avoid odors or situations

that trigger symptoms and should eat whatever reduces the nausea sensation. Unfortunately, there is no cure-all. However, reminding the mother that this is a good sign for the pregnancy (i.e., the body is responding as it should), and that it *will* end, often reassures her and lowers the worry and stress, thus helping with the nausea.

When early pregnancy is characterized by excessive vomiting (severity is often estimated by the PUQE score: pregnancy-unique quantification of emesis) and weight loss (often at least 5% prepregnant weight), usually with dehydration, electrolyte imbalances can occur. Here, "morning sickness" becomes hyperemesis gravidarum (HG). The prevalence of HG is 0.3% to 3% of pregnancies (ACOG, 2018b) and is the most frequent cause of hospital admissions early in pregnancy, increasing both worry and the economic burden. Risk factors are the same as those with NVP. Recurrence rate in a subsequent pregnancy is 15% to 81% (Grooten et al, 2016), with higher estimates from surveys in which symptoms are reported rather than those just looking at hospital admissions. Early treatment of NVP, including even preemptive, is thought to help prevent progression to HG (ACOG, 2018b).

Fetal complications of HG vary but include poor fetal growth and preterm delivery. There is an increased risk of fetal loss with gestational malnutrition, as high as 37% spontaneous fetal loss rate among women with significant weight loss and Wernicke's encephalopathy (Chiossi et al, 2006). While documented congenital anomalies are rare, chondrodysplasia punctata resulting from maternal vitamin K deficiency has been documented (Erick, 2014). Research has shown these exposed children have a 3.28-fold increase in the odds of receiving a neurodevelopmental diagnosis, including attention or sensory disorders and speech, language, and learning delays, especially if the HG started before 5 weeks of gestation (Fejzo et al, 2015). Lower insulin sensitivity in children exposed to HG has also been seen (Abramowitz et al, 2017). Maternal complications include extreme fatigue, dehydration, and malnutrition. HG is associated with guilt and a loss of self, often with a sense of dying, as well as with social isolation. It is associated with increased depression and/or anxiety but the direction of the relationship is controversial and stigmatizing the mother is not helpful (Dean et al, 2018). Other complications may include splenic avulsion (spleen is torn from its normal location, resulting in an emergency situation due to excessive bleeding), esophageal rupture, diaphragmatic tears, pneumothorax, Valsalva retinopathy, hypocalcemia, liver dysfunction, acute renal failure, rhabdomyolysis, central pontine myelinolysis, and delirium, as well as maternal posttraumatic stress syndrome and high risk of pregnancy termination when management of HG fails (Erick, 2014; Fejzo et al, 2012; Dean et al, 2018; ACOG 2018b; Abramowitz et al, 2017). Maternal deaths associated with HG have been reported (Fejzo et al, 2016). Difficulty producing breastmilk and bonding also may have to be addressed.

Hospitalization for nutrition support and hydration usually is indicated for HG. Management goals include appropriate weight gain for pregnancy, correction of fluid and electrolyte deficits, avoidance of ketosis, control of HG symptoms, and achievement of nitrogen, vitamin, and mineral balance. Because pregnancy is a condition of accelerated starvation, refeeding syndrome is seen often, especially with the provision of simple dextrose-containing intravenous fluids. Phosphorus, magnesium, and potassium must be evaluated daily because low levels may result in cardiac irregularities and respiratory failure (see Chapter 12). Another potentially serious complication is Wernicke's encephalopathy, with at least 63 cases being reported worldwide (Di Gangi et al, 2012). It is thought to be caused by thiamin depletion and, because there is little storage in the body (Frank, 2015), a deficiency can develop in as little as 2 weeks of vomiting (Selitsky et al, 2006). There is no consensus on early diagnosis, treatment, or prevention. The classic triad of nystagmus and ophthalmoplegia, mental status changes, and ataxia has been found in only 16% of known HG cases. Women in 60% of cases displayed ocular symptoms, 83% had cerebellar changes, and 52% had memory impairment (Di Gangi et al, 2012). Symptoms are often vague and nonspecific, including headaches, fatigue, abdominal discomfort, irritability, and inability to concentrate. If not treated quickly, Wernicke's encephalopathy can progress to Korsakoff syndrome, with chronic maternal memory impairment (Kloss et al, 2018). Thiamin blood levels are not useful for diagnosis. Instead, thiamin is given intravenously, and a presumptive diagnosis is made if the patient responds. ACOG recommends giving 100 mg IV thiamin with the initial rehydration fluid, followed by 100 mg/day for the next 2 to 3 days, followed by IV multivitamins (ACOG, 2018b). Correcting deficiencies of niacin and magnesium also may be helpful.

In HG, early enteral tube feeding does not consistently improve birthweight (Grooten et al, 2017). Women with severe emesis and retching have often dislodged tubes and are sometimes reluctant for replacement. During hospitalization, frequent nursing checks on tube placement add to sleep deprivation issues, which have not been fully appreciated (Erick, 2014). When enteral nutrition is not tolerated and oral intake is not sufficient, parenteral nutrition should be considered (see Chapter 11). Historically, problems with infections, as well as hyperglycemia, hepatic dysfunction, and respiratory compromise have all been seen (Worthington et al, 2017). However, with careful management, including avoiding overfeeding, adequate glucose control, and meticulous venous access care, these problems can be minimized or eliminated. Parenteral nutrition has safely been employed during pregnancy for HG, as well as GI disorders such as short bowel syndrome and Crohn's disease (Mogensen and Erick, 2017).

Women historically have been reassured that even with HG the fetus is protected, using adequate birth weight as evidence. However, given the results of the Dutch famine studies, it is known that birth weight does not necessarily predict long-term health and that there are consequences of early malnutrition, even if later resolved (Erick, 2014; Roseboom et al, 2011). HG merits early and aggressive attention and treatment.

Some women develop ptyalism gravidarum, or excess saliva. It often has an abrupt onset 2 to 3 weeks after conception and reported prevalence varies widely, from 0.08% in the United States to 35% in Turkey (Thaxter Nesbeth et al, 2016). Hormonal changes are thought to play a role but a new possible causal explanation is an increase in the half-life of endokinin B (Lowry and Woods, 2018). Salivary output can be substantial, up to 1.5 to 2.0 liters/day, and can be a source of lost electrolytes as well as dehydration (Thaxter Nesbeth et al, 2016) because the saliva is often spit into a cup or paper tissue. It may interfere with swallowing and cause distended cheek pouches and swollen salivary glands. Because the saliva is excessively thick and the tongue is often enlarged and coated, ptyalism often interferes with speech. It may increase the nausea and vomiting and often adversely affects the sense of taste. It interferes with sleep and is associated with increased depression. However, ptyalism does not appear dangerous for the fetus. Antihistamines may be helpful, as may chewing gum or sucking on hard candy, throat lozenges, lemon drops, or ice. Ptyalism ceases at delivery but may end after the first trimester for some people (Thaxter Nesbeth et al, 2016).

Oral Health

Good oral health is important throughout one's lifetime, including during pregnancy (see Chapter 24). Pregnant women can receive dental care while pregnant, with some qualifications. The National Maternal and Child Oral Health Resource Center provides guidance. Although periodontal infection is associated with preterm birth and LBW, treatment does not appear to lower that risk. However, optimal

maternal oral hygiene may lower the amount of *Streptococcus mutans* transmitted to the infant through sharing spoons or licking pacifiers, thus lowering or delaying the risk of childhood caries.

During pregnancy, increased inflammatory response to dental plaque causes gingivae to swell and bleed more easily. Rinsing with salt water (1 tsp salt in 1 cup warm water) can help soothe the irritation. Erosion of enamel may occur with increased exposure to gastric acid from vomiting or gastric reflux. Rinsing with a baking soda solution (1 tsp baking soda in 1 cup water) may help neutralize the acid (ACOG, 2013a) and tooth brushing should be avoided for at least an hour after vomiting to allow the enamel to reharden (Dragan et al, 2018).

Preexisting Medical Conditions

Many women begin pregnancy with preexisting conditions that can complicate the pregnancy and modify nutrient requirements and appropriate food sources, as well as the supplementation that is necessary. As an example, celiac disease adversely affects fertility for men and women, and the absorption of nutrients often is impaired (Freeman, 2010). Women with celiac disease have increased risk of miscarriages and preterm deliveries. Some prenatal supplements may contain gluten or wheat binders and should be avoided. Women with phenylketonuria (PKU) must be following the dietary restrictions months prior to conception to minimize damage to the fetal brain (see Chapter 42). Women with inflammatory bowel disease may have low serum vitamin B_{12} levels if there is damage to the intestines. Women with HIV infection may have higher energy needs and the interaction of nutrients with medications may have to be considered. Immigrant women may suffer with active malaria, which invades the placenta, or GI parasites, which can both decrease nutrient intakes and increase nutrient losses. Women with preexisting depression are at risk for poor pregnancy outcome and postpartum depression, putting the mother and her newborn at risk if she is unable to function optimally.

Women also may develop conditions resulting from the pregnancy that need particular attention, including HG, gallstones, or intrahepatic cholestasis of pregnancy. They also may be involved in a motor vehicle accident or other trauma that requires special care or even time in an intensive care unit (ICU). In all cases, the needs of the mother and the fetus must remain paramount. Although guidance is available for some conditions (Crozier, 2017), strong evidence-based recommendations are lacking.

Food Safety during Pregnancy

Although a pregnant woman is no more likely to be exposed to pathogens than a nonpregnant woman, she and her fetus may be at higher risk of suffering negative consequences from foodborne illnesses. In addition, because metabolically active tissues may be more susceptible to the action of toxins, along with the potential long-term effects of fetal exposure to suboptimal conditions, a pregnant woman often has questions regarding the safety of common foods and nonnutritive substances. Those food safety issues of most concern vary between populations. Box 14.5 summarizes general food safety guidelines.

However, caution is advised to not overestimate the risk of food contamination in pregnancy or the amount of control that an individual has in lowering that risk. It is critical to avoid the impression that a healthy baby is guaranteed if parents do everything right and that the mother is to blame if anything goes wrong. In addition, it is becoming increasingly apparent that maternal psychological stress is also harmful to the pregnancy (see *Clinical Insight:* Stress During Pregnancy).

BOX 14.5 General Food Safety Guidelines

Clean

- Wash hands thoroughly with soap and water, especially before and after handling food, and after using the bathroom, changing diapers, or handling pets. Do not touch mucous membranes after handling meats.
- Wash cutting boards, dishes, utensils, and countertops with hot water and soap. Washing utensils, including cutting boards, in the dishwasher is preferable.
- Wash raw fruits and vegetables thoroughly under running water, even if the skin will not be eaten.
- Do not wash or rinse meat and poultry.

Separate to Avoid Cross Contamination

- Separate raw meat, poultry, and seafood from ready-to-eat foods when shopping, preparing, and storing foods.
- Use one cutting board for raw meat, poultry, and seafood and another one for fresh fruits and vegetables.
- Place cooked food on a clean plate. The unwashed plate that held raw meat, poultry, or seafood, may be contaminated.

Cook to Proper Temperature

- Cook foods thoroughly. Use a food thermometer to check the temperature. (Color is not a reliable indicator of meat doneness.) Examples include the following:
  - Beef, pork, veal, lamb, large cuts (steaks, roasts, and chops): 145° F + 3-minute rest
  - Fish: 145° F
  - Beef, pork, veal, lamb, ground meats: 160° F
  - Egg dishes: 160° F
  - Turkey, chicken, duck (whole animal, pieces, ground): 165° F

- Cook eggs until firm.
- Reheat leftovers to at least 165° F and sauces, gravies, and soups should be boiled.

Chill to Avoid the Danger Zone

- Refrigerator should register at 40° F or below and the freezer at 0° F. Check the temperature periodically with an appliance thermometer.
- Limit the time foods are in the danger zone, the range of temperatures at which bacteria can grow quickly, usually between 40° F and 140° F.
- Defrost (and marinate) foods in the refrigerator, not on the kitchen counter.
- Refrigerate or freeze perishables (foods that can spoil or become contaminated by bacteria if left unrefrigerated) promptly.
- Use ready-to-eat, perishable foods (dairy, meat, poultry, seafood, produce) as soon as possible.
- 2-hour rule: discard perishable foods left out at room temperature for more than 2 hours. If it is a hot day (more than 90° F), shorten the time to 1 hour.

Avoid High-Risk Foods

- Avoid unpasteurized milks, including goat milk, and foods made of unpasteurized milks. Even if soft cheeses are pasteurized, hard cheeses are safer.
- Avoid raw or undercooked meats, poultry, eggs, fish, or seafood.
- Avoid unpasteurized fruit or vegetable juices. Unpasteurized juice, including cider, must be boiled (full rolling boil) for at least 1 minute.
- Avoid raw or undercooked sprouts, including alfalfa, clover, mung bean, and radish. Cooked sprouts are lower risk.
- Do not open bulging cans.
- Boil home-canned foods for 20 minutes.
- Pay attention to national food recalls, as well as cautions issued locally. Pregnancy is not the time to gamble.

Adapted from Cox JT, Phelan ST: Food safety in pregnancy, part 1: putting risks into perspective, *Contemporary Ob/Gyn* 54:44, 2009a; United States Department of Health and Human Services (USDHHS): *Keep Food Safe: Check your Steps* (website): https://www.foodsafety.gov/keep/basics/index.html, 2018.

CLINICAL INSIGHT

Stress During Pregnancy

Prenatal psychological stress is associated with shorter gestations and lower birth weights. Stress also appears to interact with poor nutrition to negatively affect fetal neurocognitive development, especially the hippocampus and memory functioning, using the same mechanisms as infectious stress (Monk et al, 2013).

All nutrients are important for neuronal and glial cell growth and development. Stress appears to alter the metabolism of many nutrients (protein, glucose, zinc, iron, chromium, choline, folate, vitamin D, B vitamins), but not others (LCPUFA, copper, iodine, vitamin A), and some nutrients (LCPUFA, protein, zinc, iron, choline) may have a role in the stress response (Monk et al, 2013; McCabe et al, 2017; Lindsay et al, 2019).

Distress can induce insulin resistance and proinflammatory cytokines, diverting amino acids to gluconeogenesis and energy production rather than protein production (Monk et al, 2013). Stress also raises the risk of hypertension, increasing uterine artery resistance and lowering nutrient delivery to the fetus. Risk of autism and schizophrenia may increase, but the timing of the insult may affect the response (Marques et al, 2013). Prenatal stress also affects placental development and placental response to fetal development in a sex-specific manner (Cao-Lei et al, 2017), as well as fetal programming, including affecting the production of genes that affect the ability to regulate stress as an adult (Georgieff et al, 2015).

Maternal and fetal immune systems communicate bidirectionally, and the fetal immune system (innate and adaptive) can be disrupted with maternal stress, as well as by exposure to toxins and malnutrition. This disruption may be sufficient to affect a child's response to vaccines but there is no consensus on the timeframe of vulnerability or on the mechanisms (Marques et al, 2013).

When studying infant neurocognitive development, psychological stress and nutritional status must be studied together to examine their bidirectional and synergistic effects, but the effects appear to differ with race and offspring sex (Lindsay et al, 2019). Maternal depression and anxiety, as well as maternal malnutrition, are associated with altered offspring brain anatomy, cognitive impairments, and neurodevelopmental disorders.

When studying intervention strategies, stress and nutrition also need to be studied together (Lindsay et al, 2019). High fat diets appear to be neuroprotective in the context of maternal stress exposure. The type of fat, specifically a low n3:n6 ratio, may be of concern, but the effect appears to vary by race and ethnicity. Prenatal supplementation with antioxidants or 1-carbon nutrients may lower the anxiogenic effects of perinatal stress in the adult offspring, at least in the rodent model. Many nutrients, including choline, lutein, B_6, B_{12}, folate, methionine, and betaine, are being studied, but the beneficial effects appear to be sex-specific.

CLINICAL INSIGHT

Stress During Pregnancy—cont'd

Current evidence is insufficient to recommend any specific diet or nutrient components to mitigate the effect of prenatal stress on neurodevelopmental outcomes in the offspring.

Often issues of psychological stress arise in the course of discussing food intake and weight gain. They would include, but are not limited to, catastrophic life events, verbal or physical abuse, unemployment, and food insecurity, as well as anxiety about the pregnancy itself. In addition, a history of adverse childhood experiences (ACEs) is also associated with lower birthweights and shorter gestational age (Smith et al, 2016), as well as increased risk in the perinatal and postnatal periods (Madigan et al, 2017). Paternal stress and trauma appear to affect sperm development, negatively affecting offspring neurodevelopment (Chan et al, 2018). Whether or not any of these historic exposures to stress are mediated, or can be altered, by nutritional interventions is unknown. A referral to a mental health professional for evaluation and treatment is warranted and good support systems appear to be helpful (Madigan et al, 2017). See Chapter 30 for more information.

Alcohol

Abundant evidence from animal studies and human experience associates maternal alcohol consumption with teratogenicity, causing a variety of problems collectively known as Fetal Alcohol Spectrum Disorders (FASDs). Fetal alcohol syndrome (FAS), the most involved of these conditions, is the leading cause of preventable birth defects, potentially affecting 5% to 10% of pregnancies worldwide (Harris et al, 2017) (see Chapter 43).

Use of any alcohol during pregnancy is associated with an increased rate of miscarriage, placenta abruption, LBW (five-fold increased risk with at least 1 drink/day), preterm delivery (twofold increased risk), and cognitive compromise (Cox and Phelan, 2009b). Epigenetic effects have also been documented (Gupta et al, 2016) and both maternal and paternal gene expression may affect a fetus' susceptibility to FAS. However, the effects on an individual are difficult to predict and even dizygotic twins can be affected differently (Sarman, 2018).

Poor nutrition can exacerbate the development of FAS. High blood alcohol concentrations can displace or reduce the transfer of nutrients across the placenta. While prenatal interventions to prevent or reverse alcohol's teratogenicity are being explored, including the use of antioxidants and other nutrients, results are not consistent and none are approved for clinical use (Gupta et al, 2016).

ACOG, the American Academy of Pediatrics (AAP), and the March of Dimes recommend that alcohol not be used during pregnancy because no safe threshold has been identified. Reduced-alcohol wines and beers contain small amounts of alcohol and also are contraindicated. Despite the multiple warnings of fetal injury caused by alcohol, some women continue to drink in pregnancy and they should be offered assistance. However, for those women who are fearful of the alcohol they consumed early in pregnancy, possibly before realizing they were pregnant, reassurance is advised.

Allergens

Restriction of the maternal diet during pregnancy and lactation is not advised as a strategy to lower the risk of infant food allergies and may be counterproductive (Renz et al, 2018). Maternal dietary proteins found in amniotic fluid and cord blood have been hypothesized to support the development of tolerance but the issue is still being debated (Jeurink et al, 2018). The mother should avoid her own allergens during pregnancy and lactation but should eat a variety of other foods, including the father's allergenic foods. Regarding peanuts, studies have shown the child has a slightly increased risk of developing peanut sensitization if a mother eats peanuts more than twice a week, but avoidance by the mother appears to be associated with even higher risk (Fleischer et al, 2013). The mother is encouraged to breastfeed exclusively for the first few months. Foods should be added to the infant's diet carefully while still receiving breastmilk, but delaying introduction of solid foods past 6 months provides no benefit. Use of probiotics by the mother or child may be beneficial, but type, timing, and dose are unknown. The roles of maternal fish oil consumption and vitamin D deficiency are also being studied but current data are conflicting and no definite dietary guidance can be given (Garcia-Larsen et al, 2018).

Artificial Sweeteners

Research on the safety of artificial sweeteners is limited, but the FDA has deemed the following safe for use in moderation, including during pregnancy and lactation: saccharin, acesulfame-K, sucralose, aspartame, neotame, advantame, steviol glycosides from stevia leaves, and extracts from monk fruit.

Food additives, including artificial sweeteners, are tested for short- and long-term toxicity; reproductive effects, including teratogenicity; and any adverse effects on an animal's reproductive organs or systems, any birth defects, and genetic toxicity (Rulis and Levitt, 2009). From that data, a safety factor is applied; usually 1/100th of the dose in which any problems have been seen. The resulting value is the acceptable daily intake (ADI), defined as the estimated amount of a food additive that someone can safely consume on average every day over a lifetime without any appreciable health risk. Monk fruit is too new for an ADI to have been determined. Current intakes of the other sweeteners listed here, except for stevia, are well below these ADI levels (Shankar et al, 2013; see Chapter 29).

Saccharin (Sweet'N Low, Sweet Twin, Sugar Twin, Necta Sweet) crosses the placenta (Cohen-Addad et al, 1986) and may accumulate in the fetus and in breastmilk, but adverse effects on the fetus and infant have not been documented (Pope et al, 2014). It has been delisted as a human carcinogen (Kroger et al, 2006; Shankar et al, 2013).

Acesulfame-K (Sunett, Sweet One) consumption by pregnant women is classified as safe, even without long-term studies during human pregnancy. It often is used in conjunction with other artificial sweeteners. It is said to not be metabolized in humans (Kroger et al, 2006). However, in mice it can appear in the amniotic fluid and breastmilk after an oral infusion (Zhang et al, 2011) and animal models have shown it can cross the placenta and increase the preference for sweets as adults (Pope et al, 2014).

Sucralose (Splenda, Nevella), a carbohydrate derived from sucrose, appears to pass through the GI tract relatively unchanged, is not bioreactive, and does not bioaccumulate (Magnuson et al, 2017). There is no evidence of harm when used during pregnancy and lactation (Pope et al, 2014). It has not been found to be teratogenic in animal studies.

Aspartame (Equal, NutraSweet, Natra Taste) is metabolized to phenylalanine, aspartic acid, and methanol in the GI tract. Studies have shown no significant effect on fertility, conception rates, embryo toxicity, fetotoxicity, or teratogenesis at the levels tested in animals (London, 1988). Its use during pregnancy and lactation has not been found to increase risk of brain tumors in children (Shankar et al, 2013). The aspartic acid does not cross the placenta in monkeys, and the methanol content is less than that of many fruit juices (Kroger et al, 2006; London, 1988; Pope et al, 2014). Although it is not absolutely contraindicated for women with PKU or for women breastfeeding an infant with PKU, it must be counted as a phenylalanine source. High circulating concentrations of phenylalanine are known to damage the fetal brain (see Chapter 42). Neotame (Newtame) is also a source of phenylalanine and aspartic acid but, because it is much sweeter, the amounts consumed are negligible and do not have to be counted (Kroger et al, 2006). Advantame is also a source of phenylalanine but at such low concentrations that it also does not need to be counted (FDA, 2014). There are no human reproductive studies on advantame, but it is sweeter than neotame, so very small amounts would likely be consumed.

Both stevia and monk fruit are plant-derived sweeteners considered generally recognized as safe (GRAS) in their purified forms. Stevia (Pure Via, Truvia, SweetLeaf) has not been found to affect fetal development, at least with short-term use. *Stevia rebaudiana* traditionally has been used by the indigenous populations of Paraguay for fertility control (Ulbricht et al, 2010). Animal studies have suggested that steviol glycosides may have adverse effects on the male reproductive system, but there are no confirming studies in humans (Kroger et al, 2006; Ulbricht et al, 2010). Caution is advised when used by pregnant or lactating women, or for use longer than 2 years, because of insufficient evidence of safety (Ulbricht et al, 2010; Pope et al, 2014). There is little information on the excretion of Rebaudioside A (the refined preparation of the active ingredient, now considered GRAS) and the other plant components, including steviol glycosides, into breastmilk, so caution is advised when nursing a newborn or a preterm infant. The ADI for stevia is the equivalent of only 9 sweetener packets/day for someone weighing 60 kg. For the extracts of *Siraitia grosvenorii*, known as Swingle fruit, Luo Han Guo, or monk fruit, there is no information available for pregnancy or lactation.

Sugar alcohols (polyols) and polydextrose, a type of dietary fiber, are both likely safe for use during pregnancy. Other sweeteners are available internationally, including thaumatin (*Thaumatococcus daniellii*), derived from the Katemfe fruit. The effect on pregnancy is unknown but is not expected to be of concern (Pope et al, 2014).

Artificial sweeteners often are found in foods with low nutrient content. Intakes may have to be limited so as not to displace the more valuable, nutrient-dense foods. Although average intakes are well below the ADI, an assessment of the diet is warranted to identify those women who may be ingesting multiple sources of artificial sweeteners. If intakes are high, alternatives should be offered.

Bisphenol-A, Phthalates, and Other Environmental Toxins

Bisphenol-A (BPA), an endocrine disruptor, is associated with recurrent miscarriages and may affect thyroid function in humans, especially in the fetus. Its function at the cellular level is still being investigated but there is evidence in mice that it acts similar to diethylstilbestrol (DES) (ACOG, 2013b). Phthalates are associated with shortened gestational length and developmental disruptions. BPA and phthalates, along with 20 other chemicals, are associated with increased risk of weight gain, insulin resistance, and type 2 diabetes later in life after developmental exposure (Barouki et al, 2012). See Table 14.2 for more examples.

There are calls to limit the use of BPA, phthalates, and other environmental toxins. Although recommendations can be made to avoid specific plastics and canned foods (BPA is used as a lining material), most people also have high exposure through air, dust, and personal care products (Sathyanarayana et al, 2013), and changing behavior does not necessarily reduce risk. In addition, having a plastic labeled

"BPA free" does not ensure safety. Most plastics under stress (exposure to boiling water, ultraviolet rays in sunlight, or microwaving) release estrogenic chemicals that may be of more concern than those plastics containing BPA (Yang et al, 2011).

Although it is known that exposure to environmental toxins can have long-term effects, it is unknown whether or how the effects vary by gender or life stage. It is also unknown how the placenta mediates exposure to toxins (ACOG, 2013b; Bloomfield, 2011). The effects may be nonlinear (i.e., low doses can be more harmful than high doses) (Barouki et al, 2012). There are also potential effects on gene expression. ACOG is calling for better research on the reproductive effects of environmental toxins and societal change regarding exposure to these toxins (ACOG, 2013b).

Much of the effect of these chemicals may be during organogenesis, so reducing preconceptual exposure is likely to be most productive. Raising concerns with a mother later in pregnancy without actually being able to change outcomes would not be helpful.

Caffeine and Energy Drinks

Caffeine crosses the placenta and increases maternal catecholamines, but it appears that intakes of less than 200 mg/day are not associated with increased risk of miscarriages, low birthweight, or preterm birth (Practice Committee, 2017). It does not decrease uterine blood flow or oxygenation. However, although there is no clear evidence of harm, the evidence also does not follow the expected dose-response curve, so the effect cannot be determined definitively. The half-life of caffeine increases during pregnancy (8.3 hours longer on average, but can be up to 16 hours longer) so the effect on the fetal brain is potentially increased (Temple et al, 2017). Smoking doubles the clearance rate but alcohol consumption decreases it.

Caffeinated beverages are not considered to be of high nutritional quality, and moderation is encouraged. See Appendix 25 for caffeine food sources. Energy drinks and energy shots are not recommended during pregnancy. They may contain very high caffeine levels (> 500 mg) and also can be highly sweetened (Temple et al, 2017). In addition, these drinks often have high levels of added nutrients and herbal products that have not been evaluated for safety during pregnancy (Procter and Campbell, 2014).

Lead and Cadmium

Contaminants in food are the exception rather than the rule in the United States, but they do occur. In high concentrations, they can pass across the placenta to the fetus (Fig. 14.7). Heavy metals are of particular concern.

Lead contamination is associated with increased risk of miscarriage, gestational hypertension, IUGR, preterm delivery, and impaired neurobehavioral development. It easily crosses the placenta by passive diffusion (Caserta et al, 2013).

In addition to old paint chips, poorly glazed dishware (often imported) and leaded crystal decanters may contain high amounts of lead. Pregnant women should avoid using dolomite as a calcium supplement because the seashells or sea coral often contain heavy metals, including lead, as a result of dumping industrial wastes in the oceans. Imported candies from many areas, including Mexico, China, and India, have also been found to contain lead (Handley et al, 2017) Spices and herbs, notably ground turmeric, have been found to be adulterated with lead chromate (Cowell et al, 2017). Lead can also be found in imported cosmetics, ceremonial powders, and medications, including kohl, henna, sindoor, ayurvedic medicines, and Mexican digestive medicines (Lin et al, 2010). It has also been found in maca root powder (*Lepidium meyenii*), often taken as a fertility enhancer (Johnson-Arbor et al, 2018).

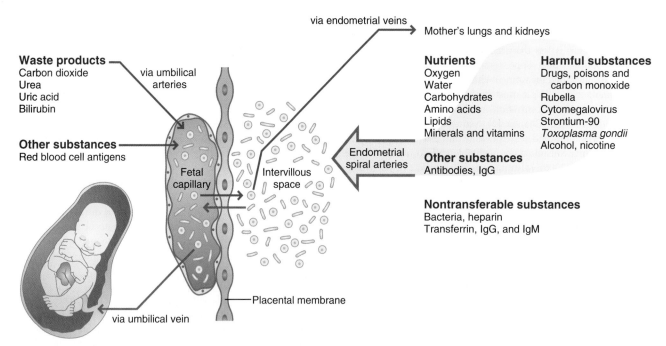

Fig. 14.7 Transfer of substances across the placental membrane. *Ig,* Immunoglobulin.

Cadmium exposure is associated with poor fetal growth (Caserta et al, 2013). It accumulates in the placenta rather than in the fetus, affecting zinc transport to the fetus and altering both the production of placental hormones and trophoblast cell migration. One source of cadmium and other heavy metals may be seaweeds grown in contaminated waters (Desideri et al, 2016).

Other potential contaminants, or sources of contamination, may be important as well, so local issues should be investigated and appropriate guidance given.

Listeria monocytogenes

Listeria monocytogenes affects 1600 Americans each year, killing 260 of them, making it the third leading cause of death resulting from food poisoning (CDC, 2018d). Pregnant women are 10 times more likely than other healthy adults to become infected with *Listeria* spp. and rates among U.S. Hispanic women are 24 times that of the general population, but the reasons for the increased susceptibility are unclear. Although the incidence of listeriosis declined 42% between 1996 and 2012 because of better food safety measures, it has plateaued since then and a better understanding of the effect of different strains, doses, genetic susceptibility, and other unknown factors is needed (Wadhwa Desai and Smith, 2017).

In studies of women who developed listeriosis during pregnancy, 10% to 20% suffered a miscarriage, 11% had a stillbirth, and 50% of them had a preterm delivery (Adams Waldorf and McAdams, 2013). Listeria can also cause neonatal meningitis, sepsis, and pneumonia. It may only cause flu-like symptoms in the mother and can mimic a urinary tract infection, but many women have no symptoms and the lack of maternal symptoms is not a reliable marker for fetal risk. Fetal transmission is not inevitable. Infections are much more likely during the third trimester (96%) than in the first (3%), but the consequences are more serious with the earlier infections. With better surveillance and more food recalls, there is now more of an awareness of an exposure, but there is little guidance on how to prevent the devastating effects if the mother is asymptomatic (Wadhwa Desai and Smith, 2017).

Listeria is a soilborne bacteria and infection results from eating contaminated foods of animal origin or raw produce. Because it can also be airborne, can tolerate high salt environments, and grows in moist environments at refrigeration temperatures, raw milk, smoked seafood, frankfurters, pâté, soft cheeses (especially if made with unpasteurized milk), and uncooked meats are likely sources. Most cases of listeriosis are associated with sporadic contamination rather than epidemics (CDC, 2018d). Because of improvements in processing, the risk of contamination in packaged cold cuts is now one fifth that of retail-sliced meats (Batz et al, 2011). Recommendations to reduce risk include using only pasteurized food products and heating precooked meat products to steaming (Box 14.6).

Mercury and Polychlorinated Biphenyls (PCBs)

Methylmercury contamination is known to affect fetal neural development disproportionately. It crosses the placenta and blood-brain barrier and accumulates in the fetus. Cord blood levels are 2 to 3 times that of maternal levels (Schofield, 2017).

Traces of methylmercury are found in most fish, but concentrations are highest in those fish that are large and predatory. Although advisories are specific to local conditions, the U.S. EPA and FDA currently recommend that all women of childbearing age avoid the consumption of those fish that surpass 1 ppm methylmercury. The methylmercury accumulates in the lean tissue, so cooking methods do not affect the mercury content of the fish (see *Focus On: Childhood Methylmercury Exposure and Toxicity* in Chapter 16).

Not everyone has found long-term problems with methylmercury consumption (Van Wijngaarden et al, 2013). Research shows that selenium may mitigate the harmful effects of mercury by a variety of potential mechanisms. However, the role of selenium in mercury poisoning is multifaceted and bidirectional, with complex interactions depending on the form of mercury, the form of selenium, the

BOX 14.6 *Listeria* Guidelines

Follow the general safety guidelines in Box 14.5, including the following:

- Avoid cross contamination with the fluid from hot dog packages.
- Keep raw meats separated from vegetables, cooked foods, and ready-to-eat foods.
- Wash fruits and vegetables thoroughly.
- Eat perishable and ready-to-eat foods (dairy, meat, poultry, seafood, produce) as soon as possible. Check for "use by" dates once/week and throw out food that has passed. Follow recommended storage times for foods.
- Wipe up spills immediately. Clean the refrigerator regularly with hot water and mild liquid detergent, rinse.

Choose lower risk foods.

- Avoid unpasteurized milk or any foods made from raw milks.
- Make sure soft cheeses (feta, Brie, Camembert, blue-veined, or Mexican style "queso blanco," "queso fresco," or Panela) are made with pasteurized milk.
- Do not eat hot dogs, luncheon meats, or deli meats unless reheated to steaming (165° F). Meats may be chilled afterward. As an alternative, cooked meats or canned meats (salmon, chicken, tuna) may be used for sandwiches.
- Do not eat refrigerated pâtés or meat spreads. Canned or shelf-stable versions may be eaten.
- Do not eat ham salad, chicken salad, or seafood salad made at the store. Instead, make them at home following general food safety guidelines.
- Do not eat refrigerated smoked seafood unless it is in a cooked dish (165° F). This includes smoked salmon, trout, whitefish, cod, tuna, and mackerel. They are often labeled "nova-style," "lox," "kippered," "smoked," or "jerky." They are found in the refrigerated section or sold at the deli counter. Canned or shelf-stable versions may be eaten.

Adapted from Cox JT, Phelan ST: Food safety in pregnancy, part 1: putting risks into perspective, *Contemporary Ob/Gyn* 54:44, 2009a; United States Department of Health and Human Services (USDHHS): *Food Safety for Pregnant Women* (website): https://www.foodsafety.gov/risk/pregnant/index.html#_Food_Poisoning_During_1, 2018.

BOX 14.7 Fish Safety Guidelines

- Do not eat shark, tilefish from the Gulf of Mexico (also called golden or white snapper, golden bass), king mackerel, marlin, orange roughy, bigeye tuna, or swordfish.
- Albacore ("white") canned tuna should be limited to 4 oz/week. See Chapter 16 for other fish that should also be limited.
- Other cooked fish and seafood may be eaten, up to 12 oz/week. See *Focus On:* Omega-3 Fatty Acids in Pregnancy and Lactation for recommended choices.
- Avoid refrigerated seafood products unless cooked before eating (165° F).
- Avoid raw or undercooked fish and seafood, including sushi and shellfish. All fish and shellfish should be cooked to 145° F.
- Observe local advisories regarding mercury and other contaminants. For access to your state's or territory's advisories, see: https://fishadvisoryonline.epa.gov/general.aspx.

Adapted from Cox JT, Phelan ST: Food safety in pregnancy, part 2: what can I eat, doctor? *Contemporary Ob/Gyn* 54:24, 2009b; United States Department of Health and Human Services (USDHHS): Food Safety for Pregnant Women (website): https://www.foodsafety.gov/risk/pregnant/index.html#_Food_Poisoning_During_1, 2018; Food and Drug Administration (FDA): Advice about Eating Fish: *What Pregnant Women & Parents Should Know*, November 2017. https://www.fda.gov/Food/ResourcesForYou/Consumers/ucm393070.htm.

organ, and the dose (Spiller, 2018). The selenium and mercury contents of fish and shellfish are now being characterized worldwide (Burger and Gochfeld, 2013). Although some have promoted a selenium:mercury ratio as a better way to characterize risk, that may be premature. Selenium appears to protect against mercury toxicity only up to a limit, and excess selenium also can be highly toxic.

Fish also can be a source of polychlorinated biphenyls (PCBs), and prenatal exposure has been associated with child neurologic deficits (Cox and Phelan, 2009b). Although no longer produced, PCBs still remain in the water systems. Although PCBs can be absorbed through the skin and lungs, they primarily enter the body from ingestion of contaminated fatty fish. Farmed and wild ocean fish can contain PCBs, but fresh water fish from the Great Lakes are often of more concern. PCBs readily pass through the placenta and breastmilk. Pregnant and nursing women should avoid eating fish from water known to be highly contaminated with PCBs. Fish from other areas should be cooked to minimize the ingestion of the fat and the skin should not be eaten.

Regarding wild versus farmed salmon, there is controversy. Farmed Atlantic salmon is higher in contaminants (PCBs, dioxins, polybrominated diphenyl ethers or PBDEs, and some pesticides) than wild Pacific salmon, but it also contains higher levels of omega-3s than wild Pacific salmon. Although no data are specific to

pregnancy, researchers conclude that the benefit (lives saved from coronary disease) from North and South American farmed sources outweighs the risk (lives lost to cancer) and is on par with the wild sources (Cox and Phelan, 2009b).

The federal guidelines regarding the consumption of commercially available fish have increased the number of fishes that should be avoided (see Chapter 16). Local fresh waters and therefore fish may also be contaminated. Questions regarding methylmercury, PCBs, and other contaminants should be directed to state natural resource departments. In addition, many fish have different local names and both availability and acceptability vary widely, so the guidance many need to be adapted to local conditions.

Most fish and seafood are low in methylmercury, and a few are particularly high in DHA (see *Focus On:* Omega-3 Fatty Acids in Pregnancy and Lactation), so consumption should be promoted. Fish may carry pathogens as well and all fish and seafood should be well cooked (Box 14.7).

Other Foodborne Pathogens and Probiotics

Brucella spp., *Salmonella* spp., and *Campylobacter jejuni* are also of particular concern for pregnant women (Procter and Campbell, 2014). Prompt diagnosis of brucellosis and maternal antibiotic treatment can save the life of the fetus. Transmission of *Brucella* spp. through breastmilk also has been reported. Cases of fetal sepsis and multiorgan failure, leading to death, have been reported with nontyphoidal *Salmonella*. *Salmonella typhi*, the bacteria that cause typhoid fever, and *Campylobacter jejuni* can cross the placenta and infect the fetus, causing miscarriage, stillbirth, or preterm labor (Dean and Kendall, 2012). In addition, other food contaminants, including *E. coli*, can affect anyone, including pregnant women. If exposed, women should be treated carefully, avoiding dehydration. To limit exposure, food recalls should be observed and careful food choices should be made. Federal guidance is available (see Chapter 8).

For a discussion of the issues regarding the microbiome, see *Clinical Insight:* The Microbiome During Pregnancy and Lactation.

CLINICAL INSIGHT

The Microbiome During Pregnancy and Lactation

The importance of the microbiome is now more appreciated, including during pregnancy. While it is now generally thought that the presence of bacteria is not necessarily a pathogenic condition, there is not yet complete consensus on that point (Manuck, 2017; Zhou and Xiao, 2018).

The microbiome of both males and females appears to play a role in conception, including the seminal fluid microbiome (Younes et al, 2018). The vaginal microbiome is known to be important in reproduction and appears to affect assisted reproductive technology (ART) results, but research is still preliminary (García-Velasco et al, 2017). It varies over time and between women, but whether, and how, the diet affects it is still unknown. The vaginal microbiome colonizes the newborn during delivery, potentially affecting immune function and neurodevelopment.

It is now known that the placenta, amniotic fluid, and fetus are not sterile and that microbes move from the maternal to the fetal environment. How that transfer occurs is not completely clear but is hypothesized to be through the blood (Prince et al, 2015), possibly through increased permeability of gingival vascular bed in gingivitis (Younes et al, 2018). Also unclear is whether the transfer can also go from the fetus to the mother (Pelzer et al, 2017). The microbiome of the placenta appears to be unique, is established early, and is more similar to the maternal oral cavity than to her gut, vaginal, or skin microbiome (Prince et al, 2015). Historically, the concern has been that transfer of bacteria to amniotic fluid could cause inflammation and therefore preterm delivery. Particular concern is raised for those women with immune suppression or dysfunction, as well as those with abnormalities in the gastrointestinal mucosal barrier. However, assuming the presence of bacteria is a normal phenomenon, questions are now being investigated regarding how these bacteria vary, what impact they have, and how they can be modified to help maternal and offspring health.

It is now known that the microbiome varies between women. It gets less diverse over the course of pregnancy and the microbiome among women with gestational diabetes mellitus (GDM) is even less diverse (Wickens et al, 2017). The consequences of the variability are not yet clear but it is known that the microbiome midpregnancy differs among women who go on to deliver preterm (Manuck, 2017) and it is speculated that *Lactobacillus* may provide an antibacterial defense over the intraamniotic infections associated with preterm birth. The microbiome may affect perinatal depression and anxiety (Rackers et al, 2018). The dietary components affecting mood, anxiety, and stress response are not completely clear but it appears a high fat diet affects the microbiome composition. In maternal obesity, an altered microbiome is associated with altered short-chain fatty acid production and gene expression, as well as poor glucose control, but whether interventions can help restrain weight gain, reduce GDM frequency, or improve insulin sensitivity is unclear (Zhou and Xiao, 2018). There is no consistent evidence that interventions affect preterm birth risk or other infant or maternal outcomes, including SGA, LGA, or premature rupture of membranes (PROM) (Jarde et al, 2018). There is some evidence that maternal supplementation with particular strains and doses may be helpful in controlling gestational weight gain, frequency of GDM, glycemic control, modulating inflammatory markers, and reducing the risk of preeclampsia, as well as preventing the development of airway inflammation in offspring (in mice) (Rodríguez-González et al, 2018). Also being investigated are the effects of the microbiome on the fetus' developing immune system and metabolic functioning. However, in the case of atopic disorders, it is not clear if maternal supplementation during pregnancy only, without lactation or infant supplementation, will lower the risk of infant eczema (Wickens et al, 2018; Garcia-Larsen et al, 2018). It is thought that the microbial colonization of the uterus, placenta, and amniotic fluid may prime the fetus to become tolerant to bacteria after birth and therefore affect the infant microbiome and long-term health (Younes et al, 2018).

Improving maternal dysbiosis may help infant health and probiotics appear to be safe when used by healthy people. Attempts to modify the maternal microbiome through the use of prebiotics and probiotics are being investigated for potential benefit during pregnancy. However, there is no evidence yet of a direct beneficial effect of probiotics on reproductive health outcomes (García-Velasco et al, 2017). The results of interventions are often inconsistent and, although most studies have been done on women with normal weight, it is unclear about the impact of prepregnant body mass index (BMI) on the microbiome or the ability to change it. The optimal combination of bacteria (most often tested are *Lactobacillus* spp. and/or *Bifidobacterium* spp.), strains, dosing, timing and duration of exposure, and routes of administration, as well as the age, baseline nutritional status of the mother, and the interaction with stress are all critical and not yet clear, nor is the relative impact of probiotic supplements compared with the consumption of fermented foods. However, there is evidence that the use of fermented milk products is associated with up to a 40% reduction in the risk of severe preeclampsia, depending on the dose (Griffin, 2015), but even just 30 mL/day appears helpful (Berti et al, 2017). Whether the bacteria must be whole or living is also unclear but there is evidence of effective host priming, even if the bacteria are dead, at least in murine studies (Pelzer et al, 2017). In addition, for many commercial products, there appears to be a lack of correlation between the label and the actual contents of the supplements (Jarde et al, 2018) and, while contamination with pathogens is uncommon, it has been reported (Sohn and Underwood, 2017). Many trials are underway and the clinical and application guidelines are still in development.

During lactation, the milk microbiome may contribute to short- and long-term infant health and also to mammary health. Mammary dysbiosis often leads to acute, subacute, or subclinical mastitis. This condition may be resistant to antibiotics and could lead to undesired early weaning. New research providing selected lactobacilli strains isolated from breastmilk show potential in treating this painful condition so that the continuation of successful breastfeeding is not jeopardized (Fernández et al, 2014).

Toxoplasma gondii

Toxoplasma gondii is a parasite that may cross the placenta, causing miscarriage or fetal death. Survivors have chorioretinitis, hearing loss, and long-term neurologic and neurocognitive deficits, but can also have rashes, hepatosplenomegaly, ascites, fever, periventricular calcifications, ventriculomegaly, and seizures (ACOG, 2015c). Rates of congenital toxoplasmosis in the United States are unknown (it is not a reportable disease) but are estimated at 400 to 4000 cases/year (Cox and Phelan, 2009a). Although present in all countries, the prevalence varies considerably. Highest rates of congenital toxoplasmosis are found in some countries in South America, the Middle East, and Africa (Torgerson and Mastroiacovo, 2013).

Symptoms are often mild, flu-like, and unrecognized, although people with immunosuppression can have chorioretinitis and encephalitis. Clinical toxoplasmosis is rare in the United States, and 90% of pregnant women who are infected have no noticeable symptoms (Cox and Phelan, 2009a). However, even without maternal symptoms, the fetus can become infected. Overall transmission rates appear to be 20% to 50% but vary by trimester, including 10% to 15% in the first trimester, 25% in the second, and over 60% in the third trimester (ACOG, 2015c). Although transmission is lowest in the first trimester, the severity is also highest and as many as 90% of those exposed will eventually develop sequelae, even without clinical signs at birth. The risk of passing the parasite to the fetus is reduced greatly if the mother has been previously exposed and is already seropositive. Although some countries (including France, Austria, Italy, Portugal, and Uruguay) routinely screen pregnant women (Oz, 2017), this is not standard practice in the United States except for those with HIV or immunosuppression (ACOG, 2015c).

Commonly women are encouraged to not handle used kitty litter when pregnant, because the cat is the definitive host for *Toxoplasma*. However, a cat passes the oocysts for only a few weeks in its lifetime. In addition, these oocysts are infective only after being exposed to the environment for at least a day. If the litter box is changed daily, there is little danger, even if the cat were infected and passing the eggs. Cats should be kept indoors and not fed raw meat.

Because the oocysts can live in the environment for years, water, dust, insects, and garden soil can also be contaminated. Fruits and vegetables must be washed, and contaminated water should not be ingested. Gloves should be used when gardening.

Meats and milks also can be infected with tissue cysts, and it is estimated that up to half the cases of toxoplasmosis occur with handling or eating undercooked or raw infected meats, especially wild game and those meats labeled "free-range" or organic (Jones and Dubey, 2012). Oysters, clams, and mussels can be contaminated through water runoff. Unpasteurized goat, camel, and donkey milk are also known sources (Oz, 2017), as are homemade cured, dried, and smoked meats. The injected salt solution that often is used in pork and chicken will kill tissue cysts, as may freezing the meat for a few days. Cooking will kill the parasite, but minimum temperatures must be achieved (Box 14.8).

BOX 14.8 *Toxoplasma* Guidelines

- Follow the general food safety guidelines from Box 14.5.
- Freeze meats for several days before cooking.
- Wash hands after handling raw meats.
- Cook meats to at least 150° F + 3-minute rest (whole cuts), 160° F (ground meats, wild game), or 165° F (poultry). These temperatures may be higher than the USDA recommends for other pathogens. Do not sample meat until it is cooked. Meats that are smoked, cured in brine, or dried may still be infectious.
- Raw oysters, mussels, and clams should not be eaten.
- Keep children's sandboxes covered when not in use.
- Wear gloves when gardening or handling sand from a sandbox. Wash hands thoroughly afterward.
- Peel or thoroughly wash fruits and vegetables before eating.
- Avoid unpasteurized milk, including goat's milk.
- Do not drink water from the environment unless it is boiled.
- Keep your cats indoors. Do not feed them raw or undercooked meats or unpasteurized milks.
- Clean the litter box daily. If possible, have someone else change the litter box. If not, wear gloves and wash hands with soap and warm water afterward.
- Do not adopt a new cat while pregnant nor handle strays, especially kittens.
- Control rodents and other potential intermediate hosts.
- If butchering wild game or venison, bury the organs so that wild cats cannot eat them and spread the infection.

Adapted from Cox JT, Phelan ST: Food safety in pregnancy, part 1: putting risks into perspective, *Contemporary Ob/Gyn* 54:44, 2009a; Jones JL, Dubey JP: Foodborne toxoplasmosis, *Clin Infect Dis* 55:845, 2012.

Guide for Eating during Pregnancy

Recommended Food Intake

The increased nutrient requirements of pregnancy can often be met by following the Daily Food Guide (Table 14.15). The USDA MyPlate Plan can be used interactively online. Although it can be a starting point, it is designed for those women with uncomplicated pregnancies. In addition, unless very nutrient-dense foods are chosen, it is likely to be deficient in iron, vitamin D, vitamin E, choline, potassium, and DHA (Center for Nutrition Policy and Promotion [CNPP], 2018). Box 14.9 provides a summary of nutritional care. Weight gain and fetal growth should be monitored and the plan modified as needed.

Fluids

Drinking 8 to 10 glasses of quality fluid daily, mainly water, is encouraged. The DRI for fluid increases slightly during pregnancy, but a woman's body size as well as climate conditions are important considerations. Adequate hydration improves the overall sense of well-being. Frequent urination is often a complaint from pregnant women. However, optimal hydration reduces risks for urinary tract infections, kidney stones, and constipation. In addition, dehydration can cause uterine irritability. Women often must be reminded to pay attention to their intake of liquids, using urine color after the first morning void as a guide.

Nutrient Supplementation During Pregnancy

Supplementation of a mother's diet during pregnancy may take the form of additional energy, protein, fatty acids, vitamins, or minerals that exceed her routine daily intake. The more compromised the nutritional status of the woman, the greater the benefit for pregnancy outcome with improved diet and nutrient supplementation. Among women in low- and middle-income countries, supplementation of both micronutrients and macronutrients, including balanced protein-energy supplements as well as lipid supplements, can improve fetal growth and birth outcomes (Vaivada et al, 2017), including a reduced risk of preterm births (Heidkamp et al, 2017). It is unclear, however, if supplementation benefits fetal growth if the maternal status is not compromised (da Silva Lopes et al, 2017). In the United States pregnant women at nutritional risk are encouraged to enroll in the Special Supplemental Nutrition Program for Women, Infants, and Children (WIC), administered by the USDA. The WIC program serves eligible pregnant women and breastfeeding (until 1 year postpartum) and nonbreastfeeding women (until 6 months postpartum), as well as infants and children (up to age 5). For women, "nutritional risk" criteria may include anemia, poor gestational weight gain, and inadequate diet, as well as a variety of preexisting medical conditions. WIC provides targeted supplemental foods, nutrition education, and breastfeeding support as well as health care referrals. Outcome studies show improved birth weights and higher mean gestational ages in infants born to WIC participants.

The goal for nutritional supplementation is to consume the necessary nutrients as food, taking advantage of the likely beneficial synergistic effects and including phytonutrients or other bioactive compounds whose effects are not yet fully appreciated. However, judicious use of dietary supplements (as a multivitamin-multimineral) is needed with undernourished women, including those with a history of bariatric surgery, teenage mothers, women with substance abuse, women with a short interval between pregnancies, women with a history of delivering an infant with LBW, and those pregnant with multiple fetuses. Preconceptual supplementation is recommended for folic acid and may be warranted for other nutrients as well. Current research is examining which micronutrients are most critical to include in the multivitamin-multimineral supplements (da Silva Lopes et al, 2017).

TABLE 14.15   Daily Food Guide: Recommended Servings for a Woman Pregnant with a Singleton or Lactating

| Food Group | PREGNANT WOMAN (NORMAL WEIGHT, 30 MINUTES EXERCISE/WEEK) | | | LACTATING WOMAN (NO FORMULA SUPPLEMENTATION) | | Serving Sizes (1) |
	First Trimester	Second Trimester	Third Trimester	Early Lactation (0-6 mos)	Later Lactation (6+ mos)	
Total daily calories	1800	2200	2400	2130	2200	
Meat and beans, oz	5	6	6.5	7	6	1 oz = 1 oz meat, poultry, or fish, 1 egg, ¼ c beans, ½ oz nuts, ¼ c tofu
Milk products, cups	3	3	3	3-4	3	1 c = 1 c milk or yogurt, 1.5 oz hard cheese, 2 c cottage cheese
Breads, grains, oz — half should be whole grains	6	7	8	8	9	1 oz = 1 slice bread, ½ c cooked starch, 1 c RTE cereal
Fruits and Vegetables (cups)	4	5	5	6	6	1 c = 1 c raw or cooked fruit or vegetable, ½ c dried fruit, 2 c leafy vegetables
Vitamin C rich	1	1	1	1	1	
Beta-carotene rich	1	1	1	1	1	
Folate rich	1	1	1	1	1	
Others	1	2	2	3	3	
Fats and oils, tsp	6	7	8	8	8	Included are those foods naturally high in fats, including olives, avocados, and nuts
Extras, calories	290	360	410	330	400	High fat or sugar foods or higher amounts of foods from the other groups
Beverages	10 c water/day (watch urine color)			8-12 glasses water or other beverage (drink to satisfy thirst)		8 oz.

(1) See the ChooseMyPlate website for more examples.
RTE, Ready to eat.
Adapted from *American College of Obstetricians and Gynecologists (ACOG):* Nutrition during Pregnancy. Patient Education Pamphlet AP001, September 2012; USDA: What is MyPlate, July 2018. https://www.choosemyplate.gov/MyPlate.

BOX 14.9   Summary of Nutritional Care During Pregnancy

1. A variety of foods, focusing on nutrient-dense food choices
2. Energy intake to allow for appropriate weight gain
3. Protein intake to meet nutritional needs, approximately an additional 25 g/day; additional 50 g/day/fetus if pregnant with more than one fetus. This often requires 20% of energy intake from protein
4. DHA from fatty fish (low in methylmercury) twice a week
5. Mineral and vitamin intakes to meet the recommended daily allowances. Folic acid supplementation is often required; iron supplementation may be necessary
6. Sodium intake that is not excessive but not less than 2300 mg/day. Iodized salt is recommended
7. Sufficient fluid intake to produce dilute urine, usually at least 2 L/day
8. Alcohol omitted
9. Omission of toxins and nonnutritive substances from food, water, and environment as much as possible

Many pregnant women have limited knowledge regarding the nutrients in the dietary supplements they have been advised to purchase. Dietary supplements are not regulated as drugs in the United States (Binns et al, 2018). There is no standard definition of what a dietary supplement labeled "prenatal vitamin" must contain and the contents vary widely. Having it be available by prescription does not imply that the supplement is better, nor safer, nor that it contains higher levels of any particular nutrient (Saldanha et al, 2017). In fact, a recent study found those prenatal supplements available over-the-counter actually contain more nutrients than many of the supplements available only by prescription. It is important to read the label on prenatal supplements because some are much more complete than others, and some include ingredients in addition to the vitamins and minerals. Women often need advice on local, suitable choices. Look for those that contain the United States Pharmacopeia (USP), Consumer Labs, or National Sanitation Foundation (NSF) seals of approval for quality (not safety or effectiveness) (see Chapter 11). A balanced prenatal supplement should contain 400 to 800 mcg of folic acid and also should contain iron unless contraindicated. Caution is advised with the use of the prenatal gummies because they seldom contain iron. Copper is recommended if the supplement also contains zinc or iron (Uriu-Adams et al, 2010). The supplement should contain 150 mcg of iodine in the form of potassium iodide, not kelp or seaweed (Leung et al, 2013). Although some contain DHA, at least as much benefit can come from including high DHA fish regularly in the diet (see *Focus On: Omega-3 Fatty Acids in Pregnancy and Lactation*).

Those supplements containing nutrient levels much higher than the DRI are not recommended because of known teratogenic effects (e.g., preformed vitamin A), as well as potential epigenetic effects. Some contain many additional ingredients, including herbal preparations, many of which have not been evaluated for safety during pregnancy and may be contraindicated, especially during the first trimester.

As a reminder, prenatal multivitamins-multiminerals may be more critical when a woman's nutritional status is at risk. For others, they may be used as insurance but should not be used as a substitute for eating well. Whether prenatal multivitamin-multimineral supplements are necessary for women living in affluent societies is debated, but their use is common. For women living in low- and middle-income conditions, prenatal supplementation has been associated with better birth outcomes (Vaivada et al, 2017).

Nutrition Education

Nutrition intervention, including medical nutrition therapy (MNT), has been effective in improving the maternal diet, reducing the risk of anemia in late pregnancy, and improving gestational weight gain, thus lowering the risk of preterm birth and improving infant head circumference size and birth weight (Blondin and LoGiudice, 2018). For low-income recipients at risk for low gain and therefore poor fetal growth and preterm delivery, results are enhanced if education is combined with balanced energy and protein supplementation and/or micronutrient supplements. Among women who are overweight and obese, dietary and lifestyle advice results in a significant reduction in the relative risk of delivering an LGA infant, with no increase in the risk of delivering an SGA baby, even if there is no effect on maternal weight gain (Dodd et al, 2015).

ACOG recommends that any woman who is overweight or obese be offered nutrition assessment and counseling, both during the preconception period and the prenatal visits (ACOG, 2014; ACOG, 2015d) and this should continue postpartum to minimize postpartum weight retention. Regarding the effectiveness of MNT on curbing excessive maternal weight gain, results are mixed but interventions can be effective (Elliott-Sale et al, 2018) and studies are ongoing. The intensity of the intervention needs to be balanced with compliance limitations, and addressing barriers must be individualized (Dodd et al, 2015). It appears that diet interventions are more effective than those focusing on physical activity or both (Walker et al, 2018). However, while exercise programs alone do not appear to affect maternal weight gain or birthweight, they do improve maternal fitness (Seneviratne et al, 2015) and may provide other long-term benefits. It is unclear whether a particular exercise dose is critical and it is also unclear if the effect of exercise varies by maternal prepregnant BMI (McDonald et al, 2016.).

All women should be given appropriate guidance on the weight gain, as well as nutrient intakes, that are expected, as recommended by the WHO (WHO, 2016b). Although energy needs increase slightly, the mother is not "eating for two" because of the hormonal and metabolic changes that occur during pregnancy, including lowering of maternal nutrient stores (Wakimoto et al, 2015). Helping a mother find acceptable concentrated sources of nutrients and minimizing the intake of high-calorie, low-nutrient foods is likely to reassure the woman who starts the pregnancy overweight or obese and/or is gaining excessively. Just routine weighing is not effective in reducing gestational weight gain, at least among women with obesity (Haby et al, 2018). However, it is certainly helpful when combined with other interventions (Goldstein et al, 2016) and mothers often want guidance.

Although repeated individual face-to-face contact with personalized advice is often done, it isn't always effective. Group meetings are sometimes helpful because of the expanded support that they provide, but in some instances women gain even more weight when participating in group education. While literature may be useful and sufficient for some, for many people just receiving printed materials is likely to not be beneficial. Although eHealth (electronic) and mHealth (mobile) interventions have potential, they have not been shown to be effective. Overall,

there is no one best intervention with optimal duration, intensity, or setting. Interventions should be adapted to local conditions and individualized. Even low levels of intensity and frequency can be helpful in giving a client small "nudges" (Walker et al, 2018).

MNT is known to be helpful during pregnancy. However, to be most effective, dietitians and nutritionists must consider all current issues. A pregnant woman may have poor weight gain and also low iron levels. Foods that address both issues at the same time should be used. She may have low calcium intake but also have GDM, thus modifying how she is counseled. She may have cultural practices that could affect her nutritional status. For example, a woman who is consistently veiled when outside of her house may be at particular risk of low vitamin D levels because of the lack of sun exposure on her skin. She may have preexisting medical conditions that must be managed, including carrying parasitic infections common in her home country. She may develop issues during pregnancy (e.g., anemia, gallstones, or GDM) but also may have medical issues that are not directly related to the pregnancy (e.g., cancer or a Crohn's disease flare-up). She may experience trauma from a motor vehicle accident or physical abuse that could require an ICU admission. She may be willing to walk more but be afraid to do so near her home or after dark. All nutritional issues must be balanced, often with little research data to give firm guidance. One should give the best advice known but be open to changes as the evidence becomes available.

In addition, cultural aspects of counseling also must be kept in mind (see Chapter 10). The beliefs and customs of the home culture of both parents are important in predicting health behaviors and should be addressed, ideally preconceptually. Acculturation of both is important, but the direction of influence can't always be predicted. For example, non-Hispanic white mothers are more likely to smoke than non-Hispanic black or Hispanic women. However, rates of smoking are higher among immigrants with higher levels of acculturation. A father's beliefs and acculturation are also important, influencing maternal health behaviors (Cheng et al, 2018). For many health behaviors, nativity appears to be more important than ethnicity.

A woman's perceived risk of abnormal weight gain may differ from the U.S. norm. Childrearing, including pregnancy and lactation, usually has strong cultural components, and it is advisable to understand the beliefs and customs of the population groups being served. Although each individual does not necessarily follow, or may not even be aware of, all the beliefs held in the culture, they may influence a person's response to nutritional suggestions. For example, a woman coming from a culture that believes that cleft lip and palate are caused by seeing an eclipse may rely on the safety pin over her abdomen to protect her and may therefore be less concerned about taking her folic acid supplements. If a woman, or a family member, is fearful that eating crabs during pregnancy will cause a miscarriage, that belief should be respected and other sources of protein can be chosen (Milman et al, 2016). A Vietnamese woman who is fearful of drinking cold orange juice immediately postpartum because of the negative effect it will have on the skin years later may be willing to warm the juice, put sugar in it, or eat kiwis for vitamin C instead. A woman from Mexico who believes that you must comply with a craving or something will be missing from the baby, will be afraid to not eat the dirt she is craving. However, she may be willing to smell the wet dirt and eat a burned tortilla, thus complying with the craving but ingesting something that is not likely to be contaminated. She may believe that "vitamins make you hungry" and so will stop taking her prenatal supplements if she feels, or has been told, she is gaining too much weight.

Families often need to be reassured that low-fat and nonfat milks contain the same levels of protein, calcium, and vitamin D as the whole milk (i.e., they are not watered down milk and therefore dangerous for pregnancy). Immigrants from countries where tap water is not potable need to be reassured that it is treated in the United States and is safe to drink, and that bottled water is not only more expensive but also often does not contain fluoride. On the other hand, an immigrant may be fearful of the prenatal care in the United States when she is not routinely screened for *Toxoplasma gondii*, as is the standard of care at home.

Cultural differences are not apparent just with immigrants. Women who follow a well-balanced vegetarian diet can certainly have a successful pregnancy, assuming food availability is not limited. However, these women may need nutritional guidance regarding protein, iron, zinc, calcium, omega-3 fatty acids, and vitamin B$_{12}$, especially as trying to eat the required volume of food becomes the limiting factor later in the pregnancy (see Chapter 10). Followers of Jehovah's Witness, because they choose not to receive blood transfusions, may need both earlier and more consistent advice on the consumption of high-iron foods to help keep their iron levels as optimal as possible, lowering their risk of severe complications even if blood loss at delivery is high. Those who practice different dietary patterns during holidays, including fasting, may need guidance on how to minimize the impact of that change on the developing fetus. Someone working nights may need ideas on how to distribute her meals to optimize glucose control.

Pregnant women are adult learners and relevant, simple, concrete messages are most effective, especially if they are memorable and motivational (Girard and Olude, 2012). Having mothers set their own goals is helpful (Haby et al, 2018). Blaming parents for their choices is not helpful and care should be taken when discussing the epigenetic consequences of actions or inactions. All people should be counseled with sensitivity, reinforcing those practices that are particularly helpful and modifying only those practices that may be harmful. One must investigate atypical dietary patterns and food sources to best fit the customs of the patient. Cultural differences should not be ignored or rejected outright. If there are some that must be modified now, it is best to explain why, how, and for how long. Otherwise, the guidance of grandmothers and cultural history will likely prevail.

Pregnancy is a time of great impact. Although historically the goal had just been a full-term, full-size newborn, now the focus has expanded to include ensuring someone biologically predisposed to be healthy from birth to old age (ACOG, 2013b). It is often a time when a mother is very receptive to doing her best for her child. Eating more fruits and vegetables, lean meats, low-fat milks, and whole grains while minimizing excess fat, sugar, and salt intakes will likely improve maternal health and birth outcomes in the short term. Animal research is showing high maternal intakes of fats and sugars during pregnancy and lactation results in altered development of the central reward system in offspring, leading to excessive intakes of these foods postnatally (Mennella, 2014). In addition, research has demonstrated that flavors familiar to the infant, from exposure through the amniotic fluid and breastmilk, are more likely to be accepted by that child when first offered, thus increasing the chance of consumption. Although this may be important nutritionally, exposure to a variety of flavors early in life when the developing brain has heightened sensitivity to environmental influences also appears to facilitate acceptance of novel foods later. Eating better during pregnancy helps develop better food habits for the mother and the rest of her family that, hopefully, will carry on past the current pregnancy, improving the entire family's health. In addition, she is likely to be having positive epigenetic effects and improving the health of future generations, as well as lowering health care costs (Simeoni et al, 2018).

POSTPARTUM PERIOD = PRECONCEPTUAL PERIOD

Reproductive health concerns do not end at delivery and the postpartum period can be considered the "fourth trimester." In addition, for

many women, the postpartum period can be considered a preconceptual period.

Excess postpartum weight retention is associated with increased risk of GDM and hypertension during a subsequent pregnancy, even in normal- and underweight women who gain appropriately in that subsequent pregnancy. Nutrition and exercise counseling should continue postpartum, with the goal of returning the mother to her prepregnant weight within 6 to 12 months and achieving healthy BMI before attempting another pregnancy. However, because less than half of postpartum women achieve their prepregnant weight by 1 year, and over a quarter of women keep at least 10 pounds, all women who are overweight or obese should be offered nutrition counseling for at least 12 to 18 months after delivery (Stang and Huffman, 2016). Intensive dietary intervention, along with objective targets for exercise such as the use of heart rate monitors or pedometers, appear most effective (Nascimento et al, 2014).

Appropriately treating or resolving medical issues such as GDM before a subsequent pregnancy will help ensure a healthy outcome for both mother and baby. Adequate stress management will minimize the adverse effects of stress hormones on offspring neurodevelopment (Huberty et al, 2017).

Nutrient stores also need to be replenished, and short interpregnancy intervals (less than 12 to 18 months) are associated with increased risk of miscarriage, preterm delivery, IUGR or LBW, stillbirth, and early neonatal death (Wu et al, 2012a), as well as maternal morbidity and mortality (Huberty et al, 2017). The nutritional demands of breastfeeding also must be considered, and for those in areas with limited resources, it may take at least 1 year to recover. The WHO recommends women delay conception at least 24 months after a live birth to reduce the risk of adverse maternal, perinatal, and neonatal outcomes, but the applicability of these recommendations to women in the United States is questioned and is being studied (Ahrens et al, 2018). Maternal depletion is theorized to operate through changes in protein and energy balance, but maternal weight is not a predictor of micronutrient status. Even in high-income countries, LBW risk increases if the interpregnancy interval is less than 6 months, and a significant proportion of low-income women in the United States are still iron deficient 2 years after delivery (Bodnar et al, 2002). Other nutrients also may be depleted for an extended period, including folate, vitamin A, and DHA, negatively affecting the subsequent pregnancy (Conde-Agudelo et al, 2012). An antioxidant-rich preconceptual diet may lower oxidative stress and improve pregnancy outcomes. Inflammation is also thought to play a role in increased risk with short interconceptual periods (Wendt et al, 2012), and those women who have no nonpregnant, nonlactating time may be at particular risk. Women who have interpregnancy food supplementation have babies with higher birthweights and lengths and maternal hemoglobin values are higher (Wakimoto et al, 2015).

It is theorized that preconceptual nutrition is as critical as nutrition during pregnancy and for many nutrients, likely more critical because of their role in placental formation and organogenesis (see Preconception and Fertility).

LACTATION

Exclusive breastfeeding is unequivocally the preferred method of infant feeding for the first 6 months of life. Many professional health organizations have endorsed this recommendation, including the Academy of Nutrition and Dietetics, the AAP, ACOG, the American Academy of Family Practitioners, Healthy People 2020, the WIC program, the U.S. Surgeon General, and the U.S. Breastfeeding Committee. These organizations recommend breastfeeding throughout the first year and beyond, as long as mutually desired by mother and child; the WHO encourages breastfeeding throughout the second year of life. Breastfeeding offers protection from GI and other infections and serves as a critical source of energy and nutrients during illness, reducing mortality among malnourished children. The development of strong immune and digestive systems in breastfed babies is thought to be due to the development of beneficial bacteria in the baby's gut, providing a healthy gut microbial population.

Mothers should be encouraged to breastfeed for as long as possible, even if it is not the full year. Nutrition from breastmilk and the protection from illness it provides are unmatched by any other substitute. In 2016 the Lancet Breastfeeding Series was released stating that, if optimal duration of a minimum of 12 months was achieved, global health care savings would be $300 billion dollars per year. Additionally, 820,000 lives per year would be saved, and 20,000 deaths from breast and ovarian cancers could be avoided (Victora et al, 2016). Women should be supported in their decision to breastfeed for any length of time, whether it is for just 2 weeks, 2 years, or longer. Breastmilk continues to provide nutrition and immunities throughout the time the mother is lactating. Many women face barriers that may prevent them from breastfeeding for as long as they would like, so support from the health care system along with family members and the community is necessary for mothers to reach their goals (Fig. 14.8).

There are many health benefits for mother and child, as shown in Box 14.10. A recent study examined the racial and socioeconomic disparities in infant feeding, noting that higher rates of breastfeeding are seen in families in which the mother is older and married, with a higher education and income. Long-term health outcomes of breastfed infants and their nonbreastfed siblings were compared and researchers noted that many of these children had similar long-term positive outcomes as their breastfed siblings or children in a comparative group. The authors concluded that a supportive breastfeeding environment and not breastfeeding alone contributes to long-term positive health outcomes of children (Colen and Ramey, 2014). Studies also have

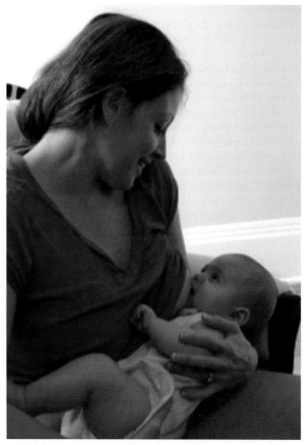

Fig. 14.8 A nursing mother and her infant enjoy the close physical and emotional contact that accompanies breastfeeding. (Courtesy Robert Raab.)

BOX 14.10 Benefits of Breastfeeding

For Infant
Decreases Incidence and Severity of Infectious Diseases
Bacterial meningitis
Bacteremia
Diarrhea
Infant botulism
Necrotizing enterocolitis
Otitis media
Respiratory tract infection
Septicemia
Urinary tract infection

Decreases Rates of Other Diseases
Asthma
Celiac disease
Crohn's disease
Food allergies
Hodgkin's disease
Hypercholesterolemia
Leukemia
Lymphoma
Overweight and obesity
Sudden infant death syndrome
Types 1 and 2 diabetes

Other Benefits
Promotes analgesia during painful procedures (heel stick for newborns)
Promotes enhanced performance on cognitive development tests
Promotes mother-child bonding
Promotes ready acceptance of solid foods

For Mother
Decreases menstrual blood loss
Decreases postpartum bleeding
Decreases risk of hormonal (breast and ovarian) cancers
Promotes earlier return to prepregnancy weight
Increases child spacing
Promotes rapid uterine involution
Decreases need for insulin in mothers with diabetes
Decreases risk of postmenopausal hip fracture and osteoporosis

For Society
Reduces health care costs
Decreases costs to public programs (i.e., WIC)
Prevents excess lost wages resulting from employee absenteeism for sick children
Supports greener environment

Reference: American Academy of Pediatrics and American College of Obstetricians and Gynecologists: *Breastfeeding handbook for physicians*, Second Edition, Elk Grove Village, Ill, 2013, American Academy of Pediatrics.

shown that levels of C-reactive protein (CRP), a key biomarker of inflammation and a predictor of increased cardiovascular and metabolic disease risk in adulthood, are significantly lower among individuals who were breastfed. Decreased concentrations corresponded to the duration of earlier breastfeeding. Researchers conclude that the longer the duration of breastfeeding, the less inflammation and lower risk for heart and metabolic diseases later in life (McDade et al, 2014).

In 1991, the WHO and the United Nations Children's Fund adopted the Baby-Friendly Hospital Initiative (BFHI), a global effort to increase the incidence and duration of breastfeeding. To become "baby-friendly," a hospital must demonstrate to an outside review board that it implements the "Ten Steps to Successful Breastfeeding," (Ten Steps) a guideline for mother-baby management in the hospital (Box 14.11). In the United States the nongovernmental agency that oversees the designation process is Baby-Friendly USA. In 2018 the WHO released their revised Implementation Guidance for the BFHI (WHO, 2018a). The original Ten Steps have been further refined to meet the current evidence and have been categorized into four focus areas: (1) critical management procedures to support breastfeeding, (2) key clinical practices to support breastfeeding, (3) coordination, and (4) quality-improvement processes. Baby-Friendly USA will be making changes to the U.S. Guidelines in Criteria to be in alignment with WHO recommendations. In a recent systematic review, the Agency for Healthcare Research and Quality (AHRQ) found that the BFHI is associated with improved rates of breastfeeding initiation and duration (Feltner et al, 2018).

The *Surgeon General's Call to Action to Support Breastfeeding* 2011 report states that breastfeeding should be promoted to all women in the United States and supported by clinicians, employers, communities, researchers, and government leaders. All are encouraged to commit to enabling mothers to meet their personal goals for breastfeeding. However, too many mothers are still not able to reach these goals. Improvement of support systems is needed for mothers to overcome challenges and barriers so often in the way of successful breastfeeding. Excess health risks associated with not breastfeeding can be found in Box 14.12.

BOX 14.11 Baby-Friendly Hospital Initiative: Ten Steps to Successful Breastfeeding

1. Have a written breastfeeding policy that is routinely communicated to all health care staff.
2. Train all health care staff in the skills necessary to implement this policy.
3. Inform all pregnant women about the benefits and management of breastfeeding.
4. Help the mother initiate breastfeeding within 1 hour of birth.
5. Show mothers how to breastfeed and how to maintain lactation, even if they are separated from their infants.
6. Give newborn infants no food or drink other than breastmilk unless medically indicated.
7. Practice rooming-in; allow mothers and infants to remain together 24 hours a day.
8. Encourage breastfeeding on demand.
9. Give no artificial teats or pacifiers (also called dummies or soothers) to breastfeeding infants.
10. Foster the establishment of breastfeeding support groups and refer mothers to them on discharge from the hospital or clinic.

Adapted from Baby-Friendly USA *The Ten Steps to Successful Breastfeeding* (website): https://www.babyfriendlyusa.org/for-facilities/practice-guidelines/10-steps-and-international-code/, 2018.

BOX 14.12 Excess Health Risks Associated with Not Breastfeeding

Outcome	Excess Risk* (%)	Comparison Groups
Among full-term infants		
Acute ear infections (otitis media)	100	EFF vs. EBF for 3 or 6 months
Eczema (atopic dermatitis)	47	EBF <3 months vs. EBF ≥3 months
Diarrhea and vomiting (gastrointestinal infection)	178	Never BF vs. ever BF
Hospitalization for lower respiratory tract diseases in the first year	257	Never BF vs. EBF ≥4 months
Asthma, with family history	67	BF, 3 months vs. ≥3 months
Asthma, no family history	35	BF, 3 months vs. ≥3 months
Childhood obesity	32	Never BF vs. ever BF
Type 2 diabetes mellitus	64	Never BF vs. ever BF
Acute lymphocytic leukemia	23	Never BF vs. 6 months
Acute myelogenous leukemia	18	Never BF vs. 6 months
Sudden infant death syndrome	56	Never BF vs. ever BF
Among preterm infants		
Necrotizing enterocolitis	138	Never BF vs. ever BF
Among mothers		
Breast cancer	4	Never BF vs. ever BF (per year of breastfeeding)
Ovarian cancer	27	Never BF vs. ever BF

*The excess risk is approximated by using the odds ratios reported in the referenced studies.
EFF, Exclusive formula feeding.
EBF, Exclusive breastfeeding.
BF, Breastfeeding.
Adapted from U.S. Department of Health and Human Services: *The Surgeon General's Call to Action to Support Breastfeeding,* Washington, DC, 2011, Office of the Surgeon General.

Contraindications

Contraindications to breastfeeding are rare, but a few conditions warrant at least a temporary interruption from either direct feeding from the breast or from feeding breastmilk. Breastfeeding is contraindicated for infants with classic galactosemia, and for mothers who have active untreated tuberculosis, are positive for human T-cell lymphotropic virus type 1 or 2, have brucellosis, use drugs of abuse (without medical supervision), have HIV (in the United States) (USDHHS, 2018a), or who take certain medications (i.e., antimetabolites and chemotherapeutic agents). Exclusive breastfeeding in HIV positive mothers on antiretroviral therapy is highly recommended throughout the world (WHO, 2016a). A mother should not breastfeed with active herpes simplex lesions on her breast; however, expressed milk can be used without concern. If a mother develops varicella 5 days before through 2 days after delivery, she should be separated from her infant but can provide her expressed milk to the infant. Mothers who have influenza should be encouraged to continue to breastfeed (CDC, 2018b). Mothers acutely infected with H1N1 influenza should separate themselves from their infants while febrile, but again, can provide their expressed milk for feedings (AAP, 2012). The use of most radioactive isotopes requires temporary cessation of breastfeeding, ranging from 6 hours to up to 1 month (Hale, 2019). Women undergoing procedures using these types of medications should consult with their health care provider to determine the specific drug used so that adequate time is allowed for clearance, but no more time than is necessary so that breastfeeding can be resumed. Clearance time varies between drugs; expressing and discarding breastmilk can help preserve milk production if extended cessation is necessary.

The CDC advises women in the United States who have HIV to refrain from breastfeeding to avoid postnatal transmission to their infants through their breastmilk. Because sanitary conditions for safe use of infant formula are available in the United States, experts believe the morbidity risk can be kept to a minimum. However, in developing countries where sanitary conditions are not as prevalent, and the rate of mortality in the infant from infectious diseases and malnutrition are high, the health risks of not breastfeeding must be considered. In addition, in areas where HIV is prevalent, exclusively breastfeeding for the first 3 months has been shown to reduce the risk of infants acquiring HIV compared with infants who receive a mixed diet of human milk and other foods, including infant formula. Six months of exclusive breastfeeding while the mother receives antiretroviral therapy has been shown to significantly reduce the postnatal acquisition of HIV (AAP, 2012).

Nutritional Requirements of Lactation

Despite the fact that breastfeeding increases the need for energy and some nutrients, human milk is made from maternal nutrient stores, so well-nourished mothers need not worry that the quality of their breastmilk will suffer from an imperfect diet. Breastmilk remains perfect for the infant even in cases of hardship and famine. Only in rare cases when mothers experience long-term, severe nutritional deficiency is their breastmilk affected. An excuse to not choose breastfeeding based on the fact that a woman enjoys drinking coffee or tea, or an occasional alcoholic beverage, is unwarranted.

Unless a vitamin-mineral deficiency is identified, or the mother has a restricted diet or an issue with malabsorption, dietary supplements are usually not necessary. A diet including a variety of whole foods, adequate in calories, should provide the woman with all the nutrients she needs. Despite this fact, many clinicians recommend the continued use of a prenatal vitamin/mineral supplement for the duration of lactation, especially if the mother remains iron deficient after birth.

Increased prolactin receptors in the breast and therefore higher maternal prolactin levels develop with early suckling stimulation and milk removal, a process enhanced with increased frequency of breastfeeding in the early neonatal period. The maternal response to her infant's hunger cues will stimulate her milk supply, averaging about 8 to 12 breastfeeds over 24 hours in the first 2 to 3 weeks. Encouraging the mother to focus on recognizing hunger cues versus watching the clock is highly recommended. The belief that more milk is made with increased fluid consumption is misguided because the body will excrete excessive fluid to maintain electrolyte balance. This actually may result in a decrease of milk production. Concern for the mother's hydration and her ability to produce an adequate milk supply is only valid during extreme conditions such as severe drought or famine. Insufficient milk supply can be as much of a problem in well-nourished women as in poorly nourished women; cross-cultural studies show it to be unrelated to maternal nutrition status. Poor maternal nutrition may affect the quantity, but not quality, of mothers' milk (Lawrence and Lawrence, 2016). Although a mother's milk maintains its quality even when nutrient intake is suboptimal, the woman feels the effects of eating poorly, possibly affecting her immune system, and feels tired with less energy. A nutritious dietary intake helps her cope with the everyday demands of caring for a new infant.

Milk composition varies according to the mother's diet. For example, the fatty acid composition of a mother's milk reflects her dietary intake. In addition, milk concentrations of selenium, iodine, and some of the B vitamins reflect the maternal diet. Breastmilk of *extremely malnourished* mothers has been shown to have lower levels of various nutrients, reflecting the foods she has available to eat. One must remember that milk composition varies widely in the concentration of macronutrients within and between individual mothers. Several factors, including length of pregnancy, mother's diet, stage of lactation, duration of feeding, and the time of day the feeding takes place, can affect the composition of human milk. Protein levels tend to fall in the early postpartum period, whereas the fat component of the milk initially may decrease and eventually increase in concentration over time. During an individual feeding, fat content typically increases significantly and can result in a much higher caloric content in the milk toward the end of the feeding (Khan et al, 2013). Fat content also may be higher when the interval between breastfeedings is closer together. When the infant "cluster feeds," the milk available in the breast is higher in fat content. When more time is allowed between feedings, the breasts fill with milk with higher water content. At the next feeding, the infant may not be able to consume all the milk available and ends up taking mainly low-fat milk.

Energy

Milk production is 80% efficient: production of 100 mL of milk (approximately 75 kcal) requires an 85-kcal expenditure (Lawrence and Lawrence, 2016). During the first 6 months of lactation, average milk production is 750 mL/day (about 24 oz), with a range of 550 to more than 1200 mL/day. Because production is a function of the frequency, duration, and intensity of infant suckling, infants who feed well are likely to stimulate the production of larger volumes of milk.

The DRI for energy during lactation is 330 kcal greater during the first 6 months of lactation and 400 kcal greater during the second 6 months of lactation over that for a nonpregnant woman. However, considering milk production usually drops to an average of 600 mL/day (approximately 20 oz/day) after other foods are introduced into the infant's diet, ingested calorie levels may have to be adjusted for the individual woman who wishes to avoid weight gain. A mother is able to draw approximately 100 to 150 kcal/day from pregnancy fat stores.

Healthy breastfeeding women can lose as much as 1 pound per week and still supply adequate milk to maintain their infants' growth. The combination of diet and exercise together, or diet alone can help women to lose weight after childbirth (Amorim Adegboye and Linne, 2013). In a study of 68 adolescent mothers and 64 adult mothers, postpartum weight loss in both groups was significantly greater in those who were exclusively breastfeeding (EBF) compared with those who did not EBF. Moreover, the infants of the mothers continued to grow according to the 2006 WHO growth standards despite their mothers' weight loss (Sámano et al, 2013). However, milk production has been shown to decrease in mothers whose intakes are suboptimal (less than 1500 to 1800 calories/day) (West and Marasco, 2009). Mothers are advised to wait until breastfeeding is well established (approximately 2 months) before consciously trying to lose weight so that an adequate milk supply can be established. Appropriate fluid intake (such as drinking for thirst) and adequate rest also are recommended. A slow weight loss of no more than about 5 pounds per month supports more permanent weight loss as well as allows for adequate energy and nutrition for new motherhood.

Protein

The DRI suggests an additional 25 g of protein a day for lactation, or 71 g of protein a day, based on an RDA of 1.1 gm/kg/day of a woman's body weight. Clinical judgment is necessary with protein recommendations because 71 g/day may be too low for a woman with a larger body size and too high for the woman with a smaller body. Women with surgical delivery and women who enter pregnancy with poor nutritional status may need additional protein. The average protein requirement for lactation is estimated from milk composition data and the mean daily volume of 750 mL, assuming 70% efficiency in the conversion of dietary protein to milk protein.

Breastmilk has a whey:casein ratio of 90:10 early in lactation, which changes to 80:20 as an average, and to 60:40 as the baby gets older. It is speculated that this ratio makes breastmilk more digestible. In contrast, the whey:casein ratio of cow's milk protein is 18:82. Cow's milk–based infant formula varies among commercial manufacturers, ranging from 18:82 whey:casein, to 52:48 whey:casein, and even up to 100% whey (see Chapter 15).

Carbohydrates

The RDA for carbohydrate is designed to provide enough calories in the diet for adequate volumes of milk and to maintain an adequate energy level during lactation. This may have to be adjusted depending on activity of the mother and the amount of breastfeeding. The woman with poor gestational weight gain may require more carbohydrates. Women who had gestational diabetes during pregnancy should continue on the MNT diet they were on during pregnancy for optimal management of blood sugar if recommended to do so by their medical provider. A modified carbohydrate diet is often implemented to meet the dietary needs in this condition.

The principal carbohydrate in human milk is lactose; however, there is no evidence that maternal intake of carbohydrates affects the level of lactose in her milk.

Lipids

Dietary fat choices by the mother can increase or decrease specific fatty acids in her milk, but not the total amount of fat in the milk. Severe restriction of energy intake results in mobilization of body fat, and the milk produced has a fatty acid composition resembling that of the mother's body fat.

There is no DRI for total lipids during lactation because it depends on the amount of energy required by the mother to maintain milk production. The recommended amounts of specific omega-6 and omega-3 LCPUFAs during lactation vary little from pregnancy; they are crucial for fetal and infant brain development. One to two servings of fish per week meet this need (herring, canned light tuna, salmon). Mothers should avoid eating predatory fish to prevent excessive levels of dietary mercury (pike, marlin, mackerel, albacore tuna, and swordfish) (AAP, 2012; see also Chapter 16). Intake of trans fats should be kept to a minimum by the nursing mother so that the potential for their appearance in her breastmilk is reduced. See *Focus On: Omega-3 Fatty Acids in Pregnancy and Lactation* for more information about including DHA in the maternal diet.

Human milk contains 10 to 20 mg/dL of cholesterol, resulting in an approximate consumption of 100 mg/day, which has been determined to be essential to the diet of the infant. The amount of cholesterol in milk does not reflect the mother's diet and decreases over time as lactation progresses.

Vitamins and Minerals

Vitamin D. The vitamin D content of breastmilk is related to maternal vitamin D intake as well as environmental conditions. Numerous case reports document marginal or significant vitamin D deficiency in infants of lactating women who are veiled, who are dark skinned, who have a BMI of more than 30, who use sunscreens heavily, or who live in latitudes with decreased sun exposure. Women with lactose intolerance who do not drink vitamin D–fortified milk or take a vitamin supplement may be at higher risk for vitamin D deficiency. Hypocalcemic rickets, including cases of dilated cardiomyopathy, have been reported in the United States in breastfed, dark-skinned infants (Brown et al, 2009).

Because of reports of clinical rickets, the AAP recommends that all infants receive 400 IU (10 mcg) of vitamin D as a daily supplement starting at birth, allowing the infant to easily achieve vitamin D sufficiency. For formula-fed infants, they may cease supplementation once the infant is consuming 1 liter of formula per day. Canada recommends 800 IU/day for adults living north of 45° N latitude, but the mother may need much higher doses (100 mcg or 4000 IU/ day) to achieve normal 25(OH)D concentrations and vitamin D adequacy in her exclusively breastfed infant. Because the antirachitic activity of human milk is low (5-80 IU/L), the lactating mother requires a significant amount of vitamin D daily from food or UV exposure. Maternal circulation allows transfer of the parent compound, Vitamin D3 itself, and not circulating 25(OH)D, into human milk. Although maternal baseline circulating 25(OH)D level may be adequate, it cannot be assumed that the vitamin D activity of the mother's milk is adequate for the infant. Because of the binding affinity to vitamin D binding protein, the circulating half-life of 25(OH)D is 3 to 4 weeks, while that of vitamin D3 is just 12 to 24 hours; the reduced affinity of vitamin D3 allows the unbound vitamin D3 to diffuse across cell membranes from blood into the milk. In order for levels for vitamin D to be sustained in both the maternal circulation as well as the milk supply, a daily dose of vitamin D is required. Recent studies have shown that a daily maternal intake of 6400 IU of vitamin D is safe and allows a mother to produce milk that will provide adequate amounts of vitamin D to her exclusively breastfed nursling, without additional supplementation directly to the infant (Hollis et al, 2015).

Calcium. Although breastfeeding mothers should be encouraged to meet their DRI for calcium from their diet, the calcium content of breastmilk is not related to maternal intake, and there is no convincing evidence that maternal change in bone mineral density is influenced by calcium intake across a broad range of intakes up to 1600 mg/day. A recent study evaluated calcium intakes of 33 Gambian lactating women during two different lactational time periods. The study found that even with suboptimal intakes, the bone mineral mobilization during lactation was recovered after lactation. They concluded that successive periods of long lactation are not associated with progressive skeletal depletion (Sawo et al, 2013).

Iodine. Adequate breastmilk iodine levels are particularly important for proper neurodevelopment in nursing infants, and required intakes are nearly double nonpregnant values. Iodine concentrations in breastmilk are considered to be adequate to meet infants' iodine nutritional needs in areas where food sources are adequate. However, mothers living in iodine-deficient areas, especially if also consuming goitrogens or exposed to perchlorate contamination, may produce milk with iodine concentrations insufficient to meet the needs of the infant. As mentioned earlier, hyper- and hypo-thyroidism can affect breastmilk production, and so mothers should choose food sources of iodine, such as iodized salt, dairy foods, seafood, and breads made with iodide. Recent recommendations from the AAP state that lactating women should ensure a daily intake of 290 mcg of iodide, which generally requires supplementation of 150 mcg/day.

Zinc. The requirements for zinc during lactation are greater than those during pregnancy. Breastmilk provides the only dietary source of zinc for exclusively breastfed infants, and it remains a potentially important source of zinc for children beyond infancy who continue to breastfeed. In the process of normal lactation, the zinc content of breastmilk drops dramatically during the first few months from 2 to 3 mg/day to 1 mg/day by the third month after birth. Zinc supplementation has not been found to affect concentrations in the breastmilk of women in developed countries but may increase the zinc content of the milk of women in developing countries with suboptimal zinc status (Sazawal et al, 2013).

Vitamin B_{12} and the Vegan Mother. For lactating mothers who follow a strict vegan diet without any animal products, a vitamin B_{12} supplement is strongly recommended. The milk of a vegan mother can be severely deficient in vitamin B_{12}, leading to a deficiency in her infant which, if not treated, can lead to growth failure and permanent damage to the nervous system. Nursing mothers who follow a strict vegetarian diet should have their infant's B_{12} levels monitored. Lactating mothers who have undergone gastric bypass surgery are also at greater risk for B_{12} deficiency (see Appendix 31).

Sodium. Sodium intake during lactation should be controlled with the inclusion of a diet composed of foods high in nutritional value, which are naturally lower in sodium. Although there is no specific recommendation or restriction for sodium in the diet of breastfeeding mothers, a relationship has been established between the sodium intake of mothers and breastfeeding success. A recent study examined whether maternal salt preference may facilitate breastfeeding. The investigators found that mothers with a preference for a low salt intake had higher rates of successful breastfeeding beyond day 7 compared with mothers with high salt preference. Mothers with high salt preference had the shortest exclusive breastfeeding duration up to postnatal day 25 (Verd et al, 2010). Future studies are warranted to determine exactly what effect maternal sodium intake has on the success of breastfeeding.

Fluids

A nursing mother may feel a need to drink simply because of increased fluid output when breastfeeding her infant. She should drink to thirst but not feel she must force fluids, which is not beneficial and may cause discomfort. The beverage of choice is water; however, water is the main component of many beverages and can be used as such in the body.

Caffeine. Caffeine is acceptable in moderate amounts (less than 300 mg daily, see Appendix 25) and does not present a problem for the healthy full-term infant. If the mother is nursing a preterm infant, however, the baby may be particularly sensitive to large intakes of caffeine. In this case the mother is advised to observe her infant closely for signs of overstimulation, such as being unusually fussy or not being able to settle easily. If so, the mother should adjust her caffeine intake accordingly. It may take a few days after reducing caffeine intake for mother to notice a difference in the baby's symptoms. There is no evidence that caffeine affects milk supply, although if a baby is overstimulated, he may not nurse well, which could lead to dysfunctional breastfeeding and eventually a lowered maternal milk supply.

Alcohol. No safe amount of alcohol has been established for the nursing mother, but recommendations include limiting intake to 0.5 g alcohol/kg maternal body weight (AAP, 2012). For a 60-kg mother, this equals approximately 2 oz liquor, 8 oz wine, or two beers per day. Peak alcohol levels occur in about ½ to 1 hour after drinking, although this varies among women depending on mother's body composition. There is no need for a mother to express and discard her milk after taking 1 to 2 drinks, thinking this will speed the elimination of alcohol from the milk, unless it is for her own comfort. As blood alcohol decreases, so does alcohol concentration in the milk. Mothers should be discriminatory about any alcohol intake when nursing a premature, young, or sick baby because this baby would be affected much more than the older, more mature baby. In addition, mothers should consider their ability to care for their children when under the influence of alcohol. If occasional alcohol intake occurs, moderation is advised at all times for breastfeeding mothers.

Box 14.13   Summary of Nutritional Care During Lactation

1. A variety of foods, focusing on nutrient-dense food choices.
2. Energy intake to allow for maintaining health and well-being; calorie level no less than 1800 kcal/day. Intentional weight loss not advised before breastfeeding is well established (approximately 2 months).
3. Protein intake to meet nutritional needs, approximately an additional 25 g/day from base level prepregnancy. This often requires 20% of energy intake from protein.
4. DHA from fatty fish (low in methylmercury) twice a week.
5. Mineral and vitamin intakes to meet the recommended daily allowances (usually met from a variety of foods in the diet). Supplements as directed from health care provider.
6. Drink to thirst; have beverages readily available during nursing and when expressing breastmilk.
7. If desired, alcoholic beverages can be consumed on occasion, in moderation. Not recommended with preterm, very young, or sick infants.
8. Omission of toxins and nonnutritive substances from food, water, and environment as much as possible.

See Table 14.15 and Box 14.13 for summaries of nutritional care during lactation.

Prenatal Breastfeeding Education

The advantages of breastfeeding should be presented throughout the childbearing years. During pregnancy, counseling on the risks of formula feeding and the process of lactation should be provided to women so that they can make an informed decision about how they will feed their baby and so that they understand how to achieve successful breastfeeding. As optimal maternity care practices become the norm in hospitals and birth centers, women should be educated on these practices in advance of delivery. Prenatal breastfeeding education is recommended strongly for women and their partners. The emotional support provided by the mother's partner contributes heavily to the success of the breastfeeding experience.

During this time the mother should identify a support person to call upon after breastfeeding begins. Because initiation and establishment of breastfeeding can seem intense and full of challenges for new mothers, it is wise for her to know who to turn to when questions or concerns arise. A knowledgeable family member or health professional, doula, peer counselor, or childbirth educator can provide the encouragement so often needed for a mother in the early postpartum period. Prenatal breastfeeding counseling with regular follow-up after delivery has been shown to have a positive effect on early initiation and sustained exclusive breastfeeding, especially among primiparous mothers, with group counseling having even more beneficial impact than individual counseling (WHO, 2017). When more complicated problems are identified, an International Board Certified Lactation Consultant (IBCLC) can intervene, which may mean the difference between early weaning and a successful breastfeeding experience.

Physiology and Management of Lactation

Mammary gland growth during menarche and pregnancy prepares the woman for lactation. Hormonal changes in pregnancy markedly increase breast, areola, and nipple size as well as significantly increase ducts and alveoli and influence mammary growth. Late in pregnancy the lobules of the alveolar system are maximally developed, and small amounts of colostrum may be released for several weeks before term and

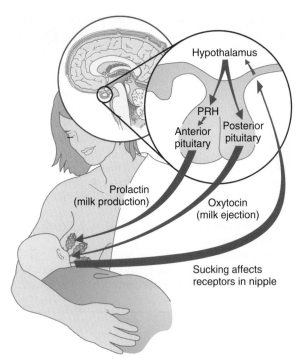

Fig. 14.9 Physiology of milk production and the let-down reflex. *PRH,* Pituitary-releasing hormone.

for a few days after delivery. After birth there is a rapid drop in circulating levels of estrogen and progesterone accompanied by a rapid increase in prolactin secretion, setting the stage for a copious milk supply.

The usual stimulus for milk production and secretion is suckling. Subcutaneous nerves of the areola send a message via the spinal cord to the hypothalamus, which in turn transmits a message to the pituitary gland, where the anterior and posterior areas are stimulated. Prolactin from the anterior pituitary stimulates alveolar cell milk production, as shown in Fig. 14.9. Women who have diabetes, who are obese, who experience stress during delivery, or who have retained placental fragments in the uterus are at risk for delayed milk production (i.e., when signs of lactogenesis are absent 72 hours after birth).

Oxytocin from the posterior pituitary stimulates the myoepithelial cells of the mammary gland to contract, causing movement of milk through the ducts and lactiferous sinuses, a process referred to as let-down. "Let-down" is highly sensitive. Oxytocin may be released by visual, tactile, olfactory, and auditory stimuli; and even by thinking about the infant. Oxytocin secretion also can be inhibited by pain, emotional and physical stress, fatigue, and anxiety.

Stages of Milk and Variations in Composition

Human milk varies in nutritional composition throughout the maternal lactational period and seems to be more sensitive to maternal factors such as body composition, diet, and parity during later lactation than during the first few months (Lawrence and Lawrence, 2016). This fluid is constantly changing to meet the needs of the growing infant; nutrient composition changes throughout the duration of lactation, but also over the course of a day, and even during a feeding.

The delivery of the placenta after the birth of a baby triggers lactogenesis I, or the beginning of milk production. Colostrum is the thick, yellowish secretion that is the first feeding for the infant. It is higher in protein and lower in fat and carbohydrate, including lactose, than mature milk. It facilitates the passage of meconium (first stool of neonate), is high in antioxidants, and is lower in water-soluble vitamins than

mature milk. Colostrum is also higher in fat-soluble vitamins, protein, sodium, potassium, chloride, zinc, and immunoglobulins than mature milk. Colostrum provides approximately 20 kcal/oz and is a rich source of antibodies. It is considered the baby's first immunization.

Transitional milk begins to be produced approximately 2 to 5 days after delivery until around 10 to 14 days postpartum. During this stage of lactogenesis II, white, creamy milk is produced in much greater quantities than colostrum, and breasts become larger and firmer. This is the time when mothers feel their milk "come in." It is important for mothers to breastfeed often during this stage (8 to 12 times/day) to avoid engorgement and allow proper emptying of the breast by the infant. This also ensures adequate fluid and nutrition for the baby during this time. This period is an extremely important time to bring in a full milk supply, which can be established by the infant only with unrestricted access to breastfeeding.

Mature milk is the final stage of milk production and usually begins to appear near the end of the second week after childbirth. Foremilk, the first milk released during a breastfeed, is high in water content to meet the baby's hydration needs. It is low in calories but high in water-soluble vitamins and protein. This milk is thinner, sometimes with a bluish color, and resembles skim milk when first released from the breast.

As the baby nurses during a breastfeed, the milk becomes creamier, indicating a higher fat content. This milk, high in fat-soluble vitamins and other nutrients, is called hindmilk. It provides satiety and the calories to ensure growth in the baby. It is important for the mother to allow the infant to empty the first breast at each feeding to obtain this hindmilk, before offering the other breast. This way, the baby is assured of obtaining the complete nutrition available from the mother's milk. Hindmilk is released as the breast is emptied and signals to the baby that a feeding is over. This mechanism helps the infant to learn when to end a feeding and may contribute to the prevention of overeating and subsequently becoming overweight later in life. The longer the mother goes between feedings, the more foremilk will be stored in the breast; however, when feedings are closer together, the baby receives more hindmilk in each feeding. Babies need a balanced diet, with sufficient amounts of foremilk and hindmilk for proper growth and development.

As the mother progresses during the lactational stage of motherhood, her breasts return to her prepregnancy size and may appear somewhat softer and smaller than earlier. This does not indicate a lower milk supply, but only her body's adjustment to established breastfeeding. A woman continues to produce nutritious mature milk, as well as enjoy the emotional and immunologic benefits, for as long as she breastfeeds. Exclusive breastfeeding is recommended for the first 6 months, followed by continued breastfeeding as complementary foods are introduced, with continuation of breastfeeding for 1 year or longer, as mutually desired by mother and child (AAP, 2012).

As mentioned previously, breastmilk is a dynamic fluid, changing throughout the lactational period of the mother. Breastmilk continues to provide an infant with needed amounts of essential nutrients well beyond the first year of life, especially protein, fat, and most vitamins. Breastfed infants tend to gain less weight and usually are leaner than are formula-fed infants in the second half of infancy, which does not seem to be the result of nutritional deficits, but rather infant self-regulation of energy intake. The nutrients most likely to be limiting in the diets of breastfed infants after 6 months of exclusive breastfeeding are minerals such as iron, zinc, and calcium. These nutrients are readily available through an age-appropriate diet consisting of meats, whole grains, dairy foods, fruits, and vegetables.

During growth spurts, or times of rapid infant development—typically around 2 weeks, again at 4 to 6 weeks, and anytime between

3 and 6 months—babies may increase their desire to nurse to meet caloric needs. If allowed to do so, this triggers an increase in the mother's prolactin level, and after a few days, she will begin to make more milk. If supplements are introduced at these times to satisfy the infant's hunger, the mother will not have the advantage of increased stimulation from the infant's suckling and will not be able to keep up her supply to meet the baby's nutritional needs. Many mothers do not understand this concept of "supply and demand" and unintentionally may sabotage their breastfeeding relationship.

Initiation of Breastfeeding

Breastfeeding is a learned skill for mother and her infant. All babies should be put skin-to-skin immediately after birth and remain in direct skin-to-skin contact until the first feed is accomplished or as long as the mother desires (WHO, 2017; WHO, 2018a). Within 48 to 96 hours after birth the breasts become fuller and firmer as the milk volumes increase. Skin-to-skin contact in the first hour improves breastfeeding exclusivity and duration and helps to regulate temperature, blood sugar, and blood pressure of the infant. This practice is recommended regardless of desired feeding method.

Exclusively breastfed babies do not need additional water because 87% of breastmilk is water. However, cases of hypernatremic dehydration in babies caused by suboptimal breastfeeding do occur. Most cases are due to lack of support for mothers who feel intimidated and overwhelmed at delivery, lack breastfeeding education, and are unaware of the consequences of dehydration. Extreme heat or hot weather also may increase the need for more frequent breastfeeding to avoid dehydration. The consequence of hypernatremic dehydration can be permanent brain damage or death. Therefore it is vital that an experienced health care professional evaluate the breastfeeding within 2 to 4 days after birth; problems identified can be addressed and a plan of care can be implemented (WHO, 2018a).

During the first days and weeks of breastfeeding, mothers should feed on demand or "on cue." Watching and listening to the infant guides a mother to know when to offer a feeding. When a mother responds to her infant's hunger cues, nursing "on demand," she provides the quantity the baby needs, as long as supplements are avoided, and pacifiers are not used to "mask" the baby's hunger. A newborn's stomach is very small and holds only about a teaspoon or two of fluid at a time, matching the small amount of colostrum available from the mother. The colostrum is very easily absorbed, and that is why the infant will give frequent hunger cues to the mother. As a newborn's stomach enlarges over the next few days and weeks, so does the mother's milk supply as long as no supplement has interfered with this process of supply and demand. Extra bottle feedings can stretch the infant's stomach so that the supply the mother has available can no longer satisfy the baby. This situation may cause a mother to feel that she does not have enough milk and has failed at breastfeeding, and possibly unnecessarily cause her to wean. It is common to breastfeed 8 to 12 times a day while the breastmilk is increasing and an adequate supply is being established. After breastfeeding has been fully established in the first few weeks, lactating women may begin to feel the strong tingling sensation in the breasts caused by oxytocin release, signaling the let-down reflex. (See earlier explanation.) This sensation automatically causes a sudden release of milk from the breasts. If this occurs when the mother is not available for her baby, firm pressure on the breasts stops milk from flowing.

As breastfeeding continues, mothers begin to settle into a pattern of feeding that is comfortable and relaxed. Although each mother-baby couplet is different, most babies become more efficient at the breast and are able to take in more milk at a feeding time, as much as several ounces in just a few minutes. This allows the feedings to become less frequent and take less time. When breastfeeding is total nourishment for the baby, some feeds may be short just to satisfy a baby's thirst, and others may last 20 to 30 minutes if the baby is very hungry. This is no cause for worry, as long as the mother continues to respond to the infant's cues. Parents should be educated about this process so that they do not get discouraged or think that the intense feeding schedule that is common in the early weeks will last for the entire breastfeeding experience.

Practice, patience, and perseverance are necessary for successful breastfeeding, along with a strong support system for the mother, including family, friends, health care personnel, her workplace, and the community around her (see Box 14.11). With learned hand expression or the help of an effective breast pump, the mother is able to express and store her milk for later use when she is away from her infant. Pump rentals or purchase may be covered by insurance or available through the WIC program. See Box 14.14 for a summary of tips for success in breastfeeding.

Breastfeeding by Women with Diabetes. Women who have insulin-dependent diabetes may experience "lactation hypoglycemia" as they increase their breastfeeding sessions. Plasma glucose levels in the lactating diabetic mother are lower because of maternal stores being used for milk production. The daily maternal insulin requirement is

---

Box 14.14 Tips for Breastfeeding Success

During your pregnancy:
- Enroll in the Special Supplemental Nutrition Program for Women, Infants, and Children (WIC) program, if eligible.
- Attend a breastfeeding class.
- Ask your medical provider about breastfeeding.
- Read about breastfeeding.
- Get 1 to 2 good nursing bras.
- Find a supportive person that can help you.

In the hospital:
- Let doctors and nurses know that you plan to breastfeed.
- Request that your baby be put skin-to skin immediately after birth.
- Breastfeed during the first hour after birth.
- Keep baby in room with you 24 hours/day.
- Avoid using bottles or pacifiers.
- Ask for an International Board Certified Lactation Consultant (IBCLC) to help with correct latch.
- Breastfeed whenever your baby shows hunger cues (8 or more times in 24 hours).
- If doctor orders supplementation, use expressed breastmilk first. Request donor milk if unable to provide mother's own milk.
- If you and your baby are separated because of illness, hand express and ask for a breast pump.
- Ask about breastfeeding support services available in your community.

During the first 2 to 3 weeks at home:
- Avoid bottles or a pacifier.
- Breastfeed whenever your baby shows hunger cues, at least 8 times a day.
- Make sure baby latches onto the breast correctly.
- Continue skin-to-skin care whenever possible.
- Watch for 6 to 8 wet and 2 to 3 messy diapers daily by end of first week.
- For questions or concerns, call the WIC Lactation Specialist or an IBCLC.
- See baby's doctor within 1-2 days for a weight check if discharged from the birthing facility before 48 hours of age. Those discharged after 48 hours of age should be seen within 2-3 days of discharge.
- If enrolled in WIC, see nutritionist to obtain nutritious foods for yourself.
- Participate in mother-to-mother support groups.

usually lower in these women, and frequent glucose monitoring must be emphasized to ensure safety for the mother and baby. Because newborns of mothers with diabetes frequently are admitted to the NICU for closer observation, more support should be offered to these mothers to ensure breastfeeding success.

Breastfeeding Preterm and Sick Infants. Breastmilk for a preterm infant is not only beneficial but also absolutely necessary to ensure protection from infection and other illnesses (see Chapter 41). A mother may be overwhelmed when her baby is delivered before the due date or is admitted to the NICU for any reason. If the baby is not strong enough for effective breastfeeding, professional help should be used so that the mother can begin milk expression, and her milk can be available for the infant's nutrition.

A mother may find that she is totally dependent on the breast pump for several days, weeks, or even months. During this time, it is important for the mother (and father) to employ skin-to-skin care of their baby to allow appropriate stimulation of prolactin production in the mother for her milk supply to be maintained. This connection with her newborn also assists in the bonding process so important in the development of a healthy, loving relationship, which is challenged by the unfortunate situation in which the mother and her family find themselves. The mother will continue to need support and encouragement throughout the baby's hospitalization, and even more so when discharge gets closer. The total transfer of care to the parents can be an even bigger challenge, and they will need much guidance and follow-up to ensure breastfeeding is successful.

In the case of adoption, a devastating prognosis, or infant death, the mother can prepare herself for a gradual decrease in her milk supply to allow for her physical health. Any milk she has in storage can be donated to a human milk bank (see *Focus On:* What Is a Human Milk Bank? in Chapter 41). This will give her comfort in knowing that the milk she produced and saved for her own baby will not be wasted but be used for another infant who may need it. Again, much support and guidance from knowledgeable professionals is necessary during these trying times.

Breastfeeding Multiples. Breastfeeding twins, triplets, or more is certainly challenging, but possible. A mother who plans to breastfeed multiples will most likely need assistance, especially in the early days. If the babies are healthy and brought home soon after birth, she can begin breastfeeding them right away and establish her milk supply with the help of at least two babies instead of one. This means a greater milk supply will be available if she responds to their hunger cues, just like with a singleton. She will be busier, no doubt, and feeding multiples during the first few weeks will be intense, to say the least. If the mother is determined to establish a good breastmilk supply early on and has the household help she needs, she can be successful. If, however, the infants are sick and must remain hospitalized for a while, she needs to use an effective breast pump to bring in her milk supply and should make her expressed breastmilk available for the babies' nutrition. A lactation consult with an IBCLC is strongly recommended in such cases.

See Table 14.16 for a summary of common problems that breastfeeding mothers may encounter, with ways to prevent or remedy these situations.

TABLE 14.16 Management of Breastfeeding Difficulties

Problem	Approaches
Inverted nipples	Breast shells with appropriate backing may be used during the last trimester of pregnancy. Before feeding the infant, roll the nipple gently between the fingers until erect. May use breast pump for 1-2 minutes before latching baby to bring nipple out.
Breast engorgement	Massage breasts prior to and during feeding, soften breasts/nipple by expressing a small amount of milk or use reverse pressure softening technique; allow baby to nurse frequently and/or express with hand or pump after feeding to relieve engorgement. Use cool compresses to ease pain after breastfeeding. Raw cabbage leaves placed on breasts for a few minutes every few hours may help to reduce swelling. Approved oral antiinflammatory medication may be used for pain.
Poor latch	Ensure proper positioning at breast; encourage baby to take a "mouth-full" of breast into his mouth; use nipple shield as last resort (use only with professional guidance).
Baby's mouth not open wide enough	Before feeding, depress the infant's lower jaw with one finger as the nipple is guided into the mouth. Elicit wide-open mouth from baby by tickling upper lip with nipple and hand expressing drops of milk from the nipple.
Sore nipples	Assess if pain is acute or chronic. Strive for proper latch (possible temporary use of nipple shields with professional guidance); limited evidence for interventions for initial nipple pain but will likely do no harm: hand express milk and allow to air dry, approved nipple ointment, breast shells with appropriate backing if extremely sensitive, hydrogel pads, approved pain meds. Check for ankyloglossia, fungal infection, or improperly fitting pump flange.
Baby sucks poorly	Stimulate sucking motions by pressing upward under the baby's chin. Use breast massage to express milk in baby's mouth and stimulate suck/swallow. Rule out infant/maternal physical or medical issues.
Baby demonstrates rooting but does not grasp the nipple; eventually cries in frustration	Interrupt the feeding, comfort the infant; the mother should take time to relax before trying again. Place baby in a comfortable position facing the breast. Express a few drops of milk on the nipple to entice the baby to latch.
Baby falls asleep while nursing	Mother may be able to awaken the infant by holding baby upright using skin-to-skin (when possible), rubbing baby's back, talking to baby, or providing similar quiet stimuli; another effort at feeding can then be made. If the baby falls asleep again, the feeding should be postponed. Use breast massage to encourage milk to flow more rapidly and stimulate infant to suck/swallow.
Plugged ducts	Firm fingertip massage in area of plug. Moist heat compresses before/during feedings on affected area. Therapeutic breast massage, frequent emptying of breast. Point baby's tongue in direction of plugged duct. Lecithin supplement may help to prevent reoccurrence. Refer to medical provider if not resolved within 72 hours.

TABLE 14.16 Management of Breastfeeding Difficulties—cont'd

Problem	Approaches
Mastitis	Signs of infection: breast is red and tender. Possible maternal fever, malaise. Maternal antibiotics may be indicated; call physician. Continue to breastfeed as comfort allows; frequent emptying of breasts with breastfeeding or expression. Breastmilk is safe for baby. Maternal rest recommended.
Thrush	Controversial diagnosis, inconclusive literature. Treatment usually includes mother and baby to prevent cross-infection/reinfection. Wash hands meticulously; sterilize items in contact with mother's breasts or baby's mouth or diaper area. Keep nipples dry. Approved nipple ointment for mother and oral medication (antifungal) for infant indicated—call physician. Breastmilk is safe for baby. Continue to treat at least 1 week after symptoms are gone to prevent return of infection. Some natural remedies may help: vinegar rinses on nipples and baby's diaper area, garlic supplements, probiotics/acidophilus, Echinacea, grapefruit seed extract—consult physician or lactation consultant.
Raynaud's Nipple vasospasms	Ensure proper latch to prevent worsening of symptoms. Keep nipples warm. May apply dry heat immediately after nursing. Use approved pain medication as needed; consider calcium channel blocker. Avoid caffeine, nicotine, and other vasoconstrictive drugs.
Perceived low milk supply	Offer breast frequently to allow infant to stimulate milk supply as desired; practice skin-to-skin care to stimulate prolactin production; express milk after/between feedings; avoid pacifiers and bottle supplementation unless advised by health care professional. Good nutrition, rest, and stress management is also advised. Watch for signs of adequate infant output (frequent wet diapers; appropriate bowel movements). Monitor baby's weight for reassurance of adequate maternal milk supply/infant intake.
True low milk supply	Ensure infant is latched correctly for maximum comfort and effectiveness; offer both breasts at every feeding—switch sides a few times during a feeding session for extra stimulation; avoid pacifiers and bottles; increase breast emptying by nursing or expression (length and frequency)—8-12 times/day; use pump for a few minutes after a breastfeed; when pumping, continue for 5 minutes after milk stops flowing to elicit additional let down; include pumping session between 1 and 5 A.M. when milk production is highest; use high-quality electric double pump (consider renting hospital grade pump); massage breast while pumping; always use correct flange size; use skin-to-skin care at each nursing session; rest/adequate nutrition/hydration; manage stress. Consider galactogogues (natural herbs or medication)—only with medical supervision (see Table 14.17). Supplementation may be necessary (human milk preferred, possibly using supplementer at breast, cup, syringe, dropper).

Consult with physician and IBCLC (International Board Certified Lactation Consultant) for expert advice.

Galactogogues

Low milk supply is a common concern among breastfeeding mothers. Whether real or perceived, mothers throughout the ages have turned to herbal remedies and medications to assist them in increasing their milk supply. Because milk supply is determined mainly by emptying the breasts regularly and effectively, this should be the first action taken to promote milk production. However, sometimes because of the effects of maternal or infant illness and hospitalization, or separation because of work or school, a mother may find that despite her efforts, her milk supply is faltering. Galactogogues also have been used in cases of adoption or relactation (reestablishing a milk supply after weaning). Galactogogues, or milk production stimulants, can be classified as medications, herbals, or foods—each with its own results. Herbals must be used with caution as many contain chemical substances that may be dangerous to the infant. A lactation consultant, registered dietitian nutritionist, or herbalist who is knowledgeable about their use in breastfeeding mothers should be consulted before using them. Standard recommended doses should not be exceeded (Hale, 2019).

Table 14.17 provides a list of common galactogogues along with possible side effects and contraindications. Medications used to increase a mother's milk supply must be prescribed by the mother's health care provider. Lactating women should tell the baby's health care provider if anything is taken to increase milk supply. Although traditional use of galactogogues suggests safety and possible efficacy, the mechanisms of action for most herbals have not been proven (Brodribb, 2018). Despite some traditional beliefs, beer and other alcoholic beverages do not increase milk supply and should not be used for this purpose.

Sustaining Maternal Milk Supply and Preservation of Successful Breastfeeding

Insufficient milk supply is rarely a problem for the well-fed, well-rested, and unstressed mother who stays in close contact with her baby. Sucking stimulates the flow of milk; thus feeding on demand should supply ample amounts of milk to the infant. Skin-to-skin care also can benefit the mother and baby by stimulating prolactin production in the mother while keeping the baby comforted and familiar with the mother. In the early days, indications of sufficient milk supply are that the baby continues to gain weight and length steadily, has at least six to eight wet diapers daily, and has frequent stools. Refer to Table 14.16 for tips on increasing milk supply.

Occasionally, however, breastfeeding complications can interfere with success. Fig. 14.10 illustrates potential problems in the mother or the infant that should be investigated if the mother feels that her milk supply is dropping or the baby is showing signs of slow growth. The cause of the problem must be identified and corrected to preserve the breastfeeding relationship and maintain the infant's growth and development. Professional assistance is available to identify and correct any complications that may interfere with successful breastfeeding. An IBCLC can be found at birth hospitals or centers, pediatric hospitals, maternal-child clinics, physicians' offices, and private practices.

Sometimes the infant may show intolerance (i.e., fussiness, loose stools) to something the mother has ingested. The mother is advised to temporarily eliminate suspected irritants until a later time when the baby is older and the GI tract more mature. Many times, food sensitivity is outgrown after a few weeks or months. Any food may be the culprit,

TABLE 14.17   Common Galactogogues

Class of Galactogogue	Specific Substance	Comments
Prescription Medications	Domperidone (*Motilium*)	Raises prolactin and proven useful as a galactogogue; few CNS effects such as depression. Associated with increase in cardiac arrhythmias (QTc prolongation).
	Metoclopramide *(Reglan/Maxeran/Maxolon)*	Raises prolactin and proven useful as a galactogogue; side effects may include headache, diarrhea, sedation, gastric upset, nausea, extrapyramidal symptoms, severe depression.
Herbals	Fenugreek (*Trigonella foenum graecum*)	Strong reputation as an effective galactogogue, but undocumented. Side effects include maple syrup odor in urine and sweat (mother and baby); may cause diarrhea, hypoglycemia, dyspnea. Not to be taken during pregnancy.
	Milk Thistle *(Silybum marianum/Silymarin)*	Reputation as a galactogogue, but undocumented. Side effects include occasional mild GI side effects, increased clearance of metronidazole.
	Cooking herbs: anise, basil, blackseed, caraway, coriander, dill, fennel seeds, moringa leaf Nonfood herbs: alfalfa, blessed thistle, nettle, goat's rue, red clover, shatavari	Historical and cultural uses as galactogogues; effectiveness undocumented. Assumed to be safe with recommended dosages (varies with specific herbs), although strengths of herbal product ingredients may vary depending on particular plant used and how processed; caution is advised for use during pregnancy. Some companies make special blends for breastfeeding mothers.
Foods/beverages	Grains, nuts, seeds: oats (not instant), barley, brown rice, beans, sesame, almonds Fruits/Vegetables: dark green leafy vegetables, apricots, dates, figs, cooked green papaya Soups made from Torbangun or Malunggay leaves	Historical and cultural uses as galactogogues; effectiveness undocumented.

Adapted from Marasco L: Inside track: increasing your milk supply with galactogogues, *J Hum Lact* 24:455, 2008; Hale TW: *Medications and mother's milk*, ed 18, Amarillo, Tex, 2019, Hale Publishing; Academy of Breastfeeding Medicine Protocol Committee (ABM): ABM Clinical Protocol #9: Use of Galactogogues in initiating or augmenting the rate of maternal milk secretion, *Breastfeeding Med* 13:307, 2018.

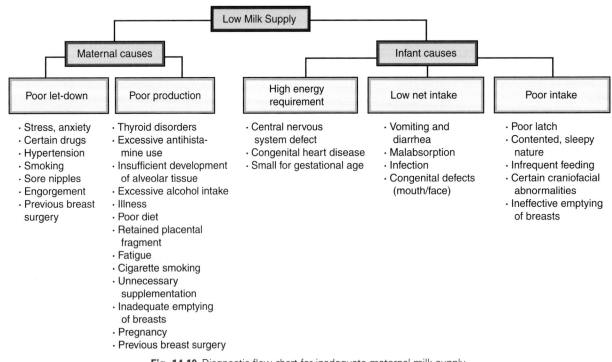

Fig. 14.10 Diagnostic flow chart for inadequate maternal milk supply.

including cow's milk protein (casein fraction), cruciferous vegetables, carbonated drinks, or even spicy foods. When suspicious foods are removed from the mother's diet, it is important to assess the nutritional quality of her diet and supplement appropriately.

Concerns During Lactation

Transfer of Drugs and Toxins into Human Milk

Almost all drugs taken by the mother appear in her milk to some degree. The amount that usually transfers is small, and only rarely does the amount transferred into the mother's milk result in clinically relevant doses in the infant. Many factors influence how medications transfer into human milk: milk/plasma ratio, molecular weight of the drug, and the protein binding and lipid solubility of the drug. Once a drug has been ingested by the infant through the mother's milk, it must travel through the baby's GI tract before absorption. There are many processes here that may disallow the drug from being metabolized in the infant's system. Caution is recommended especially for mothers who are nursing premature or ill infants as they are at a higher risk of the effects of even small amounts of medications that may come through maternal milk (Hale, 2019).

Many mothers have discontinued breastfeeding because of their need for a medication, when in fact there was a good chance that the drug could have been taken without risk to the baby. It is likely that medications penetrate colostrum more than mature milk, although even during this time, the amounts the baby is exposed to are very low. When the medication increases in the mother's plasma, it also increases in her milk. When the medication level falls in the mother's plasma, equilibrium is sought in the mother's milk, which drives the medication back into her plasma for elimination (Hale, 2019).

Centrally active drugs (anticonvulsants, antidepressants, antipsychotics) frequently penetrate milk in elevated levels based merely on their physiochemistry. When sedation, depression, or other central nervous system (CNS) effects are experienced by the mother when taking the medication, it is likely to penetrate the milk and cause similar effects in the infant. These drugs must be used with caution, and the mother should always discuss the risk-benefits of breastfeeding and her need for such medications with her health care provider.

Maternal Substance Abuse. According to the AAP, maternal substance abuse is not a categorical contraindication to breastfeeding. If a mother is well nourished and negative for HIV, even if narcotic-dependent, she should be encouraged to breastfeed as long as she is supervised in a methadone maintenance program (AAP, 2012; Academy of Breastfeeding Medicine Protocol Committee [ABM], 2015). Breastfeeding still provides many immunologic, nutritional, and bonding advantages over artificial feeding. Very little methadone is transferred into breastmilk; however, studies are mixed reporting how breastfeeding should be managed in the mother-infant dyad to lessen the risk for neonatal abstinence syndrome (Isemann et al, 2011). Growth parameters in the child should be monitored to ensure adequate development, but breastfeeding should continue to be encouraged as long as these measures are within the normal range. The long-term effect of methadone exposure beyond the neonatal period is relatively unknown. Studies have shown samples of blood and breastmilk up to 1 year show low concentrations of methadone, justifying the recommendation that mothers continue to breastfeed (Hudak et al, 2012). If a mother decides to discontinue breastfeeding, weaning slowly over 3 to 4 weeks helps to protect the infant from withdrawal symptoms.

The AAP and ACOG have provided information regarding the transfer of drugs and other chemicals into human milk (AAP, 2013). Websites that can provide more information are listed at the end of the chapter.

Environmental Toxins. There is concern about environmental toxins entering the milk of a lactating mother; however, at this time there are no established "safe" levels to aid in clinical interpretation. Despite any pollutants that may be found in human milk, the benefits of breastfeeding far outweigh the risks posed by any contaminants that may be found there. Nonetheless, mothers should take care not to allow any unnecessary exposure to pesticides and other harsh chemicals, as well as limit intake of animal fat, which can contain higher amounts of environmental contaminants. This helps safeguard against unwanted substances in human milk.

In the past, mothers were told not to lose too much weight too fast after pregnancy because it was thought that a rapid weight loss could possibly accelerate the release of toxins stored in a woman's body fat. However, this has not been proven to be true. Nonetheless, slow, steady weight loss during the postpartum period is recommended to allow a healthy return to prepregnancy weight with greater likelihood of keeping the weight off.

Overweight or Obesity

Overweight or obese lactating women can restrict their energy intake (once the milk supply is well-established) by 500 kcal per day by decreasing consumption of foods high in fat and simple sugars, but they must increase their intake of foods high in calcium, vitamin D, vitamin A, vitamin C, and omega-3 fats to provide key nutrients for their milk supply. The lactational period can be used as a time to allow natural slow weight loss in these mothers by taking advantage of the caloric demands of breastfeeding. The nutritional status of lactating women who have previously undergone bariatric surgery requires close attention because suboptimal levels of iron, vitamin A, vitamin D, vitamin K, folate, and calcium have been reported (see Chapter 20).

Women with higher prepregnant BMI values also warrant extra lactation support to prevent early weaning and to reach their breastfeeding goals. Research has shown that although intentions of the obese woman to breastfeed may be strong, there can be many psychosocial determinants that may influence her commitment and ability to initiate or continue nursing her infant. Obese women also have shown to have delayed lactogenesis II, the sudden increase in volume a few days after delivery, which could be a risk factor in not establishing a milk supply. Although obese women experience lower rates of successful breastfeeding, the association between maternal obesity and breastfeeding outcomes has not been explained fully (Hauff et al, 2014).

Exercise and Breastfeeding

The breastfeeding mother should be encouraged to resume an exercise routine a few weeks after delivery and after lactation is well established. Aerobic exercise at 60% to 70% of maximum heart rate has no adverse effect on lactation; infants gain weight at the same rate, and the mother's cardiovascular fitness improves (Lovelady, 2011). Exercise also improves plasma lipids and insulin response in lactating women.

Mothers may be reluctant to exercise because of concerns of how this affects their breastmilk and consequently the growth of their infants. Moderate aerobic exercise (45 minutes/day, 5 days/week) has not been shown to affect milk volume or its composition. Mothers who incorporate diet and exercise into their routines in an effort to lose weight during the postpartum period also have been studied and have shown no ill effects on the growth of their infants (Lovelady, 2011).

Breast Augmentation

Breast augmentation, a procedure in which an implant is inserted into the breast to enlarge it, is a common elective breast procedure. Periareolar and transareolar incisions can cause lactation insufficiency. These mothers should be encouraged to breastfeed, and their infants monitored for appropriate weight gain. Other means of augmentation, in which implants are placed between breast tissue and the chest wall, usually have no effect on the woman's ability to produce a full milk supply.

Reduction Mammoplasty

Reduction mammoplasty often is recommended for women with extremely large breasts who suffer from back, shoulder, or neck pain or poor body image. In lactating women who have had this surgery there are wide variations in milk production, from little to full production, depending on the amount of tissue removed and the type of surgical incision. These mothers also should be encouraged to breastfeed and be given anticipatory guidance and support; their infants should be monitored closely for appropriate weight gain.

Postpartum Depression

Postpartum depression (PPD) may be one of the most underdiagnosed obstetric complications in the United States. PPD leads to numerous negative consequences affecting the mother and child, including increased costs of medical care, inappropriate medical care, child abuse and neglect, discontinuation of breastfeeding, and family dysfunction. All this adversely affects early brain development in the infant (Earls, 2010), which could possibly lead to future problems.

Although effective treatment is available, fewer than half of mothers with this condition are recognized or seek help. PPD has been found to be lower in breastfeeding mothers (Xu et al, 2014). Because breastfeeding triggers the release of the hormone oxytocin, many women report feeling calm and relaxed while they are nursing. When breastfeeding is successful and things are going well, with maintenance of a good milk supply without complications, and the baby is gaining appropriate weight, the breastfeeding relationship can ward off feelings of loneliness, emptiness, or failure—common feelings in PPD. A higher circulating oxytocin level sustains a sense of calm and allows a mother to cope with the everyday stresses of new motherhood. Conversely, when things are not going well, when complications of breastfeeding and new motherhood become overwhelming, many new mothers experience signs of the "blues," which can escalate into full PPD. The "baby blues," affecting 70% to 80% of all new mothers (APO, 2015), is short lived, does not impair functioning, and can be treated with reassurance and emotional support. PPD, however, is characterized by a major depressive episode within 1 month after delivery and is experienced in 10% to 15% of women after giving birth. Symptoms are restlessness, anxiety, fatigue, and a sense of worthlessness. Some new mothers worry they will hurt themselves or their babies. Unlike the "baby blues," PPD does not go away quickly. A mother with diagnosed PPD usually requires a more intensive approach to treatment (USDHHS, 2018b).

Diet quality and overall nutritional status may affect the risk of PPD (Procter and Campbell, 2014). Many dietary components are being investigated regarding their role in minimizing PPD, including omega-3 fatty acids, folate, vitamins B_2, B_6, B_{12}, D, calcium, iron, and selenium. However, there is little evidence of benefit from supplementation. Mawson and Wang recently proposed that high levels of vitamin A compounds may be in part responsible for maternal PPD, and that breastfeeding offers protection against PPD by maintaining endogenous retinoids below a threshold concentration. Women accumulate retinoids in the liver and the breast during pregnancy in preparation of providing vitamin A to their infants. Because prolonged lactation reduces maternal stores of retinoids, this also provides a natural means of reducing potentially toxic concentrations in the mother (Mawson and Wang, 2013).

When early signs of PPD are present, and a mother stops breastfeeding, even more severe depression can affect the mother. Oxytocin

levels fall abruptly, and a mother's feelings of failure may become even more pronounced. It is critical for families to be aware and for health care providers to screen for early symptoms of PPD not only to prevent more serious symptoms of the disease but also to protect and preserve the breastfeeding relationship. Maternal-child health care providers must prepare mothers and families for expected breastfeeding challenges, advocate for a supportive environment in birthing hospitals, and promote breastfeeding as the cultural norm in the community so that the breastfeeding relationship is successfully established early in the postpartum period (Olson et al, 2014).

PPD can affect milk production, let-down, and the ability to maintain an adequate milk supply for the baby. The elevated levels of cortisol present in PPD may delay lactogenesis II. When the blues turns into a more serious form of PPD, the establishment of a healthy bond between mother and child may be affected, jeopardizing the breastfeeding relationship and potentially leading to early weaning (Wu et al, 2012b).

Medical treatment for PPD while breastfeeding includes medications such as Zoloft, Paxil, and Prozac. These should be taken immediately after a feeding to allow the maximum time for drug clearance from milk before the next feeding. Also, the mother can express and discard her milk collected when peak serum levels of the drug are present. Monoamine oxidase (MAO) inhibitors are contraindicated for treatment of PPD if the mother is breastfeeding (Hale, 2019).

Birth Control and Breastfeeding

Many women begin to think about birth control shortly after delivery and while they are breastfeeding a new baby. The mother must consider the effects of the birth control method on her nursling, as well as how it may affect her milk supply.

The Lactation Amenorrhea Method (LAM) does not involve any device or medication and is completely safe for breastfeeding mothers. LAM is an important modern contraceptive method that, when practiced correctly, has a 98% effectiveness rate 6 months postpartum (Fabic and Choi, 2013). It must be emphasized that the method is effective ONLY when three conditions are met: (1) the infant is less than 6 months old, (2) the mother is amenorrheic, and (3) the mother is fully breastfeeding (baby not receiving anything other than milk at the breast, meeting all sucking needs at the breast without a pacifier). Mothers must be very attentive to the inclusion of all these factors if they are dependent on this method to prevent pregnancy. As soon as one of these parameters is absent, the mother is advised that she should employ an additional form of birth control if pregnancy is still not desirable.

Birth control methods using a combination of progestin and estrogen come in several different forms: combination birth control pill, monthly injections, patch, and the vaginal ring. Although progestin and estrogen are approved by the AAP for use in breastfeeding mothers, it is possible that estrogen-containing contraceptives may affect a mother's milk supply and therefore a progestin-only medication (minipill) may be a better choice, at least until 6 months postpartum. A longer lasting form of progestin-only birth control is the Depo-Provera ("depo") shot that lasts at least 12 weeks but may be effective even up to a year.

A progestin-only intrauterine device (IUD) such as Mirena may have fewer side effects on a mother's milk supply. This product delivers hormones directly to the lining of the uterus, leading to only a slight increase in serum progesterone levels, less than with the minipill. The birth control implant (Norplant, Implanon) is another choice for women who wish to choose progestin-only means of birth control. The implant can last up to 5 years. Women are warned they may want to consider the pill form before using a longer-lasting form of birth control in case they are susceptible to a drop in milk supply even with progestin-only pills. This allows them to stop the pills and choose another birth control method (i.e., LAM or barrier) so that they do not have to wait for the effects of the progestin to wear off. No effect on infant growth has been noted with these medications, but for those who may be concerned about the unknown, barrier methods of birth control, an IUD without hormones (ParaGard), or LAM, ensure that no drug is secreted in breastmilk.

One other form of birth control pill, meant to be used as a last resort (breastfeeding or not), is the so-called "morning-after pill." These are also available in a combination of estrogen and progestin (Preven, Ovral), or the progestin-only form (Plan B, Plan B One-Step). Mothers should consult with their health care providers or lactation consultants if a drop in milk supply is noticed. This may be just a short-lived, temporary condition, but close follow-up can ensure that this is the case. The AAP has approved this medication for use during breastfeeding, although it should be used only in rare circumstances.

Breastfeeding during Pregnancy

Mothers may discover they are pregnant while they are still nursing a young baby or child. If the pregnancy is normal and healthy, it is considered safe to continue to breastfeed throughout the pregnancy. A mother need not worry that her milk will be any less nutritious for her nursling. She may be concerned that the act of breastfeeding will interfere with her pregnancy, but that is not a valid concern unless she experiences a difficult pregnancy and is at risk for early labor.

Increased fatigue and nausea early in pregnancy may be challenging for the expectant mother; however, if breastfeeding continues, rest and a concerted effort to maintain good nutritional intake is a must. Sore nipples are also common early in pregnancy and may be the first sign to the mother that she is pregnant. She may need to employ methods of dealing with nipple tenderness (i.e., distraction, pain management techniques) to get through this period of time if breastfeeding is to continue. Because the quantity of the milk may decrease and the taste of the milk may change early during pregnancy, the nursling may reject breastfeeding altogether and self-wean. A mother may need to provide encouragement to the baby to continue to breastfeed, especially if the baby is very young and still dependent on breast milk to fulfill the majority of nutritional needs.

Tandem Nursing

Tandem nursing is when the mother breastfeeds siblings who are not twins. As soon as the placenta is delivered, the mother will begin to produce colostrum once again. The mother should ensure that the new baby always has priority to this because it provides the protection the newborn needs. Sometimes mothers find that the nursing toddler is a help to her by preventing or relieving engorgement. In fact, with the stronger suck and intake of the toddler, the mother may begin to overproduce for the newborn. If she develops a strong let-down reflex releasing a large quantity of milk when the newborn first latches, it may cause coughing and choking. In this case the mother may want to express a small amount of milk before latching her newborn, or simply allow the toddler to nurse for a few minutes first.

Concerns of hygiene are unwarranted when a mother is nursing two siblings. The small bumps on the areola called Montgomery glands produce a natural oil that cleans, lubricates, and protects the nipple during pregnancy and breastfeeding. This oil contains an enzyme that kills bacteria so that both children are protected. In addition, more immunities will be passed on through the breastmilk itself. If, however, the mother or one child develops thrush, she is advised to limit each child to one breast temporarily.

An older baby who has weaned prior to the birth of a new sibling may express interest in breastfeeding again. Handling this situation is a delicate one and calls for special attention to the older child, whether or not the mother decides to offer the breast again.

Weaning

Weaning begins at the first introduction of anything other than mother's milk. As a breastmilk substitute or solid foods begin to be offered to the baby, the weaning process has begun. Although breastfed babies tend to accept a variety of solid foods well, because of the fact that they already have been introduced to different flavors of food through their mother's milk, this does not mean that the infant is ready to stop breastfeeding. Breastmilk is recommended for the infant throughout at least the first year of life as stated previously, and even through the second year of life by some authorities (WHO, 2018b). A mother may choose to allow baby-led weaning, which simply means she will offer breastfeeding for as long as the baby is interested. If a baby seems to be losing interest in breastfeeding while still very young (i.e., younger than 12 months), the mother can try various methods of encouraging the baby to continue to breastfeed, such as ensuring a good position at the breast, and cutting out any bottles or foods so that more nutrition will be offered through breastfeeding. An older baby may be distracted easily during nursing sessions; a quiet, darkened room may help to keep the baby focused on nursing and get back on track with breastfeeding regularly. Human milk remains a nutritious fluid for as long as it is produced by the mother; however, the breastfeeding relationship changes as the baby gets older. Babies may show a lack of desire to breastfeed at different ages, depending on many factors. As the child grows, breastfeeding becomes less of a nutritional need but more of a need for the psychological bond with their mother. Older infants may be happy to nurse three to four times a day, and toddlers may show interest only every now and then.

Some mothers may choose mother-led weaning, which is when the mother encourages the baby to stop breastfeeding. She may begin to offer other foods or beverages when the baby wants to nurse or try to distract the baby in other ways. If this method is used, the mother should ensure that the baby's emotional needs are met because this could be a trying time for mother and child. The decision is up to the mother, and her decision should be supported, although if at all possible, she should be encouraged to provide her milk throughout the first year for her health and the health of her baby.

Return to Work or School

A mother's return to work or school can be a major challenge for continued successful breastfeeding; however, it is possible and encouraged. If a nursing mother returns to work or school, it is best to wait until breastfeeding is going well and a good milk supply has been established. Babies placed in child care experience a higher chance of becoming ill when exposed to other children; however, breastmilk offers protection against germs the child is likely to be exposed to in these environments.

An exclusive diet of human milk continues to provide optimal nutrition through the baby's first 6 months. After that time, when appropriate solid foods are introduced into the baby's diet, mother's milk is the milk of choice at least through the baby's first year and beyond. The mother also experiences rewards if she is able to continue to breastfeed after her return to work or school. This helps to maintain an emotional connection with her baby because she will be reminded physically throughout the day of the need to express milk from her breasts. She also can continue to preserve the breastfeeding relationship with her baby when at home. Because of the advance in quality of breast pumps on the market today, mothers are able to express milk and maintain their supply effectively and comfortably. See Table 14.18 for breastmilk home storage guidelines.

TABLE 14.18 Home Storage of Human Milk

Type of Breastmilk	Locations and Temperatures		
	Countertop – Room Temperature (≤ 77° F or 25° C)	Refrigerator (40° F or 4° C)	Freezer (≤ 0° F or −18° C)
Freshly Expressed or Pumped	Up to 4 hours	Up to 4 days	Within 6 months is best, up to 12 months is acceptable
Thawed, Previously Frozen	1–2 hours	Up to 1 day (24 hours)	Never refreeze human milk
Leftover from a Feeding (*baby did not finish the bottle*)	Use within 2 hours after baby's last feeding or discard		

Adapted from CDC: *Proper Storage and Preparation of Breast Milk* (website): https://www.cdc.gov/breastfeeding/recommendations/handling_breastmilk. htm, 2018.

Many mothers are able to obtain breast pumps using their health insurance or through the WIC program. Federal and state laws also offer protection for the lactating worker so that she is ensured a private, clean space (other than a restroom) to express her milk while away from her baby. Mothers should talk to school personnel or their work supervisor before their maternity leave so that a plan is in place upon her return, and so that all parties involved will have an understanding of what to expect. Mothers should be made aware of federal and state provisions available to them based on employment category. A woman who expresses her milk regularly throughout the day with an effective pump can maintain a full milk supply for as long as she desires while at work or school full time. A mother facing this situation can find more help with this by discussing any questions or challenges with a lactation professional.

CLINICAL CASE STUDY 1

Carol is a 34-year-old woman who was pregnant recently for the first time, but the baby had anencephaly and died at birth. She has a sister who has spina bifida and an older brother who had a stroke when he was 14. Carol has now been tested and found to have a genetic defect known as a 677C>T polymorphism in the methylenetetrahydrofolate reductase (MTHFR) gene.

Of course, she and her husband were devastated with the loss of their first child, but they also very much want to be parents. She has gone to genetic counseling but is also coming to you to find out what she can do to lower the chances that this happens again. She is worried about using the traditional prenatal vitamin-mineral supplement because she has been cautioned that she is unable to metabolize folic acid from diet and supplements.

Nutrition Diagnostic Statement
- Altered nutrient (folic acid) metabolism related to a genetic alteration as evidenced by positive results for C>T in the MTHFR gene and family history of spina bifida and stroke.

Nutrition Care Questions
1. What advice would you give Carol about any special dietary changes?
2. Carol knows that there is a special prenatal vitamin-mineral supplement available but does not know how to obtain it. How will you help Carol find this supplement?
3. What are the risks for a successful pregnancy outcome if Carol cannot find this special prenatal supplement?
4. What other concerns do you have regarding her pregnancy?

CLINICAL CASE STUDY 2

Cecilia is 3 months postpartum after a normal labor and full-term delivery. She tells you that she is exclusively breastfeeding her baby about eight times a day but is very tired and is not getting much sleep because her baby always seems fussy between feedings—day and night. She has been determined to lose her "baby weight" and for the past 6 weeks, she has been restricting her caloric intake to around 1200 calories/day, including approximately six diet drinks every day. She reports that the pediatrician told her that the baby's weight gain has slowed over the past month and she would like her to begin supplementing the baby with formula. She is hesitant to do this because her goal is to continue breastfeeding exclusively until the baby is 6 months old, and then possibly continue until at least the baby's first birthday.

Nutrition Diagnostic Statement
- Difficulty breastfeeding related to poor maternal dietary intake as evidenced by mother's report of inappropriate diet and baby's poor weight gain

Nutrition Care Questions
1. What would you tell Cecilia regarding her concern about losing her "baby weight"?
2. What would you tell her to do to improve her dietary intake?
3. How would you address her baby's fussiness and inadequate weight gain?
4. What advice would you give her to preserve her breastfeeding and achieve her breastfeeding goals?

USEFUL WEBSITES

Academy of Breastfeeding Medicine
American Academy of Pediatrics
American College of Obstetrics and Gynecologists-Breastfeeding Page
Black Mothers' Breastfeeding Association
Carolina Global Breastfeeding Institute
Centers for Disease Control and Prevention
Food Safety for Pregnant Women
Infant Risk Center-Texas Tech University Health Sciences Center
International Board of Lactation Consultant Examiners
International Lactation Consultant Association
La Leche League
Lactation Education Resources
LactMed—a Toxnet Database
National Association of Professional and Peer Lactation Supporters of Color (NAPPLSC)
National Maternal and Child Oral Health Resource Center
Natural Medicines Comprehensive Database
Office on Women's Health: Breastfeeding
Reaching Our Sisters Everywhere
United States Breastfeeding Committee
United States Department of Agriculture; MyPlate Plan for Moms
United States Fish Consumption Advisories
United States Lactation Consultant Association
Women's Health Dietetic Practice Group
World Alliance for Breastfeeding Action (WABA)

REFERENCES

Abramowitz A, Miller ES, Wisner KL: Treatment options for hyperemesis gravidarum, *Arch Womens Ment Health* 20:363–372, 2017.

Academy of Breastfeeding Medicine Protocol Committee (ABM), Reece-Stremtan S, Marinelli KA: ABM clinical protocol #21: guidelines for breastfeeding and drug-dependent woman, *Breastfeed Med* 10(3):135–141, 2015.

Adams Waldorf KM, McAdams RM: Influence of infection during pregnancy on fetal development, *Reproduction* 146:R151–R162, 2013.

Agarwal MM: Gestational diabetes mellitus: an update on the current international diagnostic criteria, *World J Diabetes* 6:782–792, 2015.

Ahrens KA, Hutcheon JA, Ananth CV, et al: Report of the Office of Population Affairs' expert work group meeting on short birth spacing and adverse pregnancy outcomes: methodological quality of existing studies and future directions for research, *Paediatr Perinat Epidemiol* 33(1):O5–O14, 2018. doi:10.1111/ppe.12504.

American Academy of Pediatrics, Section on Breastfeeding: Breastfeeding and the use of human milk, *Pediatrics* 129:e827–e841, 2012.

American Academy of Pediatrics, American College of Obstetricians and Gynecologists: *Breastfeeding handbook for physicians*, ed 2, Elk Grove Village, IL, 2013, American Academy of Pediatrics.

American College of Obstetricians and Gynecologists: ACOG committee opinion No. 495: Vitamin D: screening and supplementation during pregnancy, *Obstet Gynecol* 118:197–198, 2011.

American College of Obstetricians and Gynecologists: ACOG Committee Opinion No. 650: physical activity and exercise during pregnancy and the postpartum period, *Obstet Gynecol* 126:e135–e142, 2015a.

American College of Obstetricians and Gynecologists: ACOG Practice Bulletin No. 148: Thyroid disease in pregnancy, *Obstet Gynecol* 125:996–1005, 2015b.

American College of Obstetricians and Gynecologists: ACOG Practice bulletin no. 151: Cytomegalovirus, parvovirus B19, varicella zoster, and toxoplasmosis in pregnancy, *Obstet Gynecol* 125:1510–1525, 2015c.

American College of Obstetricians and Gynecologists: ACOG Practice bulletin No. 156: Obesity in Pregnancy, *Obstet Gynecol* 126:e112, 2015d.

American College of Obstetricians and Gynecologists: ACOG Practice Bulletin No. 202: Gestational Hypertension and Preeclampsia, *Obstet Gynecol* 133:e1–e25, 2019.

American College of Obstetricians and Gynecologists Committee on Health Care for Underserved Women: Committee opinion no. 591: challenges for overweight and obese women, *Obstet Gynecol* 123:726–730, 2014.

American College of Obstetricians and Gynecologists' Committee on Obstetric Practice, Committee on Genetics; U.S. Food and Drug Administration: Committee Opinion No 671: perinatal risks associated with assisted reproductive technology, *Obstet Gynecol* 128:e61–e68, 2016a.

American College of Obstetricians and Gynecologists Committee on Obstetric Practice: Committee Opinion No. 722: Marijuana Use During Pregnancy and Lactation, *Obstet Gynecol* 130:e205–e209, 2017a.

American College of Obstetricians and Gynecologists Committee on Practice Bulletins—Gynecology: Practice Bulletin no. 150. Early pregnancy loss, *Obstet Gynecol* 125:1258–1267, 2015e.

American College of Obstetricians and Gynecologists, Committee on Practice Bulletins-Gynecology: Practice Bulletin No. 194: Polycystic Ovary Syndrome, *Obstet Gynecol* 131:e157–e171, 2018a.

American College of Obstetricians and Gynecologists Committee on Practice Bulletins—Obstetrics: Practice bulletin no. 130: prediction and prevention of preterm birth, *Obstet Gynecol* 120:964–973, 2012.

American College of Obstetricians and Gynecologists Committee on Practice Bulletins-Obstetrics: Practice Bulletin No. 187: Neural Tube Defects, *Obstet Gynecol* 130:e279–e290, 2017b.

American College of Obstetricians and Gynecologists, Committee on Practice Bulletins-Obstetrics: Practice Bulletin No. 189: nausea and vomiting of pregnancy, *Obstet Gynecol* 131:e15–e30, 2018b.

American College of Obstetricians and Gynecologists, Committee on Practice Bulletins—Obstetrics: Practice Bulletin No. 190: Gestational Diabetes Mellitus, *Obstet Gynecol* 131:e49–e64, 2018c.

American College of Obstetricians and Gynecologists. Committee on Practice Bulletins—Obstetrics; Society for Maternal–Fetal Medicine: Practice Bulletin No. 169: Multifetal Gestations: Twin, Triplet, and Higher-Order Multifetal Pregnancies, *Obstet Gynecol* 128:e131–e146, 2016b.

American College of Obstetricians and Gynecologists Women's Health Care Physicians, Committee on Health Care for Underserved Woman: ACOG committee opinion No. 569: Oral health care during pregnancy and through the lifespan, *Obstet Gynecol* 122:417–422, 2013a.

American College of Obstetricians and Gynecologists: *Exposure to toxic environmental agents*, Companion Document, 2013b. Available at: https://www.acog.org/-/media/Committee-Opinions/Committee-on-Health-Care-for-Underserved-Women/ExposuretoToxic.pdf.

American College of Obstetricians and Gynecologists: *FAQ 196: Marijuana and pregnancy*, 2018d. Available at: https://www.acog.org/Patients/FAQs/Marijuana-and-Pregnancy.

American College of Obstetricians and Gynecologists: *Hypertension in Pregnancy, November 2013*, 2013c. Available at: http://www.ilpqc.org/docs/htn/ACOGExecSummary/HypertensioninPregnancy.pdf.

American Diabetes Association: Standards of Medical Care in Diabetes-2018, *Diabetes Care* 42:s1, 2019.

American Pregnancy Organization: *Baby blues*, 2015. Available at: http://americanpregnancy.org/first-year-of-life/baby-blues/.

Amorim Adegboye AR, Linne YM: Diet or exercise, or both, for weight reduction in women after childbirth, *Cochrane Database Syst Rev* (7):CD005627, 2013.

Auerbach M: Commentary: Iron deficiency of pregnancy - a new approach involving intravenous iron, *Reprod Health* 15(Suppl 1):96, 2018.

Auerbach M, Adamson JW: How we diagnose and treat iron deficiency anemia, *Am J Hematol* 91:31–38, 2016.

Avilés M, Gutiérrez-Adán A, Coy P: Oviductal secretions: will they be key factors for the future ARTs? *Mol Hum Reprod* 16:896–906, 2010.

Barouki R, Gluckman PD, Grandjean P, et al: Developmental origins of non-communicable disease: implications for research and public health, *Environ Health* 11:42, 2012.

Barrett JR: Low prenatal exposures to fluoride: are there neurotoxic risks for children? *Environ Health Perspect* 125:104002, 2017.

Batz MB, Hoffman S, Morris JG: *Ranking the risks: the 10 pathogen-food combinations with the greatest burden on public health*, 2011. Available at: Available at: https://folio.iupui.edu/bitstream/handle/10244/1022/72267 report.pdf.

Belkacemi L, Nelson DM, Desai M, et al: Maternal undernutrition influences placental-fetal development, *Biol Reprod* 83:325–331, 2010.

Bellver J, Rodríguez-Tabernero L, Robles A, et al: Polycystic ovary syndrome throughout a woman's life, *J Assist Reprod Genet* 35:25–39, 2018.

Berti C, Agostoni C, Davanzo R, et al: Early-life nutritional exposures and life-long health: immediate and long-lasting impacts of probiotics, vitamin D, and breastfeeding, *Nutr Rev* 75:83–97, 2017.

Berti C, Biesalski HK, Gärtner R, et al: Micronutrients in pregnancy: current knowledge and unresolved questions, *Clin Nutr* 30:689–701, 2011.

Bilbo SD, Block CL, Bolton JL, et al: Beyond infection - Maternal immune activation by environmental factors, microglial development, and relevance for autism spectrum disorders, *Exp Neurol* 299(Pt A):241–251, 2018.

Binns CW, Lee MK, Lee AH: Problems and prospects: public health regulation of dietary supplements, *Annu Rev Public Health* 39:403–420, 2018.

Bjørke-Monsen AL, Ulvik A, Nilsen RM, et al: Impact of pre-pregnancy BMI on B vitamin and inflammatory status in early pregnancy: an observational cohort study, *Nutrients* 8(12): E776, 2016.

Blaize AN, Pearson KJ, Newcomer SC: Impact of maternal exercise during pregnancy on offspring chronic disease susceptibility, *Exerc Sport Sci Rev* 43:198–203, 2015.

Block T, El-Osta A: Epigenetic programming, early life nutrition and the risk of metabolic disease, *Atherosclerosis* 266:31–40, 2017.

Blondin JH, LoGiudice JA: Pregnant women's knowledge and awareness of nutrition, *Appl Nurs Res* 39:167–174, 2018.

Bloomfield FH: How is maternal nutrition related to preterm birth? *Annu Rev Nutr* 31:235–261, 2011.

Blumfield ML, Collins CE: High-protein diets during pregnancy: healthful or harmful for offspring? *Am J Clin Nutr* 100:993–995, 2014.

Blusztajn JK, Slack BE, Mellott TJ: Neuroprotective actions of dietary choline, *Nutrients* 9(8):E815, 2017. doi:10.3390/nu9080815.

Bø K, Artal R, Barakat R, et al: Exercise and pregnancy in recreational and elite athletes: 2016/2017 evidence summary from the IOC expert group meeting, Lausanne. Part 5. Recommendations for health professionals and active women, *Br J Sports Med* 52:1080–1085, 2018.

Bodnar LM, Cogswell ME, Scanlon KS: Low income postpartum women are at risk of iron deficiency, *J Nutr* 132:2298–1302, 2002.

Bonis C, Lorenzini F, Bertrand M, et al: Glucose profiles in pregnant women after a gastric bypass: findings from continuous glucose monitoring, *Obes Surg* 26:2150–2155, 2016.

Booth A, Camacho P: A closer look at calcium absorption and the benefits and risks of dietary versus supplemental calcium, *Postgrad Med* 125:73–81, 2013.

Bouga M, Lean MEJ, Combet E: Contemporary challenges to iodine status and nutrition: the role of foods, dietary recommendations, fortification and supplementation, *Proc Nutr Soc* 77:302–313, 2018.

Brannon PM, Picciano MF: Vitamin D in pregnancy and lactation in humans, *Annu Rev Nutr* 31:89–115, 2011.

Brannon PM, Stover PJ, Taylor CL: Integrating themes, evidence gaps, and research needs identified by workshop on iron screening and supplementation in iron-replete pregnant women and young children, *Am J Clin Nutr* 106:1703S–1712S, 2017.

Brannon PM, Taylor CL: Iron Supplementation during pregnancy and infancy: uncertainties and Implications for Research and policy, *Nutrients* 9(12): E1327, 2017. doi:10.3390/nu9121327.

Brett KE, Ferraro ZM, Yockell-Lelievre J, et al: Maternal-fetal nutrient transport in pregnancy pathologies: the role of the placenta, *Int J Mol Sci* 15:16153–16185, 2014.

Brodribb W: ABM Clinical Protocol #9: use of galactogogues in initiating or augmenting maternal milk production, second revision 2018, *Breastfeed Med* 13:307, 2018.

Broughton DE, Moley KH: Obesity and female infertility: potential mediators of obesity's impact, *Fertil Steril* 107:840–847, 2017.

Brown J, Crawford TJ, Alsweiler J, et al: Dietary supplementation with myo-inositol in women during pregnancy for treating gestational diabetes, *Cochrane Database Syst Rev* 9:CD012048, 2016.

Brown J, Nunez S, Russell M, et al: Hypocalcemic rickets and dilated cardio-myopathy: case reports and review of literature, *Pediatr Cardiol* 30: 818–823, 2009.

Burdge GC, Tan SY, Henry CJ: Long-chain *n*-3 PUFA in vegetarian women: a metabolic perspective, *J Nutr Sci* 6:e58, 2017.

Burger J, Gochfeld M: Selenium and mercury molar ratios in commercial fish from New Jersey and Illinois: variation within species and relevance to risk communication, *Food Chem Toxicol* 57:235–245, 2013.

Burton GJ: The John Hughes Memorial Lecture: stimulation of early placental development through a troph-blast-endometrial dialog, *J Equine Vet Sci* 66:14–18, 2018.

Burton GJ, Fowden AL, Thornburg KL: Placental origins of chronic disease, *Physiol Rev* 96:1509–1565, 2016.

Bustos M, Venkataramanan R, Caritis S: Nausea and vomiting of pregnancy - What's new? *Auton Neurosci* 202:62–72, 2017.

Cannarella R, Condorelli RA, Mongioṽ̈ LM, et al: Does a male polycystic ovarian syndrome equivalent exist? *J Endocrinol Invest* 41:49–57, 2018.

Cantor AG, Bougatsos C, Dana T, et al: Routine iron supplementation and screening for iron deficiency anemia in pregnancy: a systematic review for the U.S. Preventive Services Task Force, *Ann Intern Med* 162:566–576, 2015.

Cao C, Fleming MD: The placenta: the forgotten essential organ of iron transport, *Nutr Rev* 74:421–431, 2016.

Cao C, O'Brien KO: Pregnancy and iron homeostasis: an update, *Nutr Rev* 71:35–51, 2013.

Cao-Lei L, de Rooij SR, King S, et al: Prenatal stress and epigenetics, *Neurosci Biobehav* Rev, S0149-7634(16)30726-6, 2017. doi:10.1016/j.neubiorev.2017.05.016.

Cardwell MS: Eating disorders during pregnancy, *Obstet Gynecol Surv* 68: 312–323, 2013.

Carlson SE, Gajewski BJ Valentine CJ, et al: Assessment of DHA on reducing early preterm birth: the ADORE randomized controlled trial protocol, *BMC Pregnancy Childbirth* 17:62, 2017.

Caserta D, Graziano A, Lo Monte G, et al: Heavy metals and placental fetal-maternal barrier: a mini-review on the major concerns, *Eur Rev Med Pharmacol Sci* 17:2198–2206, 2013.

Castillo-Castrejon M, Powell TL: Placental nutrient transport in gestational diabetic pregnancies, *Front Endocrinol (Lausanne)* 8:306, 2017.

Catalano PM, Shankar K: Obesity and pregnancy: mechanisms of short term and long term adverse consequences for mother and child, *BMJ* 356:j1, 2017. doi:10.1136/bmj.j1.

Caudill MA: Folate bioavailability: implications for establishing dietary recommendations and optimizing status, *Am J Clin Nutr* 91:1455S–1460S, 2010.

Caudill MA, Strupp BJ, Muscalu L, et al: Maternal choline supplementation during the third trimester of pregnancy improves infant information processing speed: a randomized, double-blind, controlled feeding study, *FASEB J* 32:2172–2180, 2018.

Center for Nutrition Policy and Promotion: *Nutrients in healthy US-Style food pattern: nutrients in the pattern at each calorie level and comparison of nutrient content to the nutritional goals for that Pattern,* 2018. Available at: https://www.cnpp.usda.gov/sites/default/files/usda_food_patterns/NutrientsInHealthyUS-StyleFoodPattern.pdf.

Centers for Disease Control and Prevention: *Folic acid,* 2018a. Available at: https://www.cdc.gov/ncbddd/folicacid/index.html.

Centers for Disease Control and Prevention: *Influenza (Flu),* 2018b. Available at: https://www.cdc.gov/breastfeeding/breastfeeding-special-circumstances/maternal-or-infant-illnesses/influenza.html.

Centers for Disease Control and Prevention: *Recommendations to prevent and control iron deficiency in the United States,* 1998. Available at: https://www.cdc.gov/mmwr/pdf/rr/rr4703.pdf.

Centers for Disease Control and Prevention: *Teen pregnancy,* 2018c. Available at: https://www.cdc.gov/teenpregnancy/index.htm.

Centers for Disease Control and Prevention: *People at risk - pregnant women and newborns,* 2018d. Available at: https://www.cdc.gov/listeria/risk-groups/pregnant-women.html.

Chan JC, Nugent BM, Bale TL: Parental advisory: maternal and paternal stress can impact offspring neurodevelopment, *Biol Psychiatry* 83:886–894, 2018.

Chang S, Lodico L, Williams Z: Nutritional composition and heavy metal content of the human placenta, *Placenta* 60:100–102, 2017.

Chang T, Choi H, Richardson CR, et al: Implications of teen birth for over-weight and obesity in adulthood, *Am J Obstet Gynecol* 209:110.e1-7, 2013.

Chavarro JE, Schlaff WD: Introduction: Impact of nutrition on reproduction: an overview, *Fertil Steril* 110:557–559, 2018.

Cheang KI, Nguyen TT, Karjane NW, et al: Raspberry leaf and hypoglycemia in gestational diabetes mellitus, *Obstet Gynecol* 128:1421–1424, 2016.

Cheng ER, Taveras EM, Hawkins SS: Paternal acculturation and maternal health behaviors: influence of father's ethnicity and place of birth, *J Womens Health (Larchmt)* 27:724–732, 2018.

Chiossi G, Neri I, Cavazzuti M, et al: Hyperemesis gravidarum complicated by Wernicke encephalopathy: background, case report, and review of the literature, *Obstet Gynecol Surv* 61:255–268, 2006.

Claycombe KJ, Brissette CA, Ghribi O: Epigenetics of inflammation, maternal infection, and nutrition, *J Nutr* 145:1109S–1115S, 2015.

Cohen-Addad N, Chatterjee M, Bekersky I, et al: In utero-exposure to saccharin: a threat? *Cancer Lett* 32:151–154, 1986.

Colen CG, Ramey DM: Is breast truly best? Estimating the effects of breast-feeding on long-term child health and wellbeing in the United States using sibling comparisons, *Soc Sci Med* 109:55–65, 2014.

Colson NJ, Naug HL, Nikbakht E, et al: The impact of MTHFR 677 C/T genotypes on folate status markers: a meta-analysis of folic acid intervention studies, *Eur J Nutr* 56:247–260, 2017.

Conde-Agudelo A, Rosas-Bermudez A, Castaño F, et al: Effects of birth spacing on maternal, perinatal, infant, and child health: a systematic review of causal mechanisms, *Stud Fam Plann* 43:93–114, 2012.

Cowell W, Ireland T, Vorhees D, et al: Ground turmeric as a source of lead exposure in the United States, *Public Health Rep* 132:289–293, 2017.

Cox JT, Phelan ST: Food safety in pregnancy, part 1: putting risks into perspective, Contemporary *Ob Gyn* 54:44, 2009a.

Cox JT, Phelan ST: Food safety in pregnancy, part 2: what can I eat, doctor? *Contemporary Ob Gyn* 54:24, 2009b.

Craig JR, Jenkins TG, Carrell DT, et al: Obesity, male infertility, and the sperm epigenome, *Fertil Steril* 107:848–859, 2017.

Crider KS, Quinlivan EP, Berry RJ, et al: Genomic DNA methylation changes in response to folic acid supplementation in a population-based intervention study among women of reproductive age, *PLoS One* 6:e28144, 2011.

Crozier TME: General care of the pregnant patient in the intensive care unit, *Semin Respir Crit Care Med* 38:208–217, 2017.

Dalton LM, Ní Fhloinn DM, Gaydadzhieva GT, et al: Magnesium in pregnancy, *Nutr Rev* 74:549–557, 2016.

da Silva Lopes K, Ota E, Shakya P, et al: Effects of nutrition interventions during pregnancy on low birth weight: an overview of systematic reviews, *BMJ Glob Health* 2: e000389, 2017.

Dean C, Bannigan K, Marsden J: Reviewing the effect of hyperemesis gravidarum on women's lives and mental health, *Br J Midwifery* 26:109, 2018.

Dean C, O'Hara ME: Ginger is ineffective for hyperemesis gravidarum, and causes harm: an internet based survey of sufferers, *MIDIRS Midwifery Digest* 25:4, 2018.

Dean J, Kendall P: *Food safety during pregnancy, Fact Sheet No. 9.372,* 2012. Available at: http://extension.colostate.edu/docs/pubs/foodnut/09372.pdf.

Dekker G, Robillard PY, Roberts C: The etiology of preeclampsia: the role of the father, *J Reprod Immunol* 89:126–132, 2011.

DelCurto H, Wu G, Satterfield MC: Nutrition and reproduction: links to epigenetics and metabolic syndrome in offspring, *Curr Opin Clin Nutr Metab Care* 16:385–391, 2013.

Deputy NP, Sharma AJ, Kim SY, et al: Achieving appropriate gestational weight gain: the role of healthcare provider advice, *J Womens Health (Larchmt)* 27:552–560, 2018.

Desideri D, Cantaluppi C, Ceccotto F, et al: Essential and toxic elements in seaweeds for human consumption, *J Toxicol Environ Health A* 79:112–122, 2016.

Desrosiers TA, Siega-Riz AM, Mosley BS, et al: Low carbohydrate diets may increase risk of neural tube defects, *Birth Defects Res* 110:901–909, 2018.

Dewailly E, Rouja P, Schultz E, et al: Vitamin A intoxication from reef fish liver consumption in Bermuda, *J Food Prot* 74:1581–1583, 2011.

Dhasarathy A, Roemmich JN, Claycombe KJ: Influence of maternal obesity, diet and exercise on epigenetic regulation of adipocytes, *Mol Aspects Med* 54:37–49, 2017.

Di Gangi S, Gizzo S, Patrelli TS, et al: Wernicke's encephalopathy complicating hyperemesis gravidarum: from the background to the present, *J Matern Fetal Neonatal Med* 25:1499–1504, 2012.

Dodd JM, O'Brien CM, Grivell RM: Modifying diet and physical activity to support pregnant women who are overweight or obese, *Curr Opin Clin Nutr Metab Care* 18:318–323, 2015.

Dolin CD, Deierlein AL, Evans MI: Folic acid supplementation to prevent recurrent neural tube defects: 4 milligrams is too much, *Fetal Diagn Ther* 44(3):161–165, 2018. doi:10.1159/000491786.

Domínguez-González MR, Chiocchetti GM, Herbello-Hermelo P, et al: Evaluation of iodine bioavailability in seaweed using in vitro methods, *J Agric Food Chem* 65:8435–8442, 2017.

Dragan IF, Veglia V, Geisinger ML, et al: Dental care as a safe and essential part of a healthy pregnancy, *Compend Contin Educ Dent* 39:86–91, 2018.

Dror DK, Allen LH: Interventions with vitamins B6, B12 and C in pregnancy, *Paediatr Perinat Epidemiol* 26:55–74, 2012.

Dubois L, Diasparra M, Bédard B, et al: Adequacy of nutritional intake during pregnancy in relation to prepregnancy BMI: results from the 3D Cohort Study, *Br J Nutr* 120:335–344, 2018.

Dunlop AL, Kramer MR, Hogue CJ, et al: Racial disparities in preterm birth: an overview of the potential role of nutrient deficiencies, *Acta Obstet Gynecol Scand* 90:1332–1341, 2011.

Earls MF, Committee on Psychosocial Aspects of Child and Family health American Academy of Pediatrics: Incorporating recognition and management of perinatal and postpartum depression into pediatric practice, *Pediatrics* 126:1032–1039, 2010.

Elango R, Ball RO: Protein and amino acid requirements during pregnancy, *Adv Nutr* 7:839S–844S, 2016.

Elliott-Sale KJ, Graham A, Hanley SJ, et al: Modern dietary guidelines for healthy pregnancy; maximising maternal and fetal outcomes and limiting excessive gestational weight gain, *Eur J Sport Sci* 19(1):62–70, 2018. doi:10.1080/17461391.2018.1476591.

Englund-Ögge L, Brantsæter AL, Sengpiel V, et al: Maternal dietary patterns and preterm delivery: results from large prospective cohort study, *BMJ* 348:g1446, 2014.

Erick M: Hyperemesis gravidarum: a case of starvation and altered sensorium gestosis (ASG), *Med Hypotheses* 82:572–580, 2014.

Faas MM, Melgert BN, de Vos P: A brief review on how pregnancy and sex hormones interfere with taste and food intake, *Chemosens Percept* 3:51–56, 2010.

Fabic MS, Choi Y: Assessing the quality of data regarding use of the lactational amenorrhea method, *Stud Fam Plann* 44:205–221, 2013.

Farr A, Chervenak FA, McCullough LB, et al: Human placentophagy: a review, *Am J Obstet Gynecol* 218:401.e1–401.e11, 2018.

Feichtinger M, Stopp T, Hofmann S, et al: Altered glucose profiles and risk for hypoglycaemia during oral glucose tolerance testing in pregnancies after gastric bypass surgery, *Diabetologia* 60:153–157, 2017.

Fejzo MS, Ching C, Schoenberg FP, et al: Change in paternity and recurrence of hyperemesis gravidarum, *J Matern Fetal Neonatal Med* 25:1241–1245, 2012.

Fejzo MS, Mac Gibbon K, Mullin PM: Why are women still dying from nausea and vomiting of pregnancy? *Gynecol Obstet Case Rep* 2:2, 2016.

Fejzo MS, Magtira A, Schoenberg FP, et al: Neurodevelopmental delay in children exposed in utero to hyperemesis gravidarum, *Eur J Obstet Gynecol Reprod Biol* 189:79–84, 2015.

Fernández I, Arroyo R, Espinosa I, et al: Probiotics for human lactational mastitis, *Benef Microbes* 5:169–183, 2014.

Feltner C, Weber RP, Stuebe A, et al: *Breastfeeding programs and policies, breastfeeding uptake, and maternal health outcomes in developed countries. Comparative effectiveness Review No. 210.* (Prepared by the RTI International–University of North Carolina at Chapel Hill Evidence-based Practice Center under Contract No. 290-2015-00011-I.) AHRQ Publication No. 18-EHC014.EF. Rockville, MD: Agency for Healthcare Research and Quality; July 2018. Available at: https://effectivehealthcare.ahrq.gov/topics/breastfeeding/research.

Fisher AL, Nemeth E: Iron homeostasis during pregnancy, *Am J Clin Nutr* 106:1567S–1574S, 2017.

Fleischer DM, Spergel JM, Assa'ad AH, et al: Primary prevention of allergic disease through nutritional interventions, *J Allergy Clin Immunol Pract* 1:29–36, 2013.

Fleming TP, Watkins AJ, Velazquez MA, et al: Origins of lifetime health around the time of conception: causes and consequences. *Lancet* 391:1842–1852, 2018.

Food and Drug Administration: *How sweet it is: all about sugar substitutes*, 2014. Available at: https://www.fda.gov/ForConsumers/ConsumerUpdates/ucm397711.htm.

Frank LL: Thiamin in clinical practice, *JPEN J Parenter Enteral Nutr* 39:503–520, 2015.

Freeman HJ: Reproductive changes associated with celiac disease, *World J Gastroenterol* 16:5810–5814, 2010.

Furber CM, McGowan L, Bower P, et al: Antenatal interventions for reducing weight in obese women for improving pregnancy outcome, *Cochrane Database Syst Rev* (1):CD009334, 2013.

Garcia AH, Voortman T, Baena CP, et al: Maternal weight status, diet, and supplement use as determinants of breastfeeding and complementary feeding: a systematic review and meta-analysis, *Nutr Rev* 74:490–516, 2016.

Garcia-Larsen V, Ierodiakonou D, Jarrold K, et al: Diet during pregnancy and infancy and risk of allergic or autoimmune disease: A systematic review and meta-analysis, *PLoS Med* 15:e1002507, 2018.

García-Velasco JA, Menabrito M, Catalán IB: What fertility specialists should know about the vaginal microbiome: a review, *Reprod Biomed Online* 35:103–112, 2017.

Gatford KL, Houda CM, Lu ZX, et al: Vitamin B12 and homocysteine status during pregnancy in the metformin in gestational diabetes trial: responses to maternal metformin compared with insulin treatment, *Diabetes Obes Metab* 15:660–667, 2013.

Gaur DS, Talekar MS, Pathak VP: Alcohol intake and cigarette smoking: impact of two major lifestyle factors on male infertility, *Indian J Pathol Microbiol* 53:35–40, 2010.

Georgieff MK: Iron assessment to protect the developing brain, *Am J Clin Nutr* 106:1588S–1593S, 2017.

Georgieff MK, Brunette KE, Tran PV: Early life nutrition and neural plasticity, *Dev Psychopathol* 27:411–423, 2015.

Girard AW, Olude O: Nutrition education and counseling provided during pregnancy: effects on maternal, neonatal and child health outcomes, *Paediatr Perinat Epidemiol* 26:191–204, 2012.

Godfrey KM, Cutfield W, Chan SY, et al: Nutritional Intervention Preconception and During Pregnancy to Maintain Healthy Glucose Metabolism and Offspring Health ("NiPPeR"): study protocol for a randomised controlled trial, *Trials* 18:131, 2017a.

Godfrey KM, Reynolds RM, Prescott SL, et al: Influence of maternal obesity on the long-term health of offspring, *Lancet Diabetes Endocrinol* 5:53–64, 2017b.

Goldstein R, Teede H, Thangaratinam S, et al: Excess gestational weight gain in pregnancy and the role of lifestyle intervention, *Semin Reprod Med* 34:e14–e21, 2016.

Goodnight W, Newman R, Society of Maternal-Fetal Medicine: Optimal nutrition for improved twin pregnancy outcome, *Obstet Gynecol* 114:1121–1134, 2009.

Greenan CW, Newman RB, Wojciechowski B, et al: Achievement of body mass index specific weight gain recommendations: impact on preterm birth in twin pregnancies, *Am J Perinatol* 34:1293–1301, 2017.

Griffin C: Probiotics in obstetrics and gynaecology, *Aust N Z J Obstet Gynaecol* 55:201–209, 2015.

Grooten IJ, Koot MH, van der Post JA, et al: Early enteral tube feeding in optimizing treatment of hyperemesis gravidarum: the Maternal and Offspring outcomes after Treatment of HyperEmesis by Refeeding (MOTHER) randomized controlled trial, *Am J Clin Nutr* 106:812–820, 2017.

Grooten IJ, Roseboom TJ, Painter RC: Barriers and challenges in hyperemesis gravidarum research, *Nutr Metab Insights* 8 (Suppl 1):33–39, 2016.

Gryder LK, Young SM, Zava D, et al: Effects of human maternal placentophagy on maternal postpartum iron status: a randomized, double-blind, placebo-controlled pilot study, *J Midwifery Womens Health* 62:68–79, 2017.

Guéant JL, Namour F, Guéant-Rodriguez RM, et al: Folate and fetal programming: a play in epigenomics? *Trends Endocrinol Metab* 24:279–289, 2013.

Gupta KK, Gupta VK, Shirasaka T: An update on fetal alcohol syndrome-pathogenesis, risks, and treatment, *Alcohol Clin Exp Res* 40:1594–1602, 2016.

Haby K, Berg M, Gyllensten H, et al: Mighty mums - a lifestyle intervention at primary care level reduces gestational weight gain in women with obesity, *BMC Obes* 5:16, 2018.

Hale TW: *Medications and mothers' milk*, ed 18, Amarillo, TX, 2019, Hale Publishing.

Hamby T, Kunnel N, Dallas JS, et al: Maternal iodine excess: an uncommon cause of acquired neonatal hypothyroidism, *J Pediatr Endocrinol Metab* 31(9):1061–1064, 2018. doi:10.1515/jpem-2018-0138.

Handley MA, Nelson K, Sanford E, et al: Examining lead exposures in California through State-issued health alerts for food contamination and an exposure-based candy testing program, *Environ Health Perspect* 125:104503, 2017.

Hansen BR, Bottner WA, Ravindran A, et al: Desiderosmia (olfactory craving): a novel symptom associated with iron deficiency anemia, *Am J Hematol* 92:E93–E94, 2017.

Harris AA: Practical advice for caring for women with eating disorders during the perinatal period, *J Midwifery Womens Health* 55:579–586, 2010.

Harris BS, Bishop KC, Kemeny HR, et al: Risk factors for birth defects, *Obstet Gynecol Surv* 72:123–135, 2017.

Hauff LE, Leonard SA, Rasmussen KM: Associations of maternal obesity and psychosocial factors with breastfeeding intention, initiation, and duration, *Am J Clin Nutr* 99:524–534, 2014.

Headen I, Cohen AK, Mujahid M, et al: The accuracy of self-reported pregnancy-related weight: a systematic review, *Obes Rev* 18:350–369, 2017.

Heaney RP, Rafferty K: The settling problem in calcium-fortified soybean drinks, *J Am Diet Assoc* 106:1753, 2006.

Heidkamp R, Clermont A, Phillips E: Modeling the impact of nutrition interventions on birth outcomes in the lives saved tool (LiST), *J Nutr* 147:2188S–2193S, 2017.

Hennessy G: Marijuana and pregnancy, *Am J Addict* 27:44–45, 2018.

Hester J, Hanna-Rose W, Diaz F: Zinc deficiency reduces fertility in C. elegans hermaphrodites and disrupts oogenesis and meiotic progression, *Comp Biochem Physiol C Toxicol Pharmacol* 191:203–209, 2017.

Heyden EL, Wimalawansa SJ: Vitamin D: effects on human reproduction, pregnancy, and fetal well-being, *J Steroid Biochem Mol Biol* 180:41–50, 2018.

Holick MF: The vitamin D deficiency pandemic: Approaches for diagnosis, treatment and prevention, *Rev Endocr Metab Disord* 18:153–165, 2017.

Hollis BW, Wagner CL: New insights into the vitamin D requirements during pregnancy, *Bone Res* 5:17030, 2017.

Hollis BW, Wagner CL, Howard CR, et al: Maternal versus infant vitamin D supplementation during lactation: A randomized controlled trial, *Pediatrics* 136:625–634, 2015. doi:10.1542/peds.2019-1063.

Hovdenak N, Haram K: Influence of mineral and vitamin supplements on pregnancy outcome, *Eur J Obstet Gynecol Reprod Biol* 164:127–132, 2012.

Huberty J, Leiferman JA, Kruper AR, et al: Exploring the need for interventions to manage weight and stress during interconception, *J Behav Med* 40:145–158, 2017.

Hudak ML, Tan RC, COMMITTEE ON DRUGS, et al: Neonatal drug withdrawal, *Pediatrics* 129:e540–e560, 2012.

Hunt MG, Belfer S, Atuahene B: Pagophagia improves neuropsychological processing speed in iron-deficiency anemia, *Med Hypotheses* 83:473–476, 2014.

Hutcheon JA, Platt RW, Abrams B, et al: Pregnancy weight gain by gestational age in women with uncomplicated dichorionic twin pregnancies, *Paediatr Perinat Epidemiol* 32:172–180, 2018.

Isemann B, Meinzen-Derr J, Akinbi H: Maternal and neonatal factors impacting response to methadone therapy in infants treated for neonatal abstinence syndrome, *J Perinatol* 31:25–29, 2011.

Jacquemyn Y, Meesters J: Pregnancy as a risk factor for undertreatment after bariatric surgery, *BMJ Case Rep* 2014:bcr2013202779, 2014. doi:10.1136/bcr-2013-202779.

Jans G, Matthys C, Bel S, et al: AURORA: bariatric surgery registration in women of reproductive age - a multicenter prospective cohort study, *BMC Pregnancy Childbirth* 16:195, 2016.

Jarde A, Lewis-Mikhael AM, Moayyedi P, et al: Pregnancy outcomes in women taking probiotics or prebiotics: a systematic review and meta-analysis, *BMC Pregnancy Childbirth* 18:14, 2018.

Jellin JM, Gregory PJ, editors: *Natural medicines comprehensive database* (tm), 2018. Available at: www.naturalmedicines.com.

Jensen TK, Gottschau M, Madsen JO, et al: Habitual alcohol consumption associated with reduced semen quality and changes in reproductive hormones;

a cross-sectional study among 1221 young Danish men, *BMJ Open* 4: e005462, 2014.

Jeurink PV, Knipping K, Wiens F, et al: Importance of maternal diet in the training of the infant's immune system during gestation and lactation, *Crit Rev Food Sci Nutr* 59(8):1311–1319, 2018. doi:10.1080/10408398.2017.140 5907.

Johnson SK, Groten T, Pastuschek J, et al: Human placentophagy: effects of dehydration and steaming on hormones, metals and bacteria in placental tissue, *Placenta* 67:8–14, 2018.

Johnson-Arbor K, Vo K, Wong F, et al: Unintentional and Sequential lead exposure from a ceramic mug and maca (Lepidium meyenii), *J Med Toxicol* 14:152–155, 2018.

Jones CJ, Choudhury RH, Aplin JD: Tracking nutrient transfer at the human maternofetal interface from 4 weeks to term, *Placenta* 36:372–380, 2015.

Jones JL, Dubey JP: Foodborne toxoplasmosis, *Clin Infect Dis* 55:845–851, 2012.

Kaiser LL, Campbell CG: *Practice paper of the Academy of Nutrition and Dietetics: nutrition and lifestyle for a healthy pregnancy outcome*, 2014. Available at: https://www.eatrightpro.org/practice/position-and-practice-papers/practice-papers/practice-paper-nutrition-lifestyle-healthy-pregnancy-outcome.

Karachaliou M, Georgiou V, Roumeliotaki T, et al: Association of trimester-specific gestational weight gain with fetal growth, offspring obesity, and cardiometabolic traits in early childhood, *Am J Obstet Gynecol* 212:502. e1-14, 2015.

Kassir R, Goiset MP, Williet N, et al: Bariatric surgery and pregnancy: What outcomes? *Int J Surg* 36:66–67, 2016.

Kelleher AM, Burns GW, Behura S, et al: Uterine glands impact uterine receptivity, luminal fluid homeostasis and blastocyst implantation, *Sci Rep* 6:38078, 2016.

Kennedy DA, Lupattelli A, Koren G, et al: Safety classification of herbal medicines used in pregnancy in a multinational study, *BMC Complement Altern Med* 16:102, 2016.

Khan S, Prime DK, Hepworth AR, et al: Investigation of short-term variations in term breast milk composition during repeated breast expression sessions, *J Hum Lact* 29:196–204, 2013.

Kim T, Burn SC, Bangdiwala A, et al: Neonatal morbidity and maternal complication rates in women with a delivery body mass index of 60 or higher, *Obstet Gynecol* 130:988–993, 2017.

Kloss O, Eskin NAM, Suh M: Thiamin deficiency on fetal brain development with and without prenatal alcohol exposure, *Biochem Cell Biol* 96:169–177, 2018.

Koletzko B, Cetin I, Brenna JT, et al: Dietary fat intakes for pregnant and lactation women, *Br J Nutr* 98:873–877, 2007.

Kotelchuck M, Lu M: Father's role in preconception health, *Matern Child Health J* 21:2025–2039, 2017.

Kovacs CS: Calcium, phosphorus, and bone metabolism in the fetus and newborn, *Early Hum Dev* 91:623–628, 2015.

Kovacs CS: Maternal mineral and bone metabolism during pregnancy, lactation, and post-weaning recovery, *Physiol Rev* 96:449–547, 2016.

Kovacs CS: The role of vitamin D in pregnancy and lactation: insights from animal models and clinical studies, *Annu Rev Nutr* 32:97–123, 2012.

Kroger M, Meister K, Kava R: Low-calorie sweeteners and other sugar substitutes: a review of the safety issues, *Compr Rev Food Sci Food Saf* 5:35–47, 2006.

Kwak-Kim J, Park JC, Ahn HK, et al: Immunological modes of pregnancy loss, *Am J Reprod Immunol* 63:611–623, 2010.

Kwong W, Tomlinson G, Feig DS: Maternal and neonatal outcomes after bariatric surgery; a systematic review and meta-analysis: do the benefits outweigh the risks? *Am J Obstet Gynecol* 218:573–580, 2018.

Larqué E, Gil-Sánchez A, Prieto-Sánchez MT, et al: Omega 3 fatty acids, gestation and pregnancy outcomes, *Br J Nutr* 107(Suppl 2):S77–S84, 2012.

Lauritzen L, Carlson SE: Maternal fatty acid status during pregnancy and lactation and relation to newborn and infant status, *Matern Child Nutr* 7:41–58, 2011.

La Vecchia C: Low-calorie sweeteners and the risk of preterm delivery: results from two studies and a meta-analysis, *J Fam Plann Reprod Health Care* 39:12–13, 2013.

Lawlor DA, Wills AK, Fraser A, et al: Association of maternal vitamin D status during pregnancy with bone-mineral content in offspring: a prospective cohort study, *Lancet* 381:2176–2183, 2013.

Lawrence RA, Lawrence RM: *Breastfeeding: a guide for the medical profession*, ed 8, Maryland Heights, MO, 2016, Elsevier Mosby.

LeBlanc ES, Perrin N, Johnson JD Jr, et al: Over-the-counter and compounded vitamin D: is potency what we expect? *JAMA Intern Med* 173:585–586, 2013.

Leddy MA, Jones C, Morgan MA, et al: Eating disorders and obstetric-gynecologic care, *J Womens Health (Larchmt)* 18:1395–1401, 2009.

Lee AI, Okam MM: Anemia in pregnancy, *Hematol Oncol Clin N Am* 25: 241–259, 2011.

Lee SY, Stagnaro-Green A, MacKay D, et al: Iodine contents in prenatal vitamins in the United States, *Thyroid* 27:1101–1102, 2017.

Leese HJ, Hugentobler SA, Gray SM, et al: Female reproductive tract fluids: composition, mechanism of formation and potential role in the developmental origins of health and disease, *Reprod Fertil Dev* 20:1–8, 2008.

Legro RS: Effects of obesity treatment on female reproduction: results do not match expectations, *Fertil Steril* 107:860–867, 2017.

Lengyel CS, Ehrlich S, Iams JD, et al: Effect of modifiable risk factors on preterm birth: a population based-cohort, *Matern Child Health J* 21:777–785, 2017.

Leung AM, Pearce EN, Braverman LE: Sufficient iodine intake during pregnancy: just do it, *Thyroid* 23:7–8, 2013.

Léveillé P, Rouxel C, Plourde M: Diabetic pregnancy, maternal and fetal docosahexaenoic acid: a review of existing evidence, *J Matern Fetal Neonatal Med* 31:1358–1363, 2018.

Lewis EL, Sierra LJ, Barila GO, et al: Placental immune state shifts with gestational age, *Am J Reprod Immunol* 79:e12848, 2018.

Lin CG, Schaider LA, Brabander DJ, et al: Pediatric lead exposure from imported Indian spices and cultural powders, *Pediatrics* 125:e828–e835, 2010.

Lindsay KL, Buss C, Wadhwa PD, et al: The interplay between nutrition and stress in pregnancy: implications for fetal programming of Brain development, *Biol Psychiatry* 85(2):135–149, 2019. doi:10.1016/j.biopsych.2018.06.021.

Lisonkova S, Muraca GM, Potts J, et al: Association between prepregnancy body mass index and severe maternal morbidity, *JAMA* 18:1777–1786, 2017.

London RS: Saccharin and aspartame. Are they safe to consume during pregnancy? *J Reprod Med* 33:17–21, 1988.

Lovelady C: Balancing exercise and food intake with lactation to promote post-partum weight loss, *Proc Nutr Soc* 70:181–184, 2011.

Lowry P, Woods R: The placenta controls the physiology of pregnancy by increasing the half-life in blood and receptor activity of its secreted peptide hormones, *J Mol Endocrinol* 60:R23–R30, 2018.

Lui S, Jones RL, Robinson NJ, et al: Detrimental effects of ethanol and its metabolite acetaldehyde, on first trimester human placental cell turnover and function, *PLoS One* 9:e87328, 2014.

Luke B: Adverse effects of female obesity and interaction with race on reproductive potential, *Fertil Steril* 107:868–877, 2017.

Luke B: Nutrition for multiples, *Clin Obstet Gynecol* 58:585–610, 2015.

Luke B, Eberlein T, Newman R: *When you're expecting twins, triplets, or quads*, ed 4, New York, NY, 2017, Harper.

Lumen A, George NI: Estimation of iodine nutrition and thyroid function status in late-gestation pregnant women in the United States: Development and application of a population-based pregnancy model, *Toxicol Appl Pharmacol* 314:24–38, 2017.

Lumey LH, Stein AD, Kahn HS, et al: Cohort profile: the Dutch Hunger Winter families study, *Int J Epidemiol* 36:1196–1204, 2007.

Ma RCW, Schmidt MI, Tam WH, et al: Clinical management of pregnancy in the obese mother: before conception, during pregnancy, and postpartum, *Lancet Diabetes Endocrinol* 4:1037–1049, 2016.

Mackie FL, Cooper NS, Whitticase LJ, et al: Vitamin A and micronutrient deficiencies post-bariatric surgery: aetiology, complications and management in a complex multiparous pregnancy, *Eur J Clin Nutr* 72:1176–1179, 2018.

Madigan S, Wade M, Plamondon A, et al: Maternal Adverse Childhood Experience and Infant Health: Biomedical and Psychosocial Risks as Intermediary Mechanisms, *J Pediatr* 187:282–289.el, 2017.

Magnuson BA, Roberts A, Nestmann ER: Critical review of the current literature on the safety of sucralose, *Food Chem Toxicol* 106:324–355, 2017.

Maldonado M, Alhousseini A, Awadalla M, et al: Intrahepatic cholestasis of pregnancy leading to severe vitamin K deficiency and coagulopathy, *Case Rep Obstet Gynecol* 2017:5646247, 2017.

Manuck TA: Racial and ethnic differences in preterm birth: a complex, multifactorial problem, *Semin Perinatol* 41:511–518. 2017.

Marques AH, O'Connor TG, Roth C, et al: The influence of maternal prenatal and early childhood nutrition and maternal prenatal stress on offspring immune system development and neurodevelopmental disorders, *Front Neurosci* 7:120, 2013.

Marx W, Ried K, McCarthy AL, et al: Ginger-Mechanism of action in chemotherapy-induced nausea and vomiting: A review, *Crit Rev Food Sci Nutr* 57:141–146, 2017.

Matok I, Clark S, Caritis S, et al: Studying the antiemetic effect of vitamin B6 for morning sickness: pyridoxine and pyridoxal are prodrugs, *J Clin Pharmacol* 54:1429–1433, 2014.

Matusiak K, Barrett HL, Callaway LK, et al: Periconception weight loss: common sense for mothers, but what about for babies? *J Obes* 2014:204295, 2014.

Mawson AR, Xueyuan W: Breastfeeding, retinoids, and postpartum depression: a new theory, *J Affective Disord* 150:1129–1135, 2013.

McCabe D, Lisy K, Lockwood C, et al: The impact of essential fatty acid, B vitamins, vitamin C, magnesium and zinc supplementation on stress levels in women: a systematic review, *JBI Database System Rev Implement Rep* 15:402–453, 2017.

McDade TW, Metzger MW, Chyu L, et al: Long-term effects of birth weight and breastfeeding duration on inflammation in early adulthood, *Proc Biol Sci* 281:20133116, 2014.

McDonald SM, Liu J, Wilcox S, et al: Does dose matter in reducing gestational weight gain in exercise interventions? A systematic review of literature, *J Sci Med Sport* 19:323–335. 2016.

McDonnell SL, Baggerly KA, Baggerly CA, et al: Maternal 25(OH)D concentrations ≥40 ng/mL associated with 60% lower preterm birth risk among general obstetrical patients at an urban medical center, *PLoS One* 12: e0180483, 2017.

McGuire J, Kaplan J, Lapolla J, et al: The 2014 FDA assessment of commercial fish: practical considerations for improved dietary guidance, *Nutr J* 15:66, 2016.

McLaren DS, Kraemer K: Food sources, *World Rev Nutr Diet* 103:20–26, 2012.

Mechanick JI, Youdim A, Jones DB, et al: Clinical practice guidelines for the perioperative nutritional, metabolic, and nonsurgical support of the bariatric surgery patient—2013 update: cosponsored by American Association of Clinical Endocrinologists, the Obesity Society, and American Society for Metabolic and Bariatric Surgery, *Endocr Pract* 19:337–372, 2013.

Ménézo Y, Guérin P, Elder K: The oviduct: a neglected organ due for reassessment in IVF, *Reprod Biomed Online* 30:233–240, 2015.

Mennella JA: Ontogeny of taste preferences: basic biology and implications for health, *Am J Clin Nutr* 99:704S–711S, 2014.

Merhi ZO, Keltz J, Zapantis A, et al: Male adiposity impairs clinical pregnancy rate by in vitro fertilization without affecting day 3 embryo quality, *Obesity* 21:1608–1612, 2013.

Middleton P, Gomersall JC, Gould JF, et al: Omega-3 fatty acid addition during pregnancy. *Cochrane Database Syst Rev* 11:CD003402, 2018. doi:10.1002/14651858.CD003402.pub3.

Milagro FI, Mansego ML, De Miguel C, et al: Dietary factors, epigenetic modifications and obesity outcomes: progresses and perspectives, *Mol Aspects Med* 34:782–812, 2013.

Miller NC, Georgieff MK: Maternal nutrition and child neurodevelopment: actions across generations, *J Pediatr* 187:10–13, 2017.

Millward DJ: Identifying recommended dietary allowances for protein and amino acids: a critique of the 2007 WHO/FAO/UNU report, *Br J Nutr* 108(Suppl 2):S3–S21, 2012.

Milman N, Paszkowski T, Cetin I, et al: Supplementation during pregnancy: beliefs and science, *Gynecol Endocrinol* 32:509–516, 2016.

Mogensen KM, Erick ME. Pregnancy and Lactation. In Mueller CM, Lord LM, Marian M, et al, editors: *The ASPEN adult nutrition support core curriculum*, ed 3, Silver Spring, MD, 2017, American Society for Parenteral and Enteral Nutrition, pp 397–417.

Monash University: *International evidence-based guideline for the assessment and management of polycystic ovary syndrome* 2018, Melbourne Australia, 2018. Available at: https://www.monash.edu/__data/assets/pdf_file/0004/1412644/PCOS_Evidence-Based-Guidelines_20181009.pdf.

Monk C, Georgieff MK, Osterholm EA: Research review: maternal prenatal distress and poor nutrition—mutually influencing risk factors affecting infant neurocognitive development, *J Child Psychol Psychiatry* 54:115–130, 2013.

Mor G, Cardenas I, Abrahams V, et al: Inflammation and pregnancy: the role of the immune system at the implantation site, *Ann N Y Acad Sci* 1221:80–87, 2011.

Mora-Esteves C, Shin D: Nutrient supplementation: improving male fertility fourfold, *Semin Reprod Med* 31:293–300, 2013.

Moser G, Windsperger K, Pollheimer J, et al: Human trophoblast invasion: new and unexpected routes and functions, *Histochem Cell Biol* 150(4):361–370, 2018. doi:10.1007/s00418-018-1699-0.

Moussa HN, Hosseini Nasab S, Haidar ZA, et al: Folic acid supplementation: what is new? Fetal, obstetric, long-term benefits and risks, *Future Sci OA* 2:FSO116, 2016.

Murray-Kolb LE: Iron status and neuropsychological consequences in women of reproductive age: what do we know and where are we headed? *J Nutr* 141:747S–755S, 2011.

Myatt L, Thornburg KL: Effects of prenatal nutrition and the role of the placenta in health and disease, *Methods Mol Biol* 1735:19–46, 2018.

Myers JE: What are the metaboloc precursors which increase the risk of pre-eclampsia and how could these be investigated further, *Placenta* 60:110–114, 2017.

Nascimento SL, Pudwell J, Surita FG, et al: The effect of physical exercise strategies on weight loss in postpartum women: a systematic review and meta-analysis, *Int J Obes (Lond)* 38:626–635, 2014.

National Academies of Sciences, Engineering, and Medicine: *Harmonization of approaches to nutrient reference values: applications to young children and women of reproductive age,* Washington, DC, 2018, The National Academies Press. https://doi.org/10.17226/25148.

National Institutes of Health consensus development conference statement: diagnosing gestational diabetes mellitus, March 4-6, 2013, *Obstet Gynecol* 122:358–369, 2013.

Nelson SM, Matthews P, Poston L: Maternal metabolism and obesity: modifiable determinants of pregnancy outcome, *Human Reprod Update* 16:255–275, 2010.

Nishiyama S, Mikeda T, Okada T, et al: Transient hypothyroidism or persistent hyperthyrotropinemia in neonates born to mothers with excessive iodine intake, *Thyroid* 14:1077–1083, 2004.

Nourbakhsh M, Miller A, Gofton J, et al: Cannabinoid hyperemesis syndrome: reports of fatal cases, *J Forensic Sci* 64(1):270–274, 2018. doi:10.1111/1556-4029.13819.

Noventa M, Quaranta M, Vitagliano A, et al: May underdiagnosed nutrition imbalances be responsible for a portion of so-called unexplained infertility? From diagnosis to potential treatment options, *Reprod Sci* 23:812–822, 2016.

Nugent BM, Bale TL: The omniscient placenta: metabolic and epigenetic regulation of fetal programming, *Front Neuroendocrinol* 39:28–37, 2015.

Obeid R, Holzgreve W, Pietrzik K: Is 5-methyltetrahydrofolate an alternative to folic acid for the prevention of neural tube defects? *J Perinat Med* 41:469–483, 2013.

O'Brien KO, Ru Y: Iron status of North American pregnant women: an update on longitudinal data and gaps in knowledge from the United States and Canada, *Am J Clin Nutr* 106:1647S–1654S, 2017.

O'Donnell A, McParlin C, Robson SC, et al: Treatments for hyperemesis gravidarum and nausea and vomiting in pregnancy: a systematic review and economic assessment, *Health Technol Assess* 20:1–268, 2016.

Office of Dietary Supplements, National Institute of Health: *Dietary Supplement Fact Sheet: Iron*, 2018. Available at: https://ods.od.nih.gov/factsheets/Iron-HealthProfessional/.

Oken E, Guthrie LB, Bloomingdale A, et al: A pilot randomized controlled trial to promote healthful fish consumption during pregnancy: the food for thought study, *Nutr J* 12:33, 2013.

Olausson H, Goldberg GR, Laskey MA, et al: Calcium economy in human pregnancy and lactation, *Nutr Res Rev* 25:40–67, 2012.

Olson T, Holtslander L, Bowen A: Mother's milk, mother's tears, breastfeeding with postpartum depression, *Clin Lact* 5:9, 2014.

Orzylowska EM, Jacobson JD, Bareh GM, et al: Food intake diet and sperm characteristics in a blue zone: a Loma Linda Study, *Eur J Obstet Gynecol Reprod Biol* 203:112–115, 2016.

Otten JJ, Hellwig JP, Meyers JD: *Dietary reference intakes: the essential guide to nutrient requirements*, Washington, DC, 2006, Institute of Medicine of the National Academies, National Academies Press.

Owen CM, Goldstein EH, Clayton JA, et al: Racial and ethnic health disparities in reproductive medicine: an evidence-based overview, *Semin Reprod Med* 31:317–324, 2013.

Oz HS: Fetomaternal and pediatric toxoplasmosis, *J Pediatr Infect Dis* 12:202–208, 2017.

Parent B, Martopullo I, Weiss NS, et al: Bariatric surgery in women of childbearing age, timing between an operation and birth, and associated perinatal complications, *JAMA Surg* 152:128–135, 2017.

Parrott J, Frank L, Rabena R, et al: American society for metabolic and bariatric surgery integrated health nutritional guidelines for the surgical weight loss patient 2016 update: micronutrients, *Surg Obes Relat Dis* 13:727–741, 2017.

Patel A, Lee SY, Stagnaro-Green A, et al: Iodine content of the best-selling United States adult and prenatal multivitamin preparations, *Thyroid* 29(1):124–127, 2018. doi:10.1089/thy.2018.0386.

Paul L, Selhub J: Interaction between excess folate and low vitamin B12 status, *Mol Aspects Med* 53:43–47, 2017.

Pearce EN: Iodine nutrition: recent research and unanswered questions, *Eur J Clin Nutr* 72:1226–1228, 2018.

Pearce EN, Andersson M, Zimmermann MB: Global iodine nutrition: where do we stand in 2013? *Thyroid* 23:523–528, 2013.

Pelizzo G, Calcaterra V, Fusillo M, et al: Malnutrition in pregnancy following bariatric surgery: three clinical cases of fetal neural defects, *Nutr J* 13:59, 2014.

Pelzer E, Gomez-Arango LF, Barrett HL, et al: Review: maternal health and the placental microbiome, *Placenta* 54:30–37, 2017.

Pentieva K, Selhub J, Paul L, et al: Evidence from a randomized trial that exposure to supplemental folic acid at recommended levels during pregnancy does not lead to increased unmetabolized folic acid concentrations in maternal or cord blood, *J Nutr* 146:494–500, 2016.

Pludowski P, Holick MF, Pilz S, et al: Vitamin D effects on musculoskeletal health, immunity, autoimmunity, cardiovascular disease, cancer, fertility, pregnancy, dementia and mortality—a review of recent evidence, *Autoimmun Rev* 12:976–989, 2013.

Plumptre L, Masih SP, Ly A, et al: High concentrations of folate and unmetabolized folic acid in a cohort of pregnant Canadian women and umbilical cord blood, *Am J Clin Nutr* 102:848–857, 2015.

Pocobelli G, Yu O, Fuller S, et al: One-step approach to identifying gestational diabetes mellitus: association with perinatal outcomes, *Obstet Gynecol* 132(4):859–867, 2018. doi:10.1097/AOG.0000000000002780.

Pope E, Koren G, Bozzo P: Sugar substitutes during pregnancy, *Can Fam Physician* 60:1003–1005, 2014.

Practice Committee of the American Society for Reproductive Medicine in collaboration with the Society for Reproductive Endocrinology and Infertility: Optimizing natural fertility: a committee opinion, *Fertil Steril* 107:52–58, 2017.

Prentice AM, Mendoza YA, Pereira D, et al: Dietary strategies for improving iron status: balancing safety and efficacy, *Nutr Rev* 75:49–60, 2017.

Preston JD, Reynolds LJ, Pearson KJ: Developmental origins of health span and life span: a mini-review, *Gerontology* 64:237–245, 2018.

Prince AL, Chu DM, Seferovic MD, et al: The perinatal microbiome and pregnancy: moving beyond the vaginal microbiome, *Cold Spring Harb Perspect Med* 5:a023051, 2015. doi:10.1101/cshperspect.a023051.

Procter SB, Campbell CG: Position of the Academy of Nutrition and Dietetics: nutrition and lifestyle for a healthy pregnancy outcome, *J Acad Nutr Diet* 114:1099–1103, 2014.

Rackers HS, Thomas S, Williamson K, et al: Emerging literature in the microbiota-brain axis and perinatal mood and anxiety disorders, *Psychoneuroendocrinology* 95:86–96, 2018.

Rai D, Bird JK, McBurney MI, et al: Nutritional status as assessed by nutrient intakes and biomarkers among women of childbearing age—is the burden of nutrient inadequacies growing in America? *Public Health Nutr* 18:1658–1669, 2015.

Rao R, Georgieff MK: The nutritionally deprived fetus and newborn infant. Chapter 19, pages 277–286, in Acquired Brain Injury in the Fetus and Newborn, Shevell M, Miller S, editors: Mac Keith Press, London, 2012.

Rasmussen KM, Abrams B, Bodnar LM, et al: Recommendations for weight gain during pregnancy in the context of the obesity epidemic, *Obstet Gynecol* 116:1191–1195, 2010.

Rasmussen KM, Yaktine AL: *Weight gain during pregnancy: reexamining the recommendations*, Washington, DC, 2009, Institute of Medicine, National Research Council.

Renz H, Allen KJ, Sicherer SH, et al: Food allergy, *Nat Rev Dis Primers* 4:17098, 2018. doi:10.1038/nrdp.2017.98.

Richard K, Holland O, Landers K, et al: Review: effects of maternal micronutrient supplementation on placental function, *Placenta* 54:38–44, 2017.

Rivera JO, González-Stuart A, Ortiz M, et al: Guide for herbal product use by Mexican Americans in the largest Texas-Mexico border community, *Tex Med* 102:46–56, 2006.

Roberts JM, Bell MJ: If we know so much about preeclampsia, why haven't we cured the disease? *J Reprod Immunol* 99:1–9, 2013.

Rodríguez-González GL, Castro-Rodríguez DC, Zambrano E: Pregnancy and lactation: a window of opportunity to improve individual health, *Methods Mol Biol* 1735:115–144, 2018.

Roleda MY, Skjermo J, Marfaing H, et al: Iodine content in bulk biomass of wild-harvested and cultivated edible seaweeds: Inherent variations determine species-specific daily allowable consumption, *Food Chem* 254:333–339, 2018.

Roseboom TJ, Painter RC, van Abeelen AF, et al: Hungry in the womb: what are the consequences? Lessons from the Dutch famine, *Maturitas* 70:141–145, 2011.

Roth DE: Vitamin D supplementation during pregnancy: safety considerations in the design and interpretation of clinical trials, *J Perinatol* 31:449–459, 2011.

Roth DE, Leung M, Mesfin E, et al: Vitamin D supplementation during pregnancy: state of the evidence from a systematic review of randomised trials, *BMJ* 359:j5237, 2017.

Rulis AM, Levitt JA: FDA's food ingredient approval process: safety assurance based on scientific assessment, *Regul Toxicol Pharmacol* 53:20–31, 2009.

Saldanha LG, Dwyer JT, Andrews KW, et al: Is nutrient content and other label information for prescription prenatal supplements different from nonprescription products? *J Acad Nutr Diet* 117:1429–1436, 2017.

Saltzman E, Karl JP: Nutrient deficiencies after gastric bypass surgery, *Annu Rev Nutr* 33:183–203, 2013.

Sámano R, Martínez-Rojano H, Godínez Martínez E, et al: Effects of breastfeeding on weight loss and recovery of pregestational weight in adolescent and adult mothers, *Food Nutr Bull* 34:123–130, 2013.

Sarman I: Review shows that early foetal alcohol exposure may cause adverse effects even when the mother consumes low levels, *Acta Paediatr* 107:938–941, 2018.

Sathyanarayana S, Alcedo G, Saelens BE, et al: Unexpected results in a randomized dietary trial to reduce phthalate and bisphenol a exposures, *J Expo Sci Environ Epidemiol* 23:378–384, 2013.

Sawo Y, Jarjou LM, Goldberg GR, et al: Bone mineral changes after lactation in Gambian women accustomed to a low calcium intake, *Euro J Clin Nutr* 67:1142–1146, 2013.

Sazawal S, Black RE, Dhingra P, et al: Zinc supplementation does not affect the breast milk zinc concentration of lactation women belonging to low socioeconomic population, *J Hum Nutr Food Sci* 1:1014, 2013.

Schisterman EF, Mumford SL, Browne RW, et al: Lipid concentrations and couple fecundity: the LIFE study, *J Clin Endocrinol Metab* 99:2786–2794, 2014.

Schmidt RJ, Kogan V, Shelton JF, et al: Combined prenatal pesticide exposure and folic acid intake in relation to autism spectrum disorder, *Environ Health Perspect* 125:097007, 2017.

Schofield K: The metal neurotoxins: an important role in current human neural epidemics? *Int J Environ Res Public Health* 14:E1511, 2017.

Scolari Childress KM, Myles T: Baking soda pica associated with rhabdo-myolysis and cardiomyopathy in pregnancy, *Obstet Gynecol* 122:495–497, 2013.

Scott C, Andersen CT, Valdez N, et al: No global consensus: a cross-sectional survey of maternal weight policies, *BMC Pregnancy Childbirth* 14:167, 2014.

Scotter MJ, Thorpe SA, Reynolds SL, et al: Survey of animal livers for vitamin a content, *Food Addit Contam* 9:237–242, 1992.

Selitsky T, Chandra P, Schiavello HJ: Wernicke's encephalopathy with hyperemesis and ketoacidosis, *Obstet Gynecol* 107:486–490, 2006.

Seneviratne SN, McCowan LM, Cutfield WS, et al: Exercise in pregnancies complicated by obesity: achieving benefits and overcoming barriers, *Am J Obstet Gynecol* 212:442–449, 2015.

Shankar P, Ahuja S, Sriram K: Non-nutritive sweeteners: review and update, *Nutrition* 29:1293–1299, 2013.

Shireman TI, Kerling EH, Gajewski BJ, et al: Docosahexaenoic acid supplementation (DHA) and the return on investment for pregnancy outcomes, *Prostaglandins Leukot Essent Fatty Acids* 111:8–10, 2016.

Siega-Riz AM, Gray GL: Gestational weight gain recommendations in the context of the obesity epidemic, *Nutr Rev* 71(Suppl 1):S26–S30, 2013.

Silasi M, Cardenas I, Kwon JY, et al: Viral infections during pregnancy, *Am J Reprod Immunol* 73:199–213, 2015.

Simeoni U, Armengaud JB, Siddeek B, et al: Perinatal origins of adult disease, *Neonatology* 113:393–399, 2018.

Smith MV, Gotman N, Yonkers KA: Early childhood adversity and pregnancy outcomes, *Matern Child Health J* 20:790–798, 2016.

Sohn K, Underwood MA: Prenatal and postnatal administration of prebiotics and probiotics, *Semin Fetal Neonatal Med* 22:284–289, 2017.

Spiller HA: Rethinking mercury: the role of selenium in the pathophysiology of mercury toxicity, *Clin Toxicol (Phila)* 56:313–326, 2018.

Stagnaro-Green A, Pearce E: Thyroid disorders in pregnancy, *Nat Rev Endocrinol* 8:650–658, 2012.

Stang J, Huffman LG: Position of the Academy of Nutrition and Dietetics: obesity, reproduction, and pregnancy outcomes, *J Acad Nutr Diet* 16:677–691, 2016.

Stephenson J, Heslehurst N, Hall J, et al: Before the beginning: nutrition and lifestyle in the preconception period and its importance for future health, *Lancet* 391:1830–1841, 2018.

Stone J, Kohari KS: Higher-order multiples, *Clin Obstet Gynecol* 58:668–675, 2015.

Størdal K, Mårild K, Tapia G, et al: Fetal and maternal genetic variants influencing neonatal vitamin D status, *J Clin Endocrinol Metab* 102:4072–4079, 2017.

Szymanski LM, Satin AJ: Strenuous exercise during pregnancy: is there a limit? *Am J Obstet Gynecol* 207:179.e1-e6, 2012.

Tande DL, Ralph JL, Johnson LK, et al: First trimester dietary intake, biochemical measures, and subsequent gestational hypertension among nulliparous women, *J Midwifery Womens Health* 58:423–430, 2013.

Teas J, Pino S, Critchley A, et al: Variability of iodine content in common commercially available edible seaweeds, *Thyroid* 14:836–841, 2004.

Temel S, van Voorst SF, Jack BW, et al: Evidence-based preconceptional lifestyle interventions, *Epidemiol Rev* 36:19–30, 2014.

Temple JL, Bernard C, Lipshultz SE, et al: The safety of ingested caffeine: a comprehensive review, *Front Psychiatry* 8:80, 2017.

Thaxter Nesbeth KA, Samuels LA, Nicholson Daley C, et al: Ptyalism in pregnancy - a review of epidemiology and practices, *Eur J Obstet Gynecol Reprod Biol* 198:47–49, 2016.

Torgerson PR, Mastroiacovo P: The global burden of congenital toxoplasmosis: a systematic review, *Bull World Health Organ* 91:501–508, 2013.

Trabace L, Tucci P, Ciuffreda L, et al: "Natural" relief of pregnancy-related symptoms and neonatal outcomes: above all do no harm, *J Ethnopharmacol* 174:396–402, 2015.

Trezevant MS, Winton JC, Holmes AK: Hypercalcemia-induced pancreatitis in pregnancy following calcium carbonate ingestion, *J Pharm Pract* 32(2):225–227, 2017. doi:10.1177/0897190017745410.

Trogstad L, Magnus P, Stoltenberg C: Pre-eclampsia: risk factors and causal models, *Best Pract Res Clin Obstet Gynaecol* 25:329–342, 2011.

Ulbricht C, Isaac R, Milkin T, et al: An evidence-based systematic review of stevia by the natural standard research collaboration, *Cardiovasc Hematol Agents Med Chem* 8:113–127, 2010.

United States Department of Health and Human Services: *Recommendations for the use of antiretroviral drugs in pregnant women with HIV infection and interventions to reduce perinatal HIV transmission in the United States*, 2018a. Available at: https://aidsinfo.nih.gov/guidelines/html/3/perinatal/513/counseling-and-management-of-women-living-with-hiv-who-breast-feed.

United States Department of Health and Human Services, Office on Women's Health: *Postpartum depression*, 2018b. Available at: https://www.women-shealth.gov/mental-health/mental-health-conditions/postpartum-depression.

Uriu-Adams JY, Scherr RE, Lanoue L, et al: Influence of copper on early development: prenatal and postnatal considerations, *Biofactors* 36:136–152, 2010.

Usadi RS, Legro RS: Reproductive impact of polycystic ovary syndrome, *Curr Opin Endocrinol Diabetes Obes* 19:505–511, 2012.

Uwaezuoke SN, Eneh CI, Ndu IK: Relationship between exclusive breastfeeding and lower risk of childhood obesity: a narrative review of published evidence, *Clin Med Insights Pediatr* 11:1179556517690196, 2017.

Vaivada T, Gaffey MF, Das JK, et al: Evidence-based interventions for improvement of maternal and child nutrition in low-income settings: what's new? *Curr Opin Clin Nutr Metab Care* 20:204–210, 2017.

Van der Zee B, de Wert G, Steegers EA, et al: Ethical aspects of paternal preconception lifestyle modification, *Am J Obstet Gynecol* 209:11–16, 2013.

Vanhees K, Vonhögen IG, van Schooten FJ, et al: You are what you eat, and so are your children: the impact of micronutrients on the epigenetic programming of offspring, *Cell Mol Life Sci* 71:271–285, 2014.

Vannuccini S, Clifton VL, Fraser IS, et al: Infertility and reproductive disorders: impact of hormonal and inflammatory mechanisms on pregnancy outcome, *Hum Reprod Update* 22:104–115, 2016.

Van Wijngaarden E, Thurston SW, Myers GJ, et al: Prenatal methyl mercury exposure in relation to neurodevelopment and behavior at 19 years of age in the Seychelles Child Development Study, *Neurotoxicol Teratol* 39:19–25, 2013.

Verd S, Nadal-Amat J, Gich I, et al: Salt preference of nursing mothers is associated with earlier cessation of exclusive breastfeeding, *Appetite* 54:233–236, 2010.

Victora CG, Bahl R, Barros AJ, et al: Breastfeeding in the 21st century: epidemiology, mechanisms, and lifelong effect, *Lancet* 387:475–490, 2016.

Vitner D, Harris K, Maxwell C, et al: Obesity in pregnancy: a comparison of four national guidelines, *J Matern Fetal Neonatal Med* 32(15):2580–2590, 2019. doi:10.1080/14767058.2018.1440546.

Vricella LK: Emerging understanding and measurement of plasma volume expansion in pregnancy, *Am J Clin Nutr* 106:1620S–1625S, 2017.

Wadhwa Desai R, Smith MA: Pregnancy-related listeriosis, *Birth Defects Res* 109:324–335, 2017.

Wakimoto P, Akabike A, King JC: Maternal nutrition and pregnancy outcome—a look back, *Nutrition Today* 50:221–2229, 2015.

Walker R, Bennett C, Blumfield M, et al: Attenuating pregnancy weight gain-what works and why: a systematic review and meta-analysis, *Nutrients* 10:E944, 2018. doi:10.3390/nu10070944.

Walter JR, Perng W, Kleinman KP, et al: Associations of trimester-specific gestational weight gain with maternal adiposity and systolic blood pressure at 3 and 7 years postpartum, *Am J Obstet Gynecol* 212:499.e1-e12, 2015.

Wendt A, Gibbs CM, Peters S, et al: Impact of increasing inter-pregnancy interval on maternal and infant health, *Paediatr Perinat Epidemiol* 26:239–258, 2012.

Werner EF, Froehlich RJ: The potential role for myoinositol in the prevention of gestational diabetes mellitus, *Am J Perinatol* 33:1236, 2016.

West D, Marasco L: *The breastfeeding mother's guide to making more milk*, New York, NY, 2009, McGraw Hill.

Wickens K, Barthow C, Mitchell EA, et al: Maternal supplementation alone with Lactobacillus rhamnosus HN001 during pregnancy and breastfeeding does not reduce infant eczema, *Pediatr Allergy Immunol* 29:296–302, 2018.

Wickens KL, Barthow CA, Murphy R, et al: Early pregnancy probiotic supplementation with Lactobacillus rhamnosus HN001 may reduce the prevalence of gestational diabetes mellitus: a randomised controlled trial, *Br J Nutr* 117:804–113, 2017.

World Health Organization: *Guideline: protecting, promoting and supporting breastfeeding in facilities providing maternity and newborn services*, 2017. Available at: http://apps.who.int/iris/handle/10665/259386.

World Health Organization: Guideline: *Updates on HIV and infant feeding: the duration of breastfeeding, and support from health services to improve feeding practices among mothers living with HIV*, 2016a. Available at: https://www.ncbi.nlm.nih.gov/books/NBK379872/.

World Health Organization: *Implementation guidance: protecting, promoting and supporting breastfeeding in facilities providing maternity and newborn services – the revised baby-friendly hospital initiative*, 2018a. Available at: http://www.who.int/nutrition/publications/infantfeeding/bfhi-implementation-2018.pdf.

World Health Organization: *Infant and young child feeding*, 2018b. Available at: http://www.who.int/news-room/fact-sheets/detail/infant-and-young-child-feeding.

World Health Organization: *WHO recommendations on antenatal care for a positive pregnancy experience*, 2016b. Available at: http://www.who.int/reproductivehealth/publications/maternal_perinatal_health/anc-positive-pregnancy-experience/en/.

Worthington P, Balint J, Bechtold M, et al: When is parenteral nutrition appropriate? *JPEN J Parenter Enteral Nutr* 41:324–377, 2017.

Wu G, Imhoff-Kunsch B, Girard AW: Biological mechanisms for nutritional regulation of maternal health and fetal development, *Paediatr Perinat Epidemiol* 26:4–26, 2012a.

Wu Q, Chen HL, Xu XJ: Violence as a risk factor for postpartum depression in mothers: a meta-analysis, *Arch Womens Ment Health* 15:107–114, 2012b.

Xu F, Li Z, Binns C, et al: Does infant feeding method impact on maternal mental health? *Breastfeed Med* 9:215–221, 2014.

Yajnik CS, Deshpande SS, Jackson AA, et al: Vitamin B12 and folate concentrations during pregnancy and insulin resistance in the offspring: the Pune Maternal Nutrition Study, *Diabetologia* 51:29–38, 2008.

Yang CZ, Yaniger SI, Jordan VC, et al: Most plastic products release estrogenic chemicals: a potential health problem that can be solved, *Environ Health Perspect* 119:989–996, 2011.

Younes JA, Lievens E, Hummelen R, et al: Women and their microbes: the unexpected friendship, *Trends Microbiol* 26:16–32, 2018.

Young SL: *Craving earth: understanding pica, the urge to eat clay, starch, ice, and chalk*, New York, NY, 2011, Columbia University Press.

Young SM, Gryder LK, Cross C, et al: Effects of placentophagy on maternal salivary hormones: a pilot trial, part 1, *Women Birth* 31:e245–e257, 2018a.

Young SM, Gryder LK, Cross C, et al: Placentophagy's effects on mood, bonding, and fatigue: a pilot trial, part 2, *Women Birth* 31:e258–e271, 2018b.

Young SM, Gryder LK, David WB, et al: Human placenta processed for encapsulation contains modest concentrations of 14 trace minerals and elements, *Nutr Res* 36:872–878, 2016a.

Young SM, Gryder LK, Zava D, et al: Presence and concentration of 17 hormones in human placenta processed for encapsulation and consumption, *Placenta* 43:86–89, 2016b.

Zeisel SH, Klatt KC, Caudill MA: Choline, *Adv Nutr* 9:58–60, 2018.

Zeisel SH: Nutrition in pregnancy: the argument for including a source of choline, *Int J Womens Health* 5:193–199, 2013.

Zhang GH, Chen ML, Liu SS, et al: Effects of mother's dietary exposure to acesulfame-K in pregnancy or lactation on the adult offspring's sweet preference, *Chem Senses* 36:763–770, 2011.

Zhang S, Regnault TR, Barker PL, et al: Placental adaptations in growth restriction, *Nutrients* 7:360–389, 2015.

Zhou K, West HM, Zhang J, et al: Interventions for leg cramps in pregnancy, *Cochrane Database Syst Rev* (8):CD010655, 2015.

Zhou L, Xiao X: The role of gut microbiota in the effects of maternal obesity during pregnancy on offspring metabolism, *Biosci Rep* 38:BSR20171234, 2018. doi:10.1042/BSR20171234.

Zielińska MA, Wesołowska A, Pawlus B, et al: Health effects of carotenoids during pregnancy and lactation, *Nutrients* 9:E838, 2017. doi:10.3390/nu9080838.

Zielinski R, Searing K, Deibel M: Gastrointestinal distress in pregnancy: prevalence, assessment, and treatment of 5 common minor discomforts, *J Perinat Neonatal Nurs* 29:23–31, 2015.

15

Nutrition in Infancy

Kelly N. McKean, MS, RDN, CSP, CD
Mari O. Mazon, MS, RDN, CD

KEY TERMS

alpha-lactalbumin
arachidonic acid (ARA)
baby-led weaning
casein
casein hydrolysate
catch-up growth
colostrum

docosahexaenoic acid (DHA)
early childhood caries (ECC)
electrolytically reduced iron
growth channel
lactoferrin
lag-down growth
oligosaccharides

palmar grasp
pincer grasp
renal solute load
secretory immunoglobulin A (sIgA)
whey proteins

During the first 2 years of life, which are characterized by rapid physical and social growth and development, many changes occur that affect feeding and nutrient intake. The adequacy of infants' nutrient intakes affects their interaction with their environment. Healthy, well-nourished infants have the energy to respond to and learn from the stimuli in their environment and to interact with their parents and caregivers in a manner that encourages bonding and attachment.

PHYSIOLOGIC DEVELOPMENT

The length of gestation, the mother's prepregnancy weight, and the mother's weight gain during gestation determine an infant's birth weight. After birth, the growth of an infant is influenced by genetics and nourishment. Most infants who are genetically determined to be larger reach their growth channel, a curve of weight and length or height gain throughout the period of growth, at between 3 and 6 months of age. However, many infants born at or below the tenth percentile for length may not reach their genetically appropriate growth channel until 1 year of age; this is called catch-up growth. Infants who are larger at birth and who are genetically determined to be smaller grow at their fetal rate for several months and often do not reach their growth channel until 13 months of age. This phenomenon during the first year of life is called lag-down growth.

Growth in infancy is monitored with the routine collection and monitoring of anthropometric data, including weight, length, head circumference, and weight-for-length for age. These are plotted on the appropriate World Health Organization (WHO) growth chart shown in Appendix 3. The WHO growth charts are used for the first 2 years of life and consist of a series of percentile curves that show the distribution of body measurements in infants and children in optimal growth conditions. When the anthropometric data are plotted on the growth charts, the percentiles rank the infant by showing what percentage of the reference population the infant would equal or exceed. For example, a 7-month-old infant girl who has a weight-for-age at the 75th percentile weighs the same or more than 75% of the reference population for 7-month-old girls and weighs less than 25% of the same population. It is important to monitor growth trends over time and not focus on one measurement.

Infants may lose approximately 7% of their body weight during the first few days of life, but their birth weight usually is regained by the seventh to tenth day. Weight loss of more than 10% in the newborn period indicates need for further assessment regarding adequacy of feeding. Growth thereafter proceeds at a rapid but decelerating rate. Infants usually double their birth weight by 4 to 6 months of age and triple it by the age of 1 year. The amount of weight gained by the infant during the second year approximates the birth weight. Infants increase their length by 50% during the first year of life and double it by 4 years. Total body fat increases rapidly during the first 9 months, after which the rate of fat gain tapers off throughout the rest of childhood. Total body water decreases throughout infancy from 70% at birth to 60% at 1 year. The decrease is almost all in extracellular water, which declines from 42% at birth to 32% at 1 year of age.

The stomach capacity of infants increases from a range of 10 to 20 mL at birth to 200 mL by 1 year, enabling infants to consume more food at a given time and at less frequent intervals as they grow older. During the first weeks of life, gastric acidity decreases and for the first few months remains lower than that of older infants and adults. The rate of emptying is relatively slow, depending on the size and composition of the meal. Because peristalsis and sphincter function along the digestive tract continue to mature during infancy, newborns often

Sections of this chapter were written by Cristine M. Trahms, MS, RDN, CD, FADA.

experience regurgitation (Singendonk et al, 2014). Reducing the volume at each feeding or keeping the infant upright immediately after a feeding can help reduce the risk of regurgitation.

Fat absorption varies in the neonate. Human milk fat is well absorbed, but butterfat is poorly absorbed, with fecal excretions of 20% to 48%. The fat combinations in commercially prepared infant formula are well absorbed. The infant's lingual and gastric lipases hydrolyze short- and medium-chain fatty acids in the stomach. Gastric lipase also hydrolyzes long-chain fatty acids and is important in initiating the digestion of triglycerides in the stomach. Most long-chain triglycerides pass unhydrolyzed into the small intestine, where they are broken down by pancreatic lipase. The bile salt–stimulated lipase present in human milk is stimulated by the infant's bile salts and hydrolyzes the triglycerides in the small intestine into free fatty acids and glycerol. Bile salts, which are effective emulsifiers when combined with monoglycerides, fatty acids, and lecithin, aid in the intestinal digestion of fat.

The activities of the enzymes responsible for the digestion of disaccharides—maltase, isomaltase, and sucrase—reach adult levels by 28 to 32 weeks' gestation. Lactase activity (responsible for digesting the disaccharide in milk) reaches adult levels by birth. Pancreatic amylase, which digests starch, continues to remain low during the first 6 months after birth. If the infant consumes starch before this time, increased activity of salivary amylase and digestion in the colon usually compensate.

The neonate has functional but physiologically immature kidneys that increase in size and concentrating capacity in the early weeks of life. The kidneys double in weight by 6 months and triple in weight by 1 year of age. The last renal tubule is estimated to form between the eighth fetal month and the end of the first postnatal month. The glomerular tuft is covered by a much thicker layer of cells throughout neonatal life than at any later time, which may explain why the glomerular filtration rate is lower during the first 9 months of life than it is in later childhood and adulthood. In the neonatal period the ability to form acid, urine, and concentrate solutes is often limited. The renal concentrating capacity at birth may be limited to as little as 700 mOsm/L in some infants. Others have the concentrating capacity of adults (1200 to 1400 mOsm/L). By 6 weeks, most infants can concentrate urine at adult levels. Renal function in a normal newborn infant is rarely a concern; however, difficulties may arise in infants with diarrhea or those who are fed formula that is too concentrated.

NUTRIENT REQUIREMENTS

Nutrient needs of infants reflect rates of growth, energy expended in activity, basal metabolic needs, and the interaction of the nutrients consumed. Balance studies have defined minimum acceptable levels of intakes for a few nutrients, but for most nutrients the suggested intakes have been extrapolated from the intakes of normal, thriving infants consuming human milk. The dietary reference intakes (DRIs) for infants are shown in the inside cover of this book.

Energy

Full-term infants who are breastfed to satiety or who are fed a standard infant formula generally adjust their intake to meet their energy needs when caregivers are sensitive to the infant's hunger and satiety cues. An effective method for determining the adequacy of an infant's energy intake is to monitor carefully gains in weight, length, head circumference, and weight-for-length for age and plot these data on the WHO growth charts shown in Appendix 3. During the first year a catch-up or lag-down period in growth may occur.

If infants begin to experience a decrease in their rate of weight gain, do not gain weight, or lose weight, their energy and nutrient intake should be monitored carefully. If the rate of growth in length decreases or ceases, potential malnutrition, an undetected disease, or both should be investigated thoroughly. If the weight gain proceeds at a much more rapid rate than growth in length, the energy concentration of the formula, the quantity of formula consumed, and the amount and type of semisolid and table foods offered should be evaluated. The activity level of the infant also should be assessed. Infants who are at the highest end of the growth charts for weight-for-length, or who grow rapidly in infancy, tend to be at greater risk for obesity later in life (Druet et al, 2012).

The equations to calculate the estimated energy requirement (EER) for infants 0 to 12 months of age are in Table 15.1. The EER includes the total energy expenditure plus energy needed for growth for healthy infants with normal growth (see Chapter 2).

Protein

Protein is needed for tissue replacement, deposition of lean body mass, and growth. Protein requirements during the rapid growth of infancy are higher per kilogram of weight than those for older children or adults (Table 15.2). Recommendations for protein intake are based on the composition of human milk, and it is assumed that the efficiency of human milk use is 100%.

Infants require a larger percentage of total amino acids as essential amino acids than do adults. Histidine seems to be an essential amino acid for infants, but not for adults, and tyrosine, cystine, and taurine may be essential for premature infants (Pencharz and Ball, 2006; see Chapter 41).

Human milk or infant formula provides the major portion of protein during the first year of life. The amount of protein in human milk is adequate for the first 6 months of life, even though the amount of protein in human milk is considerably less than in infant formula. From 6 months of age the diet should be supplemented with additional sources of high-quality protein, such as yogurt, strained meats, pureed legumes, mashed egg yolk, pureed fish with low mercury content (i.e., salmon, chunk light tuna, pollock, cod, and perch), or cereal

TABLE 15.1   Equations for Calculating Estimated Energy Requirement (EER) for Infants

Age	Calculation
0-3 months	(89 × Weight of infant [kg] − 100) + 175
4-6 months	(89 × Weight of infant [kg] − 100) + 56
7-12 months	(89 × Weight of infant [kg] − 100) + 22

From Institute of Medicine: *Dietary reference intakes for energy, carbohydrate, fiber, fat, fatty acids, cholesterol, protein, and amino acids*, Washington, DC, 2002/2005, The National Academies Press.

TABLE 15.2   Protein Dietary Reference Intakes (DRIs) for Infants

Age	Grams/Day	Grams/Kilogram/Day
0-6 months	9.1	1.52
6-12 months	11	1.2

From Institute of Medicine: *Dietary reference intakes for energy, carbohydrate, fiber, fat, fatty acids, cholesterol, protein, and amino acids*, Washington, DC, 2002/2005, The National Academies Press.

mixed with formula or human milk. A complete list of low mercury seafood can be found on the Food and Drug Administration (FDA) website under "Eating fish: What pregnant women and parents need to know."

Infants may not receive adequate protein if their formula is excessively diluted for a prolonged period, or if they have multiple food allergies and are placed on a restricted diet without appropriate medical or nutritional supervision (see Chapter 25).

Lipids

Lipids provide a large proportion of infants' energy intakes in order to meet the energy demands for rapid growth. The current adequate intake is 31 g of fat per day from birth to 6 months and 30 g of fat per day for infants 7 to 12 months. This is based on the average fat intakes from breastmilk for infants from birth to 6 months and the average fat intakes from breastmilk and complementary foods for infants 7 to 12 months. Significantly lower fat intakes (e.g., with skim-milk feedings) may result in an inadequate total energy intake. An infant may try to correct the energy deficit by increasing the volume of milk ingested but usually cannot make up the entire deficit this way.

Human milk contains the essential fatty acids linoleic acid and alpha-linolenic acid, as well as the longer-chain derivatives arachidonic acid (ARA) (C20:4ω-6) and docosahexaenoic acid (DHA) (C22:6ω-3). While ARA content of human milk is mostly consistent and unaffected by the mother's diet, DHA content does reflect the mother's intakes and is found in a wide range of concentrations in human milk (Carlson and Colombo, 2016). See Chapter 14 *Focus On*: Omega-3 Fatty Acids in Pregnancy and Lactation. Infant formulas are supplemented with linoleic acid and alpha-linolenic acid, from which ARA and DHA are derived. Except for a few specialty products, standard formulas for term infants in the United States now also are supplemented with ARA and DHA, although there are no regulatory requirements for their inclusion.

Linoleic acid is essential for growth and dermal integrity. The adequate intake for infants has been set based on the average linoleic acid intake from breastmilk, or 4.4 g/day for infants younger than 6 months of age and based on the average intake from breastmilk and complementary foods, or 4.6 g/day for infants 7 months to 1 year of age. The human milk content of linoleic acid varies based on the mother's diet; its caloric contribution can range from approximately 6% to 10% of breastmilk's energy content. The Infant Formula Act of 1980 requires that at least 2.7% of infant formula's total energy be from linoleic acid. Safflower, corn, and soybean oil are good sources of linoleic acid. The current recommendation for alpha-linolenic acid is 0.5 g/day during the first year of life. This is based on the average intakes from breastmilk for infants 0 to 6 months and average intakes from breastmilk and complementary foods for infants 7 to 12 months. Flaxseed, chia seed, canola oil, and soybean oil are good sources of alpha-linolenic acid.

The concentration of DHA in human milk varies, depending on the amount of DHA in the mother's diet. DHA and ARA are the major omega-3 and omega-6 long-chain polyunsaturated fatty acids (LCPUFAs) of neural tissues, and DHA is the major fatty acid of the photoreceptor membranes of the retina. Studies looking at visual, neurodevelopmental, or growth outcomes in formula-fed term infants on DHA- or ARA-supplemented formula have shown mixed results (Jasani et al, 2017). Studies are finding that the ratio of DHA to ARA added to formula may be critical (Carlson and Colombo, 2016). The American Academy of Pediatrics (AAP) has not taken an official stand on the addition of LCPUFAs to infant formula.

Carbohydrates

Carbohydrates should supply 30% to 60% of the energy intake during infancy. Approximately 40% of the energy in human milk and 40% to 50% of the energy in infant formulas is derived from lactose or other carbohydrates. Although rare, some infants cannot tolerate lactose and require a modified formula in their diet (see Chapters 27 and 42).

The adequate intake for birth to 6 months is 60 g/day. This is based on the average carbohydrate intake from human milk. The adequate intake for 7 months to 12 months is 95 g/day. This is based on the average carbohydrate intake from human milk and complementary foods. Grains (cereal, pasta, rice), starchy vegetables (peas, corn, potatoes), and sugar from fruits provide natural sources of carbohydrates.

Botulism in infancy is caused by the ingestion of *Clostridium botulinum* spores, which germinate and produce toxins in the bowel lumen. Infant botulism has been associated with eating honey that contains the bacterial spores. Light and dark corn syrups also have been reported to contain the spores, although cases of infant botulism have not been linked to corn syrup. The spores are extremely resistant to heat treatment and are not destroyed by current methods of processing. Thus honey and corn syrup should not be fed to infants younger than 1 year of age because they have not yet developed the immunity required to resist botulism spore development.

Water

The water requirement for infants is determined by the amount lost from the skin and lungs and in the feces and urine, in addition to a small amount needed for growth. The recommended total water intake for infants, based on the DRIs, is 0.7 L/day for infants up to 6 months and 0.8 L/day for infants 6 to 12 months of age. Note that total water includes all water contained in food, beverages, and drinking water. Fluid recommendations per kilogram of body weight are shown in Table 15.3.

Because the renal concentrating capacity of young infants may be less than that of older children and adults, they may be vulnerable to developing a water imbalance. Under ordinary conditions, human milk and formula that is properly prepared supply adequate amounts of water. However, when formula is boiled, the water evaporates and the solutes become concentrated; therefore, boiled milk or formula is inappropriate for infants. In very hot and humid environments, infants may require additional water. When losses of water are high (e.g., vomiting and diarrhea), infants should be monitored carefully for fluid and electrolyte imbalances.

Water deficits result in hypernatremic dehydration and its associated neurologic consequences (e.g., seizures, vascular damage). Hypernatremic dehydration has been reported in breastfed infants who lose greater than 10% of their birth weight in the first few days of life (Panagoda et al, 2015). Because of the potential for hypernatremic dehydration, careful monitoring of volume of intake, daily weights,

TABLE 15.3 Maintenance Fluid Requirements of Infants and Children (Holliday-Segar Method)

Body Weight	Fluid Requirement
0-10 kg	100 mL/kg
11-20 kg	1000 mL + 50 mL/kg for each kg above 10 kg
>20 kg	1500 mL + 20 mL/kg for each kg above 20 kg

From Holliday MA, Segar WE. The maintenance need for water in parenteral fluid therapy. *Pediatrics* 19:823-832, 1957.

and hydration status (e.g., number of wet diapers) in all newborns is warranted.

Water intoxication results in hyponatremia, restlessness, nausea, vomiting, diarrhea, and polyuria or oliguria; seizures also can result. This condition may occur when water is provided as a replacement for milk, the formula is excessively diluted, or bottled water is used instead of an electrolyte solution in the treatment of diarrhea.

Minerals

Calcium

Breastfed infants retain approximately two thirds of their calcium intake. The recommended adequate intake (AI), the mean intake, is based on calcium intakes in healthy breastfed infants. The AI for infants 0 to 6 months of age is 200 mg/day; the AI for infants 6 to 12 months of age is 260 mg/day; formulas contain more calcium per volume than human milk to assure similar levels of calcium absorption (see Appendix 39). During the first year of life, human milk or infant formula is the major source of calcium. Cow's milk or milk alternatives are not appropriate substitutes. Calcium-fortified cereal, yogurt, tofu, and cheese are good sources of calcium.

Fluoride

The importance of fluoride in preventing dental caries has been well documented. However, excessive fluoride may cause dental fluorosis, ranging from fine white lines to entirely chalky teeth (see Chapter 24). To prevent fluorosis, the tolerable upper intake level for fluoride has been set at 0.7 mg/day for infants up to 6 months and 0.9 mg/day for infants 6 to 12 months of age. Fluoride concentration of 0.7 ppm (0.7 mg/L) in drinking water has been proposed as being optimal for safety and caries prevention (Academy of Nutrition and Dietetics [AND], 2012). Fluoride content of water supplies can be obtained through local public health departments or water utilities. Fluoride containing toothpaste should be used sparingly—just a smear on a toothbrush (American Academy of Pediatric Dentistry [AAPD], 2014).

Human milk is very low in fluoride. Infants who exclusively consume infant formula reconstituted with fluoridated water may be at increased risk of developing mild fluorosis (Centers for Disease Control and Prevention [CDC], 2015). Using water that is free of or low in fluoride, which are waters labeled "purified," "demineralized," "deionized," "distilled," or "produced through reverse-osmosis," may decrease this risk. Other dietary sources of fluoride during infancy include commercially prepared infant cereals and wet pack cereals processed with fluoridated water. Fluoride supplementation is not recommended for infants younger than 6 months of age, and after 6 months of age is recommended only if an infant is at high risk of developing dental caries and drinks insufficiently fluoridated water (AND, 2012). After tooth eruption it is recommended that fluoridated water be offered several times per day to breastfed infants, those who receive cow's milk, and those fed formulas made with water that contain less than 0.3 mg of fluoride/L (AAP, 2014b).

Iron

Full-term infants are considered to have adequate stores of iron for growth up to a doubling of their birth weight. This occurs at approximately 4 months of age in full-term infants and much earlier in prematurely born infants. Recommended intakes of iron increase according to age, growth rate, and iron stores. At 4 to 6 months of age, infants who are fed only human milk are at risk for developing a negative iron balance and may deplete their reserves by 6 to 9 months. Iron in human milk is highly bioavailable; however, breastfed infants should receive an additional source of iron by 4 to 6 months of age (AAP, 2012). For breastfed term infants, the AAP recommends iron supplementation of 1 mg/kg/day starting at 4 months of age and continuing until appropriate complementary foods have been introduced (AAP, 2014b). Complementary foods high in iron include strained meats and iron-fortified infant cereals. In addition, by 6 months of age offering one serving of vitamin C-rich foods per day enhances iron absorption from nonheme sources such as tofu, beans, peas, lentils, and eggs. Formula-fed infants receive adequate iron from formula. Cow's milk is a poor source of iron and should not be given before 12 months of age.

Iron deficiency and iron deficiency anemia are common health concerns for the older infant. Between 6 and 24 months of age, because of rapid growth, iron requirements per kilogram of body weight are higher than at any other period of life. Risk factors associated with a higher prevalence of iron deficiency anemia include low birth weight, low intake of iron-rich complementary foods, high intake of cow's milk, low socioeconomic status, and immigrant status.

Monitoring iron status is important because of the long-term cognitive effects of iron deficiency in infancy. There is consistent association between iron deficiency anemia in infancy and long-lasting poor cognition, developmental deficits, and behavioral performance (Domellöf et al, 2014). Thus it is important that this dietary advice reaches high-risk groups to prevent these significant long-term effects (see Appendix 42 and Chapter 31).

Zinc

Zinc is critical for growth and development. The AI is 2.0 mg for infants 0 to 12 months. During the first 6 months of life, human milk or infant formula provides adequate zinc. Although zinc is better absorbed from human milk than from infant formula, the zinc content of human milk decreases during the first 6 months. A dietary source of zinc becomes necessary for breastfed infants at this time. Good sources of zinc with high bioavailability include red meat, eggs, yogurt, and cheese. The presence of phytic acid makes plant sources of zinc (grains, legumes, nut products) less bioavailable. Infants who are zinc deficient can exhibit growth impairment (Terrin et al, 2015; see Appendix 47).

Vitamins

Vitamin B$_{12}$

Milk from lactating mothers who follow a strict vegan diet may be deficient in vitamin B$_{12}$, especially if the mother followed the regimen for a long time before and during her pregnancy. Vitamin B$_{12}$ deficiency has also been diagnosed in infants breastfed by mothers with pernicious anemia (Roumeliotis et al, 2012; see Chapter 32). During infancy, signs of vitamin B$_{12}$ deficiency include inadequate growth, reflux or feeding difficulties, hypotonia, developmental regression, and movement disorders (Fadilah et al, 2017; see Appendix 31). Good food sources of vitamin B$_{12}$ include animal products, including fish, meat, poultry, eggs, milk, and milk products. Vitamin B$_{12}$ is generally not present in plant foods, but some foods are fortified with vitamin B$_{12}$, such as breakfast cereals, meat substitutes, nondairy milks, and nutritional yeast products.

Vitamin D

The vitamin D content of breastmilk is correlated to the vitamin D status of the mother. Studies have shown that high maternal intakes of vitamin D, supplemented 2000 IU to 6400 IU per day, were associated with higher breastmilk vitamin D concentrations. However, infants of mothers supplemented with 2000 IU per day or more have similar serum concentrations as infants receiving a vitamin D supplement of 400 IU per day (Munns et al, 2016). The current recommended dietary allowance (RDA) for vitamin D for lactating mothers is 600 IU per day, and the tolerable upper limit is 4000 IU per day. Coupled with the AAP's recommendation to keep all infants under the age of 6 months out of direct sunlight, exclusively and partially breastfed infants are at high risk for vitamin D deficiency (AAP, 2016). For the prevention of rickets and vitamin D deficiency, a minimum vitamin D intake of 400 IU per day shortly after birth is recommended for all infants. All breastfed infants need a vitamin D supplement of 400 IU per day. Formula-fed infants who consume less than 1000 mL of formula per day also need supplementation (Antonucci et al, 2018).

There appears to be a higher risk of rickets among unsupplemented, breastfed infants and children with dark skin. Because a variety of environmental and family lifestyle factors can affect sunlight exposure and absorption of vitamin D, the AAP recommendations to provide supplemental vitamin D are appropriate for all infants. Supplementation up to 800 IU of vitamin D per day may be needed for infants at higher risk, such as premature infants, dark-skinned infants and children, and those who reside in northern latitudes or at higher altitudes (Antonucci et al, 2018; see Appendix 38).

Vitamin K

The vitamin K requirements of the neonate need special attention. Deficiency may arise because newborns do not store vitamin K and their gut bacteria is not developed enough to supply the needed amount. Low vitamin K can happen in any infant, regardless of gender or ethnicity, and results in bleeding or hemorrhagic disease. This condition is more common in breastfed infants than in formula-fed infants because human milk contains only 2.5 mcg/L of vitamin K, whereas cow's milk–based formulas contain approximately 20 times this amount. All infant formulas contain a minimum of 4 mcg of vitamin K per 100 kcal of formula. The AI for infants is 2 mcg/day during the first 6 months and 2.5 mcg/day during the second 6 months of life. This can be supplied by mature breastmilk, although perhaps not during the first week of life. For breastfed infants, vitamin K supplementation is necessary during that time to considerably decrease the risk for hemorrhagic disease. Most hospitals require that infants receive an injection of vitamin K as a prophylactic measure shortly after birth (CDC, 2017).

Supplementation

Vitamin and mineral supplements should be prescribed only after careful evaluation of the infant's intake. Commercially prepared infant formulas are fortified with all necessary vitamins and minerals; therefore formula-fed infants rarely need supplements. Breastfed infants need additional vitamin D supplementation shortly after birth, and iron by 4 to 6 months of age (see *Focus On:* Vitamin and Mineral Supplementation Recommendations for Full-Term Infants). Chapter 41 discusses the feeding of premature or high-risk infants and their special needs. Chapter 11 discusses more about dietary supplementation.

Analysis of dietary intakes of infants in the United States indicate they are generally adequate, but the likelihood of inadequacy increases beyond 1 year of age. Iron is the main nutrient of concern in the older infant, 6 to 12 months of age, with about 1 in 5 older infants below the estimated average requirement (EAR) with a general trend of consuming less iron-fortified cereal as they approach 1 year of age (Bailey et al, 2018). Supplemental iron may be necessary if unable to increase iron intake from food sources.

MILK

Human Milk

Human milk is unquestionably the food of choice for the infant. Its composition is designed to provide the necessary energy and nutrients in appropriate amounts. It contains specific and nonspecific immune factors that support and strengthen the immature immune system of the newborn and thus protect the body against infections. Human milk also helps prevent diarrhea and otitis media (AAP, 2012). Allergic reactions to human milk protein are rare. Moreover, the closeness of the mother and infant during breastfeeding facilitates attachment and bonding (see Fig. 14.11 in Chapter 14) and breastmilk provides nutritional benefits (e.g., optimal nourishment in an easily digestible and bioavailable form), decreases infant morbidity, provides maternal health benefits (e.g., lactation amenorrhea, maternal weight loss, some cancer protection), and has economic and environmental benefits (Lessen and Kavanagh, 2015; see Chapter 14).

During the first few days of life, a breastfeeding infant receives colostrum, a yellow, transparent fluid that meets the infant's needs during the first week. It contains less fat and carbohydrate, but more protein and greater concentrations of sodium, potassium, and chloride than mature milk. It is also an excellent source of immunologic substances.

Note that breastfeeding may not be appropriate for mothers with certain infections or those who are taking medications that may have untoward effects on the infant. For example, a mother who is infected with human immunodeficiency virus can transmit the infection to the infant, and a mother using psychotropic drugs or other pharmacologic drugs may pass the medication to the infant through her breastmilk (AAP, 2012; see Chapter 14).

The Academy of Nutrition and Dietetics (AND) and the AAP support exclusive breastfeeding (EBF) for the first 6 months of life and then breastfeeding supplemented by complementary foods until at least 12 months (AAP, 2012; Lessen and Kavanagh, 2015). It is important to note the ages of the infants in these recommendations; adding other foods at too young of an age decreases breastmilk intake and increases early weaning. Healthy Children 2020 objectives support breastfeeding among mothers of newborn infants (see *Focus On: Healthy Children 2020 Objectives: Nourishment of Infants*).

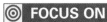 **FOCUS ON**

Healthy Children 2020 Objectives: Nourishment of Infants

Healthy People 2020 is a comprehensive set of health objectives for the United States to achieve during the second decade of the twenty-first century. Healthy People 2020 identifies a wide range of public health priorities and specific, measurable objectives. The objectives have 42 focus areas, one of which is Maternal, Infant, and Child Health. The objectives related to nourishment of infants are as follows:

GOAL: Improve the health and well-being of women, infants, children, and families.

Objective: Increase the proportion of infants who are breastfed to 81.9% in the early postpartum period, to 60.6% at 6 months, and to 34.1% at 1 year of age. Increase the proportion of infants that are exclusively breastfed to 46.2% through 3 months of age and 25.5% through 6 months of age.

Objective: Reduce the proportion of breastfed newborns who receive formula supplementation within the first 2 days of life to 14.2%.

GOAL: Promote health and reduce chronic disease risk through the consumption of healthful diets and achievement and maintenance of healthy body weights.

Objective: Eliminate very low food security among children.

Objective: Reduce iron deficiency among children ages 1-2 years to less than 14.3%.

GOAL: Prevent and control oral and craniofacial diseases, conditions, and injuries and improve access to preventive services and dental care.

Objective: Reduce the proportion of young children with dental caries in their primary teeth.

The complete text of the Healthy People 2020 Objectives can be found on the Office of Disease Prevention and Health Promotion Website under HealthyPeople.gov.

Composition of Human and Cow's Milk

The composition of human milk is different from that of cow's milk; for this reason, unmodified cow's milk is not recommended for infants until at least 1 year of age. Both provide approximately 20 kcal/oz; however, the nutrient sources of the energy are different. Protein provides about 6% of the energy in human milk and 20% of the energy in cow's milk. Human milk is 60% **whey proteins** (mainly lactalbumins) and 40% casein; by contrast, cow's milk is 20% whey proteins and 80% casein. **Casein** forms a tough, hard-to-digest curd in the infant's stomach, whereas **alpha-lactalbumin** in human milk forms soft, flocculent, easy-to-digest curds. Taurine and cystine are present in higher concentrations in human milk than in cow's milk; these amino acids may be essential for premature infants. Lactose provides 40% of the energy in human milk and only 30% of the energy in cow's milk (Lawrence and Lawrence, 2016).

Lipids provide about 50% of the energy in human and whole cow's milk. Linoleic acid, an essential fatty acid, provides 4% of the energy in human milk and only 1% to 2% in cow's milk. The cholesterol content of human milk is 10 to 20 mg/dL compared with 10 to 15 mg/dL in whole cow's milk. Less fat is absorbed from cow's milk than from human milk; a lipase in human milk is stimulated by bile salts and contributes significantly to the hydrolysis of milk triglycerides (Lawrence and Lawrence, 2016).

All of the water-soluble vitamins in human milk reflect maternal intake. Cow's milk contains adequate quantities of the B-complex vitamins, but little vitamin C. Human milk and supplemented cow's milk provide sufficient vitamin A. Human milk is a richer source of vitamin E than cow's milk.

The quantity of iron in human and cow's milk is small (0.3 mg/L). Approximately 50% of the iron in human milk is absorbed, whereas less than 10% of the iron in cow's milk is absorbed. The bioavailability of zinc in human milk is higher than in cow's milk. Cow's milk contains four times as much calcium, six times as much phosphorus as human milk, and three times the total salt content of human milk (Lawrence and Lawrence, 2016).

The much higher protein and mineral content of cow's milk results in a higher **renal solute load**, or amount of nitrogenous waste and minerals that must be excreted by the kidney. The sodium and potassium concentrations in human milk are about one third those in cow's milk, contributing to the lower renal solute load of human milk. The osmolality of human milk averages 300 mOsm/kg, whereas that of cow's milk is 350 mOsm/kg (Lawrence and Lawrence, 2016).

Antiinfective Factors

Human milk and colostrum contain antibodies and antiinfective factors that are not present in infant formulas. **Secretory immunoglobulin A (sIgA)**, the predominant immunoglobulin in human milk, plays a role in protecting the infant's immature gut from infection by keeping viruses and bacteria from invading the mucosa. Breastfeeding should be maintained until the infant is at least 3 months of age to obtain this benefit (Lawrence and Lawrence, 2016).

The iron-binding protein **lactoferrin** in human milk deprives certain iron-dependent bacteria in the gastrointestinal tract of iron and thus slows their growth. Lysozymes, which are bacteriolytic enzymes found in human milk, destroy the cell membranes of bacteria after the peroxides and ascorbic acid that are also present in human milk have inactivated them. They also have a significant role in the development of intestinal flora (Lawrence and Lawrence, 2016). Human milk enhances the growth of the bacterium *Lactobacillus bifidus*, which produces an acidic gastrointestinal (GI) environment that interferes with the growth of certain pathogenic organisms. Because of these antiinfective factors, the incidence of infections is lower in breastfed infants than in formula-fed infants.

The Microbiome and Probiotics and Prebiotics

Colonization with nonpathogenic microbiota is important for infant health and affects health and disease in later life. This colonization is necessary for normal immune system development. A disturbance in this process may contribute to immune disease such as food allergies, atopic dermatitis, and asthma. The development of gut microbiota in infancy occurs during a critical window. By 3 years of age, the human GI tract has established its normal flora or microbiome, with the majority of this occurring in the first year of life. This ecosystem in early life is influenced by such factors as mode of birth (cesarean vs. vaginal delivery), environment, human milk vs. formula feeding, introduction to solids, and use of antibiotics (Tanaka and Nakayama, 2017). Breastfeeding and introduction of whole foods can greatly assist in establishing a healthy microbiome for life.

Probiotics are microorganisms that, when administered as an oral supplement or as part of food, may confer health benefits to the host by changing the gut microbiome. Studies have looked at the effects of postnatal probiotic supplementation on the prevention of atopic disease such as asthma, eczema, and allergic rhinitis. Results have been mixed, depending on the strain of probiotics used, and whether the mother also was supplemented during pregnancy (Elazab et al, 2013).

Evidence is emerging that supplementing term infants with the probiotic *Lactobacillus reuteri* (*L. reuteri*) may decrease their risk of colic, gastroesophageal reflux, and constipation (Indrio et al, 2014). However, supplementation with *L. reuteri* does not appear to be effective in treating colic. In fact, a well-controlled study found no reduction in crying or fussiness in colicky infants receiving the probiotic. Interestingly the formula-fed infants who were given *L. reuteri* actually fussed more than formula-fed infants given placebo (Sung et al, 2014). The effectiveness of supplemental probiotic use is still under study. Although probiotics have been found generally to be safe, their content may be variable under current FDA regulation (Van den Nieuwboer et al, 2014). Similar caution should be used as when using other nutrition supplements. See Chapter 11.

Prebiotics are nondigestible food ingredients that promote the growth of the gut's bacteria. Human milk contains prebiotics in the form of oligosaccharides, which are highly abundant and unique to human milk. The addition of short-chain gluco-oligosaccharides and long-chain fructo-oligosaccharides to infant formula results in gut microflora more similar to those of human milk-fed infants (Oozeer et al, 2013). The AAP has no official stance on the addition of probiotics or prebiotics to infant formula. Some infant formulas in the United States are now supplemented with probiotics or prebiotics.

Formulas

Infants who are not breastfed are fed an infant formula based on cow's milk or a soy product. Many mothers may choose to offer a combination of breastmilk and formula feedings.

Commercial formulas made from heat-treated nonfat milk or a soy product and supplemented with vegetables fats, vitamins, and minerals are formulated to approximate, as closely as possible, the composition of human milk. They provide the necessary nutrients in an easily absorbed form. The manufacture of infant formulas is regulated by the FDA through the Infant Formula Act (FDA, 2015). By law, infant formulas are required to have a nutrient level that is consistent with these guidelines. They were most recently updated in 2015 to add minimum and maximum levels of selenium (Table 15.4). Refer to individual manufacturers' websites to obtain the most accurate information and compare the composition of various infant formulas and feeding products. Organic infant formulas are increasingly available, and they must also meet all standards required for United States Department of Agriculture Organic certification. Homemade infant formulas are not recommended.

Various products are available for infants who cannot tolerate the protein in cow's milk–based formulas. Soy-based infant formulas are recommended for (1) term infants in vegetarian families, (2) term infants with galactosemia or hereditary primary lactase deficiency, and (3) term infants with documented immunoglobulin E-associated allergy to cow's milk who are not also allergic to soy protein. In many cases, an infant may be allergic to both, and soy formula would not be appropriate. Soy-based formulas are not recommended (1) for preterm infants because of the increased risk of osteopenia and aluminum content, (2) for the prevention of colic or allergy, or (3) for infants with cow's milk protein-induced enterocolitis or enteropathy (AAP, 2014b; see Chapter 25).

The protein in soy infant formula is soy protein isolate supplemented with L-methionine, L-carnitine, and taurine. A concern raised about soy formula includes its content of phytates, which may impair the absorption of minerals and trace elements. Exposure to higher levels of phytoestrogens, isoflavones, and aluminum and their potential health consequences have also been areas of discussion. Aluminum from mineral salts is found in soy infant formulas at concentrations of 500 to 2500 ng/mL, levels that exceed aluminum concentrations in human milk of 4 to 65 ng/mL and in cow's milk formula of 15 to

TABLE 15.4　Nutrient Levels in Infant Formulas as Specified by the Infant Formula Act

Specified Nutrient Component	Minimum Level Required (per 100 kcal of Energy)
Protein (g)	1.8
Fat (g)	3.3
Percentage of calories from fat	30
Linoleic acid (mg)	300
Percentage of calories from linoleic acid	2.7
Vitamin A (IU)	250
Vitamin D (IU)	40
Vitamin E (IU)	0.7
Vitamin K (mcg)	4
Thiamin (B_1) (mcg)	40
Riboflavin (B_2) (mcg)	60
Pyridoxine (B_6) (mcg)	35
Vitamin B_{12} (mcg)	0.15
Niacin (mcg)	250
Folic acid (mcg)	4
Pantothenic acid (mcg)	300
Biotin (mcg) (nonmilk-based formulas only)	1.5
Vitamin C (Ascorbic acid) (mg)	8
Choline (mg) (nonmilk-based formulas only)	7
Inositol (mg) (nonmilk-based formulas only)	4
Calcium (mg)	60
Phosphorus (mg)	30
Magnesium (mg)	6
Iron (mg)	0.15
Zinc (mg)	0.5
Manganese (mcg)	5
Copper (mg)	60
Iodine (mg)	5
Selenium (mcg)	2
Sodium (mg)	20
Potassium (mg)	80
Chloride (mcg)	55

From Food and Drug Administration: Electronic Code of Federal Regulations: Title 21:107, Infant Formulas, Final Rule (21 CFR 107), *Fed Reg* 50:45108, 1985. *Amended Fed Reg* 80:35841, 2015.

400 mg/mL. This appears to be of no concern except for preterm infants and infants with renal failure. A systematic review with meta-analysis of infants consuming soy formula found that the patterns of growth; bone health; and metabolic, reproductive, endocrine, immune, and neurologic functions were similar to those of infants fed human milk or cow's milk-based formula (Vandenplas et al, 2014).

Infants who cannot tolerate cow's milk–based or soy products can be fed formulas made from a casein hydrolysate, which is casein that has been split into smaller components by treatment with acid, alkali, or enzymes. These formulas do not contain lactose. For infants who have severe food protein intolerances and cannot tolerate hydrolysate formulas, free amino acid–based formulas are available. Hydrolysate and free amino acid–based formulas often contain some medium-chain triglycerides (MCT) as a portion of the fat, which is helpful in certain malabsorptive conditions. Other formulas are available for children with problems such as malabsorption or metabolic disorders (e.g., phenylketonuria) (see Box 25.9 in Chapter 25).

Formulas are also available for older infants and toddlers. However, "older infant" formulas are usually unnecessary unless toddlers are not receiving adequate amounts of infant or table foods.

Whole Cow's Milk

Some parents may choose to transition their infant from formula to fresh cow's milk before 1 year of age. However, the AAP Committee on Nutrition has concluded that infants should not be fed whole cow's milk during the first year of life (AAP, 2014b). Infants who are fed whole cow's milk have been found to have lower intakes of iron, linoleic acid, and vitamin E, and excessive intakes of sodium, potassium, and protein. Cow's milk may cause a small amount of GI blood loss. When introduced at 1 year of age, only pasteurized cow's milk and milk products should be offered (AAP, 2014a).

Low-fat (1% to 2%) and nonfat milk are also inappropriate for infants during the first 12 months of life. The infants may ingest excessive amounts of protein in large volumes of milk in an effort to meet their energy needs, and the decreased amount of essential fatty acids may be insufficient for preventing deficiency (AAP, 2014b). Substitute or imitation milks such as soy, rice, oat, or nut milks are also inappropriate during the first year of life due to their low content of calories, fat, vitamins, and minerals.

Formula Preparation

Commercial infant formulas are available in ready-to-feed forms that require no preparation, as concentrates prepared by mixing with equal parts of water, and in powder form that is designed to be mixed with 2 oz of water per level scoop of powder.

Infant formulas should be prepared in a clean environment. All equipment, including bottles, nipples, mixers, and the top of the can of formula, should be washed thoroughly. Water used for mixing infant formula must be from a safe water source. If there is concern or uncertainty about the safety of tap water, bottled water may be used or cold water may be boiled for 1 minute (no longer), then cooled to room temperature for no more than 30 minutes before it is used. Boiling water will kill bacteria but will not remove toxic chemicals. Well water should be tested for nitrates before giving it to infants under 1 year of age (AAP, 2014b).

Formula may be prepared for up to a 24-hour period and refrigerated. Formula for each feeding should be warmed in a hot water bath. Microwave heating is not recommended because of the risk of burns from formula that is too hot or unevenly heated. Any formula offered and not consumed at that feeding should be discarded and not reused later, because of bacterial contamination from the infant's mouth.

Bisphenol-A (BPA) is a chemical that was present in many hard plastic bottles, such as baby bottles and reusable cups, and metal food and beverage containers, including canned liquid infant formula. Due to concerns about the potential effects of BPA on the brain, behavior, and prostate gland in fetuses, infants, and young children, BPA has not been used to make bottles, infant feeding cups, or infant formula packaging for the U.S. market since 2013.

FOOD

Infants can meet their nutrition needs from homemade or commercial infant food. Some families choose to offer a combination of both.

BOX 15.1 Directions for Home Preparation of Infant Foods

1. Select fresh, high-quality fruits, vegetables, or meats.
2. Be sure that all utensils, including cutting boards, grinder, knives, and other items, are thoroughly cleaned.
3. Wash hands before preparing the food.
4. Clean, wash, and trim the food in as little water as possible.
5. Cook the foods until tender in as little water as possible. Avoid overcooking, which may destroy heat-sensitive nutrients.
6. Do not add salt or sugar. Do not add honey to food intended for infants younger than 1 year of age.[*]
7. Add enough water for the food to be easily puréed.
8. Strain or purée the food using an electric blender, a food mill, a baby food grinder, or a kitchen strainer.
9. Pour purée into an ice cube tray and freeze.
10. When the food is frozen hard, remove the cubes and store in freezer bags.
11. When ready to serve, defrost and heat in a serving container the amount of food that will be consumed at a single feeding.

[*]*Clostridium botulinum* spores, which cause botulism, have been reported in honey; young infants do not have the immune capacity to resist this infection.

Families who would like to make their own infant food can do so easily by following the directions in Box 15.1. Home-prepared foods generally are more concentrated in nutrients than commercially prepared foods because less water is used. Salt and sugar should not be added to foods prepared for infants. Dry infant cereals are fortified with electrolytically reduced iron, which is iron that has been fractionated into small particles for improved absorption. Four level tablespoons of cereal provide approximately 5 mg of iron, or approximately half the amount the infant requires. Therefore infant cereal is usually the first food added to the infant's diet. Rice and rice products have been found to contain arsenic, but at levels that are safe to be consumed as part of a varied diet (FDA, 2016).

Most strained ("Stage 1" or "Stage 2") and junior ("Stage 3") meats are prepared with water. Strained meats, which have the highest energy density of any of the commercial baby foods, are an excellent source of high-quality protein and heme iron. Vegetable and fruit baby foods provide carbohydrates and vitamins A and C. Vitamin C is added to numerous commercial fruit products. Stage 1 fruits and vegetables are typically single-ingredient, whereas Stage 2 and Stage 3 foods may contain additional ingredients such as grain or dairy.

Baby yogurts are usually full fat and fortified with vitamin D and are good sources of calcium. They are available plain or flavored with pureed fruits or vegetables. Some may have added sweeteners, which most infants do not need in their diet. They often contain thickeners such as pectin, tapioca starch, or flour.

Various commercially prepared foods and organically grown products are available for infants. See *Focus On: Is Organic Produce Healthier?* in Chapter 8 for a discussion of organic foods. These products vary widely in their nutrient value. Foods for infants should be thoughtfully selected to meet their nutritional and developmental needs.

Previously, families were advised to delay introducing potentially allergenic foods such as dairy, peanuts, egg whites, and fish until after the first birthday. Allergy experts now say that for infants with no family history of food allergy, there is no reason to delay introducing these foods, and in fact introducing these foods before the infant's first birthday may have protective effects against developing food allergies later in life (Fleischer et al, 2013).

FEEDING

Early Feeding Patterns

Because milk from a mother with an adequate diet is designed uniquely to meet the needs of the human infant, breastfeeding for the first 6 months of life is recommended strongly. Most chronic medical conditions do not contraindicate breastfeeding.

A mother should be encouraged to nurse her infant immediately after birth. Those who care for and counsel parents during the first postpartum days should acquaint themselves with ways in which they can be supportive of breastfeeding. Ideally, counseling and preparation for breastfeeding starts in the last few months or weeks of pregnancy (see Chapter 14).

Regardless of whether infants are breastfed or formula fed, they should be held and cuddled during feedings. Once a feeding rhythm has been established, infants become fussy or cry to indicate they are hungry, whereas they often smile and fall asleep when they are satisfied (Table 15.5). Infants, not adults, should establish the feeding schedules. Feeding schedules vary widely among infants, with breastfed infants tending to feed more frequently than formula-fed infants. Initially, most infants feed every 2 to 3 hours; by 2 months of age most feed every 3 to 4 hours. By 6 months of age infants usually are able to consume enough during the day to allow the parent or caregiver to omit night feedings. Infants may feed more frequently during periods of rapid growth.

Development of Feeding Skills

At birth, infants coordinate sucking, swallowing, and breathing, and are prepared to suckle liquids from the breast or bottle but are not able to handle foods with texture. During the first year, typical infants develop head control, the ability to move into and sustain a sitting posture, and the ability to grasp, first with a palmar grasp and then with a refined pincer grasp (Fig. 15.1, *B*). They develop mature sucking and rotary chewing abilities and progress from being fed to feeding themselves using their fingers. In the second year, they learn to feed themselves independently with a spoon (Fig. 15.2).

Addition of Semisolid Foods

Developmental readiness and nutrient needs are the criteria that determine appropriate times for the addition of various foods. During the first 4 months of life, the infant attains head and neck control, and oral motor patterns progress from a suck to a suckling to the beginnings of a mature sucking pattern. For the first 6 months of life, breastmilk or infant formula is adequate as the sole source of nutrition. Table 15.6 lists developmental landmarks and their indications for semisolid and table food introduction.

Around 6 months of age, when the mature sucking movement is refined and munching movements (up-and-down chomping motions) begin, the introduction of strained or pureed foods is appropriate. To support developmental progress, pureed food is offered to the infant from a spoon, not combined with formula in a bottle and not directly from a squeezable pouch (see Fig. 15.1, *A*). The sequence in which these foods are introduced is not important; however, it is important that one single ingredient food (e.g., peaches, not peach yogurt, which has many ingredients) be introduced at a time. Introducing a single new food at a time at 2- to 7-day intervals enables parents to identify any allergic responses or food intolerances. Introducing vegetables before fruits may increase vegetable acceptance. Foods introduced may vary depending on country of origin and culture of the family.

Infants demonstrate their acceptance of new foods by slowly increasing the variety and quantity of solids they accept. Breastfed infants seem to accept greater flavor varieties than do formula-fed infants

TABLE 15.5   Hunger and Satiety Behaviors in Infants

Approximate Age	Hunger Cue	Satiety Cue
Birth through 5 months	Wakes and tosses Sucks on fist Fusses or cries Opens mouth while feeding to show wants more	Falls asleep Turns head away Seals lips together Decreases rate of sucking or stops sucking Purses lips, bites nipple, spits nipple out, or smiles and lets go
4 months through 6 months	Fusses or cries Smiles, coos, gazes at caregiver during feeding Moves head toward spoon Tries to swipe food toward mouth	Distracted or pays more attention to surroundings Turns head away Bites nipple or spits it out Decreases rate of sucking or stops sucking Obstructs mouth with hands
5 months through 9 months	Reaches for food Points to food	Rate of feeding slows down Pushes food away Keeps mouth tightly closed Changes posture Uses hands more actively
8 months through 11 months	Gets excited when food is presented Reaches for food Points to food	Clenches mouth shut Pushes food away Rate of feeding slows down Shakes head to say "no more" Plays with utensils, throws utensils
10 months through 12 months	Expresses desire for specific food with words or sounds	Hands bottle or cup to caregiver Shakes head to say "no more" Sputters with tongue and lips

Modified from U.S. Department of Agriculture: *Infant Nutrition and Feeding: a Guide for Use in the WIC And CSF Programs*, Washington DC, 2009.

(Harris and Coulthard, 2016). Parents who thoughtfully offer a variety of nourishing foods are more likely to provide a well-balanced diet and help their children learn to accept more flavors.

As oral-motor maturation proceeds, an infant's rotary chewing ability develops, indicating a readiness for more textured foods such as well-cooked mashed vegetables, casseroles, and pasta from the family menu. Learning to grasp—with the palmar grasp, then with an inferior pincer grasp, and finally with the refined pincer grasp—indicates a readiness for finger foods such as oven-dried toast or arrowroot biscuits (see Fig. 15.1, *B*). Table 15.6 presents recommendations for adding foods to an infant's diet. Foods with skins or rinds and foods that stick to the roof of the mouth (e.g., hot dogs, grapes, nut butters) may cause choking and should not be offered to young infants.

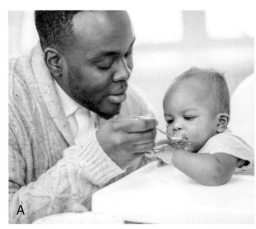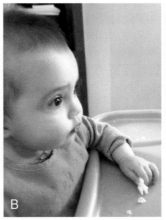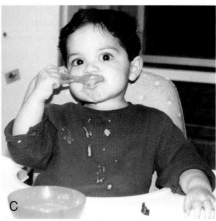

Fig. 15.1 Development of feeding skills in infants and toddlers. **A,** This 6 month old is showing hunger and readiness for the next bite by leaning into the spoon. **B,** This 8-month-old girl is using a refined pincer grasp to pick up her food. **C,** This 19-month-old boy is beginning to use his spoon independently, although he is not yet able to rotate his wrist to keep food on it. (A. From www.istockphoto.com.)

TABLE 15.6 Feeding Behaviors: Developmental Landmarks During the First 2 Years of Life

Developmental Landmarks	Age (MO)	Change Indicated	Examples of Appropriate Foods
Tongue laterally transfers food in the mouth Shows voluntary and independent movements of the tongue and lips Sitting posture can be sustained Shows beginning of chewing movements (up and down movements of the jaw)	6	Introduction of soft, mashed table food	Canned, boneless, skinless fish such as chunk light tuna or salmon (avoid albacore tuna for mercury content); mashed potatoes; well-cooked, mashed vegetables; ground meats in gravy and sauces; mashed beans or pieces of tofu; soft, diced fruit such as bananas, peaches, and pears; yogurt
Reaches for and grasps objects with palmar grasp Brings hand to mouth	6-9	Finger feeding (large pieces of food)	Oven-dried toast, teething biscuits
Approximates lips to rim of the cup	6-9	Introduction of cup for sipping liquids	Water, breastmilk, or infant formula. Juice and cow's milk are not recommended during the first year.
Voluntarily releases food (refined digital [pincer] grasp)	9-12	Finger feeding (small pieces of food)	Bits of cottage cheese, dry cereal, peas, beans, and other bite-size vegetables; small pieces of meat
Shows rotary chewing pattern	9-12	Introduction of food of varied textures from family menu	Well-cooked, chopped meats and casseroles; cooked vegetables and canned fruit (not mashed); toast; potatoes; macaroni, spaghetti; peeled ripe fruit
Understands relationship of container and its contents	9-12	Beginning of self-feeding (though messiness should be expected)	Food that when scooped adheres to the spoon, such as applesauce, cooked cereal, porridge, mashed potatoes, cottage cheese, yogurt
Shows increased movements of the jaw Shows development of ulnar deviation of the wrist	12-18	More skilled at cup and spoon feeding	Chopped fibrous meats, such as roast and steak; raw vegetables and fruit (introduced gradually)
Walks alone	12-18	May seek food and obtain food independently	Mixed textures, food from the family meal; foods of high nutritional value
Names food, expresses preferences; prefers unmixed foods Goes on food jags Appetite appears to decrease	18-24		Balanced food choices, with child permitted to develop food preferences (parents should not be concerned that these preferences will last forever)

Modified from Trahms CM, Pipes P: *Nutrition in infancy and childhood*, ed 6, New York, 1997, McGraw-Hill.

Baby-led weaning is a practice that is becoming popular among parents in industrialized, Western countries, in which parents offer finger foods that infants self-feed as first foods. Some families strictly offer finger foods whereas others choose to offer a combination of finger foods and purees from a spoon. With careful attention to the infant's developmental readiness and the food's texture and nutrition content, infants fed with baby-led weaning can achieve appropriate growth, meet nutrition needs, and avoid choking (Taylor et al, 2017). See Box 15.2 for more on baby-led weaning.

BOX 15.2 Baby-Led Weaning

Baby-led weaning is a philosophy which promotes infants self-feeding all complementary foods. Infants appropriate for this are able to sit unassisted, have a palmar grasp, and bring food to their mouth, which often happens around 6 months of age.

Special attention should be paid to minimize choking risk, and to ensure the infant meets energy and nutrient needs, specifically iron. Some general guidelines for baby-led weaning include:

- Foods should be mashable between tongue and roof of the mouth or tough enough that they do not break off, such as strips of meat
- Do not offer foods that form a crumb in mouth
- Foods should be as long as infant's fist, at least on one side
- Infants should be sitting upright and always supervised
- Never place an entire food into the infant's mouth. Infants should control how much food they put into their mouth.
- Offer the following foods at each meal:
  - Iron-rich food
  - Energy-rich food
  - Fruit or vegetable
- When an infant is ill, increase breastmilk or formula feeding frequency and offer foods that infant can easily eat.

Although baby-led weaning has been promoted as decreasing risk of childhood overweight because infants learn to self-regulate their intakes better, studies have not supported this claim.

Modified from Taylor RW, Williams SM, Fangupo LJ, et al: Effect of a baby-led approach to complementary feeding on infant growth and overweight: a randomized clinical trial, *JAMA* Pediatr 171:838–846, 2017.

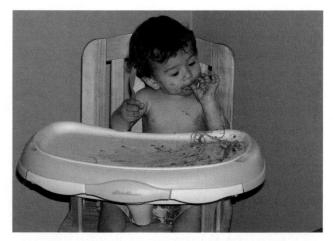

Fig. 15.3 This 14-month-old girl is learning to self-feed; it's normal to be messy.

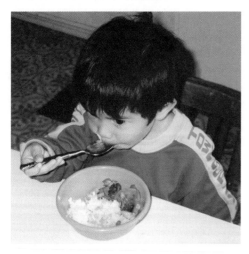

Fig. 15.2 This 2-year-old is skilled at self-feeding because he has the ability to rotate his wrist and elevate his elbow to keep food on the spoon.

During the last quarter of the first year, infants can approximate their lips to the rim of the cup and can drink if the cup is held for them. During the second year they gain the ability to rotate their wrists and elevate their elbows, thus allowing them to hold the cup themselves and manage a spoon (see Fig. 15.1, *C*). They are very messy eaters at first (Fig. 15.3), but by 2 years of age most typical children skillfully feed themselves (see Fig. 15.2).

Weaning from Breast or Bottle to Cup

The introduction of solids into an infant's diet begins the weaning process in which the infant transitions from a diet of only breastmilk or formula to a more varied one. Weaning should proceed gradually and be based on the infant's rate of growth and developmental skills. Weaning foods should be chosen carefully to complement the nutrient needs of the infant, promote appropriate nutrient intake, and maintain growth.

Many infants begin the process of weaning with the introduction of the cup at approximately 6 to 9 months of age and complete the process when they are able to ingest an adequate amount of milk or formula from a cup at 18 to 24 months of age. Parents of infants who are breastfed may choose to transition the infant directly to a cup or have an intermittent transition to a bottle before the cup is introduced.

Early Childhood Caries

Dental caries is the most common chronic disease of childhood (AAP, 2014c). **Early childhood caries (ECC)**, or "baby bottle tooth decay" is a pattern of tooth decay that involves the upper anterior and sometimes lower posterior teeth. ECC is common among infants and children who are allowed to bathe their teeth in sugar (sucrose or lactose) throughout the day and night. If infants are given sugar-sweetened beverages or fruit juice in a bottle during the day or at bedtime after teeth have erupted, the risk of dental caries increases (see Chapter 24).

To promote dental health, infants should be fed and burped and then put to bed without milk or food. Juice should not be introduced into the diet before 12 months of age unless clinically indicated. Juice should be limited to, at most, 4 oz/day for toddlers 1 through 3 years of age and only offered from a cup (Heyman and Abrams, 2017). Parents and caregivers can be taught effective oral health practices for infants, not only by dentists but also by other paraprofessionals (Edelstein, 2017).

Feeding Older Infants

Typically developing children have a natural ability to eat. They eat as much as they need, they grow in the way that is right for them, and they learn to eat the foods their parents eat. As infants transition toward family food, the parent is responsible for what is offered and when and where they eat. The child is responsible for how much and whether to eat the foods that are offered. This is known as the division of responsibility in feeding proposed by the Satter Feeding Dynamics Model. Based on what the child can do, not on how old they are, parents guide their children through transitions from nipple feeding as a young infant to eventually eating table foods at family meals (Satter, 2000). Table 15.6 highlights appropriate feeding based on developmental landmarks.

As maturation proceeds and the rate of growth slows down, infants' interest in and approach to food changes. Between 9 and 18 months of age most reduce their breastmilk or formula intake. They can become finicky about what and how much they eat.

In the weaning stage infants have to learn many skills, including the ability to chew and swallow solid food and use utensils. They learn to tolerate various textures and flavors of food, eat with their fingers, and then feed themselves with a utensil. Very young children should be encouraged to feed themselves (see *Clinical Insight:* A Look at the Food Practices of Infants and Toddlers).

CLINICAL INSIGHT

A Look at the Food Practices of Infants and Toddlers

The Feeding Infants and Toddlers Study was a national random sample of more than 2500 infants and toddlers from 4 to 24 months of age and their mothers.

- Assuming that a variety of nutritious foods are offered to infants and toddlers, parents and caregivers should encourage self-feeding without concern for compromising energy intake and nutrient adequacy (Carruth et al, 2004b).
- Parents and caregivers should offer a variety of fruits and vegetables daily; sweets, desserts, sweetened beverages, and salty snacks should be offered only occasionally. Because family food choices influence the foods offered to infants, family-based approaches to healthy eating habits should be encouraged (Fox et al, 2004).
- By 24 months of age, 50% of toddlers were described as picky eaters. When offering a new food, caregivers must be willing to provide 8 to 15 repeated exposures to enhance acceptance of that food (Carruth et al, 2004a).
- Infants and toddlers have an innate ability to regulate energy intake. Parents and caregivers should understand the cues of hunger and satiety and recognize that coercive admonitions about eating more or less food can interfere with the infant's or toddler's innate ability to regulate energy intake (Fox et al, 2006).
- On average, infants and toddlers were fed seven times per day, and the percentage of children reported to be eating snacks increased with age. Snack choices for infants and toddlers could be improved by delaying the introduction of and limiting foods that have a low nutrient content and are energy dense (Skinner et al, 2004).

At the beginning of a meal, children are hungry and should be allowed to feed themselves; when they become tired, they can be helped quietly. Emphasis on table manners and the fine points of eating should be delayed until they have the necessary maturity and developmental readiness for such training.

The food should be in a form that is easy to handle and eat. Meat should be cut into bite-size pieces. Potatoes and vegetables should be mashed so that they can be eaten easily with a spoon. Raw fruits and vegetables should be in sizes that can be picked up easily. In addition, the utensils should be small and manageable. Cups should be easy to hold, and dishes should be designed so that they do not tip over easily.

Type of Food

In general, children prefer simple, uncomplicated foods. Food from the family meal can be adapted for the child and served in child-size portions. Children younger than 6 years of age usually prefer mild-flavored foods. Because a young child's stomach is small, a snack may be required between meals. Children ages 2 to 6 years often prefer raw instead of cooked vegetables and fruits.

Infants should be offered foods that vary in texture and flavor. Infants who are accustomed to many kinds of foods are less likely to limit their variety of food choices later. To add variety to an infant's diet, vegetables and fruits can be added to cereal feedings. In order to ensure a nutritionally adequate diet, it is important to offer a variety of age appropriate foods and textures. Older infants generally reject unfamiliar foods the first time they are offered. When parents continue to offer small portions of these foods without comment, infants become familiar with them and often accept them. It may take 8 to 15 repeated exposures before acceptance of the food (Carruth et al, 2004a). It is important that fruit juice does not replace more nutrient-dense foods. If excessive amounts of juice are consumed, children may fail to thrive.

Serving Size

The size of a serving of food offered to a child is very important. At 1 year of age infants eat one third to one half the amount an adult normally consumes. This proportion increases to one half an adult portion by the time the child reaches 3 years of age and increases to about two thirds by 6 years of age. Young children should not be served a large plateful of food; the size of the plate and the amount should be in proportion to their age. A tablespoon (not a heaping tablespoon) of each food for each year of age is a good guide to follow. Serving less food than parents think or hope will be eaten helps children eat successfully and happily. They will ask for more food if their appetite is not satisfied. As soon as they are able, encourage young children to serve themselves.

Forced Feeding

Children should not be forced to eat; instead, the cause for the unwillingness to eat should be determined. A typical, healthy child eats without coaxing. Children may refuse food because they are too inactive to be hungry or too active and overtired. To avoid overfeeding and underfeeding, parents should be responsive to the cues for hunger and satiety offered by the infant. A child who is fed snacks or given a bottle too close to mealtime (within 90 minutes) is not hungry for the meal and may refuse it.

Parents who support the development of self-feeding skills respond to the infant's need for assistance and offer encouragement for self-feeding; they also allow the infant to initiate and guide feeding interactions without pressure on the infant for neatness in self-feeding or amount of food consumed. If a child refuses to eat, the family meal should be completed without comment, and the plate should be removed. This procedure is usually harder on the parent than on the child. At the next mealtime, the child will be hungry enough to enjoy the food presented.

Eating Environment

Young children should eat their meals at the family table; it gives them an opportunity to learn table manners while enjoying meals with a family group. Sharing the family fare strengthens ties and makes mealtime pleasant. However, if the family meal is delayed, the children should receive their meals at the usual time. When children eat with the family, everyone must be careful not to make unfavorable comments about any food. Children are great imitators of the people they admire; thus, if the father or older siblings make disparaging remarks about squash, for example, young children are likely to do the same.

CLINICAL CASE STUDY

Arvan is a 10-month-old East Indian infant who was born full-term and has been a generally well child. He was referred to see a registered dietitian nutritionist (RDN) due to parents' concerns about his growth and that he "isn't eating enough."

Assessment

Arvan was breastfed from birth until 6 months of age. His mother says her milk supply decreased after returning to work, so she began supplementing with standard infant formula. She says that Arvan would not finish a bottle on his own so had to be force-fed.

Solids were introduced at 6 months of age. Arvan's mother started with ragi (finger millet) mixed with formula. She says that Arvan would eat only a little bit, so again had to be force-fed with a lot of distractions so he would "eat enough."

Arvan's mother says that he is no longer breastfed, and that she and his grandparents have to chase him around the house to get him to finish a bottle of formula. Lately, the distraction feeding has not been working, and Arvan refuses to open his mouth after only taking a few bites of food. She says that parents or grandparents feed him all meals, and that she herself was fed until she was 3 years of age. She says that Arvan often will try to grab the spoon, but the family does not let him feed himself because it creates a mess.

Arvan's mother describes a typical day as the following. She says all meals take close to an hour and involve distractions, coaxing, and sometimes forcing:

7 am: 8 oz. of formula offered, usually finishes all 8 oz.

9 am: Parent or grandparent offers 2 idlis (lentil and rice cake) and ½ large banana. Arvan eats 1 idli and ¼ banana.

11:30 am: 8 oz. of formula offered, finishes about 6 oz.

Nap

1:30 pm: Parent or grandparent offers ½ cup dalia (bulgur) porridge with milk, sugar, ghee (clarified butter), and ground nuts. Arvan eats about 3 tablespoons.

3:30 pm: 8 oz. of formula of offered, finishes about 6 oz.

6:00 pm: Parent or grandparent offers ½ cup vegetable khichadi (peas, potatoes, rice, lentils). Arvan eats about ¼ cup.

8:00 pm: 8 oz. of formula offered, finishes about 6 oz.

Diet analysis: 700 kcal, 17 g protein, 500 mg calcium, 300 IU vitamin D, 11 mg iron

Anthropometrics:

Weight (without clothes or diaper): 9.2 kg (~50th percentile)

Length: 77.0 cm (~95th percentile)

Weight-for-length: between 10th and 25th percentiles

Growth history: Arvan's weight was following around the 75th percentile from birth until 6 months of age. At his 9-month well-child visit, his weight percentile had decreased to about the 50th percentile. His length has consistently followed around the 95th percentile since birth. A very gradual decrease in weight-for-length percentiles from the 25th percentile at birth is noted.

Supplements/medications: None

Laboratories: None

Estimated needs: 740 kcal, 14 g protein, 260 mg calcium, 400 IU vitamin D, 11 mg iron

Nutrition Diagnostic Statements

- Inadequate energy intake related to discordant feeding relationship as evidenced by history of force-feeding, gradual decline in weight-for-length percentile, and intakes below estimated needs.
- Inadequate vitamin D related to food and nutrition knowledge deficit about dietary sources of vitamin D and inadequate food intake as evidenced by vitamin D intake below the AI of 400 IU/d.

Intervention

- Commend Arvan's mother on providing a structured meal schedule and offering nutrition-rich, age-appropriate foods, and encourage her to continue doing so.
- Counsel Arvan's mother about typical infant serving sizes and suggest offering him smaller portions at the beginning of meals. Encourage Arvan to be the one to dictate how much or how little he will eat.
- Explore with Arvan's mother ways to help Arvan develop his self-feeding skills while minimizing mess. Finger foods, drop-mats, remove clothes during mealtimes, etc. Point out that Arvan is asserting his desire to feed himself by grabbing the spoon and refusing to be fed by others.
- Educate Arvan's mother about infant hunger and fullness cues and how to respect those cues when spoon-feeding. Suggest that Arvan be given a spoon of his own that he can practice with thick foods such as yogurt or pudding.
- Encourage Arvan's mother to share these recommendations with all family members who feed him.
- Recommend a baby/children's liquid vitamin D supplement that does not exceed 1000 IU/day.

Monitoring/Evaluation

Follow-up in 6 to 8 weeks to monitor the following:

- Weight, length, weight-for-length percentiles, with goal of preventing further decrease in weight-for-length percentile.
- Energy, protein, calcium, vitamin D, iron intakes using 3-day food record or 24-hour recall, with goal of meeting estimated needs and micronutrient DRIs
- Parent/grandparent-child feeding relationship, with goal of diminishing use of distractions, having Arvan's hunger/fullness cues respected, and encouraging self-feeding skills development

USEFUL WEBSITES

American Academy of Pediatrics
Bright Futures: Nutrition in Practice
CDC and WHO Growth Charts
Healthy People 2020: Objectives for Improving Health
University of Washington Assuring Pediatric Nutrition in the Hospital and Community

REFERENCES

Academy of Nutrition and Dietetics, Palmer CA, Gilbert JA: Position of the Academy of Nutrition and Dietetics: the impact of fluoride on health, *J Acad Nutr Diet* 112:1443–1453, 2012.

American Academy of Pediatric Dentistry: *Reference manual, clinical guidelines, guideline on fluoride therapy*, 37:176–179, 2014.

American Academy of Pediatrics, Committee on Infectious Diseases, Committee on Nutrition: Consumption of raw or unpasteurized milk and milk products by pregnant women and children, *Pediatrics* 133:175–179, 2014a.

American Academy of Pediatrics, Committee on Nutrition: *Pediatric nutrition*, ed 7, Elk Grove Village, IL, 2014b, American Academy of Pediatrics.

American Academy of Pediatrics, Council on Environmental Health, Section on Dermatology: Ultraviolet radiation—a hazard to children and adolescents, *Pediatrics* 127:588–597, 2011 (reaffirmed Sept 2016).

American Academy of Pediatrics, Section on Breastfeeding: Breastfeeding and the use of human milk, *Pediatrics* 129:e827–e841, 2012.

American Academy of Pediatrics, Section on Oral Health: Maintaining and improving the oral health of young children, *Pediatrics* 134:1224–1229, 2014c.

Antonucci R, Locci C, Clemente MG, et al: Vitamin D deficiency in childhood—old lessons and current challenges, *J Pediatr Endocrinol Metab* 31:247–260, 2018.

Bailey RL, Catellier DJ, Jun S, et al: Total usual nutrient intakes of US children (under 48 months): findings from the feeding infants and toddlers study (FITS) 2016, *J Nutr* 148:1557S–1566S, 2018.

Carlson SE, Colombo J: Docosahexaenoic acid and arachidonic acid nutrition in early development, *Adv Pediatr* 63(1):453–471, 2016.

Carruth BR, Ziegler PJ, Gordon A, et al: Prevalence of picky eaters among infants and toddlers and their caregivers' decisions about offering a new food, *J Am Diet Assoc* 104:S57–S64, 2004a.

Carruth BR, Ziegler PJ, Gordon A, et al: Developmental milestones and self-feeding behaviors in infants and toddlers, *J Am Diet Assoc* 104:S51–S56, 2004b.

Centers for Disease Control and Prevention: *Facts about vitamin K deficiency bleeding*, 2017. Available at: https://www.cdc.gov/ncbddd/vitamink/facts.html.

Centers for Disease Control and Prevention: Overview: *infant formula and fluorosis*, 2015. Available at: http://fluoridealert.org/wp-content/uploads/cdc.infant-formula-fluorosis.july2015.pdf.

Domellöf M, Braegger C, Campoy C, et al: Iron requirements of infants and toddlers, *J Pediatr Gastroenterol Nutr* 58:119–129, 2014.

Druet C, Stettler N, Sharp S, et al: Prediction of childhood obesity by infancy weight gain: an individual-level meta-analysis, *Paediatr Perinat Epidemiol* 26:19–26, 2012.

Edelstein BL: Pediatric dental-focused interprofessional interventions—rethinking early childhood oral health management, *Dent Clin N orth Am* 61:589–606, 2017.

Elazab N, Mendy A, Gasana J, et al: Probiotic administration in early life, atopy, and asthma: a meta-analysis of clinical trials, *Pediatrics* 132: e666–e676, 2013.

Fadilah A, Musson R, Ong MT, et al: Vitamin B12 deficiency in infants secondary to maternal deficiency: a case series of seven infants, *EJPN* 21:e3, 2017.

Fleischer DM, Spergel JM, Assa'ad AH, et al: Primary prevention of allergic diseases through nutritional interventions, *J Allergy Clin Immunol: In Practice* 1:29–36, 2013.

Food and Drug Administration: FDA statement on testing and analysis of arsenic in rice and rice products, 2016. Available at: https://www.fda.gov/food/metals/fda-statement-testing-and-analysis-arsenic-rice-and-rice-products.

Food and Drug Administration: Electronic Code of Federal Regulations; Title 21:107, Infant Formulas, Final Rule (21 CFR 107), *Fed Reg* 50:45108, 1985. Amended Fed Reg 80:35841, 2015.

Fox MK, Devaney B, Reidy K, et al: Relationship between portion size and energy intake among infants and toddlers: evidence of self-regulation, *J Am Diet Assoc* 106:S77–S83, 2006.

Fox MK, Pac S, Devaney B, et al: Feeding infants and toddlers study: What foods are infants and toddlers eating? *J Am Diet Assoc* 104:S22–S30, 2004.

Harris G, Coulthard H: Early eating behaviours and food acceptance revisited: breastfeeding and introduction of complementary foods as predictive of food acceptance, *Curr Obes Rep* 5:113–120, 2016.

Heyman MB, Abrams SA, American Academy of Pediatrics Section on Gastroenterology, Hepatology, and Nutrition, et al: Fruit juice in infants,

children, and adolescents: current recommendations, *Pediatrics* 139: e20170967, 2017.

Indrio F, Di Mauro A, Riezzo G, et al: Prophylactic use of a probiotic in the prevention of colic, regurgitation, and functional constipation: a randomized clinical trial, *JAMA Pediatr* 168:228–233, 2014.

Jasani B, Simmer K, Patole SK, et al. Long chain polyunsaturated fatty acid supplementation in infants born at term, *Cochrane Database Syst Rev* 3:CD000376, 2017. doi:10.1002/14651858.CD000376.pub4.

Lawrence RA, Lawrence RM. *Breastfeeding: a guide for the medical profession*, 8 ed, Philadelphia, PA, 2016, Elsevier, Inc.

Lessen R, Kavanagh K: Position of the Academy of Nutrition and Dietetics: promoting and supporting breastfeeding, *J Acad Nutr Diet* 115:444–449, 2015.

Munns CF, Shaw N, Kiely M, et al: Global consensus recommendations on prevention and management of nutritional rickets, *J Clin Endocrinol Metab* 101:394–415, 2016.

Oozeer R, van Limpt K, Ludwig T, et al: Intestinal microbiology in early life: specific prebiotics can have similar functionalities as human-milk oligosaccharides, *Am J Clin Nutr* 98:561S–571S, 2013.

Panagoda R, De Cure N, McCuaig R, et al: Neonatal hypernatraemic dehydration, *J Paediatr Child Health* 51(6):653–654, 2015.

Pencharz PB, Ball RO: Amino acid requirements of infants and children, *Nestle Nutr Workshop Ser Pediatr Program* 58:109–116, 2006.

Roumeliotis N, Dix D, Lipson A: Vitamin B12 deficiency in infants secondary to maternal causes, *CMAJ* 184:1593–1598, 2012.

Satter E: *Child of mine—feeding with love and good sense*, revised ed, Palo Alto, CA, 2000, Bull Publishing Co.

Singendonk MM, Rommel N, Omari TI, et al: Upper gastrointestinal motility: prenatal development and problems in infancy, *Nat Rev Gastroenterol Hepatol* 11:545–555, 2014.

Skinner JD, Ziegler P, Pac S, et al: Meal and snack patterns of infants and toddlers, *J Am Diet Assoc* 104:S65–S70, 2004.

Sung V, Hiscock H, Tang ML, et al: Treating infant colic with the probiotic Lactobacillus reuteri: double blind, placebo controlled randomised trial, *BMJ* 348:g2107, 2014.

Tanaka M, Nakayama J: Development of the gut microbiota in infancy and its impact on health in later life, *Allergol Int* 66:515–522, 2017.

Taylor RW, Williams SM, Fangupo LJ, et al: Effect of a baby-led approach to complementary feeding on infant growth and overweight: a randomized clinical trial, *JAMA Pediatr* 171:838–846, 2017.

Terrin G, Berni Canani R, Di Chiara M, et al: Zinc in early life: a key element in the fetus and preterm neonate, *Nutrients* 7(12):10427–10446, 2015.

Van den Nieuwboer M, Claassen E, Morelli L, et al: Probiotic and synbiotic safety in infants under two years of age, *Benef Microbes* 5:45–60, 2014.

Vandenplas Y, Castrellon PG, Rivas R, et al: Safety of soya-based infant formulas in children, *Br J Nutr* 111:1340–1360, 2014.

16

Nutrition in Childhood

Beth Ogata, MS, RDN, CD, CSP
Sharon A. Feucht, MA, RDN, CD

KEY TERMS

adiposity rebound
catch-up growth
failure to thrive (FTT)

food jags
growth channels
growth deficiency

pediatric undernutrition
primarily wasted
stunted growth

The period that begins after infancy and lasts until puberty often is referred to as the latent or quiescent period of growth—a contrast to the dramatic changes that occur during infancy and adolescence. Although physical growth may be less remarkable and proceed at a steadier pace than it did during the first year, these preschool and elementary school years are a time of significant growth in the social, cognitive, and emotional areas.

GROWTH AND DEVELOPMENT

Growth Patterns

The rate of growth slows considerably after the first year of life. Increments of change are small compared with those of infancy and adolescence. Weight typically increases an average of 1.6 to 3.9 kg (3½ lb at age 2 years to 8 ½ lb for boys 10 to 11 years) per year with only slight differences between each sex. Girls generally increase their rate of gain between 10 and 11 years, with boys starting between 11 and 12 years of age, signaling the approach of puberty. Height increase increments average 5 to 9 cm (2 to 3½ inches) per year with lower increases in late childhood until the individual growth spurt seen in puberty (Centers for Disease Control and Prevention [CDC 2017]). While growth is generally steady during the preschool and school age years, it can be erratic in individual children, with periods of no growth followed by growth spurts. These patterns usually parallel similar changes in appetite and food intake. For parents, these periods of slower (but normal) growth and decreased appetite can cause anxiety, potentially leading to mealtime struggles.

Body proportions of young children change significantly after the first year. Head growth is minimal, trunk growth slows substantially, and limbs lengthen considerably, all of which create more mature body proportions. Walking and increased physical activity lead to the legs straightening and increased muscle strength in the abdomen and back.

The body composition of preschool and school age children remains relatively constant. Fat gradually decreases during the early childhood years, reaching a minimum between 4 and 6 years of age. Children then experience the adiposity rebound, or increase in body fatness in preparation for the pubertal growth spurt. Earlier adiposity rebound (before 5 ½ years of age) has been associated with increased

adult body mass index (BMI) (Williams and Goulding, 2009). Sex differences in body composition become increasingly apparent: boys have more lean body mass per centimeter of height than girls. Girls have a higher percentage of weight as fat than boys, even in the preschool years, but these differences in lean body mass and fat do not become significant until adolescence.

Assessing Growth

A complete nutrition assessment includes the collection of anthropometric data. This includes length or stature, weight, and weight-for-length or BMI, all of which are plotted on the recommended growth charts (see Appendix 3). Other measurements that are less commonly used but that provide estimates of body composition include mid upper-arm circumference and triceps or subscapular skin folds. Care should be taken to use standardized equipment and techniques for obtaining and plotting growth measurements. Charts designed for birth to 24 months of age are based on length measurements and nude weights, whereas charts used for 2- to 20-year-olds are based on stature (standing height) and weight with light clothing and without shoes (see Chapter 5).

The proportion of weight to length or height is a critical element of growth assessment. This parameter is determined by plotting the weight-for-length on the World Health Organization (WHO) birth to 24-month growth charts, or calculating BMI and plotting it on the 2- to 20-year-old CDC growth charts. Growth measurements obtained at regular intervals provide information about an individual's growth pattern. One-time measurements do not allow for interpretation of growth status. Growth channels are not well established until after 2 years of age. Children generally maintain their heights and weights in the same growth channels during the preschool and childhood years, although rates of growth can vary within a selected period.

Growth and medical monitoring, as well as a discussion of developmental expectations, usually occur at annual well child visits with the child's primary care provider. Regular monitoring of growth enables problematic trends to be identified early and intervention initiated so that long-term growth is not compromised. Weight that increases rapidly and crosses growth channels may suggest the development of obesity (Fig. 16.1). Lack of weight gain over a period of

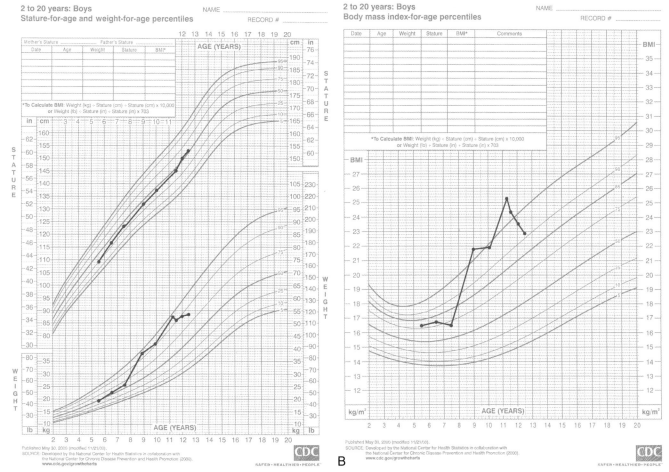

Fig. 16.1 Growth chart (A) and BMI chart (B) for an 8-year-old boy who gained excessive weight after having leg surgery and being immobilized in a body cast for 2 months. The surgery and immobilization were followed by a long period of stress caused by family problems. At the age of 11 years, he became involved in a weight management program. (Source of growth charts only: Centers for Disease Control and Prevention: Growth Charts [website]: http://www.cdc.gov/growthcharts/, 2017.)

months or weight loss may be a result of undernutrition, an acute illness, an undiagnosed chronic disease, or significant emotional or family problems (Fig. 16.2). Children evaluated by health care professionals only when they are ill may miss monitoring of growth and development.

Catch-Up Growth

A child who is recovering from an illness or undernutrition and whose growth has slowed or ceased experiences a greater than expected rate of recovery. This recovery is referred to as catch-up growth, a period during which the body strives to return to the child's normal growth channel. The degree of growth suppression is influenced by the timing, severity, and duration of the precipitating cause, such as a severe illness or prolonged nutritional deprivation.

Initial studies supported the thesis that malnourished infants who did not experience immediate catch-up growth would have permanent growth restriction. However, studies of malnourished children from developing countries who subsequently received adequate nourishment, as well as reports of children who were malnourished because of chronic disease such as celiac disease or cystic fibrosis, have shown that these children caught up to their normal growth channels after the first year or two of life when their disease was managed.

The nutritional requirements for catch-up growth depend on whether the child has overall stunted growth (height and weight are proportionally low) and is chronically malnourished, or is primarily wasted, meaning that the weight deficit exceeds the height deficit. With renourishment, expectations for weight gain vary. A chronically malnourished child may not be expected to gain more than 2 to 3 g/kg/day, whereas a child who is primarily wasted may gain as much as 20 g/kg/day.

Nutrient requirements, especially for energy and protein, depend on the rate and stage of catch-up growth. For instance, more protein and energy are needed during the initial period of very rapid weight gain and for those in whom lean tissue is the major component of the weight gain. In addition to energy, other nutrients are important, including vitamin A, iron, and zinc.

Current growth parameters are used to evaluate the child's weight in relation to age and stature and to estimate a "desirable" or goal weight. Formulas are then used to estimate the minimum and maximum energy needed for catch-up growth. After a child who is wasted catches up in weight, dietary management must change to slow the weight gain velocity and avoid excessive gain. The catch-up in linear growth peaks approximately 1 to 3 months after treatment starts, whereas weight gain begins immediately.

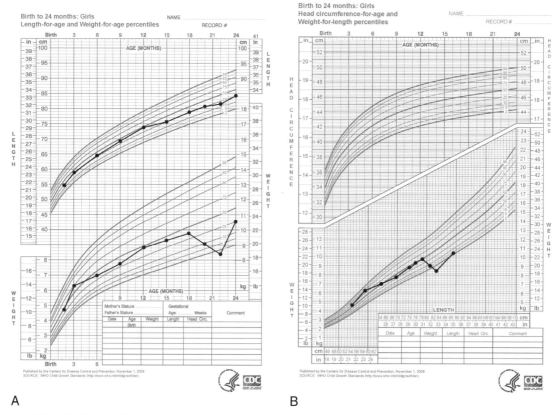

Fig. 16.2 Growth charts for a 2-year-old girl who experienced significant weight loss during a prolonged period of diarrhea and feeding problems. After being diagnosed with celiac disease, she began following a gluten-free diet and entered a period of catch-up growth. (Source of growth charts only: Centers for Disease Control and Prevention: *Growth Charts* [website]: http://www.cdc.gov/growthcharts/, 2017.)

NUTRIENT REQUIREMENTS

Because children are growing and developing bones, teeth, muscles, and blood, they need more nutritious food in proportion to their size than do adults. They may be at risk for malnutrition when they have a poor appetite for a long period, eat a limited number of foods, or dilute their diets significantly with nutrient-poor foods.

The dietary reference intakes (DRIs) are based on current knowledge of nutrient intakes needed for optimal health (see inside cover). Most data for preschool and school age children are values interpolated from data on infants and adults. The DRIs are meant to improve the long-term health of the population by reducing the risk of chronic disease and preventing nutrient deficiencies. Thus, when an intake is less than the recommended level, it cannot be assumed that a particular child is inadequately nourished.

Energy

The energy needs of healthy children are determined by basal metabolism, rate of growth, and energy expenditure of activity. Dietary energy must be sufficient to ensure growth and spare protein from being used for energy, while not allowing excess weight gain. The acceptable macronutrient distribution ranges (AMDRs) are 45% to 65% as carbohydrate, 30% to 40% as fat, and 5% to 20% as protein for 1- to 3-year-olds, with carbohydrates the same for 4- to 18-year-olds, 25% to 35% as fat, and 10% to 30% as protein (Institute of Medicine [IOM], 2005).

The DRIs for estimated energy requirement (EER) are average energy requirements based on life-stage groupings for healthy individuals of normal weight. Toddlers 13 through 35 months are grouped together; for older children the EERs are divided by sex and age (3 to 8 years and 9 to 18 years). The EER includes the total energy expenditure plus energy needed for growth (see Chapter 2). The DRIs are applied to child nutrition programs and other guidelines (Otten et al, 2006). Box 16.1 provides examples of determining EER for three children. On an individual basis, it can be useful to estimate energy requirements using kilocalories per kilogram of weight or per centimeter of height.

Protein

The need for protein decreases from approximately 1.1 g/kg in early childhood to 0.95 g/kg in late childhood (Table 16.1). Protein intake can range from 5% to 30% of total energy, depending on age. Protein deficiency is uncommon in American children, partly because of the cultural emphasis on high-protein foods. Protein intake less than the estimated average requirement (EAR) or recommended dietary allowance (RDA) is rare among children in the United States (Berryman et al, 2018). Children who are most at risk for inadequate protein intake are those on strict vegan diets, those with multiple food allergies, or those who have limited food selections because of fad diets, severe sensorimotor issues, or inadequate access to food.

Minerals and Vitamins

Minerals and vitamins are necessary for normal growth and development. Insufficient intake can cause impaired growth and result in deficiency diseases. The DRIs are listed inside the cover.

BOX 16.1 Determining Estimated Energy Requirements

(Examples using data from Box 2.1, Chapter 2)

1. For 13- to 35-month-old children:

$$EER (kcal) = (89 \times wt [kg]) - 100 + 20$$

An 18-month-old boy has a length of 84 cm and weighs 12.5 kg

$$EER (kcal) = (89 \times 12.5) - 100 + 20$$
$$EER (kcal) = 1113 - 100 + 20$$
$$EER (kcal) = 1033$$

2. For girls 3 through 8 years:

$$EER (kcal) = 135.3 - ([30.8 \times age\ in\ yrs] + PA \times ([10 \times wgt\ in\ kg] + [934 \times hgt\ in\ m]) + 20$$

A 6½-year-old girl is 112 cm tall, weighs 20.8 kg, and has moderate activity (PA coefficient of 1.31)

$$EER (kcal) = 135.3 - (30.8 \times 6.5) + 1.31 \times ([10 \times 20.8] + [934 \times 1.12]) + 20$$
$$EER (kcal) = 135.3 - 200.2 + 1.31 \times (208 + 1046.1) + 20$$
$$EER (kcal) = 135.3 - 200.2 + 1642.9 + 20$$
$$EER (kcal) = 1598$$

3. For overweight boys 3 through 18 years (weight maintenance):

$$TEE (kcal) = 114 - ([50.9 \times age\ in\ yrs] + PA \times ([19.5 \times wgt\ in\ kg] + [1161.4 \times hgt\ in\ m])$$

A 7-year, 4-month-old boy is 128.4 cm tall, weighs 33.9 kg, and has low active activity (PA coefficient of 1.12)

$$TEE (kcal) = 114 - (50.9 \times 7.25) + 1.12 \times ([19.5 \times 33.9] + [1161.4 \times 1.284])$$
$$TEE (kcal) = 114 - 39.6 + 1.12 \times (66.1 + 1491.2)$$
$$TEE (kcal) = 114 - 39.6 + 1744.2$$
$$EER (kcal) = 1819$$

EER, Estimated energy requirement; *PA*, physical activity; *TEE*, total energy expenditure.

TABLE 16.1 Protein Dietary Reference Intakes (DRIs) for Children Through Age 13 Years

Age	Grams/Day*	PROTEIN Grams/Kilogram/Day
1-3 yr	13 g/day	1.05 g/kg/day
4-8 yr	19 g/day	0.95 g/kg/day
9-13 yr	34 g/day	0.95 g/kg/day

*Recommended dietary allowance for reference individual (g/day).

Iron

Young children are at risk for iron deficiency and iron deficiency anemia, which can affect development and behavior. National Health and Nutrition Examination Survey (NHANES) data indicate that children with prolonged bottle feeding and those of Mexican American descent are at highest risk for iron deficiency (Hamner et al, 2016; Brotanek et al, 2005; Moshfegh et al, 2005). Recommended intakes must factor in the absorption rate and quantity of iron in foods, especially those of plant origin. The prevalence of iron deficiency among 1- to 5-year-olds in the United State is 7.1%, and the prevalence of iron deficiency anemia is 1.1%, with higher rates among children 1 to 2 years of age (Gupta et al, 2017).

Calcium

Calcium is needed for adequate mineralization and maintenance of growing bone in children. The RDA for calcium for children 1 to 3 years old is 700 mg/day, for children 4 to 8 years it is 1000 mg/day, and for those 9 to 18 years it is 1300 mg per day. Actual need depends on individual absorption rates and dietary factors such as quantities of protein, vitamin D, and phosphorus. Because milk and other dairy products are primary sources of calcium, children who consume limited amounts of these foods are often at risk for poor bone mineralization. Other calcium-fortified foods such as soy, rice, and nut milks and fruit juices are also good sources (see Appendix 39).

Zinc

Zinc is essential for growth; a deficiency results in growth failure, poor appetite, decreased taste acuity, and poor wound healing. Because the best sources of zinc are meat and seafood, some children may regularly have low intakes (see Appendix 47). Diagnosis of zinc deficiency, especially marginal deficiency, may be difficult because laboratory parameters, including plasma, serum erythrocyte, hair, and urine, are of limited value in determining zinc deficiency. There is a positive influence of zinc supplementation on growth and serum zinc concentrations.

Vitamin D

Vitamin D is needed for calcium absorption and deposition of calcium in the bones; other functions within the body, including prevention of chronic diseases such as cancer, cardiovascular disease, and diabetes, are important areas of current investigation. Because this nutrient also is formed from sunlight exposure on the skin, the amount required from dietary sources depends on factors such as geographic location and time spent outside (see Appendix 38).

The DRI for vitamin D for infants is 400 IU (10 mcg) per day and for children is 600 IU (15 mcg) per day. Vitamin D-fortified milk is the primary dietary source of this nutrient, and breakfast cereals and nondairy milks often are fortified with vitamin D. Dairy products such as cheese and yogurt, however, are not always made from fortified milk. Milks other than cow milk (e.g., goat, soy, almond, or rice) may not be fortified with vitamin D. For young children the current DRI for vitamin D is higher than what may be consumed from a typical diet. Supplementation may be needed after a careful assessment or measurement of vitamin D status. It is becoming more common to measure serum 25(OH) vitamin D in children; however, there is some controversy regarding what constitutes optimal levels (Rovner and O'Brien, 2008).

Vitamin-Mineral Supplements

Thirty-one percent of children under 18 years of age take a multivitamin-mineral supplement (Dwyer et al, 2013). Families with more education, higher incomes, private health insurance, and access to health care were more likely to use supplements. However, these may not be the families who are at greatest risk for having inadequate diets.

Fluoride can help prevent dental caries. If a community's water supply is not fluoridated, fluoride supplements are recommended from 6 months until 16 years of age. However, individual family practices should be assessed, including the child's primary source of fluids (e.g., drinking water, juices, or other beverages) and fluoride sources from child care, school, toothpaste, and mouthwash (see Chapter 25).

The American Academy of Pediatrics (AAP) does not support giving healthy children routine supplements of any vitamins or minerals other than fluoride. However, children at risk for inadequate nutrition who may benefit include those (1) with anorexia, inadequate appetite, or who consume fad diets; (2) with chronic disease (e.g., cystic fibrosis, inflammatory bowel disease, hepatic disease); (3) from food-insecure families or who suffer parental neglect or abuse; (4) who participate in a dietary program for managing obesity; (5) who consume a vegetarian or vegan diet without adequate calcium intake and/or dairy products and vitamin B_{12}; (6) with faltering growth (failure to thrive); (7) with developmental disabilities.

Children who routinely take a multiple vitamin or a vitamin-mineral supplement usually do not experience negative effects if the supplement contains nutrients in amounts that do not exceed the DRIs, especially the tolerable upper intake level. However, some nutrients can be "missed" by general multiple vitamin supplements. Although many children consume less than the recommended amount of calcium, children's vitamin-mineral supplements typically do not contain significant amounts of calcium. For example, among children ages 2 to 18 years who took supplements, one-third did not meet recommendations for calcium and vitamin D intakes even with supplements. In addition, supplement use was associated with increased prevalence of excessive intakes of iron, zinc, vitamin A, and folic acid (Bailey et al, 2012). In addition, an analysis of supplements marketed for infants and children indicated that available supplements do not necessarily meet recommendations for intake; for some nutrients, not enough is provided, and for others, the supplements provide excessive amounts (Madden et al, 2014). Children should not take megadoses, particularly of the fat-soluble vitamins and minerals, especially liquid and gummy vitamins, because large amounts can result in toxicity. Careful evaluation of each pediatric supplement is suggested because many types are available but incomplete. Because many vitamin-mineral supplements look and taste like candy, parents should keep them out of reach of children to avoid excessive intake of nutrients such as iron.

Complementary and integrative nutrition therapies are becoming more common for children, especially for those with special health care needs such as Down syndrome, autism spectrum disorder (ASD), or cystic fibrosis (see Chapters 33 and 43). As part of the nutrition assessment, practitioners should inquire as to the use of these products and therapies, be knowledgeable about their efficacy and safety, and help families determine whether they are beneficial and how to use them (see Chapter 11).

PROVIDING AN ADEQUATE DIET

The development of feeding skills, food habits, and nutrition knowledge parallels the cognitive development that takes place in a series of stages, each laying the groundwork for the next. Table 16.2 outlines the development of feeding skills in terms of Piaget's theory of child psychology and development.

Intake Patterns

Children's food patterns have changed over the years. Dietary studies show decreased intakes of sugars and fats in children over age 2,

---

TABLE 16.2   Feeding, Nutrition, and Piaget's Theory of Cognitive Development

Developmental Period	Cognitive Characteristics	Relationship to Feeding and Nutrition
Sensorimotor (birth-2 yr)	Neonate progresses from autonomic reflexes to a young child with intentional interaction with the environment and the beginning use of symbols. Food is used primarily to satisfy hunger, as a medium to explore the environment, and to practice fine motor skills.	Progression involves advancing from sucking and rooting reflexes to the acquisition of self-feeding skills.
Preoperational (2-7 yr)	Thought processes become internalized; they are unsystematic and intuitive. Use of symbols increases. Reasoning is based on appearances and happenstance. The child's approach to classification is functional and unsystematic. The child's world is viewed egocentrically.	Eating becomes less the center of attention and is secondary to social, language, and cognitive growth. Food is described by color, shape, and quantity, but the child has only a limited ability to classify food into "groups." Foods tend to be categorized into "like" and "don't like." Foods can be identified as "good for you," but reasons why they are healthy are unknown or mistaken.
Concrete operational (7-11 yr)	The child can focus on several aspects of a situation simultaneously. Cause-and-effect reasoning becomes more rational and systematic. The ability to classify, reclassify, and generalize emerges. A decrease in egocentrism permits the child to take another's view.	The child begins to realize that nutritious food has a positive effect on growth and health but they have a limited understanding of how or why. Mealtimes take on more of a social significance. The expanding environment increases opportunities for influences on food selection; i.e. peer influence increases.
Formal operational (11 yr and beyond)	Hypothetical and abstract thought expand. The child's understanding of scientific and theoretical processes deepens.	The concept of nutrients from food functioning at physiologic and biochemical levels can be understood. Conflicts in making food choices may be realized (i.e., knowledge of the nutritious value of foods may conflict with preferences and nonnutritive influences).

although amounts consumed are still higher than recommendations. Whole grain consumption has slightly increased. Children continue to eat the same amounts of fruit, vegetables, dairy and total meat, poultry, and seafood (Bowman et al, 2017).

In comparison to the Dietary Guidelines for Americans, most children do not meet recommendations. Those 2 to 5 years of age do consume adequate fruit, whole grains, and dairy, but all children are still low in vegetable intake (Guenther et al, 2013).

More energy comes from snacks, and portion sizes have increased. In addition, more food is consumed in environments other than the home, often leading to increased energy intake. Foods served to children 6 to 12 years of age at school supply similar amounts of energy and nutrients compared with food eaten at home (Mancino et al, 2010). Foods with low nutrient density (soft drinks, desserts, sweeteners, and salty snacks) often displace nutrient-dense foods.

Like physical growth patterns, food intake patterns are not smooth and consistent. Although subjective, appetites usually follow the rate of growth and nutrient needs. By a child's first birthday, milk consumption begins to decline. In the next year vegetable intake decreases; intakes of cereals, grain products, and sweets increase. Young children often prefer softer protein sources instead of meats that are harder to chew.

Changes in food consumption are reflected in nutrient intakes. The early preschool years show a decrease in calcium, phosphorus, riboflavin, iron, and vitamin A compared with infancy. Intakes of most other key nutrients remain relatively stable. During the early school years, a pattern of consistent and steadily increased intakes of most nutrients is seen until adolescence. In healthy children a wide variability of nutrient intake is seen at any age. Children are most likely to consume inadequate amounts of calcium, vitamin D, fiber, and potassium (Bailey et al, 2010; Kranz et al, 2012). However, clinical signs of malnutrition in American children are rare.

Factors Influencing Food Intake

Numerous influences, some obvious and others subtle, determine the food intake and habits of children. Habits, likes, and dislikes are established in the early years and carried through to adulthood. The major influences on food intake in the developing years include family environment, societal trends, the media, peer pressure, and illness or disease.

Family Environment

For toddlers and preschool children the family is the primary influence in the development of food habits. In young children's immediate environment, parents and older siblings are significant models. Food attitudes of parents, parental behavior, and food practices can be strong predictors of food likes and dislikes and diet complexity in children of primary school age. Similarities between children's and their parents' food preferences are likely to reflect genetic and environmental influences (Savage et al, 2007; Fildes et al, 2014; Larsen et al, 2015).

Contrary to common belief, young children do not have the innate ability to choose a balanced, nutritious diet; they can choose one only when presented with nutritious foods. A positive feeding relationship includes a division of responsibility between parents and children. The parents and other adults are to provide safe, nutritious, developmentally appropriate food as regular meals and snacks. The children decide how much, if any, they eat. This approach is consistent with a responsive parenting approach, allowing the parent and child to recognize hunger and satiety cues and respond appropriately (Black and Aboud, 2011). Ellyn Satter promotes this "division of responsibility" approach to feeding as well (Satter, 2000).

Eating together at family meals is becoming less common, partly because of family schedules, more time eating in front of a screen, and the decreasing amount of time available for planning and preparing family meals. School age children and adolescents who eat more dinners with their families consume more fruits and vegetables, less soda, and fewer fried foods than those who rarely eat dinner with their families (Larson et al, 2007). Family meals have other benefits, including a positive influence on nutrition beliefs and possibly prevention of excessive weight gain. Studies show these effects continue into adulthood (Chan and Sobal, 2011; Watts et al, 2018).

The atmosphere around food and mealtime also influences attitudes toward food and eating. Unrealistic expectations for a child's mealtime manners, arguments, and other emotional stress can have a negative effect. Meals that are rushed create a hectic atmosphere and reinforce the tendency to eat too fast. A positive environment is one in which sufficient time is set aside to eat, occasional spills are tolerated, and conversation that includes all family members is encouraged (Fig. 16.3).

Socioeconomic Influences

Almost one in five American children lives in a family with an income below the poverty line; in 2016 13.3 million children lived in poverty. Single-parent households predominantly headed by women have lower incomes and less money for all expenses, including food, than households headed by men; about half of children in families with a female householder were in poverty (Semega et al, 2017). This phenomenon makes these families increasingly vulnerable to multiple stressors such as marginal health and nutritional status partly because of lack of jobs, child care, adequate housing, and health insurance.

In 2016, 12.3% of U.S. households experienced food insecurity. Among households with children, 16.5% were food insecure, with both children and adults experiencing food insecurity in 8.0% of households with children (Coleman-Jensen et al, 2017). Federal food and nutrition assistance programs (including the Special Supplemental Nutrition Program [SNAP], the Special Supplemental Nutrition Program for Women, Infants and Children [WIC], and the National School Lunch Program) provide benefits to about 59% of food-insecure households (see Chapter 8). The food stamp allotment for families, based on the U.S. Department of Agriculture (USDA) Thrifty Food Plan, does not provide adequate funds to

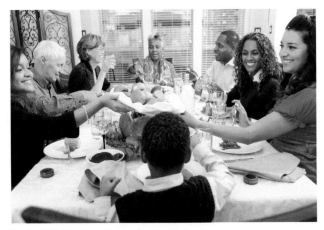

Fig. 16.3 Eating together gives meals a place of prominence in the home—meals that will not be replaced with fast foods eaten on the run. From www.istockphoto.com.

purchase food based on the government's nutrition guidelines, especially when labor is considered (Davis and You, 2010). Food insecurity also increases the risk for children younger than age 3 years to be iron deficient with anemia. Studies suggest that intermittent hunger in American children is associated with increased developmental risk (see *Focus On*: Childhood Hunger and Its Effect on Cognition and Behavior) (Rose-Jacobs et al, 2008). Even marginal food insecurity, which is often thought not to be an indicator of nutrition risk in adults, is associated with adverse health outcomes in children (Cook et al, 2013).

◎ FOCUS ON

Childhood Hunger and Its Effect on Cognition and Behavior

Food insecurity is associated with anemia, lower nutrient intake, cognitive problems, aggression, and anxiety. Children with food insecurity have poorer general health and higher rates of depression, and for adolescents, suicidal ideation and lower scores on academic tests (Gundersen and Ziliak, 2015; Hobbs and King, 2018). Specific nutrient deficiencies such as iron deficiency anemia can result in a decreased ability to pay attention and poorer problem-solving skills. With federal welfare reform legislation and in economic downturns, an increasing number of children from low-income families are at risk for limited food resources (Stang and Bayerl, 2010).

The U.S. Department of Agriculture (USDA) measures food insecurity through questions administered in a supplement to the Census Bureau's Current Population Survey. Households are divided into the following categories: high food secure (all household members had access at all times to enough food), marginal food secure (some members reported anxiety about food sufficiency or shortage of food, but no indication of changes in diet or food intake), low food secure (at least some household members reported reduced quality, variety, or desirability of diet), and very low food secure (one or more members reported multiple indications of disrupted eating patterns and reduced intake). Data from 2016 indicated that 16.5% of U.S. households with children were food-insecure. In 2016, 6.5 million children in the United States lived in food-insecure households (Coleman-Jensen et al, 2017). Groups at higher risk of food insecurity include households headed by an African American or Hispanic person and those with children (Gundersen and Ziliak, 2015).

A longitudinal study following approximately 21,000 children from kindergarten through third grade found that persistent food insecurity was predictive of impaired academic outcomes, poorer social skills, and a tendency to increased body mass index (BMI) (Ryu and Bartfeld, 2012).

Although these studies have limitations because of other factors that may affect a child's functioning (e.g., stress, family dysfunction, or substance abuse), a correlation exists between children's lack of sufficient food and their behavioral and academic functioning. As future studies provide more evidence of this relationship, it will be clear that social policies must ensure the provision of children's basic needs for optimal growth and development.

Media Messages

Food is marketed to children using a variety of techniques (television, radio and print advertising) and digital messages from a variety of devices. School age children may be exposed to in-school marketing, sponsorship, product placement, and sales promotion. Television advertising and in-school marketing are regulated to some degree. Parents report children younger than 8 years of age spend slightly more than 2 hours per day watching screens (television, mobile devices, DVDs, video games, and computers) (Rideout, 2017). Children younger than 13 years of age who watch 2 hours of television per day may view 56 to 126 food advertisements; 32% of the ads are for fast food products in the United States. Eighty percent of the food ads focus on foods high in energy or nutrients less desirable using dietary standards (Kelly et al, 2010). In another sample of television advertising to children, more than 40% of commercials were for food, with 80% to 95% for items high in saturated fat, trans fat, sugar, and sodium (Powell et al, 2013).

Screen time can be detrimental to growth and development because it encourages inactivity and passive use of leisure time. In a sample of children 4 to 11 years of age, just over one-third had low levels of active play, while two-thirds of the sample had high screen time; one-fourth of the group had both low activity levels and high screen time (Anderson et al, 2008). Television viewing with its multiple media cues to eat has been suggested as a factor contributing to excessive weight gain in school age children, especially when there is a television in the child's bedroom (Gilbert-Diamond et al, 2014). Increases in hours of television viewing are associated with rising BMIs in boys and girls, with females also affected by watching DVDs/videos and electronic games. For those already at risk with higher BMIs, limits on noneducational viewing may be part of intervention strategies (Falbe et al, 2013). Television viewing has also been inversely associated with fruit and vegetable consumption (American Public Health Association [APHA], 2017).

Preschool children are generally unable to distinguish commercial messages from regular programs; in fact, they often pay more attention to the commercials. As children get older, they gain knowledge about the purpose of commercial advertising and become more critical of its validity but are still susceptible to the messages. Media literacy education programs teach children and adolescents about the intent of advertising and media messages and how to evaluate and interpret their obvious and subtle influences. Comprehensive and consistent regulation approaches plus monitoring the use of the most common persuasive marketing techniques (premium offers, promotional characters, nutrition- and health-related claims, taste and fun appeal) is suggested (Jenkin et al, 2014). Guidance is available for health care providers and families with children through the American Academy of Pediatrics website page, Media and Young Minds (AAP, 2016).

Significant decreases have occurred in beverage and food vending in schools, but both forms of sales still occur. Elementary-age students often are given coupons to encourage their families to purchase food, whereas those in upper grades may be exposed to in-school exclusive beverage contracts and other types of marketing (Terry-McElrath et al, 2014). The USDA has established nutrition standards for snack foods and beverages available for sale in schools but does not address food marketing. Standards that can be enforced are still needed to clarify the nutrition content of all foods and beverages marketed in school settings.

Peer Influence

As children grow, their worlds expand and their social contacts become more important. Peer influence increases with age and affects food attitudes and choices. This may result in a sudden refusal of a food or a request for a currently popular food. Decisions about whether to participate in school meals may be made more on the basis of friends' choices than on the menu. Such behaviors are developmentally typical. Positive behaviors such as a willingness to try new foods can be reinforced. Parents must set limits on undesirable influences but also must be realistic; struggles over food are self-defeating.

FOCUS ON

Childhood Methylmercury Exposure and Toxicity

Mercury toxicity can cause neurologic problems, which can lead to cognitive and motor deficits. Toxicity related to prenatal exposure is documented, and there is evidence that postnatal exposure is dangerous as well (Myers et al, 2009; Oken and Bellinger, 2008). Exposure to mercury can occur through environmental contact and eating contaminated foods. Methylmercury, the most toxic form of mercury, accumulates in fish.

Public health agencies have looked at balancing the benefits of minimizing exposure to this neurotoxin with the risk of limiting intake of docosahexaenoic acid (DHA) and eicosapentaenoic acid (EPA) as well as a source of high biologic value protein. DHA and EPA are essential omega-3 fatty acids and have received much attention because of their importance in cognitive and vision development and their cardiovascular benefits (Mahaffey et al, 2008). In addition, fish advisories are available in certain states. The U.S. Environmental Protection Agency's (EPA) reference dose for methylmercury is based on body weight: 0.1 mcg/kg/day. The Food and Drug Administration (FDA) and EPA have made recommendations for fish intake by young children, as well as for women of childbearing age and pregnant and breastfeeding women (FDA, 2017). These recommendations were designed to encourage fish consumption, while limiting exposure to mercury. Current recommendations differ from previous versions by recommending minimum intake of iron. These recommendations are presented in a chart and set of frequently asked questions:

Advice About Eating Fish

What Pregnant Women & Parents Should Know

Fish and other protein-rich foods have nutrients that can help your child's growth and development.

For women of childbearing age (about 16-49 years old), especially pregnant and breastfeeding women, and for parents and caregivers of young children.

- *Eat 2 to 3 servings of fish a week from the "Best Choices" list OR 1 serving from the "Good Choices" list.*
- *Eat a variety of fish.*
- *Serve 1 to 2 servings of fish a week to children, starting at age 2.*
- *If you eat fish caught by family or friends, check for fish advisories. If there is no advisory, eat only one serving and no other fish that week.**

Use this chart!

You can use this chart to help you choose which fish to eat, and how often to eat them, based on their mercury levels. The "Best Choices" have the lowest levels of mercury.

What is a serving?

To find out, use the palm of your hand!

 For an adult 4 ounces

 For children, ages 4 to 7 2 ounces

Best Choices EAT 2 TO 3 SERVINGS A WEEK   OR   Good Choices EAT 1 SERVING A WEEK

Best Choices			Good Choices		
Anchovy	Herring	Scallop	Bluefish	Monkfish	Tilefish (Atlantic Ocean)
Atlantic croaker	Lobster, American and spiny	Shad	Buffalofish	Rockfish	Tuna, albacore/ white tuna, canned and fresh/frozen
Atlantic mackerel	Mullet	Shrimp	Carp	Sablefish	
Black sea bass	Oyster	Skate	Chilean sea bass/ Patagonian toothfish	Sheepshead	Tuna, yellowfin
Butterfish	Pacific chub mackerel	Smelt	Grouper	Snapper	Weakfish/seatrout
Catfish		Sole	Halibut	Spanish mackerel	White croaker/ Pacific croaker
Clam	Perch, freshwater and ocean	Squid	Mahi mahi/ dolphinfish	Striped bass (ocean)	
Cod	Pickerel	Tilapia			
Crab	Plaice	Trout, freshwater			
Crawfish	Pollock	Tuna, canned light (includes skipjack)			
Flounder	Salmon	Whitefish			
Haddock	Sardine	Whiting			
Hake					

Choices to Avoid HIGHEST MERCURY LEVELS

King mackerel	Shark	Tilefish (Gulf of Mexico)
Marlin	Swordfish	Tuna, bigeye
Orange roughy		

*Some fish caught by family and friends, such as larger carp, catfish, trout and perch, are more likely to have fish advisories due to mercury or other contaminants. State advisories will tell you how often you can safely eat those fish.

www.FDA.gov/fishadvice

www.EPA.gov/fishadvice

EPA United States Environmental Protection Agency

FDA U.S. FOOD & DRUG ADMINISTRATION

Illness or Disease

Children who are ill usually have a decreased appetite and limited food intake. Acute viral or bacterial illnesses are often short-lived but may require an increase in fluids, protein, or other nutrients. Chronic conditions such as asthma, cystic fibrosis, or chronic renal disease may make it difficult to obtain sufficient nutrients for optimal growth. Children with these types of conditions are more likely to have behavior problems relating to food. Children requiring special diets (e.g., those who have diabetes, food allergies, or phenylketonuria) not only have to adjust to the limits of foods allowed but also have to address issues of independence and peer acceptance as they grow older. Some rebellion against the prescribed diet is typical, especially as children approach puberty.

Feeding Preschool Children

From 1 to 6 years of age children experience vast developmental progress and acquisition of skills. One-year-old children primarily use

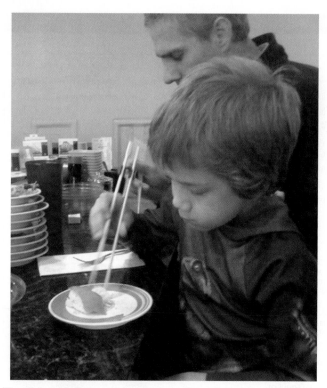

Fig. 16.4 Use of alternative eating utensils can increase a preschooler's interest in trying new foods and development of fine motor skills.

fingers to eat and may need assistance with a cup. By 2 years of age, they can hold a cup in one hand and use a spoon well but may prefer to use their hands at times. Six-year-old children have refined skills and are beginning to use a knife for cutting and spreading.

As the growth rate slows after the first year of life, appetite decreases, which often concerns parents. Children have less interest in food and an increased interest in the world around them. They can develop food jags, which can be periods when foods that were previously liked are refused, or there are repeated requests to eat the same food meal after meal. This behavior may be attributable to boredom with the usual foods or may be a means of asserting newly discovered independence. Parents may have concerns with their child's seemingly irrational food behavior. Struggles over control of the eating situation are fruitless; no child can be forced to eat. This period is developmental and temporary (Fig. 16.4).

A positive feeding relationship includes a division of responsibility between parents and children. Young children can choose a balanced nutritious diet if presented with nutritious foods. The parents and other adults provide safe, nutritious, developmentally appropriate food as regular meals and snacks; and the children decide how much, if any, they eat (Satter, 2000). Parents maintain control over what foods are offered and have the opportunity to set limits on inappropriate behaviors. Neither rigid control nor a laissez-faire approach is likely to succeed. Parents and other care providers should continue to offer a variety of foods, including the child's favorites, and not make substitutions a routine. Parents' food preferences also influence children's acceptance of foods, as children often model parents' behaviors (Wardle and Cooke, 2008).

With smaller stomach capacities and variable appetites, preschool children should be offered small servings of food four to six times a day at regular and predictable intervals. Snacks are as important as meals in contributing to the total daily nutrient intake. Carefully chosen snacks are those dense in nutrients and least likely to promote dental caries. A general starting point is to offer 1 tablespoon of each food for every year of age and to serve more food according to the child's appetite. Table 16.3 is a guide for food and portion size.

Senses other than taste play an important part in food acceptance by young children. They tend to avoid food with extreme temperatures, and some foods are rejected because of odor rather than taste. A sense of order in the food presentation often is preferred; many children do not accept foods that touch each other on the plate, and mixed dishes or casseroles with unidentifiable foods are not popular. Broken crackers may go uneaten, or a sandwich may be refused because it is "cut the wrong way."

The physical setting for meals is important. Children's feet should be supported, and chair height should allow a comfortable reach to the table at chest height. Sturdy, child-size tables and chairs are ideal, or a high chair or booster seat should be used. Dishes and cups should be unbreakable and heavy enough to resist tipping. For very young children, a shallow bowl is often better than a plate for scooping. Thick, short-handled spoons and forks allow for an easier grasp. Young children do not eat well if they are tired; this should be considered when meal and play times are scheduled.

Fruit juices and juice drinks are common beverages for young children; they frequently replace water and milk in children's diets. In addition to altering the diet's nutrient content, excessive intake of fruit juice can result in carbohydrate malabsorption and chronic, nonspecific diarrhea. This suggests that juices, especially apple and pear, should be avoided when using liquids to treat acute diarrhea. For children with chronic diarrhea, a trial of restricting fruit juices may be warranted before more costly diagnostic tests are done.

When children aged 2 to 11 years consume 100% juice, their diets have significantly higher intakes of energy, carbohydrates, vitamins C and B_6, potassium, riboflavin, magnesium, iron, and folate, and significantly lower intakes of total fat, saturated fatty acids, discretionary fat, and added sugar; this 100% juice intake does not correlate with overweight later (Nicklas et al, 2008). However, excess juice intake (12 to 30 oz/day) by young children may decrease a child's appetite, resulting in decreased food intake and poor growth. The AAP policy statement recommends limiting juice intake: no more than 4 oz per day for 1- to 3-year-olds, 4 to 6 oz per day for 4- to 6-year-olds, and 8 oz per day for 7- to 18-year-olds (Heyman and Abrams, 2017).

Large volumes of sweetened beverages, combined with other dietary and activity factors, may contribute to overweight in a child. High intake of fructose, especially from sucrose and high-fructose corn syrup in processed foods and beverages, may lead to increased plasma triglycerides and insulin resistance. In several studies, low calcium intake and obesity have been correlated with high intake of sugar-sweetened beverages in preschool children (Keller et al, 2009; Lim et al, 2009). Higher milk and lower sweetened-beverage intake is associated with improved nutrient intake, including calcium, potassium, magnesium, and vitamin A (O'Neil et al, 2009). Children should be offered milk, water, and healthy snacks throughout the day instead of sugar-sweetened choices.

Excess sodium is another concern. An increase in sodium or salt intake results in an increase in systolic blood pressure and diastolic blood pressure (Bergman et al, 2010). A reduction in the use of processed foods may be warranted for children with elevated blood pressure. The Dietary Approaches to Stop Hypertension (DASH) diet is useful for all age groups because it increases potassium, magnesium, and calcium in relation to sodium intake (see Appendix 17).

Meal time in group settings is an ideal opportunity for nutrition education programs focused on various learning activities around food (Fig. 16.5). Experiencing new foods, participating in simple food preparation, and planting a garden are activities that develop and enhance positive food habits and attitudes.

TABLE 16.3 Suggested Portion Sizes for Children*

These suggestions are not necessarily appropriate for all children (and may be inappropriate for some children with medical conditions that greatly affect nutrient needs). They are intended to serve as a general framework that can be individualized based on a child's condition and growth pattern.

	1- to 3-Year-Olds	4- to 6-Year-Olds	7- to 12-Year-Olds	Comments
Grain Products	Bread: ½ to 1 slice Rice, pasta, potatoes: ¼ to ½ cup Cooked cereal: ¼ to ½ cup Ready-to-eat cereal: ¼ to ½ cup Tortilla: ½ to 1	Bread: 1 slice Rice, pasta, potatoes: ½ cup Cooked cereal: ½ cup Ready-to-eat cereal: ¾ to 1 cup Tortilla: 1	Bread: 1 slice Rice, pasta, potatoes: ½ cup Cooked cereal: ½ cup Ready-to-eat cereal: 1 cup Tortilla: 1	Include whole grain foods and enriched grain products.

Vegetables	Cooked or pureed:
	  2-4 tablespoons
	Raw: few pieces, if child can chew well
		Cooked or pureed:
		  3-4 tablespoons
		Raw: few pieces
			Cooked or pureed: ½ cup
			Raw: ½ to 1 cup
				Include one green leafy or yellow vegetable for vitamin A, such as spinach, carrots, broccoli, or winter squash.

Fruit	Raw (apple, banana, etc.): ½ to 1 small, if child can chew well Canned: 2-4 Tablespoons Juice: 3-4 ounces	Raw (apple, banana, etc.): ½ to 1 small, if child can chew well Canned: 4-8 Tablespoons Juice: 4 ounces	Raw (apple, banana, etc.): 1 small Canned: ¾ cup Juice: 5 ounces	Include one vitamin C–rich fruit, vegetable, or juice, such as citrus juices, an orange, grapefruit sections, strawberries, melon in season, a tomato, or broccoli.
Milk and Dairy Products	Milk, yogurt, pudding: 2-4 ounces Cheese: ¾ ounce	Milk, yogurt, pudding: ½ to ¾ cup Cheese: 1 ounce	Milk, yogurt, pudding: 1 cup Cheese: 1 ½ ounces	

Meat, Poultry, Fish, Other Protein	Meat, poultry, fish: 1-2 ounces
	Eggs: ½ to 1
	Peanut butter: 1 Tablespoon
	Cooked dried beans:
	  4-5 Tablespoons
		Meat, poultry, fish: 1-2 ounces
		Eggs: 1-2
		Peanut butter: 2 Tablespoons
		Cooked dried beans:
		  4-8 Tablespoons
			Meat, poultry, fish: 2 ounces
			Eggs: 2
			Peanut butter: 3 Tablespoons
			Cooked dried beans: 1 cup	

*This is a guide to a basic diet. Fats, oils, sauces, desserts, and snack foods provide additional energy to meet the needs of a growing child. Foods can be selected from this pattern for meals and snacks.
Modified from Lowenberg ME: Development of food patterns in young children. In Trahms CM, Pipes P: *Nutrition in infancy and childhood*, ed 6, St Louis, 1997, WCB/McGraw-Hill and Harris; Harris AB et al: *Nutrition strategies for children with special needs*, 1999, USC University Affiliated Program, Los Angeles.

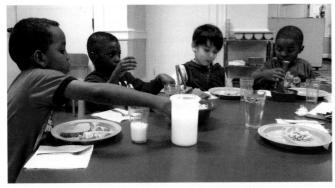

Fig. 16.5 Children who eat with each other in an appropriate environment often eat more nutritiously and try a wider variety of foods than when eating alone or at home. (Courtesy of Ana Raab.)

Feeding School Age Children

Growth from ages 6 to 12 years is slow but steady, paralleled by a constant increase in food intake. Children are in school a greater part of the day; and they begin to participate in clubs, organized sports, and recreational programs. The influence of peers and significant adults such as teachers, coaches, or sports idols increases. Except for severe

issues, most behavioral problems connected with food have been resolved by this age, and children enjoy eating to alleviate hunger and obtain social satisfaction.

School age children may participate in the school lunch program or bring a lunch from home. The National School Lunch Program (NSLP), established in 1946, is administered by the USDA. Children from low-income families are eligible for free or reduced-price meals. The School Breakfast Program (SBP), begun in 1966, is offered in many schools that participate in the lunch program. The USDA also offers the Afterschool Snacks and Summer Food Service for organized programs, the Fresh Fruit and Vegetable Program in selected schools, the Special Milk program for children not participating in school lunch, and the Child and Adult Food Care Program that reaches children in group or family child care sites (see Chapter 8).

Guidelines for the meals provided by the NSLP, SBP, and other programs are based on the IOM report, *School Meals, Building Blocks for Healthy Eating* and legislated by the 2010 Healthy, Hunger-Free Kids Act (McGuire, 2011). In addition to guidelines to align meal patterns with the Dietary Guidelines and to address other childhood health concerns, the Act makes resources and technical assistance available. Nutrition standards for the NSLP and SBP that follow the IOM recommendations and made significant changes to meal patterns were published in 2012. Some revisions and flexibility in meeting these standards have been introduced (Food and Nutrition Service, 2012; USDA, 2018).

Efforts have been made to decrease food waste by altering menus to accommodate student preferences, allowing students to decline one or two menu items and offering salad bars. Efforts to increase participation in school lunch require consistent messages that support healthful eating (Hayes et al, 2018).

School wellness policies were required by the school year 2006 to 2007 in institutions participating in school lunch and school breakfast programs. The school, including the administration, teachers, students, and food service personnel, in cooperation with families and the community, are encouraged to work together to support nutrition integrity in the educational setting (Bergman et al, 2010).

Consumption of school meals also is affected by the daily school schedule and the amount of time allotted for children to eat. One study suggested that children should have 25 minutes of seated time to increase dietary intake but also to reduce food waste (Cohen et al, 2016). Recess scheduled before lunch may increase intake of fruits, however more research is needed (Price and Just, 2015; Chapman et al, 2017; Fenton et al, 2015). A Montana "Recess Before Lunch" pilot study documented improvement in the mealtime atmosphere and students' behavior. Discipline problems on the playground, in the lunchroom, and in the classroom decreased (Montana Office of Public Instruction, 2010).

Children who require a special diet because of certain medical conditions such as diabetes, celiac disease, or documented food allergy are eligible for modified school meals. Children with developmental disabilities are eligible to attend public school from ages 3 to 21 years, and some of them need modified school meals (e.g., meals that are texture modified, or with increased or decreased energy density). To receive modified meals, families must submit written documentation by a medical professional of the diagnosis, meal modification, and rationale. For children receiving special education services, the documentation for meals and feeding can be incorporated as objectives in a child's individual education plan (IEP) (see Chapter 43).

Studies of lunches packed at home indicate that they usually provide fewer nutrients but less fat than school lunch meals. Favorite foods tend to be packed, so children have less variety. Food choices are limited to those that travel well and require no heating or refrigeration. A typical well-balanced lunch brought from home could include a sandwich with whole-grain bread and a protein-rich filling; fresh vegetables, fruit, or both; low-fat milk; and possibly a cookie, a graham cracker, or another simple dessert. Food safety measures (e.g., keeping perishable foods well chilled) must be observed when packing lunches for school.

Today many school age children are responsible for preparing their own breakfasts. It is not uncommon for children to skip this meal altogether, even children in the primary grades. Children who skip breakfast tend to consume less energy and other nutrients than those who eat breakfast (Wilson et al, 2006). Reviews of the effects of breakfast on cognition and school performance indicate a positive association between breakfast and school performance (Adolphus et al, 2016) (see *Focus On*: Breakfast: Does It Affect Learning?).

Snacks are commonly eaten by school age children, primarily after school and in the evening. As children grow older and have money to spend, they tend to consume more snacks from vending machines, fast-food restaurants, and neighborhood grocery stores. Families should continue to offer wholesome snacks at home and support nutrition education efforts in the school. In most cases, good eating habits established in the first few years help children through this period of decision making and responsibility. Developing and supporting programs and policies that ensure access to

FOCUS ON

Breakfast: Does It Affect Learning?

The educational benefits of school meal programs and especially the role of breakfast in better school performance have been debated and discussed for decades. Overall, breakfast consumption has been associated with better on-task classroom behavior (i.e., attention in class, and engagement in learning activities) regardless of nutritional and/or socioeconomic status. A literature review indicates associations between school performance and breakfast consumption, especially among children who were at nutritional risk (i.e., had wasted and stunted growth) and or were from low socioeconomic backgrounds (Adolphus et al, 2013). School-based breakfast experiments in 9- to 11-year-old and 6- to 8-year-old children found similar positive results with breakfast consumption (i.e., enhanced short-term memory, better spatial memory, and improved processing of complex visual stimuli), but other reports are less supportive (Adolphus et al, 2013). These studies suggest that brain functioning is sensitive to short-term variations in nutrient availability. A short fast may impose greater stress on young children than on adults, resulting in metabolic alterations as various homeostatic mechanisms work to maintain circulating glucose concentrations.

In addition to potential positive effects on academic performance, breakfast contributes significantly to the child's overall nutrient intake. These studies underscore the potential benefits—not only for low-income and at-risk children but also for all school children—of a breakfast at home or school meal programs that include breakfast. In 2016 14.57 million children participated in school breakfast programs (SBPs) (USDA, 2017). In 2015–2016, an additional 3.7% of students eligible for free and reduced-price school meals ate school breakfasts (Food Research and Action Center [FRAC], 2018).

better-quality food, larger quantities of food, and better living conditions for low-income children help to reduce health disparities where present.

Nutrition Education

As children grow, they acquire knowledge and assimilate concepts. The early years are ideal for providing nutrition information and promoting positive attitudes about all foods. This education can be informal and take place in the home with parents as models and a diet with a wide variety of foods. Food can be used in daily experiences for the toddler and preschooler and to promote the development of language, cognition, and self-help behaviors (e.g., labeling; describing size, shape, and color; sorting; assisting in preparation; and tasting).

More formal nutrition education is provided in preschools, Head Start programs, and public schools. Some programs such as Head Start have federal guidance and standards that incorporate healthy eating and nutrition education for the families involved. Nutrition education in schools is less standard and frequently has minimum or no requirements for inclusion in the curriculum or the training of teachers. Recommendations include policies in schools promoting coordination between nutrition education; access to and promotion of child nutrition programs; and cooperation with families, the community, and health services (Bergman et al, 2010).

Teachers attempting to teach children nutrition concepts and information should take into account the children's developmental level. The play approach, based on Piaget's theory of learning, is one method for teaching nutrition and fitness to school age children. Activities and information that focus on real-world relationships with food are most likely to have positive results. Meals, snacks, and food preparation activities provide children opportunities to practice and reinforce their nutrition knowledge and demonstrate their cognitive understanding. Involving parents in nutrition education projects can produce positive outcomes that are also beneficial in the home. Many written and electronic resources on nutrition education for children exist, including resources through the USDA's Team Nutrition and Choose MyPlate websites.

NUTRITIONAL CONCERNS

Overweight and Obesity

Overweight and obesity among children is a significant public health problem. The prevalence of obesity and overweight increased rapidly in the 1990s and 2000s, and plateaued from 2005 to 2006 and 2013 to 2014 (Hales et al, 2018). Obesity rates in some populations, for example Hispanic and non-Hispanic white children and adolescents, are continuing to increase.

NHANES (2015–2016) reported an obesity (BMI-for-age above the 95th percentile) prevalence of 16.8% in youth ages 2 to 19 years, and extreme obesity (BMI-for-age >120% of the 95th percentile) prevalence of 5.6% (Hales et al, 2018). For children 2 to 5 years of age, the prevalence of obesity decreased from 13.9% in 2003 to 2004 to 9.4% in 2013 to 2014 (Ogden et al, 2018a). Prevalence of obesity is higher among non-Hispanic black and Hispanic youth than among non-Hispanic white and non-Hispanic Asian children and adolescents (Ogden et al, 2018a). The prevalence of obesity varies by income and education level as well; obesity rates are lower in the highest income and education groups than among other groups (Ogden et al, 2018b). The Expert Committee report suggests the following terms to describe risk based on BMI: *obesity* as BMI-for-age at or above the 95th percentile and *overweight* as BMI-for-age between the 85th and 94th percentiles (Barlow and Committee, 2007), and CDC definitions also include a designation for "extreme" or "severe" obesity. Determining whether growing children are obese is difficult. Some excess weight may be gained at either end of the childhood spectrum; the 1-year-old toddler and the prepubescent child may weigh more for developmental and physiologic reasons, but this extra weight is often not permanent. BMI, a useful clinical tool for screening for overweight, has limitations in determining obesity because of variability related to sex, ethnicity, body composition, and maturation stage.

The CDC growth charts allow tracking of BMI from age 2 into adulthood; thus children can be monitored periodically, and intervention provided when the rate of BMI change is excessive. The BMI charts show the adiposity rebound, which normally occurs in children between 4 and 6 years of age (see Appendix 3). Children whose adiposity rebound occurs before 5½ years of age are more likely to weigh more as adults than those whose adiposity rebound occurs after 7 years of age. The timing of the adiposity rebound in childhood and excess fatness in adolescence are two critical factors in the development of obesity, with the latter being the most predictive of adult obesity and related morbidity (Williams and Goulding, 2009).

Although genetic predisposition is an important factor in obesity development, the increases in the prevalence of overweight children cannot be explained by genetics alone. Factors contributing to excess energy intake for the pediatric population include ready access to eating and food establishments, eating tied to sedentary leisure activities, children making more food and eating decisions, larger portion sizes, and decreased physical activity. In addition, American children snack three times a day, with chips, candy, and other low-nutrient foods providing more than 27% of their daily energy intake; this contributes 168 kcal per day (Piernas and Popkin, 2010). Many of the risk factors

for obesity are more prevalent among children from racial/ethnic minorities and families with lower socioeconomic status.

Inactivity plays a major role in obesity development, whether it results from screen time, limited opportunities for physical activity, or safety concerns that prevent children from enjoying free play outdoors. Although increased television viewing and computer and handheld game use have been associated with childhood overweight, a review suggests that the greater risk of overweight is related to television viewing plus a low activity level (Ritchie et al, 2005). The need to use automobiles for short trips limits children's opportunities to walk to local destinations, a phenomenon particularly relevant to children in the suburbs.

Obesity in childhood is not a benign condition, despite the popular belief that overweight children will outgrow their condition. The longer a child has been overweight, the more likely the child is to be overweight or obese during adolescence and adulthood. Consequences of overweight in childhood include psychosocial difficulties such as discrimination, a negative self-image, depression, and decreased socialization. Many overweight children have one or more cardiovascular risk factors such as hyperlipidemia, hypertension, or hyperinsulinemia (Daniels, 2009). An even more dramatic health consequence of overweight is the rapid increase in the incidence of type 2 diabetes in children and adolescents, which has a serious effect on adult health, development of other chronic diseases, and health care costs (see Chapter 30).

The AAP has developed guidelines for overweight screening and assessment for children from age 2 through adolescence (Barlow and Committee, 2007). In addition to growth parameters, other important information includes dietary intake and patterns, previous growth patterns, family history, physical activity, and family interactions. The U.S. Preventive Services Task Force (USPSTF) recommends obesity screening for children and adolescents 6 years and older and referral to comprehensive, intensive behavioral intervention treatment programs, if appropriate (Grossman et al, 2017).

A 2010 paper described a lower prevalence of obesity among children who were exposed to the following routines: regularly eating the evening meal as a family, obtaining adequate night-time sleep, and having limited screen-viewing time (Anderson and Whitaker, 2010). Interventions for obesity in children have had limited effect on the childhood obesity problem, especially for black, Hispanic, and Native American populations. Success is most likely to result from programs that include comprehensive behavioral components such as family involvement, dietary modifications, nutrition information, physical activity, and behavioral strategies (Barlow and Committee, 2007). Incorporating behavioral intervention in obesity treatment improves outcomes and is most effective with a team approach. Depending on the child, goals for weight change may include a decrease in the rate of weight gain, maintenance of weight, or, in severe cases, gradual weight loss (see Chapter 20). An individualized approach should be tailored to each child, with minimum use of restrictive diets or medication, except if there are other significant diseases and no other options.

Intervention strategies require family involvement and support. Incorporating motivational interviewing and stages of change theory into the comprehensive program will likely be more successful (see Chapter 13). Changes to address overweight should include the child's input, with choices and plans that modify the family's food and activity environment, not just the child's. Adequate energy and other nutrients are needed to ensure maintenance of height gain velocity and nutrient stores. The hazards of treating overweight children too aggressively include alternate periods of undereating and overeating, feelings of failure in meeting external expectations, ignoring internal cues for appetite and satiation, feelings of deprivation and isolation, an increased risk for eating disorders, and a poor or an increasingly poor self-image.

Some children with special health care needs, such as those with Down syndrome, Prader-Willi syndrome, short stature, and limited mobility, are at increased risk for being overweight. Their size, level of activity, and developmental status must be considered when estimating energy intake and providing dietary guidance to their families (see Chapter 43).

Prevention of childhood obesity is an important public health priority in the United States. The IOM has published recommendations that target families, health care professionals, industry, schools, and communities (IOM, 2012). The recommendations include schools (improved nutritional quality of food sold and served, increased physical activity, wellness education), industry (improved nutrition information for consumers, clear media messages), health care professionals (tracking BMI, providing counseling for children and families), and communities and government (better access to healthy foods, improved physical activity opportunities). Schools are a natural environment for obesity prevention, which can include nutrition and health curricula, opportunities for physical education and activity, and appropriate school meals. Efforts have resulted in school nutrition policies that limit the kinds of products sold in vending machines and food and beverages sold for fundraising. Cross-sectional data indicate that policies that limit the sale of competitive foods and beverages (foods sold outside the school meal programs) are associated with changes in consumption and availability of foods. More research is needed to understand long-term health effects of these policies (Chriqui et al, 2014). More research also is needed to develop effective prevention strategies that address the needs of diverse populations.

Families are essential for modeling food choices, healthy eating, and leisure activities for their children. Parents influence children's environment by choosing nutrient-rich foods, having family meals (including breakfast), offering regular snacks, and spending time together in physical activity, all of which can be critical in overweight prevention. Reducing sedentary behaviors can increase energy expenditure and reduce prompts to eat; the AAP recommends limiting screen time to no more than 2 hours per day (AAP, 2016). Parents exerting too much control over their child's food intake or promoting a restrictive diet may cause children to be less able to self-regulate and more likely to overeat when the opportunity is available (Ritchie et al, 2005). Health professionals should support positive parenting within the child's developmental level.

Underweight and Failure to Thrive

Weight loss, lack of weight gain, or failure to thrive (FTT) can be caused by an acute or chronic illness, a restricted diet, a poor appetite (resulting from constipation, medication, or other issues), feeding problems, neglect, or a simple lack of food. Some experts prefer the terms pediatric undernutrition or growth deficiency. Infants and toddlers are most at risk for poor growth, often as a result of prematurity, medical conditions, developmental delays, inadequate parenting, or a combination of these. Dietary practices also can contribute to poor growth, including food restrictions in preschool children stemming from parents' concerns about obesity, atherosclerosis, or other potential health problems.

A careful assessment is critical and must include the social and emotional environment of the child and any physical findings. If neglect is documented to be a contributing factor, health professionals are obligated to report the case to the local child protective services.

Because of the complexity of growth failure, an interdisciplinary team is ideal for assessments and interventions.

The provision of adequate energy and other nutrients and nutrition education should be one part of an overall interdisciplinary plan to assist children and their families. Attempts should be made to increase children's appetites and modify the environment to ensure optimal intake. Frequent small meals and snacks should be offered at regular times, using developmentally appropriate, nutrient-dense foods. This optimizes the smaller stomach capacity of the young child and provides structure and predictability for the eating environment. Families should receive support for positive parent-child interactions, with respect for the division of responsibility in feeding and avoidance of any pressure or coercion on the child's eating. Severe malnutrition may require carefully planned interventions and close monitoring to prevent refeeding syndrome.

Chronic constipation can result in poor appetite, diminished intake, and FTT. Ensuring adequate fluid and fiber intake can help relieve constipation, improve appetite, and eventually promote weight gain. Because the fiber intake of children is often low, especially in children who are picky eaters, fiber intake always should be addressed in the evaluation. Fiber can be increased by adding legumes, fruits (especially dried fruits), vegetables, high-fiber breakfast cereals, bran muffins, or all of these to the diet.

Iron Deficiency

Iron deficiency is one of the most common nutrient disorders of childhood. The highest prevalence of anemia in children occurs in those younger than 2 years of age (Gupta et al, 2017). Iron deficiency is less of a problem among older preschool and school age children.

Infants with iron deficiency, with or without anemia, tend to score lower on standardized tests of mental development and pay less attention to relevant information needed for problem solving. Poorer cognitive performance and delayed psychomotor development have been reported in infants and preschool children with iron deficiency. Deficiency can have long-term consequences, as demonstrated by poorer performance on developmental tests in late childhood and early adolescence (Lozoff et al, 2007). Iron intake should be considered during assessments of individual diets and in policy decisions intended to address the nutrition needs of low-income, high-risk children.

In addition to growth and the increased physiologic need for iron, dietary factors also play a role. For example, a 1-year-old child who continues to consume a large quantity of milk and excludes other foods may develop anemia. Some young preschool children do not eat much meat, so most of their iron is consumed in the nonheme form from fortified cereals, which is absorbed less efficiently (see Chapter 31).

Dental Caries

Nutrition and eating habits are important factors affecting oral health. An optimal nutrient intake is needed to produce strong teeth and healthy gums. The composition of the diet and an individual's eating habits (e.g., dietary carbohydrate intake, eating frequency) are significant factors in the development of dental caries (see Chapter 24).

Allergies

Food allergies during infancy and childhood are more likely when a child has a family history of allergies. Allergic symptoms are seen most often as respiratory or gastrointestinal responses as well as skin responses but may include fatigue, lethargy, and behavior changes. There can be confusion about the definitions of *food allergy*, *food intolerance*, and *food sensitivity*, and some tests for food allergies are unspecific and equivocal. See Chapter 25 for management of food allergies in children.

Attention-Deficit/Hyperactivity Disorder (ADHD) and Autism Spectrum Disorder

ADHD and Autism Spectrum Disorder are two common neurological disorders of childhood that affect behavior, socialization, and communication. Both can affect eating behaviors and nutrient intake which can manifest as food aversions, hypersensitivity to textures and flavors, and inadequate intake. See Chapter 43 for more details about assessment and MNT for these conditions.

PREVENTING CHRONIC DISEASE

The roots of chronic adult diseases such as heart disease, cancer, diabetes, and obesity are often based in childhood—a phenomenon that is particularly relevant to the increasing rate of obesity-related diseases such as type 2 diabetes. To help decrease the prevalence of chronic conditions in Americans, government and nonprofit agencies have been promoting healthy eating habits for children. Their recommendations include the Dietary Guidelines for Americans, the USDA MyPlate, the National Cholesterol Education Program (NCEP), and the National Cancer Institute Dietary Guidelines (see Chapter 10).

Cardiovascular Health

Compared with their counterparts in many other countries, American children and adolescents have higher blood cholesterol levels and higher intakes of saturated fatty acids and cholesterol. Early coronary atherosclerosis begins in childhood and adolescence. Risk factors include family history, breastfeeding and perinatal factors, nutrition and diet, physical activity, tobacco exposure, hypertension, hyper- and dyslipidemia, overweight and obesity, and diabetes. These were explored by an expert panel (National Heart Lung and Blood Institute, 2011); selected recommendations with nutrition implications are briefly summarized as follows:

For most healthy children limiting total fat to 30% of total energy, saturated fat to 7% to 10%, and dietary cholesterol to 300 mg/day is recommended. A balanced energy intake, increased intake of fruits and vegetables, and limiting "extra calories" to 5% to 15% total intake also is recommended for most children. Fiber intake of at least "age + 5 grams" (e.g., for a 4-year-old, 4 + 5 = 9 g per day) or 14 g fiber/1000 kilocalories is suggested.

For children with dyslipidemia, who are overweight or obese, or who have "risk factor clustering" or high-risk medical conditions, the Expert Panel recommends consideration of the Cardiovascular Health Integrated Lifestyle Diet (CHILD-1) as the first stage in dietary change (National Heart Lung and Blood Institute, 2011). This is a DASH-style pattern with emphasis on fat-free/low-fat dairy and increased intake of fruits and vegetables.

For all children, the approach to modifying risk factors, especially related to dietary fat intake, should be individualized (see Chapter 32).

Calcium and Bone Health

Osteoporosis prevention begins early by maximizing calcium retention and bone density during childhood and adolescence, when bones are growing rapidly and are most sensitive to diet and the important effects of physical activity (see Chapter 23). However, mean dietary intakes of calcium are lower than the AI, with 20% to 30% of pubertal girls having intakes less than 500 mg/day. One longitudinal study of white children from infancy to 8 years of age found that bone mineral content was positively correlated with intake of protein and several

minerals, suggesting that many nutrients are related to bone health in children (Bounds et al, 2005). Because food consumption surveys show that children are drinking more soft drinks and noncitrus juices and less milk, education is needed to encourage young people to consume an appropriate amount of calcium from food sources and possibly supplements (see Appendix 39).

Fiber

Education about dietary fiber and disease prevention has mainly been focused on adults, and only limited information is available on the dietary fiber intake of children. Dietary fiber is needed for health and normal laxation in children. National survey data indicate that preschool children consume a mean of 11 to 12 g/day of dietary fiber; school age children consume approximately 14 to 15 g/day (USDA, 2014). This is lower than the DRI for children, which is based on the same 14 g/1000 kcal as adults because of lack of scientific evidence for the pediatric population (Otten et al, 2006). Generally, higher fiber intakes are associated with more nutrient-dense diets in young children (Kranz et al, 2012; Papanikolaou et al, 2017).

The Gut Microbiome

The gut microbiome is an emerging topic in nutrition, including pediatric nutrition. It is clear that dietary and other factors affect the number and type of bacteria that colonize the gut. Factors that can affect the gut microbial community include dietary fiber, prebiotics, probiotics, and the use of antibiotic medication (see Chapter 1).

The gut bacteria profile seems to be associated with short- and long-term health outcomes. In addition to effects on GI disorders, research continues to explore the relationship between the gut microbiome and short- and long-term health outcomes, including obesity, digestive disorders, inflammation, and cancers (Peregrin, 2013).

Physical Activity

Children should be physically active each day, including play as well as structured activities, depending on age and developmental level. Decreased levels of physical activity are still seen in one third of children 4 to 11 years of age, with almost two thirds of the same group having high screen time (Anderson et al, 2008). Regular physical activity helps control excess weight gain and improves musculoseketal health and fitness and components of cardiovascular health (Janssen and Leblanc, 2010). Physical activity may also improve the child's mental health, blood pressure, and lipid profile (Janssen and Leblanc, 2010).

Current physical activity recommendations for those ages 6 through 17 years of age are 60 minutes or more of physical activity every day with the majority at a moderate or vigorous aerobic intensity. Children and adolescents should do vigorous intensity activity at least 3 days per week and include muscle-strengthening and bone-strengthening activity on at least 3 days per week. Information regarding activities that will meet these recommendations and are appropriate for children is available (U.S. Department of Health and Human Services [USDHHS], 2008). Strategies to increase activity in preschool and childcare settings, schools, and the community include more activity breaks, increased time outside, and improved walking/biking path infrastructure (USDHHS, 2012). Screen time (active games, exercise or dance videos, or TV exercise programs) can be a beneficial source of activity for youth. Three in 10 youth ages 9 to 18 engaged in at least 1 hour of active screen time weekdays, and 4 in 10 youth did the same on weekends (Wethington et al, 2013). MyPlate's *Eat Smart to Play Hard* materials promote the recommendation for 60 minutes of physical activity each day (Fig. 16.6). The Dietary Guidelines for Americans and MyPlate also have been applied to children and their parents.

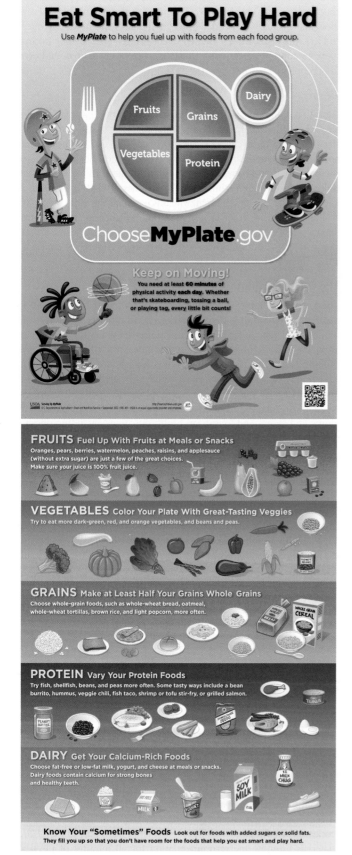

Fig. 16.6 Eat smart to play hard. (From United States Department of Agriculture: *Eat Smart to Play Hard* (website): http://www.fns.usda.gov/sites/default/files/eatsmartminiposter.pdf, 2012.)

CLINICAL CASE STUDY

Brian is a 7-year, 4-month-old white male who gained 15 pounds during the past school year. His height is 50½ inches, and his weight is 75 pounds. Brian moved to a new home and began a new school a year ago after his parents' divorce. After-school care has been provided by a retired neighbor, who loves to bake for Brian. He has few friends in the neighborhood, and his main leisure activities have been watching television and playing video games. When he gets bored, he often looks for a snack. His mother reports that they often rely on take-out and fast-food meals because of the time constraints of her full-time job, and she has gained weight herself. She recently started an aerobics class with a friend and is interested in developing healthier eating habits for herself and Brian.

After joint sessions with Brian and his mother, the following goals were identified by the family: (1) explore after-school care at the local community center, which has a physical activity component; (2) alter grocery and menu selection to emphasize the MyPlate and low-fat choices while still meeting the family's time and resource constraints; (3) begin to incorporate physical activities (Brian identified swimming and bicycling as things he would like to do) on the weekends; and (4) limit television and video games to no more than 2 hours daily.

After 4 months, Brian has enrolled in the local community center's afterschool program and participates in organized soccer and "pick-up" basketball. Weekends are a challenge. Brian and his mother have not yet incorporated physical activity into their weekend routine, and Brian finds it tough to limit screen time to 2 hours on the weekends. Brian has lost 4 pounds and is taller; he is 51 inches tall and weighs 66 pounds.

Nutrition Diagnostic Statement

- Overweight/obesity related to infrequent physical inactivity, sedentary lifestyle, and estimated excessive energy intake as evidenced by BMI-for-age above the 95th percentile.

Nutrition Care Questions

1. Calculate and plot Brian's BMI over time. Discuss the changes.
2. What recommendations should be made to prevent Brian and his mother from resuming their old habits?
3. What other activities can Brian try to help him avoid or reduce the tendency to eat when he is not hungry?
4. What would you suggest to promote a positive feeding relationship between Brian and his mother, considering his age and level of development?
5. What recommendations can you make to decrease Brian's energy intake and make it more consistent with MyPlate recommendations? Consider ideas to alter Brian's favorite recipes (e.g., his favorite meal is fried chicken with gravy, mashed potatoes, and ice cream), select healthy options from take-out or fast-food options, and modify snack options.
6. Are there any nutrient-related concerns because Brian's diet is being altered to help with weight management? Or because of his age? Or other factors?

USEFUL WEBSITES

Bright Futures in Practice: Nutrition
CDC Growth Charts
Health.gov Guidelines for Physical Activity
MyPlate Food Guidance System
National Center for Education in Maternal and Child Health
Pediatric Nutrition Dietetic Practice Group (DPG) Academy of
    Nutrition and Dietetics
USDA Food and Nutrition Service - School Meals

REFERENCES

Adolphus K, Lawton CL, Champ CL, et al: The Effects of breakfast and breakfast composition on cognition in children and adolescents: a systematic review, *Adv Nutr* 7(3):590S–612S, 2016.

Adolphus K, Lawton CL, Dye L: The effects of breakfast on behavior and academic performance in children and adolescents, *Front Hum Neurosci* 7:425, 2013.

American Academy of Pediatrics: Council on communications and media. Media and young minds, *Pediatrics* 138(5):e20162591, 2016.

American Public Health Association: *Food marketing and advertising directed at children and adolescents: implications for overweight.* Policy Statement 2003-17, 2017. Available at: https://www.apha.org/policies-and-advocacy/public-health-policy-statements/policy-database/2014/07/24/16/35/food-marketing-and-advertising-directed-at-children-and-adolescents-implications-for-overweight.

Anderson SE, Economos CD, Must A: Active play and screen time in US children aged 4 to 11 years in relation to sociodemographic and weight status characteristics: a nationally representative cross-sectional analysis, *BMC Public Health* 8:366, 2008.

Anderson SE, Whitaker RC: Household routines and obesity in US preschool-aged children, *Pediatrics* 125(3):420–428, 2010.

Bailey RL, Dodd KW, Goldman JA, et al: Estimation of total usual calcium and vitamin D intakes in the United States, *J Nutr* 140(4):817–822, 2010.

Bailey RL, Fulgoni VL, Keast DR, et al: Do dietary supplements improve micronutrient sufficiency in children and adolescents? *J Pediatr* 161(5):837–842, 2012.

Barlow SE, Expert Committee: Expert committee recommendations regarding the prevention, assessment, and treatment of child and adolescent overweight and obesity: summary report, *Pediatrics* 120(Suppl 4):S164–S192, 2007.

Bergman EA, Gordon RW, American Dietetic Association: Position of the American Dietetic Association: local support for nutrition integrity in schools, *J Am Diet Assoc* 110(8):1244–1254, 2010.

Berryman CE, Lieberman HR, Fulgoni VL, et al: Protein intake trends and conformity with the Dietary Reference Intakes in the United States: analysis of the National Health and Nutrition Examination Survey, 2001-2014, *Am J Clin Nutr* 108(2):405–413, 2018.

Black MM, Aboud FE: Responsive feeding is embedded in a theoretical framework of responsive parenting, *J Nutr* 141(3):490–494, 2011.

Bounds W, Skinner J, Carruth BR, et al: The relationship of dietary and lifestyle factors to bone mineral indexes in children, *J Am Diet Assoc* 105(5):735–741, 2005.

Bowman SA, Clemens JC, Friday JE, et al: Food patterns equivalents intakes by Americans: what we eat in America, NHANES 2003-04 and 2013-2014. In *Dietary Data Brief No. 17*, 2017, Food Surveys Research Group.

Brotanek JM, Halterman JS, Auinger P, et al: Iron deficiency, prolonged bottle-feeding, and racial/ethnic disparities in young children, *Arch Pediatr Adolesc Med* 159(11):1038–1042, 2005.

Centers for Disease Control and Prevention: *National center for health statistics. Data tables of stature for age and weight for age charts*, 2017. Available at: https://www.cdc.gov/growthcharts/clinical_charts.htm.

Chan JC, Sobal J: Family meals and body weight. Analysis of multiple family members in family units. *Appetite* 57(2):517–524, 2011.

Chapman LE, Cohen J, Canterberry M, et al: Factors associated with school lunch consumption: reverse recess and school "Brunch", *J Acad Nutr Diet* 117(9):1413–1418, 2017.

Chriqui JF, Pickel M, Story M: Influence of school competitive food and beverage policies on obesity, consumption, and availability: a systematic review, *JAMA Pediatr* 168(3):279–286, 2014.

Cohen JF, Jahn JL, Richardson S, et al: Amount of time to eat lunch is associated with children's selection and consumption of school meal entrée, fruits, vegetables, and milk, *J Acad Nutr Diet* 116(1):123–128, 2016.

Coleman-Jensen A, Rabbitt MP, Gregory CA, et al: *Household food insecurity in the United States in 2016, ERR-237*, Washington, DC, 2017, US Department of Agriculture ERS.

Cook JT, Black M, Chilton M, et al: Are food insecurity's health impacts underestimated in the U.S. population? Marginal food security also predicts adverse health outcomes in young U.S. children and mothers, *Adv Nutr* 4(1):51–61, 2013.

Daniels SR: Complications of obesity in children and adolescents, *Int J Obes (Lond)* 33(Suppl 1):S60–S65, 2009.

Davis GC, You W: The thrifty food plan is not thrifty when labor cost is considered, *J Nutr* 140(4):854–857, 2010.

Dwyer J, Nahin RL, Rogers GT, et al: Prevalence and predictors of children's dietary supplement use: the 2007 National Health Interview Survey, *Am J Clin Nutr* 97(6):1331–1337, 2013.

Expert Panel on Integrated Guidelines for Cardiovascular Health and Risk Reduction in Children and Adolescents, National Heart Lung and Blood Institute: Expert panel on integrated guidelines for cardiovascular health and risk reduction in children and adolescents: summary report, *Pediatrics* 128(Suppl 5):S213–S256, 2011.

Falbe J, Rosner B, Willett WC, et al: Adiposity and different types of screen time, *Pediatrics* 132(6):e1497–e1505, 2013.

Fenton K, Rosen NJ, Wakimoto P, et al: Eat lunch first or play first? Inconsistent associations with fruit and vegetable consumption in elementary school, *J Acad Nutr Diet* 115(4):585–592, 2015.

Fildes A, van Jaarsveld CH, Llewellyn CH, et al: Nature and nurture in children's food preferences, *Am J Clin Nutr* 99(4):911–917, 2014.

Food and Drug Administration: Advice about eating fish, from the Environmental Protection Agency and Food and Drug Administration; Revised fish advice, *Fed Regist* 82(12):6571–6574, 2017.

Food and Nutrition Service, USDA: Nutrition standards in the National School Lunch and School Breakfast Programs. Final rule, *Fed Regist* 77(17):4088–4167, 2012.

Food Research and Action Center: *School breakfast scorecard 2016–2017 school year*, 2018. Available at: https://frac.org/research/resource-library/school-breakfast-scorecard-2016-2017-school-year-february-2018.

Gilbert-Diamond D, Li Z, Adachi-Mejia AM, et al: Association of a television in the bedroom with increased adiposity gain in a nationally representative sample of children and adolescents, *JAMA Pediatr* 168(5):427–434, 2014.

Grossman DC, Bibbins-Domingo K, Curry SJ, et al: Screening for Obesity in Children and Adolescents: US Preventive Services Task Force Recommendation Statement, *JAMA* 317(23):2417–2426, 2017.

Guenther PM, Casavale KO, Reedy J, et al: Update of the Healthy Eating Index: HEI-2010, *J Acad Nutr Diet* 113(4):569–580, 2013.

Gundersen C, Ziliak JP: Food insecurity and health outcomes, *Health Aff (Millwood)* 34(11):1830–1839, 2015.

Gupta PM, Perrine CG, Mei Z, et al: Iron, anemia, and iron deficiency anemia among young children in the United States, *Nutrients* 9(8):E876, 2017.

Hales CM, Fryar CD, Carroll MD, et al: Trends in obesity and severe obesity prevalence in us youth and adults by sex and age, 2007-2008 to 2015-2016, *JAMA* 319(16):1723–1725, 2018.

Hamner HC, Perrine CG, Scanlon KS: Usual intake of key minerals among children in the second year of life, NHANES 2003-2012, *Nutrients* 8(8):E468, 2016.

Hayes D, Contento IR, Weekly C: Position of the academy of nutrition and dietetics, society for nutrition education and behavior, and school nutrition association: comprehensive nutrition programs and services in schools, *J Acad Nutr Diet* 118(5):913–919, 2018.

Heyman MB, Abrams SA, Section on Gastroenterology, Hepatology, and Committee on Nutrition: Fruit Juice in Infants, children, and adolescents: current recommendations, *Pediatrics* 139(6):e20170967, 2017.

Hobbs S, King C: The unequal impact of food insecurity on cognitive and behavioral outcomes among 5-year-old urban children, *J Nutr Educ Behav* 50(7):687–694, 2018.

Institute of Medicine, Committee on Accelerating Progress in Obesity Prevention, Glickman D: *Accelerating progress in obesity prevention: solving the weight of the nation* Washington, DC, 2012, National Academies Press.

Institute of Medicine, Panel on Macronutrients, Institute of Medicine (US). Standing Committee on the Scientific Evaluation of Dietary Reference Intakes: *Dietary reference intakes for energy, carbohydrate, fiber, fat, fatty acids, cholesterol, protein, and amino acids*, Washington, DC, 2005, National Academies Press.

Janssen I, Leblanc AG: Systematic review of the health benefits of physical activity and fitness in school-aged children and youth, *Int J Behav Nutr Phys Act* 7:40, 2010.

Jenkin G, Madhvani N, Signal L, et al: A systematic review of persuasive marketing techniques to promote food to children on television, *Obes Rev* 15(4):281–293, 2014.

Keller KL, Kirzner J, Pietrobelli A, et al: Increased sweetened beverage intake is associated with reduced milk and calcium intake in 3- to 7-year-old children at multi-item laboratory lunches, *J Am Diet Assoc* 109(3):497–501, 2009.

Kelly B, Halford JC, Boyland EJ, et al: Television food advertising to children: a global perspective, *Am J Public Health* 100(9):1730–1736, 2010.

Kranz S, Brauchla M, Slavin JL, et al: What do we know about dietary fiber intake in children and health? The effects of fiber intake on constipation, obesity, and diabetes in children, *Adv Nutr* 3(1):47–53, 2012.

Larsen JK, Hermans RC, Sleddens EF, et al: How parental dietary behavior and food parenting practices affect children's dietary behavior. Interacting sources of influence? *Appetite* 89:246–257, 2015.

Larson NI, Neumark-Sztainer D, Hannan PJ, et al: Family meals during adolescence are associated with higher diet quality and healthful meal patterns during young adulthood, *J Am Diet Assoc* 107(9):1502–1510, 2007.

Lim S, Zoellner JM, Lee JM, et al: Obesity and sugar-sweetened beverages in African-American preschool children: a longitudinal study, *Obesity (Silver Spring)* 17(6):1262–1268, 2009.

Lozoff B, Corapci F, Burden MJ, et al: Preschool-aged children with iron deficiency anemia show altered affect and behavior, *J Nutr* 137(3):683–689, 2007.

Madden MM, DeBias D, Cook GE: Market analysis of vitamin supplementation in infants and children: evidence from the dietary supplement label database, *JAMA Pediatr* 168(3):291–292, 2014.

Mahaffey KR, Clickner RP, Jeffries RA: Methylmercury and omega-3 fatty acids: co-occurrence of dietary sources with emphasis on fish and shellfish, *Environ Res* 107(1):20–29, 2008.

Mancino LT, Guthrie JF, Todd JE, et al: *How food away from home affects children's diet quality.* In. *ERR-104.* 2010, U.S. Dept. of Agriculture, Econ. Res. Serv.

McGuire S: Institute of Medicine. 2009. School meals: building blocks for healthy children. Washington, DC: the National Academies Press, *Adv Nutr* 2(1):64–65, 2011.

Montana Office of Public Instruction: *The Montana office of public instruction school nutrition pilot project - a recess before lunch policy in four Montana schools,* 2010; Available at: http://www.montana.edu/teamnutrition/documents/RBL%20pilot%20project.pdf.

Moshfegh A, Goldman J, Jaspreet A, et al: *What we eat in America, NHANES 2001-2002: usual nutrient intakes from food compared to dietary reference intakes,* Washington, DC, 2005, US Department of Agriculture, Agricultural Research Service.

Myers GJ, Thurston SW, Pearson AT, et al: Postnatal exposure to methyl mercury from fish consumption: a review and new data from the Seychelles Child Development Study, *Neurotoxicology* 30(3):338–349, 2009.

Nicklas TA, O'Neil CE, Kleinman R: Association between 100% juice consumption and nutrient intake and weight of children aged 2 to 11 years, *Arch Pediatr Adolesc Med* 162(6):557–565, 2008.

Ogden CL, Carroll MD, Fakhouri TH, et al: Prevalence of obesity among youths by household income and education level of head of household - United States 2011-2014, *MMWR Morb Mortal Wkly Rep* 67(6):186–189, 2018a.

Ogden CL, Fryar CD, Hales CM, et al: Differences in obesity prevalence by demographics and urbanization in US children and adolescents, 2013-2016, *JAMA* 319(23):2410–2418, 2018b.

Oken E, Bellinger DC: Fish consumption, methylmercury and child neurodevelopment, *Curr Opin Pediatr* 20(2):178–183, 2008.

O'Neil CE, Nicklas TA, Liu Y, et al: Impact of dairy and sweetened beverage consumption on diet and weight of a multiethnic population of head start mothers, *J Am Diet Assoc* 109(5):874–882, 2009.

Otten JJ, Hellwig JP, Meyers LD: *DRI, dietary reference intakes: the essential guide to nutrient requirements,* Washington, DC, 2006, National Academies Press.

Papanikolaou Y, Jones JM, Fulgoni VL: Several grain dietary patterns are associated with better diet quality and improved shortfall nutrient intakes in US children and adolescents: a study focusing on the 2015-2020 Dietary Guidelines for Americans, *Nutr J* 16(1):13, 2017.

Peregrin T: The inside tract: what RDs need to know about the gut microbiome, *J Acad Nutr Diet* 113(8):1019–1023, 2013.

Piernas C, Popkin BM: Trends in snacking among U.S. children, *Health Aff (Millwood)* 29(3):398–404, 2010.

Powell LM, Schermbeck RM, Chaloupka FJ: Nutritional content of food and beverage products in television advertisements seen on children's programming, *Child Obes* 9(6):524–531, 2013.

Price J, Just DR: Lunch, recess and nutrition: responding to time incentives in the cafeteria, *Prev Med* 71:27–30, 2015.

Rideout V: *The common sense census: media use by kids age zero to eight,* San Francisco, CA, 2017, Common Sense Media.

Ritchie LD, Welk G, Styne D, et al: Family environment and pediatric overweight: what is a parent to do? *J Am Diet Assoc* 105(5 Suppl 1): S70–S79, 2005.

Rose-Jacobs R, Black MM, Casey PH, et al: Household food insecurity: associations with at-risk infant and toddler development, *Pediatrics* 121(1):65–72, 2008.

Rovner AJ, O'Brien KO: Hypovitaminosis D among healthy children in the United States: a review of the current evidence, *Arch Pediatr Adolesc Med* 162(6):513–519, 2008.

Ryu JH, Bartfeld JS: Household food insecurity during childhood and subsequent health status: the early childhood longitudinal study—kindergarten cohort, *Am J Public Health* 102(11):e50–e55, 2012.

Satter E: *Child of mine: feeding with love and good sense,* Palo Alto, Calif. Berkeley, CA, 2000, Bull Publishers.

Savage JS, Fisher JO, Birch LL: Parental influence on eating behavior: conception to adolescence, *J Law Med Ethics* 35(1):22–34, 2007.

Semega J, Fontenot K, Kollar M: *Income and poverty in the United States: 2016,* Washington, DC, 2017, US Government Printing Office.

Stang J, Bayerl CT, American Dietetic Association: Position of the American Dietetic Association: child and adolescent nutrition assistance programs, *J Am Diet Assoc* 110(5):791–799, 2010.

Terry-McElrath YM, Turner L, Sandoval A, et al: Commercialism in US elementary and secondary school nutrition environments: trends from 2007 to 2012, *JAMA Pediatr* 168(3):234–242, 2014.

US Department of Agriculture, Agriculture Research Service: *Nutrient intakes from food: mean amounts consumed per individual, by gender and age, what we eat in America, NHANES 2013-2014.*

US Department of Health and Human Services: *Physical activity guidelines for Americans midcourse report: strategies to increase physical activity among youth,* Washington, DC, 2012, U.S. Department of Health and Human Services.

US Department of Health and Human Services, Office of Disease Prevention and Health Promotion: *2008 Physical activity guidelines for Americans summary,* 2008; Available at: http://www.health.gov/paguidelines/guidelines/summary.aspx.

USDA Food and Nutrition Service: *Nutrition standards for school meals,* 2019. Available at: https://www.fns.usda.gov/school-meals/nutrition-standards-school-meals.

USDA Food and Nutrition Service: *The school breakfast program,* 2017. Available at: https://www.fns.usda.gov/sbp/school-breakfast-program.

Wardle J, Cooke L: Genetic and environmental determinants of children's food preferences, *Br J Nutr* 99(Suppl 1):S15–S21, 2008.

Watts A, Berge JM, Loth K, et al: The transmission of family food and mealtime practices from adolescence to adulthood: longitudinal findings from project EAT-IV, *J Nutr Educ Behav* 50(2):141–147.e1, 2018.

Wethington H, Sherry B, Park S, et al: Active screen time among US youth aged 9-18 years, 2009, *Games Health J* 2:362–368, 2013.

Williams SM, Goulding A: Patterns of growth associated with the timing of adiposity rebound, *Obesity (Silver Spring)* 17(2):335–341, 2009.

Wilson NC, Parnell WR, Wohlers M, et al: Eating breakfast and its impact on children's daily diet. *Nutrition & Dietetics.* 63(1):15–20, 2006.

17

Nutrition in Adolescence

Nicole Larson, PhD, MPH, RDN, LD
Tashara M. Leak, PhD, RDN
Jamie S. Stang, PhD, MPH, RDN

KEY TERMS

adolescence	menarche	sexual maturity rating (SMR)
body image	peak height gain velocity	Tanner staging
disordered eating	physiologic anemia of growth	thelarche
growth spurt	pubarche	
gynecologic age	puberty	

Adolescence is one of the most exciting yet challenging periods in human development. Generally thought of as the period of life that occurs between 12 and 21 years of age, adolescence is a period of tremendous physiologic, psychological, and cognitive transformation during which a child becomes a young adult. The gradual growth pattern that characterizes early childhood changes to one of rapid growth and development, affecting physical and psychosocial aspects of health. Changes in cognitive and emotional functioning allow teens to become more independent as they mature. Peer influence and acceptance may become more important than family values, creating periods of conflict between teens and parents. Because all of these changes have a direct effect on the nutrient needs and dietary behaviors of adolescents, it is important that health care providers develop a full understanding of how these developmental changes of adolescence can affect nutritional status.

GROWTH AND DEVELOPMENT

Puberty is the period of rapid growth and development during which a child physically develops into an adult and becomes capable of reproduction. It is initiated by the increased production of reproductive hormones such as estrogen, progesterone, and testosterone and is characterized by the outward appearance of secondary sexual characteristics, such as breast development in females and the appearance of facial hair in males.

Psychological Changes

The physical growth of puberty transforms the teen body into an adult-like form, leading adults to believe that adolescent development is complete. However, the social and emotional development of adolescence lags behind. The mismatch between how teens look and how they act may lead adults to deduce that adolescents are "not acting their age." The rebellion that is associated with the teen years is actually the manifestation of their search for independence and a sense of autonomy. Food can be, and often is, used as a means of exerting autonomy. Adolescents may choose to become vegetarian as a way to differentiate themselves from their meat-eating parents or to express their moral and ethical concerns over animal welfare or the environment.

Cognitive and emotional development may vary greatly among adolescents, with some adolescents maturing faster than others. In general, adolescence is a time of impulsivity as a result of slow development in regions of the brain that govern cognitive control combined with a heightened reward response. Cognitive ability, including abstract reasoning, expands during adolescence; however, teens are more likely to base decisions on emotional as opposed to rational contexts (Steinberg, 2016). Psychosocial development can affect health and nutritional status in many ways, including the following:

- Preoccupation with body size, body shape, and body image (the mental self-concept and perception of personal body size), resulting from the rapid growth and development that has occurred, may lead to dieting and possibly disordered eating behaviors
- Diminishing trust and respect for adults as authority figures, including nutrition and health professionals
- Strong influence of peers and social media, especially around areas of body image and appearance, with the influence of a few select peers becoming more important than that of large groups as adulthood approaches
- More pronounced social, emotional, and financial independence, leading to increased independent decision making related to food and beverage intake
- Significant cognitive development as abstract reasoning is nearly complete and egocentrism decreases; however, teens may still revert to less complex thinking patterns when they are stressed
- Development of future orientation, which is required to understand the link between current behavior and chronic health risks
- Development of social, emotional, financial, and physical independence from family as teens leave home to attend college or seek employment
- Development of a core set of values and beliefs that guides moral, ethical, and health decisions

The psychosocial development of adolescents has a direct bearing on the foods and beverages they choose. Food choices are more likely to be based on taste, cost, convenience, and peer behaviors than on health benefits because these influences satisfy an adolescent's innate preference for immediate reward. Nutrition education and counseling that addresses topics adolescents care about such as improving athletic or scholastic performance and improving energy can be particularly effective in influencing health behavior change. Although many adolescents are concerned with their physical appearance, it is important to address this topic with caution and sensitivity so as not to reinforce negative biases or increase a sense of shame.

Sexual Maturity

Sexual maturity rating (SMR), also known as Tanner staging, is used to assess clinically the degree of sexual maturation during puberty (Tanner, 1962). Among males SMR is based on genital and pubic hair development (Fig. 17.1 and Table 17.1). Among females SMR is assessed by breast and pubic hair development. SMR is measured through a series of five stages, with stage 1 marking prepubertal development and stage 5 marking the completion of physical growth and development (see Appendix 4). The five stages of SMR correlate with other markers of growth and development during puberty, such as alterations in height, weight, body composition, and endocrine functioning. A thorough understanding of the relationship

between physical growth and development and SMR enables health care professionals to assess an adolescent's potential for future growth.

The timing of pubertal development is dependent on gender, ethnic/racial background, and between individuals within population subgroups. Puberty typically begins earlier for females, between the ages of 8 and 12 years, and begins between 9 and 14 years for males (Abreu and Kaiser, 2016). There is evidence that African American and Hispanic females tend to enter puberty and experience menarche earlier than non-Hispanic white females; variation in timing is notable for both thelarche (breast development stage 2) and pubarche (public hair stage 3). For example, data from the National Health and Nutrition Examination Study III (NHANES III, 1988–1994) shows that the median age of menarche is 12.2 years in African American females, 12.2 years in Hispanic females, and 12.6 years in non-Hispanic white females (Ramnitz and Lodish, 2013). Similarly, breast development occurs at a mean age of 9.5 years in African American females, 9.7 years in Hispanic females, and 10.3 years in non-Hispanic white females. Evidence regarding ethnic/racial differences in the timing of puberty for males is supported by fewer studies and is less consistent. However, NHANES III data shows that the timing of Tanner stage 2 genital development tends to be earlier for African American males (9.2 years) than for Hispanic males (10.3 years), but not different in comparison with non-Hispanic white males (10 years) (Ramnitz and Lodish, 2013).

Individual variation in the timing of puberty within population subgroups is influenced by genetic, environmental, and nutrition factors. There is strong evidence that a minimum body weight is needed for pubertal development to progress and also consistent evidence that obesity may contribute to early onset of puberty in females (Abreu and Kaiser, 2016; Li et al, 2017). An analysis of data from five cohort studies showed that the number of females with early puberty was greater in the group with a body mass index (BMI) in the 95th percentile or higher than that in the group with lower BMIs. The difference in puberty timing was specifically related to thelarche; elevated BMI was not linked to menarche (the onset of menses or menstruation). Evidence regarding an association between obesity and the onset of puberty in males is inconsistent (Li et al, 2017). Likewise, evidence regarding the influence of other specific nutritional factors is limited and, as yet, inconsistent. One example of a factor being investigated is animal foods; some research suggests that higher intake of animal foods is related to earlier sexual development, whereas vegetable protein intake has been related to later maturation (Villamor and Jansen, 2016). Evidence for the influence of other nutritional factors including prenatal nutrition, infant feeding practices, and childhood intake of fat, carbohydrate, and micronutrients is mixed (Villamor and Jansen, 2016).

In summary, many factors impact the timing of puberty and there is great variation across and within population subgroups. Secular trend data suggest that the age of pubertal development in U.S. females has declined since the late 1800s and may have continued to decline since the mid-1900s; however, data are insufficient to establish a similar trend among males and there continues to be much normal variation in timing (Abreu and Kaiser, 2016). Secular declines in the average age of menarche are likely due in part to improvements in general health and nutrition over time among the population (Ramnitz and Lodish, 2013). For individuals, it is further important to recognize that menarche increases the micronutrient requirements of females and the timing of menarche should therefore be evaluated during a full nutrition assessment.

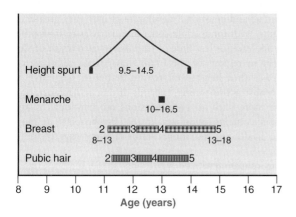

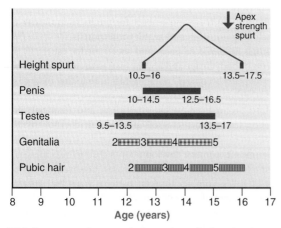

Fig. 17.1 Sequence of events during puberty in females (upper chart) and males (lower chart). Breast, genitalia, and pubic hair development are numbered 2 to 5 based on the Tanner developmental stages. (From Marshall WA, Tanner JM: Variations in the pattern of pubertal changes in males, Arch Dis Child 45:13, 1970.)

TABLE 17.1 Ratings of Sexual Maturation*

	Pubic Hair	Genitalia	Corresponding Changes
Males			
Stage 1	None	Prepubertal	
Stage 2	Small amount at outer edges of pubis, slight darkening	Beginning penile enlargement Testes enlarged to 5-mL volume Scrotum reddened and changed in texture	Increased sweat gland activity
Stage 3	Covers pubis	Penis longer Testes enlarged to 8-10 mL Scrotum enlarged	Voice changes Faint mustache and facial hair Axillary hair Beginning of peak height gain velocity (growth spurt of 6-8 inches)
Stage 4	Adult type, does not extend to thighs	Penis wider and longer Testes enlarged to 12 mL Scrotal skin darker	End of peak height gain velocity More facial hair Darker hair on legs Voice deeper Possibly severe acne
Stage 5	Adult type, spreads to thighs	Adult penis Testes enlarged to 15 mL	Significantly increased muscle mass
Females			
Stage 1	None	No change from childhood	
Stage 2	Small amount, downy, on medial labia	Breast buds	Increased sweat gland activity Beginning of peak height gain velocity (growth spurt of 3-5 inches)
Stage 3	Increased, darker, curly	Larger, but no separation of the nipple and the areola	End of peak height gain velocity Beginning of acne Axillary hair
Stage 4	More abundant, coarse texture	Larger Areola and nipple form secondary mound	Possibly severe acne Menarche begins
Stage 5	Adult, spreads to medial thighs	Adult distribution of breast tissue, continuous outline	Increased fat and muscle mass

*See Appendix 4.
Modified from Tanner JM: *Growth at adolescence*, ed 2, Oxford, 1962, Blackwell Scientific Publications.

Linear Growth

The velocity of physical growth during adolescence is much higher than that of early childhood (Fig. 17.2). On average, adolescents gain about 20% of their adult height during puberty. There is a great deal of variability in the timing and duration of growth among adolescents as illustrated in Fig. 17.3 by a group of 13-year-old students.

Linear growth occurs throughout the 4 to 7 years of pubertal development in most teens; however, the largest percentage of height is gained during an 18- to 24-month period commonly referred to as the growth spurt. The fastest rate of growth during the growth spurt is labeled the peak height gain velocity. Although growth slows after the achievement of sexual maturity, linear growth and weight acquisition continue into the late teens for females and early 20s for males and young men. Most females gain no more than 2 to 3 inches after menarche, although females who have early menarche tend to grow more after its onset than do those having later menarche. Increases in height are accompanied by increases in weight during puberty. Teens gain 40% to 50% of adult body weight during adolescence. The majority of weight gain coincides with increases in linear height. However, it should be noted that teens may gain more than 15 pounds after linear growth has ceased. Changes in body composition accompany changes in weight and height. Males gain twice as much lean tissue as females, resulting in differentiation in percent body fat and lean body mass.

Body fat levels increase from prepuberty averages of 15% for males and 19% for females, to 15% to 18% in males and 22% to 26% in females. Differences in lean body mass and body fat mass affect energy and nutrient needs throughout adolescence and differentiate the needs of females from those of males.

Deviations from the normal patterns of growth described here may occur along with chronic conditions experienced in childhood or the medications prescribed to treat common conditions. For example, the prescription of stimulant medications for the treatment of attention-deficit/hyperactivity disorder (ADHD) and inhaled corticosteroids for the treatment of asthma have been investigated due to concerns regarding appetite suppression and growth deficits (Richardson et al, 2017). Short-term studies of stimulant treatment have shown dose-dependent growth deficits of 1 to 1.4 cm/year mainly in the first 2 years of treatment. Research evidence regarding the longer-term impact of stimulants on growth is mixed; studies have reported divergent effects on growth and many studies have shown no clinically significant height deficits by adulthood. Similarly, inhaled corticosteroids are associated with mild growth suppression in the short term (0.4 to 1.5 cm/year) but no clinically significant effects on adult height. While additional research is needed to evaluate these therapies, the examples highlight the importance of addressing the impact of medication use as part of pediatric nutritional assessments.

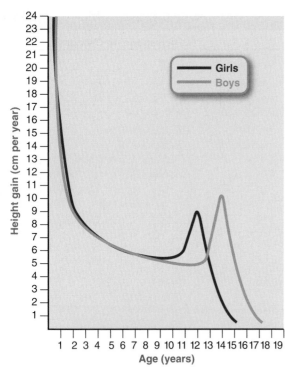

Fig. 17.2 Typical individual velocity curves for supine length or height in males and females. Curves represent the growth velocity of the typical boy and girl at any given age.

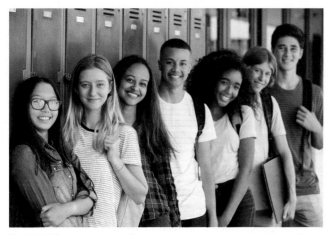

Fig. 17.3 These teens are all the same age, but their energy needs vary according to their individual growth rates. From www.istockphoto.com.

NUTRIENT REQUIREMENTS

The dietary reference intakes (DRIs) for adolescents are listed by chronologic age and gender (see inside cover). Although the DRIs provide an estimate of the energy and nutrient needs for an individual adolescent, actual need varies greatly between teens as a result of differences in body composition, degree of physical maturation, and level of physical activity. Therefore health professionals should use the DRIs as a guideline during nutritional assessment but should rely on clinical judgment and indicators of growth and physical maturation to make a final determination of an individual's nutrient and energy requirements.

Energy

Estimated energy requirements (EERs) vary greatly among males and females because of variations in growth rate, body composition, and physical activity level (PAL). EERs were established by the National Academy of Medicine, formerly the Institute of Medicine, and are calculated using an adolescent's gender, age, height, weight, and PAL, with an additional 25 kilocalories (kcal) per day added for energy deposition or growth (Institute of Medicine [IOM], 2006). To determine adequate energy intake, physical activity assessment is required. The energy requirements allow for four levels of activity (sedentary, low active, active, and very active), which reflect the energy expended in activities other than the activities of daily living. Tables 17.2 and 17.3 show the EER for each activity level based on PALs.

Adequacy of energy intake for adolescents is assessed best by monitoring weight and BMI. Excessive weight gain indicates that energy intake is exceeding energy needs, whereas weight loss or a drop in BMI below an established percentile curve suggests that energy intake is inadequate to support the body's needs. Groups of adolescents who are at elevated risk for inadequate energy intake include teens who "diet" or frequently restrict caloric intake to reduce body weight; individuals living in food-insecure households, temporary housing, or on the street; adolescents who frequently use alcohol or illicit drugs, which may reduce appetite or replace food intake; and teens with chronic health conditions such as cystic fibrosis, Crohn's disease, or muscular dystrophy.

Recent concerns about excessive energy intake among youth have centered on intake of solid fats and added sugars. The mean daily intake of solid fats and added sugars among young people ages 12 to 19 years represents 32% of total energy consumption (Bowman et al, 2016). On a given day, young people consume a mean of 38 grams of solid fats and 21.8 teaspoon equivalents of added sugars (Bowman et al, 2016). The main food and beverage sources of solid fats are milk, grain-based desserts, pizza, cheese, processed meats, and fried potatoes. Grain-based desserts are also a main source of added sugar intake along with sugar-sweetened beverages, candy and other sweet snacks, ready-to-eat cereals, dairy-based desserts, and sweeteners and syrups. Sugar-sweetened beverages are of particular concern as a source of added sugar intake; soft drinks contribute nearly 30% and fruit drinks contribute 15% of added sugars consumed by youth ages 2 to 18 years (Keast et al, 2013). NHANES data revealed that 64% of males and 61% of females consume a sugar-sweetened beverage on a given day (Rosinger et al, 2017). The proportion of energy from solid fats and added sugars is similar for foods and beverages obtained from stores (33%), schools (32%), and fast-food restaurants (35%) (Poti et al, 2014).

Counseling related to excessive energy intakes among adolescents should focus on intake of discretionary calories, especially those from added sweeteners consumed through soft drinks and candy and from solid fats consumed through snack foods and fried food. Tips should be provided for selecting nutrient-dense foods and beverages at all locations where teens spend their time.

Protein

During adolescence protein requirements vary with degree of physical maturation. The DRIs for protein intake are estimated to allow for adequate pubertal growth and positive nitrogen balance (IOM, 2006). Table 17.4 illustrates the protein requirements for adolescents. Actual protein needs are best determined based on a per kilogram of body weight method during puberty to account for differences in rates of growth and development among teens.

Insufficient protein intake is uncommon in the U.S. adolescent population. However, as with energy intake, food security issues, chronic illness, frequent dieting, and substance use may compromise

TABLE 17.2 Estimated Energy Requirements for Adolescent Males

Age	Reference Weight (kg [lb])	Reference Height (m [in])	ESTIMATED ENERGY REQUIREMENTS (KCAL/DAY)			
			Sedentary PAL*	Low Active PAL*	Active PAL*	Very Active PAL*
9	28.6 (63.0)	1.34 (52.8)	1505	1762	2018	2334
10	31.9 (70.3)	1.39 (54.7)	1601	1875	2149	2486
11	35.9 (79.1)	1.44 (56.7)	1691	1985	2279	2640
12	40.5 (89.2)	1.49 (58.7)	1798	2113	2428	2817
13	45.6 (100.4)	1.56 (61.4)	1935	2276	2618	3038
14	51.0 (112.3)	1.64 (64.6)	2090	2459	2829	3283
15	56.3 (124)	1.70 (66.9)	2223	2618	3013	3499
16	60.9 (134.1)	1.74 (68.5)	2320	2736	3152	3663
17	64.6 (142.3)	1.75 (68.9)	2366	2796	3226	3754
18	67.2 (148)	1.76 (69.3)	2383	2823	3263	3804

*PAL categories, which are based on the amount of walking per day at 2-4 mph, are as follows: *sedentary*, no additional activity; *low active*, 1.5-2.9 miles/day; *active*, 3-5.8 miles/day; and *very active*, 7.5-14 miles/day (see Table 2.3).
PAL, Physical activity level.
Data from Institute of Medicine, Food and Nutrition Board: *Dietary reference intakes for energy, carbohydrate, fiber, fat, fatty acids, cholesterol, protein, and amino acids*, Washington, DC, 2002, National Academies Press.

TABLE 17.3 Estimated Energy Requirements for Adolescent Females

Age	Reference Weight (kg [lb])	Reference Height (m [in])	ESTIMATED ENERGY REQUIREMENTS (KCAL/DAY)			
			Sedentary PAL*	Low Active PAL*	Active PAL*	Very Active PAL*
9	29.0 (63.9)	1.33 (52.4)	1390	1635	1865	2248
10	32.9 (72.5)	1.38 (54.3)	1470	1729	1972	2376
11	37.2 (81.9)	1.44 (56.7)	1538	1813	2071	2500
12	40.5 (89.2)	1.49 (58.7)	1798	2113	2428	2817
13	44.6 (91.6)	1.51 (59.4)	1617	1909	2183	3640
14	49.4 (108.8)	1.60 (63)	1718	2036	2334	3831
15	52.0 (114.5)	1.62 (63.8)	1731	2057	2362	2870
16	53.9 (118.7)	1.63 (64.2)	1729	2059	2368	2883
17	55.1 (121.4)	1.63 (64.2)	1710	2042	2353	2871
18	56.2 (123.8)	1.63 (64.2)	1690	2024	2336	2858

*PAL categories, which are based on the amount of walking per day at 2-4 mph are as follows: *sedentary*, no additional activity; *low active*, 1.5-2.9 miles/day; *active*, 3-5.8 miles/day; and *very active*, 7.5-14 miles/day (see Table 2.3).
PAL, Physical activity level.
Data from Institute of Medicine, Food and Nutrition Board: *Dietary reference intakes for energy, carbohydrate, fiber, fat, fatty acids, cholesterol, protein, and amino acids*, Washington, DC, 2002, National Academies Press.

TABLE 17.4 Protein: Estimated Average Requirements and Recommended Dietary Allowances for Adolescents

Age (yr)	EAR (g/kg/day)	RDA (g/kg/day)
9-13	0.76	0.95 or 34 g/day*
14-18 Males	0.73	0.85 or 52 g/day*
14-18 Females	0.71	0.85 or 46 g/day*

*Based on average weight for age.
EAR, Estimated average requirement; *RDA*, recommended dietary allowance.
Data from Institute of Medicine, Food and Nutrition Board: *Dietary reference intakes for energy, carbohydrate, fiber, fat, fatty acids, cholesterol, protein, and amino acids*, Washington, DC, 2002, National Academies Press.

protein intakes among adolescents. Teens who follow vegan or similarly restrictive diets are also at elevated risk for inadequate protein intake.

When protein intake is inadequate, alterations in growth and development are seen. In the still-growing adolescent, insufficient protein intake results in delayed or stunted increases in height and weight. In the physically mature teen, inadequate protein intake can result in weight loss, loss of lean body mass, and alterations in body composition. Impaired immune response and susceptibility to infection also may be seen.

Carbohydrates and Fiber

Carbohydrate requirements of adolescents are estimated to be about 130 g/day (IOM, 2006). The requirements for carbohydrates, as for most nutrients, are extrapolated from adult needs and should be used as a starting point for the determination of an individual adolescent's actual need. Adolescents who are very active or actively growing need additional carbohydrates to maintain adequate energy intake, whereas those who are inactive or have a chronic condition that limits mobility may require fewer carbohydrates. Whole grains are the preferred source of carbohydrates because these foods provide vitamins, minerals, and fiber. Intake of carbohydrate is adequate in most teens; data from the 2013–2014 What We Eat in America survey, a component of the NHANES, suggest that average daily intakes of carbohydrate are 298 g for teenage males and 220 g for females (U.S. Department of Agriculture [USDA], Agricultural Research Service [ARS], 2016b).

However, fiber intakes of youth are low because of poor intake of whole grains, fruits, and vegetables. The adequate intake (AI) values for fiber intake among adolescents are 31 g/day for males 9 to 13 years old, 38 g/day for males 14 to 18 years old, and 26 g/day for 9- to 18-year-old females. These values are derived from calculations that suggest that an intake of 14 g/1000 kcal provides optimal protection against cardiovascular disease (CVD) and cancer (IOM, 2006). Adolescents who require less energy intake because of activity restrictions may have needs that are lower than the AI values.

What We Eat in America survey data suggest that average daily intakes of fiber are 16.4 g for teenage males and 12.5 g for females (USDA, ARS, 2016b). The disparities between fiber recommendations and actual intakes suggest that more emphasis must be placed on making optimal sources of carbohydrates, including whole grains, fruits, vegetables, and legumes, readily available and appealing choices in the settings where adolescents make food choices.

Fat

DRI values for total fat intake have not been established for adolescents. Instead it is recommended that total fat intakes not exceed 30% to 35% of overall energy intake, with no more than 10% of calories coming from saturated fatty acids. Specific recommendations for intakes of omega-6 and omega-3 fatty acids have been set in an attempt to ensure that teens consume adequate essential fatty acids to support growth and development, as well as to reduce chronic disease risk later in life. The AI for omega-6 polyunsaturated fatty acids (linoleic acid) is 12 g/day for 9- to 13-year-old males, 10 g/day for 9- to 13-year-old females, 16 g/day for 14- to 18-year-old males, and 11 g/day for 14- to 18-year-old females. Estimated requirements for omega-3 polyunsaturated fatty acids (alpha-linolenic acid) among teens are 1.2 g/day for 9- to 13-year-old males, 1 g/day for 9- to 13-year-old females, 1.6 g/day for 14- to 18-year-old males, and 1.1 g/day for 14- to 18-year-old females (IOM, 2006).

Minerals and Vitamins

Micronutrient needs of youth are elevated during adolescence to support physical growth and development. The micronutrients involved in the synthesis of lean body mass, bone, and red blood cells are especially important during adolescence. Vitamins and minerals involved in protein, ribonucleic acid, and deoxyribonucleic acid synthesis are needed in the greatest amounts during the growth spurt. Needs decline after physical maturation is complete; however, the requirements for vitamins and minerals involved in bone formation are elevated throughout adolescence and into adulthood, because bone density acquisition is not completed by the end of puberty.

In general, adolescent males require greater amounts of most micronutrients during puberty, with the exception of iron. Micronutrient intakes during adolescence are often inadequate among some subgroups of teens, especially among females and young people of non-Hispanic black race (Moore et al, 2012; Papanikolaou et al, 2015). Data from the National Growth and Health Study, which followed a cohort

of more than 2300 girls over 10 years, suggest that the majority of teenage girls have inadequate intakes of calcium, magnesium, potassium, and vitamins D and E (Moore et al, 2012). The proportion of girls with inadequate intakes tends to increase with age. What We Eat in America survey data also can be used to monitor the adequacy of micronutrient intakes among U.S. adolescents. Compared with DRI recommendations this survey data suggests intakes of vitamin E and calcium are often too low among males and females (Tables 17.5 and 17.6) (USDA, ARS, 2016b).

Calcium

Because of accelerated muscular, skeletal, and endocrine development, calcium needs are greater during puberty and adolescence than during childhood or the adult years. Bone mass is acquired at much higher rates during puberty than any other time of life. In fact, females accrue approximately 37% of their total skeletal mass from ages 11 to 15 years, making adolescence a crucial time for osteoporosis prevention (IOM, 2011).

The recommended dietary allowance (RDA) for calcium is 1300 mg for all adolescents with an upper level intake of 3000 mg/day (IOM, 2011). Calcium intake declines with age during adolescence, especially among females. Research suggests that high soft drink consumption in the adolescent population contributes to low calcium intake by displacing milk consumption (Ranjit et al, 2010); conversely, adolescents who report more often having milk served at dinner tend to have lower intakes of sugar-sweetened beverages (Watts et al, 2018). Interventions to promote calcium consumption among young people should be

TABLE 17.5 Mean Intakes of Select Nutrients Compared with DRIs: Adolescent Males

	Mean Intake	9- to 13-year-old RDA/AI	14- to 18-year-old RDA/AI
Vitamin A (mcg RAE)	648	600	700
Vitamin D (µg)	6.0	15	15
Vitamin E (mg)	9.3	11	15
Thiamin (mg)	1.99	0.9	1.2
Riboflavin (mg)	2.53	0.9	1.3
Niacin (mg)	31.5	12	16
Vitamin B$_6$ (mg)	2.53	1	1.3
Folate (µg DFE)	620	300	400
Vitamin B$_{12}$ (µg)	6.50	1.8	2.4
Vitamin C (mg)	75.9	45	75
Phosphorus (mg)	1604	1250	1250
Magnesium (mg)	296	240	410
Iron (mg)	17.4	8	11
Zinc (mg)	13.7	8	11
Calcium (mg)	1186	1300	1300
Sodium (mg)	3960	1500	1500
Fiber (g)	16.4	31	38

AI, Adequate intake; *DRI,* dietary reference intake; *RDA,* recommended dietary allowance.
Data sources: U.S. Department of Agriculture (USDA), Agricultural Research Service (ARS): *Nutrient Intakes from Food and Beverages: Mean Amounts Consumed per Individual, by Gender and Age, in the United States, 2013-2014, What We Eat in America,* NHANES (website): www.ars.usda.gov/nea/bhnrc/fsrg, 2016.

TABLE 17.6 Mean Intakes of Select Nutrients Compared with DRIs: Adolescent Females

	Mean Intake	9- to 13-year-old RDA/AI	14- to 18-year-old RDA/AI
Vitamin A (mcg RAE)	507	600	700
Vitamin D (µg)	3.7	15	15
Vitamin E (mg)	6.7	11	15
Thiamin (mg)	1.35	0.9	1
Riboflavin (mg)	1.70	0.9	1
Niacin (mg)	20.5	12	14
Vitamin B_6 (mg)	1.60	1	1.2
Folate (µg DFE)	467	300	400
Vitamin B_{12} (µg)	3.90	1.8	2.4
Vitamin C (mg)	62.7	45	65
Phosphorus (mg)	1095	1250	1250
Magnesium (mg)	210	240	360
Iron (mg)	12.1	8	15
Zinc (mg)	8.6	8	9
Calcium (mg)	842	1300	1300
Sodium (mg)	2844	1500	1500
Fiber (g)	12.5	26	26

AI, Adequate intake; *DRI*, dietary reference intake; *RDA*, recommended dietary allowance.
Data sources: US Department of Agriculture (USDA), Agricultural Research Service (ARS): *Nutrient Intakes from Food and Beverages: Mean Amounts Consumed per Individual, by Gender and Age, in the United States, 2013-2014. What We Eat in America*, NHANES (website): www.ars.usda.gov/nea/bhnrc/fsrg, 2016.

BOX 17.1 Risk Factors for Iron Deficiency

Inadequate Iron Intake/Absorption/Stores
Food insecurity or living in poverty
Malabsorption diseases (e.g., celiac disease)
Unbalanced vegetarian eating styles, especially vegan diets
Restrictive diets that eliminate entire food groups
Low intakes of meat, fish, poultry, or iron-fortified foods
Low intake of foods rich in ascorbic acid
Frequent dieting or restricted eating
Chronic or significant weight loss
Meal skipping
Substance abuse
History of iron-deficiency anemia
Recent immigration from developing country
Special health care needs

Increased Iron Requirements and Losses
Heavy or lengthy menstrual periods
Rapid growth
Pregnancy (recent or current)
Inflammatory bowel disease
Chronic use of aspirin, nonsteroidal antiinflammatory drugs (e.g., ibuprofen), or corticosteroids
Participation in endurance sports (e.g., long-distance running, swimming, cycling)
Intensive physical training
Frequent blood donations
Parasitic infection

Reprinted with permission from Stang J, Story M, editors: *Guidelines for adolescent nutrition services*, Minneapolis, 2010, Center for Leadership Education and Training in Maternal and Child Nutrition, Division of Epidemiology and Community Health, School of Public Health, University of Minnesota.

initiated early and focus not only on increasing dairy product intake but also on decreasing intakes of soft drinks and increasing intakes of nondairy foods that are rich in calcium. Nondairy sources of calcium are particularly important for young people who may not consume milk for health or cultural reasons. Examples of nondairy calcium sources include calcium-fortified orange juice, soy milk, rice milk, and almond milk; calcium-fortified ready-to-eat cereals; enriched breads and other grains; some legumes (e.g., white beans) and dark green vegetables (e.g., kale, broccoli); and tofu prepared with calcium sulfate.

Iron

Iron requirements are increased during adolescence to support the deposition of lean body mass, increase in red blood cell volume, and need to replace iron lost during menses among females. Iron needs are highest during periods of active growth among all teens and are especially elevated after the onset of menses in adolescent females. The DRI for iron among females increases from 8 mg/day before age 13 (or before the onset of menses) to 15 mg/day after the onset of menses (IOM, 2006). Among adolescent males recommended intakes increase from 8 to 11 mg/day, with higher levels required during the growth spurt. Iron needs remain elevated for women after age 18 but fall back to prepubescent levels in men once growth and development are completed (IOM, 2006).

Median intakes of iron among adolescents in the United States are less than desirable. Increased needs for iron, combined with low intakes of dietary iron, place adolescent females at risk for iron deficiency and anemia. Rapid growth may temporarily decrease circulating iron levels, resulting in physiologic anemia of growth. Other risk factors

for iron deficiency anemia are listed in Box 17.1. During adolescence, iron deficiency anemia may impair the immune response, decrease resistance to infection, and decrease cognitive functioning and short-term memory (see Appendix 42).

Folate

The DRI for folate intake among adolescents is 300 mcg/day for 9- to 13-year-old males and females, increasing to 400 mcg/day for 14- to 18-year-olds (IOM, 2006). The need for folate increases during later adolescence to support accretion of lean body mass and to prevent neural tube defects among females of reproductive age. Food sources of folate should include naturally occurring folate, found in dark green leafy vegetables and citrus fruit, and folic acid found in fortified grain products (see Appendix 31).

Average intakes of folate reported in the 2013–2014 What We Eat in America survey suggest that adolescent females are at greater risk for inadequate intake than are males (USDA, ARS, 2016b). This is a cause for concern among adolescent females who have achieved menses and are sexually active, as having adequate folate status before conception is important for the prevention of birth defects such as spina bifida (see Chapter 14).

Vitamin D

Vitamin D plays an important role in facilitating calcium and phosphorus absorption and metabolism, which has important implications for bone development during adolescence (IOM, 2011). There is also some evidence that suggests vitamin D may play a role in cardiometabolic health, immunity, preventing chronic disease, and protecting against certain types of cancer; however, given the state of this evidence the current RDA is based solely on benefits for bone health (Golden and Carey, 2016). The RDA for vitamin D requirements among adolescents is 600 IU/day (15 µg/day) (IOM, 2011). See Appendix 38 for dietary sources.

A recent IOM report concluded that a serum 25(OH)D level of 20 ng/mL covers the requirement of 97.5% of the population (IOM, 2011). However, it is recommended that individuals at risk for vitamin D deficiency maintain a higher level of 30 ng/mL and there is a need for additional research to resolve ongoing debate and controversy regarding cutoff values for adequate and optimal circulating levels (Smith et al, 2017).

Based on current guidelines, there is a high prevalence of vitamin D deficiency among U.S. adolescents. Among youth ages 14 to 18 years, approximately one third have serum 25(OH)D levels below 20 ng/mL and 43% have levels between 20 to 29 ng/mL (Moore and Liu, 2017). There also have been noted declines in vitamin D status over the past two decades. NHANES data collected during the preceding few decades established that serum 25(OH)D levels decreased by 15% to 16% (Ganji et al, 2012). The reductions were especially obvious among non-Hispanic black participants and those in the highest BMI quintile.

Several factors may contribute to the recent increases and prevalence of vitamin D deficiency (Fiscaletti et al, 2017). Increased use of topical sunblock lotions has been advocated to prevent premature aging of the skin and some skin cancers, but its use also decreases vitamin D synthesis. Some evidence suggests that individuals with a higher BMI more readily sequester cutaneous vitamin D in adipose tissue, making it less bioavailable. Further, overweight youth may be less likely to engage in regular physical activity outdoors and thus have less exposure to sunlight. Other risk factors for vitamin D deficiency include malabsorption syndromes such as cystic fibrosis, long-term use of medications that increase its catabolism (e.g., corticosteroids), lactose intolerance or milk allergy, darkly pigmented skin, and residence at northern geographic latitudes where youth may spend little time outdoors during colder months. Low vitamin D intake is an important health risk for adolescents and deserves attention during nutrition assessment, education, and intervention (see Appendix 38).

Supplement Use by Adolescents

The consumption of moderate portions of a wide variety of foods is preferred to nutrient supplementation as a method for obtaining adequate nutrient intake. Despite this recommendation, studies show that adolescents do not consume nutrient-dense foods and usually have inadequate intakes of many vitamins and minerals; thus supplements such as a multivitamin may be beneficial for many adolescents (Keast et al, 2013). For most vitamins and minerals, national survey data indicate that only a small percentage of adolescents (<15%) are supplement consumers (USDA, ARS, 2017). The adolescents most likely to use supplements are those in good health with a higher household income and health insurance (Dwyer et al, 2013).

The use of herbal and other nonvitamin, nonmineral dietary supplements is not well documented. National data suggest that 5% of adolescents consume nonvitamin, nonmineral supplements; however, this estimate is based on parental report and the actual prevalence of use is likely higher as adolescents may not disclose all supplement use to their parents (Wu et al, 2013). Adolescents most likely to use nonvitamin, nonmineral supplements are those who report non-Hispanic white race, a higher household income, activity limitations resulting from chronic health conditions, long-term prescription use, or relatively heavy use of physician services. Many adolescent athletes also use or may consider the use of dietary supplements to improve sport

performance (see Chapter 22). The short- and long-term effects of such nonnutritional supplement use by adolescents are not known. Health professionals should screen adolescents for supplement use and should counsel them accordingly (see Chapter 11).

FOOD HABITS AND EATING BEHAVIORS

Food habits of concern that are seen more frequently among adolescents than other age groups include irregular consumption of meals, excessive snacking, eating away from home (especially at fast-food restaurants), dieting, and meal skipping. Many factors contribute to these behaviors, including decreasing influence of family, increasing influence of peers, exposure to various forms of media, employment outside the home, greater discretionary spending capacity, and increasing responsibilities that leave less time for adolescents to eat meals with their families. Most adolescents are aware of the importance of nutrition and the components of a healthy diet; however, they may have many barriers to overcome. Among the most challenging barriers are household food insecurity, discrimination against some ethnic/racial groups, and weight-related concerns (Larson and Story, 2015; Waxman et al, 2015).

Teens perceive taste preferences, hectic schedules, the cost and accessibility of different foods, and social support from family and friends to be key factors that affect their food and beverage choices (Berge et al, 2012). For example, parents may positively influence the food and beverage choices of teens by modeling healthy eating habits, selecting healthy foods for family meals, encouraging healthy eating, and setting limits on the consumption of unhealthy snack foods. Friends influence each other through modeling and shared activities, such as eating out at fast-food restaurants and purchasing snacks at convenience stores near school.

Developmentally, many teens lack the ability to associate current eating habits with future disease risk. Teens often are more focused on "fitting in" with their peers. They adopt health behaviors that demonstrate their quest for autonomy and make them feel more like adults such as drinking alcohol, smoking, and engaging in sexual activity. Nutrition education and counseling should focus on short-term benefits that many adolescents care about, such as improving school and sports performance and having more energy. Although appearance is also important to many adolescents, this topic needs to be discussed carefully so as to not reinforce negative biases. Messages should be positive, developmentally appropriate, and concrete. Specific skills such as choosing water, unsweetened tea, or milk over sugar-sweetened drinks; ordering broiled rather than fried meats; and choosing baked rather than fried snack foods are key concepts to discuss.

Irregular Meals and Snacking

Meal skipping is common among adolescents. Meal skipping increases throughout adolescence as teens try to sleep longer in the morning, try to lose weight through calorie restriction, and try to manage their busy lives. Breakfast is the most commonly skipped meal. National data suggest that approximately one quarter of adolescents (12 to 19 years) skip breakfast on a given day (USDA, ARS, 2016a). Breakfast skipping has been associated with poor health outcomes, including higher BMI; poorer concentration and school performance; and increased risk of inadequate nutrient intake (Burrows et al, 2017). Adolescents who skip breakfast tend to have a higher intake of added sugars and poorer intake of key nutrients (e.g., calcium, vitamin A) compared with those who eat breakfast, especially when the breakfast meal is composed of healthy foods that may be fortified such as ready-to-eat cereal.

Teens who skip meals often snack in response to hunger instead of eating a meal. Most teens (92% of males, 91% of females) consume at least one snack per day, and the majority of teens who report snacking consume two or more snacks per day (USDA, ARS, 2016c). Snack foods consumed by teens are often high in added fats, sweeteners, and sodium. Soft drinks and other sugar-sweetened beverages are consumed commonly, accounting for a substantial proportion of daily caloric intake and representing an important source of caffeine consumption (see *Focus On:* Caffeine and Substance Use by Adolescents). Daily average energy intake from sugar-sweetened beverages is 232 calories among teen boys and 162 calories among teen girls, representing 9.3% and 9.7% of total daily calories respectively (Rosinger et al, 2017). Frequent snacking may promote higher total energy intake and a higher proportion of energy provided by added and total sugars (Larson and Story, 2013). However, national data indicate that snacks also make positive contributions to intake of key nutrients. For example, 2013–2014 NHANES data for male and female adolescents indicate that foods and beverages consumed at snack occasions provide 16% to 17% of folate intake, 21% to 25% of vitamin C intake, 20% of vitamin D intake, 23% to 25% of calcium intake, and 16% to 19% of iron intake (USDA, ARS, 2016d). Because snacks are prevalent and often consumed in place of meals, teens should be encouraged to make healthy choices when choosing these snack foods and beverages. Box 17.2 provides ideas for healthy snacks or meal alternatives for teens.

Fast Foods and Convenience Foods

Convenience foods include foods and beverages from vending machines, canteens, school stores, fast-food restaurants, and convenience stores. As adolescents spend considerable amounts of time in and around schools, convenience foods available at school and in the surrounding neighborhood are likely to influence their eating patterns. National data indicate vending machines are available in 33% of middle schools and 66% of high schools (Centers for Disease Control and Prevention, 2015). About one quarter of all

middle schools and 29% of high schools have a school store where students can purchase food or beverages (Centers for Disease Control and Prevention, 2015). In addition, middle schools and high schools often have a fast-food restaurant or convenience store within walking distance. Fast-food restaurants and convenience stores are socially acceptable places for teens to eat, spend time with their friends, and even work.

BOX 17.2   Adolescent-Friendly Healthy Snacks

Unsweetened, low-fat yogurt layered with berries and granola
Oatmeal made with milk and sliced fruit
Whole grain crackers with cheese and fruit
Sliced apples dipped in peanut butter
Whole-wheat bagel or english muffin half topped with cream cheese, peanut butter or almond butter
Air-popped popcorn
Whole-wheat pita wedges topped with 1 to 2 tablespoons of hummus
Baked tortilla chips with bean dip or salsa
Baked potato topped with salsa or broccoli and melted cheese
Graham crackers and peanut or almond butter
Frozen yogurt or 100% juice bars with no added sugar
Trail mix (dried fruit with nuts and seeds)
Baby carrots with hummus
Whole grain, low sugar granola bars
Mini rice cakes or popcorn cakes with hummus
Whole-wheat tortilla wraps with turkey, cheese, lettuce, and tomato

Adapted with permission from Stang J, Story M, editors: *Guidelines for adolescent nutrition services*, Minneapolis, 2010, Center for Leadership Education and Training in Maternal and Child Nutrition, Division of Epidemiology and Community Health, School of Public Health, University of Minnesota.

◎ FOCUS ON

Caffeine and Substance Use by Adolescents

Three out of four adolescents consume caffeine on a given day, mostly from soft drinks, tea, and coffee (Branum et al, 2014). Although average caffeine intake among adolescents does not exceed the recommended daily limit of 100 mg, energy drinks are becoming increasingly popular, and the amount of caffeine in these drinks is not regulated by the Food and Drug Administration (FDA) (Branum et al, 2014; Seifert et al, 2011). The FDA has imposed a limit on caffeine of 71 mg per 12-ounce serving for soft drinks, whereas energy drinks have been found to contain nonnutritive stimulants (e.g., caffeine and guarana) in amounts that range from 2.5 to 171 mg per ounce (Terry-McElrath et al, 2014). Of further concern, at least one study has found that energy drink users are more likely than their peers to report alcohol, cigarette, and illicit drug use.

The relationship between energy drink consumption and substance abuse was explored using a 2010–2011 survey. This survey data were collected from a nationally representative sample of 21,995 secondary school students (grades 8, 10, and 12) who were participating in the Monitoring the Future study (Terry-McElrath et al, 2014). Students self-reported how many energy drinks they consumed on an average day. Substance use data were also self-reported, including frequency of alcohol, cigarette, marijuana, and amphetamine use in the past 30 days. Energy drink consumption was related to greater use of each substance for students in all grades. This research suggests that certain groups of adolescents may be particularly likely to consume energy drinks and to be substance users, and nutrition educators should inform parents and adolescents about the masking effects of caffeine in energy drinks on alcohol- and other substance-related impairments.

Highly processed convenience foods tend to be low in vitamins, minerals, and fiber, but high in calories, added fat, sweeteners, and sodium. National data suggest that many teens consume one or more item from a fast-food restaurant or the convenient snack options at school on a given day (Poti et al, 2014). Few adolescents are willing to stop purchasing such convenience foods because the low price, easy

access, and taste appeal to them. Instead of asking young people to not eat these foods, health professionals should counsel them on how to make healthy choices and work with schools to implement the USDA nutrition standards for convenience foods sold in schools (Fig. 17.4; Hayes et al, 2018). Counseling adolescents with concrete guidelines that are easy to remember, such as choosing snacks or vending and

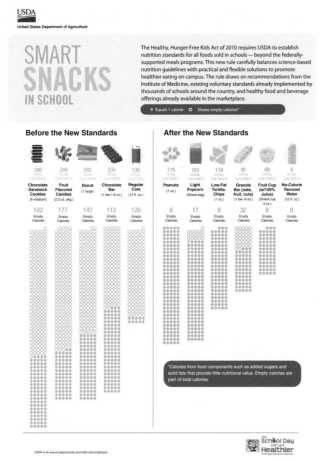

Fig. 17.4 Smart Snacks in School: U.S. Department of Agriculture nutrition standards for convenience foods sold in schools. Available at: https://www.fns.usda.gov/school-meals/tools-schools-focusing-smart-snacks.

fast-food options with fewer than 5 g of fat per serving and no more than a few grams of added sugar, can be particularly effective. Adolescents also can be encouraged to check labels to determine whether foods are made from whole grains or are high in added sweeteners or sodium.

Family Meals

The frequency with which adolescents eat meals with their families decreases with age (Child Trends, 2013). Nearly half of 12- to 14-year-olds eat meals with their families at least 6 days per week compared with just more than one third of 15- to 17-year-olds. Adolescents who eat meals with their families have been found to have better academic performance, to be less likely to engage in risky behaviors such as illicit drug use, and to be less likely to have school problems compared with peers who do not frequently engage in family meals (Goldfarb et al, 2015).

Developing healthful eating patterns at family meals during adolescence may improve the likelihood that individuals will choose to consume nutritious foods in adulthood and may protect them from the future development of overweight (Berge et al, 2015). Family meals not only allow for more communication between teens and their parents but also provide an ideal environment during which parents can model healthy food and beverage choices and attitudes toward eating. Teens who eat at home more frequently have been found to consume fewer soft drinks and more calcium-rich foods, fruit, and vegetables (Larson et al, 2013) (see *Focus On:* Family Meals and Nutritional Benefits for Teens).

FOCUS ON
Family Meals and Nutritional Benefits for Teens

When teens regularly share dinners with their families, they are more likely to have diets of higher nutritional quality, and some evidence suggests the practice may protect them against the future development of overweight in young adulthood (Berge et al, 2015). However, different schedules and difficulty finding time to eat together are common barriers to sharing the evening meal. One study examined whether there are similar benefits associated with eating breakfast together (Larson et al, 2013). Students at 20 public middle schools and high schools in the Minneapolis-St. Paul metropolitan area of Minnesota were surveyed about their dietary practices and how often they have a family meal at breakfast and at dinner. Approximately 71% of students at these schools qualified for free or reduced-price school meals and 81% represented a racial/ethnic background other than non-Hispanic white. Among these students, family breakfast meals occurred on average less often than family dinners (1.5 breakfast meals versus 4.1 dinner meals per week) and less than 10% of students ate together daily with "all or most" of their family at breakfast. However, participation in more frequent family breakfast meals was linked to several markers of better diet quality (e.g., more fruits, whole grains, and fiber) as well as lower risk for overweight. These associations were found while accounting for family dinner frequency as well as structural and organizational characteristics of families and thus suggest that although it is not always possible to eat dinner together, coming together for other meals such as breakfast can provide benefits. Health professionals should encourage families to eat together at breakfast as well as at dinner, and to provide supports for addressing challenges such as lack of time, food security, and limited food preparation skills.

Media and Advertising

The advertising of food and beverages is a multi-billion dollar business. In 2016 a total of more than $13.5 billion was spent by food, beverage, and restaurant companies on advertising their products (Harris et al, 2017). These food-related companies promote their products using a number of different techniques (e.g., contests, product placements, sponsorships, celebrity endorsements, viral marketing) and multiple forms of media; however, television is a dominant advertising medium. Of the $13.5 billion spent on advertising by food-related companies, $10 billion was spent on television advertising (Harris et al, 2017).

The high television advertising expenditures translate to the daily average of 10 to 11 food-related ads being viewed by youth. Despite recent declines in the amount of time youth spend watching television, an average of more than 2 hours per day are spent with television and the number of food-related ads appearing per hour of television programming was found to increase between 2007 and 2016. An analysis of television advertising found that just 56 of the more than 20,300 food-related companies were responsible for 85% of food-related ads viewed by youth; these companies include several that participate in the self-regulatory programs known as the Children's Food and Beverage Advertising Initiative (CFBAI) and Children's Confection Advertising Initiative (CCAI) but also a large number of companies that do not limit their child-directed advertising to healthier dietary choices. Although the CFBAI and CCAI companies were further found to have kept their pledges from 2007 to 2016 by reducing ads for less healthy products on children's television channels and media primarily directed to children under age 12 years, these improvements had limited benefits for adolescent viewers. During this period, adolescent exposure to ads for candy, sugary drinks, snack food, and fast-food brands was conversely found to increase. Most food advertisements viewed by adolescents are for products high in fat, sugar, or sodium, and fast-food restaurant advertisements are the most frequently viewed (Powell et al, 2010). Research shows that food advertising increases young people's immediate and future food choices and food brand preferences and it is not until late adolescence that a young person's ability to cope with advertising will surface (Lapierre et al, 2017). Along with ongoing efforts to limit young people's exposure to advertising for unhealthy products, media literacy education can and should be taught to teens to assist them in determining the accuracy and validity of media and advertising messages.

Dieting and Body Image

Body image concerns are common during adolescence. Many adolescents describe themselves as being overweight despite being at a healthy BMI, signifying a disturbance in their body image. Poor body image can lead to weight control issues and dieting. The Youth Risk Behavior Surveillance System data from 2017 show that 47.1% of U.S. high school students were attempting to lose weight. The prevalence of dieting was higher among female (59.9%) than male (34.0%) students. Hispanic females had the highest prevalence of dieting at 65.6%, followed by white females (58.6%), black females (55.3%), Hispanic males (45.7%), white males (30.6%), and black males (28.9%) (Kann et al, 2018).

Eating nutrient-dense foods (e.g., fruits and vegetables, lean meats and fish, low fat or nonfat dairy, legumes, nuts) to limit calories and getting regular exercise can be viewed as healthy weight loss behaviors when used in moderation and can be a starting point for nutrition education and counseling to improve eating behaviors. However, not all dieting behaviors have the potential to improve health. High-risk dieting practices are used by many adolescents and carry with them the risk of poor nutritional status and increased risk for disordered eating (see Chapter 21). The most recent available national survey data on disordered eating behaviors indicate that fasting, or refraining from eating for more than 24 hours, was practiced by 17% of female and 7% of male U.S. high school students in the past month as a means of dieting (Eaton et al, 2012). Furthermore, 6% of females and 4% of males had used diet pills to lose weight; the prevalence of this behavior was highest among Hispanic students and increased with age. The use of purging methods, including vomiting and laxative or diuretic use, was reported by 6% of females and 3% of males. White and Hispanic students were more likely to report purging behaviors than African American students. In providing adolescents with advice around healthy weight loss behaviors, it is prudent to also screen for the use of any high-risk dieting practices so that appropriate counseling regarding the harms of such practices can be provided.

NUTRITION SCREENING, ASSESSMENT, AND COUNSELING

The American Academy of Pediatrics recommends that adolescents have an annual health screening to address priority issues, including physical growth and development, social and academic competence, emotional well-being, risk reduction (e.g., for substance use, sexually transmitted infections), and violence and injury prevention (Hagan et al, 2017). The supervision of physical growth and development should involve an assessment of nutrition risk and the provision of anticipatory guidance. Nutrition screening should include the assessment of height, weight, and BMI to determine weight status; evaluation for the presence of iron deficiency anemia (females only); review of oral health (e.g., regular dental visits, intake of high-sugar foods); and assessment of physical fitness and media use, including time spent engaged with social media (Anderson and Jiang, 2018). Anticipatory guidance should further address healthy eating behaviors and building a positive body image.

Weight, height, and BMI should be plotted using the Centers for Disease Control and Prevention (CDC) National Center for Health Statistics BMI tables to determine appropriateness of weight for height (see Appendix 3). A BMI below the fifth percentile may signal the presence of chronic or metabolic disease, growth failure, or an eating disorder. A BMI at or above the 85th percentile but below the 95th percentile may indicate that an adolescent is overweight, whereas a BMI at or above the 95th percentile may indicate the presence of obesity. For some young people, a high BMI value reflects high lean body mass rather than high levels of body fat; therefore, it can be valuable to conduct further direct assessment of body fat when done in a sensitive manner and used to inform counseling that is focused on health behaviors (Hagan et al, 2017) (for additional information, see Chapter 5).

When nutrition screening indicates the presence of nutritional risk, a full assessment should be conducted. Nutrition assessment should include a complete evaluation of food intake through a 24-hour recall, dietary records, or brief food frequency questionnaire (see Chapter 4). The adequacy of energy, fiber, macronutrients, and micronutrients should be determined, as well as excessive intake of any dietary components such as sodium or sweeteners. Nutritional assessments also should include an evaluation of the nutritional environment, including parental, peer, school, cultural, and personal lifestyle factors. The attitude of the adolescent toward food and nutrition is important; helping the adolescent overcome perceived barriers to eating well through methods such as motivational interviewing is an essential component of nutrition counseling.

Teens who live in food-insecure households, temporary housing, or shelters, or who have run away from home are at especially high nutritional risk, as are adolescents who use alcohol and street drugs. It is important that health professionals working with high-risk teens develop partnerships with community-based food assistance programs to ensure that youth have access to a steady, nutritious food supply. Homeless teens, as well as those living in temporary shelters, benefit from nutrition counseling focusing on lightweight, low-cost, prepackaged foods that do not require refrigeration or cooking facilities. Dried fruit, nuts, granola bars, cereal bars, tuna in pouches, and meat jerky are foods that should be available for runaway or homeless teens.

Education and counseling should be tailored to meet any specific nutrition diagnoses identified during the assessment. An adolescent with a diagnosis of type 2 diabetes who experiences rapid weight gain requires a different type and intensity of counseling than a teen who has been diagnosed with iron deficiency anemia. Knowledge, attitude, motivation, and behavior must be addressed when guiding adolescents toward acquiring healthful food habits. For a plan to succeed the adolescent needs to be interested in making change; therefore an assessment of a teenager's desire to change is essential. Encouraging the desire to change usually requires attention, creativity, patience, and significant rapport building (see Chapter 13).

Information can be provided in various settings ranging from the classroom to the hospital (Fig. 17.5). It is valuable for clinicians to understand the change process and how to communicate it meaningfully so they can provide personalized and more effective counseling. Parents may be included in the process and are encouraged to be supportive. Recommended eating plans based on recommended energy intakes for adolescents are shown in Table 17.7.

SPECIAL TOPICS

Vegetarian Dietary Patterns

As adolescents mature, they begin to develop autonomous social, moral, and ethical values. These values may lead to vegetarian eating

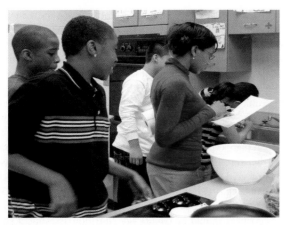

Fig. 17.5 Adolescents who help prepare nutritious meals become engaged in the healthy eating process.

practices because of concerns about animal welfare, the environment, or personal health. Concerns about body weight also motivate some adolescents to adopt a vegetarian diet because it is a socially acceptable way to reduce dietary fat. Some research has suggested that adolescents who consume vegetarian diets are less likely to be overweight or obese than their omnivorous peers (Schürmann et al, 2017). Well-planned vegetarian diets that include a variety of legumes, nuts, seeds, fruits and vegetables, and whole grains can provide adequate nutrients for adolescents (Melina et al, 2016); however, there is a need for additional research on the benefits and possible risks of vegetarian diets for young people under the age of 18 years, especially if they are overly restrictive.

Vegetarian diets that become increasingly more restrictive should be viewed with caution, because this may signal the development of disordered eating, with the vegetarian diet used as a means to hide a restriction of food intake (Melina et al, 2016). This increased risk for unhealthy weight control behaviors seems to persist even after the vegetarian eating style is discontinued, suggesting that although the

TABLE 17.7 Recommended Number of Servings for Adolescents Ages 13 and 16 Years Based on Activity Level*

	Grains (oz-eq/day)	Whole Grains (oz-eq/day)[†]	Vegetables (cups/day)	Fruit (cups/day)	Dairy (cups/day)	Seafood (oz/week)	Meat, poultry, eggs (oz/week)	Nuts, seeds, soy products (oz/week)	Oils (g/day)
Males									
13 Years									
Sedentary	6	3	2.5	2	3	8	26	5	27
Moderately Active	7	3.5	3	2	3	9	28	5	29
Active	9	4.5	3.5	2	3	10	31	5	34
16 Years									
Sedentary	8	4	3	2	3	10	31	5	31
Moderately Active	10	5	3.5	2.5	3	10	33	6	36
Active	10	5	4	2.5	3	10	33	6	51
Females									
13 Years									
Sedentary	5	3	2	1.5	3	8	23	4	22
Moderately Active	6	3	2.5	2	3	8	26	5	27
Active	7	3.5	3	2	3	9	28	5	29
16 Years									
Sedentary	6	3	2.5	1.5	3	8	23	4	24
Moderately Active	6	3	2.5	2	3	8	26	5	27
Active	8	4	3	2	3	10	31	5	31

oz-eq, one ounce-equivalent is: 1 slice (1 ounce) of bread; 1 ounce uncooked pasta or rice; ½ cup cooked rice, pasta, or cereal; 1 tortilla (6″ diameter); 1 pancake (5″ diameter); 1 ounce ready-to-eat cereal (about 1 cup cereal flakes)

*Activity level categories are defined as follows: *sedentary*, a lifestyle that includes only the light physical activity associated with typical day-to-day life; *moderately active*, a lifestyle that includes physical activity equivalent to walking about 1.5 to 3 miles per day at 3 to 4 miles per hour, in addition to the light physical activity associated with typical day-to-day life; and *active*, a lifestyle that includes physical activity equivalent to walking more than 3 miles per day at 3 to 4 miles per hour, in addition to the light physical activity associated with typical day-to-day life.

[†]Number of servings of whole grains are not in addition to but are included in the number of servings of grains.

Adapted from the U.S. Department of Agriculture (USDA): *Dietary Guidelines for Americans, 2015-2020* (website): https://health.gov/dietaryguidelines/2015/.

issues are related, vegetarian diets likely do not cause disordered eating and instead may serve as a symptom.

Vegetarian adolescents often have optimal intakes of iron, vitamin A, and fiber and low intakes of dietary cholesterol. Vegetarian diets are consistent with the Dietary Guidelines for Americans and can meet the DRIs for all nutrients. A sample eating plan to assist vegetarian adolescents in achieving adequate energy and nutrient intakes is listed in Table 17.8.

Vegan diets, which do not include animal products of any kind, do not provide natural sources of vitamin B_{12} and may be deficient in calcium, vitamin D, zinc, iron, and long-chain omega-3 fatty acids (Melina et al, 2016). Therefore vegan adolescents need to choose foods naturally high in or fortified with these nutrients. A daily multivitamin-mineral supplement is essential for vegans. Instructing adolescents and their caregivers on the planning of a well-balanced vegetarian diet and use of fortified foods can prevent potential nutrient deficiencies.

Skin Health

Skin health is impacted by the appearance of acne, which most often peaks during adolescence and affects 80% to 90% of U.S. adolescents.

Effective treatment for the condition is important because acne can significantly affect quality of life and in some cases lead to social withdrawal, anxiety, or depression. There is some research suggesting the potential value of incorporating medical nutrition therapy in the treatment of acne. For example, a recent study among 250 young adults (ages 18 to 25) in New York City found evidence that dietary factors may influence or aggravate acne development by comparing the self-reported usual dietary patterns of participants who reported no or mild acne to those with moderate to severe acne (Burris et al, 2014). Young adults with moderate to severe acne reported higher glycemic index diets, including more added sugars, total sugars, milk servings, saturated fat, and trans fatty acids and fewer servings of fish. The majority of all participants (58%) additionally reported the perception that diet aggravates or influences their acne.

The evidence from this study combined with other epidemiologic, observational, and experimental research does not demonstrate that diet causes acne but indicates it may aggravate or influence the condition to some degree (Burris et al, 2013). It is possible that medical nutrition therapy as an adjunct to dermatology therapy may be beneficial for some young people with acne. However, a number of questions

TABLE 17.8 Recommended Number of Servings for Vegetarian Adolescents Ages 13 and 16 Years Based on Activity Level*

	Grains (oz-eq/day)	Vegetables (cups/day)	Fruit (cups/day)	Dairy (cups/day)	Eggs (oz-eq/week)	Beans and peas (oz-eq/week)	Nuts and seeds (oz-eq/week)	Soy products (oz-eq/week)	Oils (g/day)
Males									
13 Years									
Sedentary	6.5	2.5	2	3	3	6	7	8	27
Moderately Active	7.5	3	2	3	3	6	7	8	29
Active	9.5	3.5	2	3	3	9	9	10	34
16 Years									
Sedentary	8.5	3	2	3	3	8	8	9	31
Moderately Active	10.5	3.5	2.5	3	4	10	10	11	36
Active	10.5	4	2.5	3	4	10	13	13	51
Females									
13 Years									
Sedentary	5.5	2	1.5	3	3	4	5	6	22
Moderately Active	6.5	2.5	2	3	3	6	7	8	27
Active	7.5	3	2	3	3	6	7	8	29
16 Years									
Sedentary	6.5	2.5	1.5	3	3	6	6	6	24
Moderately Active	6.5	2.5	2	3	3	6	7	8	27
Active	8.5	3	2	3	3	8	8	9	31

oz-eq, one ounce-equivalent is: 1 slice (1 ounce) of bread; 1 ounce uncooked pasta or rice; ½ cup cooked rice, pasta, or cereal; 1 tortilla (6″ diameter); 1 pancake (5″ diameter); 1 ounce ready-to-eat cereal (about 1 cup cereal flakes)

*Activity level categories are defined as follows: *sedentary*, a lifestyle that includes only the light physical activity associated with typical day-to-day life; *moderately active*, a lifestyle that includes physical activity equivalent to walking about 1.5 to 3 miles per day at 3 to 4 miles per hour, in addition to the light physical activity associated with typical day-to-day life; and *active*, a lifestyle that includes physical activity equivalent to walking more than 3 miles per day at 3 to 4 miles per hour, in addition to the light physical activity associated with typical day-to-day life.

Adapted from the U.S. Department of Agriculture (USDA): *Dietary Guidelines for Americans, 2015-2020* (website): https://health.gov/dietaryguidelines/2015/.

remain that must be addressed by additional research before the efficacy and clinical relevance of diet therapy can be established and evidence-based guidelines developed to guide dietitian nutritionists in practice.

Currently, the most reasonable approach to practice is to approach each young person with acne on an individual basis to determine whether dietary counseling may be beneficial. The evidence base most consistently supports guiding individuals with acne toward a healthful, low-glycemic load diet that is low in saturated fat and high in whole grains, fruit, and vegetables. An additional dietary intervention that may similarly offer multiple health benefits is to recommend increasing consumption of omega-3 fatty acids (see Appendix 26). As long as intake of calcium and vitamin D are sufficient, it may further be beneficial to recommend a diet lower in dairy but as yet the quantity of milk necessary to exacerbate acne has not been established.

Promoting Healthy Weight-Related Attitudes and Behaviors

An estimated 10% to 20% of teens engage in disordered eating behaviors, such as binge-purge behavior, compensatory exercise, laxative and diuretic abuse, and binge eating (Neumark-Sztainer et al, 2012). These behaviors do not occur with enough regularity or frequency to be diagnosed as an eating disorder, but they may have significant health implications for adolescents. Symptoms that may signal the presence of unhealthy weight-related attitudes and disordered eating behaviors include recurring gastrointestinal complaints, amenorrhea, or unexplained weight loss. Females at an overweight BMI have been found to be twice as likely to engage in disordered eating behaviors. In order to identify and intervene on these risky behaviors, it is valuable to conduct screening for disordered eating. In particular, it is important for screening questions to address body dissatisfaction, fear of weight gain, frequency of dieting and fasting, use of laxatives and diuretics, use of diet pills, fear of certain foods (e.g., foods containing fat or sugar), vomiting, bingeing, and compensatory exercise.

Adolescents are particularly vulnerable to the complications of eating disorders. The effect of malnutrition on linear growth, brain development, and bone acquisition can be persistent and irreversible. It is important for the achievement of a strong recovery that symptoms of an eating disorder are recognized by others early in the course of illness and that health professionals are involved in implementing an effective care plan so that symptoms can be quickly reduced (Vall and Wade, 2015) (see Chapter 21).

Promoting a Healthy Weight Status

Adolescent weight status is typically evaluated based on BMI (weight/height^2 [kg/m^2]) as shown in Appendix 3. Maintaining behaviors that promote a healthy weight status in adolescence is important for overall health and well-being during this period of development as well as for future adult health. Weight status is influenced by a complex set of factors, including genetics, metabolic efficiency, PAL, dietary intake, medical and behavioral health conditions, medication use, and environmental and psychosocial factors (see Chapter 20). Inadequate weight gain and underweight are concerns for some adolescents with special health care needs, but the most prevalent concern among young people this age is excess weight gain.

Among 12- to 15-year-olds and 16- to 19-year-olds in the United States, the prevalence of being at an overweight BMI, higher than the 85th percentile, is respectively 38.7% and 41.5%. The prevalence of being at an obese BMI, at or above the 95th percentile, is approximately 20.5% among both age groups; the prevalence of severe obesity (120% of the 95th percentile) is estimated to be 7% to 10%

among youth (Skinner et al, 2018). For some adolescents, a high BMI reflects high lean body mass rather than potentially unhealthy levels of body fat (Hagan et al, 2017). However, adolescents who are at an overweight BMI are more likely to have metabolic abnormalities such as elevated blood glucose, triglycerides, cholesterol, and liver enzymes. Laboratory testing and additional screening are therefore recommended for adolescents at a high BMI to assess for the presence of chronic disease risk factors and presence of diabetes and liver disease (Hagan et al, 2017). If risk factors are noted, it is recommended that aspartate aminotransferase (AST) and alanine aminotransferase (ALT) measurements be completed to assess liver function and screen for nonalcoholic steatohepatitis (see Chapter 28). It is recommended that a fasting glucose level be drawn on any overweight adolescent with two or more risk factors for CVD or with a family history of diabetes. For adolescents at an obese BMI, it is recommended that microalbumin/creatinine ratio also be assessed. Additional assessments for conditions such as sleep apnea, orthopedic disorders, polycystic ovary disease, and hormonal abnormalities should be performed based on presenting symptoms.

Current guidelines for adolescent overweight and obesity suggest a staged care, multicomponent treatment process (Box 17.3) based on a teen's BMI, age, motivation, and the presence of comorbid conditions (Hagan et al, 2017; Henry et al, 2018). Four stages are recommended, with progress through the stages based on age, biologic development, level of motivation, weight status, and success with previous stages of treatment (Hoelscher et al, 2013). Advancing to the next stage of treatment may be recommended if insufficient progress is made to improve weight status or resolve comorbid conditions after 3 to 6 months. There is evidence that counseling to promote healthy weight status is most effective when it includes group pediatric weight management sessions and family involvement (Henry et al, 2018). Regardless of the approach taken, it is critical that the focus of counseling is on making healthy lifestyle and dietary choices. Adolescents at a higher weight status need to be supported by their family and not subjected to shaming comments about their weight from health professionals, caregivers, or peers.

Bariatric surgery has been used as a treatment for producing weight loss, but concern has been expressed regarding its use in adolescents (Ryder et al, 2018). Recommendations for bariatric surgery suggest that it may be justified only by the presence of severe obesity (Kelly et al, 2013). While long-term outcome data show that bariatric surgery may lead to improvements in cardiometabolic health, difficulty in complying with dietary restrictions after surgery often leads to complications (Inge et al, 2017). Complications of bariatric surgery include dumping syndrome after high carbohydrate intake, voluntary excessive food intake, and B vitamin deficiencies caused by poor compliance with vitamin-mineral supplementation (see Chapter 20).

In summary, overweight and obesity in adolescence have short- and long-term health consequences. Adolescents who are at an overweight BMI and particularly those who experience rapid weight gain or a BMI that represents severe obesity are at higher risk for hyperlipidemia, hypertension, insulin resistance, and type 2 diabetes compared with normal weight peers (Ryder et al, 2018). Not all adolescents at higher BMIs experience metabolic abnormalities during this stage of development; however, epidemiologic studies of obesity and disease risk demonstrate that an obese BMI is associated with greater risk of premature mortality and morbidity. Premature mortality and morbidity are most often related to the presence of diabetes, hypertension, coronary heart disease, stroke, asthma, and polycystic ovary syndrome among individuals who were overweight or obese during adolescence (Reilly and Kelly, 2011).

BOX 17.3 Staged Care Treatment for Overweight and Obesity

Four treatment stages are recommended, with progress through the stages based on the adolescent's age, biologic development, level of motivation, weight status, and success with previous stages of treatment. Advancing to the next stage of treatment may be recommended if insufficient progress is made to improve weight status or resolve comorbid conditions after 3 to 6 months.

Stage 1 is appropriate for adolescents at an overweight body mass index and with no comorbid conditions and/or sexual maturity rating (SMR) of 4 or less. This stage of care consists of general nutrition and physical activity advice and can be provided by a single health care provider, including physicians, nurses, and dietitians who have training in pediatric weight management. Weight loss should be monitored monthly by the provider and not exceed 1 to 2 pounds per week. Achieve 1 hour of moderate-to-vigorous physical activity each day. Limit daily screen time to no more than 2 hours.

Guidelines for Stage 1

- Remove television and other forms of screen media from the bedroom.
- Consume five fruit and vegetable servings per day, but limit intake of juice.
- Limit eating occasions away from home with the exception of school meals.
- Participate in family meals on most days of the week.
- Consume at least three meals per day rather than frequently snacking.
- Eat mindfully, only when hungry, and only until satiated.
- Reduce consumption of most energy-dense foods and beverages and eliminate consumption of sugar-sweetened beverages.
- Select appropriate portion sizes when eating at home and away from home.

Stage 2 includes the same concepts as stage 1, but it provides more structure. This stage of obesity treatment can be provided by a single health care provider with training in motivational counseling. However, referrals for additional services such as physical therapy or counseling may be necessary for some adolescents. Stage 2 treatment is considered successful if weight maintenance or weight loss of up to 2 pounds per week is achieved. Assessment of progress should be monitored monthly.

Guidelines for Stage 2

- Monitor food and beverage intake through daily food and exercise journals or record books.
- Set goals for food and physical activity behavior changes and monitor progress toward goals.

- Limit time spent with screen media to no more than 60 minutes per day.
- Follow a structured meal plan with scheduled meal and snack times.
- Plan and monitor physical activity to ensure 60 minutes of moderate-to-vigorous activity is achieved each day.
- Reinforce successful lifestyle changes through the use of age-appropriate, nonfood rewards such as tickets to a local event or museum, jewelry, clothing, or music.

Stage 3 is more structured than stage 2. Youth with a BMI at or above the 99th percentile for age and gender may start treatment in stage 3. Treatment services are provided by a multidisciplinary team that includes a physician or pediatric nurse practitioner, a counselor (psychologist or social worker), a registered dietitian nutritionist, and an exercise physiologist or physical therapist. Stage 3 treatment is considered successful when BMI no longer exceeds the 85th percentile for age and gender; however, weight loss should be monitored to not exceed 2 pounds per week. If no improvement is seen after 3 to 6 months, or if comorbid conditions worsen, it is recommended that treatment advance to stage 4.

Guidelines for Stage 3

- The treatment program provides at least 50 hours and ideally more than 70 hours of intervention within 2 to 6 months.
- A family component and an adolescent-only component are offered.
- A highly structured meal plan is developed and monitored.
- A highly structured physical activity plan is developed and monitored.
- A formal behavior modification program is instituted by a counselor, with parental involvement as appropriate.

Stage 4 treatment is a tertiary care service and is reserved for severely obese adolescents or those who have a BMI at or above the 95th percentile for age and gender and who have significant comorbidities that require concerted intervention. This treatment stage is available only in clinical settings that employ a full range of health professionals who are trained specifically in the behavioral and medical management of pediatric obesity.

Guidelines for Stage 4

- Intensive dietary regimens, such as meal replacement, protein-sparing modified fasts, and oral medication.
- Bariatric surgery may be used.

Adapted from Spear B et al: Recommendations for treatment of child and adolescent overweight and obesity, *Pediatrics* 120:S254, 2007 and U.S. Preventative Services Task Force; Barton M: Screening for Obesity in Children and Adolescents: U.S. Preventive Services Task Force Recommendation Statement, *Pediatrics* 125:361, 2010.

Promoting Cardiovascular Health

Whereas a healthy diet during adolescence helps to prevent CVD in adulthood, the presence of hyperlipidemia and hypertension are important risk factors. Hyperlipidemia and hypertension are apparent in adolescence and have been shown to be predictive of CVD risk in later life. Components of a health screening assessment aimed at the identification and prevention of risk for CVD and other chronic diseases are listed in Table 17.9. Table 17.10 lists the classification criteria for the diagnosis of hyperlipidemia among youth. National data suggest that one in five adolescents 12 to 19 years old has elevated blood lipid levels (CDC, 2010). The prevalence of hyperlipidemia among adolescents varies according to BMI from 14% among adolescents at a BMI,85th percentile to 22% among adolescents at an overweight BMI and 43% among adolescents at an obese BMI. The prevalence of low, high-density lipoprotein (HDL) cholesterol and high triglyceride levels appeared to increase with age. Adolescent males were almost three times more likely to have low HDL cholesterol levels compared with females

at any age. These youth are considered candidates for therapeutic lifestyle counseling with emphasis on nutrition and physical activity intervention.

The National Heart, Lung, and Blood Institute (NHLBI) has recommended that all youth with elevated blood lipids be referred to a registered dietitian or nutritionist for medical nutrition therapy. The dietary recommendations for youth up to 21 years of age with elevated low-density lipoprotein (LDL) cholesterol are listed in Box 17.4, and those for elevated triglycerides and non-HDL cholesterol are listed in Box 17.5.

National screening criteria for blood pressure levels among adolescents are available through the National Heart Lung and Blood Institute through the NIH. Adolescents 13 years of age and older who have consistent systolic readings of 130-139 mm Hg or diastolic readings of 80-89 mm Hg meet the diagnostic criteria for hypertension.

Dietary counseling and weight management are integral components of hypertension treatment. The Dietary Approaches to Stop

TABLE 17.9   **Suggested Health Screening Schedule for Health Promotion and Chronic Disease Prevention**

Risk Factor	Ages 12-17 Years	Ages 18-21 Years
Family history of premature cardio-vascular disease	• Update previous family history at each visit. • Provide dietary counseling and referral based on family history as necessary.	• Assess changes in family history at least annually. • Provide dietary counseling and referral based on family history as necessary.
Eating behaviors and patterns	• Assess diet using appropriate methods. • Provide education and counseling as needed.	• Review eating behaviors and provide education to improve dietary intake and nutritional status.
Growth and weight status	• Weigh and measure teen at each visit. Plot height, weight, and BMI. Review with adolescent and parent(s). • If adolescent is overweight, provide step 1 counseling to adolescent and parent(s) and schedule follow-up visit. • If adolescent is obese, provide step 2 counseling and refer to a comprehensive weight management program.	• Weigh and measure client at each visit. Calculate BMI based on height and weight measurements. • If overweight or obese, thoroughly assess diet and physical activity patterns and provide counseling as appropriate. • If overweight or obese, refer to primary health provider for full health assessment.
Blood lipids	• Refer adolescent with family history of premature heart disease, family history of dyslipidemia, or those who are overweight/obese to primary care provider and request a blood lipid panel. • Review blood lipid levels with adolescent and parent(s). Provide nutrition counseling as appropriate. • If adolescent is overweight, provide dietary counseling in accordance with step 1. • If adolescent is obese, provide dietary counseling in accordance with step 2 and refer to comprehensive weight management program. • The addition of plant sterols or stanols at no more than 2 g/day can be recommended for teens with familial hyperlipidemia. • If dietary management is not effective, refer to primary care provider for physical examination and management of dyslipidemia by medication as needed.	• Refer adolescent with family history of premature heart disease, family history of dyslipidemia, or those who are overweight/obese to primary care provider and request a blood lipid panel. • Review blood lipid levels with adolescent and parent(s). Provide nutrition counseling as appropriate. • If client is overweight or obese, provide dietary counseling as appropriate and refer to weight management program. • The addition of plant sterols or stanols at no more than 2 g/day can be recommended for clients with familial hyperlipidemia. • If dietary management is not effective, refer to primary care provider for physical examination and management of dyslipidemia by medication as needed.
Blood pressure	• Review blood pressure results with adolescent and parent(s). • Provide counseling in accordance with the DASH diet. Request follow-up visit. • If adolescent is overweight, provide dietary counseling in accordance with step 1. • If adolescent is obese, provide dietary counseling in accordance with step 2 and refer to comprehensive weight management program. • If dietary management is not effective, refer to primary care provider for physical examination and management of hypertension by medication as needed.	• Review blood pressure results with client. • Provide counseling in accordance with the DASH diet. Request follow-up visit. • If client is overweight or obese, provide dietary counseling as appropriate and refer to weight management program. • If dietary management is not effective, refer to primary care provider for physical examination and management of hypertension by medication as needed.
Diabetes	• Refer adolescent with family history of diabetes, signs of acanthosis nigricans, symptoms consistent with diabetes, or those who are overweight/obese to a primary care provider and request a fasting blood glucose. • Review fasting blood glucose levels with adolescent and parent(s). Provide nutrition counseling as appropriate. • If adolescent is overweight, provide dietary counseling in accordance with step 1. • If adolescent is obese, provide dietary counseling in accordance with step 2 and refer to comprehensive weight management program.	• Refer client with family history of diabetes, signs of acanthosis nigricans, symptoms consistent with diabetes, or those who are overweight/obese to primary care provider and request a fasting blood glucose. • Review fasting blood glucose levels with client. Provide nutrition counseling as appropriate. • If client is overweight or obese, provide dietary counseling and refer to comprehensive weight management program.
Physical activity	• Review physical activity pattern and behaviors with adolescent and parent(s). • Reinforce need for 60 min or more of moderate-to-vigorous physical activity per day. • Reinforce limiting sedentary and screen time to no more than 2 hours per day.	• Review physical activity pattern and behaviors with client. • Reinforce need for 60 min or more of moderate-to-vigorous physical activity each day. • Reinforce limiting sedentary and screen time to no more than 2 hours per day.

DASH, Dietary Approaches to Stop Hypertension
Adapted from U.S. Department of Health and Human Services (USDHHS), National Institutes of Health (NIH), National Heart, Lung, and Blood Institute (NHLBI): *Expert panel on integrated guidelines for cardiovascular health and risk reduction in children and adolescents.* Summary report, NIH Publication No 12-7486A, October 2012.

TABLE 17.10 Classification Criteria for the Diagnosis of Hyperlipidemia in Adolescents (10- to 19-years-old)*

	Acceptable	Borderline	Unacceptable
Total cholesterol (mg/dL)	≤170	170-199	≥200
LDL cholesterol (mg/dL)	<110	110-129	≥130
Non-HDL cholesterol (mg/dL)	<120	120-144	>145
HDL cholesterol (mg/dL)	>45	40-45	<40
Triglycerides (mg/dL)	<90	90-129	>130
Apolipoprotein A-1 (mg/dL)	>120	115-120	<115
Apolipoprotein B (mg/dL)	<90	90-109	>110

*Based on the average of two measurements.
HDL, High-density lipoprotein; LDL, low-density lipoprotein.
Adapted from U. S. Department of Health and Human Services (USDHHS), National Institutes of Health (NIH), National Heart, Lung, and Blood Institute (NHLBI): *Expert panel on integrated guidelines for cardiovascular health and risk reduction in children and adolescents. Summary report*, NIH Publication No 12-7486A, October 2012.

BOX 17.4 Dietary Recommendations for Elevated Low-Density Lipoprotein Cholesterol in Adolescents

- Limit total fat intake to no more than 25% to 30% of calories.
- Limit saturated fat intake to no more than 7% of calories.
- Dietary cholesterol intake should not exceed 200 mg/day.
- Plant sterol esters and/or stanol esters can replace usual fat intake up to 2 g/day for children with familial hypercholesterolemia.
- Up to 12 g of psyllium fiber can be added to the diet each day as cereal enriched with psyllium.
- At least 1 hour of moderate to vigorous exercise should be obtained daily.
- Sedentary and/or screen time should be limited to less than 2 hours each day.

Adapted from U.S. Department of Health and Human Services, National Institutes of Health, National Heart, Lung and Blood Institute: *Expert panel on integrated guidelines for cardiovascular health and risk reduction in children and adolescents. Summary report*, NIH Publication No 12-7486A, October 2012.

BOX 17.5 Dietary Recommendations for Adolescents with Elevated Triglyceride or Non-High-Density Lipoprotein Cholesterol Levels

- Limit total fat intake to no more than 25% to 30% of calories.
- Limit saturated fat intake to no more than 7% of calories.
- Reduce intake of added and natural sugars in the diet.
- Replace simple carbohydrates with complex carbohydrate and whole grains.
- Avoid sugar-sweetened beverages.
- Increase the intake of fish high in omega-3 fatty acids.

Adapted from U.S. Department of Health and Human Services, National Institutes of Health, National Heart, Lung and Blood Institute: *Expert panel on integrated guidelines for cardiovascular health and risk reduction in children and adolescents. Summary report*, NIH Publication No 12-7486A, October 2012.

TABLE 17.11 Cardiovascular Health Integrated Lifestyle Diet (CHILD 1) Recommendations, Ages 11 to 21 Years

Primarily select fat-free unflavored milk, water, and unsweetened tea as beverage choices.
Limit or avoid sugar-sweetened beverages.
Try to consume a range of 25% to 30% of daily energy needs from total fatty acids.
Limit saturated fatty acids to 8% to 10% of daily energy needs.
Keep monounsaturated and polyunsaturated fatty acids to no more than 20% of daily energy intake.
Avoid trans fatty acids.
Limit dietary cholesterol to 300 mg/day.
Choose foods high in dietary fiber often to include a goal of 14 g fiber per 1000 kcal.
Choose naturally sweetened juices (no added sugar) and limit intake to 4 to 6 oz/day.
Limit sodium intake.
Try to eat breakfast daily.
Try to eat meals together with other family members at the same table.
Limit fast food meals.
Use the Dietary Approaches to Stop Hypertension eating plan as a guide to plan meals.
Aim to keep average energy intake close to estimated energy requirements with adjustment for growth and physical activity as needed.

Adapted from U.S. Department of Health and Human Services (USDHHS), National Institutes of Health (NIH), National Heart, Lung, and Blood Institute (NHLBI): *Expert panel on integrated guidelines for cardiovascular health and risk reduction in children and adolescents. Summary report*, NIH Publication No 12-7486A, October 2012.

Hypertension (DASH) eating pattern has been shown to be effective in reducing blood pressure in many individuals (see Chapter 32 and Appendix 17). In addition to following the DASH diet, adolescents with elevated blood pressure should be counseled to reduce sodium intake to less than 2000 mg/day and to achieve and maintain a healthy body weight.

The NHLBI has developed the CHILD 1 (Cardiovascular Health Integrated Lifestyle Diet) diet and nutrition guidelines, which integrate dietary approaches to prevent hypertension and hyperlipidemia, and promote a healthy weight (Table 17.11). These guidelines include the DASH dietary guidelines as well as recommendations for upper limits for total and saturated fatty acids and dietary cholesterol intake. The CHILD 1 guidelines recommend avoiding sweetened beverages, limiting juice intake, and increasing fiber intake to a level of 14 g/1000 kcal.

Metabolic syndrome is considered to be a clustering of risk factors that, taken together, signal a need to intensify the depth and breadth of prevention measures that are recommended. It is estimated that 3.3% of all U.S. adolescents have metabolic syndrome; the rate is much higher among adolescents at an obese BMI, among whom it is estimated to be 29.2% (Friend et al, 2013).

Preventing and Screening for Diabetes

The exact prevalence of diabetes among adolescents is not known, but it is estimated that approximately 193,000 people under the age of 20 have diabetes (CDC, 2017). Findings from the SEARCH for Diabetes in Youth Study suggest that the incidence of type 1 and type 2 diabetes is 21.7 cases and 12.5 cases respectively per 100,000 people younger than 20 years (Mayer-Davis et al, 2017). Ethnic and racial minority youth are at increased risk for both type 1 and type 2 diabetes compared with their non-Hispanic white counterparts.

The growing incidence of type 2 diabetes among adolescents is of particular public health concern. Between 2002 and 2012, the incidence of type 2 diabetes increased by 7.1% (Mayer-Davis et al, 2017). Type 2 diabetes is more common in those with a family history of diabetes and in those who have significant and rapid weight gain or obesity. Recommendations for type 2 diabetes screening, including assessment for physical signs such as acanthosis nigricans (dark, velvety patches of skin in body folds and creases), are listed in Box 17.6. The prevention of type 2 diabetes includes following the CHILD 1 dietary guidelines and additional physical activity at a level to reduce body weight (U.S. Department of Health and Human Services [USDHHS], National Institutes of Health [NIH], NHLBI, 2012).

Promoting Physical Activity

Participation in adequate physical activity is critical to the prevention of diabetes as well as the promotion of cardiovascular health, a healthy weight, high quality sleep, academic achievement, and overall well-being (National Center for Chronic Disease Prevention and Health Promotion, 2014; Physical Activity Guidelines Advisory Committee, 2018). National recommendations for physical activity are for adolescents to be active at least 60 minutes each day, including participation in vigorous activity at least 3 days each week (USDHHS, 2018). In addition, it is recommended that muscle-strengthening (e.g., working with resistance bands, lifting weights, yoga) and bone-strengthening activities (e.g., running, jumping rope, basketball) be included in the 60 minutes of physical activity at least three times a week. The Move Your Way campaign through the Office of Disease Prevention and Health Promotion was developed along with these national recommendations and

---

BOX 17.6 Recommendations for Screening Adolescents for Type 2 Diabetes Mellitus

Youth who are at an overweight or obese body mass index and exhibit two of the following risk factors are at high risk:

- First- or second-degree relative with a history of type 2 diabetes
- Member of a racial/ethnic group considered at higher risk (American Indian, African American, Latino, Asian American/Pacific Islander)
- Dyslipidemia
- Hypertension
- Acanthosis nigricans
- Polycystic ovary syndrome

Screening should begin at age 10 or the onset of puberty, whichever occurs first. Screening should occur every 2 years.

Adapted from U.S. Department of Health and Human Services, National Institutes of Health, National Heart, Lung and Blood Institute: *Expert panel on integrated guidelines for cardiovascular health and risk reduction in children and adolescents. Summary report*, NIH Publication No 12-7486A, October 2012.

---

may be a useful source of educational materials. In order to achieve these recommendations for being active and getting adequate sleep, the American Academy of Pediatrics recommends that adolescents and their parents develop limits for media use (e.g., designated media-free times, consistent limits on time spent using media and types of media) as part of a Family Media Use Plan (Council on Communications and Media, 2016). Many young people do not meet minimum recommendations for physical activity and a high proportion spend excessive amounts of time engaged with screen media. Overall, slightly less than half of U.S. high school students report being physically active for at least 60 minutes per day on 5 days or more per week; males are more active than females with 57% versus 37% meeting recommendations. Media use is also high on school days among high school students, with 43.0% reporting that they played video or computer games or used a computer for 3 or more hours per day and 20.7% reporting they watched television 3 or more hours per day.

Adolescent athletes have unique nutrient needs. Adequate fluid intake to prevent dehydration is especially critical for young athletes. Young adolescents are at higher risk for dehydration because they produce more heat during exercise but have less ability to transfer heat from the muscles to the skin. They also sweat less, which decreases their capacity to dissipate heat through the evaporation of the sweat.

Athletes who participate in sports that use competitive weight categories or emphasize body weight are at elevated risk for the development of disordered eating behaviors. A concern among female athletes is the female athlete triad relationship, a constellation of low body weight and inadequate body fat levels, amenorrhea, and osteoporosis (see Chapter 22). The female athlete triad may lead to premature bone loss, decreased bone density, increased risk of stress fractures, and infertility (De Souza et al, 2017). Nutrition assessment and education for teenage athletes should focus on obtaining adequate energy, macronutrients, and micronutrients to meet the needs for growth and development and to maintain a healthy body weight. The use of anabolic agents (such as steroids or insulin) and other ergogenic supplements should also be included in nutrition screening. National survey data show that 2.9% of U.S. high school students have taken steroids without a prescription at least once in their life, with a higher proportion of males reporting steroid use than females (3.3% vs. 2.4%) (Kann et al, 2018). Furthermore, several studies have found that athletes are more likely than nonathletes to use performance-enhancing substances (LaBotz and Griesemer, 2016).

Meeting Nutritional Needs During Pregnancy

Although birth rates among females 15 to 19 years have declined over the past few decades and reached a low of 20.3 births per 1000 adolescents in 2015, adolescent pregnancy remains a significant public health issue (Martin et al, 2018). Adolescent females who become pregnant are at particularly high risk for nutritional deficiencies because of elevated nutrient needs. Pregnant adolescents with a **gynecologic age** (the number of years between the onset of menses and current age) of less than 4 and those who are undernourished at the time of conception have the greatest nutritional needs. As with adult women, pregnant adolescents require additional folic acid, iron, zinc, and other micronutrients to support fetal growth (see Chapter 14). Calcium and vitamin D are also important nutrients in pregnancy, because both are necessary for growth and development of the adolescent mother and fetus (Young et al, 2012). Pregnant adolescents need a full nutrition assessment early in pregnancy to determine any nutrient deficiencies and to promote adequate weight gain. Weight gain recommendations for pregnancy are listed in Table 14.11 in Chapter 14. Referral to appropriate food assistance programs such as the Special Supplemental Nutrition Program for Women, Infants and Children is an important part of prenatal nutrition education.

CLINICAL CASE STUDY

Cherise is an 18-year-old white female and high school senior who saw a nurse at the school-based clinic. While taking her medical history, the school nurse noted that Cherise had frequent headaches and fatigue. Cherise's blood pressure reading fell into the 92nd percentile. The school nurse referred her to a local community clinic for a more thorough evaluation.

A physician's assistant (PA) at the community clinic took a social history and performed a physical examination on Cherise. A sexual maturity rating (SMR) stage of 5 was noted. The PA noted that Cherise's BMI had increased over the past year from the 85th to the 95th percentile for her age and gender. Her blood pressure registered at the 94th percentile. The family history revealed a strong family history of cardiovascular disease, diabetes, and renal disease. Cherise thought her father may be taking medication for his cholesterol and blood pressure, but she reported no health issues for her mother. No signs of acanthosis nigricans were noted on the physical examination.

Laboratory results show that Cherise had elevated total, non-HDL, and LDL cholesterol levels along with a marginally low HDL level. The liver enzyme and blood glucose values were at the upper end of normal. A referral was made for Cherise to see a registered dietitian nutritionist (RDN) for nutrition and exercise counseling.

The outpatient RDN reviewed Cherise's medical history, confirmed her family history of cardiovascular disease, and measured her height and weight. Cherise's BMI value plotted at the 95th percentile. The RDN completed a 24-hour dietary recall with Cherise, beginning with the last thing she had eaten that day and working backward to facilitate a complete and accurate recall. The RDN also inquired about usual dietary patterns and physical activity as well as the presence of any food allergies/intolerances and avoidances.

Cherise reported that she usually skipped breakfast because she didn't have time to eat in the morning, but she often buys a caramel macchiato from the school store at 7:15 AM. The first food Cherise ate most days was usually a snack from the vending machine at 10:30 AM, which consisted of a granola bar or a bag of chips and a juice drink. Occasionally she would purchase a la carte lunches of tacos or a burger, but generally she skipped lunch. Cherise was out of school at 2 PM each day, at which time she went to work as a clothing sales clerk at the local mall. She had a half-hour break in the late afternoon or early evening, when she would go to the food court for dinner. Her evening meal usually consisted of one to two slices of pepperoni pizza, two tacos, or one to two pieces of fried chicken with a soft drink. About half of the time she also ordered fries or nachos. When Cherise returned home from work at 10:15 PM, she usually had a snack of ice cream, tortilla chips, spicy cheese puffs, or microwave popcorn while doing her homework. A large glass of juice or lemonade usually accompanied her snack. On weekends, Cherise worked as many hours at the mall as she could, often meeting friends for pizza or fast food on her nights off. Her physical activity consisted of walking between the house and bus stop in the morning and evening, walking around school between classes, and being on her feet in the evenings at her sales job.

The RDN counseled Cherise regarding dietary changes and physical activity. A follow-up visit was scheduled 4 weeks in the future.

Cherise did not return to see the RDN for her follow-up appointment and did not keep her follow-up appointments with the PA. Five months later, she returned to see the PA at which time her health status was reassessed. Cherise's blood pressure was still at the 94th percentile and her BMI now at the 96th percentile. When counseled about her dietary habits and physical activity, Cherise reported that she had tried to follow the recommendations of the RDN but found it hard because of time constraints. She reported that she wanted to lose weight and thought she could do this because she would graduate in a few weeks and would have more time to devote to exercise and preparing food at home. The PA suggested she see the RDN again for more dietary and physical activity counseling.

The RDN reviewed the previous dietary recommendations with Cherise and suggested she attend the clinic's 12-week weight management program. Cherise attended the first five sessions of the program, then stopped. She had lost 12 pounds during the five sessions. Several months later Cherise was once again seen by the PA. Her blood pressure continued to be elevated and her BMI was plotted at the 94th percentile. When questioned about the weight loss program, Cherise reported that her mother had changed jobs and lost her health insurance benefits, so she could no longer participate in the program. The RDN connected Cherise with the local YMCA, which offered a weight management program for adults on a sliding fee scale. Five months later Cherise's BMI was assessed at 26.8 and a weight loss of 19 pounds from previous levels was noted.

Nutrition Diagnostic Statements

- Excessive energy intake (NI-1.3) related to inconsistent meal patterns and dietary history including mostly low fiber and energy-dense convenience foods as evidenced by a BMI at the 95th percentile
- Excessive fat intake (NI-5.6.2) related to a preference for convenience foods, including pizza, fried snacks, and ice cream as evidenced by elevated total and LDL cholesterol
- Inadequate physical activity (NB-2.1) related to a busy work and school schedule as evidenced by patient reported not having enough time to participate in regular physical activity
- Limited adherence to nutrition-related recommendations (NB-1.6) related to socioeconomic barriers and busy work and school schedule as evidenced by BMI up 1 percentile at follow-up visit

Nutrition Care Questions

1. How would you classify Cherise's blood pressure based on the reading at the school nurse's office?
2. How would you classify Cherise's weight based on the readings at the first visit at the community clinic? Is there any additional information you would want to know about her weight history to make your assessment?
3. Based on her family health history, what laboratory tests would you order to be consistent with the National Heart, Lung, and Blood Institute (NHLBI) recommendations?
4. What type of nutrition recommendations would be ideal for Cherise based on her blood pressure, weight gain history, and laboratory results?
5. What specific strategies would be beneficial for the RDN to recommend to Cherise regarding improving her dietary intake?
6. What strategies would you recommend for Cherise to change her level of physical activity?

USEFUL WEBSITES

American Academy of Pediatrics: Media and Children
American School Health Association
National Eating Disorder Association
School Nutrition Association

REFERENCES

Abreu AP, Kaiser UB: Pubertal development and regulation, *Lancet Diabetes Endocrinol* 4(3):254–264, 2016.
American Academy of Pediatrics, Council on Communications and Media: Media use in school-aged children and adolescents, *Pediatrics* 138(5):e20162592, 2016.

Anderson M, Jiang J: Teens, social media and technology 2018, *Pew Research Center* 2018. Available at: https://www.pewresearch.org/internet/2018/05/31/teens-social-media-technology-2018/

Berge JM, Arikian A, Doherty WJ, et al: Healthful eating and physical activity in the home environment: results from multifamily focus groups, *J Nutr Educ Behav* 44:123–131, 2012.

Berge JM, Wall M, Hsueh TF, et al: The protective role of family meals for youth obesity: 10-year longitudinal associations, *J Pediatr* 166:296–301, 2015.

Bowman SA, Friday JE, Clemens JC, et al: A comparison of food patterns equivalents intakes by Americans. *Dietary Data Brief No. 16*, September 2016.

Branum AM, Rossen LM, Schoendorf KC: Trends in caffeine intake among U.S. children and adolescents, *Pediatrics* 133:386–393, 2014.

Burris J, Rietkerk W, Woolf K: Acne: the role of medical nutrition therapy, *J Acad Nutr Diet* 113:416–430, 2013.

Burris J, Rietkerk W, Woolf K: Relationships of self-reported dietary factors and perceived acne severity in a cohort of New York young adults, *J Acad Nutr Diet* 114:384–392, 2014.

Burrows T, Goldman S, Pursey K, Lim R. Is there an association between dietary intake and academic achievement: a systematic review, *J Hum Nutr Diet* 30(2):117–140, 2017.

Centers for Disease Control and Prevention, Division of Adolescent and School Health: *Results from the School Health Policies and Practices Study 2014*, 2015. Available at: https://www.cdc.gov/healthyyouth/data/shpps/results.htm.

Centers for Disease Control and Prevention: *National diabetes statistics report, 2017*, Atlanta, GA, 2017, Centers for Disease Control and Prevention, U.S. Department of Health and Human Services. Available at: https://www.cdc.gov/diabetes/data/statistics/statistics-report.html.

Centers for Disease Control and Prevention: Prevalence of abnormal lipid levels among youths—United States, 1999 -2006, *MMWR Morb Mortal Wkly Rep* 59(2):29–33, 2010.

Child Trends: *Family meals: indicators on children and youth*, 2013. Available at: https://www.childtrends.org/wp-content/uploads/2013/05/indicator0.80414800%201369598448.html

De Souza MJ, Koltun KJ, Etter CV, et al: Current status of the female athlete triad: update and future directions, *Curr Osteoporos Rep* 15(6):577–587, 2017.

Dwyer J, Nahin RL, Rogers GT, et al: Prevalence and predictors of children's dietary supplement use: the 2007 National Health Interview Survey, *Am J Clin Nutr* 97:1331–1337, 2013.

Eaton DK, Kann L, Kinchen S, et al: Youth risk behavior surveillance—United States, 2011, MMWR Surveill Summ 61(4):1–162, 2012

Fiscaletti M, Stewart P, Munns CF: The importance of vitamin D in maternal and child health: a global perspective, *Public Health Rev* 38:19, 2017.

Friend A, Craig L, Turner S: The prevalence of metabolic syndrome in children: a systematic review of the literature, *Metab Syndr Relat Disord* 11(2):71–80, 2013.

Ganji V, Zhang X, Tangpricha V: Serum 25-hydroxyvitamin D concentrations and prevalence estimates of hypovitaminosis D in the U.S. population based on assay-adjusted data, *J Nutr* 142:498–507, 2012.

Golden NH, Carey DE: Vitamin D in health and disease in adolescents: when to screen, whom to treat, and how to treat, *Adolesc Med State Art Rev* 27:125–139, 2016.

Goldfarb SS, Tarver WL, Locher JL, et al: A systematic review of the association between family meals and adolescent risk outcomes, *J Adolesc* 44:134–149, 2015.

Hagan JF, Shaw JS, Duncan PM, editors: *Bright futures: guidelines for health supervision of infants, children, and adolescents*, ed 4, Elk Grove Village, IL, 2017, American Academy of Pediatrics.

Harris JL, Frazier W, Romo-Palafox M, et al: FACTS 2017. *Food industry self-regulation after 10 years: progress and opportunities to improve food advertising to children*. Hartford, CT. UConn Rudd Center for Food Policy & Obesity, 2017.

Hayes D, Contento IR, Weekly C: Position of the Academy of Nutrition and Dietetics, Society for Nutrition Education and Behavior, and School Nutrition Association: comprehensive nutrition programs and services in schools, *J Acad Nutr Diet* 118(5):913–919, 2018.

Henry BW, Ziegler J, Parrott JS, et al: Pediatric weight management evidence-based practice guidelines: components and contexts of interventions, *J Acad Nutr Diet* 118(7):1301–1311, 2018.

Hoelscher DM, Kirk S, Ritchie L, et al: Position of the Academy of Nutrition an d Dietetics: interventions for the prevention and treatment of pediatric overweight and obesity, *J Acad Nutr Diet* 113:1375–1394, 2013.

Inge TH, Jenkins TM, Xanthakos SA, et al: Long-term outcomes of bariatric surgery in adolescents with severe obesity (FABS-5+): a prospective follow-up analysis, *Lancet Diabetes Endocrinol* 5(3):165–173, 2017.

Institute of Medicine: *Dietary reference intakes: the essential guide to nutrient requirements*, Washington, DC, 2006, National Academies Press.

Institute of Medicine: *Dietary reference intakes for calcium and vitamin D*, Washington, DC, 2011, National Academies Press.

Kann L, McManus T, Harris WA, et al: Youth risk behavior surveillance – United States, 2017, *MMWR Surveill Summ* 67(8):1–114, 2018

Keast DR, Fulgoni VL III, Nicklas TA, et al: Food sources of energy and nutrients among children in the United States: National Health and Nutrition Examination Survey 2003 -2006, *Nutrients* 5:283–301, 2013.

Kelly AS, Barlow SE, Rao G, et al: Severe obesity in children and adolescents: identification, associated health risks, and treatment approaches: a scientific statement from the American Heart Association, *Circulation* 128:1689–1712, 2013.

LaBotz M, Griesemer BA, Council on Sports Medicine and Fitness: Use of performance-enhancing substances, *Pediatrics* 138(1):e20161300, 2016.

Lapierre MA, Fleming-Milici F, Rozendaal E, et al: The effect of advertising on children and adolescents, *Pediatrics* 140(Suppl 2):S152, 2017.

Larson N, MacLehose R, Fulkerson JA, et al: Eating breakfast and dinner together as a family: associations with sociodemographic characteristics and implications for diet quality and weight status, *J Acad Nutr Diet* 113:1601–1609, 2013.

Larson N, Story M: A review of snacking patterns among children and adolescents: what are the implications of snacking for weight status? *Child Obes* 9:104–115, 2013.

Larson N, Story M: Barriers to equity in nutritional health for U.S. children and adolescents: a review of the literature, *Curr Nutr Rep* 4(1):102–110, 2015.

Li W, Liu Q, Deng X, et al: Association between obesity and puberty timing: a systematic review and meta-analysis, *Int J Environ Res Public Health* 14(10):E1266, 2017.

Martin JA, Hamilton BE, Osterman MJ, et al: Births: final data for 2016, *Nat Vital Stat Rep* 67(1), 2018. Hyattsville, MD, National Center for Health Statistics. Available at: https://www.cdc.gov/nchs/products/nvsr.htm.

Mayer-Davis EJ, Lawrence JM, Dabelea D, et al: Incidence trends of type 1 and type 2 diabetes among youths, 2002-2012, *N Engl J Med* 376(15):1419–1429, 2017.

Melina V, Craig W, Levin S: Position of the Academy of Nutrition and Dietetics: vegetarian diets, *J Acad Nutr Diet* 116(12):1970–1980, 2016.

Moore CE, Liu Y: Elevated systolic blood pressure of children in the United States is associated with low serum 25-hydroxyvitamin D concentrations related to body mass index: National Health and Examination Survey 2007-2010, *Nutr Res* 38:64–70, 2017.

Moore LL, Singer MR, Qureshi MM, et al: Food group intake and micronutrient adequacy in adolescent girls, *Nutrients* 4:1692–1708, 2012.

National Center for Chronic Disease Prevention and Health Promotion, Division of Population Health: *Health and academic achievement*, Atlanta, GA, 2014, Centers for Disease Control and Prevention. Available at: https://www.cdc.gov/healthyschools/health_and_academics/index.htm.

Neumark-Sztainer D, Wall MM, Larson N, et al: Secular trends in weight status and weight-related attitudes and behaviors in adolescents from 1999 to 2010, *Prev Med* 54:77–81, 2012.

Papanikolaou Y, Brooks J, Reider C, et al: Comparison of inadequate nutrient intakes in non-Hispanic blacks vs. non-Hispanic whites: an analysis of NHANES 2007-2010 in U.S. children and adults, *J Health Care Poor Underserved* 26(3):726–736, 2015.

Physical Activity Guidelines Advisory Committee: *2018 Physical Activity Guidelines Advisory Committee Scientific Report*, Washington, DC, 2018, U.S. Department of Health and Human Services. Available at: https://health.gov/paguidelines/second-edition/report.aspx.

Poti JM, Slining MM, Popkin BM: Where are kids getting their empty calories? Stores, schools, and fast-food restaurants each played an important role in empty calorie intake among US children during 2009-2010, *J Acad Nutr Diet* 114:908–917, 2014.

Powell LM, Szczypka G, Chaloupka FJ: Trends in exposure to television food advertisements among children and adolescents in the United States, *Arch Pediatr Adolesc Med* 164:794–802, 2010.

Ramnitz MS, Lodish MB: Racial disparities in pubertal development, *Semin Reprod Med* 31:333–339, 2013.

Ranjit N, Evans MH, Byrd-Williams C, et al: Dietary and activity correlates of sugar-sweetened beverage consumption among adolescents, *Pediatrics* 126:e754–e761, 2010.

Reilly JJ, Kelly J: Long-term impact of overweight and obesity in childhood and adolescence on morbidity and premature mortality in adulthood: systematic review, *Int J Obes* 35:891–898, 2011.

Richardson E, Seibert T, Uli NK: Growth perturbations from stimulant medications and inhaled corticosteroids, *Transl Pediatr* 6(4):237–247, 2017.

Rosinger A, Herrick K, Gahche J, et al: Sugar-sweetened beverage consumption among U.S. youth, 2011-2014, *NCHS data brief* (271):1–8, Hyattsville, MD, 2017, National Center for Health Statistics.

Ryder JR, Fox CK, Kelly AS: Treatment options for severe obesity in the pediatric population: current limitations and future opportunities, *Obesity* 26(6):951–960, 2018.

Schürmann S, Kersting M, Alexy U: Vegetarian diets in children: a systematic review, *Eur J Nutr* 56:1797–1817, 2017.

Seifert SM, Schaechter JL, Hershorin ER, et al: Health effects of energy drinks on children, adolescents, and young adults, *Pediatrics* 127:511–528, 2011.

Skinner AC, Ravanbakht SN, Skelton JA, et al: Prevalence of obesity and severe obesity in US children, 1999-2016, *Pediatrics* 141(3):e20173459, 2018.

Smith TJ, Lanham-New SA, Hart KH: Vitamin D in adolescents: Are current recommendations enough? *J Steroid Biochem Mol Biol* 173:265–272, 2017.

Steinberg L: *Adolescence*, ed 11, New York, NY, 2016, McGraw-Hill Higher Education.

Tanner J: *Growth at adolescence*, Oxford, UK, 1962, Blackwell Scientific Publications.

Terry-McElrath YM, O'Malley PM, Johnston LD: Energy drinks, soft drinks, and substance use among United States secondary school students, *J Addict Med* 8:6–13, 2014.

U.S. Department of Agriculture, Agricultural Research Service: *Breakfast: percentages of selected nutrients contributed by foods and beverages consumed at breakfast, by gender and age, in the United States. What we eat in America, NHANES 2013-2014*, 2016a. Available at: www.ars.usda.gov/nea/bhnrc/fsrg.

U.S. Department of Agriculture, Agricultural Research Service: *Nutrient Intakes from food and beverages: mean amounts consumed per individual, by gender and age, in the United States. What we eat in America, NHANES 2013–2014*, 2016b. Available at: www.ars.usda.gov/nea/bhnrc/fsrg.

U.S. Department of Agriculture, Agricultural Research Service: *Snacks: distribution of snack occasions, by gender and age, in the United States. What we eat in America, NHANES 2013–2014*, 2016c. Available at: www.ars.usda.gov/nea/bhnrc/fsrg.

U.S. Department of Agriculture, Agricultural Research Service: Snacks: percentages of selected nutrients contributed by foods and beverages eaten at *snack occasions, by gender and age, in the United States. What we eat in America, NHANES 2013–2014*, 2016d. Available at: www.ars.usda.gov/nea/bhnrc/fsrg.

U.S. Department of Agriculture, Agricultural Research Service: *Total nutrient intakes: percent reporting and mean amounts of selected vitamins and minerals from food and beverages and dietary supplements, by gender and age. What we eat in America, NHANES 2013–2014*, 2017. Available at: www.ars.usda.gov/nea/bhnrc/fsrg.

U.S. Department of Health and Human Services, National Institutes of Health, National Heart, Lung and Blood Institute: *Expert panel on integrated guidelines for cardiovascular health and risk reduction in children and adolescents*, Summary report, October 2012. NIH Publication No 12-7486A.

U.S. Department of Health and Human Services: *Physical Activity Guidelines for Americans*, ed 2, Washington, DC, 2018, U.S. Department of Health and Human Services. Available at: https://health.gov/paguidelines/second-edition/.

Vall E, Wade TD: Predictors of treatment outcome in individuals with eating disorders: a systematic review and meta-analysis, *Int J Eat Disord* 48(7):946–971, 2015.

Villamor E, Jansen EC: Nutritional determinants of the timing of puberty, *Annu Rev Public Health* 37:33–46, 2016.

Watts AW, Miller J, Larson NI, et al: Multicontextual correlates of adolescent sugar-sweetened beverage intake, *Eat Behav* 30:42–48, 2018.

Waxman E, Popkin SJ, Galvez M: *Bringing teens to the table: a focus on food insecurity in America*. Chicago, IL, 2015, Feeding America.

Wu CH, Wang CC, Kennedy J: The prevalence of herb and dietary supplement use among children and adolescents in the United States: results from the 2007 National Health Interview Survey, *Complement Ther Med* 21:358–363, 2013.

Young BE, McNanley TJ, Cooper EM, et al: Maternal vitamin D status and calcium intake interact to affect fetal skeletal growth in utero in pregnant adolescents, *Am J Clin Nutr* 95:1103–1112, 2012.

18

Nutrition in the Adult Years

Judith L. Dodd, MS, RDN, LDN, FAND

KEY TERMS

consumer price index (CPI)
food desert
food security
functional foods
health disparities

health-related quality of life (HRQOL)
isoflavones
metabolic syndrome
nutritional genomics
phytochemicals

phytoestrogens
phytonutrients
premenstrual syndrome (PMS)
wellness

This chapter emphasizes the background and tools for encouraging adults to set nutrition-related lifestyle goals that promote positive health and reduce risk factors. Other chapters of this text provide a focus on the present and potential role of medical nutrition therapy (MNT) in the prevention and intervention for major chronic diseases and conditions that affect food and nutrition choices in the adult years, such as cardiovascular disease (CVD), diabetes, cancer, weight gain, and osteoporosis. Added to these are health-related conditions such as arthritis, Alzheimer's disease, renal disease, and inflammatory-related conditions, which research indicates have potential links to lifestyle and food and nutrition choices. The role of inflammation in chronic disease is becoming increasingly evident (see Chapter 7).

The adult years are a time for nutrition and dietetics professionals to be leaders and team members helping adults achieve and maintain positive health. The goals for Healthy People 2020 provide the framework (Centers for Disease Control and Prevention [CDC], 2017a). The evidence is convincing that decisions for a healthy lifestyle must be made early in life for health promotion and disease prevention (Academy of Nutrition and Dietetics [AND], 2013b).

SETTING THE STAGE: NUTRITION IN THE ADULT YEARS

The focus of this chapter is on nutrition and food-related behaviors for the years after adolescence but before one is deemed an "older adult," often defined as age 65 based on traditional retirement age, although this definition is in a period of change. Admittedly this is a wide range of ages, and, like all population groups, the adult years are heterogeneous. The description of what constitutes being an "older adult" is in constant flux as people change their retirement age, as life expectancy projections are adjusted, and as medical science and lifestyle alterations extend life spans and opportunities for an optimum quality of life. A life expectancy of 80 and above is a reality backed up by CDC statistics with life expectancy in 2017 at 78.8 (CDC, 2018c). Evidence continues to indicate that the adult years set the framework for quality

of life as well as life expectancy. Nutrition and food-related behaviors are key factors, and the earlier prevention becomes the goal, the better the outcome (AND, 2013b).

The dietary reference intakes (DRIs) (see inside cover) provide an overview of the nutrient recommendations for age groups under the DRI umbrella. Staying current on changes in DRI is a critical part of the nutrition and dietetics professional's tools because changes are made as research is validated. Nutrient needs in the adult life cycle are similar but, as in all life stages, are affected by gender, state of health, genetics, medications, and lifestyle choices such as eating behaviors, smoking, and physical activity level. These are markers, determined through assessment, that a nutrition and health professional can use to determine this population's needs. Other markers are less evident and include the adult's perceptions of quality of life and motivation in the areas of nutrition and health (National Institutes of Health [NIH], 2018d)

When the objectives are prevention and behavior change, such markers become critical. Research continues to indicate that positive changes at any age and lifestyle behaviors can make a difference in total health and life expectancy. Making these changes early in life, rather than later, and maintaining them throughout the adult years should be goals. Genetics always has been a consideration in assessment of nutrition status and life potential, but the evolving science of nutritional genomics has become an important marker in nutrition and dietetics practice (see Chapter 6).

SETTING THE STAGE: MESSAGES

A first step for nutrition and dietetics professionals is to recognize that many adults are prime targets for nutrition and health information that offers positive guidance that is understandable and implementable. However, this translates into growing evidence that adults can also be targets for misinformation and guidance based on promises and quick-fixes rather than evidence-based MNT. Rebekah Nagler, PhD, studied the potential role of consumer reaction to what appeared to be contradictory nutrition information or guidance. According to Nagler, confusion and backlash may make people more likely to ignore not only the contradictory information but also the widely accepted nutritional advice such as eating more fruits and vegetables. Nagler also noted that those with the greatest exposure to contradictory information expressed the most confusion with nutrition (Nagler, 2014).

As with any group, adults must be approached with strategies and guidance that fit their health and education needs as well as their capability to implement them. There needs to be an understanding that research is dynamic and ongoing. This should be firmly fixed in the minds of the messenger (the nutrition professional) and the receiver (the patient or client). It is the role of the nutrition professional to verify messaging, separating current evidence-based messages from those based on preliminary or single studies. What is reported as news or guidance to the consumer may appear to be contradictory to current practice when in fact the basis is preliminary research rather than evidence based.

The challenge to nutrition and dietetics professionals is staying current on research and guidelines while acknowledging the potential motivations of their audience or clients and their sources of information. In a technologically savvy world with instant access to nutrition and health advice by self-proclaimed as well as credentialed professionals, this becomes even more of a challenge.

Surveys support the idea that adults are seeking nutrition information and using it to make positive lifestyle changes but are finding that making these changes is a challenge. Time, lack of willpower, conflicting messages, and identifying the efficacy of the messages are cited as barriers (International Food Information Council [IFIC], 2017). The 2017 IFIC Foundation Food and Health Survey identified barriers and noted that consumer confusion is a key concern. Consumers expressed doubt about their choices and noted that they relied on their social network for advice. However, they also noted limited trust in the advice from friends and family. Trust was high for health professionals including RDNs. Interest in adopting and maintaining healthy eating behaviors and confidence for food safety was higher in the baby boomer generation and older adults than in younger adults (IFIC, 2017). As with any age grouping, knowing more about a person's food- and nutrition-related behaviors and beliefs is a critical part of determining how to reach that person with a message.

Another helpful tool for reaching adults is to review the influences of behavior and knowledge on nutrition and health. A review of the health and nutrition information in the media reinforces the idea that nutrition and health information is popular. However, consumers are selective about their personal concerns and their source of information. The IFIC Foundation Food and Health Surveys in 2013, 2015, 2017, and 2018 noted strong interest in trying to lose weight. However, in the 2017 study it was reported that the interest in weight loss benefits from adjusting food intake fall dramatically with age. For those ages 18 to 34, 40% of the respondents reported an interest. At ages 18 to 34 there was a slight drop to 38%, with 23% reported at ages 50 to 64 and 28% at ages 65 to 80 (IFIC, 2017). Changes reported include lowering the amounts of food eaten, eating more fruits and vegetables, drinking more water or low- or no-calorie beverages, including more whole grains, reducing the choice of foods higher in sugar or added sugars, and consuming smaller portions. All these changes are in line with guidance that is suggested in the Dietary Guidelines for Americans (DGA).

The interest in nutrition and in food continues to be evident in the adult years. Popular literature demonstrates a growing interest in cooking, cookbooks, supermarket RDNs, grocery store and farm-to-table events, and other food-related activities (IFIC, 2018). This is

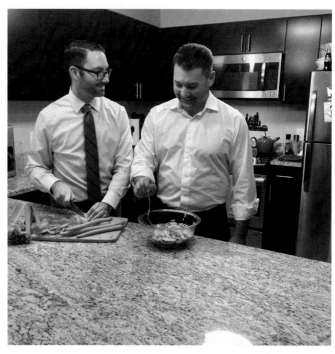

Fig. 18.1 Cooking at home can be the best way to eat balanced and nutritious meals but can also be the most challenging during the adult years due to busy schedules.

surprising because despite all this interest in cooking, Americans continue to cook less and eat fewer meals at home. Cooking at home is a challenge in the adult years due to busy schedules (Fig. 18.1).

Messages regarding the potential benefits and risks of certain foods and nutrients are being heard by consumers. These include messages on the negative effect of saturated fat, trans fatty acids, and sodium. Food companies are changing products to reflect a more health-promoting choice, and restaurants are following this lead. Proposed changes in labeling laws for both food and restaurants have added pressure as the amounts of calories, sodium, and other key nutrients become more identifiable to the consumer. A study on energy and sodium contents of menu items in U.S. chain restaurants concluded that when industry marketing indicated healthier options, it was balanced by simultaneous less-healthy changes in menu choices. For example, as lower-calorie options were offered, the appetizer menu added more fried foods to dip in high-sodium sauces with the featured drinks. It was concluded that there was no meaningful change in energy and sodium content in main entrées in a 1-year (2010–2011) time period (Wu and Sturm, 2014). As the new requirements for restaurant labeling of menu items are fully implemented, it will be interesting to see if this results in both food establishments offering healthier options and customers making healthier choices.

The nutrition and dietetics professional can be a positive influence in advocating and educating for meaningful and real changes in the food supply with a focus on prevention. However, there must be a consumer-driven effort to support these changes. To be a leader, or at least a player, the nutrition and dietetics professional must be aware of community resources and influences, available food sources, and changing food behaviors. Although this chapter focuses on adults, it's important to remember that children are affected by their adult role models, which increases the potential benefits from a focus on prevention.

INFORMATION SOURCES

Where consumers get their information is a factor to consider. The source and the appeal of the message affect how realistic and meaningful information is to the consumer. However, the scientific value and the application of evidence-based information vary. To the adult consumer, the promise of specific benefit is more important than the standard "it's good for you" message, and the scientific validity of the message may not be the determining point. The 2017 IFIC study pointed to this belief (IFIC, 2017).

Sources of information continue to change. Traditional print sources decline as digital and electronic sources increase. Use of phones for digital applications, or "apps," is a growing trend and so is creating, marketing, and evaluating apps. The AND and its affiliates have resources available to identify valid sources. Publications are available to assist in evaluating and selecting digital tools. One such book is *Bits & Bytes: A Guide to Digitally Tracking Your Food, Fitness, and Health*, coauthored by Meagan F. Moyer, MPH, RDN, LD, and the AND (Bits and Bytes, 2016). AND Dietetic Practice Group newsletters and postings frequently include reviews. An ongoing column, *CLICK*, is in the magazine *Food & Nutrition* (published by the AND) (AND CLICK, 2018). The Internet and related links are major information sources thus creating another challenge to the professional seeking to provide evidence-supported information.

Regarding believable and credible human sources of nutrition information, health professionals, including registered dietitians, doctors, and nurses, continue to be rated as the most credible (IFIC, 2017). However, when consumers were asked about the factors that affect their willingness to believe new food and health information, others in their environment, including family and friends, were named as potential influencers.

Surveys have shown an increase in the number of consumers familiar with MyPlate and in those who use food labels, shelf information, and other tools (IFIC, 2017, 2018). Popular literature indicates a growing segment of the population interested in food, cooking, cookbooks, celebrity chefs, and so on, and labels them "foodies." The Nutrition Facts panel and other label information (see Chapter 10) influence nutrition and food decisions, but there may be gaps in the interpretation. The growing lists of ingredients, unknown terminology, changing ingredients, and even the format can make nutrition labels less useful. Changes in the format and content of labels as well as front-of-package systems have been discussed for at least 10 years and are a work in progress. Changes in portion size, the Nutrition Facts panel, and the front-of-package/label claims will be in place by 2020 (U.S. Department of Health and Human Services [USDHHS], 2018b; U.S. Department of Agriculture [USDA], 2018b, 2018c).

Studies indicate that consumers will use labels and would welcome a reliable front-of-package system (Wu and Sturm, 2014). Although the movement for more labeling on menus has been met with mixed reactions, regulations will require labeling by 2020. All these efforts are additional pieces of what is a developing puzzle that involves actions at the state and regional level as well as from federal sources. A continuing theme is the need for an overall consumer-related valid message based on current, understandable evidence-based tools. Also critical to the effort is credentialed food, nutrition, and health professionals who can guide consumers to sources they can easily use to validate information.

Nutrition Information and Education for Adults

Mainstream adults in reasonable health frequently are ignored as a unique segment of the population who can benefit from nutrition assessment and education. Preventive strategies are likely to be targeted to address the formative years of prenatal, infancy, childhood, adolescence, and young adulthood. Older adults are another group likely to be the focus of health intervention strategies and quality-of-life messages as this is a growing age group. The population group in the middle of the continuum, the adult aged 25 to approximately 65, is likely to be segmented in reference to a potential or existing disease state, a life event, or a lifestyle choice. For example, adults are targeted as having or being at risk for diabetes or heart disease, in need of a medication, being pregnant, or being an athlete.

The adult who is not pregnant, an athlete, or "sick," but who seeks guidance on normal nutrition or prevention of disease, may be directed toward diets for chronic disease or weight loss. Such information may be a good fit when the information is based on science, but it can miss the mark on overall prevention goals. Fortunately, the guidance provided by such groups as the American Heart Association (AHA), the AND, the American Diabetes Association (ADA), and the American Cancer Society (ACS) tend to mirror the 2015–2020 DGA. These guidelines will continue to change with the updating of the DGA (USDHHS, 2018a). The overall focus on diet with evolving guidelines is to emphasize quality of food choices, including a message of the role of "healthy fats" (NIH, 2018c). Another change that affects how the DGA will be implemented both by consumers and food producers is the elimination of trans fats as ingredients (Food and Drug Administration [FDA], 2018a).

Several guidelines and reports are aimed at heart-healthy guidance. Heart disease remains the number one disease-related cause of death in adult men and women. The AHA released prevention guidelines in 2006 with a focus on improving overall health and achieving improved cardiovascular health of all Americans by 20% by 2020 (Lloyd-Jones et al, 2010). In November 2013 the AHA, along with the American College of Cardiology (ACC) and the National Heart, Lung, and Blood Institute (NHLBI), released four guidelines based on evidence-based reviews sponsored by NHLBI (see Chapter 32) (Harold and Jessup, 2013). The ACC/AHA recommends a diet high in vegetables, fruits, whole grains, low-fat poultry, fish, non-tropical vegetable oils, nuts, and low-fat dairy, and low in sweets, sugar-sweetened beverages, and red meat (see Chapter 32). The Dietary Approaches to Stop Hypertension (DASH) diet pattern or USDA food pattern (MyPlate) is recommended to achieve this diet. The 2015–2020 DGA is consistent with the ACC/AHA emphasizing increasing the intake of vegetables and fruit to meet the MyPlate guidance of half the plate. A 2015 study by the Produce for Better Health Foundation (PBH) noted that fruit and vegetable consumption has declined 7% over 5 years (from 2009 to 2014). Adults ages 18 to 44 (along with children of all ages) were cited as a population group showing this decrease (PBH, 2015). Nutrition messages related to consumption of fat, choices of fat sources, and choices of vegetables and fruits frame the guidance provided by the AHA, AND, ADA, and ACS as well as meet guidance provided by the DGA.

Guidelines for diabetes prevention continue to be related to healthy lifestyle guidelines of the DGA (see Chapter 29). A 2014 study indicated that research will continue to explore obesity and overweight. In a Danish study the link to being obese or overweight was a factor but there was a time difference noted. Maintaining an overweight or obese status for multiple years increased the risk more than the presence of elevated body mass index (BMI) or weight. This led to the conclusion that focusing on small weight reduction for the total population may be more beneficial than concentrating on weight loss targeted to high-risk individuals (Vistisen et al, 2014).

Health education and public health programs, along with improved research and care, have contributed to changes in morbidity and mortality of the adult population. U.S. adults are on a path to positive change, moving from knowledge to action (CDC, 2013, 2018a, 2018b, 2018c). Nutrition assessment is a critical component of MNT and guidance for prevention. The nutrition and dietetics professional should either lead or be a part of lifestyle management teams. These professionals can link MNT to food and economic and social choices, and they can frame the guidance to be useful and achievable. Nutrition education, basic cooking ability, communication, and assessment skills add other dimensions to the goal of moving adults to action. Adults in the awareness and action stages are likely to be looking for answers, often short-term fixes or reversals of a health problem rather than more realistic long-term behavior changes. For example, adults may want to know where carbohydrates fit into the total diet and whether there are "better carbs," the message on "good" or any fat now that trans fats have been almost banned, a "healthy" or "unhealthy" food or diet, whether to buy organically grown or locally grown foods, or what to do about sodium. These are issues best addressed by skilled nutrition and dietetics professionals who can provide valid current information that answers short-term questions but builds on long-term solutions.

Guidance based on science generally addresses total diet and lifestyle rather than single nutrients or foods. The concepts of *healthful eating*, *nutrient density*, and *nutritious foods* are debated by food and nutrition professionals as science and technology move forward. Unfortunately, food and nutrition debates and new research findings, often meant to clarify the evidence, are fodder for media coverage, adding to the confusion and perception of mixed messages. A search for information on choosing foods for health can result in evidence-based information such as the DGA, as well as questionable guidance based on single studies or product promotion. The combination of marketing and electronic media makes it easier to mix science with speculation and outright untruths. Adults with an interest in improving the nutritional quality of their diet may end up with unreliable advice pointing to quick-fix solutions.

The Wellness Years and Food Security

The adult years span a broad range chronologically and are complicated by physiologic, developmental, and social factors. Along with their genetic and social history, adults have accumulated the results of behaviors and risks from environmental factors. These factors shape the heterogeneity of the adult years. Nonetheless, the adult years are an ideal time for positive health promotion and disease prevention messages. In the transitions from early to middle adulthood, health and wellness may take on a new importance. This may be the result of a life event or education (an epiphany) that triggers awareness that being well and staying well are important. Examples include learning the results of a screening for blood pressure, cholesterol, or diabetes; facing the reality of death; facing the health crisis of a peer or family member; or realizing that clothes do not fit as well as they should. Regardless of the reason, the concept of wellness takes on a new meaning, and these events are teachable moments.

The Wellness Councils of America (WELCOA) describes wellness as a process that involves being aware of better health and actively working toward that goal (WELCOA, 2018). With this mindset, a state of wellness can exist at any age and can start at any point in a person's life course. Wellness is more than physical health and well-being. A state of well-being includes mental and spiritual health and encompasses the ability of a person to move through Maslow's Hierarchy of Needs (Maslow, 1970).

The ability to address nutrition needs requires food security (i.e., access to a safe, acceptable, and adequate source of food). Part of the issue of food security is quantity and part is quality. According to USDA data, in 2016, 87.7% of U.S. households were food secure,

slightly higher than in 2012. Of the remaining population, 12.3% of households were reported as food insecure (USDA, 2016).

The current economic climate has put added emphasis on food security or access and potential population inequalities. The highest levels of food insecurity are reported to be in African American, Native American, and Hispanic households (USDA, 2016).

The issues of quantity, quality, and acceptability are a part of the food security discussion. It is often more expensive to eat healthy foods than less healthy, high-calorie foods. However, limited skills in the areas of wise food purchasing and food preparation coupled with limited food access and equipment resources further complicate a person's ability to follow advice for a healthy lifestyle. This emphasizes the need for adult consumer education in basic food skills. The Supplemental Nutrition Assistance Program (SNAP), formerly known as food stamps, aims to alleviate food insecurity and eligibility, for participation is based on income level. The program includes some money for nutrition education (USDA, 2018b). SNAP, like other food and nutrition assistance programs, is being reviewed and altered not only to adjust access but also to increase the nutrition quality and types of food offered. The fact that SNAP is a program that serves the working poor as well as those who are unemployed often is overlooked. Feeding America is a website to visit for more information on food insecurity (Feeding America, 2014, 2018). Food insecurity frames the need for guidance from nutrition and dietetics professionals on food access, acceptability, and use.

Quality of Life and Work-Life Balance

Perceptions of personal health (mental and physical) relate to views on wellness and perceptions of quality of life. Health-related quality of life (HRQOL) is a concept used to measure the effects of current health conditions on a person's everyday life. To capture this and create a tool for professionals, the CDC measures population HRQOL perceptions, including the perception of "feeling healthy." Using HRQOL, one can learn about how adults relate their health to their daily performance. On average, Americans report feeling "unhealthy" approximately 6 days a month and "healthy" or "full of energy" approximately 19 days a month; adults with the lowest income levels and more chronic diseases report more "unhealthy" days (CDC, 2016b, 2016c).

To promote quality of life, adults are being urged to set a goal of "work-life" balance. This is not a new concept and fits into the need for stress reduction and relaxation as a part of a healthy lifestyle. However, the idea of balancing work time with leisure also can be a reason adults use for not exercising, not cooking, eating on the run, ignoring nutrition guidelines, or skipping meals. Leisure time can be interpreted as screen time, inactivity while watching activity, or social interaction, all of which are sedentary and may be accompanied by eating and drinking. Regardless of the reasons and the interpretations, the idea of work-life balance is a message that is receiving social media attention and an issue that often is related to multitasking and assuming multiple roles (Fig. 18.2). In the concept of wellness or prevention, there is a mental health link as well as a potential block to leading a health-promoting lifestyle, not only for adults but also for their associates, family members, and others in their sphere of influence. The pros and cons and the potential health benefits of work-life balance is a topic for worksites and for dietetic and nutrition professionals (CDC, 2017a).

The adult years offer unique opportunities to evaluate health status, build on positive factors, and change the negative factors that affect quality of life. Because adults are teachers, coaches, parents, caregivers, and worksite leaders, targeting the wellness-related attitudes and behaviors of adults potentially can have a multiplier effect. A positive wellness focus may influence the health of the adult and anyone who is in their sphere of influence.

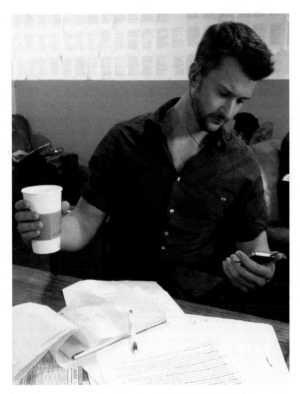

Fig. 18.2 Eating quickly without attention, when stressed or when multitasking, often results in poor nutritional intake in the adult years.

LIFESTYLE AND HEALTH RISK FACTORS

Lifestyle choices, including activity, lay the framework for health and wellness. The health of people living in the United States has continued to improve in part because of education that has led to lifestyle changes. Life expectancy has continued to increase (projected at 78.7 years), and the morbidity and mortality rates from heart disease, cancer, and stroke have dropped (CDC, 2016a, 2018c). Overall life expectancy for the African American population is 3.8 years less than that of the Caucasian population. This disparity is attributed to higher death rates from heart disease, cancer, homicide, diabetes, and perinatal conditions (CDC, 2013). These statistics point the way for increased emphasis on prevention and intervention initiatives in minority populations.

Even when the emphasis is on wellness and prevention, there is a strong link to risk factors that influence morbidity and mortality. In the United States the leading causes of death and debilitation among adults include (1) heart disease, (2) cancer, (3) chronic lower respiratory diseases, (4) cerebrovascular disease, (5) accidents (unintentional injuries), (6) Alzheimer's disease, (7) diabetes, and (8) nephritis, nephrotic syndrome, and nephrosis. Chronic diseases, including heart disease, stroke, cancer, and diabetes, are among the most costly and preventable of all health problems and account for one third of the years of potential life lost before age 65 and for 75% of the nation's medical care costs. These health issues have direct links to diet and lifestyle, but they are also affected by complex social determinants and environmental factors (Box 18.1).

The information quoted is for all adults, but when adjusting for age, the leading causes of death for young adults 18 to 44 are related to preventable causes, with suicide and homicide in the top three causes for adults under 34 years of age. Accidents or unintentional

---

BOX 18.1   A Focus on Health Disparities and Nutrition

Differences in health between populations have been observed by researchers and clinicians for a long time. Historically, those differences have been most stark when comparing the general population to racial and ethnic minorities. In 1899 American sociologist and author W. E. B. Du Bois wrote in his book *The Philadelphia Negro* about the higher death rates, prevalence of disease, and generally poorer health of urban African Americans (Williams, 2010). But what at the time was viewed by many as the result of biological and immutable differences between races, Du Bois argued and modern researchers now know is in fact the product of a complex mix of social, behavioral, environmental, and genetic contributors to health disparities, and not a fixed characteristic of any one group or race.

Health disparities are differences in the burden of disease or worse health outcomes in a group compared with the general population. Disparities can be found in the overall rate of disease incidence, prevalence, morbidity, mortality, or survival rates. According to the National Institutes of Health, groups observed to have these differences are designated health disparity populations and include racial and ethnic minorities, populations of low socioeconomic status, sexual and gender minorities, and rural or medically underserved persons (NIMHD, 2019).

The determinants of health that factor into health disparities cover many more aspects than just biology. Social determinants of health (see Chapter 8) including socioeconomic factors, psychological influences, social support, discrimination, and a variety of related components are critically important to understanding disparities. These determinants span the behavioral, physical, or built environment, and sociocultural and health care domains, and have impacts on the individual, interpersonal, community, and societal levels (NIMHD, 2017).

Nutrition is a key component in understanding and, in many cases, addressing health disparities. In many diseases in which disparities persist across groups, including hypertension, type 2 diabetes, kidney disease, and obesity, medical nutrition therapy (MNT) is critical to effective intervention. However, additional nutrition-focused research needs to be done in order to determine the most effective methods for addressing disparities in affected communities. In order to address the nonbiological aspects of disparities, simple diet-based strategies alone are not enough. Individual and community values, health literacy, and sustainability are determining factors in the long-term success of the ability of professionals to improve health disparities.

Michael J. Hahn, BA

Williams DR, Sternthal M: Understanding Racial/ethnic Disparities in Health: Sociological Contributions, *Journal of health and social behavior* 51(Suppl):S15-S27, 2010, doi:10.1177/0022146510383838.

National Institutes of Health (NIH), National Institute of Minority Health and Health Disparities (NIMHD) "HDPulse - Health Disparities Resources." https://hdpulse.nimhd.nih.gov/. Published 2019. Accessed September 30, 2019.

National Institutes of Health (NIH), National Institute of Minority NIH, NIMHD. "NIMHD Research Framework." https://www.nimhd.nih.gov/docs/framework-factsheet.pdf. Published 2017.

---

injuries play a different role in younger adults. Accidents are the fifth leading cause of death and debilitation among all adults but moves up to first place for adults under 44, with emphasis on ages 25 to 44 (CDC, 2016a, 2018b, 2018c). Presumably the other leading causes of death, involving chronic diseases and those more diet related, can be important prevention teaching points at younger ages. Add to the list osteoporosis and new links to such health issues as Alzheimer's disease or arthritis as health problems that affect health care costs and loss of quality of life and that have a potential lifestyle and nutrition link (CDC, 2018a).

Overweight and obesity are either precursors to or complications in all of these diseases. The prevalence of overweight, as measured by a BMI of 25 or more, has increased at all ages but appears to be holding steady and even showing slight decline. It is important when looking at the overall health of adults to consider elevated BMI as a major risk factor but to move to the next phase of total assessment to identify the health profile. Hypertension, hyperlipidemia, and elevated blood glucose often are seen together with or without obesity, known as the metabolic syndrome (see Chapter 29). Increasing numbers of obese and overweight adults have been linked to an increase in the number of cases of metabolic syndrome. There is a genetic link to this syndrome but lifestyle is a major issue. Evidence suggests that it is possible to delay or control the risk factors associated with metabolic syndrome with lifestyle changes, including health-promoting diet and exercise patterns, with the help of health professionals (NIH, 2018c; CDC, 2018a, 2016b).

Obesity and overweight directly link with calorie imbalance. An estimated less than half of U.S. adults participate in regular physical activity, with one fourth reporting no activity. Many health risks in the adult years, including coronary artery disease, certain types of cancer, hypertension, type 2 diabetes, depression, anxiety, and osteoporosis have a relationship with lack of participation in regular physical activity and poor eating behaviors. One cannot achieve positive health without a combination of physical activity and food choices that fit personal needs for energy balance and nutrition.

On the other end of the weight spectrum is chronic underweight, frequently accompanied by undernutrition. Anorexia nervosa is the extreme condition, found in both genders across the age span. An unhealthy weight or unhealthy concern about body weight not only affects overall health but in women also can affect fertility and the ability to conceive.

HEALTH DISPARITIES AND GLOBAL HEALTH

Eliminating disparities that increase the health risks for affected populations is a major goal of effective health policy. Health disparities (see Box 18.1) related to inadequate access to safe and affordable food are often based on race, ethnicity, gender, education, income level, and geographic location. Inadequate access to care is a disparity that has a major effect on a person's wellness. Chronic diseases and obesity have been shown to be more of a burden to racial minorities and women (CDC, 2016b, 2018a). There is a higher incidence of heart disease, diabetes, and obesity or overweight in low-income, African American, and Hispanic populations (CDC, 2018a). These same population groups have limited access to preventive care, nutrition education, and guidance (USDHHS, 2018a, 2018b). Research and public policy aimed at addressing the social determinants and structural discrimination that contribute to these health disparities is imperative to improving health for all.

World Health

The problems associated with chronic diseases are similar in other countries (World Health Organization [WHO], 2017). Also cited are infectious diseases such as human immunodeficiency virus, tuberculosis, and tropical diseases as barriers to global achievement of positive health status. Eight United Nations Millennium Development Goals seek to reduce the number of people who suffer from hunger and to increase access to safe water and sanitation. However, obesity has been cited as being of epidemic proportions globally, with

at least 2.8 million people dying each year as a result of being overweight or obese.

WHO: Key Facts (WHO, 2018)

- Worldwide, obesity has tripled since 1975.
- In 2016, more than 1.9 billion adults 18 years and older were overweight. Of these, 650 million were obese.
- 39% of adults aged 18 years and over were overweight and 13% were obese.
- Most of the worlds population live in countries where overweight or obesity kill more people than underweight.
- 41 million children under the age of 5 were overweight or obese in 2016.
- Over 340 million children and adolescents aged 5-19 were overweight or obese in 2016.

This condition, once associated with higher-income countries, is now listed by WHO as prevalent in low- and middle-income countries. The growing international problem of obesity is a point for consideration and involvement.

Access to a safe and affordable food supply goes beyond the borders of the United States. The quality and quantity of food and lifestyle factors are concerns that require more than provision of food. A newer and growing emphasis on food lifestyles is identifying "food deserts." CDC defines food deserts as areas that lack access to affordable fruits, vegetables, whole grains, low-fat dairy, and other foods that make up the full range of a healthy diet (CDC, 2017b). USDA expands the definition with a focus on limited access to supermarkets, supercenters, and other sources of affordable and healthy foods, noting food deserts can occur in rural or urban settings. Knowing the potential of access to healthy foods, knowing the limitations, and working to expand this access is a critical part of assisting adults and families in meeting nutrition goals. The USDA Food Access Research Atlas and Economic Research Services Outlook are starting points for nutrition and dietetic professionals (USDA, 2016, 2018a).

NUTRITIONAL FACTORS AFFECTING ADULT WOMEN AND MEN

Women's Health

The reproductive years constitute a significant stage of a woman's life. Many issues that affect the health of women are related to the monthly hormonal shifts associated with menses. Osteoporosis, heart disease, and some cancers are disease states that are affected by specific hormones. Pregnancy and breastfeeding have an effect on a woman's health (see Chapter 14). Breastfeeding helps control weight, lower the risk for diabetes, and improves bone health. Therefore encouraging women to breastfeed is a potential prevention strategy for the future health of the mother and infant.

Shifts of estrogen and progesterone hormones trigger the female reproductive cycle and affect health. Associated with menses is a complex set of physical and psychological symptoms known as premenstrual syndrome (PMS). Reported symptoms vary but are described as general discomfort, anxiety, depression, fatigue, breast pain, and cramping. Such symptoms are reported to occur approximately 1 week to 10 days before the onset of menses and increase in severity into menses. Currently, there is no single cause or intervention identified for PMS. Hormone imbalance, neurotransmitter synthesis defects, and low levels of certain nutrients (i.e., vitamin B_6 and calcium) have been implicated (NIH, Office of Dietary Supplements [ODS], 2018c, 2018d, 2018f). A diet high in sodium and refined carbohydrates has been implicated, but the evidence is not complete enough to make recommendations (NIH, ODS, 2018d). A greater emphasis on a plant-based diet of whole grains, fruits, vegetables, lean or low-fat protein sources, and low-fat dairy or soy beverages is a reasonable intervention and may cause relief in some women. Exercise and relaxation techniques have been reported as lessening the symptoms.

When menses end, either because of age or surgical removal of reproductive organs, women have unique health and nutrition concerns. Perimenopause and menopause generally begin in the late 40s. However, genetics, general health, and the age that menses began can alter the timing of this marker. Typically, estrogen production decreases around age 50, when endogenous estrogen circulation decreases approximately 60%. The effects include a cessation of menses and the loss of the healthful benefits of estrogen. Even after the ovaries cease production, a weaker form of estrogen continues to be produced by the adrenal glands, and some is stored in adipose tissue.

As estrogen decreases, symptoms associated with menopause may occur. The onset of menopause and the reported side effects vary. Some women experience a gradual decline in the frequency and duration of menses, whereas others experience an abrupt cessation. The symptoms most often reported include low energy levels and vasomotor symptoms (hot flashes). Bone, heart, and brain health are affected. The decrease in circulating estrogen limits the body's ability to remodel bones, resulting in a decrease of bone mass. Lower levels of circulating estrogen also affect blood lipid levels, increasing total cholesterol and low-density lipoprotein (LDL) cholesterol levels and decreasing high-density lipoprotein (HDL) levels. Brain function, particularly memory, also is affected but the memory loss associated with menopause is often temporary.

Managing menopause promotes emphasis on plant-based foods for the benefits of phytoestrogens, soluble fiber, and other components. Having sufficient calcium, vitamin D, vitamin K, and magnesium, and using the DRI as the guideline are important for protecting bone health. Although soy (isoflavones) continues to be rumored by the popular press as a way to control hot flashes, current research is not definitive (NIH, NCCIH, 2016). A study of American women published in *Menopause* found that only women who are able to produce the soy metabolite equol get relief from hot flashes by eating soy (Newton et al, 2015). Of 357 study participants 34% were equol producers. The authors warned that a readily available test for the metabolite must be developed, and more randomized studies are needed to be able to make any recommendations that soy be a treatment for hot flashes.

Heart disease, cancer, and stroke continue to be the leading causes of death in women (CDC, 2017b). Again, although genetics are a factor, lifestyle is a major predictor and complicating factor.

Weight is a risk factor for heart disease and some cancers. Weight gain is an issue for women, with a 35% prevalence of obesity in American women aged 20 to 74 years compared with 33% in the same aged men. One half of non-Hispanic African American women and two fifths of Hispanic women are obese, compared with one third of non-Hispanic white women (CDC, 2016b, 2018b). Physical activity with aerobic endeavors and resistance and weight-bearing exercise is protective for bone, cardiovascular, and emotional health. The key nutrition message is one of balanced food intake with nutrient-dense foods that are low in fat. However, once again personal assessment and tailoring to meet individual needs are a critical part of success in weight loss and maintenance.

Men's Health

The leading causes of death among American men include heart disease, prostate and lung cancers, and unintentional injuries. For the adult man, a diet that supports reducing the risk for heart disease is especially important because men develop heart disease at a younger age than women. Regular exercise and activity are important. Along with contributing to cardiovascular health, weight-bearing exercise has a positive effect on bone health.

Another issue in adult men is iron intake. Unless adult men are diagnosed with iron deficiency anemia and require additional iron, they should not seek additional iron from multivitamin or mineral supplements, enriched sports drinks, or energy bars. Excessive iron intake is problematic because it is an oxidant in the body; men and postmenopausal women do not have menstruation, pregnancy, or lactation to get rid of excess iron.

Like women, today's male population also is affected by obesity and the risk factors that come with excess weight such as diabetes, heart disease, and orthopedic problems. The ACS reports that one in seven men will have prostate cancer in his lifetime but only one in 36 will die of this disease. Obesity may play a role in these cancers. Some studies indicate that foods high in lycopene, an antioxidant found in tomatoes and other fruits and vegetables, may provide a protective role in lowering the risk factors for developing prostate cancer. Although this is still being studied, it is an emerging area for nutrition and diet in lowering risk factors and an area for dietetic and nutrition professionals to continue to explore. Such factors as how the food high in lycopene is prepared may have an effect on the usefulness of the lycopene (ACS, 2018).

INTERVENTIONS, NUTRITION, AND PREVENTION

Adults are in the ideal life cycle phase for health promotion and disease prevention nutrition advice because of the combination of life experience and influence. This group has the potential to shape personal lifestyle choices and influence others. The tools are in place, including the DGA, MyPlate, and the Nutrition Facts panel on food labels (see Chapter 10).

The vegetarian diet or a more plant-based diet and the Mediterranean diet have become popular with health and nutrition professionals and the public. The motivation is both personal health and health of the planet and support the recommendations of the DGA.

Implementation of positive choices and moving people along the continuum of a healthy lifestyle are other issues. Studies indicate consumers are aware of the concerns associated with lifestyle and diet but have a limited interest in making sustainable changes (IFIC, 2017, 2018). Consumers are aware of the implied promises for good health that come with messages from the media, friends, and health professionals; however, they are unlikely to move from awareness to action without motivation stronger than a message or promise. One perception of consumers is that eating healthful foods means giving up foods they like or having to eat foods that do not have the taste they prefer. A total diet approach of making gradual changes to food and lifestyle choices may help. The Small Steps: Big Rewards program is an example of such an approach with a goal of preventing type 2 diabetes (NIH, National Diabetes Education Program, 2018b).

The steps to prevention and health promotion, even when small, are personal responsibilities that cannot be legislated. Americans have many choices: what and where they eat, where they receive their information, and what they include or exclude from their lifestyle. Adults value choice and food selection as a right, even if it leads to poor health, chronic disease, or death. Some messages are directed at reaching adults where they live and work. For the working adult population, much of the day is tied to a worksite. There are increasing efforts in the private and public sectors to promote positive work site nutrition-related behaviors and programs.

FOOD TRENDS AND PATTERNS

Where one eats, who prepares it, and how much is consumed are patterns of behavior and choice. There is no stereotypical "adult" lifestyle. Adults may be single or partnered, with or without children, and working outside the home or at home. The sit-down family meals at home have given way to eating on the run, take-out, and drive-through. Too little time for planning or preparation and limited cooking skills can lead to reliance on processed foods, speed-scratch cooking (combining processed with fresh ingredients), or more food prepared out of the home. Today's economic climate and changing dietary recommendations present new challenges. The nutrient-dense approach is essential because energy needs decrease as age increases. Reaching men and women with an understandable and relevant message, especially heads of households or gatekeepers, is critical.

The consumer price index (CPI) estimates that Americans spend more than half of their food dollars away from home. This is an amount that continues to increase and that fluctuates by month. The CPI for food measures the average change over time in the prices paid by urban consumers, using a representative market basket of consumer goods and services. The Economic Research Service (ERS) of the USDA follows these expenditures and manages the data set. This is a valuable resource for monitoring expenditures and planning for meaningful interventions (USDA, 2018a).

Changing food patterns and the use of more processed and purchased foods can result in an increase in dietary sodium, fat, and sweeteners and a decrease in use of basic foods such as fruits, vegetables, and whole grains. Portion sizes (either the amount presented, or the amount eaten) replace serving sizes (what is recommended as a serving by the DGA or other source), as others determine what is considered a "meal" or "snack." Portions have continued to increase in size in the United States.

Dietary changes have affected nutrition and already are reflected in the current concerns for weight and nutrient imbalances. The 2015 DGA and MyPlate (see Chapter 10) can be viewed as attempts to put more emphasis on basic foods that are nutrient dense rather than calorie dense and on total amounts of foods per day rather than numbers of servings. The most current information is reflected in the information used to shape the 2015 DGA but stay tuned as the 2020 DGA will change (Health.Gov, 2018).

Adult diets are likely to be higher in total fat than the 30% of total calories recommended in the 2015 DGA and include a predominance of carbohydrates as added sugar and refined grains. Fruit and vegetable guidelines are not being met, although increases are being noted. Although chicken and fish servings have increased, animal sources outweigh plant-based protein sources. Health guidelines continue to move in the direction of increasing plant-based foods. Key nutrients that may be in short supply are calcium, magnesium, and potassium; the antioxidants vitamins A, C, and E; and vitamin D (USDHHS, 2018a). Accessing information building to the 2015 DGA (Scientific Report of the 2015 DGA Advisory Committee) will give a clearer picture (Health.Gov, 2018).

NUTRITIONAL SUPPLEMENTATION

A position of the AND (formerly the American Dietetic Association) is that the best nutritional strategy for promoting optimal health and reducing the risk of chronic disease is to choose a variety of nutrient-rich foods. Additional nutrients from fortified foods and supplements help people meet their nutritional needs as specified by science-based nutrition standards such as the DRI (AND, 2009a). In making this statement, the AND puts food first but leaves the door open for those with specific nutrient needs, identified through assessment by a dietetics or health professional, to be nutritionally supplemented.

Traditionally, one thinks of vitamins and minerals, fiber, and protein as nutrient supplements, generally in a pill, capsule, or liquid form. The DRIs are the standards used with most adults. However, food fortification is another form of nutrient supplementation. The level of fortified foods (such as energy bars, sports drinks, smoothies, or ingredients for fortification) in the marketplace puts another layer of potential nutrient sources in the mix with traditional supplements. Less traditional supplements such as herbals and other natural dietary "enhancers" are added to the array of supplements available to consumers. Information continues to build on the safety of some of the ingredients used to fortify or supplement. Examples include the 2014 report on the safety of caffeine added to foods and supplements and the ongoing updates from the NIH, ODS, and National Center for Complementary and Integrative Health (IOM, 2014; NIH, 2016; NIH, NCCIH, 2018a).

Either because of choice, access, or health-related issues, Americans may not meet the dietary recommendations for promoting optimal health. Several segments of the adult population fall into high-risk groups who are unlikely to meet their nutrient needs because of life stage (e.g., pregnancy), alcohol or drug dependency, food insecurity, chronic illness, recovery from illness, or choosing a nutritionally restrictive diet or lifestyle. Other persons with special needs include those with food allergies or intolerances that eliminate major food groups, persons using prescription drugs or therapies that change the way the body uses nutrients, those with disabilities that limit their ability to enjoy a varied diet, and those who are just unable or unwilling because of time or energy to prepare or consume a nutritionally adequate diet. These adults potentially need a nutritional supplement (AND, 2009a, 2013b).

FUNCTIONAL FOODS

Articles and news reports have attributed many benefits to what are known as functional foods. In the 1980s the Japanese government created a class of foods they labeled as functional, meaning that they had health benefits beyond nutrition. Here in the United States the FDA has not yet defined functional foods, but the AND defines them as "whole foods along with fortified, enriched, or enhanced foods that have a potentially beneficial effect on health when consumed as part of a varied diet on a regular basis at effective levels based on significant standards of evidence." Adults interested in attaining and maintaining wellness are frequently interested in altering dietary patterns or choosing these foods for added health benefits. The desire for fewer calories and multiple health benefits, especially when children are in the home, is driving the growth in the U.S. functional foods market. Sloan describes this drive for real-food solutions, for "healthy" foods as a reminder to consumers of the long-term value of staying healthy (Sloan, 2012). Eight out of ten Americans are making an effort to eat healthfully, and 42% are concerned about the nutrient content of the foods they buy. One result is an increase in sales of functional foods and beverages. Sloan notes that young adults, ages 18 to 24, are the top users of functional foods and beverages. This increase in sales of these foods and beverages is related to the search for healthier foods from familiar staples with better health profiles as well as options for individual nutrients (Sloan, 2012).

In a 2013 position paper on functional foods, the AND notes all food is functional at some level, but there is growing evidence of components in food beyond traditional nutrients (AND, 2013a). Examples of large classes of functional foods are conventional foods, such as whole grains, fruits, vegetables, and nuts, as well as modified foods like sports drinks, bars, yogurt, cereal, and orange juice. These are examples of foods believed to have benefits beyond their usual nutrient value (AND, 2013a; IFIC, 2018). Functional foods can include whole foods as well as those that are fortified, enriched, or enhanced by the addition of food components or nutrients.

Providing this information to the segment of the adult population looking for ways to enhance health not only gains the adults' attention but also takes nutrition guidance to a higher level. Research continues to provide information on dietary patterns and components of foods that may have added benefits for health. Helping to lower blood cholesterol or control blood glucose, serving as an antioxidant or scavenger against harmful components, promoting a healthy gastrointestinal tract, or stimulating activity of detoxification enzyme systems in the liver are examples of benefits being reported and researched for validity.

Phytochemicals or phytonutrients (from the Greek word *phyto*, meaning "plant") are biologically active and naturally occurring chemical components in plant foods. In plants, phytochemicals act as natural defense systems for their host and offer protection against microbial invasions or infections. They also provide color, aroma, and flavor, with more than 2000 plant pigments identified. These include flavonoids, anthocyanins, and carotenoids. Functional foods have become a favorite topic of the consumer press, which often exaggerate the benefit of the food (see *Focus On:* Chocolate: A Functional Food?). As part of human consumption, phytonutrients can have antioxidant, detoxification, and antiinflammatory functions in the body.

◎ FOCUS ON

Chocolate: A Functional Food?

Chocolate can be considered a healthy food, as long as it is eaten in moderation. White chocolate is generally the cocoa butter portion with added sugar and flavorings and does not possess the same health benefits as milk or dark chocolate. Some facts about chocolate are the following:

- Chocolate is a plant food, made from beans harvested from a cocoa tree. Once the beans are removed from a pod, they are fermented, dried, roasted, and then ground. This produces a liquid, which is pressed to separate the cocoa butter from the solids. The end result is a cake that is then ground to make cocoa powder.
- Cocoa butter contains saturated fat, but research indicates the effect on blood cholesterol is neutral and may even be positive. However, it is a calorie source.
- Chocolate is a source of flavonoids, naturally occurring compounds that serve as antioxidants. Known as polyphenols, these are the same antioxidants found in tea, red wine, and some fruits and vegetables. These compounds give chocolate its rich color as well as potential health benefits. Dark chocolate has the most flavonoids.
- It is believed flavonoids help the body repair damage to cells and may even provide a protective shield.

- Chocolate is also a source of plant sterols, B vitamins, magnesium, and potassium, all with potential heart-health benefits.
- Chocolate can potentially improve mood because cocoa is believed to have a positive effect on boosting endorphin and serotonin levels in the brain.
- There are some potential negatives along with the potential of an allergic reaction:

  Cocoa is a source of oxalates. For some this can be a trigger for certain types of kidney stones.

  Caffeine is present in chocolate with dark chocolate taking the lead and milk chocolate at about one third the amount of the dark chocolate. This is a stimulant with varying effects based on your health and the amount consumed.

  Dark chocolate is a source of tyramine, also present in red wine, and some fermented and aged foods. Still under investigation but worth noting is the potential for triggering migraine headaches.

  Chocolate is often in foods with excessive calories. Added sugar and fat in popular chocolate desserts, candies, and beverages bring to light the ongoing theme. Keep the portions real for your personal needs.

Soy is another example of a food with value beyond quality protein but like others, research is still being collected and evaluated. The potential health benefits of soy products or components of soy include the potential of reducing the risk for heart disease and certain types of cancer and reducing vasomotor symptoms (hot flashes) in menopausal females. Note that soy itself, as a plant, has no cholesterol and is a source of isoflavones, a phytoestrogen or plant estrogen. In 1999 the FDA approved a food label claim for soy, addressing its potential role in reducing the risk of heart disease. This was reevaluated in 2013 when FDA Model guidelines noted the following:

1. 25 grams of soy protein a day, as part of a diet low in saturated fat and cholesterol, may reduce the risk of heart disease.
2. Diets low in saturated fat and cholesterol that include 25 g of soy protein a day may reduce the risk of heart disease (FDA, 2018c).

The ACS concludes that cancer survivors may safely consume up to three servings daily (ACS, 2014; McCullough, 2012). Soy continues to be considered a quality protein with potential of added health benefits (NIH, NCCIH, 2016).

One cannot address dietary guidance without considering the issues of functional components and functional foods. Rather than isolating and promoting food components, current thinking supports the emphasis on food as a package and as a first source for nutrients and potential enhancers. In the big picture it is the person's health status, lifestyle choices, and genetics that form the potential for wellness, but dietary enhancement is a tool that gains attention and helps the person move forward on the wellness continuum.

ADULT HEALTH NEXT STEPS

The objectives for this chapter are to introduce direction for the well adult. This is a segment of the population who already may be a candidate for MNT, but the intent is to focus on resources for prevention and wellness. A 2013 position of the AND, The Role of Nutrition in Health Promotion and Chronic Disease Prevention, was a rallying point. In this position the statement was made that primary prevention is the most affordable method to prevent chronic disease (AND, 2013b). Prevention strategies include MNT because the line between being "healthy" and being "well" relates to control, maintenance, and, for the adult, taking personal responsibility for setting a path as early as possible in the life cycle. However, an important strategy is selecting nutrient-dense foods, a point made in the 2015 DGA and emphasized in a 2016 practice paper of the AND (AND, 2016).

CLINICAL CASE STUDY

Aileen is a 28-year-old African American woman who lives in a suburb of Chicago with her husband and 12-year-old daughter. She is 5 ft, 10 in tall and currently weighs 165 pounds. In the past 2 years she has gained 10 pounds. At a recent neighborhood health fair at the YMCA, Aileen's blood glucose and blood pressure screening results were higher than they had been a year ago but were still in a good range. She has a family history of heart disease and diabetes and recognizes that her weight gain is an issue. Both she and her husband work full time and blending their schedules with that of their daughter is hectic. They have one car needed by her husband for work. Aileen travels mostly by bus and does all the cooking and shopping. They have a kitchen with a range, oven, microwave, and refrigerator/freezer. She describes her food shopping habits as chaotic and last minute, often stopping at the local convenience store since the distance to the nearest supermarket is 5 miles by car. They eat out (fast food or take-out) for most lunches and at least two dinners a week. They have no regular activity or exercise. As a family, they have the minimum health insurance with a large copayment; thus they do not have an ongoing health care routine.

Aileen made an appointment with a locally based health care source. She asked for dietary counseling and was asked to bring a 1-day food recall for the registered dietitian. She reported the following: breakfast: egg and sausage on a bagel, coffee; midmorning: low-fat snack bar from vending machine with coffee; lunch: double burger with cheese on a bun and large fries, ketchup, and extra pickles, diet soda; dinner: frozen dinner that included chicken, rice, and corn. She had an iceberg lettuce salad with diet ranch dressing "to add something green." Beverage was a diet soda. During the evening she had a dish of chocolate ice cream and sweet tea. She reports that in her coffee she likes two packets of sugar and some nondairy creamer.

Nutrition Diagnostic Statements

- Altered nutrition related laboratory values related to busy schedule, reduced access to a supermarket, consumption of high sodium and high glycemic convenience foods and recent weight gain as evidenced by elevated blood glucose and blood pressure.
- Physical inactivity related to time constraints and busy schedule as evidenced by report of no regular exercise in daily routine.

Nutrition Care Questions

1. What social, lifestyle, and nutrition triggers are likely to be identified by the dietitian?
2. What foods should Aileen consider including in her diet to build a prevention-related meal plan?
3. Plan a meal pattern and two sample meals that illustrate your recommendations, including at least one at-home and away-from-home breakfast, lunch, and dinner.

USEFUL WEBSITES

Academy of Nutrition and Dietetics (Formerly the American Dietetic Association)
American Cancer Society
American Diabetes Association
American Heart Association
Centers for Disease Control and Prevention
Dietary Guidelines for Americans
Food and Agriculture Organization
Healthy People 2020
Institute of Food Technologists
Institute of Medicine
International Food Information Council Food Insights
National Institutes of Health (NIH) Office of Dietary Supplements
U.S. Department of Agriculture: Agricultural Research Service
U.S. Department of Agriculture: MyPlate
U.S. Department of Health and Human Services
Wellness Councils of America
World Health Organization

REFERENCES

Academy of Nutrition and Dietetics, Moyer MF: *Bits and Bytes: a guide to digitally tracking your food, fitness, and health*, Chicago IL, 2016, Academy of Nutrition and Dietetics.

Academy of Nutrition and Dietetics: *CLICK: APP REVIEWS, food & nutrition*, 2018, Academy of Nutrition and Dietetics. On-going publication.

Academy of Nutrition and Dietetics, Crowe KM, Francis C: Position of the academy of nutrition and dietetics: functional foods, *J Acad Nutr Diet* 113:1096–1103, 2013a.

Academy of Nutrition and Dietetics, Slawson DL, Fitzgerald N, et al: Position of the academy of nutrition and dietetics: the role of nutrition in health promotion and chronic disease prevention, *J Acad Nutr Diet* 113:972–979, 2013b.

Academy of Nutrition and Dietetics, American Dietetic Association, Marra MV, Boyar AP: Position of the American Dietetic Association: nutrient supplementation, *J Am Diet Assoc* 109:2073–2085, 2009a.

Centers for Disease Control and Prevention: *Leading causes of death, United States*, 2016a. Available at: https://www.cdc.gov/nchs/fastats/leading-causes-of-death.htm.

Centers for Disease Control and Prevention: *Adult obesity facts*, 2016b. Available at: http://www.cdc.gov/obesity/data/adult.html.

Centers for Disease Control and Prevention: *Chronic disease prevention and health promotion*, 2018a. Available at: https://www.cdc.gov/chronicdisease/index.htm.

Centers for Disease Control and Prevention: *FastStats A to Z*, 2018b. Available at: http://www.cdc.gov/nchs/fastats/; https://www.cdc.gov/nchs/.

Centers for Disease Control and Prevention: *FastStats: life expectancy*, 2018c. Available at: https://www.cdc.gov/nchs/fastats/life-expectancy.htm.

Centers for Disease Control and Prevention: *Health, United States 2016*, 2017a Available at: http://www.cdc.gov/nchs/hus.htm.

Centers for Disease Control and Prevention: *Health-related quality of life (HRQOL)*, 2016b. Available at: http://www.cdc.gov/hrqol/.

Centers for Disease Control and Prevention: *Health-related quality of life (HRQOL): CDC's healthy days measures used in the America's health rankings*, 2016c. Available at: http://www.cdc.gov/hrqol/featured-items/healthy-days.htm.

Centers for Disease Control and Prevention: *Heart disease facts*, 2017b. Available at: http://www.cdc.gov/heartdisease/facts.htm.

Centers for Disease Control and Prevention: *Vital and health statistics series 10:259: summary health statistics for the U.S. population: national health interview survey, 2012*, 2013. Available at: http://www.cdc.gov/nchs/data/series/sr_10/sr10_259.pdf.

Feeding America: *The state of hunger in America*, 2019. Available at: https://www.feedingamerica.org/hunger-in-america.

Feeding America: *Supplemental nutrition assistance program (SNAP)*, 2018. Available at: http://feedingamerica.org/how-we-fight-hunger/programs-and-services/public-assistance-programs/supplemental-nutrition-assistance-program/snap-myths-realities.aspx.

Food and Drug Administration: *Label claims*, 2018c. Available at: https://www.fda.gov/food/labelingnutrition/ucm2006873.htm.

Harold JG, Jessup M: ACC/AHA special report: new ACC/AHA prevention guidelines: building a bridge to even stronger guideline collaborations, *Circulation* 128:2852–2853, 2013.

Health.Gov: *Scientific report of the 2015 dietary guidelines Advisory Committee*, 2018. Available at: http://www.health.gov/dietaryguidelines/2015-scientific-report.

Institute of Medicine: *Caffeine in food and dietary supplements: examining safety - workshop summary*, 2014. Available at: http://www.nationalacademies.org/hmd/Reports/2014/Caffeine-in-Food-and-Dietary-Supplements-Examining-Safety.aspx.

International Food Information Council: *Good food, good flavor, good health: blending the benefits of flavor and health through herbs and spices*, update 2018. Available at: https://foodinsight.org/good-food-good-flavor-good-health-blending-the-benefits-of-flavor-and-health-through-herbs-and-spices/.

International Food Information Council: *2018 IFIC foundation food and health survey*, Washington DC, 2018. Available at: https://www.foodinsight.org/2018.food-and-health-survey.

International Food Information Council: *2017 IFIC foundation food and health survey*, also 2013, 2015. Washington, DC, 2017. Available at: https://www.foodinsight.org/2017-food-and-health-survey.

Lichtenstein AH, American Heart Association Nutrition Committee, Appel LJ, et al: Diet and lifestyle recommendations revision 2006: a scientific statement from the American Heart Association Nutrition Committee, *Circulation* 114:82–96, 2006.

Lloyd-Jones DM, Hong Y, Labarthe D, et al: Defining and setting national goals for cardiovascular health promotion and disease reduction: the American Heart Association's strategic Impact Goal through 2020 and beyond, *Circulation* 121:586–613, 2010.

Maslow AH: *Motivation and personality*, ed 2, New York, NY, 1970, Harper.

McCullough M: *The bottom line on soy and breast cancer risk, American Cancer Society*, 2012. Available at: http://www.cancer.org/cancer/news/expertvoices/post/2012/08/02/the-bottom-line-on-soy-and-breast-cancer-risk.aspx.

Nagler RH: Adverse outcomes associated with media exposure to contradictory nutrition messages. *J Health Commun* 19:24–40, 2014.

National Institutes of Health, National Center for Complementary and Integrative Health: *Soy*, 2016. Available at: https://nccih.nih.gov/health/soy/ataglance.htm.

National Institutes of Health, National Center for Complementary and Integrative Health: 2018a. Available at: nccih.nih.gov/.

National Institutes of Health, National Diabetes Education Program: *NDEP Strategic Plan*, 2018b. Available at: www.niddk.nih.gov/health-information/communication-programs/ndep.

National Institutes of Health, National Heart, Lung, and Blood Institute: *Metabolic Syndrome*, 2018c. Available at: http://www.nhlbi.nih.gov/health/health-topics/topics/ms/.

National Institutes of Health, Medline: *Fat*, 2018c. Available at: https://medlineplus.gov/dietaryfats.html.

National Institutes of Health, Office of Dietary Supplements: *Nutrient recommendations: dietary reference intakes*, 2018d. Available at: https://ods.od.nih.gov/Health_Information/Dietary_Reference_Intakes.aspx.

National Institutes of Health, Office of Dietary Supplements: *Dietary supplements: what you need to know*, 2018f. Available at: http://ods.od.nih.gov/.

Newton KM, Reed SD, Uchiyama S, et al: A cross-sectional study of equol producer status and self-reported vasomotor symptoms, *Menopause* 2015;22(5):489–495.

Produce for Better Health: *State of the plate*. Available at: https://fruitsandveggies.org/.

Sloan AE: Top 10 functional food trends, *Food Technol* 68, 2012.

U.S. Department of Agriculture, Economic Research Service: *Food Price Outlook*, 2018a. Available at: http://www.ers.usda.gov/data-products/food-price-outlook/summary-findings.aspx.

U.S. Department of Agriculture, Economic Research Service: *Food security status of U.S. households in 2016*, 2016. Available at: http://www.ers.usda.gov/topics/food-nutrition-assistance/food-security-in-the-us/key-statistics-graphics.aspx#foodsecure.

U.S. Department of Agriculture, Economic Research Service: *Supplemental Nutrition Assistance Program (SNAP)*, 2018b. Available at: https://www.fns.usda.gov/snap/supplemental-nutrition-assistance-program-snap.

U.S. Department of Agriculture, National Agricultural Library: *Food labeling*, 2018c. Available at: https://www.nal.usda.gov/fnic/food-labeling.

U.S. Department of Health and Human Services: *Health care*, 2018b, HHS.gov. Available at: http://www.hhs.gov/healthcare/index.html.

U.S. Department of Health and Human Services: *Healthfinder.gov, 2018c. Available at:* http://www.healthfinder.gov.

Vistisen D, Witte DR, Tabák AG, et al: Patterns of obesity development before the diagnosis of type 2 diabetes: the Whitehall II cohort study, *PLOS Med* 11:e1001602, 2014.

Wellness Council of America: *The 7 benchmarks of success*, Omaha, NE, 2018. Available at: https://www.welcoa.org/.

World Health Organization: *10 Facts on obesity*, 2017. Available at: http://www.who.int/features/factfiles/obesity/en/index.html.

World Health Organization: *World health statistics report*, 2018. Available at: http://www.who.int/gho/publications/world_health_statistics/en/.

Wu HW, Sturm R: Changes in the energy and sodium content of main entrées in US Chain Restaurants from 2010 to 2011, *J Acad Nutr Diet* 114:209–219, 2014.

19

Nutrition in Aging

Janice L. Raymond, MS, RDN, CSG
Lindsey Callihan, MS, RDN, CSG

KEY TERMS

achlorhydria
activities of daily living (ADLs)
age-related macular degeneration (AMD)
Blue Zones
cataract
constipation
culture change in long-term care
Dining Practice Standards
dysgeusia
dysphagia
food first
functionality
geriatrics

gerontology
glaucoma
home- and community-based services
  (HCBS) waivers
hospice care
hyposmia
instrumental activities of daily living (IADLs)
long-term services and supports (LSS)
Mini Nutrition Assessment (MNA)
Minimum Data Set (MDS)
National Pressure Ulcer Advisory Panel
  (NPUAP)

palliative care
polypharmacy
pressure injury
presbyopia
quality of life
Resident Assessment Instrument (RAI)
sarcopenia
sarcopenic obesity
sedentary death syndrome (SeDS)
senescence
skilled nursing facility (SNF)
xerostomia

THE OLDER POPULATION

In 2017 there were an estimated 962 million people age 60 or older in the world. This is 13% of the global population. Europe has the greatest percentage population age 60 and older at 25%. The number of older persons worldwide is projected to be 1.4 billion in 2030 and could rise to 3.1 billion in 2100 (United Nations World Population Aging Report, 2017). Population aging, now a global phenomenon, is no longer limited to developed, higher-income countries.

Today, one in seven Americans is age 65 or older. They are living longer, healthier, and more functionally fit lives than ever before. Fig. 19.1 shows older adults involved in physical activities. Those born today can expect to live an average of 80 years. Women who reach age 65 can expect to live an additional 20.4 years, and men, 17.8 years. By the year 2050 the population older than age 65 will grow from approximately 44 million to 84 million, increasing from 14% to 21% of the population. The fastest-growing segment is those older than age 85, currently 6 million and increasing to 18 million in 2050. Members of minority groups also will increase from 21% to more than 39% of the older population (Colby and Ortman, 2014; Ortman et al, 2014) (Figs. 19.2 and 19.3).

The year 2030 marks an important demographic turning point in U.S. history according to the U.S. Census Bureau's 2017 National Population Projections. By 2030, all baby boomers will be older than age 65. This will expand the size of the older population so that one in every five residents will be retirement age.

A few years ago no state had more people older than age 65 than those younger than 18. Growth in the older-than-65 population will equal 3.5 times the U.S. growth as a whole. This demographic shift has enormous social, economic, and political implications (Ortman et al, 2014).

Women live longer than men. The older-than-65 female/male ratio is 129:100; it increases to 200:100 among those older than age 85. More than 71% of older men are married, whereas only 45% of older women are married (Ortman et al, 2014). Almost half (45%) of women over age 75 live alone; thus more men die married and most women die unmarried.

Classification

Everyone knows people older than themselves, but those considered "old" depends a lot on one's own age. Today gray hair color, wrinkles, retirement, or age 65 no longer defines old. Yet qualifying as an "older adult" is based on the minimum eligibility age of 65 in many federal programs. The U.S. Census Bureau uses a stratified system to define this generation-spanning age group; those aged 65 to 74 are the young old; 75 to 84, old; and 85 or older, oldest old. Some consider today's new old to be those in their 90s. The more than 100,000 centenarians alive today are no longer considered unique, and many of them still live independently (see *Focus On:* Centenarians . . . Life in the Blue Zone).

Portions of this chapter written by Nancy S. Wellman, PhD, RDN, FAND, and Barbara J. Kamp, MS, RDN.

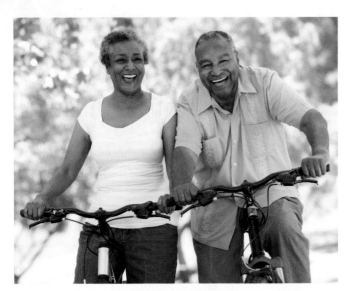

Fig. 19.1 Active older adults.

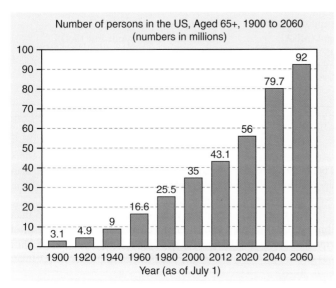

Fig. 19.2 Population ages 65 and older: 1900 to 2060.

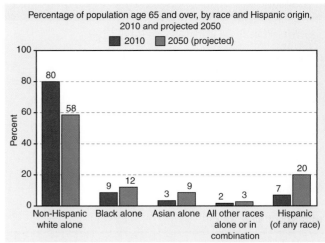

Fig. 19.3 Population age 65 and over, by race and Hispanic origin, 2010 and projected 2050. Note: The term non-Hispanic white alone is used to refer to people who reported being white and no other race and who are not Hispanic. The term black alone is used to refer to people who reported being black or African American and no other race, and the term Asian alone is used to refer to people who reported only Asian as their race. The use of single-race populations in this chart does not imply that this is the preferred method of presenting or analyzing data. The U.S. Census Bureau uses a variety of approaches. The race group "All other races alone or in combination" includes American Indian and Alaska Native alone; Native Hawaiian and other Pacific Islander alone; and all people who reported two or more races. Reference population: These data refer to the resident population. (U.S. Census Bureau: 2010 Census Summary File 1; Table 4. http://www.census.gov/prod/cen2010/doc/sf1.pdf, 2011.)

GERONTOLOGY, GERIATRICS, AND THE SPECTRUM OF AGING

Gerontology is the study of normal aging, including factors in biology, psychology, and sociology. Geriatrics is the study of the chronic diseases frequently associated with aging, including diagnosis and treatment. Although medical nutrition therapy commonly has been practiced in hospitals and long-term care facilities, nutrition services have moved out of hospitals and into homes and communities where the focus is on health promotion, risk reduction, and disease prevention.

NUTRITION IN HEALTH PROMOTION AND DISEASE PREVENTION

In aging adults, nutrition care is not limited to disease management or medical nutrition therapy but has broadened to have a stronger focus on healthy lifestyles and disease prevention. Without increased emphasis on better diets and more physical activity at all ages, health care expenditures will rise exorbitantly as the population ages. It is never too late to emphasize nutrition for health promotion and disease prevention. Older Americans, more than any other age group, want health and nutrition information and are willing to make changes to maintain their independence and quality of life. They often need help in improving self-care behaviors and they want to know how to eat healthier, exercise safely, and stay motivated.

Nutrition may include three types of preventive services. In primary prevention, the emphasis is on nutrition in health promotion and disease prevention. Pairing healthy eating with physical activity is equally important.

Secondary prevention involves risk reduction and slowing the progression of chronic nutrition-related diseases to maintain functionality and quality of life. Functionality as related to strength and mobility is perceived as a positive way to discuss fitness versus disability and dependence.

In tertiary prevention, care/case management and discharge planning often involve chewing and appetite problems, modified diets, and functional limitations. Complex cases often are influenced by nutrition issues that must be addressed; care managers can benefit from consulting with dietitians. In some circumstances dietitians are the case managers.

THEORIES ON AGING

Gerontologists study aging and have diverse theories about why the body ages. No single theory can fully explain the complex processes of aging (Park and Festini, 2017). A good theory integrates knowledge

FOCUS ON

Centenarians . . . Life in the Blue Zone

Centenarians are a growing segment of older adults in the United States and in other developed nations, including Japan. The worldwide estimate of centenarians is 450,000. The U.S. Census Bureau estimated for 2009 there were about 65,000 centenarians and that there will be more than 1 million by 2050. As with the aging population as a whole, women represent 85% of the long lived. A new group of individuals older than age 110, supercentenarians, have sufficient numbers to merit dedicated research.

What is known about extremely long-lived individuals? Centenarians generally have delays in functional decline. They also tend to either never develop a chronic disease or develop one late in life. Much has been written about longevity in the southern Japanese of Okinawa. The ongoing Okinawa Centenarian Study suggests that low caloric intake may produce fewer destructive free radicals. This intake plus an active lifestyle, natural ability to combat the stresses of life, and a genetic predisposition favor a healthy, functional, longer life.

The National Institute on Aging has identified communities around the world where people are living longer and living measurably better. They called these areas, where people reach the age of 100 at rates 10 times greater than in the United States, the Blue Zones. One such community is Okinawa. Others include the Nicoya Peninsula in Costa Rica, Ikaria in Greece, and Sardinia in Italy. Only one Blue Zone exists in the United States, the Loma Linda community in California. Residents of Loma Linda boast the longest life spans in America, living on average a decade longer than other Americans. These Blue Zone groups have been found to have common characteristics related to food: very little animal protein and four to six servings of fruits, vegetables, legumes, and nuts. However, eating wisely is only part of what seems to be a prescription for long life. The people of these communities don't smoke and make regular low-intensity exercise part of their daily routine (e.g., gardening, walking). They are people who can articulate their purpose in life, are spiritually fulfilled, and have strong social networks.

In the New England Centenarian Study, independent function to at least age 90 was identified as a predominant feature of those who live to 100 or more. Other important factors are that few centenarians are obese, they rarely smoke, and while alcohol is part of the traditional diet in all but the Loma Linda group, it is consumed in moderation or not at all. At least 50% of centenarians have first-degree relatives or grandparents who also achieved very old age, and many have exceptionally old siblings (Buettner and Skemp, 2016).

TABLE 19.1 Predetermination and Accumulated Damage Theories on Aging

Theory	Description
Predetermination: Built-in mechanism determines when aging begins and time of death	
Pacemaker theory	"Biologic clock" is set at birth, runs for a specified time, winds down with aging, and ends at death.
Genetic theory	Life span is determined by heredity.
Rate of living theory	Each living creature has a finite amount of a "vital substance," and, when it is exhausted, the result is aging and death.
Oxygen metabolism theory	Animals with the highest metabolisms are likely to have the shortest life spans.
Immune system theory	Cells undergo a finite number of cell divisions that eventually cause deregulation of immune function, excessive inflammation, aging, and death.
Accumulated damage: Systemic breakdown over time	
Crosslink/glycosylation theory	With time, proteins, DNA and other structural molecules in the body make inappropriate attachments, or crosslinks, to each other, leading to decreased mobility, elasticity, and cell permeability.
Wear-and-tear theory	Years of damage to cells, tissues, and organs eventually take their toll, wearing them out and ultimately causing death.
Free radical theory	Accumulated, random damage caused by oxygen radicals slowly causes cells, tissues, and organs to stop functioning.
Somatic mutation theory	Genetic mutations caused by oxidizing radiation and other factors accumulate with age, causing cells to deteriorate and malfunction.
Telomere length	Telomeres protect and cap linear chromosome ends. Short telomeres have been associated with many age-related conditions.

DNA; Deoxyribonucleic acid.

and tells how and why phenomena are related. Broadly, theories can be grouped into two categories: predetermined (genetic) and accumulated damage. A loss of efficiency comes about as some cells wear out, die, or are not replaced. Identification of the mechanisms that affect aging could lead to interventions that slow or alter aging. Most likely several theories explain the heterogeneity in older populations (Table 19.1).

PHYSIOLOGIC CHANGES

Aging is a normal biologic process. However, it involves some decline in physiologic function. Organs change with age. The rates of change differ among individuals and within organ systems. It is important to distinguish between normal changes of aging and changes caused by chronic diseases like heart disease, diabetes, and arthritis.

The human growth period draws to a close at about age 30, when senescence begins. Senescence is the organic process of growing older and displaying the effects of increased age. Disease and impaired function are not inevitable parts of aging. Nevertheless, certain systemic changes occur as part of growing older. These changes result in varying degrees of efficiency and functional decline. Factors such as genetics, illnesses, socioeconomics, and lifestyle determine how aging progresses for each person. Indeed, one's outward expression of age may or may not reflect one's chronologic age, and ageist stereotypes should be eliminated. The oldest woman to have finished a marathon was Gladys Burrill in 2012 who was 93—and she didn't start running marathons until her mid-80s. Jaring Timmerman began competitive swimming at 79 and broke records in 2014 at age 104.

Body Composition

Body composition changes with aging. Fat mass, visceral fat, and intermuscular fat increase, whereas lean muscle mass decreases (Santanasto et al, 2017). Sarcopenia is defined as age-related loss of skeletal muscle function and muscle mass. It is known to increase risk for falls and decrease quality of life. International clinical guidelines on the diagnosis and management of sarcopenia were recently published

(Dent et al, 2018). Included is a measurement tool that would standardize diagnosis of sarcopenia, something that has thus far not been agreed on. Also included is a recommendation for rapid screening using gait speed. Treatment recommendations for sarcopenia include the prescription of resistance-based physical activity, and a conditional recommendation for protein supplementation/a protein-rich diet. The proposed term "skeletal muscle function deficit" best describes the variety of muscular conditions that contribute to clinically meaningful mobility impairment (Correa-de-Araujo and Hadley, 2014). All losses are important because of the close connection between muscle mass and strength. By the fourth decade of life, evidence of sarcopenia is detectable, and the process accelerates after approximately age 75. Prevention strategies deserve emphasis because of the strong relationships of sarcopenia to functional decline, disability, hospitalization, institutionalization, and mortality (Litchford, 2014).

Sarcopenic obesity is the loss of lean muscle mass in older persons with excess adipose tissue. Together the excess weight and decreased muscle mass exponentially compound to further decrease physical activity, which in turn accelerates sarcopenia. An extremely sedentary lifestyle in obese persons is a major detractor from quality of life.

Sedentary lifestyle choices can lead to **sedentary death syndrome (SeDS)**, a phrase coined by the President's Council on Sports, Fitness, and Nutrition. It describes the life-threatening health problems caused by a sedentary lifestyle. Sedentary lifestyle can be defined as a level of inactivity below the threshold of the beneficial health effects of regular physical activity or, more simply, burning fewer than 200 calories in physical activity per day.

Although no amount of physical activity can stop the biological aging process, there is evidence that exercise can minimize the physiologic effects of a sedentary lifestyle and increase the time a person remains active by limiting the development and progression of chronic disease. There is emerging evidence that suggests both psychological and cognitive benefits from regular exercise in older adults. According to the American College of Sports Medicine, the exercise prescription for older adults should include aerobic exercise, muscle strengthening exercise, and flexibility exercise. The Centers for Disease Control and Prevention (CDC) quantifies the amount of exercise older adults need and the National Institute on Aging (NIA) has a guide for physical activity (CDC, 2013; NIA, 2010).

A summary of the World Health Organization (WHO) recommendations for exercise for people age 65 years and older (Taylor, 2014) are as follows:

1. At least 150 min of moderate-intensity aerobic activity per week, or at least 75 min of vigorous-intensity aerobic activity or an equivalent combination.
2. Aerobic activity should be performed in bouts of at least 10 min duration.
3. For additional health benefits, undertake up to 300 min of moderate-intensity or 150 min of vigorous-intensity aerobic activity or an equivalent combination per week.
4. People with poor mobility should do balance exercises to prevent falls on 3 or more days.
5. Muscle-strengthening activities should be done on 2 or more days.
6. If older adults are unable to do the recommended amounts of physical activity due to health conditions, they should be as physically active as they are able.

Taste and Smell

Sensory losses affect people to varying degrees, at varying rates, and at different ages. Genetics, environment, and lifestyle are part of the decline in sensory competence. Age-related alterations to the sense of taste, smell, and touch can lead to poor appetite, limited food choices, and lower nutrient intake. Some **dysgeusia** (altered taste),

loss of taste, or **hyposmia** (decreased sense of smell) are attributable to aging. Thinning of epithelium and decline in the regeneration of olfactory receptor cells leads to dysfunction (Schiffman, 2009). Medications may play as big a role as aging in this population. Other causes include conditions such as Bell's palsy, head injury, diabetes, liver or kidney disease, hypertension, neurologic conditions including Alzheimer's disease and Parkinson's disease, and zinc or niacin deficiency. Untreated mouth sores, tooth decay, poor dental or nasal hygiene, and cigarette smoking also can decrease these senses.

Because taste and smell sensation thresholds are higher, older adults may be tempted to overseason foods, especially to add more salt, which may have a negative effect in many older adults. Because taste and smell stimulate metabolic changes such as salivary, gastric acid, and pancreatic secretions and increases in plasma levels of insulin, decreased sensory stimulation may impair these metabolic processes as well.

Hearing and Eyesight

While hearing loss is not the only condition that impedes a caregiver's ability to communicate with their patients, there is no question that the communication barriers it imposes are among the most impactful. For millions of older Americans, many of whom are among the oldest-old, hearing loss strips away the opportunity for clinicians and caregivers to share information simply by speaking. As hearing worsens, the exchange and flow of information slows to a trickle, and conversation and discussion simply stop. The consequences are known to be broadly negative for patients and caregivers alike.

The WHO (March 2018) has estimated that 360 million people worldwide have hearing loss that is moderate or higher in severity (what the WHO refers to as "disabling" hearing loss). In the United States, an estimated 40 million people (Lin et al, 2011) have bilateral hearing loss that is severe enough to constantly inhibit conversation. Hearing loss is exceedingly more prevalent among the elderly. There is widespread consensus the prevalence will increase as the population ages. The most common cause is the aging process. So-called age-related loss affects both ears equally, increases in severity over time, and is not preventable. Other causes include loud noise (noise-induced hearing loss), drug-induced loss (there are a number of ototoxic medications), hearing loss that has hereditary roots, and loss that is disease and illness-related (National Institute on Deafness and Other Communicative Disorders, National Institutes of Health, 2013a).

Levels of severity. Hearing loss is typically defined using one of four levels of severity. Individuals with mild loss have difficulty hearing normal conversation, especially in environments with background noise. As the hearing loss progresses to the moderate level, speech-sounds are increasingly difficult to hear with any clarity. In the absence of hearing aids, words have to be spoken in a raised voice at a close distance to be heard. For those with severe hearing loss, speech becomes largely unintelligible and even the most sophisticated hearing aids grow ineffective. Those who have profound loss are functionally deaf and rely mainly on sign language and lip reading to converse with others. As a condition that typically worsens with age, the higher levels of loss are more prevalent among those who have reached their 70s or 80s.

Impact. There is substantial evidence that higher levels of hearing loss have a broadly detrimental impact on the individual's physical and cognitive functioning, psychological health, self-esteem, and overall satisfaction with their quality of life. Recent research has shown an association between hearing loss and a decline in both cognitive and physical functioning. A study at Johns Hopkins University (Chien and Lin, 2012) found that older adults with hearing loss experience a rate of decline in thinking and in memory that is 30% to 40% faster than among those with normal hearing. Other studies have shown that hearing loss is associated with dementia, physical decline, and an increased frequency of falls. Studies reporting on the alienating effects of hearing loss have found that it is a source of loneliness, isolation, depression, anxiety, and paranoia, and that it leads to marked decrease in satisfaction with family life. Hearing loss causes the individual to feel embarrassed, upset, lonely, and withdrawn; and they may appear confused, uncaring, and difficult. Studies have shown that hearing loss causes feelings of dependence, frustration, and guilt, that it induces behaviors that include bluffing and being demanding, and that it often results in decreased self-esteem (Ciorba, 2012).

Hearing loss by gender. Researchers at Johns Hopkins have reported that the prevalence of hearing loss is significantly higher among males. However, while the prevalence among males is especially pronounced in the younger age groups, it diminishes as age increases. In all, males account for 70% of those with hearing loss between the ages of 30 and 69, but only 51% among those in their 70s, and only 38% among those over the age of 80.

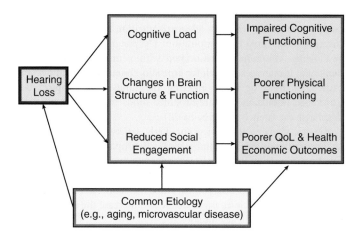

Treatment. Apart from surgical implants in the most severe cases, hearing aids are the only form of treatment. But while the technology has advanced significantly in recent years, adoption and use remains extremely low.

Box 19.1 illustrates how speech is distorted by hearing loss, in this case the loss that occurs (and worsens) as we age (Presbycusis).

BOX 19.1 Missing Sounds by Hearing Loss Severity

Level of Hearing Loss	Spoken Sentence	Missing Sounds
Normal Hearing	I am your dietitian and I will be helping you manage your congestive heart failure with small, manageable dietary changes.	
Mild	I am your dietitian and I will be helping you manage your conge tive heart ailure wi mall, manageable dietary change	K, f, s, th
Moderate	I am your dietitian and I will be el ing you mana e your con e tive eart ailure wi mall, mana eable dietary ane	Above plus ch, p, h, g, sh
Severe	m y u d e t t n n d w e e n y u m n e y u c n e t ve e t u e w m, m n e e d e t y ne	Above plus i, o, a, r, b, l, v

Hearing loss can be difficult to spot. It is easy to imagine that a patient's hearing loss is easy to identify and detect. As it turns out, that is often not the case. It is not uncommon, for instance, for patients to hide their hearing loss by engaging in a number of "bluffing" behaviors that can give caregivers a false sense of having communicated effectively.

If a patient has hearing loss, the caregiver's "speaking behaviors" can help. When working with an elderly patient population, the chances are very high of encountering patients with varying levels of hearing loss. One of the findings of the National Council on Disability was that most clinicians and caregivers do not have a practical understanding of how to communicate effectively with patients who have hearing loss, and they often do not appreciate the medical necessity of employing appropriate methods of communication to ensure the effectiveness of their care.

In all cases, it is important to keep in mind that correct speaking behaviors should be employed regardless of whether the patient is using a hearing aid or an assistive listening device.

KEY SPEAKING BEHAVIORS

- Stand in front of the patient and as near to them as possible.
- Make sure the patient can see your mouth as you talk.
- Speak clearly, slowly, and "mouth" your words more than you would with patients who have normal hearing.
- Speak up and ask the patient if a different volume level would be helpful (in some cases talking louder not only doesn't help, but can make matters worse).
- Look directly at the patient (don't look down, at a computer screen, etc.).
- Choose your words more carefully (esoteric words will be harder for the patient to understand).
- Be patient—you may be asked to repeat yourself (you may be asked to do so repeatedly).

While it is tempting to yell to be heard, it is usually not a good idea. Yelling can be irritating and raises concerns about patient privacy and often does not make speech any easier to understand. If speech sounds garbled, yelling only makes the garbled speech louder, not clearer.

For some patients, the only recourse will be to write messages down for them to read. Whiteboards are used most often and although this is a cumbersome process requiring patience, it is often the only solution.

Age-related macular degeneration (AMD) is a disease of the retina that affects central vision and can lead to blindness in older people. AMD is the leading cause of legal blindness in Americans age 65 and older. It affects more than 1.75 million individuals in the United States. It is expected to increase to more than 5 million by 2050 (American Optometric Association [AOA], 2014). Smoking, race (it is more common in Caucasians), and family history are known risk factors (Chew et al, 2014; National Eye Institute, 2014). As the population ages, AMD is becoming a more significant public health problem. AMD occurs when the macula, the center part of the retina, degrades. The result is central vision loss. The macular pigment is composed of two chemicals, lutein and zeaxanthin. A diet rich in fruits and vegetables may help delay or prevent the development of AMD. Micronutrition supplementation often is used in the treatment of AMD (Aslam et al, 2014; Korobelnik, 2017).

Presbyopia is a loss of elasticity in the crystalline lens that causes an inability to focus clearly at close distances and results in the need for reading glasses. This becomes apparent around the fourth decade of life (AOA, 2014). As it worsens, poor vision interferes with shopping, cooking, and eating.

Glaucoma is damage to the optic nerve resulting from high pressure in the eye. It is the second most common cause of vision loss, affecting approximately 3 million Americans. Hypertension, diabetes, and cardiovascular disease (CVD) increase the risk of glaucoma.

A cataract is a clouding of the lens of the eye. Approximately half of Americans 65 and older have some degree of clouding of the lens. The most common treatment is surgery; the clouded lens is removed and replaced with a permanent prosthetic lens. A diet high in beta carotene, selenium, lutein, omega-3 fat, and vitamins C and E may delay cataract development (AOA, 2014). Studies show that a high sodium intake may increase risk of cataract development. Ultraviolet (UV) radiation exposure is related directly to 5% of worldwide cataracts. When the UV index is 3 and above, protective sunglasses are recommended.

Immunocompetence

Age-related alterations in the immune system include both cellular and serologic changes that cause dysfunction in the response to foreign and self-antigens. Immune response is slower and less efficient. The mechanisms of age-related changes in immune function are not fully understood but likely depend on genetics, environmental factors, and lifestyle choices (Keenan, 2018). Maintaining good nutritional status promotes good immune function.

Oral

Diet and nutrition can be compromised by poor oral health (see Chapter 24). Tooth loss, use of dentures, and xerostomia (dry mouth) can lead to difficulties in chewing and swallowing. Decreases in taste sensation and saliva production make eating less pleasurable and more difficult. Oral diseases and conditions are common among people who grew up without the benefit of community water fluoridation and other fluoride products. However, the percentage of Americans age 65 and older who are missing all of their natural teeth (edentulous) is falling. Missing, loose, or decayed teeth or poor-fitting, painful dentures are common problems that make it difficult to eat some foods. People with these mouth problems often prefer soft, easily chewed foods and avoid some nutritionally dense options such as whole grains, fresh fruits and vegetables, and meats.

The nutrition-related consequences of polypharmacy, taking five or more medications or over-the-counter drugs daily, are significant. More than 400 commonly used medications can cause dry mouth. Preparing foods that are moisture-rich such as hearty soups and stews, adding sauces, and pureeing and chopping foods can make meals easier to eat. In addition, those with poor oral health may benefit from fortified foods with increased nutrient density (see *Focus On: Food First!*).

Gastrointestinal

Some gastrointestinal (GI) changes are considered to be normal consequences of aging though some changes can be attributed to other clinical causes and should be evaluated (Box 19.2). GI changes can negatively affect a person's nutrient intake, starting in the mouth. As a normal consequence of aging, taste and smell changes occur in the older adult including decreased ability to taste salt, bitter, sweet, and sour. Additionally, changes in salivation due to natural aging or medication side effects can further alter taste sensations and cause challenges for older adults.

Age- and disease-related changes in swallow function, including reduction of oral and esophageal muscle mass and connective tissue elasticity, can cause delay in the swallow processes of older adults. Increased oropharyngeal phase of swallowing (see Chapter 39),

---

BOX 19.2 Gastrointestinal (GI) Changes with Aging

Head: Decreased velocity of neuronal conduction to GI tract, decreased hunger sensations

Nose/Mouth: Decreased taste, smell, changes in dentition, decreased saliva

Neck: Increased oropharyngeal phase, delayed opening of esophageal sphincter, decreased peristaltic pressure in esophagus

Stomach: Increased and more rapid satiety, reduced peristalsis and gastric contractile force increase in gastric pH

Intestines: Decreased absorption of carbohydrate, protein, triglyceride, folate, B_{12}, D, calcium; increased absorption of vitamins A and C, cholesterol

Lower intestines: Decreased rectal wall elasticity, decreased colonic motility, constipation

---

delayed opening of the esophageal sphincter, and decreased peristaltic pressure in the esophagus can all contribute to challenges in functional swallow, which may threaten adequate nutrition and make one more susceptible to choking or aspiration. Dysphagia, a dysfunction in swallowing, commonly is associated with neurologic diseases and dementia. It increases the risk for aspiration pneumonia, an infection caused by food or fluids entering the lungs (see Chapter 33). Thickened liquids and texture-modified foods can help people with dysphagia eat safely (see Appendix 20).

Gastric changes also can occur. Early satiety due to age-related changes in the stomach in combination with impaired gastric mucosal function leads to an inability to resist damage and can result in ulcers, cancer, and infections. Gastritis causes inflammation and pain, delayed gastric emptying, and discomfort. These affect the bioavailability of nutrients such as calcium, B_{12}, and zinc and increase the risk of developing a chronic deficiency disease.

Achlorhydria is the insufficient production of stomach acid. Sufficient stomach acid and intrinsic factor are required for the absorption of vitamin B_{12}. Although substantial amounts are stored in the liver, B_{12} deficiency does occur. Symptoms can often be misdiagnosed because they mimic Alzheimer's disease or other chronic conditions and include extreme fatigue, dementia, confusion, and tingling and weakness in the arms and legs (see Chapter 39). It has become common practice to use calcium carbonate antacids as a way to supplement calcium intake, though this is contraindicated in the elderly who are already at risk for inadequate gastric acid.

Constipation is defined as having fewer bowel movements than usual, having difficulty or excessive straining at stool, painful bowel movements, hard stool, or incomplete emptying of the bowel. It is one of the most common disorders in the U.S. population, and its prevalence increases with age. Primary causes include insufficient fluids, lack of physical activity, and low intake of dietary fiber. Studies have also shown that distinct physiologic changes affecting colonic motility occur in older people. They include myenteric dysfunction, increased collagen deposits in the left colon, reduced inhibitory nerve input to the colon's muscle layer, and increased binding of plasma endorphins to intestinal receptors (see Chapter 27).

Diminished anal sphincter pressure or degeneration of the internal anal sphincter and loss of rectal wall elasticity are age-related changes. Constipation also is caused by some medications commonly used in older people such as narcotics and antidepressants that actually slow intestinal transit. Diuretics can cause decreased stool moisture, another contributing factor in constipation.

The incidence of diverticulosis increases with age. Half of the population older than age 60 develop it, but only 20% of them have clinical manifestations. The most common problems with diverticular disease are lower abdominal pain and diarrhea (see Chapter 27).

Each of these changes in the GI could have substantial impact on the overall nutrition of the older adult as limitations in ability to consume adequate food quantity coupled with decreased nutrient absorption can result in undernutrition.

Cardiovascular

CVD, including heart disease and stroke, is the leading cause of death in all genders in all racial and ethnic groups and is not necessarily a disease of aging. CVD age-related changes are extremely variable and are affected by environmental influences such as smoking, exercise, and diet. Changes can include decreased arterial wall compliance, decreased maximum heart rate, decreased responsiveness to beta-adrenergic stimuli, increased left ventricle muscle mass, and slowed ventricular relaxation. Often the end result of hypertension and artery disease is chronic heart failure. One in nine hospital admissions in the United States include the diagnosis of heart failure. A low-sodium diet and fluid restriction are commonly prescribed for this condition. These diet restrictions in conjunction with other side effects of heart failure often lead to decreased nutrient consumption. See Chapter 32 for discussion of the multifaceted approach required to manage CVD in older adults.

Renal

Age-related changes in renal function vary tremendously. Some older adults experience little change, whereas others can have devastating, life-threatening change. On average glomerular filtration rate, measured in creatinine clearance rates, declines by approximately 8 to 10 mL/min/1.73m^2 per decade after age 30 to 35. The resulting increase in serum creatinine concentrations should be considered when determining medication dosages. The progressive decline in renal function can lead to an inability to excrete concentrated or dilute urine, a delayed response to sodium deprivation or a sodium load, and delayed response to an acid load. Renal function is also affected by dehydration, diuretic use, and medications, especially antibiotics (see Chapter 34).

Neurologic

There can be significant age-related declines in neurologic processes. Cognition, steadiness, reaction time, coordination, gait, sensations, and **activities of daily living (ADLs)** (toileting, bathing, eating, dressing) often decline with age, but the velocity of the decline varies greatly from one individual to another and is dependent on disease as much as on aging. On average, the brain loses 5% to 10% of its weight between the ages of 20 and 90, but most, if not all, neurons are functional until death unless a specific pathologic condition is present (Galvin and Sadowsky, 2012).

It is important to make the distinction between normal, age-related decline and impairment from conditions such as dementia, a disease process (Galvin and Sadowsky, 2012). Memory difficulties do not necessarily indicate dementia, Alzheimer's disease, Parkinson's disease, or any mental disorder (see Chapters 39 and 40). Many changes in memory can be attributed to environmental factors, including stress, chemical exposure, and inadequate food and fluid, rather than to physiologic processes. Urinary tract infections are associated with changes in cognition that mimic dementia but are reversible with treatment (Beveridge et al, 2011). However, even mild cognitive impairment may affect eating, chewing, and swallowing, thus increasing the risk of malnutrition (Lopes da Silva et al, 2014). The greatest risk factor for developing dementia is in fact advanced age.

Pressure Injuries

Pressure injuries, formerly called pressure sores and before that, bedsores or decubitus ulcers, develop from continuous pressure that impedes capillary blood flow to skin and underlying tissue. Several factors contribute to the formation of pressure injuries, but impaired mobility, poor circulation, obesity, and urinary incontinence are key.

Older adults with neurologic problems, those heavily sedated, and those with dementia are often unable to shift positions to alleviate pressure. Paralysis, incontinence, sensory losses, and rigidity can contribute to the problem. Notably malnutrition and undernutrition (inadequate energy intake) set the stage for its development and can delay wound healing. The escalating chronic nature of pressure injury in nonambulatory or sedentary individuals requires vigilant attention to nutrition.

The National Pressure Injury Advisory Panel (NPIAP), formerly National Pressure Ulcer Advisory Panel (NPUAP), is an independent not-for-profit professional organization dedicated to the prevention and management of pressure injuries. The NPIAP Board of Directors is composed of leading multidisciplinary experts who share a commitment to the prevention and management of pressure injuries.

The mission of the National Pressure Injury Advisory Panel (NPIAP) is to provide interprofessional leadership to improve patient outcomes in pressure injury prevention and management through education, public policy and research. NPIAP provides vital publications for medical, nursing and nutrition professionals working in all healthcare settings.

The 2019 *International Clinical Practice Guideline for the Prevention and Treatment of Pressure Injuries (CPG)* presents recommendations and summarizes the supporting evidence for pressure injury prevention and treatment. The new edition was developed as a four-year collaboration between the National Pressure Injury Advisory Panel (NPIAP), the European Pressure Ulcer Advisory Panel (EPUAP) and the Pan Pacific Pressure Injury Alliance (PPPIA). It provides a detailed analysis and discussion of available research, critical evaluation of the assumptions and knowledge in the field, recommendations for clinical practice, important implementation considerations, a description of the methodology used to develop the guideline, and acknowledgment of the many experts formally involved in the development process. The guideline may be purchased at www.guidelinesales.com.

Several classification systems describe pressure injuries. The six stages of injury, based on the depth of the sore and level of tissue involvement, are described in Table 19.2. As wound nutrition tends to equal whole-body nutrition, coordinated efforts of a multidisciplinary treatment team are important. The benefits of specific levels of energy (30-35 kcal/kg) and protein (1.25-1.5 g/kg) for prevention of pressure injuries in patients at risk of malnutrition recommended in the previous guidelines are now considered inconclusive. The 2019 guidelines focus on individualized assessment by the RDN rather than standardized prescriptions. However the recommendation above for calories and protein remain for individuals with existing pressure injuries. Additionally, a high calorie, high protein supplement is recommended for those with a pressure injury who are malnourished and unable to meet their needs through diet alone. Recommendations for a protein supplement high in arginine, zinc and antioxidants was included for stage II, III and IV pressure injuries (European Pressure Ulcer Advisory Panel, National Pressure Injury Advisory Panel and Pan Pacific Pressure Injury Alliance, 2019).

QUALITY OF LIFE

Quality of life is a general sense of happiness and satisfaction with one's life and environment. Health-related quality of life is the personal sense of physical and mental health and the ability to react to factors in the physical and social environments. To assess health-related quality of life, common measures and scales, either general or disease-specific, can be used. Because older age often is associated with health problems and decrease in functionality, quality-of-life issues become relevant.

Depression

Psychological changes often manifest as depression, and its extent can vary widely from person to person. Among older persons depression

TABLE 19.2 Pressure Injury Stages

Deep Tissue Injury

Deep Tissue Pressure Injury: Persistent nonblanchable deep red, maroon, or purple discoloration

Intact or nonintact skin with localized area of persistent nonblanchable deep red, maroon, or purple discoloration or epidermal separation revealing a dark wound bed or blood-filled blister. Pain and temperature change often precede skin color changes. Discoloration may appear differently in darkly pigmented skin. This injury results from intense and/or prolonged pressure and shear forces at the bone-muscle interface. The wound may evolve rapidly to reveal the actual extent of tissue injury or may resolve without tissue loss. If necrotic tissue, subcutaneous tissue, granulation tissue, fascia, muscle, or other underlying structures are visible, this indicates a full thickness pressure injury (unstageable, stage 3 or stage 4). Do not use Deep Tissue Pressure Injury (DTPI) to describe vascular, traumatic, neuropathic, or dermatologic conditions.

Stage 1

Stage 1 Pressure Injury: Nonblanchable erythema of intact skin

Intact skin with a localized area of nonblanchable erythema, which may appear differently in darkly pigmented skin. Presence of blanchable erythema or changes in sensation, temperature, or firmness may precede visual changes. Color changes do not include purple or maroon discoloration; these may indicate deep tissue pressure injury, heralding sign of risk.

Stage 2

Stage 2 Pressure Injury: Partial-thickness skin loss with exposed dermis

Partial-thickness loss of skin with exposed dermis. The wound bed is viable, pink or red, moist, and may also present as an intact or ruptured serum-filled blister. Adipose (fat) is not visible and deeper tissues are not visible. Granulation tissue, slough, and eschar are not present. These injuries commonly result from adverse microclimate and shear in the skin over the pelvis and shear in the heel. This stage should not be used to describe moisture associated skin damage (MASD) including incontinence associated dermatitis (IAD), intertriginous dermatitis (ITD), medical adhesive related skin injury (MARSI), or traumatic wounds (skin tears, burns, abrasions).

Stage 3

Stage 3 Pressure Injury: Full-thickness skin loss

Full-thickness loss of skin, in which adipose (fat) is visible in the ulcer and granulation tissue and epibole (rolled wound edges) are often present. Slough and/or eschar may be visible. The depth of tissue damage varies by anatomic location; areas of significant adiposity can develop deep wounds. Undermining and tunneling may occur. Fascia, muscle, tendon, ligament, cartilage, and/or bone are not exposed. If slough or eschar obscures the extent of tissue loss, this is an unstageable pressure injury.

Stage 4

Stage 4 Pressure Injury: Full-thickness skin and tissue loss

Full-thickness skin and tissue loss with exposed or directly palpable fascia, muscle, tendon, ligament, cartilage, or bone in the ulcer. Slough and/or eschar may be visible. Epibole (rolled edges), undermining, and/or tunneling often occur. Depth varies by anatomic location. If slough or eschar obscures the extent of tissue loss this is an unstageable pressure injury.

Unstageable

Unstageable Pressure Injury: Obscured full-thickness skin and tissue loss

Full-thickness skin and tissue loss in which the extent of tissue damage within the ulcer cannot be confirmed because it is obscured by slough or eschar. If slough or eschar is removed, a stage 3 or stage 4 pressure injury will be revealed. Stable eschar (i.e., dry, adherent, intact without erythema, or fluctuance) on the heel or ischemic limb should not be softened or removed.

National Pressure Ulcer Advisory Panel (NPUAP) announces a change in terminology from pressure ulcer to pressure injury and updates the stages of pressure injury. April 2016.

often is caused by other conditions such as heart disease, stroke, diabetes, cancer, grief, or stress. Depression in older people frequently is undiagnosed or misdiagnosed because symptoms are confused with other medical illnesses. Untreated depression can have serious side effects for older adults. It diminishes the pleasures of living, including eating; it can exacerbate other medical conditions; and it can compromise immune function. Depression is associated with decreased appetite, weight loss, and fatigue. Nutritional care plays an important role in addressing this condition (see Chapter 40). Providing nutrient- and calorie-dense foods, additional beverages, texture-modified foods, and favorite foods at times when people are most likely to eat the greatest quantity can be very effective. In that comorbidities lead to polypharmacy and concern regarding drug-drug interactions, providers may choose to omit antidepressants, which leaves the depression untreated.

Given the untoward consequences of unintentional weight loss with aging and the lack of Food and Drug Administration–approved medications for appetite stimulation in older adults, food and nutritional interventions along with the treatment of underlying conditions that contribute to weight loss, such as poor dentition, deserve greater attention. One antidepressant, mirtazapine (Remeron), has helped increase appetite and weight gain in depressed elderly patients. With appropriate monitoring for side effects, mirtazapine may be a drug of choice for older persons experiencing weight loss and depression (Rudolph, 2009) and could potentially decrease gastroparesis, nausea, and vomiting (Malamood et al, 2017).

Food and nutrition contribute to one's physiologic, psychological, and social quality of life (Raymond, 2019). A measure of nutrition-related quality of life has been proposed to document quality-of-life outcomes for individuals receiving medical nutrition therapy. Effective strategies to improve eating and thereby improve nursing home residents' quality of life are well established but could be more widely implemented (Bernstein and Munoz, 2012) (see *New Directions:* Culture Change).

✳ NEW DIRECTIONS

Culture Change

Culture Change in Long-Term Care

The Pioneer Network was formed in 1997 by a small group of prominent professionals (including dietitians) working in long-term care to advocate for person-directed care. This group called for a radical change in the culture of aging so that when our grandparents, parents—and ultimately we—go to a nursing home or other community-based setting, it is to thrive, not to decline. This movement, away from institutional provider-driven models to more humane consumer-driven models that embrace flexibility and self-determination, has come to be known as the *culture change movement*. The belief is that the quality of life and living for older Americans is rooted in a supportive community and cemented by relationships that respect each individual regardless of age, medical condition, or limitations.

The mission of the Pioneer Network is to:
- Create communication, networking, and learning opportunities
- Build and support relationships and community
- Identify and promote transformations in practice, services, public policy, and research
- Develop and provide access to resources and leadership

Values and Principles
- Know each person.
- Each person can and does make a difference.
- Relationship is the fundamental building block of a transformed culture.
- Respond to spirit, as well as mind and body.
- Risk-taking is a normal part of life.
- Put person before task.
- All elders are entitled to self-determination wherever they live.
- Community is the antidote to institutionalization.
- Do unto others as you would have them do unto you.
- Promote the growth and development of all.
- Shape and use the potential of the environment in all its aspects: physical, organizational, psycho/social/spiritual.
- Practice self-examination, searching for new creativity and opportunities for doing better.
- Recognize that culture change and transformation are not destinations but a journey, always a work in progress.

Functionality

Functionality and functional status are terms used to describe physical abilities and limitations in, for example, ambulation. Functionality, the ability to perform self-care, self-maintenance, and physical activities, correlates with independence and quality of life. Disability rates among older adults are declining, but the actual number considered disabled is increasing as the size of the aging population grows. Limitations in ADLs (toileting, bathing, eating, dressing) and instrumental activities of daily living (IADLs) such as managing money, shopping, telephone use, travel and transportation, housekeeping, preparing meals, taking medications correctly, and other individual self-performance skills needed in everyday life, are used to monitor physical function (Federal Interagency Forum on Aging-Related Statistics, 2012).

Many nutrition-related diseases affect functional status in older individuals. Inadequate nutrient intake may hasten loss of muscle mass and strength, which can have a negative effect on performing ADLs. Among the older adults who have one or more nutrition-related chronic diseases, impaired physical function may cause greater disability, with increased morbidity, nursing home admissions, or death.

Frailty and Failure to Thrive

The four syndromes known to be predictive of adverse outcomes in older adults that are prevalent in patients with frailty or "geriatric failure to thrive" include impaired physical functioning, malnutrition, depression, and cognitive impairment. Symptoms include weight loss, decreased appetite, poor nutrition, dehydration, inactivity, and impaired immune function. Interventions should be directed at easily remediable contributors in the hope of improving overall functional status. Optimal management requires a multidisciplinary, multifaceted approach. Occupational therapists and speech therapists are essential to comprehensive care management. Nutrition interventions, especially those rectifying protein-energy malnutrition, are essential but often difficult to implement in an older person who is disinterested in eating. Because overall diet quality has been shown to be associated inversely with prevalent and future frailty status in a large cohort of community-living older men, more attention to the total dietary intakes when advancing age is critical (Galvin and Sadowsky, 2012). Liberalization of overly restrictive diet prescriptions is often key to improving calorie intake and dietary quality (Raymond, 2019). It is important to recognize when failure to thrive is actually normal end of life. Spiritual support is an important component of the care.

Weight Maintenance

Obesity

The prevalence of obesity in all ages has increased during the past 25 years in the United States; older adults are no exception. Obesity rates are greater among those ages 65 to 74 than among those age 75 and older. Obesity is a major cause of preventable disease and premature death. Both are linked to increased risk of coronary heart disease, type 2 diabetes, endometrial, colon, postmenopausal breast, and other cancers, asthma and other respiratory problems, osteoarthritis, and disability. Obesity causes a progressive decline in physical function, which may lead to increased frailty. Overweight and obesity can lead to a decline in IADLs.

Weight loss therapy that maintains muscle and bone mass is recommended for obese older adults because it improves physical function and quality of life and reduces the multiple medical complications associated with obesity. Weight maintenance, not weight loss, should be the goal in the very old because extra weight is actually a benefit. Normal BMI standards are not appropriate for the very old since they have not been validated in this population.

Weight loss of no more than 10% of total body weight over 6 months should be the initial goal in those who are appropriate for weight intervention. Mild calorie restriction and increased activity should be encouraged (see Chapter 20).

Having a higher body weight after age 70 may be health protective. A study reviewed data from two long-term studies and found that adults who were overweight averaged a 13% lower risk of death from any cause over 10 years, compared with those who were in the optimal BMI range (Flicker et al, 2010). Those who were underweight were 76% more likely to die, although the obese had the same mortality risk as those of within the optimal BMI range. The researchers concluded that the body mass index (BMI) thresholds for overweight and obese may be overly restrictive for older adults. Notably, the researchers also found that being sedentary increased the risk of death in men by 28%; in women, the risk was doubled.

Underweight and Malnutrition

The actual prevalence of underweight among older adults is low; women older than age 65 are three times as likely as their male counterparts to be underweight (Winter et al, 2014). However, many older adults are at risk for undernutrition and malnutrition (Federal Interagency Forum on Aging-Related Statistics, 2012). Among those hospitalized, 40% to 60% are malnourished or at risk for malnutrition, 40% to 85% of nursing home residents have malnutrition, and 20% to 60% of home care patients are malnourished. Many community-residing older persons consume fewer than 1000 kcal/day, an amount not adequate to maintain good nutrition. Some causes of undernutrition include medications, depression, decreased sense of taste or smell, poor oral health, chronic diseases, dysphagia, and other physical problems that make eating difficult. Social causes may include living alone, inadequate income, lack of transportation, and limitations in shopping for and preparing food.

Health care professionals frequently overlook protein-energy malnutrition (PEM). The physiologic changes of aging, as well as changes in living conditions and income, contribute to the problem. Symptoms of PEM often are attributed to other conditions, leading to misdiagnosis. Some common symptoms are confusion, fatigue, and weakness. Older adults with low incomes, who have difficulty chewing and swallowing meat, who smoke, or who engage in little or no physical activity are at increased risk of developing PEM.

Strategies to decrease PEM include increased caloric and protein intake. Strategies to improve intake in a long-term care community should be individualized based on the specific situation. Nutrition risk screening is an important first step (see Chapter 4).

In community settings older adults should be encouraged to eat energy-dense and high-protein foods. Federal food and nutrition services are also available for the many who reside at home (see sections below and *Focus On:* Food First!). Diets should be individualized rather than restricted to offer more choices and honor personal preference (Dorner and Friedrich, 2018). Simple, practical approaches, such as adding gravies and creams, can increase calories and soften foods for easier chewing.

◎ FOCUS ON

Food First!

There are many reasons for practitioners to consider changing from the use of commercially manufactured nutritional supplements to nutrient-dense real food. Although commercial nutritional supplements are convenient to use and provide high calories and high protein, people like to eat food and drink fluids that taste good, provide a variety of flavors, and are familiar to them. Food is more than a can of milk protein with added vitamins and minerals, it is culture, tradition, and part of life celebrations. The smell of food and appearance on a plate is part of the overall eating experience.

Fortified foods at meals and snack time in lieu of commercially prepared supplements can satisfy the most demanding palate because they can be flexible and individualized. Virtually any food can be calorie enhanced; many can be protein enhanced.

Fortified food programs have been known by a variety of names: Every Bite Counts, Nutrition Intervention Program, Enhanced Food Program, Super Foods, or Food Fortification Program. Today, thanks to the Dining Practice Standards published in 2011 and adopted by the Centers for Medicare and Medicaid, **Food First!** is the term of choice for this approach. Traditionally, fortified food programs have focused on adding calories and protein to a couple of foods on the menu each day. For example, cream is added to hot cereal and powdered milk is added to milk (double-strength milk). This approach can lead to lack of variety and food fatigue. A program approach to fortifying food will provide more flexibility and ultimately be more successful.

Digna Cassens, MHA, RDN

Modified from www.flavorfulfortifiedfood.com.

When difficulties meeting nutritional needs arise in the older adult, there may be a question as to the benefits of placing a feeding tube and administering artificial nutrition. Though this can be an option for some older adults with significant swallowing difficulties who are cognitively intact, it is the position of the American Geriatrics Society (2014) that feeding tubes are not recommended for adults with advanced dementia. In older adults with advanced dementia, feeding tubes have been associated with increased agitation, use of chemical and physical restraints, tube-related complications including hospital visits, risk of aspiration, and greater likelihood of new pressure injury development. For those with advanced dementia, it is recommended that close attention be paid to assistance at meals, individual-centered approaches to eating and should include a focus on altering the environment to maximize oral intake for the older adult with advanced dementia.

NUTRITION SCREENING AND ASSESSMENT

Simple and easy-to-use nutrition screening tools have been validated (Skipper et al, 2012). However, the physical and metabolic changes of aging can yield inaccurate results. Examples are anthropometric measurements: height, weight, and BMI. A meta-analysis of BMI and all-cause mortality concluded that being overweight was not associated with an increased risk of mortality in older populations. The mortality risk increased in underweight older people, those with a BMI of less than 23 (Winter et al, 2014).

With aging, fat mass increases and height decreases as a result of vertebral compression. An accurate height measure may be difficult in those unable to stand up straight, the bed bound, those with spinal deformations such as a dowager's hump, and those with osteoporosis. Measuring arm span or knee height may give more accurate measurements (see Appendix 11). BMIs based on questionable heights are inaccurate and result is misdiagnosis of malnutrition. Clinical judgment is needed for accuracy.

The Mini Nutritional Assessment (MNA) includes two forms: a screening Short Form (MNA-SF) and the full assessment (Kaiser et al, 2009). The validated MNA-SF is the most widely used screening method to identify malnutrition in noninstitutionalized older adults (see Chapter 4). It includes six questions and a BMI evaluation, or a calf circumference if a BMI is not possible. The MNA-SF is being used as a screening assessment tool in long-term care and is especially useful in the short stay units.

NUTRITION NEEDS

Many older adults have special nutrient requirements because aging affects absorption, utilization, and excretion of nutrients (Bernstein and Munoz, 2012). The dietary reference intakes (DRIs) separate the cohort of people age 50 and older into two groups, ages 50 to 70 and 71 and older. The current U.S. Dietary Guidelines are for adults in general and can be found in Chapter 10. They emphasize intake of whole grains, fruit and vegetables, legumes, nuts, and low-fat dairy and suggest minimizing intake of foods low in solid fats and added sugars, and processed meat. Other studies show that older persons have low intakes of calories, total fat, fiber, calcium, magnesium, zinc, copper, folate, and vitamins B_{12}, C, E, and D. When challenged by decreased appetite, early satiety, and reduced access to food, meeting recommendations can become difficult for the older adult. It is very important to consider these and other factors which inhibits one's ability to meet estimated needs including socioeconomic status, disease state and overall health, ability to chew and swallow, and ability to taste. It is the position of the Academy of Nutrition and Dietetics that estimated needs for older adults should be met with individualized nutrition care plans based on nutritional status, medical condition, and personal preference and that restrictive diets specific to disease state should be thoroughly evaluated based on risk and benefit to each individual (Table 19.3).

There is no predictive equation specific to older adults. However, the Mifflin-St. Jeor energy equation can be used to assess calorie needs in healthy older or obese adults (see Chapter 2) though it can often overestimate an older individual's needs. A quick energy estimate is provided in the table below. Certain disease states such as end-stage

TABLE 19.3   Nutrient Needs Change with Aging

Nutrient	Changes with Aging	Practical Solutions
Energy	Basal metabolic rate decreases with age because of changes in body composition. Energy needs decrease 3% per decade in adults.	Encourage nutrient-dense foods in amounts appropriate for caloric needs.
Protein 0.8 g/kg minimum	Minimal change with age but research evidence is growing that the current RDA is too low. Researchers are suggesting 1.0–1.2 gm/kg.	Protein intake should not be routinely increased; excess protein could unnecessarily stress aging kidneys.
Carbohydrates 45%–65% total calories Men 30 g fiber Women 21 g fiber	Constipation may be a serious concern for many.	Emphasize complex carbohydrates: legumes, vegetables, whole grains, fruits to provide fiber, essential vitamins, minerals. Increase dietary fiber to improve laxation especially in older adults.
Lipids 20%–35% total calories	Heart disease is a common diagnosis.	Overly severe restriction of dietary fats alters taste, texture, and enjoyment of food; can negatively affect overall diet, weight, and quality of life. Emphasize healthy fats rather than restricting fat.
Vitamins and minerals	Understanding vitamin and mineral requirements, absorption, use, and excretion with aging has increased but much remains unknown.	Encourage nutrient-dense foods in amounts appropriate for caloric needs. Oxidative and inflammatory processes affecting aging reinforce the central role of micronutrients, especially antioxidants.
Vitamin B_{12} 2.4 mg	Risk of deficiency increases because of low intakes of vitamin B_{12}, and decline in gastric acid, which facilitates B_{12} absorption.	Those 50 and older should eat foods fortified with the crystalline form of vitamin B_{12} such as in fortified cereals or supplements.
Vitamin D 600-800 IU*	Risk of deficiency increases as synthesis is less efficient; skin responsiveness as well as exposure to sunlight decline; kidneys are less able to convert D_3 to active hormone form. As many as 30% to 40% of those with hip fractures are vitamin D insufficient.	Supplementation may be necessary and is inexpensive. A supplement is indicated in virtually all institutionalized older adults.
Folate 400 µg	May lower homocysteine levels; possible risk marker for atherothrombosis, Alzheimer's disease, and Parkinson's disease.	Fortification of grain products has improved folate status. When supplementing with folate, must monitor B_{12} levels.
Calcium 1200 mg	Dietary requirement may increase because of decreased absorption; only 4% of women and 10% of men age 60 and older meet daily recommendation from food sources alone.	Recommend naturally occurring and fortified foods. Supplementation may be necessary. However, in older women, high intakes may be occurring with supplements.
Potassium 4700 mg	Potassium-rich diet can blunt the effect of sodium on blood pressure.	Recommend meeting potassium recommendation with food, especially fruits and vegetables.
Sodium 1500 mg	Risk of hypernatremia caused by dietary excess and dehydration. Risk of hyponatremia caused by fluid retention.	Newer evidence based on direct health outcomes is inconsistent with the recommendation to lower dietary sodium in the general population, including older adults, to 1500 mg per day. More research is needed.†
Zinc Men 11 mg Women 8 mg	Low intake associated with impaired immune function, anorexia, loss of sense of taste, delayed wound healing, and pressure ulcer development.	Encourage food sources: lean meats, oysters, dairy products, beans, peanuts, tree nuts, and seeds, especially pumpkin seeds.
Water	Hydration status can easily be problematic. Dehydration causes decreased fluid intake, decreased kidney function, increased losses caused by increased urine output from medications (laxatives, diuretics). Symptoms: electrolyte imbalance, altered drug effects, headache, constipation, blood pressure change, dizziness, confusion, dry mouth and nose.	Encourage fluid intake of at least 1500 mL/day or 1 mL per calorie consumed. Risk increases because of impaired sense of thirst, fear of incontinence, and dependence on others to get beverages. Dehydration is often unrecognized; it can present as falls, confusion, change in level of consciousness, weakness or change in functional status, or fatigue.

*National Research Council: *Dietary Reference Intakes for Calcium and Vitamin D*, Washington, DC, 2011, The National Academies Press.
†National Research Council: *Sodium intake in populations: assessment of evidence*, Washington, DC, 2013, The National Academies Press.
Baum J, Il-Young K, Wolfe R: Protein Consumption and the Elderly: What Is the Optimal Level of Intake? Nutrients. 2016 Jun; 8(6): 359. Published online 2016 Jun 8. doi: 10.3390/nu8060359.

BOX 19.3 Nutrition Needs for Older Adults

Quick Calorie Estimate

Healthy older adult	18-22 kcal/kg women
	20-24 kcal/kg men
Weight gain for underweight or older adult experiencing unintended weight loss	25-40 kcal/kg
Pressure injury	30-35 kcal/kg

Quick Protein Estimate

Healthy older adult	1.0-1.2 g/kg
Dialysis or pressure injury	1.2-1.5 g/kg

Quick Fluid Estimate

Healthy older adult	25-30 kcal/kg or 1 ml/kcal
Congestive heart failure or edema	25 ml/kg
Infection or fluid loss from draining wounds	35 kcal/kg

Adapted from: *Nutrition Care of the Older Adult: A Handbook for Nutrition Throughout the Continuum of Care*, 3rd Ed. Dietetics in Health Care Communities Dietetic Practice Group; Kathleen C. Niedert, RDN, CSG, LD, FADA, Editor-in-Chief; Marla P. Carlson, Editor

renal disease on dialysis, pressure injuries, and congestive heart failure warrant adjustments to estimated needs to ensure adequate calorie, protein, and fluid needs are met. As with any energy estimation, it is important to continue to monitor weight and conduct nutrition-focused physical assessments often to ensure estimates are adequate for each individual (Box 19.3).

MEDICARE BENEFITS

The federal Medicare program covers most of the health care costs of those 65 and older and persons with disabilities. However, this federally funded health insurance program does not cover the cost of residential/institutional long-term care. A portion of payroll taxes and monthly premiums deducted from Social Security payments finance Medicare.

Medicare benefits are provided in four parts. Part A covers inpatient hospital care, some skilled nursing care for specific "skilled services", hospice care, and some home health care costs for limited periods of time. It is premium free for most citizens. Part B has a monthly premium that helps pay for physicians and physician surrogates, outpatient hospital care, and some other care not covered by Part A (physical and occupational therapy, for example). Part C allows private insurers, including health maintenance organizations (HMOs) and preferred provider organizations (PPOs), to offer health insurance plans to Medicare beneficiaries. These must provide the same benefits the original Medicare plan provides under Parts A and B. Part C HMOs and PPOs also may offer additional benefits, such as dental and vision care. Part D provides prescription drug benefits through private insurance companies.

The **2010 Affordable Care Act** (see Chapter 9) changed Medicare to include an annual wellness visit and a personalized prevention assessment and plan with no copayment or deductible. Prevention services include referrals to education and preventive counseling or community-based interventions to address risk factors. Expansion of medical nutrition therapy reimbursement for registered dietitians/nutritionists was anticipated, however major changes have been made to the original legislation now calling this into question. More universal access to nutrition services has implications for aging healthier and promoting quality of life and independence.

Medicaid, for qualified low-income individuals, finances a variety of long-term care services via multiple mechanisms, including Medicaid State Plans and home- and community-based services (HCBS) waivers, Section 1915 (c). Both provide service to nursing home–appropriate older adults to help prevent or decrease nursing home or institutionalization. States may offer an unlimited variety of services under this waiver. These programs may provide traditional medical services (dental, skilled nursing) and nonmedical services (meal delivery, case management, environmental modifications). States have the discretion to choose the number of older persons served and the services offered.

Program of All-Inclusive Care for the Elderly (PACE) is a comprehensive managed care system for people over 55 who are nursing home eligible and who meet low income criteria. The program is funded through Medicare and Medicaid. Coordinated preventive, primary, acute, and long-term care services allow older adults to remain in their homes for as long as possible (Thomas and Burkemper, 2013). The PACE model is based on the belief that it is better for the well-being of older adults with chronic care needs to be served in the community whenever possible. PACE is multidisciplinary and includes dietitian services. There are more than 100 PACE Programs nationwide.

PACE Programs and HCBS waivers reflect federal commitments to delay or avoid nursing home placement whenever possible. The U.S. Administration on Aging is now under the new umbrella of the U.S Administration on Community Living. Terms such as "aging in community," "communitarian alternatives," "age-friendly living," "care circles," and especially "long-term services and supports" (LSS) (versus "long-term care") are indicative of the transformations taking place in the more positive approaches to aging (Bernstein et al, 2012; Rudolph, 2009).

NUTRITION SUPPORT SERVICES

U.S. Department of Health and Human Services Older Americans Act (OAA) Nutrition Program

The OAA was originally enacted in 1965 and approved for a 3-year reauthorization in 2015 by unanimous vote by the Senate. The OAA Nutrition Program is the largest, most visible federally funded community-based nutrition program for older persons (Lloyd and Wellman, 2015). Primarily a state-run program, it has few federal regulations and considerable variation in state-to-state policies and procedures. Goals of the OAA include supporting seniors' independence and helping prevent hospitalization and nursing care with funding extending to 56 state agencies, over 200 tribal organizations, and over 20,000 local service providers. Nutrition program funding is distributed based on a formula which considers each state's population of older adults over age 60. This nutrition program provides congregate and home-delivered meals (usually 5 days per week using Meals on Wheels), nutrition screening, education, and counseling, as well as an array of other supportive and health services. The OAA Nutrition Program, available to all persons age 60 and older regardless of income, successfully targets those in greatest economic and social need, with particular attention to low-income minorities and rural populations. Generally, a higher proportion of older adults who receive OAA services have a higher percent of food insecurity and functional limitations compared with those who do not utilize services (Vieira et al, 2017). Particular attention is paid to those individuals who are members of minority groups, live in rural areas, have low income, have limited English proficiency, and are at risk for institutional care.

More than half of the OAA annual budget supports the nutrition program, which provides about 219 million congregate and home-delivered meals to 2.4 million older adults annually (U.S. Administration on Aging, 2019). According to the ACL and U.S.

Administration on Aging, 91% of participants stated that home-delivered meals have helped them stay in their own homes and more than 60% of participants indicate that home-delivered meals provide one half or more of their total intake for the day. Home-delivered meals have grown to more than 61% of all meals served and almost half of the programs have waiting lists. To receive home-delivered meals, an individual must be assessed to be home bound, frail, or isolated, though the benefits may also extend to caregivers, spouses, and people with disabilities.

At congregate sites, the nutrition program provides access and linkages to other community-based services. It is the primary source of food and nutrients for many program participants and presents opportunities for active social engagement and meaningful volunteer roles. The meals provided are required to be nutritionally dense, supply more than 33% of the recommended dietary allowances (an OAA requirement), and provide 40% to 50% of daily intakes of most nutrients (Lloyd and Wellman, 2015).

The OAA Nutrition Program is closely linked to HCBS through cross-referrals within the Aging Network. Because older adults are being discharged earlier from hospitals and nursing homes, many require a care plan that includes home-delivered meals and other nutrition services (e.g., nutrition screening, assessment, education, counseling, and care planning). Many states are creating programs to provide necessary medical, social, and supportive HCBS, including home-delivered meals, nutrition education, and counseling services. States are being encouraged to help older adults and people with disabilities live in their homes and fully participate in their communities by the ACL. Its role is to build the capacity of the national aging and disability networks to better serve older persons, caregivers, and individuals with disabilities.

U.S. Department of Agriculture (USDA) Food Assistance Programs

For low-income adults, research suggests evidence of lower caloric intake, poorer dietary quality, greater risk of hypoglycemia, lower medication adherence, and difficulty paying bills at the end of the month when finances diminish. Several USDA food and nutrition assistance programs are available to older adults after participants meet certain criteria as all USDA programs are means tested. A recent study suggests that older adults dually enrolled in Medicare and Medicaid services who receive SNAP benefits had reduced hospitalization and emergency department visits compared with those that did not utilize these benefits (Samuel et al, 2018). This could have significant implications on the general health of older adult populations, though the majority of U.S. adults who are eligible for SNAP benefits do not participate. Additional information on USDA food assistance programs can be found in Chapter 9.

Commodity Supplemental Food Program

The Commodity Supplemental Food Program (CSFP) strives to improve the health of low-income Americans by supplementing their diets with nutritious USDA commodity foods. It provides food and administrative funds to states but not all states are enrolled. In states which administer CSFP, services are offered in diverse locations such as public health, nutrition services, or agriculture departments. Eligible populations include adults age 60 and older with incomes less than 130% of the poverty level. Local CSFP agencies determine eligibility, distribute food, and provide nutrition education. The food packages do not provide a complete diet but may be good sources of nutrients frequently lacking in low-income diets and can include dry milk, juice, oats, dry cereal, rice, pasta, peanut butter, dry beans, canned meat/poultry/fish, and canned fruits and vegetables.

Seniors Farmers' Market Nutrition Program

The Seniors Farmers' Market Nutrition Program (SFMNP) is administered by state departments of agriculture, aging and disability services, or federally recognized Native American tribal governments. Not all states operate SFMNP on a statewide basis. SFMNP provides coupons to low-income older individuals to purchase fresh unprepared fruits, vegetables, honey, and herbs at farmers' markets, roadside stands, and community-supported agriculture (CSA) programs. It provides eligible older adults with local, seasonal access to fresh fruits and vegetables as well as nutrition education and information. The SFMNP serves low-income older adults who are generally at least 60 years old and who have incomes not more than 185% of the U.S. poverty guidelines.

Medicaid and Nutrition Services

Older adults who meet certain income criteria may qualify for additional support from Medicaid agencies and Medicaid health plans. Many states use HCBS waivers to support low-income older adults and an increasing number of states are creating LSS to more broadly support older adult communities. Practices supporting the nutrition-related needs of older adults are growing in popularity as states understand the broader implications of addressing these needs. Some Medicaid-based health plans are also increasing their involvement with nutrition professionals, assisting plan members in SNAP enrollment and utilizing assessment data to monitor nutrition-related needs and outcomes (Center for Healthcare Strategies, 2019).

COMMUNITY AND RESIDENTIAL FACILITIES FOR OLDER ADULTS

The report *Long-Term Care Providers and Services Users in the United States, 2015-2016* found that 65,600 paid, regulated long term services providers served over 8.3 million people (Harris-Kojetin et al, 2016). This is in an increase of 7,100 service providers since 2013. Long term care services were provided by 4,600 adult day services, 12,200 home health agencies, 4,300 hospices, 15,600 nursing homes and 28,900 assisted living and similar residential care communities. Each day, there are more than 286,300 enrolled adult day service participants, 1,347,600 skilled nursing facilities (SNFs) residents (for those requiring a higher level of medical care), and 811,500 residential care residents. In 2015, approximately 1,426,000 patients received services from hospices, a 14% increase from 2013.

People move to residential facilities, generally known as assisted living, when they can no longer safely live alone because they have some cognitive impairment requiring supervision or need help with ADLs because of immobility. Care is provided in ways that promote maximum independence and dignity. Assisted living care's annual cost is generally quite a bit less than nursing homes. Residents are encouraged to maintain active social lives with planned activities, exercise classes, religious and social functions, and opportunities to travel outside the facility. These communities are now required in some states to provide therapeutic diets but in those states without such regulation residents have difficulty getting special requirements met for services such as texture modified meals.

Comprehensive state regulations for food and nutrition services in assisted living care is not yet widespread, but there is growing consensus that it should be regulated. Emphasizing that food and nutrition matter at every age, it is essential that support for nutrition and quality of life extend beyond food availability and safety. Dietitian expertise is needed for nutrition assessment and care planning to meet special needs such as type and amounts of macronutrients and micronutrients, texture modifications, and quality of food choices and presentation.

Only about 3% or 1.4 million older adults live in the approximately 15,700 nursing homes (Harris-Kojetin et al, 2019). The percentage of the population that lives in nursing homes increases dramatically with age, especially for those older than age 85. However, the overall percentage has declined since 1990, likely because of healthier aging, the federal cost-containment policy to delay residential placement in nursing homes by providing more aging services in the community, as well as the increased availability and use of hospice. The percentage increases with age, ranging from 1% for persons age 65 to 74 years to 3% for persons age 75 to 84 years and 10% for persons age 85. The cost of nursing home care differs by state with the most expensive reported in Alaska where a semiprivate room is more than $23,000 per month and the least expensive is Oklahoma at about $4500 per month (Seniorliving.org).

SNFs are federally regulated by the Centers for Medicare and Medicaid Services; assisted living centers, by each state. More residents are in SNFs for short-stay, post-acute care, thus more comprehensive medical nutrition therapy is now needed. Nutritional care is directed toward identifying and responding to changing physiologic and psychological needs over time that protect against avoidable decline (Box 19.4).

BOX 19.4	**Types of Residential Housing**
Independent Living Facility (IL or ILF)	Apartment style, condominium, or freestanding home living for independent seniors.
Assisted Living Facility (AL or ALF)	Apartment style housing that offers organized social interaction and support services as needed. Health care services are available by outside providers who visit the facility periodically. Meals are offered and assistance with medication management and some physical assistance with activities of daily living and transportation can be offered.
Skilled Nursing Facility (SNF) Nursing Home	Accredited establishment that offers 24-hour care and access to in-house health care providers and nursing, assistance with activities of daily living, meals and snacks, and organized social activities. Many SNFs also provide rehabilitative services where patients can receive therapy and healthcare services to recover from an injury or illness with the goal of returning to a more independent setting.
Continuous Care Retirement Community (CCRC)	These communities combine all levels of care onto one property and include housing and services for independent, assisted, and skilled living.
Rehabilitation Hospital	Hospital-like setting which provides extended acute care for patients requiring stabilization before transferring to an SNF or more independent setting. These hospitals bridge the gap for patients requiring advanced therapy but who are not appropriate to stay in a general hospital or transfer to a SNF.
Adult Family Home (AFH)	Traditional home in a residential neighborhood which supports needs of its residents by assisting with activities of daily living, meals, and personal care. Most states require licensing and are inspected on a regular basis, though some states do not require licensing of these facilities. Nursing care may be available on site. AFHs typically house between 2 and 9 residents at a time.

The culture change movement in long-term care (LTC) has led to the creation of the Dining Practice Standards (DPS). The DPS were published by the Pioneer Network's Dining Clinical Task Force, a multidisciplinary group of LTC and nutrition experts. These guidelines were agreed to by Centers for Medicare and Medicaid Services (CMS) and over a dozen professional groups, including the Academy of Nutrition and Dietetics (AND). The guidelines provide evidence-based support for resident-centered dining, for liberalized diets, for food first, and for decreased dependence on medical nutritional supplements. CMS has subsequently incorporated the DPS into the survey process.

In 1987 Congress passed reform legislation as part of the Omnibus Reconciliation Act (OBRA) to improve the quality of care in SNFs by strengthening standards that must be met for Medicare/Medicaid reimbursement. Since that time SNFs have been required by CMS to conduct periodic assessments to determine the residents' needs; to provide services that ensure residents maintain the highest practical, physical, mental, and psychological well-being; and to ensure that no harm is inflicted. This is accomplished using the Minimum Data Set (MDS), which is part of the federally mandated process for clinical assessment of residents of LTC facilities licensed under Medicare or Medicaid. Section K of the MDS is specific to nutrition and is generally the responsibility of the dietitian to complete but can be done by nursing staff (Fig. 19.4). This form documents "triggers" that may place a resident at nutrition risk and therefore requires an intervention. This assessment must be done at admission and if there is a significant change in the resident's condition such as weight loss or skin breakdown. Reassessment is required quarterly and annually. The entire process is known as the Resident Assessment Instrument (RAI). It provides the individual assessment of each resident's functional capabilities and helps identify problems and develop a care plan.

High nutrition risk individuals must be identified and assessed monthly by the dietitian. High risk is defined as:
- Significant weight loss defined as 5% of body weight in 1 month or 10% of body weight in 6 months
- Nutrition support (tube feedings or parenteral nutrition)
- Dialysis patients
- Wounds or pressure injuries

Palliative Care and Hospice

During the course of a disease process there are multiple services and approaches that can ease symptoms and focus on keeping one comfortable. Palliative care is an approach to care that can be initiated at any point during a person's life or illness and can be provided in conjunction with curative treatment. Palliative care focuses on providing relief from symptoms and alleviating the stress of illness and disease management. Teams of specially trained health professionals work alongside a patient's other providers to give an extra layer of support for achieving the goal of improved quality of life for both the patient and family. Palliative care services can be provided in outpatient or inpatient settings, long term care communities, or at home and may be covered by Medicare, Medicaid, or private insurances. Though the palliative care approach is best to initiate at the diagnosis of a disease, there are many benefits to starting care at any point during the progression of a particular disease.

Hospice care is a service which provides extra support to a terminally ill individual and to the family. Hospice care is covered under Medicaid, Medicare, and most private insurance plans and HMOs. A patient must meet specific criteria to be eligible for hospice care including diagnosis of a terminal illness with an estimate of 6 months or less life expectancy. Once enrolled in services, hospice develops a care plan and care team to meet a patient's individual needs. Hospice teams can include the patient's personal physician, hospice physician, nurses, home health aides, social workers, clergy, trained volunteer, speech/physical/occupational therapists, and dietitians. The team helps provide relief of pain and symptoms, emotional support to both the patient and family, medical equipment and medications, and bereavement care and counseling to family and friends. Hospice care can be provided in the home in conjunction with private caregivers or in hospice centers, hospitals, and long-term care communities. For many, this extra level of support can ease the transition, provide comfort, and increase quality of life for the patient and family alike. For more on palliative and hospice care, see Chapter 35.

Section K	Swallowing/Nutritional Status

K0100. Swallowing Disorder

Signs and symptoms of possible swallowing disorder

↓ Check all that apply

☐	A.	Loss of liquids/solids from mouth when eating or drinking
☐	B.	Holding food in mouth/cheeks or residual food in mouth after meals
☐	C.	Coughing or choking during meals or when swallowing medications
☐	D.	Complaints of difficulty or pain with swallowing
☐	Z.	None of the above

K0200. Height and Weight - While measuring, if the number is X.1-X.4 round down; X.5 or greater round up

☐☐ inches	A. **Height** (in inches). Record most recent height measure since admission
☐☐☐ pounds	B. **Weight** (in pounds). Base weight on most recent measure in last 30 days; measure weight consistently, according to standard facility practice (e.g., in a.m. after voiding, before meal, with shoes off, etc.)

K0300. Weight Loss

Enter Code ☐	Loss of 5% or more in the last month or loss of 10% or more in last 6 months 0. **No** or unknown 1. **Yes, on** physician-prescribed weight-loss regimen 2. **Yes, not on** physician-prescribed weight-loss regimen

K0500. Nutritional Approaches

↓ Check all that apply

☐	A.	Parenteral/IV feeding
☐	B.	Feeding tube - nasogastric or abdominal (PEG)
☐	C.	Mechanically altered diet - requires change in texture of food or liquids (e.g., pureed food, thickened liquids)
☐	D.	Therapeutic diet (e.g., low salt, diabetic, low cholesterol)
☐	Z.	None of the above

K0700. Percent Intake by Artificial Route - Complete K0700 only if K0500A or K0500B is checked

Enter Code ☐	A. **Proportion of total calories the resident received through parenteral or tube feeding** 1. **25% or less** 2. **26-50%** 3. **51% or more**
Enter Code ☐	B. **Average fluid intake per day by IV or tube feeding** 1. **500 cc/day or less** 2. **501 cc/day or more**

Fig. 19.4 The Minimum Data Set, Section K version 3.0. (From the Centers for Medicare and Medicaid Services, Baltimore, MD.)

CLINICAL CASE STUDY

MF is an 86-year-old white female resident in a skilled nursing facility with unintentional weight loss. She was admitted 3 months ago from the hospital after a hip fracture. She had been residing in an independent living facility for several years. She reports she has been eating poorly because of difficulty moving around, being generally uncomfortable, and states, "If I am not active, I don't need to eat so much." Intake is less than 50% of regular diet. No problems chewing or swallowing are noted after a speech language pathologist's evaluation. Admission weight was 112 pounds; current weight is 95 pounds. Self-reported height is 5' 3"; Hgb/Hct is normal; total cholesterol is 135; and Mini Nutrition Assessment score is 5. Hip scans show slow fracture healing and no improvement in bone density; currently she is being supplemented with calcium 1000 mg/day and vitamin D 600 IU/day. Blood pressure is 128/80 with furosemide (Lasix); other medications are lorazepam (Ativan), fentanyl transdermal patch (Duragesic), senna (Senokot-S), docusate (Colace), and mirtazapine (Remeron).

Nutrition Diagnostic Statement

- Unintentional weight loss related to food intake of less than 50% of meals with limited physical activity as evidenced by severe weight loss of 17 lbs/14% of body weight over three months.

Continued

CLINICAL CASE STUDY—cont'd

Nutrition Care Questions

1. Comment on the appropriateness of and use for each medication. Would you suggest any changes or additional medications?
2. What strategies could you use to help improve this resident's food and fluid intake?
3. What suggestions are appropriate to promote fracture healing and increase bone density?
4. Do you suspect that this client is constipated? What would you recommend in terms of food choices to deal with this?

USEFUL WEBSITES

Administration for Community Living
Administration on Aging
American Association of Retired Persons
American Geriatrics Society
American Society on Aging
Centers for Medicare and Medicaid Services
Meals on Wheels Association of America
National Association of Nutrition and Aging Services Programs
National Institute on Aging
National Institutes of Health Senior Health
National Study of Long-Term Care Providers (NSLTCP)
Older Americans Act Nutrition Program
Pioneer Network

REFERENCES

American Dietetic Association: Individualized nutrition approaches for older adults in health care communities, *J Am Diet Assoc* 110:1549–1553, 2010.

American Geriatrics Society Ethics Committee and Clinical Practice and Models of Care Committee: American Geriatrics Society Feeding Tubes in Advanced Dementia Position Statement, *J Am Geriatr Soc* 62(8):1590–1593, 2014.

American Optometric Association: *Glossary of common eye & vision conditions-presbyopia*, 2014. Available at: http://www.aoa.org/patients-and-public/eye-and-vision-problems/glossary-of-eye-and-vision-conditions/presbyopia.

Aslam T, Delcourt C, Holz F, et al: European survey on the opinion and use of micronutrition in age-related macular degeneration: 10 years on from the Age-Related Eye Disease Study, *Clin Ophthalmol* 8:2045–2053, 2014.

Bernstein M, Munoz N, Academy of Nutrition and Dietetics: Position of the Academy of Nutrition and Dietetics: food and nutrition for older adults: promoting health and wellness, *J Acad Nutr Diet* 112:1255–1277, 2012.

Beveridge LA, Davey PG, Phillips G, et al: Optimal management of urinary tract infections in older people, *Clin Interv Aging* 6:173–180, 2011.

Buettner D, Skemp S: Blue Zones: lessons from the World's Longest Lived, *Am J Lifestyle Med* 10(5):318–321, 2016.

Center for Health Care Strategies: *Providing home- and community-based nutrition services to low-income older adults: promising health plan practices*, 2018. Available at: www.chcs.org/media/HSBC-Nutrition-ServicesBrief_042318_updated.pdf.

Centers for Disease Control and Prevention: *The State of Aging and Health in America 2013*, Atlanta, GA, 2013, US Dept of Health and Human Services. Available at: http://www.cdc.gov/features/agingandhealth/state_of_aging_and_health_in_america_2013.pdf.

Chew EY, Clemons TE, Agrón E, et al: Ten-year follow-up of age-related macular degeneration in the Age-Related Eye Disease Study: AREDS report no. 36, *JAMA Ophthalmol* 132:272–277, 2014.

Chien W, Lin FR: Prevalence of hearing aid use among older adults in the United States, *Arch Intern Med* 172:292–293, 2012.

Ciorba A, Bianchini C, Pelucchi,S, et al: The impact of hearing loss on quality of life of elderly adults, *Clin Interv Aging*. 7:159–63, 2012.

Colby SL, Ortman JM: *The baby boom cohort in the United States: 2012 to 2060*, 2014. Available at: http://www.census.gov/prod/2014pubs/p25-1141.pdf.

Correa-de-Araujo R, Hadley E: Skeletal Muscle Function Deficit: a new terminology to embrace the evolving concepts of sarcopenia and age-related muscle dysfunction, *J Gerontol A Biol Sci Med Sci* 69:591–594, 2014.

Dent E, Morley JE, Cruz-Jentoft AJ, et al: International clinical practice guidelines for sarcopenia (ICFSR): screening, diagnosis and management, *J Nutr Health Aging* 22:1148-1161, 2018.

Dorner B, Friedrich EK: Position of the Academy of Nutrition and Dietetics: individualized nutrition approaches for older adults: long-term care, post-acute care, and other settings, *J Acad Nutr Diet* 118(4):724-735, 2018.

European Pressure Ulcer Advisory Panel, National Pressure Injury Advisory Panel and Pan Pacific Pressure Injury Alliance: *Prevention and treatment of pressure ulcers/injuries Quick Reference Guide* 2019. Available at: http://internationalguideline.com/guideline.

Federal Interagency Forum on Aging-Related Statistics: *Older Americans 2012: key indicators of well-being*, Washington, DC, 2012, U.S. Government Printing Office.

Flicker L, McCaul KA, Hankey GJ, et al: Body mass index and survival in men and women aged 70 to 75, *J Am Geriatr Soc* 58:234–241, 2010.

Galvin JE, Sadowsky CH: Practical guidelines for the recognition and diagnosis of dementia, *J Am Board Fam Med* 25:367–382, 2012.

Harris-Kojetin L, Sengupta M, Lendon J, et al: *Long-term care services in the United States: 2015-2016*, Hyattsville, MD, 2019, National Center for Health Statistics.

Kaiser MJ, Bauer JM, Ramsch C, et al: Validation of the mini nutritional assessment short-form (MNA-SF): a practical tool for identification of nutritional status, *J Nutr Health Aging* 13:782–788, 2009.

Keenan C and Allan R: Epigenomic drivers of immune dysfunction in aging, *Aging Cell*. Available at: https://doi.org/10.1111/acel.12878 2018.

Korobelnik JF, Rougier MB, Delyfer MN, et al: Effect of dietary supplementation with lutein, zeaxanthin, and ω-3 on macular pigment: a randomized clinical trial, *JAMA Ophthalmol* 135(11):1259–1266, 2017.

Li-Korotky HS: Age-related hearing loss: quality of care for quality of life, *Gerontologist* 52:265–271, 2012.

Lin FR, Niparko JK, Ferrucci L. Hearing loss prevalence in the United States, *Arch Intern Med* 171(20):1851–1852, 2011.

Litchford MD: Counteracting the trajectory of frailty and sarcopenia in older adults, *Nutr Clin Pract* 29:428–434, 2014.

Lloyd JL, Wellman NS: Older Americans Act Nutrition Programs: a community-based nutrition program helping older adults remain at home, *J Nutr Gerontol Geriatr* 34:90–109, 2015.

Lopes da Silva S, Vellas B, Elemans S, et al: Plasma nutrient status of patients with Alzheimer's disease: systematic review and meta-analysis, *Alzheimers Dement* 10:485–502, 2014.

Malamood M, Roberts A, Kataria R, et al. Mirtazapine for symptom control in refractory gastroparesis, *Drug Des Devel Ther* 11:1035–1041, 2017. doi:10.2147/DDDT.S125743.

National Eye Institute, National Institute of Health: *Age-Related Macular Degeneration*, 2014. Available at: https://www.nei.nih.gov/eyedata/amd.asp.

National Institute on Aging: *Exercise & physical activity: your everyday guide from the National Institute on Aging*, 2010. Available at: http://www.nia.nih.gov/health/publication/exercise-physical-activity/introduction.

National Institute on Deafness and Other Communicative Disorders, National Institutes of Health: *Age-related hearing loss*, 2013a. Available at: http://www.nidcd.nih.gov/health/hearing/Pages/presbycusis.aspx.

Ortman JM, Velkoff VA, Hogan H: *An aging nation: the older population in the United States*, 2014. Available at: http://www.census.gov/prod/2014pubs/p25-1140.pdf?eml=gd&utm_medium=email&utm_source=govdelivery.

Park DC, Festini SB: Theories of memory and aging: a look at the past and a glimpse of the future, *J Gerontol B Psychol Sci Soc Sci* 72(1):82–90, 2017.

Raymond JL: The art and science of nutrition for healthy aging. *Health Progress* 100:20–22, 2019.

Rudolph DM: Appetite stimulants in long term care: a literature review, *Internet J Adv Nurs Pract* 11(1):1–8, 2009.

Samuel LJ, Szanton SL, Cahill R, et al: Does the Supplemental Nutrition Assistance Program affect hospital utilization among older adults? The case of Maryland, *Popul Health Manag* 21(2):88–95, 2018.

Santanasto AJ, Goodpaster BH, Kritchevsky SB, et al: Body composition remodeling and mortality: the Health aging and body composition study, *J Gerontol* 72(4):513–519, 2017.

Schiffman SS: Effects of aging on the human taste system, *Ann N Y Acad Sci* 1170:725–729, 2009.

Skipper A, Ferguson M, Thompson K, et al: Nutrition screening tools: an analysis of the evidence, *J Parenter Enteral Nutr* 36:292–298, 2012.

Taylor D: Physical activity is medicine for older adults, *BMJ* 90:26–32, 2014.

Thomas DR, Burkemper NM: Aging skin and wound healing, *Clin Geriatr Med* 29(2):xi–xx, 2013.

Thomas KS, Mor V: Providing more home-delivered meals is one way to keep older adults with low care needs out of nursing homes, *Health Aff (Millwood)* 32:1796–1802, 2013.

United Nations. *World Population Ageing Report*, United Nations, NY, 2017. Available at: https://www.un.org/en/development/desa/population/publications/pdf/ageing/WPA2017_Report.pdf.

U.S. Administration on Aging: Nutrition Services (OAA Title IIIC), 2019. Available at: https://fas.org/sgp/crs/misc/R43414.pdf.

Vieira ER, Vaccaro JA, Zarini GG, et al: Health indicators of US older adults who received or did not receive meals funded by the Older Americans Act, *J Aging Res,* October 2017. https://doi.org/10.1155/2017/2160819.

Winter JE, MacInnis RJ, Wattanapenpaiboon N, et al: BMI and all-cause mortality in older adults: a meta-analysis, *Am J Clin Nutr* 99:875–890, 2014.

World Health Organization. *Deafness and hearing loss,* March 2018. Available at: https://www.who.int/en/news-room/fact-sheets/detail/deafness-and-hearing-loss.

PART IV

Nutrition for Weight Management

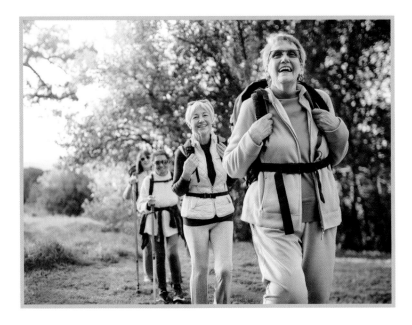

The chapters in this section reflect the evolution of nutritional science, from the identification of nutrient requirements and the practical application of this knowledge to the concepts that relate nutrition to the prevention of chronic and degenerative diseases and to optimization of health and performance.

The relationship between nutrition and dental disease has long been recognized. In more recent decades the possibility of nutrition therapy to prevent and treat bone disease has become an active area of research and we are now aware that the inflammatory process is a factor that nutrition can modulate.

Healthy lifestyles, good nutrition, and physical activity are foundations of health, fitness, and disease prevention. Understanding the role of nutrition in sports and in optimizing performance has led to dietary and exercise practices generally applicable to a rewarding, healthy lifestyle.

Increased access to highly processed and calorically dense foods has led to an overabundant intake of energy for many individuals. Efforts to reduce body weight, widely pursued with varying degrees of enthusiasm and diligence, are often disheartening, making the knowledge presented here so important. Frustration with dieting and stress often lead to eating disorders, which are increasing in frequency and require attention and understanding from the nutrition professional.

20

Nutrition in Weight Management

Lucinda K. Lysen, RDN, RN, BSN
Dorene Robinson, RDN, CDN
Rebecca Rudel, MPH, RDN, CNSC

KEY TERMS

abdominal fat	hyperphagia	night-eating syndrome (NES)
activity thermogenesis (AT)	hyperplasia	nonalcoholic fatty liver disease (NAFLD)
adipocyte	hypertrophy	nonexercise activity thermogenesis (NEAT)
adiposity rebound	hypophagia	nutritional genomics
android fat distribution	incretin	obesity
bariatric surgery	insulin	obesogen
body mass index (BMI)	intermittent fasting (IF)	overweight
brown adipose tissue (BAT)	intragastric balloon (IGB)	resting metabolic rate (RMR)
carbohydrate-insulin theory of obesity	ketogenic diet	self-help programs
commercial weight loss centers	ketones	sensory-specific satiety
comorbidities	ketosis	set point theory
essential fat	laparoscopic sleeve gastrectomy (LSG)	storage fat
fat mass	lean body mass (LBM)	semivolatile organic compounds (SVOCs)
fat-free mass (FFM)	leptin	telehealth
gastric banding	lipogenesis	underweight
gastric bypass	lipoprotein lipase (LPL)	vagus nerve
ghrelin	meal replacements	very low-calorie diets (VLCDs)
gynoid fat distribution	medically supervised weight loss programs	visceral adipose tissue (VAT)
Health at Every Size; HAES®	metabolic syndrome (MetS)	white adipose tissue (WAT)
hormone-sensitive lipase (HSL)	morbid obesity	yo-yo effect

Body weight is the sum of bone, muscle, organs, body fluids, and adipose tissue. Some or all of these components are subject to normal change as a reflection of growth, reproductive status, variation in physical activity, and the effects of aging. Consistent body weight is orchestrated by neural, hormonal, and chemical mechanisms as well as individual genetic polymorphisms that balance energy intake and expenditure within fairly precise limits. Abnormalities of these complex mechanisms can result in weight fluctuations.

On one end of the weight spectrum is underweight. Although the inability to gain weight can be a primary problem, low body weight is usually secondary to a disease state, an eating disorder, or a psychiatric disorder. In the elderly or in children, unintentional weight loss can be especially detrimental and should be addressed early to prevent malnutrition or other undesirable consequences including poor growth, depressed immune function, hormone imbalance, delayed healing, and loss of bone density. Most crucial is the in utero development of the fetus. Babies deprived of nutrition before birth and who have low birth weight may be primed for accelerated growth after birth when exposed to a nutrient-rich environment (that can sometimes start with excessive intake of infant formula). Furthermore, inadequate passage of nutrients across the placenta and low birth weight eventually can lead to an increased risk of developing obesity and diabetes (Apovian, 2011).

On the other end of the spectrum, and more common, are the conditions of overweight and obesity.

WEIGHT MANAGEMENT AND OBESITY: ITS FOUNDATION IN NUTRITIONAL MEDICINE

The growing amount of attention over the last four decades to the field of weight management and obesity has largely been brought about by the historical findings of a handful of researchers. In the forefront—beginning in the 1970s—was George L. Blackburn, MD, PhD, who, along with Bruce Bistrian, MD, PhD, at Harvard Medical School, and a number of other highly respected colleagues, provided the foundation for what eventually became the field of nutritional medicine. Publications highlighting the inadequate nutrition management of hospitalized patients put this topic and nutritional medicine on the "world map." Despite the fact that Dr. Blackburn and his group found that many of the hospitalized patients were shockingly malnourished (Blackburn et al, 1977), they also discovered that the patients were often not underweight but instead, were overweight or even obese. This led to Dr. Blackburn's development of nutritional liquid and solid diets, supplementing patients with protein to encourage loss of body fat while saving muscle and improving nutritional status. The protein-sparing modified fast, which spared protein and protected organs, became the basis of the very low–carbohydrate diet for weight loss in obese patients (Blackburn, 1973). With obesity reaching epidemic proportions over the years, scientific research expanded, diet and weight loss programs grew dramatically and the specialties of weight management and obesity quickly grew into a billion-dollar industry. Over time, Dr. Blackburn's ongoing landmark studies and cutting edge findings in weight management and obesity brought him recognition around the world, earning him the title " Father of Obesity" (Table 20.1: The Story of George L. Blackburn, MD, PhD). The growing population of obese individuals and the plethora of evidence that it is associated with chronic disease has motivated intense research on the subject and resulted in obesity as a specialty in nutritional medicine. Obesity meets the criteria to be classified as a "disease," which has made it reimbursable by insurance companies for medical treatment, and in many cases, for nutritional management by Registered Dietitian Nutritionists.

TABLE 20.1 The Story of George L. Blackburn, MD, PhD

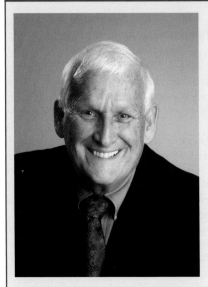

The evolution of the field of obesity and nutritional medicine and the premise on which we practice as nutrition professionals today is largely based upon the countless research and scientific findings and the decades of contributions from the work of George L. Blackburn, MD, PhD.

Dr. Blackburn was born in McPherson, Kansas, and attended the University of Kansas, where he received his baccalaureate degree in chemistry and doctor of medicine degree. After completing his surgical internship and residency at the Fifth Harvard Surgical Service, Boston City Hospital, he attended the Massachusetts Institute of Technology where he received his PhD in nutritional biochemistry. His thesis was entitled "A New Concept and Its Application for Protein-Sparing Therapies During Semistarvation." This research was the foundation for Dr. Blackburn's milestone studies identifying the high prevalence of protein-calorie malnutrition in general surgical and medical patients. Dr. Blackburn was among the very first to recognize that up to 50% of hospitalized medical and surgical patients suffered from moderate to severe malnutrition. To address these challenges, he pioneered the formulation of intravenous hyperalimentation and introduced some of the first novel disease-specific formulas. It was then, at the New England Deaconess Hospital, Harvard Medical School, that he established the first multidisciplinary nutrition support service in the world, for the safe delivery of total parenteral nutrition. Dr. Blackburn always felt that building bridges and bringing minds together among health care professionals to share knowledge and ideas would lead to the most successful patient outcomes.

Dr. Blackburn, along with Harvard colleague Bruce Bistrian, MD, PhD, was the first to demonstrate that it was possible during weight loss to promote the loss of body fat while preserving lean tissue. The work of Dr. Blackburn's research on amino acid therapy as a means of preserving lean tissue during times of stress and starvation evolved into his development of the protein-sparing modified fast diet, and the first carefully regimented medically supervised weight loss program of its kind.

Dr. Blackburn was the first surgeon in New England to perform a Roux-en-Y gastric bypass for morbidly obese patients in 1973. He formed a multidisciplinary team to care for his weight loss surgery patients—similar to the nutrition support service. In 2004 and 2009 he organized and chaired the first evidence-based guidelines for weight loss surgery, catalyzing the formation of accreditation bodies and standards for certification of weight loss surgery centers and providers across the United States.

Dr. Blackburn was a founder of the American Society for Parenteral and Enteral Nutrition and served as its second president. He played a key role in the development of the North American Association for the Study of Obesity— now the Obesity Society. He was a member of the Beth Israel Deaconess Medical Center Department of Surgery for 45 years. He established and, for 25 years, directed the Harvard Medical School CME course "Practical Approaches to the Treatment of Obesity"—which is now the Harvard "Blackburn Course in Obesity Medicine." He authored over 400 original peer-reviewed research publications, nine books, and hundreds of educational documents, guidelines, and reports. Throughout his career, he taught hundreds of medical students, residents, postdoctoral research fellows, registered dietitians, dietetic technicians, nurses, and pharmacists who practice his teachings around the world. In 1992 Dr. Blackburn was nominated for and selected as an honorary member of the American Dietetic Association—now the Academy of Nutrition and Dietetics.

Inseparable from his efforts for over four decades to expand our knowledge in nutrition and metabolism was Dr. Blackburn's identification and unceasing support of the critical role the dietitian plays in patient management. During his lifetime, Dr. Blackburn elevated dietitians as "nutrition experts". He stressed that the role of the registered dietitian was to assess and monitor nutrition status; provide nutrition counseling, care, and therapy; and is the obvious liaison between medical professionals and health care providers. The central role of the dietitian on Dr. Blackburn's nutrition teams was a model that influenced physicians and administrators and other health care professionals to follow suit, opening doors for dietitians everywhere.

Shortly after Dr. Blackburn's death in 2017, Caroline Apovian, MD, Professor of Medicine and Pediatrics, Boston University School of Medicine, and 2018 president of the Obesity Society, reflected on Dr. Blackburn's tremendous accomplishments during an interview. She said, "George Blackburn was truly the father of nutrition and obesity medicine. His energy and enthusiasm were incredible. He is someone who not only encouraged me to do my best work, but also countless other colleagues and friends. He was a great man whom I and many others will deeply miss."

Many thanks to Barb Ainsley, DTR, Administrative Associate and former Administrative Assistant to Dr. George Blackburn, Center for the Study of Nutrition Medicine, Feihe Nutrition Lab, Beth Israel New England Deaconess Medical Center, Boston, for her assistance in preparation of this section.

George L. Blackburn, MD, PhD, "Father of Nutritional and Obesity Medicine" (1936-2017)
by Barbara Ainsley, DTR and Lucinda K. Lysen, RDN, RN, BSN

BODY WEIGHT COMPONENTS

Body weight often is described in terms of its composition, and different models have been advanced to estimate body fat. Assessment of body composition is discussed in detail in Chapter 5. Traditionally, a two-compartment model divides the body into fat mass, the fat from all body sources including the brain, skeleton, intramuscular fat, and adipose tissue, and fat-free mass (FFM), which includes water, protein, and mineral components (Fig. 20.1). The proportions of FFM are relatively constant from person to person.

Although *FFM* often is used interchangeably with the term lean body mass, it is not exactly the same. Lean body mass (LBM) includes water, bones, organs and skeletal muscle. LBM is higher in men than in women and represents the largest component of resting metabolic rate (RMR). Minimizing the loss of LBM is desirable during the weight loss process. Water, which makes up 60% to 65% of body weight, is the most variable component of LBM, and the state of hydration can induce fluctuations of several pounds.

Body Fat

Total body fat is the combination of "essential" and "storage" fats, usually expressed as a percentage of total body weight that is associated with optimum health. Muscle and even skeletal mass adjust to some extent to support the burden of excess adipose tissue.

Essential fat, necessary for normal physiologic functioning, is stored in small amounts in the bone marrow, heart, lung, liver, spleen, kidneys, muscles, and the nervous system. In men, approximately 3% of body fat is essential. In women, essential fat is higher (12%) because it includes body fat in the breasts, pelvic regions, and thighs that supports the reproductive process.

Storage fat is the energy reserve, primarily as triglycerides (TGs), in adipose tissue. This fat accumulates under the skin and around the internal organs to protect them from trauma. Most storage fat is "expendable." The fat stores in adipocytes are capable of extensive variation. This allows for the changing requirements of growth, reproduction, aging, environmental and physiologic circumstances, the availability of food, and the demands of physical activity. Total body fat (essential fat plus storage fat) as a percentage of body weight associated with the average individual is between 18% and 24% for men and 25% and 31% for women. On the other extreme, "elite fit" men are as low as 2% to 5% body fat and women 10% to 13%.

Adipose Tissue Composition

Adipose tissue exerts a profound influence on whole-body homeostasis. Adipose tissue is located primarily under the skin, in the mesenteries

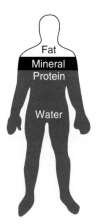

Fig. 20.1 The components of fat-free mass in the body.

and omentum, and behind the peritoneum. This is often referred to as visceral adipose tissue (VAT). Although it is primarily fat, adipose tissue also contains small amounts of protein and water. White adipose tissue (WAT) stores energy as a repository for TGs, cushions abdominal organs, and insulates the body to preserve heat. Carotene gives WAT a slight yellow color. Small amounts of brown adipose tissue (BAT) can be found in a substantial proportion of adults as well as in infants. Unlike WAT, BAT is made of small droplets and many more iron containing mitochondria, which makes it brown. In adults BAT is activated via cold exposure helping to regulate body temperature, however BAT is not activated in thermoneutral conditions. A general activation of BAT continues to interest drug manufactures as a potential obesity therapy, but for the present BAT plays only a minor part in human energy metabolism (Tam et al, 2012).

Adipocyte Size and Number

The mature fat cell (adipocyte) consists of a large central lipid droplet surrounded by a thin rim of cytoplasm, which contains the nucleus and the mitochondria. These cells can store fat equal to 80% to 95% of their volume. Gains in weight and adipose tissue occur by increasing the number of cells, adding the size of cells as lipid, or a combination of the two.

Hyperplasia (increased number of cells) occurs as a normal growth process during infancy and adolescence. Cell number increases in lean and obese children into adolescence, but the number increases faster in obese children. In teens and adults, increases in fat cell size are more common, but hyperplasia also can occur after the fat content of existing cells has reached capacity.

During normal growth, the greatest percentage of body fat (approximately 25%) is set by 6 months of age. In lean children, fat cell size then decreases; this decrease does not occur in obese children. At the age of 6 years in lean children, adiposity rebound occurs, especially in girls, with an increase in body fat. An early adiposity rebound occurring before 5 ½ years old is predictive of a higher level of adiposity at 16 years of age and in adulthood; a period of later rebound is correlated with healthy adult weight (Hughes et al, 2014).

With hypertrophy (increased cell size), fat depots can expand as much as 1000 times at any age, as long as space is available. In a classic study, Björntorp and Sjöström (1971) demonstrated, using weight loss as a result of trauma, illness, or starvation, that fat cell size decreases but cell numbers remain the same.

Fat Storage

Most stored fat comes directly from dietary TGs. The fatty acid composition of adipose tissue mirrors the fatty acid composition of the diet. Even excess dietary carbohydrate and protein are converted to fatty acids in the liver by the comparatively inefficient process of lipogenesis. Under conditions of relative energy balance, little dietary carbohydrate is converted to fat for storage. In conditions of positive energy balance, carbohydrate oxidation increases while TGs are preferentially stored and de novo-lipogenesis from carbohydrate occurs when more carbohydrate is present than can be either oxidized or stored as (liver or muscle) glycogen (Song et al, 2018).

Semivolatile organic compounds (SVOCs) accumulate in adipose tissues from exposure to toxins, chemicals, and pesticides. When adipose tissue is mobilized during weight loss, SVOCs are released (see *Clinical Insight:* What's in That Fat When You Lose It?). The effect of SVOCs on the developing fetal brain is not yet known (see Chapter 14), which adds to the health concern about obese pregnant women who lose weight.

What's in That Fat When You Lose It?

The role of toxins in obesity development and later fat loss is becoming increasingly concerning as the emerging evidence forms a plausible link between toxins and obesity. Exposure to toxins comes from two main sources: the environment (external or exogenous toxins), which includes environmental pollutants such as pesticides, industrial compounds, solvents, detergents, plasticizers, cosmetic additives, chemical additives, colorings, preservatives, flavorings, microbial toxins such as aflatoxins from peanuts, mycotoxins from molds, and bisphenol-A found in plastic baby bottles, toys, and especially dental sealants; and "lifestyle chemicals," such as alcohol, over-the-counter (OTC) drugs, and prescription drugs. It can be byproducts from food preparation such as acrylamide from French fries, nitrosamines from cold cuts and sausages, polycyclic aromatic hydrocarbons (PCAHs) from charbroiled meats, trans fats from partial hydrogenation of fats and advanced glycosylated end products (AGEs) in foods in which the glucose molecule is brought to high temperatures. Toxins can also originate from the gut (i.e., breakdown products of metabolism, including hormones, internal toxins such as metabolites of yeast [d-arabinitol], or gut bacteria).

Studies show that these toxins, which are often fat soluble and have an affinity for adipose tissue, are often stored in the body's depot fat. Their presence is linked to inflammation, development of type 2 diabetes, and a suppressed resting metabolic rate (post-weight loss). In the case of weight or fat loss, the release of these toxins can interfere with the body's functioning, placing a burden on the liver and even its ability to continue to lose more fat (La Merrill et al, 2013; Lee et al, 2018; Tremblay et al, 2004).

With increasing exposure, toxins may alter metabolism, disrupt endocrine function, damage the mitochondria, increase inflammation and oxidative stress, lower thyroid hormones, and alter circadian rhythms and the autonomic nervous system. These all interfere with key weight control mechanisms in the body. Using a comprehensive approach to obesity, including the assessment and treatment of toxin-mediated effects, may result in more effective body fat and weight management. Lifestyle modifications may be helpful, including reducing exposure to toxins and supporting mobilization and elimination of stored and external toxins; however, the specific mechanisms of support, including promoting normoglycemia and ingestion of cruciferous vegetables and fibrous foods, are still under investigation (Lee et al, 2017).

Sheila Dean, DSc, RDN, LDN, CCN, IFMCP

Lipoprotein Lipase

Dietary TG is transported to the liver by chylomicrons. Endogenous TGs synthesized in the liver from free fatty acids (FFA) travel as part of very-low-density lipoprotein particles. The enzyme **lipoprotein lipase (LPL)** moves lipid from the blood into the adipose cell by hydrolyzing TGs into FFA and glycerol. Glycerol proceeds to the liver; fatty acids enter the adipocyte and are reesterified into TGs. When needed by other cells, TGs are hydrolyzed once again to fatty acids and glycerol by **hormone-sensitive lipase (HSL)** within the adipose cell; they then are released into the circulation.

Hormones affect LPL activity in different adipose tissue regions. Estrogens stimulate LPL activity in the gluteofemoral adipocytes, and thus promote fat storage in this area for childbearing and lactation. In the presence of sex steroid hormones, a normal distribution of body fat exists. With a decrease in sex steroid hormones—as occurs with menopause or gonadectomy—central obesity tends to develop.

REGULATION OF BODY WEIGHT

Body weight is the product of genetic effects (DNA), epigenetic effects (heritable traits that do not involve changes in DNA), and the environment (Kaplan, 2018). Body weight regulation is usually described in terms of a homeostatic biological feedback system acting on energy intake and energy expenditure to maintain or "defend" a stable body weight. Similarly, **set point theory** originally arose to explain the intractable tendency to regain weight after weight loss. Body weight regulation is asymmetric in that there is little defense against weight gain while conversely both hunger and adaptations in various components of energy expenditure can make weight loss harder.

Observational studies do not provide consistent evidence for a biological control of body weight (Müller et al, 2018). While the complete picture of body weight regulation is not clear, much of what is known falls into the realm of appetite regulation. Adaptation to energy restriction (a drop in RMR beyond what is expected from changes in body weight and composition) is well known, but highly variable and less understood.

Because the precision of appetite control is undermined in the prevailing obesogenic environment that includes psychosocial, behavioral, and environmental factors that affect eating behavior (and therefore energy intake), new models of body weight regulation which also address these missing factors have been called for (Belfort-DeAguiar and Seo, 2018; Hall et al, 2014).

Hunger, Appetite, and Satiety

Satiety is associated with the postprandial state when excess food is being stored. Hunger is associated with the postabsorptive state when those stores are being mobilized. Physical triggers for hunger are much stronger than those for satiety, which external cues for eating can override.

When either overfeeding or underfeeding occurs in children they exhibit spontaneous **hypophagia** (undereating) or **hyperphagia** (overeating) accordingly. Adults, however, are less consistent in naturally compensating for overeating, which can result in body weights slowly creeping up over time. Unexplained weight loss in adults is often a symptom of other factors including stress or underlying disease. See *Focus On: Signals from a Host of Hormones* and Table 20.2 for further information and detail on the neurochemicals and hormones involved in appetite and satiety.

Metabolic Rate and Voluntary Activity

The RMR (see Chapter 2) explains 60% to 70% of total energy expenditure. RMR declines with age. When the body is deprived of adequate energy from starvation or voluntary energy restriction, RMR drops, therefore conserving energy. The more severe the energy restriction, the greater the potential reduction in RMR; up to 15% with very-low-calorie diets (VLCDs). This suppression of RMR is beyond what is attributable to weight loss (which consists of both LBM and fat mass) and is a form of adaptation to energy scarcity. Most but not all reviews of the subject find RMR normalizes post-weight loss with maintenance level energy intakes (Ostendorf et al, 2018). Ongoing suppression of RMR may result from extreme approaches to weight loss.

Activity thermogenesis (AT) is the energy expended in voluntary activity, the most variable component of energy expenditure. Under normal circumstances physical activity accounts for 15% to 30% of total energy expenditure. **Nonexercise activity thermogenesis (NEAT)** is the energy expended for all activity that is not sleeping, eating, or sports-like exercise. It includes going to work, typing, doing yard work, toe-tapping, even fidgeting (see Chapter 2). NEAT varies as much as 2000 kcal/day between individuals, and it has been theorized to have untapped potential value in weight management. Proponents of NEAT

TABLE 20.2   Regulatory Factors Involved in Eating and Weight Management

Brain Neurotransmitters	Characteristics and Function
Norepinephrine and dopamine	Released by the sympathetic nervous system (SNS) in response to dietary intake; mediates the activity of areas in the hypothalamus that govern feeding behavior. Fasting and semistarvation lead to decreased SNS activity and increased adrenal medullary activity with a consequent increase in epinephrine, which fosters substrate mobilization. Dopaminergic pathways in the brain play a role in the reinforcement properties of food.
Serotonin, neuropeptide Y, and endorphins	Decreases in serotonin and increases in neuropeptide Y have been associated with an increase in carbohydrate appetite. Neuropeptide Y increases during food deprivation; it may be a factor leading to an increase in appetite after dieting. Preferences and cravings for sweet, high-fat foods observed among obese and bulimic patients involve the endorphin system.
CRF Orexin (hypocretin)	Involved in controlling adrenocorticotropic hormone release from the pituitary gland; CRF is a potent anorexic agent and weakens the feeding response produced by norepinephrine and neuropeptide Y. CRF is released during exercise. Orexin is a neurotransmitter produced by the hypothalamus that has a weak resemblance to secretin produced in the gut and is an appetite stimulant and central regulator of glucose and energy homeostasis.

Gut Hormones	Characteristics and Function
Incretins	Gastrointestinal peptides increase the amount of insulin released from the beta cells of the pancreas after eating, even before blood glucose levels become elevated. They also slow the rate of absorption by reducing gastric emptying and may directly reduce food intake. Incretins also inhibit glucagon release from the alpha cells of the pancreas. (See GLP-1 and GIP.)
CCK	Released by the intestinal tract when fats and proteins reach the small intestine, receptors for CCK have been found in the gastrointestinal tract and the brain. CCK causes the gallbladder to contract and stimulates the pancreas to release enzymes. At the brain level, CCK inhibits food intake.
Bombesin	Released by enteric neurons; reduces food intake and enhances the release of CCK.
Enterostatin	A portion of pancreatic lipase involved specifically with satiety after the consumption of fat.
Adiponectin	An adipocytokine secreted by the adipose tissue that modulates glucose regulation and fatty acid catabolism. Levels of this hormone are inversely correlated with BMI. The hormone plays a role in metabolic disorders such as type 2 diabetes, obesity, and atherosclerosis. Levels drop after gastric bypass surgery for up to 6 months.
Glucagon	Increased secretion of glucagon is caused by hypoglycemia, increased levels of norepinephrine and epinephrine, increased plasma amino acids, and cholecystokinin. Decreased secretion of glucagon occurs when insulin or somatostatin is released.
Apolipoprotein A-IV	Synthesized and secreted by the intestine during lymphatic secretion of chylomicrons. After entering the circulation, a small portion of apolipoprotein A-IV enters the CNS and suppresses food consumption.
Fatty acids	Free fatty acids, triglycerides, and glycerol are factors that also affect uptake of glucose by peripheral tissues.
GLP-1 and GIP	Released by intestinal mucosa in the presence of meals rich in glucose and fat; stimulate insulin synthesis and release; GLP-1 decreases glucagon secretion, delays gastric emptying time, and may promote satiety; examples of incretin hormones.
Insulin	Acts in the CNS and the peripheral nervous system to regulate food intake and is involved in the synthesis and storage of fat. It is possible that obese persons with insulin resistance or deficiency have a defective glucose disposal system and a depressed level of thermogenesis. The greater the insulin resistance, the lower the thermic effect of food. Fasting insulin levels increase proportionally with the degree of obesity; however, many obese persons have insulin resistance because of a lack of response by insulin receptors, impaired glucose tolerance, and associated hyperlipidemia. These sequelae can usually be corrected with weight loss.
Leptin	An adipocytokine secreted by the adipose tissue, correlated with percent of body fat. Primary signal from energy stores; in obesity loses the ability to inhibit energy intake or to increase energy expenditure. Compared with men, women have significantly higher concentrations of serum leptin.
Resistin	An adipocytokine expressed primarily in adipocytes; antagonizes insulin action.
Ghrelin	Produced primarily by the stomach; acts on the hypothalamus to stimulate hunger and feeding. Ghrelin levels are highest in lean individuals and lowest in the obese. Increased levels are seen in people who are dieting, and suppressed levels are noted after gastric bypass, possibly counteracted by adiponectin.
PYY$_{3-36}$	Secreted by endocrine cells lining the small bowel and colon in response to food; a "middle man" in appetite management. PYY seems to work opposite from ghrelin; it induces satiety.
IL-6 and TNF-α	Both are gut hormones. Cytokines secreted by adipose tissue and participate in metabolic events. Impair insulin signals in muscle and liver. Levels are proportional to body fat mass (Thomas and Schauer, 2010).
Oxyntomodulin	Secreted from L-cells in small intestine in response to a meal. Exerts its biologic effects through activation of GLP-1 and glicentin-related pancreatic peptide (GRPP) (Bray and Bouchard, 2014).

TABLE 20.2   Regulatory Factors Involved in Eating and Weight Management—cont'd

Brain Neurotransmitters	Characteristics and Function
GLP-2	Produced in the L-cells of small intestines and in neurons of CNS. Is an intestinal growth factor. Inhibits gastric emptying and acid secretion while stimulating intestinal blood flow. Decreases gastric acid secretion and gastric emptying and increases mucosal growth (Bray and Bouchard, 2014).
FGF-21	Expressed in the liver and secreted mainly during fasting and after feeding a ketogenic diet. Can decrease body weight without affecting food intake. Increases insulin sensitivity, decreases gluconeogenesis, and increases glucose uptake in adipocytes (Bray and Bouchard, 2014).
Other Hormones	**Characteristics and Function**
Thyroid hormones	Modulate the tissue responsiveness to the catecholamines secreted by the SNS. A decrease in triiodothyronine lowers the response to SNS activity and diminishes adaptive thermogenesis. Women should be tested for hypothyroidism, particularly after menopause. Weight regain after weight loss may be a function of a hypometabolic state; energy restriction produces a transient, hypothyroid, hypometabolic state.
Visfatin	An adipocytokine protein secreted by visceral adipose tissue that has an insulin-like effect; plasma levels increase with increasing adiposity and insulin resistance.
Adrenomedullin	A new regulatory peptide secreted by adipocytes as a result of inflammatory processes.

BMI, Body mass index; *CCK*, cholecystokinin; *CNS*, central nervous system; *CRF*, corticotropin-releasing factor; *GIP*, glucose-dependent insulinotropic peptide; *GLP-1*, glucagon-like peptide 1; *IL-6*, interleukin-6; PYY_{3-36}, peptide YY3-36; *SNS*, sympathetic nervous system; *TNF-α*, tumor necrosis.
Thomas S, Schauer P: Bariatric surgery and the gut hormone response, *Nutr Clin Pract* 25:175, 2010; Bray GA, Bouchard C: *Handbook of obesity*, ed 3, Boca Raton, Fla, 2014, CRC Press.

suggest standing and ambulating for 2.5 hours per day, and reengineering work, school, and home environments to support a more active lifestyle (Garland et al, 2011). However, passive compensation, by reducing other forms of physical activity, may prove to balance off increases in NEAT (O'Neal et al, 2017) and there is presently no evidence showing that strategies promoting NEAT are effective for weight loss or obesity treatment (Chung et al, 2018).

◎ FOCUS ON

Signals from a Host of Hormones

A host of hormones—insulin, leptin, adiponectin, and ghrelin, among others—communicate with the hypothalamus to regulate a person's food intake. These regulatory hormones govern feeding in response to signals originated in affected body tissues.

Insulin controls the amount of glucose in the blood by moving it into the cells for energy. **Leptin**, which is produced mainly by fat cells, contributes to long-term fullness by sensing the body's overall energy stores. Adiponectin is also made by fat cells and helps the body respond better to insulin by boosting metabolism. **Ghrelin**, the hunger hormone, tells the brain when the stomach is empty, prompting hunger pangs.

The stomach communicates with the brain via the **vagus nerve**, part of the autonomic nervous system that travels from the brain to the stomach. When filled with food or liquid, the stomach's stretch receptors send a message to the brain indicating satiety (Guo et al, 2018). Gastric bypass surgery reduces the stomach to the size of an egg, and triggers a sharp drop in ghrelin levels, which lessens hunger and oral intake. Traditional dieting, however, tends to boost ghrelin levels.

OVERWEIGHT AND OBESITY

Overweight and obesity occur as a result of an imbalance between total energy intake (food and beverages consumed) and total energy expenditure. Despite this seemingly straightforward model, the factors which act to dysregulate energy balance are complex. Lifestyle, environmental, and genetic factors have a multifaceted interaction with psychological, cultural, and physiologic influences. Over the years, many hypotheses have evolved however no single theory can completely explain all manifestations of obesity or apply consistently to all persons.

Prevalence

The United States leads the world as far as the total number of persons with obesity. When looked at as a percentage of the population however, the United States ranks 19th after the Oceania Islands, the Middle East, and South America. According to the World Health Organization (WHO), worldwide obesity has nearly tripled since 1975 (WHO, 2018).

In the United States the estimates of overweight and obesity among adults and children are based on measured weights and heights from the National Health and Nutrition Examination Survey (NHANES), conducted by the National Center for Health Statistics, Centers for Disease Control and Prevention (CDC) (Figs. 20.2 and 20.3). The 2015–2016 NHANES findings were that the prevalence of obesity was 39.8% in adults and 18.5% in youth. The prevalence of obesity remains higher among African American and Hispanic populations. The prevalence of obesity by state (based on the ongoing Behavioral Risk Factor Surveillance Study and published by the CDC) can be seen in Fig. 20.4.

ELEMENTS OF ENERGY BALANCE DYSREGULATION

Genetics

With the exception of rare monogenic types of obesity (as in Prader-Willi's syndrome and Bardet-Biedl's syndrome), more and more research shows that the development of obesity involves a complex interaction with numerous genetic variants and environmental factors related to energy intake and expenditure (Goodarzi, 2018). Hormonal and neural factors involved in weight regulation include short-term and long-term "signals" that determine satiety and feeding activity. Small defects in their expression or interaction may contribute significantly to weight gain. **Nutritional genomics** is the study of the

---

✳ NEW DIRECTIONS

Partnership for a Healthier America Addressing Childhood Obesity

Because the number of obese children in the United States has tripled since 1980, and obesity now rivals smoking as the largest cause of preventable death and disease, a foundation was launched in the spring of 2010 to address this serious epidemic of childhood obesity. This foundation, Partnership for a Healthier America, has as its mission the simple concept that children should have good, nutritious food to eat and the chance to be physically active every day to become healthy adults.

The objectives of the partnership are to support the national goal of solving the childhood obesity challenge "within a generation" set by former First Lady Michelle Obama, who historically has served as Honorary Chairperson of the organization. The Partnership brings together the public and private sectors, organizations, business and thought leaders, the media, and states and local communities to make meaningful and measurable commitments for fighting childhood obesity. The plan has four pillars:

* Offering parents the tools and information they need to make healthy choices for their children
* Introducing healthier food into the nation's schools
* Ensuring that all families have access to healthy, affordable food in their communities
* Increasing opportunities for children to be physically active, both in and out of school

The partnership aims to support, unite, and inspire families from every corner of the United States to implement and sustain the four-pillar plan.

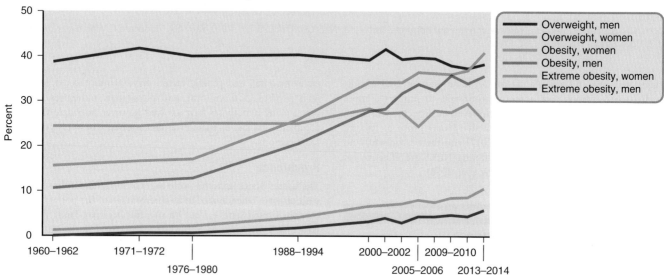

NOTES: Age-adjusted by the direct method to the year 2000 U.S. Census Bureau estimates using age groups 20–39, 40–59, and 60–74.
Overweight is body mass index (BMI) of 25 kg/m² or greater but less than 30 kg/m²; obesity is BMI greater than or equal to 30; and extreme obesity is BMI greater than or equal to 40. Pregnant females were excluded from the analysis.
SOURCES: NCHS, National Health Examination Survey and National Health and Nutrition Examination Surveys.

Fig. 20.2 Trends in adult overweight, obesity, and extreme obesity among men and women aged 20–74; United States 1960–1962 through 2013–2014.

interactions between dietary components and the instructions in a cell or genome, and the resulting changes in metabolites that affect gene expression (Camp and Trujillo, 2014) (see Chapter 6).

The number and size of fat cells, regional distribution of body fat, and RMR also are influenced by genes. Studies of twins confirm that genes determine 50% to 70% of the predisposition to obesity. Although numerous genes are involved, several have received much attention—the *Ob* gene, the *adiponectin (ADIPOQ)* gene, the "fat mass and obesity associated" gene or *FTO* gene, and the *beta3-adrenoreceptor* gene. The *Ob* gene produces leptin (Ferguson, 2010). The *beta3-adrenoreceptor* gene, located primarily in the adipose tissue, is thought to regulate RMR and fat oxidation in humans.

Nutritional and/or lifestyle choices can either activate or inhibit these obesity-triggering genes. Thus the formula for successful long-term weight management could necessitate the behavioral application of individual genetics. Genetic research is currently drawing significant attention from private interests invested in capitalizing on genetic-based "individualized medicine and nutrition" (Loos, 2018). Despite hundreds of "obesity genes" having been identified, however, we are only at the point of being able to apply genetic information to a few individual treatments. One such treatment is congenital leptin deficiency, which can be treated with daily injections of recombinant human leptin (Choquet, 2011). Well known obesity researcher Claude Bouchard, PhD, recently explained that regardless of the growing body of genetic research, "it is hard to see how we can [yet] anchor a prevention or treatment strategy on our genes," and that, "despite all the noise surrounding this [obesity gene] issue, it still comes down to changing your behavior. It's diet and exercise" (Endocrine Today, 2018) (see *Clinical Insight:* Randomized Controlled Trial Matching Diet to Genetic Predisposition Fails to Improve Weight Loss).

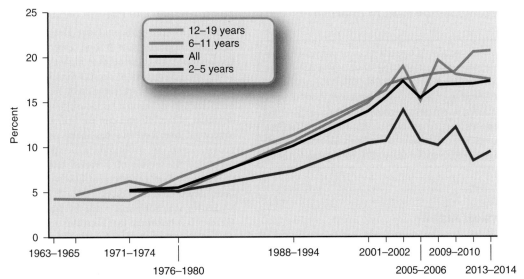

Trends in obesity among children and adolescents aged 2–19 years, by age: United States, 1963–1965 through 2013–2014

NOTES: Obesity is defined as body mass index (BMI) greater than or equal to the 95th percentile from the sex-specific BMI-for-age 2000 CDC Growth Charts.
SOURCES: NCHS, National Health Examination Surveys II (ages 6–11) and III (ages 12–17); and National Health and Nutrition Examination Surveys (NHANES) I–III, and NHANES 1999–2000, 2001–2002, 2003–2004, 2005–2006, 2007–2008, 2009–2010, 2011–2012, and 2013–2014.

Fig. 20.3 Trends in children and adolescents aged 2–19 years, by age: United States, 1963–1965 through 2013–2014.

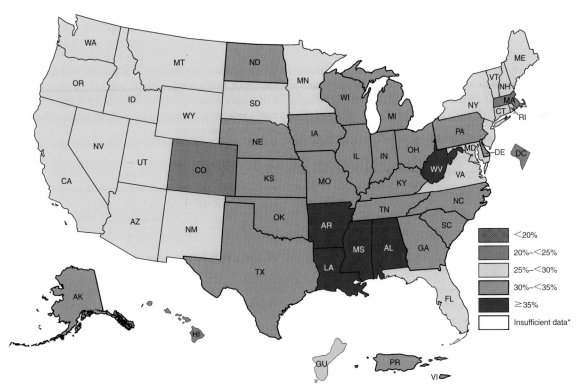

Fig. 20.4 CDC Obesity Prevalence Map Prevalence of obesity among U.S. adults in 2017. (Centers for Disease Control and Prevention [CDC] Behavioral Risk Factor Surveillance System Survey, 2017.)

CLINICAL INSIGHT

Randomized Controlled Trial Matching Diet to Genetic Predisposition Fails to Improve Weight Loss

The first randomized controlled trial (RCT) to test if genetic predisposition improved weight loss in response to a healthy low-fat vs. healthy high-fat diet showed no difference in weight loss (Gardner et al, 2018). Will personalized medicine and nutrition eventually become the prevailing approach to treatment of disease—including overweight and obesity? This almost certainly will be the case. However, according to a number of scientific papers, the hype surrounding personalized medicine using nutritional genomics remains ahead of the science (Caulfield, 2015; Endocrine Today, 2018; Mozaffarian, 2016).

Inadequate Physical Activity

The view that inactivity is a major factor in the development of overweight and obesity is debated. It is true that lack of regular physical activity is a fact for Americans of all ages. Only 21% of adults meet the recommended levels of weekly physical activity (150 minutes per week of moderate-intensity aerobic activity and two sessions of muscle strengthening) for general health. Meanwhile 250 to 300 minutes of moderate-intensity aerobic activity per week is recommended for weight loss and weight loss maintenance (Chin et al, 2016). However, researchers pushing back on the physical activity emphasis point out that "you can't outrun a bad diet," and argue that avoiding sugary drinks, fast food, and overeating in general will save far more calories than people will expend hitting weekly physical activity targets (Fulton, 2016; Malhotra et al, 2015).

Medication Usage and Weight Gain

Although weight gain can be due to disease, clinicians also should consider the possibility that the patient's medication may be contributing. Diabetes medications, thyroid hormone replacement, psychotropics, antidepressants, steroids, and antihypertensive medications can be problematic. The use of such medications must be considered carefully, and alternatives with less deleterious effects selected when possible (Appendix 13).

Sleep, Stress, and Circadian Rhythms

Lack of adequate sleep alters the endocrine regulation of hunger and appetite. Hormones that affect appetite are activated and may promote excessive energy intake. Recurrent sleep deprivation can modify the amount, composition, and distribution of food intake and may be contributing to the obesity epidemic. It is estimated that more than 50 million Americans suffer from sleep deprivation. Others may have shift work or exposure to bright light at night, increasing the disruption of circadian rhythms and enhancing the prevalence of obesity (Garaulet et al, 2013).

There is also a relationship between inadequate sleep, disrupted circadian rhythm, genes, and the development of metabolic syndrome. Stress is another factor. The adrenal hormone cortisol is released when an individual is under stress. Cortisol stimulates insulin release to maintain blood glucose levels in the "fight-or-flight" response; increased appetite eventually follows. Chronic stress with constantly elevated cortisol levels can also lead to appetite changes.

Cortisol levels are typically high in the early morning and low around midnight. Individuals with night-eating syndrome (NES) may have a delayed circadian rhythm of meal intake due to genetically programmed neuroendocrine factors, including altered cortisol levels (Stunkard and Lu, 2010).

Taste, Satiety, and Portion Sizes

Food and its taste elements evoke pleasure responses. The endless variety and reasonable cost of food (especially highly processed food) in the United States contributes to higher calorie intake; people eat more when offered a variety of choices than when a single food is available. Normally, as foods are consumed, they become less desirable; this phenomenon is known as sensory-specific satiety. The opposite situation is the "all-you-can-eat buffet," in which the diner reaches satiety for one food but has many choices remaining for the next course. From an evolutionary perspective sensory-specific satiety promoted the intake of a varied and nutritionally balanced diet; the modern food environment however provides too many (energy-dense, low-nutrient) choices.

Leptin is a hormone, made by fat cells, that decreases appetite. Ghrelin is a hormone that increases appetite in response to the time elapsed since the last meal. Levels of leptin, the appetite suppressor, are lower in individuals with a lower body weight and higher in the obese because they correlate to one's total adipose tissue. However, for reasons yet to be elucidated, people with obesity are seemingly resistant to the appetite-suppressing effects of leptin and are sometimes referred to as leptin resistant.

Passive overeating is partly the result of excessive portion sizes that are now accepted as normal. The portions and calories that restaurants and fast-food outlets commonly serve in one meal can often exceed a person's energy needs for the entire day.

Obesogens

Endocrine disrupting chemicals (EDCs) are exogenous chemicals that can interfere with any aspect of hormone action. Most EDCs are persistent organic pollutants (POPs), which are manufactured chemicals in the environment (water, food, and food packaging), that are becoming increasingly implicated in bodyweight dysregulation. The original "obesogen hypothesis" (Grün and Blumberg, 2006) pertained to fetal EDC exposure leading to obesity in later life. Most EDCs are lipophilic and stored in adipose tissue. Some EDCs have 3- to 8-year half-lives in the human body. Higher exposure levels may be associated with insulin resistance, expansion of fat storage, alterations in satiety and appetite regulation, greater reductions in RMR with weight loss, and a lesser increase in RMR with weight gain (Liu, 2018). Examples of suspected obesogens are bisphenol-A (BPA) and phthalates (in food containers and packaging), organochlorine and organophosphate (banned pesticides), and perfluoroalkyl substances (industrial marine applications) (Nappi, 2016). (See *Clinical Insight:* What's in that Fat When You Lose It?)

Viruses and Pathogens

In the last two decades, at least 10 adipogenic pathogens have been identified, including viruses, scrapie agents (spongiform encephalopathies from sheep or goats), bacteria, and gut microflora. Whether "infectobesity" is a relevant contributor to the obesity epidemic remains to be determined. A human adenovirus, adenovirus-36 (Ad-36), is capable of inducing adiposity in experimentally infected animals by increasing the replication, differentiation, lipid accumulation, and insulin sensitivity in fat cells and reducing leptin secretion and expression. A growing number of studies have found higher levels of Ad-36 antibodies in subjects with obesity (Ponterio and Gnessi, 2015). To date, three meta-analyses have shown an association between Ad-36 infection and obesity in both adults and children (Tambo and Pace, 2016).

Gut Microflora and Diet

Researchers studying the microbiome have proposed that the gut may have a bigger role in energy balance than previously thought. A number of theories attempt to explain how this complicated process might work (Krajmalnik-Brown et al, 2012). Essentially, indigestible complex polysaccharides promote and maintain a healthy microbiome. A highly processed-food diet (essentially devoid of indigestible polysaccharides) begins and reinforces a downward spiral of inflammation, increased tendency to store fat, as well as appetite and satiety dysregulation.

Assessment

Overweight and obesity are defined as abnormal or excessive fat accumulation that may impair health (WHO, 2018). Body mass index (BMI) is calculated by the formula: weight (in kilograms)/height (in meters)^2. It is possible to be overweight based on BMI but not be "overfat" or obese. It is also possible to have a healthy BMI but still have excessive body fat. In fact, normal weight obesity (NWO) allows patients at greater risk for cardiovascular disease (CVD) and coronary artery disease (CAD) to go unnoticed by their physicians (Ashraf and Baweja, 2013). These situations occur because BMI is only a proxy for adiposity rather than a direct measurement. However, because BMI is derived from readily available measurements of height and weight it is the most convenient clinical approach to estimate body fat. The National Institutes of Health (NIH) guidelines classify individuals with a BMI of ≥25 as overweight and those with a BMI of ≥30 as obese (Table 20.3). Based on percent body fat content obesity is ≥25% in men and ≥30% in woman. See Chapter 5 for a detailed discussion of body fat assessment.

Because BMI is a crude proxy for body fat, and also fails to account for body fat distribution, morbidity and mortality studies using BMI consistently produce "J" shaped curves, which at first seem to suggest that lower BMIs are as unhealthy as the higher BMIs (class II obesity or above). When waist-to-hip ratio (WHR) or weight-to-height ratio (WHtR) are substituted for BMI however, both demonstrate positive (linear) relationships with mortality (Carmienke et al, 2013). Similarly, A Body Shape Index (ABSI), which incorporates waist circumference (WC) with height and weight into one formula, has also been shown to be a better mortality predictor than BMI alone (Krakauer and Krakauer, 2014).

When WC and percentage of fat are both high, they are significant predictors of heart failure and other risks associated with obesity. WC is a strong correlate of insulin sensitivity index in older adults (Huth et al, 2016). A WHR of more than 0.8 for women and 1 for men is associated with high risk for cardiovascular events. Similarly, WC ≥ 40 inches in men and ≥35 inches in women signifies increased risk, equivalent to a BMI of 25 to 34.

Health Risks and Longevity

In most people, obesity can be viewed as metabolically unhealthy. Chronic diseases such as heart disease, type 2 diabetes, hypertension, stroke, gallbladder disease, infertility, sleep apnea, hormonal cancers, and osteoarthritis tend to worsen as the degree of obesity increases (Fig. 20.5; see Table 20.3).

There is a subset of obese persons who present as metabolically healthy. This subgroup, the metabolically healthy obese (MHO), has appropriate insulin sensitivity and absence of diabetes, dyslipidemia, and hypertension (Boonchaya-anant and Apovian, 2014). There is currently no universal definition of MHO. However, the idea that MHO might be benign and not require treatment is debatable. In long-term follow-up MHO adults were at increased risk for all-cause mortality and CVD (Kramer et al, 2013). Researchers are urging that treatment of MHO not be ignored until metabolic symptoms occur (Atkinson and Macdonald, 2018).

Inflammation

Obesity is now recognized as a chronic and systemic inflammatory disease whereas it was once believed that excess adipose stores were inert. Adipose tissue is involved in the secretion of a wide range of active substances (tumor necrosis factor, interleukin-6, C-reactive protein [CRP], etc.), most but not all (adiponectin) involved in inflammatory actions. The overall result underlies development of hyperlipidemia, metabolic syndrome, diabetes mellitus, muscle protein loss, CVD, stroke, and some cancers (Bueno et al, 2014; Grimble, 2010; Rocha and Folco, 2011).

Irrespective of the growing body of data on the systemic inflammatory systems set off by obesity, the precise trigger is yet to be determined. One theory is that nutrient overload in adipocytes

TABLE 20.3 Classification of Overweight and Obesity

Classification of Overweight and Obesity by BMI, Waist Circumference, and Associated Disease Risk*

Disease Risk* Relative to Normal Weight and Waist Circumference

	BMI (kg/m²)	Obesity Class	Men ≤102 cm (≤40 in) Women ≤ 88 cm (≤ 35 in)	> 102 cm (>40 in) > 88 cm (>35 in)
Underweight	<18.5		—	—
Normal[+]	18.5-24.9		—	—
Overweight	25.0-29.9		Increased	High
Obesity	30.0-34.9	I	High	Very High
	35.0-39.9	II	Very High	Very High
Extreme Obesity	≥40	III	Extremely High	Extremely High

* Disease risk for type 2 diabetes, hypertension, and CVD.
[+] Increased waist circumference can also be a marker for increased risk even in persons of normal weight.
From National Institutes of Health, National Heart, Lung, and Blood Institute: Clinical Guidelines on the Identification, Evaluation, and Treatment of Overweight and Obesity in Adults: Evidence Report, NIH Publication No. 98-4083, 1998.

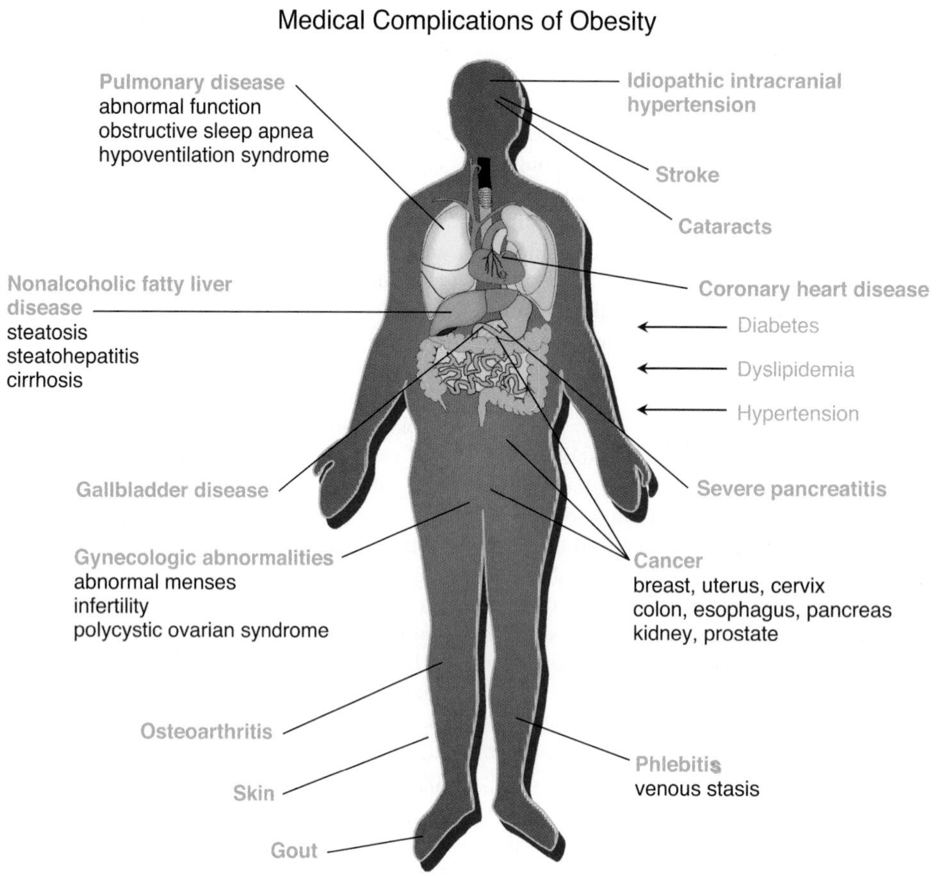

Medical Complications of Obesity

Pulmonary disease
abnormal function
obstructive sleep apnea
hypoventilation syndrome

Idiopathic intracranial hypertension

Stroke

Cataracts

Nonalcoholic fatty liver disease
steatosis
steatohepatitis
cirrhosis

Coronary heart disease

Diabetes

Dyslipidemia

Hypertension

Gallbladder disease

Severe pancreatitis

Gynecologic abnormalities
abnormal menses
infertility
polycystic ovarian syndrome

Cancer
breast, uterus, cervix
colon, esophagus, pancreas
kidney, prostate

Osteoarthritis

Skin

Phlebitis
venous stasis

Gout

Fig. 20.5 The medical complications of obesity are extensive. (Reprinted with permission from Delichatsios HK: Obesity assessment in the primary care office, Harvard Medical School. 23rd Annual International Conference-Practical approaches to the treatment of obesity, Boston, June 18-20 2009).

induces intracellular stress, which results in activation of inflammatory cascades (Ellulu et al, 2017). As discussed earlier, other factors implicated in the development of inflammation include microbiome-derived endotoxins, environmental chemicals, viruses, saturated fats, and chronic overeating. A dietary change to an antiinflammatory diet and regular physical activity can reduce obesity-related inflammation. (For discussion of inflammation, see Chapter 7.)

Nonalcoholic fatty liver disease (NAFLD) is associated with overweight and obesity and may progress to end-stage liver disease (see Chapter 28). Obesity is also a risk factor for various cancers, infertility, poor wound healing, and poor antibody response to hepatitis B vaccine. Thus the costs of obesity are staggering. The CDC estimates the direct cost of care for obesity at $147 billion (CDC, 2008). The Internal Revenue Service issued a rule in 2002 qualifying obesity as a disease, allowing taxpayers to claim weight loss expenses as a medical deduction if undertaken to treat an existing disease.

The U.S. government recognizes the immense effect of obesity on the health and financial well-being of its citizens. Healthy People 2020 objectives also identify the implications of overweight and obesity (see Chapter 8). The objectives include targets to increase the proportion of adults who are at a healthy weight and to reduce the proportion of adults, children, and adolescents who are obese. Overweight adolescents often become obese adults; obese individuals are at increased risk for comorbidities of type 2 diabetes, hypertension, stroke, certain cancers, infertility, and other conditions.

Fat Deposition and the Metabolic Syndrome

Regional patterns of fat deposit are controlled genetically and differ between and among men and women. Two major types of fat deposition are excess subcutaneous truncal-abdominal fat (the apple-shaped android fat distribution) and excess gluteofemoral fat in thighs and buttocks (the pear-shaped gynoid fat distribution). The android shape is more common among men. Gynoid fat deposition in women during child-bearing years is utilized to support the demands of pregnancy and lactation. Women with the gynoid type of obesity do not develop the impairments of glucose metabolism in those with an android deposition (Wajchenberg, 2013). Postmenopausal women more closely follow the male pattern of abdominal fat stores, sometimes referred to as "belly fat."

Abdominal fat is an indicator of fat surrounding internal organs or visceral fat. According to a major study done through the Brigham and Women's Hospital in Boston over 7 years and including more than 3000 people (Framingham Study patients were used), those with higher amounts of abdominal fat, versus fat in other parts of the body, were found to have higher risks of cancer and heart disease (Britton et al, 2013). Many other reputable scientific studies have been performed, validating the findings repeatedly.

Visceral obesity, or excessive VAT under the peritoneum and in the intraabdominal cavity, is correlated highly with insulin resistance and diabetes. Metabolic syndrome (MetS) consists of three or more of the following abnormalities: waist circumference ≥102 cm (40 in) in men and ≥88 cm (35 in) in women, serum TGs ≥150 mg/dL, high-density lipoprotein (HDL) level less than 40 mg/dL in men and less than 50 mg/dL in women, blood pressure 135/85 mm Hg or higher, or fasting glucose 100 mg/dL or higher. Increased visceral fat is a risk factor for CAD, dyslipidemia, hypertension, stroke, type 2 diabetes, and MetS (Wajchenberg, 2013). By the same token, VAT and low cardiorespiratory fitness (CRF) levels are associated with a deteriorated cardiometabolic risk profile. Achieving a low level of VAT and a high level of CRF is an important target for cardiometabolic health.

Weight Discrimination

Widespread bias and discrimination based on weight have been documented in education, employment, and health care. Like other forms of prejudice, this stems from a lack of understanding of the chronic, complex, and sometimes intractable nature of obesity and its medical consequences. The United States is the first (and only) country that currently classifies obesity as a disease; the disease classification was necessary in order for insurance to cover obesity treatment within the U.S. health care system (Müller and Geisler, 2017). The vast majority of the United States does not consider obesity a protected class and therefore weight-based employment discrimination does not have a basis for a legal claim (Pomeranz and Puhl, 2013). Both adults and children with a larger body size experience adverse social, educational, and psychological consequences as a result of weight bias. They also face discrimination from healthcare providers and this can affect their willingness to seek medical care. It is essential to break down the barriers caused by ignorance and indifference. Patient support groups help to correct the negative effect of this type of discrimination.

MANAGEMENT OF OBESITY IN ADULTS

In 1998 the National Heart, Lung, and Blood Institute (NHLBI) in collaboration with National Institute of Diabetes and Digestive and Kidney Diseases (NIDDK) issued the *Clinical Guidelines on the Identification, Evaluation, and Treatment of Overweight and Obesity in Adults: Evidence Report*. It was the first federal clinical practice guidelines to deal with overweight and obesity issues developed using evidence-based medicine methodology. The guidelines provided the scientific evidence behind the recommendations for weight loss and weight loss maintenance as well as practical strategies for implementing the recommendations. The 1998 clinical guidelines were partially updated in 2013 addressing five specific questions and published in three major medical journals (NHLBI, 2014). The five areas addressed in 2013 were as follows: (1) what are the expected health benefits of weight loss as a function of the amount and duration of weight loss, (2) are current WC and BMI cut points appropriate (defined obesity) for certain population subgroups, (3) which diets—among a handful of popular diets—are effective for weight loss, (4) what is the efficacy and effectiveness of comprehensive lifestyle approaches to weight loss and weight loss maintenance, and (5) what is the efficacy and safety of bariatric surgical procedures.

Before the NHLBI evidence report clinicians focused almost entirely on weight loss via caloric restriction, exercise was not routinely recommended, and weight loss maintenance was generally overlooked. The strategies for weight loss (and weight loss maintenance)

analyzed, reviewed, and outlined in the NHLBI report were dietary therapy (CR), physical activity, behavior therapy (self-monitoring, stress management, stimulus control, problem-solving, contingency management, cognitive restructuring, and social support), combined therapy (dietary, physical activity, and behavioral therapies), pharmacotherapy, and surgery. Today, a chronic disease-prevention model incorporates these interdisciplinary therapies and lifestyle interventions from physicians, dietitians, exercise specialists, and behavior therapists.

Goals of Treatment

The goal of obesity treatment is to achieve enough weight loss to significantly improve overall health. Achieving a moderate loss is beneficial. Obese persons who lose 5% to 10% of initial body weight are likely to improve their blood glucose, blood pressure, and cholesterol levels and reduce various markers of systemic inflammation. Since continual, gradual weight gain is the norm, choosing to maintain present body weight is also beneficial (but also requires vigilance and effort).

Despite the recognition that moderate weight loss is beneficial and may be more easily achievable, patients usually have self-defined goal weights that are considerably higher. Therefore health professionals need to encourage their patients to target more realistic initial weight loss goals.

In general, weight loss after age 65 is not advised; actuarial tables show no benefit and possible harm due to loss of LBM. In fact, in the obese older adult, sarcopenia (loss of muscle mass) is the strongest predictor of disability and inability to perform daily activities. A BMI below 23 is considered below desirable in older adults (see Chapter 19).

Rate and Extent of Weight Loss

Reduction of body weight involves the loss of both protein and fat. The relative proportions of each depend on initial body composition and to some degree by the rate of weight reduction. Strength training can help minimize loss of lean tissue in some subjects. Steady weight loss over a longer period favors reduction of fat stores, limits the loss of vital protein tissues, and minimizes the decline in resting energy expenditure (REE) that can accompany severe energy restriction. Recommended calorie deficit guidelines result in a loss of approximately 0.5 to 1 pound per week for persons with a BMI of 27 to 35, and 1 to 2 pounds per week for those with BMIs greater than 35. These energy deficits need to be individually calculated, and continually adjusted with weight loss in order to maintain the targeted calorie deficits and therefore weekly rates of weight loss (Byrne et al, 2012). When these deficits are maintained, they will lead to an approximately 10% weight loss in 6 months (Academy of Nutrition and Dietetics [AND], 2016). For the next 6 months the focus changes from weight loss to weight maintenance. After this phase, further weight loss may be considered.

Even with the same caloric intake, rates of weight reduction vary. Men reduce weight faster than women of similar size because of their higher LBM and RMR. The heavier person expends more energy than one who is less obese and loses faster on a given calorie intake than a lighter person.

Many people who do not lose weight when following a prescribed energy restriction may be consuming more energy than they report and may also overestimate their physical activity levels. Underreporting of energy intake is the norm and is shown to increase with BMI. Underreporting of estimated intake has been extensively studied; it impacts the reliability of epidemiologic studies and creates the illusion of resistance to weight loss during energy restriction (Dhurandhar et al, 2015).

Lifestyle Modification

Behavior modification is the cornerstone of lifestyle intervention. It focuses on restructuring a person's environment, dietary intake, and physical activity by using goal setting, stimulus control, cognitive restructuring, and relapse prevention. It also provides feedback on progress and places the responsibility for change and accomplishment on the patient.

Stimulus control involves identifying stimuli that may encourage incidental eating and identifying and limiting exposure to high-risk situations. Examples of stimulus control strategies include learning to shop carefully for healthy foods, shopping when not hungry, keeping high-calorie foods out of the house, limiting the times and places of eating, and consciously avoiding situations in which overeating occurs.

Problem solving is the process of defining a problem, generating possible solutions, evaluating and choosing the best solution, implementing the new behavior, evaluating outcomes, and reevaluating alternative solutions if needed.

Cognitive restructuring teaches patients to identify, challenge, and correct the negative thoughts that frequently undermine their efforts to lose weight and keep it off. A cognitive therapy program that underscores the inextricable connection between emotions and eating, and how to manage that connection successfully using positive long-term mental strategies, has been developed and found useful (Beck, 2011).

Self-monitoring with daily food and activity records is positively associated with greater weight loss. Adding the place and time of food intake, as well as accompanying thoughts and feelings, adds complexity (which reduces compliance) but may help identify the physical and emotional settings in which eating occurs. Physical activity can be tracked in minutes, miles, or calories expended. Self-monitoring can also provide insight into the occurrence of relapses and how they can be prevented.

A comprehensive program of lifestyle modification produced a loss of approximately 10% of initial weight in 16 to 26 weeks in a review of randomized controlled trials, including the Diabetes Prevention Program. Long-term continued patient-therapist contact significantly improves weight-loss maintenance (AND, 2016).

Email and phone consults appear to be useful methods for contact and support as part of structured behavioral weight loss and weight loss maintenance programs. Multiple strategies for behavior therapy often are needed. Self-monitoring with mobile device apps (see Box 4.5 in Chapter 4), pharmacotherapy, targeted educational interventions from the web, meal replacements, and telephone interventions have taken over the weight loss industry. Body monitoring—a new monitoring method to measure weight change—involves wearing a device that tracks body processes like temperature, movement, acceleration, heating fluctuations, and so on—and records calorie burn. Combined with a food log entered into the system, a person can adjust food intake based upon data provided by the system.

Telehealth programs, which provide interaction with health care professionals through visual and verbal communication via phone and computer screens, are exploding in health care, while saving tremendous costs and time. Telehealth is now being used as an effective vehicle with dietitians for one-on-one and group consults and for providing nutrition education programs.

Dietary Modification Recommendations

Weight loss programs should combine a nutritionally balanced dietary regimen with exercise and lifestyle modification. Selecting the appropriate treatment strategy depends on the goals and health risks of the patient. When these approaches fail to bring about the desired reduction in body fat, sometimes medication may be added. For morbid obesity (BMI ≥40) surgical intervention may be necessary.

Treatment options include the following:
- A balanced reduced-calorie macronutrient adjusted eating plan, increased physical activity, and lifestyle modification
- A balanced reduced-calorie macronutrient adjusted eating plan, increased physical activity, lifestyle modification, and pharmacotherapy
- Surgery plus an individually prescribed eating regimen, physical activity, and lifestyle modification program
- Prevention of weight regain via actively balancing energy intake and output
- Mindset interventions via cognitive restructuring

Restricted-Energy Eating Plan

A balanced, restricted-energy eating plan is the most widely prescribed method of weight reduction. The diet should be nutritionally adequate and meet but not exceed energy needs for weight reduction. A caloric deficit of 500 to 1000 kcal daily usually meets this goal for subjects ≥30 BMI. The prescribed energy level varies with the individual's body size and activities. For example, for a 500-calorie deficit the initial daily energy prescription for a 5′5″, age 35, 30-BMI female would be approximately 1400 calories, or approximately 1700 calories for a 40-BMI female of the same height and age. Regardless of the level of CR, healthful eating and regular physical activity should be daily goals. All means possible (coaching, motivational interviewing, cognitive restructuring, etc.) should be utilized by the health care team to support healthy lifestyle changes.

All reduced calorie diets (low-fat, low-carbohydrate, balanced) produce similar (long-term) weight loss which means recommendations can be tailored to individual preferences (Hall, 2017; Johnston, 2014). In all cases subjects should be encouraged to consume predominantly whole foods options (fresh, unprocessed vegetables, fruits, beans [legumes], and whole grains plus a variety of seafood, poultry, and lean meats).

The recommended dietary allowance (RDA) for protein is based on maintenance level energy requirements and is not applicable to the situation of energy restriction. Too little attention to protein intake during energy restriction results in undesirable effects on LBM and underlying REE. Protein prescription of 1.2 g per kg appears to be necessary to minimize the loss of LBM, prevent reduced REE, and preserve bone mineral density in situations of energy restriction (Drummen et al, 2018; Leidy, 2015; Westerterp-Plantenga et al, 2012). However, higher levels of protein also tend to blunt improvements in insulin resistance in individuals with insulin resistance.

Alcohol and foods high in sugar, especially beverages, should be limited to small amounts. Alcohol makes up 10% of the diet for many regular drinkers and contributes 7 kcal/g. Heavy drinkers who consume 50% or more of daily calories from alcohol may have a depressed appetite, whereas moderate users tend to gain weight with the added alcohol calories. Habitual use of alcohol may result in lipid storage, weight gain, or obesity.

There is no evidence that using nonnutritive sweeteners reduces food intake or enhances an individual's weight loss. A recent meta analysis of the available studies on nonnutritive sweeteners concluded that the literature does not clearly support the intended benefits of nonnutritive sweeteners for weight management, and observational data suggest that routine intake of nonnutritive sweeteners may be associated with increased BMI and cardiometabolic risk. Further research is needed to fully characterize the long-term risks and benefits of nonnutritive sweeteners (Azad et al, 2017).

Vitamin and mineral supplements that meet age-related requirements usually are recommended when there is a daily intake of less than 1200 kcal for women and 1800 kcal for men, or when it is difficult to choose foods that will meet all nutrient needs at the restricted energy intake.

Weight Loss Programs

Commercial and Self-Help Programs

Millions of Americans turn to commercial weight loss centers (NutriSystems, Jenny Craig, etc.) (Table 20.4) or self-help programs (diet book or Internet-based) in search of permanent weight loss each year. Commercial weight loss centers usually require the use of proprietary prepackaged meals. Prepackaged diets allow subjects to avoid food preparation and reduce the number of choices about food (and what to eat) throughout the day. Some provide classes on behavior modification and healthy eating.

Some brands of meal replacements are available over the counter (OTC) in drug stores, supermarkets, or via home delivery (e.g., Weight Watchers, SlimFast, HMR, etc.). The goal of using these foods is to provide structure and replace other higher calorie foods. Per serving, most meal replacements include 10 to 20 g of protein, various amounts of carbohydrate, 0 to 10 g of fat, up to 5 g of fiber, and 25% to 30% of RDAs for vitamins and minerals. Usually drinks or shakes are milk (casein or whey), pea protein, rice protein, or soy based; are high in calcium; and have 150 to 250 kcal per serving. They are frequently ready to use, portion controlled, or made with a purchased powder. People who have difficulty with self-selection or portion control may use meal replacements as part of a comprehensive weight management program. Substituting one or two daily meals or snacks with meal replacements is a successful weight loss and weight maintenance strategy (AND, 2016). Meal replacements are also utilized in medically supervised weight loss programs (see Very-Low-Calorie Diets).

The Internet has spawned a new generation of web-based weight loss options including Diet.com, NutriSystem.com, SparkPeople.com, SouthBeach.com, MyFitnessPal, and WeightWatchers.com. A handful of randomized controlled clinical trials have attempted to address whether personalization improves outcomes from these programs. However, results have been mixed and it remains to be determined (Collins et al, 2012). Apart from Weight Watchers, there is not a strong base of evidence behind the major commercial and self-help weight loss programs. The Federal Trade Commission (FTC) requires program advertisements to voluntarily include the phrase "results not typical," but has insufficient resources to further protect consumers from misleading advertising. More controlled trials are needed to assess the efficacy of commercial programs, therefore it is important to evaluate all weight loss programs for sound nutritional and behavioral practices.

Very-Low-Calorie Diets

Diets providing ≤800 kcal are classified as very-low-calorie diets (VLCDs). Little evidence suggests that an intake of fewer than 800

TABLE 20.4 Popular Weight Loss Diets*
Atkins Diet
Blood Type Diet
Caveman Diet
Detox Diet
Flat Belly Diet
Flexitarian
Glycemic Index Diet
HCG Diet
Intermittant fasting
Jenny Craig
LA Weight Loss
Mayo Clinic Diet
Medifast Diet
NutriSystem Diet
Nutritarian Diet
Raw Food Diet
South Beach Diet
The 17-Day Diet
The 5:2 Diet
The 8-Hour Diet
The Fast Diet
The Ketogenic Diet
The Mediterranean Diet
The Paleo Diet
Vegan Diet

*The Academy of Nutrition and Dietetics has a page on their website devoted to evaluating weight loss and fad diets https://www.eatright.org/health/weight-loss/fad-diets

calories daily is of any advantage. An example of a significant exception to this would be the hospitalized patient on a metabolic unit who is monitored carefully, is less than 65 years old, and has a condition such as congestive heart failure secondary to obesity. In such a case, immediate and rapid weight loss is considered life saving.

VLCDs are hypocaloric but relatively rich in protein (0.8 to 1.5 g per kg per day). They are designed to include a full complement of vitamins, minerals, electrolytes, and essential fatty acids, but not calories, and they are usually given for a period of 12 to 16 weeks as part of a medically supervised comprehensive lifestyle-modification program requiring regular medical monitoring and attendance of weekly group classes. Their major advantage (with patient compliance) is rapid weight loss.

Physicians often refer patients that would benefit medically (Fig. 20.6) from rapid weight loss (e.g., severe obstructive sleep apnea, congestive heart failure, and severe obesity with multiple comorbidities) to VLCD programs. Because of potential side effects, prescription of these diets is reserved for persons with a BMI of ≥30 (or ≥27 with at least one comorbidity) for whom other diet programs have been unsuccessful.

An OTC VLCD that first became popular in the early 1970s resulted in several deaths related to its low-quality, incomplete protein profile. The high-quality protein formulations used in medically supervised programs provide efficacy and safety for those with morbid obesity. Adverse side effects to VLCDs include higher risk for gallstones, cold intolerance, fatigue, weakness, lightheadedness, constipation or diarrhea, hair loss, dry skin, menstrual changes,

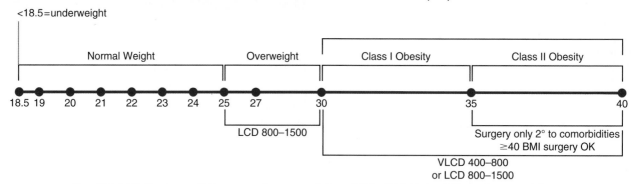

Fig. 20.6 BMI Continuum & Treatment Recommendations (NIH). 1998 National Heart, Lung, and Blood Institute - National Institute of Diabetes and Digestive and Kidney Diseases: Clinical Guidelines on the Identification, Evaluation, and Treatment of Overweight and Obesity in Adults: Evidence Report.

and gout; some of these may be related to triiodothyronine (thyroid) deficiency (see Chapter 30). Emerging data seem to indicate that as fat stores diminish, molecules are released that can affect further weight loss (see *Clinical Insight:* What's in That Fat When You Lose It?).

The current literature indicates that even though there is significantly greater weight loss with VLCDs in the short term (up to 13% greater than low calorie diets, or LCDs, with behavioral counseling), there are on average no significant differences in the long term (Gudzune et al, 2015). Weight loss maintenance requires ongoing vigilance and permanent lifestyle changes—that target a reduced weight net-energy-balance—regardless of the methods employed to lose weight (Hall et al, 2011).

Popular Diets and Practices

Each year, new books (or websites) promising weight loss find their way to the consumer through the popular press and media. Some of the programs are sensible and appropriate, whereas others emphasize fast results with minimum effort. Some of the proposed diets would lead to nutritional deficiencies over an extended period; however, the potential health risks are seldom realized because the diets usually are abandoned after a few weeks. Diets that emphasize fast results with minimum effort encourage unrealistic expectations, setting the dieter up for failure, subsequent guilt, and feelings of helplessness about managing a weight problem.

Online commercial diet programs have grown dramatically in the past decade. A programmed approach, for people on the run who carry their phones and computers, with a product line offered and accessibility to counselors and health professionals, has made the business of diets a multibillion-dollar industry. One on one and group online counseling, phone access to discuss weight loss progress and setbacks, and delivery of "to-your-door" foods and meals are some of the enticing aspects of joining these programs. Consumers continue to need proper guidance to separate the good, sound diet programs from the bad. Popular diets come and go; some are reviewed or described by various websites (see Table 20.4).

Intermittent Fasting

Traditionally, fasting has been considered primarily the act of willingly abstaining from food, drink, or both, for a set period of time and has been used at different times of the year in religious observances for centuries. Applying intermittent fasting (IF) type regimes as an approach to weight loss has recently been popularized by various diet books which claim there are metabolic advantages to IF leading to faster, or more, weight loss.

In the popular literature IF encompasses a variety of approaches including (1) limiting eating to the same 8 hours daily, (2) an alternating pattern of under- and overeating days, (3) fasting 2 days per week and eating normally the other 5 days, and (4) having regular splurge days (in the middle of stretches of fasting).

While there are multiple studies pertaining to IF in the scientific literature, most are studying biomarkers of cardiovascular disease or longevity and have not looked at weight loss as an outcome. Additionally, many have no control or comparison groups. Reviews of studies that have compared IF with a constant-calorie-restriction group (Davis et al, 2016; Harris et al, 2018; Headland et al, 2016) find no differences in weight loss, body composition, or insulin sensitivity.

Some popular IF regimes have been criticized for promoting an unhealthy "anything goes" diet on nonfasting days, which seems to border on encouragement for binging and/or disordered eating. Diet quality, however, becomes more—not less—important during any ongoing period of energy restriction.

In summary, IF is no more effective than other approaches to calorie restriction and the effects of using IF for weight loss maintenance have yet to be studied.

Low-Carbohydrate and Ketogenic Diets

When carbohydrate intake is less than 50 g per day, ketosis provides the brain and skeletal muscles with an alternate energy source in the form of ketones derived from lipolysis (the breakdown of fat). Ketones are believed to improve satiety (suppress appetite), at least initially.

Low-carbohydrate and ketogenic diets provide rapid initial weight loss from diuresis secondary to the carbohydrate restriction; early weight loss may be ≥60% water. This diuretic effect is a result of depleted liver and muscle glycogen which holds three to four times its weight in water.

In a classic energy-nitrogen balance method study comparing an 800-calorie ketogenic diet with an 800-calorie mixed diet, subjects did lose weight more rapidly at the beginning of the ketogenic diet period, however the extra weight loss was due solely to excess water losses. Both diets led to the same amount of body fat and protein (LBM) losses (Yang and Van Itallie, 1976). A recent much shorter version of this type of study by the NIH also found no advantage to the ketogenic diet (Hall et al, 2015).

The impact of a ketogenic diet on the microbiome and overall nutrient intake are two areas of concern. A recent study on the effect of a ketogenic diet on the gut microbiota found a bacterial group supposed to be involved in the exacerbation of the inflammatory condition of the gut mucosa associated with the ketogenic diet pattern (Tagliabue et al, 2017). The recommended upper limit for dietary fat is 35% of calorie intake per the dietary reference intakes, which are intended to ensure adequate micronutrients and shield against preventable diseases (see Appendix 19 on the ketogenic diet).

High-protein (rather than high-fat) variants of low-carbohydrate and ketogenic diets include the Zone and South Beach Diets, which restrict carbohydrates to no more than 40% of total calories, with fat and protein each providing 30% of total calories. These diets are considered moderate choices within the low-carbohydrate category and include generous amounts of fiber and fresh fruits and vegetables, and they stress the kind of fat, with emphasis on monounsaturated and polyunsaturated fat and limitation of saturated fat. For more information about a ketogenic diet and the conditions for which it has been studied, see Appendix 19.

Unanswered questions about the ketogenic diet include:

- What are the long-term (1 year or longer) effects, is it safe?
- Do the diet's health benefits extend to higher risk individuals with multiple health conditions and the elderly? For which disease conditions do the benefits of the diet outweigh the risks?
- As fat is the primary energy source, what is the effect of such a high-fat diet that includes so much saturated fat?
- Is the high fat, moderate protein intake on a ketogenic diet safe for disease conditions that interfere with normal protein and fat metabolism, such as heart, kidney, and liver diseases?
- Is a ketogenic diet too restrictive for periods of rapid growth?
- Is the ketogenic diet safe and is it effective for athletes?

The carbohydrate-insulin theory of obesity is the foundation of low-carbohydrate and ketogenic diets. The basic theory is that carbohydrates stimulate insulin secretion causing increased fat storage, which increases appetite and suppresses metabolism resulting in weight gain. Low carbohydrate intake does decrease insulin secretion (Abassi, 2018). The insulin theory however, only describes postprandial energy metabolism while ignoring the rest of the 24-hour energy metabolism picture. Insulin levels don't remain elevated, and overnight—in the fasting state—fat oxidation increases, reducing fat stores. A net gain in fat stores only occurs with positive energy balance. Recent carefully controlled metabolic laboratory studies appear to have invalidated the insulin theory of obesity (Hall et al, 2015; Hall and Guo, 2017). A recent systematic review of high quality randomized controlled trials (RCTs) comparing low-carbohydrate with isoenergetic (having the same total calories) balanced diets found essentially no difference in weight loss, measures of glycemic control, blood pressure, or blood lipid between the two diets (Naude et al, 2014).

Very-Low-Fat (High-Carbohydrate) Diets

Very-low-fat (high-carbohydrate) diets contain less than 10% of calories from fat, such as the original Dr. Dean Ornish's Program for Reversing Heart Disease and the Pritikin Program. Ten percent of energy from fat however is well below the current acceptable macronutrient distribution range (AMDR) for fat which is 20% to 35% of total calorie intake (National Academy of Sciences Institute of Medicine, 2005).

TABLE 20.5   Acceptable Macronutrient Distribution Ranges (AMDR)% of Total Calorie Intake

	2005	Previous Guidelines
Protein	10% to 35%	10% to 35%
Carbohydrate	45% to 65%	50% or more
Fat	20% to 35%	30% or less

NAS IOM: Dietary Reference Intakes for Energy, Carbohydrate, Fiber, Fat, Fatty acids, Cholesterol, Protein, and Amino Acids (Macronutrients), *The National Academies Press.* 2005.

Less than 20% fat may negatively impact essential fatty acid intake and fat-soluble nutrient absorption (Table 20.5). Less restrictive and more popular variations of these diets do allow fat as 20% of total energy intake. Weight loss on these diets is due solely to energy restriction. Because fat provides more than two times the energy per gram as protein or carbohydrate (9 kcal versus 4 kcal), limiting fat is theoretically the most efficient way to decrease calories. The unforeseen consequence of severe fat restriction however is compensatory intake of sugar and/or processed carbohydrates which can trigger metabolic syndrome.

Balanced Lower Calorie Diets

Balanced-nutrient reduction diets are less common among so-called "popular" diets. The full document of the (2015–2020) Dietary Guidelines for Americans outlines the details of three eating plans in its appendices that qualify: the Healthy U.S.-Style Eating Pattern, Healthy Mediterranean-Style Eating Pattern, and Healthy Vegetarian Eating Pattern.

Reduced-energy diets for weight management should be nutritionally sound, not harmful, and feasible to maintain over time. This requires sustainability in terms of ease of adherence, using readily available and affordable foods, and social and cultural acceptability (Naude et al, 2014). The U.S. Department of Agriculture (USDA) supported a scientific review of popular diets to assess their efficacy for weight loss and weight maintenance, as well as their effect on metabolic parameters, mental well-being, and reduction of chronic disease. A summary is shown in Table 20.6.

Over-the-counter medications and herbal supplements for weight loss have been popular for many years. With some exceptions, the majority of these supplements have limited data with regard to their efficacy and safety, and many of the most effective supplements for weight loss (caffeine and ephedra) have significant cardiovascular and neurologic risks or have been banned by the Food and Drug Administration (FDA) (e.g., ephedra). Dietitians should be aware of popular supplements in order to best serve clients and patients. According to the FDA, a high percentage of weight loss products are adulterated and contain illegal drugs and stimulants that are not listed on the label. See Table 20.7 for popular nutritional supplements used for weight loss. Reliable information on dietary supplements can be obtained from the NIH Office of Dietary Supplements website as well as consumer warnings on recalled and banned products from the FDA's website (see Chapter 11).

Physical Activity

Physical activity is the most variable component of energy expenditure (see Chapter 2). Increases in energy expenditure through exercise and other forms of physical activity are important components of interventions for weight loss and its maintenance. By increasing LBM in proportion to fat, physical activity helps to balance the loss of LBM

TABLE 20.6 Results of U.S. Department of Agriculture Scientific Review of Popular Diets

Area	Finding
Weight loss	Diets that reduce caloric intake result in weight loss; all popular diets result in short-term weight loss if followed.
Body composition	All low-calorie diets result in a loss of body fat. In the short term, high-fat, low-carbohydrate, and ketogenic diets cause a greater loss of body water than body fat.
Nutritional adequacy	• High-fat, low-carbohydrate diets are low in vitamins E and A, thiamin, B_6, and folate; and the minerals calcium, magnesium, iron, and potassium. They are also low in dietary fiber. • Very-low-fat diets are low in vitamins E and B_{12} and the mineral zinc. • With proper food choices, a moderate-fat, balanced-nutrient reduction diet is nutritionally adequate.
Metabolic parameters	• Low-carbohydrate diets cause ketosis and may significantly increase blood uric acid concentrations. • Blood lipid levels decline as body weight decreases. • Energy restriction improves glycemic control. • As body weight declines, blood insulin and plasma leptin levels decrease. • As body weight declines, blood pressure decreases.
Hunger and compliance	No diet was optimal for reducing hunger.
Effect on weight maintenance	Controlled clinical trials of high-fat, low-carbohydrate, low-fat, and very-low-fat diets are lacking; therefore no data are available on weight maintenance after weight loss or long-term health benefits or risk.

From Freedman M et al: Popular diets: a scientific review, *Obes Res* 9(Suppl 1):1S, 2001.

TABLE 20.7 Nonprescription Weight Loss Products

Product	Claim	Effectiveness	Safety
Alli: OTC version of prescription drug orlistat (Xenical)	Decreases absorption of dietary fat	Effective; weight loss amounts typically less for OTC versus prescription	FDA investigating reports of liver injury, pancreatitis
Bitter orange (synephrine)	Increases calories burned	Insufficient reliable evidence to rate	Possibly unsafe, increase in heart rate and blood pressure
Chitosan	Blocks absorption of dietary fat	Ineffective for weight loss	Possibly safe, may cause bloating
Chromium	Increases calories burned, decreases appetite, and builds muscle	Insufficient reliable evidence to rate	Likely safe
Conjugated linoleic acid (CLA)	Reduces body fat and builds muscle	Ineffective for weight loss	Possibly safe
Ephedra (Ma Huang)	Decreases appetite and increases fat burned	Possibly effective	Unsafe due to cardiovascular risk and banned by FDA
Green tea extract	Increases calorie and fat metabolism and decreases appetite	Ineffective for weight loss	Possibly safe
Guar gum	Blocks absorption of dietary fat and increases feeling of fullness	Ineffective for weight loss	Likely safe but increased gastrointestinal distress
Hoodia gordonii	Decreases appetite	Insufficient reliable evidence to rate	Insufficient information, high risk of mislabeling
Senna	Cathartic; laxative, causes diarrhea	Insufficient reliable evidence to rate	Likely unsafe, stimulant laxative
Raspberry ketones	Increases lipolysis	Insufficient reliable evidence to rate	Likely unsafe especially for hypertension
Garcinia cambogia	Blocks enzymes in body which convert glucose to fat. Also increases serotonin in brain, limiting appetite and providing extra energy	Ineffective for weight loss (Esteghamati, 2015)	Reports of liver damage associated

FDA, Food and Drug Administration; *OTC,* over the counter.
Adapted from Natural Medicines in the Clinical Management of Obesity, Natural Medicines Comprehensive Database (website): http://naturaldatabase.therapeuticresearch.com:80/ce/ceCourse.aspx?s=ND&cs=&pc=09%2D32&cec=1&pm=; Scott GN: *Is raspberry ketone effective for weight loss?* http://www.medscape.com/viewarticle/775741, 2012.
Additional information from https://www.ncbi.nlm.nih.gov/pmc/articles/PMC4386228/; Esteghamati A, Mazaheri T, Vahidi Rad M, Noshad S. Complementary and alternative medicine for the treatment obesity: a critical review. *Int J Endocrinol Metab* 2015; 13:e19678; Pittler MH, Ernst E. Guar gum for body weight reduction: meta-analysis of randomized trials. *Am J Med* 2001; 110:724. Up to Date Obesity in adults: Drug Therapy

and reduction of RMR that inevitably accompany intentional weight reduction. Other positive side effects of increased activity include strengthening cardiovascular integrity, increasing sensitivity to insulin, and expending additional energy and therefore calories.

The CDC's Physical Activity Guidelines for Americans suggest a minimum of 150 minutes of physical activity weekly, with two sessions of weight training, to achieve health benefits. However, recent studies have shown that adhering to physical activity guidelines without adhering to a calorie-restricted diet will lead to only minimal or modest weight loss; proper nutritional intake is crucial for weight loss. For weight maintenance or prevention of weight gain, 200 to 300 minutes of weekly physical activity may be more effective. The majority of participants in the National Weight Control Registry (NWCR) who have kept off at least 10% of their weight for at least a year report 1 hour per day of physical activity (at least 420 minutes per week).

Overweight and obese adults should gradually increase to optimal levels of physical activity. Even if an overweight or obese adult is unable to achieve this level of activity, there is evidence that significant health benefits can be realized by participating in at least 30 minutes of daily activity of moderate intensity. Targeting these levels of physical activity can improve health-related outcomes and facilitate long-term weight control.

Aerobic exercise and resistance training should be recommended. Resistance training increases LBM, raising the RMR and one's ability to use more of the energy intake, and increases bone mineral density, especially for women (see Chapter 23). Aerobic exercise is important for cardiovascular health through elevated RMR, calorie expenditure, energy deficit, and loss of fat. In addition to the physiologic benefits of exercise, other benefits include relief of boredom, increased sense of control, and improved sense of well-being. The whole family can get involved in pleasurable exercise activities (Fig. 20.7).

The recommendations for exercise from the American College of Sports Medicine differ for weight loss versus weight maintenance. Physical activity of fewer than 150 minutes per week has a minimal effect on weight loss, whereas physical activity of greater than 150 minutes per week usually results in modest weight loss (defined as 2 to 3 kg), and physical activity between 225 and 420 minutes per week is

likely to result in the greatest weight loss (5 to 7.5 kg). However, this high volume of physical activity may not be practical for the general population. Research on maintaining weight indicates that moderate to vigorous physical activity of 150 to 250 minutes per week, at an energy equivalent of 1200 to 2000 kcal per week (about 12 to 20 miles per week of jogging or running) is sufficient to prevent weight gain (Swift et al, 2014). However, obese individuals who have successfully lost weight may require a substantial amount of physical activity to maintain weight loss.

Failure to meet the recommended levels of aerobic physical activity leads to nearly $117 billion in annual health care costs and 10% of all premature deaths, according to the Department of Health and Human Services 2018 physical fitness report in the *Journal of the American Medical Association* (Piercy et al, 2018).

Pharmaceutical Management

Appropriate pharmacotherapy can augment diet, physical activity, and behavior therapy as treatment for patients with a BMI of 30 or higher or patients with 27 or higher who also have significant risk factors or disease. These agents can decrease appetite, reduce absorption of fat, or increase energy expenditure. As with any drug treatment, physician monitoring for efficacy and safety is necessary. Pharmacotherapy is not a "magic pill"; dietitians should collaborate with other health professionals regarding the use of FDA–approved pharmacotherapy. Not all individuals respond, but for patients who do respond, weight loss of approximately 2 to 20 kg can be expected usually during the first 6 months of treatment. Medication without lifestyle modification is less effective.

As of April, 2018, five long-term weight loss drugs were listed as approved by the FDA: orlistat (Xenical), liraglutide (Saxenda, Victoza), lorcaserin (Belviq), naltrexone-bupropion (Contrave), and phentermine-topiramate (Qsymia) (Table 20.8 for mechanisms of action and common side effects of prescription weight loss drugs).

The choice of weight loss drug is determined by the physician in partnership with the patient. In general, medications can be categorized as central nervous system (CNS)-acting agents and non-CNS-acting agents. Some CNS-acting agents focus on the brain, increasing the availability of norepinephrine. Drug Enforcement Agency Schedule II anorexic agents such as amphetamines have a high potential for abuse and are not recommended for obesity treatment. Other CNS-acting agents act by increasing serotonin levels in the brain. Two such drugs, fenfluramine (commonly used in combination with phentermine, known as "fen-phen") and dexfenfluramine, were removed from the market in 1997 after concerns were raised regarding the possible side effects of cardiac valvulopathy, regurgitation, and primary pulmonary hypertension. Common side effects of many CNS-acting agents are dry mouth, headache, insomnia, and constipation.

Vitamins and supplements may be helpful in addressing a patient's nutrition concerns while trying to lose weight. OTC and natural weight loss products hold varying degrees of safety and efficacy. See Table 20.7 for additional information.

Nondiet Approach

The nondiet approach (also known as Health at Every Size; HAES®) is described as a weight-neutral approach that proposes that the body will attain its natural weight if the individual eats healthfully, becomes attuned to hunger and satiety cues, and incorporates physical activity. Advocates for this approach promote size acceptance, respect for the diversity of body shapes and sizes, and promotion of intuitive eating. The approach is described as focusing on achieving health rather than attaining a certain weight.

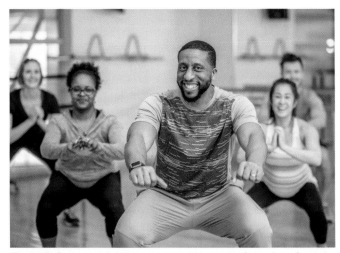

Fig. 20.7 Group activity classes help build community and can increase motivation to exercise.

TABLE 20.8   Prescription Drugs Approved for Obesity Treatment*

Weight Loss Drug	Approved For	How It Works	Common Side Effects
Orlistat Sold as Xenical by prescription; over-the-counter version sold as Alli	Xenical: adults and children ages 12 and older Alli: adults only	Inhibits gastrointestinal lipase, which reduces the amount of fat absorbed from food by approximately 1/3—up to 150 to 200 calories less per day.	Stomach pain, gas, diarrhea, and leakage of oily stools Lowered fat-soluble vitamin absorption; supplements are typically recommended and should be taken >2 hours apart from drug Note: Rare cases of severe liver injury reported. Should not be taken with cyclosporine.
Lorcaserin Sold as Belviq	Adults	Acts on the serotonin receptors in the brain. This may help you eat less and feel full after eating smaller amounts of food.	Headaches, dizziness, feeling tired, nausea, dry mouth, cough, and constipation. Should not be taken with selective serotonin reuptake inhibitors (SSRIs) and monoamine oxidase inhibitor (MAOI) medications
Phentermine-topiramate Sold as Qsymia	Adults	A mix of two drugs: phentermine (suppresses your appetite and curbs your desire to eat) and topiramate (used to treat seizures or migraine headaches). May make you feel full and make foods taste less appealing.	Tingling of hands and feet, dizziness, taste alterations (particularly with carbonated beverages), trouble sleeping, constipation, dry mouth, and increased heart rate Note: Sold only through certified pharmacies. May lead to birth defects. Do not take Qsymia if you are pregnant or planning a pregnancy.
Other appetite suppressant drugs (drugs that curb your desire to eat), which include phentermine benzphetamine diethylpropion phendimetrazine Sold under many names	Adults	Increase chemicals in the brain that affect appetite. Make you feel that you are not hungry or that you are full. Note: Only FDA approved for a short period of time (up to 12 weeks).	Dry mouth, difficulty sleeping, dizziness, headache, feeling nervous, feeling restless, upset stomach, diarrhea, and constipation

*Note: *Metformin, used for type 2 diabetes, is a prescription drug which has been used by physicians as an "off-label" treatment of obesity.*
Adapted from www.niddk.nih.gov Mar 3, 2014.
Padwal R, Li SK, Lau DC: Long-term pharmacotherapy for obesity and overweight, *Cochrane Database of Syst Rev* (4):CD004094, 2003.
Perrault L: Obesity in adults: Drug Therapy. In Post TW, editor: *UpToDate*, Waltham, MA, 2018, UpToDate.

A fat-acceptance movement responding to weight bias and stigma, which persist both within and outside of the health care system, preceded the nondiet movement (see section on Weight Stigma and Social Justice). Advocates for this approach generally feel that CR is harmful (leading to eating disorders, body dissatisfaction, low self-esteem, and psychological harms). Nondiet advocates do not believe that obesity in and of itself is a risk factor for chronic disease and and assert that the medical community is complicit in the "medicalization and pathologizing of fatness" (Ulian et al, 2018a). Nondiet advocates believe that obesity is natural (genetically determined) and unrelated to energy balance, and they point to relapse data as proof that attempts to lose weight often do not work.

To date there have been 10 studies (described in 15 research papers) using a nondiet approach published between 1999 and 2016. Among these 10 studies were a total of 697 subjects who were almost exclusively white women ages 30 to 50. Two of six papers reported a significant improvement in total and low-density lipoprotein (LDL) cholesterol (Bacon et al, 2002; Mensinger et al, 2016), and one paper reported a significant improvement in high-density lipoprotein (HDL) (Carroll et al, 2007). Two of three papers reported a small change in systolic or diastolic blood pressure (Bacon et al, 2002; Carroll et al, 2007). Only one study (which provided supervised exercise) reported a clinically and statistically significant change in body mass, 3.6% loss of initial body weight (3.5 kgs) (Ulian et al, 2015). Only three trials have compared a nondiet approach with traditional weight loss interventions (Bacon et al, 2002; Mensinger et al, 2016; Steinhardt et al, 1999).

The nondiet studies do consistently show improvements in psychological variables (self-esteem, quality of life, and depression). When behavioral-type weight loss studies collect data on psychological variables (self-esteem, body image, health-related quality of life) they consistently report improvements as well (Blaine et al, 2007; Lasikiewicz et al, 2014). Furthermore, in contrast to the idea that intentional weight loss precipitates mood disturbance, reductions in depressive symptoms are consistent via any active treatment (lifestyle modification, exercise, nondiet, etc.) (Fabricatore et al, 2011).

A 5% weight loss leads to clinically significant improvements in metabolic variables. On average professional weight loss interventions induce a 9.5% weight loss from baseline and maintain 54% of the loss at 1 year (Ramage et al, 2014). Weight regain data from clinical weight loss interventions however are not randomizable (applicable) to the general population. The most recent available data (collected via the NHANES) found that 36.6% of 14,306 U.S. adults were maintaining at least a 5% weight loss (Kraschnewski et al, 2010).

While young women with body image disturbance are at higher risk for the development of eating disorders, intentional weight loss programs, when administered by a trained and empathetic professional, do not appear to increase the incidence of eating disorders. In fact, some studies report increased body satisfaction and a healthier relationship with food in addition to weight loss (National Task Force on the Prevention and Treatment of Obesity, 2000; Palavras et al, 2017; Wadden et al, 2004).

Well-designed behavioral weight loss interventions are able to reduce weight, improve metabolic profiles, and improve psychological outcomes. Behavioral programs vary but typically address: (1) emotional eating triggers; (2) balanced nutrition; (3) social support; and (4) exercise, and sometimes also include cognitive restructuring via exploration of dysfunctional thoughts regarding weight, body shape, or dieting.

Pursuing weight loss, or not, is an individual choice. For individuals who choose not to focus on weight, a nondiet approach can lead to improved body image and psychological variables. The effects on metabolic variables and the quality of dietary intake are unclear (Leblanc et al, 2012; Ulian, 2018b) and passive weight loss is not an expected an outcome.

Bariatric Surgery

Bariatric surgery is currently considered the only long-term effective treatment for extreme or class III obesity with a BMI of 40 or greater, or a BMI of 35 or greater with comorbidities. According to the American Society for Metabolic and Bariatric Surgery, 228,000 bariatric surgeries were done in 2017 with an increase of 16% from 2015. Sleeve gastrectomy and Roux-en-Y gastric bypass (RYGB) are the two most common bariatric surgeries in the United States, with 58.1% and 18.7% performed, respectively. The laparoscopic adjustable gastric banding (LAGB) and biliopancreatic diversion with duodenal switch (BPD/DS) are still done, but prevalence is decreasing; with LAGB making up 3.4% of bariatric surgeries, and BPD/DS, 0.6% (American Society for Metabolic and Bariatric Surgery [ASMBS], 2016).

Before any extremely obese person is considered for surgery, failure of a comprehensive program that includes calorie reduction, exercise, lifestyle modification, psychological counseling, and family involvement must be demonstrated. Failure is defined as an inability of the patient to reduce body weight by one third and body fat by one half, and an inability to maintain any weight loss achieved. Such patients have intractable morbid obesity and should be considered for surgery.

If surgery is chosen, the patient is evaluated extensively with respect to physiologic and medical complications, psychological problems such as depression or poor self-esteem, and motivation. Behavioral counseling, especially in the postoperative period, can improve weight loss (Stewart and Avenell, 2016). Postoperative follow-up requires evaluation at regular intervals by the surgical team and a registered dietitian nutritionist (RDN). In addition, behavioral or psychological support is necessary. Studies indicate some positive physiologic changes in liver fibrosis, BMI, branched chain amino acid production, and reversal of insulin-induced increases in brain glucose metabolism (Abdennour et al, 2014; Tuulari et al, 2013).

Sleeve Gastrectomy, Gastric Bypass, and Laparoscopic Adjustable Gastric Banding

Weight loss surgery procedures reduce the amount of food that can be eaten at one time and produce early satiety (Fig. 20.8). The new stomach capacity may be as small as 30 mL or approximately 2 tablespoons. After surgery the patient's diet progresses from clear liquid to full liquid to puree, soft, and finally to a regular diet as tolerated, with emphasis on protein and fluid intake (Table 20.9). The results of gastric surgery are more favorable than those from the intestinal bypass surgery practiced during the 1970s. On average, the reduction of excess body weight after gastric restriction surgery correlates to approximately 30% to 40% of initial body weight. In addition to the greater absolute weight loss observed, the gastric bypass tends to have sustainable results with significant resolution of hypertension, type 2 diabetes mellitus, osteoarthritis, back pain, dyslipidemia, cardiomyopathy, nonalcoholic steatohepatitis, and sleep apnea. However, late complications may be seen, such as vitamin deficiencies, electrolyte problems, or even intestinal failure. Patients should be nutritionally assessed regularly (see Appendices 11 and 12). Thirty-day major complication rates for all bariatric procedures have been found to be 1.15% anastomotic leak, 0.37% myocardial infarction, and 1.17% pulmonary embolism (Chang et al, 2018).

The laparoscopic sleeve gastrectomy (LSG) initially was used for patients with a BMI greater than 60 as a precursor to the BPD/DS, but it is now used as a stand-alone procedure and currently is the most popular bariatric surgery in the United States. The sleeve gastrectomy involves removing approximately 80% of the stomach, creating a long, thin gastric pouch by stapling or sewing the stomach longitudinally. The pyloric sphincter is left intact (Meek et al, 2016). Complications associated with the LSG can include gastric bleeding, stenosis, leak, and reflux. One of the most common complications from sleeve gastrectomy involves acid reflux, occurring in 20% to 30% of patients (Braghetto et al, 2012). Occasionally, RYGB is necessary to resolve reflux complications (Weiner et al, 2011) (see Fig. 20.6).

Gastric bypass involves reducing the size of the stomach with the stapling procedure but then connecting a small opening in the upper portion of the stomach to the small intestine by means of an intestinal loop. The original operation in the late 1960s evolved into the RYGB. Because use of the lower part of the stomach is omitted, the gastric bypass patient may have dumping syndrome as food empties quickly into the duodenum (see Chapter 26). The tachycardia, sweating, and abdominal pain are so uncomfortable that they motivate the patient to make the appropriate behavioral changes and refrain from overeating and choosing less healthful foods, such as sugar-sweetened beverages. Eventually the pouch expands to accommodate 4 to 5 oz at a time. Sometimes gastric bypass surgery can lead to bloating of the pouch, nausea, and vomiting. A postsurgical food record noting the tolerance for specific foods in particular amounts helps in devising a program to avoid these episodes.

Up to 16% of patients may experience postoperative complications (Beebe and Crowley, 2015). These include anastomotic leaks, strictures, perforation, gastric fistulas, bowel obstructions, wound infections, respiratory failure, and intractable nausea and vomiting.

Laparoscopic adjustable gastric banding (LAGB), the band creating the reduced stomach pouch, can be adjusted so that the opening to the rest of the stomach can be made smaller or enlarged. The band, filled with saline, has a tube exiting from it to the surface of the belly just under the skin; this allows for the injection of additional fluid or reduction of fluid into the band. Rates of lap-band placement have been decreasing across the United States, with some bariatric centers and surgeons no longer performing the procedure. Many patients are drawn to the band

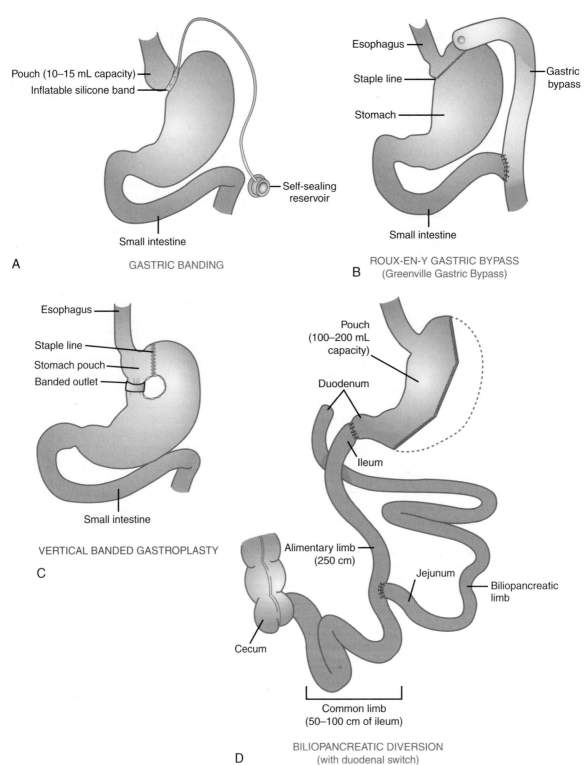

Fig. 20.8 Bariatric surgeries. Dietitians in Nutrition Support newsletter, June 2014, P. 10, Vol. 6, No. 3.

as an option as it is reversible; however, many practitioners and researchers find the complications outweigh the benefits (Ibrahim et al, 2017).

Bariatric surgery places an individual at risk for malnutrition that requires lifelong follow-up and monitoring by the multidisciplinary team. Nutritional status should be frequently evaluated by an RDN. Monitoring should include an assessment of total body fat loss and a full micronutrient assessment. Pre- and postsurgical micronutrient assessment should include thiamine, vitamin B_{12}, folate, iron, vitamin D, calcium, other fat-soluble vitamins, zinc, and copper. In many cases, a liquid multivitamin mineral supplement is used. Recommended vitamin supplementation after bariatric surgery can be found in Table 20.10 (Parrott et al, 2017).

TABLE 20.9 Diet Progression After Sleeve Gastrectomy and Roux-en-Y Gastric Bypass

Stage of Diet	Duration	Foods Allowed
Clear Liquids	Start within 24 hours after surgery. Duration 2-3 meals	Sugar-free clear liquids, such as water, unsweetened decaffeinated tea, sugar-free gelatin, sugar-free popsicles, broth
Stage 2 – Full Liquid Diet	A few days to 1 week	Protein drink, fat-free (skim) milk, unsweetened nondairy milk, strained cream soups
Stage 3 – Pureed	A few weeks to about 1 month	Foods that are the consistency of a smooth paste or thick liquid, without any solid pieces. Examples include low-fat cottage cheese, low-fat or fat-free ricotta cheese, blended meats, fish, eggs, beans, fruits, and vegetables
Stage 4 – Soft foods	About 1 month	Ground or finely diced meats, canned or soft fresh fruit, cooked vegetables without skin, eggs, beans
Stage 5 – Solid foods	Start about 8 weeks post surgery	Gradually incorporate firmer, diced, or chopped foods.

https://www.mayoclinic.org/tests-procedures/gastric-bypass-surgery/in-depth/gastric-bypass-diet/art-20048472

TABLE 20.10 Recommended Vitamin Supplementation After Bariatric Surgery

Supplement	Recommendation
Thiamine	At least 12 mg daily, and preferably a dose of 50 mg thiamine from a B-complex supplement or multivitamin once daily
Vitamin B$_{12}$	350-500 μg orally by disintegrating tablet, sublingual, or liquid daily OR nasal spray as directed by manufacturer OR 1000 μg monthly parenterally
Folate (Folic Acid)	400-800 μg daily from a multivitamin. Women of childbearing age should take 800-1000 μg daily.
Iron	Post-RYGB, LSG, and BPD/DS patients should take at least 45-60 mg elemental iron cumulatively daily (from multivitamin and other supplements). Those with low risk of deficiency, such as males with LAGB procedures, should take at least 18 mg from their multivitamin daily. Oral supplementation should be in divided doses, separately from calcium supplement, acid-reducing medications, and foods high in phytates and polyphenols.
Calcium	LAGB, LSG, RYGB: 1200-1500 mg daily BPD/DS: 1800-2400 mg daily Calcium should be given in divided doses to enhance absorption. Calcium carbonate should be taken with meals to increase absorption, calcium citrate has good absorption when taken with meals and also on an empty stomach.
Vitamin D	Dosage of vitamin D is based on 25(OH)D levels. 3000 IU daily of vitamin D is recommended until 25(OH)D levels are >30 ng/L.
Vitamins A, E, and K	LAGB: vitamin A 5000 IU and vitamin K 90-120 μg daily RYGB and LSG: vitamin A 5000-1000 IU and vitamin K 90-120 μg daily BPD/DS: vitamin A 1000 IU and vitamin K 300 μg daily All weight loss surgeries: vitamin E 15 mg daily Special attention should be paid to postsurgical supplementation of vitamins A and K in pregnant women.
Zinc	BPD/DS: Multivitamin with minerals containing 200% of the RDA (1622 mg/d) RYGB: Multivitamin with minerals containing 100%-200% of the RDA (8-22 mg/d) LSG/LAGB: Multivitamin with minerals containing 100% of the RDA (8-11 mg/d) To minimize the risk of copper deficiency in post-WLS patients, it is recommended that the supplementation protocol contain a ratio of 8-15 mg of supplemental zinc per 1 mg of copper.
Copper	BPD/DS or RYGB: 200% of the RDA (2 mg/d) LSG or LAGB: 100% of the RDA (1 mg/d) Copper gluconate or sulfate is the recommended source of copper for supplementation.

BPD/DS, Biliopancreatic diversion with duodenal switch; *LAGB*, laparoscopic adjustable gastric banding; *LSG*, laparoscopic sleeve gastrectomy; RDA, recommended dietary allowance; *RYGB*, Roux-en-Y gastric bypass; *WLS*; weight loss surgery.

Bariatric surgery is increasing in popularity as a treatment of extreme obesity for the adolescent population. Similar preoperative requirements exist; however, the age and cognitive emotional maturity of the patient need to be taken into consideration given the lifelong nutritional, psychological, and physical ramifications.

Non-Surgical Weight Loss Procedures

Surgical management of weight continues to evolve. Select bariatric surgery centers across the United States have started utilizing the intragastric balloon (IGB). The IGB, which is made of silicone, is endoscopically placed in the stomach for 6 months. During the

6 months in which the balloon resides in the stomach, patients are expected to learn and develop healthy eating habits that persist after the balloon has been removed. Complications include abdominal pain, nausea, esophagitis, flatulence, and gastric ulcer. An IGB can increase weight loss by 14.25% (Saber et al, 2017). There is currently insufficient evidence regarding the IGB's efficacy or safety. The Aspire Assist is a gastrostomy tube placed during gastroscopy. Patients can aspirate contents of a meal approximately 20 minutes after eating, thus decreasing caloric absorption.

Maintaining Reduced Body Weight

Energy requirements for weight maintenance after weight reduction are lower than at the original weight because smaller bodies have smaller energy requirements. Most studies show that the RMR of reduced weight subjects versus stable-weight-controls (of the same height, weight, and gender) are not different (Clamp et al, 2018). A follow-up study of participants in *The Biggest Loser* television show (who lost significant amounts of weight) found that after weight regain, RMR remained suppressed (Fothergill et al, 2016). These results open questions about possible long-term effects of extreme energy restriction—especially coupled with extreme levels of physical activity—on eventual RMR. People who have lost weight will always have reduced energy requirements due to reduced body mass, which necessitates permanent lifestyle changes to maintain the net energy balance supporting their reduced body weight (Hall et al, 2011).

The NWCR consists of more than 5000 individuals who have been successful in long-term weight loss maintenance. The purpose of establishing the NWCR is to identify the common characteristics of those who succeed in long-term weight loss maintenance. There is very little similarity in how these individuals lost weight, but there are some common behaviors they all have for keeping the weight off. Lifestyle modification and a sense of self-efficacy appear to be essential. To maintain weight loss, NWCR participants report the following:

1. Eating a relatively low-fat (24%) diet
2. Eating breakfast almost every day
3. Weighing themselves regularly, usually once per day to once per week
4. Engaging in high levels (60 to 90 minutes per day) of physical activity

A national weight loss registry is contributing to our understanding of those tactics that lead to long term success. Dietary restriction of fat, frequent self-weighing, and ongoing leisure time physical activity were factors associated with maintaining weight loss (Thomas et al, 2014). Support groups are valuable for obese persons who are maintaining a new lower weight; they help individuals facing similar problems. Two self-help support groups are Overeaters Anonymous (OA) and Take Off Pounds Sensibly (TOPS). These groups are inexpensive, continuous, include a "buddy system," and encourage participation on a regular basis, or as often as needed. Weight Watchers programs offer free lifelong maintenance classes for those who have reached and are maintaining their goal weights.

Interestingly, "boring" and "monotonous" diets can provide a strategy for reducing food intake. Diets that are repetitious (without change from meal to meal) are a useful consideration for controlling intake, because people tend to overeat when they have many mealtime choices. This can be a particular problem in a society where one in three meals is eaten away from home. Restaurants and vending trucks or machines generally offer many options, most high in calories (see *Focus On:* Restaurant and Vending Machine Nutrition Labeling).

Overall, a common sense approach is needed. Some phrases can be shared with individuals who are trying to maintain their weight loss, including the following: (1) The best diet is "make it, don't buy it," (2) "Easy does it"—use moderation at all meals and snacks, and (3) "Avoid drinking your calories."

◎ FOCUS ON

Restaurant and Vending Machine Nutrition Labeling

When the Affordable Care Act was signed into law in 2010, restaurant labeling laws were included as part of the legislation for health care reform (Federal Register, 2014). Because many Americans eat one third of their calories away from home, the intent of this public health effort was to provide consumers with the food label as an educational tool to make healthier eating choices when dining out. It took 8 years to bring this to fruition, with many delays and interruptions due to government and industry controversies.

In 2018, the FDA enacted the following legislation:

1. In restaurants and in similar food establishments with greater than 20 locations serving the same menu, all menu items must list the calorie content of foods.
2. Vending machine labeling operators who own or operate 20 or more vending machines must disclose their vending machine calorie information, subject to certain exemptions as determined by the FDA.

Although other data like fat, saturated fat, cholesterol, sodium, total carbohydrates, sugar, fiber, and total protein were eliminated during the many years it took to get this legislation enacted, we can now finally provide—through this labeling—an educational tool to the public for making more informed food choices. It is up to us, as nutrition professionals, to be persistent and work with our legislators on the enactment of future nutrition labeling rules and education. For more detailed information about timing and implementation of the labeling rule, you may contact www.fda.gov.

Plateau Effect

A common experience for the person in a weight reduction program is arrival at a weight plateau, as weight loss slows and eventually seems to stop. Recent research explains that the plateau effect is mainly due to a lack of ongoing energy deficit. Subjects tend to maintain an energy deficit for only about 6 weeks, then gradually return to their baseline energy intake. This means a state of equilibrium has been reached at which the energy intake is equal to energy expenditure. To move out of this phase, reestablishing an energy deficit is required.

There are several factors that reduce RMR and total energy expenditure (TEE) during energy restriction and weight loss, including: energy restriction—RMR can decrease at the onset of energy restriction by as much as 15% within 2 weeks, which varies with the magnitude of energy restriction; loss of metabolically active body tissue—weight loss consists of both LBM and fat, and less of either (but especially LBM) reduces RMR; the cost of physical activity is also less because a body that weighs less requires less energy expenditure to move around; and the thermic effect of food is generally about 10% of energy intake, which is automatically less with energy restriction. These are not the major factors stalling weight loss however; it is necessary to reestablish an energy deficit.

Weight Cycling

Repeated bouts of weight loss and regain, known as weight cycling or the yo-yo effect, occurs in men and women and is common in overweight and lean individuals. Research is mixed on whether weight cycling results in increased body fatness and weight with the end of each cycle. Undesirable psychological effects are less disputed.

WEIGHT MANAGEMENT IN CHILDREN AND ADOLESCENTS

About one third of U.S. children ages 2 to 19 are overweight or obese (State of Obesity, 2018). Childhood obesity increases the risk of obesity in adulthood. For the child who is obese after 6 years of age, the probability of obesity in adulthood is significantly greater if either the mother or the father is obese.

The BMI tables for determining childhood obesity are available for use by health care practitioners (see Appendix 8). High preschool BMI is consistently associated with adult obesity, central obesity, and early onset MetS (Lloyd et al, 2012).

Children or adolescents with a BMI in the 85th percentile or higher with complications of obesity, or with a BMI in the 95th percentile or higher with or without complications, should be carefully assessed for genetic, endocrinologic, and psychological conditions, and secondary complications such as hypertension, dyslipidemias, type 2 diabetes, sleep apnea, and orthopedic problems.

Assessment involves investigating all of the social and environmental factors, including family dynamics, that influence eating and activity habits as well as readiness for change. The primary goal of treatment is to achieve healthy eating and activity, not to achieve an ideal body weight (IBW). For children aged 2 to 5, the goal is prolonged weight maintenance or slowing of the rate of weight gain, which allows for a gradual decline in BMI as children grow in height. This is an appropriate goal in the absence of any secondary complication of obesity. However, if secondary complications are present, children in this age group may benefit from weight loss if their BMI is at the 95th percentile or higher. For children aged 6 and older, prolonged weight maintenance is appropriate if their BMI is between the 85th and 95th percentile and if they have no secondary complications. If a secondary complication is present, or if the BMI is at the 95th percentile or above, weight loss may be advised. Comprehensive, intensive behavioral interventions should be offered (Kaiser Permanente, 2012).

If the weight appropriate for the child's or teen's anticipated adult height has already been reached, maintenance at that weight should be the lifetime goal. The child who already exceeds an optimal adult weight can safely experience a slow weight loss of 10 to 12 pounds per year until the optimal adult weight is reached. Balanced micronutrient intake for children includes 45% to 60% of kilocalories from carbohydrates, 25% to 40% from fat, and 10% to 35% from protein. New directions in childhood obesity research since the turn of the 21st century have uncovered 25(OH)D deficiency (defined as a level less than or equal to 57 nmol/L or 20 ng/mL). This has been manifested by a lack of sun exposure and the increase in use of sunscreen—blocking the skin's absorption of ultraviolet light. Low vitamin D is predominant in obese children. The accompanying proinflammatory association with diabetes and atherogenic pathways has prompted recommendations to test kindergarten and first grade children. Children with low levels of vitamin D could have the systemic inflammatory mediators and reduced insulin sensitivity pathways inhibited by vitamin D supplementation (Reyman et al, 2014).

The child or adolescent who needs to reduce weight requires attention from family and health professionals. This attention should be directed to all the areas mentioned previously, with family modification of eating habits and increased physical activity. The program should be long term, over the entire growth period of the child and perhaps longer.

Inactivity often is coupled with sedentary hobbies, excessive TV watching, or prolonged sitting in front of a computer or game screen. Some theorize that physical inactivity appears to be the result of fatness rather than its cause (Metcalf et al, 2011), however others have postulated that environmental factors, such as a decrease in active commuting, high school physical education, and outdoor play, are contributing factors as well (Bassett et al, 2015). Additional research is required, however it is possible that factors other than inactivity may be more important in obesity development in children (see *New Directions:* Partnership for a Healthier America Addressing Childhood Obesity).

EXCESSIVE LEANNESS OR UNINTENTIONAL WEIGHT LOSS

Almost eclipsed by the attention focused on obesity is the need for some people to gain weight. The term underweight is applicable to those who are 15% to 20% or more below accepted weight standards. Because underweight is often a symptom of disease, it should be assessed medically. A low BMI, less than 18.5 in adults, a BMI of less than 5% for children, and less than 23 in older adults, is associated with greater mortality risk than that of individuals with optimal BMI. Undernutrition may lead to under functioning of the pituitary, thyroid, gonads, and adrenals. Other risk factors include loss of energy and susceptibility to injury and infection, as well as a distorted body image and other psychological problems (see Chapter 21).

Cause

Underweight or unintentional weight loss can be caused by (1) inadequate oral food and beverage intake, with insufficient quantities to match activity; (2) excessive physical activity, as in the case of compulsive athletic training; (3) inadequate capacity for absorption and metabolism of foods consumed; (4) a wasting disease that increases the metabolic rate and energy needs, as in cancer, acquired immune deficiency syndrome (AIDS), or hyperthyroidism; or (5) excess energy expenditure during psychological or emotional stress.

Assessment

Assessing the cause and extent of underweight before starting a treatment program is important. A thorough history and pertinent medical tests usually determine whether underlying disorders or food insecurity are causing the underweight. From anthropometric data such as arm muscle and fat areas, it is possible to determine whether health-endangering underweight really exists (see Appendix 11). Assessment of body fatness is useful, especially in dealing with the patient who has an eating disorder. Biochemical measurements indicate whether malnutrition accompanies the underweight (see Chapter 5 and Appendix 11).

Management

Any underlying cause of unintentional weight loss or low BMI must be the first priority. A wasting disease or malabsorption requires treatment. Nutrition support and dietary changes are effective, along with treatment of the underlying disorder (Table 20.11).

TABLE 20.11 Nutrition Management of Unintentional Weight Loss

Concern	Tips
Anxiety, stress, depression	Antidepressants can help; monitor choice to be sure they do not contribute to weight fluctuations. Ensure adequacy of physical activity as well as folate, B6, B12 and essential fatty acids. See Chapter 40.
Cancer	Gastrointestinal cancers are especially detrimental. Some treatments and medications can cause loss of appetite, as can the cancer itself. See Chapter 35.
Celiac disease	Ensure that all gluten-containing foods and ingredients are eliminated from the diet.
Changes in activity level or dietary preparation methods	Avoid skipping meals; prepare foods with high energy density; add snacks between meals.
Diabetes, new onset	See a physician; monitor medications and ensure adequate intake. See Chapter 29.
Dysphagia or chewing difficulties	Alter food and liquid textures accordingly to improve chewing and swallowing capability. See Chpater 39.
Hyperthyroidism	Too much thyroxine can cause weight loss. See Chapter 30.
Inflammatory bowel disease	Small frequent protein and calorie rich meals, low residue, may need enteral or parenteral nutrition. See Chapter 27.
Intestinal ischemia	Needs medical intervention and potentially enteral or parenteral feedings. See Chapters 12, 26, and 27.
Medications	Some medications can cause weight loss; check with physician; add protein and calorie rich meals and snacks, manage GI side effects like nausea, constipation and diarrhea.
Nausea and vomiting	Infections, other illnesses, hormonal changes, and some medications cause nausea and vomiting; small, frequent meals; serve liquids between meals instead of with meals to reduce fullness. See Chapters 26 and 35.
Pancreatitis and cystic fibrosis	Monitor for sufficiency of pancreatic enzyme replacement, easy to digest, small frequent meals and snacks, lower fat if steatorrhea is present. See Chapters 28 and 33.
Food insecurity	Provide resources for food assistance programs

If the cause of the underweight is inadequate oral food and beverage intake, activity should be limited, and psychological counseling initiated if necessary. If the cause is food insecurity, provide local resources for food assistance.

Appetite Enhancers

The FDA has approved orexigenic agents that include corticosteroids, cyproheptadine, loxiglumide (cholecystokinin antagonist), megestrol acetate, mirtazapine, dronabinol, oxoglutarate, anabolic agents (testosterone or Anadrol), Oxandrin (oxandrolone or oxandrolona), and growth hormone. Use of orexigenic agents for weight loss in seniors is saved for those whose conditions are refractory to usual treatments. One third of older adults, especially women, exhibit weight loss in combination with depression. Mirtazapine is an effective antidepressant that is well tolerated and increases appetite. It is particularly effective in elderly patients with dementia-related weight loss (Fox et al, 2009). Dronabinol is used for chemotherapy-induced nausea and vomiting in cancer and AIDS patients; it has been shown to induce weight gain in patients with dementia. For older adults, moderate amounts of alcohol can also help to increase appetite.

High-Energy Diets

A careful history may reveal inadequacies in dietary habits and nutritional intakes. Meals should be scheduled and eaten when relaxed instead of hastily planned or quickly eaten. The underweight person frequently must be encouraged to eat, even if not hungry.

The secret is to individualize the program with readily available foods that the individual enjoys, with a plan for regular eating times throughout the day. In addition to meals, snacks are usually necessary to adequately increase the energy intake. High-calorie liquids taken with meals or between meals are often effective in those who have loss of appetite or early satiety. Everyday foods can be fortified to increase the calories and protein (see *Focus On:* Food First! in Chapter 19).

The energy distribution of the diet should be approximately 30% of the kilocalories from fat, with the majority from monounsaturated or polyunsaturated sources and at least 12% to 15% of the kilocalories from protein. In addition to an intake according to estimated energy requirements for the present weight, 500 to 1000 extra kcals per day should be planned. If 2400 kcal maintains the current weight, 2900 to 3400 kcal would be required for weight gain.

The intake should be increased gradually to avoid gastric discomfort, discouragement, electrolyte imbalances, and cardiac dysfunction. Step-up plans are outlined in Table 20.12. In underweight children, nonnutritional factors, insufficient caloric intake, excessive nutrient losses, and abnormal energy metabolism may contribute to growth failure and morbidity. Thus adequate nutritional support should be an integral part of the management plan. Lipid-based nutrient supplements are fortified products that are often ready-to-use therapeutic foods or highly concentrated supplements that can be administered at "point of service" or emergency settings (Chaparro and Dewey, 2010).

TABLE 20.12 Suggestions for Increasing Energy Intake

Additional Foods		kcal	Protein (g)
Plus 500 kcal (Served Between Meals)			
A. whole grain fruit and nut cereal		270	5
1 banana		80	
1 c whole milk		160	8
	Total	510	13
B. Milkshake made with 1/2 cup ice cream		145	3
1 tablespoon peanut butter		90	4
1 medium banana		105	8
1 cup whole milk		160	8
	Total	500	23
C. 6 graham cracker squares		165	3
2 T peanut butter		172	8
1 c orange juice		122	
2 T raisins		52	
	Total	511	11
Plus 1000 kcal (Served Between Meals)			
A. 8 oz fruit on the bottom Greek whole milk yogurt		260	18
1 slice whole grain bread		70	3
2 oz cheese		226	14
1 medium apple		87	
¼ of 14-inch cheese pizza		306	16
1 small banana		81	1
	Total	1030	52

Additional Foods		kcal	Protein (g)
B. Instant breakfast with whole milk		280	15
1 c cottage cheese		239	31
½ c pineapple		95	
1 c apple juice		117	
6 graham cracker squares		165	3
1 pear		100	1
	Total	996	50
Plus 1500 kcal (Served Between Meals)			
A. 2 slices whole grain bread		140	6
2 T peanut butter		180	8
1 T jam		110	
6 whole grain crackers		120	3
8 oz fruit on the bottom Greek whole milk yogurt		260	18
3/4 c roasted peanuts		630	28
½ c apricot nectar		70	
	Total	1510	63
B. 1 medium fruit muffin		350	6
2 tsp. butter		70	
4 oz fruit on the bottom Greek whole milk yogurt		130	10
whole grain fruit and nut cereal		272	5
1 banana		80	
1 c whole milk		160	8
1 bagel		260	10
2 T cream cheese		100	2
2 T jam		110	
	Total	1530	40

Source: US Department of Agriculture Food Data Central. https://fdc.nal.usda.gov

CLINICAL CASE STUDY

Norma is a 45-year-old Latina woman who has tried numerous weight loss programs. She has followed strict diets and has never exercised in previous weight loss attempts. She was prescribed lisinopril but forgets to take it regularly. Her blood pressure is 160/90, she is 5 ft 4 in, and she weighs 195 lb. Her lowest body weight was 130 lb at age 30, maintained for 2 years by increasing physical activity and reducing portions and between meal snacking. Since that time her weight has slowly increased to its current level, which Norma reports as her highest ever weight. She reports struggling with motivation and falling back on old habits of not watching portions and eating in front of the TV. Physical activity often falls off when life gets busy and Norma reports putting the needs of others in her family before her own. She tried numerous diets as teenager, when she weighed 170 lb for 3 years but had a hard time staying on them due to the abundance of food at family and social gatherings. What guidelines would you offer to Norma at this time?

Nutrition Diagnostic Statements

• Excessive kcal intake related to difficulty with motivation for health behavior changes as evidence by gradual weight gain of 65 lbs over 15 years and current BMI of 33.5.

• Physical inactivity related to busy schedule and not prioritizing self-care as evidenced by not being physically active for many years and steady weight gain.

Nutrition Care Questions

1. How would you address the concern that she is not taking her medication regularly?
2. What dietary recommendations would you have for Norma?
3. Which macro- and micronutrients would you discuss with Norma (e.g., total fat, saturated fat, protein, sodium, potassium, calcium)?
4. How would you bring up exercise and what would you recommend for Norma?
5. What would you recommend if she wanted to take a dietary supplement for weight loss?

USEFUL WEBSITES

America on the Move
American Society of Bariatric Surgery
Calorie Restriction Society
Healthy Kids, Healthy Future
International Obesity Task Force
Let's Move!
National Heart, Lung, and Blood Institute: Identification, Evaluation, and Treatment of Overweight and Obesity in Adults
National Weight Control Registry
Obesity Week
The Obesity Society
Shape Up America
Weight Control Information Network: National Institute of Diabetes and Digestive and Kidney Disease

REFERENCES

Abbasi J: Interest in the ketogenic diet grows for weight loss and type 2 diabetes, *JAMA* 319:215–217, 2018.

Abdennour M, Reggio S, Le Naour G, et al: Association of adipose tissue and liver fibrosis with tissue stiffness in morbid obesity: links with diabetes and BMI loss after gastric bypass, *J Clin Endocrinol Metab* 99(3):898–907, 2014.

Raynor HA, Champagne CM: Academy of Nutrition and Dietetics, American Dietetic Association: Position of the Academy of Nutrition and Dietetics: interventions for the treatment of overweight and obesity in adults, *J Acad Nutr Diet* 116(1):129–147, 2016.

American Medical Association: *Press release: AMA adopts new policies,* June 18, 2013.

American Society for Metabolic and Bariatric Surgery: *Estimate of bariatric surgery numbers, 2011-2016,* 2016. Available at: https://asmbs.org/resources/estimate-of-bariatric-surgery-numbers.

Apovian C: Is the secret in the strands? Proceedings of the 25th International Conference of Practical Approaches to the Treatment of Obesity, *Harv Med Sch* 407–411, June 16-18, 2011.

Ashraf MJ, Baweja P: Obesity: the 'huge' problem in cardiovascular diseases, *Mo Med* 110(6):499–504, 2013.

Atkinson RL, Macdonald IA: Editors' note: omitting obesity treatment leads to poor outcomes, even in those who appear to be metabolically healthy, *Intl J Obes* 42:285, 2018.

Azad MB, Abou-Setta AM, Chauhan BF, et al: Nonnutritive sweeteners and cardiometabolic health: a systematic review and meta-analysis of randomized controlled trials and prospective cohort studies, *CMAJ* 189(28):E929–E939, 2017. Available at: https://doi.org/10.1503/cmaj.161390.

Bacon L, Keim NL, Van Loan MD, et al: Evaluating a 'non-diet' wellness intervention for improvement of metabolic fitness, psychological well-being and eating and activity behaviors. *Int J Obes Relat Metab Disord* 26:854–865, 2002.

Bassett DR, John D, Conger SA, et al: Trends in physical activity and sedentary behaviors of United States youth, *J Phys Act Health* 12(8):1102–1111, 2015.

Beck JS: *Cognitive behavior therapy: the basics and beyond*, ed 2, New York, NY, 2011, Guilford.

Beebe ML, Crowley N: Can hypocaloric, high-protein nutrition support be used in complicated bariatric patients to promote weight loss? *Nutr Clin Pract* 30:522–529, 2015.

Belfort-DeAguiar R, Seo D: Food cues and obesity: overpowering hormones and energy balance regulation, *Curr Obes Rep* 7:122-129, 2018.

Björntorp P, Sjöström L: Number and size of adipose tissue fat cells in relation to metabolism in human obesity, *Metabolism* 20:703–713, 1971.

Blackburn GL, Bistrian BR, Maini BS, et al. Nutritional and metabolic assessment of the hospitalized patient, *J Parenter Enteral Nutr* 1(1):11–22, 1977.

Blackburn GL, Bistrian BR, Maini BS, et al. Nutrition and Metabolic Assessment of the Hospitalized Patient, *JPEN* 1(1):11–22, 1977.

Blackburn GL, Flatt JP, Clowes GH: Protein-sparing therapy during period of starvation with sepsis or trauma, *Annals of Surgery* 177(5):588.

Blaine BE, Rodman J, Newman JM: Weight loss treatment and psychological well-being: a review and meta-analysis, *J Health Psychol* 12(1):66–82, 2007.

Boonchaya-anant P, Apovian CM: Metabolically healthy obesity—does it exist? *Curr Atheroscler Rep*, 16:441, 2014.

Braghetto I, Csendes A, Lanzarini E, et al: Is laparoscopic sleeve gastrectomy an acceptable primary bariatric procedure in obese patients? Early and 5-year postoperative results, *Surg Laparosc Endosc Percutan Tech* 22(6):479–486, 2012.

Bray GA, Bouchard C: *Handbook of obesity*, ed 3, Boca Raton, Fl, 2014, CRC Press.

Britton KA: Abdominal fat linked to raised heart, cancer risks, *J Am Coll Cardio,* July 10, 2013.

Bueno AC, Sun K, Martins CS, et al: A novel ADIPOQ mutation (p.M40K) impairs assembly of high-molecular-weight adiponectin and is associated with early-onset obesity and metabolic syndrome, *J Clin Endocrinol Metab* 99;E683–E693, 2014.

Byrne NM, Wood RE, Schutz Y, et al: Does metabolic compensation explain the majority of less-than-expected weight loss in obese adults during a short-term severe diet and exercise intervention? *Int J Obes (Lond)* 36:1472–1478, 2012.

Camp KM, Trujillo E: Position of the Academy of Nutrition and Dietetics: nutritional genomics, *J Acad Nutr Diet* 114:299–312, 2014.

Carmienke S, Freitag MH, Pischon T, et al: General and abdominal obesity parameters and their combination in relation to mortality: a systematic review and meta-regression analysis, *Eur J Clin Nutr* 67(6):573–585, 2013.

Carroll S, Borkoles E, Polman R: Short-term effects of a non-dieting lifestyle intervention program on weight management, fitness, metabolic risk, and psychological well-being in obese premenopausal females with the metabolic syndrome, *Appl Physiol Nutr Metab* 32(1):125–142, 2007.

Caulfield T: The obesity gene and the (misplaced) search for a personalized approach to our weight gain problems, *Wake Forest J Law Policy* 5(1):125–145, 2015.

Centers for Disease Control and Prevention: *Overweight and obesity trends, 2008.* Available at: https://www.cdc.gov/obesity/adult/causes.html.

Chan DC, Watts GF, Gan SK, et al: Effect of ezetimibe on hepatic fat, inflammatory markers, and apolipoprotein B-100 kinetics in insulin-resistant obese subjects on a weight loss diet, *Diabetes Care* 33:1134–1139, 2010.

Chang SH, Freeman NLB, Lee JA, et al: Early major complications after bariatric surgery in the USA, 2003-2014: a systematic review and meta-analysis, *Obes Rev* 19:529–537, 2018.

Chaparro CM, Dewey KG: Use of lipid-based nutrient supplements (LNS) to improve the nutrient adequacy of general food distribution rations for vulnerable sub-groups in emergency settings, *Matern Child Nutr* 6 (Suppl 1):1–69, 2010.

Chin SH, Kahathuduwa CN, Binks M: Physical activity and obesity: what we know and what we need to know, *Obes Rev* 17(12):1226–1244, 2016.

Choquet H, Meyre D: Genetics of obesity: what have we learned? *Curr Genomics.* 12:169-179, 2011.

Chung N, Park MY, Kim J, et al: Non-exercise activity thermogenesis (NEAT): a component of total daily energy expenditure, *J Exerc Nutrition Biochem* 22(2):23–30, 2018.

Clamp LD, Hume DJ, Lambert EV, et al: Successful and unsuccessful weight-loss maintainers: strategies to counteract metabolic compensation following weight loss, *J Nutr Sci* 28(7):e20, 2018.

Collins CE, Morgan PJ, Jones P, et al: A 12-week commercial web-based weight-loss program for overweight and obese adults: randomized controlled trial comparing basic versus enhanced features, *J Med Internet Res* 14(2):e57, 2012.

Davis CS, Clarke RE, Coulter SN, et al: Intermittent energy restriction and weight loss: a systematic review, *Eur J Clin Nutr* 70:292–299, 2016.

Dhurandhar NV, Schoeller D, Brown AW, et al: Energy balance measurement: when something is NOT better than nothing. *Int J Obes (Lond)* 39(7):1109–1113, 2015.

Dietary guidelines for Americans, 2015-2020, ed 8, December 2015, U.S. Department of Health and Human Services and U.S. Department of Agriculture. Available at: http://health.gov/dietaryguidelines/2015/guidelines/.

Drummen M, Tischmann L, Gatta-Cherifi B, et al: Dietary protein and energy balance in relation to obesity and co-morbidities, *Front Endocrinol (Lausanne)* 6;9:443, 2018.

Ellulu MS, Patimah I, Khaza'ai H, et al: Obesity and inflammation: the linking mechanism and the complications, *Arch Med Sci* 13(4):851–863, 2017.

Endocrine Today: *Understanding genetics of obesity will require larger studies, effect sizes,* March 23, 2018: Available at: https://www.healio.com/endocrinology/obesity/news/online/%7B2dd78204-08a8-4093-a633-8528cfd8c7c6%7D/understanding-genetics-of-obesity-will-require-larger-studies-effect-sizes?page=4.

Fabricatore AN, Wadden TA, Higginbotham AJ, et al: Intentional weight loss and changes in symptoms of depression: a systematic review and meta-analysis, *Int J Obes (Lond)* 35:1363–1376, 2011.

Federal Register: *Food labeling: nutrition labeling of standard menu items in restaurants and similar retail food establishments,* 2014. Available at: https://www.federalregister.gov/regulations/0910-AG57/food-labeling-nutrition-labeling-of-standard-menu-items-in-restaurants-and-similar-retail-food-estab.

Ferguson JF, Phillips CM, Tierney AC, et al: Gene-nutrient interactions in the metabolic syndrome: single nucleotide polymorphisms in ADIPOQ and ADIPOR1 interact with plasma saturated fatty acids to modulate insulin resistance, *Am J Clin Nutr* 91:794–801, 2010.

Fothergill E, Guo J, Howard L, et al: Persistent metabolic adaptation 6 years after "The Biggest Loser" competition, *Obesity (Silver Spring)* 24:1612–1619, 2016.

Fox CB, Treadway AK, Blaszczyk AT, et al: Megestrol acetate and mirtazapine for the treatment of unplanned weight loss in the elderly, *Pharmacotherapy* 29(4):383–397, 2009.

Fulton JE: *The state of physical activity in America,* 2016. Available at: https://health.gov/paguidelines/second-edition/meetings/1/The-State-of-Physical-Activity-in-America.pdf.

Garaulet M, Ordovás JM, Madrid JA: The chronobiology, etiology and pathophysiology of obesity, *Int J Obes (Lond)* 34:1667–1683, 2010.

Gardner CD, Trepanowski JF, Del Gobbo LC, et al: Effect of low-fat vs low-carbohydrate diet on 12-month weight loss in overweight adults and the association with genotype pattern or insulin secretion: the dietfits randomized clinical trial, *JAMA* 319(7):667–679, 2018.

Garland T, Schutz H, Chappell MA, et al: The biological control of voluntary exercise, spontaneous physical activity and daily energy expenditure in relation to obesity: human and rodent perspectives, *J Exp Biology* 214:206–229, 2011.

Goodarzi MO: Genetics of obesity: what genetic association studies have taught us about the biology of obesity and its complications, *Lancet diabetes Endocrinol* 6:223–236, 2018.

Grimble RF: The true cost of in-patient obesity: impact of obesity on inflammatory stress and morbidity, *Proc Nutr Soc* 69:511–517, 2010.

Grün F, Blumberg B: Environmental obesogens: organotins and endocrine disruption via nuclear receptor signaling, *Endocrinology* 147(Suppl 6):S50–S55, 2006.

Gudzune KA, Doshi RS, Mehta AK, et al: Efficacy of commercial weight-loss programs: an updated systematic review, *Ann Intern Med* 162(7):501–512, 2015.

Guo J, Brager DC, Hall KD: Simulating long-term human weight loss dynamics in response to calorie restriction, *Am J Clin Nutr* 558–565, 2018.

Hall KD, Bemis T, Brychta R, et al: Calorie for calorie, dietary fat restriction results in more body fat loss than carbohydrate restriction in people with obesity, *Cell Metab* 22:427–436, 2015.

Hall KD, Guo J: Obesity energetics: body weight regulation and the effects of diet composition, *Gastroenterology* 152(7):1718-1727.e3, 2017.

Hall KD, Hammond RA, Rahmandad H: Dynamic interplay among homeostatic, hedonic, and cognitive feedback circuits regulating body weight, *Am J Public Health* 104:1169–1175, 2014.

Hall KD, Sacks G, Chandramohan D, et al: Quantification of the effect of energy imbalance on bodyweight, *Lancet* 378(9793):826–837, 2011.

Hall KD: A review of the carbohydrate—insulin model of obesity, *Eur J Clin Nutr* 323–326, 2017.

Harris L, McGarty A, Hutchison L, et al: Short-term intermittent energy restriction interventions for weight management: a systematic review and meta-analysis, *Obes Rev* 19(1):1–13, 2018.

Headland M, Clifton PM, Carter S, et al: Weight-loss outcomes: a systematic review and meta-analysis of intermittent energy restriction trials lasting a minimum of 6 months, *Nutrients* 8(6):E354, 2016.

Hughes AR, Sherriff A, Ness AR, et al: Timing of adiposity rebound and adiposity in adolescence, *Pediatrics* 134:e1354–e1361, 2014.

Huth C, Pigeon É, Riou Mν̀a: Fitness, adiposopathy, and adiposity are independent predictors of insulin sensitivity in middle-aged men without diabetes, *J Physiol Biochem* 72(3):435–444, 2016.

Ibrahim AM, Thumma JR, Dimick JB: Reoperation and medicare expenditures after laparoscopic gastric band surgery, *JAMA Surg* 152(9):835–842, 2017.

Johnston BC, Kanters S, Bandayrel K, et al: Comparison of weight loss among named diet programs in overweight and obese adults a meta-analysis. *JAMA* 312(9):923–933, 2014.

Kaiser Permanente: *Weight management in children and adolescents screening and intervention guide,* 2012. Available at: https://wa.kaiserpermanente.org/static/pdf/public/guidelines/weight-adolescent.pdf.

Kaplan, L: *Treating obesity: A 2018 overview. Blackburn course in obesity medicine.* Harvard Medical School, June 2018. Available at: https://obesity.hmscme.com.

Krajmalnik-Brown R, Ilhan ZE, Kang DW, et al: Effect of gut microbes on nutrient absorption and energy regulation, *Nutr Clin Pract* 27:201–214, 2012.

Krakauer NY, Krakauer JC: Dynamic association of mortality hazards with body shape, *PLoS One* 9:e88793, 2014.

Kramer CK, Zinman B, Retnakaran R: Are metabolically healthy overweight and obesity benign conditions? A systematic review and meta-analysis, *Ann Intern Med* 159(11):758–769, 2013.

Kraschnewski JL, Boan J, Esposito J, et al: Long-term weight loss maintenance in the United States, *Int J Obes* 34;1644–1654, 2010.

La Merrill M, Emond C, Kim MJ, et al: Toxicological Function of Adipose Tissue: Focus on persistent organic pollutants, *Environ Health Perspect* 121:162–169, 2013.

Lasikiewicz, N, Myrissa K, Hoyland A, et al: Psychological benefits of weight loss following behavioral and/or dietary weight loss interventions. A systematic research review, *Appetite* 72:123–137, 2014.

Leblanc V, Provencher V, Bégin C, et al: Impact of a Health-At-Every-Size intervention on changes in dietary intakes and eating patterns in premenopausal overweight women: results of a randomized trial, *Clin Nutr* 31(4):481–488, 2012.

Lee YM, Jacobs DR Jr, Lee DH: Persistent organic pollutants and type 2 diabetes: a critical review of review articles, *Front Endocrinol (Lausanne)* 9:712, 2018.

Lee YM, Kim KS, Jacobs DR Jr, et al: Persistent organic pollutants in adipose tissue should be considered in obesity research, *Obes Rev* 18(2):129–139, 2017.

Leidy HJ, Clifton PM, Astrup A, et al: The role of protein in weight loss and maintenance, *Am J Clin Nutr* 101:1320S–1329S, 2015.

Liu G, Dhana K, Furtado JD, et al: Perfluoroalkyl substances and changes in body weight and resting metabolic rate in response to weight-loss diets: a prospective study, *PLos Med* 15(2):e1002502, 2018.

Lloyd LJ, Langley-Evans SC, McMullen S: Childhood obesity and risk of the adult metabolic syndrome: a systematic review, *Int J Obes* 36:1–11, 2012

Loos RJ. The genetics of adiposity, *Curr Opin Genet Dev* 50:86–95, 2018.

Malhotra A, Noakes T, Phinney S: It is time to bust the myth of physical inactivity and obesity: you cannot outrun a bad diet, *Br J Sports Med* 49(15):967–968, 2015.

Meek CL, Lewis HB, Reimann F, et al: The effect of bariatric surgery on gastrointestinal and pancreatic peptide hormones, *Peptides* 77:28–37, 2016.

Mensinger JL, Calogero RM, Stranges S, et al: A weight-neutral versus weight-loss approach for health promotion in women with high BMI: a randomized-controlled trial, *Appetite* 105:364–374, 2016.

Metcalf BS, Hosking J, Jeffery AN, et al: Fatness leads to inactivity, but inactivity does not lead to fatness: a longitudinal study in children (EarlyBird 45), *Arch Dis Child* 96:942–947, 2011.

Mozaffarian D: Dietary and policy priorities for cardiovascular disease, diabetes, and obesity a comprehensive review, *Circulation* 133(2):187–225, 2016.

Müller MJ, Geisler C: Defining obesity as a disease, *Nature* 71:1256–1258, 2017.

Müller MJ, Geisler C, Heymsfield SB, et al: Recent advances in understanding body weight homeostasis in humans, *F1000Research* 7:F1000 Faculty Rev-1025, 2018.

Nappi F, Barrea L, Di Somma C, et al: Endocrine aspects of environmental "Obesogen" pollutants, *Int J Envir Res Pub Health* 13:765, 2016.

NAS IOM: Dietary Reference Intakes for Energy, Carbohydrate, Fiber, Fat, Fatty acids, Cholesterol, Protein, and Amino Acids (Macronutrients), *The National Academies Press*. 2005. Available at: https://www.nal.usda.gov/sites/default/files/fnic_uploads/energy_full_report.pdf.

National Task Force on the Prevention and Treatment of Obesity: Dieting and the development of eating disorders in overweight and obese adults, *Arch Intern Med* 160(17):2581–2589, 2000.

Naude CE, Schoonees A, Senekal M, et al: Low carbohydrate versus isoenergetic balanced diets for reducing weight and cardiovascular risk: a systematic review and meta-analysis, *PLOS One* 9(7):e100652, 2014.

NHLBI: Expert Panel Report: Guidelines (2013) for the management of overweight and obesity in adults, *Obesity* 22(suppl 2):S41–S410, 2014. NIH Publication No. #98-4083.

O'Neal TJ, Friend DM, Guo J, et al: Increases in physical activity result in diminishing increments in daily energy expenditure in Mice, *Curr Biol* 27:423–430, 2017.

Ostendorf DM, Melanson EL, Caldwell AE, et al: No consistent evidence of a disproportionately low resting energy expenditure in long-term successful weight-loss maintainers, *Am J Clin Nutr* 108(4):658–666, 2018.

Palavras MA, Hay P, Filho CA, et al: The efficacy of psychological therapies in reducing weight and binge eating in people with bulimia nervosa and binge eating disorder who are overweight or obese-a critical synthesis and meta-analyses. *Nutrients* 9(3):E299, 2017 doi:10.3390/nu9030299.

Parrott J, Frank L, Rabena R, et al: American society for metabolic and bariatric surgery integrated health nutritional guidelines for the surgical weight loss patient 2016 update: micronutrients, *Surg Obes Relat Dis* 13(5):727–741, 2017.

Piercy KL, Troiano RP, Ballard RM, et al: The physical activity guidelines for Americans, *JAMA* 2020:2020–2028, 2018.

Pomeranz JL, Puhl RM: New developments in the law for obesity and discrimination protection, *Obesity* 21:469–471, 2013.

Ponterio E, Gnessi L: Adenovirus 36 and obesity: an overview, *Viruses* 7:3719–3740, 2015.

Ramage S, Farmer A, Eccles KA, et al: Healthy strategies for successful weight loss and weight maintenance: a systematic review, *Appl Physiol Nutr Metab* 39:1–20, 2014.

Reyman M, Verrijn Stuart AA, van Summeren M, et al: Vitamin D deficiency in childhood obesity is associated with high levels of circulating inflammatory mediators, and low insulin sensitivity, *Int J Obes (Lond)* 38(1):46–52, 2014.

Rocha VZ, Folco EJ: Inflammatory concepts of obesity, *Int J Inflam* 2011:529061, 2011.

Saber AA, Shoar S, Almadani MW, et al: Efficacy of first-time intragastric balloon in weight loss: a systematic review and meta-analysis of randomized controlled trials, *Obes Surg* 27:277–287, 2017.

Song Z, Xiaoli AM, Yang F: Regulation and metabolic significance of De Novo Lipogenesis in Adipose Tissues, *Nutrients* 10(10):E1383, 2018.

State of Obesity: *The state of childhood obesity*, 2018. Available at: https://stateofobesity.org/childhood-obesity-trends/.

Steinhardt MA, Bezner JR, Adams TB: Outcomes of a traditional weight control program and a nondiet alternative: a one-year comparison, *J Psychol* 133(5):495–513, 1999.

Stewart F, Avenell A: Behavioural Interventions for severe obesity before and/or after bariatric surgery: a systematic review and meta-analysis, *Obes Surg* 26:1203–1214, 2016.

Stunkard A, Lu XY: Rapid changes in night eating: considering mechanisms, *Eat Weight Disord* 15:e2–e8, 2010.

Swift DL, Johannsen NM, Lavie CJ, et al: The role of exercise and physical activity in weight loss and maintenance, *Prog Cardiovasc Dis* 56(4):441–447, 2014.

Tagliabue A, Ferraris C, Uggeri F, et al: Short-term impact of classical ketogenic diet on gut microbiota in GLUT1 Deficiency Syndrome: a 3-month prospective observational study, *Clin Nutr ESPEN* 17:33–37, 2017.

Tam CS, Lecoultre V, Ravussin E: Brown adipose tissue: mechanisms and potential therapeutic targets, *Circulation* 125(22):2782–2791, 2012.

Tambo A, Pace NP: The Microbial hypothesis: contributions of adenovirus infection and metabolic endotoxaemia to the pathogenesis of obesity, *Int J Chron Dis* 2016:7030795, 2016.

Thomas JG, Bond DS, Phelan S, et al, Weight-loss maintenance for 10 years in the National Weight Control Registry, *Am J Prev Med* 46:17–23, 2014.

Tremblay A, Pelletier C, Doucet E, et al: Thermogenesis and weight loss in obese individuals: a primary association with organochlorine pollution, *Int J Obes Relat Metab Disord* 28:936–939, 2004.

Tuulari JJ, Karlsson HK, Hirvonen J, et al: Weight loss after bariatric surgery reverses insulin-induced increases in brain glucose metabolism of the morbidly obese, *Diabetes* 62:2747–2751, 2013.

Ulian MD, Benatti FB, de Campos-Ferraz PL, et al: The effects of a "Health At Every Size®"-based approach in obese women: a pilot-trial of the "Health and Wellness in Obesity" study, *Front Nutr* 2:34, 2015.

Ulian MD, Aburad L, da Silva Oliveira MS, et al: Effects of Health At Every Size® interventions on health-related outcomes of people with overweight and obesity: a systematic review, *Obes Rev* 19:1659–1666, 2018a.

Ulian MD, Pinto AJ, de Morais Sato P, et al: Effects of a new Health at Every Size-based intervention for the management of obesity, *PLoS ONE* 13(7):e0198401, 2018b.

Wadden TA, Sarwer DB: Behavioral assessment of candidates for bariatric surgery: a patient-oriented approach, *Surg Obes Relat Dis* 2:171–179, 2006.

Wajchenberg BL: Subcutaneous and visceral adipose tissue: their relation to the metabolic syndrome, *Endocr Rev* 21(6):697–738, 2013.

Westerterp-Plantenga MS, Lemmens SG, Westerterp KR: Dietary protein – its role in satiety, energetics, weight loss and health, *Br J Nutr* 108(52):S105–S112, 2012.

Weiner RA, Theodoridou S, Weiner S: Failure of laparoscopic sleeve gastrectomy—further procedure? *Obes Facts* 4 (Suppl 1):42–46, 2011.

WHO: *Obesity and overweight fact sheet*. 2018. Available at: http://www.who.int/mediacentre/factsheets/fs311/en/.

Yang MU, Van Itallie TB: composition of weight lost during short-term weight reduction. Metabolic responses of obese subjects to starvation and low-calorie ketogenic and nonketogenic diets, *J Clin Invest* 58:722–730, 1976.

21

Nutrition in Eating Disorders

Janet E. Schebendach, PhD, RDN
Justine Roth, MS, CEDRD

KEY TERMS

anorexia nervosa (AN)
avoidant/restrictive food intake disorder (ARFID)
binge
binge eating disorder (BED)
bulimia nervosa (BN)

cognitive-behavioral therapy (CBT)
Diagnostic and Statistical Manual of Mental Disorders, fifth edition (DSM-5)
diet-induced thermogenesis (DIT)
family-based therapy (FBT)

other specified feeding or eating disorder (OSFED)
purging
refeeding syndrome (RFS)
Russell's sign

Feeding and eating disorders (EDs) are characterized by a persistent disturbance of eating or eating-related behavior that results in significantly impaired physical health and psychosocial functioning. Diagnostic criteria (Box 21.1) are published in the *Diagnostic and Statistical Manual of Mental Disorders, fifth edition (DSM-5)* (American Psychiatric Association [APA], 2013). Revised DSM-5 criteria are available for anorexia nervosa (AN), bulimia nervosa (BN), and binge eating disorder (BED); new criteria have been established for other specified feeding or eating disorder (OSFED), avoidant/restrictive food intake disorder (ARFID), pica, and rumination disorder.

Anorexia Nervosa

Essential features of anorexia nervosa (AN) include persistent energy intake restriction; intense fear of gaining weight or of becoming fat or persistent behavior that interferes with maintenance of appropriate weight; and a disturbance in self-perceived weight or shape. The two diagnostic subtypes are restrictive eating only (AN-R) and restrictive eating interspersed with binge eating or purging (AN-BP); crossover between the subtypes is possible over the course of illness. The DSM-5 allows clinicians to document a severity rating for a case of AN: mild, moderate, severe, and extreme. Severity ratings are differentiated based on current body mass index (BMI, adults) or BMI percentile (children/adolescents); however, the rating may be increased at the clinician's discretion to reflect clinical symptoms, degree of functional disability, and the need for supervision. In the general population, lifetime prevalence of AN is about 1% in women and less than 0.5% in men (Hay et al, 2014). Presentation typically occurs during adolescence or young adulthood, but prepubertal and late-onset (after age 40) cases have been described. Although AN occurs across culturally and socially diverse populations, increased prevalence occurs in postindustrialized, high-income countries. Within the United States, presentation of weight concerns among individuals with EDs may vary across cultural and ethnic groups (Becker, 2016; Sala, 2013). Body image dissatisfaction, dangerous weight control behaviors, and EDs are emerging issues for lesbian, gay, bisexual, transgender and queer (LGBTQ) youth (McClain and Peebles, 2016), but prevalence and incidence rates for AN in these populations are not currently reported. Risk and prognostic factors associated with AN include genetic, physiologic, environmental, and temperamental characteristics (Table 21.1). The crude mortality rate is about 5% per decade with death attributed to medical complications directly related to AN or suicide (APA, 2013).

Bulimia Nervosa

Features of bulimia nervosa (BN) include recurrent episodes of binge eating followed by inappropriate compensatory behaviors in an effort to prevent weight gain, and self-evaluation that is unduly influenced by body shape and weight (APA, 2013). A binge consumption is an episode of uncontrollable eating of an excessive amount of food in a discrete period of time. Inappropriate compensatory mechanisms include self-induced vomiting, misuse of laxatives, diuretics, fasting, and excessive exercise. An individual may employ one or more methods. The DSM-5 includes four levels of severity ratings based on frequency of inappropriate compensatory behaviors: mild, moderate, severe, extreme. Although the default level of severity is based on the frequency of these episodes, the level of severity may be increased at the clinician's discretion to reflect other symptoms and the degree of functional disability. Lifetime prevalence of BN is approximately 2% in women and 0.5% in men (Hay et al, 2014). Initial presentation typically occurs during adolescence or young adulthood; prepubertal and late onset (after age 40) cases are uncommon. Diagnostic crossover from BN to AN occurs in 10% to 15% of cases. However, individuals who cross over to AN often revert back to BN, and some experience multiple crossovers between these disorders. BN occurs at similar frequencies in industrialized countries (APA, 2013). The prevalence of BN is similar among ethnic groups (APA, 2013). Risk and prognostic factors associated with BN include genetic, physiologic, environmental, and temperamental characteristics (see Table 21.1). BN is associated with a significantly elevated risk for mortality (all-cause and suicide), with a crude mortality rate of approximately 2% per decade (APA, 2013).

BOX 21.1   American Psychiatric Association (DSM-5) Diagnostic Criteria

Anorexia Nervosa (AN)

A. Restriction of energy intake relative to requirements, leading to a significantly low body weight in the context of age, sex, developmental trajectory, and physical health. *Significantly low weight* is defined as a weight that is less than minimally normal, or for children and adolescents, less than that minimally expected.

B. Intense fear of gaining weight or of becoming fat, or persistent behavior that interferes with weight gain, even though at a significantly low weight.

C. Disturbance in the way in which one's body weight or shape is experienced, undue influence of body weight or shape on self-evaluation, or persistent lack of recognition of the seriousness of the current low body weight.

Specify whether:

1. Restricting type: During the last 3 months, the individual has not engaged in recurrent episodes of binge eating or purging behavior (i.e., self-induced vomiting or the misuse of laxatives, diuretics, or enemas). This subtype describes presentations in which weight loss is accomplished primarily through dieting, fasting, and/or excessive exercise.

2. Binge-eating/purging type: During the last 3 months, the individual has engaged in recurrent episodes of binge eating or purging behavior (i.e., self-induced vomiting or the misuse of laxatives, diuretics, or enemas).

Specify current severity:

The minimum level of severity is based, for adults, on current body mass index (BMI) (see below) or, for children and adolescents, on BMI percentile. The ranges below are derived from World Health Organization categories for thinness in adults; for children and adolescents, corresponding BMI percentiles should be used. The level of severity may be increased to reflect clinical symptoms, the degree of functional disability, and the need for supervision.

Mild: BMI $\geq$17 kg/m^2
Moderate: BMI 16-16.99 kg/m^2
Severe: BMI 15-15.99 kg/m^2
Extreme: BMI <15 kg/m^2

Bulimia Nervosa (BN)

A. Recurrent episodes of binge eating at least once a week for 3 months. An episode of binge-eating is characterized by both of the following:

1. Eating, in a discrete period of time (e.g., within any 2-hour period), an amount of food that is definitely larger than what most individuals would eat in a similar period of time under similar circumstances.

2. A sense of lack of control over eating during the episode (e.g., a feeling that one cannot stop eating or control what or how much one is eating).

B. Recurrent inappropriate compensatory behaviors in order to prevent weight gain, such as self-induced vomiting; misuse of laxatives, diuretics, or other medications; fasting; or excessive exercise.

C. The binge eating and inappropriate compensatory behaviors both occur, on average, at least once a week for 3 months.

D. Self-evaluation is unduly influenced by body shape and weight.

E. The disturbance does not occur exclusively during episodes of AN.

Specify current severity:

The minimum level of severity is based on the frequency of inappropriate compensatory behaviors (see below). The level of severity may be increased to reflect other symptoms and the degree of functional disability.

Mild: An average of 1-3 episodes of inappropriate compensatory behaviors per week.

Moderate: An average of 4-7 episodes of inappropriate compensatory behaviors per week.

Severe: An average of 8-13 episodes of inappropriate compensatory behaviors per week.

Extreme: An average of 14 or more episodes of inappropriate compensatory behaviors per week.

Binge Eating Disorder (BED)

A. Recurrent episodes of binge eating. An episode of binge-eating is characterized by both of the following:

1. Eating, in a discrete period of time (e.g., within any 2-hour period), an amount of food that is definitely larger than what most individuals would eat in a similar period of time under similar circumstances.

2. A sense of lack of control over eating during the episode (e.g., a feeling that one cannot stop eating or control what or how much one is eating).

B. The binge-eating episodes are associated with three (or more) of the following:

1. Eating more rapidly than normal.

2. Eating until feeling uncomfortably full.

3. Eating large amount of food when not physically hungry.

4. Eating alone because of feeling embarrassed by how much one is eating.

5. Feeling disgusted with oneself, depressed, or very guilty afterward.

C. Marked distress regarding binge eating is present.

D. The binge eating occurs, on average, at least once a week for 3 months.

E. The binge eating is not associated with the recurrent use of inappropriate compensatory behavior as in bulimia nervosa and does not occur exclusively during the course of BN or AN.

Specify current severity:

The minimum level of severity is based on the frequency of episodes of binge eating (see below). The level of severity may be increased to reflect other symptoms and the degree of functional disability.

Mild: 1-3 binge-eating episodes per week.
Moderate: 4-7 binge-eating episodes per week.
Severe: 8-13 binge-eating episodes per week.
Extreme: 14 or more binge-eating episodes per week.

Other Specified Feeding and Eating Disorder

This category applies to presentations in which symptoms characteristic of a feeding and eating disorder that cause clinically significant distress or impairment in social, occupational, or other important areas of functions predominate but do not meet the full criteria for any of the disorders in the feeding and eating disorders diagnostic class. The other specified feeding and eating disorder category is used in situations in which the clinician chooses to communicate the specific reason that the presentation does not meet the criteria for any specific feeding and eating disorder. This is done by recording "other specified feeding or eating disorder" followed by the specific reason (e.g., "bulimia nervosa of low frequency"). Examples of presentations that can be specified using the "other specified" designation include the following:

1. Atypical AN: All of the criteria for AN are met, except that despite significant weight loss, the individual's weight is within or above the normal range.

2. BN (of low frequency and/or limited duration): All of the criteria from BN are met, except that the binge eating and inappropriate compensatory behaviors occur, on average, less than once a week and/or for less than 3 months.

3. BED (of low frequency and/or limited duration): All of the criteria for BED are met, except that the binge eating occurs, on average, less than once a week and/or for less than 3 months.

4. Purging disorder: Recurrent purging behavior to influence weight or shape (e.g., self-induced vomiting; misuse of laxatives, diuretics, or other medications) in the absence of binge eating.

5. Night eating syndrome: Recurrent episodes of night eating, as manifested by eating after awakening from sleep or by excessive food consumption after the evening meal. There is awareness and recall of the eating. The night eating is not better explained by external influences such as changes in the individual's sleep-wake cycle or by local social norms. The night eating causes significant distress and/or impairment in functioning. The disordered pattern of eating is not better explained by BED or another mental disorder, including substance use, and is not attributable to another medical disorder or to the effect of medication.

BOX 21.1 American Psychiatric Association (DSM-5) Diagnostic Criteria—cont'd

Unspecified Feeding or Eating Disorder

This category applies to presentations in which symptoms characteristic of a feeding and eating disorder that cause clinically significant distress or impairment in social, occupational, or other important areas of functioning predominate but do not meet the full criteria for any of the disorders in the feeding and eating disorders diagnostic class. The unspecified feeding and eating disorder category is used in situations in which the clinician chooses *not* to specify the reason that the criteria are not met for a specific feeding and eating disorder, and includes presentations in which there is insufficient information to make a more specific diagnosis (e.g., in emergency room settings).

Avoidant/Restrictive Food Intake Disorder*

A. An eating or feeding disturbance (e.g., apparent lack of interest in eating or food; avoidance based on the sensory characteristics of food; concern about aversive consequences of eating) as manifested by persistent failure to meet appropriate nutritional and/or energy needs associated with one (or more) of the following:
   1. Significant weight loss (or failure to achieve expected weight gain or faltering growth in children).
   2. Significant nutritional deficiency.
   3. Dependence on enteral feeding or oral nutritional supplements.
   4. Marked interference with psychosocial functioning.
B. The disturbance is not better explained by lack of available food or by an associated culturally sanctioned practice.
C. The eating disturbance does not occur exclusively during the course of AN or BN, and there is no evidence of a disturbance in the way in which one's body weight or shape is experienced.
D. The eating disturbance is not attributable to a concurrent medical condition or not better explained by another mental disorder. When the eating disturbance occurs in the context of another condition or disorder, the severity of the eating disturbance exceeds that routinely associated with the condition or disorder and warrants additional clinical attention.

Pica

A. Persistent eating of nonnutritive, nonfood substances over a period of at least 1 month.
B. The eating of nonnutritive, nonfood substances is inappropriate to the developmental level of the individual.
C. The eating behavior is not part of a culturally supported or socially normative practice.
D. If the eating behaviors occur in the context of another mental disorder (e.g., intellectual disability [intellectual developmental disorder], autism spectrum disorder, schizophrenia) or medical condition (including pregnancy), it is sufficiently severe to warrant additional clinical attention.

Rumination Disorder

A. Repeated regurgitation of food over a period of at least 1 month. Regurgitated food may be rechewed, reswallowed, or spit out.
B. The repeated regurgitation is not attributable to an associated gastrointestinal or other medical condition (e.g., gastroesophageal reflux, pyloric stenosis).
C. The eating disturbance does not occur exclusively during the course of AN, BN, BED, or avoidant/restrictive food intake disorder.
D. If the symptoms occur in the context of another mental disorder (e.g., intellectual disability [intellectual developmental disorder] or another neurodevelopmental disorder), they are sufficiently severe to warrant additional clinical attention.

*A change to criterion A has been proposed. The stem includes the clause, "as manifested by persistent failure to meet appropriate nutritional and/or energy needs;" however, criterion A.4 does not describe a manifestation of a nutritional problem. The APA proposes to delete the clause in the stem, so that marked psychosocial impairment alone would satisfy criterion A.
American Psychiatric Association: *Diagnostic and Statistical Manual of Mental Disorders*, ed 5, Arlington, VA, 2013, American Psychiatric Association.

TABLE 21.1 Risk and Prognostic Factors Associated With Anorexia Nervosa and Bulimia Nervosa

Diagnosis	Temperament	Environment	Genetic and Physiologic
AN	Obsessional traits in childhood Anxiety disorders	Cultures/settings that value thinness Occupations/avocations that encourage thinness, (e.g., modeling, elite athletics)	First-degree biological relative with AN, BN, bipolar disorder, or depressive disorder Higher concordance rates in monozygotic vs. dizygotic twins Functional imaging studies indicate a range of brain abnormalities but unclear if changes are primary anomalies or secondary to malnutrition
BN	Weight concerns Low self-esteem Depressive symptoms Social anxiety disorder Overanxious disorder of childhood	Internalization of thin body ideal Increased weight concerns Childhood sexual abuse Childhood physical abuse	Childhood obesity/large body size Early pubertal maturation Genetic vulnerabilities

AN, Anorexia nervosa; *BN*, bulimia nervosa.
American Psychiatric Association: *Diagnostic and Statistical Manual of Mental Disorders*, ed 5, Arlington, VA, American Psychiatric Association, 2013.

Binge Eating Disorder

A major change in the DSM-5 is the official recognition of binge eating disorder (BED) as a clinical disorder. Although BED was included in the DSM-IV (APA, 2000), those criteria were established only for research purposes. The essential feature of BED is recurrent episodes of binge eating without inappropriate compensatory measures (such as purging) intended to prevent weight gain. BED diagnostic criteria include four levels of severity ratings (mild, moderate, severe, and extreme) that are based on the frequency of binge episodes. The level of severity may be increased at the clinician's discretion to reflect other symptoms as well as the degree of functional disability. The lifetime prevalence of BED is approximately 3.5% in women and 2% in men (Hay et al, 2014). BED occurs at similar frequencies in most industrialized countries. In the United States, prevalence rates appear comparable among Caucasians, Latinos, Asians, and African Americans. BED is more prevalent among individuals seeking weight loss treatment than in the general population. Crossover from BED to other EDs is uncommon. Binge eating disorder appears to run in families, which may reflect additive genetic influences (APA, 2013); less is known about temperamental and environmental risk and prognostic factors.

Other Specified Feeding or Eating Disorder

Other specified feeding or eating disorder (OSFED) applies to atypical AN (restrictive eating in the presence of normal weight), atypical BN and atypical BED (episodes are less frequent or of limited duration), purging disorder (i.e., recurrent purging in the absence of binge eating), and night eating syndrome. Treatment of subclinical AN, BN, and BED is similar to that used for full criteria presentation, but the frequency of therapeutic interventions (e.g., psychotherapy, nutrition therapy, medical management) and the treatment setting (e.g., inpatient hospitalization, day hospital/partial hospitalization, intensive outpatient treatment, outpatient treatment) may differ. Patients with a purging disorder and night eating syndrome often benefit from psychotherapeutic approaches used in the treatment of BN and BED.

Avoidant/Restrictive Food Intake Disorder

Patients with avoidant/restrictive food intake disorder (ARFID) exhibit restrictive/avoidant eating behaviors that result in significant weight loss, impaired growth, nutritional deficiencies, and reliance on enteral feedings/supplements, as well as impaired psychosocial functioning (Norris et al, 2016). These restrictive eating behaviors are not associated with body image dissatisfaction or fear of weight gain. Compared with patients with AN and BN, these individuals tend to be younger and have higher proportion of males; be selective (picky) eaters since early childhood; have fears of choking or vomiting; and avoid foods based on their appearance, texture, and smell (Fisher et al, 2014).

CLINICAL CHARACTERISTICS AND MEDICAL COMPLICATIONS

Although EDs are classified as psychiatric illnesses, they are associated with significant medical complications, morbidity, and mortality. Numerous physiologic changes result from the dysfunctional behaviors associated with AN, BN, and BED. Some are minor changes related to excessive or inadequate nutrient intake; some are pathologic alterations with long-term consequences; a few represent potentially life-threatening conditions.

Anorexia Nervosa

Initially, individuals with AN may simply appear underweight. As the disease progresses, patients appear increasingly cachectic and prepubescent in their appearance (Fig. 21.1). Common physical findings at this stage include lanugo (i.e., a soft, downy hair growth on the face and extremities), dry skin and hair, cold intolerance, cyanosis of the extremities, edema, and primary or secondary amenorrhea. The degree of symptomatology varies person to person and with duration of illness; for example, some women with anorexia experience amenorrhea, some do not.

Cardiovascular complications may include bradycardia, orthostatic hypotension, cardiac arrhythmias, and pericardial effusion. Protein-energy malnutrition (PEM) with resultant loss of lean body mass is associated with reduced left ventricular mass and systolic dysfunction; however, cardiac function is largely reversible with nutritional rehabilitation and weight restoration.

Gastrointestinal complications secondary to starvation include delayed gastric emptying, decreased small bowel motility, and

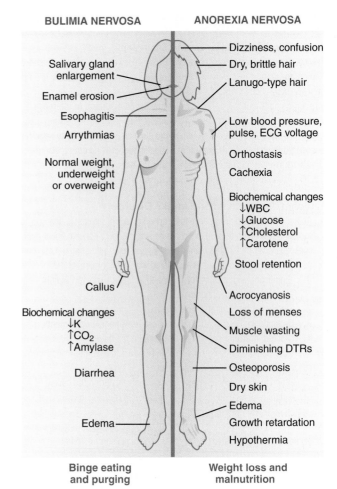

Fig. 21.1 Physical and clinical signs and symptoms of bulimia nervosa and anorexia nervosa. *DTRs,* Deep tendon reflexes; *ECG,* electrocardiogram; *WBC,* white blood cell.

constipation. Complaints of abdominal bloating and a prolonged sensation of abdominal fullness complicate the refeeding process. Lactose intolerance may develop secondary to malnutrition and will usually resolve after weight gain. Oral enzyme supplements and lactose-free dairy products may be beneficial during the refeeding process. A nationwide study conducted in Sweden found a positive association between celiac disease (CD) and AN both before and after CD diagnosis (Marild et al, 2017); this bidirectional association may be attributed to misdiagnosis, shared risk factors, and shared genetic susceptibility.

Osteopenia, osteoporosis, and increased risk of bone fractures occur in males and females with AN (Westmoreland et al, 2016). Adolescents with AN have decreases in biochemical markers of both bone formation and resorption, indicative of reduced bone turnover, whereas adults with AN have decreased bone formation and increased resorption markers, indicative of an uncoupling of bone turnover, both of which lead to reductions in bone mineral density (BMD) (Robinson et al, 2017). In a sample of predominantly female adults, osteopenia was diagnosed in 25.9% of AN-R patients and 34.8% of AN-BP patients and osteoporosis was diagnosed in 34.3% of AN-R and 21.1% of AN-BP patients (Mehler et al, 2018). Although weight gain and resumption of menses in AN patients are associated with increased spine and hip BMD, permanent deficits are likely. No specific therapies are currently approved for treatment of osteoporosis secondary to AN.

Patients with AN have thyroid hormones levels consistent with the nonthyroidal illness syndrome: thyroxin (T4) and triiodothyronine (T3) are low or low normal, reverse T3 is elevated, and thyroid-stimulating hormone (TSH) is normal or elevated (Winston, 2012). This syndrome is likely an adaptive response to conserve energy during chronic undernutrition, and these abnormalities typically normalize with weight gain.

Abnormal liver function tests may occur in AN (Mehler et al, 2018). Hepatic changes are generally asymptomatic and self-limiting, but rare cases of liver damage and liver failure have been reported. Elevated enzymes that result from malnutrition will improve during nutritional rehabilitation. Less frequently, elevated liver transaminases secondary to steatosis may occur during the refeeding process (Westmoreland et al, 2016).

Renal complications include renal insufficiency, decreased renal concentrating ability, increased urine output, proteinuria, and hematuria. In general, these symptoms ameliorate with adequate hydration and treatment of malnutrition (Campbell and Peebles, 2014).

Hematologic abnormalities include anemia, leukopenia, and thrombocytopenia. Anemia reportedly occurs in 20% to 40% of malnourished AN patients, yet iron deficiency is not typically found (Mehler et al, 2018; Westmoreland et al, 2016).

Bulimia Nervosa

Clinical signs and symptoms of BN are more difficult to detect because patients are usually of normal weight and secretive in behavior. When vomiting occurs, there may be clinical evidence such as (1) scarring of the dorsum of the hand used to stimulate the gag reflex, known as Russell's sign (Fig. 21.2); (2) parotid gland enlargement; and (3) erosion of dental enamel with increased dental caries resulting from the frequent presence of gastric acid in the mouth.

Gastrointestinal symptoms occur in individuals with BN who use vomiting as a purging method (Westmoreland et al, 2016). These include sore throat, dysphagia, gastrointestinal reflux, esophagitis, mild hematemesis (vomiting of blood), and more serious but considerably less frequent complications like Mallory-Weiss esophageal tears, esophageal rupture, and acute gastric dilation or rupture. Symptoms associated with laxative misuse vary with type, dose, and duration of use. Patients may present with diarrhea, abdominal cramping, rectal bleeding, and rectal prolapse. Abuse of stimulant laxatives (i.e., those containing bisacodyl, cascara, or senna) can damage intestinal nerve fibers in the bowel wall, whereby the colon becomes increasingly dependent on these stimulants to propulse fecal material; this results in cathartic colon syndrome (Westmoreland et al, 2016). Cessation of laxatives, particularly of the stimulant type, may result in severe rebound constipation that requires ongoing medical management.

Self-induced vomiting and abuse of stimulant laxatives account for 90% of the purging behaviors found in BN (Westmoreland et al, 2016). Vomiting results in decreased potassium (hypokalemia), decreased chloride, and increased bicarbonate, resulting in metabolic alkalosis. Excessive laxative abuse initially results in hyperchloremic metabolic acidosis; however, this reverts to a state of metabolic alkalosis after a chronic volume depleted state evolves (Westmoreland et al, 2016). Hypokalemia also occurs secondary to laxative misuse. Hypokalemia from purging is associated with increased risk of atrial and ventricular arrhythmias (Trent et al, 2013).

Individuals with BN may experience menstrual irregularity, leading to the mistaken belief that they are unable to conceive. Unplanned pregnancies, miscarriages, and babies born with a lower birthweight and smaller head circumference are documented in BN patients (Koubaa et al, 2013; Linna et al, 2013). It is unknown if negative outcomes are associated with malnutrition, inadequate prenatal care, or another mechanism specific to bulimic behavior.

Binge Eating Disorder

The predominant feature of BED is episodes of excessive eating. In many cases, but not all, this binge eating results in overweight or obesity, yet causes greater functional impairment, decreased quality of life, and greater levels of psychiatric comorbidity (depression and anxiety) than obesity without BED (Kornstein et al, 2016). Ingestion of large amounts of food may cause considerable upper and lower gastrointestinal distress. Symptoms include abdominal pain, fullness, delayed gastric emptying, bloating, acid regurgitation, heartburn, dysphagia, nausea, diarrhea, constipation, fecal urgency, fecal incontinence, and anal blockage. BED is associated with an increased lifetime risk of type 2 diabetes, hypertension, and metabolic syndrome (Kornstein et al, 2016).

TREATMENT APPROACH

Treatment of EDs requires a multidisciplinary approach that includes psychiatric, psychological, medical, and nutrition interventions, ideally provided at a level of care appropriate to the severity of the illness. Levels of care offered by facilities in the United States include inpatient hospitalization, residential treatment, partial or day hospitalization, intensive outpatient treatment, and outpatient treatment (APA, 2006; Steinglass et al, 2016). Treatment guidelines and policy statements on the necessary components of treatment are available from the APA (APA, 2006; APA, 2012), the Society for Adolescent Health and Medicine (SAHM) (SAHM, 2015), the American Academy of Pediatrics (Rosen and American Academy of Pediatrics Committee on Adolescence, 2010), the Academy of Nutrition and Dietetics (Ozier et al, 2011), and the Royal Australian and New Zealand College of Psychiatrists (Hay et al, 2014).

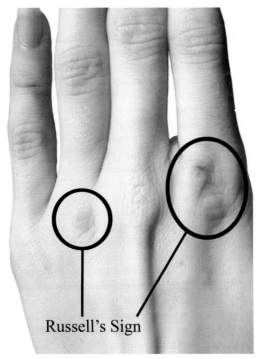

Russell's Sign

Fig. 21.2 Russell's sign. Calluses on the knuckles or the back of the hand resulting from repeated self-induced vomiting over a long period of time.

Inpatient hospitalization may be provided on a psychiatric or medical unit that utilizes a behavioral protocol developed for ED patients. Specialized residential treatment programs also provide 24-hour care but are less likely to admit the medically or psychiatrically unstable patient because of their location outside of a hospital setting. That said, some residential treatment programs are adding acute medical stabilization units to their facility. Partial and day hospital programs typically provide 6 to 8 hours of specialized multidisciplinary treatment 5 to 7 days per week, depending on an individual patient's need for supervision. Intensive outpatient treatment programs provide several hours of multidisciplinary care each week. This may be scheduled in the late afternoon or early evening so that the patient can attend after school or work. The least intensive treatment setting is outpatient care. Psychotherapist, medical doctor, and registered dietitian nutritionist (RDN) appointments are typically scheduled at different times and locations; this necessitates a coordinated effort at communication among all clinicians. The APA (2006, 2012) level of care guidelines recommends that the treatment setting be selected in accordance with a patient's medical status, suicidality, body weight, motivation to recover, presence of comorbid conditions, need for supervision and structure, ability to control compulsive exercising, and purging behavior.

PSYCHOLOGIC MANAGEMENT

EDs are complex psychiatric illnesses that require psychological assessment and ongoing treatment. Evaluation of the patient's cognitive and psychological stage of development, family history, family dynamics, and psychopathologic condition is essential for the development of a comprehensive psychosocial treatment program.

The long-term goals of psychosocial interventions in AN are (1) to help patients understand and cooperate with their nutritional and physical rehabilitation, (2) to help patients understand and change behaviors and dysfunctional attitudes related to their EDs, (3) to improve interpersonal and social functioning, and (4) to address psychopathologic and psychological conflicts that reinforce or maintain eating-disordered behaviors (APA, 2006).

In the acute stage of illness, malnourished AN patients are obsessive and negativistic, making it difficult to conduct formal psychotherapy. It is therefore recommended that intensive, highly structured psychological therapies be initiated after the medical and cognitive effects of acute starvation have been stabilized (Hay et al, 2014).

Behavioral management is often used for individuals with low weight and restrictive eating behaviors (Attia and Walsh, 2009; Steinglass et al, 2016). These protocols encourage the achievement of normal weight and healthy eating through the use of reinforcements for healthy behavioral choices. Treatment typically includes the supervision of all meals and snacks, as well as postmeal psychological support for "having eaten" and monitoring to prevent compensatory behaviors like vomiting, standing, and exercising. Behavioral management can be used in inpatient, residential, and outpatient treatment settings; however, effectiveness depends on consistency of expectations and supervision, which can be more challenging on an outpatient basis.

Once acute malnutrition has been corrected and weight restoration is underway, the AN patient is more likely to benefit from psychotherapy. Psychotherapy can help the patient understand and change core dysfunctional thoughts, attitudes, motives, conflicts, and feelings related to the ED. Associated psychiatric conditions, including deficits in mood, impulse control, and self-esteem, as well as relapse prevention, should be addressed in the psychotherapeutic treatment plan.

No consensus has been reached on the best overall approach to psychotherapy in AN; however, studies suggest that family-based therapy (FBT) is the treatment of choice in adolescents with relatively brief AN (Gur et al, 2018). FBT for AN is a 3-phase manualized outpatient treatment consisting of 10 to 20 sessions conducted over 6 to 12 months (Lock and Le Grange, 2013). Phase 1 aims to empower parents to play an active role in the weight restoration of their adolescent; it focuses on the dangers associated with severe malnutrition and emphasizes the need for parents to take immediate action to reverse this. In phase 1, the FBT therapist assists parents in refeeding their child using parental coaching techniques. In phase 2, the parents are encouraged to help their adolescent gradually resume control over eating again. Phase 3 begins once the adolescent is able to maintain a stable weight ≥95% of ideal body weight (IBW) independently. At this point, the focus of treatment shifts toward the establishment of a healthy adolescent identity, increased adolescent autonomy, and the development of appropriate parental boundaries. It is noteworthy that FBT certification is limited to licensed mental health professionals and that the RDN plays no formal role in the FBT process.

If FBT is contraindicated, then enhanced cognitive behavioral therapy (CBT-E) may be an effective alternative for adolescents, and a good option for adults with AN (Fairburn, 2008). Two versions of CBT-E are available: focused (the core treatment) and broad (includes clinical perfectionism, core low self-esteem, and interpersonal difficulties modules). Treatment intensities include a 20-session version for patients with a BMI >17.5 and a 40-session version for patients with a BMI between 15.0 and 17.5. CBT-E is a manualized therapy provided by psychotherapists on inpatient units as well as in outpatient settings. CBT-E typically includes the self-monitoring of food intake and eating behaviors (binge eating, purging, restricting). The role of the RDN in CBT-E is minimal and will vary with the treatment setting (i.e., greater involvement on inpatient units). On an outpatient basis, consultation with a nutritionist may be limited to patients with complicated diet issues (e.g., diabetes mellitus, CD, vegan diet) and challenging work/sleep schedules (e.g., individuals who work overnight shifts).

Classic cognitive behavioral therapy (CBT) is a 20-session structured therapy that includes behavioral and cognitive interventions. CBT directs the client toward modifying dysfunctional thinking and behavior (see Chapter 13). Current data suggest that CBT is the recommended treatment for BN and BED, with interpersonal therapy (IPT) considered a strong treatment alternative (Gurr et al, 2018). CBT consists of three distinct and systematic phases of treatment: (1) establishing a regular eating pattern, (2) evaluating and changing beliefs about shape and weight, and (3) preventing relapse. Similar to CBT-E, classic CBT is manualized psychotherapeutic intervention provided by a trained psychotherapist. The role of the RDN is limited to patients with comorbid medical diagnoses and eating issues that require more advanced nutrition training.

Dialectical behavioral therapy (DBT), a skill-based therapy that focuses on mindfulness, distress tolerance, emotion regulation, and interpersonal effectiveness, may be helpful in BN cases in which comorbid psychiatric disorders (e.g., depression and mood disorders, personality disorders, and substance abuse disorders), self-injurious behaviors (e.g., cutting), and greater impulsivity are manifested (Berg and Wonderlich, 2013). In some instances, an antidepressant medication (typically a selective serotonin reuptake inhibitor [SSRI] such as fluoxetine) is prescribed adjunctive to psychotherapy.

Technology-based assessments and interventions are being tested in patients with EDs (Ellison et al, 2016). Smartphone "apps" like *Recovery Record* and Rise UP + Recover have been specifically developed

BOX 21.2 Recovery Apps

New technology offers eating disorder recovery focused tools in the form of applications or "apps." The distinction between a "fitness app" and an eating disorder recovery app is significant for the treatment of those with eating disorders. While they may both focus on logging and recording, eating disorder apps discourage the tracking of calories and activity and rather promote the self-monitoring of thoughts and feelings around food intake. Utilizing a self-monitoring platform on a smart phone offers several advantages over paper monitoring as many people keep their phones on them majority of the time. Using the apps may be more convenient which lends itself to real-time monitoring, accuracy, and more consistency in records.

The following apps provide helpful tools to support the efforts of eating disorder recovery:

1. Recovery Record: This app allows you to connect with multiple treatment team members for a real-time tracking and monitoring setting. It provides personalized coping strategies, meal plans, tracking of feelings, urges to use behaviors as well as components of cognitive-behavioral–based interventions.

2. Rise UP + Recover: This app has a comparable self-monitoring feature that allows for recording of intake, emotions, and "target behaviors" such as bingeing and purging. It does not allow for an interactive experience with your treatment team, but you can export meal data and share with others through email. Users can also share motivational quotes, images, and affirmations.

Fairburn CG, Rothwell ER: Apps and eating disorders: a systemic clinical appraisal, *Int J Eat Disord* 48:1038, 2015.
Juarascio AS, Manasse SM, et. al. Review of smartphone applications for the treatment of eating disorders. *Eur Eat Disord Rev* 23:1, 2014.

to complement face-to-face psychotherapy and medical nutrition therapy (MNT) for EDs (Box 21.2).

Validated instruments and questionnaires are available for screening and diagnosis of patients with EDs. The Eating Disorder Examination - 17.0D (Fairburn et al, 2014) is a structured interview that takes approximately 1 hour to administer by a trained clinician; it can be used to diagnose DSM-5 AN, BN, BED, and OSFED in individuals ages 14 and up. The Eating Disorder Assessment for DSM-5 (EDA-5) is an interview-based semistructured interview that takes approximately 15 minutes to administer by a clinician with modest training; it can be accessed at www.eda5.org to diagnose DSM-5 AN, BN, BED, ARFID, OSFED, pica, and rumination disorder in adults (Sysko et al, 2015). Self-report measures may be used for screening purposes. Representative instruments include the Eating Attitudes Test (Eat-26), Eating Disorder Inventory, and the Eating Disorder Examination-Questionnaire (APA, 2006). The SCOFF (Morgan et al, 1999), a brief and effective screening tool that is easy to administer and score, is highlighted in Box 21.3.

BOX 21.3 The SCOFF Questionnaire*

1. Do you make yourself sick because you feel uncomfortably full?
2. Do you worry you have lost control over how much you eat?
3. Have you recently lost more than one stone (14 lb) in a 3-month period?
4. Do you believe yourself to be fat when others say you are too thin?
5. Would you say that food dominates your life?

* Two or more "yes" answers suggest the presence of an eating disorder.
From Morgan JF, Reid F, Lacey JH: *BMJ* 4:1467, 1999.

NUTRITION MANAGEMENT

Roles and responsibilities of the RDN in the treatment of individuals with EDs include assessment, intervention, monitoring, evaluation, and care coordination. Although AN, BN, and BED have different presenting features, similarities exist in the assessment and management of these disorders.

Nutrition Assessment

Nutrition assessment should include a thorough diet history, as well as the evaluation of biochemical, energy metabolism, and anthropometric markers of nutritional status.

Diet History

The diet history should include assessment of energy; macronutrient, micronutrient, and fluid intakes; energy density; diet variety; and an evaluation of eating attitudes, behaviors, and habits (see Chapter 4). Patients with a shorter duration of illness should be queried about their premorbid diet and eating habits as this may be a useful benchmark by which to gauge recovery.

Anorexia Nervosa

Patients with restricting type AN typically eat fewer than 1200 kcal/day. Patients with binge-purge type AN have more variable diet patterns, and energy intake should be assessed across the spectrum of restriction and binge eating. Although the early literature often described AN patients as carbohydrate "phobic" (Russell, 1967), more recent studies suggest greater dietary fat avoidance (Forbush and Hunt, 2014). Percent of calories contributed by protein may be in the average to above-average range, but adequacy of protein intake becomes marginalized as caloric intake decreases. A vegetarian or vegan diet may not contain adequate high-biologic value protein in the presence of low calorie intake.

Inadequate calories, limited diet variety, and poor food group representation increase risk for deficient micronutrient intakes. In general, micronutrient intake parallels macronutrient intake, and AN patients who consistently restrict dietary fat are at greater risk for diets that are deficient in essential fatty acids and fat-soluble vitamins. Based on a 30-day diet history, Hadigan et al (2000) found that more than 50% of 30 AN patients failed to meet recommended dietary allowances (RDA) for vitamin D, calcium, folate, vitamin B12, magnesium, copper, and zinc (see inside cover for dietary reference intake [DRIs]). Abnormal fluid intake is common, and the diet history should query patients about types, amounts, and rationale for fluid consumption. Some individuals restrict fluid intake because they find it difficult to tolerate feelings of fullness afterward; others drink excessive amounts to feel full and suppress appetite. Extremes in fluid restriction or ingestion may require monitoring of urine specific gravity and serum electrolytes. Many AN patients consume excessive amounts of artificially sweetened beverages and artificial sweeteners. Use of these products should be addressed during the course of nutrition therapy.

Bulimia Nervosa

Chaotic eating, ranging from restriction to normal eating to binge eating, makes it difficult to assess total energy intake in BN. The caloric content of a binge, the degree of caloric absorption after a purge, and the extent of calorie restriction between binge episodes must be evaluated. Patients with BN assume that vomiting is an efficient mechanism for eliminating calories consumed during binge episodes; however, this is a common misconception. In a study of the caloric content of foods ingested and purged in a feeding laboratory, it was determined that, as a group, BN subjects consumed a mean of 2131 kcal during a binge

BOX 21.4 Determination of Average Daily Energy Intake in the Individual with Bulimia Nervosa (BN)

1. Keep a record of patient intake for 7 days.
2. Out of the 7 days, determine the number of nonbinge days (which may include restrictive and normal intake days).
3. Approximate the total caloric content for the week.
4. Determine the number of binge days.
5. Determine the approximate caloric content of the binge days and then deduct 50% of the caloric content of binges that are purged (vomited).
6. Finally, average the caloric intake over the 7-day period. Determination of this average energy intake, as well as the range of intake, will be useful information for the assessment process.

BOX 21.5 Assessment of Eating Attitudes, Behaviors, and Habits

1. Eating attitudes
   A. Food aversions
   B. Safe, risky, forbidden foods
   C. Magical thinking
   D. Binge trigger foods
   E. Ideas on appropriate amounts of food
   F. Refusal to eat a food item that does not have a nutrition facts label
2. Eating behaviors
   A. Ritualistic behaviors
   B. Unusual food combinations
   C. Atypical use of condiments (e.g., mustard, lemon juice, vinegar) and seasonings (e.g., black pepper)
   D. Atypical use of eating utensils and use of utensils to consume a finger food (e.g., using a knife and fork to eat a muffin)
   E. Excessive use of artificial sweeteners
3. Eating habits
   A. Intake pattern
      (1) Number of meals and snacks
      (2) Time of day, including times when eating may be restricted (e.g., patients will not permit themselves to eat before or after a certain time in the day).
      (3) Duration of meals and snacks
      (4) Eating environment—where and with whom
      (5) How consumed—sitting or standing or while looking at a screen
   B. Food group avoidance; particularly those with higher energy density
   C. Diet variety from all food groups, including those with a low energy density content
   D. Fluid consumption:
      Restricted vs. excessive
      Types: caloric, noncaloric, beverage water, alcohol

and vomited only 979 kcal afterward (Kaye et al, 1993). As a rule of thumb, RDNs can estimate that about 50% of energy consumed during a binge is retained.

In a similar manner, patients misusing laxatives believe that catharsis will prevent the absorption of food and calories; however, laxatives do not act on the small intestine, where the majority of absorption occurs. In a laboratory study that was conducted by Bo-Linn et al (1983), two BN participants ate a standardized diet and took their regular daily dose of laxatives (35 and 50 tablets, accordingly). Results indicated that despite outputs of 4 to 6 L of diarrhea per day, these participants decreased calorie absorption by only 12%. Because of day-to-day variability, a 24-hour recall is not a particularly useful assessment tool. To assess energy intake, it is helpful to estimate daily food consumption over the course of a week using the method outlined in Box 21.4.

Nutrient intake in patients with BN varies with the cycle of binge eating and restriction, and it is likely that overall diet quality and micronutrient intake is inadequate. A 14-day dietary intake study of 50 BN patients revealed that at least 50% of participants consumed less than two thirds of the RDA for calcium, iron, and zinc on nonbinge days. Furthermore, 25% of participants had inadequate intakes of zinc and iron when overall intake (i.e., binge and nonbinge days) was assessed (Gendall et al, 1997). Even when the diet appears adequate, nutrient loss occurs secondary to purging, thus making it difficult to assess true adequacy of nutrient intake. Use of vitamin and mineral supplements also should be determined but, once again, retention after purging must be considered.

Eating Behavior

Characteristic attitudes, behaviors, and eating habits seen in AN and BN are shown in Box 21.5. Food aversions, common in this population, include red meat, baked goods, desserts, full-fat dairy products, added fats, fried foods, and caloric beverages. Patients with EDs often incorrectly regard specific foods or groups of foods as absolutely "good" or absolutely "bad." Irrational beliefs and dichotomous thinking about food choices should be identified and challenged throughout the treatment process.

In comparison to healthy individuals, patients with AN exhibit characteristic mealtime behaviors that include staring at food, tearing food, nibbling/picking, dissecting food, napkin use, inappropriate utensil use, hand fidgeting, eating latency, and nibbling/picking latency (Gianini et al, 2015). In the assessment process, the RDN may discover unusual or ritualistic behaviors the patient practices, unusual food combinations, and excessive use of spices, vinegar, lemon juice, and artificial sweeteners. Meal spacing and length of time allocated for a meal also should be determined. Many patients save their self-allotted food ration until late in the day; others are fearful of eating past a

certain time of day. AN patients often eat in an excessively slow manner. This may be a tactic to avoid food intake, but it also may be an effect of starvation (Keys, 1950). Time limits for meal and snack consumption frequently are incorporated into behavioral treatment plans and FBT.

Many BN patients eat quickly, reflecting their difficulties with satiety cues. In addition, BN patients may identify foods they fear will trigger a binge episode. The patient may have an all-or-nothing approach to "trigger" foods. Although the patient may prefer avoidance, assistance with reintroduction of controlled amounts of these foods at regular times and intervals is helpful.

Patients may feel a sense of shame about particular food and eating practices, so these behaviors may not be identified during the initial assessment period. The assessment process continues during subsequent meetings and, in some cases, will not be complete until the RDN has observed the patient during a meal time.

Biochemical Assessment

The marked cachexia of AN may lead one to expect many biochemical indices of malnutrition (see Chapter 5), but this is rarely the case. Compensatory mechanisms are remarkable, and laboratory abnormalities may not be observed until the illness is far advanced.

Significant alterations in visceral protein status are less common than expected in AN. Indeed, adaptive phenomena that occur in chronic starvation are aimed at the maintenance of visceral protein metabolism at the expense of the somatic compartment. Although serum albumin is usually normal (Mehler et al, 2018; Barron et al, 2017; Achamrah et al, 2017), when hypoalbuminemia does occur, it is associated with a poorer prognosis (Winston, 2012). Prealbumin is a more sensitive marker of malnutrition, and a low serum prealbumin level may be associated with the development of serious complications of refeeding (i.e., hypophosphatemia and hypoglycemia) in extremely underweight individuals (Gaudiani et al, 2014) (see Appendix 12).

Despite typical consumption of a very low-fat, low-cholesterol diet, malnourished AN patients often manifest elevated total cholesterol, low-density lipoprotein (LDL) cholesterol, and high-density lipoprotein (HDL) cholesterol levels (Winston, 2012). Although the cause is unclear and cardiovascular risk is uncertain, the bulk of available evidence suggests that lipid abnormalities improve or normalize after recovery and a low-fat, low-cholesterol diet is not warranted during the weight restoration process. If hyperlipidemia predates the development of AN, or a strong family history of hyperlipidemia is identified, the patient can be reassessed after nutritional rehabilitation. Lipid profiles routinely are included in laboratory assessments; however, a fasting lipid profile is not warranted until the patient is restored to a healthy and stable body weight.

Individuals with BN also may have elevated lipid levels, but the validity of the test must be questioned if the patient is actively binge eating. Furthermore, some BN patients cannot comply with the abstinence period required for a fasting lipid profile. Patients with BN eat chaotically, consuming a high-fat, high-calorie diet during binge episodes, and a low-fat, low calorie diet during intermittent periods of restriction. An inaccurate lipid profile may lead to the unnecessary prescription of a restricted diet, which in turn may exacerbate binge eating episodes and reinforce an all-or-nothing approach to eating. If hyperlipidemia predates the development of BN, or if a strong family history of hyperlipidemia is identified, the patient should be reassessed after eating behavior and diet are stabilized (see Chapter 32).

Hypoglycemia results from a deficit of precursors that are needed for gluconeogenesis and glucose production. Patients with mild hypoglycemia are often asymptomatic; however, severe hypoglycemia is associated with increased risk of the refeeding syndrome (Gaudiani et al, 2014) and hospitalization may be warranted (Winston, 2012; see Chapter 12).

Vitamin and Mineral Deficiencies

Despite obviously deficient diets, surprisingly few studies address biochemical markers of micronutrient status in patients with EDs. Laboratory values are not always accurate in assessing micronutrient deficiencies because blood values in many cases do not reflect the full extent of depletion of total body nutrient stores. The decreased need for micronutrients in a catabolic state, possible use of vitamin supplements, and the selection of micronutrient-rich foods may afford some degree of protection in low weight patients; however, the shift from catabolic to anabolic processes may precipitate micronutrient deficiencies during refeeding and weight restoration. Study findings conflict, but zinc, copper, vitamin C, vitamin A, vitamin D, riboflavin, folate, and vitamin B6 deficiencies have been reported in AN (Mehler et al, 2018; Barron et al, 2017; Achamrah et al, 2017). Thiamin deficiency, prevalent among low-weight AN patients, may be exacerbated by increased carbohydrate intake during refeeding, and a thiamin supplement may be warranted (Winston, 2012). Given that assays for some vitamins and trace elements may not always be readily available, and that the relationship between blood concentrations and whole-body status is unclear, it may be more practical to prescribe a prophylactic vitamin/mineral supplement during refeeding and weight restoration (Winston, 2012).

Hypercarotenemia, attributed to mobilization of lipid stores, catabolic changes caused by weight loss, and metabolic stress, may occur in AN; excessive dietary intake of carotenoids is less likely (Winston, 2012). Hypercarotenemia resolves during weight restoration and measurement of serum carotene levels is unnecessary.

Iron requirements are decreased in AN secondary to amenorrhea and the overall catabolic state. At treatment onset, the hemoglobin level may be falsely elevated as a result of dehydration resulting in hemoconcentration. Malnourished patients may also have fluid retention, and associated hemodilution may falsely lower the hemoglobin level.

Low zinc levels in patients with AN have been reported by some investigators (Barron et al, 2017) but not by others (Achamrah et al, 2017). Zinc deficiency may result from inadequate energy consumption and transition to a vegetarian diet. Although zinc deficiency may be associated with altered taste perception and weight loss, there is no evidence that deficiency causes or perpetuates symptoms of AN. Supplemental zinc is purported to enhance food intake and weight gain in AN patients, but there is limited evidence to support this claim (Lock and Fitzpatrick, 2009).

Low 25-hydroxy vitamin D (25[OH]D) levels have been reported in low-weight AN patients (Mehler et al, 2018; Modan-Moses et al, 2014). Although vitamin D and calcium contribute to healthy bone development, there is no evidence to suggest that calcium or vitamin D supplementation increases BMD in AN (Robinson et al, 2017). Nevertheless, some researchers suggest routine assessment of 25(OH) D levels (Mehler et al, 2018; Modan-Moses et al, 2014). To date, adequate energy intake and normalization of body weight are the primary agents of bone health in AN. Supplements, like calcium and vitamin D, are variably prescribed among treatment programs and clinicians.

Fluid and Electrolyte Balance

Vomiting and laxative and diuretic use can result in significant fluid and electrolyte imbalances in patients with EDs (Trent et al, 2013). Baseline potassium, chloride, sodium, and CO_2 levels should be obtained in patients with purging and restricting behaviors, with monitoring based on symptomatology.

Urine concentration is sometimes decreased, and urine output increased in semistarvation. Edema can occur in response to malnutrition and refeeding. An increase in extracellular water frequently occurs in AN patients with a BMI less than 15 to 16 kg/m2 (Rigaud et al, 2010). Although fluid retention usually dissipates with refeeding, limiting sodium intake to 2 g/day may be helpful (Rigaud et al, 2010). Depletion of glycogen and lean tissue is accompanied by obligatory water loss that reflects characteristic hydration ratios. For example, the obligatory water loss associated with glycogen depletion may be in the range of 600 to 800 mL. Varying degrees of fluid intake, ranging from restricted to excessive, may affect electrolyte values in patients with EDs (see Chapter 3).

Energy Expenditure

Metabolic adaptation to starvation occurs in malnourished AN patients (Kosmiski et al, 2014) and results in reduced resting energy expenditure (REE) in the range of 50% to 93% of predicted values (Haas et al, 2018b). Weight loss, decreased lean body mass, energy restriction, low T_3, and decreased leptin levels have been implicated in the pathogenesis of this hypometabolic state. At the completion of refeeding, REE reportedly increases to 94% to 119% of predicted values (Haas et al, 2018b). In addition to increased REE, AN patients often exhibit exaggerated diet-induced thermogenesis (DIT) in response to refeeding and this metabolic resistance to weight gain may contribute to the high calorie prescriptions needed during nutritional rehabilitation (Kosmiski et al, 2014). Findings on REE in BN patients are contradictory, with investigators finding reduced levels, normal levels, and elevated levels of REE at baseline (de Zwaan et al, 2002). Proposed causes of a decreased REE include metabolic adaptation to intermittent periods of dietary restraint and fasting interfaced with binge eating and purging, as well as a history of weight suppression. Increased REE may be caused by a preabsorptive release of insulin that activates the sympathetic nervous system during binge eating. Patients with BN may also find it difficult to fast for the requisite 10- to 12-hour period before REE testing. Although baseline and follow-up measurements of REE may be useful during the nutritional rehabilitation process (Mehler et al, 2010), access to indirect calorimetry equipment is often limited. Handheld calorimeters are readily available, but data on their accuracy in this patient population are limited (Hipskind et al, 2011; see Chapter 2).

Anthropometric Assessment

Patients with AN have PEM, characterized by significantly depleted adipose and somatic protein stores but a relatively intact visceral protein compartment. These patients meet the criteria for a diagnosis of severe PEM. A goal of nutritional rehabilitation is restoration of body fat and fat-free mass. Although these compartments do regenerate, the extent and rate vary.

Body composition studies of eating disordered patients have utilized underwater weighing, dual-energy x-ray absorptiometry (DEXA) equipped with body composition software, and skinfold thicknesses. Imaging techniques such as computed tomography (CT) and magnetic resonance imaging (MRI) also have been used to obtain detailed measurements of specific regions or tissues (e.g., visceral adipose fat) or fat infiltration of tissues. Total body protein assessment using in vivo neutron activation analysis (IVNAA) has recently been described in adolescents with AN (Haas et al, 2018a). Most body composition methodologies are limited to the research setting. Bioelectrical impedance analysis (BIA) is more clinically available, but shifts in intracellular and extracellular fluid compartments in patients with severe EDs may affect the accuracy of body fat estimate (see Chapter 5 and Appendix 11).

Careful assessment of height and weight are essential components of clinical management in all ED diagnostic groups. In AN and ARFID, weight restoration, followed by weight maintenance (adults) or age-appropriate weight gain (children/adolescents), is critical for recovery. In BN, cessation of binge/purge episodes with concurrent weight maintenance is the primary treatment goal. In BED, cessation of binge eating along with weight stabilization (size acceptance) or weight loss may be recommended (Grilo, 2017).

In hospitalized/residential treatment, an early morning, preprandial, gowned body weight measurement is recommended. The patient should be advised to empty bowel and bladder before weight assessment. Urine specific gravity can be checked if water loading is suspected. Patients may resort to deceptive tactics (water loading, hiding heavy objects like rolls of coins and marine diving weights on their person, and holding urine and bowel content) to reach a mandated weight goal. Frequency of weight checks varies among treatment programs but is typically every 1 to 3 days; known versus blind weight protocols also vary. On an outpatient basis, a gowned weight should be obtained on the same scale, at approximately the same time of day, at least once a week in early treatment. If the patient is seeing multiple health care professionals, only one should be weighing the patient.

Body weight, as a metric for assessment and a goal for recovery, is measured and monitored throughout treatment. However, "healthy" or "ideal" reference weights, like the Metropolitan Life Insurance Company tables and the Hamwi* method, provide widely varying and empirically unsupported results. Due to these limitations, BMI has

become increasingly accepted in the management of ED patients (see Chapter 5 and Appendix 11). In AN, four categories of BMI severity ratings, based on the World Health Organization categories for thinness in adults, have been incorporated into the DSM-5 (APA, 2013).

Delayed growth and stunting can occur in adolescents with AN. Height and weight data should be obtained from the primary medical record and replotted on the National Center Health Statistics (NCHS) weight-for-age and height-for-age percentiles growth chart and the BMI-for-age percentiles growth chart to determine whether linear growth has deviated from premorbid trajectories. Age at pubertal onset and current pubertal stage provide information about actual versus expected development. Assessment of a deficit in linear growth and potential for catch-up should be determined by a pediatrician or adolescent medicine specialist. In the older patient, a height deficit is likely permanent. In all age groups, height should be carefully measured using a stadiometer rather than a scale-anchored measuring rod (see Appendix 5).

BMI should be calculated and plotted on the NCHS BMI-for-age percentiles growth chart. The BMI percentile does not, however, describe how far an adolescent's BMI deviates from the norm. The BMI z-score is therefore recommended to assess the degree of deviation from the median, as well as to categorize the degree of malnutrition (SAHM, 2015). Median BMI, defined as the 50th percentile BMI for age and sex, can also be used to compare the adolescent to the reference population. Percent median BMI (current BMI/50th percentile, BMI for age and sex x 100) is also used to categorize mild, moderate, and severe degrees of malnutrition (SAHM, 2015). For adolescents, weight recovery is typically defined as 95% of the median BMI (Garber et al, 2016). BMI-for-age data tables providing the 50th percentile BMI value (median BMI) are available at the Centers for Disease Control and Prevention (CDC) website using the search term "growth charts."

Rate of weight gain in AN may be affected by hydration status, glycogen stores, metabolic factors, and changes in body composition (Box 21.6). Rehydration and replenished glycogen stores contribute to

---

*Hamwi Method for women: 100 lb for the first 5 feet of height plus 5 lb per inch for every inch over 5 feet plus 10% for a large frame and minus 10% for a small frame. For men: 106 lb for the first 5 feet of height plus 6 lb per inch for every inch over 5 feet plus 10% for a large frame and minus 10% for a small frame.

> ### BOX 21.6 Factors Affecting Rate of Weight Gain in Anorexia Nervosa
>
> 1. Fluid balance
>   A. Polyuria seen in semistarvation
>   B. Edema
>   (1) Starvation
>   (2) Refeeding
>   C. Hydration ratios in tissues
>   (1) Glycogen: 3-4:1
>   (2) Protein stores: 2-3:1
> 2. Metabolic rate
>   A. Resting energy expenditure (REE): Low weight: REE 30% to 40% below predicted value for height, weight, age, gender
>   Refeeding: progressive increases in REE
>   Weight restoration: REE normalizes
>   B. Postprandial energy expenditure (PPEE)
>   Under normal metabolic conditions: PPEE approx. 10% greater than REE
>   In AN: PPEE may be 30% to 40% greater than REE
>   Duration of exaggerated response varies among individuals
>   C. Respiratory quotient
> 3. Energy cost of tissue gained
>   A. Fat-free mass
>   B. Adipose tissue
> 4. Previous obesity associated with decreased metabolic resistance to weight gain
> 5. Physical activity: time standing, volitional activity, fidgeting behavior

weight gain during the first few days of refeeding. Thereafter, weight gain results from increased lean and fat stores. A general assumption is that someone has to increase or decrease caloric intake by 3500 kcal to cause a 1-lb change in body weight, but the true energy cost depends on the type of tissue gained. More energy is required to gain fat versus lean tissue, but weight gain may be a mix of fat and lean tissues. In adult women with AN, short-term weight restoration has been associated with a significant increase in truncal fat and central adiposity; this distribution, however, appears to normalize within 1 year of weight maintenance (Mayer et al, 2009). Short-term weight restoration in adolescent females has been associated with and without central adiposity (de Alvaro et al, 2007; Franzoni et al, 2013).

MEDICAL NUTRITION THERAPY AND COUNSELING

Treatment of an ED may begin at one of five levels of care: outpatient, intensive outpatient, partial or day treatment, inpatient, or residential. The RDN is an essential part of the treatment team at all levels of care; roles and responsibilities of caring for individuals with EDs are summarized in Table 21.2.

TABLE 21.2 Roles and Responsibilities of Registered Dietitian Nutritionists Caring for individuals with Eating Disorders

Nutrition Assessment:	**Specific Activities:**
Identify nutrition problems that relate to medical and physical condition, including eating disorder symptoms and behaviors.	Eating patterns
	Core eating attitudes
	Core attitudes regarding body weight and shape
	Assess behavioral-environmental symptoms:
	Food restriction
	Binge eating
	Preoccupation
	Rituals
	Secretive eating
	Affect and impulse control
	Vomiting or other purging behaviors
	Excessive exercise
	Anthropometric assessment:
	Measure height, weight, calculate BMI
	Obtain height and weight history
	Adolescents and young adults up to age 20:
	Plot on NCHS growth charts
	Assess growth patterns
	Calculate BMI z-score, percent of median BMI
	Assess degree of malnutrition:
	Adults: BMI
	Adolescents: BMI z-scores and percent of median BMI
	Interpret biochemical data and assess risk of refeeding syndrome
	Apply diagnosis, plan intervention, coordinate with treatment team
Nutrition Intervention:	Ensure diet quality, regular eating pattern, increased amount and variety of foods, normal perceptions of hunger and satiety, provide suggestions about supplement use
Calculate and monitor energy and macronutrient intake to establish expected rates of weight change, and body composition and health goals. Guide goal setting to normalize eating patterns for nutrition rehabilitation and weight restoration or maintenance as appropriate.	Provide a structured meal plan
	Provide psychological support and positive reinforcement
	Counsel patients and caregivers on food selection with consideration given to individual preferences, health history, physical factors, psychological factors, and resources
Nutrition Monitoring and Evaluation:	Monitor rate of weight gain
Monitor nutrient intake and adjust as needed.	Upon weight restoration, adjust food plan for weight maintenance
	Communicate progress with the treatment team
	Adjust treatment plan as needed
Care Coordination:	Work collaboratively with the treatment team, delineate roles and tasks, communicate nutrition needs across treatment settings (i.e., inpatient, day patient, outpatient)
Provide counsel to team about protocols to maximize tolerance of feeding regimen or nutrition recommendations, guidance about supplements to ensure maximum absorption, minimize drug nutrient interactions, and referral for continuation of care as needed.	Function as a resource and educator for other health care professionals and family members
	Advocate for evidence-based treatment and access to care
Advanced Training:	Use advanced knowledge and skills relating to nutrition
Seek specialized training in other counseling techniques, such as cognitive behavioral therapy, dialectical behavioral therapy, and motivational interviewing.	Seek supervision and case consultation from a licensed health professional to gain and maintain proficiency in eating disorders treatment

BMI, Body mass index; *NCHS*, National Center for Health Statistics.
Adapted from: Ozier AD, Henry BW: Position of the American Dietetic Association: Nutrition intervention in the treatment of eating disorders. *J Acad Nutr Diet*, 111:1236, 2011.

BOX 21.7 Guidelines for Medical Nutrition Therapy for Anorexia Nervosa

1. Caloric prescription
   A. Initial prescription
      APA (2006): 30 to 40 kcal/kg/day (approx. 1000 to 1600 kcal/day)
      Higher kcal prescriptions require monitoring for refeeding syndrome (RFS)
      Types of feedings: meal based, liquid supplements, tube feedings; total parenteral nutrition (TPN) (rare)
   B. Weight gain phase:
      Assess for individualized versus standardized approach
      Progressive increases in kcal prescription to promote desired rate of weight gain
      Late treatment: 70 to 100 kcal/kg/day (APA, 2006); approx. 3000 to 4000 kcal/day for females and 4000 to 4500 kcal/day for males
   C. Weight maintenance phase:
      Adults: 40 to 60 kcal/kg/day
      Children/adolescents: kcal intake sufficient for normal growth and development
2. Macronutrient intake
   A. Protein
      15% to 20% kcal
      Minimum intake = Recommended dietary allowance (RDA) in g/kg ideal body weight
      Promote high biologic value sources; avoid vegetarian diets
   B. Carbohydrate
      50% to 60% kcal
      Decrease carbohydrate to 40% kcal if blood glucose is elevated or patient has RFS
      Provide insoluble fiber for treatment of constipation.
   C. Fat
      Hospitalized/day treatment patients: 30% kcal
      Outpatients: progressively increase dietary fat until a 30% fat kcal diet is attained.
      Include sources of essential fatty acids
3. Micronutrient intake:
   A. 100% RDA multivitamin/mineral supplement.
   B. Avoid supplemental iron during initial phase of refeeding and if patient is constipated.
   C. Assess need for additional thiamin supplement.
   D. Assess need for additional calcium supplementation.
4. Energy density
   A. Promote intake of energy dense foods and beverages
      If nutrient intake is assessed by computer analysis, calculate a Dietary Energy Density Score (DEDS): DEDS = kcal intake divided by weight (g) of food and beverage
   B. Goal for DEDS: ≥1.0
5. Diet variety
   A. Promote intake of a wide variety of foods and beverages within all food groups.
   B. Pay particular attention to the variety of complex carbohydrates, caloric beverages, and added fats.

In AN, the chosen level of care is determined by the severity of malnutrition, degree of medical and psychiatric instability, duration of illness, growth failure, and ability to manage recovery in the home. In some instances, treatment begins on an inpatient unit but is stepped down to a less intensive level of care as weight restoration progresses. In other instances, treatment begins on an outpatient basis; however, if progress is absent or considered inadequate, care is stepped up to a more intensive level.

In BN, treatment typically begins and continues on an outpatient basis. On occasion a patient with BN may be directly admitted to an intensive outpatient or day treatment program. However, inpatient hospitalization is relatively uncommon and generally is of short duration and for the specific purpose of fluid and electrolyte stabilization.

Anorexia Nervosa

Guidelines for MNT for AN are summarized in Box 21.7. Goals for nutrition rehabilitation include restoration of body weight and normalization of eating patterns and behaviors. Although MNT is an essential component of treatment, guidelines are based largely on clinical experience rather than scientific evidence (Rocks et al, 2014).

Refeeding may occur in a variety of settings including inpatient medical units, inpatient psychiatric units, residential programs, day treatment/partial hospitalization, and outpatient settings. For adolescents engaged in FBT, the family home is the primary setting for refeeding. Refeeding may include combinations of meal-based feedings, liquid calorie supplements, tube feedings (continuous or bolus); parenteral nutrition (PN) is rarely used and not recommended unless no other form of refeeding is possible (Garber et al, 2016).

Weight restoration for medically unstable, severely malnourished (BMI <15 kg/m² in adult and <70% median BMI in adolescents), or growth-impaired adolescents may require supervised weight gain in a specialized inpatient unit or residential treatment program. A few programs incorporate weight stabilization, weight gain, and weight maintenance phases into their treatment programs, but most initiate weight shortly after admission. Treatment includes a targeted rate of expected weight gain. The APA (2006) recommends a targeted weight gain of 2 to 3 lbs. per week, others, including the SAHM, consider this rate of weight gain too conservative (SAHM, 2015; Garber et al, 2012; Golden et al, 2013; Katzman, 2012; Kohn et al, 2011).

Initial calorie prescriptions, and subsequent caloric adjustments, are also not widely agreed upon. The current standard of care for refeeding is to "start low" (approximately 1200 kcal/day) and "advance slow" (200 kcal increases every other day), the purpose of which has been to minimize the risk of refeeding syndrome, which is defined below (Garber et al, 2016). The tendency for conservative refeeding approaches to result in slower rates of weight gain and longer hospitalizations has prompted some treatment programs to use more aggressive "standardized" approaches to refeeding, which includes a higher initial calorie prescription and more rapid advancement during the refeeding process. An example of a standardized approach described by Haynos et al (2016) is provided in Table 21.3. This type of protocol may be safe and effective in clinical settings that include a highly skilled eating disorder treatment team. In a clinical setting that is less specialized, it may be safer to prescribe an initial diet in accordance with the APA practice guideline (2006) recommendation of 30 to 40 kcal/kg of body weight per day (approximately 1000 to 1600 kcal/day) followed by progressive calorie increases (e.g., 200 kcal) at a frequency that will promote a consistent rate of weight gain. A systematic review of feeding approaches in AN conducted by Garber et al (2016) resulted in the following evidence-based conclusions: (1) lower calorie refeeding is too conservative in mildly (80% to 89% median BMI) and moderately (70% to 79% median BMI) malnourished adolescents; (2) there is insufficient evidence to support changing the current standard of care for refeeding (i.e., start low, go slow) in severely malnourished adolescents (<70% median BMI) and adults (BMI <15 kg/m²).

Risk of hypophosphatemia and complications associated with the refeeding syndrome (RFS) may present during the first few weeks of nutritional rehabilitation. Manifestations of RFS include fluid and electrolyte imbalance; cardiac, neurologic, and hematologic complications;

TABLE 21.3 Example of a Standardized Refeeding Protocol for Hospitalized Patients with Anorexia Nervosa

Days Since Admission	Meal Prescription (kcal)	Liquid Supplement (Ensure Plus) Prescription (kcal)	Total Prescription (kcal)
0	1800	0	1800
7	2200	0	2200
9	2220	350	2550
12	2600	350	2950
15	2600	700	3300
17	3000	700	3700

Haynos A, Snipes C, et al. *Int J Eat Disord* 49:50, 2016.

and sudden death. Risk for the development of RFS may depend more on the degree of malnutrition rather than caloric intake and rate of weight gain (Agostino et al, 2013; Garber et al, 2012; Golden et al, 2013; Kohn et al, 2011). At-risk individuals must be monitored carefully with daily measurements of serum phosphorus, potassium, and magnesium for the first 5 to 7 days of refeeding, and every other day for several weeks thereafter. Supplemental phosphorus, magnesium, and potassium may be given orally or intravenously. In some instances, prophylactic supplementation is provided to high-risk individuals; in other cases, supplementation is based on serum levels. Thiamin (B1) supplementation may be required at the onset and throughout the course of nutritional rehabilitation. Plasma glucose levels must be closely monitored for hypo- and hyperglycemia (Boateng et al, 2010). A systematic review of approaches to refeeding was conducted by Garber et al (2016). A position statement on the management of RFS in hospitalized adolescents is available from the SAHM (2014), and guidelines for identification of adults at high risk for RFS are available from the National Institute for Health and Clinical Excellence (NICE) (NICE, 2009).

Later in the course of weight restoration, caloric prescriptions in the range of 70 to 100 kcal/kg of body weight per day (approximately 3000 to 4000 kcal/day) may be needed, and male patients may require as much as 4000 to 4500 kcal/day (APA, 2006). Changes in REE, DIT, and the type of tissue gained contribute to high energy requirements. Patients who require extraordinarily high energy intakes should be questioned or observed for discarding of food, vomiting, exercising, and excessive physical activity, including fidgeting.

After the goal weight is attained, the caloric prescription may be slowly decreased to promote weight maintenance. Weight maintenance requirements are generally higher than expected and are usually in the range of 2200 to 3000 kcal/day. Caloric prescriptions may remain at higher levels in adolescents with the potential for continued growth and development.

AN patients receiving care in less-structured environments, such as an outpatient treatment program or a private nutrition practice, may be challenging and resistant to following formalized meal plans. A practical approach is the addition of 200 to 300 calories per day to the patient's typical (baseline) energy intake; however, the RDN must be mindful that these patients tend to overestimate their energy intake (Schebendach et al, 2012).

Once the energy prescription is calculated, a reasonable distribution of macronutrients must be determined. Patients may express multiple food aversions. Extreme avoidance of dietary fat is common, but continued omission will make it difficult to provide concentrated sources of energy needed for weight restoration. A dietary fat intake of at least 30% of calories is recommended. This can be accomplished easily when AN patients are treated on inpatient units or in day

hospital programs. On an outpatient basis, however, small, progressive increases in the dietary fat prescription may elicit more cooperation and less resistance. Although some patients will accept small amounts of added fat (such as salad dressing, mayonnaise, or butter), many do better when the fat content is less obvious (as in cheese, peanut butter, granola, and snack foods). Encouraging the gradual change from fat-free products (fat-free milk) to low-fat products (1% or 2% milk) and finally to full-fat items (whole milk) is also acceptable to some patients.

Protein intake in the range of 15% to 20% of total calories is recommended. To ensure adequacy the minimum protein prescription should equal the RDA for age and sex in gram per kilogram (g/kg) IBW (see inside cover). Vegetarian diets often are requested but should be discouraged during the weight restoration phase of treatment.

Carbohydrate intake in the range of 50% to 60% of calories are generally well tolerated. A lower carbohydrate diet (e.g., 40% of calories) may be indicated for a hyperglycemic patient. Constipation is a common problem in early treatment, and food sources of insoluble fiber may be beneficial (see Appendix 28).

Although vitamin and mineral supplements are not universally prescribed, the potential for increased needs during the later stages of weight gain must be considered. Prophylactic prescription of a vitamin and mineral supplement that provides 100% of the RDA may be reasonable, but iron supplementation may be contraindicated early in treatment (Royal College of Psychiatrists, 2005). Owing to the increased risk of low BMD, calcium and vitamin D–rich foods should be encouraged; there is no consensus on the use of calcium and vitamin D supplements in this population.

Delayed gastric emptying and resultant early satiety with complaints of abdominal distention and discomfort after eating are common in AN. In early treatment intake is generally low and can be tolerated in three meals per day. However, as the caloric prescription increases, between-meal feedings become essential. The addition of an afternoon or evening snack may relieve the physical discomfort associated with larger meals, but some patients express feelings of guilt for "indulging" between meals. Commercially available, defined-formula liquid supplements containing 30 to 45 calories per fluid ounce often are prescribed once or twice daily. Patients are fearful that they will become accustomed to the large amount of food required to meet increased caloric requirements; thus use of a liquid supplement is appealing because it can easily be discontinued when the goal weight is attained. The consumption of meals, snacks, and liquid supplements must be supervised during intake and immediately after (1-hour period) intake to prevent purging.

Claims of lactose intolerance, food allergies, and gluten sensitivity complicate the refeeding process. These may be legitimate or simply a covert means of limiting food choice. To the extent possible, all claims should be verified by prior or current medical testing. Lactose intolerance secondary to malnutrition may occur but typically resolves during the course of weight restoration. If medically warranted, lactose-free whole milk products and the prescription of an oral enzyme supplement before meals and snacks can be easily accommodated.

Food allergies and a gluten-free diet are far more challenging. Many patients claim to be vegetarians; however, the adoption of this dietary practice usually occurs in close proximity to the onset of AN. Many treatment programs prohibit vegetarian diets during the weight restoration phase of treatment; others allow a lacto-ovo vegetarian diet. The relationship of social, cultural, and family influences and religious beliefs relative to the patient's vegetarian status must be explored.

Institutions vary with respect to their menu-planning protocol. In some institutions the meal plan and food choices are fixed initially without patient input; as treatment progresses and weight is restored, the patient generally assumes more responsibility for menu planning. In other inpatient programs the patient participates in menu planning from the beginning of treatment. Some institutions have established guidelines that the patient must comply with to maintain the "privilege" of menu planning. Guidelines may require a certain type of milk (e.g., whole vs. low-fat) and the inclusion of specific types of foods such as added fats, animal proteins, desserts, and snacks. A certain number of servings from the different food groups may be prescribed at different calorie levels.

Meal planning methods vary among treatment programs, but data to suggest that one method is superior to another is lacking. Some programs use food group exchanges, others customize their approach. Regardless of the method, AN patients find it difficult to make food choices and plan menus. The RDN can be extremely helpful in providing a structured meal plan and guidance in the selection of nutritionally adequate meals and a varied diet. In a study of recently weight-restored, hospitalized AN patients, those who selected more energy-dense foods and a diet with greater variety had better treatment outcomes during the 1-year period immediately after hospital discharge, and this effect was independent of total caloric intake (Schebendach et al, 2008).

In an outpatient setting, the treatment team has less control over energy intake, food choice, and macronutrient distribution. Under these circumstances the RDN must use counseling skills to begin the process of developing a plan for nutritional rehabilitation. AN patients are typically precontemplative and, at best, ambivalent about making changes in eating behavior, diet, and body weight; some are defiant and hostile on initial presentation. Motivational interviewing and CBT techniques may be useful in the nutrition counseling of AN patients (Ozier et al, 2011); the reader is referred to Fairburn (2008) for a thorough review of CBT techniques.

Effective nutritional rehabilitation and counseling must ultimately result in weight gain and improved eating attitudes and behaviors. A comprehensive review of nutrition counseling techniques can be found in Chapter 13 and in Herrin and Larkin (2013) and Stellefson Myers and Caperton-Kilburn (2017).

Avoidant/Restrictive Food Intake Disorder

Patients with ARFID restrict/avoid their food intake to the extent that it is clinically significant; however, food restriction is not associated with shape and weight concerns. Patients may have sensory problems related to appearance, taste, smell, color, or texture of food. Others have a fear of swallowing/vomiting and they may have difficulty with solid foods or foods with a lumpy texture. There are currently no evidence-based guidelines specific to ARFID (Kohn, 2016). Since ARFID is associated with reluctance to normalize eating behaviors, behavioral management may be the first-line treatment. Behavioral management

should include: (1) an individualized assessment of the restrictive behaviors that includes a detailed history of symptoms that interfere with normal eating and food choice, (2) a plan that specifically reinforces the successful eating of restricted foods, and (3) a plan that specifically reinforces the reversal of avoidant/restrictive behaviors (Steinglass et al, 2016). Treatment needs to include individualized goals appropriate for specific symptoms. For example, discomfort with oral sensations may require graded exposure to novel foods, and fear of choking or vomiting may require specific swallowing exercises targeted to these symptoms (Steinglass et al, 2016), and collaboration with occupational therapists who specialize in feeding disorders may be necessary. The Nine Item Avoidant/Restrictive Food Intake Disorder Screen (NIAS) may useful in the assessment of ARFID-related eating behaviors in this patient population (Zickgraf and Ellis, 2018)

Bulimia Nervosa

Guidelines for MNT in BN are summarized in Box 21.8. BN is described as a state of dietary chaos characterized by periods of uncontrolled, poorly structured eating, followed by periods of restrained food intake. The RDN's role is to help develop a reasonable plan of controlled eating while assessing the patient's tolerance for structure.

During the initial onset of BN, much of the patient's eating and purging behavior is aimed at weight loss. Later in the process, the behaviors may be habitual and out of control. Even if the patient is legitimately overweight, immediate goals must be interruption of the binge-and-purge cycle, restoration of normal eating behavior, and stabilization

---

BOX 21.8 Guidelines for Medical Nutrition Therapy of Bulimia Nervosa

1. Caloric prescription for weight maintenance
   A. If metabolic rate appears normal, provide dietary reference intake (DRI) for energy (approximately 2200 to 2400 kcal/day).
   B. If there is strong evidence of a hypometabolic rate:
      Start at 1600 to 1800 kcal/day
      Increase in 100 to 200 kcal/week increments up to 2200 to 2400 kcal/day
   B. Monitor body weight and adjust caloric prescription for weight maintenance.
   C. Avoid low-calorie diets as these may exacerbate bingeing and purging behaviors.
2. Macronutrients
   A. Protein
      (1) 15% to 20% kcal
      (2) Minimum: recommended dietary allowance (RDA) in g/kg of ideal body weight
      (3) High biological value sources
   D. Carbohydrate
      (4) 50% to 60% kcal
      (5) Provide insoluble fiber sources for treatment of constipation
   E. Fat
      (6) 30% kcal
      (7) Provide source of essential fatty acids
3. Micronutrients
   A. 100% RDA multivitamin/mineral supplement
   B. Avoid supplemental iron if patient is constipated
4. Energy density
   C. Provide foods with a range of energy densities
   D. Provide an overall diet with an energy density of approximately 1.0
5. Diet variety
   E. Promote intake of a wide variety of foods and beverages within all food groups

of body weight. Attempts at dietary restraint for the purpose of weight loss typically exacerbate binge-purge behavior in BN patients.

Patients with BN have varying degrees of metabolic efficiency, which must be taken into account when prescribing the baseline diet. Assessment of REE along with clinical signs of a hypometabolic state, such as a low T_3 level and cold intolerance, are useful in determining the caloric prescription. If a low metabolism is suspected, a caloric prescription of 1600 to 1800 calories daily is a reasonable place to start; however, this prescription should be titrated upwards, in 100 to 200 calorie per week increments, to stimulate the metabolic rate. Ultimately, a weight maintenance diet of 2200 to 2400 kcal/day is attainable and well tolerated. If a patient is willing and able to provide a detailed diet history or a 7-day food record, the initial caloric prescription can also be calculated by the method described in Box 21.4.

Body weight should be monitored with a goal of stabilization; however, BN patients need a great deal of encouragement to follow weight maintenance versus weight loss diets. They must be reminded that attempts to restrict caloric intake may only increase the risk of binge eating and that their pattern of restrained intake followed by binge eating has not facilitated weight loss in the past.

A balanced macronutrient intake is essential for the provision of a regular meal pattern. This should include sufficient carbohydrates to prevent craving and adequate protein and fat to promote satiety. In general, a balanced diet providing 50% to 60% of the calories from carbohydrate, 15% to 20% from protein, and approximately 30% from fat is reasonable.

Adequacy of micronutrient intake relative to the caloric prescription, macronutrient distribution, and diet variety should be assessed. A multivitamin and mineral preparation may be prescribed to ensure adequacy, particularly in the initial phase of treatment.

Bingeing, purging, and restrained intake often impair recognition of hunger and satiety cues. The cessation of purging behavior coupled with a reasonable daily distribution of calories at three meals and prescribed snacks can be instrumental in strengthening these biologic cues. Many patients with BN are afraid to eat earlier in the day because they are fearful that these calories will contribute to caloric excess if they binge later. They also may digress from their meal plans after a binge, attempting to restrict intake to balance out the binge calories. Patience and support are essential in this process of making positive changes in their eating habits.

When the BN patient is receiving CBT, the RDN may assist the CBT therapist in the phase 1 goal of establishing a regular meal pattern. The RDN and the psychotherapist must, however, maintain active communication to avoid overlap in the counseling sessions. If the BN patient is engaged in a type of psychotherapy other than CBT, the RDN should incorporate more CBT skills into the nutrition counseling sessions (Herrin and Larkin, 2013; Stellefson Meyers and Caperton-Kilburn, 2017).

Patients with BN are typically more receptive to nutrition counseling than AN patients and less likely to present in the precontemplation stage of change. Suggested strategies for nutrition counseling at the precontemplation, contemplation, preparation, action, and maintenance stages are given in Table 21.4 (see Chapter 13).

TABLE 21.4 Counseling Strategies Using the Stages of Change Model in Eating Disorders	
Stage of Change	**Counseling Strategies**
Precontemplation	Establish rapport. Assess nutrition knowledge, beliefs, attitudes. Conduct thorough review of food likes and dislikes, safe and risky foods, forbidden foods (assess reason), binge and purge foods. Assess physical, anthropometric, metabolic status. Assess level of motivation. Use motivational interviewing techniques. Decisional balance: weigh costs and benefits of maintaining current status versus costs and benefits of change.
Contemplation	Identify behaviors to change; prioritize. Identify barriers to change. Identify coping mechanisms. Identify support systems. Discuss self-monitoring tools: food and eating behavior records. Continue motivational interviewing technique.
Preparation	Implement nutrition-focused CBT. Implement self-monitoring tools: food and eating behavior records. Determine list of alternative behaviors to bingeing and purging.
Action	Develop a plan of healthy eating. Reinforce positive decision making, self-confidence, and self-efficacy. Promote positive self-rewarding behaviors. Develop strategies for handling impulsive behaviors, high-risk situations, and "slips." Continue CBT. Continue self-monitoring.
Maintenance and relapse	Identify strategies; manage high-risk situations. Continue positive self-rewarding behaviors. Reinforce coping skills and impulse-control techniques. Reinforce relapse prevention strategies. Determine and schedule follow-up sessions needed for maintenance and reinforcement of positive changes in eating behavior and nutrition status.

CBT, Cognitive behavioral therapy.
Modified from Stellefson Myers E: *Winning the war within: nutrition therapy for clients with anorexia or bulimia nervosa,* Dallas, 2006, Helm Publishing.

Binge Eating Disorder

Strategies for treatment of BED include nutrition counseling and dietary management, individual and group psychotherapy, and medication management. Size-acceptance (HAES; Health At Every Size), improved body image, increased physical activity, and improved health and nutrition are treatment goals for BED. Some treatment programs focus primarily on nutrition counseling and weight loss. Unfortunately, behavioral weight loss therapy may be effective in attaining short-term rather than long-term weight loss in these individuals (Wilson, 2011). Results of a 6-month combined CBT and dietary counseling intervention (provided by RDs) conducted in obese BED patients indicated improved psychological functioning and a significant decrease in binge eating episodes, but no clinically meaningful weight loss (Masheb et al, 2016). MNT counseling for the BED patient requires ongoing communication with the psychotherapist and a clear intervention goal (i.e., nutrition counseling based on wellness and size-acceptance or behavioral weight loss treatment). Guided self-help CBT (Fairburn, 1995) is also a treatment option (Striegel-Moore et al, 2010).

Orthorexia Nervosa

Numerous studies have provided evidence for the condition of orthorexia nervosa (ON), an eating pattern characterized by an obsession for and fixation on healthy eating. It is currently not categorized as an eating disorder, and the current scientific debate is whether this is a behavioral or lifestyle phenomenon or a true mental disorder. Although being aware of and concerned with the nutritional quality of the food eaten is not a problem in and of itself, people can become fixated on so-called healthy eating (often characterized as clean eating) and actually damage their own well-being by adherence to strict food rules. While ON is not clinically defined and is not included in the DSM-5, the National Eating Disorders Association states that it is currently being treated by eating disorder experts who treat ON as a variety of anorexia and/or obsessive-compulsive disorder (Esposito and Fierstein, 2018).

Preliminary criteria for the diagnosis of ON were proposed in 2004 (Donini et al, 2004). Since that time diagnostic criteria have been proposed for the condition (Dunn and Bratman, 2016). A recent large cross-sectional study (Strahler et al, 2018) explored whether ON is of epidemiologic and clinical relevance, and whether it can be distinguished from other mental health disorders and healthy lifestyle features. They confirmed the epidemiologic and clinical relevance of orthorexic behaviors but found strong conceptual overlap with other mental health problems and ultimately challenged the idea that ON is a distinct mental health disorder category.

Monitoring Nutritional Rehabilitation

Guidelines for patient monitoring are indicated in Box 21.9. The health professional, patient, and family must be realistic about

---

BOX 21.9   Patient Monitoring

1. Body weight
   A. Establish treatment goal weight and body mass index (BMI)
   B. Determine:
      a. Acceptable rate of weight gain in anorexia nervosa (AN)
      b. Maintenance weight in bulimia nervosa (BN)
   C. Children and adolescents:
      c. Plot weight on National Center for Health Statistics (NCHS) weight-for-age percentile growth chart
      d. Determine weight percentile
   D. Monitor weight:
      (1) Inpatient and partial hospitalization
         a. Frequency: Inpatient: daily or every other day; partial hospitalization: varies with diagnosis, age of patient, phase of treatment (i.e., daily, several times per week, once per week)
         b. Gowned
         c. Morning weight
         d. Preprandial
         e. Postvoid
         f. Same scale
         g. Check urine specific gravity if fluid loading is suspected
         h. Additional random weight checks if fluid loading is suspected
      (2) Outpatient treatment:
         a. Once every 1 to 2 weeks in early treatment, less frequently in mid- to late treatment
         b. Gowned
         c. Postvoid
         d. Same time of day
         e. Same scale
         f. Check urine specific gravity if fluid loading is suspected
2. Height
   A. Measure baseline height using a stadiometer
   B. Children and adolescents:
      (1) Plot height on NCHS stature-for-age percentile growth chart
      (2) Determine height percentile

      (3) Assess for growth impairment
      (4) Monitor height every 1 to 2 months in patients with growth potential
3. BMI:
   A. Adults: calculate BMI using Centers for Disease Control and Prevention (CDC) online calculator for adults: https://www.cdc.gov/healthyweight/assessing/bmi/adult_bmi/english_bmi_calculator/bmi_calculator.html
   B. Children and adolescents:
      (1) Calculate BMI, BMI percentile, and BMI z-score using CDC online calculator for children and adolescents at https://www.cdc.gov/healthyweight/bmi/calculator.html
      (2) Plot BMI on NCHS body mass index-for-age percentile chart
      (3) Determine median BMI (50th percentile BMI for age and sex) using CDC Data Table of BMI-for-age charts
      (4) Calculate percent median BMI [(current BMI/median BMI) x 100]
4. Outpatient diet monitoring
   A. AN
   Daily food record to include:*
      (1) Food
      (2) Fluid: caloric, noncaloric, alcohol
      (3) Artificial sweeteners
      (4) Eating behavior: time, place, how eaten, with whom
      (5) Dietary energy density
      (6) Diet variety
   B. BN
   Daily food record to include:*
      (1) Food
      (2) Fluid: caloric, noncaloric, alcohol
      (3) Artificial sweeteners
      (4) Eating behavior: time, place, how eaten, with whom
      (5) Emotions and feelings when eating
      (6) Foods eaten at a binge
      (7) Time and method of purge
      (8) Dietary energy density
      (9) Diet variety
      (10) Exercise

*Consider having patient monitor intake with an app (see Box 21.2).

treatment, which is often a long-term process. Although outcomes may be favorable, the course of treatment is rarely smooth and linear, and clinicians must be prepared to monitor progress with patience and compassion.

Nutrition Education

Patients with EDs may appear knowledgeable about food and nutrition. Despite this, nutrition education is an essential component of their treatment plan. Indeed, some patients spend significant amounts of time reading nutrition-related information, but their sources may be unreliable, and their interpretation potentially distorted by their illness. Malnutrition may impair the patient's ability to assimilate and process new information. Early and middle adolescent development is characterized by the transition from concrete to abstract operations in problem solving and directed thinking, and normal developmental issues must be considered when teaching adolescents with EDs (see Chapter 17).

Nutrition education materials must be assessed thoroughly to determine whether language and subject matter are bias free and appropriate for AN and BN patients. For example, literature provided by many health organizations promotes a low-fat diet and low-calorie lifestyle for the prevention and treatment of chronic disease. This material is in direct conflict with a treatment plan that encourages increased caloric and fat intake for the purpose of nutritional rehabilitation and weight restoration.

Although the interactive process of a group setting may have advantages, these topics can also be effectively incorporated into individual counseling sessions. Topics for nutrition education are suggested in Box 21.10.

Prognosis

The course and outcome of AN are highly variable. Some individuals fully recover, some have periods of recovery followed by relapse, and others are chronically ill for many years (APA, 2013). Although approximately 70% of individuals with BN achieve remission, those who have not achieved remission after 5 years of illness may demonstrate a chronic course (Keel and Brown, 2010).

BOX 21.10   Topics for Nutrition Education

Guidelines for recovery: energy, macronutrient, vitamin, mineral, and fluid intakes
Impact of malnutrition on adolescent growth and development
Physiologic and psychological consequences of malnutrition
Set point theory and the determination of a healthy body weight
Impact of energy restriction on the metabolic rate
Ineffectiveness of vomiting, laxatives, and diuretics in long-term weight control
Causes of bingeing and purging, and techniques to break the cycle
Changes in body composition that occur during weight restoration
Exercise and energy balance
What does "healthy eating" mean to you?
Challenging food rules
Emotional undereating and overeating
Intuitive eating: how to get in touch with hunger and satiety cues
Meal planning strategies for recovery and maintenance of a healthy body weight
Social and holiday dining
Interpreting food labels
Strategies for food shopping

SUMMARY

The clinical care of patients with EDs requires a collaborative treatment team at all levels of care. Specialized treatment programs (inpatient, day patient, outpatient) typically provide ready access to mental health professionals who can assist and support the RDN in the management of this challenging patient population. When the team consists of independent practitioners, communication and professional support may be more challenging. In this case the RDN may benefit from membership in an organization of eating disorder professionals that provides ongoing educational opportunities, as well as mentorship, support, and case supervision.

CLINICAL CASE STUDY 1

Anorexia Nervosa

Melissa is in her second week of hospitalization in an inpatient eating disorder specialized hospital unit. She is a 15-year-old Hispanic female who immigrated to the Unites States 6 years ago. Her parents report preoccupation with her body and food intake beginning at 12 years of age. Upon admission, Melissa's weight is 78 pounds, her height is 62.25 inches, and her body mass index (BMI) is 14.2.

Patient began menses at the age of 12 and, due to typical adolescent developmental changes, reported feeling uncomfortable in her body. At this time, she measured 58 inches and weighed 93 pounds, 76th percentile BMI for age). She learned she could restrict through seeing her mom diet at home and began counting her calories. She would aim for less than 1000 calories per day and began walking for 30 to 60 minutes daily. After 6 months, halfway through her sixth-grade year, Melissa had dropped to 82 pounds and did not grow in height during this time; she dropped to the 46th percentile (BMI for age) and stopped menstruating. Melissa's parents began worrying and started to adapt a Maudsley/family-based therapy approach that included eating all meals at home with them. She would continue to restrict at school and exercise as much as she could but was able to gain weight back and by the beginning of 7th grade was up to 105 pounds and grew 2 inches.

Melissa continued to be monitored by her pediatrician and entered high school with a height of 61 inches and weighed 112 pounds. Entering high school, Melissa quickly became stressed with the high demand of her classes and began restricting again, this time down to approximately 500 to 800 calories per day. By January of this year Melissa's weight had dropped to 89 pounds, so she began outpatient treatment. Her typical daily intake before admission was 1 cup coffee in the morning with an apple. For lunch she had salad that she packed from home with 3 ounces of sliced turkey on it and a ½ cup of brown rice with balsamic vinegar. For dinner she had two pieces of Laughing Cow cheese with steamed vegetables in her room, telling her parents she had too much work to do to sit at the table. If she got hungry at night, she would have an individual bag of fat-free popcorn. She also reported 60 to 90 minutes of walking or running per day at the gym after school. Since her first onset of menses, Melissa was getting her period on average 4 to 5 times per year; however, it has now been 6 months since her last period. Melissa denies any purging or laxative abuse. At her most recent pediatrician appointment, Melissa lost another 2 pounds since the week prior, and her heart rate was 68. The doctor recommended inpatient hospitalization for refeeding.

Continued

CLINICAL CASE STUDY 1

Anorexia Nervosa—cont'd

Since being in the hospital, Melissa has struggled with eating 100% of her meals and has been caught hiding food in her napkin and spilling her supplements out in the garbage when staff is not looking. The staff report she is consuming on average 60% to 75% of her three meals and two snacks. She reports fearing any foods high in fat such as cheese, fried foods, desserts of any kind, meat, oils, and potato chips.

Medical history: Amenorrhea, hypokalemia

Current medications: MVI with trace minerals, thiamine daily

Inpatient calorie prescription: 3000 kcal/day + 8 fl oz Ensure Plus

B/P: 89/58

Pulse: 58

Laboratory Values:

Test	Result	Reference Range
Sodium	129	135-147 mEq/L
Potassium	3.3	3.5-5.2 mEq/L
Chloride	94	95-107 mEq/L
Calcium	8.2	8.7-10.7 mg/dL
CO_2	32	22- 29 mmol/L
Glucose	65	60- 69 mg/dL (fasting)
BUN	23	8-21 mg/dL
Creatinine	1.2	0.65-1.00 mg/dL
Phosphorous	3.2	2.5-4.6 mg/dL
Magnesium	2.2	1.7-2.3
Cholesterol	240	<200

Nutrition Diagnostic Statement

- Underweight related to abnormal eating pattern as evidenced by restrictive caloric intake and excessive exercise in the setting of a 14.2 BMI for age.

Nutrition Care Questions

1. List the essential criteria for the diagnosis of anorexia nervosa (AN). Indicate Melissa's AN subtype.
2. What indications supporting hospitalization did Melissa meet before her admission?
3. Would you classify Melissa as malnourished? What criteria did you use to make this determination?
4. What are the significant physical findings from a nutrition-focused physical examination of Melissa? What are some other symptoms commonly seen in AN?
5. Assess Melissa's laboratory values and indicate what other values also may be altered in her condition.
6. What are the primary nutrition therapy goals for Melissa? How will these goals change as treatment progresses?
7. Plot anthropometric data on National Center for Health Statistics (NCHS) weight-for-age, height-for-age, and BMI-for-age percentiles charts for females, age 2 to 20 years. Calculate BMI, BMI percentile, BMI z-score, and percentile median BMI. Based on these criteria, what is Melissa's initial treatment goal weight and BMI? How often would you recommend reassessing these goals?
8. What are some behavioral or psychological treatment approaches that could be used to help Melissa?

CLINICAL CASE STUDY 2

Bulimia Nervosa

Kristin is a 34-year-old white female who has come to see you in your outpatient private practice. Her chief complaint is that she feels "out of control and wants to stop bingeing."

Kristin currently is employed as a marketing director at a company in New York City. She describes her life to be very stressful: working approximately 50 to 55 hours per week in the office and has several social engagements in the evenings. She reports an "unhealthy" relationship with food since she was a teenager, when she was a "yoyo dieter," and would take various diet pills to lose weight. Her weight as a teenager fluctuated between slightly underweight to normal. Kristin began to purge in college after some of her friends introduced her to the idea of vomiting. Later, after moving to New York City and becoming stressed with life events, she began to purge more often after what she describes as "binges."

Currently Kristin reports skipping breakfast most days but has a large cup of coffee, black, with five packets of artificial sweetener. She has a snack around 10 AM of a handful of almonds and sometimes a fruit. She usually goes to the gym during her lunch hour, where she does 45 to 55 minutes of cardio. For lunch Kristin has two hardboiled eggs, a piece of toast, and a diet soda. A few times per week after client lunches Kristin feels stressed that she ate "fear foods," so she binges on cookies or candy and afterward purges in her private bathroom. In the afternoon Kristin usually has another coffee or diet soda and a protein bar. After work Kristin goes home with plans of eating a normal dinner but, after ordering takeout from the local Chinese, Italian, or sushi restaurant, binges on approximately 2000 to 3000 calories' worth of food before purging.

Kristin has a hard time at social events that occur several times a week and binges or purges after them as well. In total Kristin estimates she is binge/purging

five times per week, sometimes twice per day. Kristin is frustrated with the binge/purge cycle she is caught in and is requesting guidance for a meal plan.

Medical history: Dental caries requiring three root canals and two implants; irritable bowel syndrome with constipation

Current medications: Fluoxetine 40 mg, Colace 100 mg once daily

Height: 5'5", weight: 138 lb (BMI: 23.0)

Laboratory data:

Test	Result	Reference Range
Sodium	139	135-147 mEq/L
Potassium	3.3	3.5-5.2 mEq/L
Chloride	94	95-107 mEq/L
Calcium	8.2	8.7-10.7 mg/dL
CO_2	29	22-29 mmol/L
Glucose	85	60-99 mg/dL (fasting)
BUN	15	8-21 mg/dL
Creatinine	1.2	0.65-1.00 mg/dL
Phosphorous	3.6	2.5-4.6 mg/dL
Magnesium	2.2	1.7-2.3
Amylase	105	25-100 units/L
Cholesterol	210	<200 mg/dL
Bicarbonate	16.5	18.0-23.0 mmol/L

Nutrition Diagnostic Statement

- Disordered eating pattern (NB-1.5) related to bingeing and purging as evidenced by a pattern of restrictive eating, bingeing, and self-induced vomiting.

CLINICAL CASE STUDY 2
Bulimia Nervosa—cont'd

Nutrition Care Questions

1. What are the medical complications Kristin is experiencing secondary to her bingeing and purging? What are some others she could develop if she does not stop?
2. Discuss which laboratory values are abnormal.
3. What are your main goals for nutrition therapy while working with Kristin?
4. How might you approach meal planning with Kristin?
5. How might you help Kristin talk about her fear foods and set goals for including them in her diet without bingeing on them?
6. What techniques would be helpful for Kristin to challenge her urges to binge and purge during stressful work situations?

USEFUL WEBSITES

Academy for Eating Disorders
American Psychiatric Association
National Association of Anorexia Nervosa and Associated Disorders
National Eating Disorders Association
Health at Every Size Community Website
International Association of Eating Disorder Professionals (IAEDP)
Maudsley Parents – Family Based Treatment for Eating Disorders
National Association of Anorexia Nervosa and Associated Disorders
International Size Acceptance Association
Society for Adolescent Health and Medicine
Training Institute for Child and Adolescent Eating Disorders

REFERENCES

Achamrah N, Coëffier M, Rimbert A, et al: Micronutrient status in 153 patients with anorexia nervosa, *Nutrients* 9:E225, 2017.

Agostino H, Erdstein J, Di Meglio G: Shifting paradigms: continuous nasogastric feeding with high caloric intakes in anorexia nervosa, *J Adolesc Health* 53:590–594, 2013.

American Psychiatric Association: *Diagnostic and statistical manual of mental disorders*, ed 5, Arlington, VA, 2013, APA Press.

American Psychiatric Association: *Practice guidelines for the treatment of patients with eating disorders*, ed 3, Washington, DC, 2006, APA Press.

American Psychiatric Association: *Guide watch*, Washington DC, 2012, APA Press.

American Psychiatric Association: *Diagnostic and statistical manual for mental disorders*, ed 4, Washington, DC, 2000, APA Press, text revision.

Attia E, Walsh BT: Behavioral management for anorexia nervosa, *N Engl J Med* 360:500–506, 2009.

Becker AE: Eating problems in special populations cultural considerations. In *Handbook of assessment and treatment of eating disorders*, Arlington, VA, 2016, American Psychiatric Association Publishing.

Barron LJ, Barron RF, Johnson JCS, et al: A retrospective analysis of biochemical and haematological parameters in patients with eating disorders, *J Eat Disord* 5:32, 2017.

Berg KC, Wonderlich SA: Emerging psychological treatments in the field of eating disorders, *Curr Psychiatry Rep* 15:407, 2013.

Boateng AA, Sriram K, Meguid MM, et al: Refeeding syndrome: treatment considerations based on collective analysis of literature case reports, *Nutrition* 26:156–167, 2010.

Bo-Linn GW, Santa Ana CA, Morawski SG, et al: Purging and calorie absorption in bulimic patients and normal women, *Ann Intern Med* 99:14–17, 1983.

Campbell K, Peebles R: Eating disorders in children and adolescents: state of the art review, *Pediatrics* 134:582–592, 2014.

de Alvaro MT, Muñoz-Calvo MT, Barrios V, et al: Regional fat distribution in adolescents with anorexia nervosa: effect of duration of malnutrition and weight recovery, *Eur J Endocrinol* 157:473–479, 2007.

de Zwaan M, Aslam Z, Mitchell JE: Research on energy expenditure in individuals with eating disorders: a review, *Int J Eat Disord* 32:127–134, 2002.

Donini LM, Marsili D, Graziani MP, et al: Orthorexia nervosa: a preliminary study with a proposal for diagnosis and an attempt to measure the dimension of the phenomenon, *Eat Weight Disord* 9:151–157, 2004

Dunn TM, Bratman S: On orthorexia nervosa: a review of the literature and proposed diagnostic criteria, *Eat Behav* 21:11–17, 2016.

Ellison JM, Wonderlich SA, Engel SG: Application of modern technology in eating disorder assessment and Intervention. In *Handbook of assessment and treatment of eating disorders*, Arlington, 2016, American Psychiatric Association Publishing.

Esposito S, Fierstein D. *The signs and symptoms of orthorexia*, 2018, National Eating Disorders Association. Available at: https://www.nationaleatingdisorders.org/blog/when-does-healthy-eating-become-dangerous.

Fairburn CG: *Cognitive behavior therapy and eating disorders*, New York, NY, 2008, Guilford Press.

Fairburn CG: *Overcoming binge eating*, New York, NY, 1995, Guilford Press.

Fairburn CG, Cooper Z, O'Connor M: *Eating disorder examination*, Edition 17.0D, April 2014, The Center for Research on Dissemination at Oxford. Available at: https://www.credo-oxford.com/pdfs/EDE_17.0D.pdf.

Fairburn CG, Rothwell ER: Apps and eating disorders: a systematic clinical appraisal, *Int J Eat Disord* 48:1038–1046, 2015.

Fisher MM, Rosen DS, Ornstein RM, et al: Characteristics of avoidant/restrictive food intake disorder in children and adolescents: a "new disorder" in DSM-5, *J Adolesc Health* 55:49–52, 2014.

Forbush KT, Hunt TK: Characterization of eating patterns among individuals with eating disorders: what is the state of the plate? *Physiol Behav* 134:92–109, 2014.

Franzoni E, Ciccarese F, Di Pietro E, et al: Follow-up of bone mineral density and body composition in adolescents with restrictive anorexia nervosa: role of dual-energy X-ray absorptiometry, *Eur J Clin Nutr* 68:247–252, 2013.

Garber AK, Michihata N, Hetnal K, et al: A prospective examination of weight gain in hospitalized adolescents with anorexia nervosa on a recommended refeeding protocol, *J Adolesc Health* 50:24–29, 2012.

Garber AK, Sawyer SM, Golden NH, et al: A systematic review of approaches to refeeding in patients with anorexia nervosa, *Int J Eat Disord* 49:293–310, 2016.

Gaudiani JL, Sabel AL, Mehler PS: Low prealbumin is a significant predictor of medical complications in severe anorexia nervosa, *Int J Eat Disord* 47:148–156, 2014.

Gendall KA, Sullivan PE, Joyce PR, et al: The nutrient intake of women with bulimia nervosa, *Int J Eat Disord* 21:115–127, 1997.

Gianini L, Liu Y, Wang Y, et al: Abnormal eating behavior in video-recorded meals in anorexia nervosa, *Eat Behav* 19:28–32, 2015.

Gur E, Latzer Y, Stein D: Editorial: new developments in the psychology, neuropsychology and psychotherapy of eating disorders, *Isr J Psychiatry Relat Sci* 55:3–7, 2018.

Golden NH, Keane-Miller C, Sainani KL, et al: Higher caloric intake in hospitalized adolescents with anorexia nervosa is associated with reduced length of stay and no increased rate of refeeding syndrome, *J Adolesc Health* 53:573–578, 2013.

Grilo CM: Psychological and behavioral treatments for binge-eating disorder, *J Clin Psychiatry* 78(Suppl 1):20–24, 2017.

Hadigan CM, Anderson EJ, Miller KK, et al: Assessment of macronutrient and micronutrient intake in women with anorexia nervosa, *Int J Eat Disord* 28:284–292, 2000.

Haas V, Kent D, Kohn MR, et al: Incomplete total body protein recovery in adolescent patients with anorexia nervosa, *Am J Clin Nutr* 107:303–312, 2018a.

Haas V, Stengel A, Mähler A, et al: Metabolic barriers to weight gain in patients with anorexia nervosa: a young adult case report, *Front Psychiatry* 9:199, 2018b.

Hay P, Chinn D, Forbes D, et al: Royal Australian and New Zealand College of Psychiatrists clinical practice guidelines for the treatment of eating disorders, *Aust N Z J Psychiatry* 48:977–1008, 2014.

Haynos AF, Snipes C, Guarda A, et al: Comparison of standardized versus individualized caloric prescriptions in the nutritional rehabilitation of inpatients with anorexia nervosa, *Int J Eat Disord* 49:50–58, 2016.

Herrin M, Larkin M: *Nutrition counseling in the treatment of eating disorders,* ed 2, New York, NY, 2013, Routledge.

Hipkind P, Glass C, Charlton D, et al: Do handheld calorimeters have a role in assessment of nutrition needs in hospitalized patients? A systematic review of literature, *Nutr Clin Pract* 26:426–433, 2011.

Juarascio AS, Manasse SM, Goldstein SP, et al. Review of smartphone applications for the treatment of eating disorders, *Eur Eat Disord Rev* 23:1–11, 2015.

Katzman DK: Refeeding hospitalized adolescents with anorexia nervosa: is "start low, advance slow" urban legend or evidence based? *J Adolesc Health* 50:1–2, 2012.

Kaye WH, Weltzin TE, Hsu LK, et al: Amount of calories retained after binge eating and vomiting, *Am J Psychiatry* 150:969–971, 1993.

Keel PK, Brown TA: Update on course and outcome in eating disorders, *Int J Eat Disord* 43:195–204, 2010.

Keys A: *The biology of human starvation* (vols 1 and 2), Minneapolis, 1950, University of Minnesota Press.

Kohn JB: What is ARFID? *J Acad Nutr Diet* 116:1872, 2016.

Kohn MR, Madden S, Clarke SD: Refeeding in anorexia nervosa: increased safety and efficiency through understanding the pathophysiology of protein calorie malnutrition, *Curr Opin Pediatr* 23:390–394, 2011.

Kornstein SG, Kunovac JL, Herman BK, et al. Recognizing binge-eating disorder in the clinical setting: a review of the literature, *Prim Care Companion CNS Disord* 18(3):1, 2016.

Kosmiski L, Schmiege SJ, Mascolo M, et al: Chronic starvation secondary to anorexia nervosa is associated with an adaptive suppression of resting energy expenditure, *J Clin Endocrinol Metab* 99:908–914, 2014.

Koubaa S, Hällström T, Hagenäs L, et al: Retarded head growth and neurocognitive development in infants of mothers with a history of eating disorders: longitudinal cohort study, *BJOG* 120:1413–1422, 2013.

Linna MS, Raevuori A, Haukka J, et al: Reproductive health outcomes in eating disorders, *Int J Eat Disord* 46:826–833, 2013.

Lock J, Le Grange D. *Treatment manual for anorexia nervosa, a family-based approach,* ed 2, New York, NY, 2013, The Guilford Press.

Lock JD, Fitzpatrick KK: Anorexia nervosa, *BMJ Clin Evid* 2009:1011, 2009.

Masheb RM, Dorflinger LM, Rolls BJ, et al: Binge abstinence is associated with reduced energy intake after treatment in patients with binge eating disorder and obesity, *Obesity (Silver Spring)* 24:2491–2496, 2016.

McClain Z, Peebles R: Body image and eating disorders among lesbian, gay, bisexual, and transgender youth, *Pediatr Clin North Am* 63(6):1079–1090, 2016.

Mårild K, Størdal K, Bulik CM, et al: Celiac disease and anorexia nervosa: A nationwide study, *Pediatrics* 139(5):e20164367, 2017.

Mayer LE, Klein DA, Black E, et al: Adipose tissue distribution after weight restoration and weight maintenance in women with anorexia nervosa, *Am J Clin Nutr* 90:1132–1137, 2009.

Mehler PS, Blalock DV, Walden K, et al: Medical findings in 1,026 consecutive adult inpatient-residential eating disordered patients, *Int J Eat Disord* 51:305–313, 2018.

Mehler PS, Winkelman AB, Andersen DM, et al: Nutritional rehabilitation: practical guidelines for refeeding the anorectic patient, *J Nutr Metab*, 2010:625782, 2010.

Modan-Moses D, Levy-Shraga Y, Pinhas-Hamiel O, et al: High prevalence of vitamin D deficiency and insufficiency in adolescent inpatients diagnosed with eating disorders, *Int J Eat Disord* 48:607–614, 2014.

Morgan JF, Reid F, Lacey JH: The SCOFF questionnaire: assessment of a new screening tool for eating disorders, *BMJ* 319:1467–1468, 1999.

National Institute for Health and Clinical Excellence: *Guideline for the management of refeeding syndrome* (adults), ed 2, United Kingdom, 2009, NHS Foundation Trust.

Norris ML, Spettigue WJ, Katzman DK: Update on eating disorders: current perspectives on avoidant/restrictive food intake disorder in children and youth, *Neuropsychiatr Dis Treat* 12:213–218, 2016.

Ozier AD, Henry BW, American Dietetic Association: Position of the American Dietetic Association: nutrition intervention in the treatment of eating disorders, *J Am Diet Assoc* 111:1236–1241, 2011.

Rigaud D, Boulier A, Tallonneau I, et al: Body fluid retention and body weight change in anorexia nervosa patients during refeeding, *Clin Nutr* 29:749–755, 2010.

Robinson L, Micali N, Misra M: Eating disorders and bone metabolism in women, *Curr Opin Pediatr* 29:488–496, 2017.

Rocks T, Pelly F, Wilkinson P: Nutrition therapy during initiation of refeeding in underweight children and adolescent inpatients with anorexia nervosa: a systematic review of the evidence, *J Acad Nutr Diet* 114:897–907, 2014.

Rosen DS, American Academy of Pediatrics Committee on Adolescence: Identification and management of eating disorders in children and adolescents, *Pediatrics* 126:1240–1253, 2010.

Russell GF: The nutritional disorder in anorexia nervosa, *J Psychosom Res* 11:141–149, 1967.

Sala M, Reyes-Rodríguez ML, Bulik CM, et al: Race, ethnicity, and eating disorder recognition by peers, *Eat Disord* 21:423–436, 2013.

Schebendach JE, Porter KJ, Wolper C, et al: Accuracy of self-reported energy intake in weight-restored patients with anorexia nervosa compared with obese and normal weight individuals, *Int J Eat Disord* 45:570–574, 2012.

Schebendach JE, Mayer LE, Devlin MJ, et al: Dietary energy density and diet variety as predictors of outcome in anorexia nervosa, *Am J Clin Nutr* 87:810–816, 2008.

Society for Adolescent Health and Medicine, Golden NH, Katzman DK, et al: Position paper of the Society for Adolescent Health and Medicine: medical management of restrictive eating disorders in adolescents and young adults, *J Adolesc Health* 56:121–125, 2015.

Society for Adolescent Health and Medicine: Refeeding hypophosphatemia in hospitalized adolescents with anorexia nervosa: a position statement of the Society for Adolescent Health and Medicine, *J Adolesc Health* 55:455–457, 2014.

Steinglass J, Mayer L, Attia E: Treatment of restrictive eating and low-weight conditions, including anorexia nervosa and avoidant/restrictive food intake disorder. In *Handbook of Assessment and Treatment of Eating Disorders.* Arlington, 2016, American Psychiatric Association Publishing.

Stellefson Myers E: *Winning the war within: nutrition therapy for clients with anorexia or bulimia nervosa,* Dallas, 2006, Helm Publishing.

Stellefson Myers E, Caperton-Kilburn C: *Winning the war within: nutrition therapy for clients with eating disorders,* ed 3, Dallas, 2017, Helm Publishing.

Strahler J, Hermann A, Walter B, et al: Orthorexia nervosa: a behavioral complex or a psychological condition? *J Behav Addict* 7(4):1143–1156, 2018.

Striegel-Moore RH, Wilson GT, DeBar L, et al: Cognitive behavioral guided self-help for the treatment of recurrent binge eating, *J Consult Clin Psychol* 78:312–321, 2010.

Sysko R, Glasofer DR, Hildebrandt T, et al: The eating disorder assessment for DSM-5 (EDA-5): development and validation of a structured interview for feeding and eating disorders, *Int J Eat Disord* 48(5):452–463, 2015.

Trent SA, Moreira ME, Colwell CB, et al: ED management of patients with eating disorders, *Am J Emerg Med* 31:859–865, 2013.

Westmoreland P, Krantz MJ, Mehler PS: Medical complications of anorexia nervosa and bulimia, *Am J Med* 129:30–37, 2016.

Wilson GT: Treatment of binge eating disorder, *Psychiatr Clin North Am* 34:773–783, 2011.

Winston AP: The clinical biochemistry of anorexia nervosa, *Ann Clin Biochem* 49:132–343, 2012.

Zickgraf HF, Ellis JM: Initial validation of the Nine Item Avoidant/Restrictive Food Intake Disorder Screen (NIAS): a measure of three restrictive eating patterns, *Appetite* 123:32–42, 2018.

22

Nutrition in Exercise and Sports Performance

Lisa Dorfman, MS, RDN, CSSD, CCMS, LMHC, FAND

KEY TERMS

actomyosin
adenosine diphosphate (ADP)
adenosine triphosphate (ATP)
aerobic metabolism
anabolic effects
anaerobic metabolism
androgenic effects
anorexia athletica (AA)
athletic energy deficit (AED)
creatine phosphate (CP)
dehydration
dehydroepiandrosterone (DHEA)
eating, exercise, and body image (EEBI)
    disorders
ergogenic aid

exercise related transient abdominal
    pain (ETAP)
fat adaptation strategy
female athlete triad (FAT)
glycemic index
glycogen
glycogen loading (glycogen
    supercompensation)
glycogenolysis
glycolysis
high-intensity interval training (HIIT)
hypohydration
human growth hormone (HGH)
lactic acid
metabolic equivalents (METs)

microbiome
mitochondria
muscle dysmorphia (MD)
myoglobin
nutrition periodization
oxidative phosphorylation
pseudoanemia
relative energy deficit in sports (RED-S)
respiratory exchange ratio (RER)
reactive oxygen species (ROS)
sports anemia
thermoregulation
Vo$_2$max

Optimal athletic performance is the culmination of genetics, proper training, adequate nutrition, hydration, desire, and adequate rest. Nutrition is especially important to recreational and competitive athletes regardless of age or gender. Understanding sport-specific physiologic requirements for training and competition is integral to obtaining sufficient energy, optimal levels of macronutrients and micronutrients, and adequate levels of fluids. A balanced dietary intake is vital for supporting energy needs and stamina for training hard, achieving target performance, body composition and weight goals, adequate recovery, and reducing the incidence of illness and injury. In some cases, the use of supplements and sports foods is also helpful (Hosseinzadeh et al, 2017; International Olympic Committee [IOC], 2018; Mielgo-Ayuso et al, 2015).

BIOENERGETICS OF PHYSICAL ACTIVITY

Exercise nutrition requires essential elements from food to fuel muscle contractions, build new tissue, preserve lean muscle mass, optimize skeletal structure, repair existing cells, maximize oxygen transport, maintain favorable fluid and electrolyte balance, and regulate metabolic processes.

The human body must be supplied continuously with energy to perform its many complex functions. Three metabolic systems supply energy for the body: one dependent on oxygen (oxidative phosphorylation or aerobic metabolism) and the other two independent of oxygen (creatine phosphate and anaerobic glycolysis or anaerobic metabolism). The use of one system over the other depends on the duration, intensity, and type of physical activity.

Adenosine Triphosphate: Ultimate Energy Source

Regardless of the energy system used to generate power for exercise, the body relies on a continuous supply of fuel through adenosine triphosphate (ATP), found within the mitochondria of the body. The energy produced from the breakdown of ATP provides the fuel that activates muscle contraction. The energy from ATP is transferred to the contractile filaments (myosin and actin) in the muscle, which form an attachment of actin to the cross-bridges on the myosin molecule, thus forming actomyosin. Once activated the myofibrils slide past each other and cause the muscle to contract.

Although ATP is the main currency for energy in the body, it is stored in limited amounts. Approximately 3 oz of ATP is stored in the body at any one time (McArdle et al, 2014). This provides only enough energy for several seconds of exercise, and yet ATP must be resynthesized continually to provide a constant energy source. When ATP loses a phosphate, thus releasing energy, the resulting adenosine diphosphate (ADP) is combined enzymatically with another high-energy phosphate from creatine phosphate (CP) to resynthesize ATP. The concentration of high-energy CP in the muscle is five times that of ATP.

Creatine kinase is the enzyme that catalyzes the reaction of CP with ADP and inorganic phosphate. This is the fastest and most immediate means of replenishing ATP, and it does so without the use of oxygen (anaerobic). Although this system has great power, it is time limited because of the limited concentration of CP found in the muscles (see Creatine later in the chapter).

The energy released from this ATP-CP system will support an all-out exercise effort of only a few seconds, such as in a power lift, tennis serve, or sprint. If the all-out effort continues for longer than 8 seconds, or if moderate exercise is to proceed for longer periods, an additional source of energy must be provided for the resynthesis of ATP. The production of ATP carries on within the muscle cells through either the anaerobic or aerobic pathways.

Anaerobic or Lactic Acid Pathway

The next energy pathway for supplying ATP for more than 8 seconds of physical activity is the process of glycolysis. In this pathway the energy in glucose is released without the presence of oxygen. Lactic acid is the end product of glycolysis. Without the production of lactic acid, glycolysis would shut down. The coenzyme called nicotinic acid dehydrogenase (NAD) is in limited supply in this pathway. When NAD is limited, the glycolytic pathway cannot provide constant energy. By converting pyruvic acid to lactic acid, NAD is freed to participate in further ATP synthesis. The amount of ATP furnished is relatively small; the process is only 30% efficient. This pathway contributes energy during an all-out effort lasting up to 60 to 120 seconds. Examples are a 440-yard sprint and many sprint-swimming events (Powers et al, 2018).

Although this process provides immediate protection from the consequences of insufficient oxygen, it cannot continue indefinitely. When exercise continues at intensities beyond the body's ability to supply oxygen and convert lactic acid to fuel, lactic acid accumulates in the blood and muscle, lowers the pH to a level that interferes with enzymatic action, and causes fatigue. Lactic acid can be removed from the muscle, transported into the bloodstream, and converted to energy in muscle, liver, or brain. Otherwise, it is converted to glycogen. Conversion to glycogen occurs in the liver and to some extent in muscle, particularly among trained athletes.

The amount of ATP produced through glycolysis is small compared with that available through aerobic pathways. Substrate for this reaction is limited to glucose from blood sugar or the glycogen stored in the muscle. Liver glycogen contributes but is limited.

Aerobic Pathway

Production of ATP in amounts sufficient to support continued muscle activity for longer than 90 to 120 seconds requires oxygen. If sufficient oxygen is not present to combine with hydrogen in the electron transport chain, no further ATP is made. Thus the oxygen furnished through respiration is of vital importance. Here, glucose can be broken down far more efficiently for energy, producing 18 to 19 times more ATP. In the presence of oxygen, pyruvate is converted to acetyl coenzyme A (CoA), which enters the mitochondria. In the mitochondria acetyl CoA goes through the Krebs cycle, which generates 36 to 38 ATP per molecule of glucose (Fig. 22.1).

Aerobic metabolism is limited by the availability of a continuous and adequate supply of oxygen, and the availability of coenzymes. At the onset of exercise and with the increase in exercise intensity, the ability of the cardiovascular system to supply adequate oxygen is a limiting factor, and this is largely due to the level of conditioning. The aerobic pathway provides ATP by metabolizing fats and proteins. A large amount of acetyl CoA, which enters the Krebs cycle and provides enormous amounts of ATP, is provided by beta-oxidation of fatty acids. Proteins may be catabolized into acetyl CoA or Krebs cycle intermediates, or they may be directly oxidized as another source of ATP.

Energy Continuum

A person who is exercising may use one or more energy pathways. For example, at the beginning of any physical activity, ATP is produced anaerobically. As exercise continues, the lactic acid system produces

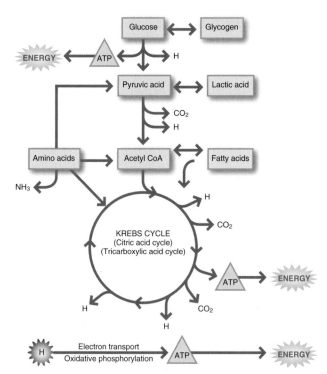

Fig. 22.1 Production of ATP for exercise.

ATP for exercise. If the person continues to exercise and does so at a moderate intensity for a prolonged period, the aerobic pathway will become the dominant pathway for fuel. On the other hand, the anaerobic pathway provides most of the energy for short-duration, high-intensity exercise such as sprinting; the 200-meter swim; or high-power, high-intensity moves in basketball, football, or soccer. However, all of the ATP-generating pathways are turned on at the onset of exercise (Powers et al, 2018).

Other factors that influence oxygen capabilities and thus energy pathways are the capacity for intense exercise and its duration. These two factors are inversely related. For example, an athlete cannot perform high-power, high-intensity moves over a prolonged period. To do this, the athlete would have to decrease the intensity of the exercise to increase its duration (Fig. 22.2).

The aerobic pathway cannot tolerate the same level of intensity as duration increases because of the decreased availability of oxygen and accumulation of lactic acid. As the duration of exercise increases, power output decreases. The contribution of energy-yielding nutrients must be considered also. As the duration of exercise lengthens, fats contribute more as an energy source. The opposite is true for high-intensity exercise; when intensity increases, the body relies increasingly on carbohydrates as substrate (Powers et al, 2018).

FUELS FOR CONTRACTING MUSCLES

Protein, fat, and carbohydrate are possible sources of fuel for ATP generation and therefore muscle contraction. The glycolytic pathway is restricted to glucose, which can originate in dietary carbohydrates or stored glycogen, or it can be synthesized from certain amino acids through the process of gluconeogenesis. The Krebs cycle is fueled by three-carbon fragments of glucose; two-carbon fragments of fatty acids; and carbon skeletons of specific amino acids, primarily alanine and the branched-chain amino acids. All these

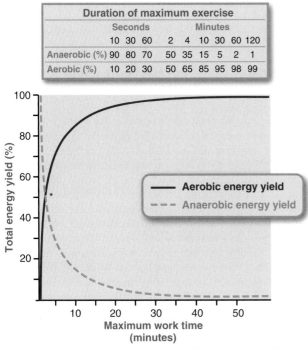

Fig. 22.2 Relative contribution of aerobic and anaerobic energy during maximum physical activity of various durations. Note that 90 to 120 seconds of maximum effort requires 50% of the energy from each of the aerobic and anaerobic processes. This is also the point at which the lactic acid pathway for energy production is at its maximum.

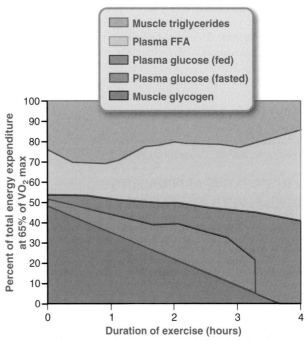

Fig. 22.3 Principle Energy Source and Exercise Duration.

substrates can be used during exercise; however, the intensity and duration of the exercise determine the relative rates of substrate use (Powers et al, 2018).

Intensity

The intensity of the exercise is important in determining what fuel will be used by contracting muscles. High-intensity, short-duration exercise has to rely on anaerobic production of ATP. Because oxygen is not available for anaerobic pathways, only glucose and glycogen can be broken down anaerobically for fuel. When glycogen is broken down anaerobically, it is used 18 to 19 times faster than when broken down aerobically. Persons who are performing high-intensity workouts or competitive races may run the risk of running out of muscle glycogen before the event or exercise is done as a result of its high rate of use (Powers et al, 2018).

Sports that use the anaerobic and aerobic pathways also have a higher glycogen-use rate and, like anaerobic athletes, athletes in these sports also run the risk of running out of fuel before the race or exercise is finished. Sports such as basketball, football, soccer, tennis, and swimming are good examples; glycogen usage is high because of the intermittent bursts of high-intensity sprints and running drills. In moderate-intensity sports or exercise such as jogging, hiking, aerobic dance, gymnastics, cycling, and recreational swimming, approximately half of the energy for these activities comes from the aerobic breakdown of muscle glycogen, whereas the other half comes from circulating blood glucose and fatty acids.

Moderate- to low-intensity exercise such as walking is fueled primarily by the aerobic pathway; thus a greater proportion of fat can be used to create ATP for energy. Fatty acids cannot supply all the ATP during high-intensity exercise because fat cannot be broken down fast enough to provide the energy. Also, fat provides less energy per

liter of oxygen consumed than does glucose (4.65 kcal/L of O_2 versus 5.01 kcal/L of O_2). Therefore when less oxygen is available in high-intensity activities, there is a definite advantage for the muscles to be able to use glycogen because less oxygen is required.

In general, glucose and fatty acids provide fuel for exercise in proportions depending on the intensity and duration of the exercise and the fitness of the athlete. Exertion of extremely high intensity and short duration draws primarily on reserves of ATP and CP. High-intensity exercise that continues for more than a few seconds depends on anaerobic glycolysis (Powers et al, 2018). During exercise of low-to-moderate intensity (60% of maximum oxygen uptake [Vo_2max]), energy is derived mainly from fatty acids. Carbohydrate becomes a larger fraction of the energy source as intensity increases until, at an intensity level of 85% to 90% Vo_2max, carbohydrates from glycogen are the principal energy source, and the duration of activity is limited (Fig. 22.3) (Powers et al, 2018).

Duration

The duration of a training session determines the substrate used during the exercise bout. For example, the longer the time spent exercising, the greater the contribution of fat as the fuel. Fat can supply up to 60% to 70% of the energy needed for ultraendurance events lasting 6 to 10 hours. As the duration of exercise increases, the reliance on aerobic metabolism becomes greater, and a greater amount of ATP can be produced from fatty acids. However, fat cannot be metabolized unless a continuous stream of some carbohydrates is also available through the energy pathways. Therefore muscle glycogen and blood glucose are the limiting factors in human performance of any type of intensity or duration (Powers et al, 2018).

Effect of Training

The length of time an athlete can oxidize fatty acids as a fuel source is related to the athlete's conditioning, as well as the exercise intensity. In addition to improving cardiovascular systems involved in oxygen delivery, training increases the number of mitochondria and the levels of enzymes involved in the aerobic synthesis of ATP, thus increasing the capacity for fatty acid metabolism. Increases in mitochondria with aerobic training are seen mainly in the type IIA (intermediate fast-twitch) muscle fibers. However, these fibers quickly lose their aerobic capacity with the cessation of aerobic training, reverting to the genetic baseline.

These changes from training result in a lower **respiratory exchange ratio (RER)**, also called respiratory quotient, which is CO_2 eliminated/ O_2 consumed; lower blood lactate and catecholamine levels, and a lower net muscle glycogen breakdown at a specific power output. These metabolic adaptations enhance the ability of muscle to oxidize all fuels, especially fat (Powers et al, 2018).

AN INTEGRATIVE APPROACH TO WORKING WITH ATHLETES

Performance nutrition is not limited to exercise physiology or diet alone but integrates six core areas of study: the role of optimal overall health and longevity, optimal growth, peak physiologic function, energy balance and body composition, nutrition enhancement, and safety.

Genetics and individualized differences, exercise environments, and life stress also can affect the athlete's microbiome and tolerance of specific nutrients. It appears that exercise is linked with modifying the brain-gut-microbe axis, diet microbe host metabolic interactions, neuroendocrine and neuroimmune interactions. There is evidence to suggest that stress, both physiologic and emotional, can modulate the composition of gut microbiota and vice versa; the microbiota can act like an endocrine organ secreting serotonin, dopamine, or other neurotransmitters and control the hypothalamic-pituitary-adrenal (HPA) axis in athletes (Clark and Mach, 2017). See Chapter 30 for more information about the HPA axis.

Although a direct relationship between exercise and gut microbial composition or function has not been established, there are several mechanisms by which physical activity might modify the microbiota and impact immune status, gut function, the incidence of upper respiratory infections (URI), mood, and sports performance (Clark and Mach, 2017; Foster et al, 2017; Hart, 2018; O'Sullivan et al, 2015). It is estimated that 20% to 60% of athletes are impacted by the stress of excessive exercise, especially endurance training and inadequate recovery and 20% to 50% of athletes suffer from gastrointestinal symptoms, which have been shown to increase with exercise intensity (Clark and Mach, 2017; Lamprecht et al, 2012). (see *Clinical Insight*.)

Training and dietary programs that aim to balance the systematic stressors that athletes experience, together with personalized diet plans to improve performance, can reduce exercise-related stress symptoms and improve gut microbiota, inflammation, and performance. One study demonstrated this with the Irish international rugby football team during World Cup training camp. The study found that when monitoring diet and exercise under extreme training condition and comparing to controls, professional athletes had lower levels of inflammatory cytokines and increased fecal microbial diversity suggesting that exercise plays a protective and positive role in nourishing the microbiota (O'Sullivan et al, 2015).

In order to find solutions for potential nutrient deficiencies, dietitians must integrate anthropometric, biochemical, and dietary data and feedback from athletes to determine how additional factors such as alterations in gut microbiota, food allergies or intolerances, dietary preferences or aversions, and/or disease processes may affect the overall absorption, assimilation, digestion, metabolism, and transport of specific macronutrients, micronutrients, or fluids, and ultimately affect performance potential.

A sports dietitian also needs to be able to critically evaluate health claims, advise on special dietary modifications, and recommend evidence informed nutritional supplements to enhance physical performance and exercise training responses.

NUTRITIONAL REQUIREMENTS OF EXERCISE

Energy

The most important component of successful sports training and performance is to ensure adequate calorie intake to support energy expenditure and maintain strength, endurance, muscle mass, and overall health. Energy and nutrient requirements vary with age, gender, weight, height, training/sport type, frequency, intensity, and duration. Other influencing factors include typical diet, history of restrictive and disordered eating; and endocrine and environmental conditions such as heat, cold, and altitude. Data suggests that a negative energy balance is common in endurance athletes, weight making and esthetic sports (wrestling, gymnastics, skating, dancing), and athletes with a larger body size, especially during high-volume training (Rogerson, 2017). Estimating energy intake is also challenging to accomplish, especially in sports that are less well studied (Powers et al, 2018).

Individuals who participate in an overall fitness program (i.e., 30 to 40 min/day, three times per week) can generally meet their daily nutritional needs by following a normal diet providing 25 to 35 kcal/kg/day or roughly 1800 to 2400 calories a day. However, energy requirements for athletes training 90 minutes a day may require 45 to 50 kcal/kg/day, and in certain sports even more (Thomas et al, 2016).

For example, the 50-kg athlete engaging in more intense training of 2 to 3 hours/day five to six times a week or high-volume training of 3 to 6 hours in one to two workouts per day 5 to 6 days a week may expend up to an additional 600 to 1200 calories a day above and beyond resting energy expenditure, thus requiring 50 to 80 kcal/kg/day or roughly 2500 to 4000 kcal/day. For elite athletes or athletes with larger bodies, daily calorie needs can reach 150 to 200 kcal/kg, or roughly 7500 to 10,000 calories a day, depending on the volume and intensity of different training phases.

Estimation of Energy Requirements

Resting metabolic rate (RMR) or resting energy expenditure (REE) can be measured using indirect calorimetry or estimated by using predictive equations. Indirect calorimetry involves using a handheld device such as the MedGem calorimeter or metabolic cart typically used in exercise physiology or research settings to measure a person's oxygen consumption to determine RMR or basal metabolic rate (BMR). Measuring RMR or BMR is more accurate than using prediction equations.

Predictive equations are used to estimate RMR/BMR when technical equipment, such as a metabolic cart, is not available. The Cunningham equation has been shown to be the best predictor of RMR or REE for active men and women followed by the Harris-Benedict equation. DeLorenzo developed an equation that also has been shown to be accurate specifically with male strength and power athletes such as those in water polo, judo, and karate (Academy of Nutrition and Dietetics [AND], 2014; Jagim et al, 2018). If the sports dietitian has body composition data including percent body fat, the REE can be calculated as shown in Box 22.1.

Once REE has been calculated, the total energy expenditure (TEE) can be estimated using energy expenditure from physical activity. Because metabolic equipment is expensive, requires considerable training to use, and is not practical outside research settings, indirect methods can be employed and include heart rate monitors, pedometers, or accelerometers.

BOX 22.1 Calculating RMR from Body Composition Data

RMR (calories/day) = 500 + (22 x LBM in kilograms)

RMR = resting metabolic rate
LBM = lean body mass

BOX 22.2 Calculating Daily Energy Requirements for Athletes

Cunningham Equation

RMR or REE (resting energy expenditure in kcalories/day) = 500 + [22 x lean body mass (LBM) in kilograms (kg)]

For example:

175-pound (79.5kg) athlete with 10% body fat

Kg of fat = fat weight = 79.5 kg x.10 = 7.9 kg fat.

LBM = total weight – fat weight = 79.5 – 7.9 = 71.6 kg of LBM

REE = 500 + (22 x 71.6kg LBM) = 2075 calories.

To Determine EEPA—Energy Expended for Physical Activity

Can use:

Calories expended in a day using: http://www.cdc.gov/nccdphp/dnpa/physical/pdf/PA_Intensity_table_2_1.pdf

Or

Can use:

Specific caloric expenditures for different weights using: http://www.nutribase.com/exercala.htm

Or

Can multiply REE by the activity factor using:

1.200 = sedentary (little or no exercise)

1.375 = lightly active (about 30 minutes of moderate training, 1-3 days/week)

1.550 = moderately active (45 minutes of moderate training, 3-5 days/week)

1.725 = very active (training for 1 hour, 6-7 days/week)

1.900 = extra active (very hard training, including weight lifting, 2-3 days/week)

Or METs (Metabolic Equivalents)

Example METs = 4.5. Weight of individual: 80 kg.

Amount of energy expended = 0.0175 kcal/kg/minute x 80 kg x 4.5 = 6.3 kcal/min.

Walking for 30 minutes at 4 mph for an 80 kg individual = 189 kcal.

METs Calculation source: http://www.globalrph.com/metabolic_equivalents.htm

To continue the example:

The EEPA for this 175-pound athlete who is training hard would be the following:

REE (2075 kcalories) x activity factor (1.9) = 3942 *total* kcalories for basal energy expenditure (BEE) and EEPA

To continue the example:

Thermic effect of food (TEF) = the total kcalories for REE and EEPA x 10% = 3942 x 0.1 = 394 kcalories

Total daily energy requirements = total kcalories (3942) + TEF (394 kcalories) = 4336 kcalories.

Total daily energy requirements = 4336 kcalories

Thompson J, Manore MM. Predicted and measured resting metabolic rate of male and female endurance athletes. *J Am Diet Assoc.* 1996 Jan; 96(1):30-4.

Other indirect methods are to use a daily activity factor as a base to which is added calories expended in exercise, which are calculated by multiplying the calories expended per minute of exercise times the amount of time spent in that activity, known as metabolic equivalents (METs) of task (Powers et al, 2018). One MET is defined as the amount of oxygen consumed while sitting quietly in a chair at rest and equivalent to 3.5 mL O_2 per kg body weight x min, while the energy cost of an activity is (mL O_2/kg/min) x 3.5 (Jetté et al, 1990) A recent study, however, suggests that the standardized MET value overestimated observed resting oxygen consumption (VO_2) in 114 healthy men, resulting in underestimations of the maximal MET and energy cost of running (Ázara et al, 2017).

Heart rate monitoring to estimate energy expenditure is based on the assumption that there is a linear relationship between heart rate and VO_2. Using heart rate to calculate intensity is not necessarily accurate since increases may be due to not only energy demand but also factors such as stress, medications, caffeine, and dehydration. Pedometers measure ambulatory distance covered, which is a limitation of the method because it does not consider other types of physical activities such as weight lifting, cycling, or yoga. Accelerometers have the advantage of measuring all activities, are easy to wear, and can give feedback for long periods of time. Other personal fitness devices have been developed in recent years, although no method is as accurate as measuring directly with a metabolic cart. A method for calculating TEE using activity factors provided is shown in Box 22.2.

Meeting caloric needs for many fitness-minded or elite, intensely training individuals can be a challenge regardless of the accuracy of the formulas used to predict energy needs.

For high school and college athletes, disruptive sleep patterns and accommodating academic, social, and training schedules often lead to skipped meals, high frequency of unplanned snacking, use of sport shakes and bars in lieu of whole food meals, and late-night snacking while studying or socializing online or with friends. Adult athletes with family and work responsibilities and religious obligations such as fasting, Lent, or celebrating Ramadan may also have additional challenges when juggling daily training schedules with carpools, work deadlines, and accommodating family's eating schedules, which may ultimately compromise the quantity, quality, and timing of meals and greatly affect energy, strength levels, and overall health.

In elite athletes, consuming enough food at regular intervals without compromising performance is challenging, particularly when athletes are traveling abroad, or are at the mercy of airport food, foreign foods and schedules, unfamiliar training facilities, delays, and unforeseen events such as weather-postponed games and competition schedules. All athletes regardless of age and lifestyle demands can be better prepared by packing snacks and ready-to-eat meals, which are essential for keeping energy intakes adequate to support overall health and performance.

Meeting the daily energy needs and the appropriate macronutrient distribution for active individuals may necessitate the use of formulated sports bars, drinks, and convenience foods and snacks in addition to whole foods and meals. While whole foods are preferred over convenience or packaged foods, dietitian nutritionists need to be open minded and flexible in accommodating athletes' lifestyles and eating behaviors when designing meal plans for maximum sport performance.

WEIGHT MANAGEMENT

One goal of a performance-targeted diet is to help an athlete reach an optimum body size and weight/body fat distribution to achieve greater athletic success. Although exercise performance is influenced by weight/body composition, these physical measures are not the only performance criteria for optimal sports outcomes. Optimal weight, BMI, and body composition measures for athletic performance have yet to be determined, therefore sports performance may be the best indicator to determine an athlete's optimal body composition and weight at their age for best performance (Carl et al, 2017).

Regardless of age, ultimately, an athlete's optimal competitive body weight and relative body fatness should be determined based on individual health and level of performance. For young athletes there are no established recommendations regarding body composition in children and adolescents. For master-level athletes older than 40 years, chronic training has been shown to preserve body fat levels similar to that of young, healthy individuals in an exercise mode-specific manner (McKendry et al, 2018).

In some sports, athletes may be pressured to lose weight and body fat to improve their power-to-weight ratio (as for running, distance cycling, and triathlons), achieve a desirable body composition for aesthetic sports (i.e., gymnastics, figure skating, dancing, cheerleading, and diving) or compete in a specific weight class (as for wrestling, lightweight rowing, sailing, martial arts, horse racing [jockeys], and boxing), in spite of having an appropriate weight for overall health (Larson-Meyer et al, 2018; Manore, 2015).

Athletes' body-fat percentages vary depending on sex and sport as assessed in one study of 898 male and female athletes from 21 sports (Schneiter et al, 2014). When no standard exists, experts agree athletes should remain above a certain minimal body fat. While the estimated minimal level of body fat compatible with health is 5% for males and 12% for females, optimal body-fat percentages for an athlete may be much higher to achieve optimal success in their respective sports and need to be established on an individual basis. The highest optimal weight can be calculated using a value at the highest end of the range satisfactory for health: 10% to 22% body fat for males and 20% to 32% for females (Turocy et al, 2011).

Weight Loss

In efforts to maximize performance or meet weight criteria determined by specific sports—whether to "make a lower weight" in sports such as martial arts, sailing, rowing, or wrestling, or reach a higher weight for power lifting, football, or baseball—many athletes alter normal energy intake to either gain or lose weight (Carl et al, 2017). Although such efforts are sometimes appropriate, weight reduction or weight gain programs may involve elements of risk, especially when the pressure to lose or gain weight is expected in an unrealistically short amount of time. For some young athletes, achievement of an unrealistically low weight or conversely a high weight with the use of weight gainer or other supplements can jeopardize growth and development.

The goal weight of an athlete is based on optimizing health and performance and should be determined by the athlete's best previous performance weight and body composition. Adequate time should be allowed for a slow, steady weight loss of approximately 1 to 2 pounds each week over several weeks. Weight loss should be achieved during off-season or preseason when competition is not a priority. A weight loss planning guide can be found online at the *AND Sports Nutrition Care Manual*.

The National Athletic Trainers Association (NATA) suggests the lowest safe weight should be calculated at no lower than the weight determined by the low reference body fat composition delineated by sex and age. The lowest safe weight can be defined as the lowest weight

TABLE 22.1 Body Fat (%) Standards by Sex and Age

Body Fat Standard	Males	Females
Lowest reference body fat for adults	5	12
Lowest reference body fat for adolescents	7	14
Healthy body fat ranges	10-22	20-32

sanctioned by the governing body at which a competitor may compete (Turocy et al, 2011). When no standard exists, participants would be required to remain above a certain minimal body fat. (Turocy et al, 2011; Table 22.1).

In 1997 specific rules and guidelines were implemented by the National Collegiate Athletic Association (NCAA) to ensure safe weight control practices in wrestling, applied early in the competitive season and conducted on a regular basis to ensure prevention of dehydration and other weight-cutting behaviors. In 2006 the National Federation of State High School Associations adopted similar standards for determining body weights, although they are not accepted or enforced universally.

Weight Gain

Athletes are often motivated to gain lean muscle mass for power and team sports. An athlete's stage of development, genetic factors, and type of training, diet, and motivation are all factors that influence weight gain and muscle development (Carl et al, 2017). The healthiest strategy for weight gain is to increase muscle mass by consuming sufficient calories and macronutrients. The rate of weight gain will be dependent on the athlete's genetic makeup, degree of positive energy balance, number of rest and recovery sessions per week, and exercise type (Hall et al, 2012).

Weight gain should be gradual to avoid excess body fat deposition, which is not conducive to optimal performance. An excess of 2 pounds per week may result in increased body fat. Male athletes can target a reasonable gain of 0.5 lb to 1.0 lb of lean mass per week, whereas females can expect a gain 0.25 lb to 0.75 pounds of lean mass per week. Increased energy intake should always be combined with strength training to induce muscle growth.

Nutrient-dense, high-calorie foods such as nuts and nut butters and avocados are a great addition to meals and snacks. Smoothies and nut butter sandwiches can add healthy fats, protein, and vitamins and minerals. Other foods such as beans and lentils, lean meats, and dairy can also be incrementally added to daily calorie needs to achieve an additional 250 to 500 calories per day.

WEIGHT MANAGEMENT AND AESTHETICS

Disordered Eating

Although drive, perfection, and attention to detail are the hallmarks of talented athletes, they are also some of the personality traits associated with the development of eating disorders (see Chapter 21). Disordered eating behaviors among athletes can be difficult to detect given the tendencies of athletes to maintain rigid nutritional requirements, follow intense training schedules, and push through fatigue and pain.

Disordered eating behaviors specifically in athletes have been termed anorexia athletica (AA), where the ultimate goal is to perform at one's best as opposed to thinness in and of itself. Athletes who are more vulnerable to AA are those who participate in "lean-build" sports, such as cross country running, swimming, gymnastics, cheerleading, dance, yoga, and wrestling, who may think they need to be a certain weight or body type, often far less than what it is realistic to attain and maintain to be competitive. This desire to be unrealistically light or lean may lead to restrictive eating, bingeing and purging, and excessive training far beyond what is required for their sport.

Female Athlete Triad

Chronic dieting by female athletes can lead to the female athlete triad (FAT), which consists of three interrelated health disorders: low energy availability with or without an eating disorder, osteoporosis, and amenorrhea. The prevalence of FAT for athletes participating in lean-requiring versus non–lean-requiring sports has been shown to range from 1.5% to 6.7% and from 0% to 2.0% respectively (Gibbs et al, 2013). For example, it has been shown that student and professional female dancers consume only 70% to 80% of the recommended dietary allowance (RDA) for total daily energy intake (Mountjoy et al, 2014).

The low energy intake of athletic energy deficit (AED), also known as relative energy deficit in sports (RED-S), can lead to an increase in bone fractures, lifelong consequences for bone and reproductive health, impaired judgment, decreased coordination, decreased concentration, irritability, depression, and decreased endurance performance in developing adolescent girls and even young men (Ackerman et al, 2018). Evidence suggests it is energy availability that regulates reproductive function in women, not exercise or body composition, and that ensuring adequate calorie intake is imperative to the overall health of the athletic woman (Ackerman et al, 2019; De Souza et al, 2014). Low energy intake paired with ovarian suppression or amenorrhea has been associated with poor athletic performance.

Muscle Dysmorphia

Although many studies suggest females are more susceptible to disordered eating behaviors than males, results from descriptive data from project EAT (Eating Among Teens) revealed that males in a weight-related sport are comparable to females in the same category. In fact, as the media's portrayal of the male physique has been increasingly muscular and unattainable, men have become more dissatisfied with their bodies and more vulnerable to eating, exercise, and body image (EEBI) disorders.

Muscle dysmorphia (MD), also known as "bigorexia" or reverse AN, is a disorder in which individuals are preoccupied with their bodies not being muscular enough or big enough. It is marked by symptoms that are similar to and the opposite of AN symptomatology.

AA and MD experience grossly distorted perceptions of their bodies, which in the case of MD, often leads to maladaptive eating, exercise, and substance use behaviors, including preoccupation with diet and excessively high protein intakes. In addition there is anabolic steroid, diet pill, caffeine, and over-the-counter supplement abuse, especially of those reputed for fat-burning, ergogenic, or thermogenic effects. Last, the athlete exercises excessively, especially weight lifting, in an attempt to increase body satisfaction and attain the "perfect" lean and muscular physique. As with other EEBI, MD can lead to social, occupational, and relationship impairments (Box 22.3).

Research suggests that this preference for a muscular physique is already evident in boys as young as 6 years old and may affect up to

---

BOX 22.3 Body Image and Eating Disorders in Athletes

Anorexia Athletica

Exercising beyond the requirements for good health

Obsessive dieting; fear of certain foods

Obsessive or compulsive exercising; overtraining

Won't eat with teammates, tries to hide dieting

Stealing time from work, school, and relationships to exercise

Focusing on challenge and forgetting that physical activity can be fun

Defining self-worth in terms of performance

Rarely or never being satisfied with athletic achievements

Always pushing on to the next challenge

Justifying excessive behavior by defining self as an athlete or insisting that the behavior is healthy

Desire to keep losing more pounds despite already low body weight

Mood swings; angry outbursts

Menstrual periods stop

http://www.eatingdisordersonline.com/explain/anorexiathleticasigns.php

Muscle Dysphoria

Primarily male eating disorder

Getting bigger is on the mind constantly. This includes thinking about diet, working out, or appearance

See themselves as looking small or "puny" even though they typically appear normal or very muscular to others

Constant concerns with body fat percentage

Hide physique with baggy clothing since never feel "good enough" and is source of shame

Workouts take precedence over other significant events or time spent with family and friends

Fear that missing one workout session will set them back or stymie progress

Workout even when injured

Common to abuse anabolic steroids to enhance their appearance

Missing workout or eating a "forbidden" food item can trigger extreme anxiety and crush self-esteem

Individual might add additional workout sessions, skip meals, or use some means to punish themselves for diet cheating

Frequently accompanying symptoms of depression

http://www.eatingdisordersonline.com/lifestyle/general/recognizing-muscle-dysmorphia-bigorexia

---

95% of college-age American men who are dissatisfied with some aspect of their body and up to 25% of college men engaging in negative body talk (Engeln et al, 2013; Murray et al, 2012). Many studies suggest that bodybuilders display higher MD prevalence rates and more MD features than other resistance training athletes, with prevalence rates ranging from 3.4% to 53.6% within this population (Cerea et al, 2018).

MACRONUTRIENTS

According to the position of the AND, Dietitians of Canada, and the American College of Sports Medicine (ACSM), most recreational athletes do not need to eat a diet that is substantially different than the U.S. Dietary Guidelines for Americans to attain and maintain optimal health (Kerksick et al, 2017). Individuals engaging in a general fitness

TABLE 22.2   A Nutrition Periodization Program

Cycle	Training Goal/Dietary Recommendation
Preseason training	Preparation load cycles followed by recovery cycles
	Higher or lower energy needs depending on weight goals
	Greater protein needs for lean muscle mass development
Competitive season	Peak cycles with recovery; energy needs depending on expenditure; higher carbohydrate needs to support high-intensity competition; protein and fat needs relative to weight maintenance, recovery and overall health
Postseason training	Active rest-transition cycle of conditioning and recovery; energy to support but not exceed needs; emphasis on more lax dietary guidelines for mental and emotional competitive break

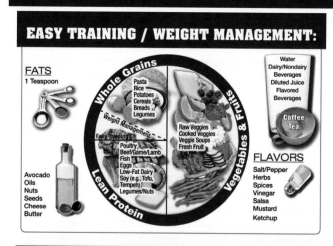

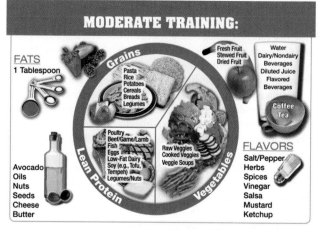

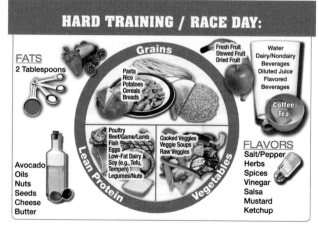

Fig. 22.4 The Athlete's Plate adjusted for training and competition. United States Olympic Committee Sport Dietitians and University of Colorado Sport Nutrition Graduate Program, My Plate for Athletes.

program of moderate activity typically can meet their macronutrient needs by consuming a normal balanced diet of 45% to 55% of calories from carbohydrates (3 to 5 g/kg/day), 10% to 15% from protein (0.8 to 1 g/kg/day), and 25% to 35% from fat (0.5 to 1.5 g/kg/day).

Nutrition Periodization

The composition of the athlete's diet is dependent on training phase: preseason, season, off-season; sport type including intensity and duration of training; and weight and body composition goals. Competitive athletes involved in moderate- to high-volume training will however require greater amounts of carbohydrates, protein, and fat to meet macronutrient needs for training and seasonal requirements and goals, whether it is gaining mass, improving speed, and/or improving endurance. Specific macronutrient recommendations should be used when counseling a competitive or elite athlete to maximize performance, a concept known as nutrition periodization.

Nutrition periodization is a term to describe dietary modification to match specific training patterns during in and off seasons as well as pre- and postcompetition periods, which are marked by different nutritional needs. Periodization involves different training cycles, including load, recovery peak, and conditioning that are implemented according to the athlete's sports demands and competition schedules (Kerksick et al, 2017; Table 22.2).

Strategies and Tools for Eating Guides in Athletes

According to the United States Olympic Committee (USOC), sports dietitians, and other sports nutrition experts, keeping guidelines simple for athletes is imperative for compliance.

The USOC dietitians created the Athlete's Plate as a guide for eating for athletes based on easy, moderate, and hard training regimens (Fig. 22.4). This tool helps athletes who play a sport for more than 5 hours a week modify servings and portion sizes from each food group based on their training.

CARBOHYDRATE

Adequate glycogen stores are important, particularly for endurance athletes, for maintaining high work rate and preventing fatigue. Carbohydrates are one of two main fuels used for sport activity. The first source of glucose for the exercising muscle is its own glycogen store. When this is depleted, glycogenolysis and then gluconeogenesis (both in the liver) maintain the glucose supply. Glycogen depletion can result from inadequate carbohydrate intake after training sessions, especially multiple training sessions, or may also be a gradual process, occurring over repeated days of heavy training in which muscle glycogen breakdown exceeds its replacement. Glycogen depletion can also occur during high-intensity exercise that is repeated several times during competition or training.

During endurance exercise that exceeds 90 minutes, such as marathon running, muscle glycogen stores become progressively smaller. When they drop to critically low levels, high-intensity exercise cannot be maintained. In practical terms the athlete is exhausted and must either stop exercising or drastically reduce the pace. Athletes often refer to this as "hitting the wall."

Historically, a high-carbohydrate or glycogen loading (glycogen supercompensation) diet was used to guide athletes to enhance and maximize glycogen stores and be able to continue endurance performance, but this approach has its benefits and drawbacks (McArdle et al, 2014). The 7-day carbohydrate-loading approach combined muscle-specific depletion training with a low-carbohydrate diet for 4 days followed by a high-carbohydrate diet and little to no training for 3 days before competition. Normal muscle typically contains about 1.7 g glycogen per 100 g of muscle; supercompensation packs up to 5 g glycogen per 100 g of muscle. Although this may be beneficial for the endurance athlete training or competing over 60 minutes, it has not been shown to benefit those in higher-intensity, shorter-duration activities. The negative effects of the additional weight of 2.7 g of water for each gram of glycogen can be a hindrance to performance, making it a heavy fuel. A modified approach of gradual exercise tapering along with more modified increases in carbohydrate intake may minimize the negative outcomes associated with classical loading (McArdle et al, 2014).

Experts now agree that habitual carbohydrate regimens for competitive athletes are not advantageous, instead recommending periodizing carbohydrate intake depending on the intensity and duration of training sessions; training block goals; and glycogen supercompensation before competition (Casazza et al, 2018).

Effects of Training Low, Competing High

Numerous studies conducted over the past 40 to 50 years have consistently directed to carbohydrates as the primary macronutrient for sustaining and improving physical performance. In recent years, with the advent of techniques that better allow scientists to measure the metabolism of key nutrients such as proteins/amino acids and studies on alternative feeding regimens such as ketogenic diets, performance diets have become more personalized. Considering the athlete's preferences, genetic makeup, dietary history, and training regimen requires a periodization approach optimizing nutrient needs for performance (Kanter, 2018).

Research suggests that training low, competing high, and a nutritional periodization approach, can increase the rate of fat oxidation while attenuating the rate of muscle glycogenolysis during submaximal exercise.

Studies have investigated the impact of short-term, 1- to 2-week diet-training interventions that increase endogenous muscle glycogen and lipids and alter patterns of substrate utilization during exercise. Otherwise known as the fat adaptation strategy or "train low" approach, well-trained endurance athletes consume a high-fat, low-cholesterol diet for up to 2 weeks while undertaking their normal training and then immediately follow this by a high-carbohydrate diet and tapering of exercise 1 to 3 days before an endurance event.

Recent studies have also examined the proposal that adaptation to a low-carbohydrate (<25% energy), high-fat (>60% energy) (LCHF) diet to increase muscle fat utilization during exercise could enhance performance in trained individuals by reducing reliance on muscle glycogen. Studies suggest a LCHF for 5 days retools the muscle to enhance fat-burning capacity with changes that persist in spite of acute strategies to restore carbohydrate availability (i.e., glycogen supercompensation, carbohydrate intake during exercise). In addition, a 2- to 3-week exposure to minimal carbohydrate (<20 g/day) intake achieves adaptation to high blood ketone concentrations (Burke, 2015). However, in one study with elite endurance racewalkers, in contrast to training with diets providing chronic or periodized high carbohydrate availability, adaptation to an LCHF diet impaired performance despite a significant improvement in peak aerobic capacity (Burke et al, 2017).

While recent research suggests an athlete's need for protein and some fats may be higher than once believed, and dietary protein and fat can provide necessary energy to perform physical activity, carbohydrate is the substrate most efficiently metabolized by the body and the only macronutrient that can be broken down rapidly enough to provide energy during periods of high-intensity exercise (Kanter, 2018).

Carbohydrate Recommendations

The amount of carbohydrate required depends on the athlete's total daily energy expenditure, type of sport, gender, and environmental conditions, with the ultimate goal of providing adequate energy for performance and recovery and a protein sparing effect.

Recommendations should provide for daily carbohydrate intake in grams relative to body mass and allow flexibility for the athlete to meet these targets within the context of energy needs and other dietary goals. Carbohydrate intake of 5 to 7 g/kg/day can meet general training needs, and 7 to 10 g/kg/day will likely suffice for endurance athletes, although elite athletes training 5 to 6 hours a day may need as much as 12 g/kg/day or a range of 420 to 720 g of carbohydrates a day for the 60-kg athlete (AND, 2014; Powers et al, 2018).

Carbohydrates are especially important not only as an overall contributor to meeting daily calorie needs but also as ergogenic aids in a more time-specific approach, also known as nutritional periodization, designed to enhance and maximize performance for competition, especially more than 90 minutes in length.

Food Timing
Pretraining Carbohydrates

The pretraining or preevent meal serves two purposes: (1) it keeps the athlete from feeling hungry before and during the exercise, and (2) it maintains optimal levels of blood glucose for the exercising muscles. A preexercise meal can improve performance compared with exercising in a fasted state. Athletes who train early in the morning before eating or drinking risk developing low liver glycogen stores, which can impair performance, particularly if the exercise regimen involves endurance training.

Carbohydrate meals before exercise can enhance liver glycogen stores. In addition to allowing for personal preferences and psychological factors, the preevent meal should be high in carbohydrate, nongreasy, and readily digested. Fat should be limited because it delays gastric emptying time and takes longer to digest. A meal eaten 3½ to 4 hours before competition should be limited to 25% of the kilocalories from fat. Closer to the event, the fat content should be less than 25% (Box 22.4).

Exercising with a full stomach may cause indigestion, nausea, and vomiting. Thus the pregame meal should be eaten 3 to 4 hours before an event and can provide up to 200 to 350 g of carbohydrates for athletes exercising more than 90 minutes, although each athlete has to make an individual determination based on personal tolerance as to the amount and source before exercise (≤4 g/kg) (Potgieter, 2013). Allowing time for partial digestion and absorption provides a final addition to muscle glycogen, additional blood sugar, and

For athletes who compete in events such as track or swimming meets or soccer, basketball, volleyball, and wrestling tournaments all day, nutritious, easy-to-digest food and fluid choices may be a challenge. The athlete should consider the amount of time between eating and performance when choosing foods during all-day events. Suggested precompetition menus include the following:

1 Hour or Less Before Competition—About 100 to 150 kcal
One of these choices:
Fresh fruit such as a banana or orange slices
Half of a sports or breakfast bar
Corn tortilla or small plain arepa
1 small naan, roti chapati, or makai
1 slice of bread, ½ plain bagel or ½ English muffin
1 small pita, lavash, or sangak
Crackers such as rice crackers, saltines, or Melba toast
Small box of plain rice or flake cereal or hot cereal packet-quinoa, oatmeal, rice.
8 to 12 oz of a sports drink

2 to 3 Hours Before Competition—About 300 to 400 kcal
One of these choices:
½ of turkey or hummus sandwich on pita with ½ banana
½ bagel with low-sugar jelly and 1 banana
2 pancakes with light or sugar-free syrup and berries
32 fluid oz of a sports drink, endurance drink
1 low-sugar smoothie with berries, banana, and 1 scoop (< or = 20 g) of protein, which can be plant-based, whey, or egg whites
1 sports energy bar, 1 cup sports beverage, 1 cup water
1 clear broth soup, plain baked or sweet potato or yuca w/yogurt topping

3 to 4 Hours Before Competition—About 600 to 700 kcal
One of these selections:
Scrambled eggs/egg whites with 2 waffles or toast and banana
1 pita pocket with hummus, pureed fruit or pea soup, crackers, fruit
1 to 6-in turkey sub with lettuce, tomato, and small bag baked chips
1 3-oz grilled chicken breast with small baked potato, roll, and water
1 to 2 cups pasta, 2 to 3 oz chicken breast, 1 small roll
Miso soup, 1 sushi roll or 4 to 5 pieces sashimi with rice
1 20-oz sport shake with protein scoop, 1 sports bar, 1 banana, water

also relatively complete emptying of the stomach. To avoid gastrointestinal (GI) distress, the carbohydrate content of the meal should be reduced when the meal is close to the exercise time. For example, 4 hours before the event, the athlete consume 4 g of carbohydrate per kilogram of body weight, whereas 1 hour before the competition the athlete would consume 1 g of carbohydrate per kilogram of body weight.

Commercial liquid formulas providing an easily digested high-carbohydrate fluid are popular with athletes and probably leave the stomach faster. Foods high in fiber, fat, and lactose cause GI distress for some (e.g., bloating, gas, or diarrhea) and should be avoided before competition. Athletes should always use what works best for them by experimenting with foods and beverages during practice sessions and planning ahead to ensure they have these foods available when they compete.

Types of Carbohydrate

Even though the effects of different sugars on performance, substrate use, and recovery have been studied extensively, the optimal type of carbohydrate for the athlete is still subject to debate by sports performance experts (Colombani et al, 2013). The glycemic index represents the ratio of the area under the blood glucose curve resulting from the ingestion of a given quantity of carbohydrate and the area under the glucose curve resulting from the ingestion of the same quantity of white bread or glucose (see Appendix 28).

While preexercise consumption of a low-glycemic-index (LGI) carbohydrate meal is generally recommended, the results from subsequent exercise performance has been inconsistent (Burdon et al, 2017). A recent meta-analysis indicated that while the endurance performance following an LGI meal was superior to that following a high-glycemic-index (HGI) meal, subgroup analyses demonstrated that the effect did not vary across outcome measures (exercise to exhaustion, time trial, and work output) or athletic status (trained or recreational participants) (Wang et al, 2017).

Pretraining Fasting

Some athletes either rise too early for workouts to consume a meal or snack or feel nauseous when consuming food before exercise. An overnight fast causes a drop in liver glycogen, causing glycogenolysis to maintain the supply of glucose to the brain. Although a modest fall in blood sugar may not affect the average individual, it may affect the physical and cognitive performance of athletes fasting longer than 12 to 24 hours. Although some evidence suggests a metabolic advantage of endurance training in a fasted state to increase fat oxidation in trained muscles, other evidence supports the intake of nutrients, primarily carbohydrates, before, during, and after training sessions (Pinckaers et al, 2017; Pons et al, 2018).

Personalizing the preexercise fuel prescription for athletes is critical, because the wrong food or fluid may impact a morning run or an elite competition.

Training Fuel During Exercise

Carbohydrates consumed during endurance exercise lasting longer than 1 hour ensure the availability of sufficient amounts of energy during the later stages of exercise, improve performance, and may delay fatigue. Carbohydrate ingestion for exercise duration less than 60 minutes does not appear to be warranted (Thomas et al, 2016).

The type of carbohydrates consumed may affect performance during exercise. Because glucose and fructose are absorbed by the intestine via different transporters (SGLT1 and GLUT5), their combination in sports products appears to allow for greater absorption of carbohydrate resulting in higher rates of oxidation (Rosset et al, 2017). Recent research suggests that compared with water, a solution containing fructose attenuates thermoregulatory responses compared with glucose (Suzuki et al, 2014). Glucose ingestion during exercise was shown to spare endogenous protein and carbohydrates in fed cyclists without glycogen depletion; thus consuming an exogenous carbohydrate during endurance exercise helped to maintain blood glucose and improve performance (McArdle et al, 2014). (See Fig. 22.5).

The form of carbohydrate consumed does not appear to be a factor physiologically, although some athletes prefer to use a sports drink, whereas others prefer to eat solid food or gel and drink water. Studies have also shown that frequent contact with carbohydrate-containing beverages with the mouth and oral cavity through a mouth rinse during short high-intensity workouts can stimulate parts of the brain and

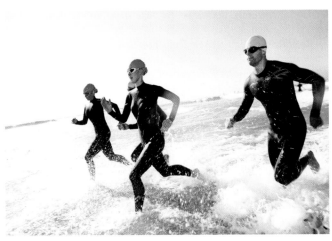

Fig. 22.5 A triathlon is a high-intensity endurance sport during which both carbohydrates and fats are used as fuels, the amount depending on the speed and length of the event. (Photo©istock.com).

nervous system to reduce perceived exertion and increase work intensity (Peart, 2017).

If a sports drink with carbohydrates is consumed during exercise, the rate of carbohydrate ingestion recommended is approximately 25 to 30 g every 30 minutes, an amount equivalent to 1 cup of a 4% to 8% carbohydrate solution taken every 15 to 20 minutes. This ensures that 1 g of carbohydrate is delivered to the tissues per minute at the time fatigue sets in. It is unlikely that a carbohydrate concentration of less than 5% is enough to help performance, but solutions with a concentration greater than 10% often are associated with abdominal cramps, nausea, and diarrhea.

Combining protein and carbohydrates in a sport fluid or snack also may improve performance, muscle protein synthesis and net balance, and recovery. Amino acids ingested in small amounts, alone or in conjunction with carbohydrates before or after exercise, appear to improve net protein balance and may stimulate protein synthesis during exercise and postexercise recovery (Australian Institute of Sport [AIS], 2014). Adding protein to carbohydrate beverages/gel during exhaustive endurance exercise has been shown to suppress markers of muscle damage 12 to 24 hours postexercise and decreases muscle soreness (Jäger et al, 2017).

Postworkout and Recovery Fuel

Dietary strategies that can enhance recovery from the negative effects of exercise can help promote effective physiologic adaptation, muscle conditioning after exercise, and enable a faster return to training. The resulting improvement in training efficiency may lead to significant performance benefits and sport career longevity by supporting repetitive training and competition and helping to maintain immune status and long-term health (Lynch, 2013).

Identifying the precise optimal quantity of carbohydrate to maximize glycogen repletion has been shown to be challenging due to the number of confounding variables, including the type and timing of the ingested carbohydrate, the training status of the participants, and the duration of the postexercise recovery period (Alghannam et al, 2018). It has been demonstrated that carbohydrate ingestion at a rate of 1.2 g/kg body weight/hour during the postexercise recovery period results in a 150% greater glycogen response relative to lower

amounts. In addition, because 1.6 g/kg bodyweight/hour does not further stimulate muscle glycogen resynthesis, it is considered the optimal amount to maximize muscle glycogen repletion (Alghannam et al, 2018).

The consumption of carbohydrates with a high glycemic index appears to result in higher muscle glycogen levels 24 hours after exercise compared with the same amount of carbohydrates provided as foods with an LGI (Cermak and van Loon, 2013). Adding approximately 5 to 9 g of protein with every 100 g of carbohydrate eaten after exercise may further increase glycogen resynthesis rate, provide amino acids for muscle repair, and promote a more anabolic hormonal profile (Sousa et al, 2014).

Many athletes find it difficult to consume food immediately after exercise. Usually when body or core temperature is elevated, appetite is depressed, and it is difficult to consume carbohydrate-rich foods. Many athletes find it easier and simpler to drink their carbohydrates and ingest easy-to-eat, carbohydrate-rich foods such as fruit pops, bananas, oranges, melon, or apple slices, or consume a sports recovery shake or bar.

Supplemental sport shakes, drinks, and energy bars may offer an easy-to-carry, easy-to-consume, and easy-to-digest meal-replacement. These products are often fortified with 33% to 100% of the dietary reference intakes (DRIs) for vitamins and minerals; provide varying amounts and types of carbohydrates, protein, and fat; and are ideal for athletes on the run. They can be used pericompetitively, while traveling, at work, in the car, or throughout the day at multievent meets such as track and field, swimming, diving, or gymnastics.

Many fitness-minded and athletic individuals use these products, generally recognized as safe, as a convenient way to enhance their diets. However, if they are substituted in the place of whole foods on a regular basis, they can deprive the athlete of a well-balanced diet. They also may contain excesses of sugars, fats, and protein and banned substances such as stimulants and other botanicals prohibited by United States Anti-Doping Agency (USADA) in and out of competition.

PROTEIN

The current RDA is 0.8 g/kg bodyweight, and the acceptable macronutrient distribution range for protein for people 18 years and older is 10% to 35% of total calories. Reports of food intake in athletes and nonathletes consistently indicate that protein represents from 12% to 20% of total energy intake or 1.2 to 2 g/kg/day. The exception to the rule is small, active women who may consume a low-energy intake in conjunction with their exercise or training program.

Recent studies suggest and support higher protein requirements than the RDA and increase with high training volumes in order to maintain energy balance, protein balance, and muscle mass (Jäger et al, 2017). Factors affecting the protein needs of athletes include age, gender, lean body mass, fitness level, training regimen, and phase of competition.

Protein for Muscle Hypertrophy

Resistance training (RT) and diet consistently appear to play a role in postworkout muscle protein synthesis. The metabolic basis for muscle growth appears to be a balance between muscle protein synthesis (MPS) and prevention of catabolism, especially the balance of myofibrillar protein or contractile protein synthesis, in which dietary protein plus exercise plays an important role. RT enhances the anabolism by 40% to 100% over and above resting levels and dietary protein response for up to 24 hours when protein is consumed immediately before and at least within 24 hours after (Tipton and Phillips, 2013). Studies have also suggested that preexercise feedings of amino acids in combination with carbohydrates can achieve maximal rates of MPS, but proteins and amino acids during this time have not been shown to improve performance (Jäger et al, 2017).

For athletes interested in muscle hypertrophy, protein consumed within the recommended range for resistance-training athletes of 1.2 to 2 g of protein per kilogram of body weight is recommended. Research shows that a minimum of 30 g of high-quality protein at each meal that contains 2.5 g leucine per meal will optimally stimulate protein synthesis. Research suggests the anabolic response to resistance exercise and protein ingestion works just as well with whole food proteins as with nutritional supplement proteins, although convenience often makes the difference because taking a high-protein shake or bar to training is more practical than carrying a chicken breast. After resistance exercise, between 20 and 25 g of a high-quality protein maximizes the response of MPS, whereas no difference appears to occur between the ingestion of 20 g of protein and 40 g, suggesting that more is not better, at least in young, resistance-trained males. Better responses have been reported from spreading protein intake throughout the day 0.3g/kg every 3 to 5 hours (Jäger et al, 2017).

Several studies in people engaged in RT show that consuming some protein before sleep can increase the rate of protein synthesis during the night and/or augment muscle mass and strength. Participants in these studies consumed a bedtime drink containing 27.5 or 40 g of the milk protein casein, which increased circulating amino acid levels throughout the night. Some studies show increased MPS when plasma levels of amino acids are raised (Jäger et al, 2017; National Institutes of Health [NIH] Office of Dietary Supplements [ODS], 2017). Preworkout ingestion of essential amino acids also appears to enhance the MPS response.

Although the inclusion of carbohydrates does not seem to have an impact on protein synthesis, it may have an impact on the prevention of breakdown. Fat content of postworkout fuel also may have a positive impact. Whole milk may increase utilization of available amino acids for protein synthesis (Elliot et al, 2006).

FAT

Fat is an essential component of an athlete's diet as a concentrated source of food energy, supplying 9 kcal/g. Essential fatty acids are necessary for cell membranes, skin health, hormones, and transport of fat-soluble vitamins. The body has total glycogen stores (muscle and liver) equaling approximately 2600 calories, whereas each pound of body fat supplies about 3500 calories. This means that an athlete weighing 74 kg (163 lb) with 10% body fat has 16.3 lb of fat and thus carries energy worth about 57,000 calories depending on the individual's metabolic rate.

The greater use of fat as an energy source to spare muscle glycogen has been shown to improve performance in ultraendurance events. Improved fat oxidation can be achieved through long slow duration exercise, fasting, acute preexercise intake of fat/ketones, and high-fat low-carbohydrate diets (Bytomski, 2018). Exercise intensity and duration are important determinants of fat oxidation.

Fat oxidation rates decrease when exercise intensity becomes high. A high-fat diet has been shown to compromise high-intensity performance even when a high-fat diet regimen is followed by carbohydrate loading before high-intensity performance (McArdle et al, 2014). The mode and duration of exercise also can affect fat

oxidation; running increases fat oxidation more than cycling (Rosenkilde et al, 2015).

Recently very high-fat ketogenic diets have become popular in athlete communities, with mixed performance results. In one study, researchers examined the impact of adaptation to a ketogenic, low-carbohydrate diet during 3 weeks of intensified training in world-class endurance athletes. All groups consumed identical calories and protein (40 cal/kg and 2.2 g/kg) and constant high-carbohydrate, periodized high-carbohydrate, or low-carbohydrate diets. Both high-carbohydrate groups improved performance after intensified training but showed no improvement for the low-carbohydrate high-fat group (Burke et al, 2017).

While ketone bodies have also been suggested to have positive effects on exercise metabolism and performance as an alternative fuel source, sparing muscle glycogen, there is limited information in recreational and/or elite athletes.

Fats, Inflammation, and Sports Injury

When athletes are injured, they want to heal and get back to training as soon as possible. Specific foods at the right time can help to provide energy for rehabilitation, rebuild strength, and ensure a complete, healthy, and faster recovery.

Increased oxidative stress and inflammatory responses among individuals performing strenuous exercise, elite athletes, or military personnel have been consistently reported. Stress to muscle leads to inflammation, bruising, and tissue breakdown. Failure to decrease inflammation can lead to scar tissue, poor mobility, and delayed recovery times. The inflammatory stage is affected by foods, especially by the types of dietary fat consumed. A diet high in trans fats, saturated fats, and some omega-6 vegetable oils has been shown to promote inflammation and impact the gut microbiota, whereas a diet high in monounsaturated fat and essential omega-3 fats has been shown to be antiinflammatory (see Chapter 7 and Appendix 26).

Omega-3 polyunsaturated fatty acids have been shown to decrease the production of inflammatory eicosanoids, cytokines, and reactive oxygen species; to possess immunomodulatory effects; and to attenuate inflammatory diseases. While human data is inconclusive as to whether supplementation is effective in attenuating the inflammatory, immunomodulatory response to exercise, animal studies assessing the effectiveness of supplementation on exercise metabolism and endurance exercise performance have produced very promising findings (Shei et al, 2014).

Diets supplemented with omega-3 fats have been shown to reduce postexercise delayed-onset muscle soreness and inflammation and promote healing (Jouris et al, 2011). There is also evidence to suggest a strong connection between omega-3 status and neuroprotection and supplementation to accelerate recovery from traumatic brain injury, including concussion (Michael-Titus and Priestley, 2014; Rawson et al, 2018).

Supplemental omega-3 fat has been recommended during the inflammation stage after injury, especially when the diet is deficient. However, some concern exists regarding the sources of omega-3 fat supplements and fish oils, because some have been found to be contaminated with mercury and polychlorinated biphenyls (PCBs), toxins dangerous to humans (see *Focus On:* Omega-3 Fatty Acids in Pregnancy and Lactation in Chapter 14).

Plant-based foods are also good sources of alpha linolenic acid (ALA), an omega-3 fatty acid. However, the conversion in the body of ALA to the more active forms of omega-3 fatty acids, docosahexaenoic acid (DHA) and eicosapentaenoic acid (EPA), is very low. Plant-based foods rich in ALA include spinach, broccoli, tomatoes, green peas, flaxseeds, chia seeds, walnuts, almonds, and tofu. Wheat germ, free-range beef, poultry, and some eggs are also good sources of omega-3 fats when the animals are fed omega-3–rich food (see Appendix 26).

Monounsaturated fats such as olive, peanut, canola, and sesame oils, as well as avocado oil, also inhibit and reduce inflammation by interfering with proinflammatory compounds such as leukotrienes, which are produced naturally by the body.

FLUID

Maintaining fluid balance requires the constant integration of input from hypothalamic osmoreceptors and vascular baroreceptors so that fluid intake matches or modestly exceeds fluid loss (McArdle et al, 2014). Proper fluid balance maintains blood volume, which in turn supplies blood to the skin for body temperature regulation. Because exercise produces heat, which must be eliminated from the body to maintain appropriate temperatures, regular fluid intake is essential. Any fluid deficit that is incurred during an exercise session can potentially compromise the subsequent exercise bout.

The body maintains appropriate temperatures by **thermoregulation**. As heat is generated in the muscles during exercise, it is transferred via the blood to the body's core. Increased core temperature results in increased blood flow to the skin; in cool-to-moderate ambient temperatures, heat is then transferred to the environment by convection, radiation, and evaporation.

Environmental conditions have a large effect on thermoregulation. When ambient temperatures range from warm to hot, the body must dissipate the heat generated from exercise, as well as the heat absorbed from the environment. When this occurs, the body relies solely on the evaporation of sweat to maintain appropriate body temperatures. Thus maintaining hydration becomes crucial when ambient temperatures reach or exceed 36° C (96.8° F). The hotter the temperature, the more important sweating is for body-heat dissipation. Exercise in the heat also affects blood flow and alters the stress response, with modest changes in circulating leukocytes and cytokines. A critical threshold for elevation of body temperature is 3.5° C (6° F), above which the systemic inflammatory response leads to heatstroke (Tyler et al, 2016).

Humidity affects the body's ability to dissipate heat to a greater extent than air temperatures. As humidity increases, the rate at which sweat evaporates decreases, which means more sweat drips off the body without transferring heat from the body to the environment. Combining the effects of a hot, humid environment with a large metabolic heat load produced during exercise taxes the thermoregulatory system to its maximum. Ensuring proper and adequate fluid intake is key to reducing the risk of heat stress.

Fluid Balance

Body fluid balance is regulated by mechanisms that reduce urinary water and sodium excretion, stimulate thirst, and control the intake and output of water and electrolytes. In response to dehydration, antidiuretic hormone (ADH or vasopressin) and the renin-angiotensin II–aldosterone system increase water and sodium retention by the kidneys and provoke an increase in thirst. These hormones maintain the osmolality, sodium content, and volume of extracellular fluids, and play a major role in the regulation of fluid balance (see Chapter 3).

Water losses throughout the course of the day include those from sweat and the respiratory tract, plus losses from the kidneys and GI tract. When fluid is lost from the body in the form of sweat, plasma volume decreases and plasma osmolality increases. The kidneys, under hormonal control, regulate water and solute excretion in excess of the obligatory urine loss. However, when the body is subjected to hot environments, hormonal adjustments occur to maintain body function. Some of these adjustments include the body's conservation of water and sodium and the release of ADH by the pituitary gland to increase water absorption from the kidneys. These changes cause the urine to become more concentrated, thus conserving fluid and making the urine a dark gold color. This feedback process helps to conserve body water and blood volume.

At the same time, aldosterone is released from the adrenal cortex and acts on the renal tubules to increase the resorption of sodium, which helps maintain the correct osmotic pressure. These reactions also activate thirst mechanisms in the body. However, in situations in which water losses are increased acutely, such as in athletic workouts or competition, the thirst response can be delayed, making it difficult for athletes to trust their thirst to ingest enough fluid to offset the volume of fluid lost during training and competition. A loss of 1.5 to 2 L of fluid is necessary before the thirst mechanism kicks in, and this level of water loss already has a serious effect on temperature control. Athletes need to rehydrate on a timed basis rather than as a reaction to thirst, enough to maintain the preexercise weight.

Imbalance between fluid intake and fluid loss during prolonged exercise may increase the risk for **dehydration**. It is estimated that more than 50% to 55% of athletes in professional sports, collegiate sports, high school sports, and youth sports arrive at workouts dehydrated (McDermott et al, 2017; Hew-Butler et al, 2018). Dehydration may enhance the development of hyperthermia, heat exhaustion, and heat stroke. The reasons for dehydration vary. In one study, approximately 66% of collegiate athletes, more men than women, were found to be dehydrated pretraining, due to individual hydration habits, lack of hydration before early morning practices, or lack of knowledge regarding proper hydration before and after training (Volpe et al, 2009). **Hypohydration** is particularly common in weight class sports. One study found the prevalence of elite wrestlers, judokas, boxers, and taekwondo athletes on competition day was 89% (Pettersson et al, 2013).

Urine specific gravity is a noninvasive test that assesses the hydration level of athletes. It measures the concentration of all chemical particles in the urine and looks at the ratio of the density of urine compared with the density of water. The specific density of water would be 1.000. Ideally, urine specific gravity results will fall between 1.002 and 1.030 when the kidneys are functioning normally and the athlete is hydrated. Specific gravity results above 1.010 can indicate mild dehydration. The higher the number, the more dehydrated the athlete is. The best sample for a urine specific gravity test contains 1 to 2 ounces of urine first thing in the morning, when the urine is the most concentrated.

Men appear to have higher sweat rates that may lead to more fluid loss during exercise compared with women. Studies also have shown that men have higher plasma sodium levels and a higher prevalence of hypernatremia than women after prolonged exercise, which suggests larger fluid losses in men. In contrast, it also is reported that women have an increased risk for overdrinking, which could lead to exercise-associated hyponatremia. This was demonstrated in a recent endurance study that compared female and male walkers. The study demonstrated a significantly larger change in body mass in men than in women, a higher incidence of dehydration in the men (27% of the men vs. 0% of the women showed postexercise hypernatremia), and a significantly lower fluid intake and higher fluid loss in the men compared with females (Eijsvogels et al, 2013).

Body water is lost as a consequence of thermoregulatory sweating, and when fluid intake is insufficient to replace sweat losses, hypohydration occurs. It is well established that a 2% body mass loss can impair endurance performance, especially in hot/humid environments, however, the impact of hypohydration on an athlete's performance during team sport competition is less clear (Nuccio et al, 2017). The effect of hydration status on team sport performance has been studied mostly in soccer, basketball, cricket, and baseball, with mixed results (Nuccio et al, 2017). Hypohydration typically impaired performance at higher levels (3% to 4%) and when the method of dehydration involved heat stress. Increased subjective ratings of fatigue and perceived exertion consistently accompanied hypohydration.

Sweat losses in team sports can be significant due to repeated bursts of high-intensity activity, as well as the large body size of athletes, equipment and uniform requirements, and environmental heat stress often present during training and competition. Significant hypohydration of >2% has been reported most consistently in soccer. Mean sweating rates from 1.0 to 2.9 L/h have been reported for college and professional American football players, with several studies reporting 3.0 L/h or more in some larger players (Davis et al, 2016). Although American football, rugby, basketball, tennis, and ice hockey have reported high sweating rates, fluid balance disturbances have generally been mild, with a mean <2%, probably due to ample drinking opportunities.

Although, for years, studies have shown that substantial fluid and body mass losses greater than 2% of total body weight were related to an impaired exercise performance, one study shows otherwise (Wall et al, 2013). High-intensity prolonged exercise may increase the discrepancy between fluid intake and losses. In one study, increased body temperature and dehydration up to 3% in well-trained male cyclists had no effect on a 25-km cycling time-trial performance in hot conditions in well-trained men who were blinded to their hydration status (Wall et al, 2013).

Daily Fluid Needs

Fluid intake recommendations for sedentary individuals vary greatly because of the wide disparity in daily fluid needs created by body size, physical activity, and environmental conditions. The DRI for water and electrolytes identifies the adequate intake for water to be 3.7 L/day for men (130 oz/day, 16 cups of fluid/day) and 2.7 L/day for women (95 oz/day, approximately 12 cups/day) (Institute of Medicine [IOM], 2005). Approximately 20% of the daily water need comes from water found in fruits and vegetables; the remaining 80% is provided by beverages, including water, juice, milk, coffee, tea, soup, sports drinks, and soft drinks. When individuals work, train, and compete in warm environments, their fluid needs can increase greatly (McArdle et al, 2014).

Fluid Replacement

Controversy exists among experts as to how to assess fluid needs because there is no scientific consensus regarding the best method to assess hydration status. Recreational sports typically result in hypotonic fluid losses, which increase relative concentrations of blood and urine. Field measures to assess body hydration status include body mass measurements, urine specific gravity and color, and taste sensation. Each has its limitations (McArdle et al, 2014).

Several position statements and recommendations are published by a variety of professional organizations that address fluid and electrolyte replacement before, during, and after exercise. A summary of these recommendations can be found in Box 22.5.

Although specific recommendations differ slightly, the intent is to keep athletes well hydrated. These strategies will help prevent hypohydration, maximize safety during exercise, and optimize physical performance (McDermott et al, 2017).

Fluid Absorption

The speed at which fluid is absorbed depends on a number of different factors, including the amount, type, temperature, and osmolality of the fluid consumed and the rate of gastric emptying. Because glucose is absorbed actively in the intestines, it can markedly increase sodium and water absorption. A carbohydrate-electrolyte solution potentially enhances exercise capacity, especially in endurance athletes, by elevating blood sugar, maintaining high rates of carbohydrate oxidation, preventing central fatigue, and reducing perceived exertion (McDermott et al, 2017).

Early studies indicate that water absorption is maximized when luminal glucose concentrations range from 1% to 3% (55 to 140 mM); however, most sports drinks contain two to three times this quantity without causing adverse GI symptoms for most athletes. To determine the concentration of carbohydrate in a sports drink, the grams of

---

BOX 22.5 Summary of Guidelines for Proper Hydration

General Guidelines

Monitor fluid losses: Weigh in before and after practice, especially during hot weather and the conditioning phase of the season.

Do not restrict fluids before, during, or after the event.

Do not rely on thirst as an indicator of fluid losses.

Drink early and at regular intervals throughout the activity.

Avoid alcohol before, during, or after exercise because it may act as a diuretic and prevent adequate fluid replenishment.

Discourage caffeinated beverages a few hours before and after physical activity because of their diuretic effect.

Before Exercise

Drink approximately 400 to 600 mL (14 to 22 oz) of water or sports drink 2 to 3 hours before the start of exercise.

During Exercise

Drink 150 to 350 mL (6 to 12 oz) of fluid every 15 to 20 min, depending on race speed, environmental conditions, and tolerance; no more than 1 C (8 to 10 oz) every 15 to 20 min, although individualized recommendations must be followed.

After Exercise

Drink 25% to 50% more than post workout weight loss to ensure hydration 4 to 6 hours after exercise.

Drink 450 to 675 mL (16 to 24 oz) of fluid for every pound of body weight lost during exercise.

If an athlete is participating in multiple workouts in 1 day, then 80% of fluid loss must be replaced before the next workout.

Electrolyte Replacement

Sodium: 0.5 to 0.7 g/L in activity longer than 1 hour to enhance palatability and the drive to drink, to reduce the risk of hyponatremia, and to minimize risk of muscle cramps.

carbohydrate or sugar in a serving are divided by the weight of a serving of the drink, which is usually 240 g, the approximate weight of 1 cup of water. A 6% carbohydrate drink contains 14 to 16 g of carbohydrate per 8 oz (1 cup).

Cold water is preferable to warm water because it attenuates changes in core temperature and peripheral blood flow, decreases sweat rate, speeds up gastric emptying, and is absorbed more quickly. In one recent study, sweating response was influenced by water temperature and voluntary intake volume. Cool tap water at 60° F appeared to replace fluids better in dehydrated individuals compared with warmer fluids (Hosseinlou et al, 2013).

Burdon et al. (2013) showed that, although ingestion of cold beverages is preferable, an ergogenic benefit was also seen from the effect of ice slush ingestion and mouthwash on thermoregulation and endurance performance in the heat. Another study compared ice slush to cold water in moderately active males while running and showed prolonged time to exhaustion and reduced rectal temperature, supporting possible sensory and psychological effects of ice slush beverages either consumed or used as a mouthwash. Precooling with an ice slushy solution also may have more beneficial effects over cold fluid ingestion during exercise and performance (Dugas, 2011).

Children

Children differ from adults in that, for any given level of dehydration, their core temperatures rise faster than those of adults, probably because of a greater number of heat-activated sweat glands per unit skin area than in adolescents or adults. Children sweat less even though they achieve higher core temperatures. Sweat composition also differs between children and adults: adults have higher sodium and chloride concentrations but lower lactate, hydrogen, and potassium concentrations. Children also take longer to acclimate to heat than adolescents and adults (McArdle et al, 2014).

Because young children often do not drink enough when offered fluids freely during exercise in hot and humid climates, and because they participate in physical activities less than 60 minutes in duration, often little attention is paid to their hydration. Children who participate in sports activities must be taught to prevent dehydration by drinking above and beyond thirst and at frequent intervals, such as every 20 minutes. As a general rule, a child 10 years of age or younger should drink until thirst is satiated and then should drink an additional half a glass (3 to 4 oz or ⅓ to ½ cup) of fluid.

Older children and adolescents should follow the same guidelines; however, they should consume an additional cup of fluid (8 oz). When relevant, regulations for competition should be modified to allow children to leave the playing field periodically to drink. One of the hurdles to getting children to consume fluids is to provide fluids they like. Providing a sports drink or slushy ice drink as described in the previous section that will maintain the drive to drink may be the key to keeping child athletes hydrated.

Older Athletes

Hydration is especially important for masters athletes (older than 40 years), especially during the first 5 days of heat acclimatization. Hypohydration (water loss exceeding water intake with a body water deficit) in older individuals can affect circulatory and thermoregulatory function to a greater extent and may be caused by the lower skin blood flow, causing core temperature to rise. Because the thirst drive is reduced in older adults, they need to drink adequately before exercise, well before they become thirsty (McDermott et al, 2017). Although older adults can restore fluid losses, this occurs at a slower rate than younger adults.

Hydration at High Altitudes

Unacclimated individuals undergo a plasma volume contraction when acutely exposed to moderately high altitude. This is the result of increased renal sodium and water excretion and decreased voluntary sodium and water intake. Respiratory losses are increased by high ventilatory rates and typically dry air. The result is an increase in serum hematocrit and hemoglobin, which increases the oxygen-carrying capacity of the blood, but at the cost of reduced blood volume, stroke volume, and cardiac output. Fluid requirements increase as a result. With acclimation, red blood cell production increases and plasma and blood volumes return to pre–high altitude levels.

Electrolytes

The replacement of electrolytes as well as water is essential for complete rehydration (Table 22.3).

Sodium

It is important to include sodium in fluid-replacement solutions, especially with excessive intake of plain water (McArdle et al, 2014) for events lasting more than 2 hours; sodium should be added to the fluid to replace losses and to prevent hyponatremia. Rehydration with water alone dilutes the blood rapidly, increases its volume, and stimulates urine output. Blood dilution lowers sodium and the volume-dependent part of the thirst drive, thus removing much of the drive to drink and replace fluid losses.

Water-soluble electrolytes such as sodium can move rapidly across the proximal intestines. During prolonged exercise lasting more than 4 to 5 hours, including sodium in replacement fluids increases palatability and facilitates fluid uptake from the intestines. Sodium and carbohydrate are actively transported from the lumen to the bloodstream.

Water replacement in the absence of supplemental sodium can lead to decreased plasma sodium concentrations. As plasma sodium levels fall below 130 mEq/L, symptoms can include lethargy, confusion, seizures, or loss of consciousness. Exercise-induced hyponatremia may

TABLE 22.3 Comparison of the Sweat Electrolyte Losses* and Sports Drink Content

Electrolyte	Sweat Loss mg/L	Standard Sport Drink mg/L	Endurance Specific Sport Drink mg/L
Sodium	900-2600	230-1700	800-1110
Potassium	150	80-125	390-650
Magnesium	8.3-14.2	0	10-815
Chloride	900-1900	0	390-1550
Calcium	28	0-100	24-275
Iron	0.1-0.4	0	0
Phosphorus	40	0	0
Zinc	0.36-.0.48	0	0-5

*Dependent on exercise duration, intensity, ambient temperature, hydration status before and during exercise

Baker A: Nutrition for Sports 22: Sweat mineral losses. http://www.arniebakercycling.com/pubs/Free/NS%20Sweat.pdf.

Kenefick RW, Cheuvront SN: Hydration for recreational sport and physical activity, *Nutr Rev* 70 (Suppl 2):S137, 2012.

result from fluid overloading during prolonged exercise over 4 hours. Hyponatremia is associated with individuals who drink plain water in excess of their sweat losses or who are less physically conditioned and produce a saltier sweat.

Guidelines recommend the consumption of sodium during exercise to replace losses in sweat; however, the effects of sodium on thermoregulation are less clear. In one double-blind, randomized-sequence, crossover study, 11 endurance athletes underwent 2 hours of endurance exercise at 60% heart rate reserve with 1800 mg of sodium supplementation during one trial and placebo during the other trial. A progressive intensity time-to-exhaustion test was performed after the 2-hour steady state exercise as an assessment of exercise performance. High-dose sodium supplementation did not appear to impact thermoregulation, cardiovascular drift, or physical performance in trained, endurance athletes (Earhart et al, 2015).

Potassium

As the major electrolyte inside the body's cells, potassium works in close association with sodium and chloride in maintaining body fluids, as well as generating electrical impulses in the nerves, muscles, and heart. Potassium balance is regulated by aldosterone and its regulation is precise. Although aldosterone acts on sweat glands to increase the resorption of sodium, potassium secretion is unaffected. Loss of potassium from skeletal muscle has been implicated in fatigue during athletic events. There is little loss of potassium through sweat, and in a recent study exercise intensity has been shown to have a minimal impact on sweat potassium losses in practice and can be easily replaced by diet (Baker et al, 2019).

VITAMINS AND MINERALS

Many micronutrients play an important role in the regulation of processes that support sports performance, ranging from energy production to the manufacture of new cells and protein. A deficiency in one or more of these nutrients may lead to impairment either directly or by reducing the athlete's ability to train effectively (i.e., iron deficiency, anemia) or stay away from illness or injury (i.e., calcium and vitamin D) and bone health. Suboptimal nutrient intakes and deficiencies may also have a profound impact on performance (Maughan et al, 2018).

While all athletes are encouraged to follow sports nutrition strategies that optimize dietary intake to support optimal health and performance, many fall short of meeting 100% of the recommended dietary allowance (RDA) for micronutrients. In one study of Dutch elite and sub elite athletes, micronutrient intakes of 553 athletes showed that nonusers of supplements were at risk for low intakes of vitamins B_1, B_2, B_3 and vitamins A, C, and selenium (Wardenaar et al, 2017).

High training volume, exercise performed in stressful conditions including hot conditions and altitude, or training with substandard diets may promote excessive losses of micronutrients because of increased catabolism or excretion (Lukaski, 2004). Para athletes (athletes with disabilities) are a high-risk group for inadequate dietary intake leading to deficiencies in energy, carbohydrate, protein, iron, and vitamin D, which can impair sports performance (Scaramella et al, 2018).

Training and work schedules, low-nutrient snacks, infrequent nutrient-dense meals, and overall low calorie intakes may cause inadequate intakes of vitamins and minerals. Athletes who adopt popular diets that eliminate whole food groups such as meat, dairy, grains, or fruits, as in the case of vegans, or those following a Paleo or ketogenic diet, run the risk of poor micronutrient intake. Micronutrients such as calcium, zinc, iron, vitamin B_{12}, and others will be of concern.

Description of vitamin metabolism and resulting physical performance is very limited. Assessments of vitamin intake, biochemical measures of vitamin status, and determination of resulting physical performance involves systematic protocols that obtain, verify, and interpret evidence of nutrition related problems, as well as their causes and significance. A complete assessment is required; however, very few studies have provided this information.

In 2010 numerous dietary vitamin and mineral deficiencies were reported in elite female athletes, including folate (48%), calcium (24%), magnesium (19%), and iron (4%) (Heaney et al, 2010). A 2014 report also highlighted the risk of injury in female athletes with iron, vitamin D, and calcium deficiencies (McClung et al, 2014). A 2013 study of male athletes showed significant deficiencies in vitamin A (44% of group), vitamin C (80% of group), vitamin D (92% of group), folate (84% of group), calcium (52% of group), and magnesium (60% of group) (Wierniuk and Włodarek, 2013).

Without a doubt, impaired micronutrient status affects exercise and work performance. Some of the deficiency signs and symptoms associated with exercise have been summarized in this section (Table 22.4).

B Vitamins

Increased energy metabolism creates a need for more of the B vitamins, including thiamin, riboflavin, niacin, pyridoxine, folate, biotin, pantothenic acid, and choline, which serve as part of coenzymes involved in regulating energy metabolism by modulating the synthesis and degradation of carbohydrates, protein, fat, and bioactive compounds.

Some athletes who have poor diets, and athletes such as wrestlers, jockeys, figure skaters, gymnasts, or rowers who consume low-calorie diets for long periods of time may be prone to deficiencies. A B-complex vitamin supplement to meet the RDA may be appropriate (Thomas et al, 2016). However, there is no evidence that supplementing the well-nourished athlete with more B vitamins increases performance.

The intake of folate could potentially be low in athletes whose consumption of whole grains, whole fruits, and vegetables is low. Likewise a deficiency of vitamin B_{12} could develop in a vegetarian athlete after several years of a strict vegan intake; thus a vitamin B_{12} supplement may be warranted. However, while correcting folate and vitamin B_{12} deficiencies with a supplement may be warranted for a safeguard for health, supplementation for either vitamin has not been shown to improve performance.

Antioxidants

Antioxidants have been studied individually and collectively for their potential to enhance exercise performance or to prevent exercise-induced muscle tissue damage. Cells continuously produce free radicals and reactive oxygen species (ROS) as a part of metabolic processes. The rate of VO_2 during exercise may increase 10- to 15-fold, or as much as 100-fold in active peripheral skeletal muscles. This oxidative stress increases the generation of lipid peroxides and free radicals, and the magnitude of stress depends on the ability of the body's tissues to neutralize ROS (see Chapter 7).

Free radicals are neutralized by antioxidant defense systems that protect cell membranes from oxidative damage. These systems include catalase; superoxide dismutase; glutathione peroxidase; antioxidant

TABLE 22.4 Ergogenic Aids

Ergogenic Aid	Reported Action/Claim	Research on Ergogenic Effects	Side Effects
Antioxidants	Minimize free radical damage to muscle, reducing fatigue inflammation soreness	Small clinical trials; does not directly improve performance	May hinder some physiologic and physical exercise induced adaptations
Arginine	Increases blood flow and O_2 delivery to muscle; increases HGH secretion	Limited clinical trials with conflicting results; little or no effect on vasodilation, blood flow, or exercise metabolites.	Diarrhea and nausea
Beetroot or beet juice	Enhances NO bioavailability; dilates blood vessels in exercising muscle, reduces O_2 use, improves energy production	Acute performance benefits seen 2-3 hours following ingestion of 310-560 mg; prolonged periods also may benefit performance; 4%-25% improvement in exercise time to exhaustion; enhances type II muscle fiber function resulting in 3%-5% improvement of HIIT team sport 12-40 min duration. Performance gains harder to obtain in highly trained athletes	GI upset in some athletes
Beta alanine	Increases carnosine synthesis, augments buffering capacity in muscle reducing muscle fatigue and loss of force in high intensity exercise	Daily consumption of approx. 65 mg/kg BM ingested in split dose, 0.8-1.6 every 3-4 hours over 10-12 weeks may have small performance benefits during continuous and intermittent exercise of 30 s-10 min	Skin rash, transient paresthesia
Betaine	Increases creatine production, blood nitric acid levels or water retention in cells	Limited clinical trials in men with conflicting results; potential but modest strength and power improvements with bodybuilders and cyclists	No safety concerns reported for 2-5 g/day up to 15 days
Citrulline	Dilates blood vessels to increase delivery of O_2 and nutrients to skeletal muscle	Few clinical trials with conflicting results	Few safety concerns reported for up to 9 g for 1 day or 6 g/day for up to 16 days
HMB (beta-hydroxy-beta-methylbutyrate)	Metabolite of EAA leucine; anticatabolic; enhances recovery by stimulating protein and glycogen synthesis	3 g in 2 divided doses shown to improve performance; may increase upper-body strength and lean body mass and minimize muscle damage; decreases muscle catabolism	No safety concerns reported for dose of 3 g/day for up to 2 months
Collagen hydrolysate/gelatin and vitamin C	Increased collagen production, thickened cartilage, decreased joint pain	Gelatin and collagen supplements are low risk; increased collagen production, decreased pain recovery from injury reported; dose 5-15 g gelatin with 50 g vitamin C; collagen hydrolysate dose is 10 g/day	
Curcumin	Antiinflammatory, decrease muscle damage, DOMS	Conflicting results—reductions in DOMS, CK, and inflammatory cytokines (TNF-α, IL-8) following eccentric contraction, however not seen following endurance exercise	Up to 5 g/day dose, none reported
Chondroitin sulfate	Builds and grows cartilage	No studies that it is effective in treating arthritis or joint damage or helps torn ligaments or cartilage	None
Glucosamine	Serves as nonsteroidal antiinflammatory drug alternative	Readily absorbed; benefit in reducing pain and need for medication	None reported
Creatine	Increases lean mass and strength, enhances recovery from intense exercise; enhances adaptive response to exercise; increases intracellular water; enhances recovery from DOMS; decreased risk/enhanced recovery from TBI	Well studied, shows benefit for high-intensity intermittent activity, variation in response, greater impact with those with low stores (i.e., vegan, vegetarian, or low meat eaters); recommended dose of creatine monohydrate is 20 g/day for 5 days followed by 3-5 g/day to increase and maintain levels	No negative effect up to 4 years; weight gain due to water retention not suitable for weight dependent sports; anecdotal reports of nausea, diarrhea, stiffness, heat intolerance
Omega 3 fatty acids	Improved cognitive processing, decreased risk, enhanced recovery from TBI; reduced symptoms or enhanced recovery from DOMS	Few data on TBI, animal studies show structural damage and cognitive decline reduced; benefits to muscle damage inconsistent; may increase protein synthesis in muscle	Low risk but possible bleeding GI problems or increased LDL
Probiotics	Decrease severity or duration of GI distress; decreased incidence duration and severity of URTI	Modest benefits to athletes w/GI issues or traveling to regions which GI issues more likely; most studies report reduced incidence of URTI but specific recommendations/strains difficult to ascertain	Dosing regimens of 10 (9) to 4 x 10 (10) for 4-21 weeks

Continued

TABLE 22.4 Ergogenic Aids—cont'd

Ergogenic Aid	Reported Action/Claim	Research on Ergogenic Effects	Side Effects
COQ₁₀	Cofactor for ATP production; electron transport in mitochondria; reduces fatigue	Mixed: double-blinded, placebo, crossover trial, 100 mg/d for 2 months, lift loads of 75 g/kg of body weight 5x/30 s improved mean power; may improve in those with mitochondrial disorders or CoQ deficiency	
Sodium bicarbonate/ sodium citrate	Buffers lactic acid production; delays fatigue	High level of intraindividual variability in performance; increases body's ability to buffer lactic acid during sub max exercise for events lasting 1-7 min	Stomach distress: bloating, diarrhea; dangerous in high doses; alkalosis; dosing with small carbohydrate meal may reduce GI upset
Sodium phosphate	Buffer	Some; increases VO₂max and anaerobic threshold by 5%-10%; improves endurance	Stomach distress
Creatine	Improves strength, power, and intermittent sprint performance; accelerates training recovery	Increases muscle free creatine, phosphocreatine; performance effect seen in sprint/power through endurance by enhancing muscle glycogen storage; stimulates muscle anabolism, muscle relaxation; effects may fade after 2 months supplementation; consume with CHO to increase levels to greater extent	Weight gain 0.8%-2.9%; watch with weight-sensitive sports; unknown long term

ALA, α-Lipoic acid; *ATP*, adenosine triphosphate; *BM*, body mass; *CF*, cardiorespiratory fitness; *CHO*, cholesterol; *CK*, creatine kinase; *DOMS*, delayed onset muscle soreness; *EAA*, essential amino acid; *GH*, growth hormone; *GI*, gastrointestinal; *HIIT*, high-intensity interval training; *HGH*, human growth hormone; *HMB*, β-hydroxy-β-methylbutyrate; *IL-8*, interleukin-8; *LDL*, low-density lipoprotein; *NO*, nitric oxide; *TBI*, traumatic brain injury; *TNF-α*: tumor necrosis factor alpha; *URTI*, upper respiratory tract infection.

vitamins A, E, and C; selenium; and phytonutrients such as carotenoids (see Chapter 7). Susceptibility to oxidative stress varies from person to person, and the effect is influenced by diet, lifestyle, environmental factors, and training. Antioxidant nutrients may enhance recovery from exercise by maintaining optimal immune response and lowering lipid peroxidation.

Although large-dose antioxidant supplementation attenuates exercise-induced ROS production and consequential oxidative damage, studies suggest oversupplementation may block necessary cellular adaptations to exercise (Sureda et al, 2013). Further research is needed to assess the response to supplementation with varying degrees of exercise duration and intensity (Sureda et al, 2013).

A diet rich in fruits and vegetables can ensure an adequate intake of antioxidants, and prudent use of an antioxidant supplement may provide insurance against a suboptimal diet and the increased stress from exercise. Research has also shown the positive benefits of phytonutrients with antiinflammatory and antioxidant effects, which may help with posttraining inflammation. Examples include anthocyanins in purple and red fruits and vegetables, and quercetin found in red onions, blueberries, tomatoes, apples, black tea, and purple grapes. Compounds found in tart cherry juice help to reduce inflammation, muscle damage, and oxidative stress (Rawson et al, 2018).

Vitamin D

Over the past few years, vitamin D has been shown to play an increasingly important role in sports performance beyond its role in calcium absorption and use in bone formation (Todd et al, 2015). As a secosteroid hormone, upon activation to 1,25-hydroxy vitamin D₃, vitamin D responsive gene expression is altered with more than 1000 responsive genes affecting MPS, muscle strength, muscle size, reaction time, balance coordination, endurance, inflammation, and immunity, all of which are important to athletic performance (Box 22.6).

Vitamin D deficiency may be more common in athletes than previously thought, especially in specific groups (Shuler et al, 2012). The prevalence appears to vary by sport, training location, time of year, and skin color (Rawson et al, 2018). Research has shown that more than 75% of Caucasians and 90% of African Americans and Latinos are possibly vitamin D deficient according to set values. It is possible that up to 77% of athletes who live in northern climates with little winter sunlight and who are indoor athletes (94% of basketball players and 83% of gymnasts) may be affected by deficiencies of vitamin D (Sikora-Klak et al, 2018). One recent study showed vitamin D deficiency is quite common among National Basketball Association (NBA) Draft Combine participants, affecting 73.5% (Grieshober et al, 2018). Outdoor athletes may not have an advantage over indoor athletes; in a National Football League (NFL) study, 81% of Caucasian and African

BOX 22.6 Vitamin D and Athletic Performance

Vitamin D Potential Impact on Athletic Performance

Positive effect on muscle strength, power, and mass
Increased force and power output of skeletal muscle tissue
May influence maximal oxygen uptake (VO₂max)
Improved skeletal muscle function and bone strength
Potentially increased size and number of type II muscle fibers
Decreased recovery time from training
Increase testosterone production

From Dahlquist DT et al: Plausible ergogenic effects of vitamin D on athletic performance and recovery, *J Int Soc Sports Nutr*, 12:33, 2015.

American players may be at risk for deficiency. Blood tests can better determine deficiency states.

Although the specific amount of vitamin D needed to reverse deficiency states has not been determined, partly because it depends on the extent of deficiency, athletes should be tested and guided by a health professional if diagnosed with a deficiency (see Chapter 5 and Appendices 12 and 38).

After a detailed assessment, recommendations for attaining and maintaining optimal vitamin D levels can be individualized to the athlete's current 25(OH)D concentration, dietary intake, lifestyle habits and clinical symptoms. The recommendation for fair-skinned individuals is to obtain 5 minutes and for dark-skinned individuals, 30 minutes of sunlight exposure to arms, legs, and back several times a week without sunscreen (see Appendix 38). Short-term, high-dose "loading" regimens for rapid repletion under the care of a physician also may be beneficial (Todd et al, 2015).

MINERALS

Although 12 minerals have been shown to be designated as essential nutrients, iron, calcium, magnesium, and copper have biochemical functions with the potential to affect athletic performance.

Iron

Iron is critical for sport performance because, as a component of hemoglobin, it is instrumental in transporting oxygen from the lungs to the tissues. It performs a similar role in myoglobin, which acts within the muscle as an oxygen acceptor to hold a supply of oxygen readily available for use by the mitochondria. Iron is also a vital component of the cytochrome enzymes involved in the production of ATP. Iron adequacy can be a limiting factor in performance because deficiency limits aerobic endurance and the capacity for work. Even partial depletion of iron stores in the liver, spleen, and bone marrow, as evidenced by low serum ferritin levels, may have a detrimental effect on exercise performance, even when anemia is not present (see Chapter 31).

Sports anemia is a term applied to at least three different conditions: hemodilution, iron deficiency anemia, and foot-strike anemia. Athletes at risk are the rapidly growing male adolescent; the female athlete with heavy menstrual losses; the athlete with an energy-restricted diet; distance runners who may have increased GI iron loss, hematuria, hemolysis caused by foot impact, and myoglobin leakage; and those training with heavy sweating in hot climates. Recent research suggests that anemia may be common in female athletes, especially adolescent and premenopausal females, long-distance runners, and vegetarians, who should be screened periodically to assess their iron status. One retrospective analysis of routine blood test data taken from 2009 to 2015 from elite level runners and triathletes 21 to 36 years old showed a higher incidence of at least 1 episode of iron deficiency in 60% of female triathletes, 55.6% of female runners, 37.5% of male triathletes, and 31.3% of male runners compared with values reported for endurance athletes (20% to 50% females, 0% to 17% males) (Coates et al, 2017). In another study of 2749 collegiate athletes, 2.2% of females indicated iron deficiency anemia and 30.9% indicated iron deficiency without anemia. For male athletes, 1.2% indicated iron deficiency anemia and 2.9% indicated iron deficiency without anemia (Parks et al, 2017)

Heavy endurance training also can cause a transient decrease in serum ferritin and hemoglobin. This condition, known as pseudoanemia, is characterized by reduced hemoglobin levels resulting from expanding blood volumes that are almost those of clinical anemia but return to pretraining normal levels. Performance does not appear to deteriorate and the pseudoanemia may in fact improve aerobic capacity and performance (McArdle et al, 2014).

Some athletes, especially long-distance runners, experience GI bleeding that is related to the intensity and duration of the exercise, the athlete's ability to stay hydrated, how well the athlete is trained, and whether they have taken ibuprofen before the competition. Iron loss from GI bleeding can be detected by fecal hemoglobin assays.

It is possible that using serum hemoglobin as the determining factor for identifying anemic athletes who may benefit from iron supplementation with performance improvement is not the best biomarker. Nonanemic athletes (with normal serum hemoglobin) who are supplemented with iron have shown improved performance. Optimal levels of serum ferritin, which is the most common index of body iron status associated with performance, and thus a better marker, may also be inadequate, because athletes supplemented with iron to achieve higher than "normal" serum ferritin levels have also shown improved performance (DellaValle, 2013). Some athletes experience iron deficiency without anemia and have normal hemoglobin levels but reduced levels of serum ferritin (20 to 30 ng/mL; see Chapter 5).

Athletes should be assessed for their iron status using serum hemoglobin and serum ferritin at the beginning of and during the training season. This is especially important in those suspected to have sickle cell trait (SCT) because their rate of sudden death is 10 to 30 times higher than in non-SCT athletes. Typically deaths have occurred early in the season, during exhaustive drills in hot weather without adequate warmup time (Harris et al, 2012). In 2010 the NCAA instituted a universal screening program to test for SCT in all Division I athletes; however, in athletes at the high school level, and in the NBA, NFL, Navy, Marines, and Air Force, testing is not required (Jung et al, 2011).

Although male athletes have been reported to consume at least the RDA for iron, female athletes tend to consume somewhat less for a variety of reasons, including low energy intake, lower intake of animal products, or adherence to a vegetarian or vegan diet (Rogerson, 2017). Increasing dietary intake of iron or supplementation is the only way to replace iron losses and improve status (Farrokhyar, 2015).

Who should be supplemented and with how much iron remains to be answered. Given the evidence suggesting iron's role in overall health and physical performance, there is no debate that athletes with clinical deficiency should be identified and treated. Whether those with subclinical deficiency should be treated with iron supplementation remains controversial. Individuals with normal status typically do not benefit from supplementation, and concerns regarding unregulated doses and overload should be considered.

Calcium

Suboptimal levels of dietary calcium intake are seen in athletes. Because low levels of calcium intake have been shown to be a contributing factor in osteoporosis, young female athletes, especially those who have had interrupted menstrual function, may be at risk for decreased bone mass. Strategies to promote the resumption of menses include estrogen replacement therapy, promotion of optimal weight status, and reduced training. Regardless of menstrual history, most female athletes need to increase their calcium, vitamin D_3, and magnesium intake. Dairy and nondairy options such as fortified almond, flax, and soy beverages, yogurts and cheeses, calcium-fortified fruit juices, and tofu made with calcium sulfate are good sources (see Appendix 39).

Magnesium

Magnesium is an essential mineral that supports more than 300 enzymatic reactions including glycolysis, fat and protein metabolism, and ATP hydrolysis, and is a regulator of neuromuscular, immune, and hormonal functions. Although hypomagnesemia has been seen in athletes, possibly caused by excessive sweating while training and transient redistribution of magnesium indicating a release from one storage area to an active site, levels return to normal within 24 hours after exercise (Malliaropoulos et al, 2013).

True magnesium deficiency has been shown to impair athletic performance, causing muscle spasms and increased heart rate and VO$_2$ during submaximal exercise. For deficient athletes, supplemental magnesium has been shown to improve performance by improving cellular function, although in athletes with adequate status, performance outcomes are mixed (Kass et al, 2013). In one recent study with female volleyball players, magnesium supplementation improved alactic (does not produce any lactic acid) anaerobic metabolism, even though the players were not magnesium deficient (Setaro et al, 2014). In another study with young men participating in a strength training program for 7 weeks, daily magnesium intake of 8 mg/kg of body weight resulted in increases in muscle strength and power, whereas marathon runners with adequate stores did not seem to benefit (Moslehi et al, 2013). As with most nutrients, supplementation does not seem to improve performance in those who are not deficient. Food sources of magnesium include whole grains, nuts, beans, and leafy greens. See Appendix 43 for sources of magnesium.

In a 2017 meta-analysis, no significant improvements in the supplementation group were observed regarding isokinetic peak torque extension, muscle, or muscle power, nor does the evidence support a beneficial effect of supplementation on muscle fitness in most athletes and physically active individuals who have a relatively high Mg status (Wang et al, 2017).

CLINICAL INSIGHT

Gastrointestinal Issues in Athletes

Gut issues are a common problem, affecting about 45% to 85% of athletes, 30% to 50% on a regular basis and in 70% of runners (Jeukendrup, 2017a; Koon et al, 2017; ter Steege et al, 2012). Issues can affect the upper GI tract, such as reflux, heart burn, chest pain, nausea, vomiting, gastritis, peptic ulcers, bleeding, or **exercise related transient abdominal pain (ETAP)**, also known as "stitches," or the lower GI tract, such as gas, bloating, excessive urge to defecate, diarrhea, hemorrhoids, and colitis.

Genetic and individualized differences, exercise environments, and life stressors can affect the athlete's gut function, **microbiome**, and tolerance of specific foods. Although a direct relationship between exercise and gut microbial composition or function has not been established, there are several mechanisms by which physical activity might modify the microbiota and impact immune status, gut function, the incidence of upper respiratory infections (URI), mood, and sports performance (Clark and Mach, 2017; Foster et al, 2017; Hart, 2018; O'Sullivan et al, 2015).

It appears that exercise impacts the brain-gut-microbe axis, diet microbe host metabolic interactions, neuroendocrine and neuroimmune interactions; and an individual athlete's response to physical stress. It is thought that the microbiota can act like an endocrine organ secreting serotonin, dopamine, or other neurotransmitters that can modify the stress response in athletes. There is also evidence to suggest that exercise-induced stress, both physiologic and emotional, can modulate the composition of gut microbiota and vice versa (Clark and Mach, 2017).

Additionally, changes in mechanical forces seen with endurance sports, (i.e., long-distance running and triathlon) include altered GI blood flow and GI motility, along with neuroendocrine changes from training. ETAP may be possibly due to irritation of the peritoneum although gastric or diaphragm ischemia, muscular cramping, and stretching of the visceral ligaments of the solid organs have also been proposed (Koon et al, 2017).

Other factors such as the athlete's pretraining and/or precompetition diet, climate changes, cool to very hot/humid conditions, emotional stress due to competition, dehydration, nonsteroidal antiinflammatory drug (NSAID) use, and whether or not the athlete has evacuated before exercise (bowel movement) may also add to GI distress.

It is estimated that 20% to 60% of athletes are impacted by the stress of excessive training, especially endurance training along with inadequate recovery, and the impacts have also been shown to increase with exercise intensity (Clark and Mach, 2017; Lamprecht et al, 2012). Educating athletes on best pretraining and precompetition fueling; applying a periodization trial and error with simple plain, low fiber, low fat, spice free solid or liquid, whole or sport food with varying amounts and types of carbohydrate sources and blends is one strategy for eliminating potential GI issues.

Assessment tools used to rule out food-related issues include (1) a thorough dietary analysis including an analysis of foods, fluids, alcohol use, and supplements consumed before, during, and after training; (2) food sensitivity or allergy testing to determine whether food intolerances to gluten, lactose, or other foods or herbals exist; (3) a bowel function and chronic GI disease history and functional comprehensive stool test; (4) a history of overall fluid intake and possible dehydration because of changes in training climate; and (5) a history of infections and antibiotic use.

Training and dietary programs that aim to balance the systematic stressors that athletes experience together with personalized diet plans to improve performance can reduce exercise-related stress symptoms and improve gut function and athletic performance. One study that supports this is with an Irish rugby football team during World Cup training camp. Compared with controls, monitoring diet and exercise while training under extreme training conditions was found to lower levels of inflammatory cytokines and increase fecal microbial diversity. This suggests that exercise can play a protective and positive role in nourishing the microbiota when athletes are nutritionally well fed and training incorporates adequate recovery (O'Sullivan et al, 2015). This supports a body of research that suggests that the GI system is highly adaptable. The rate of gastric emptying and perceptions of fullness can be decreased or "trained," and the diet can play an important role (Jeukendrup, 2017a).

Nutritional strategies for overcoming GI issues include an elimination diet or low FODMAP diet, and/or a competition-day diet that is individualized to the athlete based on their tolerance of foods. Another strategy is to offer a high-carbohydrate diet, as this can increase the activity of glucose-1 transporters (SGLT1) in the intestine allowing greater carbohydrate uptake and oxidation during exercise (Jeukendrup, 2017b; Koon et al, 2017).

ERGOGENIC AIDS

Athletes are always looking for an edge, such as a new technique, a training regimen, or gear that might help them improve athletic performance, increase strength and speed, or hasten recovery after training. Many athletes test the latest trendy diet or supplement to achieve sports success in spite of whether it supports optimal health or, at worst, leads to the risk of illness, injury, or a failing drug doping blood test. Unfortunately, many athletes are misinformed about the best way to achieve sports performance with diet alone (Kanter, 2018).

Ergogenic aids include any training technique, mechanical device, nutrition practice, pharmacologic method, or physiologic technique that can improve exercise performance capacity and training adaptations. Many athletes devote substantial time and energy striving for optimal performance and training and turn to ergogenic aids, especially dietary supplements (Larson-Meyer et al, 2018).

The Food and Drug Administration (FDA) regulates dietary supplement products and ingredients in addition to labeling, product claims, package inserts, and accompanying literature. The Federal Trade Commission (FTC) regulates dietary supplement advertising. (See Chapter 11 for a definition of a dietary supplement as defined by the Dietary Supplement Health and Education Act [DSHEA] of 1994.)

According to the law, dietary supplement manufacturers are allowed to publish information about the benefits of dietary supplements in the form of advertisements, including structure and function claims. This results in a great deal of printed material that can be confusing to athletes at the point of sale of nutritional products. In addition, athletes are bombarded with advertisements and testimonials from other athletes and coaches about the effects of dietary supplements on performance.

The use of ergogenic aids in the form of dietary supplements is widespread in all sports (Garthe and Maughan, 2018). Many athletes, whether recreational or professional, use some form of dietary supplementation to improve athletic performance or to assist with weight loss (Knapik et al, 2016; Larson-Meyer et al, 2018).

According to one survey, 88% of collegiate athletes report using one or more nutritional supplements (Buell et al, 2013). A recent meta-analysis of 159 studies suggested that it is difficult to generalize about dietary supplement use by athletes because of the lack of homogeneity among studies (Knapik et al, 2016). Data has suggested that elite athletes use dietary supplements more than nonelite athletes, use is similar for men and women, and appears to change little over time. Additionally, a larger proportion of athletes use dietary supplements compared with the general U.S. population.

Surveys show reasons for supplement use are varied and differ between genders. Women athletes often take supplements for their health, or to overcome an inadequate diet, whereas men may take supplements to improve speed, agility, strength, and power, and also use them to help build body mass and reduce weight or excess body fat. In one study, 75% of adolescent athletes reported taking supplements, males for sports performance enhancement and better muscle development and function, whereas females reported taking supplements for immune system improvement (Zdešar Kotnik et al, 2017). See Table 22.5 for discussion of ergogenic aids commonly used by athletes.

TABLE 22.5 Commonly Used Banned and Recreational Drugs Used by Athletes

Ergogenic Drug	Goals of Use	Athletic Effect	Adverse Effects
Alcohol	Reduce stress and inhibition; most widespread used drug in sport (88% of intercollegiate athletes)	No benefits	Dependence producing; twofold higher risk of injury; cardiovascular/liver disease; worsens left ventricular dysfunction; decreases amino acid, glucose utilization; decreases energy, hypoglycemia; dehydration; decreases skeletal muscle capillary density, cross-sectional area; inhibits sarcolemmal calcium channel actions, impairs excitation-contraction coupling and diminishes performance; decreases muscle oxidative capability; compromises blood coagulation/fibrinolysis/postexercise perturbations in clotting factors; positive energy balance, obesity; increases HR and VO_2, reductions in power output
Nicotine	CNS psychostimulant	Mixed: Enhances brain norepinephrine and dopamine; higher doses enhance serotonin and opiate exerting calming and depressing effect, increases pain tolerance; increases muscle blood flow, lipolysis; may improve cognitive function, learning memory, and reaction time and fine motor abilities; delays central fatigue	Addictive; may lead to development of respiratory, cardio, and skin diseases and tobacco-related cancers if smoked; increases heart rate and blood pressure, cardiac stroke volume and output, and coronary blood flow; increases skin temperature
Tetrahydrocannabinol (marijuana, cannabis)	Diminish nerves/pre competition stress, and anxiety; relax/decrease inhibition; improve sleep	No positive effect	Increases HR and BP at rest; physical work capacity decreases by 25%; decrease in standing steadiness, reaction time, psychomotor performance
Anabolic androgenic steroids	Gain muscle mass and strength	Increase muscle mass and strength, especially when combined with strength training and high-protein diets	Multiple organ systems including infertility, gynecomastia, female virilization, hypertension, atherosclerosis, physeal closure, aggression, depression, suicidal ideation

Continued

TABLE 22.5   Commonly Used Banned and Recreational Drugs Used by Athletes—cont'd

Ergogenic Drug	Goals of Use	Athletic Effect	Adverse Effects
Androstenedione	Increases testosterone to gain muscle mass and strength	Increase muscle strength and size	Tendopathy, rhabdomyolysis; tendon rupture
DHEA	Increases testosterone to gain muscle mass and strength	No measurable effect	Increases estrogens in men; impurities in preparation
Human growth hormone	Increase muscle mass, strength, and definition	Decreases subcutaneous fat and increases lipolysis; increases muscle mass and strength; improves wound healing; stimulates testosterone production	Acromegaly, glucose intolerance, physeal closure, increased lipids, myopathy
Stimulants (ephedrine alkaloids, amphetamines, cocaine)	Increases weight loss; fatigue delay	Increases metabolism, no clear performance benefit, although may benefit power, endurance, strength, or speed; reduces tiredness; increases alertness and aggression	Muscle and joint pain; misjudgment in time orientation; tremors; cerebral vascular accident, arrhythmia, myocardial infarction, seizure, psychosis, hypertension, death
Arimidex, (anastro-zole); selective estrogen receptor modulators (SERMs) like tamoxifen	Cancer drug used to decrease estrogen levels associated with testosterone use	None; increase testosterone, luteinizing hormone secretion; increase muscle strength and size; prevent bone loss	Side effects associated with taking these agents; early fatigue; increased bone resorption and decreased BMD (hip, lumber spine)
Ghrelin mimetics (GHRP6 and GHRP2)	Increase GH secretion	Increase muscle mass; stimulate glycogenesis; anabolic effects on muscle mass	GH-associated side effects (see above)
Glucocorticoids	Alleviate pain; reduce tiredness	No improvement	Growth suppression, osteoporosis, avascular necrosis of femoral head; tendon or facial rupture (by local injections) osteoarthritis

BMD, Bone mineral density, *BP*, blood pressure; *CNS*, central nervous system; *DHEA*, dehydroepiandrosterone; *GH*, growth hormone; *HR*, heart rate.
Refs: Pesta, D et al 2013; Nikolopoulios, D et al 2011, Rogol A 2010; Hoffman J et al 2009.

The biggest concern for athletes is the use of drugs prohibited in sport and the possibility that a supplement may contain something that will result in a positive drug test, which may also apply to supplemental sport food products such as drinks, shakes, and bars. In fact a wide range of stimulants, steroids, and other agents that are included in the World Anti-Doping Agency's (WADA) prohibited list have been identified in supplements. This may occur either intentionally or unintentionally by the manufacturers in the preparation of the raw ingredients or in the formulation of the finished product. In some cases, the amount of product may be exceptionally higher or lower than the therapeutic dose (Table 22.6). The FDA has identified sports supplements and ergogenic aids among the highest risk for adulteration with drugs and baned substances (see Chapter 11).

Research suggests that all too often, physically active individuals, including high-level athletes, obtain nutrition information from coaches, fellow athletes, trainers, advertisements, and the Internet rather than well-informed and educated sports dietitians, physicians, and accredited exercise professionals (Morente-Sánchez and Zabala, 2013).

Information on the efficacy and safety of many of these products used by athletes is limited or completely lacking. Sports nutritionists need to be on the forefront of information; know how to evaluate the scientific merit of articles and advertisements about exercise and nutrition products so that they can separate marketing hype from scientifically based training and nutrition practices (see Chapter 11). Certification programs such as National Sanitation Foundation (NSF) for Sport and Informed Choice can help guide dietitians and athletes to selecting certified safe sport supplements.

NSF for Sport is a program that focuses primarily on the sports supplement manufacturing and sourcing process, provides preventive measures to protect against adulteration of products, verifies label claims against product contents, and identifies athletic banned substances in the finished product or ingredients. The program, designed for manufacturers and their products, includes product testing for more than 180 banned substances, label content confirmation, formulation and label review, and production facility and supplier inspections, as well as ongoing monitoring in line with substance prohibitive lists. The program is recognized by the NFL, National Football League Players Association (NFLPA), Major League Baseball (MLB), Major League Baseball Players Association

TABLE 22.6   Foods High in Branched-Chain Amino Acids

Branched-Chain Amino Acid	Food Sources
Leucine	Meat, dairy, nuts, beans, brown rice, soy, and whole wheat
Isoleucine	Meat, chicken, eggs, fish, almonds, chickpeas, soy protein, and most seeds
Valine	Meat, dairy, soy protein, grains, peanuts, and mushrooms

(MLBPA), Professional Golfers Association (PGA), Ladies Professional Golf Association (LPGA), and Canadian Centre for Ethics in Sports (CCES).

Informed Choice is also a quality assurance program for sports nutrition products, suppliers to the sports nutrition industry, and supplement manufacturing facilities. Its testing capability for supplements/ingredients includes the analysis of over 146 substances that are considered prohibited in sport and substances that pose a threat with respect to product contamination. These substances include drugs of abuse, anabolic agents, stimulants, beta-2-agonists, masking agents, and so on. Testing methods used for a range of substances from these categories have been validated and accredited to the ISO 17025 standard in supplements/ingredients in each of the relevant matrices: powders, bars, liquids, capsules, tablets, and so on, with defined method capabilities/reporting limits.

POPULAR ERGOGENIC AIDS

Creatine

As an amino acid, creatine is produced normally in the body from arginine, glycine, and methionine. Most dietary creatine comes from meat, but half is manufactured in the liver and kidneys. For meat eaters, dietary intake of creatine is approximately 1 g daily (Kreider et al, 2017). The body also synthesizes approximately 1 g of creatine per day, for a total production of approximately 2 g daily (Kreider et al, 2017).

In normal, healthy persons approximately 40% of muscle creatine exists as free creatine; the remainder combines with phosphate to form creatine phosphate (CP). Approximately 2% of the body's creatine is broken down daily to creatinine before excretion by the kidneys. The normal daily excretion of creatinine is approximately 2 g for most persons. Those with lower levels of intramuscular creatine, such as vegetarians, may benefit from creatine supplementation (McArdle et al, 2014).

Creatine monohydrate is one of the most popular supplements used by strength and power athletes. Supplementation elevates muscle creatine levels and facilitates the regeneration of CP, which helps to regenerate ATP. A variety of synthetic creatine supplements have been developed, including creatine malate, pyruvate, citrate, and many more with marketing claims of greater performance enhancement and absorption. Creatine monohydrate is not only the most extensively studied but the most clinically effective form of creatine for use in nutritional supplements in terms of muscle uptake and ability to increase high-intensity exercise capacity (Kreider et al, 2017).

Numerous reviews identify performance benefits with repeated bouts of high-intensity exercise less than 150 s in duration with the greatest impact in less than 30 s (Lanhers et al, 2017). Classical loading consists of an initial loading phase of 15 to 20 g per day for 4 to 7 days, followed by a maintenance dose of 2 to 5 g per day. However, alternative dosing methods also have been shown to effectively increase creatine stores and result in strength gains. Regimens without the loading include a dose of 0.3 g/kg body weight for 5 to 7 days, followed by maintenance dose of 0.03 g/kg body weight for 4 to 6 weeks. However, with this regimen creatine stores increase more slowly, and it may take longer to see the strength training effects (Hall and Trojian, 2013).

As creatine is one of the most researched supplements, numerous studies support the use and effectiveness of creatine for short-term, maximum output exercise such as weight lifting, running a 100-m sprint, swinging a bat, or punting a football. When creatine stores in the

muscles are depleted, ATP synthesis is prevented and energy can no longer be supplied at the rate required by the working muscle. Improved athletic performance has been attributed to this ATP resynthesis.

Creatine supplementation increases body mass or muscle mass during training. It may improve submaximal exercise performance for high-intensity interval training (HIIT), which promotes fitness similar to endurance training. A 2013 study on swimmers showed creatine supplementation improved swimming performance and reduced blood lactate levels after intermittent sprint swimming bouts (Dabidi Roshan et al, 2013).

Studies are conflicting on creatinine's effect on aerobic performance. In a double-blind, placebo-controlled study 16 male amateur soccer players, consuming 20 g of creatine per day, or a placebo, for 7 days, experienced no beneficial effect on physical measures obtained during a 90-minute soccer test (Williams et al, 2014).

Creatine absorption appears to be stimulated by insulin. Therefore ingesting creatine supplements in combination with carbohydrate, amino acids, or protein can increase muscle creatine concentrations. Once creatine is taken up by the muscles, it is trapped within the muscle tissue. It is estimated that once creatine stores in the muscle are elevated, it generally takes 4 to 6 weeks for creatine stores to return to baseline (Kreider et al, 2017).

Few data exist on the long-term benefits and risks of creatine supplementation. Because of the long-term risks, the American Orthopedic Society for Sports Medicine, the ACSM, and the American Academy of Pediatrics (AAP) advise children and adolescents younger than 18 years and pregnant or nursing women to never take creatine supplements. While a few case studies have reported that individuals purportedly taking creatine with or without other supplements presented with high creatinine levels and/or renal dysfunction, there appears to be no compelling evidence that supplementation negatively affects renal function in healthy or clinical populations (Kreider et al, 2017; Williamson and New, 2014).

Beta-Alanine

Intermittent bouts of high-intensity interval training (HIIT) deplete energy substrates and allow for metabolite accumulation. Studies suggest that supplementation with beta-alanine may improve endurance performance as well as lean body mass (Kern and Robinson, 2011). Because of its relationship with carnosine, beta-alanine appears to have ergogenic potential. Carnosine is believed to be one of the primary acid buffering substances in muscle. Although carnosine is synthesized from two amino acids, beta-alanine and histidine, its synthesis appears to be limited by the availability of beta-alanine, thus taking supplemental beta-alanine can increase carnosine levels and reduce lactic acid build up in the muscles (Trexler et al, 2015; Peeling et al, 2018).

This proposed benefit would help increase an athlete's capacity for training and increase time to fatigue. Supplementing with beta-alanine has been associated with improved strength, anaerobic endurance, body composition, and performance on various measures of anaerobic power output.

Daily supplementation with 3.2 to 6.4 g (approx. 65mg/kg body mass) for a minimum of 2 to 4 weeks can increase muscle carnosine content about 65% above resting levels; extended to 10 to 12 weeks, 80% above resting levels and improving tolerance for exercise bouts lasting 30 seconds to 10 minutes. However, the correlation between muscle changes and magnitude of performance benefits are yet to be determined. The only reported side effect is paresthesia (tingling), but studies indicate this can be attenuated by using divided lower doses (1.6 g) or using a sustained-release formula (Trexler et al, 2015).

Caffeine

Research on the physiologic benefits of caffeine on performance is extensive in areas of strength, endurance, rates of perceived effort, hydration, and recovery. The ergogenic benefits include:

(1) affecting the central nervous system (CNS) and cognitive performance
(2) mobilizing fat and sparing glycogen during exercise
(3) increasing intestinal absorption and oxidation of carbohydrates
(4) speeding up resynthesis of muscle glycogen in recovery
(5) reducing perceived exertion and pain of training.

Caffeine contributes to endurance performance, apparently because of its ability to enhance mobilization of fatty acids and thus conserve glycogen stores. Caffeine also may directly affect muscle contractility, possibly by facilitating calcium transport. It could reduce fatigue as well by reducing plasma potassium accumulation, which contributes to fatigue. An energy-enhancing effect is seen with up to 3 mg/kg body mass or about 200 mg caffeine for the 150-lb athlete (Spriet, 2014). Unwanted side effects of overconsuming caffeine that may limit performance are headaches, insomnia, GI irritation, reflux, shakiness, heart palpitations, and increased urination. Previous reports showed that caffeine combined with ephedra resulted in serious illness and death, and the combination was banned from use in dietary supplements by the FDA in 2004. Safety data from 50 trials determined that the use of ephedra or ephedrine combined with caffeine has been associated with a 2.2- to 3.6-fold increases in odds of psychiatric, autonomic, or GI symptoms, and heart palpitations (Shekelle et al, 2003).

Consumer demand for caffeine has resulted in greater accessibility and acceptance of a variety of beverages beyond coffee and tea. An emerging trend in sports nutrition is the intake of caffeine-containing energy drinks and drink shots for performance.

The growing availability and consumption of energy drinks with caffeine among all age groups is of concern, especially among young athletes because excessive amounts of caffeine have been shown to disrupt adolescent sleep patterns, exacerbate psychiatric disease, cause physiologic dependence, increase the risk of subsequent addiction and risk-taking behaviors, raise blood pressure, and cause dehydration, vomiting, irregular and rapid heartbeat, convulsions, coma, and death. Altered sleep patterns from excessive caffeine use can lead to poor performance, delayed reaction times, and increased risk for injuries.

Energy drinks consumed with alcohol are another growing concern among health experts, and in 2010 the FDA declared caffeine an "unsafe food additive" to alcoholic beverages, effectively banning premixed alcoholic energy drinks.

There are concerns and safety issues regarding another similar supplement, citrus aurantium L. (bitter orange) extracts, which are also used for weight loss/weight management, sports performance, appetite control, energy, and mental focus and cognition, and which contain p-synephrine as the primary protoalkaloid, as they have similar structural aspects as ephedrine (Stohs, 2017).

Nitrates and Beet Juice

Several studies suggest that inorganic nitrates may alter the physiologic responses to exercise and enhance performance by increasing vasodilation and glucose uptake and reducing blood pressure and the O_2 cost of submaximal exercise (Peeling et al, 2018). Because the consumption of nitrate salts may result in the production of harmful nitrogenous compounds, researchers have explored using natural nitrate-rich foods such as beetroot juice and powders. A dose of dietary nitrate, approximately 0.5 L of beetroot juice, has been shown to increase plasma nitrite, which peaks within 3 hours and remains elevated for 6 to 9 hours before returning to baseline (Wylie et al, 2013).

In one study, supplementing the diet with 0.5 L of beetroot juice per day for 4 to 6 days reduced the steady state cost of submaximal exercise by 5% and extended the time to exhaustion during high-intensity cycling by 16%, which has been confirmed in other exercise populations, including rowers and team sports. Although the mechanistic bases for the effects are unclear, evidence suggests mitochondrial efficiency and contractile function may be enhanced (Wylie et al, 2013). Other positive effects include increased NO_2 and vasodilation and reduced VO_2 at less than or equal to VO_2max intensity while improving the relationship between watts required and VO_2 level, increasing time-to-exhaustion at less than or equal to VO_2max intensity (Domínguez et al, 2017; Mills et al, 2017).

It has been recommended to consume nitrate immediately before, during, and after long-duration endurance exercise because of peak and maintenance level times. A daily dose of the supplement has been shown to keep plasma nitrite elevated (Jones et al, 2013). Although there is a possibility that uncontrolled high doses of nitrate salts may be harmful to health, natural sources found in beetroot, spinach, lettuce, and celery are likely to promote health.

PERFORMANCE ENHANCEMENT SUBSTANCES AND DRUGS: DOPING IN SPORT

The use of performance enhancement substances is not a new phenomenon in sports. As early as 776 bc the Greek Olympians were reported to use substances such as dried figs, mushrooms, and strychnine to perform better. Their use is prevalent in amateur and professional athletes, receiving even greater attention with use by high-profile accomplished athletes such as Lance Armstrong, disqualification of some professional athletes for failed drug tests, and the seizure of companies caught with tainted supplements (Pope et al, 2014).

Since 2004, the WADA has had a list of banned drugs for athletes who compete and a strategy to detect drugs such as anabolic steroids, erythropoietin (EPO), human growth hormone (HGH), and insulin-like growth factor (IGF-1). WADA annually updates its prohibited list of supplements suspected of (1) illegally enhancing athletic performance, (2) representing an actual or potential health risk to the athlete, or (3) violating the spirit of the sport.

As the number of individuals participating in different sports increases, so does the variety of doping agents. According to WADA, the rate of use has been fairly consistent, suggesting a prevalence of approximately 2% of elite athletes. Rates derived from self-reports have ranged from 1.2% to 26%. Between 10% and 24% of male athletes have reported they would use doping if it would help them achieve better results without the risk of consequences, with an additional 5% to 10% indicating potential doping behavior regardless of health hazards.

Reasons given for using banned substances include achievement of athletic success by improving performance, financial gain, improving recovery, prevention of nutritional deficiencies, and the idea that others use them or the "false consensus effect."

Steroids

Androgenic-anabolic steroids (AASs) categorize all male sex steroid hormones, their synthetic derivatives, and their active metabolites used to enhance athletic performance and appearance. AAS use was reported in the 1950 Olympics and was banned in 1976. Steroids may be used as oral or intramuscular preparations.

The legal and illegal use of these drugs is increasing as a result of society's preoccupation with increasing muscle strength, size, and libido. Originally designed for therapeutic uses to provide enhanced anabolic potency, nontherapeutic use of AAS is increasing among adolescents and females. Anecdotal evidence suggests widespread use of anabolic steroids among athletes (20% to 90%), especially at the professional and elite amateur levels. Use among high school boys is approximately 5% to 10%; rates among college athletes are slightly higher.

Anabolic effects of AAS include increased muscle mass; increased bone mineral density; increased blood cell production; decreased body fat; increased heart, liver, and kidney size; vocal cord changes; and increased libido. Anabolic steroids increase protein synthesis in skeletal muscles and reverse catabolic processes; however, increased muscle mass and strength are observed only in athletes who maintain a high-protein, high-calorie diet during steroid administration. Androgenic effects are the development of secondary sexual characteristics in men, changes in genital size and function, and growth of auxiliary pubic and facial hair. Some adverse effects associated with steroid use are irreversible, especially in women.

Although steroid use has some valid medical uses (e.g., the treatment of delayed puberty, or body wasting resulting from disease), it also has adverse physical and emotional consequences in adolescents, such as arrested bone growth, internal organ damage, feminization in males, and masculinization in females. It also is associated with other high-risk behaviors, such as the use of other illicit drugs, reduced involvement in school, poor academic performance, engaging in unprotected sex, aggressive and criminal behavior, and suicidal ideation and attempted suicide.

Erythropoietin

EPO is used commonly to promote the body's production of red blood cells in patients with bone marrow suppression, such as patients with leukemia, those who are receiving chemotherapy, or those with renal failure (see Chapters 34 and 35). In athletes, injections increase the serum hematocrit and oxygen-carrying capacity of the blood, and thus enhance Vo_2max and endurance. EPO use as an ergogenic aid is difficult to detect because it is a hormone produced by the kidneys, although newer blood tests can detect its use. Typically, athletes with elevated hematocrit have been banned from endurance sports for suspected EPO misuse; however, despite its ban by the IOC, it is still commonly abused. Drastically high hematocrit combined with exercise-induced dehydration can lead to thick or viscous blood, which can lead to coronary or cerebral vascular occlusions, heart attack, or stroke. EPO also can cause elevated blood pressure or elevated potassium levels.

Human growth hormone (HGH) has many functions in the body, and it is produced naturally throughout life. It stimulates protein synthesis, enhances carbohydrate and fat metabolism, helps to maintain sodium balance, and stimulates bone and connective tissue turnover. HGH production decreases with age after the peak growth years. The amount secreted is affected by diet, stress, exercise, nutrition, and medications. HGH is banned by the IOC; however, it continues to be used by athletes. Potential side effects include skin changes, darkening of moles, adverse effects on glucose and lipid metabolism, and the growth of bones as evidenced by development of a protruding jaw and boxy forehead.

Prohormones and Steroids

Prohormones are popular among bodybuilders, many of whom believe that these prohormones are natural boosters of anabolic hormones. Androstenedione, 4-androstenediol, 19-nor-4-androstenedione, 19-nor-4-androstenediol, 7-keto dehydroepiandrosterone (DHEA), and 7-keto DHEA are naturally derived precursors to testosterone and other anabolic steroids.

Androstenedione

Androstenedione is a prehormone, an inactive precursor to female estrogen and male testosterone. It has about one-seventh of the activity of testosterone and is a precursor that directly converts to testosterone by a single reaction. It is produced naturally in the body from either DHEA or 17-alpha-hydroxyprogesterone. Some researchers have found that taking androstenedione elevates testosterone more than DHEA does; however, the induced increase lasts only several hours and remains at peak levels for just a few minutes. Acute or long-term administration of testosterone precursors does not effectively increase serum testosterone levels and fails to produce any significant changes in lean body mass, muscle strength, or performance improvement (Smurawa and Congeni, 2007).

Adverse reactions occur in male and female athletes, including muscle tightness and cramps, increased body weight, acne, GI problems, changes in libido, amenorrhea, liver damage, and stunted growth in adolescents. Consumption of a prohormone supplement can alter a patient's hypothalamic-pituitary-gonadal axis. Andro-related hormones may elevate abnormally estrogen-related hormones and alter elevations of serum estrogen, which is thought to increase the risk for developing prostate or pancreatic cancers. A significant decline in high-density lipoprotein (HDL) occurs, leading to an increased cardiovascular disease risk. Therefore taking androstenedione may be irresponsible because of the potential risks associated with long-term use. Until there is scientific support for its use, androstenedione should not be sold under the assumption that it is either an effective or a safe athletic ergogenic aid. Clearly, adolescents and women of childbearing age should not use it. In 1998 androstenedione was added to the list of banned substances by the IOC and several amateur and professional organizations, including the NFL and the NCAA.

Dehydroepiandrosterone (DHEA) is a weak androgen and product of dehydroandrosterone-3-sulfate (DHEA-S) and is used to elevate testosterone levels. It is a precursor to more potent testosterone and dihydrotestosterone. Although DHEA-S is the most abundant circulating adrenal hormone in humans, its physiologic role is poorly understood. DHEA has been labeled the "fountain of youth" hormone because its levels peak during early adulthood. The decline with aging has been associated with increased fat accumulation and risk of heart disease. Several studies have suggested a positive correlation between increased plasma levels of DHEA and improved vigor, health, and well-being in persons who range in age from 40 to 80 years. By decreasing cortisol output from the liver by 50%, DHEA could have an anabolic effect.

DHEA supplementation does not increase testosterone levels or increase strength in men, but it may increase testosterone levels in women with a virilizing effect. Because DHEA can take several different hormonal pathways, the one that it follows depends on several factors, including existing levels of other hormones. It can take several routes in the body and interact with certain enzymes along the sex-steroid pathway. Thus it can turn into less desirable byproducts of testosterone, including dihydrotestosterone, which is associated with male-pattern baldness, prostate enlargement, and acne.

The benefits of taking DHEA for sports performance have not been clearly established, and the effects of chronic DHEA ingestion are not known. Long-term safety has not been established, and there are concerns that chronic use in men may worsen prostate hyperplasia or even promote prostate cancer. DHEA is not recommended for athletic use because it can alter the testosterone-epitestosterone ratio so that it exceeds the 6:1 limit set by the IOC, the USOC, the NFL, and the NCAA.

CLINICAL CASE STUDY

Jose is a 32-year-old Hispanic male and former college athlete who has been competing in long-distance triathlon and marathon events for the past year. He complains of low energy as training and racing duration increases and is plagued by gut issues—gas and bloating after meals, nausea, and vomiting during races. He also suffers from sleep issues, waking up frequently during the night. He works full time at a stressful job as manager of an electrical contracting firm and trains in swimming, cycling, and running 10 to 12 hours/week.

Assessment

His height is 5 ft, 9 in and his weight is 174 lb. His body composition analysis as measured using the International Society for the Advancement of Kinanthropometry (ISAK) method was 6.8% (10.4 lb. body fat, 164 lb. [74kg] fat free mass [FFM]. He is satisfied with his body fat percentage but would like to reduce his weight, if possible, to lighten up for the running portion of his events.

A urine specific gravity test determined hydration status on three visits: 1.035, 1.025, and 1.030

Cholesterol levels were 250 mg/dL, high-density lipoprotein (HDL) 50 mg/dL, low-density lipoprotein (LDL) 170 mg/dL, triglycerides 160 mg/dL; all other values were within normal limits.

Using the Cunningham equation to calculate resting energy expenditure (REE):

$$500 + (22 \times FFM \text{ [kg]}) \quad 500 + (22 \times 74) = 2128 \text{ REE}$$

Day off training: Activity factor 1.2 = approximately 2553 calories

1-2 hours steady state training: Activity factor 1.4 = approx. 2979 calories

3-4 hours steady state training: Using Activity factor 1.6 = approx. 3404 calories

4-6 hours training steady state: Using 1.73 Activity factor = approx. 4581 calories

Current Diet

Breakfast 1 hour before workout

12 oz coffee with 1 oz coffee creamer

3 eggs, fried with onions, 2 slices bacon, 2 slices ham

1 corn tortilla with cheese

Analysis: 570 calories, 30 grams fat (49%), 40 grams carbs (28%) 570 mg cholesterol

Workout: 2000-yard swim, 2-hour bicycle ride, 4-mile run

During swim portion of workout (less than 1 hour): nothing

During cycle portion of workout: 2 hours

2 electrolyte pills every 20 minutes on bike—total 12 pills

Each pill contains: 40 mg Na—480 mg sodium

3 16 oz bottles fluid:

- 1 ×170 calories, 32 g cholesterol, 10 g protein
- 1 bottle high carbohydrate, hypertonic sports drink with maltodextrin—270 cal, 54 g carb, 7 g sugar and protein, 220 mg Na, 25 mg caffeine
- Water

1 gel pack every 30 minutes = 6 packs

Double latte with caffeine 110 cal, 27g carbs, 200 mg Na

During run portion of workout (less than 1 hour): nothing

Total workout fuel: 1100 calories, 248 g carbohydrates (124 g/hr cycling, 900 mg Na)

Immediately after workout: nothing

Breakfast

Coffee with half-and-half

1 plain bagel, cream cheese, jelly

Banana

12 ounces milk

Snack: none

Lunch

2-6 oz chicken breasts grilled with skin, 2 cups black beans and white rice, ½ cup fried plantains

Snack: high-protein sports bar

Dinner

1 onion soup with melted cheese

12 oz grilled steak

1 c yellow rice

Sautéed mushrooms

Dietary Analysis

3041 calories, 216 g protein (2.77 g/kg) (28%), 249 g carbohydrates (3.15 g/kg) (33%), 13.5% saturated fat, 1172 mg cholesterol, 5634 mg Na recommended dietary allowance (RDA): 64% potassium, 85% Ca and folate, 26% vitamin C, 30% vitamin E, 13% vitamin K, dietary fluid intake = 9 cups

Nutrition Diagnostic Statements

- Inadequate energy intake (NI-1.2) related to knowledge deficit about kcal needs for exercise performance as evidenced by diet low in calories (3041 calories [4141 with sport fuel] vs. 4581 calories required.
- Inadequate carbohydrate intake (NI-5.8.1) related to knowledge deficit about carbohydrate needs for sports performance as evidenced by intake of 249 g carbohydrates (3.15 g/kg) (33%) (497 g sport fuel), vs. a minimum of 5 to 7 g/kg = 395-553 g
- Excess fat intake (NI-5.5.2) related to knowledge deficit about fat needs for exercise performance as evidenced by total fat intake of 38% total calories, saturated fat and cholesterol 1172 mg
- Other assessments:
  - Low in antioxidants
  - Excessive fat in preworkout breakfast
  - Excessive in sport fuel carbohydrates and sodium for 2-hour bike portion of ride
  - Excessive in mealtime calories and protein
  - Questionable whether athlete can tolerate fructo-, oligo-, di-, and monosaccharides and polyols (FODMAPs) foods (i.e., onions, beans, mushrooms, cream cheese, dairy [lactose], sport fuel sources of high fructose corn syrup [HFCS], and gluten). See Chapter 27 for more information about FODMAPs.

Interventions

- Increase meal frequency and calories while modifying fat, saturated fat, and cholesterol
- Increase plant-based tolerable sources of protein and complex carbohydrates
- Modify amounts of animal protein at mealtime to 4 to 5 oz. (30 to 35 g)
- Improve leafy green vegetable intake via juicing or cooked versions if whole food vegetables not desired or tolerated
- Improve intake of antioxidant rich fruits and fruit juices without added sugar since fruits and fruit juices have ample amounts of sugar and excess fructose can cause gastrointestinal (GI) distress in some athletes.

Recommendations

Prebiotic/probiotic rich foods to support gut health; Some RDN's recommend enzymes before meals but the use is controversial in traditional medicine as evidence is based on expert opinion vs. clinical trials.

Adjust amount of sport fuel intake to decrease amount of sugar consumed during training/competition. Decrease electrolyte supplementation as excess amounts can cause GI distress in some athletes and is typically unnecessary since sports drinks already contain sodium and other electrolytes.

CLINICAL CASE STUDY—cont'd

Consider reducing carbohydrate-fortified liquids and/or changing carbohydrate source (i.e., as different beverages offer different simple and complex sugar sources and tolerability is individualized).

Include meditation or yoga on day off from training and/or prayer or meditation 5 to 10 minutes a day for relaxation

Laboratory and Integrative Approaches

Follow-up lipid profile after 9 to 12 weeks on modified fat, saturated fat, and cholesterol diet

Nutrition Care Questions

1. Calculate calorie and macronutrient needs using Cunningham equation and guidelines provided in chapter.
2. Assess what eating/lifestyle behaviors may be affecting this athlete's energy levels (i.e., sleep, stress, portion sizes at meal time).
3. Calculate training/race day/recovery fuel formulas for preworkout, workout calories, carbohydrates, and sodium.
4. List issues that appear to be a valid reason to initiate FODMAPs and elimination diet.

USEFUL WEBSITES

Academy of Dietetics and Nutrition (AND)
Australian Institute of Sport
Board Certification Specialists in Sports Dietetics (CSSD)
Collegiate and Professional Sports Dietitians Association (CPSDA)
International Society for Sports Nutrition (ISSN)
Sports Nutrition Care Manual
United States Olympic Committee Sports Dietitian Registry (USOC)

Resources, Fact Sheets, Books, Programs, and Guides

Academy of Nutrition and Dietetics. Sports Nutrition: A Practice Manual for Professionals.
Banned Substances Control Group
Informed Choice
International Society of Sports Nutrition
National Sanitation Foundation (NSF), Certified for Sport
Sports Nutrition: A Handbook for Professionals, 6th Edition
Sports, Cardiovascular and Wellness Nutrition Dietetic Practice Group (SCAN), Academy of Nutrition and Dietetics
United States Olympic Committee (USOC), Sports Nutrition Performance

Supplement Education/Certification Information

Drug-Free Sport
Examine.com
Natural Medicines Database
NSF Certification for Sports Supplements
Informed Choice Sports Supplement Certification
Taylor Hooton Foundation

Company-Sponsored Websites for Research/Handouts

EAS Academy
Gatorade Sports Science Institute
Office of Dietary Supplements, National Institutes of Health
Sport Science
Whey Protein Institute

REFERENCES

Academy of Nutrition and Dietetics: *Sports Nutrition Care Manual (SNCM)*, 2014. Available at: http://www.nutritioncaremanual.org/about-sncm.
Ackerman KE, Holtzman B, Cooper KM, et al. Low energy availability surrogates correlate with health and performance consequences of Relative Energy Deficiency in Sport, *Br J Sports Med* 53(10):628–633, 2019.
Alghannam AF, Gonzalez JT, Betts JA. Restoration of muscle glycogen and functional capacity: role of post-exercise carbohydrate and protein co-ingestion, *Nutrients* 10(2):E253, 2018. doi:10.3390/nu10020253.
Australian Institute of Sport: *Supplements: executive summary*, 2014. Available at: http://www.ausport.gov.au/ais/nutrition/supplements.
Ázara HM, Farinatti PTV, Midgley AW, et al: Standardized MET value underestimates the energy cost of treadmill running in men, *Int J Sports Med* 38(12):890–896, 2017. doi:10.1055/s-0043-115739.
Baker LB, Ungaro C, De Chavez PJ, et al: Exercise intensity effects on total sweat electrolyte losses and regional vs. whole-body sweat [Na$^+$], [Cl$^-$], and [K$^+$], *Eur J Appl Physiol* 119(2):361–375, 2019. doi:10.1007/s00421-018-4048-z.
Buell JL, Franks R, Ransone J, et al: National Athletic Trainers' Association position statement: evaluation of dietary supplements for performance nutrition, *J Athl Train* 48:124–136, 2013.
Burdon CA, Hoon MW, Johnson NA, et al: The effect of ice slushy ingestion and mouthwash on thermoregulation and endurance performance in the heat, *Int J Sport Nutr Exerc Metab* 23:458–469, 2013.
Burdon CA, Spronk I, Cheng HL, O'Connor HT: Effect of glycemic index of a pre-exercise meal on endurance exercise performance: a systematic review and meta-analysis. *Sports Med* 47(6):1087–1101, 2017. doi:10.1007/s40279-016-0632-8.
Burke LM: Re-examining high-fat diets for sports performance: did we call the 'nail in the coffin' too soon? *Sports Med* 45(Suppl 1):S33–S49, 2015. doi:10.1007/s40279-015-0393-9.
Burke LM, Ross ML, Garvican-Lewis LA, et al: Low carbohydrate, high fat diet impairs exercise economy and negates the performance benefit from intensified training in elite race walkers, *J Physiol* 595(9):2785–2807, 2017. doi:10.1113/JP273230.
Bytomski JR: Fueling for Performance, *Sports Health* 10(1):47–53, 2018.
Carl RL, Johnson MD, Martin TJ: *Council on Sports Medicine and Fitness*, Promotion of healthy weight-control practices in young athletes, *Pediatrics* 140(3):e20171871, 2017. doi:10.1542/peds.2017-1871.
Casazza GA, Tovar AP, Richardson CE, et al: Energy availability, macronutrient intake, and nutritional supplementation for improving exercise performance in endurance athletes, *Curr Sports Med Rep* 17(6):215–223, 2018. doi:10.1249/JSR.0000000000000494.
Cerea S, Bottesi G, Pacelli QF, et al: Muscle dysmorphia and its associated psychological features in three groups of recreational athletes, *Sci Rep* 8(1):8877, 2018. doi:10.1038/s41598-018-27176-9.
Cermak NM, van Loon LJ: The use of carbohydrates during exercise as an ergogenic aid, *Sports Med* 43:1139–1155, 2013.
Clark A, Mach N: The Crosstalk between the Gut Microbiota and Mitochondria during Exercise, *Front Physiol* 8:319, 2017. doi:10.3389/fphys.2017.00319.
Coates A, Mountjoy M, Burr J: Incidence of iron deficiency and iron deficient anemia in elite runners and triathletes, *Clin J Sport Med* 27(5):493–498, 2017. doi:10.1097/JSM.0000000000000390.
Colombani PC, Mannhart C, Mettler S: Carbohydrates and exercise performance in non-fasted athletes: a systematic review of studies mimicking real-life, *Nutr J* 12:16, 2013.
Dabidi Roshan V, Babaei H, Hosseinzadeh M, et al: The effect of creatine supplementation on muscle fatigue and physiological indices following intermittent swimming bouts, *J Sports Med Phys Fitness* 53:232–239, 2013.

Davis JK, Baker LB, Barnes K, et al: Thermoregulation, fluid balance, and sweat losses in American football players, *Sports Med* 46(10):1391–1405, 2016. doi:10.1007/s40279-016-0527-8.

DellaValle DM: Iron supplementation for female athletes: effects on iron status and performance outcomes, *Curr Sports Med Rep* 12:234–239, 2013.

De Souza MJ, Nattiv A, Joy E, et al: 2014 Female Athlete Triad Coalition consensus statement on treatment and return to play of the female athlete triad: 1st International Conference held in San Francisco, CA, May 2012, and 2nd International Conference held in Indianapolis, IN, May 2013, *Clin J Sport Med* 24:96–119, 2014.

Domínguez R, Cuenca E, Maté-Muñoz JL, et al: Effects of beetroot juice supplementation on cardiorespiratory endurance in athletes. A systematic review, *Nutrients* 9(1):E43, 2017. doi:10.3390/nu9010043.

Dugas J: Ice slurry ingestion increases running time in the heat, *Clin J Sport Med* 21:541–542, 2011.

Earhart EL, Weiss EP, Rahman R, et al: Effects of oral sodium supplementation on indices of thermoregulation in trained, endurance athletes, *J Sports Sci Med* 14(1):172–178, 2015.

Eijsvogels TM, Scholten RR, van Duijnhoven NT, et al: Sex difference in fluid balance responses during prolonged exercise, *Scand J Med Sci Sports* 23:198–206, 2013.

Elliot TA, Cree MG, Sanford AP, et al: Milk ingestion stimulates net muscle protein synthesis following resistance exercise, *Med Sci Sports Exerc* 38(4):667–674, 2006.

Engeln R, SladeK MR, Waldron H: Body talk among college men: content, correlates, and effects, *Body Image* 10:300–308, 2013.

Farrokhyar F, Tabasinejad R, Dao D, et al: Prevalence of vitamin D inadequacy in athletes: a systematic-review and meta-analysis, *Sports Med* 45:365–378, 2015.

Foster JA, Rinaman L, Cryan JF: Stress & the gut-brain axis: regulation by the microbiome, *Neurobiol Stress* 7:124–136, 2017. doi:10.1016/j.ynstr.2017.03.001.

Garthe I, Maughan RJ: Athletes and supplements: prevalence and perspectives, *Int J Sport Nutr Exerc Metab* 28(2):126–138, 2018. doi:10.1123/ijsnem.2017-0429.

Gibbs JC, Williams NI, De Souza MJ: Prevalence of individual and combined components of the female athlete triad, *Med Sci Sports Exerc* 45:985–996, 2013.

Grieshober JA, Mehran N, Photopolous C, et al: Vitamin D insufficiency among professional basketball players: a relationship to fracture risk and athletic performance, *Orthop J Sports Med* 6(5):2325967118774329, 2018. doi:10.1177/2325967118774329.

Hall KD, Heymsfield SB, Kemnitz JW, et al: Energy balance and its components: implications for body weight regulation, *Am J Clin Nutr* 95(4):989–994, 2012. doi:10.3945/ajcn.112.036350.

Hall M, Trojian TH: Creatine supplementation, *Curr Sports Med Rep* 12:240–244, 2013.

Harris KM, Haas TS, Eichner ER, et al: Sickle cell trait associated with sudden death in competitive athletes, *Am J Cardiol* 110:1185–1188, 2012.

Hart G: Gut microbiota, IgG-guided elimination diet and sports performance, *BAOJ Nutrition* 4:052, 2018.

Heaney S, O'Connor H, Gifford J, et al: Comparison of strategies for assessing nutritional adequacy in elite female athletes' dietary intake, *Int J Sport Nutr Exerc Metab* 20:245–256, 2010.

Hew-Butler TD, Eskin C, Bickham J, et al: Dehydration is how you define it: comparison of 318 blood and urine athlete spot checks, *BMJ Open Sport Exerc Med* 4(1):e000297, 2018. doi:10.1136/bmjsem-2017-000297.

Hosseinzadeh J, Maghsoudi Z, Abbasi B, et al: Evaluation of dietary intakes, body composition, and cardiometabolic parameters in adolescent team sports elite athletes: a cross-sectional study, *Adv Biomed Res* 6:107, 2017. doi:10.4103/2277-9175.213667.

Hosseinlou A, Khamnei S, Zamanlu M: The effect of water temperature and voluntary drinking on the post rehydration sweating, *Int J Clin Exp Med* 6:683–687, 2013.

Institute of Medicine: *Dietary reference intakes for water, potassium, sodium, chloride, and sulfate*, Washington, DC, 2005, National Academies Press.

International Olympic Committee: IOC consensus statement: dietary supplements and the high-performance athlete, *Int J Sport Nutr Exerc Metab* 28(2):104–125, 2018. doi:10.1123/ijsnem.2018-0020.

Jagim AR, Camic CL, Kisiolek J, et al: Accuracy of resting metabolic rate prediction equations in athletes, *J Strength Cond Res* 32(7):1875–1881, 2018.

Jäger R, Kerksick CM, Campbell BI, et al. International Society of Sports Nutrition Position Stand: protein and exercise, *J Int Soc Sports Nutr* 14:20, 2017. doi:10.1186/s12970-017-0177-8.

Jetté M, Sidney K, Blümchen G: Metabolic equivalents (METS) in exercise testing, exercise prescription, and evaluation of functional capacity, *Clin Cardiol* 13(8):555–565, 1990.

Jeukendrup AE: Training the gut for athletes, *Sports Med* 47(Suppl 1):101–110, 2017a. doi:10.1007/s40279-017-0690-6.

Jeukendrup AE: Periodized nutrition for athletes, *Sports Med* 47(Suppl 1):51–63, 2017b. doi:10.1007/s40279-017-0694-2.

Jones AM, Vanhatalo A, Bailey SJ: Influence of dietary nitrate supplementation on exercise tolerance and performance, *Nestle Nutr Inst Workshop Ser* 75:27–40, 2013.

Jouris KB, McDaniel JL, Weiss EP: The effect of omega-3 fatty acid supplementation on the inflammatory response to eccentric strength exercise, *J Sports Sci Med* 10:432–438, 2011.

Jung AP, Selmon PB, Lett JL, et al: Survey of sickle cell trait screening in NCAA and NAIA institutions, *Phys Sportsmed* 39:158–165, 2011.

Kanter M: High-quality carbohydrates and physical performance: expert panel report, *Nutr Today* 53(1):35–39, 2018. doi:10.1097/NT.0000000000000238.

Kass LS, Skinner P, Poeira F: A pilot study on the effects of magnesium supplementation with high and low habitual dietary magnesium intake on resting and recovery from aerobic and resistance exercise and systolic blood pressure, *J Sports Sci Med* 12:144–150, 2013.

Kenefick RW, Cheuvront SN: Hydration for recreational sport and physical activity, *Nutr Rev* 70(Suppl 2):S137–S142, 2012.

Kerksick CM, Arent S, Schoenfeld BJ, et al: International society of sports nutrition position stand: nutrient timing, *J Int Soc Sports Nutr* 14:33, 2017. doi:10.1186/s12970-017-0189-4.

Kern BD, Robinson TL: Effects of β-alanine supplementation on performance and body composition in collegiate wrestlers and football players, *J Strength Cond Res* 25:1804–1815, 2011.

Knapik JJ, Steelman RA, Hoedebecke SS, et al: Prevalence of dietary supplement use by athletes: systematic review and meta-analysis, *Sports Med* 46(1):103–123, 2016. doi:10.1007/s40279-015-0387-7.

Koon G, Atay O, Lapsia S: Gastrointestinal considerations related to youth sports and the young athlete, *Transl Pediatr* 6(3):129–136, 2017. doi:10.21037/tp.2017.03.10.

Kreider RB, Kalman DS, Antonio J, et al: International Society of Sports Nutrition position stand: safety and efficacy of creatine supplementation in exercise, sport, and medicine, *J Int Soc Sports Nutr* 14:18, 2017 doi:10.1186/s12970-017-0173-z.

Lamprecht M, Bogner S, Schippinger G, et al: Probiotic supplementation affects markers of intestinal barrier, oxidation, and inflammation in trained men; a randomized, double-blinded, placebo-controlled trial, *J Int Soc Sports Nutr* 9(1):45, 2012. doi:10.1186/1550-2783-9-45.

Lanhers C, Pereira B, Naughton G, et al: Creatine supplementation and upper limb strength performance: a systematic review and meta-analysis, *Sports Med* 47(1):163–173, 2017. doi:10.1007/s40279-016-0571-4.

Larson-Meyer DE, Woolf K, Burke L: Assessment of nutrient status in athletes and the need for supplementation, *Int J Sport Nutr Exerc Metab* 28(2):139–158, 2018. doi:10.1123/ijsnem.2017-0338.

Lukaski HC: Vitamin and mineral status: effects on physical performance, *Nutrition* 20(7-8):632–644, 2004.

Lynch S: The differential effects of a complex protein drink versus isocaloric carbohydrate drink on performance indices following high-intensity resistance training: a two arm crossover design, *J Int Soc Sports Nutr* 10:31, 2013.

Malliaropoulos N, Tsitas K, Porfiriadou A, et al: Blood phosphorus and magnesium levels in 130 elite track and field athletes, *Asian J Sports Med* 4:49–53, 2013.

Manore MM: Weight management for athletes and active individuals: a brief review, *Sports Med* 45(Suppl 1):S83–S92, 2015. doi:10.1007/s40279-015-0401-0.

Maughan RJ, Shirreffs SM, Vernec A: Making decisions about supplement use, *Int J Sport Nutr Exerc Metab* 28(2):212–219, 2018. doi:10.1123/ijsnem.2018-0009.

McArdle WD, Katch FI, Katch VL: *Exercise physiology: nutrition, energy, and human performance*, ed 8, Philadelphia, PA, 2014, Lippincott Williams & Wilkins.

McClung JP, et al: Female athletes: a population at risk of vitamin and mineral deficiencies affecting health and performance, *J Trace Elem Med Biol* 28:388–392, 2014.

McDermott BP, Anderson SA, Armstrong LE, et al: National athletic trainers' association position statement: fluid replacement for the physically active, *J Athl Train* 52(9):877–895, 2017. doi:10.4085/1062-6050-52.9.02.

Mckendry J, Breen L, Shad BJ, et al: Muscle morphology and performance in master athletes: a systematic review and meta-analyses, *Ageing Res Rev* 45:62–82, 2018. doi:10.1016/j.arr.2018.04.007.

Michael-Titus AT, Priestley JV: Omega-3 fatty acids and traumatic neurological injury: from neuroprotection to neuroplasticity? *Trends Neurosci* 37:30–38, 2014.

Mielgo-Ayuso J, Maroto-Sánchez B, Luzardo-Socorro R, et al: Evaluation of nutritional status and energy expenditure in athletes, *Nutr Hosp* 26;31(Suppl 3):227–336, 2015. doi:10.3305/nh.2015.31.sup3.8770.

Mills CE, Khatri J, Maskell P, et al: It is rocket science - why dietary nitrate is hard to 'beet'! Part II: further mechanisms and therapeutic potential of the nitrate-nitrite-NO pathway, *Br J Clin Pharmacol* 83(1):140–151, 2017. doi:10.1111/bcp.12918.

Morente-Sánchez J, Zabala M: Doping in sport: a review of elite athletes' attitudes, beliefs, and knowledge, *Sports Med* 43:395–411, 2013.

Moslehi N, Vafa M, Sarrafzadeh J, et al: Does magnesium supplementation improve body composition and muscle strength in middle-aged overweight women? A double-blind, placebo-controlled, randomized clinical trial, *Biol Trace Elem Res* 153:111–118, 2013.

Mountjoy M, Sundgot-Borgen J, Burke L, et al: The IOC consensus statement: beyond the Female Athlete Triad—Relative Energy Deficiency in Sport (RED-S), *Br J Sports Med* 48:491–497, 2014.

Murray SB, Rieger E, Hildebrandt T, et al: A comparison of eating, exercise, shape, and weight related symptomatology in males with muscle dysmorphia and anorexia nervosa, *Body Image* 9:193–200, 2012.

National Institutes of Health [NIH], Office of Dietary Supplements: *Dietary supplements for exercise and athletic performance*, 2017. Available at: https://ods.od.nih.gov/factsheets/ExerciseAndAthleticPerformance-Health-Professional/.

Nuccio RP, Barnes KA, Carter JM, et al: Fluid balance in team sport athletes and the effect of hypohydration on cognitive, technical, and physical performance, *Sports Med* 47(10):1951–1982, 2017. doi:10.1007/s40279-017-0738-7.

O'Sullivan O, Cronin O, Clarke SF, et al: Exercise and the microbiota, *Gut Microbes* 6(2):131–136, 2015. doi:10.1080/19490976.2015.1011875.

Parks RB, Hetzel SJ, Brooks MA: Iron deficiency and anemia among collegiate athletes: a retrospective chart review, *Med Sci Sports Exerc* 49(8):1711–1715, 2017. doi:10.1249/MSS.0000000000001259.

Peart DJ: Quantifying the effect of carbohydrate mouth rinsing on exercise performance, *J Strength Cond Res* 31(6):1737–1743, 2017. doi:10.1519/JSC.0000000000001741.

Peeling P, Binnie MJ, Goods PSR, et al: Evidence-based supplements for the enhancement of athletic performance. *Int J Sport Nutr Exerc Metab* 28(2):178–187, 2018. doi:10.1123/ijsnem.2017-0343.

Pesta DH, Angadi SS, Burtscher M, et al: The effects of caffeine, nicotine, ethanol, and tetrahydrocannabinol on exercise performance, *Nutr Metab (Lond)* 10:71, 2013.

Pettersson S, Ekström MP, Berg CM: Practices of weight regulation among elite athletes in combat sports: a matter of mental advantage? *J Athl Train* 48:99–108, 2013.

Pinckaers PJ, Churchward-Venne TA, Bailey D, et al: Ketone bodies and exercise performance: the next magic bullet or merely hype? *Sports Med* 47(3):383–391, 2017. doi:10.1007/s40279-016-0577-y.

Pons V, Riera J, Capó X, et al: Calorie restriction regime enhances physical performance of trained athletes, *J Int Soc Sports Nutr* 9;15:12, 2018. doi:10.1186/s12970-018-0214-2.

Pope HG Jr, Wood RI, Rogol A, et al: Adverse health consequences of performance-enhancing drugs: an Endocrine Society scientific statement, *Endocr Rev* 35:341–375, 2014.

Potgieter S: Sport Nutrition: a review of the latest guidelines for exercise and sport nutrition from the American College of Sport Nutrition, the International Olympic Committee and the International Society for Sports Nutrition. *South Afr J Clin Nutr* 26(1):6–16, 2013. doi:10.1080/16070658.2013.11734434.

Powers SK, Howley ET: *Exercise physiology: theory and application to fitness and performance*, ed 10, New York, NY, 2018, McGraw-Hill Education.

Rawson ES, Miles MP, Larson-Meyer DE: Dietary supplements for health, adaptation, and recovery in athletes, *Int J Sport Nutr Exerc Metab* 28(2):188–199, 2018. doi:10.1123/ijsnem.2017-0340.

Rogerson D: Vegan diets: practical advice for athletes and exercisers, *J Int Soc Sports Nutr* 14:36, 2017. doi:10.1186/s12970-017-0192-9.

Rosenkilde M, Reichkendler MH, Auerbach P, et al: Changes in peak fat oxidation in response to different doses of endurance training, *Scand J Med Sci Sports* 25(1):41–52, 2015.

Rosset R, Lecoultre V, Egli L, et al: Postexercise repletion of muscle energy stores with fructose or glucose in mixed meals, *Am J Clin Nutr* 105(3):609–617, 2017. doi:10.3945/ajcn.116.138214.

Smurawa TM, Congeni JA: Testosterone precursors: use and abuse in pediatric athletes, *Pediatr Clin North Am* 54(4):787–796, 2007.

Scaramella J, Kirihennedige N, Broad E: Key nutritional strategies to optimize performance in para athletes, *Phys Med Rehabil Clin N Am* 29(2):283–298, 2018. doi:10.1016/j.pmr.2018.01.005.

Setaro L, Santos-Silva PR, Nakano EY, et al: Magnesium status and the physical performance of volleyball players: effects of magnesium supplementation, *J Sports Sci* 32:438–445, 2014.

Shei RJ, Lindley MR, Mickleborough TD: Omega-3 polyunsaturated fatty acids in the optimization of physical performance, *Mil Med* 179 (Suppl 11):144–156, 2014. doi:10.7205/MILMED-D-14-00160.

Shekelle PG, Hardy ML, Morton SC, et al: Efficacy and safety of ephedra and ephedrine for weight loss and athletic performance: a meta-analysis, *JAMA* 289(12):1537–1545, 2003.

Shuler FD, Wingate MK, Moore GH, et al: Sports health benefits of vitamin d, *Sports Health* 4:496–501, 2012.

Sikora-Klak J, Narvy SJ, Yang J, et al: The effect of abnormal vitamin D levels in athletes, *Perm J* 22:17–216, 2018. doi:10.7812/TPP/17-216.

Sousa M, Teixeira VH, Soares J: Dietary strategies to recover from exercise-induced muscle damage, *Int J Food Sci Nutr* 65:151–163, 2014.

Spriet LL: Exercise and sport performance with low doses of caffeine, *Sports Med* 44(Suppl 2):S175–S184, 2014.

Stohs SJ: Safety, efficacy, and mechanistic studies regarding citrus aurantium (bitter orange) extract and p-synephrine, *Phytother Res* 31(10):1463–1474, 2017. doi:10.1002/ptr.5879.

Sureda A, Ferrer MD, Mestre A, et al: Prevention of neutrophil protein oxidation with vitamins C and E diet supplementation without affecting the adaptive response to exercise, *Int J Sport Nutr Exerc Metab* 23:31–39, 2013.

Suzuki A, Okazaki K, Imai D, et al: Thermoregulatory responses are attenuated after fructose but not glucose intake, *Med Sci Sports Exerc* 46:1452–1461, 2014.

ter Steege RW, Geelkerken RH, Huisman AB, et al: Abdominal symptoms during physical exercise and the role of gastrointestinal ischaemia: a study in 12 symptomatic athletes, *Br J Sports Med* 46:931–935, 2012.

Thomas DT, Erdman KA, Burke LM: Position of the Academy of Nutrition and Dietetics, Dietitians of Canada, and the American College of Sports Medicine: Nutrition and Athletic Performance, *J Acad Nutr Diet* 116(3):501–528, 2016. doi:10.1016/j.jand.2015.12.006.

Tipton KD, Phillips SM: Dietary protein for muscle hypertrophy, *Nestle Nutr Inst Workshop Ser* 76:73–84, 2013.

Todd JJ, Pourshahidi LK, McSorley EM, et al: Vitamin D: recent advances and implications for athletes, *Sports Med* 45(2):213–229, 2015.

Trexler ET, Smith-Ryan AE, Stout JR, et al: International society of sports nutrition position stand: Beta-Alanine, *J Int Soc Sports Nutr* 12:30, 2015. doi:10.1186/s12970-015-0090-y.

Turocy PS, DePalma BF, Horswill CA, et al: National Athletic Trainers' Association position statement: safe weight loss and maintenance practices in sport and exercise, *J Athl Train* 46:322–336, 2011.

Tyler CJ, Reeve T, Hodges GJ, et al: The effects of heat adaptation on physiology, perception and exercise performance in the heat: a meta-analysis, *Sports Med* 46(11):1699–1724, 2016. doi:10.1007/s40279-016-0538-5.

Volpe SL, Poule KA, Bland EG: Estimation of prepractice hydration status of National Collegiate Athletic Association Division I athletes, *J Athl Train* 44:624–629, 2009.

Wall BA, Watson G, Peiffer JJ, et al: Current hydration guidelines are erroneous: dehydration does not impair exercise performance in the heat, *Br J Sports Med* 49(16):1077–1083, 2013.

Wang R, Chen C, Liu W, et al: The effect of magnesium supplementation on muscle fitness: a meta-analysis and systematic review, *Magnes Res* 30(4):120–132, 2017. doi:10.1684/mrh.2018.0430.

Wardenaar F, Brinkmans N, Ceelen I, et al: Micronutrient intakes in 553 dutch elite and sub-elite athletes: prevalence of low and high intakes in users and non-users of nutritional supplements, *Nutrients* 9(2):E142, 2017. doi:10.3390/nu9020142.

Wierniuk A, Włodarek D: Estimation of energy and nutritional intake of young men practicing aerobic sports, *Rocz Panstw Zakl Hig* 64:143–148, 2013.

Williams J, Abt G, Kilding AE: Effects of creatine monohydrate supplementation on simulated soccer performance, *Int J Sports Physiol Perform* 9: 503–510, 2014.

Williamson L, New D: How the use of creatine supplements can elevate serum creatinine in the absence of underlying kidney pathology, *BMJ Case Rep* Sep 19, 2014. pii: bcr2014204754. doi:10.1136/bcr-2014-204754.

Wylie LJ, Mohr M, Krustrup P, et al: Dietary nitrate supplementation improves team sport-specific intense intermittent exercise performance, *Eur J Appl Physiol* 113:1673–1684, 2013.

Zdešar Kotnik K, Jurak G, Starc G, et al: Faster, stronger, healthier: adolescent-stated reasons for dietary supplementation, *J Nutr Educ Behav* 49(10):817–826.e1, 2017. doi:10.1016/j.jneb.2017.07.005.

23

Nutrition and Bone Health

Karen Chapman-Novakofski, PhD, RDN, LDN
Rickelle Richards, PhD, MPH, RDN

KEY TERMS

7-dehydrocholesterol
25-hydroxy vitamin D (calcidiol)
1,25-dihydroxy vitamin D_3 (calcitriol)
bisphosphonates
bone densitometry
bone mineral content (BMC)
bone mineral density (BMD)
bone modeling
bone remodeling
bone resorption
calcium homeostasis
calcitonin

cancellous bone
collagen
cortical bone
estrogen agonists
estrogen receptor (ER)
hydroxyapatite
hyponatremia
osteoblast
osteocalcin
osteoclast
osteocytes
osteoid

osteomalacia
osteopenia
osteoporosis
parathyroid hormone (PTH)
peak bone mass (PBM)
primary osteoporosis
sarcopenia
secondary osteoporosis
selective estrogen receptor modulator
   (SERM)
trabecular bone

INTRODUCTION

Adequate nutrition is essential for the development and maintenance of the skeleton. Although diseases of the bone such as osteoporosis and osteomalacia (a condition of impaired mineralization caused by vitamin D and calcium deficiency) have complex causes, the development of these diseases can be minimized by providing adequate nutrients throughout the life cycle. Of these diseases, osteoporosis is the most common and destructive of productivity and quality of life. As true of many chronic diseases, signs and symptoms of osteoporosis become more evident in older age.

As more adults reach older ages, osteoporosis with resulting hip, wrist, and vertebral fractures has become more significant in cost, morbidity, and mortality in the United States. Prevention and treatment are equally important to the quality of life.

BONE STRUCTURE AND BONE PHYSIOLOGY

Bone is a term used to mean both an organ, such as the femur, and a tissue, such as trabecular bone tissue. Each bone contains bone tissues of two major types, trabecular and cortical. These tissues undergo bone modeling during growth (height gain) and bone remodeling after growth ceases.

Bone mass is a generic term that refers to bone mineral content (BMC). Bone mineral density (BMD) describes the mineral content of bone per unit of bone. Neither BMC nor BMD provides information on the microarchitectural (three-dimensional) structural quality of bone tissue (i.e., index of risk of fracture).

Composition of Bone

Bone consists of an organic matrix or osteoid, primarily collagen fibers, in which salts of calcium and phosphate are deposited in combination with hydroxyl ions in crystals of hydroxyapatite. The cable-like tensile strength of collagen and the hardness of hydroxyapatite combine to give bone its great strength. Other components of the bone matrix include osteocalcin, osteopontin, and several other matrix proteins.

Types of Bone Tissue

Approximately 80% of the skeleton consists of compact or cortical bone tissue. Shafts of the long bones contain primarily cortical bone, which consists of osteons or Haversian systems that undergo continuous but slow remodeling, and both contain an outer periosteal layer of compact circumferential lamellae and an inner endosteal layer of trabecular tissue. The remaining 20% of the skeleton is trabecular or cancellous bone tissue, which exists in the knobby ends of the long bones, the iliac crest of the pelvis, the wrists, scapulas, vertebrae, and the regions of bones that line the marrow. Trabecular bone is less dense than cortical bone as a result of an open structure of interconnecting bony spicules that resemble a sponge in appearance.

The elaborate interconnecting components (columns and struts) of trabecular bone add support to the cortical bone shell of the long bones and provide a large surface area that is exposed to circulating fluids from the marrow and is lined by a disproportionately larger number of cells than cortical bone tissue. Therefore trabecular bone tissue is much more responsive to estrogens or the lack of estrogens than cortical bone tissue (Fig. 23.1). The loss of trabecular bone tissue late in life is largely responsible for the occurrence of fractures, especially those of the spine (vertebral fractures).

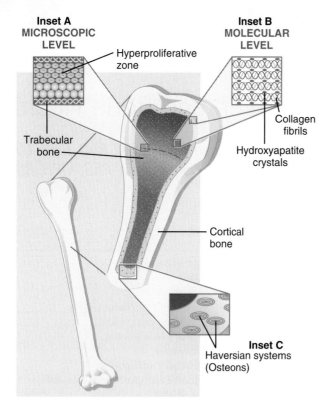

Fig. 23.1 Schematic diagram of the structure of a long bone (hemisection of a long bone, such as the tibia). The ends of the long bones contain high percentages of trabecular (cancellous) bone tissue, whereas the shaft contains predominately cortical bone tissue. *Inset A* includes an enlarged section (approximately 100-fold) of the growth plate (epiphysis) and the subjacent hyperproliferative zone containing cartilage cells stacked like coins. *Inset B* includes a section of collagen molecules (triple helices) surrounded by mineralized deposits (dark spheroids) at a magnification of approximately 1,000,000-fold. These collagen-mineral complexes exist in both trabecular and cortical bone tissues. *Inset C* shows the cross-section of half of the midshaft of a long bone (magnification 10-fold). This section of cortical bone tissue contains vertical Haversian systems (osteons) that run parallel with the shaft axis; many are required to extend this system from one end of the shaft to the other. At the center of each osteon is a canal that contains an artery that supplies bone tissues with nutrients and oxygen, a vein for removing wastes, and a nerve for returning afferent relays to the brain. (Copyright John J. B. Anderson and Sanford C. Garner.)

Bone Cells

Osteoblasts are responsible for the formation or production of bone tissue, and osteoclasts govern the resorption or breakdown of bone (also see Bone Modeling and Bone Remodeling later in this chapter). The functions of these two cell types are listed in Table 23.1.

Two other important cell types also exist in bone tissue, osteocytes and bone-lining cells (inactive osteoblasts), both of which are derived from osteoblasts. The origin of the osteoblasts and osteoclasts is from primitive precursor cells found in bone marrow, stimulated by hormones and growth factors as part of their differentiation to become mature, functional bone cells.

Cartilage

In the embryo, cartilage forms the first temporary skeleton, until it develops into a mature bone matrix. In the adult, cartilage is found as flexible supports in areas such as the nose and ear. Cartilage is not bone, and it is neither vascularized nor calcified.

TABLE 23.1 Functions of Osteoblasts and Osteoclasts

Osteoblasts	Osteoclasts
Bone Formation	**Bone Resorption**
Synthesis of matrix proteins: • Collagen type 1 (90%); • Osteocalcin and others (10%)	Degradation of bone tissue via enzymes and acid (H^+) secretion
Mineralization	
Communication: Secretion of cytokines that act on osteoblasts	Communication: Secretion of enzymes that act on osteoclasts

Calcium Homeostasis

Bone tissue serves as a reservoir of calcium and other minerals. Calcium homeostasis refers to the process of maintaining a constant serum calcium concentration. The serum calcium is regulated by complex mechanisms that balance calcium intake and excretion with bodily needs. When calcium intake is not adequate, homeostasis is maintained by drawing on mineral from the bone to keep the serum calcium ion concentration at its set level (approximately 8.5 to 10 mg/dL). Homeostasis can be accomplished by drawing from two major skeletal sources: readily mobilizable calcium ions in the bone fluid or osteoclastic resorption from the bone tissue itself. The daily turnover of skeletal calcium ions (transfers in and out of bone) supports the dynamic activity of bone tissue in calcium homeostasis.

Serum calcium concentration is regulated by two calcium-regulating hormones—parathyroid hormone (PTH) and 1,25 dihydroxy vitamin D3 (calcitriol). If serum calcium levels fall, PTH will increase reabsorption from the kidney and bone, and calcitriol will increase gut absorption and initiate osteoclastic activity for bone breakdown. Increased serum calcium, hypercalcemia, occurs primarily due to hyperparathyroidism. Serum calcium includes free calcium (formerly called ionized calcium) and albumin-bound calcium.

Bone Modeling

Bone modeling is the term applied to the growth of the skeleton. Bone formation and resorption are not linked as they are in remodeling. In long bones, growth occurs both at terminal epiphyses (growth plates that undergo hyperproliferation) and circumferentially in lamellae; at each location, cells undergo division and contribute to the formation of new bone tissue (see Fig. 23.1). Although we typically consider bone modeling complete by the time mature height is achieved, bone modeling can occur later in life, especially in response to physical activity. Bone modeling results in the formation of new bone, but it does not remove or repair old bone as is seen in bone remodeling (Langdahl et al, 2016).

During the growth period, formation exceeds the resorption of bone. Peak bone mass (PBM) is reached by 30 years of age or so (Fig. 23.2). The long bones stop growing in length by approximately age 18 in females and age 20 in males, but bone mass continues to accumulate for a few more years by a process known as consolidation (i.e., filling-in of osteons in the shafts of long bones). The age when BMD acquisition ceases is variable and depends on diet and on physical activity, genetics, and hormonal influences.

PBM is greater in men than in women because of men's larger frame sizes. The greater height of most males accounts for the greater PBM. The variation in BMD within an ethnicity is greater than among ethnicities. Genetics, skeletal size, and presence or absence of chronic

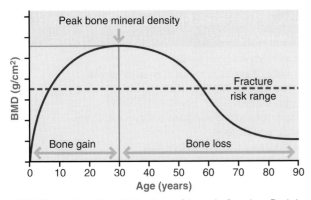

Fig. 23.2 The early gain and later loss of bone in females. Peak bone mineral density (BMD) is typically achieved by age 30. Menopause occurs at approximately age 50 or within a few years. Postmenopausal women typically enter the fracture risk range after age 60. Men have a more gradual decline in BMD, which starts at 50 years. (Copyright John J. B. Anderson and Sanford C. Garner.)

disease influence BMD, and social, environmental, and personal factors also influence probability of fracture risk (Leslie, 2012).

Bone Remodeling

Bone is a dynamic organ both during growth and maintenance. **Bone remodeling** is a process in which bone is continuously resorbed through the action of the osteoclasts and reformed through the action of the osteoblasts. The remodeling process is initiated by the *activation* of preosteoclastic cells in the bone marrow. Interleukin (IL)-1 and other cytokines released from bone-lining cells act as the triggers in the activation of precursor stem cells in bone marrow. The preosteoclast cells from the bone marrow migrate to the surfaces of bone while differentiating into mature osteoclasts. The osteoclasts then cover a specific area of trabecular or cortical bone tissue. Acids and proteolytic enzymes released by the osteoclasts form small cavities on bone surfaces and *resorb* both bone mineral and matrix on the surface of trabecular bone or cortical bone. The resorptive process is rapid, and it is

completed within a few days, whereas the refilling of these cavities by osteoblasts is slow (i.e., on the order of 3 to 6 months or even as long as 1 year or more in older adults).

The *rebuilding* or *formation* stage involves secretion of collagen and other matrix proteins by the osteoblasts, also derived from precursor stem cells in bone marrow. Collagen polymerizes to form mature triple-stranded fibers, and other matrix proteins are secreted. Within a few days, salts of calcium and phosphate begin to precipitate on the collagen fibers, developing into crystals of hydroxyapatite. Approximately 4% of the total bone surface is involved in remodeling at any given time as new bone is renewed continually throughout the skeleton. Even in the mature skeleton, bone remains a dynamic tissue. Normal bone turnover is illustrated in Fig. 23.3.

When the resorption and formation phases are in balance, the same amount of bone tissue exists at the completion of the formation phase as at the beginning of the resorption phase. The benefit to the skeleton of this remodeling is the renewal of bone without any microfractures. With aging, osteoclastic resorption becomes relatively greater than formation by osteoblasts. This imbalance between formation and resorption is referred to as "uncoupling" of the osteoblastic and osteoclastic activity.

Because of the uncoupling of cell activity, age is an important determinant of BMD. Cortical bone tissue and trabecular bone tissue undergo different patterns of aging. Loss of cortical bone occurs around age 50, with an increase in cortical porosity in both genders. Trabecular bone loss may begin much earlier. In men trabecular bone loss reflects thinning of the trabecula. In women, the trabecular bone loss appears to be because of trabecula loss entirely (Farr and Khosla, 2015).

OSTEOPENIA AND OSTEOPOROSIS

This loss of bone can continue throughout aging, eventually leading to osteopenia or osteoporosis. However, it is important to remember that not all older persons have poor bone health, and that bone disease can occur in younger people, although rarely. Differences between normal and osteoporotic bone—both trabecular and cortical tissues—are shown in Fig. 23.4.

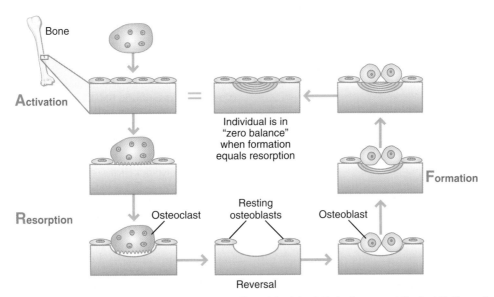

Fig. 23.3 Normal bone turnover in healthy adults. (Copyright John J. B. Anderson and Sanford C. Garner.)

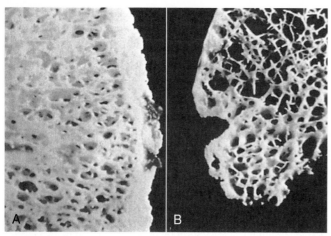

Fig. 23.4 Difference between normal bone **(A)** and osteoporotic bone **(B)**. (From Maher AB et al: *Orthopedic nursing*, Philadelphia, 1994, Saunders.)

Prevalence

The prevalence of osteoporosis depends on the diagnostic criteria. Prevalence estimates using BMD T-scores of <2.5 at the femur neck and/or spine suggest that 10.3% of adults over 50 years in the United States have osteoporosis (Wright et al, 2014). When the Fracture Risk Assessment Tool (FRAX) calculations are used as the diagnostic criteria, 11.6% of men and 13.0% of women over age 50 were predicted to have osteoporosis. When identified low trauma fracture is a diagnosis, with or instead of the low T-score or FRAX score, the osteoporosis prevalence estimates increase to 16% of men and 29.9% of women over 50 years (Wright et al, 2017).

Types of Osteoporosis

Osteoporosis is considered to have a broad spectrum of variant forms. Primary osteoporosis occurs as a result of the natural aging process. BMD declines both with age and with the loss of estrogen after menopause. For women, primary osteoporosis is more likely 10 to 15 years after menopause, and in men, around age 65 to 80 (Ji and Yu, 2015). However, lifestyle factors and genetics also influence if and when osteoporosis may occur. Secondary osteoporosis results when an identifiable drug or disease process causes loss of bone tissue (Box 23.1).

Causes and Risk Factors

Osteoporosis is a complex, heterogeneous disorder and many risk factors contribute during a lifetime. Low BMD is common to all types of

osteoporosis, but an imbalance between bone resorption and formation results from an array of factors characteristic of each form of this disease. Risk factors for osteoporosis include age, race, gender, and factors noted in Box 23.2.

Alcohol

Excessive alcohol consumption is a risk factor for developing osteoporosis, probably because of toxic effects on osteoblasts. Moderate alcohol intake seems to have no detrimental effect on bone, and some studies show a modest positive effect. Three or more drinks per day is associated with increased risk of falling and may pose other threats to bone health (Abrahamsen et al, 2014).

Body Weight

There is a strong correlation between BMD and BMI suggesting that a BMI of <21 kg/m² is associated with low BMD and greater fracture risk in women.

Cigarette Smoking

There are direct and indirect cellular effects on bone caused by smoking, as well as possible hormonal changes and lower dietary calcium absorption. Smoking may also be associated with lower body weight, decreased physical activity, and poor diet (Abrahamsen et al, 2014).

Ethnicity

Osteoporosis is a multifactorial disease, and determining the role of ethnicity in osteoporosis, BMD, bone strength, bone quality, and fracture incidence is difficult. While genetics have made strides in determining the role of ethnicity or race in these outcomes, the blending of ethnicities and races also makes definitive statements elusive. In addition, ethnicity has an influence on many lifestyle factors that could also affect these outcomes, such as diet and physical activity. A related issue is body frame size, often associated with an ethnic group (Rivadeneira and Uitterlinden, 2017).

Limited Weight-Bearing Exercise

Accrual and maintenance of healthy bone requires exposure to weight-bearing pressures throughout the lifespan. Immobility in varying degrees is well recognized as a cause of bone loss. Invalids confined to bed or persons unable to move freely are commonly affected. Astronauts living in conditions of zero gravity for only a few days experience bone loss, especially in the lower extremities; appropriate exercise is a feature of their daily routines.

Loss of Menses

Acceleration of bone loss coincides with menopause, either natural or surgical, at which time the ovaries stop producing estrogen. In association with the decline in estrogen, more bone sites are undergoing resorption and for a longer time, with bone formation diminished. Compensatory mechanisms for the efflux of calcium from bone during this period of enhanced resorption include decreased renal calcium reabsorption, decreased intestinal calcium absorption, and reduced PTH secretion (Drake et al, 2015).

Any interruption of menstruation for an extended period results in bone loss. The amenorrhea that accompanies excessive weight loss seen in patients with anorexia nervosa or in hypothalamic amenorrhea, which occurs in individuals who participate in high-intensity sports or dance, is often associated with lifetime low bone density, compromised bone architecture, and increased fracture risk (Chou and Mantzoros, 2018).

Nutrients

Many nutrients and several nonnutrients have been implicated as causal risk factors for osteoporosis. Poor calcium and vitamin D intake have been linked to poor bone health, osteoporosis, and fracture risk. Vitamin C assists in the formation of collagen, which is necessary for healthy bones. Other nutrients that may play a role include protein (when it is too high or too low), vitamins A, B_6, B_{12}, E, and K, as well as thiamin (Abrahamsen et al, 2014).

Medications

A number of medications contribute adversely to osteoporosis, either by interfering with calcium absorption or by actively promoting calcium loss from bone (Box 23.3). For example, corticosteroids affect vitamin D metabolism and can lead to bone loss. Excessive amounts of exogenous thyroid hormone can promote loss of bone mass over time.

Sarcopenia

Sarcopenia is defined as a loss of skeletal muscle, with associated decline in muscle function. This results in increased risk for falls and disability. Sarcopenia is associated with low bone mass, osteoporosis, and hip fractures in most studies (Oliveira and Vaz, 2015).

BOX 23.3   Medications that Increase Calcium Loss and Promote Risk of Osteoporosis

Aluminum-containing antacids
Corticosteroids
Cyclosporine
Heparin
Lasix and thiazide diuretics
Lithium
Medroxyprogesterone acetate
Methotrexate
Phenobarbital
Phenothiazine derivatives
Phenytoin (Dilantin)
Thyroid hormone
Tetracycline

Diagnosis and Monitoring

Bone densitometry measures bone mass on the basis of tissue absorption of photons produced by x-ray tubes. Dual-energy x-ray absorptiometry (DEXA) (see Chapter 5) is available in most hospitals and many clinics for the measurement of the total body and regional skeletal sites such as the lumbar vertebrae and the proximal femur (hip). Results of DEXA measurements are commonly expressed as T-scores. When the BMD T-score is 2.5 standard deviations (SDs) below the mean, a diagnosis of osteoporosis is made; between 1 and 2.5 SD is considered low bone mass or osteopenia; and within 1 SD of the adult mean is considered normal.

Definitions

When BMD falls sufficiently below healthy values (1 SD according to World Health Organization [WHO] standards) low bone mass or osteopenia exists. Osteoporosis occurs when the BMD becomes so low (greater than 2.5 SDs below healthy values) that the skeleton is unable to sustain ordinary strains. However, the National Osteoporosis Foundation (NOF) states that the WHO BMD diagnostic classification should not be applied to premenopausal women, men younger than 50 years of age, or children. Clinical assessment and ethnically adjusted Z-scores are thought to be more reflective of the norms in other groups.

Ultrasound Measurements of Bone

Ultrasound instruments measure the velocity of sound waves transmitted through bone and broadband ultrasound attenuation (BUA). Measurements at the calcaneus (heel) correlate fairly well with BMD measurements at this same skeletal site. However, ultrasound measurements are considered screening tools, whereas DEXA measurements are considered diagnostic.

Fracture Risk Assessment

The WHO Collaborating Centre for Metabolic Bone Disease, housed at the University of Sheffield, United Kingdom, developed an algorithm to predict fracture by using femoral head BMD and clinical indicators of low bone mass (Kanis et al, 2011). This uses economic modeling to guide the most cost-effective instances to begin medications (Borgström et al, 2011). Vertebral fractures that are confirmed by x-rays are a strong predictor of future vertebral fractures, as well as fractures at other sites (Kanis et al, 2011).

In the United States the National Bone Health Alliance recognizes FRAX as a means to diagnose osteoporosis risk; however, experiencing previous fractures and BMD testing are other tools that can be used (Siris et al, 2014). Several additional screening measures have been developed and suggested by the U.S. Preventative Services Task Force as being moderately accurate at predicting osteoporosis (Curry, 2018). See Table 23.2.

Bone Markers

Enzymes or degradation products in serum or urine have been used for research and are beginning to be used more often to monitor drug treatment effectiveness. For bone formation, serum osteocalcin, serum bone alkaline phosphatase, and serum procollagen type I N-terminal propeptide (P1NP) are often used. For bone resorption, serum and urine C-telopeptide of type 1 collagen and urine N-telopeptide of type 1 collagen are used. Formation markers are useful in monitoring the effectiveness of anabolic medications, whereas resorptive markers are useful for monitoring antiresorptive medications (Chapurlat and Confavreux, 2016).

TABLE 23.2	**Screening Tools for Osteoporosis**		
Tool Name Abbreviation	**Full Name**	**Authors**	**Variables Used**
FRAX	Fracture Risk Assessment Tool	Kanis et al, 2011	Gender, age, BMI, parental history of hip fracture, tobacco smoking, use of oral glucocorticoids, causes of secondary osteoporosis, alcohol
ORAI	Osteoporosis Risk Assessment Instrument	Cadarette et al, 2000	Age, weight, estrogen
OSIRIS	Osteoporosis Index of Risk	Sedrine et al, 2002	Age, weight, estrogen, previous fracture
OST	Osteoporosis Self-Assessment Tool	Richy et al, 2004	Age, weight
SCORE	Simplified Calculated Risk Estimation Score	Von Mühlen, et al, 1999	Age, weight, previous fracture, rheumatoid arthritis, estrogen, race

BMI, Body mass index

CLINICAL INSIGHT

Postmenopausal Women at High Risk for Hip Fracture

It is important to identify women who are at risk of developing osteoporosis as early as possible so that measures can be taken to monitor bone status and to prevent further bone loss. Because low bone mineral density (BMD) is a major risk factor for osteoporosis, its assessment is clinically useful. Assessment of bone status based on the existence of one or more risk factors such as age, height, weight, smoking status, alcohol consumption, drug use, calcium intake, exercise, frame size, and selected bone markers is not sufficiently accurate. BMD as measured by bone densitometry is more clinically useful. Typically, total body BMD and the regional sites such as the proximal femur and lumbar vertebrae are measured by dual-energy x-ray absorptiometry.

A BMD measurement of an at-risk woman entering menopause (before becoming estrogen deficient) serves as a baseline for subsequent measurements as the individual becomes increasingly estrogen deficient and loses bone mass. This information helps physicians and patients make decisions about the need for and use of drug therapy such as bisphosphonates, parathyroid hormone drugs, and estrogen agonist or antagonists. For men or women on long-term glucocorticosteroid therapy, a BMD measurement may indicate the need for treatment with a bone-preserving medication or calcitonin.

NUTRITION AND BONE

Energy

Calories do not have a direct effect on bone; rather, inadequate calories leading to low body weight or too many calories leading to overweight both have effects on bone. Being underweight is considered a risk factor for osteoporosis, while being overweight may be protective. While BMI and BMD are positively correlated, and fracture risk for hip and spine is lower in obese versus nonobese, fracture risk is higher in obese individuals at the proximal humerus, upper leg, and ankle (Fassio et al, 2018).

Protein

Both protein and calcium are important components of PBM, especially before puberty. Adequate protein intake, with adequate calcium intake, is needed for optimal bone health. Protein intakes greater than the recommended dietary allowance (RDA) may be beneficial in older adults to slow the loss of BMD, reduce the risk of hip fracture, and promote bone health, providing that calcium intakes are also adequate (Rizzoli et al, 2018). However, very-high-protein diets used specifically for weight loss have been linked to decreased BMD (Campbell and Tang, 2010).

Minerals

Calcium

Calcium intake in the primary prevention of osteoporosis has received much attention. The Institute of Medicine (IOM) dietary reference intakes (DRIs) for calcium and vitamin D are given as RDAs. The RDA for calcium from preadolescence (age 9 years) through adolescence (up to 19 years) was increased to 1300 mg/day for both genders (IOM, 2011). The RDAs for calcium in adults, pregnant and lactating women, and children are listed on the inside cover.

The Dietary Guidelines for Americans identified calcium as an underconsumed nutrient (U.S. Department of Health and Human Services and U.S. Department of Agriculture, 2015). Food sources are recommended first for supplying calcium needs because of the co-ingestion of other essential nutrients that aid in absorption. In the United States the primary source of calcium is dairy foods. However, calcium fortification of nondairy foods such as nondairy milks and other beverages, juices, breakfast cereals, bread, and some crackers is common.

Calcium bioavailability from foods is generally good, and the amount of calcium in the food is more important than its bioavailability. However, the order of concern relative to calcium absorption efficiency is first the individual's need for calcium, second the amount consumed because absorption efficiency is inversely related to amount consumed, and third the intake of absorption enhancers or inhibitors. For example, absorption from foods high in oxalic and phytic acid (certain vegetables and legumes) is lower than from dairy products.

The amount of calcium in foods varies with the brand, serving size, and fortification. Read the Nutrition Facts label to determine the amount of calcium per serving. Multiply the daily value (DV) percentage by 10 to determine the milligrams of calcium. For example, a 20% DV equals 200 mg of calcium (see Chapter 12). Labeling for "excellent" (>200 mg/serving) and "good" (100 to 200 mg/serving) sources of calcium are regulated by the Food and Drug Administration (FDA) (FDA, 2013).

Reaching RDA levels of calcium from foods should be the first goal, but if insufficient amounts of calcium from foods are consumed, supplements of calcium are recommended to reach the age-specific RDA. An increasing percentage of the population is taking calcium supplements. Persons who should take supplements include those not meeting the RDA on most days, those taking corticosteroids, those with low bone mass or osteoporosis, women who are perimenopausal or postmenopausal (see *Clinical Insight*, Postmenopausal Women at High Risk for Hip Fracture), and those who are lactose intolerant. Calcium carbonate is the most common form of calcium supplement. It should be taken with food because an acidic environment enhances absorption. For those with achlorhydria, which is a growing concern due to the increase in use of acid-blocking drugs, calcium citrate may

TABLE 23.3 Upper Limit for Calcium Intake

Age	Amount, mg
Birth to 6 months	1000
7-12 months	1500
1-8 years	2500
9-18 years	3000
19-50 years	2500
Over 50 years	2000

be more appropriate because it does not require an acidic environment for absorption and does not further reduce the acidity of the stomach.

Calcium supplementation absorption is optimal when taken as individual doses of 500 mg or less. Many formulations include vitamin D, because the likelihood of needing vitamin D is high if calcium supplementation is needed. Choosing a supplement that has the United States Pharmacopeia designation increases the likelihood that the supplement quantity is consistent with the label, and that good manufacturing practices are used.

Calcium supplementation increases the risk of reaching the upper limit of safety (UL). Other sources of calcium include water and medications, especially antacids. The UL for each age group is listed in Table 23.3.

Phosphate

The body's reserve of phosphorus is found in the bone as hydroxyapatite. Phosphate salts are available in practically all foods either naturally or because of processing. In healthy adults, the urinary phosphorus excretion approximately equals intake.

The impact of higher dietary phosphorus or a low calcium: phosphorus ratio on bone health is unresolved. Researchers have found both a negative effect and no effect, with limitations in the ability to determine dietary phosphorus noted as a complicating issue (Anderson et al, 2017; Calvo and Tucker, 2013).

Trace Minerals

Many trace elements are beneficial for bone health, such as boron, copper, manganese, magnesium, selenium, and zinc. However, cadmium, cobalt, and lead are detrimental. The role of fluoride in bone health is unclear (Zofkova et al, 2017).

Vitamins
Vitamin A

Vitamin A consumption consists of both retinol (animal sources) and carotenoids (plant sources). Some research has linked high dietary intake of retinol to greater risk of osteoporosis and hip fracture. In contrast, carotenoids, the precursors to vitamin A found only in plants, has shown beneficial effects. Although the research is not definitive, generally carotenoids are thought to be safe and beneficial (Tanumihardjo, 2013).

Vitamin D

In 2008 the FDA amended the label health claim regulations concerning calcium and osteoporosis so that they could also include vitamin D because of increasing recognition that vitamin D plays a pivotal role in calcium uptake and therefore bone homeostasis (FDA, 2013). While the main function of vitamin D is to maintain serum calcium and phosphorus levels within a constant range, vitamin D is important in stimulating intestinal calcium transport. Vitamin D also stimulates activity of osteoclasts in bone. In both these areas the net desired effect is to increase calcium availability.

An individual's vitamin D status depends mostly on sunlight exposure, and secondarily on dietary intake of vitamin D. The synthesis of vitamin D by skin exposed to sunlight varies considerably as a result of many factors, including skin color, sunscreen use, environmental latitude, season of the year, time of day, and age (Holick, 2014). The skin of older individuals is less efficient at producing vitamin D following exposure to ultraviolet (UV) light because lower amounts of 7-dehydrocholesterol are present in the skin (Gallagher, 2013). In addition, older adults typically have little exposure to the outdoors and therefore less sunlight. Those who live at northern latitudes in the United States and Canada are at increased risk of osteoporosis because of limited UV light during winter months (Holick, 2014).

The few foods that naturally contain vitamin D are egg yolks; fatty fish such as salmon, mackerel, catfish, tuna, and sardines; cod liver oil; and some mushrooms (see Appendix 38). The vitamin D content of fish varies, as does the content in UV-exposed mushrooms. Fluid milk in the United States is fortified with vitamin D at a standardized level of 400 IU per quart, whereas other foods, including juices, cereals, yogurt, and margarines, may be fortified in varying amounts. The RDAs for vitamin D across the life cycle are shown inside the cover. The UL is 100 µg (4000 IU) for everyone older than 8 years, and lower levels for younger children (see inside cover). From any source, vitamin D must be hydroxylated in the kidney before becoming the physiologically active calcitriol.

To prevent rickets, the American Academy of Pediatrics and other global health professionals recommend that all infants who are exclusively breastfed be supplemented with 400 IU of vitamin D. Infants who are both formula and breastfed should also be supplemented until they are consistently taking 1 liter (1 quart) of formula a day. Experts further recommend continuing the supplementation until 1 year of age, when children begin drinking vitamin D–fortified milk (Munns et al, 2016; Wagner and Greer, 2008).

The older adult is at increased risk for vitamin D deficiency because of the decreased synthesis of vitamin D by the skin and decreased exposure to sunlight, increased body fat, and decreased renal function that decreases the hydroxylation of vitamin D to its active form (Gallagher, 2013; Pourshahidi, 2015). In general, daily vitamin D intake of 20 mcg (800 IU) is recommended for seniors to reach serum 25-hydroxy vitamin D (calcidiol) levels higher than 20 ng/mL, thus preventing vitamin D insufficiency (Gallagher, 2013). The most common blood test for vitamin D status is serum 25-hydroxy vitamin D level, and the normal range is considered to be 20 to 50 ng/mL (Wisse, 2016).

Vitamin K

Vitamin K is an essential micronutrient for bone health. Its role in posttranslational modification of several matrix proteins, including osteocalcin, is well established (Hamidi et al, 2013). Vitamin K may also contribute to favorable bone health through decreasing bone resorption and increasing collagen content in bone cells (Hamidi et al, 2013). Following bone resorption, osteocalcin is released and enters the blood. In this way, osteocalcin serves as a serum bone marker for predicting the risk of a fracture (see Appendix 37).

Most of the vitamin K intake in the United States is from green leafy vegetables, with about one third from fats and oils. Although menaquinones, a form of vitamin K, are formed in the gut by bacteria, the influence of this source on vitamin K status appears to be weak. Many older adults have inadequate intakes of vitamin K, primarily because their consumption of dark-green leafy vegetables is so low. It is important to consider the vitamin K intake in older persons who may also be taking blood-thinning medications (vitamin K antagonists). Rather than having these patients avoid vitamin K in foods and thus jeopardize their bone status, it is better to have the vitamin K daily intake be consistent and regulate the vitamin K antagonist medication. Because it is difficult for older adults to consume a consistent amount of vitamin K in their diet each day, a supplemental form of vitamin K is recommended for those on blood-thinning medications (Mahtani et al, 2014). In fact, it has been shown that therapeutic international normalized ratio (INR) ranges from blood-thinning medication can be achieved with vitamin K in low-dose supplementation and when fluctuations are few (Mahtani et al, 2014).

Other Dietary Components

Several other dietary factors have been associated with bone health, but their relative quantitative importance is not clear.

Alcohol

Although previously mentioned as a risk factor, low to moderate consumption of wine and beer may be beneficial to bone health. High alcohol intake is associated with lower bone density, higher prevalence of osteoporosis, and increased risk of fracture, although associated poor lifestyle factors and comorbid conditions increase the difficulty of interpreting results (Gaddini et al, 2016).

Caffeine

The relationship of consumption of caffeine to osteoporosis has not been clearly established. Whereas coffee intake was associated with a modestly increased risk of bone fracture in women, the opposite was true for men, where higher coffee intake was associated with a decreased risk in a meta-analysis of nine cohort and six case-control studies (Lee et al, 2014). However, a systematic review concluded that up to 400 mg/day of caffeine in healthy adults is not associated with adverse health effects, including bone (Wikoff et al, 2017). Interpretation of the caffeine content of coffee or other beverages is difficult because of variation due to brewing, portion size, and other beverage additions.

Dietary Fiber

Fiber includes a variety of different compounds, and so intake of "fiber" as a category can produce different effects on bone. Prebiotics are a form of fiber that has beneficial effects on calcium absorption and may have beneficial effects on bone health in humans (Wallace et al, 2017). The bioavailability of calcium in plant foods high in oxalates or phytates may be low. The overall impact on BMD, osteoporosis, and fracture risk has not been well studied.

Soy and Isoflavones

Epidemiologic studies have reported the prevalence of hip fracture to be lower in older Asian women who have a diet high in soy and isoflavones compared with older Caucasian women. Human studies have been inconclusive concerning the role of isoflavones on bone health, possibly because of differing study designs, doses, lengths of study, differences in participants, and other dietary or exercise components (Zheng et al, 2016). Soy protein has not been shown to be more beneficial to bone health than other protein sources (Shams-White et al, 2018).

High Acid or Alkaline Diets

Higher acid diets include those high in protein, dairy, and grains. It is theorized that these higher acid diets might increase calcium excretion and have a detrimental effect on bone. The theory also supports a converse beneficial effect of an alkaline diet (high in fruits and vegetables) on bone. Several meta-analyses, experimental studies, observational studies, and reviews have not supported either the negative effect of higher acid diets on bone or the positive effects of an alkaline diet on bone. Higher protein intake may, in fact, have a positive effect on bone (Cuenca-Sánchez et al, 2015; Hanley and Whiting, 2013; Remer et al, 2014).

Sodium

In a recent meta-analysis study, a high-sodium diet was found to increase osteoporosis risk (Fatahi et al, 2018). This association may be attributable to increased calcium excretion (Fatahi et al, 2018). Although the calciuric effect of sodium has been speculated, there seem to be no adverse effects with adequate calcium and vitamin D intake (Ilich et al, 2010). On the opposite end of the spectrum, because sodium is found abundantly in bone, hyponatremia, or low serum sodium, may increase an older adult's osteoporosis risk (Hannon and Verbalis, 2014).

Vegetarian Diets

Research has shown lower BMD among vegetarians compared with omnivores; however, the potential impact on osteoporosis risk is relatively small (Ho-Pham et al, 2009). Vegans and some vegetarians may consume less protein, vitamin D, vitamin B_{12}, and calcium compared with omnivores, thus increasing osteoporosis risk; however, vegan and vegetarian diets also typically include higher levels of other nutrients that may have positive effects on bone (Tucker, 2014). A study done in children concluded that a well-planned vegetarian diet that included dairy and egg intake did not lead to significantly lower bone mass and found some evidence that the lacto-ovo-vegetarian diet was protective against bone abnormalities (Ambroszkiewicz et al, 2018)

Prevention of Osteoporosis and Fractures

The increasing longevity of the population emphasizes the need for prevention of osteoporosis. Universal guidelines apply to everyone. Consuming adequate amounts of calcium and vitamin D, lifelong muscle strengthening and weight-bearing exercise, avoidance of tobacco, moderate or no intake of alcohol, and steps to avoid falls are all part of the holistic approach to a lifestyle that promotes bone health (North American Menopause Society [NAMS], 2010).

Exercise

To preserve bone health through adulthood, the American College of Sports Medicine recommends weight-bearing aerobic activity with high bone-loading force (such as intensive walking, jogging, or ascending/descending stairs) three to five times per week, resistance training two to three times per week, and balance exercises (Chodzko-Zajko et al, 2009; Garber et al, 2011). Regular walking and swimming appear to have minor benefits on BMD in older individuals (Beck et al, 2017).

Diet

The NOF recommends universal guidelines for all adults for the prevention of osteoporosis that includes adequate calcium and vitamin D, and a balanced diet of low-fat dairy, fish, fruits, and vegetables. Although the NOF recommends the same amount of calcium intake as the IOM, the NOF recommends higher amounts of vitamin D than the IOM for those 50 years and older (800 to 1000 IU/day). If these intake goals are not reached by food, supplements should be considered. In addition, achieving and maintaining a healthy weight and consuming a lower sodium diet is recommended for optimal bone health for women.

TREATMENT OF OSTEOPOROSIS

Medical Nutrition Therapy

Calcium (1000 to 1200 mg/day) and vitamin D_3 (800 IU/day) are typically recommended for patients being treated with one of the bone drugs, either antiresorptive or anabolic; ideally patients should achieve these nutrients levels from dietary sources, but if necessary, supplemental forms can be used (Gallagher, 2013; Rizzoli et al, 2014). These amounts are considered both safe and sufficient for bone formation.

Because of the range of nutrients involved in bone health, a healthy diet emphasizing the key nutrients seems most promising in achieving an intake for optimal bone health (Higgs et al, 2017). The registered dietitian nutritionist should evaluate the client's diet for all bone-related nutrients and tailor recommendations based on personal preferences, cultural differences, nutrient recommendations, need for supplements, and strategies that enhance quality of life (Dorner et al, 2018).

Exercise

For those with osteoporosis, recommendations include daily balance exercises, weight-bearing aerobic exercise 5 or more days a week, resistance training 2 or more days a week, and limiting twisting or other activities leading to poor alignment of the spine (Giangregorio et al, 2015). It is important to note that each client's situation with osteoporosis is unique and, therefore, should be evaluated by a health professional to determine appropriate exercises based on the client's specific medical history (Giangregorio et al, 2015).

FDA-Approved Drugs for Prevention and Treatment of Osteoporosis

Most medications approved for the prevention of osteoporosis when BMD is low or there is a high risk of fracture are also approved for the treatment of osteoporosis. These include bisphosphonates (alendronate, risedronate, ibandronate, zoledronic acid), peptide hormones (teriparatide and calcitonin), estrogen (in the form of menopausal hormone therapy), estrogen agonists or selective estrogen receptor modulators (SERMs), and a biologic agent (denosumab). However, because of potential side effects, nonestrogen treatment is recommended, especially if menopausal symptom relief is not a goal.

The bisphosphonates act as antiresorbers on osteoclasts to reduce their bone-degradative activities. They act by inhibiting osteoclast-mediated bone resorption. Possible side effects include gastrointestinal problems and rare cases of jaw necrosis. Teriparatide is a form of PTH that works by increasing osteoblast number and function. Calcitonin is used to inhibit osteoclastic bone resorption by blocking the stimulatory effects of PTH on these cells. Calcitonin can be administered by nasal spray. It improves BMD, especially of the lumbar spine, and it may reduce the recurrence of fractures in patients with osteoporosis. Estrogen agonists or antagonists used to be referred to as selective estrogen receptor modulators (SERMS) are able to stimulate estrogen receptors (ER) in bone tissue and yet have very little effect on the ERs of the breast or uterus. Two examples of these drugs are tamoxifen and raloxifene. The most common side effect is hot flashes. The biologic agent denosumab works by preventing the formation of osteoclasts. Possible side effects include joint and muscle pain.

For those with osteoporosis (men and women), often a bisphosphonate or denosumab (women) is prescribed. Because long-term effects are not clear, treatment is suggested for 5 years rather than lifelong. Patient preferences, risk of falling, other comorbidities, and the costs and benefits of medication should be discussed between client and physician to develop individualized care (Qaseem et al, 2017).

INTEGRATIVE APPROACHES

The most common integrative interventions for bone health include an anti-inflammatory diet, calcium and bone supportive micronutrients such as boron, magnesium and vitamin K and nutritive herbs such as nettle (*Urtica dioica*). Inflammation is a risk factor in many chronic diseases, including osteoporosis. Diet has been shown to be a contributing factor in inflammation and may accelerate bone loss, especially in women (Veronese et al, 2017) (See Chapter 7 and Appendix 22). Dietary supplements containing calcium and other bone support nutrients (covered in this chapter) are a common integrative intervention. For more information about safely recommending dietary supplements, see Chapter 11. Nettle is an anti-inflammatory herb and is a rich source of calcium, about 1400 mg per 100 grams dried herb or 430 mg cooked fresh herb (Suliburska, 2012) (Bauman, 2018). Because this plant contains tiny stinging hairs under the leaves, they must be thoroughly macerated, dried or cooked before eating. Nettles are commonly made into an infusion (¼ cup dried herb to 1 quart of cold water, soaked overnight) or used in soups, casseroles, homemade pesto and egg dishes. The Natural Medicines Database lists potential side effects as diarrhea and skin rash, however this is rare as most of the negative side effects are due to consuming fresh nettles with the stinging hairs in tact. Nettles are not recommended in pregnancy or lactation (Natural Medicines Database, 2019).

CLINICAL CASE STUDY

Grace, a 70-year-old white woman of Northern European ancestry, developed lactose intolerance during her early 50s when she had a serious gastrointestinal infection. She currently is retired, lives alone, and stays indoors most of each day watching television. Approximately 3 years ago at age 67, she had dual-energy x-ray absorptiometry (DEXA) measurements that showed that she had low bone mineral density (BMD) values of her proximal femur and lumbar vertebrae (both values were classified as osteoporotic). Her height and weight at the time were 5'5" and 120 pounds. Her FRAX assessment was a 9.7% of fracture in the next 10 years. Her physician recommended that she start taking supplements of calcium (1000 mg/day) and vitamin D (800 units/day) because of her lactose intolerance and her lack of consumption of all dairy products. Because of the fragility of her bones, her exercise should focus on posture, balance, gait, coordination, and hip and trunk stabilization.

Grace took the supplements regularly for a year when a second set of DEXA measurements revealed that she had practically maintained her BMD values of 1 year earlier, with only a small decline in BMD. However, her continuing low measurements concerned her physician, and he ordered laboratory tests of calcium-regulatory hormones to see if she had any hormonal complications. These tests showed that her parathyroid hormone and 25-hydroxy vitamin D concentrations fell in the upper half of the normal range for each variable. Other routine measurements such as serum calcium and phosphate were normal. After discussion of her high risk of an osteoporotic fracture, her physician decided to place Grace on a bisphosphonate drug in addition to calcium and vitamin D.

After 1 year on the new therapy and continuation of the calcium and vitamin D, her BMD values (her third set of DEXA measurements) actually increased a few percentage points, even though they remained within the classification of osteoporosis. She and her physician decided to continue this for another 4 years before reevaluating her condition.

Nutrition Diagnostic Statement
- Inadequate calcium and vitamin D intake related to avoidance of dairy products as evidenced by diet history revealing less than 20% of estimated requirements.

Nutrition Care Questions
1. How would you classify Grace's calcium intake at the initial visit with her physician (who did not take a diet history or estimate her calcium intake)? Her vitamin D intake? Her exposure to sunlight?
2. What would you have recommended to improve her calcium intake from foods so that she could reduce her supplemental calcium to 500 mg/day? Why would you recommend foods to provide calcium rather than supplements? Could you make similar recommendations for improving her intake of vitamin D from foods?
3. Design a set (3 days minimum) of daily menus that provide approximately 800 mg of calcium from foods alone, which, coupled with a 500-mg supplement, would provide a total of 1300 mg, the current adequate intake for calcium. Similarly, design these same meals to include 400 units of vitamin D, with another 400 units coming from supplements.

REFERENCES

Abrahamsen B, Brask-Lindemann D, Rubin KH, et al: A review of lifestyle, smoking and other modifiable risk factors for osteoporotic fractures, *Bonekey Rep* 3:574, 2014.

Ambroszkiewicz J, Chełchowska M, Szamotulska K, et al: The assessment of bone regulatory pathways, bone turnover, and bone mineral density in vegetarian and omnivorous children, *Nutrients* 10(2):E183, 2018. doi:10.3390/nu10020183.

American College of Sports Medicine, Chodzko-Zajko WJ, Proctor DN, et al: American College of Sports Medicine position stand. Exercise and physical activity for older adults, *Med Sci Sports Exerc* 41(7):1510–1530, 2009.

Anderson JJB, Adatorwovor R, Roggenkamp K, et al: Lack of influence of calcium/phosphorus ratio on hip and lumbar bone mineral density in older Americans: NHANES 2005-2006 cross-sectional data, *J Endocr Soc* 1(5):407–414, 2017.

Bauman H, Perez J: Food as medicine: stinging nettle. American Botanical Council, *HerbalGram* 15(7), 2018. Available at: http://cms.herbalgram. org/heg/volume15/07July/FAM_Nettle.html.

Beck BR, Daly RM, Singh MA, et al: Exercise and Sports Science Australia (ESSA) position statement on exercise prescription for the prevention and management of osteoporosis, *J Sci Med Sport* 20(5):438–445, 2017.

Borgström F, Ström O, Kleman M, et al: Cost-effectiveness of bazedoxifene incorporating the FRAX® algorithm in a European perspective, *Osteoporos Int* 22(3):955–965, 2011.

Cadarette SM, Jaglal SB, Kreiger N, et al: Development and validation of the Osteoporosis Risk Assessment Instrument to facilitate selection of women for bone densitometry, *CMAJ* 162:1289–1294, 2000.

Campbell WW, Tang M: Protein intake, weight loss, and bone mineral density in postmenopausal women, *J Gerontol A Biol Sci Med Sci*, 65:1115–1122, 2010.

Calvo MS, Tucker KL: Is phosphorus intake that exceeds dietary requirements a risk factor in bone health? *Ann N Y Acad Sci* 1301:29–35, 2013.

Chapurlat RD, Confavreux CB: Novel biological markers of bone: From bone metabolism to bone physiology, *Rheumatology (Oxford)* 55:1714–1725, 2016.

Chou SH, Mantzoros C: Bone metabolism in anorexia nervosa and hypothalamic amenorrhea, *Metabolism* 80:91–104, 2018.

Cuenca-Sánchez M, Navas-Carrillo D, Orenes-Piñero E: Controversies surrounding high-protein diet intake: satiating effect and kidney and bone health, *Adv Nutr* 15;6(3):260–266, 2015.

Curry SJ, US Preventive Services Task Force: Screening for Osteoporosis to Prevent Fractures: US Preventive Services Task Force Recommendation Statement, *JAMA* 319(24):2521–2531, 2018.

Dorner B, Friedrich EK: Position of the Academy of Nutrition and Dietetics: individualized nutrition approaches for older adults: long-term care, post-acute care, and other settings, *J Acad Nutr Diet* 118(4):724–735, 2018.

Drake MT, Clarke BL, Lewiecki EM: The pathophysiology and treatment of osteoporosis, *Clin Ther* 37(8):1837–1850, 2015.

Farr JN, Khosla S: Skeletal changes through the lifespan—from growth to senescence, *Nat Rev Endocrinol* 11: 513–521, 2015.

Fassio A, Idolazzi L, Rossini M, et al: The obesity paradox and osteoporosis, *Eat Weight Disord* 23:293–302, 2018.

Fatahi S, Namazi N, Larijani B, et al: The association of dietary and urinary sodium with bone mineral density and risk of osteoporosis: a systematic review and meta-analysis, *J Am Coll Nutr* 4:522–532, 2018.

FDA (Food and Drug Administration). *Guidance for industry: a food labeling guide*, 2013. Available at: https://www.fda.gov/media/81606/download.

Gaddini GW, Turner RT, Grant KA, et al: Alcohol: A simple nutrient with complex actions on bone in the adult skeleton, *Alcohol Clin Exp Res* 40(4):657–671, 2016.

Gallagher JC: Vitamin D and aging, *Endocrinol Metab Clin North Am* 42(2):319–332, 2013.

Garber CE, Blissmer B, Deschenes MR, et al: American College of Sports Medicine position stand. Quantity and quality of exercise for developing and maintaining cardiorespiratory, musculoskeletal, and neuromotor fitness in apparently healthy adults: guidance for prescribing exercise, *Med Sci Sports Exerc* 43(7):1334–1359, 2011.

Giangregorio LM, McGill S, Wark JD, et al: Too Fit To Fracture: outcomes of a Delphi consensus process on physical activity and exercise recommendations for adults with osteoporosis with or without vertebral fractures, *Osteoporos Int* 26(3):891–910, 2015.

Hamidi MS, Gajic-Veljanoski O, Cheung AM: Vitamin K and bone health, *J Clin Densitom* 16(4):409–413, 2013.

Hanley DA, Whiting SJ: Does a high dietary acid content cause bone loss, and can bone loss be prevented with an alkaline diet? *J Clin Densitom* 16(4):420–425, 2013.

Hannon MJ, Verbalis JG: Sodium homeostasis and bone *Curr Opin Nephrol Hypertens* 23(4):370–376, 2014.

Higgs J, Derbyshire E, Styles K: Nutrition and osteoporosis prevention for the orthopaedic surgeon: a wholefoods approach, *EFORT Open Rev* 23;2(6):300–308, 2017.

Holick MF: Sunlight, ultraviolet radiation, vitamin D and skin cancer: how much sunlight do we need? *Adv Exp Med Biol.* 810:1–16, 2014.

Ho-Pham LT, Nguyen ND, Nguyen TV: Effect of vegetarian diets on bone mineral density: a Bayesian meta-analysis, *Am J Clin Nutr* 90(4):943–950, 2009.

Ilich JZ, Brownbill RA, Coster DC: Higher habitual sodium intake is not detrimental for bones in older women with adequate calcium intake, *Eur J Appl Physiol* 109:745–755, 2010.

Institute of Medicine (US) Committee to Review Dietary Reference Intakes for Vitamin D and Calcium; Editors: A Catharine Ross, Christine L Taylor, Ann L Yaktine, and Heather B Del Valle. Washington (DC): National Academies Press (US); 2011.

Ji MX, Yu Q: Primary osteoporosis in postmenopausal women, *Chronic Dis Transl Med* 1(1):9–13, 2015.

Kanis JA, Hans D, Cooper C, et al: Interpretation and use of FRAX in clinical practice, *Osteoporos Int* 22(9):2395–2411, 2011.

Langdahl B, Ferrari S, Dempster DW: Bone modeling and remodeling: potential as therapeutic targets for the treatment of osteoporosis, *Ther Adv Musculoskelet Dis* 8:225–235, 2016.

Lee DR, Lee J, Rota M, et al: Coffee consumption and risk of fractures: a systematic review and dose-response meta-analysis, *Bone* 63:20–28, 2014.

Leslie WD: Ethnic differences in bone mass: clinical implications, *J Clin Endocrinol Metab* 97:4329-4340, 2012.

Mahtani KR, Heneghan CJ, Nunan D, et al: Vitamin K for improved anticoagulation control in patients receiving warfarin, *Cochrane Database Syst Rev* (5):CD009917, 2014.

Munns CF, Shaw N, Kiely M, et al: Global consensus recommendations on prevention and management of nutritional rickets, *J Clin Endocrinol Metab* 101(2):394–415, 2016.

National Osteoporosis Foundation: Clinician's Guide to Prevention and Treatment of Osteoporosis. Cosman F, de Beur SJ, LeBoff MS, Lewiecki EM, Tanner B, Randall S, Lindsay R; National Osteoporosis Foundation. *Osteoporos Int* 25(10):2359–2381, 2014. doi:10.1007/s00198-014-2794-2. Epub 2014 Aug 15. Erratum in: Osteoporos Int. 2015 Jul;26(7):2045-7.

Natural Medicines Database: *Stinging nettle.* TRC Natural Medicines, October, 2019. Available at: https://naturalmedicines.therapeuticresearch. com/databases/food,-herbs-supplements/professional.aspx?productid= 664.

North American Menopause Society: Management of osteoporosis in postmenopausal women: 2010 position statement of the North American Menopause Society, *Menopause* 17:25–54, 2010.

Oliveira A, Vaz C: The role of sarcopenia in the risk of osteoporotic hip fracture, *Clin Rheumatol* 34(10):1673–1680, 2015.

Qaseem A, Forciea MA, McLean RM, et al: Treatment of low bone density or osteoporosis to prevent fractures in men and women: a clinical practice guideline update from the American College of Physicians, *Ann Intern Med* 166(11):818–839, 2017.

Pourshahidi LK: Vitamin D and obesity: current perspectives and future directions, *Proc Nutr Soc* 74(2):115–124, 2015.

Remer T, Krupp D, Shi L: Dietary protein's and dietary acid load's influence on bone health, *Crit Rev Food Sci Nutr* 54(9):1140–1150, 2014.

Richy F, Gourlay M, Ross PD, et al: Validation and comparative evaluation of the osteoporosis self-assessment tool (OST) in a Caucasian population from Belgium, *QJM* 97:39–46, 2004.

Rivadeneira F, Uitterlinden AG: Scrutinizing the genetic underpinnings of bone strength, *J Bone Miner Res* 32(11):2147–2150, 2017.

Rizzoli R, Abraham C, Brandi ML: Nutrition and bone health: turning knowledge and beliefs into healthy behaviour, *Curr Med Res Opin* 30(1):131–141, 2014.

Rizzoli R, Biver E, Bonjour JP, et al: Benefits and safety of dietary protein for bone health-an expert consensus paper endorsed by the European Society for Clinical and Economical Aspects of Osteopororosis, Osteoarthritis, and Musculoskeletal Diseases and by the International Osteoporosis Foundation, *Osteoporos Int* 29(9):1933–1948, 2018. doi:10.1007/s00198-018-4534-5.

Sedrine WB, Chevallier T, Kvasz A, et al: Development and assessment of the Osteoporosis Index of Risk (OSIRIS) to facilitate selection of women for bone densitometry, *Gynecol Endocrinol* 16:245–250, 2002.

Shams-White MM, Chung M, Fu Z, et al: Animal versus plant protein and adult bone health: a systematic review and meta-analysis from the National Osteoporosis Foundation, *PLoS One* 13(2):e0192459, 2018.

Siris ES, Adler R, Bilezikian J, et al: The clinical diagnosis of osteoporosis: a position statement from the National Bone Health Alliance Working Group, *Osteoporos Int* 25(5):1439–1443, 2014.

Suliburska J, Kaczmarek K: Herbal infusions as a source of calcium, magnesium, iron, zinc and copper in human nutrition, *Int J Food Sci Nutr* 63(2):194-198.

Tanumihardjo SA: Vitamin A and bone health: the balancing act, *J Clin Densitom* 16(4):414–419, 2013.

Tucker KL. Vegetarian diets and bone status. *Am J Clin Nutr* 100 (Suppl 1):329S–335S, 2014.

U.S. Department of Health and Human Services, U.S. Department of Agriculture: *2015–2020 Dietary guidelines for Americans*, ed 8, December 2015. Available at: https://health.gov/dietaryguidelines/2015/guidelines/.

Von Mühlen D, Visby Lunde A, Barrett-Connor E, et al: Evaluation of the simple calculated osteoporosis risk estimation (SCORE) in older Caucasian women: the Rancho Bernardo study, *Osteoporos Int* 10:79–84, 1999.

Veronese N, Stubbs B, Koyanagi A, et al: Pro-inflammatory dietary pattern is associated with fractures in women: an eight-year longitudinal cohort study, *Osteoporos Int* 1:143–151, 2018.

Wagner CL, Greer FR, American Academy of Pediatrics Section on Breastfeeding, American Academy of Pediatrics Committee on Nutrition: Prevention of rickets and vitamin D deficiency in infants, children, and adolescents, *Pediatrics* 122:1142–1152, 2008.

Wallace TC, Marzorati M, Spence L, et al: New frontiers in fibers: Innovative and emerging research on the gut microbiome and bone health, *J Am Coll Nutr* 36(3):218–222, 2017.

Wikoff D, Welsh BT, Henderson R, et al: Systematic review of the potential adverse effects of caffeine consumption in healthy adults, pregnant women, adolescents, and children, *Food Chem Toxicol* 109:585–648, 2017.

Wisse B, for the US National Library of Medicine, US National Institute of Health and Human Services, NIH, Updated 2016. Available at: https://medlineplus.gov/ency/article/003569.htm.

Wright NC, Looker AC, Saag KG, al: The recent prevalence of osteoporosis and low bone mass in the United States based on bone mineral density at the femoral neck or lumbar spine, *J Bone Miner Res* 29(11):2520–2526, 2014.

Wright NC, Saag KG, Dawson-Hughes B, et al: The impact of the new National Bone Health Alliance (NBHA) diagnostic criteria on the prevalence of osteoporosis in the USA, *Osteoporos Int* 28(4):1225–1232, 2017.

Zheng X, Lee SK, Chun OK: Soy isoflavones and osteoporotic bone loss: A review with an emphasis on modulation of bone remodeling, *J Med Food* 19(1):1–14, 2016.

Zofkova I, Davis M, Blahos J: Trace elements have beneficial, as well as detrimental effects on bone homeostasis, *Physiol Res* 66(3):391–402, 2017.

24

Nutrition for Oral and Dental Health

Janice L. Raymond, MS, RDN, CSG

Portions of this chapter were written by Diane Rigassio Radler, PhD, RDN.

KEY TERMS

anticariogenic	dentin	lingual caries
calculus	early childhood caries (ECC)	periodontal disease
candidiasis	edentulism	plaque
cariogenic	enamel	remineralization
cariogenicity	fermentable carbohydrate	root caries
cariostatic	fluoroapatite	stomatitis
coronal caries	fluorosis	Streptococcus mutans
demineralization	gingiva	xerostomia
dental caries	gingival sulcus	xylitol
dental erosion	hydroxyapatite	

Diet and nutrition play key roles in tooth development, integrity of the gingiva (gums) and mucosa, bone strength, and the prevention and management of diseases of the oral cavity. Diet has a local effect on tooth integrity; the type, form, and frequency of foods and beverages consumed have a direct effect on the oral pH and microbial activity, which may promote dental decay. Nutrition systemically affects the development, maintenance, and repair of teeth and oral tissues.

Nutrition and diet affect the oral cavity, but the reverse is also true: that is, the status of the oral cavity may affect one's ability to consume an adequate diet and achieve nutritional balance. Indeed, there is a lifelong synergy between nutrition and the integrity of the oral cavity in health and disease related to the known roles of diet and nutrients in the growth, development, and maintenance of the oral cavity structure, bones, and tissues (Touger-Decker and Mobley, 2013).

NUTRITION FOR TOOTH DEVELOPMENT

Primary tooth development begins at 2 to 3 months' gestation. Mineralization begins at approximately 4 months' gestation and continues through the preteen years. Therefore maternal nutrition must supply the preeruptive teeth with the appropriate building materials. Inadequate maternal nutrition consequently affects tooth development.

Teeth are formed by the mineralization of a protein matrix. In dentin, protein is present as collagen, which depends on vitamin C for normal synthesis. Vitamin D is essential to the process by which calcium and phosphorus are deposited in crystals of hydroxyapatite, a naturally occurring form of calcium and phosphorus that is the mineral component of enamel and dentin. Fluoride added to the hydroxyapatite provides unique caries-resistant properties to teeth in prenatal and postnatal developmental periods.

Diet and nutrition are important in all phases of tooth development, eruption, and maintenance (Fig. 24.1). Posteruption diet and nutrient intake continue to affect tooth development and mineralization, enamel development and strength, and eruption patterns of the remaining teeth. The local effects of diet, particularly fermentable carbohydrates and eating frequency, affect the production of organic acids by oral bacteria and the rate of tooth decay as described later in this chapter.

DENTAL CARIES

Dental caries (described below) remains the most common chronic disease in both children and adults despite the fact that it is preventable (National Institute of Dental and Craniofacial Research website). Unfortunately, differences are evident in caries prevalence; approximately 20% to 25% of U.S. children have 80% of the dental caries. Trends in dental caries have demonstrated that children who come from homes in which parents have a college education have fewer caries than children from homes in which parents have less than a college education (Centers for Disease Control and Prevention [CDC], 2017). These differences, or health disparities, may happen as a result of lack of access to care, cost of care not reimbursed by third-party payers (e.g., insurance, Medicaid), lack of knowledge of preventive dental care, or a combination of factors. The CDC cites the percent of U.S. children aged 5 to 19 with untreated dental caries between 2011 and 2014 was 18.6%. The percent of U.S. adults aged 20 to 44 during that same time frame was 31.6%.

Pathophysiology

Dental caries is an oral infectious disease in which organic acid metabolites lead to gradual demineralization of tooth enamel, followed

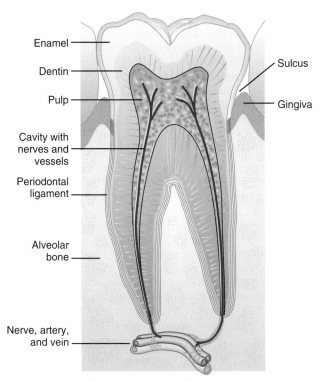

Fig. 24.1 Anatomy of a tooth.

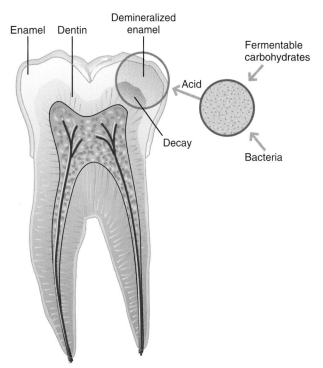

Fig. 24.2 Formation of dental caries.

by rapid proteolytic destruction of the tooth structure. Caries can occur on any tooth surface. The cause of dental caries involves many factors. Four factors must be present simultaneously: (1) a susceptible host or tooth surface; (2) microorganisms such as *Streptococcus* or *Lactobacillus* in the dental plaque or oral cavity; (3) fermentable carbohydrates in the diet, which serve as the substrate for bacteria; and (4) time (duration) in the mouth for bacteria to metabolize the fermentable carbohydrates, produce acids, and cause a drop in salivary pH to less than 5.5. Once the pH is acidic, which can occur within minutes, oral bacteria can initiate the demineralization process. Fig. 24.2 shows the formation of dental caries.

Susceptible Tooth

The development of dental caries requires the presence of a tooth that is vulnerable to attack. The composition of enamel and dentin, the location of teeth, the quality and quantity of saliva, and the presence and extent of pits and fissures in the tooth crown are some of the factors that govern susceptibility. Alkaline saliva has a protective effect and acidic saliva increases susceptibility to decay.

The Oral Microbiome

The microbiome plays an important role in our health and well-being. The oral cavity represents one of the most diverse microbial communities in the human body made up of at least 700 species (Duran-Pinedo and Frias-Lopez, 2015). Microorganisms from the oral cavity are the etiologic agents for a number of infectious diseases, including dental caries, periodontal disease, alveolar osteitis (also known as dry socket that occurs after a tooth is extracted), and tonsillitis. Several studies have linked oral diseases to systemic and chronic diseases including cardiovascular disease, preterm birth, diabetes, pneumonia, and even cancer (Whitmore and Lamont, 2014). The big question in this relationship is whether the changes in the oral microbiota are the cause or the consequence of the pathologic process.

A number of acid-producing species of bacteria have been associated with dental caries. Streptococcus mutans is the most prevalent, followed by *Lactobacillus casein* and *Streptococcus sanguis*. *Bifidobacterium*, *Propionibacterium*, and *Scardovia* have also been associated with caries. In juxtaposition, some bacteria help maintain homeostasis through ammonia production from arginine and urea. For example, *Streptococcus salivarius*, one of the major alkali producers in the mouth, expresses the urease gene under acidic pH and in the presence of excessive carbohydrates (Duran-Pinedo and Frias-Lopez, 2015). Genetic variations of the type and quantity of bacteria present in the oral cavity contribute to an individual's increased risk for caries and periodontal disease, but the quantity and quality of oral hygiene contributes directly to the risk of oral infectious disease.

Substrate

Fermentable carbohydrates, those carbohydrates susceptible to the actions of salivary amylase, are the ideal substrate for bacterial metabolism. The acids produced by their metabolism cause a drop in salivary pH to less than 5.5, creating the environment for decay. Bacteria are always present and begin to reduce pH when they have exposure to fermentable carbohydrates.

Because the Dietary Guidelines for Americans and the MyPlate Food Guidance system support a diet high in carbohydrates, it is important to be aware of the cariogenicity of foods. Cariogenicity refers to the caries-promoting properties of a diet or food. The cariogenicity of a food varies, depending on the form in which it occurs, its nutrient composition, when it is eaten in relation to other foods and fluids, the duration of its exposure to the tooth, and the frequency with which it is eaten (Box 24.1). Individuals should be aware of the form of food consumed and the frequency of intake to integrate positive diet and oral hygiene habits to reduce risk of oral disease.

Fermentable carbohydrates are found in three of the five MyPlate food groups: (1) grains, (2) fruits, and (3) dairy. Although some vegetables may contain fermentable carbohydrates, little has been reported about the cariogenicity, or caries-promoting properties, of vegetables. Examples of grains and starches that are cariogenic by nature of their fermentable carbohydrate composition include crackers, chips, pretzels, hot and cold cereals, and breads.

All fruits (fresh, dried, and canned) and fruit juices may be cariogenic. Fruits with high water content, such as melons, have a lower cariogenicity than others, such as bananas and dried fruits. Fruit drinks, sodas, ice teas, and other sugar-sweetened beverages; desserts; cookies; candies; and cake products may be cariogenic. Dairy products sweetened with fructose, sucrose, or other sugars can also be cariogenic because of the added sugars; however, dairy products are rich in calcium, and their alkaline nature may have a positive influence, reducing the cariogenic potential of the food.

Like other sugars (glucose, fructose, maltose, and lactose), sucrose stimulates bacterial activity. The causal relationship between sucrose and dental caries has been established (Moynihan and Kelly, 2014). All dietary forms of sugar, including honey, molasses, brown sugar, agave, and corn syrup solids, have cariogenic potential and can be used by bacteria to produce acids that erode enamel.

Caries Promotion by Individual Foods

It is important to differentiate between cariogenic, cariostatic, and anticariogenic foods. Cariogenic foods are those that contain fermentable carbohydrates, which, when in contact with microorganisms in the mouth, can cause a drop in salivary pH to 5.5 or less and stimulate the caries process.

Cariostatic foods do not contribute to decay, are not metabolized by microorganisms, and do not cause a drop in salivary pH to 5.5 or less within 30 minutes. Examples of cariostatic foods are protein foods such as eggs, fish, meat, and poultry; most vegetables; fats; and sugarless gums. According to the American Dental Association (ADA) (ADA, 2014), sugarless gum may help to reduce decay potential because of its ability to increase saliva flow and because it uses noncarbohydrate sweeteners.

Anticariogenic foods are those that, when eaten before an acidogenic food, prevent plaque from recognizing the acidogenic food. Examples are aged cheddar, Monterey Jack, and Swiss because of the casein, calcium, and phosphate in the cheese. The five-carbon sugar alcohol, xylitol, is considered anticariogenic because bacteria cannot metabolize five-carbon sugars in the same way as six-carbon sugars such as glucose, sucrose, and fructose. It is not broken down by salivary amylase and is not subject to bacterial degradation. Salivary stimulation leads to increased buffering activity of the saliva and subsequent increased clearance of fermentable carbohydrates from tooth surfaces. Another anticariogenic mechanism of xylitol gum is that it replaces fermentable carbohydrates in the diet. *S. mutans* cannot metabolize xylitol and is inhibited by it. The antimicrobial activity against *S. mutans* and the effect of gum chewing on salivary stimulation are protective. Consumers should be advised to look for chewing gum in which xylitol is listed as the first ingredient.

Remineralization is mineral restoration of the hydroxyapatite in dental enamel. Casein phosphopeptide-amorphous calcium phosphate (CPP-ACP) is a substance that promotes remineralization of enamel surfaces (Cochrane et al, 2012). It is currently available as an ingredient trademarked as Recaldent (Cadbury Enterprises, Australia) in some brands of chewing gum. A randomized prospective study on its efficacy in a specific population with early caries showed no effect (Beerens et al, 2017).

Factors Affecting Cariogenicity of Food

Cariogenicity also is influenced by the volume and quality of saliva; the sequence, consistency, and nutrient composition of the foods eaten; dental plaque buildup; and the genetic predisposition of the host to decay.

Form and Consistency

The form and consistency of a food have a significant effect on its cariogenic potential and pH-reducing or buffering capacity. Food form determines the duration of exposure or retention time of a food in the mouth, which, in turn, affects how long the decrease in pH or the acid-producing activity will last. Liquids are rapidly cleared from the mouth and have low adherence (or retentiveness) capabilities. Solid foods such as crackers, chips, pretzels, dry cereals, and cookies can stick between the teeth (referred to as the *interproximal spaces*) and have high adherence (or retention) capability.

Consistency also affects adherence. Chewy foods such as gum drops and marshmallows, although high in sugar content, stimulate saliva production and have a lower adherence potential than solid, sticky foods such as pretzels, bagels, or bananas. High-fiber foods with few or no fermentable carbohydrates, such as popcorn and raw vegetables, are cariostatic.

Exposure

The duration of exposure may be best explained with starchy foods, which are fermentable carbohydrates subject to the action of salivary amylase. The longer starches are retained in the mouth, the greater their cariogenicity. Given sufficient time, such as when food particles become lodged between the teeth, salivary amylase makes additional substrate available as it hydrolyzes starch to simple sugars. Processing techniques, either by partial hydrolysis or by reducing particle size, make some starches rapidly fermentable by increasing their availability for enzyme action.

Sugar-containing candies rapidly increase the amount of sugar available in the oral cavity to be hydrolyzed by bacteria. Sucking on hard candies such as lollipops or sugared breath mints results in prolonged sugar exposure in the mouth. Simple carbohydrate-based snacks and dessert foods (e.g., potato chips, pretzels, cookies, cakes, and doughnuts) provide gradually increasing oral sugar concentrations for a longer duration because these foods often adhere to the tooth surfaces and are retained for longer periods than candies. In school-age children, more frequent snacking on carbohydrate-containing foods was associated with greater incidence of dental caries (Garcia et al, 2017).

Nutrient Composition

Nutrient composition contributes to the ability of a substrate to produce acid and to the duration of acid exposure. Dairy products, by virtue of their calcium- and phosphorus-buffering potential, are considered to have low cariogenic potential. Evidence suggests that cheese and milk, when consumed with cariogenic foods, help to buffer the acid pH produced by the cariogenic foods. Because of the anticariogenic properties of cheese, eating cheese with a fermentable

TABLE 24.1 Nutrition Messages Related to Oral Health for 3- to 10-Year-Old Children and Their Caregivers

Message	Rationale
Eat starchy, sticky, or sugary foods with nonsugary foods.	The pH will rise if a nonsugary item that stimulates saliva is eaten immediately before, during, or after a challenge.
Combine dairy products with a meal or snack.	Dairy products (nonfat milk, yogurt) enhance remineralization and contain calcium.
Combine fibrous foods such as fresh fruits and vegetables with fermentable carbohydrates.	Fibrous foods induce saliva production and buffering capacity.
Space eating occasions at least 2 hours apart and limit snack time to 15-30 minutes.	Fermentable carbohydrates eaten sequentially one after another promote demineralization.
Limit bedtime snacks.	Saliva production declines during sleep.
Limit consumption of acidic foods such as sports drinks, juices, and sodas.	Acidic foods promote tooth erosion that increases risk for caries.
Combine proteins with carbohydrates in snacks. Examples: tuna and crackers, apples and cheese	Proteins act as buffers and are cariostatic.
Combine raw and cooked or processed foods in a snack.	Raw foods encourage mastication and saliva production, whereas cooked or processed foods may be more available for bacterial metabolism if eaten alone.
Encourage use of xylitol- or sorbitol-based chewing gum and candies immediately after a meal or snack.*	Five minutes of exposure is effective in increasing saliva production and dental plaque pH.
Recommend sugar-free chewable vitamin and mineral supplements and syrup-based medication.	Sugar-free varieties are available and should be suggested for high caries risk groups.
Encourage children with pediatric GERD to adhere to dietary guidelines.	GERD increases risk for dental erosion and thus increases risk for caries.

*Gum is not recommended for children younger than 6 years old.
GERD, Gastroesophageal reflux disease.
Modified from Mobley C: Frequent dietary intake and oral health in children 3 to 10 years of age, *Building Blocks* 25:17, 2001.

carbohydrate, such as dessert at the end of a meal, may decrease the cariogenicity of the meal and dessert (Ravishankar et al, 2012).

Nuts, which do not contain a significant amount of fermentable carbohydrates and are high in fat and dietary fiber, are cariostatic. Protein foods such as seafood, meats, eggs, and poultry, along with other fats such as oils, margarine, butter, and seeds, are also cariostatic.

Sequence and Frequency of Eating

Eating sequence and combination of foods also affect the caries potential of the substrate. Bananas, which are cariogenic because of their fermentable carbohydrate content and adherence capability, have less potential to contribute to decay when eaten with cereal and milk than when eaten alone as a snack. Milk, as a liquid, reduces the adherence capability of the fruit. Crackers eaten with cheese are less cariogenic than when eaten alone.

The frequency with which a cariogenic food or beverage is consumed determines the number of opportunities for acid production. Every time a fermentable carbohydrate is consumed, a decline in pH is initiated within 5 to 15 minutes, causing caries-promoting activity. Small, frequent meals and snacks, often high in fermentable carbohydrate, increase the cariogenicity of a diet more than a diet consisting of three meals and minimal snacks. Eating several cookies at once, followed by brushing the teeth or rinsing the mouth with water, is less cariogenic than eating a cookie several times throughout a day. Table 24.1 lists messages that can be given to children to reduce the risk of developing dental caries.

The Decay Process

The carious process begins with the production of acids as a byproduct of bacterial metabolism taking place in the dental plaque. Decalcification of the surface enamel continues until the buffering action of the saliva is able to raise the pH above the critical level. See Box 24.2 for prevention guidelines and the Practice Paper of the Academy of Nutrition and Dietetics on Oral Health and Nutrition (Mallonee et al, 2014).

Plaque is a sticky, colorless mass of microorganisms and polysaccharides that forms around the tooth and adheres to teeth and gums. It harbors acid-forming bacteria and keeps the organic products of their metabolism in close contact with the enamel surface. As a cavity develops, the plaque blocks the tooth, to some extent, from the buffering and remineralization action of the saliva. In time the plaque combines with calcium and hardens to form calculus.

An acidic pH is also required for plaque formation. Soft drinks (diet and regular), sports beverages, citrus juices and "ades" (such as Gatorade and Powerade, etc.), and chewable vitamin C supplements have high acid content and may contribute to erosion (Tedesco et al, 2012). Research using National Health and Nutrition Examination Survey III data reported significantly more dental caries in children

---

BOX 24.2 Caries Prevention Guidelines

Brush at least twice daily, preferably after meals.
Rinse mouth after meals and snacks.
Chew sugarless gum for 15-20 min after meals and snacks.
Floss twice daily.
Use fluoridated toothpastes.
Pair cariogenic foods with cariostatic foods.
Snack on cariostatic and anticariogenic foods such as cheese, nuts, popcorn, and vegetables.
Limit between-meal eating and drinking of fermentable carbohydrates.

(ages 2 to 10 years) who consumed large amounts of carbonated soft drinks or juices compared with children who had high consumption of water or milk (Sohn et al, 2006). Other beverages and foods contribute to dental erosion, a loss of minerals from tooth surfaces by a chemical process in the presence of acid (Garcia et al, 2017). The current popular practice of drinking fruited water is a hazard to dental enamel. Fruited waters like water with lemon or other citrus added have been shown to have pH levels as low as 3. Regular tap water has a pH of 6 to 8.

Roles of Saliva

Salivary flow clears food from around the teeth as a means to reduce the risk of caries. The bicarbonate-carbonic acid system, calcium, and phosphorus in saliva also provide buffering action to neutralize bacterial acid metabolism. Once buffering action has restored pH above the critical point, remineralization can occur. If fluoride is present in the saliva, the minerals are deposited in the form of fluoroapatite, which is resistant to erosion. Salivary production decreases as a result of diseases affecting salivary gland function (e.g., Sjögren's syndrome); as a side effect of fasting; as a result of radiation therapy to the head and neck involving the parotid gland; normally during sleep and aging; with the use of medications associated with reduced salivary flow; or with xerostomia, dry mouth caused by inadequate saliva production. An estimated 400 to 500 medications currently available by prescription or over the counter may cause dry mouth. The degree of xerostomia may vary but may be caused by medications such as those to treat depression, hypertension, anxiety, human immunodeficiency virus (HIV), and allergies.

Caries Patterns

Caries patterns describe the location and surfaces of the teeth affected. Coronal caries affects the crown of the tooth, the part of the tooth visible above the gum line, and may occur on any tooth surface. Although the overall incidence of decay in the United States has declined, many states report 40% to 70% of children having some decay by age 8 (CDC, 2017).

Root caries, occurring on the root surfaces of teeth secondary to gingival recession, affects a large portion of the older population. Root caries is a dental infection that is increasing in older adults, partly because this population is retaining their natural teeth longer. The gums recede in older age, exposing the root surface. Other factors related to the increased incidence of this decay pattern are lack of fluoridated water, poor oral hygiene practices, decreased saliva, frequent eating of fermentable carbohydrates. Dementia appears to increase risk of dental caries, which is likely related to a decline in self-care and motor skills (Brennan and Strauss, 2014). Management of root caries includes dental restoration and nutrition counseling. Poor oral health from caries, pain, or edentulism often adversely affects dietary intake and nutritional status in older adults. (See Chapter 19.)

Lingual caries, or caries on the lingual side (surface next to or toward the tongue) of the anterior teeth, is seen in persons with gastrointestinal reflux, bulimia, or anorexia-bulimia (see Chapter 21). Frequent intake of fermentable carbohydrates, combined with regurgitation or induced vomiting of acidic stomach contents, results in a constant influx of acid into the oral cavity. The acid contributes to erosion of tooth surfaces that can result in tooth sensitivity and dental caries. The pattern of erosion may be indicative of erosion from reflux versus from foods or beverages (Schlueter et al, 2012).

Fluoride

Fluoride is an important element in bones and teeth (Palmer and Gilbert, 2012). Used systemically and locally, it is a safe, effective public health measure to reduce the incidence and prevalence of dental caries (ADA, 2014; CDC, 2017). Water fluoridation began in 1940; by 1999 the CDC listed water fluoridation as one of the top 10 greatest public health achievements of the 20th century because of its influence on decreasing the rate of dental caries (CDC, 2017). The effect of fluoride on caries prevention continues with water fluoridation, fluoridated toothpastes, oral rinses, and dentifrices, as well as beverages made with fluoridated water. Optimal water fluoridation concentrations (0.7 to 1.2 ppm) can provide protection against caries development without causing tooth staining (ADA, 2014). Despite the positions from the ADA and the Academy of Nutrition and Dietetics (AND), and the data from the CDC on fluoride for oral health, there is a controversy over the use of topical fluoride on teeth and systemic fluoridation in water supplies. Arguments against widespread fluoride use include claims that it can be carcinogenic and toxic; however, consumers should be urged to read the evidence.

Mechanism of Action

There are four primary mechanisms of fluoride action on teeth: (1) when incorporated into enamel and dentin along with calcium and phosphorus, it forms fluoroapatite, a compound more resistant to acid challenge than hydroxyapatite; (2) it promotes repair and remineralization of tooth surfaces with early signs of decay (incipient carious lesions); (3) it helps to reverse the decay process while promoting the development of a tooth surface that has increased resistance to decay; and (4) helps to deter the harmful effects of bacteria in the oral cavity by interfering with the formation and function of microorganisms.

Food Sources

Most foods, unless prepared with fluoridated water, contain minimal amounts of fluoride, except for brewed tea, which has approximately 1.4 ppm (Morin, 2006). Fluoride may be added unintentionally to the diet in a number of ways, including through the use of fluoridated water in the processing of foods and beverages. Fruit juices and drinks, particularly white grape juice produced in cities with fluoridated water, may have increased fluoride content; however, because of the wide variation in fluoride content, it is difficult to estimate amounts consumed.

Supplementation

Health professionals should consider a child's fluid intake as well as food sources and the availability of fluoridated water in the community before prescribing fluoride supplements. Because bones are repositories of fluoride, bone meal, fish meal, and gelatin made from bones are potent sources of the mineral. In communities without fluoridated water, dietary fluoride supplements may be recommended for children ages 6 months to 16 years.

Fluoride can be used topically and systemically. When consumed in food and drink, it enters the systemic circulation and is deposited in bones and teeth. Systemic sources have a topical benefit as well by providing fluoride to the saliva. A small amount of fluoride enters the soft tissues; the remainder is excreted. The primary source of systemic fluoride is fluoridated water; food and beverages supply a smaller amount. Table 24.2 contains a schedule of fluoride supplementation.

Fluoride supplements are not recommended for formula-fed infants or for breastfed infants living in fluoridated communities if these infants receive drinking water between feedings. If the infant does not drink water between feedings or drinks bottled water when on a diet of only breastmilk, fluoride supplementation is recommended according to established guidelines. Fluoride supplements must be prescribed by the child's health care provider; they are not available as over-the-counter supplements (ADA, 2014).

TABLE 24.2 Dietary Fluoride Supplement Schedule

	FLUORIDE ION LEVEL IN DRINKING WATER (ppm)*		
Age	<0.3 ppm	0.3-0.6 ppm	>0.6 ppm
Birth-6 mo	None	None	None
6 mo-3 yr	0.25 mg/day[†]	None	None
3-6 yr	0.50 mg/day	0.25 mg/day	None
6-16 yr	1.0 mg/day	0.50 mg/day	None

*1 ppm = 1 mg/L.
[†]2.2 mg of sodium fluoride contains 1 mg of fluoride ion.
Approved by The American Dental Association, The American Academy of Pediatrics, and The American Academy of Pediatric Dentistry, 1994.

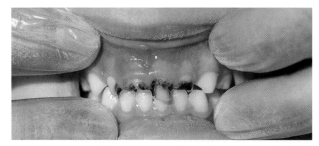

Fig. 24.3 Early childhood caries. (From Swartz MH: *Textbook of physical diagnosis, history, and examination*, ed 5, Philadelphia, 2006, Saunders.)

Topical fluoride sources include toothpastes, gels, and rinses used by consumers daily, along with more concentrated forms applied by dental professionals in the form of gels, foams, and rinses. Frequent fluoride exposure via topical fluorides, fluoridated toothpastes, rinses, and fluoridated water is important in maintaining an optimal concentration of fluoride, but excess intake should be avoided.

Excess Fluoride

Fluorosis occurs when too much fluoride is provided during tooth development and can range from mild to severe and present on teeth from unnoticeable to very apparent dark spots on teeth. Causes of mild fluorosis from excessive fluoride intake include misuse of dietary fluoride supplements, ingestion of fluoridated toothpastes and rinses, or excessive fluoride intake secondary to fluoride in foods and beverages processed in fluoridated areas and transported to other areas. Topical fluorides, available as fluoridated toothpastes and mouthwashes, are effective sources of fluoride that can be used in the home, school, or dental office. Caries prevention efforts in preschool children include diet modification, water fluoridation, or supplements in nonfluoridated areas, and supervised tooth brushing with fluoridated toothpaste (ADA, 2014).

Children younger than 6 years of age should not use fluoridated mouthwashes, and older children should be instructed to rinse, but not swallow, mouthwash. No more than a pea-size amount of toothpaste should be placed on a child's toothbrush to reduce the risk of accidental fluoride. Fluoride is most effective when given from birth through ages 12 to 13, the period when mineralization of unerupted permanent teeth occurs.

EARLY CHILDHOOD CARIES

Early childhood caries (ECC), often called "baby-bottle tooth decay," describes a caries pattern in the maxillary anterior teeth of infants and young children. Characteristics include rapidly developing carious lesions in the primary anterior teeth and the presence of lesions on tooth surfaces not usually associated with a high caries risk. Because tooth decay remains a common oral disease of childhood, caries is a primary marker for a child's oral health. Good behavioral habits and child nutrition patterns must be encouraged, beginning in infancy.

Pathophysiology and Incidence

Often ECC follows prolonged bottle-feeding, especially at night, of juice, milk, formula, or other sweetened beverages. The extended contact time with the fermentable carbohydrate–containing beverages, coupled with the position of the tongue against the nipple, which causes pooling of the liquid around the maxillary incisors, particularly

during sleep, contributes to the decay process. The mandibular anterior teeth usually are spared (Fig. 24.3) because of the protective position of the lip and tongue and the presence of a salivary duct in the floor of the mouth. In general, children from low-income families and minority populations experience the greatest amount of oral disease, the most extensive disease, and the most frequent use of dental services for pain relief; yet these children have the fewest overall dental visits (CDC, 2017).

Nutrition Care

Management of ECC includes diet and oral hygiene education for parents, guardians, and caregivers. Messages should be targeted to counter the health habits that contribute to this problem: poor oral hygiene, failure to brush a child's teeth at least daily, frequent use of bottles filled with sweetened beverages, and lack of fluoridated water. Dietary guidelines include removal of the bedtime bottle and modification of the frequency and content of the daytime bottles. Bottle contents should be limited to water, formula, or milk. Infants and young children should not be put to bed with a bottle. Teeth and gums should be cleaned with a gauze pad or washcloth after all bottle feedings. All efforts should be made to wean children from a bottle by 1 year of age. Educational efforts should be positive and simple, focusing on oral hygiene habits and promotion of a balanced, healthy diet. Between-meal snacks should include cariostatic foods. When foods are cariogenic, they should be followed by tooth brushing or rinsing the mouth. Parents and caregivers need to understand the causes and consequences of ECC and how they can be avoided.

CARIES PREVENTION

Caries prevention programs focus on a balanced diet, modification of the sources and quantities of fermentable carbohydrates, and the integration of oral hygiene practices into individual lifestyles. Meals and snacks should be followed with brushing, rinsing the mouth vigorously with water. Positive habits should be encouraged, including snacking on anticariogenic or cariostatic foods, chewing sugarless gum after eating or drinking cariogenic items, and having sweets with meals rather than as snacks. Despite the potential for a diet that is based on the dietary guidelines to be cariogenic, with proper planning and good oral hygiene a balanced diet low in cariogenic risk can be planned (see Fig. 24.4 for a sample diet).

Practices to avoid include sipping sugar-sweetened and low-pH beverages for extended periods. Adding lemon and other fruits to water has become a common practice but this lowers the pH and in general should be avoided. Frequent snacking and eating sugared breath mints or hard candies is discouraged. Over-the-counter chewable or liquid medications and vitamin preparations, such as chewable vitamin C or liquid cough syrup, may contain sugar and contribute to caries risk. Patients with dysphagia may use thickening agents in

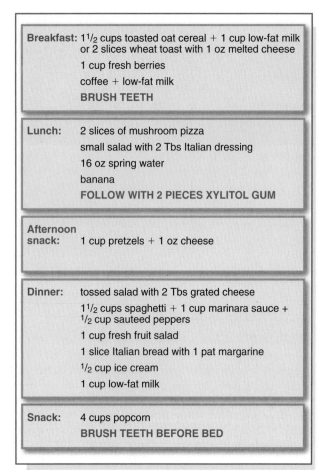

Breakfast: 1½ cups toasted oat cereal + 1 cup low-fat milk or 2 slices wheat toast with 1 oz melted cheese
1 cup fresh berries
coffee + low-fat milk
BRUSH TEETH

Lunch: 2 slices of mushroom pizza
small salad with 2 Tbs Italian dressing
16 oz spring water
banana
FOLLOW WITH 2 PIECES XYLITOL GUM

Afternoon snack: 1 cup pretzels + 1 oz cheese

Dinner: tossed salad with 2 Tbs grated cheese
1½ cups spaghetti + 1 cup marinara sauce + ½ cup sauteed peppers
1 cup fresh fruit salad
1 slice Italian bread with 1 pat margarine
½ cup ice cream
1 cup low-fat milk

Snack: 4 cups popcorn
BRUSH TEETH BEFORE BED

Fig. 24.4 A balanced diet plan with low cariogenic risk.

beverages or liquid foods (soups) to reduce the risk of aspiration. Good oral hygiene should be emphasized in these situations because the thickening agent may contain fermentable carbohydrate and can be sticky, and the type of dysphagia may contribute to inadequate clearing of food from the oral cavity.

Fermentable carbohydrates such as candy, crackers, cookies, pastries, pretzels, snack crackers, chips, and even fruits should be eaten with meals. Notably, "fat-free" snack and dessert items and "baked" chips and snack crackers tend to have a higher simple sugar concentration than their higher-fat-containing counterparts.

TOOTH LOSS AND DENTURES

Tooth loss (**edentulism**) and removable prostheses (dentures) can have a significant effect on dietary habits, masticatory function, olfaction, and nutritional adequacy. As dentition status declines, masticatory performance is compromised and may have a negative effect on food choices, resulting in decreased intake of meat, whole grains, fruits, and vegetables (Tsakos et al, 2010). This problem is more pronounced in older adults, whose appetite and intake may be compromised further by chronic disease, social isolation, and the use of multiple medications (see Chapter 19).

Dentures must be checked periodically by a dental professional for appropriate fit. Changes in body weight or changes in alveolar bone over time possibly may alter the fit of the dentures. This is a common problem in the elderly that interferes with eating. Counseling on appropriate food choices and textures is advocated.

Nutrition Care

Full dentures replace missing teeth but are not a perfect substitute for natural dentition. Before and after denture placement, many individuals may experience difficulty biting and chewing. The foods found to cause the greatest difficulty for persons with complete dentures include fresh whole fruits and vegetables (e.g., apples and carrots), hard-crusted breads, and whole muscle meats. Therefore dietary assessment and counseling related to oral health should be provided to the denture wearer. Simple guidelines should be provided for cutting and preparing fruits and vegetables to minimize the need for biting and reduce the amount of chewing. The importance of positive eating habits must be stressed as a component of total health. Overall, guidelines that reinforce the importance of a balanced diet should be part of the routine counseling given to all patients.

OTHER ORAL DISORDERS

Oral diseases extend beyond dental caries. Deficiencies of several vitamins (riboflavin, folate, B_{12}, and C) and minerals (iron and zinc) may be detected first in the oral cavity because of the rapid tissue turnover of the oral mucosa. Periodontal disease is a local and systemic disease. Select nutrients play a role, including vitamins A, C, and E; folate; beta-carotene; and the minerals calcium, phosphorus, and zinc (see Chapter 5).

Oral cancer, often a result of tobacco and alcohol use, can have a significant effect on eating ability and nutritional status. This problem is compounded by the increased caloric and nutrient needs of persons with oral carcinomas. In addition, surgery, radiation therapy, and chemotherapy are modalities used to treat oral cancer that also can affect dietary intake, appetite, and the integrity of the oral cavity. Some but not all problems affecting the oral cavity are discussed here with relevant nutrition care. Patients may try over-the-counter natural products to prevent or treat oral disease or conditions (see *Clinical Insight:* Natural Products in Oral Health).

PERIODONTAL DISEASE

Pathophysiology

Periodontal disease is an inflammation of the gingiva with infection caused by oral bacteria and subsequent destruction of the tooth attachment apparatus. Untreated disease results in a gradual loss of tooth attachment to the bone. Progression is influenced by the overall health of the host and the integrity of the immune system. The primary causal factor in the development of periodontal disease is plaque. Plaque in the **gingival sulcus**, a shallow, V-shaped space around the tooth, produces toxins that destroy tissue and permit loosening of the teeth. Important factors in the defense of the gingiva to bacterial invasion are (1) oral hygiene, (2) integrity of the immune system, and (3) optimal nutrition. The defense mechanisms of the gingival tissue, epithelial barrier, and saliva are affected by nutritional intake and status. Healthy epithelial tissue prevents the penetration of bacterial endotoxins into subgingival tissue.

Nutritional Care

Deficiencies of vitamin C, folate, and zinc increase the permeability of the gingival barrier at the gingival sulcus, increasing susceptibility to periodontal disease. Severe deterioration of the gingiva is seen in individuals with scurvy or vitamin C deficiency. Vitamins A and E, beta-carotene, and protein have a role in maintaining gingival and immune system integrity, and there is now evidence that some antioxidants can mediate the inflammation associated with periodontal

CLINICAL INSIGHT

Natural Products in Oral Health

Natural products include herbal and dietary supplements and probiotics (National Center for Complementary and Integrative Health [NCCIH], 2015). The following lists some herbal and dietary supplements that may be used to prevent or treat oral health issues. See Chapter 11 for more information about the efficacy and safety of natural products before choosing to use them in addition to or in place of conventional therapy.

Oral Use(s)	Natural Product	Use	Considerations
Mucositis	Hyaluronic acid	Topically (oral gel)	
	German chamomile	Oral rinse	May cause allergic reaction in individuals sensitive to the daisy family.
	Glutamine	Oral rinse	
	Iodine	Oral rinse (in chemotherapy treatment)	
	Kaolin	Oral rinse (in radiation treatment)	
	Aloe	Oral rinse	Only the gel should be ingested. Avoid whole leaf and aloe latex.
Mucosal lesions	Slippery elm	Topically (lozenges)	
Periodontal disease	Coenzyme Q$_{10}$	Systemically	
	Xylitol	In chewing gum or in place of fermentable carbohydrate	

Natural Medicines Comprehensive Database (www.naturaldatabase.com).

disease (Najeeb et al, 2016). When periodontal disease causes pain and avoidance of foods, nutrient intake may be limited and should be monitored (Staudte et al, 2012). Modified food textures may be beneficial to minimize nutrient deficits. The roles of calcium and vitamin D relate to the link between osteoporosis and periodontal disease, in which bone loss may be the common denominator.

In societies in which malnutrition and periodontal disease are prevalent, poor oral hygiene is also usually evident. In such instances it is difficult to determine whether malnutrition is the cause of the disease or one of many contributing factors, including poor oral hygiene, heavy plaque buildup, insufficient saliva, or coexisting illness.

Management strategies for the patient or client with periodontal disease follow many of the same guidelines as for caries prevention listed in Box 24.2. Severe periodontal disease may be treated surgically. Diet adequacy is particularly important before and after periodontal surgery, when adequate nutrients are needed to regenerate tissue and support immunity to prevent infection. Adequacy of calories, protein, and micronutrients should be part of the postoperative care plan.

ORAL MANIFESTATIONS OF SYSTEMIC DISEASE

Acute systemic diseases such as cancer and infections, as well as chronic diseases such as diabetes mellitus, autoimmune diseases, and chronic kidney disease, are characterized by oral manifestations that may alter the diet and nutritional status. Cancer therapies, including irradiation of the head and neck region, chemotherapy, and surgeries to the oral cavity, have a significant effect on the integrity of the oral cavity and on an individual's eating ability, which may consequently affect nutrition status (see Chapter 35).

If the condition of the mouth adversely affects one's food choices, the person with chronic disease may not be able to follow the optimal diet for medical nutrition therapy. For example, poorly controlled diabetes may manifest in xerostomia or candidiasis, which may then affect the ability to consume a diet to appropriately control blood sugar, further deteriorating glucose control.

In addition, many medications alter the integrity of the oral mucosa, taste sensation, or salivary production. Phenytoin (Dilantin) may cause severe gingivitis. Many of the protease inhibitor drugs used to treat HIV and acquired immune deficiency syndrome (AIDS) are associated with altered taste and dry mouth. Reduced saliva contributes to increased caries risk and also may alter the ability to form a bolus and swallow foods, especially dry foods that crumble with mastication. Care should be taken to assess the effects of medication on the oral cavity and minimize these effects using alterations in diet or drug therapy.

Diabetes Mellitus

Diabetes is associated with several oral diseases, many of which occur only in periods of poor glucose control. These include burning mouth syndrome, periodontal disease, candidiasis, dental caries, and xerostomia. The microangiopathic conditions seen in diabetes, along with altered responses to infection, contribute to risk of periodontal disease in affected persons. Tooth infection, more common in those with diabetes, leads to deterioration of diabetes control (Al-Khabbaz, 2014).

Fungal Infections

Oropharyngeal fungal infections may cause a burning, painful mouth and dysphagia. The ulcers that accompany viral infections such as herpes simplex and cytomegalovirus cause pain and can lead to reduced oral intake. Very hot and cold foods or beverages, spices, and sour or tart foods may cause pain and should be avoided. Consumption of temperate, moist foods without added spices should be encouraged. Small, frequent meals followed by rinsing with lukewarm water or brushing to reduce the risk of dental caries are helpful. Once the type and extent of oral manifestations are identified, a nutrition care plan can be developed. Oral high calorie–high protein supplements in liquid or pudding form may be needed to meet nutrient needs and optimize healing.

Head and Neck Cancers

Head, neck, and oral cancers can alter eating ability and nutrition status because of the surgeries and therapies used to treat these cancers.

TABLE 24.3   Effects of Oral Infections

Location	Problem	Effect	Diet Management
Oral cavity	Candidiasis, KS, herpes, stomatitis	Pain, infection, lesions, altered ability to eat, dysgeusia	Increase kilocalorie and protein intake; administer oral supplements; provide caries risk reduction education
	Xerostomia	Increased caries risk, pain, difficulty with mastication, lack of saliva to form bolus, tendency of food to stick, dysgeusia	Moist, soft, nonspicy foods; "smooth" cool or warm foods and fluids; caries risk reduction education
Esophagus	Candidiasis, herpes, KS, cryptosporidiosis	Dysphagia, odynophagia	Try oral supplementation first; if that is unsuccessful, initiate NG feedings using a silastic feeding tube or PEG
	CMV, with or without ulceration	Dysphagia, food accumulation	PEG

CMV, Cytomegalovirus; *KS,* Kaposi's sarcoma; *NG,* nasogastric; *PEG,* percutaneous endoscopic gastrostomy.

Surgery, depending on the location and extent, may alter eating or swallowing ability, as well as the capacity to produce saliva. Radiation therapy of the head and neck area and chemotherapeutic agents can affect the quantity and quality of saliva and the integrity of the oral mucosa. Thick, ropy saliva is often the result of radiation therapy to the head and neck area, causing xerostomia. Dietary management focuses on the recommendations described earlier for xerostomia, along with modifications in food consistency after surgery (see Chapters 35 and 39).

HIV Infection and AIDS

Viral and fungal infections, stomatitis, xerostomia, periodontal disease, and Kaposi's sarcoma are oral manifestations of HIV that can cause limitations in nutrient intake and result in weight loss and compromised nutrition status. These infections often are compounded by a compromised immune response, preexisting malnutrition, and gastrointestinal consequences of HIV infection (see Chapter 36). Viral diseases, including herpes simplex and cytomegalovirus, result in painful ulcerations of the mucosa.

Stomatitis, or inflammation of the oral mucosa, causes severe pain and ulceration of the gingiva, oral mucosa, and palate, which makes eating painful. Candidiasis on the tongue, palate, or esophagus can make chewing, sucking, and swallowing painful (odynophagia), thus compromising intake. Table 24.3 outlines the effects of associated oral infections.

Xerostomia

Xerostomia (dry mouth) is seen in poorly controlled diabetes mellitus, Sjögren's syndrome, other autoimmune diseases, and as a consequence of radiation therapy and certain medications (Box 24.3). Xerostomia from radiation therapy may be more permanent than that from other causes. Radiation therapy procedures to spare the parotid gland should be implemented when possible to reduce the damage to the salivary gland. Efforts to stimulate saliva production using the medication pilocarpine and citrus-flavored, sugar-free candies may ease eating difficulty.

Individuals without any saliva at all have the most difficulty eating; artificial salivary agents may not offer sufficient relief. Lack of saliva impedes all aspects of eating, including chewing, forming a bolus, swallowing, and sensing taste; causes pain; and increases the risk of dental caries and infections. Dietary guidelines focus on the use of moist foods without added spices, increased fluid consumption with and between all meals and snacks, and judicious food choices.

Problems with chewy (steak), crumbly (cake, crackers, rice), dry (chips, crackers), and sticky (peanut butter) foods are common in persons with severe xerostomia. Alternatives should be suggested, or the foods should be avoided to avert dysphagia risk. Drinking water with a lemon or lime twist or citrus-flavored seltzers or sucking on frozen tart grapes, berries, or sugar-free candies may help. Because these foods or beverages may contain fermentable carbohydrate or contribute to reduced pH, good oral hygiene habits are important in reducing the risk of tooth decay and should be practiced after all meals and snacks.

BOX 24.3   Medications that May Cause Xerostomia

Antianxiety agents	Diuretics
Anticonvulsants	Narcotics
Antidepressants	Sedatives
Antihistamines	Serotonin reuptake inhibitors
Antihypertensives	Tranquilizers

CLINICAL CASE STUDY

Gina is a 74-year-old white woman with a history of type 2 diabetes, hypertension, and arthritis. She states that her dentist told her she has xerostomia and periodontal disease and will need multiple tooth extractions and a full maxillary (upper) and partial mandibular (lower) denture. Because of the condition of her teeth she consumes soft foods and lots of diet soda because her mouth always feels dry. She takes glyburide for glucose control, amlodipine (Norvasc) for blood pressure control, and glucosamine and chondroitin to alleviate her arthritis. She is 5'1" and weighs 176 lb. She lives alone but receives assistance with food shopping and cooking from her family and friends. She occasionally conducts self-monitoring fasting glucose via fingerstick and states that her usual reading is 150 mg/dL.

Nutrition Diagnostic Statements

- Chewing difficulty related to poor dentition and xerostomia as evidenced by patient report and choice of soft foods.
- Altered nutrition-related laboratory value (glucose) related to diabetes and high glycemic diet as evidenced by hyperglycemia and periodontal disease.

Nutrition Care Questions

1. What are the cultural, educational, socioeconomic, and environmental influences affecting dental and nutritional health?
2. What are the diet counseling recommendations for the dental conditions (anticipated extractions, dry mouth, full and partial dentures)?
3. List an appropriate intervention for each of the diagnostic statements. How would you evaluate the impact of your intervention?
4. What would you assess at your follow-up (monitoring) appointment with Gina?

USEFUL WEBSITES

American Academy of Pediatric Dentistry
American Academy of Periodontology
American Dental Association
American Dental Hygienists Association
Diabetes and Oral Health
National Institute of Dental and Craniofacial Research
Oral Health America
Surgeon General Report on Oral Health
World Health Organization on Oral Health

REFERENCES

Al-Khabbaz AK: Type 2 diabetes mellitus and periodontal disease severity, *Oral Health Prev Dent* 12:77–82, 2014.

American Dental Association: *ADA Fluoridation Policy & Statements*, 2014. Available at: https://www.ada.org/en/public-programs/advocating-for-the-public/fluoride-and-fluoridation/fluoride-clinical-guidelines.

Beerens MW, Ten Cate JM, Buijs MJ, et al: Long-term remineralizing effect of MI Paste Plus on regression of early caries after orthodontic fixed appliance treatment: a 12-month follow-up randomized controlled trial, *Eur J Orthod* 40:457–464, 2017.

Brennan LJ, Strauss J: Cognitive impairment in older adults and oral health considerations: treatment and management, *Dent Clin North Am* 58(4):815–828, 2014.

Centers for Disease Control and Prevention: *National oral health surveillance system*, 2017. Available at: https://www.cdc.gov/oralhealthdata/overview/nohss.html.

Cochrane NJ, Shen P, Byrne SJ, et al: Remineralisation by chewing sugar-free gums in a randomised, controlled in situ trial including dietary intake and gauze to promote plaque formation, *Caries Res* 46:147–155, 2012.

Duran-Pinedo AE, Frias-Lopez J: Beyond microbial community composition: functional activities of the oral microbiome in health and disease, *Microbes Infect* 17:505–516, 2015.

Garcia RI, Kleinman D, Holt K, et al: Healthy futures: engaging the oral health community in childhood obesity prevention - conference summary and recommendations, *J Public Health Dent* 77(Suppl 1):S136–S140, 2017.

Mallonee LFH, Boyd LD, Stegeman C: Practice paper of the Academy of Nutrition and Dietetics on Oral Health and Nutrition, *JAND* 114:958, 2014.

Morin K: Fluoride: action and use, *MCN Am J Matern Child Nurs* 31:127, 2006.

Moynihan PJ, Kelly SA: Effect on caries of restricting sugars intake: systematic review to inform WHO guidelines, *J Dent Res* 93:8–18, 2014.

Najeeb S, Zafar MS, Khurshid Z, et al: The role of nutrition in periodontal health: an update, *Nutrients* 8(9):E530, 2016.

National Center for Complementary and Integrative Health: *Complementary, alternative, or integrative health: what's in a name?* 2015. Available at: https://nccih.nih.gov/health/integrative-health#types.

Palmer CA, Gilbert JA: Position of the Academy of Nutrition and Dietetics: the impact of fluoride on health, *J Acad Nutr Diet* 112:1443–1453, 2012.

Ravishankar TL, Yadav V, Tangade PS, et al: Effect of consuming different dairy products on calcium, phosphorus and pH levels of human dental plaque: a comparative study, *Eur Arch Paediatr Dent* 13:144–148, 2012.

Schlueter N, Jaeggi T, Lussi A: Is dental erosion really a problem? *Adv Dent Res* 24:68–71, 2012.

Sohn W, Burt BA, Sowers MR: Carbonated soft drinks and dental caries in the primary dentition, *J Dent Res* 85:262–266, 2006.

Staudte H, Kranz S, Völpel A, et al: Comparison of nutrient intake between patients with periodontitis and healthy subjects, *Quintessence Int* 43:907–916, 2012.

Tedesco TK, Gomes NG, Soares FZ, et al: Erosive effects of beverages in the presence or absence of caries simulation by acidogenic challenge on human primary enamel: an in vitro study, *Eur Arch Paediatr Dent* 13:36–40, 2012.

Touger-Decker R, Mobley C: Position of the Academy of Nutrition and Dietetics: oral health and nutrition, *J Acad Nutr Diet* 113:693–701, 2013.

Tsakos G, Herrick K, Sheiham A, et al: Edentulism and fruit and vegetable intake in low-income adults, *J Dent Res* 89:462–467, 2010.

Whitmore SE, Lamont RJ: Oral bacteria and cancer, *PLoS Pathog* 10:e1003933, 2014.

PART V

Medical Nutrition Therapy

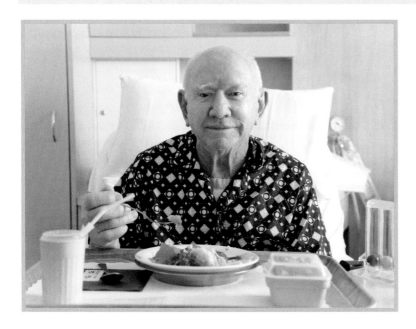

This section contains chapters that reflect the evolution of nutritional science, from the identification of nutrient requirements and the practical application of this knowledge, to the concepts that relate nutrition to the prevention of chronic and degenerative diseases and optimization of health. The role of nutrition in reducing inflammation, a major contributor to chronic disease, supports the awareness of diet in disease prevention and management.

Medical nutrition therapy (MNT) includes assessment, nutrition diagnosis, interventions, monitoring, and evaluation of disease. In some cases, MNT is a powerful preventive measure. The list of diseases amenable to nutrition intervention continues to increase, especially because many diseases and illnesses are now known to have a genetic component and a connection with the nutrient-gene expression pathway.

Sophisticated feeding and nourishment practices place an increased responsibility on those who provide nutrition care. The nutrition-related disorders included in this section can be managed by changes in dietary practices based on current knowledge. The goal of MNT is to move the individual from the continuum of disease toward better nutritional health and overall well-being.

25

Medical Nutrition Therapy for Adverse Reactions to Food: Allergies and Intolerances

L. Kathleen Mahan, MS, RDN, CD
Kathie Madonna Swift, MS, RDN, LDN, FAND

KEY TERMS

adverse reactions to food
allergen
allergen immunotherapy (AIT)
anaphylaxis
antibodies
antigen
antigen-presenting cell (APC)
atopic dermatitis
"atopic march"
atopy
basophils
B-cells
B-regulatory (B-reg) cells
component resolved diagnostics (CRD)
cow's milk protein allergy (CMPA)
cross-reactivity
cytokines
diamine oxidase (DAO)
dendritic cells (DCs)
double-blind, placebo-controlled food
    challenge (DBPCFC)
dual-allergen hypothesis
dysbiosis
elimination diet
eosinophilic esophagitis (EoE)
eosinophilic gastroenteritis (EGE)
eosinophils
epigenetic

epitope
FAILSAFE diet
Food Allergen Labeling and Consumer
    Protection Act (FALCPA)
food allergen–specific serum IgE testing
food allergy
food and symptom record
food autoimmune or immune reactivity
food-dependent, exercise-induced
    anaphylaxis (FDEIA)
food intolerance
food protein–induced enterocolitis
    syndrome (FPIES)
food protein–induced proctocolitis or
    proctitis (FPIP)
food sensitivity
galactose-α-1, 3-galactose (alpha-gal)
granulocyte
gut-associated lymphoid tissue (GALT)
histamine
histamine-N-methyltransferase (HNMT)
increased intestinal permeability or
    "leaky gut"
IgE-mediated reactions
immunoglobulin (Ig)
inflammatory mediators
latex-fruit syndrome or latex-food
    syndrome

lipid transfer protein syndrome (LTPS)
lymphocyte
mast cells
microbiome
non–IgE-mediated reactions
oral allergy syndrome (OAS)
oral food challenge (OFC)
oral tolerance
pollen-food allergy syndrome (PFAS)
prebiotics
precautionary allergen labeling (PAL)
probiotics
sensitivity-related illness (SRI)
sensitization
six-food elimination diet (SFED)
skin-prick test (SPT)
step up 2-4-6-food elimination diets
systemic nickel allergy syndrome (SNAS)
T-cells
Th cells
Th1 cells
Th2 cells
T-regulatory (T-reg) cells
T-suppressor cells
tyramine

Adverse reactions to food are common and implicated in many conditions as a result of the involvement of major organ systems, including the dermatologic, respiratory, gastrointestinal, and neurologic systems. The management of adverse reactions to food is complex because of the diverse response by which the body reacts to food and food components and the multifaceted nature of the mechanisms involved. The clinical relevance of adverse reactions to food should be carefully assessed and evaluated using the nutrition care process (Fig. 25.1).

DEFINITIONS

Adverse reactions to food encompass food allergies and food intolerances, both of which can involve multiple systems, cause diverse symptoms, and negatively impact health.

Food allergy is defined as an adverse health effect arising from a specific immune response that occurs reproducibly on exposure to a given food. A food is defined as "any substance—whether processed, semiprocessed, or raw—that is intended for human consumption, and

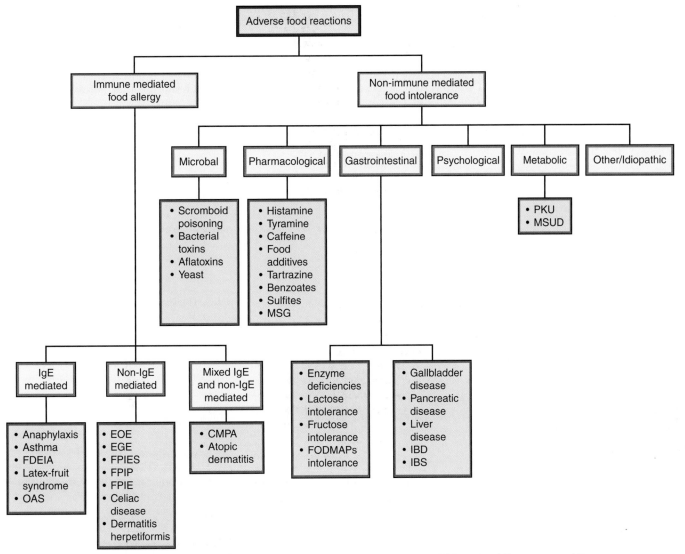

Fig. 25.1 Adverse reactions to food. *CMPA*, Cow's milk protein allergy; *EGE*, eosinophilic gastroenteritis; *EoE*, eosinophilic esophagitis; *FDEIA*, food-dependent, exercise-induced anaphylaxis; *FODMAPs*, fructo-, oligo-, di-, monosaccharides, and polyols syndrome; *FPIE*, food protein–induced enteropathy; *FPIES*, food protein–induced enterocolitis syndrome; *FPIP*, food protein–induced proctocolitis; *IBD*, inflammatory bowel disease; *MSUD*, maple syrup urine disease; *OAS*, oral allergy syndrome; *PKU*, phenylketonuria.

includes drinks, chewing gum, food additives and dietary supplements." The components within foods that trigger immunologic reactions are called antigens, and most often are glycoproteins that interact with immune cells and initiate the development of a food allergy (National Academies of Sciences, Engineering, and Medicine [NASEM], 2017).

Symptoms can range from urticaria to life-threatening anaphylaxis. Food allergy elicits reactions to foods that include the following:

- Reactions that elicit production of specific immunoglobulins such as IgE
- Reactions that result from release of inflammatory mediators in response to IgE produced against nonfood materials such as inhaled pollens or latex
- Reactions that result from inflammatory mediators released from granulocytes such as eosinophils in the digestive tract
- Reactions that affect the digestive system (enteropathies) due to proteins in milk or soy

- Gastrointestinal disorders such as celiac disease (gluten sensitive enteropathy) which has an immune component

Food intolerance is an adverse reaction to a food or food component that lacks an identified immunologic pathophysiology. It results from the body's inability to digest, absorb, or metabolize a food or component of the food. These nonimmune mediated reactions are caused by metabolic, toxicologic, pharmacologic, microbial, and undefined mechanisms (Sicherer and Sampson, 2018). For example, an individual can be intolerant to milk because of an inability to digest the carbohydrate lactose or intolerant to histamine-containing foods due to enzyme deficiencies or other mechanisms (Table 25.1).

Other terms are used by clinicians, researchers, patients, and the media but are not formally accepted by major food allergy organizations. The term **food sensitivity** is used when it is unclear whether the reaction is immunologically related or due to a biochemical or physiologic defect (Joneja, 2013). **Food autoimmune or immune reactivity** has been proposed by Vojdani to refer to the concept that when the

TABLE 25.1   Some Examples of Food Intolerances

Cause	Associated Food(s)	Symptoms
Gastrointestinal Disorders		
Enzyme Deficiencies		
Lactose intolerance (lactase deficiency)	Foods containing lactose and mammalian milk	Bloating, flatulence, diarrhea, abdominal pain
Glucose-6 phosphate dehydrogenase deficiency	Fava or broad beans	Hemolytic anemia
Fructose intolerance	Foods containing fructose or sucrose	Bloating, flatulence, diarrhea, abdominal pain
FODMAPs intolerance	Foods containing fructo-, oligo-, di-, and monosaccharides and polyols	Bloating, flatulence, diarrhea, cramping, abdominal pain
Diseases		
Cystic fibrosis	Symptoms may be precipitated by many foods, especially high-fat foods	Bloating, loose stools, abdominal pain, malabsorption
Gallbladder disease	Symptoms may be precipitated by high-fat foods	Abdominal pain after eating
Pancreatic disease Inflammatory bowel disease	Symptoms may be precipitated by eating	Anorexia, nausea, dysgeusia, and other gastrointestinal symptoms
Inborn Errors of Metabolism		
Phenylketonuria	Foods containing phenylalanine	Elevated serum phenylalanine levels, mental retardation
Galactosemia	Foods containing lactose or galactose	Vomiting, lethargy, failure to thrive
Psychological or Neurologic Reactions		
Psychological or neurologic disorder	Symptoms may be precipitated by any food	Wide variety of symptoms involving any system
Reactions to Pharmacologic Agents in Foods		
Phenylethylamine	Chocolate, aged cheeses, red wine	Migraine headaches
Tyramine	Aged cheeses, brewer's yeast, red wine, canned fish, chicken liver, bananas, eggplant, tomatoes, raspberries, plums	Migraine headaches, cutaneous erythema, urticaria, and hypertensive crisis in patients taking monoamine oxidase inhibitors (MAOIs)
Histamine and histamine releasing agents	Aged cheeses, fermented foods (e.g., sauerkraut, yogurt, kefir), processed meats (e.g., sausage, bologna, salami), canned and smoked fish, red beans, soybeans, citrus, avocado, eggplant, olives, tomatoes and tomato products, chocolate, cocoa, tea, yeast, many spices, many food additives and preservatives, shellfish, egg whites, avocado, strawberries, pineapple, spinach, nuts, peanuts, alcohol	Dizziness, flushing, hives, erythema, runny nose, headaches, decreased blood pressure, nausea, vomiting, shortness of breath, edema, urticaria, eczema, pruritus
Reactions to Food Additives		
Artificial colors: tartrazine or FD&C yellow #5 and other azo dyes	Artificially colored yellow or yellow-orange foods, soft drinks, some medicines	Hives, rash, asthma, nausea, headaches
Benzoates: benzoic acid or sodium benzoate	Processed foods as antimicrobial preservatives; color preservatives; bleaching agents Naturally occurring in berries, cinnamon and other spices, tea Dishes with spicy sauces and curry powder, avocado, dried fruits, some carbonated drinks, alcoholic mixers, milk shake syrup, some canned foods like beans, flavored chips, salad dressing	Hives, rash, asthma, angioedema, nasal congestion, headache, contact dermatitis, diverse digestive tract symptoms
Butylated hydroxyanisole (BHA); butylated hydroxytoluene (BHT)	Processed foods: used as antioxidants; also used in food packaging materials	Skin reactions such as hives
Monosodium glutamate (MSG)	Processed foods (canned foods, chips, gravy, flavor packets for instant soups, etc.) added as a flavor enhancer; often used in Asian cuisine. Naturally occurring glutamic acid is found in aged cheeses like Parmesan, fish sauce, mushrooms, spinach, marmite	Facial numbness, tingling and numbness in hands and feet, dizziness, balance problems, visual disturbances, headaches, asthma, flushing, diverse digestive tract symptoms

TABLE 25.1	Some Examples of Food Intolerances—cont'd	
Cause	**Associated Food(s)**	**Symptoms**
Nitrates and nitrites	Processed foods containing sodium nitrite, sodium nitrate, potassium nitrite and potassium nitrate; commonly found in cured meats, canned meats, smoked fish, pate, pickled meats	Flushing, hives, migraine, other headaches, digestive tract symptoms
Salicylates	Naturally occurring in a variety of fruits, vegetables, and spices	Angioedema, asthma, hives; people sensitive to aspirin at higher risk for developing intolerance
Sulfites Sodium sulfite, potassium sulfite, sodium metabisulfite, potassium metabisulfite, sodium bisulfite, potassium bisulfite, sulfur dioxide	Shrimp, avocado, instant potatoes, instant mashed potatoes, French fries, sausage, canned fruits and vegetables, dried fruits and vegetables, acidic juices, wine, beer, cider, colas, fresh fruits and vegetables treated with sulfites to prevent browning, and many other processed foods	Acute asthma and anaphylaxis in people with asthma; reactions in skin and mucous membranes
Reactions to Microbial Contamination or Toxins in Foods *Proteus, Klebsiella,* or *Escherichia coli* bacteria cause histidine to break down to a histamine	Unrefrigerated scombroid fish (tuna, bonito, mackerel); heat-stable toxin produced	Scombroid fish poisoning (itching, rash, vomiting, diarrhea); anaphylactic-type reaction

body's normal tolerance of friendly antigenic substances (autoantigens produced by the individual's immune system) is disrupted because of disease, injury, shock, trauma, drugs, or blood transfusion, the ingestion of foods containing antigenic substances with a composition similar to those of the body's autoantigens can result in the production of antibodies that react to the food antigens and the body's own tissues (Vojdani, 2015a). **Sensitivity-related illness (SRI)** has also been proposed as a condition that occurs when an individual is exposed to some type of toxin or stressor and then becomes sensitive to a food,

inhalant, or chemical, although the mechanisms are unclear (Genuis, 2010) (Box 25.1).

PREVALENCE

There is evidence that adverse food reactions are more prevalent than in the past, with a dramatic increase in food allergies in recent decades. It is estimated that 10.8% of U.S. adults have at least one food allergy, as evidenced from symptoms typical of an IgE-mediated reaction. But

BOX 25.1   Adverse Reactions to Foods: Definitions

- **Adverse food reactions:** encompass food allergies and food intolerances, both of which can result in distressing symptoms and adversely affect health
- **Allergens:** the components in foods that trigger adverse immunologic reactions; most often are specific proteins, glycoprotein, or haptens that can interact with the body's immune cells in a way that leads to development of a food allergy
- **Atopy:** a condition of genetic predisposition to produce excessive IgE antibodies in response to an allergen that results in the development of typical symptoms such as asthma, rhinitis, conjunctivitis, or eczema
- **Cross-reactivity:** when an antibody reacts not only with the original allergen but also with a similar allergen; occurs when a food allergen shares structural or sequence similarity with a different food allergen or aeroallergen (i.e., a pollen), which may then trigger an adverse reaction similar to that triggered by the original food allergen; cross-reactivity is common, for example, among different shellfish and different tree nuts, and in pollen-food allergy syndrome (PFAS)
- **Desensitization:** a state of clinical and immunologic nonresponsiveness to a food allergen that can be induced by careful, medical-guided administration of gradually increasing amounts of the allergen over a short period of time (hours to days); the maintenance of such desensitization usually requires continued regular exposure to the allergen
- **Dual-allergen exposure:** hypothesis that environmental exposure to food allergens through the skin or exposure to airborne particles early in life can lead to sensitization and allergy, and that the oral consumption of these same

foods during a developmentally appropriate period, also early in life, results in tolerance
- **Food allergy:** an adverse immune-mediated reaction to a food, usually a food protein or specific glycoprotein that the person has been sensitized to, and which, when eaten, causes the release of inflammatory mediators or chemicals that act on body tissues and result in symptoms. The reaction can be either IgE-mediated or non–IgE-mediated and occurs reproducibly upon exposure to that food
- **Food autoimmune or immune reactivity:** the concept that when the body's normal tolerance of friendly antigenic substances (autoantigens produced by an individual's body) is disrupted because of disease, injury, shock, trauma, surgery, drugs, blood transfusion, or environmental triggers, the ingestion of foods containing antigenic substances with a composition similar to those of the body's autoantigens can result in the production of antibodies that react to the food antigens and the body's own tissues (Vojdani, 2015)
- **Food intolerance:** an adverse reaction to a food or food component that lacks an identified immunologic pathophysiology
- **Food sensitivity:** a term often used to describe a reaction when it is unclear whether it is immunologically mediated or not
- **Oral tolerance:** the process that allows an individual to eat food that is "foreign" without any ill effects or reactions to it
- **Sensitivity-related illness:** the concept that an individual who is exposed to some type of toxicant or insult may then, by as yet unclear mechanisms, become sensitive to a food, inhalant, or chemical (Genuis, 2010)

Source: IOM Global Report: Finding a Path to Safety in Food Allergy: Assessment of the Global Burden, Causes, Prevention, Management and Public Policy.

only about half of those food allergic adults have been diagnosed by a physician. Of even more interest is the estimate that 19% believe they have a food allergy (Gupta et al, 2019). In Australia it may be as high as 10% (Renz et al, 2018). There are also documented worldwide increases in food allergy in rapidly emerging areas of Asia, such as China. Estimates suggest that 20% of the population alter their diet due to perceived adverse food reactions (Turnbull et al, 2015).

However, there are gaps in the precise prevalence of adverse food reactions due to misuse of the terms "food allergy" and "food intolerance," variations in study design and methodologies, and inflated self-reporting. Geographic variations; diet exposure effects; differences in age, race, and ethnicity; and other factors also complicate data reporting. Despite the lack of precise prevalence data, there is agreement that changes in diet, lifestyle, and environmental influences, interacting with genetic predisposition and microbiome alterations, can be implicated in the escalation of adverse food reactions and the parallel rise in other chronic disorders such as asthma and autoimmune diseases (Sicherer and Sampson, 2018; NASEM, 2017).

ETIOLOGY

Adverse food reactions illustrate the critical importance of appreciating "biochemical uniqueness" as a core clinical concept in nutrition assessment. Numerous factors have been identified that play a role in influencing immune- and nonimmune-mediated responses to food or food components and their ultimate interpretation by the body as either "friend" or "foe," including:

Individual Factors
Age
Genetics and epigenetics
Early life factors (maternal nutrition, birth delivery method, breast or formula feeding)
Immunocompetence and personal differences in immune function
Intestinal and skin barrier defects
Microbiome
Increased hygiene
Use of medications (e.g., antacids, nonsteroidal antiinflammatory medications)
Underlying disease
Presence of chronic stress
Environmental influences (toxin and chemical exposures sometimes referred to as the exposome)
Food-related factors
Modern westernized diet
Prenatal perinatal, and maternal nutrition
Allergen type, dose, and route of exposure
Microbial products and contamination with microorganisms
Food matrix (proteins, lipids, and glycosylated sugars)
Cooking temperature
Epithelial barrier insulting agent (alcohol, additives, toxins, unknown ingredients) (Sampson et al, 2018).

Genetics and Epigenetics

It has been recognized for more than a century that genetics plays a role in allergies and asthma. Familial aggregations and heritability estimates from twin studies provide initial evidence for genetic predisposition for food allergy, although among siblings, an increased rate of sensitization does not equate to clinical reactivity. A number of monogenic disorders associated with atopy and food allergy have been identified; however, the genetics of food allergy have shifted from identifying a single change or polymorphism in a gene to the inclusion of a multitude of contributing genetic and nongenetic risk factors (Carter and Frischmeyer-Guerrerio, 2018).

Genetic mechanisms that play a role in pathogenesis of food allergy are multifactorial and complex. The expression of food allergy is influenced by the environment, gene-environment interactions, and epigenetic modification of the genome ("epigenome"). The epigenome is largely established in utero and is relevant to early life origins of allergic disease (NASEM, 2017; Carter and Frischmeyer-Guerrerio, 2018).

More recently, genome wide association studies (GWASs) identified genes associated with food allergies. One GWAS study examined 1500 children with food allergies in Germany and the United States. This study examined more than five million genetic variations or single nucleotide polymorphisms (SNPs) in each child in the study and compared the frequency of these SNPs with the control subjects. In addition to the large number of subjects, unlike other studies, the researchers also included an oral food challenge to confirm the allergy diagnosis. The study identified five genetic risk loci for food allergies, and four of them showed a strong association with loci for atopic dermatitis (hereditary eczematous rash), asthma, and other chronic inflammatory and autoimmune diseases. The SERPINB gene cluster on chromosome 18 was pinpointed as a specific genetic risk locus for food allergies. The genes in this particular cluster are expressed in the skin and mucous membrane of the esophagus, which are involved in maintaining epithelial barrier integrity (Marenholz et al, 2017).

Another GWAS study included a meta-analysis of two phenotypes, peanut allergy and food allergy, and examined seven studies from Canadian, American, Australian, German, and Dutch populations. Multiple genes were identified as risk factors for peanut allergy and food allergy and are involved in epigenetic regulation of gene expression (Asai et al, 2018).

Unlike other diseases, the number of identified loci for food allergies is relatively small. Most of the identified candidate genes encode for products influencing immune mechanisms toward a Th2 inflammatory shift. It is hypothesized that genetic predispositions in the context of certain environmental influences such as intestinal viral infection may result in immune system dysfunction and result in food allergy (NASEM, 2017). (See Chapters 6 and 7).

PATHOPHYSIOLOGY OF FOOD ALLERGY

Major advances in research are providing further insights into the mechanisms leading to food allergies. A basic understanding of the immune system is essential since the mechanisms entail multiple molecules involved in immune regulation.

IMMUNE SYSTEM BASICS

Antibodies are specialized immune proteins that are produced in response to the introduction of an antigen (an allergen, toxin, or foreign substance) into the body. Because of their association with the immune system, antibodies are referred to as immunoglobulins (Ig). Five distinct classes of antibodies have been identified: IgA, IgD, IgE, IgG, and IgM. Each Ig has a specific function in immune-mediated reactions (Box 25.2).

The production of antibodies is a major function of the immune system and is carried out by a particular type of lymphocyte (white blood cell). There are two important groups of lymphocytes: B-cells arising from stem cells in the bone marrow, and T-cells, also originated from stem cells but later transported to the thymus gland where they mature, hence the name T-cells. Monocytes and macrophages are primarily phagocytes that engulf foreign material, break it apart, and display specific molecules of the material on their surfaces, making

BOX 25.2 The Immunoglobulins

IgA

Found in two forms—serum IgA and secretory IgA (sIgA). The latter is present in mucus secretions in the mouth, respiratory and gastrointestinal tracts, vagina, and colostrum in mammalian milk. It includes a "secretory piece" in its structure that protects it from protein-destroying enzymes in the digestive tract so that it survives in an active form as a "first-line" defense against antigens entering from the external environment. Serum IgA, which does not have the secretory piece, is in the second highest amount in circulation, exceeded only by IgG.

IgD

Found in small amounts in the tissues that line the belly and chest; involved in immunoglobulin class switching. Signals B cells to be activated. Suggestion that IgD-producing B cells are auto reactive lymphocytes and may be involved in autoimmune disease. Its role in allergy is probably minimal.

IgE

The classic allergy antibody of hay fever, asthma, eczema, food-induced allergy, food-induced anaphylaxis, pollen-food allergy syndrome (PFAS), and latex-fruit allergy. Immediate allergic reactions usually involve IgE and are the most clearly understood mechanisms.

IgG

The only antibody that crosses the placenta from mother to baby and is the most common antibody in the blood. Defends against pathogens and persists long after the threat is over. Four subtypes include IgG1, IgG2, IgG3, and IgG4. Food protein–specific IgG antibodies tend to rise in the first few months after the introduction of a food and then decreases even though the food may continue to be consumed. It appears to be part of the process of development of tolerance to food. A rise in antigen-specific IgG4 accompanied by a drop in IgE often indicates tolerance of the food. People with inflammatory bowel disorders such as untreated celiac disease or ulcerative colitis often have high levels of IgG and IgM (Stapel et al, 2008), possibly indicating the passage of food molecules as "foreign invaders" into circulation.

IgM

The largest antibody, a first-line defender that can mop up many antigens at one time. It is produced by the fetus in utero and its level rises in the presence of an in utero infection.

Stapel SO, Asero R, Ballmer-Weber BK, et al: Testing for IgG4 against foods is not recommended as a diagnostic tool: EAACI Task Force Report, *Allergy* 63:793–796, 2008.

them **antigen-presenting cells (APC)**. The antigenic component displayed on the surface is an **epitope** and is recognized by T-cells.

T-cells are a diverse group of lymphocytes with several different roles in the immune response under different circumstances, and they secrete different sets of **cytokines** (chemical messengers). **Th cells** are helper cells that adjust the system. **Th1 cells** regulate the activities of the B-cells to produce antibodies and direct damage to target cells, resulting in the destruction of antigens. This function is useful in defending against bacteria, viruses, and other pathogenic cells. **Th2 cells** mediate the allergic response by regulating the production by B-cells of IgE sensitized to food or other allergens. Other T-cells are **T-regulatory cells (T-reg cells)** and **T- suppressor cells** that regulate the immune response so that there is tolerance of the foreign but safe molecule.

Also involved in allergic reactions are **granulocytes**, cells that contain intracellular granules, which act as storage depots for defense chemicals or inflammatory mediators that, when released, not only protect the body from invading pathogens but also can produce allergic symptoms. Granulocytes called **mast cells** are located in the lungs, skin, tongue, and linings of the nose and intestinal tract, and those called **basophils** are in the circulation. Of importance in non-IgE mediated allergy are **eosinophils**, another form of granulocytes that are in blood and tissues and, when stimulated by cytokines produced by Th2 cells, migrate to the site of an allergic reaction.

When granulocytes degranulate they release **inflammatory mediators**, such as histamine, chymase, and tryptase and, in the case of mast cells, there is de novo synthesis of lipid metabolites of arachidonic acid—prostaglandins, leukotrienes, and plasma activating factor (PAF). Each of these mediators has a specific effect on local tissues and at other sites, resulting in the symptoms of an allergic reaction—vasodilation, increased vascular permeability leading to angioedema, nociceptive (painful) nerve activation causing itchiness, smooth muscle constriction, mucous secretion, and acute diarrhea.

Allergic Response

The pathophysiology of the allergic response can be described in three phases: the breakdown of oral tolerance, allergen sensitization, and reactivity to allergens leading to allergy symptoms.

Breakdown of oral tolerance. Humans are exposed to thousands of foreign molecules daily from food and the environment. Exposure to these foreign molecules in the digestive tract through ingested substances is usually followed by immune regulation or suppression, such that the substance or food is recognized as "foreign but safe," which is a prerequisite for the development of tolerance to a food or food component. **Oral tolerance** is the mechanism by which potentially antigenic substances do not trigger an immune response and is the normal physiologic response to ingested antigens (Tordesillas and Berin, 2018). The development of immunologic and clinical tolerance is thus critical to preventing food allergies and other chronic inflammatory diseases. Oral tolerance is mediated by several immune cells, including APCs such as **dendritic cells (DCs)** and macrophages, and regulatory T-cells (T_reg cells) (Bauer et al, 2015). Tolerance is acquired with innate and adaptive immune responses acting in a coordinated manner to mount a response to antigen exposure. It is a process that starts in utero and persists throughout life (Renz et al, 2018).

The gut microenvironment supports and promotes expansion of the regulating activity of T-reg cells through multiple processes including the presence of retinoic acid (from vitamin A) and microbial metabolites, such as short-chain fatty acids. B-cells also inhibit hostile immune reactivity. **B-regulatory (B-reg) cells** act mainly through interleukin-10 (IL-10), an antiinflammatory cytokine to reduce infection and allergic inflammation and to promote tolerance. A breakdown in the tolerogenic process leads to a shift away from T-reg cell induction to the generation of proallergic Th2 cells and results in sensitization to food allergens (Renz et al, 2018; Sampson et al, 2018).

Sensitization. **Sensitization** to food antigens can take place in the gastrointestinal tract, oral cavity, skin, and occasionally in the respiratory tract (Sampson et al, 2018). Gastrointestinal (GI) function is key to the maintenance of oral tolerance, and avoidance of allergic sensitization and allergic response, since the vast majority of food proteins are broken down by gastric acid and digestive enzymes in the stomach and intestine.

Recognized as being increasingly essential to this function of the GI tract is the presence of the gut **microbiome**, the collection of different types of microbes (bacteria, bacteriophage, fungi, protozoa, and viruses) that live inside the gut. The intestinal microbiome is responsible for regulating the expansion of T-reg cells and Th1 and Th2 type cells to promote immune balance. (Russler-Germain et al, 2017). Dysbiosis occurs when there is an imbalance in the microbial ecosystem, which can contribute to increased intestinal permeability or "leaky gut," and the increased likelihood that intact food proteins and peptides will pass through the intestinal lumen and reach the lymphoid tissue, leading to immune sensitization and possibly reactivity (Plunkett and Nagler, 2017). The gut-associated lymphoid tissue (GALT) is the largest mass of lymphoid tissue in the body and antigen penetration and presentation to the GALT drives food sensitization (Fritscher-Ravens et al, 2014). Other conditions such as GI disease, malnutrition, fetal prematurity, and immunodeficiency also may be associated with increased gut permeability and risk of development of food allergy. Disruptions in the microbiome and the intestinal wall barrier are the result of various factors, including cesarean delivery, formula feeding, antibiotics, chronic stress, infections, and alterations in the microbiome due to disease (see Chapters 1 and 27 for further discussion of the microbiome).

Additional forces driving tolerance breakdown and potential sensitization might arise outside the intestine, as there is evidence that food allergen entry can occur through scratched, broken, and inflamed skin (Renz et al, 2018). Like the gut, the skin microbiome consists of thousands of microbial organisms and their byproducts that inhabit the skin. A harmonious balance of the gut-skin-microbiota is now thought to be vital to a well-functioning immune system.

Reaction. The third phase of the allergic response is reactivity whenever an allergen to which the immune system is now sensitized enters the body again. Because individuals can develop immunologic sensitization as evidenced by the production of allergen-specific IgE (sIgE) or other immune cell sensitization without having allergic symptoms upon subsequent exposure to those foods, an IgE-mediated or non–IgE-mediated food allergy requires the presence of not only loss of tolerance and sensitization but also the presence of clinical symptoms due to the release of inflammatory mediators already discussed (NASEM, 2017) (Fig. 25.2).

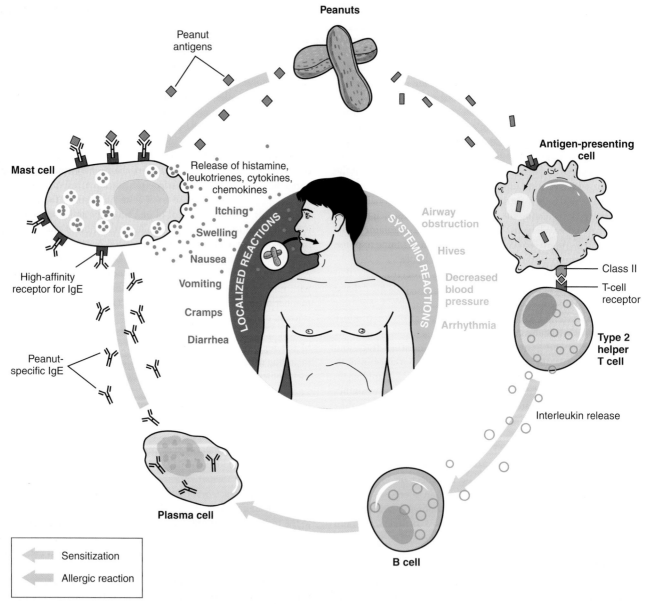

Fig. 25.2 Sensitization process and IgE-mediated allergic reaction.

IgE-mediated reactions occur when sIgE produced in response to the presence of the allergen attaches to matching sIgE antibodies on the mast cell or basophil, forming a "bridge" between them. This bridging activates the mast cell or basophil by a series of energy-requiring processes resulting in the cell's degranulation and release of the inflammatory mediators, and the appearance of allergic symptoms.

IgE-mediated food allergic reactions are rapid in onset, occurring within minutes to a few hours of exposure through either inhalation, skin contact, or ingestion. A wide range of symptoms are attributed to this type of reaction, and usually involve the GI, dermatologic, or respiratory systems and can range from mild hives to life-threatening multiple organ anaphylaxis (Fig. 25.3).

Non–IgE-mediated reactions are based on the activation of cells other than IgE, such as eosinophils, and their degranulation and release of mediators. Non–IgE-mediated reactions are present in delayed or chronic reactions to food allergen ingestion. See Table 25.2 for a comparison of IgE- and non–IgE-mediated allergic reactions.

IgE-Mediated Food Allergies

Although any food can cause an allergic reaction, a small number of foods cause the vast majority of IgE-mediated food allergies. Foods

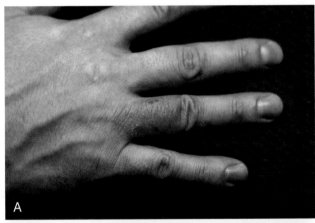

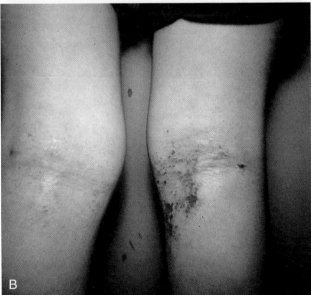

Fig. 25.3 A and **B**, Atopic eczema: An IgE-mediated skin reaction to a food allergen, commonly seen on the hands, back of knees, and the inside of elbows. A, From www.istockphoto.com.

that are more likely to induce an allergic response vary by country and region of the world according to a population's eating habits. In the United States the common allergenic foods are cow's milk, eggs, peanuts, tree nuts, fish, shellfish, wheat, and soy (NASEM, 2017). Among U.S. adults with food allergies the five most common food allergies are shellfish (2.9%), peanut (1.8%), milk (1.9%), tree nuts (1.2%), and fin fish (0.9%) (Gupta et al, 2019). In other countries, for example, Japan, egg, cow's milk, wheat, shellfish, fruit, and buckwheat account for approximately 75% of food allergies (Matsuo et al, 2015).

The main IgE-mediated allergic reactions are food-induced anaphylaxis; food-dependent, exercise-induced anaphylaxis (FDEIA); cow's milk protein allergy (CMPA); oral allergy syndrome (OAS), which recently is recognized as being two syndromes, pollen-food allergy syndrome (PFAS) and lipid transfer protein syndrome (LTPS); latex-fruit or latex-food syndrome; and systemic nickel allergy syndrome (SNAS).

Food-Induced Anaphylaxis

Food-induced **anaphylaxis** is an acute, systemic, often severe, and sometimes fatal immune response that usually occurs within a limited period following exposure to a food antigen. Multiple organ systems are affected. Symptoms include respiratory distress, abdominal pain, nausea, vomiting, cyanosis, arrhythmia, hypotension, angioedema, urticaria, diarrhea, shock, cardiac arrest, and death.

The vast majority of anaphylactic reactions to foods in adults in North America involve peanuts, tree nuts, fish, and shellfish. In children, peanuts and tree nuts are the most common causes of anaphylactic reactions, but anaphylactic reactions to cow's milk and eggs have been reported. Peanuts are the most common food allergen in fatal anaphylactic reactions (Turnbull et al, 2015).

People with known anaphylactic reactions to food allergens should carry and be prepared to use epinephrine via a portable injectable device (often called an EpiPen) at all times. Epinephrine is the drug of choice to reverse an allergic anaphylactic reaction. Delayed use of epinephrine has been associated with an increased risk of biphasic reactions, in which a recurrence of symptoms 4 to 12 hours after the initial anaphylactic reaction may be fatal. See Simons (2014) for management of an anaphylactic reaction and the website for Food Allergy Research and Education (FARE). Immediate coordination of care and referral to a physician specializing in allergy medicine is essential for patient safety. If you witness a severe allergic response or anaphylaxis, call 911 immediately and be prepared to administer cardiopulmonary resuscitation (CPR) if necessary.

FOOD-DEPENDENT, EXERCISE-INDUCED ANAPHYLAXIS (FDEIA)

Food-dependent, exercise-induced anaphylaxis (FDEIA) is a rare distinct form of allergy in which an offending food triggers an IgE-mediated anaphylactic reaction only when the sensitized individual exercises within 2 to 4 hours after eating, or occasionally, before eating the food. Signs of developing anaphylaxis are urticaria (hives), pruritus (itching), and erythema (reddening) followed by breathing difficulty and GI symptoms. The ingestion of the food is not problematic in the absence of exercise, and exercise is not problematic in the absence of consumption of the food. FDEIA appears to be more common in adolescents and young adults, and in those with known food allergy or a history of anaphylaxis. Shellfish, seafood, certain fruits, cow's milk, celery, a gliadin component in wheat, and other foods have been reported as offending agents (Asaumi and Ebisawa, 2018).

In FDEIA, the combination of a sensitizing food and exercise precipitates symptoms, possibly related to increased GI permeability and absorption, blood-flow redistribution, and increased osmolality.

TABLE 25.2   Comparison of IgE- and Non–IgE-Mediated Allergic Reactions

Characteristics/ Target Organ	IgE Mediated	Non–IgE-Mediated	Mixed IgE- and Non–IgE-Mediated
Mechanism	Th2 activation stimulates production of IgE by activated B-cell lymphocytes. Allergen binds with the receptors on sensitized IgE antibodies on mast cells or basophils. Upon binding, chemical inflammatory mediators are released.	T-cells and sometimes eosinophils are associated with triggering release of inflammatory mediators and development of symptoms.	A combination of IgE and non-IgE mechanisms
Timing	Quick onset First phase: immediate reaction—minutes to 1 hour* Late biphasic phase: may occur several hours (4 to 6) after initial reaction (e.g., alpha gal)	Delayed onset: >2 hours; often 4 to 6 hours; relapsing	Delayed onset: >2 hours; often 4 to 6 hours
Volume Required for Reaction	Small	Sometimes larger	Sometimes larger
Systemic	Anaphylaxis Food-associated exercise induced anaphylaxis (FEIA) NSAID-associated, aspirin-associated, or alcohol-associated food-induced anaphylaxis	NA	NA
Skin	Generalized urticaria Acute contact urticaria Angioedema Rash Itching Flushing	Contact dermatitis Dermatitis herpetiformis	Atopic dermatitis (eczema) (see Fig. 25.3)
Gastrointestinal Tract	Immediate gastrointestinal (GI) hypersensitivity or spasm Oral allergy syndrome (OAS) or pollen-food allergy syndrome (PFAS) Abdominal pain Nausea Vomiting Belching Bloating Diarrhea Constipation	Food protein–induced enteropathy syndromes (FPIES) Food protein–induced proctocolitis (FPIP) Celiac disease Eosinophilic esophagitis (EoE) Eosinophilic gastritis Eosinophilic gastroenteritis (EGE)	NA
Respiratory	Acute rhinitis (stuffy nose) Rhinorrhea (runny nose) Asthma Bronchospasm Laryngeal edema	NA	Asthma
Cardiovascular	Hypotension Dizziness or fainting	NA	NA

* In contrast to typical food anaphylaxis that occurs within minutes to 2 hours following ingestion of the trigger food, IgE-mediated alpha-gal-related reactions to mammalian meat, with the same anaphylaxis symptoms are delayed, occurring 3 to 8 hours after ingestion.
NA, Not applicable.
Sources: National Academies of Sciences, Engineering, and Medicine (NASEM), Institute of Medicine (IOM) *Finding a path to safety in food allergy: Assessment of the global burden, causes, prevention, management, and public policy.* Washington, DC: The National Academies Press, 2017 p. 40.
Renz H, Allen KJ, Sicherer SH, et al: Food allergy, Nature Reviews-Disease Primers, vol 4: Article number 17098, published online Jan 4, 2018.
Joneja JV: *The health professional's guide to food allergies and intolerances,* Chicago, IL, 2013, Academy of Nutrition and Dietetics.

Additional factors such as concomitant ingestion of nonsteroidal antiinflammatory drugs (NSAIDs) or alcohol can act as accelerants to the reaction (Wauters et al, 2018). The prevalence and causative agents and effective methods of diagnosis in FDEIA continue to be explored.

Galactose-α-1,3-Galactose Anaphylaxis (Alpha-Gal)

An unusual form of anaphylaxis is the delayed anaphylaxis response to mammalian meat (most commonly beef, lamb, pork, bison, buffalo,

and venison). It involves IgE antibodies that the individual forms against the oligosaccharide galactose-α-1,3-galactose ("alpha-gal"), which is typically introduced into the person during bites from ticks, most commonly the lone star tick. The lone star tick is most commonly seen in the southeast United States but its range is spreading to the Midwest from Texas to Iowa and in New England. Other ticks common in Europe or Australia can introduce alpha-gal into a person through their bite (Commins et al, 2016). Other ectoparasites such as cestodes, nematodes, and scabies in sub-Saharan

Africa can introduce alpha-gal and cause subsequent reactions (Commins, 2016).

About 4 to 6 weeks after the tick bite, the subsequent ingestion of mammalian meat, which contains alpha-gal for which there is now an IgE antibody in the previously bitten person, can lead to reactions that unlike usual immediate IgE-mediated reactions are delayed for several hours. The unique delay in the reaction is probably due to slow absorption of the complex lipids in the meat that harbor the antigen. The fattier the red meat, the more likely the reaction. High-fat dairy ice cream can also occasionally cause a reaction (Wilson and Platts-Mills, 2018).

Intradermal testing with commercially available beef, pork, and lamb extracts can be done safely and correlates well with clinically relevant alpha-gal allergy. In many cases alpha-gal allergy is not lifelong, and red meat can be reintroduced into the diet with medical supervision after 18 to 24 months of avoidance of red meat.

Fruit and Vegetable Allergies: Pollen-Food Allergy Syndrome (PFAS) and Lipid Transfer Protein Syndrome (LTPS)

What used to be called oral allergy syndrome (OAS) is now more accurately referred to as two different syndromes: pollen-food allergy syndrome (PFAS) and lipid transfer protein syndrome (LTPS) (Muluk and Cingi, 2018). Both syndromes are IgE-mediated reactions characterized by oropharyngeal symptoms of itchy mouth; scratchy throat; swelling of the lips, mouth, uvula, or tongue; and throat tightness. Itchy ears are sometimes reported. PFAS is usually a milder reaction confined just to the oral cavity. Symptoms are rapid and appear within 5 to 30 minutes after ingestion of the allergen-containing food and most often subside within 30 minutes. In LTPS the reaction not only affects the oral cavity but also can become systemic with hives, wheezing, vomiting, diarrhea, and low blood pressure, or even anaphylaxis. LTPS is a primary allergy and potentially more severe, requiring different management and even possible prescription of an epinephrine auto-injector device (ADI) (Turner and Campbell, 2014; Turner et al, 2015).

In PFAS the reaction results from contact with food allergen proteins similar to those in pollens (usually birch, ragweed, mugwort, or other grasses) that the person has already been sensitized to through the respiratory system. It is a situation of cross-reactivity between an inhaled and an ingested protein allergen that causes a reaction in the previously sensitized individual. PFAS is common in those with pollen allergies. The primary sensitization is to the pollen, not the food (Turner and Campbell, 2014; Turner et al, 2015).

The proteins resulting in PFAS are heat labile and are changed during cooking. Hence, it is the raw fruit or vegetable that causes the reaction; the cooked version can usually be consumed with no problems. Because reactions are immediate after ingestion of the raw food, most individuals can identify the food culprit. However, if it is not obvious from a thorough clinical history, use of component resolved diagnostic (CRD) testing or skin-prick testing (Table 25.3) can be useful.

LTPS is common in Mediterranean countries where lipid transfer protein (LTP) is a widely cross-reacting allergen in plant foods. In southern Europe LTPS is associated with higher risk of severe systemic reaction, but the reason for this is unknown. Because of this it is important to diagnose LTPS correctly and not misdiagnose it for the milder PFAS. The most frequently implicated foods, cooked or raw, include peaches, apples, pears, apricots, plums, cherries, walnuts, and hazelnuts (Asero et al, 2018; Venter et al, 2018). Box 25.3 lists foods and pollens associated with PFAS and LTPS.

Latex-Fruit or Latex-Food Syndrome

Natural rubber latex (NRL) or *Hevea brasiliensis*, used in latex rubber gloves, balloons, bottle nipples, children's rubber toys, elastic bands, exercise bands, and many other articles in the environment, contains many proteins that can be highly allergenic. An NRL-allergic reaction is IgE-mediated and is often seen in health care workers (8% to 17%), other workers using latex rubber gloves such as hairdressers or house cleaners, those working in the latex industry, and in those undergoing multiple surgical procedures in which they have been exposed to latex rubber surgical gloves and appliances (68% of children with spina bifida for example) (American Latex Allergy Association, 2018). Symptoms of NRL allergy include all the usual symptoms of an IgE-mediated allergy: urticaria, angioedema, runny nose, sneezing, headache, reddened and itchy eyes, sore throat, abdominal cramps, and even anaphylaxis.

It is estimated that 50% to 70% of people with latex allergies have IgE antibodies that can cross-react with antigens from foods, mostly fruits, and cause allergic symptoms of the latex-fruit syndrome or latex-food syndrome. Symptoms of latex-food allergy vary, with many being similar to those with NRL allergy, including anaphylaxis. Sensitization occurs from skin contact with latex, and the food allergy reaction is an IgE-mediated reaction to the latex cross-reacting proteins found in the food.

For those with NRL documented allergy, but with no symptoms after consumption of associated foods, it is important to keep in mind that every NRL-allergic individual reacts differently to foods with latex cross-reacting allergens. The most frequently reported foods in latex-food allergic reactions are avocado, banana, chestnut, kiwi, and mango, but other foods can be problematic (Joneja, 2013). Many latex products, especially powdered latex gloves, where inhalation of the powder increases the risk of becoming sensitized, are now banned from health care settings, making the occurrence of this latex-food allergic reaction less common. However, there are still many NRL-containing products in use (American Latex Allergy Association, 2018).

Many clinicians advise NRL-allergic individuals to avoid foods that have cross-reactivity in the interest of safety. However, it cannot be assumed that the NRL-allergic person will react to these foods, or that there will not be other NRL allergen-containing foods that may cause a reaction. Management is based on an elimination diet that begins with avoidance of foods known to be reactive for that individual. With the development of CRD testing (see Table 25.3), the problematic link between specific components of the latex protein and certain fruits is being elucidated.

Systemic Nickel Allergy Syndrome (SNAS)

Allergy to the mineral nickel begins as a contact dermatitis. It is more common in women and increases in incidence with advancing age. The individual is sensitized through prolonged skin or mucous membrane contact with nickel, usually from jewelry, buttons, metal studs, clips, watchbands, or occupations where metal contact is frequent. In this cell-mediated reaction lymphocytes produce cytokines at the site of nickel contact, which cause the itching, redness, and scaling of contact dermatitis. It is a delayed and chronic reaction that occurs with every subsequent contact with nickel at that site.

It is now recognized that the individual with nickel contact dermatitis can develop a secondary response of eczema or dermatitis even when the skin is not in contact with nickel, and it appears that this systemic nickel allergy syndrome (SNAS) in the sensitized individual is to nickel present in an ingested food.

Diagnosis of contact allergy to nickel is made using an atopy patch test (see Table 25.3), where the allergen (usually nickel sulfate) in the patch is left on the skin for up to 72 hours. After 48 hours the area

TABLE 25.3   Tests Used in the Assessment of Adverse Reactions to Foods

Skin Tests

Skin testing (scratch, prick, or puncture)	A drop of antigen is placed on the skin, and the skin is then scratched or punctured to allow penetration of the antigen to reach sensitized IgE; assesses presence of antigen-specific IgE (sIgE) and sensitization	Screening test; cannot be relied upon as sole diagnostic tool; negative results confirm absence of IgE-mediated sensitivity; positive results only confirm presence of sIgE-mediated sensitization and not necessarily food allergy; need to be combined with thorough health history of food-symptom relationship
Atopy patch test	Small pads soaked with allergen are applied to unbroken skin for 48 hours and read at 72 hours	Variable sensitivity and specificity; used to assess delayed or non-IgE reactions; no clinical value in diagnosis of food allergy; combined with skin prick testing (SPT) or sIgE may have value in the diagnosis of atopic dermatitis (Hammond and Lieberman, 2018) or eosinophilic esophagitis (Spergel et al, 2012)

Blood Tests

ImmunoCAP ImmunoCap ISAC Immulite	Test for allergen-specific IgE in serum (sIgE); serum is mixed with food on a paper disk and then washed with radioactively labeled IgE. Used for assessing IgE-mediated reactions; ISAC tests for a panel of 100 foods or more	High sensitivity, but low specificity for food allergy; detectable sIgE by itself not diagnostic of food allergy, but larger. sIgE values correlate with increased likelihood of food allergy; most reliable for these foods: eggs, wheat, cow's milk, peanuts, and soy; has the potential for over diagnosing by detecting sensitization to foods that may not be clinically relevant
Molecular Allergen Analysis (MAA); Component-resolved diagnostic (CRD) testing	Measures sIgE to specific components of protein antigens in food, not to the whole food extract; augments accuracy of conventional sIgE testing	Identifies clinically relevant sIgE from irrelevant sIgE with prognostic benefit for clinical reaction and severity; especially useful in assessing peanut allergy, pollen-food allergy syndrome (PFAS), and lipid transfer protein syndrome (LTPS)
Basophil activation test (BAT)	Using fresh whole blood, measures basophil response to an allergen in a test tube and can be an in-vitro surrogate for an oral food challenge (OFC) (Hoffmann et al, 2015).	Mimics an allergic reaction, not just sensitization; becoming more widely used to test for sesame or peanut allergy (Appel et al, 2018); potentially can distinguish between those sensitized and those clinically allergic
Mast cell activation test (MCAT)	Using plasma, measures mast cell response to allergenic cross-linking sIgE on mast cell similar to BAT	Still experimental; may be used in testing for peanut allergy (Gomes-Belo et al, 2018)
Serum IgG4	Blood testing for food-specific IgG4	Not validated for diagnostic use; tends to indicate previous exposure to the food and tolerance, not allergic reaction; may be more useful as a ratio IgG4/IgE in EoE diagnosis; may be useful in CRD testing
Leukocyte activation testing • Antigen leukocyte cellular antibody test (ALCAT) • Mediator release test (MRT)	Allergen is mixed with whole blood serum leukocyte suspension. Lysed leukocytes, primarily neutrophils, are assessed using DNA released; indicates release of inflammatory mediators and positive response to the food allergen	Measures non–IgE-mediated immune responses; indicates response to foods by innate immune cells; becoming more validated for diagnostic use (Ali et al, 2017; Garcia-Martinez et al, 2018)

Other Tests—Not Recommended

Applied kinesiology, also called muscle strength testing	Subject's arm is extended and vial with the test food is placed in the subject's hand, and the muscle strength in the opposite arm is tested by placing light pressure on the arm; test is considered positive if muscle strength weakens and arm moves more easily	Nonstandardized; may result in false-positive or false-negative results; not reliable and not validated for diagnostic use (Hammond and Lieberman, 2018)
Sublingual testing	Drops of allergen extract are placed under the tongue and symptoms are recorded	May result in false-positive results; not validated for diagnostic use
Provocation testing and neutralization	Subcutaneous injection of allergen extract elicits symptoms; this is then followed by injection of a weaker or stronger preparation to neutralize symptoms; often the pulse increased by 16 beats per minute is considered a positive test	Not validated for diagnostic use; neutralization may cause severe adverse reaction in those with true IgE-mediated food allergy

<table>
<tr><td colspan="2">**BOX 25.3** **Potential Foods and Pollens Involved in Pollen-Food Allergy Syndrome (PFAS) and Lipid Protein Transfer Syndrome (LPTS)**</td></tr>
<tr><td>Almonds</td><td>B</td></tr>
<tr><td>Apple</td><td>B</td></tr>
<tr><td>Apricot</td><td>B</td></tr>
<tr><td>Banana</td><td>R</td></tr>
<tr><td>Carrot</td><td>B, G</td></tr>
<tr><td>Celery</td><td>B</td></tr>
<tr><td>Chamomile</td><td>R</td></tr>
<tr><td>Cherry</td><td>B</td></tr>
<tr><td>Cucumber</td><td>R</td></tr>
<tr><td>Echinacea</td><td>R</td></tr>
<tr><td>Fennel</td><td>B</td></tr>
<tr><td>Fig</td><td>B, G</td></tr>
<tr><td>Green pepper</td><td>B</td></tr>
<tr><td>Hazelnut</td><td>B</td></tr>
<tr><td>Kiwi</td><td>B</td></tr>
<tr><td>Melon</td><td>R, G</td></tr>
<tr><td>Mung beans</td><td>B</td></tr>
<tr><td>Nectarine</td><td>B</td></tr>
<tr><td>Oranges</td><td>R, G</td></tr>
<tr><td>Parsley</td><td>B</td></tr>
<tr><td>Parsnip</td><td>B</td></tr>
<tr><td>Peanut</td><td>G</td></tr>
<tr><td>Peach</td><td>B</td></tr>
<tr><td>Pear</td><td>B</td></tr>
<tr><td>Plum</td><td>B</td></tr>
<tr><td>Potato</td><td>B</td></tr>
<tr><td>Prune</td><td>B</td></tr>
<tr><td>Pumpkin seed</td><td>B</td></tr>
<tr><td>Soy</td><td>B</td></tr>
<tr><td>Strawberry</td><td>B</td></tr>
<tr><td>Sunflower seeds</td><td>R</td></tr>
<tr><td>Tomato</td><td>G</td></tr>
<tr><td>Walnut</td><td>B</td></tr>
<tr><td>Zucchini</td><td>R</td></tr>
</table>

B, Birch pollen; *G*, grass pollen; *R*, ragweed pollen.
Sources: Joneja JV: *The health professional's guide to food allergies and intolerances*, Chicago, 2013, Academy of Nutrition and Dietetics, p 311. American College of Asthma, Allergy and Immunology, (ACAAI), 2018. Ferreira F, Gadermaier G and Wallner M: Tree Pollen Allergens in Global Atlas of Allergy, 2014.

under the patch is observed for redness, itchiness, or blister. Because the reaction is delayed, it may take 2 to 3 days to develop.

If, after removal of skin contact with nickel, the dermatitis persists, and there are also GI symptoms, allergy to ingested nickel in food is suspected. Dietary elimination of nickel and challenge with food nickel is the only way to determine whether nickel in food is the cause of the continuing chronic eczema and GI symptoms. A low-nickel diet (a nickel-free diet is impossible) is followed for 4 weeks until the symptoms subside. This is followed with a challenge of a high nickel food with observation (often for several weeks) of reoccurrence of symptoms (Joneja, 2013).

Nickel occurs naturally in all foods and may also be introduced through processing (metal containers) or cooking (metal utensils).

Some foods such as oats and oatmeal, cocoa, green lentils, soy beans, dried legumes, and some seeds are very high in nickel compared with others such as dairy products, many fish, and most vegetables (Joneja, 2013). It is also recommended that adding a probiotic supplement of *Lactobacillus reuteri* makes the low-nickel diet more effective in improving the GI symptoms (Randazzo et al, 2014).

An increasing number of studies are suggesting that the severity of nickel-related contact dermatitis can be reduced by oral exposure to nickel (Joneja, 2013; Di Gioacchino et al, 2014). There may be an initial worsening of the dermatitis, but prolonged exposure can reduce the clinical symptoms. The subject of nickel-contact dermatitis and nickel allergy and achievement of tolerance is complex and confusing and in need of more research.

Non–IgE-Mediated Reactions

Non–IgE-mediated allergic reactions to food continue to be elucidated. These are associated with delayed or chronic reactions, are often referred to as cell mediated, and are present in the eosinophilic GI diseases, food protein–induced enterocolitis syndrome (FPIES) and food protein–induced proctocolitis or proctitis (FPIP), and SNAS.

Eosinophilic Gastrointestinal Diseases (EGID)

Eosinophilic gastrointestinal diseases (EGID) are a group of GI disorders in which the accumulation of eosinophils (granulocytes capable of releasing inflammatory mediators) is present. These disorders include eosinophilic esophagitis, eosinophilic gastritis, eosinophilic gastroenteritis, eosinophilic enteritis, and eosinophilic colitis.

Eosinophilic esophagitis (EoE) and eosinophilic gastroenteritis (EGE) are the most studied, and are characterized by infiltration of the esophagus, stomach, or intestines with eosinophils. The conditions reflect a Th2 inflammation pattern. It is now thought that both conditions are mainly non–IgE-mediated allergic reactions, although there still may be an IgE-mediated component to the reaction. Almost half of the patients who present with EGID have atopic features (NASEM, 2014).

Eosinophilic Esophagitis (EoE)

Symptoms of EoE vary depending on the age of the person and may include early satiety and inability to manage varied food textures in young children, to reflux-like symptoms and vomiting in school-age children, and to dysphagia, refusal to eat, and food impaction in teenagers and adults. Because it is non-IgE mediated, as of yet there are no specific tests to identify the food triggers. EoE is most commonly treated with off-label use of swallowed topical corticosteroids (TCS), but the long-term efficacy and safety of this treatment is not yet established. Elimination diets are helpful and should be used if at all possible (Renz et al, 2018; Groetch et al, 2017).

The only way to know for certain that symptoms are caused by EoE is by esophageal tissue biopsy including the presence of eosinophils, and the use of an elimination diet for a period of time with resolution of the symptoms and histology normalization, followed by recurrence of symptoms and abnormal esophageal histology with reintroduction of the eliminated food (Groetch et al, 2017).

Ideally the reintroduction of each food is followed with an esophageal tissue biopsy; however, because biopsy is intrusive, time sensitive, and not always available, the Pediatric Eosinophilic Esophagitis Symptom Score (PEESS, v. 2.0) is used, especially with children. Use of this questionnaire with children 2 to 18 years of age has shown that reported symptoms of dysphagia most closely correlate with tissue markers of eosinophil activity; fewer reports of dysphagia correlate with improvement of EoE. The PEESS is available at www.jaci-inpractice.org (Martin et al, 2015).

The goals for treatment of EoE are resolution of clinical symptoms and esophageal eosinophilic inflammation, maintenance of remission to prevent potential complications such as esophageal strictures or fibrosis, correction and prevention of nutritional deficiencies, prevention of treatment-related complications, and maintenance of quality of life (Groetch et al, 2017).

An elimination diet or elemental diet presently is used to identify trigger foods and begin treatment of EoE. An elemental diet has been found to be the most effective therapy with a histologic (tissue level) disease remission rate of 90.8% in children and adults and was as effective as steroid treatment in EoE symptom resolution (Arias et al, 2014). However, this diet is difficult to implement and maintain long-term, so a less aggressive elimination diet is now recommended (Molina-Infante and Lucendo, 2018; Groetch et al, 2017).

Since the most common food triggers in EoE are cow's milk, wheat/gluten, and chicken eggs in children and adults in the United States, Spain, and Australia, many EoE dietary treatment programs use the step up 2-4-6-food elimination diets. This approach begins with a two-food (cow's milk and wheat/gluten) elimination diet. If after 6 weeks of strict adherence to this diet there is no remission of symptoms, a four-food elimination diet (cow's milk, wheat/gluten, egg, and soy) is started. If there is still no resolution, a six-food elimination diet (SFED) (cow's milk, wheat/gluten, egg, soy, peanuts/nuts, and fish/seafood) is implemented. This step up 2-4-6 approach usually results in prompt recognition of the majority of responders, reducing the number of endoscopies and costs, and shortening the diagnostic process (Molina-Infante and Lucendo, 2018). See Box 25.4 for guidelines for the step up 2-4-6 approach for elimination diets. An elemental diet consisting of an amino acid–based formula free of peptides or intact proteins may be a useful supplement, especially in young children, where the elimination diet may be difficult to implement without causing hunger, nutritional inadequacy, frustration, and abandonment of the diet.

Once problematic foods are identified, a tailored elimination diet that the patient is able to follow lifelong has been shown to be very effective in inducing remission in the majority of patients with EoE

BOX 25.4 Step Up 2-4-6 Approach to Foods Elimination

Food—Animal Milk and Wheat/Gluten Elimination Diet

You can consume all these kinds of foods for 6 weeks, preferably raw, fresh, or uncooked:

- Vegetables, tubers (potato), and legumes
- Meat (excepting processed or precooked meats, like sausages and hamburgers)
- Fish and seafood (excepting processed or precooked fish)
- Egg
- Fruit
- Nuts

You cannot consume for 6 weeks any food known to trigger allergic symptoms such as itchy mouth, scratchy throat, hives, skin rash, or asthma.

Avoid as much as possible eating out to have a better control of foods.

Try to always pick fresh, raw whole foods and avoid those cooked with sauces or fried in pans where potential contamination with breaded and/or wheat sources is likely.

You can drink coffee, tea (without animal milk), tonic water, soda, cola, fruit juice, wine, gin, vodka, and rum. Beer and whiskey are forbidden since they are gluten-containing drinks.

You can have coffee with soy, rice, almond, walnut, nut, or quinoa drinks.

Gluten-free products for those with celiac disease are allowed provided they do not contain milk (they can contain egg or soy).

Animal Milk

As a general rule, you should avoid all foods you are not fully sure to be safe.

Foods to Avoid:

- All cow's, goat's, and sheep's milk (whole, low-fat, skim, butter milk, evaporated, condensed, powdered, formula milk, hot cocoa)
- Milk products (all kind of cheeses, yogurt, butter, margarine, ice creams, milkshakes, custard, creme caramel, and rice or tapioca pudding)
- Foods that may contain milk (biscuits, cookies, doughnuts, muffins, pancakes, waffles, crackers, cream desserts, sweets, candies, chocolate with milk, sausages, ham, pork sausage)

Foods Allowed:

Milks made of soy, rice, spelt, quinoa, almond, cashews, or other nuts.

Wheat/Gluten

Foods to Avoid:

All products containing wheat, barley, rye, oats, spelt, triticale, semolina, and kamut. This wide range of products may include:

- Wheat-containing: bread, toast, biscuits, cookies, doughnuts, muffins, pretzels, pancakes, waffles, crackers, cream desserts, sweets, candies, pasta, cream, soups, sauces, malted food, and breaded or floured vegetables.
- Beer, whiskey

Be sure to avoid foods that contain any of the following information:

- Flour or floured, farina, wheat enriched, malted or malt added, breaded.
- Starch, fiber, protein, vegetable protein, semolina, hydrolyzed protein, malt, malt extract, couscous, yeast, spices, flavorings.

Foods Allowed:

All products allowed for celiac patients provided they do not contain milk or milk protein.

Food—Animal Milk, Wheat/Gluten, Egg, and Legumes Elimination Diet

You can consume all these kinds of foods for 6 weeks, preferably raw, fresh, or uncooked:

- Vegetables and tubers (potato)
- Meat (excepting processed or precooked meats, like sausages and hamburgers)
- Fish and seafood (excepting processed or precooked fish)
- Fruit
- Nuts

The same instructions apply as with the 2-food elimination diet but with the additional **elimination of two more food groups: egg and legumes.**

Egg

Foods to Avoid:

All products containing egg, baked goods, pasta, cakes, biscuits, cookies, doughnuts, muffins, pretzel, pancakes, waffles, crackers, cream desserts, sweets, candies, processed meat, goose liver, mayonnaise, food coated and wrapped in bread, breaded or creamed vegetables, processed meat, sauces.

BOX 25.4   Step Up 2-4-6 Approach to Foods Elimination—cont'd

Be sure to avoid foods that contain any of the following information:

- Albumin, apovitellin, binder, coagulant, cholesterol-free egg substitute, dried egg, egg white, egg yolk, egg lecithin, egg lysosome, eggnog, egg wash, globulin, lecithin, livetin, lysozyme, meringue, meringue powder, simplesse, surimi, ovalbumin, ovomucin, ovomucoid, ovomucin, ovomucoid, ovotransferrin, ovovitellin, powdered egg, trailblazer, vitellin, whole egg.

Legumes
Foods to Avoid:

Soy, lentils, pea, chickpeas, beans, peanuts, lupin, guar gum, carob bean, alfalfa.
Be sure to avoid foods that contain any of the following information:

- Hydrolyzed vegetable protein, plant protein, vegetable gum, and vegetable starch. These products are usually present in canned or processed foods.
- Oil made with any of the aforementioned legumes.
- African and Asian ethnic foods often contain soy and peanuts.

Food—Animal Milk, Wheat/Gluten, Egg, Legumes, Nuts, and Fish/Seafood Elimination Diet

You can consume all these kinds of foods for 6 weeks, preferably raw, fresh, or uncooked:

- Vegetables and tubers (potato)
- Meat (excepting processed or precooked meats, like sausages and hamburgers)
- Fruit

The same instructions apply as with the 4-food elimination diet but with the **additional elimination of two more food groups: nuts and fish/seafood.**

Nuts
Foods to Avoid:

Almond, artificial nuts, Brazil nut, beechnut, butternut, cashew, chestnut, chinquapin nut, coconut, filbert/hazelnut, gianduja (a chocolate-nut mixture), ginkgo nut, hickory nut, litchi/lychee/lychee nut, macadamia nut, marzipan/almond paste, nangai nut, natural nut extract (e.g., almond, walnut), nut butters (e.g., cashew butter), nut meal, nut meat, nut milk (e.g., almond milk, cashew milk), nut paste (e.g., almond paste), nut pieces, pecan, pesto, pili nut, pine nut (also referred to as Indian, pignoli, pigñolia, pignon, piñon, and pinyon nut), pistachio, praline, shea nut, walnut.

Be sure to avoid foods that contain any of the following information:

- Oil made with any of the aforementioned nuts.
- African and Asian ethnic foods often contain nuts.
- Tree nut proteins may be found in cereals, crackers, cookies, candy, chocolates, energy bars, flavored coffee, frozen desserts, marinades, barbecue sauces, and some cold cuts, such as mortadella. Some alcoholic beverages may contain nut flavoring.

Fish/Seafood
Foods to Avoid:

- All kinds of fish (anchovies, bass, catfish, cod, flounder, grouper, haddock, hake, halibut, herring, mahi-mahi, perch, pike, pollock, salmon, scrod, swordfish, sole, snapper, tilapia, trout, tuna)
- All kinds of shellfish (crab, lobster, prawns, shrimps) and mollusks (cockles, mussels, octopus, oyster, snails, squid).

Be sure to avoid foods that contain any of the following information:

- Vegetable protein, plant protein, vegetable gum, and vegetable starch. These products are usually present in canned or processed foods.
- Oil or gelatin made with any of the aforementioned fish or seafood products.
- African and Asian ethnic foods usually contain fish and seafood and are considered high-risk.

See also "How to Read a Label" in Table 25.5.
Adapted from: Molina-Infante J, Lucendo AJ: Dietary therapy for eosinophilic esophagitis, *J Allergy Clin Immunol* 142:41, 2018.

---

and offering potential for long-term treatment (Lucendo et al, 2013; Groetch et al, 2017).

Eosinophilic Gastroenteritis (EGE)

EGE is an uncommon disease characterized by eosinophilic infiltration of the GI tract in the absence of any secondary causes for the eosinophils, and the etiology and pathophysiology are unclear. The stomach and duodenum are most commonly affected, but it can involve any segment including the rectum. Symptoms vary depending on the portion of the GI tract involved, and the localized or widespread infiltration by eosinophils. Abdominal pain and nausea and vomiting are the most frequent presenting symptoms in children and adults. Adolescents may present with growth retardation, failure to thrive, and delayed puberty or amenorrhea.

EGE can occur at any age, but it is most commonly seen in those 30 to 40 years of age, and is possibly more prevalent in females (Zhang and Li, 2017; Alhmoud et al, 2016). Symptoms can easily be mistaken for other functional GI disorders. In patients with GI symptoms and a history of atopic conditions such as asthma, atopic dermatitis, allergic rhinitis, or PFAS there is high degree of clinical suspicion of EGE (Zhang and Li, 2017, NASEM, 2017). Tests for allergen-specific IgE are of no value in the identification of offending foods.

There is no consensus on the optimal treatment strategy for EGE because of a lack of large, randomized, controlled trials to clearly establish standard guidelines (Zhang and Li, 2017). However, since a high proportion of cases of EGE are associated with food allergy, an elimination or elemental diet can be recommended as a first step. The use of dietary treatment not only has been effective in reducing the need for corticosteroids, but also has improved the poor growth associated with the disease.

A proposed therapeutic strategy is to first have the patient follow an elimination diet avoiding specific airborne and food allergens. If this is not feasible or fails to achieve improvement, then glucocorticoid therapy is recommended, including starting with topical delivery and then considering systemic delivery (Zhang and Li, 2017).

Elimination diet therapy would be similar to that for EoE, beginning with an elemental diet if possible (exclusive feeding with amino acid–based formulas) or the empiric step up 2-4-6-food elimination diets. See Box 25.4 for guidelines for eliminating these foods from the diet. However, the high level of restriction and need for multiple endoscopies have hampered the implementation of elimination diets in clinical practice. Corticosteroids continue to be a widely used, clinically effective treatment.

Food Protein–Induced Enterocolitis Syndrome (FPIES)

Another non–IgE-mediated immune reaction to food is food protein–induced enterocolitis syndrome (FPIES), with the major criterion being vomiting 1 to 4 hours after ingestion of a food but with the absence of IgE-mediated skin or respiratory symptoms. FPIES is characterized by delayed repetitive vomiting (up to 10 times in an episode) after ingestion of the food, and the infant is pale, lethargic, and limp. Severe dehydration and hypovolemic shock may occur, and there may be an episode of diarrhea 1 to 5 hours later. Symptoms usually resolve within 24 hours and the child is well in between episodes (Leonard et al, 2018).

Chronic FPIES is characterized by chronic or intermittent delayed vomiting, usually in infants less than 4 months of age who are consuming cow's milk or soy formula regularly. The infant also exhibits chronic diarrhea, poor weight gain, and possibly failure to thrive. Chronic FPIES is usually diagnosed after an episode of acute FPIES when a history confirms that the symptoms have been chronic. When the trigger food is removed, the chronic FPIES resolves, but can reappear as an acute episode when the food is eaten again, usually accidentally. Oral food challenges (Table 25.4) may be needed if the diagnosis is not clear.

FPIES usually presents in infants when formula or solid foods are introduced between 2 and 7 months of age. Infants less than 2 months of age diagnosed with cow's milk or soy FPIES are more likely to present with diarrhea, bloody stools, and failure to thrive, in addition to vomiting, compared with those presenting

TABLE 25.4 Allergen Avoidance Guidelines

	Sources	Other Terms	Nutrients Involved	Alternatives
Milk *	Butter/many margarines or fat spreads, cheese, any mammalian milk (cow/sheep/goat), evaporated/condensed milk, cream, ghee, yogurt, ice creams, custard, dairy desserts, and manufactured food using any milk-based ingredient	Casein, caseinates, curd, lactoglobulin, lactose, milk solids, whey, buttermilk, milk sugar, whey sugar, whey syrup sweetener	Vitamin A, vitamin D, riboflavin, pantothenic acid, cyanocobalamin, calcium, magnesium, phosphate	Under 2 years: Extensively hydrolyzed (casein/whey) Hydrolyzed rice formulas# Amino acid–based formulas## Over 2 years Calcium-enriched, milk-free alternative drinks may be considered: • Rice milk (in some countries rice not allowed <4.5 years due to high arsenic content) • Soy milk • Oat milk • Chufa milk • Potato milk • Almond milk • Coconut milk • Pea milk Other foods: Milk-free versions of spreading fats/margarine, cheese, yogurts, ice cream, and cream
Egg **	Egg white and yolk, cakes, biscuits, specialty breads, mayonnaise	Albumin, dried egg, egg powder, egg protein, frozen egg, globulin, lecithin, livetin, ovalbumin, ovomucin, ovovitellin, pasteurized egg, vitellin	Riboflavin, biotin, protein, vitamin A, cyanocobalamin, vitamin D, vitamin E, pantothenic acid, selenium, iodine, folate	Egg replacers Adjust recipes with extra liquid or fruit purees Variety of egg-free products such as mayonnaise, cakes, muffins, puddings, and omelet mix
Wheat ***	Bread, breakfast cereals, pasta, cakes, biscuits, crackers, cold cooked meat, pies, batter, flour, cake flour, enriched flour, high-gluten flour, high-protein flour, graham flour, semolina, couscous, bottled sauces and gravies	Bran, cereal filler, farina, farro, starch, wheat, durum wheat, semolina, spelt, kamut, wheat bran, wheat gluten, wheat starch, wheat germ oil, hydrolyzed wheat protein, triticale, bulgur wheat, einkorn wheat, emmer wheat	Fiber, thiamine, riboflavin, niacin, calcium, iron, folate if fortified	Corn, rice, potato, cassava, yam, quinoa, millet, chickpea, sago, tapioca, amaranth, buckwheat Wheat-free and/or gluten-free foods, barley, rye, and regular oats may be tolerated by some individuals with wheat allergy or intolerance; however, they contain gluten Gluten-free oats may be tolerated by some individuals with celiac disease Use of alternative grains should be individualized and based on tolerance as determined by clinician and/or dietitian.

TABLE 25.4 Allergen Avoidance Guidelines—cont'd

	Sources	Other Terms	Nutrients Involved	Alternatives
Fish	All types of white and fatty fish, anchovy, (Worcestershire sauce), aspic, Caesar salad, Gentleman's Relish, kedgeree, caponata, fish sauce, paella, bouillabaisse, gumbo Some people may tolerate canned fish Fish oil capsules may cause reactions in highly sensitized individuals	Surimi Caviar	All fish: protein, iodine Fish bones: calcium, phosphorus, fluoride Fatty fish: vitamins A and D, omega-3 fatty acids	
Shellfish	Crayfish, crab, lobster, shrimp, prawns		Similar nutrients to white fish. Crab and mussels: good sources of omega-3, selenium, zinc, iodine, and copper	
Mollusks	Clams, mussels, oysters, octopus, squid, snails, scallops	Health food preparations such as green-lipped mussel extract, oyster sauce	Varying amounts of protein (scallop), calcium (clam), zinc (oysters), and iron (clam)	
Peanut****	Peanuts, defatted peanuts, peanut flakes, expeller-pressed peanut oil, peanut flour, peanut butter, peanut snacks, satay sauce May contain peanut: sprouts, confectionery, frozen desserts, Asian dishes (Indonesian, Malaysian, Thai, and Chinese), trail mix, energy or sports bars, rice crackers, cereal bars, cookies, brownies, nut toppings on ice cream, vegetarian/vegan foods, breakfast cereals, pesto sauce may sometimes contain peanut	Arachis oil, hypogeaia, peanut protein, groundnut, earth nut, monkey nut, mandelonas, mixed nuts	Vitamin E, niacin, magnesium	
Tree nut Almond, hazelnut, walnut, cashew nut, pecan nut, Brazil nut, pistachio nut, macadamia nut, Queensland nut	Similar foods as peanut Amaretto contains almond flavor Worcester sauce (walnuts) Korma sauce (almonds)	Hazelnut: filbert, cob nut Macadamia: Queensland nut, candle nut Pecan: Hickory nut Note: Nutmeg, coconut, pine nut, and palm nut are not classified as nuts	Depends on type of nut	
Sesame seed	Sesame seeds, sesame oil, halva, tahini, hummus, seeded bread/rolls, gomashio, Asian foods made with sesame oil, Greek, Iranian, Lebanese, and Turkish food, Aqua Libra is sometimes made with sesame	Gomasio—sesame seed and salt seasoning	Protein, fats, vitamin E, calcium, potassium, phosphorus, vitamin B and iron Avoidance has no significant effect on nutrition	

Continued

TABLE 25.4 Allergen Avoidance Guidelines—cont'd

	Sources	Other Terms	Nutrients Involved	Alternatives
Celery/celeriac	Primary allergy: celery and celeriac in its raw, cooked, juiced, canned, and dried (celery spice) form		Fiber Avoidance has no significant effect on nutrition	In PFAS and LTPS, dried celery/celeriac may be tolerated
Mustard	Mustard Mustard seed Curry powder Pizza Sauces, marinades, dressings		Mainly fat and protein Avoidance has no significant effect on nutrition	
Soy*****	Soy beans, soy flour, soy nuts, soy sauce, shoyu sauce, soy products (soy cheese, soy fiber, soy ice cream), meat substitutes, breads, vegetarian/vegan foods, Asian cuisine, processed meat (e.g., hot dogs), peanut butter, foods labeled as "diet" and "high-protein" or "low-fat," sport or energy bars	Edamame Tofu Miso Natto Soy protein/gum/starch Texturized (or hydrolyzed) vegetable protein Soy flavoring Soy lecithin Chee-fan Ketjap	Thiamin, riboflavin, pyridoxine, folate, calcium, phosphorus, magnesium, iron, zinc, protein, fiber	Cow's milk Rice milk (in some countries rice not allowed <4.5 years due to high arsenic content) Oat milk Chufa milk Potato milk Almond milk Coconut milk Pea milk Meat, fish, poultry, or other soy-free vegetarian alternatives
Lupin	Often used in Europe in pastries, bread, pizza, and lupin-seeded breads		Protein, fat, fiber, thiamin, riboflavin and vitamin E Avoidance has no significant effect on nutrition	

* Goat and sheep milk proteins are similar to cow milk protein, and those with cow milk allergy could experience similar symptoms with ingestion of these alternatives. All mammalian milk should be avoided initially. Goat milk is not recommended as a cow milk substitute because it has a high renal solute load and is very low in folic acid compared with cow milk.

** People with allergy to chicken egg may also be allergic to other types of eggs, such as goose, turkey, duck, or quail eggs. All should be avoided initially.

*** Note that nonfood products such as cosmetics, supplements, and medications can contain wheat ingredients and may cause an adverse reaction.

**** There is a high risk of contamination of utensils when eating out at Asian, Chinese, Mexican, Thai, Mediterranean, and Indian restaurants. Nonfood products such as cosmetics,
supplements, and medications can contain peanut ingredients and may cause an adverse reaction.

***** Several studies indicate that individuals who are soy allergic frequently tolerate soy lecithin and soy oil. There is a high risk of soy cross-contamination when eating out, especially at Asian restaurants. Nonfood products such as cosmetics, supplements, and medications can contain soy ingredients.

\# Partially hydrolyzed: nonhypoallergenic; contains partially digested proteins that have a molecular weight greater than extensively hydrolyzed formula. May cause a reaction in one third to one half of individuals with a cow's milk protein allergy.

\#\# Free amino acid–based infant formula: hypoallergenic; peptide-free formula that contains essential and nonessential amino acids. Usually tolerated by those allergic to extensively
hydrolyzed formulas.

LTPS, Lipid transfer protein syndrome; *PFAS*, pollen-food allergy syndrome.

Sources: Venter C, Groetch M, Netting M, Meyer R: A patient-specific approach to develop an exclusion diet to manage food allergy in infants and children, *Clin Exp Allergy* 48:121, 2018.

Joneja JV: *The Health Professional's Guide to Food Allergies and Intolerances*, Chicago, 2013, Academy of Nutrition and Dietetics.

later (Nowak-Węgrzyn et al, 2017). A Japanese cohort reported FPIES symptoms in 10% of infants after breastfeeding, presumably because of the problematic food protein in the breastmilk from maternal ingestion. Similarly an Australian report found this in 5% of infants (Nomura et al, 2011; Mehr et al, 2017).

Symptoms consistent with FPIES may present in older children and adults with delayed vomiting, often after the ingestion of fish, shellfish, or egg (Leonard et al, 2018). Studies from various countries show that the most common food triggers are cow's milk, soy, and grains (oats/rice) in the United States and South Korea, fish in Italy and Spain, and rice in Australia (Mehr et al, 2017).

The pathophysiology of FPIES is not well understood, but it is thought that a reaction to a consumed food protein leads to gut inflammation, which causes increased intestinal permeability and a fluid shift resulting in vomiting, diarrhea, abdominal pain, and possibly shock (Leonard et al, 2018). Food-specific IgE antibodies have no

TABLE 25.5 Food Challenge Protocols

Double-blind, placebo-controlled food challenge	Allergen is disguised and given orally and patient monitored for reaction; patient and physician blinded; also tested with placebo.	"Gold standard" for food allergy testing.
Single-blind food challenge	Suspect food is disguised from patient and orally given by physician in a clinical setting.	Less time-consuming than DBPCFC; may be used in instances in which patient experiences symptoms secondary to fear or aversion to suspect food.
Open oral food challenge	Suspect food is orally given to patient in undisguised, natural form in gradual doses under medical supervision.	Less time-consuming than DBPCFC; should not be used in instances in which patient experiences symptoms secondary to fear or aversion to suspect food.

value in the diagnosis; a thorough history followed with a specific food elimination diet and an oral food challenge (OFC) of the suspected food under medical supervision is the only way at present to make a FPIES diagnosis. It is challenging because FPIES mimics many other GI inflammatory disorders.

Treatment of FPIES focuses on removal of the offending food(s) and management of vomiting, dehydration, and shock. For infants with cow's milk or soy FPIES, breastfeeding or use of an extensively hydrolyzed casein formula is encouraged. If cow's milk or soy FPIES exists in the formula-fed infant, supervised introduction of one or the other (soy or cow's milk) formula can be considered. See Table 25.4 for cow's milk-free and soy-free formulas. Maternal avoidance of a breastfeeding infant's FPIES triggers is not recommended if the infant is thriving and asymptomatic (Nowak-Węgrzyn et al, 2017). Mothers should avoid trigger food(s) if a reaction occurs after breastfeeding or if the infant is failing to thrive. If symptoms still do not resolve, discontinuing breastfeeding and introducing an extensively hydrolyzed formula (EHF) should be considered. See Nowak-Węgrzyn et al (2017) for feeding guidelines.

Nutritional adequacy, feeding skill development, and diet expansion is vital to any infant's nutrition and development, especially in those with multiple food FPIES or feeding issues. FPIES patients should be monitored regularly for the development of tolerance and eventually diet expansion, with medically supervised oral food challenges (Table 25.5).

Food Protein–Induced Proctitis or Proctocolitis (FPIP)

In food protein–induced proctocolitis or proctitis or (FPIP), bloody and mucus-laden stools are seen in an otherwise apparently healthy baby, often at about 2 months of age. Parents are concerned when they see flecks of blood in their baby's stool, but it is usually slight and further development of anemia is rare. Common trigger foods are cow's milk protein or soy protein from infant formula, and their removal from the infant's diet usually solves the problem. In the case of the breastfed infant, the mother should remove these foods from the diet and continue to breastfeed. For the formula-fed infant, it becomes necessary to switch to an EHF, such as any of those listed in Table 25.4. However, sometimes the infant requires an elemental formula, examples of which are also listed in Table 25.4 and in Chapter 15. The bleeding usually disappears within 3 days of implementing a formula change or change in the breastfeeding mother's diet. In most cases the FPIP resolves itself by the time the baby is 1 to 2 years old, and offending foods can be introduced with monitoring of the baby's stool for blood (Meyer et al, 2018; NASEM, 2017).

FOOD INTOLERANCES

Food intolerances are adverse reactions to food that result in clinical symptoms caused by nonimmunologic mechanisms including microbial, pharmacologic, GI, metabolic, psychological and behavioral, or idiosyncratic. They are believed to be far more common than food allergies and are usually triggered by small-molecular weight chemical substances such as food additives and biologically active components of food such as biogenic amines. Symptoms induced by food intolerances are often similar to those of food allergy and may include GI, cutaneous, respiratory, and neurologic manifestations. Clinically, it is important to distinguish food intolerance from immune-mediated food allergy because food allergies can cause life-threatening anaphylactic reactions, whereas food intolerances do not (see Table 25.2).

Gastrointestinal Manifestations

Lactose Intolerance

Intolerance to the disaccharide lactose is the most common adverse reaction to food, and most cases result from a genetically influenced reduction of intestinal lactase. It is estimated that about 70% of the world's population has low production of lactase (hypolactasia) (Ugidos-Rodríguez et al, 2018). Symptoms of lactose intolerance, abdominal bloating and cramping, flatulence, and diarrhea, usually appear several hours (even up to 24) after lactose ingestion and last for several hours. Because some of the GI symptoms are similar, lactose intolerance is often confused with allergy to cow's milk. However, most individuals who are allergic to cow's milk also have symptoms in other organ systems, including the respiratory tract, skin, and, in severe cases, systemic anaphylactic reactions. Deficiencies of lactase and other carbohydrate-digesting enzymes and their management are discussed further in Chapter 27.

FODMAPs Intolerance

Maldigestion and malabsorption of the fructo-, oligo-, di-, and mono-saccharides and polyols (FODMAPs) appear to be becoming more common. Humans lack the hydrolase enzymes necessary to break down the bonds in the fructose polymer chains, so in many individuals, intake of large quantities of FODMAPs will lead to bloating, diarrhea, cramping, and flatulence. FODMAPs intolerance appears to be more common in individuals who have an underlying functional GI disorder, such as irritable bowel syndrome and small intestine bacterial overgrowth (SIBO). See Chapter 27 for more information about FODMAPs.

Gluten Intolerance

Nonceliac gluten intolerance (or sensitivity) is a condition that is being diagnosed more frequently. It is best defined as intestinal or extraintestinal symptoms that occur when gluten-containing grains are included in the diet, which resolve when the offending grains are removed from the diet. It can easily be confused with a food allergy, but it is not an allergic reaction, at least not based on our present understanding

(DeGeeter and Guandalini, 2018). It remains controversial whether gluten proteins found in wheat, rye, and barley are the cause of symptoms for those with gluten intolerance.

There is some research suggesting that fructan intolerance may be the cause of symptoms for some people, not the gluten proteins (Igbinedion et al, 2017). Because of this, the term nonceliac wheat sensitivity (NCWS) is often used to describe this condition. This is different than the other gluten-related disorder, celiac disease, which is an autoimmune reaction that occurs in the presence of gluten proteins in the diet. See Chapter 27 for a discussion of celiac disease and its dietary management.

Pharmacologic

An adverse reaction to a food may be the result of a response to a pharmacologically active component in that food. A wide range of allergy-like symptoms can result from ingestion of biogenic amines such as histamine and tyramine. Salicylates, monosodium glutamate, or food additives such as benzoates can also cause reactions.

Histamine

Histamine is a biogenic amine produced endogenously with very important functions. It is released as the first inflammatory mediator in an allergic reaction or in a physical defense reaction. When it is released and reaches a certain level, it can cause vasodilation, erythema, increased permeability of cell membranes, digestive tract upset, pruritus (itching), urticaria (hives), angioedema (tissue swelling), hypotension, tachycardia (heart racing), chest pain, nasal congestion (rhinitis), runny nose (rhinorrhea), conjunctivitis (watery, reddened, irritated eyes), headache, panic, fatigue, confusion, and irritability.

Everyone has a level of histamine that is tolerated, and when that level is exceeded in the body the symptoms of excessive histamine develop. Basal levels of 0.3 to 1 ng/mL are considered normal

(Joneja, 2017). Individuals can have increased levels of histamine due to stress, hormonal changes, and GI impairment, including inflammation or infection. Some people are more sensitive to histamine than others, usually because of a genetically determined inability to catabolize or break down histamine fast enough to keep the levels low so that histamine-induced symptoms are not triggered. One percent of the U.S. population suffers from histamine intolerance, and 80% of those sufferers are middle-aged (Maintz and Novak, 2007).

Symptoms of excessive histamine may be indistinguishable from those of food allergy because of histamine's mediator function in allergic reactions. However, histamine intolerance does not have an IgE-based mechanism as food allergy does. In histamine intolerance there is excessive histamine for the following reasons: (1) certain foods naturally contain large amounts of histamine, or its precursor histidine (which through fermentation becomes histamine), which then causes a reaction in the histamine sensitive individual; (2) some individuals are not able to deactivate or metabolize histamine in a timely manner because of a deficiency of the enzymes diamine oxidase (DAO) or histamine-N-methyltransferase (HNMT); or (3) there is the presence of other amines that also influence the histamine reaction.

Foods with a high histamine content include fermented foods, sauerkraut, aged cheeses, processed meats and fish, alcoholic beverages (beer and wine), and leftovers. Strawberries, citrus fruits, pineapple, tomatoes, spinach, egg whites, fish, shellfish, and some food additives (e.g., tartrazine) and preservatives (e.g., benzoates) stimulate histamine release from mast cells. The mechanisms for this reaction are not clear. Histamine intolerance or sensitivity may be suspected when an allergic cause for symptoms has been ruled out (Joneja, 2017). With true histamine intolerance, treatment with a histamine-restricted diet (Box 25.5) can be very helpful. The diet should be implemented for 6 weeks, with the patient keeping records of intake and symptoms followed by evaluation of progress in reduction in symptoms.

BOX 25.5 Histamine-Restricted Diet

General Description

This eating plan is designed to remove foods that contain high levels of histamine and foods and food additives that release histamine in the body. It is a test diet for people with high histamine levels and associated symptoms for which other treatments have been of little value.

Food Sources of Histamine

Histamine is present in large quantities in fermented foods. Microbial enzymes convert the amino acid histidine (present as a constituent of all proteins) to histamine in a biochemical process known as decarboxylation.

Any foods that have been subjected to microbial fermentation in their manufacture, for example: Continental sausages such as bologna, salami, pepperoni, wieners, most cheeses, soy sauce, miso, sauerkraut, alcoholic beverages, "dealcoholized" beverages, and vinegars contain histamine.

Foods that have been exposed to microbial contamination will contain histamine: the level is determined by the rapidity of action of microbial metabolism. Histamine levels will rise to a reactive level long before any signs of spoilage occur in the food. This is particularly important in fish and shellfish. Bacteria in the gut will start to convert histidine to histamine as soon as the fish dies. The longer the fish remains ungutted, the higher the level of histamine in the flesh.

Some foods, such as eggplant (aubergine), pumpkin, tomato, olives, and spinach, contain high levels of histamine naturally.

In addition, a number of food additives such as certain food dyes (e.g. tartrazine) and preservatives (e.g. benzoates) are known to mediate the release of histamine. Some of these, for example, benzoates, occur naturally in foods,

especially fruits, and have the same ability to release histamine as the food additive.

The histamine-restricted diet excludes all the foods, which are known to contain high levels of histamine, and chemicals that can release histamine when they enter the body.

Histamine-Restricted Diet

Avoid the following foods during the 4 week trial elimination period.

Meat, Poultry, Fish

- Fish and shellfish whether fresh, frozen, smoked, or canned, if processing is unknown
  - If the fish is freshly caught, gutted and cooked within ½ hour, it may be eaten
- Egg
  - A small quantity of cooked egg in a baked product such as pancakes, muffins, or cakes is allowed
- Processed, smoked, and fermented meats such as luncheon meat, sausage, hot dog or wiener, bologna, salami, pepperoni, smoked ham, cured bacon

Milk and Milk Products

- All fermented milk products, including:
  - Cheese:
    - Any kind of fermented cheese such as cheddar, Colby, blue cheese, Brie, Camembert, feta, Romano, and so on.

BOX 25.5 Histamine-Restricted Diet—cont'd

- Cheese products such as processed cheese, cheese slices, cheese spreads
- Cottage cheese
- Ricotta cheese made with microbial culture (read label)
- Yogurt
- Buttermilk
- Kefir
    - Any milk product that is curdled rather than fermented is allowed (e.g., paneer)

Fruits
- Citrus (orange, grapefruit, lemon, lime)
- Cherries
- Strawberries
- Apricots
- Raspberries
- Pineapple
- Cranberries
- Prunes
- Loganberries
- Dates
- Raisins
- Currants (fresh or dried)

Vegetables
- Tomatoes, tomato sauces, ketchup
- Spinach
- Eggplant
- Pumpkin
- Olives
- Pickles, relishes, and other foods containing vinegar

Food Additives
- Tartrazine and other artificial food colors

- Preservatives, especially benzoates, sulfites, and butylated hydroxyanisole (BHA), butylated hydroxytoluene (BHT)
    - Note: Many medications and vitamin pills contain these additives; ask your pharmacist to recommend additive-free supplements and medications

Seasonings
- Cinnamon
- Cloves
- Thyme
- Chili powder
- Anise
- Vinegar (except distilled)
- Curry powder
- Nutmeg

Miscellaneous
- Fermented soy products (such as soy sauce, miso)
- Fermented foods (such as sauerkraut)
- Tea (regular or green)
- Chocolate, cocoa, and cola drinks
- Alcoholic beverages of all types
- "Dealcoholized" beverages (e.g., beer, ale, wine, etc.)

This diet excludes all:
- Foods with naturally high levels of histamine
- Fermented foods
- Artificial food colors, especially tartrazine
- Benzoates including food sources of benzoates, benzoic acid, and sodium benzoate
- Sulfites
- BHA and BHT

Source: Joneja, JA: Histamine Intolerance: a Comprehensive Guide for Healthcare Professionals, 2017, e-published.

Tyramine

Tyramine is a biogenic amine formed from the amino acid tyrosine that is found naturally in some foods, plants, and animals. Like histamine, it can also be produced in foods as a result of fermentation, curing, aging, or spoilage of produce, dairy products, and meats. Because of the rate and extent of these processes, the tyramine content of foods varies widely. Examples of foods high in tyramine are aged cheeses, soy sauce, aged meats, pickled fish, tofu, sauerkraut, and tap beer.

Tyramine can have pharmacologic activity and can cause a rise in blood pressure. Because of this the body produces monoamine oxidase (MAO), an enzyme that guards against the build up of too much tyramine and other amines in the body, including monoamine neurotransmitters (e.g., norepinephrine, dopamine, and serotonin), and changes them into harmless compounds that can be excreted from the body safely. MAO is present in the GI tract, the liver, nerve endings, and the brain. An individual can develop an intolerance to tyramine when there is too much tyramine present in the diet, or when there is not enough MAO activity to keep its level in check. Intolerance is evidenced by blood pressure changes. Large amounts of tyramine can cause the release of excess norepinephrine, which constricts the blood vessels, causing blood pressure to rise, sometimes to a dangerously high level, known as a hypertensive crisis.

Ingestion of tyramine-containing foods also may cause migraine headaches or chronic hives in tyramine-sensitive individuals, with the response being dose dependent (Skypala et al, 2015b).

Tyramine intolerance can develop in some individuals who are taking the medication monoamine oxidase inhibitors (MAOIs), which interfere with the breakdown of tyramine. Fortunately, these medications are not prescribed as frequently today as in the past.

Other Amines and Food Additives

When histamine or tyrosine are present in foods, other biogenic amines such as lesser known putrescine, cadaverine, tryptamine, 2-phenylethylamine, spermine, and spermidine may also be present. Like histamine and tyramine, they are mainly produced by microbial decarboxylation of amino acids in the foods and can cause reactions.

Some food components are actually added to foods, and they also appear to be able to cause reactions, although they are poorly understood. Food additives such as salicylates, carmine (cochineal extracts), artificial food dyes and colorings such as FD&C yellow #5, and preservatives such as benzoic acid, sodium benzoate, butylated hydroxyanisole (BHA), butylated hydroxytoluene (BHT), nitrates, sulfites, and monosodium glutamate (MSG) can cause adverse reactions in certain individuals (Vojdani and Vojdani, 2015).

Sulfites are widely used as preservatives and antioxidants in many food products. Reactions to sulfites, including sodium metabisulfite and sodium sulfite, result in a diverse range of symptoms in sulfite-sensitive individuals. These can include dermatitis, urticaria, hypotension, abdominal pain, diarrhea, and life-threatening asthmatic and anaphylactic reactions (Vally and Misso, 2012). The mechanisms remain unclear.

Adverse reactions to MSG were originally reported as the "Chinese restaurant syndrome" because of its use in Chinese cooking. Complaints of headache, nausea, flushing, abdominal pain, and asthma occurred after ingestion. MSG is widely distributed in the food supply (e.g., bouillon, meat tenderizers, canned food, frozen food, condiments) and occurs naturally in tomatoes, Parmesan cheese, mushrooms, and other foods. Results from double-blind, placebo-controlled food challenges (DBPCFCs) found symptoms from MSG to not be persistent, clear, consistent, or serious (Geha et al, 2000; Williams and Woessner, 2009).

However, more recent data in animals and humans have indicated that MSG consumption may be a contributing factor to increased risk of overweight, independent of physical activity and total energy intake (He et al, 2011). Considering the ongoing debate about this common flavoring agent as an obesogenic agent, nutrition practitioners should be aware of MSG sensitivity (Savcheniuk et al, 2014).

A diet that is being used for those individuals with suspected intolerances to dietary amines, salicylate, and food additives is the FAILSAFE diet, a diet "free of additives, low in salicylates, amines, and flavor enhancers" designed by the Royal Prince Alfred Hospital in Australia. This diet is intended to be used for the investigation and management of people with suspected food intolerance. The FAILSAFE diet excludes strong-tasting and smelling foods and environmental chemicals, in particular:

1. **About fifty artificial food additives,** including colors (like tartrazine, sunset yellow), flavors, preservatives, and antioxidants (sulfites, nitrates, benzoates, sorbates, parabens).
2. **Salicylates (aspirin)** and polyphenols (natural flavors, colors, and preservatives) found in a wide range of fruits and vegetables.
3. **Neurotransmitters in food:** free glutamates (MSG) and amines (histamine, serotonin, dopamine, phenylethylamine, tyramine, and others) found in aged proteins and fermented foods like cheese, chocolate, game, and aged meat.
4. **Aromatic (strong-smelling and tasting) chemicals** found in perfumes, cleaning products, commercial cosmetics, and scented and colored toiletries, especially mint and menthol products.
5. **Some pharmaceutical drugs,** including aspirin, NSAIDS and other COX II inhibitors including ibuprofen, and the methyl-salicylates found in decongestants and antiinflammatory creams.

   Practicalities of the diet can be found at www.FAILSAFEdiet.com.

Microbial Contamination and Toxins

Food toxicity or food poisoning results from microbial contamination of food and causes myriad symptoms, including nausea, vomiting, diarrhea, abdominal pain, headache, and fever, many of which can be confused with an allergic reaction. It is estimated that in the United States 9.4 million people per year are affected by foodborne illness, with 31 known pathogens identified (Scallan et al, 2011). Fortunately, most episodes are self-limiting and should be distinguished from food allergy or intolerance from a thorough history. If the cause of the symptoms cannot be determined to be a food toxin or microbial contamination, then a single food elimination diet followed by a challenge of that food may be necessary (see Table 25.4).

Psychogenic and Behavioral Factors

Evidence for the role of food allergy or intolerance in various disorders such as anxiety, depression, migraine headache, attention/deficit-hyperactivity disorder, and mood disorders is emerging. Increased intestinal permeability, dysbiosis, neurotransmitter production by the gut, and gut immune system response are currently being investigated as contributing factors (see Chapters 27 and 40). If a food-symptom relationship cannot be shown for the food intolerance, but food avoidance is perceived as helpful because of the patient's personal experience, appropriate medical nutrition therapy may include food elimination and other therapeutic interventions.

MEDICAL NUTRITION THERAPY

Assessment

A thorough history and timeline including perinatal, prenatal, and birth history (e.g., vaginal or C-section), early feeding practices (breastfed vs. formula), childhood illnesses, past and current medical history, medications (for example, antibiotics, proton-pump inhibitors, etc.) dietary supplements (including probiotics), exercise patterns, and lifestyle factors (stress, sleep, relationships), along with a comprehensive diet history and food habits, helps to determine possible root causes contributing to adverse food reactions.

Anthropometric measurements are also essential as a component of nutritional assessment. The infant's and child's anthropometric data should be plotted on a growth chart and evaluated over time (see Appendix 4). Because decreased weight-for-height measurements may be related to malabsorption or food avoidance due to allergy or intolerance, patterns of growth and their relationship to the onset of symptoms should be explored (Meyer et al, 2014).

A nutrition-focused physical examination is also important in assessing the patient with adverse food reactions. Clinical signs of malnutrition should be assessed and monitored with ongoing dietary therapy (see Chapter 5 and Appendix 11).

A 7- to 14-day food and symptom record is extremely useful for uncovering adverse food reactions (Fig. 25.4). The food and symptom record should include the time the food is eaten, the quantity and type of food, all food ingredients if possible, the time symptoms appear relative to the time of food ingestion, and any supplements or medications taken before or after the onset of symptoms. Other influences such as stress, physical exercise, urine and bowel elimination, and sleep patterns, along with environmental factors, provide valuable information in piecing together the factors that affect adverse food reactions. The more thorough the information obtained about the adverse reaction, the more useful the record. For example, a reaction that appears to be caused by a food actually may be caused by a pet or a chemical or another environmental factor. A patient may prefer to use an app designed to track this type of data (see Chapter 4). The comprehensive food and symptom record is used to assess nutritional adequacy and also serves as a tool for future therapeutic interventions.

DIAGNOSIS

Diagnosis of adverse food reactions requires identification of the suspected food or food ingredient, proof that the food ingestion causes the adverse response, and verification of an immune or nonimmune-mediated response. The detailed food and symptom record as part of a comprehensive nutrition assessment is also a diagnostic tool. This information may be followed with appropriate immunologic testing by a physician; however, tests for food allergy are not completely definitive and should always be used in conjunction with a comprehensive physical examination, clinical history, and nutrition assessment (Boyce et al, 2010; Skypala et al, 2015). See Table 25.3 for a complete description of tests used in diagnosis of food allergy.

3-DAY FOOD JOURNAL

Name: _____

It is important to keep an accurate record of your usual food and beverage intake as a part of your treatment plan. Please complete this Food Journal for three consecutive days including one weekend day.

- *Do not change your eating behavior at this time, as the purpose of this food record is to analyze your present eating habits*
- *Record information as soon as possible after the food as been consumed*
- *Please describe all foods and beverages consumed as accurately and in as much detail possible including estimated amounts, brand names, cooking method, etc.*
- *Record the amount of each food or beverage consumed using standard measurements such as 8 ounces, 1/2 cup, 1 teaspoon, etc.*
- *Included any added items, for example: tea with 1 tsp honey, potato with 2 tsps butter, etc.*
- *List all beverages and types, including water, coffee, tea, sports drinks, sodas/ diet sodas, etc.*
- *Please comment on any noted emotional or physical symptoms including hunger level, stress, bloating, fatigue, adverse reaction experienced, etc.*
- *Include comments about eating habits and environment such as reasons for skipping a meal, when a meal was eaten at a restaurant, etc. and any additional details that may be important*
- *Each day please note all bowel movements, describe their consistency (regular, loose, firm, etc.), frequency, and any additional information*
- *If desired, an online site or app such as myfitness pal, www.fitday.com, etc. can be used—be sure to send me your login username and password.*

Date: _____	Food and beverages	Comments or symptoms
Breakfast Time: _____		
Snack		
Lunch Time: _____		
Snack		
Dinner Time: _____		
Elimination Description	Time: _____	Time: _____	Time: _____

From: Swift Clinic, 2018

Fig. 25.4 Food and symptom diary.

Immunologic Testing

Skin-Prick Test

In **skin-prick tests (SPT)** drops of standard food extracts are placed on the skin of the arm or back. The skin is then scratched or pricked with a lancet with each drop of extract. The areas of application are then observed for the development of the classic "wheal and flare" reaction. In theory, if the underlying mast cells have attached sIgE, inflammatory mediators are released. The wheal and flare reaction results from the action of the mediators, especially histamine, on the surrounding tissue. These skin-prick tests are the most economic immunologic tests of an Ig-E mediated reaction, providing results within 15 to 30 minutes. Comparison with the positive control (histamine) and the negative control (saline) provide parameters necessary for accurate readings (Fig. 25.5). All skin-prick tests are compared with the control wheal. Test wheals that are 3 mm greater than the negative control usually indicate a positive result.

Negative skin-prick tests have good negative predictive accuracy and strongly suggest the absence of an IgE sensitization and therefore an IgE-mediated reaction. Positive skin-prick test results, however, indicate only IgE sensitization and the possibility of a food allergy reaction. In the patient with a suspected food allergy, the skin-prick test is useful in supporting the diagnosis. For children younger than 2 years of age, the skin test is reserved to confirm immunologic mechanisms after symptoms have been confirmed by a positive test result from a

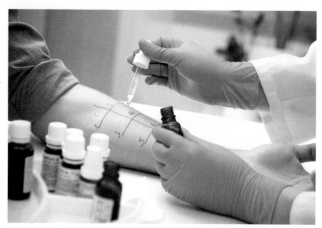

Fig. 25.5 A skin-prick test showing the wheal and flare of the reaction to the allergen. From www.istockphoto.com

supervised food challenge, or when the history of the reaction is impressive.

All foods that test positive must correlate with a strong exposure history or be proven to cause allergic reactions through food challenges before they can be considered allergenic (see Table 25.4). The most common food allergens in the United States (milk, egg, peanut, soy, wheat, shellfish, fish, and tree nuts) account for most of the positive food skin-prick tests (NASEM, 2017).

Serum Antibody Tests

Food allergen–specific serum IgE testing is used to identify foods that may be causing the allergic response. The two systems in use are ImmunoCAP or ImmunoCAP ISAC system, and the Immulite system. They are similar in that they measure for the presence of IgE antibodies sensitized to various allergens. This type of test provides a quantitative assessment of sIgE antibodies; higher levels of antibodies are often, but not always, predictors of clinical symptoms. It is a fairly effective test, as shown by testing known food-allergic children whose food allergies had been previously proven with DBPCFCs (NASEM, 2017).

Test results should be followed with either food elimination and challenge, or DBPCFCs to complete the diagnostic process. It should be noted that ImmunoCap or Immulite results or skin-testing results for IgE sensitization may remain positive even after the child has resolved the food allergy, and the food can be eaten without symptoms.

Component resolved diagnostics (CRD) testing is emerging as a useful tool in assessing food allergy. CRD involves testing for IgE sensitized to specific component proteins in foods and not just the whole protein extract. The aim of the test is based on the understanding that some proteins within a food may be more potent in causing an allergic reaction than others within the same food. For example, clinically relevant proteins may resist digestion, and IgE immune responses against such proteins may have a greater diagnostic value for systemic allergy than immune responses against more labile proteins that degrade easily and are not systemically absorbed and therefore will not cause a reaction. Much research is being done using CRD to determine which components of peanut protein are likely to cause anaphylaxis or a severe allergic response to peanuts and which will not (NASEM, 2017) (see Table 25.3).

Other Tests

A number of laboratory tests are now available that attempt to identify an individual's specific adverse reactions to foods. Some of these tests measure IgA, IgG, and IgG4 levels and are not considered reliable. Others (ALCAT and MRT) measure the amount of cytokines released by lymphocytes and granulocytes upon degranulation in response to food antigen exposure and may be useful identifying food intolerances that are not IgE mediated (Garcia-Martinez et al, 2018). Continued scientific investigation into the validity of various types of food reactivity testing is warranted (Vojdani, 2015b; see Table 25.3).

Nonimmunologic tests that may be useful in diagnosing food intolerance versus food allergy include:

- a comprehensive metabolic profile with complete blood count and differential
- stool tests for inflammatory markers, ova, parasites, or occult blood
- breath hydrogen tests for intestinal bacterial imbalance and SIBO
- genetic tests for celiac disease and gluten sensitivity, or for histamine intolerance

INTERVENTION

Elimination Diets

The elimination diet, which entails both an elimination phase and a systematic food challenge or food reintroduction phase, is the most useful tool in both the diagnosis and management of adverse food reactions. With the elimination diet, suspect foods are eliminated from the diet for a specified period determined by the nutrition assessment (usually 2 to 8 weeks), which is then followed by a reintroduction or food challenge phase. All forms (i.e., cooked, raw, frozen) of a suspected food trigger are removed from the diet, and a food and symptom record (see Fig. 25.4) is kept during the elimination phase. This record is used to ensure that all forms of suspected foods have been eliminated from the diet, to evaluate the nutritional integrity of the diet, and to document reactions when suspected foods are reintroduced.

Diets must be personalized and may entail excluding only one or two suspect foods at a time to see if there is improvement in symptoms, or it may mean eliminating several foods if multiple foods are suspected. This would entail a more limited diet such as the SFED, as shown in Box 25.4, but again the diet should be individualized as much as possible. The elimination of multiple foods can compromise nutritional integrity, especially if the individual is already at nutritional risk due to symptoms that affect dietary intake (e.g., eosinophilic esophagitis) (Skypala and McKenzie, 2018).

Elemental formulas, medical foods, or hypoallergenic formulas also may be used for additional nutrition support when using an elimination diet. An elemental formula provides high-quality calories in an easily digestible, hypoallergenic form and helps to optimize nutritional intake. These products are usually reserved for highly restrictive diets. A hydrolyzed infant formula (HF) or EHF may be required for the allergic infant who is not being completely breastfed, and who needs to avoid several foods as the diet is expanded (see Table 25.4).

After the designated elimination phase, foods are systematically reintroduced into the diet one at a time to determine any adverse reactions while the person is carefully monitored. If symptoms persist with careful avoidance of suspect foods, other causes for the symptoms should be considered. If a positive result has been obtained on a skin-prick test or sIgE blood test and symptoms improve unequivocally with the elimination of the food, that food should be excluded from the diet until an OFC is appropriate. The OFC will further prove or disprove a food-symptom relationship. If symptoms improve with the elimination of multiple foods, then multiple food challenges will be necessary.

An oral food challenge (OFC) is conducted in a supervised medical setting once symptoms have resolved, and when the person is not taking certain medications, such as antihistamines. Foods are challenged one at a time on different days while the person is carefully observed in a medical setting for the recurrence of symptoms (see Table 25.5). The form of the challenged food may be important in the nutritional assessment of adverse food reactions. For example, if someone is allergic to milk or eggs, they may be able to tolerate baked (heat-denatured) forms of these proteins but not the unbaked form (Venter et al, 2018).

Allergic individuals and their families need guidelines and suggestions for avoiding allergenic foods and ingredients, substituting permissible foods for restricted foods in meal planning and preparation, and selecting nutritionally adequate replacement foods.

Care providers and school personnel working with the food-allergic child must be trained to read labels carefully before purchasing or serving food. The Food Allergy and Anaphylaxis Network, a non-profit organization created to support children with food allergies, has worked with board-certified allergists and dietitians to develop an excellent education program for parents and day-care or school programs.

To help identify and avoid offending foods, allergy-specific lists that describe foods to avoid, state key words for ingredient identification, and present acceptable substitutes are useful and necessary in counseling (see Table 25.4).

Food ingredients to be avoided may be hidden in the diet in unfamiliar forms. When a person ingests a hidden allergen, the most common reason is that the "safe" food was contaminated. This may happen as a result of using shared serving utensils, such as at an ice cream stand (e.g., where the same scoop and rinsing water is used for both ice cream and dairy-free sorbet), salad bar, or deli (e.g., where the meat slicer may be used to slice meat and cheese). Another practice may be using the same oil to fry potatoes and fish or using the same toaster for gluten and nongluten breads (Box 25.6). Manufacturing plants or restaurants may use the same equipment to produce two different products (e.g., peanut butter and almond butter) and despite cleaning, traces of an allergen may remain on the equipment between uses.

The unknowing ingestion of an allergenic food can also occur when one product is used to make a second product, and only the

---

BOX 25.7 **Allergen Labeling of Foods**

Since January 1, 2006, the updated **U.S. Food Allergen Labeling and Consumer Protection Act (FALCPA)** requires the top allergens to be clearly listed by manufacturers as an ingredient or following the ingredient list on food labels. This includes ingredients in any amount and also mandates specific ingredients to be listed, such as the type of nut or seafood.

Requirements of the Law

- **Top eight allergens must be clearly listed** by manufacturers as an ingredient or following the ingredient list on food labels of any food product containing allergens
- Applies to all packaged foods sold in the United States
- Does not apply to U.S. Department of Agriculture (USDA)-regulated products, including meat, poultry products, and some egg products
- Does not list sources of possible contamination
- Does not apply to prescription medication or alcoholic beverages
- Does not apply to foods packaged or wrapped after being ordered by the consumer

Top Allergens

- Any ingredient containing or derived from the top eight allergens—milk, eggs, fish, shellfish, tree nuts, peanuts, wheat, or soybeans
- For tree nuts, fish, and shellfish, the specific type must be listed (e.g., walnut, pecan, shrimp, tuna)

Reading the Food Label

- Ingredients may be included within the food's ingredient list directly or in parentheses following the name, if an ingredient does not clearly identify the allergen
- Following the list of ingredients all food allergens may be listed in a "Contains" statement
- Manufacturers may voluntarily list potential unintended allergens that may be present due to cross contamination in a clear way that does not interfere with the required food ingredient list. This is called precautionary allergen label (PAL).

Note: In 2013 the FDA issued a final rule defining "gluten-free" for food labeling. This final rule requires that items labeled "gluten-free" meet a defined standard for gluten content.
Note: It is being proposed that sesame be added to the list of top allergens required on labels.

---

ingredients of the second product are listed on the food label. An example is the listing of mayonnaise as an ingredient in a salad dressing without specifically listing egg as an ingredient of the mayonnaise. Labels must be read thoroughly to ensure that ingredients have not changed in the processing of the food. The U.S. Food Allergen Labeling and Consumer Protection Act (FALCPA) and the precautionary allergen labeling (PAL) regulations are described in Box 25.7.

MONITORING AND EVALUATION

The nutritional adequacy of the diet should be monitored on a regular basis when implementing elimination diets. An ongoing evaluation of the patient's food and symptom records is essential since the omission of foods from the diet can affect the nutritional status of the individual.

Individuals, especially children with multiple food allergies, that limit their dietary intake or those who are already on restricted diets for other reasons (e.g., vegan, ketogenic, intermittent fasting) are at the greatest risk of nutritional compromise. Malnutrition and poor

---

BOX 25.6 **Reasons for Accidental Exposure to Allergens**

- Common serving utensils used to serve different foods when some may contain the allergen
- Grocery store bulk bins contaminated with an allergen from another product bin
- Manufacture of two different food products using the same equipment without proper cleaning in between
- Misleading or inaccurate labels (e.g., nondairy creamers that contain sodium caseinate)
- Ingredients added for a specific purpose are listed on the label only in general terms of their purpose rather than as a specific ingredient (e.g., egg white that is simply listed as an "emulsifier")
- Addition of an allergenic product to a second product that bears a label listing only the ingredients of the second product (e.g., mayonnaise, without noting eggs)
- Switching of ingredients by food manufacturers (e.g., a shortage of one vegetable oil prompting substitution with another)
- A child being offered a food by an individual who is uneducated about the allergy

growth may occur in children who consume improperly planned and nutritionally inadequate elimination diets for long periods of time (Keller et al, 2012). Nutritional shortcomings with elimination diets depend on which foods are being excluded.

When foods are removed from the diet, alternative nutrient sources must be provided. For example, a child with cow's milk allergy may have lower intakes of calcium, zinc, and vitamins D and B$_2$, whereas when eggs are omitted, other foods must provide choline, vitamin D, protein, and energy (Skypala and McKenzie, 2018) (Table 25.6). Dietary supplementation, including vitamins and minerals, may also need to be considered to support nutritional integrity, especially when multiple foods are excluded.

Because food is an important part of a person's culture, the social aspects of eating can make adherence to an elimination diet challenging. Nutritional issues can also arise due to increased anxiety and stress encountered with changes in lifestyle associated with elimination diets. In addition, the plethora of online sources of information and social media now available can contribute to increased confusion about what is best to eat (Skypala and McKenzie, 2018). Continued personalized dietary support from an experienced registered dietitian nutritionist (RDN) is needed to optimally guide patients managing food allergies and intolerances and to minimize the effect of dietary and lifestyle changes on family and social life. Strategies listed in Box 25.8 can help families and individuals cope with adverse food reactions and still maintain quality of life.

TABLE 25.6	**Suggested Replacements for Foods Excluded in an Elimination Diet**		
Food Excluded	**Nutrients Provided by That Food**	**Substitute Foods/Foods with Similar Nutrients**	**Comments on Problematic Substitutes**
Cow's milk	Energy, protein, calcium, B vitamins, iodine. In the United States milk is commonly fortified with vitamins A and D.	Infants: extensively hydrolyzed formula/amino acid formula Children >2 yrs and adults: plant-based milk substitutes with added calcium and vitamin D and protein (e.g., soy milk, almond, cashew, coconut and other nut milks, oat milk, rice milk, and hemp milk). Plant foods such as legumes, broccoli, and dark leafy vegetables and some grains, provide B vitamins and calcium. Fish, containing bones, and tofu set with calcium compounds are also sources of calcium. For some individuals, especially those excluding other foods in addition to milk, supplements may be necessary to meet requirements for energy, protein, and calcium.	Rice milk naturally contains inorganic arsenic, which may be a problem, and in the United Kingdom is not recommended for children under the age of 5 years. Goat or sheep milk products, or mozzarella cheese made from buffalo milk, are not suitable for those with cow's milk allergy or lactose intolerance.
Eggs	Energy, protein, B vitamins (thiamin, riboflavin, niacin, B$_6$, biotin), selenium, vitamin D	These nutrients are widely found in other animal products such as meat, seafood, vitamin D–fortified milk, and other fortified foods. Egg replacement products are available for cooking and baking. These products provide a similar consistency if a recipe calls for eggs but do not provide much nutrition. Products made from algae, yeast, pea, or soy will have more nutrition than those derived from potato starch. Potato starch is a good source of resistant starch for gut microbes.	
Peanuts (legume) and tree nuts	Energy, protein, healthy fats, a range of vitamins and minerals depending on the type of nut, including B vitamins (folic acid, thiamin, B$_6$), vitamin E, calcium, selenium, magnesium	Other nuts that do not cause symptoms may be eaten (professional advice should determine which nuts are safe). Individuals with pollen-food allergy syndrome (PFAS) can often tolerate problematic nuts when roasted. Seeds eaten in quantity will provide a similar nutrient profile to nuts, and healthy fats can be obtained from avocados and high-quality vegetable oils.	
Fruits and vegetables	Fiber, a variety of phytonutrients, which act as antioxidants, a variety of vitamins and minerals depending on the fruit or vegetable, including B vitamins (folic acid, thiamin, riboflavin), vitamin C, beta-carotene, calcium, iron, and magnesium	Only those foods that cause symptoms should be excluded, ensuring that a variety of other plant foods are consumed. Individuals with PFAS can usually tolerate problematic foods when they cooked or processed.	

TABLE 25.6	Suggested Replacements for Foods Excluded in an Elimination Diet—cont'd		
Food Excluded	**Nutrients Provided by That Food**	**Substitute Foods/Foods with Similar Nutrients**	**Comments on Problematic Substitutes**
Seafood	Protein, calcium (fish bones), iodine, vitamins A and D, vitamin B$_{12}$, omega-3 fatty acids	Individuals with seafood allergy are rarely allergic to all seafood. People with fish allergy may be able to eat shellfish, and those allergic to shellfish may tolerate fin fish. Even those with shellfish allergy may be tolerant of other types of shellfish (e.g., an individual allergic to prawns [crustaceans] may be able to eat mollusks, e.g. clams, mussels, scallops, or oysters). Flaxseeds/linseeds are also a source of omega-3 fatty acids, as are some animal products to a limited extent. Iodine is added to iodized table salt. Sea greens, milk, and eggs are other sources of iodine.	
Soy and other legumes	Energy, protein, fiber, B vitamins, calcium, magnesium, iron, and zinc	Soy and other legumes, along with nuts, are significant sources of protein in plant-based diets. Whole grains are also an important source. It is important that only those foods causing symptoms are avoided.	
Wheat	Energy, protein, fiber, B vitamins (folic acid, niacin, pantothenic acid, riboflavin, thiamin, B$_6$), iron, magnesium, phosphorous, selenium, zinc	A variety of nonwheat flours are available for cooking and baking, such as oat, barley, rye, amaranth, buckwheat, millet, quinoa, rice, sorghum, tapioca, and teff. Milk and eggs provide energy, protein, calcium, and B vitamins. Fiber can be obtained from other plant foods. Good sources of iron are meat/fish/poultry and some plant foods. Iron supplementation may be necessary. Those avoiding both milk and wheat, especially if vegetarian or vegan, may need supplements of B vitamins, calcium, iron, and trace minerals.	The grains barley, oat, and rye must also be avoided when gluten also needs to be also be eliminated. Fiber can be obtained from other whole grains and plant foods.

PREVENTION OF FOOD ALLERGIES

Intensive research is being focused on prevention strategies for allergic disease, with emphasis on potential genetic, epigenetic, environmental, and modifiable lifestyle risk factors. There is growing interest in the role of microbiome-based therapies in an attempt to promote immunologic tolerance and the central role that nutritional interventions play in manipulating the microbiome. Primary food allergy prevention aims to reduce the infant's risk of sensitization to food allergens, whereas secondary prevention aims to prevent the clinical expression of allergic disease in individuals who are either allergen sensitized or who already manifest other allergic disorders such as eczema or asthma. Allergy prevention guidelines have gradually shifted away from prolonged allergen avoidance to a greater focus on the early introduction of complementary or "solid foods" into the diets of infants (Heine, 2018; West, 2017).

The Canadian Healthy Infant Longitudinal Development (CHILD) study is one of the largest longitudinal studies, involving more than 1000 Canadian mothers and infants, to advance knowledge about the genetic and environmental determinants of atopic diseases (CHILD study, 2018). Data from this study and others have contributed to guidelines on prevention and interventions that appear to reduce the risk of developing food allergy (Box 25.9). A number of hypotheses have been proposed for the prevention of food allergy that warrant further examination.

Microbial Exposure Hypotheses

The interplay between the gut microbiome and environmental microbial burden plays a major role in the immunologic events that lead to food allergy (Heine, 2018). The microbial hypothesis proposes that a decrease in early childhood exposure to microbes impairs the development of immune regulation and oral tolerance. It incorporates two earlier concepts referred to as the "hygiene hypothesis" and the "old friends hypothesis." These hypotheses assume that immune dysregulation is due to reduced microbial exposure and a lack of fecal microbial diversity.

The hygiene hypothesis was proposed by Dr. David Strachan in 1989 and posits that the increasing incidence of both allergic and autoimmune diseases could be explained by a lack of early childhood exposure to infectious agents which suppressed immune system development. A protective effect against developing allergic rhinitis was observed with an increasing number of siblings in a household. This was related to the shared exposure of common pathogens transmitted through direct contact with other siblings. However, the International Scientific Forum on Home Hygiene (IFH; https://www.ifh-homehygiene.org) proposes that the term hygiene hypothesis be abandoned and instead recommends a "targeted hygiene" framework to maximize protection against pathogen exposure while allowing the spread of essential microbes between family members (Bloomfield et al, 2016).

The old friends hypothesis, proposed by Dr. Graham Rook in 2003, maintains that microbe exposure present in primate evolution and hunter-gatherer times was vital to keeping the human immune system in balance and preventing overreactions, which is an underlying cause of allergies. It is hypothesized that another protective effect in reducing the risk of asthma and allergic disease is growing up in a rural environment with exposure to pets and animals versus urban living, although results examining the relationship between animal exposure and food allergies are inconsistent. Changes in lifestyle and environment, such

---

BOX 25.8   Strategies for Coping with Food Allergy

Food Substitutions

Try to substitute item-for-item at meals. For example, if the family is eating pasta for dinner, substitution of a gluten-free pasta may be better accepted for the gluten-sensitive or wheat-allergic person than a dissimilar item.

Dining Out and Eating Away from Home

Eating meals away from home can be risky for individuals with food allergies. Whether at a fancy restaurant or a fast-food establishment, inadvertent exposure to an allergen can occur, even among the most knowledgeable individuals. Here are some precautions to take:

- Bring "safe" foods along to make eating out easier. For breakfast, bring along an appropriate milk if others will be having cereal with milk.
- Alert the wait staff to the potential severity of the food allergy or allergies.
- Question the wait staff carefully about ingredients.
- Always carry medications.

Special Occasions

Call the host family in advance to determine what foods will be served. Offer to provide an acceptable dish that all can enjoy.

Grocery Shopping

Be informed about what foods are acceptable and read labels carefully. Product ingredients change over time; continue to read the labels on foods, even if they were previously determined to be "safe" foods. Allow for the fact that shopping will take extra time.

Label Reading

Labeling legislation (see Box 25.7) makes it easier to identify certain potential allergens from the ingredient list on food labels. For example, when food manufacturers use protein hydrolysates or hydrolyzed vegetable protein, they must now specify the source of protein used (e.g., hydrolyzed soy or hydrolyzed corn). Although reactions to food colors or food dyes are rare, individuals who suspect

an intolerance will find them listed separately on the food label, rather than categorized simply as "food color."

Early Feeding

- Exclusive breastfeeding for 4 to 6 months
- If exclusive breastfeeding is not possible, use whey-based, partially hydrolyzed formula

Introduction of Complementary Foods

- From 4 months, early introduction of potential food allergens (peanut, egg, and others) in infants at high risk of developing food allergies

Microbiome-Modifying Interventions

- Human milk oligosaccharides
- Prebiotics (e.g., fructo-oligosaccharides and galacto-oligosaccharides)
- Probiotics (e.g., *Lactobacillus rhamnosus*)

Immune Modulating Nutrients

- Maternal omega-3 polyunsaturated fatty acid supplementation (docosahexaenoic acid (DHA) and eicosapentaenoic acid (EPA)
- Vitamin D

General

- Strengthen immunity by increasing connection to natural environments, pets, and farms
- Strengthen immunity by regular exercise
- Consume fermented food or other probiotic preparations to strengthen immune system
- Use antibiotics only when necessary; the majority of microbes are useful and help build healthy immune function
- Do not smoke; parental and family smoking around infants and children can increase risk of asthma

Sources: Heine RG: Food allergy prevention and treatment by targeted nutrition, *Ann Nutr Metabol* 72(suppl 3):34, 2018.
Haahtela T et al: The biodiversity hypothesis and allergic disease: world allergy organization position statement, *World Allergy Organ J* 6:3, 2013.

BOX 25.9   Recommendations to Promote Oral Tolerance and Prevent Allergy

- Support breastfeeding and delay introduction of solid foods until 4 to 6 months.
- Strengthen immunity by increasing connection to natural environments, pets, and farms.
- Strengthen immunity by regular physical exercise.
- Use antibiotics only when necessary; the majority of microbes are useful and help build healthy immune function.
- Consume fermented food or other probiotic preparations to strengthen immune system.
- Do not smoke: parental and family smoking around infants and children can increase risk of asthma.

From Haahtela T et al: The biodiversity hypothesis and allergic disease: world allergy organization position statement, *World Allergy Organ J* 6:3, 2013.

as rapid urbanization, highly processed diet, and excessive antibiotic use, have had profound effects that likely contribute to the onset and rise in allergic disease due to immune system aberrations from a lack of early microbial exposure and diversity. Other environmental factors contributing to the microbial exposure hypothesis include route of delivery at birth and immunizations (Bloomfield et al, 2016).

Route of Delivery

When an infant is born by cesarean delivery, the infant is not exposed to the microbial wash of the mother's vagina. Vaginally delivered infants have bacterial communities reflecting the mother's vaginal microbiota, whereas infants born by cesarean delivery have bacterial communities similar to those found on the skin (Dominguez-Bello et al, 2010). Studies examining mode of delivery and risk of food allergy have yielded conflicting results, although one systematic review did find an association between increased risk of developing food allergy or food sensitization in children delivered by cesarean section (Marrs et al. 2013).

Antibiotic Use

It is well established that antibiotics can cause perturbations in the gut microbiota. Infants can be exposed to antibiotics prenatally, at birth, or postnatally. Some infants may have multiple exposures over time, when their microbiome is still being shaped. A link between antibiotic use in early life and food allergies has been demonstrated although the relationship, including timing and frequency of exposure, needs further exploration (NASEM, 2017).

Prebiotics and Probiotics

Considering the importance of the microbiome in immune system regulation, the role of prebiotics and probiotics in allergy prevention continues to be an exploding area of investigation. A **prebiotic** is a substrate that is selectively utilized by host microorganisms conferring a health benefit (Hill et al, 2014). Breastmilk contains human milk oligosaccharides (HMO), which are nondigestible carbohydrates with prebiotic properties that provide the substrate for specific early microbial colonization. Prebiotics have been added to infant formulas, which were previously devoid of oligosaccharides, as they may decrease the incidence of atopic dermatitis. The role of HMO remains an active area of investigation (Heine, 2018).

Probiotics are live microorganisms that, when administered in adequate amounts, confer a health benefit on the host (Hill et al, 2014). Infants with allergies have been shown to have a microbial composition with lower numbers of *Bifidobacteria* compared with healthy infants (Heine, 2018). The administration of probiotics in the last weeks of pregnancy and to infants during the first few months of life is associated with a significant reduction in atopic eczema. However, the effect of the individual probiotic strain, dose, timing, food matrix, and environmental factors that affect colonization need to be explored further since results have been varied (International Scientific Association for Probiotics and Prebiotics, 2016).

The Synergy in Microbiota Research (SyMBIOTA) project is one of the largest infant microbiome studies in the world (CHILD study, 2018). It examines relationships between the infant microbiome and variations in this internal ecosystem such as antibiotic use, presence of pets, and food sensitization, that affect health and disease (Kozyrskyj, 2015; NASEM, 2017). The data suggest that lower species richness in microbiota of infants might be a predictor of food sensitization (i.e., milk, egg, peanut) even when adjustments for delivery mode, antibiotic use, and breastfeeding are considered (Azad et al, 2015). They also found that sensitization occurred after changes in microbiota diversity and richness and that this ratio could be a potential predictor of food sensitization.

Allergen Avoidance Hypothesis

Allergen exposure at conception and during pregnancy and lactation continues to be a focus of research since this is the time of the origin of the infant's immune system development. Maternal diet during pregnancy and lactation has a profound influence on the child's health (Venter et al, 2017). Avoidance of allergenic foods during pregnancy and the early postnatal period was a traditional approach for allergy prevention. However, high-quality studies on maternal diets conclude that the evidence is not strong enough to recommend changing the diet of pregnant and breastfeeding women to prevent food allergies in infants at normal or high risk of food allergies (NASEM, 2017). Thus elimination diets during pregnancy and lactation for the purpose of allergy prevention are not warranted.

Breastfeeding

Breastfeeding is one of the main influences on the infant gut microbiota development. Human milk is a nutritional matrix with a host of bioactive compounds, including growth factors and maternal antibodies that impact immune responses. There are many well-documented benefits of breastfeeding including protection against infections, obesity, and chronic diseases, and it is associated with a fecal microbiota high in beneficial *Bifidobacteria*. Many studies have examined the association between breastfeeding and the development of food allergy and the data is inconsistent. Infants who are exclusively breastfed can express clinical manifestations of food allergy, including FPIES as already described, and multiple food intolerances of infancy (Heine, 2018). The use of a hypoallergenic maternal elimination diet that

eliminates allergens such as cow's milk can be helpful if allergic symptoms are present in the infant. However, maternal dietary restrictions during pregnancy and lactation for the sole purpose of allergy prevention are not recommended (Heine, 2018). The exact role of breastfeeding in allergy prevention remains unclear, and it appears that it may not reliably confer a protective effect against food allergies, although more research is needed. At least 6 months of exclusive breastfeeding is recommended for all infants regardless of family allergy risk (see Box 25.9).

Infant Formulas

The use of infant formulas to prevent allergy in high-risk infants who are unable to exclusively breastfeed is being explored. A systematic review and meta-analysis was conducted by Boyle et al. to determine whether use of a hydrolyzed formula reduces the risk of allergic disease in high-risk infants (Boyle et al, 2016). Their conclusion, along with other systematic reviews, found that there is not sufficient evidence to support the use of hydrolyzed cow's milk formulas—partially hydrolyzed formulas (PHF) or EHF—over breastmilk for the prevention of food allergy and food sensitization. In addition, the evidence is not strong enough to conclude that hydrolyzed formulas reduce the risk of food allergy and food sensitization compared with standard formulas (NASEM, 2017).

Dual Allergen Hypothesis

The **dual allergen hypothesis** proposes that allergic sensitization to foods may occur from a disrupted skin barrier early in life, as occurs in infantile eczema. The loss of skin barrier integrity increases environmental exposure to low doses of food allergens through the skin. Data suggests that loss of function of filaggrin, a protein important for epithelial structure, along with a compromised skin barrier, increases the risk for food sensitization from the environment (Renz et al, 2018).

The hypothesis also postulates that oral exposure to these same allergens through consumption of the allergenic foods early in life leads to oral tolerance and prevents the development of sensitization and allergy even with subsequent exposures (Renz et al, 2018). This hypothesis is also thought to explain the "atopic march," a pattern that describes a process in which atopic disorders progress over time from eczema (i.e., atopic dermatitis) to asthma to multiple allergic disorders including food allergy (NASEM, 2017).

The dual allergen hypothesis was born out of the observation that infants with eczema have a high risk of developing IgE-mediated food allergies. Supporting this hypothesis are data suggesting that early dietary introduction of peanut products may confer protection against peanut allergy.

However, many questions remain about the mechanisms by which sensitization and tolerance occur, and about the elements of the immune system that represent the most important contributors to the severity of food allergy or the establishment of tolerance.

Timing of Introduction of Solids and Infant Feeding

Earlier food allergy prevention strategies recommended delayed introduction of common allergenic foods into the infant's diet. There is now direct evidence from randomized controlled trials that the paradigm is shifting from avoidance to controlled exposure (West, 2017). Although the "optimal" period for introduction of complementary foods for allergy prevention is not known, a "window period" between 4 to 6 months of age when solids are introduced is recommended by most international guidelines for the induction of tolerance (Heine, 2018; West, 2017). The Australian HealthNuts study, the Learning Early About Peanut (LEAP), and Enquiring About Tolerance (EAT) are some of the key studies that assess early versus late introduction of complementary foods for allergy prevention and provide insights on the best timing of the dietary introduction of food allergens in high-risk infants (Fleischer et al, 2015; Heine, 2018; West, 2017; DuToit et al, 2015) (see Box 25.9).

The pivotal LEAP trial provides strong evidence that early introduction of peanuts (from 4 to 11 months of age) increases protection against peanut allergy in infants who are at high risk (defined by early-onset eczema and/or egg allergy) (NASEM, 2017; West, 2017; Heine, 2018; Togias et al, 2017).

The role of diet diversity in early life feeding practices may be another influential factor in food allergy prevention. Increased diversity of complementary foods, increased vegetables and fruit, and more home-prepared meals in the first year of life have been associated with a reduced risk of food allergy (NASEM, 2017; Du Toit et al, 2018).

Many questions remain on the best strategies to optimize infant feeding regimens and support the most favorable "tolerogenic" microenvironment in the gut during the period of food allergen introduction, since the immunomodulatory capacity of the GI tract is influenced by multiple factors (West, 2017; Renz et al, 2017).

Nutritional Immunomodulation

A balanced immune system is essential to health, and nutrition is a major factor that impacts immunocompetence. The immunoregulatory network is orchestrated by a variety of nutrients such as vitamin D, folate, and omega-3 fatty acids, and is influenced not only by dietary intake but also by digestive dynamics and microbial interplay.

Vitamin D

Vitamin D has received increased recognition for its role in immune regulation, as several studies have provided evidence that vitamin D deficiency is associated with food allergy. Evidence suggests vitamin D helps promote immunoregulation through induction of T_{reg} cells and T-cell differentiation. A shift to Th2 responses occurs with low or vitamin D–deficient conditions (Renz et al, 2018). A few studies have also examined the effect of maternal vitamin D status, cord blood, 25(OH)D_3 levels, and the development of food allergy, with conflicting reports. Multiple genes are involved in vitamin D metabolism and regulatory pathways, and future studies that consider genetic polymorphisms will help clarify the relationship between vitamin D and food allergy (Jones et al, 2015; NASEM, 2017).

Fatty Acids

The role of dietary fats in allergy development has been the subject of investigation, with the omega-3 fatty acids being the most extensively studied. The amount of omega 3-fatty acids in the U.S. diet has decreased over time along with a corresponding increase in omega-6 fatty acids intake, and this imbalance is thought to be a critical nutrition factor in the prevalence of chronic disease, including allergic disorders (Heine, 2018).

Omega-3 fatty acids have antiinflammatory and immunomodulatory effects. Some studies suggest that maternal consumption of fish oil (a source of omega-3 fatty acids) in pregnancy protects against the development of asthma, eczema, and allergic sensitization in the infant, whereas others do not show these results (Palmer et al, 2013). Controversy and questions remain regarding the relationship between omega-3 fatty acid content of the maternal diet and whether this confers a protective effect against development of childhood food allergy. Further studies are needed to elucidate the role of fatty acids in allergy prevention and their role in the inflammatory cascade (see Chapter 7).

Folate

There is renewed interest in folate as a dietary methyl donor that alters gene expression and impacts immune function through epigenetic mechanisms (Brown et al, 2014). Folate exposure in utero can affect DNA methylation during fetal development and influence transcriptional activity and may be involved in T-cell differentiation. Most studies to date have focused on asthma, with a very limited number examining the relationship of folate to food allergy and food sensitization. The significant role that folate plays in methylation of key regulatory genes and its potential in allergic predisposition warrants further investigation.

Other Nutrients

Few studies have examined the relationship between maternal dietary antioxidant intake (beta-carotene, vitamins C and E, copper, and zinc) during pregnancy and the risk of developing food allergy. In addition, nutrient assessment of individuals with food allergies and intolerances has not been thoroughly examined in research and is an avenue ripe for exploration (NASEM, 2017).

Future Directions

There are a number of areas that are being intensely studied as potential therapeutics for food allergy.

Immunotherapy

The concept of allergen immunotherapy (AIT), which aims to provide desensitization in a systematic stepwise process, was first described in the early 1900s. It is a procedure inducing tolerance to a specific allergen by repetitive administration of small amounts of an allergen, and it has been effective in respiratory allergy and venom hypersensitivity. Three main clinical immunotherapy concepts have emerged since then, including oral immune therapy (OIT), sublingual immune therapy (SLIT) and epicutaneous immunotherapy (EPIT). Ongoing studies of these methods have identified benefits and limitations of each, including side effects and adverse reactions.

The effectiveness of the therapies in food allergy remains under investigation, including the potential of combination therapies such as OIT plus immune modulation with probiotics or traditional Chinese medicine (Sicherer and Sampson, 2018). A growing body of evidence supports the use of AIT for subsets of patients with food allergies; however, biomarkers that are predictive of favorable outcomes and strategies to improve the safety and efficacy of AIT are needed (Feuille and Nowak-Węgrzyn, 2018).

Genetics and Omics

The potential of genetic data and "omics" technologies such as epigenomics, proteomics, transcriptomics, metabolomics, microbiomics, and exposomics is now being recognized (see Chapter 6). For example, metabolomics can provide data on the metabolic pathway activity associated with egg and peanut allergy, whereas microbiomics can identify microbial risk factors that are influencing gut physiology. Other "omics" approaches can provide measurements of proteins involved in food allergy immune responses and environmental exposures (exposomics) contributing to food allergy prevalence. Data derived from "omics" approaches will provide robust sets of biological and environmental data that will be used to better inform our understanding of food allergy, and open new avenues for both the prevention and treatment of this disease (Dhondalay et al, 2018).

Future Innovations

Innovative approaches such as modification of relevant food allergens (to make them less allergenic while maintaining their immunogenicity) or combining other therapies (e.g., probiotic supplementation during food challenges) to increase efficacy and/or safety will continue to dominate the food allergy landscape (Neerven and Savelkoul, 2017).

USEFUL WEBSITES

Allergy Aware Canada
American Academy of Allergy, Asthma and Immunology
The Asthma and Allergy Foundation of America
Food Allergy Research Education
International Network for Diet and Nutrition in Allergy

REFERENCES

Alhmoud T, Hanson JA, Parasher G: Eosinophilic gastroenteritis: an underdiagnosed condition, *Dig Dis Sci* 61:2585–2592, 2016.

Ali A, Weiss TR, McKee D, et al: Efficacy of individualized diets in patients with irritable bowel syndrome: a randomized controlled trial, *BMJ Open Gastroenterol* 4:e000164, 2017.

American Latex Allergy Association: *What is a latex allergy?* Available at: https://www.allergyhome.org/.

Appel MY, Nachshon L, Elizur A, et al: Evaluation of the basophil activation test and skin prick testing for the diagnosis of food allergy, *Clin Exp Allergy* 48(8):1025–1034, 2018.

Asai Y, Eslami A, van Ginkel CD, et al: Genome-wide association study and meta-analysis in multiple populations identifies new loci for peanut allergy and establishes C11orf30/EMSY as a genetic risk factor for food allergy, *J Allergy Clin Immunol* 141:991–1001, 2018.

Asaumi T, Ebisawa M: How to manage food dependent exercise induced anaphylaxis (FDEIA), *Curr Opinion in Allergy Clin Immunol* 18:243–247, 2018.

Asero R, Piantanida M, Pinter E, Pravettoni V: The clinical relevance of lipid transfer protein, *Clin Exp Allergy* 48:6–12, 2018.

Azad MB, Konya T, Guttman DS, et al: Infantile gut microbiota and food sensitization: associations in the first year of life, *Clin Exp Allergy* 45:632, 2015.

Bauer RN, Manohar M, Singh AM, Jay DC, Nadeau KC: The future of biologics: applications for food allergy, *J Allergy Clin Immunol* 135:312–323, 2015.

Bloomfield SF, Rook GA, Scott EA, et al: Time to abandon the hygiene hypothesis: new perspectives on allergic disease, the human microbiome, infectious disease prevention and the role of targeted hygiene, *Perspect Public Health* 136:213–224, 2016.

Boyce JA, Jones SM, Sampson RA, et al: Guidelines for the diagnosis and management of food allergy in the United States: Report of the NIAID-sponsored Expert Panel, *J Allergy Clin Immunol* 126(Suppl 6):S1–S58, 2010.

Boyle RJ, Ierodiakonou D, Khan T, et al: Hydrolysed formula and risk of allergic or autoimmune disease: systematic review and meta-analysis, *BMJ* 8:352, 2016.

Brown SB, Reeves KW, Bertone-Johnson ER: Maternal folate exposure in pregnancy and childhood allergy: a systematic review, *Nutr Rev* 72:55–64, 2014.

Carter CA, Frischmeyer-Guerrerio PA, The genetics of food allergy, *Curr Allergy Asthma Rep* 18(1):2, 2018.

CHILD Study: *What is the CHILD study?* (website). 2018. http://childstudy.ca/about/.

Commins SP: Invited commentary: Alpha-Gal allergy: tip of the iceberg to a pivotal immune response, *Curr Allergy Asthma Rep* 16:61, 2016.

Commins SP, Jerath MR, Cox K, et al: Delayed anaphylaxis to alpha-gal, an oligosaccharide in mammalian meat, *Allergol Int* 65:16, 2016.

DeGeeter C, Guandalini S: Food sensitivities: fact versus fiction, *Gastroenterol Clin North Am* 47:895–908, 2018.

Dhondalay GP, Rael E, Acharya S, et al: Food allergy and omics, *J Allergy Clin Immunol* 141:20–29, 2018.

Di Gioacchino M, Ricciardi L, De Pità, O, et al: Nickel oral hyposensitization in patients with systemic nickel allergy syndrome, *Ann Med* 46:31–37, 2014.

Dominguez-Bello MG, Costello EK, Contreras M, et al: Delivery mode shapes the acquisition and structure of the initial microbiota across multiple body habitats in newborns, *Proc Natl Acad Sci USA* 107:1197T, 2010.

Du Toit G, Roberts G, Sayre PH, et al: Randomized trial of peanut consumption in infants at risk for peanut allergy, *N Engl J Med* 372:803–813, 2015.

Du Toit G, Sampson HA, Plaut M, et al: Food allergy: update on prevention and tolerance, *J Allergy Clin Immunol* 141:30–40, 2018.

FAILSAFEdiet.com. *About Food Intolerance.* Available at: https://www.slhd.nsw.gov.au/rpa/allergy/resources/default.html.

Ferreira F, Gadermaier G, Wallmer M: Tree pollen allergens. In Akdis C, Agache I, editors: *Global atlas of allergy, European academy of allergy and clinical immunology*, 2014. Available at: http://www.eaaci.org/GlobalAtlas/GlobalAtlasAllergy.pdf.

Feuille EJ, Nowak-Wegrzyn A: Allergen-specific immunotherapies for food allergy. *Allergy Asthma Immunol Res* 10:189–206, 2018.

Fleischer DM, Sicherer S, Greenhawt M, et al: Consensus communication on early peanut introduction and the prevention of peanut allergy in high-risk infants, *J Allergy Clin Immunol* 136:258–261, 2015.

Food Allergy Research & Education (FARE): *About anaphylaxis.* Available at: https://www.foodallergy.org/life-food-allergies/anaphylaxis.

FPIES Foundation: About food protein-induced enterocolitis syndrome. Available at: http://fpiesfoundation.org/about-fpies-3/.

Fritscher-Ravens A, Schuppan D, Ellrichmann M, et al: Confocal endomicroscopy shows food-associated changes in the intestinal mucosa of patients with irritable bowel syndrome, *Gastroenterology* 147:1012-1020.e4, 2014.

Garcia-Martinez I, Weiss TR, Yousaf MN, Ali A, Mehal WZ: A leukocyte activation test identifies food items which induce release of DNA by innate immune peripheral blood leucocytes, *Nutr Metab (Lond)* 15:26, 2018.

Geha RS, Beiser A, Ren C, et al: Multicenter, double-blind, placebo-controlled, multiple-challenge evaluation of reported reactions to monosodium glutamate, *J Allergy Clin Immunol* 106:973–980, 2000.

Genuis SJ: Sensitivity related illness: the escalating pandemic of allergy, intolerance and chemical sensitivity, *Sci Total Environ* 408:6047–6061, 2010.

Gomes-Belo J, Hannachi F, Swan K, et al: Advances in food allergy diagnosis, *Curr Pediatr Rev* 14(3):139–149, 2018.

Groetch M, Venter C, Skypala I, et al: Dietary therapy and nutrition management of eosinophilic esophagitis: a work group report of the American Academy of Allergy, Asthma and Immunology, *J Allergy Clin Immunol Pract* 5:312-324.e9, 2017.

Gupta RS, Warren CM, Smith BM et al: Prevalence and severity of food allergies among US adults, *JAMA Network Open*, 2(1):e185630, 2019.

Haahtela T, Holgate S, Pawankar R, et al: The biodiversity hypothesis and allergic disease: world allergy organization position statement, *World Allergy Org J* 6:3, 2013.

Hammond C, Lieberman JA: Unproven diagnostic tests for food allergy, *Immunol Allergy Clin North Am* 38:153–163, 2018.

He K, Du S, Xun P, et al: Consumption of monosodium glutamate in relation to incidence of overweight in Chinese adults: China Health and Nutrition Survey (CHNS), *Am J Clin Nutr* 93:1328–1336, 2011.

Heine RG: Food allergy prevention and treatment by targeted nutrition, *Ann Nutr Metab* 72(Suppl 3):33–45, 2018.

Hill C, Guarner F, Reid G et al: The Interantional Scientific Association for Probiotics and Probiotics consensus statement on the scope and appropriate use of the term probiotic, *Nature Rev Gastroenterol Hepatol*, 11:506–514, 2014.

Hoffmann HJ, Santos AF, Mayorga C, et al: The clinical utility of basophil activation testing in diagnosis and monitoring of allergic disease, *Allergy* 70:1393–1405, 2015.

Igbinedion SO, Ansari, J, Vasikaran A, et al: Non-celiac gluten sensitivity: All wheat is not celiac, *World J Gastroenterol* 23:7201–7210, 2017.

International Scientific Association for Probiotics and Prebiotics: *Prebiotics* (website): https://4cau4jsaler1zglkq3wnmje1-wpengine.netdna-ssl.com/wp-content/uploads/2016/01/Prebiotics_Infographic_rev1029.pdf.

International Scientific Forum on Home Health (IFH): *Home Hygiene & Health* (website): https://www.ifh-homehygiene.org/.

Joneja JV: *The health professional's guide to food allergies and intolerances*, Chicago, IL, 2013, Academy of Nutrition and Dietetics.

Joneja JV: *Histamine intolerance: a comprehensive guide for healthcare professionals*, Berrydale Books, 2017. Published online - ed: how do we list that?

Jones AP, D'Vaz N, Meldrum S, et al: 25.hyroxyvitamin D3 status is associated with developing adaptive and innate immune responses in the first 6 months of life, *Clin Exp Allergy* 45:220–231, 2015.

Keller MD, Shuker M, Heimall J, et al: Severe malnutrition resulting from use of rice milk in food elimination diets for atopic dermatitis, *Isr Med Assoc J* 14:40–42, 2012.

Kozyrskyj A. 2015. *Infant gut microbial markers of food sensitization at age 1.* Presented at Committee Workshop, August 31, 2015. Washington, DC.

Leonard SA, Pecora V, Fiocchi AG, et al: Food protein-induced enterocolitis syndrome: a review of the new guidelines, *World Allergy Organ J* 11:4, 2018.

Lucendo AJ, Arias Á, González-Cervera J, et al: Empiric 6-food elimination diet induced and maintained prolonged remission in patients with adult eosinophilic esophagitis: a prospective study on the food cause of the disease, *J Allergy Clin Immunol* 131:797–804, 2013.

Maintz L, Novak N: Histamine and histamine intolerance, *Am J Clin Nutr* 85:1185–1196, 2007.

Marenholz I, Grosche S, Kalb B, et al: Genome-wide association study identifies the SERPINB gene cluster as a susceptibility locus for food allergy, *Nat Commun* 8:1056, 2017.

Marrs T, Bruce KD, Logan K, et al: Is there an association between microbial exposure and food allergy? a systematic review, *Pediatr Allergy Immunol* 24:311-320.e8, 2013.

Martin LJ, Franciosi JP, Collins MH, et al. Pediatric eosinophilic esophagitis symptom scores (PEESS v2.0) identify histologic and molecular correlates of the key clinical features of disease, *J Allergy Clin Immunol* 135:1519-1528.e8, 2015.

Matsuo H, Yokooji T, Taogoshi T: Common food allergens and their IgE-binding epitopes, *Allergol Int* 64:332–343, 2015.

Mehr S, Frith K, Barnes EH, et al: Food protein-induced enterocolitis syndrome in Australia: a population-based study, 2012-2014, *J Allergy Clin Immunol*, 140:1323–1330, 2017.

Meyer R, De Koker C, Dziubak R, Venter C, et al. Malnutrition in children with food allergies in the UK. *J Hum Nutr Diet* 27:227–235, 2014.

Meyer R, Groetch M, Venter C: When should infants with cow's milk protein allergy use an amino acid formula? A practical guide, *J Allergy Clin Immunol Pract* 6:383–399, 2018.

Molina-Infante J, Lucendo AJ: Dietary therapy for eosinophilic esophagitis, *J Allergy Clin Immunol* 142:41–47, 2018.

Muluk NB, Cingi C: Oral allergy syndrome, *Am J Rhinol Allergy* 32:27–30, 2018.

National Academies of Sciences, Engineering, and Medicine (NASEM), Institute of Medicine (IOM) *Finding a path to safety in food allergy: assessment of the global burden, causes, prevention, management, and public policy*, Washington, DC, 2017, The National Academies Press. http://nap.edu/23658.

Neerven RJJV, Savelkoul H: Nutrition and allergic diseases, *Nutrients* 9:E762, 2017.

Nomura I, Morita H, Hosokawa S, et al: Four distinct subtypes of non-IgE- mediated gastrointestinal food allergies in neonates and infants, distinguished by their initial symptoms, *J Allergy Clin Immunol* 127(3):685–688.e8, 2011.

Nowak-Wegrzyn A, Chehade M, Groetch M, et al: International consensus guidelines for the diagnosis and management of food protein-induced enterocolitis syndrome: Executive Summary-Workgroup Report of the Adverse Reactions to Foods Committee, American Academy of Allergy, Asthma and Immunology, *J Allergy Clin Immunol* 139:1111–1126, 2017.

Palmer DJ, Sullivan T, Gold MS, et al: Randomized controlled trial of fish oil supplementation in pregnancy on childhood allergies, *Allergy* 68:1370–1376, 2013. http://www.phadia.com/fr/5/Produits/ImmunoCAP-Allergens/Occupational-Allergens/Allergens/Latex/.

Plunkett, CH, Nagler, CR: Influence of the microbiome on allergic sensitization to food, *J Immunol* 198:581–589, 2017.

Randazzo CL, Pino A, Ricciardi L, et al: Probiotic supplementation in systemic nickel allergy syndrome patients: study of its effects on lactic acid bacteria population and on clinical symptoms, *J Appl Microbiol* 118:202–211, 2014.

Renz H, Allen KJ, Sicherer SH, et al: Food allergy, *Nat Rev Dis Primers* 4:17098, 2018.

Renz H, Holt PG, Inouye M, et al: An exposome perspective: early life events and immune development in a changing world, *J Allergy Clin Immunol* 140:24–40, 2017.

Russler-Germain EV, Rengarajan S, Hsieh CS: Antigen-specific regulatory T-cell responses to intestinal microbiota, *Mucosal Immunol* 10:1375–1386, 2017.

Sampson HA, O'Mahoney L, Burks AW, et al: Mechanisms of food allergy, *J Allergy Clin Immunol* 141:11, 2018.

Savcheniuk OA, Virchenko OV, Falalyeyeva TM, et al: The efficacy of probiotics for monosodium glutamate-induced obesity: dietology concerns and opportunities for prevention, *EPMA J* 5:2, 2014.

Scallan E, Hoekstra RE, Angulo FJ, et al: Foodborne illness acquired in the United States - major pathogens, *Emerg Infect Dis* 17:7–15, 2011.

Sicherer SH, Sampson HA: Food allergy: a review and update on epidemiology, pathogenesis, diagnosis, prevention, and management, *J Allergy Clin Immunol* 141:41–58, 2018.

Simons FE: Anaphylaxis, in European Academy of Allergy and Clinical Immunology, Global Atlas of Allergy, *Eur Acad Allergy Clin Immunol* 191–196, 2014.

Skypala IJ, Venter C, Meyer R, et al: The development of a standardised diet history tool to support the diagnosis of food allergy, *Clin Transl Allergy* 5:7, 2015.

Skypala IJ, McKenzie R: Nutritional issues in food allergy, *Clin Rev Allergy Immunol* 2018. doi:10.1007/s12016-018-8688-x. [e-pub ahead of print]

Skypala IJ, Williams M, Reeves L, et al: Sensitivity to food additives, vaso-active amines and salicylates: a review of the evidence, *Clin Transl Allergy*, 5:34, 2015b.

Spergel JM, Brown-Whitehorn TF, Cianferoni A, et al: Identification of causative foods in children with eosinophilic esophagitis treated with an elimination diet, *J Allergy Clin Immunol* 130:461–467, 2012.

Stapel SO, Asero R, Ballmer-Weber BK, et al: Testing for IgG4 against foods is not recommended as a diagnostic tool: EAACI Task Force Report, *Allergy* 63:793–796, 2008.

Swift KM, Lisker I: Current concepts in nutrition: the science and art of the elimination diet, *Altern Complement Ther* 18:251, 2012.

Togias A, Cooper SF, Acebal M, et al: Addendum guidelines for the prevention of peanut allergy in the United States: report of the National Institute of Allergy and Infectious Diseases–sponsored expert panel, *J Allergy Clin Immunol* 139:29–44, 2017.

Tordesillas L, Berin M: Mechanisms of oral tolerance, *Clin Rev Allergy Immunol* 55:107–117, 2018.

Turnbull JL, Adams HN, Gorard DA: Review article: the diagnosis and management of food allergy and food intolerances, *Aliment Pharmacol Ther* 41:3–25, 2015.

Turner PJ, Campbell DE: A food allergy syndrome by any other name? *Clin Exp Allergy* 44:1458–1460, 2014.

Turner PJ, Dawson TC, Skypala IJ, et al: Management of pollen food and oral allergy syndrome by health care professionals in the United Kingdom, *Ann Allergy Asthma Immunol* 114:427–428, 2015.

Ugidos-Rodríguez S, Matallana-González MC, Sánchez-Mata MC: Lactose malabsorption and intolerance: a review, *Food Funct* 9:4056–4068, 2018. doi:10.1039/c8fo00555a.

Vally H, Misso NL: Adverse reactions to the sulphite additives, *Gastroenterol Hepatol Bed Bench* 5:16–23, 2012.

Venter C, Brown KR, Maslin K, et al: Maternal dietary intake in pregnancy and lactation and allergic disease outcomes in offspring, *Pediatr Allergy Immunol* 28:135–143, 2017.

Venter C, Goretch M, Netting M, et al: A patient-specific approach to develop an exclusion diet to manage food allergy in infants and children, *Clin Exp Allergy* 48:121–137, 2018.

Vojdani A: Molecular mimicry as a mechanism for food immune reactivities and autoimmunity, *Altern Ther Health Med* 21(Suppl 1):S34–S45, 2015a.

Vojdani A: The evolution of food immune reactivity testing: why immunoglobulin G or immunoglobulin A antibody for food may not be reproducible from one lab to another, *Altern Ther Health Med* 21(Suppl 1):S8–S22, 2015b.

Vojdani A, Vojdani C: Immune reactivity to food coloring, *Altern Ther Health Med* 21(Suppl 1):S52–S62, 2015.

Wauters RH, Banks TA, Lomasney EM: Food-dependent exercise-induced anaphylaxis, *BMJ Case Rep* 2018. Available at: http://dx.doi.org/10.1136/bcr-2017-222370.

West C: Introduction of complementary foods to infants, *Ann Nutr Metab* 70(Suppl 2):47–54, 2017.

Williams AN, Woessner KM: Monosodium glutamate 'allergy': menace or myth? *Clin Exp Allergy* 39:640–646, 2009.

Wilson JM, Platts-Mills TAE: Meat allergy and allergens, *Mol Immunol* 100:107–112, 2018.

Zhang M, Li Y: Eosinophilic gastroenteritis: a state-of-the-art review, *J Gastroenterol Hepatol* 32:64–72, 2017.

26

Medical Nutrition Therapy for Upper Gastrointestinal Tract Disorders

DeeAnna Wales VanReken, MS, RDN, CD, IFNCP

KEY TERMS

achalasia
achlorhydria
achylia gastrica
acid pocket
atrophic gastritis
Barrett's esophagus (BE)
bezoar
Billroth I (gastroduodenostomy)
Billroth II (gastrojejunostomy)
cannabinoid hyperemesis syndrome
dumping syndrome
duodenal ulcer
dyspepsia
dysphagia
endoscopy
esophagectomy

esophagitis
esophagogastroduodenoscopy (EGD)
functional dyspepsia
gastrectomy
gastric pull-up
gastric ulcer
gastritis
gastroesophageal reflux (GER)
gastroesophageal reflux disease (GERD)
gastroparesis
heartburn
Helicobacter pylori
hematemesis
hiatal hernia
lower esophageal sphincter (LES)
melena

mucosa-associated lymphoid tissue (MALT)
Nissen fundoplication
odynophagia
parietal cells
parietal cell vagotomy
peptic ulcer disease
pyloroplasty
Rome IV criteria
Roux-en-Y
scintigraphy
stress ulcer
upper esophageal sphincter (UES)
vagotomy
vagotomy, truncal
vagus nerve

The upper gastrointestinal tract is the portion of the alimentary canal containing the esophagus, stomach, and duodenum. Along with those segments, the oral cavity will also be included as relevant in this chapter.

Digestive disorders of both the upper and lower gastrointestinal (GI) tract, are among the most common problems in health care (see Chapter 27). Between 60 and 70 million people are affected by all digestive diseases, with over 48 million ambulatory care visits made annually in the United States alone (National Institutes of Health [NIH], 2014). As digestive disorders are the leading cause of all emergency department visits, 8.8% or more than 12,000 patients presented with stomach and abdominal pain, cramps, and spasms in 2015 alone (Centers for Disease Control and Prevention [CDC], 2015). More than 20 million diagnostic and surgical procedures involving the GI tract are performed each year (CDC, 2015). Dietary habits and specific foods can play an important role in the onset, treatment, and prevention of many GI disorders. Medical nutrition therapy is integral in the prevention and treatment of malnutrition and deficiencies that can develop from a GI tract disorder. Diet and lifestyle modifications can improve a patient's quality of life by alleviating GI symptoms and decreasing the number of health care visits and costs associated with GI disease.

Gail Cresci, PhD, RDN, LD, CNSC and Arlene Escuro, MS, RDN, CNSC were the authors of this chapter for the 14th edition.

THE ESOPHAGUS

The esophagus is a muscular tube with an average length of 25 cm in adults (Fig. 26.1), with the single but important function of delivering solids and liquids from the mouth to the stomach. It is lined with nonkeratinized stratified squamous epithelium, and submucosal glands secrete mucin, bicarbonate, epidermal growth factor, and prostaglandin E_2, which protect the mucosa from gastric acid.

The top of the esophagus is connected to the pharynx, and the bottom of the esophagus is connected to the stomach at the cardia. It is highly muscular, with muscles arranged in a way to facilitate the passage of food. As a bolus of food is moved voluntarily from the mouth to the pharynx, the upper esophageal sphincter (UES) relaxes, the food moves into the esophagus, and peristaltic waves move the bolus down the esophagus; the lower esophageal sphincter (LES) relaxes to allow the food bolus to pass into the stomach. The esophageal transit time takes an average of 5 seconds when in an upright position, and up to 30 seconds when in a supine position (la Roca-Chiapas and Cordova-Fraga, 2011).

The normal esophagus has a multitiered defense system that prevents tissue damage from exposure to gastric contents, including LES contraction, normal gastric motility, esophageal mucus, tight cellular junctions, and cellular pH regulators. Musculoskeletal disorders and motility disorders may result in dysphagia. For example, achalasia is characterized by a failure of esophageal neurons, resulting in a loss of ability to relax the LES and have normal peristalsis.

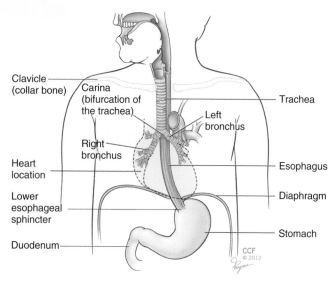

Fig. 26.1 Normal esophagus. (Cleveland Clinic, Cleveland, Ohio.)

Gastroesophageal Reflux Disease (GERD) and Esophagitis

Etiology

Gastroesophageal reflux (GER) is considered a normal physiologic process that occurs several times a day in healthy infants, children, and adults. GER generally is associated with transient relaxation of the LES independent of swallowing, which permits gastric contents to enter the esophagus. Limited information is known about the normal physiology of GER in infants, but regurgitation and spitting up, as the most visible symptom, is reported to occur daily in 50% of all infants (Lightdale and Gremse, 2013).

Gastroesophageal reflux disease (GERD) is a more serious, chronic form of GER, with symptoms or complications resulting from the reflux of gastric contents into the esophagus or beyond, and even into the oral cavity (including larynx) or lung. Symptoms are defined to include heartburn (painful, burning sensation that radiates up behind the sternum of fairly short duration) and/or regurgitation, at least once a week. Prevalence is worldwide, may be increasing over time, and varies by geographic location. The following prevalence estimates were published in a 2014 review of existing epidemiologic studies: North America 18% to 28%; Europe 9% to 26%; Middle East 9% to 33%; Australia 12%; East Asia 3% to 8% (El-Serag et al, 2014).

Esophagogastroduodenoscopy (EGD) uses a fiberoptic endoscope to directly visualize and examine the esophagus, stomach, and duodenum to classify severity of disease (see Focus On: Endoscopy and Capsules). GERD can be classified as nonerosive disease (NERD), indicating the presence of symptoms without abnormalities or erosions, or erosive disease (ERD), with symptoms and erosions present. ERD generally is associated with more severe and prolonged symptoms compared with NERD (Katz et al, 2013).

Some patients experience GERD symptoms primarily in the evening (nocturnal GERD), which has a greater impact on quality of life compared with daytime symptoms. Nocturnal GERD is associated significantly with severe esophagitis (inflammation of the esophagus) and Barrett's esophagus (an intestinal metaplasia described in further detail later in this chapter) and can lead to sleep disturbance. Patients with ERD are more likely to be men, and women are more likely to have NERD. There is a definite relationship between GERD and obesity. Several meta-analyses suggest an association between body mass index (BMI), waist circumference, weight gain, and the presence of symptoms and complications of GERD. GERD is frequent during pregnancy, usually manifesting as heartburn, and may begin in any trimester. Significant predictors of heartburn during pregnancy are increasing gestational age, heartburn before pregnancy, and parity (Katz et al, 2013) (see Chapter 14). One Korean study also found a significant association between degree of psychosocial stress and reflux esophagitis severity (Song et al, 2013).

Chest pain may be a symptom of GERD, and distinguishing cardiac from noncardiac chest pain is required before considering GERD as a cause of chest pain. Although the symptoms of dysphagia can be associated with uncomplicated GERD, its presence warrants investigation for a potential complication, including an underlying motility disorder, stricture, or malignancy. Patients with disruptive GERD (daily or more than weekly symptoms) have an increase in time off work and decrease in work productivity, and a decrease in physical functioning (Katz et al, 2013).

Pathophysiology

The pathophysiology of GERD is complex. Box 26.1 describes possible mechanisms involved in GERD. Three components make up the esophagogastric junction: the LES, the crural diaphragm, and the anatomic flap valve. This junction acts as an antireflux barrier. The LES is a 3- to 4-cm segment of circular smooth muscle at the distal end of the esophagus. The resting tone of this muscle can vary among healthy individuals, ranging from 10 mm Hg to 35 mm Hg relative to the intragastric pressure. The most common mechanism for reflux is transient LES relaxations, which are triggered by gastric distention and serve to enable gas venting from the stomach. On average, transient LES relaxations persist for about 20 seconds, which is significantly longer than the typical swallow-induced relaxation (Bredenoord et al, 2013).

For reflux to take place, pressure in the proximal stomach must be greater than the pressure in the esophagus. Patients with chronic respiratory disorders, such as chronic obstructive pulmonary disease (COPD), are at risk for GERD because of frequent increases in intraabdominal pressure. A chronically increased pressure also is seen during pregnancy and in overweight and obese people.

Hypersensitivity to acid can occur in people with erosive esophagitis and in those with normal mucosa. A factor contributing to increased esophageal sensitivity to acid is impaired mucosal barrier function. In a systematic review, the overall rate of gastric emptying

---

BOX 26.1 Possible Mechanisms Involved in Gastroesophageal Reflux Disease (GERD)

- Decreased salivation
- Transient lower esophageal sphincter (LES) relaxation
- Reduced LES pressure
- Impaired esophageal acid clearance
- Increased esophageal sensitivity
- Acid pocket
- Increased intraabdominal pressure
- Delayed gastric emptying

Data from Beaumont H et al: The position of the acid pocket as a major risk factor for acidic reflux in healthy subjects and patients with GORD, *Gut* 59:441, 2010; Bredenoord AJ et al: Gastroesophageal reflux disease, *Lancet* 381:1933, 2013; Penagini R, Bravi I: The role of delayed gastric emptying and impaired esophageal motility, *Best Pract Res Clin Gastroenterol* 24:831, 2010.

PATHOPHYSIOLOGY AND CARE MANAGEMENT ALGORITHM

Esophagitis

ETIOLOGY

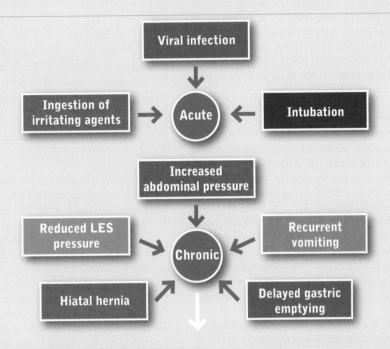

Viral infection

Ingestion of irritating agents → **Acute** ← Intubation

Increased abdominal pressure

Reduced LES pressure → **Chronic** ← Recurrent vomiting

Hiatal hernia → ← Delayed gastric emptying

PATHOPHYSIOLOGY

Reflux of gastric acid and/or intestinal contents through the lower esophageal sphincter (LES) and into the esophagus

MANAGEMENT

Behavioral Modification

Avoid:
- Eating within 3-4 hours of bedtime
- Lying down after meals
- Tight-fitting clothing
- Cigarette smoking
- Excess stress

Medical/Surgical Management

- Proton pump inhibitors
- Histamine-2 receptor antagonists
- Antacids
- Prokinetic agents
- Fundoplication

Nutrition Management

Goal:
Decrease exposure of esophagus to gastric contents
Avoid:
- Large meals
- Excess intake of dietary fat
- Alcohol, mint, coffee, and chocolate

Goal:
Decrease acidity of gastric secretions
Avoid:
- Coffee
- Alcohol

Goal:
Prevent pain and irritation
Avoid:
- Any food that the patient feels exacerbates symptoms, especially hot and spicy foods

was delayed in patients with GERD (Penagini and Bravi, 2010). However, a relationship between delayed gastric emptying and increased reflux could not be seen in this study, suggesting that impaired emptying of the stomach as a whole is not an important determinant of GER.

Good peristaltic function is an important defense mechanism against GERD, as prolonged acid clearance correlates with the severity of esophagitis and the presence of complications such as Barrett's esophagus. An occurrence during the postprandial period known as acid pocket is a layer of unbuffered, highly acidic gastric juice at the esophagogastric junction, ready to reflux due to the absence of peristaltic contraction in the proximal stomach.

Prolonged acid exposure can result in esophagitis, esophageal erosions, ulceration, scarring, stricture, and in some cases dysphagia (see *Pathophysiology and Care Management Algorithm*: Esophagitis). Acute esophagitis may be caused by reflux, ingestion of a corrosive agent, viral or bacterial infection, intubation, radiation, or eosinophilic infiltration. Eosinophilic esophagitis (EoE) is characterized by an isolated, severe eosinophilic infiltration of the esophagus manifested by GERD-like symptoms that may be caused by an immune response (see Chapter 25).

The severity of the esophagitis resulting from the GER is influenced by the composition, frequency, and volume of the gastric reflux; the health of the mucosal barrier; length of exposure of the esophagus to the gastric reflux; and the rate of gastric emptying. Symptoms of esophagitis and GERD may impair the ability to consume an adequate diet and interfere with sleep, work, social events, and the overall quality of life (Table 26.1).

Barrett's esophagus (BE) is a precancerous condition in which the normal squamous epithelium of the esophagus is replaced by an abnormal columnar-lined epithelium known as specialized intestinal metaplasia (tissue that is similar to the intestinal lining). The exact cause of BE is unknown, but GERD is a risk factor for the condition. The prevalence of BE is between 0.5% and 2% but is estimated to affect 1.6% to 6.8% of the general population (Runge et al, 2015). People with BE are at increased risk for a cancer called esophageal adenocarcinoma, with incidence rising dramatically over the past 40 years and speculated to continue to rise during coming decades (Thrift and Whiteman, 2012). Risk factors for BE include prolonged history of

TABLE 26.2   Types of Hiatal Hernia

Type 1 (sliding hiatal hernia)	Most common type; gastroesophageal junction is pushed above the diaphragm, causing a symmetric herniation of the proximal stomach
Type 2 (true paraesophageal hernia)	Fundus slides upward and moves above the gastroesophageal junction
Type 3 (mixed paraesophageal hernia)	Combined sliding and paraesophageal herniation
Type 4 (complex paraesophageal hernia)	Less common form; intrathoracic herniation of other organs, such as the colon, and small bowel into the hernia sac

GERD-related symptoms (more than 5 years), middle age, white male, obesity, smoking, and family history of BE or adenocarcinoma of the esophagus. Estrogen may be protective and account for the lower incidence of BE in females (Asanuma et al, 2016).

Abnormalities in the body such as hiatal hernia may also contribute to GER and esophagitis. The esophagus passes through the diaphragm by way of the esophageal hiatus or ring. The attachment of the esophagus to the hiatal ring may become compromised, allowing a portion of the upper stomach to move above the diaphragm. Table 26.2 describes the four types of hiatal hernia in greater detail. The most common symptom of hiatal hernia is heartburn. When acid reflux occurs with a hiatal hernia, the gastric contents remain above the hiatus longer than normal. The prolonged acid exposure increases the risk of developing more serious esophagitis. Fig. 26.2 illustrates a hiatal hernia (*A*), and postsurgical reduction (*B*). As the hiatal hernia enlarges, regurgitation may be more prominent, especially when lying down or when bending over. Epigastric pain occurs in the upper middle region of the abdomen after large, energy-dense meals. Weight reduction and decreasing meal size can reduce the negative consequences of hiatal hernia.

Patients with type 3 (mixed paraesophageal) hiatal hernia may present with severe chest pain, retching, vomiting, and hematemesis (vomiting of blood), as these hernias can twist and cause strangulation in the chest, resulting in a surgical emergency. Some patients can present with iron deficiency anemia without acute bleeding because the diaphragm becomes so irritated that the patient may develop chronic blood loss.

TABLE 26.1   Clinical Symptoms Associated with Gastroesophageal Reflux Disease (GERD)

Dental corrosion	Slow, progressive tooth surface loss associated with acid regurgitation
Dysphagia	Difficulty initiating a swallow (oropharyngeal dysphagia) or sensation of food being hindered or "sticks" after swallowed (esophageal dysphagia)
Heartburn (pyrosis)	Painful, burning sensation that radiates up behind the sternum of fairly short duration
Odynophagia	Painful swallowing
Regurgitation	Backflow of gastric content into the mouth not associated with nausea or retching
Noncardiac chest pain	Unexplained substernal chest pain resembling a myocardial infarction without evidence of coronary artery disease
Extraesophageal symptoms	Chronic cough, hoarseness, reflux-induced laryngitis, or asthma

Data from Bredenoord AJ et al: Gastro-esophageal reflux disease, *Lancet* 381:1933, 2013; Katz PO et al: Guidelines for the diagnosis and management of gastroesophageal reflux disease, *Am J Gastroenterol* 108:308, 2013.

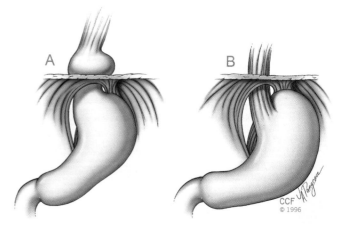

Fig. 26.2 A, Hiatal hernia. **B,** Postsurgical reduction of hiatal hernia. (Cleveland Clinic, Cleveland, Ohio.)

Medical and Surgical Management

The primary medical treatment of esophageal reflux is suppression of acid secretion. The aim in acid-suppression therapy is to raise the gastric pH above 4 during periods when reflux is most likely to occur. Proton pump inhibitors (PPIs), which decrease acid production by the gastric parietal cell, have been associated with superior healing rates and decreased relapses (Katz et al, 2013). Milder forms of reflux are managed by H_2 receptor (a type of histamine receptor on the gastric parietal cell) antagonists and antacids, which buffer gastric acid in the esophagus or stomach to reduce heartburn. Prokinetic agents, which increase propulsive contractions of the stomach, may be used in persons with delayed gastric emptying. A trial of baclofen, a gamma-amino butyric acid (GABA) agonist, can be considered in patients with objective documentation of continued symptomatic reflux despite optimal PPI therapy (Katz et al, 2013). However, there have not been long-term data published regarding efficacy of baclofen in GERD. Refer to Table 26.3 for medications commonly used

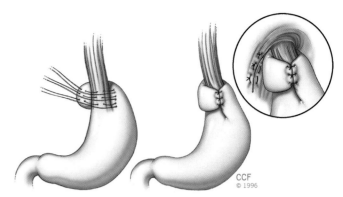

Fig. 26.3 Nissen fundoplication. (Cleveland Clinic, Cleveland, Ohio.)

in upper GI disorders. See Appendix 13 for more information about these medications.

Of patients with severe GERD, 5% to 10% do not respond to medical therapy. The Nissen fundoplication was first described as a treatment for severe reflux esophagitis in 1956 and is still the most commonly performed antireflux surgery (Fig. 26.3). During this procedure, which can be done using either open or a laparoscopic technique, the fundus or top portion of the stomach is wrapped 360 degrees around the lower esophagus and sutured in place to limit reflux (see Fig. 26.3). Surgical therapy is considered for individuals for whom medical management has been unsuccessful, those who opt for surgery to avoid lifelong need for medication to control symptoms, those experiencing more serious complications (BE, peptic stricture), and those who have extraesophageal manifestations that include both laryngeal and pulmonary symptoms (throat-clearing, hoarseness, postnasal drip, cough, shortness of breath, asthma) (Yates and Oelschlager, 2015). As many as 18% of those undergoing surgery will need a repeat operation due to fundoplication failure. Unfortunately, for these patients, quality of life scores decrease and there is less improvement of dysphagia with the second procedure, leading surgeons to consider more invasive surgeries such as Roux-en-Y or short colon interposition (Wilshire et al, 2016). Surgical approaches in children are reserved for those who have intractable symptoms unresponsive to medical therapy or who are at risk for life-threatening complications of GERD (Lightdale and Gremse, 2013). Refer to Box 26.2 for dietary guidelines after Nissen fundoplication.

Lifestyle Modifications and Medical Nutrition Therapy

The first step in symptom management of GERD should consist of changes in lifestyle, including diet. A recent small clinical trial found improvements in NERD participants with the addition of psyllium fiber into the diet three times daily for a total of 12.5 grams soluble fiber per day. Those enrolled in the study were selected if they previously ate a low (<20 g/day) fiber diet at baseline. During the study, no other dietary changes were made, and PPIs, H_2 blockers, or prokinetics were not allowed. The result demonstrated that dietary fiber increased the LES pressure and decreased total reflux episodes in participants (Morozov et al, 2018). Besides diet, other important factors that trigger reflux symptoms are caffeine, alcohol, tobacco, and stress. Initial recommendations should focus on meal size and content. Eating small rather than large meals reduces the probability that gastric contents will reflux into the esophagus.

Certain foods can lower LES pressure, including coffee and carminatives such as peppermint, but more research is needed to

---

TABLE 26.3 Common Medications Used in the Treatment of Upper Gastrointestinal Tract Disorders

Type of Medication	Common Names	Medication Function
Antacids	Magnesium, calcium, or aluminum bound to carbonate, hydroxide, or phosphate	Buffers gastric acid
Antigas	Simethicone	Lowers surface tension of gas bubbles
Antidiarrheal	Diphenoxylate Loperamide Opium preparations	Decreased gastrointestinal (GI) tract motility to induce lower stool volume output
Antidumping	Acarbose	Delays carbohydrate digestion by inhibiting alpha-glycoside hydrolase, which interferes with conversion of starch to monosaccharides
Antisecretory	Octreotide (somatostatin analog) Somatostatin	Inhibits release of insulin and other gut hormones; slows rate of gastric emptying and small intestine transit time; and increases intestinal water and sodium absorption
H_2 blocker	Cimetidine Ranitidine Famotidine Nizatidine	Blocks the action of histamine on parietal cells, decreasing the production of acid
Prokinetic	Metoclopramide Erythromycin Domperidone	Increases contractility of the stomach and shortens gastric emptying time
Proton pump inhibitor (PPI)	Omeprazole Lansoprazole Esomeprazole Pantoprazole Dexlansoprazole Rabeprazole	Inhibits acid secretion

BOX 26.2 Dietary Guidelines After a Nissen Fundoplication

1. Start clear liquid diet after surgery.
2. Advance oral diet to soft, moist, solid foods. Starting solids could be before leaving the hospital or written in hospital discharge instructions.
3. Follow soft, moist foods diet for about 2 months. Foods must be soft to pass through the esophagus.
4. Consume small, frequent meals.
5. Swallow small bites of food and chew thoroughly to allow an easy passage through the esophagus and avoid use of straw to consume liquids. Drink slowly.
6. Avoid foods and beverages that may cause backflow of stomach contents. This consists of citrus fruits and juices, tomato, pineapple, alcohol, caffeine, chocolate, carbonated beverages, peppermint or spearmint, fatty or fried foods, spicy foods, vinegar or vinegar-containing foods.
7. Avoid dry foods that are hard to pass through the esophagus, such as bread, steak, raw vegetables, rolls, dry chicken, raw fruits, peanut butter, other dry meats, or anything with skin, seeds, or nuts.
8. Avoid any food that may cause discomfort.
9. After 2 months, start to incorporate new foods into the diet. Try one new food item or beverage at a time. By 3–6 months, patient should be able to tolerate most foods.
10. Consult doctor or dietitian if having difficulty eating or losing weight.

BOX 26.3 Nutrition Care Guidelines for Reducing Gastroesophageal Reflux and Esophagitis

1. Nutrition Recommendations:
   - Avoid large, high-fat meals and decrease greasy foods.
   - Avoid eating 2 to 3 hours before lying down.
   - Avoid chocolate, mint, tomatoes, and tomato products.
   - Avoid caffeine-containing foods and beverages.
   - Avoid alcoholic beverages.
   - Avoid acidic and highly spiced foods.
   - Consume a well-balanced diet with adequate fiber.
   - Consider weight loss if overweight or obese.
   - Choose smaller, more frequent meals rather than three larger meals each day.
2. Lifestyle Recommendations:
   - Elevate the head of bed by 6 to 8 inches for individuals who have reflux episodes at night.
   - Quit smoking and avoid secondhand smoke and alcoholic beverages.
   - Reduce overall stress levels when possible.
   - Wear loose-fitting clothing around the stomach area, as tight or constricting clothing can worsen reflux.

Data from National Digestive Diseases Information Clearinghouse: *Gastroesophageal Reflux (GER) and Gastroesophageal Reflux Disease (GERD) in Adults* (website): http://digestive.niddk.nih.gov/; Song et al, 2013.

establish their clinical significance in GERD when used in normal or small amounts (Jarosz and Taraszewska, 2014; Dossett et al, 2017). Fermented alcoholic beverages (such as beer and wine) stimulate the secretion of gastric acid and should be limited. Carbonated beverages enhance gastric distention, which increases transient LES relaxations. Highly acidic foods such as citrus juices and tomatoes should be avoided because they cause pain when the esophagus is already inflamed.

The role of spices in the pathologic conditions related to upper GI disorders is not clear. When study participants with GERD were initially exposed to a capsaicin-containing red pepper sauce, an increase in both heartburn sensation and an enhancement of secondary peristalsis (triggered by esophageal distention on intake of food or beverage) occurred. However, repeating the same exposure led to a reversal of these effects, and may indicate lowered protection for the esophagus due to delayed acid clearance in those with GERD (Yi et al, 2016). Chewing gum has been shown to increase salivary secretions, which help raise esophageal pH, but studies have not demonstrated its efficacy compared with other lifestyle measures. Limiting or avoiding aggravating foods may improve symptoms in some individuals. Thus recommendations are to have a generally healthy diet and to avoid food items that, in the experience of the patient, trigger symptoms.

Obesity is a contributing factor to GERD and hiatal hernia because it increases intragastric pressure, and weight reduction may reduce acid contact time in the esophagus, leading to decreased reflux symptoms. Advising patients who have reflux episodes at night to elevate the head of the bed by 6 to 8 inches using blocks under bed posts is recommended. Further, frequent bending over should be avoided. Use of loose-fitting garments in the waist area is also thought to decrease the risk of reflux.

A few recent studies have shown an improvement of GERD symptoms with a low sugar and/or low carbohydrate diet. One small study conducted in Taiwan found statistical differences in symptoms of GERD patients based on whether a 500 mL liquid meal provided

84.8 grams versus 178.8 grams of carbohydrates, while both contained equal amounts of protein and fat. Acid-reducing medications were prohibited during the study period. Endoscopy examinations, 24-hour pH monitoring, and reflux symptoms were recorded and included but were not limited to heartburn, acid regurgitation, and abdominal discomfort. For the participants in the low-carbohydrate group, shorter acid reflux periods and fewer acid-reflux symptoms were demonstrated (Wu et al, 2018). Although there are limited studies exploring the impact of the low-carbohydrate diet on resolution of GERD symptoms, promising results such as these warrant further research.

Use of tobacco products is contraindicated with reflux. Cigarette smoking should be stopped because it is associated with decreased LES pressure and decreased salivation, thus causing prolonged acid clearance. Smoking tobacco products also compromises GI integrity and increases the risk of esophageal and other cancers. Lifestyle changes to treat GERD in infants may involve a combination of feeding changes and positioning therapy. Modifying the maternal diet if infants are breastfed, changing formulas, and reducing the feeding volume while increasing the frequency of feedings may be effective strategies to address GERD in infants. Thickened feedings appear to decrease observed regurgitation rather than the actual number of reflux episodes. Little is known about the effect of thickening formula on the history of infantile reflux or the potential allergenicity of commercial thickening agents (Lightdale and Gremse, 2013).

Identification and treatment of the mechanism underlying the GERD is the first line of therapy. A combined approach of lifestyle changes, nutrition, exercise, and stress reduction can be effective in reducing symptoms in some patients. Boxes 26.3 and 26.4 contain information about diet and lifestyle modifications and integrative approaches to help reduce symptoms of GERD.

According to the National Health Interview Survey (NHIS), which is published every 5 years, complementary and integrative medicine (CIM) use is more prevalent in those with gastrointestinal (GI) conditions versus those without. A follow-up study to the most recent report found that 42% of respondents with GI conditions saw a practitioner for or used CIM within the previous year, while only 28% of those without GI conditions used CIM. Of those who reported having GI conditions, 3% used at least one CIM modality to address the problem. GI conditions, as defined by the NHIS, were limited to one or more of the following: abdominal pain, nausea and/or vomiting, liver conditions, digestive allergies, stomach or intestinal illness, and acid reflux/heartburn. The most common CIM modalities used were paired into groups as follows (Dossett et al, 2014):

- Herbs and nonvitamin nonmineral supplements, including zinc, glutamine, deglycyrrhizinated licorice, and aloe gel
- Manipulative therapies: chiropractic, osteopathic, massage, craniosacral therapy
- Mind-body therapies: hypnosis, biofeedback, meditation, imagery, progressive relaxation
- Mind-body exercise: yoga, tai chi, qi gong
- Special diets: vegetarian or vegan, macrobiotic, Atkins, Pritikin, Ornish, or dietary counseling
- Movement therapy: Feldenkrais, Alexander technique, Pilates, Trager psychological integration
- Other: acupuncture, Ayurveda, chelation, energy healing, homeopathy, naturopathy, traditional healers

Among these, herbs and supplements, mind-body therapies, and manipulative therapies were the top three respondents reported using to address a GI condition, and 47% used 3 or more modalities. Overwhelmingly, 80% reported that they perceived CIM therapy to be helpful, but only 70% informed their medical provider about using CIM. While the NHIS acknowledges some important details about the use of CIM and GI conditions, the data are self-reported, and the conditions were limited to those included in the survey. The follow-up study is important because it reveals a significant number of individuals who are integrating CIM modalities with traditional treatment for GI disorders (Dossett et al, 2014).

With many patients using integrative medicine to treat upper GI conditions, including acid reflux/heartburn, it is important for the nutrition professional to be aware of the most common modalities being used. Acupuncture, mind-body therapies, herbs and dietary supplements, and nutrition and lifestyle interventions are all popular and have varying degrees of evidence to support their use. While acupuncture, weight loss, and elevating the head of the bed have good evidence, there is also reasonable evidence to support mind-body modalities and dietary modifications (Dossett et al, 2017; Eherer et al, 2012; Jarosz and Taraszewska, 2014, Maradey-Romero et al, 2014). Further study is needed, and specific recommendations should be tailored to the individual by a well-trained professional using evidence-based data from reliable sources, as many patients may look to anecdotal evidence that is not founded in scientific research (Cowan, 2014).

Surgery of the Esophagus

The primary indication for an esophagectomy is esophageal cancer or BE with high-grade dysplasia. A patient undergoing esophagectomy often presents with dysphagia, decreased appetite, side effects from chemotherapy, and weight loss. Esophagectomy requires that there be another conduit in place to transport food from the oropharynx to the rest of the GI tract for digestion and absorption. Placement of an enteral feeding tube preoperatively, or at the time of surgery, provides enteral access for patients who will experience eating challenges and a slow transition back to a normal diet. The enteral route of nutrition is preferred; however, if the GI tract is not functional, parenteral nutrition (PN) must be provided (see Chapter 12).

Medical Nutrition Therapy

Nutrition assessment of an esophagectomy candidate includes evaluation of treatment plans, history of weight loss, and the ability to swallow solid foods and liquids. Generally, the only esophagectomy patients screened at low nutrition risk preoperatively are those with BE with high-grade dysplasia, or those who are asymptomatic.

Preoperative phase. Swallowing difficulty (dysphagia) is the commonly identified problem in patients awaiting an esophagectomy. Dietary modifications may range from regular food with adequate chewing and slow eating to soft foods or to pureed or blenderized foods. Patients may also benefit from the addition of nutrient-dense, high-protein smoothies and nutritive beverages made from whole foods and healthy fats to maximize energy and protein intake before surgery. If the oral dietary modifications do not prevent further weight loss, nutrition support from a nasoenteric feeding tube inserted in the preoperative patient may be necessary.

Postoperative phase. A gastric pull-up procedure (Fig. 26.4) involves removal of a segment of or the entire esophageal tract and replacing it with the stomach tissue. Complications after this procedure include increased risk of aspiration, dysphagia, anastomosis leak, wound infection, and stricture at the anastomosis site. A jejunostomy feeding tube may be placed at surgery to provide postoperative nutrition until adequate oral intake is achieved. The tube feeding schedule is changed eventually from continuous to cyclical feedings at night as the patient is transitioned to an oral diet during the day.

Transition to oral intake postoperatively proceeds from clear liquids to a soft, moist foods diet. The patient is advised to eat small frequent meals with limited fluids at mealtimes. Some patients may experience dumping syndrome if food passes into the small intestine too quickly. The symptoms of dumping syndrome include abdominal pain, nausea, diarrhea, weakness, and dizziness. Box 26.5 lists dietary guidelines after esophageal surgery to prevent dumping syndrome (see Dumping Syndrome later in this chapter for more details).

Head and Neck Cancer

Pathophysiology

Cancers of the upper aerodigestive tract, collectively referred to as head and neck cancers, comprise malignancies of the oral cavity (lips and

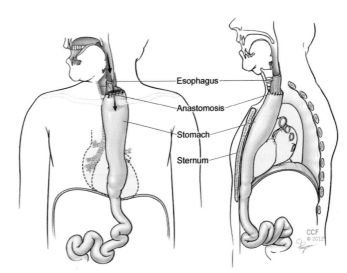

Fig. 26.4 Gastric pull-up. (Cleveland Clinic, Cleveland, Ohio.)

BOX 26.5 Nutrition Guidelines After Esophagectomy

1. Enteral nutrition is provided through a jejunostomy feeding tube after esophagectomy.
2. A patient cannot eat or drink anything by mouth until instructed by the doctor.
3. Once an oral diet is allowed, patient is provided with specific guidelines on how to taper the tube feedings and advance the oral diet (from sips of clear liquids to very moist, tender foods).
4. It may take several weeks to taper the tube feedings and adjust to oral diet. When tube feeding is discontinued, the patient should continue to flush the jejunostomy tube daily. A patient will continue to adjust to oral feedings for about 3 months.
5. During the 3-month transition:
   - Eat six small meals per day and include sources of protein and fat at every small meal.
   - Choose very tender, moist foods that can be easily cut with the side of fork or spoon and use sauces or gravies to moisten food.
   - Gradually increase the volume and variety of foods at each meal.
   - Avoid skins, seeds, nuts, tough or dry meats, breads and rolls, peanut butter, fried and greasy foods, raw vegetables, cooked corn and peas, and raw fruits.
   - Avoid items that can cause heartburn and stomach reflux such as caffeine, citrus fruits, pineapples, tomatoes, carbonated beverages, mints, and alcohol.
   - Drink no more than 4 fluid ounces of water or other liquids with meals. Drink fluids about 30 minutes before or after the meal and sip slowly.
   - Avoid concentrated sweets and sugars.
   - Eat slowly and chew foods thoroughly.
6. After 3 months, more food should be added back into the diet. Try one new food or beverage at a time.
7. After 6 months, a patient should be eating normally. It is still advised to eat frequent small meals.

inside of the mouth, including the front portion of the tongue and the roof and floor of the mouth), the oropharynx (back portion of the tongue and the part of the throat behind the oral cavity), the larynx, and the esophagus. The patient diagnosed with head and neck cancer faces unique challenges in maintaining adequate nutrition. The disease and the treatments, especially surgery and chemo- and radiation therapy, have significant impact on upper digestive tract function, and oral intake is often insufficient during and after therapy. Approximately 35% to 60% of all patients with head and neck cancer are malnourished at the time of diagnosis due to intake difficulties, tumor burden, and cachexia (Alshadwi and Nadershah, 2013). Dysphagia is a hallmark of head and neck cancer; it occurs as a result of mechanical obstruction, sensory impairment, or odynophagia (painful swallowing). In these patients there is a high prevalence of alcohol abuse and long-term tobacco use, which are also associated with chronic malnutrition (Schoeff et al, 2013).

Medical Nutrition Therapy

Depending on the tumor site, the surgical procedure may significantly alter the anatomy and lead to scarring that can negatively affect swallowing. The patient is likely to be restricted from oral intake while healing from the surgery. Placement of a gastrostomy tube is the most common approach to ensure safe delivery of adequate nutrition, but the optimal timing is not defined. Many clinicians may place them prophylactically before the start of radiation or surgical resection to prevent complications from malnutrition (Marian et al, 2017).

Although the goal is eventual transition to oral feeding, some patients will require additional enteral nutrition (EN) because of structural and sensory deficits.

Aggressive prophylactic swallowing therapy is a recent development in the treatment of dysphagia in patients with head and neck cancer. This approach focuses on maintaining or regaining function rather than simply accommodating dysfunction (reliance on feeding tube) and empowers patients to progress carefully with oral intake despite imperfect swallowing (Schoeff et al, 2013).

THE STOMACH

The stomach accommodates and stores meals, mixes food with gastric secretions, and controls emptying into the duodenum. Gastric volume is approximately 50 mL when empty but can expand to approximately 4 L. Gastric parietal cells (acid-producing cells) produce 1.5 to 2 L of acid daily, resulting in a pH between 1 and 2 (see Chapter 1 for a detailed discussion of normal stomach function).

The mucosa of the stomach and duodenum is protected from proteolytic actions of gastric acid and pepsin by a coating of mucus secreted by glands in the epithelial walls from the lower esophagus to the upper duodenum. The mucosa also is protected from bacterial invasion by the digestive actions of pepsin and hydrochloric acid (HCl). Prostaglandins play an important role in protecting the gastroduodenal mucosa by stimulating the secretion of mucus and bicarbonate and maintaining blood flow during periods of potential injury.

Dyspepsia and Functional Dyspepsia
Pathophysiology

Dyspepsia (indigestion) refers to nonspecific, persistent upper abdominal discomfort or pain. It affects an estimated 20% to 40% of the general population and significantly reduces quality of life (Ford and Moayyedi, 2013). The underlying causes of dyspepsia may include GERD, peptic ulcer disease, gastritis, gallbladder disease, or other identifiable pathologic conditions.

Functional gastrointestinal disorders (FGIDs), now known as disorders of gut-brain interaction (DGBI), have been diagnosed and classified using standards defined by the Rome criteria since its inception in the late 1980s. The most recent update using current scientific data was released in May 2016 and is known as the Rome IV criteria. According to these criteria, functional dyspepsia (FD) is defined as an umbrella term to include patients with postprandial distress syndrome (PDS) and epigastric pain syndrome (EPS) (Schmulson and Drossman, 2017). Symptoms can include postprandial fullness and early satiety, but also may cause patients to perceive epigastric discomfort and/or burning after meals. The syndromes can overlap and are considered gastroduodenal disorders that occur in the absence of any organic, systemic, or metabolic disease likely to explain the symptoms (Talley and Ford, 2015). The word discomfort is important to emphasize, as many patients will not complain of pain but rather of burning and pressure or fullness in the epigastric area, with a frequent complaint of early satiety. Belching, abdominal bloating, and nausea can also be present in both syndromes, but vomiting is considered an unusual occurrence (Schmulson and Drossman, 2017).

Medical Nutrition Therapy

Current treatments for FD have generally ignored the potential role of diet. The possible effect of specific foods and macronutrients and other dietary habits to induce or exacerbate FD symptoms has been poorly studied, and often there are conflicting results (Lacy et al, 2012). However, one more recent study demonstrated spicy, pickled, and high-fat foods as catalysts, inducing symptoms the most in patients with this condition (Akhondi-Meybodi et al, 2015). Using a food and symptom diary during a clinical evaluation of a patient with FD and assessing symptoms associated with eating patterns is useful. Dietary modifications such as consuming smaller meals with a reduction in dietary fat may be promising in FD therapy. Helping the patient identify problematic foods also can be helpful.

Gastritis and Peptic Ulcers

Pathophysiology

Gastritis is a nonspecific term literally meaning inflammation of the stomach. It can be used to describe symptoms relating to the stomach, an endoscopic appearance of the gastric mucosa, or a histologic change characterized by infiltration of the epithelium with inflammatory cells such as polymorphonuclear cells (PMNs). Acute gastritis refers to rapid onset of inflammation and symptoms. Chronic gastritis may occur over a period of months to decades, with reoccurring symptoms. Symptoms include nausea, vomiting, malaise, anorexia, hemorrhage, and epigastric pain. Prolonged gastritis may result in atrophy and loss of stomach parietal cells, with a loss of HCl secretion (achlorhydria) and intrinsic factor, resulting in pernicious anemia (see Chapter 31).

Helicobacter pylori Gastritis

Helicobacter pylori is a gram-negative bacteria that is somewhat resistant to the acidic environment in the stomach. *H. pylori* infection is responsible for most cases of chronic inflammation of the gastric mucosa and peptic ulcer, gastric cancer, and atrophic gastritis (chronic inflammation with deterioration of the mucous membrane and glands), resulting in achlorhydria and loss of intrinsic factor (Dos Santos and Carvalho, 2015).

H. pylori is a known underlying cause of noncardia gastric cancer and responsible for deaths from peptic ulcer (Axon, 2014). An updated classification of gastric cancers was adopted in part because of the role of *H. pylori*, which is a strong risk factor for noncardia gastric cancer. Traditionally, gastric cancer was considered a single disease, but scientists now classify it by its location in either the top inch of the stomach near the esophagus (gastric cardia) or the rest of the stomach (noncardia).

Developed countries have seen a decrease in *H. pylori* infections in recent years because of increased information, testing, and effective treatment. Risk factors for this infection are higher in less-developed countries with lower standard of living, poor education, and reduced lifespan. In these communities, the prevalence of reinfection is also higher, leading to an ongoing public health problem. The revelation that treating *H. pylori* infection decreases the risk for some cancers but may increase the risk of other cancers (esophageal) is also prompting more research and knowledge that treatment must be more widespread (Axon, 2014).

While prevalence of *H. pylori* infection correlates with geography and socioeconomic status of the population and begins during childhood, it is often not diagnosed until adulthood. *H. pylori* is spread through contaminated food and water and is correlated with lower levels of hygiene. More than half of the world population is infected and prevalence ranges from as low as 18.9% in Switzerland, to 24.6%–35.6% in the United States and Australia, to as high as 87.7% in Nigeria (Hooi et al, 2017). *H. pylori* infection does not resolve spontaneously, and risks of complications increase with the duration of the infection. Other risk factors contributing to pathology and disease severity include patient age at onset, specific strain and concentration of the

organism, genetic factors related to the host, and the patient's lifestyle and overall health.

In the first week after *H. pylori* infection, many PMNs and a few eosinophils infiltrate the gastric mucosa. These are replaced gradually with the mononuclear cells. The presence of lymphoid follicles is called mucosa-associated lymphoid tissue (MALT). MALT may become autonomous to form a low-grade, B-cell lymphoma called MALT lymphoma. *H. pylori* can cause duodenitis if it colonizes gastric tissue that may be present in the duodenum.

Treating *H. pylori* with antibiotics can cause PMNs to disappear within a week or two, but a mild gastritis can persist for several years, as the reduction in mononuclear cells is slow. In countries where *H. pylori* is common, so is gastric cancer. Because *H. pylori* can cause peptic ulcer and gastric cancer, antibiotic treatment is favored when it is diagnosed. Box 26.6 includes information about integrative approaches for *H. pylori*.

BOX 26.6 Integrative Approaches to *Helicobacter Pylori* and Associated GI Disease

Typical medical treatment for *H. pylori* is with "triple therapy" (TT) that combines two antimicrobial drugs (clarithromycin and amoxicillin or metronidazole) with proton pump inhibitor (PPI) for 1 to 2 weeks with an 80% to 85% success rate (Sarkar et al, 2016; Oh et al, 2016). Unfortunately, adverse events such as *Clostridium difficile* infection (CDI) or pseudomembranous colitis can occur with the change in gut flora due to TT treatment. One small randomized controlled trial (RCT) employed a 4-week comparison of standard medical treatment alone versus standard medical treatment with a probiotic added to demonstrate an eradication rate of 100% in the probiotic group versus 90% in the control. The effect was thought to be due to lowered imbalance of microbiota during treatment, thus leading to better tolerated treatment completion (Oh et al, 2016). Whereas this particular study was very small, a much larger meta-analysis reviewed similar comparison data from 6997 participants from 45 RCTs to find eradication rates of 82.31% in the probiotic group versus 72.08% in the control group (Zhang et al, 2015). Probiotics species (*Lactobacillus, Bifidobacterium*) have been studied for prevention, management, and eradication of *H. pylori* (Zhu et al, 2014). Further study on specific strains and larger clinical trials is warranted to investigate the role of probiotic therapy and whether it should be included as a standard of care in medical treatment moving forward.

Food also provides an interesting alternative to standard therapy. Emerging research on the synergy of food combinations that may inhibit the growth of *H. pylori* suggests that green tea, broccoli sprouts, black currant oil, and kimchi (fermented cabbage) help with *H. pylori* eradication (Kennan et al, 2010). Recent studies have also demonstrated anti–*H. pylori* potential and significant inhibition of the bacteria's growth by n-3 polyunsaturated fatty acids (PUFAs) in both in vitro and in vivo models. A decrease in growth and associated inflammation of *H. pylori* has been shown with administration of docosahexaenoic acid (DHA). Although some results showed fish oil as less effective than aspects of TT treatment, and omega-3s would not be a standalone therapy, data suggests, when combined with standard TT treatment, that PUFAs and DHA could have potential to damper recurrence rates (Park et al, 2015).

Because of the known relationship between *H. pylori* and peptic ulcers, eradication of the bacteria is a primary focus of treatment for those who test positive for it. Dietary polyphenols are being reviewed in a variety of studies to determine efficacy in combination with conventional treatment for peptic ulcers. Piper betel, curcumin, gallic acid, apple, grape, pomegranate and green tea polyphenols, and quercetin represent only a few compounds being investigated. These bioactive compounds are only a starting point for the direction of future research and clinical trials needed to determine the role of food as a part of the treatment for peptic ulcer disease (Farzaei et al, 2015).

Non-*Helicobacter pylori* Gastritis

Aspirin and nonsteroidal antiinflammatory drugs (NSAIDs) are corrosive; both inhibit prostaglandin synthesis, which is essential for maintaining the mucus and bicarbonate barrier in the stomach. Thus chronic use of aspirin or other NSAIDs, steroids, alcohol, erosive substances, tobacco, or any combination of these factors may compromise mucosal integrity and increase the chance for acquiring acute or chronic gastritis. Eosinophilic gastroenteritis (EGE) also may contribute to some cases of gastritis. Poor nutrition and general poor health may contribute to the onset and severity of the symptoms and can delay the healing process.

Medical Treatment

Treatment for gastritis involves removing the inciting agent (e.g., pathogenic organism, NSAIDs). Noninvasive methods for diagnosing *H. pylori* include a blood test for *H. pylori* antibodies, a urea breath test, or a stool antigen test. Endoscopy is a common invasive diagnostic tool (see *Focus On*: Endoscopy and Capsules for more details about this procedure). Antibiotics and PPIs are the primary medical treatments.

Side effects of chronic acid suppression either from disease or chronic use of PPIs are a current topic of interest in medical research. First approved in 1989, PPIs reduce gastric acid production by binding irreversibly to the hydrogen/potassium ATPase enzyme on gastric parietal cells and are now one of the most commonly prescribed medications in the United States. While they are generally well-tolerated medications and are considered safe, there have been some emerging concerns regarding long-term use over the past several years. This is especially true for those taking the medication for longer than intended, or when no longer indicated, as they are now widely available over the counter. A Mayo Clinic review found that the association between each of the health concerns and long-term PPI use varies between likely causative, unlikely causative, and unclear association. For hypomagnesemia, vitamin B_{12} deficiency, and small intestinal bacterial overgrowth (SIBO) the association is *likely causative,* whereas community acquired pneumonia (CAD) is *unlikely causative,* and bone fractures, *Clostridium difficile* infection, chronic kidney disease, and dementia have an *unclear association* (Nehra et al, 2018). See Appendix 13 for nutrients of concern for those taking these medications.

Peptic Ulcers

Etiology

Normal gastric and duodenal mucosa is protected from the digestive actions of acid and pepsin by the secretion of mucus, the production of bicarbonate, the removal of excess acid by normal blood flow, and the rapid renewal and repair of epithelial cell injury. Peptic ulcer disease occurs when open sores (peptic ulcers) form as a result of the breakdown of the normal defense and repair mechanisms, and are differentiated as either gastric or duodenal, depending on location. Typically, more than one of the mechanisms must be malfunctioning for symptomatic peptic ulcers to develop. Peptic ulcers typically show evidence of chronic inflammation and repair processes surrounding the lesion.

The primary causes of peptic ulcers are *H. pylori* infection, gastritis, use of aspirin, other NSAIDs and corticosteroids, and severe illness (see Stress Ulcers later in this chapter and *Pathophysiology and Care Management Algorithm:* Peptic Ulcer). Life stress may lead to behaviors that increase peptic ulcer risk. Although excessive use of concentrated forms of ethanol can damage gastric mucosa, worsen symptoms of peptic ulcers, and interfere with ulcer healing, alcohol consumption in moderation does not cause peptic ulcers in healthy people. Use of

tobacco products also is linked with peptic ulcer risk because tobacco decreases bicarbonate secretion and mucosal blood flow, exacerbates inflammation, and is associated with additional complications of *H. pylori* infection. Other risk factors include gastrinoma and Zollinger-Ellison's syndrome (see Chapter 28).

◎ FOCUS ON

Endoscopy and Capsules

The esophagogastroduodenoscopy (EGD) procedure allows the mucosa of the upper gastrointestinal (GI) tract to be viewed, photographed, and biopsied. Also known as an endoscopy, the procedure involves insertion of a flexible tube into the esophagus with a light and camera on the distal end. It can be passed through the esophagus and into the stomach or upper small bowel. Inflammation, erosions, ulcerations, changes in the blood vessels, and destruction of surface cells can be identified. These changes can then be correlated with chemical, histologic, and clinical findings to formulate a diagnosis. This may be useful when physicians suspect certain conditions, such as complicated gastroesophageal reflux disease (GERD) strictures, Barrett's esophagus (BE), esophageal varices, or gastroduodenal ulcers or celiac disease.

EGD also can be used for a number of therapeutic purposes, such as cauterization at ulcer sites, dilation or deployment of stents in areas of stricture, and placement of percutaneous feeding tubes. Endoscopy may be used in long-term monitoring of patients with chronic esophagitis and gastritis because of the possibility that they will develop premalignant lesions or carcinoma.

Capsule endoscopy can be used to view segments of the GI tract that are not accessible by standard EGD, to screen for abnormalities or bleeding, check pH, and measure the time it takes to pass through different segments of the GI tract. In this procedure, capsules containing a miniaturized video camera, light, and radio transmitter that can be swallowed and the signal transmitted to a receiver worn on the waist of the patient, allowing wireless capsule endoscopy. The procedure is less invasive than normal endoscopy and provides the advantage of being able to observe, record, and measure GI function as the patient is ambulatory.

Unfortunately, the images from capsule endoscopy can be blurred by rapid intestinal transit or limited in number after battery failure in cases of slow transit. In addition, reviewing the thousands of images obtained after each capsule endoscopy can be very time consuming. Prototypes of the newest generation of capsule endoscopy allow the physician to magnetically guide the capsule to a specific location by having the patient lie on a special table. Future generations of capsule endoscopy are on the drawing boards to hopefully allow therapeutic measures to be accomplished in the small bowel via capsule endoscopy.

The incidence and number of surgical procedures related to peptic ulcers has decreased markedly in the past 3 decades because of recognition of symptoms and risk factors, and earlier screening for *H. pylori*. Uncomplicated peptic ulcers in either the gastric or duodenal region may present with signs similar to those associated with dyspepsia and gastritis.

Abdominal discomfort is the most common symptom of peptic ulcers and can be felt anywhere between the navel and the breastbone. This discomfort is usually described as a dull or burning pain that occurs when the stomach is empty (between meals or during the night), and may be briefly relieved by eating food, in the case of duodenal ulcers, or by taking antacids. In both types of peptic ulcers, the symptoms last for minutes to hours and come and go for several days or weeks. Other symptoms include bloating, burping, nausea, vomiting, poor appetite, and weight loss. Some people experience only mild symptoms or none at all.

Peptic ulcers also may have "emergency symptoms," in which medical assistance should be sought immediately. These include sharp, sudden, persistent, and severe stomach pain, bloody or black stools (melena), bloody vomit (hematemesis), or vomit that looks like coffee grounds. These symptoms could be signs of a serious problem, such as:

- Acute or chronic GI bleed: when acid or a peptic ulcer breaks a blood vessel.

- GI perforation: when a peptic ulcer burrows completely through the stomach or duodenal wall, potentially penetrating an adjacent organ (e.g., pancreas)
- GI obstruction: when a peptic ulcer blocks the path of food trying to leave the stomach.

If or when these problems occur, immediate medical attention is necessary, as complications of hemorrhage and perforation contribute significantly to the morbidity and mortality of peptic ulcers.

PATHOPHYSIOLOGY AND CARE MANAGEMENT ALGORITHM

Peptic Ulcer

ETIOLOGY

H. pylori infection → Peptic Ulcer ← Stress

Aspirin and other NSAIDs → Peptic Ulcer ← Gastritis

PATHOPHYSIOLOGY

Erosion through muscularis mucosa into submucosa or muscularis propria

MANAGEMENT

Medical Management

- If *H. pylori* positive, use antibiotics
- Reduce or withdraw use of NSAIDs
- Use sucralfate, antacids
- Suppress acid secretion with proton pump inhibitors or H$_2$-receptor antagonists

Behavioral Management

- Avoid tobacco products
- Reduce stress

Nutrition Management

Decrease consumption of:
- Alcohol
- Spices, particularly red and black pepper when inflamed
- Coffee and caffeine

Increase consumption of:
- Omega-3 and Omega-6 fatty acids
- Fermented foods (yogurt, fermented cabbage, miso)
- Cooked, non-spicy, soft foods that are easy to digest

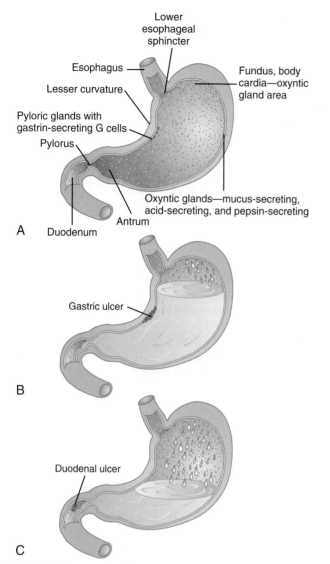

Fig. 26.5 A, Diagram showing a normal stomach and duodenum; **B,** a gastric ulcer; **C,** a duodenal ulcer.

Gastric versus Duodenal Ulcers

Pathophysiology

Although gastric ulcers can occur anywhere in the stomach, most occur along the lesser curvature (Fig. 26.5). Gastric ulcers typically are associated with widespread gastritis, inflammatory involvement of parietal cells, and atrophy of acid- and pepsin-producing cells occurring with advancing age. In some cases, gastric ulceration develops despite relatively low acid output. Antral hypomotility, gastric stasis, and increased duodenal reflux are associated commonly with gastric ulcers, and when present, may increase the severity of the gastric injury. The incidence of hemorrhage and overall mortality is higher with a gastric ulcer than a duodenal ulcer.

A duodenal ulcer is characterized by increased acid secretion throughout the entire day accompanied with decreased bicarbonate secretion. Most duodenal ulcers occur within the first few centimeters of the duodenal bulb, in an area immediately below the pylorus. Gastric outlet obstruction occurs more commonly with duodenal ulcers than with gastric ulcers, and gastric metaplasia (e.g., replacement of duodenal villous cells with gastric-type mucosal cells) may occur with duodenal ulcer related to *H. pylori*.

Medical and Surgical Management of Ulcers

Regardless of the type of ulcer, the first intervention is to evaluate the patient endoscopically and resuscitate as needed. Control acute bleeding if present.

Peptic ulcers. *H. pylori* is the primary cause of gastritis and peptic ulcers, thus its diagnosis if present, and treatment, should be the first medical intervention. At the first endoscopy, diagnostic biopsies should be taken for *H. pylori*. Treatment of *H. pylori* infection entails eradication of this organism with the appropriate antibiotic and acid-suppressive regimen. Although surgical intervention is less prevalent, emergent and elective procedures and surgeries are still required for peptic ulcer complications. Interventions can range from endoscopic, open, and laparoscopic procedures to treat individual lesions, to partial gastrectomy and occasionally selective vagotomies.

Stress ulcers. Stress ulcers may occur as a complication of metabolic stress caused by trauma, burns, surgery, shock, renal failure, or radiation therapy. A primary concern with stress ulceration is the potential for significant GI hemorrhage. Gastric ischemia associated with GI hypoperfusion, oxidative injury, reflux of bile salts and pancreatic enzymes, microbial colonization, and mucosal barrier changes also have been implicated. Although stress ulcerations usually occur in the fundus and body of the stomach, they also may develop in the antrum, duodenum, or distal esophagus. Typically shallow, and causing oozing of blood from superficial capillary beds, stress ulcer lesions also may occur deeper, eroding into the submucosa, causing massive hemorrhage or perforation.

Stress ulcers that bleed can be a significant cause of morbidity in the critically ill patient (see Chapter 37). Although current prevention and treatment include sucralfate, acid suppressants, and antibiotics as needed, high-quality evidence to guide clinical practice in effective treatments is limited. Efforts to prevent gastric ulcers in stressed patients have focused on preventing or limiting conditions leading to hypotension and ischemia and coagulopathies. Avoiding NSAIDs and large doses of corticosteroids is also beneficial.

Providing oral or enteral feeding, when possible, increases GI vascular perfusion and stimulates secretion and motility. A meta-analysis of studies in critically ill patients that received an H_2-receptor antagonist for stress ulcer prevention found this therapy to be preventative only in patients who did not receive enteral feeding. In fact, for patients receiving enteral feeding, H_2-receptor antagonist therapy may increase the risk of pneumonia and death (Chanpura and Yende, 2012). Further research is needed to prospectively test the effect of enteral feeding on the risk of stress ulcer prophylaxis.

Medical Nutrition Therapy

In persons with atrophic gastritis, vitamin B_{12} status should be evaluated because lack of intrinsic factor and gastric acid results in malabsorption of this vitamin (see Chapter 31). Low acid states may influence absorption of iron, calcium, and other nutrients because gastric acid enhances bioavailability. In the case of refractory iron deficiency anemia, other causes may be the presence of *H. pylori* and gastritis. Eradication of *H. pylori* has resulted in improved absorption of iron and increased ferritin levels (Hershko and Camaschella, 2014).

For several decades dietary factors have gained or lost favor as a significant component in the cause and treatment of dyspepsia, gastritis, and peptic ulcer disease. There is little evidence that specific dietary factors cause or exacerbate gastritis or peptic ulcer disease. Protein foods temporarily buffer gastric secretions, but they also stimulate secretion of gastrin, acid, and pepsin. Milk or cream, which in the early days of peptic ulcer management was considered important in coating the stomach, is no longer considered medicinal.

The pH of a food has little therapeutic importance, except for patients with existing lesions of the mouth or the esophagus. Most foods are considerably less acidic than the normal gastric pH of 1 to 3. The pH of orange juice and grapefruit is 3.2 to 3.6, and the pH of commonly used soft drinks ranges from approximately 2.8 to 3.5. On the basis of their intrinsic acidity and the amount consumed, fruit juices and soft drinks are not likely to cause peptic ulcers or appreciably interfere with healing. Some patients express discomfort with ingestion of acidic foods, but the response is not consistent among patients, and in some, symptoms may be related to heartburn. The dietary inclusion of "acidic foods" should be individualized based on the patient's perception of their effect.

Consumption of large amounts of alcohol may cause at least superficial mucosal damage and may worsen existing disease or interfere with treatment of the peptic ulcer. Modest consumption of alcohol does not appear to be pathogenic for peptic ulcers unless coexisting risk factors are also present. On the other hand, beers and wines significantly increase gastric secretions and should be avoided in symptomatic disease.

Coffee and caffeine stimulate acid secretion and also may decrease LES pressure; however, neither has been strongly implicated as a cause of peptic ulcers outside of the increased acid secretion and discomfort associated with their consumption.

When very large doses of certain spices are fed orally or placed intragastrically without other foods, they increase acid secretion and cause small, transient superficial erosions, inflammation of the mucosal lining, and altered GI permeability or motility. Small amounts of chili pepper or its active component, capsaicin, may increase mucosal protection by increasing production of mucus. The burning sensation in the gut when capsaicin is consumed is due to transient receptor potential vanilloid-1 (TRPV1) receptors throughout the GI tract, and repeated exposure can desensitize the receptor. Larger amounts of capsaicin may not be as well tolerated and could cause superficial mucosal damage, especially when consumed with alcohol, as TRPV1 receptors can also be stimulated by ethanol (Patcharatrakul and Gonlachanvit, 2016). Another spice, curcumin, through its antiinflammatory activity that inhibits the NF-κB pathway activation may be a chemopreventive candidate against *H. pylori*–related cancer (Sarkar et al, 2016) (see Chapter 12).

Overall, a high-quality diet without nutrient deficiencies may offer some protection and may promote healing. Persons being treated for gastritis and peptic ulcer disease should be advised to avoid foods that exacerbate their symptoms and to consume a nutritionally complete diet with adequate dietary fiber from fruits and vegetables.

Carcinoma of the Stomach

Although the incidence and mortality have fallen dramatically over the last 50 years in many regions, gastric cancer is still the second most common cause of cancer death worldwide, with varying incidence in different parts of the world and among various ethnic groups (Nagini, 2012). Despite advances in diagnosis and treatment, the 5-year survival rate of stomach cancer is only 20%.

Etiology

The cause of gastric cancer is multifactorial, but more than 80% of cases have been attributed to *H. pylori* infection. In addition, diet, lifestyle, genetic, socioeconomic, and other factors contribute to

gastric carcinogenesis. A Western diet, high in processed meats, fat, starches, and simple sugars, is associated with an increased risk of gastric cancer compared with a diet high in fruits and vegetables (Bertuccio et al, 2013). Other factors that may increase the risk of gastric cancer include alcohol consumption, excess body weight, smoking, intake of highly salted or pickled foods, or inadequate amounts of micronutrients. Certain cooking practices also are associated with increased risk of gastric cancer, including broiling of meats, roasting, grilling, baking, and deep frying in open furnaces, sun drying, salting, curing, and pickling, all of which increase the formation of carcinogenic N-nitroso compounds. Polycyclic aromatic hydrocarbons such as benzo[a]pyrene formed in smoked food have been incriminated in many areas of the world (Nagini, 2012).

Pathophysiology

Stomach cancer refers to any malignant neoplasm that arises from the region extending between the gastroesophageal junction and the pylorus. Because symptoms are slow to manifest themselves and the growth of the tumor is rapid, carcinoma of the stomach frequently is overlooked until it is too late for a cure. Loss of appetite, strength, and weight frequently precede other symptoms. In some cases, achylia gastrica (absence of HCl and pepsin) or achlorhydria (absence of HCl in gastric secretions) may exist for years before the onset of gastric carcinoma. Malignant gastric neoplasms can lead to malnutrition as a result of excessive blood and protein losses or, more commonly, because of obstruction and mechanical interference with food intake.

Medical and Surgical Management

Most cancers of the stomach are treated by surgical resection; thus, part of the nutritional considerations includes partial or total gastrectomy, a resection or removal of the stomach. Some patients may experience difficulties with nutrition after surgery.

Medical Nutrition Therapy

The dietary regimen for carcinoma of the stomach is determined by the location of the cancer, the nature of the functional disturbance, and the stage of the disease. The patient with advanced, inoperable cancer should receive a diet that is adjusted according to tolerance, preference, and comfort. Anorexia is almost always present from the early stages of disease. In the later stages of the disease, the patient may tolerate only a liquid diet. If a patient is unable to tolerate oral feeding, consideration should be given to using an alternate route, such as a gastric or intestinal enteral tube feeding, or if this is not tolerated or feasible, parenteral feeding. The nutritional support for the patient should be in accordance with the patient's goals of care (see Chapter 12).

Gastric Surgeries

Because of increased recognition and treatment for *H. pylori* and acid secretion, gastric surgeries are performed less frequently. However, partial or total gastrectomy may still be necessary for patients with ulcer disease that does not respond to therapy, or for those with malignancy. Gastric surgeries performed for weight loss or bariatric surgeries are more common. These surgeries, such as Roux-en-Y gastric bypass, gastric banding, sleeve gastrectomy, vertical banding gastroplasty, and jejunoileal bypass are designed to induce weight loss though volume restriction, malabsorption, or both (see Chapter 20).

Types of Surgeries

A total gastrectomy involves removal of the entire stomach, whereas only a portion of the stomach is removed with a subtotal or partial

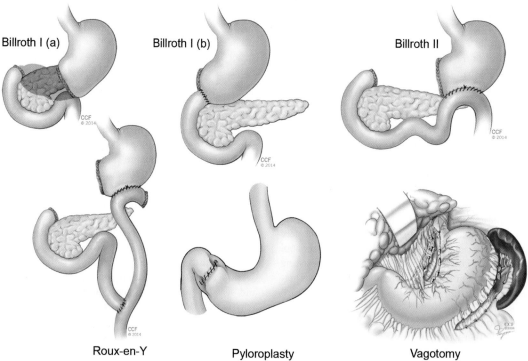

Fig. 26.6 Gastric surgical procedures [Billroth I (A: preoperative and B: postoperative), Billroth II, Roux en Y, pylorplasty, vagotomy].

gastrectomy. A gastrectomy is accompanied by a reconstructive proce-dure. A total gastrectomy is performed for malignancies that affect the middle or upper stomach. The total stomach is removed, and a Roux-en-Y reconstruction is performed to maintain GI tract continu-ity. With a Roux-en-Y, the jejunum is pulled up and anastomosed to the esophagus. The duodenum is then connected to the small bowel so that bile and pancreatic secretions can flow into the intestine. Billroth I (gastroduodenostomy) involves removal of the pylorus and/or an-trum, and an anastomosis of the proximal end of the duodenum to the distal end of the remnant stomach. A Billroth II (gastrojejunostomy) involves removal of the stomach antrum and an anastomosis of the remnant stomach to the side of the jejunum, which creates a blind duodenal loop (Fig. 26.6).

The vagus nerve is responsible for not only motility, but also stimulation of parietal cells in the proximal stomach, therefore a va-gotomy often is performed to eliminate gastric acid secretion. Truncal vagotomy, complete severing of the vagus nerve on the distal esopha-gus, decreases acid secretion by parietal cells in the stomach and de-creases their response to the hormone gastrin. A parietal cell vagot-omy (partial or selective) divides and severs only the vagus nerve branches that affect the proximal stomach where gastric acid secretion occurs, whereas the antrum and pylorus remain innervated. Vagotomy at certain levels can alter the normal physiologic function of the stom-ach, small intestine, pancreas, and biliary system. Vagotomy proce-dures commonly are accompanied by a drainage procedure (antrec-tomy or pyloroplasty) that aids with gastric emptying.

Postoperative Medical Nutrition Therapy

Oral intake of fluids and foods is initiated as soon as GI tract function returns (typically 24 to 72 hours postoperatively). Small frequent feed-ings of ice or water are normally initiated, followed by liquids and easily digested solid foods, after which the patient can progress to a regular diet. Although this is the common postoperative diet interven-tion, there is limited evidence supporting this practice. In fact, some studies suggest beginning a regular diet of tolerated foods as the first diet to improve patient tolerance (Warren et al, 2011). If the patient is unable to tolerate an oral diet for an extended period of time (e.g., 5 to 7 days), then enteral feeding should be considered if appropriate feed-ing access is available, and if not, PN should be considered.

Understanding the surgery performed and the patient's resulting anatomy is paramount to providing proper nutritional care. Nutri-tional complications after gastric surgeries are varied (Table 26.4). Complications such as obstruction, dumping, abdominal discomfort, diarrhea, and weight loss may occur, depending on the nature and extent of the disease and surgical interventions (see Fig. 26.6). Patients may have difficulty regaining normal preoperative weight because of inadequate food intake related to (1) early satiety, (2) symptoms of dumping syndrome (see later in this chapter), or (3) nutrient malab-sorption.

Patients with certain gastric surgeries, such as Billroth II, result in a mismatch in timing of food entry into the small intestine and the re-lease and interaction with bile and pancreatic enzymes, contributing to impaired nutrient digestion and absorption. Patients who are lactose tolerant before gastric surgery may experience relative lactase defi-ciency, either because food enters the small intestine further down-stream from adequate lactase presence, or because the rate of transit through the proximal small intestine is increased. Because of the com-plications of reflux or dumping syndrome associated with traditional gastrectomies, other procedures are used, including truncal, selective, or parietal cell vagotomy; pyloromyotomy; antrectomy; Roux-en-Y esophagojejunostomy; loop esophagojejunostomy; and pouches or reservoirs made from jejunal or ileocecal segments.

TABLE 26.4 Gastric Surgery–Related Nutrition Complications

Surgical Procedure	Potential Complications
Vagotomy	Impairs motor function of stomach
Total gastric and truncal vagotomy	Gastric stasis and poor gastric emptying
Total gastrectomy	Early satiety, nausea, vomiting
	Weight loss
	Inadequate bile acids and pancreatic enzymes available because of anastomotic changes
	Malabsorption
	Protein-energy malnutrition
	Anemia
	Dumping syndrome
	Bezoar formation
	Vitamin B_{12} deficiency
	Metabolic bone disease
Subtotal gastrectomy with vagotomy	Early satiety
	Delayed gastric emptying
	Rapid emptying of hypertonic fluids

Cresci G et al: *Nutrition essentials of general surgery*, ed 5, Lippincott Williams & Wilkins, 2013, Table 3–13, p 72; Rollins, CJ (2015): Chapter 23, Drug-Nutrient Interactions with Gastrointestinal Drugs. In *The Health Professional's Guide to Gastrointestinal Nutrition* (pp. 296–311). Chicago IL: Cathy Immartino.

Some chronic nutritional complications that can occur after gastric surgery include anemia, osteoporosis, and select vitamin and mineral deficiencies resulting from inadequate intake and or malabsorption. Iron deficiency may be attributed to loss of acid secretion because gastric acid normally facilitates the reduction of iron compounds, allowing their absorption. Rapid transit and diminished contact of dietary iron with sites of iron absorption can also lead to iron deficiency.

Vitamin B_{12} deficiency may cause a megaloblastic anemia (see Chapter 31). If the amount of gastric mucosa is reduced, intrinsic factor may not be produced in quantities adequate to allow for complete vitamin B_{12} absorption, and pernicious anemia may result. Bacterial overgrowth in the proximal small bowel or the afferent loop contributes to vitamin B_{12} depletion because bacteria compete with the host for use of the vitamin. Therefore after gastrectomy patients should receive prophylactic vitamin B_{12} supplementation (injections) or take synthetic oral supplementation.

Dumping Syndrome
Etiology

The dumping syndrome is a complex GI and vasomotor response to the presence of large quantities of hypertonic foods and liquids in the proximal small intestine. Dumping syndrome usually occurs as a result of surgical procedures that allow excessive amounts of liquid or solid foods to enter the small intestine in a concentrated form. Milder forms of dumping may occur to varying degrees in persons without surgical procedures, and most of the symptoms can be reproduced in normal individuals by infusing a loading dose of glucose into the jejunum. Dumping may occur as a result of total or partial gastrectomy, manipulation of the pylorus, fundoplication, vagotomy, and some gastric bypass procedures for obesity. As a result of better medical management of peptic ulcers, use of selective vagotomies, and newer surgical

procedures to avoid complications, classic dumping is encountered less frequently in clinical practice.

Pathophysiology

Symptoms can be divided into two types or stages of dumping of solids and liquids into the small intestine, and characteristics and symptom severity vary between patients:

- Early dumping (within 10 to 30 minutes postprandially) is characterized by GI and vasomotor symptoms, which include abdominal pain, bloating, nausea, vomiting, diarrhea, headache, flushing, fatigue, and hypotension. These symptoms likely occur because of the rapid influx of hyperosmolar contents into the duodenum or small intestine. A subsequent fluid shift from the intravascular compartment to the intestinal lumen occurs, resulting in small intestine distention, potentially causing cramps and bloating.
- Late dumping (1 to 3 hours postprandially) results in symptoms that are predominantly vasomotor and include perspiration, weakness, confusion, shakiness, hunger, and hypoglycemia. Late dumping is likely the result of reactive hypoglycemia. Rapid delivery, as well as hydrolysis and absorption of carbohydrates, produces an exaggerated rise in insulin level and a subsequent decline in blood glucose. The rapid changes in blood glucose and the secretion of gut peptides, glucose insulinotropic polypeptide, and glucagon-like polypeptide-1 appear to be at least partly responsible for the late symptoms (Deloose et al, 2014).

Medical Management

Medical intervention typically involves dietary changes as the initial treatment, and they are usually effective. However, in 3% to 5% of patients, severe dumping persists despite dietary change. In these patients, medications may be used to slow gastric emptying and delay transit of food through the GI tract. Some, such as acarbose, inhibit alpha glycoside hydrolase and interfere with carbohydrate absorption, and octreotide, a somatostatin analog, inhibits insulin release (see Table 26.3 for common medications). Rarely, surgical intervention is used to treat dumping syndrome.

Medical Nutrition Therapy

Patients with dumping syndrome may experience weight loss and malnutrition caused by inadequate intake, malabsorption, or a combination of both. The prime objective of nutrition therapy is to restore nutrition status and quality of life. Because they are digested more slowly, proteins and fats are better tolerated than carbohydrates, particularly simple carbohydrates. Simple carbohydrates such as lactose, sucrose, fructose, glucose, and dextrose are hydrolyzed rapidly and should be limited, but complex carbohydrates (starches) can be included in the diet.

Liquids leave the stomach and enter the jejunum rapidly; thus, some patients have trouble tolerating liquids with meals. Patients with severe dumping may benefit from limiting the amount of liquids taken with meals and drinking liquids between meals without solid food. Reclining (approximately 30 degrees) after meals may also minimize severity of symptoms.

The use of soluble fiber supplements, particularly pectin or gums (e.g., guar) can be beneficial in managing dumping syndrome because of fiber's ability to form gels with carbohydrates and fluids and delay GI transit. Patients may need to be taught about portion sizes of foods, especially of carbohydrate foods such as juices, soft drinks, desserts, and milk. The exchange list given in Appendix 18 can be used to calculate carbohydrate intake and teach about carbohydrate control.

BOX 26.7 Basic Guidelines for Dumping Syndrome

1. Eat six to eight small meals throughout the day.
2. Limit fluids to 4 ounces (½ cup) at a meal, just enough to rinse food down.
3. Drink remaining fluids at least 30 to 40 minutes before and after meals.
4. Eat slowly and chew foods thoroughly. Some may benefit from soft, ground, or pureed foods, or those that are already broken down, such as ground meats.
5. Avoid extreme temperatures of foods (very hot or very cold).
6. Use seasonings and spices as tolerated (may want to avoid pepper, hot sauce).
7. Lie down or recline for at least 30 minutes after eating.
8. Limit simple carbohydrate foods and liquids with more than 12 grams of sugar per serving. Examples: fruit juice, Gatorade, Powerade, Kool Aid, sweet tea, sucrose, honey, jelly, corn syrup, cookies, pie, doughnuts. Increase complex carbohydrate foods such as whole grains and foods made with them, and potatoes.
9. Choose foods that are higher in soluble fiber. Some examples of these foods include apples, oats, beets, carrots, and beans.
10. Include a protein-containing food at each meal.
11. Add a serving of fat such as olive oil, nut butter, or avocado to meals as tolerated to encourage slower gastric emptying. Minimize fried foods, chips, cookies, hot dogs, and other greasy foods.
12. Milk and dairy products may not be tolerated in the lactose intolerant. Introduce these slowly in the diet if they were tolerated preoperatively.
13. Avoid sugar alcohols such as sorbitol, xylitol, mannitol, and maltitol, as these may exacerbate symptoms.

University of Virginia Health System. Anti-Dumping Diet, https://uvahealth.com/services/digestive-health/images-and-docs/dumping-syndrome.pdf; Cresci GA (2015): Chapter 14, Gastrointestinal Tract Surgery. In *The Health Professional's Guide to Gastrointestinal Nutrition* (pp.168–181). Chicago IL: Cathy Immartino.

Postgastrectomy patients often do not tolerate lactose, but small amounts (e.g., 6 g or less per meal) may be tolerated at one time. Patients typically do better with cheeses or unsweetened yogurt than with fluid milk. Nondairy milks are also useful when necessary. Vitamin D and calcium supplements may be needed when intake is inadequate. Commercial lactase-containing products are available for those with significant lactose malabsorption (see Chapter 27 for further discussion of lactose intolerance and its management).

When steatorrhea (greater than 7% of dietary fat in the stool) exists, reduced-fat formulas or pancreatic enzymes may be beneficial. Box 26.7 provides general nutrition guidelines for patients with dumping syndrome after gastric surgery; however, each diet must be adjusted based on a careful dietary and social history from the patient.

GASTROPARESIS

Etiology

Gastroparesis is a syndrome of delayed gastric emptying without evidence of mechanical obstruction and is a complex and potentially debilitating condition. The nature of gastroparesis is complex in part because gastric motility is orchestrated by a variety of chemical and neurologic factors. Viral infection, diabetes, and surgeries are the most common causes for gastroparesis; however, more than 30% of cases are idiopathic. Numerous classes of clinical conditions are associated with gastroparesis, including acid-peptic diseases, gastritis, postgastric surgery, disorder of gastric smooth muscle, psychogenic disorders, long-term uncontrolled diabetes, and neuropathic disorders.

Pathophysiology

Clinical symptoms may include abdominal bloating, decreased appetite and anorexia, nausea and vomiting, fullness, early satiety, halitosis, and postprandial hypoglycemia. The gold-standard measure of gastric emptying rate is scintigraphy, a nuclear test of gastric emptying. This consists of the patient ingesting a radionucleotide-labeled meal (such as an egg labeled ^{90m}technetium), and scintigraphic images are taken over time (generally 4 hours) to assess the rate of gastric emptying. Gastric emptying is abnormal when greater than 50% of the meal is retained after 2 hours of study or when greater than 10% of the meal is retained after 4 hours.

Medical Management

Numerous symptoms of gastroparesis can affect oral intake, and the management of these symptoms generally improves nutrition status. Treatment of nausea and vomiting is perhaps the most vital, and prokinetics and antiemetics are the primary medical therapies (see Table 26.3). Metoclopramide and erythromycin are medications that may be used to promote gastric motility. SIBO, appetite, ileal brake (the slowing effect of intestinal transit of undigested food, often fat, reaching the ileum), or formation of a bezoar (concentration of undigested material in the stomach) are other factors that may affect nutritional status. In a select patient population, implantation of gastric pacemakers may be advantageous to improve gastric emptying (Ross et al, 2014).

Bezoar formation may be related to undigested food such as cellulose, hemicellulose, lignin and fruit tannins (phytobezoars), or medications (pharmacobezoars) such as cholestyramine, sucralfate, enteric-coated aspirin, aluminum-containing antacids, and bulk-forming laxatives. Treatment of bezoars includes enzyme therapy (such as papain, bromelain, or cellulase), lavage, and sometimes endoscopic therapy to mechanically break up the bezoar. Most patients respond to some combination of medication and dietary intervention; however, unresponsive and more severe cases may benefit from placement of an enteral tube into the small intestine, such as a nasoenteric small bowel feeding tube (for less than 4-week need) or percutaneous endoscopic gastrostomy with jejunal extension (PEG/J) (for more than 4-week need). The latter allows for nutrition to bypass the stomach while providing an alternative route for venting of gastric secretions, which may relieve nausea and vomiting.

Medical Nutrition Therapy

The primary dietary factors that affect gastric emptying include volume, liquids versus solids, hyperglycemia, fiber, fat, and osmolality. Generally, patients benefit from smaller, more frequent meals, as larger volumes of food that create stomach distention could delay gastric emptying and increase satiety. Patients with gastroparesis often continue to empty liquids, as they empty, in part, by gravity and do not require antral contraction.

Shifting the diet to more pureed and liquefied foods is often useful. A number of medications (such as narcotics and anticholinergics) slow gastric emptying and should be avoided if possible. Moderate to severe hyperglycemia (serum blood glucose more than 200 mg/dL) may acutely slow gastric motility, with long-term detrimental effects on gastric nerves and motility. Laboratory data considered in initial assessment include glycosylated hemoglobin A1C (if diabetes is present), ferritin, vitamin B_{12}, and 25-OH vitamin D (see Chapter 29).

Fiber, particularly pectin, can slow gastric emptying and increase risk of bezoar formation in patients who are susceptible. It is prudent to advise patients to avoid high-fiber foods and fiber supplements.

The size of the fibrous particles, not the amount of fiber, is more important in bezoar risk (e.g., potato skins versus bran). This and the resistance to chewing are factors in bezoar formation. Examination of the patient's dentition is very important because patients who have missing teeth, a poor bite, or are edentulous are at greater risk. Even people with good dentition have swallowed and passed food particles up to 5 to 6 cm in diameter (potato skins, seeds, tomato skins, peanuts).

Although fat is a powerful inhibitor of stomach emptying primarily mediated by cholecystokinin, many patients tolerate fat well in liquid form. Fat should not be restricted in patients who are struggling to meet their daily caloric needs.

⊚ FOCUS ON

New GI Disorders Classified by Rome IV Criteria

With the updated Rome criteria, some important additions have been included, as they fit the new definition of disorders of gut-brain interaction (DGBIs) due to their effect on the central nervous system (CNS). These conditions are of important note given the ongoing use of opioids for pain management, and also given the more recent legalization and increased use of marijuana in some states. The new diagnoses include:

- Narcotic bowel syndrome (NBS) or opioid-induced gastrointestinal (GI) hyperalgesia is classified as a centrally mediated disorder of GI pain. Ironically, narcotics can lead to more discomfort in those with functional GI disorders, who present with chronic or frequent pain nausea, bloating, periodic vomiting, abdominal distention, and constipation. Over time, pain can worsen or incompletely resolve with increased doses of narcotics.
- Opioid-induced constipation is classified as a bowel disorder and considered the most common adverse side effect of chronic opioid use, and is treated with medications when severe.
- **Cannabinoid hyperemesis syndrome** is classified as a gastroduodenal disorder and included with other nausea and vomiting disorders. It is a syndrome of cyclic vomiting associated with cannabis use, with a common report of symptom improvement with hot bathing, and relief of symptoms with cessation of cannabis use.

International Foundation for Functional Gastrointestinal Disorders: *Narcotic Bowel Syndrome* (website), 2018. https://www.iffgd.org/other-disorders/narcotic-bowel-syndrome.html. Schmulson and Drossman, 2017; Sorrenson CJ, DeSanto K et al: Cannabinoid Hyperemesis Syndrome: Diagnosis, Pathophysiology, and Treatment – a Systematic Review, *J Med Toxicol* 13(1):71-87, 2017.

CLINICAL CASE STUDY

Suzie is a 55-year-old female who is referred to the outpatient clinic with dumping syndrome that has started to interfere with her daily life. She travels for work, and keeping up with her busy schedule has become more difficult with symptoms at unpredictable times when she needs to be driving or in a meeting. A nutrition consultation with a registered dietitian specializing in gastrointestinal disorders is requested by her thoracic surgeon to help with relief of symptoms.

Nutrition Assessment

- *Medical History:* a short bout with dumping syndrome in 2014 after a Nissen fundoplication for a hiatal hernia that resolved a short period after surgery. After a minor hernia repair surgery to redo the fundoplication in early 2018, she began experiencing it again but with more severity. Symptoms include sudden weakness, shakiness, and hunger. She has occasional nausea during episodes, but no vomiting. Suzie also has a new diagnosis of gastroparesis, discovered before her second fundoplication. Upon discovering this, her surgeon also did a pyloroplasty during her second fundoplication surgery to try and help with gastroparesis, and she will have another gastric emptying study in 3 months. Other history includes elevated blood pressure that she reports controlling with diet, heartburn, and blood glucose levels within normal limits unless she is having a dumping episode, when it dips as low as 30 mg/dL. She also reports occasional numbness and tingling in her hands and feet.
- *Medications:* Reglan, Tums, and Omeprazole.
- *Nutrition History:* Suzie travels for work as a sales manager and is on the road constantly, eating mostly packaged and prepared foods on the go, and frozen dinners at home since she lives alone and does not enjoy cooking. Immediately after her fundoplication surgery she ate only soft foods but has recently graduated to some more–normal texture foods after ok from her surgeon to do so. She is unable to determine any food triggers for her dumping with her food journal and has not documented how soon an episode happens after eating. She tries to eat 6 smaller meals per day because her doctor told her

this would be better. She also stays well hydrated, drinking at least one 24-ounce water bottle with each meal. She met with a registered dietitian once but says the dietician did not specialize in this condition, so it was not as helpful as she would have hoped. She is mostly vegetarian but occasionally has fish or chicken. She says she is not opposed to eating meat but mostly avoids cooking it. She is open to nutrition recommendations and arrives at the appointment ready to learn.

- *Dietary recall:*
  - Breakfast: She has coffee with cream and one slice of toast with butter or jam before leaving to drive to an adjacent city for a few hours for meetings.
  - Snack: In the car, she has a cooler packed with applesauce, peach cups, or a banana, of which she selects one or two for a snack midmorning.
  - Lunch: She stops at a grocery store deli and has her favorite on-the-go meal, a large plate of macaroni and cheese, or sometimes has a chef salad now that her doctor has allowed her to eat regular-texture foods again. She eats the meal in her car most days.
  - Snack: In the afternoon she eats another of her cooler items, and occasionally has a string cheese that she picked up at the grocery store deli.
  - Dinner: Frozen meal of Michelina's fettuccine Alfredo, which she describes as high protein. She may alternate out with another frozen pasta meal if she wants some variety, but the nutrition is about the same, according to her.
- *Anthropometrics:* Height: 170.2 cm (67 inches); Weight: 66.4 kg (146 lb); body mass index (BMI): 22.9 kg/m^2
- *Usual Body Weight:* 68.2 kg (150 lbs); weight change: 2.6% decrease in 3 months (clinically insignificant)
- *Nutrition Focused Physical Assessment:* No evidence of muscle or fat loss; no lower or upper extremity edema. Tongue is sore and inflamed. Her nails are brittle and her skin is very pale.
- *Functional Capacity:* Unable to exercise over the past few months due to fatigue and low energy. She is feeling more forgetful lately as well and has to write everything down.

Continued

CLINICAL CASE STUDY—cont'd

- *Laboratory Data:* Blood glucose: 70–100 mg/dL at fasting laboratory draws, only drops low temporarily during dumping episodes; blood pressure: 144/92 (H); gastric emptying study results: 78% of gastric contents left in the stomach after 4 hours.

Nutrition Diagnostic Statements

- Food- and nutrition-related knowledge deficit (P) related to lack of prior relevant nutrition-related education (E) as evidenced by (S) intake of many refined carbohydrate foods in the setting of dumping syndrome
- Undesirable food choices (P) related to lack of prior exposure to nutrition-related information (E) as evidenced by (S) elevated blood pressure, intake of high-sodium foods

Nutrition Care Questions

1. What dietary changes would you recommend for Suzie?
2. What changes would recommend for Suzie about her eating pattern?
3. Would you recommend any micronutrient testing or supplementation? If so, which ones?
4. How would you prioritize education needs for Suzie?
5. Would you do any coordination of care with Suzie's doctor about anything you learned?

Monitoring and Evaluation

- What would you monitor at a 1-month follow up with Suzie?
- What would you measure at a 3-month follow up with Suzie?
- What would you evaluate at a 6-month follow up with Suzie?

USEFUL WEBSITES

American College of Gastroenterology
American Gastroenterological Association
The Gastroparesis and Dysmotilities Association
International Foundation for Functional Gastrointestinal Disorders
National Digestive Diseases Information Clearinghouse

REFERENCES

Akhondi-Meybodi M, Aghaei MA, Hashemian Z: The role of diet in the management of non-ulcer dyspepsia, *Middle East J Dig Dis* 7:19–24, 2015.

Alshadwi A, Nadershah M, Carlson ER, et al: Nutritional considerations for head and neck cancer patients: a review of the literature, *J Oral Maxillofac Surg* 71(11):1853–1860, 2013.

Asanuma K, Iijima K, Shimosegawa T: Gender difference in gastro-esophageal reflux diseases, *World J Gastroenterol* 22:1800–1810, 2016.

Axon A: Helicobacter pylori and public health, *Helicobacter* 19(Suppl 1): 68–73, 2014.

Bertuccio P, Rosato V, Andreano A, et al: Dietary patterns and gastric cancer risk: a systematic review and meta-analysis, *Ann Oncol* 24:1450–1458, 2013.

Bredenoord AJ, Pandolfino JE, Smout AJPM: Gastroesophageal reflux disease, *Lancet* 381:1933, 2013.

Centers for Disease Control (CDC): *NAMCS and NHAMCS web tables* (website), 2015. http://www.cdc.gov/nchs/ahcd/web_tables.htm.

Chanpura T, Yende S: Weighing risks and benefits of stress ulcer prophylaxis in critically ill patients, *Crit Care* 16:322, 2012.

Cowan RP: CAM in the real world: you may practice evidence-based medicine, but your patients don't, *Headache* 54(6):1097–1102, 2014.

Deloose E, Bisschops R, Holvoet L, et al: A pilot study of the effects of the somatostatin analog pasireotide in postoperative dumping syndrome, *Neurogastroenterol Motil* 26:803–809, 2014.

Dos Santos AA, Carvalho AA: Pharmacological therapy used in the elimination of Helicobacter pylori infection: a review, *World J Gastroenterol* 21: 139–154, 2015.

Dossett ML, Cohen EM, Cohen J: Integrative medicine for Gastrointestinal disease, *Prim Care* 44(2):265–280, 2017.

Dossett ML, Davis RB, Lembo AJ, et al: Complementary and alternative medicine use by U.S. adults with gastrointestinal conditions: results from the 2012 National Health interview survey, *Am J Gastroenterol* 109(11):1705–1711, 2014.

Eherer AJ, Netolitzky F, Högenauer C et al: Positive effect of abdominal breathing exercise on Gastroesophageal reflux disease: a randomized, controlled study, *Am J Gastroenterol* 107(3):372–378, 2012.

El-Serag HB, Sweet S, Winchester CC, et al: Update on the epidemiology of Gastro-oesophageal reflux disease: a systematic review, *Gut* 63(6):871–880, 2014.

Farzaei MH, Abdollahi M, Rahimi R: Role of dietary polyphenols in the management of peptic ulcer, *World J Gastroenterol* 21(21):6499–6517, 2015.

Ford AC, Moayyedi P: Dyspepsia, *Curr Opin Gastroenterol* 29:662–668, 2013.

Hershko C, Camaschella C: How I treat unexplained refractory iron deficiency anemia, *Blood* 123:326–333, 2014.

Hooi JKY, Lai WY, Ng WK et al: Global prevalence of Helicobacter pylori infection: systematic review and meta-analysis, *Gastroenterology* 153(2):420–429, 2017.

Jarosz M, Taraszewska A: Risk factors for gastroesophageal reflux disease: the role of diet, *Prz Gastroenterol* 9(5):297–301, 2014.

Katz MH: Failing the acid test: benefits of proton pump inhibitors may not justify the risks for many users, *Arch Intern Med* 170:747–748, 2010.

Keenan JI, Salm N, Hampton MB, et al: Individual and combined effects of foods on Helicobacter pylori growth, *Phytother Res* 24:1229–1233, 2010.

la Roca-Chiapas JM, Cordova-Fraga T: Biomagnetic techniques for evaluating gastric emptying, peristaltic contraction and transit time, *World J Gastrointest Pathophysiol* 15:65–71, 2011.

Lacy BE, Talley NJ, Locke GR III, et al: Review article: current treatment options and management of functional dyspepsia, *Aliment Pharmacol Ther* 36:3–15, 2012.

Lightdale JR, Gremse DA, Section on Gastroenterology, Hepatology, and Nutrition: Gastroesophageal reflux: management guidance for the pediatrician, *Pediatrics* 131:e1684–e1695, 2013.

Maradey-Romero C, Kale H, Fass R: Nonmedical therapeutic strategies for nonerosive reflux disease, *J Clin Gastroenterol* 48(7):584–589, 2014.

Marian M, Mattox T, Williams V: Chapter 33: Cancer. In Mueller CM, edtior: *The ASPEN adult nutrition support core curriculum,* ed 3, Silver Spring, MD, 2017, American Society for Parenteral and Enteral Nutrition, pp 651–674.

Morozov S, Isakov V, Konovalova M: Fiber-enriched diet helps to control symptoms and improves esophageal motility in patients with non-erosive Gastroesophageal reflux disease, *World J Gastroenterol* 24(21):2291–2299, 2018.

Nagini S: Carcinoma of the stomach: a review of epidemiology, pathogenesis, molecular genetics and chemoprevention, *World J Gastrointest Oncol* 4:156–169, 2012.

Nehra AK, Alexander JA, Loftus CG, et al: Proton pump inhibitors: review of emerging concerns, *Mayo Clin Proc* 93(2):240–246, 2018.

NIH National Institute of Diabetes and Digestive and Kidney Diseases: *Digestive diseases statistics for the United States.* Available at: https://www.niddk.nih.gov/health-information/health-statistics/digestive-diseases, 2014.

Oh B, Kim BS, Kim JW, et al: The effect of probiotics on gut microbiota during the Helicobacter pylori eradication: randomized controlled trial, *Helicobacter* 21(3):165–174, 2016.

Park JM, Jeong M, Kim EH, et al: Omega-3 Polyunsaturated fatty acids intake to regulate Helicobacter pylori-associated gastric diseases as nonantimicrobial dietary approach, *Biomed Res Int* 2015:712363, 2015.

Patcharatrakul T, Gonlachanvit S: Chili peppers, curcumins, and prebiotics in gastrointestinal health and disease, *Curr Gastroenterol Rep* 18(4):19, 2016.

Penagini R, Bravi I: The role of delayed gastric emptying and impaired oesophageal body motility, *Best Pract Res Clin Gastroenterol* 24:831–845, 2010.

Ross J, Masrur M, Gonzalez-Heredia R, et al: Effectiveness of gastric neurostimulation in patients with Gastroparesis, *JSLS* 18:pii:e2014.00400, 2014.

Runge TM, Abrams JA, Shaheen NJ: Epidemiology of Barrett's Esophagus and Esophageal Adenocarcinoma, *Gastroenterol Clin North Am* 44(2):203–231, 2015.

Sarkar A, De R, Mukhopadhyay AK: Curcumin as a potential therapeutic candidate for Helicobacter pylori associated diseases, *World J Gastroenterol* 22(9):2736–2748, 2016.

Schmulson MJ, Drossman DA: What Is new in Rome IV, *J Neurogastroenterol Motil* 23:151–163, 2017.

Schoeff SS, Barrett DM, Gress CD, et al: Nutritional management of head and neck cancer patients, *Pract Gastroenterol* 121:43, 2013.

Song EM, Jung HK, Jung JM: The association between reflux esophagitis and psychosocial stress, *Dig Dis Sci* 58:471–477, 2013.

Talley NJ, Ford AC: Functional dyspepsia, *N Engl J Med* 373:1853–1863, 2015.

Thrift AP, Whiteman DC: The incidence of esophageal adenocarcinoma continues to rise: analysis of period and birth cohort effects on recent trends, *Ann Oncol* 23:3155–3162, 2012.

Warren J, Bhalla V, Cresci G: Postoperative diet advancement: surgical dogma vs evidence-based medicine, *Nutr Clin Pract* 26:115–125, 2011.

Wilshire CL, Louie BE, Shultz D, et al: Clinical outcomes of reoperation for failed antireflux operations, *Ann Thorac Surg* 101(4):1290–1296, 2016.

Wu KL, Kuo CM, Yao CC, et al: The effect of dietary carbohydrate on Gastroesophageal reflux disease, *J Formos Med Assoc*, 117:973–978, 2018.

Yates RB, Oelschlager BK: Surgical treatment of gastroesophageal reflux disease, *Surg Clin North Am* 95(3):527–553, 2015.

Yi CH, Lei WY, Hung JS, et al: Influence of capsaicin infusion on secondary peristalsis in patients with gastroesophageal reflux disease, *World J Gastroenterol* 22(45):10045–10052, 2016.

Zhang MM, Qian W, Qin YY, et al: Probiotics in Helicobacter pylori eradication therapy: a systematic review and meta-analysis, *World J Gastroenterol* 21(14):4345–4357, 2015.

Zhu R, Chen K, Zheng YY, et al: Meta-analysis of the efficacy of probiotics in Helicobacter pylori eradication therapy, *World J Gastroenterol* 20:18013–18021, 2014.

Medical Nutrition Therapy for Lower Gastrointestinal Tract Disorders

DeeAnna Wales VanReken, MS, RDN, CD, IFNCP
Rachel E. Kay, MS, RDN, CD, CNSC
Carol S. Ireton-Jones, PhD, RDN, LD, CNSC, FASPEN, FAND

KEY TERMS

aerophagia
antibiotic-associated diarrhea (AAD)
Clostridium difficile (C. difficile) infection (CDI)
celiac disease (CD)
colitis, collagenous
colitis, lymphocytic
colitis, microscopic
colostomy
constipation
Crohn's disease
dermatitis herpetiformis
diarrhea
dietary fiber
diverticulitis
diverticulosis
enterocutaneous fistula (ECF)
eructation
fecal microbiota transplant (FMT)
fistula
flatulence
flatus
FODMAPs

fructose malabsorption
glutamine
gluten
gluten intolerance
gluten-sensitive enteropathy
gluten sensitivity
high-fiber diet
high-output stoma (HOS)
hypolactasia
ileal J-pouch
ileal pouch anal anastomosis (IPAA)
ileostomy
inflammatory bowel disease (IBD)
insoluble fiber
intestinal ostomy
irritable bowel syndrome (IBS)
Koch pouch
lactose intolerance
medium-chain triglycerides (MCTs)
microbiota
neurogenic bowel
oral rehydration solution (ORS)
osmotic agents

ostomy
ostomy, end
ostomy, loop
polyp
pouchitis
prebiotic
primary constipation
probiotic
proctocolectomy
refractory celiac disease
Rome IV criteria
short-bowel syndrome (SBS)
short-chain fatty acids (SCFAs)
small intestinal bacterial overgrowth (SIBO)
soluble fiber
S-pouch
steatorrhea
stimulant laxatives
stool softeners
synbiotics
tropical sprue
ulcerative colitis (UC)
W-pouch

The lower gastrointestinal (GI) tract is defined as the portion of the alimentary canal including the jejunum and ileum of the small intestine, as well as the entire large intestine. Dietary interventions for diseases of this part of the digestive system have typically been focused on methods to alleviate symptoms and to correct nutrient deficiencies. A comprehensive nutritional assessment should be performed to determine the nature and severity of the GI problem to determine the best approach for each individual. Information obtained should include a history of weight trends, medications and supplements, presence of GI and other symptoms that may affect oral intake or fluid loss, and potential signs and symptoms of micronutrient deficiencies.

COMMON INTESTINAL PROBLEMS

It is important to understand some of the common GI processes that occur in healthy people before discussing diseases relating to the lower

GI tract. Dietary ramifications such as intestinal gas, flatulence, constipation, and diarrhea are often considered in the management of more serious GI disorders.

Intestinal Gas and Flatulence
Pathophysiology
The daily volume of human intestinal gas is about 200 mL, and it is derived from complex physiologic processes, including aerophagia (swallowed air) and bacterial fermentation by the intestinal tract. Intestinal gases include carbon dioxide (CO_2), oxygen (O_2), nitrogen (N_2), hydrogen (H_2), and sometimes methane (CH_4), and are either expelled through eructation (belching) or passed rectally as flatus. Detectable levels of CH_4 produced via anaerobic fermentation by human enteric microflora of both endogenous and exogenous carbohydrates have been found in 30% to 62% of healthy adult individuals (Sahakian et al, 2010). This remains compelling, as abnormal CH_4 production has been considered in the pathogenesis of several intestinal disorders, including colon cancer, inflammatory bowel disease (IBD), irritable bowel syndrome (IBS), and diverticulosis (Triantafyllou et al, 2014).

Portions of this chapter were written by Gail Cresci, PhD, RDN, LD, CNSC and Arlene Escuro, MS, RDN, CNSC.

When patients complain about "excessive gas" or *flatulence*, they may be referring to increased volume or frequency of belching or passage of rectal gas. They may also complain of abdominal distention or cramping associated with the accumulation of gases in the upper or lower GI tract. The amount of air swallowed increases with eating or drinking too fast, smoking, chewing gum, sucking on hard candy, using a straw, drinking carbonated drinks, and wearing loose-fitting dentures. Foods that produce gas in one person may not cause gas in someone else, depending on the mix of microorganisms in the individual's colon. Inactivity, decreased motility, aerophagia, dietary components, and certain GI disorders can alter the amount of intestinal gas and individual symptoms.

Normally, the concentration of bacteria in the small intestine is significantly lower than that found in the colon. Various conditions can lead to overgrowth of bacteria in the small intestine, causing bloating, distention, nausea, diarrhea, or other symptoms. In a normally functioning bowel, factors such as gastric acid, intestinal peristalsis, the ileocecal valve, bile acids, the enteric immune system, and pancreatic enzyme secretion all work in concert to prevent the overgrowth of bacteria within the small intestine.

Medical Nutrition Therapy

When evaluating a patient, clinicians must investigate and differentiate between increased production of gas and gas that is not being passed. It is also important to consider why a patient may have new or increased symptoms or if gas is accompanied by other symptoms such as constipation, diarrhea, or weight loss. Keeping a food diary to track eating habits and symptoms may help identify specific foods or behaviors that may be contributing to gas production. Careful review of the diet and the amount of burping or gas passed may help relate specific foods to symptoms and determine the severity of the problem. Eating behaviors to consider could include whether a patient is chewing food well, eating slowly or under stressful conditions, and eating large amounts of raw foods that could be contributing to excess gas.

If milk or milk products are causing gas, a patient is evaluated for lactose intolerance (see detailed discussion later in this chapter for more in-depth discussion on this condition) and advised to avoid milk products for a short time to see if symptoms improve. Recent viral or GI infection may induce temporary or even permanent impairment in the ability to digest lactose. If intake is desired or difficult to avoid for some reason, lactase tablets, drops, and lactose-free milk products are available to help digest lactose and reduce gas.

Inactivity, constipation, intestinal dysmotility, or partial bowel obstruction may contribute to the inability to move normal amounts of gas produced. Further, a sudden change in diet, such as a drastic increase in fiber intake, also can alter gas production. Specific foods that contain raffinose (a complex sugar resistant to digestion), such as beans, cabbage, broccoli, Brussels sprouts, asparagus, and some whole grains can increase gas production. Changes in the intestinal flora occur over time after an increase in dietary fiber. A gradual introduction of fiber with adequate fluid consumption appears to reduce complaints of gas. Box 27.1 outlines foods that may cause increase in gas production.

Constipation

Constipation is a major problem worldwide. In the United States, chronic constipation leads to 8 million visits to medical providers per year (Wald, 2016). Its exact prevalence is difficult to ascertain because only a minority of patients suffering from constipation seek health care. Reports of its prevalence have varied widely, ranging from 0.7% to 29% in children and from 2.5% to 79% in adults (Forootan et al, 2018; Rajindrajith et al, 2016). This worldwide variation in prevalence

> **BOX 27.1   Foods That May Increase Intestinal Gas Production**
>
> 1. Beans (legumes)
> 2. Vegetables such as broccoli, cauliflower, cabbage, Brussels sprouts, onions, mushrooms, artichokes, and asparagus
> 3. Fruits such as pears, apples, and peaches
> 4. Whole grains such as whole wheat and bran
> 5. Sodas: fruit drinks especially apple juice and pear juice; and other drinks that contain high-fructose corn syrup, a sweetener made from corn
> 6. Milk and milk products as well as soft cheese, ice cream, and yogurt
> 7. Packaged foods such as bread, cereal, and salad dressing that contain small amounts of lactose (milk sugar).
> 8. Sugar-free candies and gums that contain sugar alcohols such as sorbitol, mannitol, erythritol, and xylitol
>
> From National Institute of Diabetes and Digestive and Kidney Diseases: *Digestive Diseases A-Z* (website): http://digestive.niddk.nih.gov/.

rates arises from factors such as cultural diversity; genetic, environmental, and socioeconomic conditions; and different health care systems. Constipation has a significant impact on quality of life, and it contributes to health care financial burden. Female gender in adults, advancing age, high body mass index, and low socioeconomic status seem to be associated with a higher prevalence of constipation (Forootan et al, 2018).

Etiology

Constipation is defined as difficulty with defecation characterized by infrequent bowel movements or dyschezia (painful, hard, or incomplete evacuations). Normal bowel movement frequency can range from three times per day to three times per week. Stool weight is used most frequently in medical practice and clinical descriptions as an objective measure of the amount or volume of stool. A volume of as little as 200 g daily is considered normal in healthy children and adults. The Bristol Stool Scale (Fig. 27.1) was first developed in Bristol, England, in the 1990s and has been modified over time but remains a useful reference for clinicians and patients to identify stool form or consistency (Lewis and Heaton, 1997).

The causes of constipation are varied and may be multifactorial. Inadequate fiber intake has been cited as the primary culprit since the early 1970s, but treatment of the underlying disorder should always be the primary course of action. It is also important to understand symptom patterns and classification of constipation to tailor therapy based on the underlying pathophysiology. Box 27.2 outlines factors and conditions known to cause constipation.

Pathophysiology

Constipation is categorized as either primary or secondary. **Primary constipation**, also known as idiopathic or functional constipation, is caused by physical or functional problems when no underlying disorder can be identified (Barco et al, 2015). The different subtypes of primary constipation can be categorized as follows (Andrews and Storr, 2011):

- Normal-transit constipation: This is most common form of chronic constipation seen by clinicians and is also known as functional constipation. Stool passes through the colon at a rate of about 5 days in persons with normal-transit constipation. In functional constipation, patients report symptoms they believe to be consistent with constipation such as the presence of hard stools or a perceived difficulty with defecation. However, on testing, stool transit is not delayed, and the stool frequency is often within the

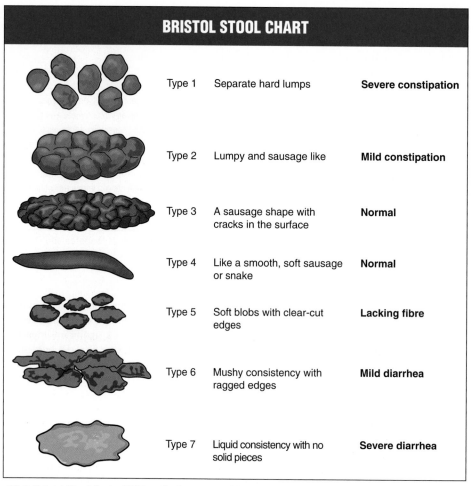

BRISTOL STOOL CHART

	Type 1	Separate hard lumps	**Severe constipation**
	Type 2	Lumpy and sausage like	**Mild constipation**
	Type 3	A sausage shape with cracks in the surface	**Normal**
	Type 4	Like a smooth, soft sausage or snake	**Normal**
	Type 5	Soft blobs with clear-cut edges	**Lacking fibre**
	Type 6	Mushy consistency with ragged edges	**Mild diarrhea**
	Type 7	Liquid consistency with no solid pieces	**Severe diarrhea**

Fig. 27.1 Bristol Stool Scale (Wikimedia Commons: File: BristolStoolChart.png (website), https://commons.wikimedia.org/wiki/File:BristolStoolChart.png, Updated June 18, 2018).

BOX 27.2　Causes of Constipation

Lifestyle and Diet
Lack of fiber in diet
Low total calorie and fluid intake
Iron and calcium supplements
Lack of exercise
Immobility
Laxative abuse
Postponing urge to defecate

Dysmotility Disorders
Chronic intestinal pseudoobstruction
Hypothyroidism
Colonic inertia
Gastroparesis
Hirschsprung disease
Chagas disease
Metabolic and endocrine abnormalities such as diabetes

Neurologic Diseases
Amyotrophic lateral sclerosis
Multiple sclerosis
Muscular dystrophy
Parkinson's disease

Friedrich ataxia
Cerebral palsy
Para- or quadriplegia
Spinal cord injury
Cerebrovascular disease
Brain trauma

Pelvic Floor Disorders
Pregnancy
Dyssynergic defecation

Chronic Use of Opiates
Oncology patients
Chronic pain patients
Narcotic bowel syndrome

Other Gastrointestinal Disorders
Diseases of the upper gastrointestinal tract
Diseases of the large bowel resulting in:
　Failure of propulsion along the colon (colonic inertia)
　Anorectal malformations or outlet obstruction
Irritable bowel syndrome (IBS) Small Intestinal Bacteria Overgrowth (SIBO)
Anal fissure

Data from Andrews CN, Storr M, 2011; Longstreth GF et al, 2006; Schiller LR: Nutrients and constipation: cause or cure? *Pract Gastroenterol* 32:4, 2008.

BOX 27.3 **Rome IV Diagnostic Criteria for Functional Constipation**

Criteria fulfilled for the last 3 months, with symptom onset at least 6 months before diagnosis
1. Must include two or more of the following:
   a. Straining during more than 25% of defecations
   b. Lumpy or hard stools (Bristol stool scale 1 to 2) in more than 25% of defecations
   c. Sensation of incomplete evacuation for more than 25% of defecations
   d. Sensation of anorectal obstruction/blockage for more than 25% of defecations
   e. Manual maneuvers to facilitate more than 25% of defecations (i.e., digital evacuation, support of the pelvic floor)
   f. Fewer than three defecations per week
2. Loose stools are rarely present without the use of laxatives.
3. There are insufficient criteria for irritable bowel syndrome.

Sood R, Ford AC: Diagnosis: rome IV criteria for FGID's – an improvement or more of the same? *Nat Rev Gastroenterol Hepatol* 13:501–502, 2016.

normal range. Patients may experience bloating and abdominal pain or discomfort. Symptoms of functional constipation typically respond with dietary fiber alone or with the addition of an osmotic agent. The Rome IV criteria for the diagnosis of functional constipation is outlined in Box 27.3 (Sood and Ford, 2016).

- Slow transit constipation: This subtype causes infrequent bowel movements (typically less than once per week). Often patients do not feel the urge to defecate but may complain of associated bloating and abdominal discomfort. Slowing of intestinal contents occurs more commonly in the rectosigmoid colon and results in decreased water content in the stool and reduced propulsive action. Treatment typically uses an aggressive laxative regimen. When severe and not resolved by other less invasive treatment options, select patients with slow transit constipation may also be considered for surgical procedures such as subtotal colectomy and ileorectal anastomosis.
- Anorectal dysfunction: This subtype is a result of pelvic floor muscle laxity, impaired rectal sensation, and decreased luminal pressure in the anal canal. Frequently, laxatives are highly ineffective in anorectal dysfunction. The use of biofeedback therapy to retrain the muscles can be used by patients with constipation caused by problems in the anorectal muscles. It uses a combination of diaphragmatic muscle training, simulated defecation, and manometric or electromyogram (EMG) guided anal sphincter and pelvic muscle relaxation, with a goal of improving recto-anal coordination and sensory awareness (Lee et al, 2014). The measurements are displayed on a video screen as line graphs, and sounds indicate when the patient is using the correct muscles.

Secondary constipation can result from a wide variety of factors. The most common of these are lack of dietary fiber, inactivity, or low fluid intake. Other causes can include but are not limited to medications, lifestyle, mechanical blockages caused by cancers, adhesions, and strictures, psychogenic factors such as anxiety, depression, dementia, or eating disorders, or metabolic abnormalities such as electrolyte imbalance and diabetes. Conditions such as obesity, pregnancy, irritable bowel syndrome (IBS), small intestinal bacteria overgrowth (SIBO), or celiac disease can also contribute to secondary constipation and should be considered in clinicians addressing the problem (Barco et al, 2015). Neurogenic bowel is a type of bowel dysfunction caused by nerve malfunction after spinal cord injury or nerve diseases including but not limited to multiple sclerosis (MS) or amyotrophic lateral sclerosis (ALS) that damages nerves associated with controlling the lower colon. The two main types of neurogenic bowel include reflex (spastic) bowel or flaccid bowel, which both lead to constipation for various reasons (Cedars Sinai, 2018)

IBS may also be associated with chronic constipation. A low FODMAP diet is often helpful. More information on IBS and a low FODMAP diet is found later in this chapter.

Medical Management for Adults

A thorough and meticulous history is most helpful in ruling out constipation secondary to medications or other underlying medical illness. After this is done, the first approach to treat mild and functional constipation is to ensure adequate dietary fiber and fluid intake, exercise, and heeding the urge to defecate. Patients who depend on laxatives are encouraged to work with a medical professional and consider a transition to something milder such as magnesium citrate when medically appropriate and reducing the laxative dose until withdrawal is complete.

When constipation persists despite lifestyle and dietary modifications, medications that promote regular bowel movements may be prescribed. Agents used in the treatment of constipation are categorized broadly as either stool softeners or stimulants.

- **Stool softeners** (i.e., docusate sodium) are anionic surfactants with an emulsifying detergent-like property that increases the water content in stool to make bowel movements easier to pass.
- **Osmotic agents** such as magnesium hydroxide, sorbitol, lactulose, and polyethylene glycol contain poorly absorbed or nonabsorbable sugars and work by pulling fluid into the intestinal lumen.
- **Stimulant laxatives** such as bisacodyl and senna increase peristaltic contraction and bowel motility and act to prevent water absorption. Chronic use of laxatives is associated with abdominal cramping and fluid imbalance.

Lubiprostone (Amitiza) is a medication that has been approved by the FDA for idiopathic constipation and to treat IBS with constipation in adults. The drug is a chloride channel activator that increases intestinal fluid secretion and mobility without altering sodium or potassium electrolytes (Bailes and Reeve, 2013). It increases spontaneous bowel movements but is contraindicated in patients with suspected or known mechanical GI obstruction. It is recommended that patients take 1500 to 2000 mL of fluids per day and a high-fiber diet in addition to the medication (Pronsky et al, 2015). Further data on efficacy of any medication should be evaluated as nutrition intervention, positioning for defecation, and physical therapy may be equally as effective.

Medical Management for Infants and Children

Constipation is often especially troubling in infants and young children. Approximately 3% to 5% of all pediatric visits are related to chronic constipation. Some patients have symptoms that persist for 6 months or more. Constipation in this life stage may be related to inadequate intake of fiber or fluid, side effects of medication, inactivity, or disordered bowel motility. Historically, a high-fiber diet has been recommended for children with constipation, but few studies document benefit (Kranz et al, 2012). A thorough history and physical examination, parent-child education, behavioral and nutritional intervention, and appropriate use of laxatives often lead to dramatic improvement.

Medical Nutrition Therapy

Primary nutrition therapy for constipation in otherwise healthy people is consumption of adequate amounts of fluids and dietary fiber, soluble and insoluble. Fiber increases colonic fecal fluid, microbial mass (which accounts for 60% to 70% of stool weight), stool weight and frequency, and the rate of colonic transit. With adequate intake of fluid, fiber may soften stools and make them easier to pass. Dietary reference intakes (DRIs) recommend consumption of 14 g dietary fiber per 1000 kcal, or 25 g for adult women and 38 g for adult men. Typical intake of dietary fiber in the United States is only about 16.2 g/day (Grooms et al, 2013).

BOX 27.4 Guidelines for High-Fiber Diets

1. Increase consumption of whole-grain breads and cereals to 6 to 11 servings daily.
2. Increase consumption of vegetables, legumes, fruits, nuts, and seeds to 5 to 8 servings daily.
3. Consume high-fiber cereals, granolas, and legumes to bring fiber intake to 25 g in women or 38 g in men or more daily.
4. Increase consumption of fluids to at least 2 L (or about 2 qt) daily.

Note: Following these guidelines may cause an increase in stool weight, fecal water, and gas. The amount that causes clinical symptoms varies among individuals, depending on age and presence of gastrointestinal (GI) disease, malnutrition, or resection of the GI tract.

Dietary fiber refers to edible plant materials not digested by the enzymes in the GI tract and is categorized as soluble or insoluble. **Soluble fiber** forms a gel, acting to slow digestion and does not generally have a laxative effect. **Insoluble fiber** absorbs water to add bulk to stool and accelerate fecal transit through the intestines (Barco et al, 2015). Fiber consists of cellulose, hemicellulose, pectins, gums, lignins, starchy materials, and oligosaccharides that are partially resistant to digestive enzymes. Both types of fiber are readily available in a whole foods diet that includes a variety of whole grains, fruits, vegetables, legumes, seeds, and nuts.

A high-fiber therapeutic diet may have to exceed 25 to 38 g/day. The **high-fiber diet** in Box 27.4 provides more than the amount of fiber typically recommended. It is important to assess dietary fiber intake before making recommendations for fiber supplementation. If a patient is already taking 25 to 30 g of dietary fiber daily, fiber supplementation is unlikely to be helpful. If less than this amount is being consumed, fiber should be added slowly in graduated doses to eventually reach 25 to 30 g per day. Amounts greater than 50 g/day are not necessary and may increase abdominal distention and excessive flatulence due to fermentation by the colonic flora.

Bran and fiber supplements may be helpful in persons who cannot or will not eat sufficient amounts of fiber-containing foods. Several of these commercial fiber supplements can be added to cereals, yogurts, fruit sauces, juices, or soups. Cooking does not destroy fiber, but the structure may change. Recommending the consumption of adequate daily fluid intake is also very important in facilitating the effectiveness of a high-fiber intake. Gastric obstruction and fecal impaction may occur when boluses of fibrous gels or bran are not consumed with sufficient fluid to disperse the fiber.

Increasing dietary fiber for laxation is unlikely to provide relief for patients with serious dysmotility syndromes, neuromuscular disorders, chronic opioid use, pelvic floor disorders, or other serious GI disease. In conditions such as neuromuscular disorders or with chronic opioid use, a specific laxative medication regimen or gut motility stimulator medication (i.e. methylnaltrexone) may be a necessary part of disease management.

Diarrhea

Diarrhea is defined by the World Health Organization as the passage of three or more loose or liquid stools per day. Diarrhea occurs when there is accelerated transit of intestinal contents through the small intestine, decreased enzymatic digestion of foodstuffs, decreased absorption of fluids and nutrients, increased secretion of fluids into the GI tract, or exudative losses.

Pathophysiology

- Diarrhea may be related to inflammatory disease; infections with fungal, bacterial, or viral agents; medications; overconsumption of sugars or other osmotic substances; an allergic response to a food;

or insufficient or damaged mucosal absorptive surface. There are many different subtypes of diarrhea associated with various medical conditions and/or surgeries.

- Exudative diarrheas are always associated with mucosal damage, leading to an outpouring of mucus, fluid, blood, and plasma proteins, with a net accumulation of electrolytes and water in the gut. Prostaglandin and cytokine release may be involved. Diarrhea associated with Crohn's disease, ulcerative colitis (UC), and radiation enteritis is often exudative.
- Osmotic diarrheas occur when osmotically active solutes are present in the intestinal tract and are poorly absorbed. An example is the diarrhea that accompanies dumping syndrome in someone that consumes a beverage containing simple sugars after having various GI-tract resections such as a Billroth II procedure (gastrojejunostomy).
- Secretory diarrheas are the result of active intestinal secretion of electrolytes and water by the intestinal epithelium, resulting from bacterial exotoxins, viruses, and increased intestinal hormone secretion. Unlike osmotic diarrhea, fasting does not relieve secretory diarrhea.
- Malabsorptive diarrheas result when a disease process impairs digestion or absorption to the point that nutrients, such as fat, appear in the stool in increased amounts. Excess fat in the stool is called **steatorrhea**. Diarrhea occurs because of the osmotic action of these nutrients and the action of the bacteria on the nutrients that pass into the colon. Malabsorptive diarrhea occurs when there is not enough healthy absorptive area or inadequate production or interrupted flow of bile and pancreatic enzymes, or there is rapid transit, such as in IBD or after extensive bowel resection. Box 27.5 lists diseases and conditions associated with malabsorption and diarrhea.
- Medication-induced diarrheas are frequent in hospitalized and long-term care patients. Medications that cause diarrhea do so by different mechanisms. For example, medications such as lactulose (used in the management of hepatic encephalopathy) and sodium polystyrene sulfonate with sorbitol (used to treat hyperkalemia) create increased bowel movements as part of their mechanism of action. Some antibiotics have direct effects on GI function. Examples include erythromycin, which acts as a motilin agonist and increases lower GI motility, as well as clarithromycin and clindamycin, which increase GI secretions.

In those with underlying illnesses such as human immunodeficiency virus (HIV) and other immune deficiency states, the causes of diarrhea are often multifactorial and can include side effects of medications, proliferation of opportunistic organisms, and GI manifestations of the disease itself (Pavie et al, 2012) (see Chapter 36). Increased risk of opportunistic infection is also associated with use of antineoplastic agents (such as chemotherapy) or in those with malnutrition.

Antibiotic-Associated Diarrhea

The human intestinal tract is home for trillions of bacteria **microbiota** (Fig. 27.2). In the normal GI tract, commensal gut microbiota ferment sloughed intestinal cells and undigested foodstuffs to gases and short-chain fatty acids (SCFAs). Absorption of SCFAs facilitates absorption of electrolytes and water from the colon. Broad-spectrum antibiotics decrease the number of commensal bacteria in the bowel and may result in decreased fermentation byproducts, reducing the absorption of electrolytes and water, thereby causing diarrhea.

Some antibiotics allow proliferation of opportunistic pathogenic microorganisms normally suppressed by competitive microorganisms in the GI tract. The toxins produced by some opportunistic microorganisms can cause colitis and increased secretion of fluid and

BOX 27.5   Diseases and Conditions Associated With Malabsorption

Inadequate Digestion
Pancreatic insufficiency
Gastric acid hypersecretion
Gastric resection

Altered Bile Salt Metabolism with Impaired Micelle Formation
Hepatobiliary disease
Interrupted enterohepatic circulation of bile salts
Bacterial overgrowth
Drugs that precipitate bile salts

Genetic Abnormalities of Mucosal Cell Transport
Disaccharidase deficiency
Monosaccharide malabsorption
Specific disorders of amino acid malabsorption
Abetalipoproteinemia
Vitamin B_{12} malabsorption
Celiac disease

Inflammatory or Infiltrative Disorders
Crohn's disease
Amyloidosis
Scleroderma
Tropical sprue
Gastrointestinal allergy
Infectious enteritis
Whipple disease
Intestinal lymphoma
Radiation enteritis
Drug-induced enteritis
Endocrine and metabolic disorders
Short-bowel syndrome (SBS)

Abnormalities of Intestinal Lymphatics and Vascular System
Intestinal lymphangiectasia
Mesenteric vascular insufficiency
Chronic congestive heart failure

Data from Beyer PL: Short bowel syndrome. In Coulston AM et al, editors: *Nutrition in the prevention and treatment of disease*, ed 1, San Diego, 2001, Academic Press; Branski D et al: Chronic diarrhea and malabsorption, *Pediatr Clin North Am* 43:307, 1996; Fine KD: Diarrhea. In Mitra AD et al: Management of diarrhea in HIV-infected patients, *Int J STD AIDS* 12:630, 2001; Podolsky DK: Inflammatory bowel disease, *N Engl J Med* 347:417, 2002; Sundarum A et al: Nutritional management of short bowel syndrome in adults, *J Clin Gastroenterol* 34:207, 2002.

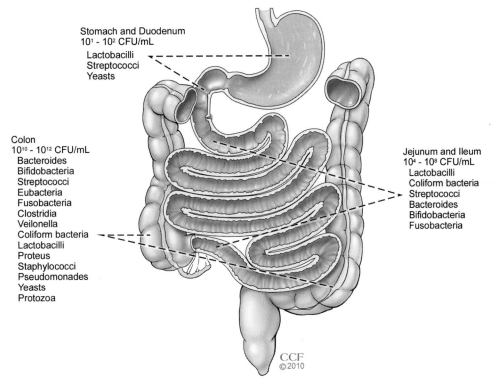

Stomach and Duodenum
10^1 - 10^2 CFU/mL
Lactobacilli
Streptococci
Yeasts

Colon
10^{10} - 10^{12} CFU/mL
Bacteroides
Bifidobacteria
Streptococci
Eubacteria
Fusobacteria
Clostridia
Veilonella
Coliform bacteria
Lactobacilli
Proteus
Staphylococci
Pseudomonades
Yeasts
Protozoa

Jejunum and Ileum
10^4 - 10^8 CFU/mL
Lactobacilli
Coliform bacteria
Streptococci
Bacteroides
Bifidobacteria
Fusobacteria

CCF
©2010

Fig. 27.2 The human gut microbiota (Illustration by David Schumick, BS, CMI. Cleveland Clinic Center for Medical Art & Photography ©2015. All rights reserved. CCF, Cleveland Clinic Foundation).

electrolytes. A rise in antibiotic use has led to an increase in antibiotic-associated diarrhea (AAD) and overgrowth of *Clostridium difficile* with resultant *Clostridium Difficile (C. Difficile) infection (CDI).*

C. difficile is a spore-forming organism, and the spores are resistant to common disinfectant agents. The spore-forming ability of *C. difficile* allows the organism to be spread inadvertently to other patients by health care providers (iatrogenic infection) if strict infection control procedures are not followed. The presence of this infection is detected by analysis of a stool sample for the presence of the toxin produced by the organisms. Clindamycin, penicillin, and cephalosporins are associated most often with the development of *C. difficile* infection. Its occurrence depends on the number of antibiotics used, the duration of exposure to antibiotics, and the patient's age and overall health. Chronic suppression of stomach acid with proton pump inhibitor medications during broad-spectrum antibiotic therapy also may increase susceptibility to CDI (Tarig et al, 2017; Trifan et al, 2017).

C. difficile was historically considered a nosocomial (hospital-acquired) diarrheal infection associated with antibiotic exposure. More recently, its prevalence has increased to include a higher incidence in populations previously considered at low risk (DePestel and Aronoff, 2013). *C. difficile* may cause colitis, secretory diarrhea, severe dilation of the colon (toxic megacolon), perforation of the bowel wall, peritonitis, or even death (Pattani et al, 2013). Adding further complication to eradicating CDI, resistant strains are less susceptible to treatment with antimicrobials and cause a more severe form of the disease with increased health care costs and higher mortality (O'Keefe, 2010).

According to the Centers for Disease Control and Prevention (CDC), *C. difficile* was estimated to cause almost 500,000 infections in the United States in 2011 alone. Of those, 83,000 patients presented with at least one recurrence, and almost 29,000 died within 30 days of the initial diagnosis. Prescribing unnecessary or incorrect antibiotics occurs in 30% to 50% of hospitalized patients who receive them. This oversight is thought to be an important contributor to increased risk for this life-threatening infection (CDC, 2015). Fortunately, with increased infection risk protocols, greater precautions with antibiotic use, and clinician awareness, there was an 8% decrease in CDI from 2011 to 2014 (CDC, 2018). See Fig. 27.3 infographic reviewing important details.

Medical Management

Because diarrhea is a symptom, not a disease, the first step in medical treatment is to identify and treat the underlying problem. The next goal is to manage fluid and electrolyte replacement. In cases of severe diarrhea, restoring fluid and electrolytes is first priority. Electrolyte losses, especially potassium and sodium, should be corrected early by using oral glucose electrolyte solutions with added potassium. Oral rehydration solutions (ORS) work because they contain concentrations of sodium and glucose that are optimal for interaction with the sodium-glucose transport (SGLT) proteins in the intestinal epithelial cells (see Chapter 1).

With intractable diarrhea, especially in an infant or young child, parenteral feeding may be required. Parenteral nutrition (PN) may even be necessary if exploratory surgery is anticipated, or if the patient is not expected to resume full oral intake within 5 to 7 days (see Chapter 12).

Supplementation with probiotics, defined below, shows some promise to prevent AAD and CDI and research is ongoing, but there are inadequate data to recommend probiotics as a primary treatment for CDIs (Pattani et al, 2013) (see *Focus On:* Probiotics and Prebiotics and the Gut Microbiota). Currently, the best treatment for refractory CDI is to employ fecal microbiota transplant (FMT). With the concept of the human gut microbiota as an organ, FMT may be considered an organ transplant. In this procedure, the gut microbiota of the person infected with *C. difficile* is replaced with healthy donor stool, typically from a family member with similar dietary and living habits. A recent study found a >90% success rate in participants receiving FMT for eradication of CDI, with no disease recurrence after procedure (Konturek et al, 2016).

◎ FOCUS ON

Probiotics and Prebiotics and the Gut Microbiota

Some gastrointestinal conditions such as *Clostridium difficile* infection (CDI), small intestinal bacterial overgrowth (SIBO), antibiotic-associated diarrhea, and perhaps inflammatory bowel disease may result or have exacerbated symptoms when there are alterations to the colonies of microorganisms that exist in the small or large intestines. Exposure to broad-spectrum antibiotics causes dramatic alterations to gut microbiota, placing the patient at risk for overgrowth of potentially pathogenic microbes and opportunistic gastrointestinal (GI) infections.

A probiotic is defined by the Food and Agriculture Organization of the United Nations and the World Health Organization (FAO/WHO) as "live nonpathogenic organisms (bacteria or yeast) which when administered in adequate amounts confer a health benefit on the host." To be a probiotic, meaning "for life," a live microbial strain must meet very stringent criteria. According to the FAO/WHO, these criteria include being safe for human consumption, being a live and viable organism with strain identification, being of human origin, being resistant to acid and bile, being able to survive the upper intestinal tract environment and reach the distal intestine (ileum and colon) to attach to the intestinal epithelium, and being able to colonize the distal intestine, confer health benefit to the host, and have scientifically proven health benefits (Cresci and Izzo, 2017). Unfortunately, such a regulatory framework does not exist in the United States at present. Therefore because of these strict criteria, some supplements termed "probiotics" are not truly probiotics and their use may be misleading to clinicians and consumers.

Certain strains of bacteria have been identified as probiotics. These may be available in supplement form (e.g., capsules, powders) or included in fermented food products (e.g., yogurts, kefir). The exact dose, means for delivery, or the duration of viability are uncertain, probably vary for different probiotic strains, and may depend on the condition to be treated. It has been suggested that probiotics may restore the balance of intestinal microbes and improve symptoms and prevent or treat conditions in which a gut dysbiosis has occurred, such as antibiotic-associated diarrhea (Pattani et al, 2013). *Saccharomyces boulardii*, a probiotic yeast, has been shown to reduce recurrence in those with CDI when high-dose oral vancomycin was also used (Cresci and Izzo, 2017). Certain types of probiotics may be effective in reducing the duration of enterovirus-induced acute infectious diarrhea in pediatric and adult patients and in those with inflammatory bowel disease (IBD).

Like probiotics, prebiotics have strict criteria for their classification. Prebiotics, undigested polysaccharides, and sloughed proteins are the food source for the commensal gut microbiota.

A prebiotic is defined as "a selectively fermented ingredient that allows specific changes, both in the composition and activity in the gut microbiota, that confer benefits upon host well-being and health" (Cresci and Izzo, 2017). Importantly, prebiotics must be resistant to gastric acidity, to hydrolysis by mammalian enzymes, and to GI absorption; must be fermented in the GI tract by the gut microbiota; and must be selective in the stimulation of the gut microbiota growth and activity that contribute to health and well-being. Prebiotics are naturally occurring or synthetic sugars and are not available to all gut microbial species. Upon reaching the distal intestine (ileum and colon), prebiotics are fermented by the gut microbiota to yield short-chain fatty acids (SCFAs) and gases (carbon dioxide, hydrogen, and methane). SCFAs (acetate, propionate, butyrate) serve many biologic roles, including aiding with water and electrolyte absorption, decreasing intraluminal pH, altering cell proliferation and differentiation, and modifying intestinal immune and inflammatory processes (Cresci and Izzo, 2017). Although probiotics have reported safety issues with select clinical conditions, prebiotics carry few safety concerns. However, like probiotics, prebiotics may also contribute to GI discomfort (bloating, gas) if introduced too rapidly into the diet.

Because there is promise in theory and in select studies for improving gut dysbiosis with supplements, further studies evaluating the optimal dose, timing, duration, and indications for probiotics, prebiotics, and their combinations, are warranted. Regular intake of food sources of prebiotics and probiotics can also encourage increased microbial diversity in the gut, reducing reliance on supplements when appropriate.

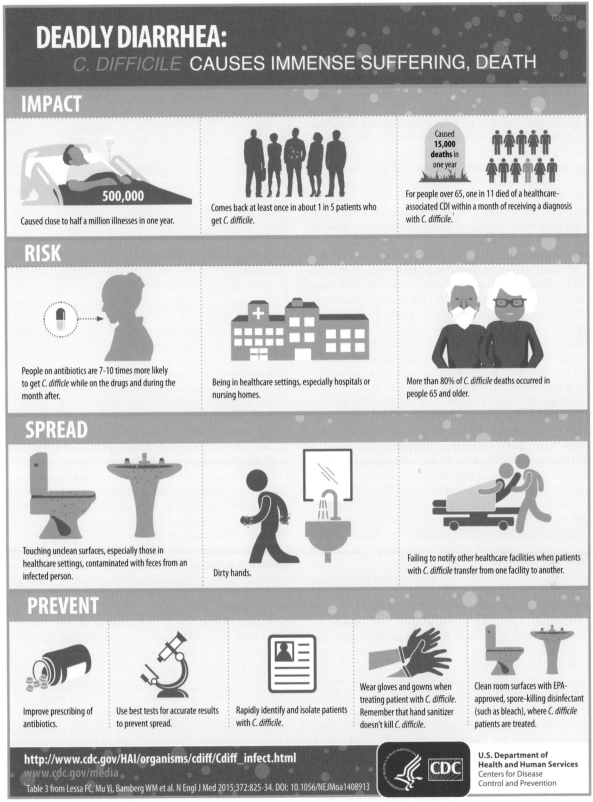

DEADLY DIARRHEA:
C. DIFFICILE CAUSES IMMENSE SUFFERING, DEATH

IMPACT

500,000
Caused close to half a million illnesses in one year.

Comes back at least once in about 1 in 5 patients who get *C. difficile.*

Caused **15,000 deaths** in one year
For people over 65, one in 11 died of a healthcare-associated CDI within a month of receiving a diagnosis with *C. difficile.*[1]

RISK

People on antibiotics are 7-10 times more likely to get *C. difficile* while on the drugs and during the month after.

Being in healthcare settings, especially hospitals or nursing homes.

More than 80% of *C. difficile* deaths occurred in people 65 and older.

SPREAD

Touching unclean surfaces, especially those in healthcare settings, contaminated with feces from an infected person.

Dirty hands.

Failing to notify other healthcare facilities when patients with *C. difficile* transfer from one facility to another.

PREVENT

Improve prescribing of antibiotics.

Use best tests for accurate results to prevent spread.

Rapidly identify and isolate patients with *C. difficile.*

Wear gloves and gowns when treating patient with *C. difficile.* Remember that hand sanitizer doesn't kill *C. difficile.*

Clean room surfaces with EPA-approved, spore-killing disinfectant (such as bleach), where *C. difficile* patients are treated.

http://www.cdc.gov/HAI/organisms/cdiff/Cdiff_infect.html
www.cdc.gov/media
[1] Table 3 from Lessa FC, Mu Yi, Bamberg WM et al. N Engl J Med 2015;372:825-34. DOI: 10.1056/NEJMoa1408913

CDC

U.S. Department of Health and Human Services
Centers for Disease Control and Prevention

Fig. 27.3 Deadly Diarrhea: *C. Difficile* causes immense suffering, death (CDC, 2015).

Products that combine probiotic microorganisms and a prebiotic fiber source have been described as synbiotics for their synergistic effects. A recent review evaluated efficacy nuf probiotics, prebiotics, and synbiotics for improvements in the microbiota for a variety of disorders. Synbiotics were found effective for hepatic encephalopathy, improved high-density lipoprotein (HDL) and fasting glucose, but also demonstrated positive results for treating infectious diarrhea in children (Patel and DuPont, 2015).

There is a long history of safe use of many strains of "live active cultures" in foods in healthy humans. However, the body of evidence is limited on the use of large doses of concentrated probiotic supplements, especially of specific strains that exhibit greater resistance to gastric acid or have increased ability to proliferate in the GI tract. Limited safety data support the use of concentrated probiotic supplements in patients with immunocompromised states or critical illness, or when probiotics are administered directly into the small intestine, as with jejunal feeding tubes, but research in this area continues (Stavrou et al, 2015). A number of case reports exist of hospitalized patients receiving concentrated strains of probiotics that have become septic because of infection in the bloodstream with the very same strain of probiotic being administered. In a review of cases of adverse events related to probiotic administration in hospitalized patients, 25% of adverse events resulted in patient death (Whelan and Myers, 2010). Many of these case reports do indicate the culprit probiotic was a non-pathogenic yeast, and since then product label warnings against providing this supplement to critically ill patients have been instated to avoid such complications. In a large double-blind, randomized study of a high-dose multispecies probiotic administered via jejunal feeding tube in patients with severe acute pancreatitis, there were significantly more deaths in those who received probiotics compared with those receiving the inactive placebo, and a reduced risk of infectious complications was not demonstrated in the probiotic group (Besselink et al, 2008). Although this historical study was concerning and provides warning before administering live cultures to critically ill patients, there were study flaws and limitations, which lead to questions whether the increased mortality was solely the result of probiotic supplementation; further study is needed in this area.

Probiotic preparations hold promise as an adjunctive or primary treatment in several gastrointestinal conditions, but research is ongoing on modifying the microbiota and there remain inadequate data thus far to make large generalizations regarding probiotic safety for all populations (Bafeta et al, 2018). In contrast, as an emerging area of scientific research, there is also a movement to determine how manipulating the microbiota can confer benefit to the host (Walsh et al, 2014). To learn more and follow this exciting area of nutrition research, the International Scientific Association for Probiotics and Prebiotics (https://isappscience.org/) is an excellent resource.

Medical Nutrition Therapy

All nutrition interventions related to diarrhea must be viewed within the context of the underlying pathologic condition responsible for the diarrhea. Replacement of necessary fluids and electrolytes is the first step, using ORS, soups and broths, vegetable juices, and isotonic liquids. Restrictive diets, such as the BRAT diet made up of bananas, rice, applesauce, and toast, are nutrient poor; no evidence indicates that they are necessary during acute diarrheal illness. Although there is limited research to support doing so, some clinicians also recommend a progression of starchy carbohydrates such as cereals, breads, and low-fat meats, followed by small amounts of vegetables and fruits, followed by fats. The goal with this progression is to limit large amounts of hyperosmotic carbohydrates that may be maldigested or malabsorbed, foods that stimulate secretion of fluids, and foods that speed the rate of GI transit.

Sugar alcohols, lactose, fructose, and large amounts of sucrose may worsen osmotic diarrheas. IBS may also be associated with diarrhea or a mix of constipation and diarrhea. Several diet changes within the low FODMAP diet similar to the foods mentioned above may improve symptoms (see Irritable Bowel Syndrome in this chapter). Because the activity of the disaccharidases and transport mechanisms decrease during inflammatory and infectious intestinal disease, sugars may have to be limited, especially in children. Malabsorption is only one potential cause of diarrhea, and diarrhea may occur without significant

TABLE 27.1 Food to Limit in a Low-Fiber (Minimal-Residue) Diet

Food	Comments
Lactose (in lactose malabsorbers)	6 to 12 g is normally tolerated in healthy lactase-deficient individuals but may not be in some individuals.
Insoluble fiber (quantities >20 g)	Modest amounts (10 to 15 g) may help maintain normal consistency of gastrointestinal (GI) contents and normal colonic mucosa in healthy states and GI disease.
Sorbitol, mannitol, and xylitol (excess, >10 g/day)	Well tolerated in moderate amounts; large amounts may cause hyperosmolar diarrhea.
Fructose (excess, 20 to 25 g/meal)	
Sucrose (excess, >25 to 50 g/meal)	
Caffeine	Increases GI secretions, colonic motility
Alcoholic beverages (especially wine and beer)	Increase GI secretions

malabsorption of macronutrients (carbohydrate, fat, and protein). Absorption of most nutrients occurs in the small intestine; diarrhea related to colonic inflammation or disease preserves the absorption of most ingested nutrients.

Minimal fiber and low-residue diets are rarely indicated (Table 27.1). Patients are encouraged to resume a regular diet as tolerated that contains moderate amounts of soluble fiber. The metabolism of soluble fiber and resistant starches by colonic bacteria leads to production of short-chain fatty acids (SCFAs), which in physiologic quantities serve as a substrate for colonocytes, facilitate the absorption of fluid and salts, and may help to regulate GI motility.

Fibrous material tends to slow gastric emptying, moderate overall GI transit, and pull water into the intestinal lumen. Providing fiber to patients with diarrhea does increase the volume of stool, and in some cases (such as small intestinal bacterial overgrowth [SIBO]) initially can increase gas and bloating. Modest intake of prebiotic components and soluble fibers such as pectin or gum slows transit through the GI tract.

Several probiotics have been studied for preventing AAD. Currently, of those tested, *Saccharomyces boulardii* and *Lactobacillus*-based formulations appear to be most effective in reducing AAD (Pattani et al, 2013). A more recent meta-analysis specifically found *Saccharomyces boulardii* to be effective in reducing risk of AAD in both children and adults without adverse side effects, but also encouraged caution in patients who are immunocompromised or with life-threatening illnesses managed in the intensive care unit (ICU) setting (Szajewska and Kotodziej, 2015). Studies are still needed to find the optimal combination of probiotics and/or prebiotics, testing for dosing schedules, and concentrations.

Severe and chronic diarrhea is accompanied by dehydration and electrolyte depletion. If also accompanied by prolonged infectious, immunodeficiency, or inflammatory disease, malabsorption of vitamins, minerals, and protein or fat also may occur, and nutrients may have to be replaced parenterally or enterally. In some forms of infectious diarrhea, loss of iron from GI bleeding may be severe enough to cause anemia. Nutrient deficiencies themselves cause mucosal changes such as decreased villi height and reduced enzyme secretion, further contributing to malabsorption. As the diarrhea begins to resolve, the addition of more normal amounts of fiber to the diet may help to restore normal mucosal function, increase electrolyte and water absorption, and increase the firmness of the stool.

Food in the lumen is needed to restore the compromised GI tract after disease and periods of fasting. Early refeeding after rehydration reduces stool output and shortens the duration of illness. Micronutrient replacement or supplementation also may be useful for acute diarrhea, probably because it accelerates the normal regeneration of damaged mucosal epithelial cells.

Treating Diarrhea in Infants and Children

Acute diarrhea is most dangerous and a leading cause of mortality in infants and small children, who are easily dehydrated by large fluid losses. Provision of extra fluids, including breastmilk, can prevent dehydration, but in the most severe cases replacement of fluid and electrolytes must be aggressive and immediate. Since 1978, the World Health Organization (WHO) has recommended a standard oral rehydration solution (ORS) for this acute situation as a way for parents to be able to participate in their children's care at home with a reduced need for IV hydration or hospitalization. The standard WHO-recommended ORS historically had an osmolarity of 311 mOsm/L and contained specific concentrations of sodium (90 mEq), potassium (20 mEq/L), chloride (80 mEq/L), and glucose (20 g/L) (Suh et al, 2010).

For over 25 years, the standard solution was used, decreasing the mortality rate from 5 million to 1.3 million deaths annually (WHO, 2002). While incredibly effective at rehydrating, reducing fecal volume or duration of illness was still an important concern, leading to research and development of a new solution. The result of this work came to fruition in 2003, when the WHO made a change to recommend a new lower osmolality solution at 245 mOsm/L with decreased concentrations of both glucose (13.5 g/L) and sodium (75 mEq/L), as it was shown to result in greater water absorption in children with noncholera diarrhea (Suh et al, 2010; WHO 2002; WHO 2006).

Overall, when reduced-osmolarity ORS is used for children with acute diarrhea, it results in decreased need for intravenous therapy, significant reduction in stool output, and decreased vomiting compared with standard WHO-recommended ORS (Atia and Buchman, 2009). Commercial solutions such as Pedialyte, Infalyte, Lytren, Equalyte, and Rehydralyte typically contain less glucose and slightly less salt than the WHO-ORS formulation and are available in pharmacies, often without a prescription. Oral rehydration therapy is less invasive and less expensive than intravenous rehydration and, when used with children, allows parents to assist with their children's recovery. However, close attention must be paid to the actual electrolyte content, as many so-called ORS are not useful for rehydration. See Table 27.2 for ORS recipes that can be used to create the formula at home. Commercial sports drinks (i.e., Gatorade) without the added salt are not recommended.

A substantial proportion of children 9 to 20 months of age can maintain adequate intake when offered either a liquid or a semisolid diet continuously during bouts of acute diarrhea. Even during acute diarrhea, the intestine can absorb up to 60% of the food eaten. Some practitioners have been slow to adopt the practice of early refeeding after severe diarrhea in infants despite evidence that "resting the gut" is actually more damaging.

Gastrointestinal Strictures and Obstruction
Pathophysiology

Patients with gastroparesis, adhesions, hernias, metastatic cancers, dysmotility, or volvulus are prone to obstruction, which can result in partial or complete blockage of movement of food or stool through the intestines. Obstructions may be partial or complete and may occur in the stomach (gastric outlet obstruction), small intestine, or large intestine. Symptoms include bloating, abdominal distention and pain, nausea, and vomiting.

Obstructions are not usually caused by foods in an otherwise healthy individual, and researchers have not found that eating, diet, and nutrition play a role in causing or preventing the frequency of obstructive symptoms in this population. However, when sections of the GI tract are partially obstructed or not moving normally, foods may contribute to obstruction. In these individuals with a compromised GI tract, it is believed that fibrous plant foods can contribute to obstruction because the fiber in the foods may not be completely chewed to pass through narrowed segments of the GI tract.

Medical Nutrition Therapy

Most clinicians would recommend patients prone to obstructions to chew food thoroughly and avoid excessive fiber intake, limiting intake to foods with less than 3 grams of fiber per serving or no more than 10 grams per day. A patient with a partial bowel obstruction may be able to tolerate a restricted-fiber diet and liquids, depending on the location of the stricture or obstruction in the GI tract. A more proximal (closer to the mouth) blockage may require a semisolid or liquid diet. However, the more distal (closer to the anus) the blockage, the less likely altering the consistency of the diet will help. Symptoms are more severe during complete obstruction. Patients may be intolerant of oral intake and of their own secretions leading to progressive dehydration, electrolyte imbalance, and systemic toxicity. Initial treatment consists of aggressive fluid resuscitation, nasogastric decompression, and administration of analgesics and antiemetics.

Patients with complete bowel obstruction may require surgical intervention. In some cases, enteral feeding beyond the point of obstruction may be feasible, but if enteral feeding is not possible for a prolonged period, PN may be needed. Working with the patient and physician is necessary to determine the nature, site, and duration of the obstruction so that nutrition therapy can be individualized.

DISEASES OF THE SMALL INTESTINE

Celiac Disease (Gluten-Sensitive Enteropathy)

The prevalence of celiac disease (CD) has been underestimated in the past and now is considered to affect 0.3% to 0.9% of the population in the United States and varies by race and ethnicity, with a marked predominance among non-Hispanic whites. Worldwide incidence of CD is about 1% (Leonard et al, 2017). The onset and first occurrence of symptoms may appear any time from infancy to adulthood. The disease may become apparent when an infant begins eating gluten-containing cereals. In some, it may not appear until adulthood, when it may be triggered or unmasked during GI surgery, stress, pregnancy, or viral infection. It may be discovered as a result of evaluation for

TABLE 27.2 Oral Rehydration Solution (ORS) Recipes*	
2 cups Gatorade, 2 cups water, ¾ tsp salt	28 g glucose, 82 mEq Na, 1.5 mEq K
or	
1 quart water, ¾ tsp salt, 6 tsp sugar	24 g glucose, 76 mEq Na, 0 mEq K

*Each makes 1 liter and should be made fresh every 24 hours.
Data from Krenitsky J, McCray S: *University of Virginia Health System Nutrition Support Traineeship Syllabus,* Charlottesville, VA, 2010, University of Virginia Health System; Recipes from Parrish CR: The clinician's guide to short bowel syndrome, *Pract Gastroenterol* 29:67, 2005.

another suspected problem (such as constipation, abdominal pain, unexplained anemia).

Etiology

The presentation in young children is likely to include the more "classic" GI symptoms of diarrhea, steatorrhea, malodorous stools, abdominal bloating, fatigue, and poor weight gain. An increasing number of patients are being diagnosed with extraintestinal symptoms (such as headache, brain "fog," anemia, reduced bone-mineral density, chronic fatigue, dental enamel hypoplasia, elevated liver enzymes). A recent study found that only 34% of pediatric patients presented with classic symptoms of CD and 43% of patients had nonclassic symptoms (Almallouhi et al, 2017). CD frequently is misdiagnosed as IBS, lactase deficiency, gallbladder disease, or other disorders not necessarily involving the GI tract, because the presentation and onset of symptoms vary so greatly.

Patients may present with one or more of a host of conditions associated with CD: anemias, generalized fatigue, weight loss or failure to thrive, osteoporosis, vitamin or mineral deficiencies, and (although rare) GI malignancy. Dermatitis herpetiformis, yet another manifestation of CD, presents as an itchy skin rash; its presence is diagnostic of CD. Box 27.6 lists conditions associated with CD. Persons who are diagnosed late in life, who cannot or will not comply with the diet, or who were diagnosed as children but told they would grow out of it, are at a higher risk for experiencing long-term complications from CD (Nachman et al, 2010).

Pathophysiology

CD, or gluten-sensitive enteropathy, is characterized by a combination of four factors: (1) genetic susceptibility, (2) exposure to gluten,

(3) an environmental "trigger," and (4) an autoimmune response. Gluten refers to specific peptide fractions of proteins (prolamins) found in wheat (glutenin and gliadin), rye (secalin), and barley (hordein). A small number of those with CD may also react to the avenin protein in oats (Pinto-Sanchez et al, 2017). These peptides are generally more resistant to complete digestion by GI enzymes and may reach the small intestine intact. In a normal, healthy intestine, these peptides are harmless, as the intestinal barrier is intact and prevents translocation from the intestine. However, in persons with CD these peptides travel from the intestinal lumen, across the intestinal epithelium, and into the lamina propria, where they can trigger an inflammatory response that results in flattening of intestinal villi and elongation of the crypt cells (secretory cells), along with a more general systemic immune response (Sams and Hawks, 2014) (Fig. 27.4). The "triggers" that cause a genetically predisposed individual to develop CD are not well understood, but stressors (e.g., illness, inflammation) are thought to play a role.

When CD remains untreated, the immune and inflammatory response eventually results in atrophy and flattening of villi. Over time, the process can cause enough damage to the intestinal mucosa to compromise normal secretory, digestive, and absorptive functions, leading to impaired micronutrient and macronutrient absorption (Kupfer and Jabri, 2012). Cells of the villi become deficient in the disaccharidases and peptidases needed for digestion and also in the carriers needed to transport nutrients into the bloodstream. The disease primarily affects the proximal and middle sections of the small bowel, although the more distal segments also may be involved (Sams and Hawks, 2014).

The term gluten sensitivity is used commonly to describe persons with nonspecific symptoms, without the immune response characteristic of CD or the consequential intestinal damage. Gluten intolerance,

---

BOX 27.6 Symptoms and Conditions Associated With Celiac Disease

Nutritional
Anemia (iron or folate, rarely B$_{12}$)
Osteomalacia, osteopenia, fractures (vitamin D deficiency, inadequate calcium absorption)
Coagulopathies (vitamin K deficiency)
Dental enamel hypoplasia
Delayed growth, delayed puberty, underweight
Lactase deficiency

Extraintestinal
Fatigue, malaise (sometimes despite lack of anemia)
Arthritis, arthralgia
Dermatitis herpetiformis
Infertility, increased risk of miscarriage
Hepatic steatosis, hepatitis
Neurologic symptoms (ataxia, polyneuropathy, seizures); may be partly nutrition related
Psychiatric syndromes

Associated Disorders
Autoimmune diseases: type 1 diabetes, thyroiditis, hepatitis, collagen vascular disease
Gastrointestinal malignancy
IgA deficiency

IgA, Immunoglobulin A.
Kupfer SS, Jabri B: Pathophysiology of celiac disease, *Gastrointest Endosc Clin N Am* 22:639, 2012.

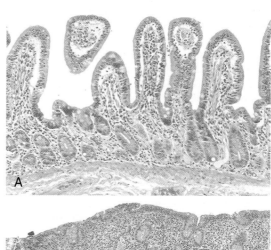
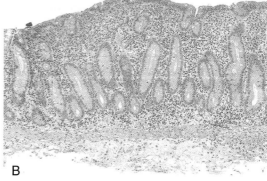

Fig. 27.4 CD (gluten-sensitive enteropathy). **A,** Peroral jejunal biopsy specimen of diseased mucosa shows severe atrophy and blunting of villi, with a chronic inflammatory infiltrate of the lamina propria. **B,** Normal mucosal biopsy. (From Kumar V et al: *Robbins and Cotran pathologic basis of disease,* ed 7, Philadelphia, 2005, Saunders.)

also called nonceliac gluten sensitivity, describes individuals who have symptoms after ingesting gluten-containing foods. Symptoms may be isolated in the gastrointestinal tract such as nausea, abdominal cramps, or diarrhea; or may be extraintestinal in nature such as brain fog or generalized pain. Patients who experience these symptoms should be advised against following a gluten-free (GF) diet without having a workup to exclude or confirm a diagnosis of CD because (1) testing to diagnose CD requires ongoing exposure to gluten in the diet, (2) there may be a different underlying medical condition for which a GF diet is not the treatment, and (3) a GF diet can be expensive and restrictive. Non-celiac gluten-sensitivity or wheat sensitivity includes a reaction to gluten as well as other components of wheat such as fructan (a FODMAP) (Gibson, 2017b).

Assessment

The diagnosis of CD is made from a combination of clinical, laboratory, and histologic evaluations. Persons suspected of having CD should be evaluated for the overall pattern of symptoms and family history. Blood screening for certain antibodies should be completed if symptoms and/or family history may indicate CD. If serology is positive, a biopsy of the small intestine is the gold standard for confirming diagnosis of CD. An intestinal biopsy positive for CD generally shows villous atrophy, increased intraepithelial lymphocytes, and crypt cell hyperplasia. However, biopsy is not used for initial screening because of its cost and invasiveness.

Elevated blood levels of certain autoantibodies are found in people with CD. To screen for CD several serologic tests are evaluated. These tests evaluate levels of serum immunoglobin A (IgA) antibodies to tissue transglutaminase (tTG IgA), which has a sensitivity of 73.9% to 100% and specificity of 77.8% to 100% (Leonard et al, 2017). There is a higher incidence of IgA deficiency in patients with CD; thus physicians often measure total IgA levels when serologic findings are normal, but the overall clinical picture suggests CD (see *Clinical Insight: Antibody Testing for Celiac Disease and Gluten Sensitivity*). Because dietary change alters diagnostic results, initial evaluation should be done *before* the person has eliminated gluten-containing foods from his or her diet. Serologic tests also may be used to monitor the response of a newly diagnosed patient treated with a GF diet. Certain genetic testing is becoming increasingly more common to evaluate for HLA DQ2 or HLA DQ8 carrier status. It is important to know as clinicians that a positive result from these tests does not indicate presence of CD, nor does it exclude it. Approximately 25% of the Caucasian population is positive for HLA DQ2, but less than 5% of these people develop CD (May-Ling Tjon et al, 2010).

Lifelong, strict adherence to a GF diet is the only known treatment for CD (see Box 27.7 for a list of safe, questionable, and unsafe choices on the GF diet). The GF diet diminishes the autoimmune process, and the intestinal mucosa usually reverts to normal or near normal. Within 2 to 8 weeks of starting the GF diet, most patients report that their clinical symptoms have abated. Histologic, immunologic, and functional improvements may take months to years, depending on the duration of the disease, age of the subject, and degree of dietary compliance. With strict dietary control, levels of the specific antibodies usually become undetectable within 6 to 12 months in most persons. Marked gut improvement and a return to normal histologic findings occurs in the majority of patients after an average of 2 years (Hutchinson et al, 2010). Patients who are able to follow the GF diet closely have a better overall response (see *Pathophysiology and Care Management Algorithm: Celiac Disease*).

In some individuals, recovery may be slow or incomplete. A small percentage of patients are "nonresponders" to diet therapy. Inadvertent gluten intake is the most common offender, but another coexisting disorder may be present (such as pancreatic insufficiency, IBS, bacterial overgrowth, fructose intolerance, other food allergies or GI maladies, or unknown causes). For nonresponders, intensive interviewing to identify a source of gluten contamination or treatment of another underlying disease may resolve the symptoms. Diagnosis of refractory celiac disease is made when patients do not respond or respond only temporarily to a GF diet, and all external causes have been ruled out, including inadvertent gluten ingestion. Patients with refractory celiac disease may respond to steroids, azathioprine, cyclosporine, or other medications classically used to suppress inflammatory or immunologic reactions.

Several novel treatments for CD are being studied for their potential as alternative therapies. Researchers seek to treat CD by reducing gluten exposure (by digestion with added enzymes), decreasing uptake of gluten (by tightening junctions between intestinal epithelial cells), altering the immune response to gluten, or repairing intestinal injury.

Medical Nutrition Therapy

Elimination of gluten peptides from the diet is the only treatment for CD presently. The diet omits all dietary forms of wheat, rye, and barley, which are the major sources of the prolamin fractions.

CLINICAL INSIGHT

Antibody Testing for Celiac Disease and Gluten Sensitivity

There are two different types of antibodies considered in celiac disease diagnosis: those which are "antigluten," and those which are "antiself" (autoimmune). "Antigluten" antibodies are the antigliadin immunoglobulin G (IgG) and immunoglobulin A (IgA). Ig stands for "immunoglobulin" or "antibody." In celiac disease, the autoimmune antibodies are antiendomysial IgA and antitissue transglutaminase IgA (tTG IgA).

The tTG IgA test is highly sensitive and specific. It correlates well with biopsy, is inexpensive, not subjective, and can be performed on a single drop of blood. However, it can be falsely positive in a patient who has other autoimmune conditions, such as type 1 diabetes. For those with a negative tTG IgA test, IgA deficiency should be considered.

Antigliadin antibodies IgG and IgA recognize a small piece of the gluten protein called gliadin. Antigliadin IgG has good sensitivity, while antigliadin IgA has good specificity. Their combined use provides a screening test for celiac disease.

Many normal individuals without celiac disease will have an elevated antigliadin IgG. It is estimated that 0.2% to 0.4% of the general population has selective IgA deficiency, while 2% to 3% or more of people with celiac disease are IgA deficient.

If a celiac panel is only positive for antigliadin IgG, this is not highly suggestive for celiac disease if the patient has a normal total IgA level. An antigliadin IgG level three to four times the upper limit of normal for that laboratory is highly suggestive of a condition where the gut is abnormally permeable ("leaky") to gluten. This can happen with food allergies, cystic fibrosis, parasitic infections, Crohn's disease, and other types of autoimmune gastrointestinal (GI) diseases. These antibodies may also be slightly elevated in individuals with no obvious disease (Kelly et al, 2015).

Ruth Leyse-Wallace, PhD, RDN

BOX 27.7   The Basic Gluten-Free Diet

Foods	Safe Choices	Avoid
Grains and flours	Amaranth, arrowroot, bean flours (such as garbanzo or fava bean), buckwheat, corn (maize) or cornstarch, flax, Job's tears, millet, potato, quinoa, ragi, rice, and wild rice sorghum, soybean (soya), tapioca, teff	Wheat (bulgur, couscous, durum, farina, graham, kamut, semolina, spelt, triticale, emmer, farro, wheat germ), rye, barley, oats (except pure, uncontaminated oats), low-gluten flour. Caution: "wheat free" does not necessarily mean "gluten free."
Cereals—hot or dry	Cream of rice, cream of buckwheat, hominy, gluten-free dry cereals, grits	Those with wheat, rye, oats (except gluten-free oats), barley, barley malt, malt flavoring, wheat germ, bran
Potatoes, rice, starch	Any plain potatoes, sweet potatoes and yams, all types of plain rice, rice noodles, 100% buckwheat soba noodles, gluten-free pasta, polenta, hominy, corn tortillas, parsnips, yucca, turnips	Battered or deep-fried French fries (unless no other foods have been fried in the same oil), pasta, noodles, wheat starch, stuffing, flour tortillas, croutons. Labels for commercial potato or rice products with seasonings should be reviewed.
Crackers, chips, popcorn	Rice wafers or other gluten-free crackers, rice cakes; plain corn chips, corn tortilla chips, potato chips, and other root (taro, beet, sweet potato, or vegetable, etc.) or grain (amaranth, quinoa) chips, plain popcorn	Gluten-free crackers, graham crackers, rye crisps, matzo, croutons, pretzels, some chips with flavorings
Desserts	Sorbet, popsicles, Italian ice, ice creams, puddings without gluten ingredients	Ice cream with bits of cookies, "crispies," pretzels, pie crust, cookies, cakes, ice cream cones, and pastries made from gluten-containing flours
Milk and yogurt	Any plain, unflavored milk or yogurt, buttermilk, cream, half and half	Malted milk, yogurts with added "crunchies" or toppings. Some flavored milks and yogurts.
Cheese	Cheese (all styles including blue cheese and Gorgonzola), processed cheese (i.e., American), cottage cheese	Some cheese spreads or sauces
Eggs	All types of plain, cooked eggs	Eggs Benedict (sauce usually made with wheat flour)
Meat, fish, shellfish, poultry	Any fresh, plain untreated meat, fish, shellfish, or poultry; fish canned in brine, vegetable broth, or water	Breaded or battered meats. Some commercially treated, preserved, or marinated meats, luncheon meats, fish, shellfish; self-basting or cured poultry (check labels)
Beans and legumes	Any plain frozen, fresh, dried, or canned (no flavorings or sauces added) beans: garbanzo beans, kidney beans, lentils, pinto beans, edamame, lima, black beans, etc.	Those with added sauces
Soy products and meat analogs or alternatives	Plain tempeh, tofu, edamame, some miso	Seitan; 3-grain tempeh, traditional soy sauce (contains wheat), many meat analogs and imitation seafood, some miso
Nuts and seeds	Any plain (salted or unsalted) nuts, seeds or nut butters, coconut	Nut butters with gluten-containing ingredients
Fruits and juices	Any plain fresh, canned, frozen fruits or juices, plain dried fruit	Dried fruit dusted with flour, pie filling thickened with flour
Vegetables	Any plain, fresh, canned or frozen vegetables including corn, peas, lima beans, etc.	Vegetables in gluten-containing sauce or gravy
Soups	Homemade soups with known allowed ingredients	Check labels on all commercial soups
Condiments, jams, and syrups	Ketchup, mustard, salsa, wheat-free soy sauce, mayonnaise, vinegar (except malt vinegar), jam, jelly, honey, pure maple syrup, molasses	Malt vinegar, soy sauce, many gravies and sauces, marinades, some salad dressings
Seasonings and flavorings	Any plain herb or spice; salt; pepper; brown or white sugar; or artificial sweetener (i.e., Equal, Sweet-N-Low, Splenda)	Seasoning mixes and bouillon with gluten ingredients
Fats	Butter, margarine, all pure vegetable oils (including canola), mayonnaise, cream	Some salad dressings and sandwich spreads
Baking ingredients	Yeast, baking soda, baking powder, cream of tartar, regular chocolate baking chips	See grains and flours; Check label on grain sweetened, carob or vegan chocolate chips
Beverages	Coffee, tea, pure cocoa powder, sodas, some soy or rice milks	Malted beverages, some flavored instant coffee mixes, some herbal teas, some soy or rice milks
Alcohol	Wine, all distilled liquor, including vodka, tequila, gin, rum, whiskey, and pure liqueurs, gluten-free beers, hard ciders	Beer, ale, lager, gluten-removed beers, some drink mixes
Candies	Check labels—many are gluten-free	Candy from bulk food bins, licorice

CD, Celiac disease.
Adapted from Parrish CR et al: *University of Virginia Health System Nutrition Support Traineeship Syllabus*, Charlottesville, Va, 2010, University of Virginia Health System.

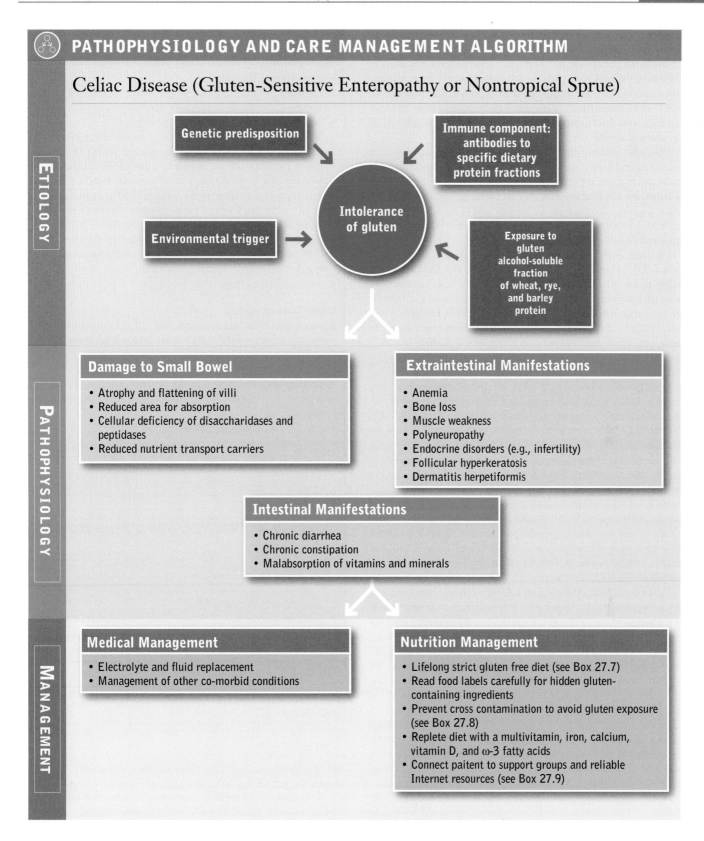

PATHOPHYSIOLOGY AND CARE MANAGEMENT ALGORITHM

Celiac Disease (Gluten-Sensitive Enteropathy or Nontropical Sprue)

ETIOLOGY

Genetic predisposition

Immune component: antibodies to specific dietary protein fractions

Intolerance of gluten

Environmental trigger

Exposure to gluten alcohol-soluble fraction of wheat, rye, and barley protein

PATHOPHYSIOLOGY

Damage to Small Bowel

- Atrophy and flattening of villi
- Reduced area for absorption
- Cellular deficiency of disaccharidases and peptidases
- Reduced nutrient transport carriers

Extraintestinal Manifestations

- Anemia
- Bone loss
- Muscle weakness
- Polyneuropathy
- Endocrine disorders (e.g., infertility)
- Follicular hyperkeratosis
- Dermatitis herpetiformis

Intestinal Manifestations

- Chronic diarrhea
- Chronic constipation
- Malabsorption of vitamins and minerals

MANAGEMENT

Medical Management

- Electrolyte and fluid replacement
- Management of other co-morbid conditions

Nutrition Management

- Lifelong strict gluten free diet (see Box 27.7)
- Read food labels carefully for hidden gluten-containing ingredients
- Prevent cross contamination to avoid gluten exposure (see Box 27.8)
- Replete diet with a multivitamin, iron, calcium, vitamin D, and ω-3 fatty acids
- Connect paitent to support groups and reliable Internet resources (see Box 27.9)

In general, patients should be assessed for nutrient deficiencies before supplementation is initiated. In all newly diagnosed patients, the clinician should consider checking levels of ferritin, folate, vitamin B_{12}, and 25-OH vitamin D. If patients present with more severe symptoms, such as diarrhea, weight loss, malabsorption, or signs of nutrient deficiencies (e.g., night-blindness, neuropathy, or prolonged prothrombin time), other vitamins such as fat-soluble vitamins (A, E, K) and minerals (zinc) should be checked.

The healing of the intestinal mucosa that occurs after initiation of a GF diet improves nutrient absorption, and many patients who eat well-balanced GF diets do not need nutritional supplementation. However, most specialty GF products are not fortified with iron, folate, and other B vitamins like other grain products, so the diet may not be as complete without at least partial supplementation. Anemia should be treated with iron, folate, or vitamin B_{12}, depending on the nature of the anemia. Patients with malabsorption may benefit from a bone-density scan to assess for osteopenia or osteoporosis. Calcium and vitamin D supplementation are likely to be beneficial in these patients. Electrolyte and fluid replacement is essential for those dehydrated from severe diarrhea.

Those who continue to have malabsorption should take a general vitamin-mineral supplement to at least meet DRI recommendations. Lactose and fructose intolerance sometimes occur secondary to CD. A low-lactose or low-fructose diet may be useful in controlling symptoms, at least initially. Once the GI tract returns to more normal function, lactase activity also may return, and the person can incorporate lactose and dairy products back into the diet.

In general, many fruits, vegetables, non–gluten containing grains, meats, and dairy products are safe to eat on a GF diet. Oats were once thought to be questionable for persons with CD; however, extensive studies have shown that they are safe in the GF diet as long as they are pure, uncontaminated oats (Pinto-Sanchez et al, 2017). However, a very small population of patients with CD may not tolerate even GF oats. In general, patients do not need to be advised against including GF oats in their diet unless they have demonstrated intolerance to GF oats.

Flours made from corn, potatoes, rice, soybean, tapioca, arrowroot, sorghum, garbanzo beans, nuts (such as almond flour), amaranth, quinoa, millet, teff, and buckwheat can be substituted in recipes. Patients can expect differences in textures and flavors of common foods using the substitute flours, and new recipes can be palatable once the adjustment is made. Blends of more than one type of GF flour often results in the best recipe outcome. In GF baked goods, gums such as xanthan, guar, and cellulose (from nongluten grains) can be used to provide the elasticity needed to trap leavening gases in baked goods.

A truly GF diet requires careful scrutiny of the labels of all bakery products and packaged foods. Gluten-containing grains are not only used as primary ingredients in many products but also may be added during processing or preparation of foods. For example, hydrolyzed vegetable protein can be made from wheat, soy, corn, or mixtures of these grains.

In the United States there is now a GF labeling law that went into effect in September 2014 (Food and Drug Administration and Health and Human Services, 2013). This law states that all food carrying a GF claim also must contain less that 20 ppm gluten (i.e., below 20 mg gluten per kg of food), including from cross-contact. Thompson discusses the law in detail (Thompson, 2015). Recent studies on the gluten content of labeled GF food in the United States showed that 95% to 99% of the products tested contained less than 20 ppm gluten (Sharma et al, 2015).

The diet for the person with CD requires a major lifestyle change because of the change from traditional grains in the diet. A tremendous number of foods made with wheat (in particular breads, cereals, pastas, and baked goods) are a common part of a Western diet. However, there is increasing awareness among food companies and restaurants of the expanding demand for GF foods, and food businesses are responding. The individual and family members should be taught about label reading, safe food additives, food preparation, sources of cross-contamination (such as toasters, condiment jars, bulk bins, and buffets), and hidden sources of gluten (such as medications and communion wafers) to be compliant with the diet. Box 27.8 provides sources of hidden gluten and cross-contamination. Eating in cafeterias, restaurants, buffets, pot lucks, street markets, at friends' homes, and at social events can be challenging, especially initially.

To avoid misinterpretation of information, newly diagnosed patients should be started with an in-depth instruction from a registered

dietitian nutritionist (RDN) on the GF diet, along with reliable resources for further guidance and support. Persons with CD usually require several educational or counseling sessions and often benefit from a support group (American Gastroenterological Association [AGA], 2015) (see Box 27.9 for CD resources).

Tropical Sprue

Tropical sprue is an acquired diarrheal syndrome with malabsorption that occurs in many tropical areas. In addition to diarrhea and malabsorption, anorexia, abdominal distention, and nutritional deficiency as evidenced by night blindness, glossitis, stomatitis, cheilosis, pallor, and edema can occur. Anemia may result from iron, folic acid, and vitamin B_{12} deficiencies.

BOX 27.8 Hidden Gluten Exposure and Cross-Contamination

Hidden Gluten Exposure

Unfortunately, gluten is not always obvious. Review the list below for some "unsuspected" products that may contain gluten.

- Over-the-counter and prescription medications
  The labeling requirements of the Food Allergen and Consumer Protection Act of 2004 (FALCPA) **do not** apply to medications (see Box 25.7 in Chapter 25). Check with your pharmacist or call the manufacturer to determine whether there is any gluten in your medications.
  Note: Dietary supplements are covered under FALCPA regulations, so wheat must be clearly listed if it is an ingredient in a vitamin, mineral, or herbal supplement.
- Communion wafers: GF alternatives are available
- Toothpaste, mouthwash, and cosmetics, especially shampoo and lipstick
- Children's modeling dough

Cross-Contamination

Below are some of the most common sources of gluten contamination. A few crumbs that may not even be seen can cause damage to the intestine, so it is best to avoid these situations:

- Toasters used for gluten-containing foods
  Keep two toasters at home and designate one as GF. Alternatively, there are now bags available that are designed to hold a piece of bread in the toaster.
- Bulk bins. Prepackaged food is a safer bet.
- Condiment jars (peanut butter, jam, mayonnaise, etc.)
  It is best to keep a separate GF jar for commonly used items and be sure to label it clearly. At the very least, make sure everyone in the house knows not to "double-dip."
- Buffet lines
  Other customers may use one serving utensil for multiple items. Food from one area may be spilled into another food container. It may be safer to order from the menu.
- Deep-fried foods
  Oil is typically used over and over to fry foods. It is highly likely that French fries (or other GF foods) are fried in the same oil as battered and breaded foods such as fried chicken.
- Strainers/colanders
  Colanders used to drain gluten-containing pasta may hold onto residual gluten proteins, as they are very difficult to thoroughly clean.

GF, Gluten free.

Adapted from Parrish CR et al: *University of Virginia Health System Nutrition Support Traineeship Syllabus,* Charlottesville, Va, 2010, University of Virginia Health System.

Pathophysiology

The diarrhea of tropical sprue appears to be an infectious type, although the precise cause and the sequence of pathogenic events remain unknown. The syndrome may include bacterial overgrowth, changes in GI motility, and cellular changes in the GI tract. Identified intestinal organisms may differ from one region of the tropics to the next. As in CD, the intestinal villi may be abnormal, but the surface cell alterations are much less severe. The gastric mucosa is atrophied and inflamed, with diminished secretion of hydrochloric acid and intrinsic factor (Langenberg et al, 2014).

Medical Treatment

Treatment of tropical sprue typically includes use of broad-spectrum antibiotics, folate, vitamin B_{12}, fluid, and electrolytes.

Medical Nutrition Therapy

Nutrition management includes restoration and maintenance of fluids, electrolytes, macronutrients, and micronutrients, and introduction of a diet that is appropriate for the extent of malabsorption (see Diarrhea earlier in this chapter). Along with other nutrients, B_{12} and folate supplementation may be needed if deficiency is identified. Nutritional deficiency increases susceptibility to infectious agents, further aggravating the condition.

INTESTINAL BRUSH-BORDER ENZYME DEFICIENCIES

Intestinal enzyme deficiency states involve deficiencies of the brush-border disaccharidases that hydrolyze disaccharides at the mucosal cell membrane. Disaccharidase deficiencies may occur as (1) rare congenital defects such as the sucrase, isomaltase, or lactase deficiencies seen in the newborn; (2) generalized forms secondary to diseases that damage the intestinal epithelium (e.g., Crohn's disease or CD); or, most commonly, (3) a genetically acquired form (e.g., lactase deficiency) that usually appears after childhood but can appear as early as 2 years of age. For this chapter, only lactose malabsorption is described in detail (see Chapter 42 for a discussion of inborn metabolic disorders).

Lactose Intolerance

Lactose intolerance is the syndrome of diarrhea, abdominal pain, flatulence, or bloating occurring after lactose consumption. Secondary lactose intolerance can develop as a consequence of infection of the small intestine, gastrointestinal surgeries, inflammatory disorders, HIV, or malnutrition. In children it is typically secondary to viral or bacterial infections. Lactose malabsorption is commonly associated with other GI disorders, such as IBS.

Etiology

High concentrations of the brush-border enzyme, lactase, is present in the small bowel of all newborn mammals. After weaning, about 75% of the world's population dramatically decreases the synthesis of this enzyme despite continued exposure to lactose (Levitt et al, 2013). These people are termed to be lactase nonpersistent. The majority of adults of Asian, African, Latino, and Native American descent are lactase nonpersistent, whereas the majority of Caucasians are lactase persistent. Lactose malabsorption or intolerance has been reported to be low in children younger than age 6 but increases throughout childhood, peaking at age 10 to 16 years.

While evidence indicates that lactose intolerance increases slightly with increasing adult age or varies by race or gender, the difference may be more closely aligned with a dose specific effect, body size, and genetic differences versus lactose intolerance (Lapides and Savaiano, 2018). However, even in adults who retain a high level of lactase levels with age (75% to 85% of white adults of Western European heritage), the quantity of lactase is about half that of other saccharidases such as sucrase, alpha-dextrinase, or glucoamylase. The decline of lactase is known as hypolactasia (see *Focus On:* Lactose Intolerance: NOT an Uncommon Anomaly).

Pathophysiology

When large amounts of lactose are consumed, especially by persons who have little remaining lactase enzyme or with concurrent GI problems, loose stools or diarrhea can occur. As is the case with any malabsorbed sugar, lactose may act osmotically and increase fecal water, as well as provide a substrate for rapid fermentation by intestinal bacteria, which may result in bloating, flatulence, and cramps. Malabsorption of lactose is due to a deficiency of lactase, the enzyme that digests the sugar in milk. Lactose that is not hydrolyzed into galactose and glucose in the upper small intestine passes into the colon, where bacteria ferment it to SCFAs, carbon dioxide, and hydrogen gas.

Medical Treatment

Lactose malabsorption is diagnosed by (1) an abnormal hydrogen breath test or (2) an abnormal lactose tolerance test. During a hydrogen breath test, the patient is given a standard dose of lactose after fasting, and breath hydrogen is measured. If lactose is not digested in the small intestine, it passes into the colon, where it is fermented by the gut microbiota to SCFAs, CO_2, and hydrogen. Hydrogen is absorbed into the bloodstream and is exhaled through the lungs. The breath hydrogen test shows increased levels 60 to 90 minutes after lactose ingestion.

During a lactose tolerance test, a dose of lactose is given, and if the individual has sufficient lactase enzyme, blood sugar rises, reflecting the digestion of lactose to galactose and glucose. If the individual is lactose intolerant (lactase deficient), blood sugar will not rise because

Lactose Intolerance: NOT an Uncommon Anomaly

When lactose intolerance was first described in 1963, it appeared to be an infrequent occurrence, arising only occasionally in the white population. Because the capacity to digest lactose was measured in people from a wide variety of ethnic and racial backgrounds, it soon became apparent that disappearance of the lactase enzyme shortly after weaning, or at least during early childhood, was actually the predominant (normal) condition in most of the world's population. With a few exceptions, the intestinal tracts of adult mammals produce little, if any, lactase after weaning (the milks of pinnipeds—seals, walruses, and sea lions—do not contain lactose).

The exception of lactose tolerance has attracted the interest of geographers and others concerned with the evolution of the world's population. A genetic mutation favoring lactose tolerance appears to have arisen approximately 10,000 years ago, when dairy farming was first introduced. Presumably, it would have occurred in places where milk consumption was encouraged because of some degree of dietary deprivation and in groups in which milk was not fermented before consumption (fermentation breaks down much of the lactose into monosaccharides). The mutation would have selectively endured, because it would promote greater health, survival, and reproduction of those who carried the gene.

It is proposed that the mutation occurred in more than one location and then accompanied migrations of populations throughout the world. It continues primarily among whites from northern Europe and in ethnic groups in India, Africa, and Mongolia. The highest frequency (97%) of lactose tolerance occurs in Sweden and Denmark, suggesting an increased selective advantage in those able to tolerate lactose related to the limited exposure to ultraviolet light typical of northern latitudes. Lactose favors calcium absorption, which is limited in the absence of vitamin D produced by skin exposure to sunlight.

Dairy farming was unknown in North America until the arrival of Europeans, but the native peoples of North America did have a source of dairy in their diets. Thus Native Americans and those of non-European descent are among the 65% of the world's population who tolerate milk poorly, if at all (Silberman and Jin, 2019). This has practical implications with respect to group feeding programs such as school breakfasts and lunches. However, many lactose-intolerant people are able to digest milk in small to moderate amounts (Shaukat et al, 2010).

TABLE 27.3 Lactose Content of Common Foods

Product	Serving Size	Approximate Lactose Content (grams)
Milk (nonfat, 1%, 2%, whole), chocolate milk, acidophilus milk, buttermilk	1 cup	10-12
Butter, margarine	1 tsp	trace
Cheese	1 ounce	0-2
Cheddar, sharp	1 ounce	0
American, Swiss, Parmesan	1 ounce	1
Bleu cheese	1 ounce	2
Cottage cheese	½ cup	2-3
Cream (heavy), whipped cream	½ cup	3-4
Cream cheese	1 ounce	1
Evaporated milk	1 cup	24
Half-and-half	½ cup	5
Ice cream	½ cup	6
Ice milk	½ cup	9
Nonfat dry milk powder (unreconstituted)	1 cup	62
Sherbet, orange	½ cup	2
Sour cream	½ cup	4
Sweetened condensed milk, undiluted	1 cup	40
Yogurt, cultured, low-fat*	1 cup	5-10

*Note: Although most yogurt does contain lactose, yogurt with live cultures is generally well tolerated by those with lactose intolerance.

the lactose is not absorbed; it passes into the colon and GI symptoms may appear. The lactose tolerance test was based originally on an oral dose of lactose equivalent to the amount in 1 quart of milk (50 g). Recently doses lower than 50 g of lactose have been used to approximate more closely the usual consumption of lactose from milk products.

Demonstrated lactose malabsorption does not always indicate a person will be symptomatic. Many factors play a role, including the amount of lactose ingested, the residual lactase activity, the ingestion of food in addition to lactose, the ability of the gut microbiota to ferment lactose, and the sensitivity of the individual to the lactose fermentation products (Misselwitz et al, 2013). Consumption of small amounts should be of little consequence because the SCFAs are readily absorbed and the gases can be absorbed or passed. Larger amounts, usually greater than 12 g/day, consumed in a single food (the amount typically found in a cup or 240 mL of milk) may result in more substrate entering the colon than can be disposed of by normal processes. Because serving sizes of milk drinks are increasing and more than one source of lactose may be consumed in the same meal, the amounts of lactose consumed may be more important than in years past (Misselwitz et al, 2013).

Medical Nutrition Therapy

Management of lactose intolerance requires dietary change. The symptoms are alleviated by reduced consumption of lactose-containing foods (see Table 27.3 for common foods containing lactose). Those

who avoid dairy products may need calcium and vitamin D supplementation unless they are diligent about including nondairy sources of these nutrients. A completely lactose-free diet is not necessary in lactase-deficient persons. Most lactose maldigesters can consume some lactose (up to 12 g/day) without major symptoms, especially when taken with meals or in the form of cheeses or fermented dairy products (Misselwitz et al, 2013).

Many adults with intolerance to moderate amounts of milk eventually adapt to and tolerate 12 g or more of lactose in milk (equivalent to one cup of full-lactose milk) when introduced gradually, in increments, over several weeks. Incremental or continuous exposure to increasing quantities of fermentable sugar can lead to improved tolerance, not as a consequence of increased lactase enzyme production but by altered gut microbiota composition. This has been shown with lactulose, a nonabsorbed carbohydrate that is biochemically similar to lactose (Lomer, 2015). Individual differences in tolerance may relate to the state of colonic adaptation. Regular consumption of milk by lactase-deficient individuals may increase the threshold at which diarrhea occurs.

Lactase enzyme in tablets or liquid or in milk products treated with lactase enzyme (e.g., Lactaid) are available for lactose maldigesters who have discomfort with milk ingestion. Commercial lactase preparations may differ in their effectiveness. Fermented milk products, such as aged cheeses and yogurts, are well tolerated because their lactose content is low. Tolerance of yogurt may be the result of a microbial galactosidase in the bacterial culture that facilitates lactose digestion in the intestine. The presence of galactosidase depends on the brand and processing method. Because this microbial enzyme is sensitive to freezing, frozen yogurt may not be as well tolerated. Although the addition of probiotics may change this, evidence is lacking (Morelli, 2014). Lactose-free or reduced lactose enteral nutrition formulas are widely available for hospitalized and long-term feeding tube patients (see Chapter 12 and Appendix 16).

Fructose Malabsorption

Dietary fructose exists in three forms: (1) the monosaccharide, (2) sucrose, a disaccharide of fructose and glucose, and (3) in chains as fructans. Consumption of fructose in the United States, especially from fruit juices, fruit drinks, and high-fructose corn syrup (HFCS) in soft drinks and confections, has increased significantly in recent years. The human small intestine has a limited ability to absorb fructose, compared with the ability to absorb glucose rapidly and completely.

Etiology

Although fructose malabsorption is common in healthy people, its appearance depends on the amount of fructose ingested. Absorption of fructose is improved when it is ingested with glucose (such as in sucrose) because glucose absorption stimulates pathways for fructose absorption. Although some degree of fructose malabsorption may be normal, those with coexisting GI disorders may be more likely to experience GI symptoms after fructose ingestion. Patients with IBS and visceral hypersensitivity may be more sensitive to gas, distension, or pain from fructose malabsorption, whereas those with small bowel bacterial overgrowth (SIBO) may experience symptoms from normal amounts of fructose.

Pathophysiology

Breath hydrogen testing has revealed that up to 75% of healthy people will incompletely absorb a large quantity of fructose (50 g) taken alone (Putkonen et al, 2013).

Fructose coexists in food with other poorly absorbed carbohydrates, which have been given the umbrella term FODMAPs. In one recent study, restricting FODMAPs in the diet demonstrated global symptom relief in those with fructose or lactose intolerance, with the benefit indicating possible relationship to changes in intestinal host or microbiome metabolism (Wilder-Smith et al, 2017).

Medical Nutrition Therapy

People with fructose malabsorption and those patients with GI conditions that experience symptoms of fructose malabsorption may not have problems with foods containing balanced amounts of glucose and fructose but may need to limit or avoid foods containing large amounts of free fructose. Pear, apple, mango, and Asian pear are notable in that they have substantially more "free fructose" (more fructose than glucose). In addition, most dried fruits and fruit juices may pose a problem in larger amounts because of the amount of fructose provided per serving. Foods sweetened with HFCS (as opposed to sucrose) are also more likely to cause symptoms. The degree of fructose intolerance and tolerance to the symptoms of fructose malabsorption are so variable that intake of these foods must generally be individualized with each patient (see Table 27.7 for a list of foods high in fructose content).

INFLAMMATORY BOWEL DISEASE

Inflammatory bowel disease (IBD) is a chronic and relapsing disorder of the gastrointestinal tract. It is characterized by chronic intestinal inflammation and is categorized into two major forms as either Crohn's disease or ulcerative colitis (UC). Crohn's disease and UC are relatively rare disorders, but they result in frequent use of health care resources. The prevalence and incidence is increasing as IBD emerges

as a global disease, though it remains most prominent in industrialized nations (Lewis et al, 2017). It is also becoming more prevalent in older adults (Ye et al, 2015).

Contrary to older data used in estimates from 1999, in 2015 the CDC found that 3.1 million (1.3%) of adults in the United States had ever been given a diagnosis of IBD. Of these, there were a higher percentage of individuals at ages 45 to 64 (1.5%) and ≥65 (1.7%) compared with younger age groups. Hispanics and non-Hispanic whites had a higher prevalence than non-Hispanic blacks. Level of education, employment, and socioeconomic status were also correlated with those who had received an IBD diagnosis (Dahlhamer et al, 2016).

While the onset of IBD occurs most often in patients 15 to 30 years of age, for some it occurs later in adulthood. IBD occurs more commonly in developed areas of the world, but in the United States it is more prevalent in those living in poverty (incomes <100% vs. ≥400% of the federal poverty level). The disease has a higher prevalence for those living outside the central city of a metropolitan statistical area. Factors having no impact on prevalence included region of residence, sex, current marital status, or health insurance coverage type (Dahlhamer et al, 2016). Reasons for the varied prevalence of IBD are not entirely clear but emerging research is investigating many aspects of the increased inflammatory and proliferative state, including etiology, epidemiology, and nutritional factors.

Crohn's disease and UC share some clinical characteristics, including diarrhea, fever, weight loss, anemia, food intolerances, malnutrition, growth failure, and extraintestinal manifestations (arthritic, dermatologic, and hepatic). In both forms of IBD, the risk of malignancy increases with the duration of the disease. Although malnutrition can occur in both forms of IBD, it is more of a lifelong concern in patients with Crohn's disease than with UC. The features that distinguish the forms of the disease in terms of genetic characteristics, clinical presentation, and treatment are discussed in Table 27.4.

Etiology

The cause of IBD is not completely understood and there is no known cure, but the most widely accepted pathogenesis involves complex interaction of the GI immunologic system of the host, and genetic and environmental factors. Emerging research is also investigating the role of the microbiota and its potential role in the disease (Nishida et al, 2018). Genetic susceptibility is now recognized to be diverse, with a number of possible gene mutations that affect risk and characteristics of the disease. The diversity in the genetic alterations among individuals may help explain differences in the onset, aggressiveness, complications, location, and responsiveness to different therapies as seen in the clinical setting. The major environmental factors include resident and transient microorganisms in the GI tract and dietary components.

The genes affected (e.g., C677T mutation related to methylenetetrahydrofolate reductase) normally play a role in the reactivity of the host GI immune system to luminal antigens such as those provided by intestinal flora and the diet. In animal models, inflammatory disease does not occur in the absence of gut microbiota. Normally, when an antigenic challenge or trauma occurs, the immune response is initiated; it is then turned off and continues to be held in check after the challenge resolves. In IBD however, increased antigen exposure, decreased host defense mechanisms, and/or decreased tolerance to some components of the gut microbiota occurs. Inappropriate inflammatory response and an inability to suppress it play primary roles in the disease. For example, two genes, NOD$_2$/CARD$_{15}$ and the autophagy gene ATG16L1 have been linked to one functional pathway of bacterial sensing, invasion, and elimination. Failure of these genes to come together can lead to impaired autophagy and persistence of bacteria, resulting in abnormal immune responses (Bossuyt and Vermeire, 2016).

The Western diet may also be a contributing factor for development of IBD (Lewis et al, 2017). In epidemiologic studies, factors

TABLE 27.4 Ulcerative Colitis versus Crohn's Disease

	Ulcerative Colitis	Crohn's Disease
Presentation	Bloody diarrhea	Perianal disease, abdominal pain (65%), mass in abdomen
Gross pathology	Rectum always involved	Rectum may not be involved
	Moves continuously, proximally from rectum	Can occur anywhere along gastrointestinal tract Not continuous: "skip lesions"
	Thin wall	Thick wall
	Few strictures	Strictures common
	Diffuse ulceration	Cobblestone appearance
Histopathology	No granulomas	Granulomas
	Low inflammation	More inflammation
	Deeper ulcers (hence named ulcerative)	Shallow ulcers
	Pseudopolyps Abscesses in crypts	Fibrosis
Extraintestinal manifestations	Sclerosing cholangitis	Erythema nodosum
	Pyoderma gangrenosum	Migratory polyarthritis Gallstones
Complications	Toxic megacolon	Malabsorption
	Cancer	Cancer
	Strictures and fistulas are very rare	Strictures or fistulas Perianal disease

associated with of the development of IBD include increased sucrose intake, lack of fruits and vegetables, a low intake of dietary fiber, increased consumption of red meat and alcohol, altered omega-6/omega-3 fatty acid ratios and insufficient vitamin D intake (Hlavaty et al, 2015). Dietary interventions to modify these factors during IBD flares are still under investigation (Owczarek et al, 2016).

Pathophysiology

Crohn's disease. Chrohn's disease may involve any part of the GI tract, but approximately 50% to 60% of cases involve the distal ileum and the colon. Only the small intestine or only the colon is involved in 15% to 25% of cases. Some unique features of Crohn's disease include segments of inflamed bowel that may be separated by healthy segments, and transmural mucosal involvement that affects all layers of the mucosa. Crohn's disease is also characterized by abscesses, fistulas, fibrosis, submucosal thickening, localized strictures, narrowed segments of bowel, and partial or complete obstruction of the intestinal lumen.

Ulcerative colitis. Ulcerative colitis disease activity is limited to only the large intestine and rectum. The disease process is continuous and is normally limited to the mucosa. Bleeding is more common in UC as well. See Fig. 27.5 (A–C) and Table 27.4 to compare and contrast further.

The inflammatory response (e.g., increased cytokines and acute-phase proteins, increased GI permeability, increased proteases, and increased oxygen radicals and leukotrienes) results in GI tissue damage. In IBD either the regulatory mechanisms are defective or the factors perpetuating the immune and acute-phase responses are enhanced, leading to tissue fibrosis and destruction. The clinical course of the disease may be mild and episodic or severe and unremitting (see *Pathophysiology and Care Management Algorithm:* Inflammatory Bowel Disease).

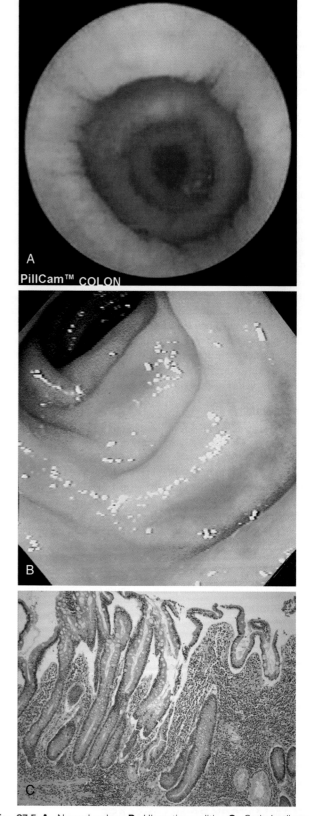

Fig. 27.5 A, Normal colon. **B,** Ulcerative colitis. **C,** Crohn's disease. (*A,* From Fireman Z, Kopelman Y: The colon—the latest terrain for capsule endoscopy. *Dig Liver Dis* 39[10]:895-899, 2007. *B,* From Black JM, Hawks JH: *Medical surgical nursing: clinical management for positive outcomes,* ed 8, St Louis, 2009, Saunders. *C,* From McGowan CE, Lagares-Garcia JA, Bhattacharya B: Retained capsule endoscope leading to the identification of small bowel adenocarcinoma in a patient with undiagnosed Crohn's disease, *Ann Diagn Pathol* 13[6]:390-393, 2009.)

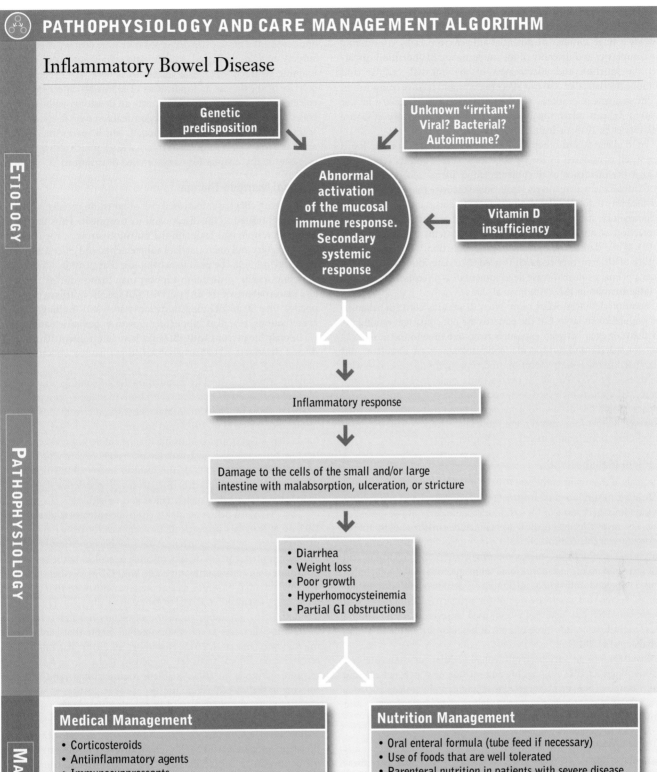

PATHOPHYSIOLOGY AND CARE MANAGEMENT ALGORITHM

Inflammatory Bowel Disease

ETIOLOGY

Genetic predisposition

Unknown "irritant" Viral? Bacterial? Autoimmune?

Abnormal activation of the mucosal immune response. Secondary systemic response

Vitamin D insufficiency

PATHOPHYSIOLOGY

Inflammatory response

Damage to the cells of the small and/or large intestine with malabsorption, ulceration, or stricture

- Diarrhea
- Weight loss
- Poor growth
- Hyperhomocysteinemia
- Partial GI obstructions

MANAGEMENT

Medical Management

- Corticosteroids
- Antiinflammatory agents
- Immunosuppressants
- Antibiotics
- Anticytokine medications

Surgical Management

- Bowel resection that can result in short bowel syndrome (SBS)

Nutrition Management

- Oral enteral formula (tube feed if necessary)
- Use of foods that are well tolerated
- Parenteral nutrition in patients with severe disease or obstruction
- Supplement with folate, B_6, B_{12}, Vitamin D, iron (if needed), and ω-3 fatty acids
- Consider use of prebiotics and probiotics (especially VSL#3)
- Modify fiber intake according to symptoms
- Test for food intolerances

Diet is an environmental factor that may trigger relapses of IBD. Foods, microbes, individual nutrients, and incidental contaminants provide a huge number of potential antigens, especially considering the complexity and diversity of the modern diet. Malnutrition can affect the function and effectiveness of the mucosal, cellular, and immune barriers; diet also can affect the type and relative composition of the resident microflora. Several nutrients, such as dietary fats or vitamin D, can affect the intensity of the inflammatory response (Hlavaty et al, 2015; Sadeghian et al, 2016).

Food allergies and other immunologic reactions to specific foods have been considered in the pathogenesis of IBD and its symptoms, though the incidence of documented food allergies, compared with food intolerances, is relatively small. Some theorize that intestinal wall permeability to food molecules and cell fragments is likely increased in inflammatory states, which would allow the potential for increased interaction of antigens with host immune systems (Michielan et al, 2015). While damage to epithelial barrier function is a characteristic feature of IBD, further research is needed to determine whether this plays a primary role in disease development or as a secondary response to inflammation in IBD (Antoni et al, 2014).

Food intolerances occur more often in persons with IBD than in the population at large, but the patterns are not consistent among individuals or even between exposures from one time to the next. Reasons for specific and nonspecific food intolerances are abundant and are related to the severity, location, and complications associated with the disease process. Partial GI obstructions, malabsorption, diarrhea, altered GI transit, increased secretions, food aversions, and associations are but a few of the problems experienced by persons with IBD. However, neither food allergies nor intolerances fully explain the onset or manifestations in all patients (see Chapter 25).

Medical Management

The goals of treatment in IBD are to induce and maintain remission and to improve nutrition status. Treatment of the primary GI manifestations appears to correct most of the extraintestinal features of the disease as well. The most effective medical agents include corticosteroids, antiinflammatory agents (aminosalicylates), immunosuppressive agents (cyclosporine, azathioprine, mercaptopurine), antibiotics (ciprofloxacin and metronidazole), and monoclonal tumor necrosis factor antagonists (anti-TNF), and infliximab, adalimumab, certolizumab, and natalizumab, agents that inactivate one of the primary inflammatory cytokines. Anti-TNF has historically been used in severe cases of Crohn's disease and fistulas, but more recently it has shown promise in UC as well (Mao et al, 2017).

Investigations of various treatment modalities for the acute and chronic stages of IBD are ongoing and include new forms of existing drugs as well as new agents targeted to regulate production and activity of cytokines, eicosanoids, or other mediators of the inflammatory and acute-phase response (Monteleone et al, 2014).

Surgical Management

In Crohn's disease, surgery may be necessary to repair strictures (narrowing of the GI lumen) or remove portions of the bowel when medical management fails. Approximately 50% to 70% of persons with Crohn's disease undergo surgery related to the disease. Surgery does not cure Crohn's disease, and recurrence often occurs within 1 to 3 years of surgery. The chance of needing subsequent surgery in the patient's life is about 30% to 70%, depending on the type of surgery and the age at the first operation. Major resections of the intestine may result in varying degrees of malabsorption of fluid and nutrients. In extreme cases patients may have extensive or multiple resections, resulting in short-bowel syndrome (SBS) and dependence on PN to maintain adequate nutrient intake and hydration (see Chapter 12).

With increased efficacy of pharmaceutical therapies for UC, the percentage of patients who undergo a colectomy to remove the colon and resolve the disease has decreased over time (Barnes et al, 2019). If surgery remains indicated, inflammation does not occur in the remaining GI tract. Whether a colectomy is necessary depends on the severity of the disease and indicators of increased cancer risk. After a colectomy for UC, surgeons may create an ileostomy with an external collection pouch and an internal abdominal reservoir fashioned with a segment of ileum or an ileoanal pouch, which spares the rectum, to serve as a reservoir for stool. The internal Koch pouch also may be used (see later in this chapter for more detailed description).

Medical Nutrition Therapy

Persons with IBD are at increased risk of nutrition problems for a host of reasons related to the disease and its treatment. Thus the primary goal is to restore and maintain the nutrition status of the individual. Foods, dietary and micronutrient supplements, and enteral and parenteral nutrition may be used to accomplish that mission. Oral diet and the other means of nutrition support may change during remissions and exacerbations of the disease. Diet and specific nutrients play a supportive role in maintaining nutrition status and limiting symptom exacerbations, as well as supporting growth in pediatric patients.

In daily life persons with IBD may have intermittent "flares" of the disease characterized by partial obstructions, nausea, abdominal pain, bloating, or diarrhea. Foods that are responsible for some GI symptoms in a normal, healthy population (gas, bloating, diarrhea) are likely to be triggers for the same symptoms in patients with mild stages of IBD or those in remission. Many report specific, individualized food intolerances (Hou et al, 2014) and are sometimes advised to eliminate foods they suspect are responsible for the intolerance. Often, the patient becomes increasingly frustrated as the diet becomes progressively limited and symptoms still do not resolve. Since malnutrition is a significant risk in patients with IBD, an overly restrictive diet only increases the likelihood of malnutrition and weight loss.

There is a great deficit of quality controlled dietary clinical trials for IBD. Because of this, no single dietary regimen for reducing symptoms or decreasing flares has been found to be conclusively effective. Though limited, current dietary research is exploring the specific carbohydrate diet, antiinflammatory diet, low FODMAPs diet, and others, and any potential they may have to help patients with IBD (Kakodkar et al, 2015; Olendzki et al, 2014; Prince et al, 2016; Braly et al, 2017; Suskind, 2016). An important aspect of dietary research is the impact of how the diet acts as an environmental factor that can affect the microbiome (Lee et al, 2015; Nishida et al, 2018). Far more dietary research and clinical trials are needed to make any specific dietary recommendations for IBD, but there is an exciting trend of interest brewing in the scientific community (Lee et al, 2016).

The ability of nutrition support as either PN or enteral nutrition (EN) to induce remission of IBD has been debated for several years. Evaluation is confounded by the natural course of IBD with exacerbations and remissions and by the genetic diversity of the patients. EN is not as effective as corticosteroid therapy to induce remission in adults with Crohn's disease. For children, however, EN is far more effective than the placebo and should be considered as a primary therapy. EN can also be used to reverse malnutrition that can occur with Crohn's, and to encourage growth in the pediatric population (Palmer et al, 2017). Children can also benefit from EN, either as sole source of nutrition or supplemental to an oral diet, to reduce dependence on steroids that may affect growth and bone disease. Complete bowel rest using PN is not necessarily required but may be used in those with inadequate functioning bowel, or for 1 to 2 weeks before surgery in malnourished patients (Palmer et al, 2017). EN has the potential to feed the intestinal epithelium and alter GI flora and is the preferred route of nutrition support in patients with adequate bowel length. EN may temper some elements of the inflammatory process, serve as a valuable source of nutrients needed for restoration of GI defects, and be steroid sparing (Richman and Rhodes, 2013). Available evidence does not support the use of EN as a first-line therapy in those with UC, but tolerance has been demonstrated during acute flares (Palmer et al, 2017).

Overall, patients and caretakers must be very committed when using EN formulas or tube feeding because it takes 4 to 8 weeks before one sees the clinical effects. Timely nutritional support is a vital component of therapy to restore and maintain nutritional health. Malnutrition compromises digestive and absorptive function by increasing the permeability of the GI tract to potential inflammatory agents. EN is always the preferred route over PN when nutrition support is medically indicated in IBD. PN is not as nutritionally complete, has increased risk of infectious complications, and is more expensive than EN. However, PN may be required in patients with persistent bowel obstruction, fistulas, and major GI resections that result in SBS where EN is not possible.

Energy needs of patients with IBD are not increased (unless weight gain is desired). Generally, when disease activity increases basal metabolic rate, physical activity is greatly curtailed, and overall energy needs, are not substantially changed. Protein requirements may be increased, depending on the severity and stage of the disease and the restoration requirements. Inflammation and treatment with corticosteroids induce a negative nitrogen balance and cause a loss of lean muscle mass. Protein losses also occur in areas of inflamed and ulcerated intestinal mucosa via defects in epithelial tight junctions (see Chapter 37). To maintain positive nitrogen balance, 1.3 to 1.5 g/kg/day of protein is recommended.

Supplemental vitamins, especially folate, B_6, and B_{12}, may be needed, as well as minerals such as iron and trace elements to replace stores or for maintenance because of maldigestion, malabsorption, drug-nutrient interactions, or inadequate intake (Owczarek et al, 2016). Diarrhea can aggravate losses of zinc, potassium, and selenium. Patients who receive intermittent corticosteroids may need supplemental calcium and vitamin D. Patients with IBD are at increased risk of osteopenia and osteoporosis; 25-OH vitamin D levels and bone density should be monitored routinely and vitamin D supplemented appropriately (Hlavaty et al, 2015). Omega-3 fatty acid supplements in Crohn's disease significantly reduce disease activity. Use of omega-3 fatty acids or fish oil supplements in UC appears to result in a significant medication-sparing effect, with reductions in disease activity and increased time in remission reported (Farrukh and Mayberry, 2014). Use of foods and supplements containing prebiotics and probiotic supplements continues to be investigated for their potential to alter the gut microbiota; and further research is indicated (Sinagra et al, 2013; Nishida et al, 2018).

During acute and severe exacerbations of the disease, the diet is tailored to the individual but usually includes reduced fiber intake and decaffeinated, low-sugar beverages for adequate hydration (Academy of Nutrition and Dietetics [AND], 2019). In people with rapid intestinal transit, extensive bowel resections, or extensive small bowel disease, absorption may be compromised. Here, excessive intake of lactose, fructose, or sorbitol may contribute to abdominal cramping, gas, and diarrhea; and high fat intake may result in steatorrhea. However, the incidence of lactose intolerance is no greater in patients with IBD than in the general population. Patients with IBD who tolerate lactose should not necessarily restrict lactose-containing foods because they can be a valuable source of high-quality protein, calcium, and vitamin D.

Patients with strictures or partial bowel obstruction benefit from a reduction in dietary fiber or limited food particle size. Small, frequent feedings may be tolerated better than large meals. Small amounts of isotonic (having the same solute concentration as bodily fluids), liquid oral supplements, may be valuable in restoring intake without provoking symptoms. In cases in which fat malabsorption is likely, supplementation with foods made with medium-chain triglycerides (MCTs) may be useful in adding calories and serving as a vehicle for fat-soluble nutrients but must be introduced slowly to avoid GI distress. However, these products are expensive and may be less effective than more basic treatments.

The information on IBD availble to the general public is sometimes inaccurate or exaggerated, or it may pertain only to one individual's situation and not to another's. A critical component of patient education for IBD pertains to helping with the evaluation of nutrition information. Patients' participation in the management of their disease may help to reduce not only the symptoms of the disease but also the associated anxiety level.

Microbiota. Probiotic foods and supplements have been investigated as potential therapeutic agents for IBD because of their ability to modify the gut microbiota and potentially modulate gut inflammatory response. Multistrain probiotic supplements (e.g., VSL#3) have been shown to be beneficial in maintaining disease remission in patients with UC who had pouchitis, inflammation in the ileal pouch surgically formed after colectomy (Shen et al, 2014). Specific probiotic supplements appear to be useful for induction and extension of remissions in pediatric and adult UC (Ghouri et al, 2014; Shen et al, 2014).

Although probiotics appear useful in UC, probiotic studies have not demonstrated significant improvement in Crohn's disease activity in adults or pediatric patients, nor do probiotic supplements appear to prolong remission in Crohn's disease (Ghouri et al, 2014). Due to many confounding factors to research including, but not limited to, medication use (antibiotics, proton-pump inhibitors, antidiarrheals), variability in probiotic quality, and differences in dietary intake among participants, it has yet to be established whether probiotics could be of benefit as part of the routine treatment in IBD (Abraham and Quigley, 2017).

Regular intake of prebiotic foods such as oligosaccharides, fermentable fibers, and resistant starches can beneficially affect the gut microbiota, feeding *Lactobacillus* and *Bifidobacteria,* thus providing competition to and theoretically suppression of pathogenic or opportunistic microbiota. In addition, fermentation of prebiotics leads to increased production of SCFAs, theoretically creating a more acidic and less favorable environment for opportunistic bacteria.

Use of probiotics and prebiotics may prevent SIBO in predisposed individuals and may be used to treat diarrhea. Additional study is needed to identify the dose, the most effective prebiotic and probiotic foods, the form in which they can be used for therapeutic and maintenance purposes, and their relative value compared with other therapies (Ghouri et al, 2014).

Microscopic Colitis

Injury of the colon caused by UC, Crohn's disease, infections, radiation injury, and ischemic insult to the colon presents with abnormalities such as edema, redness, bleeding, or ulcerations that are visible on colonoscopy examination. Unlike the colitis of IBD, microscopic colitis is characterized by inflammation that is not visible by inspection of the colon during colonoscopy and is apparent only when the colon's lining is biopsied and then examined under a microscope. Patients with microscopic colitis can have diarrhea for months or years before the diagnosis is made. The cause of microscopic colitis is unknown.

Pathophysiology

There are two types of microscopic colitis. In lymphocytic colitis, there is an accumulation of lymphocytes within the lining of the colon.

In collagenous colitis, there is also a layer of collagen (like scar tissue) just below the lining. Some experts believe that lymphocytic colitis and collagenous colitis represent different stages of the same disease. Symptoms include chronic, watery diarrhea, mild abdominal cramps, and pain. More than 30% of patients report weight loss. Microscopic colitis appears more frequently in patients aged 60 to 70 years, and collagenous colitis occurs more frequently in females (Ohlsson, 2015).

Medical Nutrition Therapy

Research is underway to determine possible effective treatments for microscopic colitis, including corticosteroids and immunosuppressive agents. Medical nutrition therapy is supportive with efforts to maintain weight and nutrition status, avoid symptom exacerbation, and maintain hydration, similar to that for IBD.

Irritable Bowel Syndrome

Irritable bowel syndrome (IBS) is a functional gastrointestinal disorder defined by the American College of Gastroenterology (ACG) IBS Task Force as "abdominal discomfort associated with altered bowel habits" (Ford et al, 2014). The Rome IV criteria for IBS and its subtypes are used to define the diagnosis based on the presence of GI symptoms (Box 27.10). IBS is a condition characterized by unexplained abdominal discomfort or pain that is associated with changes in bowel habits (Schoenfeld, 2016). Other common symptoms include gas, bloating, diarrhea and constipation, and increased GI distress associated with psychosocial distress. These symptoms may be vague and transient, making IBS a diagnosis of exclusion. It is classified as a functional disorder because tests show no histologic abnormalities and, therefore, diagnosis depends on symptoms. The diagnostic criteria also include a refining of subtypes of IBS based on predominant stool patterns (Table 27.5).

Research is underway to better define IBS, which may be reflected in a new name for this challenging disease process.

An estimated 10% to 20% of the United States population has IBS, with twice as many women as men being affected, although this may be a factor of reporting (Koff and Mullin, 2012). There are between 2.4 and 3.5 million annual physician visits for IBS in the United States alone. IBS is the most common disorder diagnosed by gastroenterologists and accounts for 20% to 40% of visits (International Foundation for Functional Gastrointestinal Disorders [IFFGD], 2014). Patients with IBS often miss school and work days, resulting in decreased productivity, increased health care costs, and decreased quality of life as a result of their symptoms.

Etiology

No specific marker or test is diagnostic for IBS. Lactulose breath testing has been used to measure breath hydrogen and methane levels resulting from an overgrowth of bacteria in the small intestine, and this has been correlated with some cases of IBS (Rezaie et al, 2017). When assessing a patient for IBS, the clinician must carefully review medication records because numerous over-the-counter and prescribed medications can cause abdominal symptoms such as pain and changes in bowel habits. In addition, the symptoms of IBS overlap with or are similar to other GI diseases such as CD, IBD, functional dyspepsia, and functional constipation. IBS may be present with CD and IBD. Rectal bleeding, iron deficiency anemia, unintentional weight loss, and family history should also be considered when assessing symptoms as they are not common for patients with IBS (Ireton-Jones, 2017; Chey et al, 2015).

Pathophysiology

The pathophysiology of IBS is not completely understood. Several factors are presumed to play a role in the etiology of IBS, including

---

BOX 27.10 Rome IV Criteria for Diagnosing Irritable Bowel Syndrome (IBS)

Rome IV Criteria for Diagnosing IBS*:
Recurrent abdominal pain, on average, at least 1 day/week in the last 3 months, associated with two or more of the following criteria:
- Related to defecation
- Associated with a change in frequency of stool
- Associated with a change in form (appearance) of stool

*Criteria fulfilled for the last 3 months with symptom onset at least 6 months before diagnosis.
Data from: Lacy BE, et al. Bowel Disorders. *Gastroenterology.* 2016;150:1393-1407; Rome III Diagnostic Criteria for Functional Gastrointestinal Disorders. http://www.romecriteria.org/assets/pdf/19_RomeIII_apA_885-898.pdf; https://irritablebowelsyndrome.net/clinical/new-rome-iv-diagnostic-criteria/.

TABLE 27.5 Subtypes of Irritable Bowel Syndrome (IBS) Based on Stool Patterns

Type	Symptoms
IBS with predominant constipation (IBS-C)	Stool type 1 and 2 more than 25% Stool type 6 and 7 less than 25%
IBS with predominant diarrhea (IBS-D)	Stool type 1 and 2 less than 25% Stool type 6 and 7 more than 25%
IBS with mixed bowel habits (IBS-M)	Stool type 1 and 2 more than 25% Stool type 6 and 7 more than 25%
Unsubtyped IBS	Meet criteria for IBS but bowel habits cannot be categorized into IBS-C, D, or M

Data from Lacy BE, et al. Bowel Disorders, *Gastroenterology* 150:1393-1407, 2016.

---

nervous system alterations (abnormal GI motility and visceral hypersensitivity), gut flora alterations, genetics, and psychosocial stress (Chey et al, 2015). Research traditionally has focused on intestinal motility; however, studies of small-bowel and colonic motility show inconsistent results with changes in the intestinal microbiome playing a large role in the development of IBS (Dupont, 2014).

Sensation in the GI tract results from stimulation of various receptors and sensory nerves in the gut wall, which transmit signals to the spinal cord and brain. Alterations in areas of the brain involved in pain modulation, autonomic nervous system dysregulation, and impaired brain-gut communication result in hyperalgesia (increased sensation to pain in the gut), visceral hypersensitivity, and altered motility (Chey et al, 2015; Anastasi et al, 2013). Dysregulation of serotonin concentrations in the GI tract has been correlated with the type of IBS a patient experiences; low serotonin concentrations are associated with constipation or a sluggish gut and higher serotonin concentrations are associated with diarrhea or increased peristalsis in the intestine (Kanazawa et al, 2011; Stasi et al, 2014).

Often SIBO is seen with IBS; however, additional studies are needed to understand whether SIBO is directly connected to IBS or is a separate entity. Although treatment of SIBO usually includes antibiotic and or herbal therapy, the low FODMAP diet is also recommended concomitantly.

Psychological conditions, such as depression and anxiety, often are observed in patients with IBS. Although it is unclear whether stress is a cause of IBS, it is known to trigger and exacerbate symptoms (Staudacher, 2017). It is not unusual for patients with

IBS to link their symptoms with lifetime or daily stress (Fadgyas-Stanculete et al, 2014).

Medical Management

The first step in the management of IBS and other functional GI disorders includes validating the reality of the patient's complaints and establishing an effective clinician-patient relationship. Care should be tailored to help the patient manage the symptoms and the factors that may trigger them. Nutrition therapy using the FODMAP elimination diet should be a primary consideration for IBS. Gibson noted that the high quality of evidence for the FODMAP elimination diet supports its use as first-line therapy (Gibson, 2017b). Drug therapy is aimed at management of symptoms associated with GI motility, visceral hypersensitivity, or psychological issues. Combination herbal remedies may be employed as well and have been found to be as effective as antibiotic treatment (Mullin et al, 2014). The treatment option is usually determined by the predominant bowel pattern and the symptoms that most disrupt the patient's quality of life (Table 27.6).

Medical Nutrition Therapy

The goals of nutrition therapy for IBS are to ensure adequate nutrient intake and explain the potential roles of foods in the management of symptoms. First-line therapy to treat IBS is the implementation of the FODMAP elimination diet or low FOODMAP diet, which is defined later in this chapter. Because the symptoms may have been ongoing for a period of time, a thorough nutrition assessment should be completed initially. This should include (1) assessment of nutritional status-body weight status, loss or gain, and food intake; (2) review of current medications for IBS and other medications; (3) review of GI symptoms (duration, severity, frequency); (4) review of supplement intake (vitamins, minerals, fats, pre- and probiotics, herbals); and (5) review of use of mind-body therapies and the results achieved (Ireton-Jones, 2017; Mullin et al, 2014). Presence of CD should be ruled out as well as any disease associated with symptoms such as delayed gastric emptying or bleeding, which are not key signs of IBS.

The FODMAPs Elimination Diet

A diet low in fermentable oligo, di, & monosaccharides and polyols (FODMAP) has been shown to be an effective therapy in the management of GI symptoms in patients with IBS. FODMAPs are made up of the fermentable carbohydrate portion of plant based foods. When metabolized by gut bacteria, FODMAPs increase gas production and and cause intestinal dysmotility (Ireton-Jones, 2017; Chey et al, 2015; Mullin, 2014; Shepherd and Gibson, 2006). In addition, these foods increase luminal water content and fluid status in the GI tract. When these are limited or eliminated, symptoms are also reduced or eliminated in up to 70% of people with IBS (Gibson, 2017a). This has been demonstrated in children as well (Chumpitazi et al, 2015).

The low FODMAPs diet limits foods that contain lactose, fructose, fructo-oligosaccharides (fructans), galacto-oligosaccharides (galactans), and polyols or sugar alcohols (sorbitol, xylitol, mannitol, isomaltase, and maltitol). These short-chain carbohydrates are poorly absorbed in the small intestine, are highly osmotic, and are rapidly fermented by bacteria in the small and large intestine, resulting in gas, pain, and diarrhea in sensitive individuals. FODMAPs have a cumulative impact on GI symptoms. A threshhold level for acceptable amounts of FODMAPs has not been well defined and is likely patient specific. Patients may tolerate small amounts, but symptoms can develop if they consume quantities that surpass their threshold. Lactulose breath testing, ordered by a physician, can be useful to demonstrate the presence of SIBO by measuring increases in breath hydrogen and methane (Rezaie et al, 2017). These gases are increased when gut bacteria metabolize FODMAPs, especially in the small intestine.

Nutrition intervention begins with elimination of all high FODMAPs foods from the diet for a trial period of approximately 6 weeks although symptoms may improve within 2 weeks (Ireton-Jones, 2017; Barrett, 2017; Catsos, 2017; Gibson, 2011). The challenge or reintroduction phase begins after the elimination phase with a slow, methodical, or controlled reintroduction of one FODMAPs category at a time to observe for symptoms and identify the most challenging foods (Vakil, 2018). The goal is to eventually reduce or eliminate GI symptoms by creating a diet that includes FODMAPs at the most tolerable intake level, and with use of alternative foods. It does not present a cure but a dietary approach to improve symptoms and quality of life.

The key to the successful FODMAP elimination diet is to work with an RDN who is very knowledgeable of the diet principles. There are many "lists" of low FODMAP foods available, and they can be confusing and challenging for the patient who is trying to follow the low FODMAP diet on their own. For this reason, no specific list of low FODMAP foods is provided in this chapter. Monash University is a reliable source for FODMAP content of foods (Gibson, 2017b). The Monash FODMAPs app, available on both iPhone and Android, is constantly being updated and an excellent resource for clinicians and clients. Monash University has other resources on the low FODMAP diet as well.

TABLE 27.6 Medical and Herbal Treatment Options for Irritable Bowel Syndrome (IBS) Symptoms

Symptom	Treatment
Abdominal pain and discomfort	Antispasmodic agents Tricyclic antidepressants Serotonin-directed agents (selective serotonin reuptake inhibitors, serotonin-3 receptor antagonists, or serotonin-4 receptor agonists) Digestive enzymes Peppermint oil Melatonin
Constipation	Fiber supplements: psyllium husk, soluble, nonfermentable Stool softeners Laxatives (osmotic, i.e., Mg; stimulant, i.e., senna)
Diarrhea	Antidiarrheal agents (loperamide, diphenoxylate with atropine) Soluble fiber supplements
Small intestinal bacterial overgrowth (SIBO)	Antibiotics Herbal treatments including berberine and oregano Elemental diet (2-week therapy) Digestive enzymes
Global symptoms and/or overall well-being	Psychotherapy (cognitive behavioral therapy, relaxation therapy, gut-directed hypnotherapy) Complementary and integrative medicine (acupuncture, meditation, stress reduction) Probiotics Prebiotics (use with caution if bloating is present)

Data from Chey W, Kurlander J, Eswaran S: Irritable bowel syndrome: a clinical review, *JAMA* 313(9):949–958, 2015; Mullin G, Shepherd SJ, Roland CB, et al: Irritable bowel syndrome: contemporary nutrition management strategies, *JPEN J Parenter Enteral Nutr* 38(7):781–799, 2014.

Nutritional deficiencies that can arise with the low FODMAPs diet include folate, thiamin, vitamin B_6, and fiber (from limiting cereals and breads), as well as calcium and vitamin D (if avoiding all dairy products in addition to lactose). An RDN can provide appropriate food substitutions to ensure an adequate diet. Patients may wish to stay on a low FODMAP diet to manage their symptoms; however, it is important to add other foods in the reintroduction phase, as these may have fibers and other key nutrients which will enhance overall health.

Several qualified dietitians have written cookbooks and have websites dedicated to assisting clients with the low FODMAP diet. Two of these are Patsy Catsos, MS, RDN and Kate Scarlata, RDN. A training course has been established at the University of Michigan called FOOD: The Main Course to Digestive Health, and also at Monash University (available online).

Diverticular Disease

Diverticular disease is one of the most common medical conditions among industrialized societies. Diverticulosis is characterized by the formation of sac-like outpouchings or pockets (diverticula) within the colon that form when colonic mucosa and submucosa herniate through weakened areas in the muscle. The prevalence of diverticulosis is difficult to determine given that most individuals remain asymptomatic. This condition becomes more common as people age, particularly in people older than age 60 (Feuerstein and Falchuk, 2016). Diverticulitis is a complication of diverticulosis that indicates inflammation of one or more diverticulum. It often represents a flare-up of diverticulosis, and after it subsides into a period of remission, it reverts to the state of diverticulosis.

Etiology

The cause of diverticulosis has not been elucidated clearly. Epidemiologic studies have implicated low-fiber diets in the development of diverticular disease, but the evidence is ambiguous regarding high- versus low-fiber diets and diverticular disease with regard to prevention and treatment. Low-fiber diets reduce stool volume, predisposing individuals to constipation and increased intracolonic pressures, which suggests that diverticulosis occurs as a consequence of pressure-induced damage to the colon. However, while dietary fiber intake has been shown as inversely related to the risk of developing the disease, a large recent study failed to show a direct correlation between low-fiber diets and diverticulosis. In that study, higher-fiber diets were associated with a higher prevalence of diverticulosis. The American Gastroenterology Association recommends increasing fiber after a diverticulitis attack but even it states that the recommendation is conditional based on weak evidence (Feuerstein and Falchuk, 2016).

More recent research has started to explore theories including genetic differences, diet, motility, microbiome, and inflammation (Feuerstein and Falchuk, 2016). Other studies have focused on the role of decreased levels of the neurotransmitter serotonin in causing decreased relaxation and increased spasms of the colon muscle. Studies have found links between diverticular disease and diets high in red meat and fat, obesity, vitamin D insufficiency, lack of exercise, smoking, and certain medications, including nonsteroidal antiinflammatory drugs such as aspirin and steroids (Maguire et al, 2015; Feuerstein and Falchuk, 2016).

Pathophysiology

Evolving pathophysiologic mechanisms in diverticulosis and diverticulitis suggest chronic inflammation, alterations in colonic microbiota, disturbed colonic sensorimotor function, and abnormal colon motility have interrelated roles in the development of diverticular disease (Feuerstein and Falchuk, 2016). Complications of diverticular disease range from painless, mild bleeding and altered bowel habits to diverticulitis. Acute diverticulitis includes a spectrum of inflammation, abscess formation, bleeding, obstruction, fistula, and sepsis from perforation (rupture).

Medical and Surgical Treatment

Treatment typically includes antibiotics and adjustment of oral intake as tolerated. Patients with severe cases of diverticulitis with acute pain and complications often require a hospital stay and treatment with intravenous (IV) antibiotics and a few days of bowel rest (clear liquids only, no solid foods). Surgery is reserved for patients with recurrent episodes of diverticulitis and complications when there is little or no response to medication. Surgical treatment for diverticulitis removes the diseased part of the colon: most commonly, the left or sigmoid colon.

Medical Nutrition Therapy

Historically, it has been common in clinical practice to recommend avoidance of nuts, seeds, hulls, corn, and popcorn to prevent symptoms or complications of diverticular disease. However, newer studies have found no association between nut, corn, or popcorn consumption and diverticular bleeding (Feuerstein and Falchuk, 2016). In fact, an inverse relationship between nut and popcorn consumption and the risk of diverticulitis was demonstrated, suggesting a protective effect.

During an acute episode of diverticulitis or diverticular bleeding, oral intake is usually reduced until symptoms subside. Complicated cases may necessitate bowel rest and require PN. Once oral intake is resumed it is prudent to begin a low-fiber diet (10 to 15 g/day) as the diet is being advanced, followed by a gradual return to a high-fiber diet.

Although there is conflicting evidence regarding fiber intake and diverticular disease, in symptomatic uncomplicated diverticular disease (SUUD), increasing fiber did demonstrate a reduction in abdominal symptoms and prevention of acute diverticulitis (Carabotti et al, 2017). A high-fiber diet in combination with adequate hydration promotes soft, bulky stools that pass more swiftly and require less straining with defecation. Recommended intakes of dietary fiber, preferably from foods, are 25 g/day for adult women and 38 g/day for men.

Fiber intake should be increased gradually because it may cause bloating or gas. If a patient cannot or will not consume the necessary amount of fiber, methylcellulose or psyllium fiber supplements have been used with good results. A high-fiber diet, sometimes with fiber supplementation, is advocated in asymptomatic diverticulosis to reduce the likelihood of disease progression, prevent the recurrence of symptom episodes, and prevent acute diverticulitis. Adequate fluid intake should accompany the high fiber intake. A recent systematic review involving 11 (mostly uncontrolled) studies of probiotic use for the treatment of diverticular disease concluded that the evidence did not show a clear benefit (Lahner et al, 2016; Feuerstein and Falchuk, 2016).

Intestinal Polyps and Colorectal Cancer

In the United States, colorectal cancer (CRC) is the fourth most common cancer in adults and the second leading cause of cancer death. It is estimated that there were 140,250 new cases of CRC in 2018, and the incidence is more common in men than women and among those of African American descent (National Cancer Institute, 2018).

Etiology

About 85% of CRCs are considered to be sporadic, whereas about 15% are familial. Familial adenomatous polyposis (FAP) accounts for less than 1% of CRCs. It is a hereditary syndrome characterized by the development of hundreds to thousands of polyps in the colon and rectum during the second decade of life. Almost all patients with FAP will develop CRC if they are not identified and treated at an early stage.

An evaluation of the association of major known risk factors for CRC with colorectal polyp risk by histology type, quantified the impact of lifestyle modifications on the prevention of polyps (Fu et al, 2012). Several lifestyle factors, including cigarette smoking, obesity, high intake of red meat, low intake of fiber, low intake of calcium, and low vitamin D levels were found to be independently associated with the risk of polyps. Additionally, use of nonsteroidal antiinflammatory drugs has shown to be protective. The risk of polyps increased progressively with an increasing number of these adverse lifestyle factors (Bostick, 2015; Fu et al, 2012).

Pathophysiology

Polyps are established precursors of CRCs and defined as a mass that arises from the surface of the intestinal epithelium and projects into the intestinal lumen. Factors that increase the risk of CRC include family history, chronic IBD, FAP, adenomatous polyps, and several dietary components. Patterns of dietary practices rather than specific nutrients may be more predictive of the risk of developing CRC.

Medical Management

The treatment of a colorectal polyp is removal, usually by colonoscopy. Large polyps often require surgery for complete removal, even if the presence of cancer is not confirmed before resection. Patients diagnosed with CRC may require moderate to significant interventions, including medications, radiation therapy, chemotherapy, surgery, and EN and/or PN support.

Medical Nutrition Therapy

Recommendations from national cancer organizations include sufficient exercise; weight maintenance or reduction; modest and balanced intake of lipids; adequate intake of fiber and optimal micronutrients from fruits, vegetables, legumes, and whole grains; and limited use of alcohol. Supplements are normally encouraged if the diet is not adequate in calories, protein, or micronutrients. The diet for cancer survivors typically follows these prevention guidelines (see Chapter 35).

NUTRITIONAL CONSEQUENCES OF INTESTINAL SURGERY

Small Bowel Resections and Short-Bowel Syndrome

Short-bowel syndrome (SBS) can be defined as inadequate absorptive capacity resulting from reduced length or decreased functional bowel after resection. A loss of 70% to 75% of small bowel usually results in SBS, defined as 100 to 120 cm of small bowel without a colon, or 50 cm of small bowel with the colon remaining. A more practical definition of SBS is the inability to maintain nutrition and hydration needs with normal fluid and food intake, regardless of bowel length, as adaptation to bowel resections can vary widely among those who have had them.

Patients with SBS often have complex fluid, electrolyte, and nutritional management issues. Consequences of SBS include malabsorption of micronutrients and macronutrients, frequent diarrhea, steatorrhea, dehydration, electrolyte imbalances, weight loss, and growth failure in children (Limketkai, 2017). Other complications include gastric hypersecretion, oxalate renal stones, and cholesterol gallstones. Individuals who eventually need long-term PN have increased risk of catheter infection, sepsis, cholestasis, and liver disease, and reduced quality of life associated with chronic intravenous nutrition support (DiBaise, 2014).

Etiology

The most common reasons for major resections of the intestine in adults include Crohn's disease, radiation enteritis, mesenteric infarct, malignant disease, and volvulus. In the pediatric population most cases of SBS result from congenital anomalies of the GI tract, atresia, volvulus, or necrotizing enterocolitis (Shatnawei et al, 2010).

Pathophysiology

Duodenal resection. Resection of the duodenum (approximately 10 to 15 inches) is rare, which is fortunate because it is the preferred site for absorption of key nutrients such as iron, zinc, copper, and folate. The duodenum is a key player in the digestion and absorption of nutrients, because it is the portal of entry for pancreatic enzymes and bile salts (see Chapter 1).

Jejunal resections. The jejunum (6 to 10 feet) is also responsible for a large portion of nutrient absorption. Normally most digestion and absorption of food and nutrients occurs in the first 100 cm of small intestine, which also includes the duodenum. Jejunal enterohormones play key roles in digestion and absorption. Cholecystokinin (CCK) stimulates pancreatic secretion and gallbladder contraction, and secretin stimulates secretion of bicarbonate from the pancreas. Gastric inhibitory peptide slows gastric secretion and gastric motility, whereas vasoactive inhibitory peptide inhibits gastric and bicarbonate secretion (see Chapter 1). What remains to be digested or fermented and absorbed are small amounts of sugars, resistant starch, lipids, dietary fiber, and fluids. After jejunal resections, the ileum typically adapts to perform the functions of the jejunum. The motility of the ileum is comparatively slow, and hormones secreted in the ileum and colon help to slow gastric emptying and secretions. Because jejunal resections result in reduced surface area and faster intestinal transit, the functional reserve for absorption of micronutrients, excess amounts of sugars (especially lactose), and lipids is reduced.

Ileal resections. Significant resections of the ileum, especially the distal ileum, produce major nutritional and medical complications. The distal ileum is the only site for absorption of bile salts and the vitamin B_{12}-intrinsic factor complex. The ileum also absorbs a major portion of the 7 to 10 L of fluid ingested and secreted into the GI tract daily (see Chapter 1). The ileocecal valve, at the junction of the ileum and cecum, maximizes nutrient absorption by controlling the rate of passage of ileal contents into the colon and preventing reflux of colonic bacteria, which may decrease risk for SIBO.

Although malabsorption of bile salts may appear to be benign, it creates a cascade of consequences. If the ileum cannot "recycle" bile salts secreted into the GI tract, hepatic production cannot maintain a sufficient bile salt pool or the secretions to emulsify lipids. The gastric and pancreatic lipases are capable of digesting some triglycerides to fatty acids and monoglycerides, but, without adequate micelle formation facilitated by bile salts, lipids are poorly absorbed. This can lead to malabsorption of fats and fat-soluble vitamins A, D, E, and K. In addition, malabsorption of fatty acids results in their combination with calcium, zinc, and magnesium to form fatty acid–mineral soaps, thus leading to their malabsorption as well. To compound matters, colonic absorption of oxalate is increased, leading to hyperoxaluria and increased frequency of renal oxalate stones. Relative dehydration and concentrated urine, which are common with ileal resections, further increase the risk of stone formation (see Chapter 34).

Colon Resections

The colon (approximately 5 ft long) is responsible for reabsorbing 1 to 1.5 L of electrolyte-rich (particularly sodium and chloride) fluid each day but is capable of adapting to increase this capacity to 5 to 6 L daily. Preservation of colon is key to maintaining hydration status.

However, if the patient has any colon left, malabsorption of bile salts can act as a mucosal irritant, increasing colonic motility with fluid and electrolyte losses. Consumption of high-fat diets with ileal resections and retained colon also may result in the formation of hydroxy fatty acids, which also increase fluid loss. Cholesterol gallstones occur because the ratio of bile acid, phospholipid, and cholesterol in biliary secretions is altered. Dependence on PN increases the risk of biliary "sludge," secondary to decreased stimulus for evacuation of the biliary tract (see Chapters 12 and 28).

Medical and Surgical Management of Resections

The first step in management is assessment of the remaining bowel length from patient surgical and health records or interview. Assessment should quantify dietary intake, as well as stool and urine output, over 24 hours. Medications and hydration status should be assessed. Medications may be prescribed to slow GI motility, decrease secretions, increase absorption with the remaining bowel, or treat bacterial overgrowth. The primary "gut slowing" medications include loperamide and occasionally narcotic medications, such as tincture of opium and liquid codeine. Somatostatin and somatostatin analogs; growth hormone; and other hormones with antisecretory, antimotility, or trophic actions have been studied for use to slow motility and secretions. Further, glucagon-like peptide analog, Teduglutide, carries the unique ability to enhance absorptive capacity in an attempt to reduce or eliminate the need for PN (Kim and Keam, 2017). Surgical procedures such as creation of reservoirs ("pouches") to serve as a form of colon, intestinal lengthening, and intestinal transplant have been performed to help patients with major GI resections. Intestinal transplant is very complex and is reserved for gut failure, or when patients develop significant complications from PN.

Medical Nutrition Therapy

Most patients who have significant bowel resections require PN initially to restore and maintain nutrition status. The duration of PN and subsequent nutrition therapy will be based on the extent of the bowel resection, the health of the patient, and the condition of the remaining GI tract. In general, older patients with major ileal resections, patients who have lost the ileocecal valve, and patients with residual disease in the remaining GI tract do not do as well. Enteral feeding provides a trophic stimulus to the GI tract; PN is used to restore and maintain nutrient status.

The more extreme and severe the problem, the slower the progression to a normal diet. Small, frequent mini meals (six to ten per day) are likely to be better tolerated than larger feedings. Tube feeding may be useful to maximize intake when a patient would not typically eat, such as during the night (see Chapter 12). Because of malnutrition and disuse of the GI tract, the digestive and absorptive functions of the remaining GI tract may be compromised, and malnutrition will delay postsurgical adaptation. The transition to more normal foods may take weeks to months, and some patients may never tolerate normal concentrations or volumes of foods and always require supplemental PN to maintain adequate fluid and nutritional status.

Maximum adaptation of the GI tract may take 1 to 2 years after surgery. Adaptation improves function, but it does not restore the intestine to normal length or capacity. Complex, intact nutrients (vs. elemental/ pre-digested formulas) are the most important stimuli of the GI tract. Other nutritional measures also have been studied as a means of hastening the adaptive process and decreasing malabsorption, but their evidence for use is limited. For example, the amino acid gluta-mine is the preferred fuel for small intestinal enterocytes and thus may be valuable in enhancing adaptation. Nucleotides (in the form of purines, pyrimidine, ribonucleic acid) also may enhance mucosal

adaptation, but unfortunately they are often lacking in parenteral and enteral nutritional products. SCFAs (e.g., butyrate, propionate, acetate), carbohydrate fermentation byproducts of commensal gut microbiota, are major fuels for the colonic epithelium.

Patients with jejunal resections and an intact ileum and colon will have a good chance of adapting quickly to a normal diet with a balance of protein, fat, and carbohydrate that is satisfactory. Six small feedings with avoidance of lactose, large amounts of concentrated sweets, and caffeine may help to reduce the risk of bloating, abdominal pain, and diarrhea. Because the typical American diet may be nutritionally lacking, and the intake of some micronutrients may be marginal, patients should be advised that the quality of the diet is of utmost importance. A multivitamin and mineral supplement may be required to meet nutritional needs.

Patients with ileal resections require increased time and patience in the advancement from PN to EN. Because of losses, fat-soluble vitamins, calcium, magnesium, and zinc may have to be supplemented. Dietary fat may have to be limited, especially in those with little remaining colon. Small amounts at each feeding are more likely to be tolerated and absorbed.

MCT products add to the caloric intake and serve as a vehicle for lipid-soluble nutrients. Because boluses of MCT oil (e.g., taken as a medication in tablespoon amounts) may add to the patient's diarrhea, it is best to divide the doses equally in feedings throughout the day. Fluid and electrolytes, especially sodium, should be provided in small amounts and frequently.

In patients with SBS an oral diet or EN plus the use of gut-slowing medications should be maximized to prevent dependence on PN. Frequent meals, removal of osmotic medications and foods, use of oral hydration therapies, and other interventions should be pursued. In some cases, overfeeding in an attempt to compensate for malabsorption results in further malabsorption, not only of ingested foods and liquids but also of the significant amounts of GI fluids secreted in response to food ingestion. Patients with an extremely short bowel may depend on parenteral solutions for at least part of their nutrient and fluid supply. Small, frequent snacks provide some oral gratification for these patients, but typically they can supply only a portion of their fluid and nutrient needs (see Chapter 12 for discussion of home PN).

Small Intestine Bacterial Overgrowth

Small intestinal bacterial overgrowth (SIBO) is a syndrome characterized by overproliferation of bacteria normally found in the large intestine within the small intestine. In a normally functioning bowel, a number of physiologic processes limit the number of bacteria in the small intestine. Among these, gastric acid, bile, and pancreatic enzymes have bacteriostatic and bactericidal action within the small bowel. Normal intestinal peristalsis leads to bowel motility that effectively "sweeps" bacteria into the distal bowel. The ileocecal valve prevents retrograde migration of the large numbers of colonic bacteria into the small intestine. SIBO also has been referred to as "blind loop syndrome" because one cause of bacterial overgrowth can result from stasis of the intestinal tract as a result of obstructive disease, strictures, adhesions (scar tissue), radiation enteritis, or surgical procedures that leave a portion of bowel without normal flow (a blind loop or Roux limb).

Etiology

Frequently, more than one of the normal homeostatic defenses listed previously must be impaired before small intestine bacteria overproliferate to the point that symptoms develop. Chronic use of antibiotics or medications that suppress gastric acid allow more ingested bacteria to survive and pass into the small bowel. Liver diseases or chronic pancreatitis can decrease the production or flow into the bowel of bile and pancreatic enzymes that control bacterial growth. Gastroparesis, narcotic medications, or bowel dysmotility disorders decrease peristalsis and can impair the ability to propel bacteria to the distal bowel. Surgical resection of the distal ileum and ileocecal valve can result in retrograde proliferation of colonic bacteria. Research also demonstrates that SIBO is a common problem for patients with IBS-D (diarrhea predominant) (Palmer et al, 2017).

Pathophysiology

Although symptoms vary depending on the amount and type of bacteria present in the small intestine, the most common symptoms of SIBO include gas, bloating, nausea, constipation, diarrhea, abdominal pain and discomfort (especially after eating), and weight loss. Bacteria within the small bowel also deconjugate bile salts, resulting in impaired formation of micelles and thus impaired fat digestion and steatorrhea. Carbohydrate malabsorption occurs because of injury to the brush border secondary to the toxic effects of bacterial products and consequent enzyme loss (Palmer et al, 2017). The expanding numbers of bacteria use the available vitamin B_{12} and other nutrients for their own growth, and the host becomes deficient. Bacteria within the small bowel produce folate as a byproduct of their metabolism, and vitamin B_{12} deficiency with normal or elevated serum folate is common. Bloating and distention also are reported frequently in SIBO, resulting from the action of bacteria on carbohydrates with production of hydrogen and methane within the small bowel.

D-lactic acidosis or D-lactate encephalopathy is a rare complication of SIBO in SBS patients with the colon in continuity and ileocecal valve removed. In these individuals, malabsorption of a large carbohydrate load can lead to excess carbohydrates being delivered to the bacteria in the colon. A lower colonic pH, induced by a large production of lactate and SCFAs, promotes growth of acid-resistant bacteria that go on to produce D-lactate. Because of the lack of D-lactate dehydrogenase, humans cannot metabolize D-lactate and symptoms of D-lactic acidosis develop. These can range from lethargy to altered mental status, ataxia, and slurred speech to aggression and coma (Htyte et al, 2011; White, 2015).

Medical Treatment

The most common pathway for medical diagnosis of SIBO is a lactulose breath test which measures levels of breath hydrogen and methane. Higher levels correlate with bacterial overgrowth in the small intestine (Rezaie et al, 2017; Palmer et al, 2017). A more invasive, small bowel aspirate and culture is the traditional gold standard. Testing for SIBO in patients with SBS may present more challenges. Some clinicians treat based on symptomatology reports in combination with preexisting risk factors. Treatment is directed toward control of the bacterial growth by administration of antibiotics or herbs or the use of an elemental diet. Historically, the most favored antibiotics have included rifaximin, metronidazole, ciprofloxacin, amoxicillin/clavulanate, or doxycycline. Treatment may involve cycling of several antibiotics until improvement of symptoms is observed (Rezaie et al, 2016). Unfortunately, recurrences can occur, warranting further treatment (Palmer et al, 2017). Typically, a 7- to 10-day course of antibiotics is successful, but some patients may require 1 to 2 months of treatment (Bohm et al, 2013). The antibiotic should be rotated to prevent bacterial resistance. There is some evidence that specific herbal preparations may be as beneficial as antibiotic therapies in the treatment of SIBO (Mullin, 2014). Research is ongoing with regard to pairing probiotics and antibiotic therapies.

Medical Nutrition Therapy

Dietary modification should target alleviation of symptoms and correction of nutrient deficiencies. With bacterial overgrowth in the small intestine, carbohydrates reaching the site where microbes are harbored serve as fuel for their proliferation, with subsequent increased production of gases and organic acids. A low FODMAP diet (previously discussed in IBS section) has the most evidence for reducing GI symptoms in SIBO. If the patient exhibits more severe carbohydrate sensitivity, a more restrictive specific carbohydrate diet (SCD) or a combination of both could be tried. In extreme cases, medically supervised elemental diets may be recommended along with the antibiotics until remission is achieved. Close support and monitoring of a trained nutrition professional is always recommended as an adjunct to medical treatments as noted above. More information can be found at Monash University at https://www.monash.edu, https://www.katescarlata.com, and SIBO Center for Digestive Health at https://sibocenter.com/category/sibo-diets/.

An assessment of the medical problem and the patient's dietary intake is necessary, as vitamin B_{12} may be lost in fermentation; the diet may lack key dietary nutrients; or the absence or removal of greater than 60 cm of the terminal ileum has occurred, putting the patient at risk for deficiencies. A routine intramuscular vitamin B_{12} may be required. If bile salts are being degraded, as in the case of blind loop syndrome, MCTs may be helpful if they provide a source of lipid and energy. Deficiencies of fat-soluble vitamins A, D, and E are of concern if fat malabsorption is present, and a water miscible version of these critical fat-soluble nutrients should be considered.

Fistula

A fistula is an abnormal passage of an organ to another organ, skin, or wound. An enterocutaneous fistula (ECF) is an abnormal passage from a portion of the intestinal tract to the skin or to a wound (e.g., colocutaneous fistula between the large intestine and the skin).

Etiology

Fistulas may occur in any part of the GI tract but are most common in the small and large intestine. ECF can be classified several ways: by volume of output per day, cause (surgical vs. spontaneous), site of origin, and number of fistula tracts. Surgery accounts for the majority of ECF development and usually manifests 7 to 10 days postoperatively. Fistulas of the intestinal tract can be serious threats to nutrition status because large amounts of fluids and electrolytes are lost, and malabsorption and sepsis can occur. Box 27.11 lists conditions associated with fistula development.

Medical Treatment

Wound care, resuscitation, source control, and the use of nutrition support during the healing phase are the primary approaches for

---

BOX 27.11   Conditions Associated With Fistula Development

Bowel resection for cancer
Bowel resection for inflammatory bowel disease
Surgery for pancreatitis
Surgery on radiated bowel
Emergent surgery
Surgical wound dehiscence
Inflammatory bowel disease (Crohn's disease or ulcerative colitis)
Radiation enteritis
Bowel ischemia
Diverticular disease

Data from Frantz D et al: Gastrointestinal disease. In Mueller CM et al, editors: The ASPEN Adult Nutrition Support Core Curriculum, ed 2, Silver Spring, Md, 2012, American Society for Parenteral and Enteral Nutrition.

medical treatment (Bhutiani et al, 2017). A fistulogram is considered the gold standard for identifying the location and route of the fistulous tract. Fluid and electrolyte balance must be restored, infection must be brought under control, and aggressive nutrition support may be necessary to permit spontaneous closure or to maintain optimal nutritional status before surgical closure.

Medical Nutrition Therapy

Nutrition management of patients with ECF can be very challenging. Initial management may include keeping the patient *nil per os* (NPO) as fistula output is quantified and administering nutritional support during the initial workup phase. PN, EN, oral diet, or a combination is used in patients with ECF. The decision regarding which route to feed patients with ECF depends on several factors, including the origin of the fistula, the presence of obstructions or abscesses, the length of functional bowel, the likelihood of fistula closure, the ability to manage fistula output, and the patient's overall medical condition (see Chapter 12).

Intestinal Ostomies

The word ostomy, derived from the Latin word *ostium*, refers to mouth or opening. An intestinal ostomy is a surgically created opening between the intestinal tract and the skin and is specifically named according to the site of origin along the intestinal tract. About 100,000 people in the United States undergo operations that result in a colostomy or ileostomy each year (Sheetz et al, 2014). The high incidence of ostomy is due in part to the increasing prevalence of CRC and diverticular surgeries in the United States. Ostomies are created for many reasons; Table 27.7 lists indications for the creation of ostomies.

Colostomies and ileostomies can be categorized as either loop or end ostomies. A loop ostomy is formed when a loop of bowel is brought up to the skin, and an incision is made on one side. The distal end is sutured to the skin, whereas the proximal side of the loop is everted back on itself (Martin and Vogel, 2012). The result is a stoma with two openings: the proximal (functional) limb from which the effluent or stool is discharged, and the distal limb, which may connect to the anus and secrete mucus. A loop ostomy is used most often when a

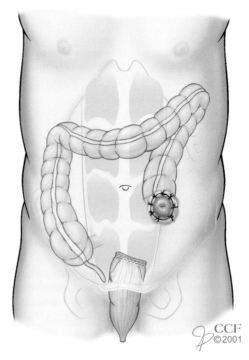

Fig. 27.6 Colostomy. (Cleveland Clinic, Cleveland, Ohio, USA.)

temporary ostomy is formed. An end ostomy is created when the bowel is cut and the end is brought through the skin to create the stoma. End and loop ostomies are potentially reversible. The output from an ileostomy is termed effluent, whereas output from a colostomy is stool.

Colostomy

A colostomy is a surgically created opening from the colon to the skin when a portion of the large intestine is removed or bypassed (Fig. 27.6). It can originate from any part of the colon: ascending, transverse, descending, or sigmoid. It typically starts functioning 2 to 5 days after surgery and the amount and type of output varies slightly, depending on the amount of remaining colon. Stool from a colostomy on the left side of the colon is firmer than that from a colostomy on the right side, with stool output ranging from 200 to 600 mL/day. Patients with sigmoid colostomies have elimination patterns similar to their preoperative states, usually one to two soft stools daily.

Ileostomy

An ileostomy is a surgically created opening from the distal small bowel (most often the terminal ileum) to the skin when the entire colon, rectum, and anus are removed or bypassed (Fig. 27.7). Typically, a new ileostomy will start functioning within 24 hours after surgery, and the effluent is initially bilious in color and watery (Willcutts and Touger-Decker, 2013). Stoma output increases initially to about 1200 mL per 24 hours for the first 1 to 2 weeks. As the bowel adapts over the next 2 to 3 months, the effluent thickens (semiliquid to porridge-like consistency) and output drops to less than a liter per day.

Medical Management

Management of a new ostomy patient involves maintenance of nutritional and hydration status, meticulous skin care, and adequate

TABLE 27.7 Potential Indications for Creation of Intestinal Ostomy	
Ileostomy	**Colostomy**
Crohn's disease	Colon cancer
Ulcerative colitis	Rectal cancer
FAP	Diverticulitis
Colon cancer	Rectal trauma
Rectal cancer	Radiation proctitis
Bowel perforation	Distal obstruction
Bowel ischemia	Fecal incontinence
Rectal trauma	Complex fistula
Fecal incontinence	
Fecal diversion	
Colonic dysmotility	
Toxic colitis	
Anastomotic leak	
Distal obstruction	
Enterocutaneous fistula	

FAP, Familial adenomatous polyposis.

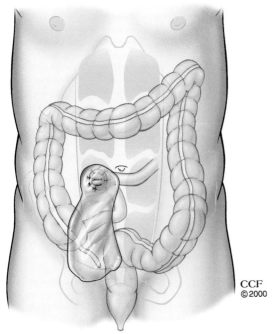

Fig. 27.7 Ileostomy. (Cleveland Clinic, Cleveland, Ohio, USA.)

containment of the fecal stream using a pouching system in the hospital and as the patient transitions to home (McDonough, 2013). It is very helpful when a patient is evaluated by an enterostomal therapist (a nurse who specializes in the care of stomas) before surgery to mark the most appropriate site for an ostomy. This minimizes potential skin and pouch system problems. A poorly constructed ostomy can cause skin excoriation and difficulty with pouch application and may significantly affect patient quality of life (QoL). A well-functioning ostomy is associated with a superior QoL. In those patients who express concerns regarding suboptimal QoL, social restrictions, psychosexual issues, and fear of the ostomy appliance leaking seem to be the major limiting factors (Charua-Guindic et al, 2011).

Medical Nutrition Therapy

Traditional recommendations for postoperative feeding of patients with either a colostomy or ileostomy was to hold feeding until the bowel started to "function" or put out stool or effluent. However, there is evidence that an oral diet or tube feeding can start early after surgery for any type of fecal diversion stoma that was created during an elective surgery. The AND and the United Ostomy Associations of America recommend a low-fiber diet for approximately 6 to 8 weeks after surgery (AND, 2014; United Ostomy Associations of America, 2011). This advice is based on the premise that the bowel is edematous and therefore at risk for being damaged and or becoming obstructed after surgery. Most patients transition to a normal diet with a gradual increase in dietary fiber intake after 6 weeks.

Vitamin B_{12} and bile salts or fat malabsorption are normally not a concern with a distal ileostomy. Greater than 100 cm of ileum must be resected before steatorrhea or fat-soluble vitamin deficiency occurs, and greater than 60 cm must be resected before vitamin B_{12} absorption is compromised (Parrish and DiBaise, 2014).

Controlling flatus and odor is a common concern for the colostomy patient rather than for a patient with an ileostomy. Many patients

elect to limit foods that have the potential to increase flatus or cause increased odor of stool output. A patient must experiment with how different foods affect output. Deodorants are available, and ostomy appliances are made with odor-barrier material and can include charcoal filters that vent and deodorize gas.

Another concern for an ileostomy is the potential for intestinal blockage or obstruction at the stoma site resulting from narrowing of the intestinal lumen at the point where the ileum is brought through the abdominal wall. Patients are instructed to chew their food very well to reduce the chance of blockage. Ileostomy patients with higher volumes of watery effluent are encouraged to incorporate thickening foods to help thicken stoma output. The patient may have to experiment because thickened output may be desirable at times but can cause discomfort if output is thickened too much. Refer to Table 27.8 for the effects of various foods on ostomy output.

TABLE 27.8	Foods That Affect Ostomy Output	
Gas-Forming Foods	**Odor-Producing Foods**	**Foods That May Control Odor**
Broccoli	Asparagus	Buttermilk
Brussels sprouts	Beans	Cranberry juice
Cabbage	Broccoli	Orange juice
Cauliflower	Brussels sprouts	Yogurt
Garlic	Cabbage	Parsley
Onions	Cauliflower	Spinach
Fish	Garlic	Tomato juice
Eggs	Onions	
Carbonated beverages	Fish	
Alcoholic beverages	Eggs	
Dairy products	Some vitamins	
Legumes (dried beans)	Strong cheese	
Chewing gum		
Foods That May Thicken Stool	**Foods That May Cause Obstruction**	**Foods That May Cause Diarrhea**
Pasta	Apple peel	Alcoholic beverages
White bread	Orange	Caffeinated fluids
White rice	Pineapple	Chocolate
Potatoes	Grapes	Whole grains
Cheese	Dried fruits	Bran cereals
Pretzels	Raw cabbage	Fresh fruits
Creamy peanut butter	Raw celery	Grape juice
Applesauce	Chinese vegetables	Prune juice
Banana	Corn	Raw vegetables
Marshmallow	Mushrooms	Spicy foods
Tapioca	Coconut	Fried foods
	Popcorn	High-fat foods
	Nuts	Foods high in refined sugar or sorbitol

Data from Academy of Nutrition and Dietetics: *Nutrition Care Manual, Ileostomy* (website): http://nutritioncaremanual.org/, 2018.
McDonough MR: A dietitian's guide to colostomies and ileostomies, *Support Line* 35(3):3, 2013; United Ostomy Associations of America: Diet and Nutrition Guide (website): http://www.ostomy.org/ostomy_info/pubs/OstomyNutritionGuide.pdf, 2011; Willcutts K et al: Ostomies and fistulas: a collaborative approach, *Pract Gastroenterol* 29:63, 2005.

Maintenance of adequate fluid and electrolyte status is an important nutrition-related issue in managing a patient with colostomy or ileostomy. Patients with an ileostomy must recognize the symptoms of dehydration and understand the importance of maintaining adequate fluid intake throughout the day. In addition, patients may have to increase their salt, potassium, and magnesium intake resulting from losses in ileostomy output.

Ostomy output may become acutely or chronically elevated, and this is much more common with an ileostomy. The generally accepted definition of a high-output stoma (HOS) is output that exceeds 2000 mL/day over 3 consecutive days, at which point water, sodium, and magnesium depletion are expected (Baker et al, 2011). There are multiple potential causes of HOS, including IBD, *Clostridium difficile*, intraabdominal sepsis, partial or intermittent obstruction, medication-related causes, drinking too much fluid (especially hypertonic/hyperosmotic fluids), or surgery that results in less than 200 cm of residual small bowel and no colon (Parrish and DiBaise, 2014).

Management of HOS includes assessment and correction of depleted electrolytes and minerals; initiation of an ORS sipped throughout the day; avoidance of hypertonic, simple sugar–containing liquids and foods; restriction of foods high in insoluble fiber; separation of solids and liquids at meals; and consumption of smaller meals, more often (up to six to eight per day) (McDonough, 2013; Parrish and DiBaise, 2014). Malnutrition can occur in cases of persistent HOS, and many patients must increase their intake to maintain their nutritional status. Meeting the increased nutritional demand may not be possible via oral means for some patients, and nutrition support via enteral tube feeding may become necessary. Antidiarrheal and antisecretory medications are the two major classes of medications recommended to reduce output in HOS.

Restorative Proctocolectomy with Ileal Pouch Anal Anastomosis

Restorative proctocolectomy with ileal pouch anal anastomosis (IPAA) has evolved as the surgical treatment of choice for patients with medically refractory UC and FAP. For UC patients requiring a colectomy, the majority elect to have an IPAA. This procedure involves removal of the entire colon and rectum (proctocolectomy) while preserving the anal sphincter, followed by creation of a reservoir using a portion of the distal ileum (ileal pouch). This pouch is then reconnected (pouch-anal anastomosis) to the preserved anal canal in which the diseased mucosa has been removed, thus maintaining continence and voluntary function. This offers a cure for the disease processes and avoids a permanent ileostomy.

Construction usually requires use of the distalmost 30 to 40 cm of ileum, with pouch configuration determined by the number of bowel limbs used. The most common pouch is the ileal J-pouch, which uses two limbs of bowel (Fig. 27.8) to create a "J"-shaped reservoir out of the patient's own small intestine. It is the preferred ileal pouch because of the efficiency of construction and optimal functional results by allowing a more normal route of defecation. Alternatives to the J-pouch configuration include three- and four-limbed pouches, such as an S-pouch or W-pouch. These alternative configurations are rarely performed because of the complexity of construction. The final decision as to which type is used remains at the discretion of the surgeon.

With any pouch surgery the recovery is longer than in those who have a conventional ileostomy because of the two-stage procedure. There will be a period of adaptation of the new reservoir after the ileostomy is closed. Initially, there could be up to 15 bowel movements a

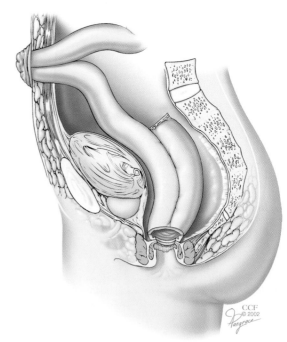

Fig. 27.8 J-pouch. (Cleveland Clinic, Cleveland, Ohio, USA.)

day with some problems of control and the need to get up several times at night. Eventually, most patients experience four to six bowel movements daily, have good control, and are not troubled by nighttime incontinence. This improves over time as the pouch capacity gradually increases.

A Koch pouch is a type of appliance-less ileostomy that uses an internal reservoir with a one-way valve, constructed from a loop of intestine that is attached to the abdominal wall with a skin-level stoma. Patients must insert a tube or catheter into the stoma to open the valve and allow drainage of the ileostomy contents. The technical difficulties of surgical construction and the potential for complications has led to decreased use of the Koch pouch in favor of the ileal J-pouch.

Medical Management

Acute and chronic complications can necessitate removal of the ileal pouch and eventual construction of a permanent ileostomy. Pouchitis is a nonspecific inflammation of the mucosal tissue forming the ileal pouch and is the most frequent long-term complication of IPAA in patients with UC. The cause of pouchitis is not entirely clear, but it may be related to bacterial overgrowth, unrecognized Crohn's disease, immunologic changes, bile salt malabsorption, or insufficient SCFA production. The usual presenting symptoms include increased stool frequency, urgency, incontinence, nocturnal seepage, abdominal cramps, and pelvic discomfort. Pouchitis may be classified based on the cause, disease duration and activity, and response to medical therapy. In the majority of patients the etiology of pouchitis is not clear and thus termed as idiopathic pouchitis (Zezos and Saibil, 2015).

Pouch endoscopy is the main modality in the diagnosis and differential diagnosis in patients with pouch dysfunction. Antibiotic therapy is the mainstay of treatment for active pouchitis. Some patients may develop dependency on antibiotics, requiring long-term maintenance therapy. The evidence for the use of probiotics in maintenance treatment of pouchitis is controversial. There may be roles for postoperative probiotic supplementation to prevent pouchitis and in maintaining remission in antibiotic-dependent pouchitis (Shen et al, 2014). Clinical expert-generated guidelines concur that the probiotic called VSL#3 can be effective for preventing recurrence of pouchitis (Ciorba, 2012; Shen et al, 2014).

Medical Nutrition Therapy

Patients who have undergone an IPAA procedure usually require supplemental vitamin B_{12} injections. The cause of vitamin B_{12} deficiency may be multifactorial: (1) reduced absorptive capacity due to distal ileal resection (main site of vitamin B_{12} absorption); (2) bacterial overgrowth is a well-known phenomenon in patients with an ileal pouch, and anaerobic bacteria can bind vitamin B_{12} in its free and intrinsic forms, leading to a decreased concentration available for absorption; and (3) insufficient B_{12} intake. The anemia experienced by patients after IPAA can also be due to iron deficiency because of impaired absorption, decreased oral intake, increased requirements, and blood loss.

Patients with a pouch often describe specific food sensitivities that may require diet alteration, even more so than do patients with permanent ileostomy (United Ostomy Associations of America, 2011). Problems often reported include obstructive symptoms and increased stool output, frequency, and gas. The incidence of obstruction may be avoided by limiting insoluble fibers, chewing thoroughly, and consuming small meals frequently throughout the day. Patients may try to experiment with timing of meals by eating larger meals earlier in the day and limiting the amount of food and fluid intake toward the end of the day to minimize sleep interruptions. The same dietary measures that are used to reduce excessive stool output (reduced caffeine, lactose avoidance if lactase-deficient, and limitation of foods high in simple sugars, fructose, and sorbitol) will likely reduce stool volume and frequency in patients with IPAA.

CLINICAL CASE STUDY

Jimmy is a 76-year-old male with a recent emergent small bowel resection due to a ruptured mesh hernia causing traumatic injury to his small intestine. He had a difficult postoperative course complicated by *Clostridium difficile* infection, clinically involuntary weight loss, diarrhea, and dehydration. At his readmission for *C. difficile* infection, a nutrition consult was received for management of diarrhea and hydration status, and to assess for any nutrient malabsorption.

Nutrition Assessment

- Anatomy: During surgery, 100 cm of the small intestine was removed, including the ileocecal valve (ICV). The majority of the colon remains intact.
- Oral intake history: Decline in appetite and oral intake since surgery due to very poor appetite and diarrhea. Before admission Jimmy was eating ¼ of his usual meals with ½ of the usual snacks and taking one oral nutrition supplement per day. Fluids: drinks coffee, iced tea, and water, and estimates he is taking in 3 to 4 cups per day.
- Current intake: In the hospital, Jimmy is eating 50% of meals provided, tolerating snacks, and sipping up to 500 mL of commercial electrolyte beverage per day. He reports never feeling hungry, is apathetic about eating, and reports not wanting to "overdo it" for fear of more bathroom trips.
- Weight and body mass index (BMI): Height: 177.8 cm (70 inches), Weight: 75 kg (165 lb), BMI: 23.7 kg/m²
- Usual body weight (UBW): 100 kg (220 lb): 25% weight loss × 3 months (clinically significant loss)
- Physical examination: pale skin; dark eye sockets; slight depression at temples; scapula pronounced; noted losses at quadriceps, gastrocnemius, and triceps; no edema noted
- Functional capacity: low energy level over past 3 months, unable to garden or cook meals, which he previously enjoyed, fatigued and tired all the time, memory slightly decreased
- Medications: started loperamide 2 mg before meals and bedtime, senior multivitamin, potassium chloride (KCl) sustained-release tablet, lisinopril dose reduced due to weight loss, statin discontinued due to cholesterol levels normalized within a few months of surgery
- 24-hour urine and stool output: 650 mL and 2200 mL
- Pertinent labs: high serum sodium (147), low serum potassium (3.0 mEq/L), low normal serum magnesium (1.3), high blood urea nitrogen (BUN): 7.6 mmol/L, stool toxin analysis for *C difficile*: positive
- Current diet: General diet

Nutrition Diagnostic Statements

- Severe protein calorie malnutrition related to poor appetite as evidenced by energy intake 25% to 50% × 3 months, involuntary weight loss at 25% × 3 months, subcutaneous fat loss, muscle loss, and decline in strength and functional capacity
- Suboptimal protein-energy intake related to altered gastrointestinal (GI) function as evidenced by diarrhea, involuntary weight loss at 25% × 3 months, UBW 220 lbs

Interventions

- Estimated energy needs: 2625 to 3000 calories/day (35 to 40 kcal/kg/day)
- Estimated protein needs: 115 to 150 g protein/day (1.5 to 2.0 g protein/kg/day)
- Nutrition goal(s): Oral intake to meet estimated needs, decrease stool output to the point where patient's hydration is maintained; maintain optimal micronutrient status.
- Replace electrolyte and fluid losses. Monitor fluid balance.
- Continue general diet with moderate insoluble fiber until diarrhea is under control, reduce simple sugars in the diet. Patient to make high-salt, high-starch, low-simple sugar food choices from the menu. Encourage separation of beverages at mealtimes.
- Provide salty/starchy snacks between meals. Encourage "thickening foods," such as boiled white rice, pasta, noodles, bread, potatoes, banana, oatmeal, applesauce, peanut butter, cheese, and tapioca pudding.
- Sip 2 L of oral rehydration solution (ORS) between meals as an alternative to commercial electrolyte beverage.
- Avoid caffeinated and hypertonic fluids.
- Consider trial of soluble fiber supplement to slow down transit time and thicken stool.
- Continue antidiarrheal medications with dosage adjusted by physician depending on volume and consistency of stool.
- Diet education: Discuss with patient and family nutrition management of micronutrient status, including intake of water-miscible versions of fat-soluble vitamins, and vitamin B_{12} shots monthly, and maintaining adequate weight and hydration status with changed bowel length.
- Recommend outpatient follow up with nutrition professional specializing in GI nutrition.
- Evaluate micronutrient status.

Monitoring and Evaluation

- Monitor oral intake via calorie counts with a goal of meeting 75% to 100% of estimated energy and protein needs.
- Monitor stool and urinary output and weight trends to assess need for home intravenous fluids (HIVF) or home parenteral nutrition (HPN) if weight and fluid status do not stabilize with increased intake and ORS.

USEFUL WEBSITES

Celiac Disease Foundation
Celiac Sprue Association
Crohn's and Colitis Foundation of America
Gluten Intolerance Group
International Scientific Association for Probiotics and Prebiotics
Monash University Low FODMAP Diet
National Institute of Diabetes and Digestive and Kidney Diseases
Nutrition in Immune Balance (NiMBAL)
United Ostomy Associations of America, Inc.
University of Virginia GI Nutrition Support Team
USDA Food Composition Databases
Wound, Ostomy and Continence Nurses Society

REFERENCES

Abraham BP, Quigley EMM: Probiotics in inflammatory bowel disease, *Gastroenterol Clin North Am* 46(4):769–782, 2017.

Academy of Nutrition and Dietetics (AND): *Ileostomy nutrition therapy* (website), 2018. http://nutritioncaremanual.org/index.cfm.

Academy of Nutrition and Dietetics (AND): *Inflammatory bowel disease (IBD) and Crohn's disease nutriiton therapy*, 2019. https://www.nutritioncaremanual.org/index.cfm.

Almallouhi E, King KS, Patel B, et al: Increasing incidence and altered presentation in a population-based study of pediatric celiac disease in North America, *J Pediatr Gastroenterol Nutr* 65:432–437, 2017.

Andrews CN, Storr M: The pathophysiology of chronic constipation, *Can J Gastroenterol* 25(Suppl B):16B–21B, 2011.

Anastasi JK, Capili B, Chang M: Managing irritable bowel syndrome, *Am J Nurs* 113:42–52, 2013.

Antoni L, Nuding S, Wehkamp J, et al: Intestinal barrier in inflammatory bowel disease, *World J Gastroenterol* 20(5):1165–1179, 2014.

Atia AN, Buchman AL: Oral rehydration solutions in non-cholera diarrhea: a review, *Am J Gastroenterol* 104:2596–2604, 2009.

Bafeta A, Koh M, Riveros C, et al: Harms reporting in randomized controlled trials of interventions aimed at modifying microbiota: a systematic review, *Ann Intern Med*, 169(4):240–247, 2018.

Baker ML, Williams RN, Nightingale JM: Causes and management of a high-output stoma, *Colorectal Dis* 3:191–197, 2011.

Barco KT, Alberino MJ, Roberts KM, et al: Chapter 6: Common gastrointestinal symptoms. In Matarese LE, Mullin GE, Raymond JL, editors: *The health professional's guide to gastrointestinal nutrition*, Chicago IL, 2015, Cathy Immartino, pp 63–78.

Barnes EL, Jiang Y, Kappelman MD, et al: Decreasing colectomy rate for ulcerative colitis in the united states between 2007 and 2016: a time trend analysis, *Inflamm Bowel Dis* izz247, 2019. Available at: https://doi.org/10.1093/ibd/izz247.

Barrett JS. How to institute the low-FODMAP Diet. *J Gastroenterol Hepatol* 32(Suppl 1):8–10, 2017.

Besselink MG, van Santvoort HC, Buskens E, et al: Probiotic prophylaxis in predicted severe acute pancreatitis: a randomised, double-blind, placebo-controlled trial, *Lancet* 371:651–659, 2008.

Bhutiani N, Benns MV, Pappas S, et al: Surgical alteration of the gastrointestinal tract. In Mueller CM, editor: *The ASPEN adult nutrition support core curriculum*, ed 3, Silver Spring, MD, 2017, American Society for Parenteral and Enteral Nutrition.

Bohm M, Siwiec RM, Wo JM: Diagnosis and management of small intestinal bacterial overgrowth, *Nutr Clin Pract* 28:289–299, 2013.

Bostick RM: Effects of supplemental vitamin D and calcium on normal colon tissue and circulating biomarkers of risk for colorectal neoplasms, *J Steroid Biochem Mol Biol* 148:86–95, 2015.

Bossuyt P, Vermeire S: Treat to target in inflammatory bowel disease, *Curr Treat Options Gastroenterol* 14:61–72, 2016.

Braly K, Williamson N, Shaffer ML, et al: Nutritional adequacy of the specific carbohydrate diet in pediatric inflammatory bowel disease, *J Pediatr Gastroenterol Nutr* 65(5):553–538, 2017.

Centers for Disease Control and Prevention (CDC): *Healthcare-associated infections - clinicians* (website), 2015. https://www.cdc.gov/hai/organisms/cdiff/cdiff_clinicians.html.

Centers for Disease Control and Prevention (CDC): *Healthcare-associated infections (HAI) progress report* (website), 2018. https://www.cdc.gov/hai/surveillance/progress-report/index.html.

Carabotti M, Annibale B, Severi C et al: Role of fiber in symptomatic uncomplicated diverticular disease: a systematic review, *Nutrients* 9(2):pii: E161, 2017.

Catsos P: *The IBS elimination diet and cookbook*. In Catsos P, editor: New York, 2017, Harmony Books.

Cedars Sinai: *Neurogenic bowel* (website). 2018. https://www.cedars-sinai.org/health-library/diseases-and-conditions/n/neurogenic-bowel.html.

Charúa-Guindic L, Benavides-León CJ, Villanueva-Herrero JA, et al: Quality of life in ostomized patients, *Cir Cir* 79:149–155, 2011.

Chey W, Kurlander J, Eswaran S: Irritable bowel syndrome: a clinical review, *JAMA* 313(9):949–958, 2015.

Chumpitazi BP, Cope JL, Hollister EB, et al: Randomised clinical trial: gut microbiome biomarkers are associated with clinical response to a low FODMAP diet in children with the irritable bowel syndrome, *Aliment Pharmacol Ther* 42:418–427, 2015.

Ciorba MA: A gastroenterologist's guide to probiotics, *Clin Gastroenterol Hepatol* 10:960–968, 2012.

Cresci G, Izzo KM: Gut microbiota. In Mueller CM editor: *ASPEN adult nutrition support core curriculum*, ed 3, Silver Spring, MD, 2017, American Society for Parenteral Enteral Nutrition.

Dahlhamer JM, Zammitti EP, Ward BW, et al: Prevalence of Inflammatory Bowel Disease Among Adults Aged >/= 18 years – United States, 2015. *MMWR Morb Mortal Wkly Rep* 65(42):1166–1169, 2016.

DePestel DD, Aronoff DM: Epidemiology of Clostridium difficile infection, *J Pharm Pract* 26(5):464–475, 2013.

DiBaise JK: Short bowel syndrome and small bowel transplantation, *Curr Opin Gastroenterol* 30:128–133, 2014.

Dupont HL: Review article: evidence for the role of gut microbiota in irritable bowel syndrome and its potential influence on therapeutic targets, *Aliment Pharmacol Ther* 2014;39(10):1033–1042.

Fadgyas-Stanculete M, Buga AM, Popa-Wagner A, et al: The relationship between irritable bowel syndrome and psychiatric disorders: from molecular changes to clinical manifestations, *J Mol Psychiatry* 2(1):4, 2014.

Farrukh A, Mayberry JF: Is there a role for fish oil in inflammatory bowel disease? *World J Clin Cases* 2:250–252, 2014.

Feuerstein JD, Falchuk KR: Diverticulosis and Diverticulitis, *Mayo Clin Proc* 91(8):1094–1104, 2016.

Food and Drug Administration, Health and Human Serices: *Food labeling; gluten-free labeling of foods*, August 2013.

Ford AC, Moayyedi P, Lacy B, et al. American College of Gastroenterology monograph on the management of irritable bowel syndrome and chronic idiopathic constipation, *Am J Gastroenterol* 109:S2–S26, 2014.

Forootan M, Bagheri N, Darvishi M: Chronic constipation: a review of literature, *Medicine (Baltimore)* 97(20):e10631, 2018.

Fu Z, Shrubsole MJ, Smalley WE, et al: Lifestyle factors and their combined impact on the risk of colorectal polyps, *Am J Epidemiol* 176:766–776, 2012.

Ghouri YA, Richards DM, Rahimi EF, et al: Systematic review of randomized controlled trials of probiotics, prebiotics, and synbiotics in inflammatory bowel disease, *Clin Exp Gastroenterol* 7:473–487, 2014.

Gibson PR: Food intolerance in functional bowel disorders, *J Gastroenterol Hepatol* 26(Suppl 3):128–131, 2011.

Gibson PR: History of the low FODMAP diet, *J Gastroenterol Hepatol* 32(Suppl 1):5–7, 2017a.

Gibson PR: The evidence base for efficacy of the low FODMAP diet in irritable bowel syndrome: is it ready for prime time as a first-line therapy? *J Gastroenterol Hepatol* 32(Suppl 1):32–35, 2017b.

Grooms KN, Ommerborn MJ, Pham DQ, et al: Dietary fiber intake and cardiometabolic risks among US adults, NHANES 1999-2010, *Am J Med* 126:1059–1067, 2013.

Halmos EP: When the low FODMAP diet does not work, *J Gastroenterol Hepatol* 32(Suppl 1):69–72, 2017.

Hlavaty T, Krajcovicova A, Payer J: Vitamin D therapy in inflammatory bowel diseases: who, in what form, and how much? *J Crohns Colitis* 9:198–209, 2015.

Hou JK, Lee D, Lewis J: Diet and Inflammatory Bowel Disease: Review of patient-targeted recommendations, *Clin Gastroenterol Hepatol* 12:1592–1600, 2014.

Htyte N, White L, Sandhu G, et al: An extreme and life-threatening case of recurrent D-lactate encephalopathy, *Nephrol Dial Transplant* 26:1432–1435, 2011.

Hutchinson JM, West NP, Robins GG, et al: Long-term histological follow-up of people with coeliac disease in a UK teaching hospital, *QJM* 103:511–517, 2010.

International Foundation for Functional Gastrointestinal Disorders (IFFGD): *About irritable bowel syndrome (IBS)* (website), 2014. http://www.aboutIBS.org.

Ireton-Jones C: The low FODMAP diet: fundamental therapy in the management of irritable bowel syndrome, *Curr Opin Clin Nutr Metab Care* 20(5):414–419, 2017.

K Bailes B, Reeve K: Constipation in older adults, *Nurse Pract* 38:21–25, 2013.

Kakodkar S, Farooqui AJ, Mikolatis SL, et al: The specific carbohydrate diet for inflammatory bowel disease: a case series, *J Acad Nutr Diet* 115(8):1226–1232, 2015.

Kanazawa M, Hongo M, Fukudo S: Visceral hypersensitivity in irritable bowel syndrome, *J Gastroenterol Hepatol* 26(Suppl 3):119–121, 2011.

Kelly CP, Bai JC, Liu E, et al: Advances in diagnosis and management of celiac disease, *Gastroenterology* 148(6):1175–1186, 2015.

Kim ES, Keam SJ: Teduglutide: a review in short bowel syndrome, *Drugs* 77(3):345–352, 2017.

Koff A, Mullin GE: Nutrition in irritable bowel syndrome. In Mullin GE, Matarese LE, Palmer M, editors: *Gastrointestinal and liver disease nutrition desk reference*, Boca Raton, Fla, 2012, CRC Press.

Konturek PC, Koziel J, Dieterich W et al: Successful therapy of Clostridium difficile infection with fecal microbiota transplantation, *J Physiol Pharmacol* 67(6):859–866, 2016.

Kranz S, Brauchla M, Slavin JL, et al: What do we know about dietary fiber intake in children and health? The effects of fiber intake on constipation, obesity, and diabetes in children, *Adv Nutr* 3:47–53, 2012.

Kupfer SS, Jabri B: Pathophysiology of celiac disease, *Gastrointest Endosc Clin N Am* 22:639–660, 2012.

Lacy BE, Mearin F, Chang L, et al: Bowel disorders, *Gastroenterology* 150:1393–1407, 2016.

Lahner E, Bellisario C, Hassan C, et al: Probiotics in the treatment of diverticular disease: a systematic review, *J Gastrointestin Liver Dis* 25:79–86, 2016.

Langenberg MC, Wismans PJ, van Genderen PJ: Distinguishing tropical sprue from celiac disease in returning travellers with chronic diarrhoea: a diagnostic challenge? *Travel Med Infect Dis* 12:401–405, 2014.

Lapides RA, Savaiano DA: Gender, age, race and lactose intolerance: Is there evidence to support a differential symptom response? A scoping review, *Nutrients* 10(12):pii: E1956, 2018.

Lee D, Albenberg L, Compher C, et al: Diet in the pathogenesis and treatment of inflammatory bowel diseases, *Gastroenterology*, 148(6):1087–1106, 2015.

Lee YY, Erdogan A, Rao SS: How to perform and assess colonic manometry and barostat study in chronic constipation, *J Neurogastroenterol Motil* 20:547–552, 2014.

Leonard M, Sapone A, Catassi C, et al: Celiac disease and nonceliac gluten sensitivity: a review, *JAMA* 318:647–656, 2017.

Levitt M, Wilt T, Shaukat A: Clinical implications of lactose malabsorption versus lactose intolerance, *J Clin Gastroenterol* 47:471–480, 2013.

Lewis JD, Albenberg L, Lee D, et al: The importance and challenges of dietary intervention trials for inflammatory bowel disease, *Inflamm Bowel Dis* 23(2):181–191, 2017.

Lewis SJ, Heaton KW: Stool form scale as a useful guide to intestinal transit time, *Scand J Gastroenterol* 32(9):920–924, 1997.

Limketkai BN, Hurt RT, Palmer LB: Short bowel syndrome. In Mueller CM editor: *The ASPEN adult nutrition support core curriculum*, ed 3, Silver Spring, MD, 2017, American Society for Parenteral Enteral Nutrition.

Lomer MC: Review article: the aetiology, diagnosis, mechanisms and clinical evidence for food intolerance, *Aliment Pharmacol Ther* 41:262–275, 2015.

Longstreth GF, Thompson WG, Chey WD, et al: Functional bowel disorders, *Gastroenterology* 130:1480–1491, 2006.

Maguire LH, Song M, Strate LL, et al: Association of geographic and seasonal variation with diverticulitis admissions, *JAMA Surg* 150:74–77, 2015.

Mao EJ, Hazlewood GS, Kaplan GG, et al: Systematic review with meta-analysis: comparative efficacy of immunosuppressants and biologics for reducing hospitalisation and surgery in Crohn's disease and ulcerative colitis, *Aliment Pharmacol Ther* 45(1):3–13, 2017.

Martin ST, Vogel JD: Intestinal stomas: indications, management, and complications, *Adv Surg* 46:19–49, 2012.

May-Ling Tjon J, van Bergen J, Koning F: Celiac disease: how complicated can it get? *Immunogenetics* 62(10):641–651, 2010.

McDonough MR: A dietitian's guide to colostomies and ileostomies, *Support Line* 35(3):3–12, 2013.

Michielan A, D'Incà R: Intestinal permeability in inflammatory bowel disease; pathogenesis, clinical evaluation, and therapy of Leaky Gut, *Mediators Inflamm* 2015:628157, 2015.

Misselwitz B, Pohl D, Frühauf H, et al: Lactose malabsorption and intolerance: pathogenesis, diagnosis and treatment, *United European Gastroenterol J* 1:151–159, 2013.

Monteleone G, Caruso R, Pallone F: Targets for new immunomodulation strategies in inflammatory bowel disease, *Autoimmun Rev* 13:11–14, 2014.

Morelli L: Yogurt, living cultures, and gut health, *Am J Clin Nutr* 99(Suppl 5):1248S–1250S, 2014.

Mullin G, Shepherd SJ, Roland CB, et al: Irritable bowel syndrome: contemporary nutrition management strategies, *JPEN J Parenter Enteral Nutr* 38(7):781–799, 2014.

Nachman F, del Campo MP, González A, et al: Long-term deterioration of quality of life in adult patients with celiac disease is associated with treatment noncompliance, *Dig Liver Dis* 42:685–691, 2010.

National Cancer Institute: *SEER cancer statistics review* (CSR) 1975-2015: *cancer stat facts: colorectal cancer* (website), 2018. https://seer.cancer.gov/statfacts/html/colorect.html.

Nishida A, Inoue R, Inatomi O, et al: Gut microbiota in the pathogenesis of inflammatory bowel disease, *Clin J Gastroenterol* 11(1):1–10, 2018.

Ohlsson B: New insights and challenges in microscopic colitis, *Therap Adv Gastroenterol* 8:37–47, 2015.

O'Keefe SJ: Tube feeding, the microbiota, and Clostridium difficile infection, *World J Gastroenterol* 16:139–142, 2010.

Olendzki BC, Silverstein TD, Persuitte GM, et al: An anti-inflammatory diet as treatment for inflammatory bowel disease: a case series report, *Nutr J* 13:5, 2014.

Owczarek D, Rodacki T, Domagała-Rodacka R, et al: Diet and nutritional factors in inflammatory bowel diseases, *World J Gastroenterol* 22:895–905, 2016.

Palmer LB, Janas R, Sprang M: Gastrointestinal disease. In Mueller CM editor: *The ASPEN adult nutrition support core curriculum*, ed 3, Silver Spring, MD, 2017, American Society for Parenteral Enteral Nutrition.

Parrish CR, DiBaise JK: Short bowel syndrome in adults- Part 2: nutrition therapy for short bowel syndrome in the adult patient, *Pract Gastroenterol* 138(10):40–51, 2014.

Patel R, DuPont HL: New approaches for bacteriotherapy: prebiotics, new-generation probiotics, and synbiotics, *Clin Infect Dis* 60(Suppl 2):S108–S121, 2015.

Pattani R, Palda VA, Hwang SW, et al: Probiotics for the prevention of antibiotic-associated diarrhea and Clostridium difficile infection among hospitalized patients: systematic review and meta-analysis, *Open Med* 7(2):e56–e67, 2013.

Pavie J, Menotti J, Porcher R, et al: Prevalence of opportunistic intestinal parasitic infections among HIV-infected patients with low CD4 cells counts in France in the combination antiretroviral therapy era, *Int J Infect Dis* 16(9):e677–e679, 2012.

Pinto-Sánchez MI, Causada-Calo N, Bercik P, et al: Safety of adding oats to a gluten-free diet for patients with celiac disease: systematic review and meta-analysis of clinical and observational studies, *Gastroenterology* 153:395–409, 2017.

Prince AC, Myers CE, Joyce T, et al: Fermentable carbohydrate restriction (Low FODMAP diet) in clinical practice improves functional Gastrointestinal symptoms in patients with inflammatory bowel disease, *Inflamm Bowel Dis* 22(5):1129–1136, 2016.

Pronsky ZM, Elbe D, Ayoob K: lubiprostone (Amitza). In Crowe JP, Epstein S, editors: *Food medication interactions*, ed 18, Birchrunville, PA, 2015, Food Medication Interactions, p 208.

Rajindrajith S, Devanarayana NM, Crispus Perera BJ, et al: Childhood constipation as an emerging public health problem, *World J Gastroenterol* 22(30):6864–6875, 2016.

Rezaie A, Buresi M, Lembo A, et al: Hydrogen and Methane-based breath testing in Gastrointestinal Disorders: the North American Consensus, *Am J Gastroenterol* 111:775–784, 2017.

Rezaie A, Pimentel M, Rao SS: How to test and treat small intestinal bacterial overgrowth: an evidence-based approach, *Curr Gastroenterol Rep* 18(2):8, 2016.

Richman E, Rhodes JM: Review article: evidence-based dietary advice for patients with inflammatory bowel disease, *Aliment Pharmacol Ther* 38:1156–1171, 2013.

Sadeghian M, Saneei P, Siassi F, et al: Vitamin D status in relation to Crohn's disease: a meta-analysis of observational studies, *Nutrition* 32:505–514, 2016.

Sahakian AB, Jee SR, Pimentel M: Methane and the gastrointestinal tract, *Dig Dis Sci* 55(8):2135–2143, 2010.

Sams A, Hawks J: Celiac disease as a model for the evolution of multifactorial disease in humans, *Hum Biol* 86:19–36, 2014.

Schoenfeld PS: Advances in IBS 2016: a review of current and emerging data, *Gastroenterol Hepatol (N Y)*, 12(8 Suppl 3):1–11, 2016.

Sharma GM, Pereira M, Williams KM: Gluten detection in foods available in the United States – a market survey, *Food Chem* 169:120–126, 2015.

Shatnawei A, Parekh NR, Rhoda KM, et al: Intestinal failure management at the Cleveland clinic, *Arch Surg* 145:521–527, 2010.

Shaukat A, Levitt MD, Taylor BC: Systematic review: effective management strategies for lactose intolerance, *Ann Intern Med* 152:797–803, 2010.

Sheetz KH, Waits SA, Krell RW, et al: Complication rates of ostomy surgery are high and vary significantly between hospitals, *Dis Colon Rectum* 57:632–637, 2014.

Shen J, Zuo ZX, Mao AP: Effect of probiotics on inducing remission and maintaining therapy in ulcerative colitis, Crohn's disease, and pouchitis: meta-analysis of randomized controlled trials, *Inflamm Bowel Dis* 20(12):2526–2528, 2014.

Shepherd SJ, Gibson PR: Fructose malabsorption and symptoms of irritable bowel syndrome: guidelines for effective dietary management, *J Am Diet Assoc* 106:1631–1639, 2006.

Silberman ES, Jin J. Lactose Intolerance, *JAMA* 322(16):1620, 2019.

Sinagra E, Tomasello G, Cappello F, et al: Probiotics, prebiotics and symbiotics in inflammatory bowel diseases: state-of-the-art and new insights, *J Biol Regul Homeost Agents* 27:919–933, 2013.

Sood R, Ford AC: Diagnosis: rome IV criteria for FGID's – an improvement or more of the same? *Nat Rev Gastroenterol Hepatol* 13:501–502, 2016.

Stasi C, Bellini M, Bassotti G, et al: Serotonin receptors and their role in the pathophysiology and therapy of irritable bowel syndrome, *Tech Coloproctol* 18:613–621, 2014.

Staudacher HM: Nutritional, microbiological and psychosocial implications of the low FODMAP diet, *J Gastroenterology Hepatology* 32(Suppl 1):16–19, 2017.

Stavrou G, Giamarellos-Bourboulis EJ, Kotzampassi K: The role of probiotics in the prevention of severe infections following abdominal surgery, *Int J Antimicrob Agents* 46(Suppl 1):S2–S4, 2015.

Suh JS, Hahn WH, Cho BS: Recent advances of oral rehydration therapy (ORT), *Electrolyte Blood Press* 8(2):82–86, 2010.

Suskind DL: The specific carbohydrate diet: what is it and is if it's right for you. In *Nutrition in immune balance (NIMBAL) therapy*, ed 1, USA, 2016, Nimbal Publishing, LLC.

Szajewska H, Kotodziej M: Systematic review with meta-analysis: *Saccharomyces boulardii* in the prevention of antibiotic-associated diarrhoea, *Aliment Pharmacol Ther* 42(7):793–801, 2015.

Tariq R, Singh S, Gupta A, et al: Association of gastric acid suppression with recurrent Clostridium difficile infection: a systematic review and meta-analysis, *JAMA Intern Med* 177(6):784–791, 2017.

Thompson T: The gluten-free labeling rule: what registered dietitian nutritionists need to know to help clients with gluten-related disorders, *J Acad Nutr Diet* 115:13–16, 2015.

Triantafyllou K, Chang C, Pimentel M: Methanogens, methane and gastrointestinal motility, *J Neurogastroenterol Motil* 20:31–40, 2014.

Trifan A, Stanciu C, Girleanu I, et al: Proton pump inhibitors therapy and risk of Clostridium difficile infection: systematic review and meta-analysis, *World J Gastroenterol* 23(35):6500–6515, 2017.

United Ostomy Associations of America: *Diet and nutrition guide* (website), 2011. https://www.ostomy.org/diet-nutrition/.

Vakil N: Dietary Fermentable Oligosaccharides, Disaccharides, Monosaccharides and Polyols (FODMAPs) and Gastrointestinal disease, *Nutr Clin Pract* 33(4):468–475, 2018.

Wald A: Constipation: advances in diagnosis and treatment, *JAMA* 315:185–191, 2016.

Walsh CJ, Guinane CM, O'Toole PW, et al: Beneficial modulation of the gut microbiota, *FEBS lett* 588(2014):4120–4130, 2014.

Whelan K, Myers CE: Safety of probiotics in patients receiving nutritional support: a systematic review of case reports, randomized controlled trials, and nonrandomized trials, *Am J Clin Nutr* 91:687–703, 2010.

White L: D-Lactic Acidosis: More Prevalent Than We Think? *Pract Gastroenterol, Nutr Issues Gastroenterol* 45:26–45, 2015.

Wikimedia Commons: *File: BristolStoolChart.png* (website), https://commons.wikimedia.org/wiki/File:BristolStoolChart.png. Updated June 18, 2018.

Wilder-Smith CH, Oleson SS, Materna A, et al: Predictors of response to a low-FODMAP diet in patients with functional gastrointestinal disorders and lactose or fructose intolerance, *Aliment Pharmacol Ther* 45(8): 1094–1106, 2017.

Willcutts K, Touger-Decker R: Nutritional management for ostomates, *Top Clin Nutr* 28:373–383, 2013.

World Health Organization: Essential Medicines and Health Products Information Portal - A World Health Organization resource, *WHO Drug Information* 16(2), 2002. Available at: https://apps.who.int/medicinedocs/en/. Updated 2017.

World Health Organization: *Oral rehydration salts* (website), 2006. http://www.who.int/maternal_child_adolescent/documents/fch_cah_06_1/en/. Updated 2018.

Ye Y, Pang Z, Chen W, et al: The epidemiology and risk factors of inflammatory bowel disease, *Int J Clin Exp Med* 8:22529–22542, 2015.

Zezos P, Saibil F: Inflammatory pouch disease: The spectrum of pouchitis, *World J Gastroenterol* 21:8739–8752, 2015.

Medical Nutrition Therapy for Hepatobiliary and Pancreatic Disorders

Jeanette M. Hasse, PhD, RDN, LD, CNSC, FADA
Laura E. Matarese, PhD, RDN, LDN, CNSC, FADA, FASPEN, FAND

KEY TERMS

acalculous cholecystitis
alcoholic liver disease
aromatic amino acids (AAAs)
ascites
bile
branched-chain amino acids (BCAAs)
calculi
cholangitis
cholecystectomy
cholecystitis
choledocholithiasis
cholelithiasis
cholestasis
cirrhosis
detoxification
dry weight
encephalopathy
end stage liver disease (ESLD)

fasting hypoglycemia
fatty liver
fulminant liver disease
hemochromatosis
hepatic encephalopathy
hepatic failure
hepatic osteodystrophy
hepatic steatosis
hepatitis
hepatorenal syndrome
icteric
jaundice
Kayser-Fleischer ring
Kupffer cells
nonalcoholic fatty liver disease
  (NAFLD)
nonalcoholic steatohepatitis (NASH)
oxidative deamination

pancreaticoduodenectomy (Whipple
  procedure)
pancreatic islet autotransplantation
pancreatitis
paracentesis
portal hypertension
portal systemic encephalopathy
postcholecystectomy syndrome
primary biliary cirrhosis (PBC)
primary sclerosing cholangitis (PSC)
secondary biliary cirrhosis
steatorrhea
transamination
varices
Wernicke encephalopathy
Wilson's disease

The liver is of primary importance; one cannot survive without a liver. The liver and pancreas are essential to digestion and metabolism. Although it is important, the gallbladder can be removed, and the body will adapt comfortably to its absence. Knowledge of the structure and functions of these organs is vital. When they are diseased, the necessary medical nutrition therapy (MNT) is complex.

PHYSIOLOGY AND FUNCTIONS OF THE LIVER

Structure

The liver is the largest gland in the body, weighing approximately 1500 g. The liver has two main lobes: the right and left. The right lobe is further divided into the anterior and posterior segments; the right segmental fissure, which cannot be seen externally, separates the segments. The externally visible falciform ligament divides the left lobe into the medial and lateral segments. The liver is supplied with blood from two sources: the hepatic artery, which supplies approximately one third of the blood from the aorta; and the portal vein, which supplies the other two thirds and collects blood drained from the digestive tract.

Approximately 1500 mL of blood per minute circulates through the liver and exits via the right and left hepatic veins into the inferior vena cava. The liver has a system of blood vessels and a series of bile ducts.

Bile, which is formed in the liver cells, exits the liver through a series of bile ducts that increase in size as they approach the common bile duct. Bile is a thick, viscous fluid secreted from the liver, stored in the gallbladder, and released into the duodenum when fatty foods enter the duodenum. It emulsifies fats in the intestine and forms compounds with fatty acids to facilitate their absorption.

Functions

The liver has the ability to regenerate itself. Only 10% to 20% of functioning liver is required to sustain life, although removal of the liver results in death, usually within 24 hours. The liver is integral to most metabolic functions of the body and performs more than 500 tasks. The main functions of the liver include (1) metabolism of carbohydrate, protein, and fat; (2) storage and activation of vitamins and minerals; (3) formation and excretion of bile; (4) conversion of ammonia to urea; (5) metabolism of steroid hormones; (6) detoxification of substances such as drugs, alcohol, and organic compounds; and (7) acting as a filter and flood chamber.

The liver plays a major role in carbohydrate metabolism. Galactose and fructose, products of carbohydrate digestion, are converted into glucose in the hepatocyte (liver cell). The liver stores glucose as glycogen (glycogenesis) and then returns it to the blood when glucose levels become low (glycogenolysis). The liver also produces "new" glucose (gluconeogenesis) from precursors such as lactic acid, glycogenic amino acids, and intermediates of the tricarboxylic acid (TCA) cycle.

Important protein metabolic pathways occur in the liver. Transamination (transfer of an amino group from one compound to another) and oxidative deamination (removal of an amino group from an amino acid or other compound) are two such pathways that convert amino acids to substrates that are used in energy and glucose production as well as in the synthesis of nonessential amino acids. Blood-clotting factors such as fibrinogen and prothrombin, as well as serum proteins including albumin, alpha-globulin, beta-globulin, transferrin, ceruloplasmin, and lipoproteins, are formed by the liver.

Fatty acids from the diet and adipose tissue are converted in the liver to acetyl-coenzyme A by the process of beta-oxidation to produce energy. Ketones also are produced. The liver synthesizes and hydrolyzes triglycerides, phospholipids, cholesterol, and lipoproteins as well.

The liver is involved in the storage, activation, and transport of many vitamins and minerals. It stores all the fat-soluble vitamins in addition to vitamin B_{12} and the minerals zinc, iron, copper, and manganese. Hepatically synthesized proteins transport vitamin A (retinol binding protein), iron (transferrin), zinc (metallothionein), and copper (ceruloplasmin) in the bloodstream. Carotene is converted to vitamin A, folate to 5-methyl tetrahydrofolic acid, and vitamin D to an active form (25-hydroxycholecalciferol, calcitriol) by the liver.

In addition to functions of nutrient metabolism and storage, the liver forms and excretes bile. Bile salts are metabolized and used for the digestion and absorption of fats and fat-soluble vitamins. Bilirubin is a metabolic end product from red blood cell destruction; it is conjugated and excreted in the bile.

Hepatocytes detoxify ammonia by converting it to urea, 75% of which is excreted by the kidneys. The remaining urea finds its way back to the gastrointestinal tract (GIT). The liver also metabolizes steroid hormones. It inactivates and excretes aldosterone, glucocorticoids, estrogen, progesterone, and testosterone. It is responsible for the detoxification of substances, including drugs and alcohol, as well as toxins such as pollutants, chemicals, pesticides and herbicides, bioactive compounds, and biological poisons such as those from toxic mushrooms. Finally, the liver acts as a filter and flood chamber by removing bacteria and debris from blood through the phagocytic action of specialized macrophages called Kupffer cells located in the sinusoids and by storing blood backed up from the vena cava as in right heart failure.

Assessment of Liver Function

Biochemical markers are used to evaluate and monitor patients having or suspected of having liver disease. Enzyme assays measure the release of liver enzymes, and other tests measure liver function. Screening tests for hepatobiliary disease include serum levels of bilirubin, alkaline phosphatase (Alk Phos), aspartate amino transferase (AST), and alanine aminotransferase (ALT). Table 28.1 elaborates common laboratory tests for liver disorders (see also Appendix 12).

TABLE 28.1 Common Laboratory Tests Used to Test Liver Function

Laboratory Test	Comment
Hepatic Excretion	
Total serum bilirubin	When increased, may indicate bilirubin overproduction or impaired hepatic uptake, conjugation, or excretion
Indirect serum bilirubin	Unconjugated bilirubin; increased with excessive bilirubin production (hemolysis), immaturity of enzyme systems, inherited defects, drug effects
Direct serum bilirubin	Conjugated bilirubin; increased with depressed bilirubin excretion, hepatobiliary disease, intrahepatic or benign postoperative jaundice and sepsis, and congenital conjugated hyperbilirubinemia
Cholestasis	
Serum alkaline phosphatase	Enzyme widely distributed in liver, bone, placenta, intestine, kidney, leukocytes; mainly bound to canalicular membranes in liver; increased levels suggest cholestasis but can be increased with bone disorders, pregnancy, normal growth, and some malignancies
γ-Glutamyl transpeptidase (GGT)	Enzyme found in high concentrations in epithelial cells lining bile ductules in the liver; also present in kidney, pancreas, heart, brain; increased with liver disease, but also after myocardial infarction, in neuromuscular disease, pancreatic disease, pulmonary disease, diabetes mellitus, and during alcohol ingestion
Hepatic Serum Enzymes	
Alanine aminotransferase (ALT, formerly SGPT, serum glutamic pyruvic transaminase)	Located in cytosol of hepatocyte; found in several other body tissues but highest in liver; increased with liver cell damage
Aspartate aminotransferase (AST, formerly SGOT, serum glutamic oxaloacetic transaminase)	Located in cytosol and mitochondria of hepatocyte; also in cardiac and skeletal muscle, heart, brain, pancreas, kidney; increased with liver cell damage
Serum lactic dehydrogenase	Located in liver, red blood cells, cardiac muscle, kidney; increased with liver disease but lacks sensitivity and specificity because it is found in most other body tissues
Serum Proteins	
Prothrombin time (PT)	Most blood coagulation factors are synthesized in the liver; vitamin K deficiency and decreased synthesis of clotting factors increase prothrombin time and risk of bleeding
International Normalized Ratio (INR)	A standardized way to report PT levels so that levels from different laboratories can be compared

TABLE 28.1 Common Laboratory Tests Used to Test Liver Function—cont'd

Laboratory Test	Comment
Serum albumin	Main export protein synthesized in the liver and most important factor in maintaining plasma oncotic pressure; hypoalbuminemia can result from expanded plasma volume or reduced synthesis as well as increased losses as occurs with protein-losing enteropathy, nephrotic syndrome, burns, gastrointestinal bleeding, exfoliative dermatitis
Serum globulin	Alpha$_1$ and alpha$_2$-globulins are synthesized in the liver; levels increase with chronic liver disease; limited diagnostic use in hepatobiliary disease, although the pattern may suggest underlying cause of liver disease (e.g., elevated immunoglobulin [Ig]G suggests autoimmune hepatitis, elevated IgM suggests primary biliary cirrhosis, elevated IgA suggests alcoholic liver disease)
Markers of Specific Liver Diseases	
Serum ferritin	Major iron storage protein; increased level sensitive indicator of genetic hemochromatosis
Ceruloplasmin	Major copper-binding protein synthesized by liver; decreased in Wilson's disease
Alpha-fetoprotein	Major circulating plasma protein; increased with hepatocellular carcinoma
Alpha$_1$-antitrypsin	Main function is to inhibit serum trypsin activity; decreased levels indicate alpha$_1$-antitrypsin deficiency, which can cause liver and lung damage
Markers for Viral Hepatitis	
Anti-HAV IgM (antibody to hepatitis A virus)	Marker for hepatitis A; indicates current or recent infection or convalescence
HBsAg (hepatitis B surface antigen)	Marker for hepatitis B; positive in most cases of acute or chronic infection
Anti-HBc (antibody to hepatitis B core antigen)	Antibody to hepatitis B core antigen; marker for hepatitis B; denotes recent or past hepatitis infection
Anti-HBs (antibody to hepatitis B surface antigen)	Antibody to HBsAg; marker for hepatitis B; denotes prior hepatitis B infection or hepatitis B vaccine; protective
HBeAg (hepatitis Be antigen)	Marker for hepatitis B; transiently positive during active virus replication; reflects concentration and infectivity of virus
Anti-HBe (antibody to hepatitis Be antigen)	Marker for hepatitis B; positive in all acute and chronic cases; positive in carriers; not protective
HBV-DNA (hepatitis B deoxyribonucleic acid)	Measures hepatitis B viral load
Anti-HCV (antibody to hepatitis C virus)	Marker for hepatitis C; positive 5-6 weeks after onset of hepatitis C virus; not protective; reflects infectious state and is detectable during and after treatment
HCV-RNA (hepatitis C virus ribonucleic acid)	Measures hepatitis C viral load
Anti-HDV	Marker for hepatitis D; indicates infection; not protective
Miscellaneous	
Ammonia	Liver converts ammonia to urea; may increase with hepatic failure and portal-systemic shunts

Data from Wedemeyer H, Pawlotsky JM: Acute viral hepatitis. In Goldman L et al, editors: *Goldman's Cecil medicine*, ed 24, Philadelphia, 2012, Elsevier Saunders. Pawlotsky JM, Mchuthinson J: Chronic viral and autoimmune hepatitis. In Goldman L et al, editors: *Goldman's Cecil medicine*, ed 24, Philadelphia, 2012, Elsevier Saunders. Woreta TA, Alqahtani SA: Evaluation of abnormal liver tests, *Med Clin North Am* 98:1, 2014. Martin P, Friedman LS: Assessment of liver function and diagnostic studies. In Friedman LS, Keeffe B, editors: *Handbook of liver disease*, ed 3, Philadelphia, 2012, Elsevier Saunders; 2012. Khalili H et al: Assessment of liver function in clinical practice. In Gines P et al, editors: *Clinical gastroenterology: chronic liver failure*, New York, 2011, Springer.

Physical examination as well as diagnostic procedures (e.g., endoscopy) or abdominal imaging tests (e.g., abdominal ultrasound, magnetic resonance imaging, or computed tomography scan) can be used to diagnose or evaluate patients for liver disease. A liver biopsy is considered the gold standard to assess the severity of hepatic inflammation and fibrosis (scar tissue).

DISEASES OF THE LIVER

Diseases of the liver can be acute or chronic, inherited or acquired. The following section provides a brief overview of viral hepatitis, nonalcoholic fatty liver disease (NAFLD), alcoholic liver disease, cholestatic liver diseases, inherited disorders, and other liver diseases.

Viral Hepatitis

Viral **hepatitis** is a widespread inflammation of the liver and is caused by various hepatitis viruses, including A, B, C, D, and E (Fig. 28.1 and Table 28.2). Hepatitis A and E are the infectious forms, mainly spread by fecal-oral route. Hepatitis B, C, and D exist in the serum and are spread by blood and body fluids (Pawlotsky, 2016). Infectious agents such as Epstein-Barr virus, cytomegalovirus, and herpes simplex virus also can cause an acute hepatitis.

The clinical manifestations of acute viral hepatitis are divided into four phases. The first phase, the incubation phase, often is characterized by nonspecific symptoms such as malaise, loss of appetite, nausea, and right upper quadrant pain (Pawlotsky, 2016). This is followed by the preicteric phase, in which the nonspecific symptoms continue. In addition, about

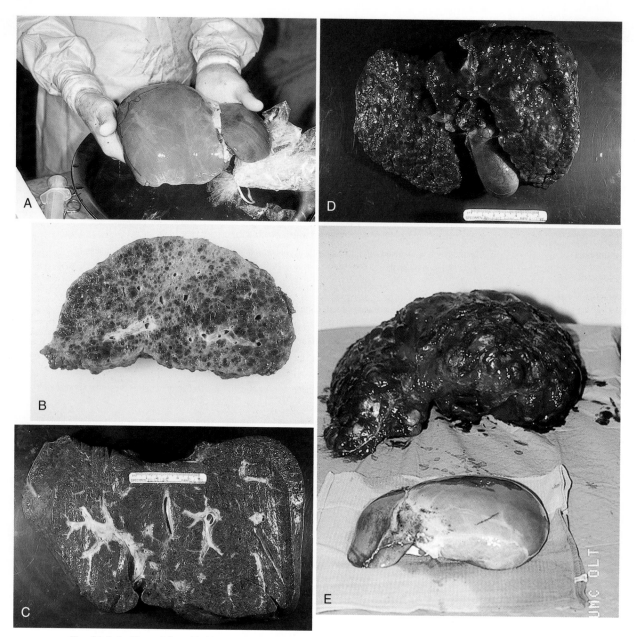

Fig. 28.1 A, Normal liver. **B,** Liver with damage from chronic active hepatitis. **C,** Liver with damage from sclerosing cholangitis. **D,** Liver with damage from primary biliary cirrhosis. **E,** Liver with damage from polycystic liver disease *(background)* and normal liver *(foreground)*. (Courtesy Baylor Simmons Transplant Institute, Baylor University Medical Center, Dallas, TX.)

10% to 20% of patients can have immune-mediated symptoms such as fever, arthralgia, arthritis, rash, and angioedema in the preicteric phase. The third phase is the icteric phase, in which jaundice (a yellowing of the skin, mucous membranes, and the eyes) appears and the nonspecific symptoms worsen and weight loss, dysgeusia (distortion of taste), and pruritus (itchy skin) may develop. Finally, during the convalescent or recovery phase, jaundice and other symptoms begin to subside.

Complete spontaneous recovery is expected in all of hepatitis A cases, in nearly 99% of acute hepatitis B cases acquired as an adult, but in only 20% to 50% of acute hepatitis C cases. Chronic hepatitis usually does not develop with hepatitis E (Pawlotsky, 2016). Vaccines exist only for hepatitis A and B; however, recent advances have resulted in effective antiviral drugs to treat chronic hepatitis B and C.

Nonalcoholic Fatty Liver Disease

Nonalcoholic fatty liver disease (NAFLD) is a spectrum of liver disease ranging from steatosis to steatohepatitis and cirrhosis. It involves the accumulation of fat droplets in the hepatocytes and can lead to inflammation, fibrosis, cirrhosis, and even hepatocellular carcinoma. Causes of NAFLD can include drugs, inborn errors of metabolism, and acquired metabolic disorders (type 2 diabetes mellitus, lipodystrophy, jejunal ileal bypass, obesity, and malnutrition). However, NAFLD is associated most commonly with obesity, type 2 diabetes mellitus, dyslipidemia, and metabolic syndrome (Chalasani, 2016). Insulin resistance with hyperinsulinism and elevated nonesterified fatty acid levels in hepatocytes characterize metabolic defects associated with NAFLD.

TABLE 28.2 Types of Viral Hepatitis

Virus	Transmission	Comments
Hepatitis A	Fecal-oral route; is contracted through contaminated drinking water, food, and sewage.	Anorexia is the most frequent symptom, and it can be severe. Other common symptoms include nausea, vomiting, right upper quadrant abdominal pain, dark urine, and jaundice (icterus). Recovery is usually complete, and long-term consequences are rare. Serious complications may occur in high-risk patients; subsequently, great attention must be given to adequate nutritional intake.
Hepatitis B and C	HBV and HCV are transmitted via blood, blood products, semen, and saliva. For example, they can be spread from contaminated needles, blood transfusions, open cuts or wounds, splashes of blood into the mouth or eyes, or sexual contact.	HBV and HCV can lead to chronic and carrier states. Chronic active hepatitis also can develop, leading to cirrhosis and liver failure.
Hepatitis D	HDV is rare in the United States and depends on HBV for survival and propagation in humans.	HDV may be a coinfection (occurring at the same time as HBV) or a superinfection (superimposing itself on the HBV carrier state). This form of hepatitis usually becomes chronic.
Hepatitis E	HEV is transmitted via the oral-fecal route.	HEV is rare in the United States (typically only occurs when imported), but it is reported more frequently in many countries of southern, eastern, and central Asia; northern, eastern, and western Africa; and Mexico. Contaminated water appears to be the source of infection, which usually afflicts people living in crowded and unsanitary conditions. HEV is generally acute rather than chronic.
Hepatitis G/GB	HGV and a virus labeled GBV-C appear to be variants of the same virus.	Although HGV infection is present in a significant proportion of blood donors and is transmitted through blood transfusions, it does not appear to cause liver disease.

HBV, Hepatitis B virus; *HCV*, hepatitis C virus; *HDV*, hepatitis D virus; *HEV*, hepatitis E virus; *HGV*, hepatitis G virus.

The initial stage of NAFLD is steatosis, which is characterized by the simple accumulation of fat within the liver. Some patients will progress to nonalcoholic steatohepatitis (NASH), which is an inflammatory condition associated with hepatocyte injury with or without fibrous tissue in the liver. NASH can develop into chronic liver disease and NASH cirrhosis up to 20% of the time. The progression to cirrhosis (permanent damage and scaring) is variable depending on age and the presence of obesity and type 2 diabetes mellitus, which contribute to a worsening prognosis (Chalasani, 2016).

The treatment suggestions for NAFLD from the American Association for the Study of Liver Diseases (AASLD) include lifestyle change (diet and exercise), weight loss, insulin-sensitizing drugs such as thiazolidinediones, and vitamin E (Chalasani, 2016). Based on the AASLD panel, a 3% to 5% weight loss can improve steatosis, but up to 10% weight loss may be needed to improve NASH and fibrosis. The AASLD recommendations state that pioglitazone (an oral antihyperglycemia medication used to treat diabetes mellitus) may be considered for NASH treatment, but not NAFLD. Vitamin E (800 IU/day of alpha-tocopherol) is considered first-line treatment for biopsy-proven NASH in patients without diabetes mellitus (Chalasani, 2016). Because disease progression and hepatocellular injury appears to be linked to oxidative stress, Vitamin E, as an antioxidant, is thought to be beneficial (Chalasani et al, 2018). Omega-3 fatty acids could be considered to treat hypertriglyceridemia in individuals with NAFLD (Chalasani et al, 2018). Emerging data suggest drinking moderate amounts of unsweetened coffee is protective against chronic liver disease, NAFLD, and hepatocellular carcinoma (Morisco et al, 2014; Chen et al, 2014; Setiawan et al, 2015).

Alcoholic Liver Disease

Alcoholic liver disease is one of the most common liver diseases in the United States, with 1% of North Americans having alcoholic liver disease. Forty percent of deaths from cirrhosis are attributed to alcohol (Chalasani, 2016). Acetaldehyde is a toxic byproduct of alcohol metabolism that causes damage to mitochondrial membrane structure and function. Acetaldehyde is produced by multiple metabolic pathways, one of which involves alcohol dehydrogenase (see *Focus On: Metabolic Consequences of Alcohol Consumption*).

◎ FOCUS ON

Metabolic Consequences of Alcohol Consumption

Ethanol is metabolized primarily in the liver by alcohol dehydrogenase. This results in acetaldehyde production with the transfer of hydrogen to nicotinamide adenine dinucleotide (NAD), reducing it to NADH. The acetaldehyde then loses hydrogen and is converted to acetate, most of which is released into the blood.

Many metabolic disturbances occur because of the excess of NADH, which overrides the ability of the cell to maintain a normal redox state. These include hyperlacticacidemia, acidosis, hyperuricemia, ketonemia, and hyperlipemia. The tricarboxylic acid (TCA) cycle is depressed because it requires NAD. The mitochondria, in turn, use hydrogen from ethanol rather than from the oxidation of fatty acids to produce energy via the TCA cycle, which leads to a decreased fatty acid oxidation and accumulation of triglycerides. In addition, NADH may actually promote fatty acid synthesis. Hypoglycemia also can occur in early alcoholic liver disease secondary to the suppression of the TCA cycle, coupled with decreased gluconeogenesis resulting from ethanol.

Several variables predispose some people to alcoholic liver disease. These include amount and duration of alcohol intake, genetic polymorphisms of alcohol-metabolizing enzymes, gender (females more than males), simultaneous exposure to other drugs, infections with hepatotropic viruses, immunologic factors, obesity, and poor nutrition status. The pathogenesis of alcoholic liver disease progresses in three stages (Fig. 28.2): hepatic steatosis (Fig. 28.3), alcoholic hepatitis, and finally cirrhosis.

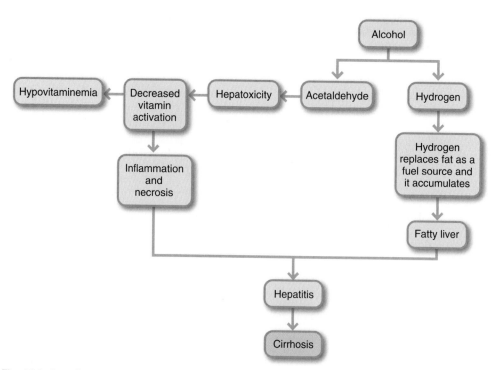

Fig. 28.2 Complications of excessive alcohol consumption stem largely from excess hydrogen and from acetaldehyde. Hydrogen produces fatty liver and hyperlipemia, high blood lactic acid, and low blood sugar. The accumulation of fat, the effect of acetaldehyde on liver cells, and other factors as yet unknown lead to alcoholic hepatitis. The next step is cirrhosis. The consequent impairment of liver function disturbs blood chemistry, notably causing a high ammonia level that can lead to coma and death. Cirrhosis also distorts liver structure, inhibiting blood flow. High pressure in vessels supplying the liver may cause ruptured varices and accumulation of fluid in the abdominal cavity. Response to alcohol differs among individuals; in particular, not all heavy drinkers develop hepatitis and cirrhosis.

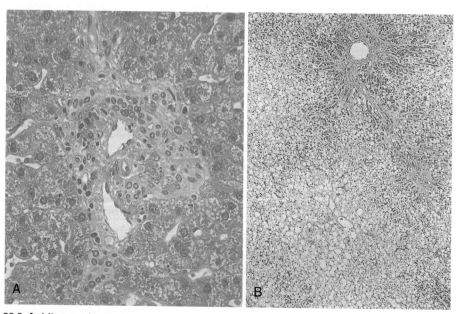

Fig. 28.3 A, Microscopic appearance of a normal liver. A normal portal tract consists of the portal vein, hepatic arteriole, one to two interlobular bile ducts, and occasional peripherally located ductules. **B,** Acute fatty liver. This photomicrograph on low power exhibits fatty change involving virtually all the hepatocytes, with slight sparing of the liver cells immediately adjacent to the portal tract (*top*). (From Kanel G, Korula J, editors: *Atlas of liver pathology,* Philadelphia, 1992, Saunders.)

Fatty infiltration, known as hepatic steatosis or fatty liver, is caused by a culmination of these metabolic disturbances: (1) an increase in the mobilization of fatty acids from adipose tissue; (2) an increase in hepatic synthesis of fatty acids; (3) a decrease in fatty acid oxidation; (4) an increase in triglyceride production; and (5) a trapping of triglycerides in the liver. Hepatic steatosis is reversible with abstinence from alcohol. Conversely, if alcohol abuse continues, cirrhosis can develop. Patients with alcoholic fatty liver disease usually are asymptomatic but can have symptoms such as fatigue, poor appetite, right upper quadrant discomfort, or hepatomegaly.

Alcoholic hepatitis generally is characterized by an enlarged liver (hepatomegaly), modest elevation of serum transaminase levels (ALT and AST), increased serum bilirubin concentrations, normal or depressed serum albumin concentrations, or anemia. Patients also may have abdominal pain, anorexia, nausea, vomiting, weakness, diarrhea, weight loss, or fever. Some patients can develop jaundice, coagulopathy, ascites (abdominal fluid retention), or mental impairment

(encephalopathy). If patients discontinue alcohol intake, hepatitis may resolve; however, the condition often progresses to the third stage.

Clinical features of alcoholic cirrhosis, the third stage, vary. Symptoms can mimic those of alcoholic hepatitis; or patients can develop complications of cirrhosis such as gastrointestinal bleeding, hepatic encephalopathy, or portal hypertension (elevated blood pressure in the portal venous system caused by the obstruction of blood flow through the liver). Patients with alcoholic cirrhosis often develop ascites, the accumulation of fluid, serum protein, and electrolytes within the peritoneal cavity caused by increased pressure from portal hypertension and decreased production of albumin (which maintains serum colloidal osmotic pressure). A liver biopsy usually reveals micronodular cirrhosis, but it can be macronodular or mixed. Prognosis depends on abstinence from alcohol and the degree of complications already developed. Ethanol ingestion creates specific and severe nutritional abnormalities (see *Clinical Insight:* Malnutrition Related to Alcoholic Liver Disease).

CLINICAL INSIGHT

Malnutrition Related to Alcoholic Liver Disease

Several factors contribute to the malnutrition common in individuals with chronic alcoholic liver disease:

1. Alcohol can replace food in the diet of moderate and heavy drinkers, displacing the intake of adequate calories and nutrients. In light drinkers, it is usually an additional energy source, or empty calories. Although alcohol yields 7.1 kcal/g, when it is consumed in large amounts it is not used efficiently as a fuel source. When individuals consume alcohol on a regular basis but do not fulfill criteria for alcohol abuse, they are often overweight because of the increased calories (alcohol addiction). This is different from the heavy drinker who replaces energy-rich nutrients with alcohol (alcohol substitution).

2. In the person with alcoholism, impaired digestion and absorption are related to pancreatic insufficiency, as well as morphologic and functional alterations of the intestinal mucosa. Acute and chronic alcohol intake impairs hepatic amino acid uptake and synthesis into proteins, reduces protein synthesis and secretion from the liver, and increases tissue catabolism in the gut.

3. Use of lipids and carbohydrates is compromised. An excess of reduction equivalents (e.g., nicotinamide adenine dinucleotide phosphate [NADH]) and

impaired oxidation of triglycerides result in fat deposition in the hepatocytes and an increase in circulating triglycerides. Insulin resistance is also common.

4. Vitamin and mineral deficiencies occur in alcoholic liver disease as a result of reduced intake and alterations in absorption, storage, and ability to convert the nutrients to their active forms. Steatorrhea resulting from bile acid deficiency is also common in alcoholic liver disease and affects fat-soluble vitamin absorption. Vitamin A deficiency can lead to night blindness. Thiamin deficiency is the most common vitamin deficiency in people with alcoholism and is responsible for Wernicke encephalopathy. Folate deficiency can occur as a result of poor intake, impaired absorption, accelerated excretion, and altered storage and metabolism. Inadequate dietary intake and interactions between pyridoxal-5-phosphate (active coenzyme of vitamin B_6) and alcohol reduce vitamin B_6 status. Deficiency of all B vitamins and vitamins C, D, E, and K is also common. Hypocalcemia, hypomagnesemia, and hypophosphatemia are not uncommon among people with alcoholism; furthermore, zinc deficiency and alterations in other micronutrients can accompany chronic alcohol intake.

Cholestatic Liver Diseases

Cholestatic liver diseases refer to conditions affecting the bile ducts.

Primary Biliary Cirrhosis

Primary biliary cirrhosis (PBC) is a chronic cholestatic disease caused by progressive destruction of small and intermediate-size intrahepatic bile ducts. The extrahepatic biliary tree and larger intrahepatic ducts are normal. Ninety-five percent of patients with PBC are women. The disease progresses slowly, eventually resulting in cirrhosis, portal hypertension, the need for liver transplantation, or death (Fogel and Sherman, 2016).

PBC is an autoimmune disorder that typically presents with an elevation of serum levels of Alk Phos and gamma glutamyl transferase (GGT) with physical symptoms of pruritus and fatigue. Several nutritional complications from cholestasis (a blockage of bile flow) can occur with PBC, including osteopenia, hypercholesterolemia, and fat-soluble vitamin deficiencies.

Primary Sclerosing Cholangitis

Primary sclerosing cholangitis (PSC) is characterized by fibrosing inflammation of segments of intra- and extrahepatic bile ducts. This

progressive disease can be characterized by three syndromes. The first is cholestasis with biliary cirrhosis, followed by recurrent cholangitis (inflammation of the bile ducts) with large bile duct strictures, and finally cholangiocarcinoma (gall bladder cancer) (Fogel and Sherman, 2016). Like PBC, PSC is considered an autoimmune disorder. In patients with PSC, about two thirds also have inflammatory bowel disease (especially ulcerative colitis), and men are more likely than women (2:1) to have PSC (Fogel and Sherman, 2016). Patients with PSC are also at increased risk of fat-soluble vitamin deficiencies resulting from steatorrhea associated with this disease. Hepatic osteodystrophy may occur from vitamin D and calcium malabsorption, resulting in secondary hyperparathyroidism, osteomalacia, or rickets. Known fat-soluble vitamin deficiencies should be treated, and calcium supplementation could be considered. Treatment of PSC is moderately successful with administration of cholestyramine, ursodeoxycholic acid, rifampin, or phenobarbital (Fogel and Sherman, 2016).

Inherited Disorders

Inherited disorders of the liver include hemochromatosis, Wilson's disease, alpha$_1$-antitrypsin deficiency, and cystic fibrosis. Porphyria, glycogen storage disease, and amyloidosis are metabolic diseases with a genetic component.

Hemochromatosis

Although iron overload can be associated with other conditions, hereditary hemochromatosis is an inherited disease of iron overload usually associated with the gene HFE (Martin, 2015; Bacon, 2015). Patients with hereditary hemochromatosis absorb and store excessive iron from the gut in the liver heart, pancreas, joints, and endocrine organs (Bacon, 2015; see Chapter 30). Increased transferrin saturation (at least 45%) and ferritin (more than two times normal) suggest hemochromatosis. Hepatomegaly, esophageal bleeding, ascites, impaired hepatic synthetic function, abnormal skin pigmentation, glucose intolerance, cardiac involvement, hypogonadism, arthropathy, and hepatocellular carcinoma may develop. Early diagnosis includes clinical, laboratory, and pathologic testing, including elevated serum transferrin levels. Life expectancy is normal if phlebotomy (or regular blood donation) is initiated before the development of cirrhosis or diabetes mellitus. Patients with hemachromotosis should avoid dietary supplements that contain iron, avoid cooking in cast iron pans, and should limit foods high in iron such as liver and red meats (see Appendix 42).

Wilson's Disease

Wilson's disease is an autosomal-recessive disorder associated with impaired biliary copper excretion (Kaler and Schilsky, 2015). Copper accumulates in various tissues, including the liver, brain, cornea, and kidneys. Kayser-Fleischer rings are greenish-yellow pigmented rings encircling the cornea just within the corneoscleral margin, formed by copper deposits. Patients can present with acute, fulminant (occurring suddenly with great severity), or chronic active hepatitis and neuropsychiatric symptoms. Low serum ceruloplasmin levels, elevated copper concentration in a liver biopsy, and high urinary copper excretion confirm the diagnosis.

Copper-chelating agents (such as D-penicillamine, trientine, or tetrathiomolybdate) (Kaler and Schilsky, 2015) and zinc supplementation (150 mg elemental zinc daily given in three divided doses to inhibit intestinal copper absorption and binding in the liver) are used to treat Wilson's disease once it is diagnosed (Schilsky, 2017). Vitamin B_6 supplementation should be considered when penicillamine is given to prevent vitamin B_6 deficiency (Kaler and Schilsky, 2015). Ongoing intravenous copper chelation is required to prevent relapses and liver failure; liver transplantation corrects the metabolic defect. A low-copper diet is no longer required but may be helpful in the initial phase of treatment. High-copper foods include organ meats, shellfish, chocolate, nuts, and mushrooms. For a comprehensive list of copper content of food, refer to the U.S. Department of Agriculture National Nutrient Database. If this disease is not diagnosed until onset of fulminant failure, survival is not possible without liver transplantation.

Alpha$_1$-Antitrypsin Deficiency

Alpha$_1$-antitrypsin deficiency is an inherited disorder that can cause liver and lung disease. Alpha$_1$-antitrypsin is a glycoprotein found in serum and body fluids; it inhibits serine proteinases. Cholestasis or cirrhosis is caused by this deficiency, and there is no treatment except liver transplantation.

Other Liver Diseases

Liver disease can be caused by several conditions other than those already discussed. Liver tumors can be primary or metastatic, benign or malignant. Hepatocellular carcinoma (HCC) usually develops in cirrhotic livers with highest risk in individuals with hepatitis B virus (HBV), hepatitis C virus (HCV), or NAFLD (Kelly and Venook, 2015). The liver also can be affected by rheumatic diseases such as rheumatoid arthritis, systemic lupus erythematosus, polymyalgia, temporal arteritis, polyarteritis nodosa, systemic sclerosis, and Sjögren syndrome (see Chapter 38). When hepatic blood flow is altered—as in acute ischemic and chronic congestive hepatopathy, Budd-Chiari syndrome, and hepatic venoocclusive disease—dysfunction occurs. Individuals with hepatic or portal vein thromboses should be evaluated for a myeloproliferative disorder. Parasitic, bacterial, fungal, and granulomatous liver diseases also occur. Finally, cryptogenic cirrhosis is any cirrhosis for which the cause is unknown.

Classifying Liver Disease According to Duration

Liver disease can be classified according to the time of onset and duration of the disease. Liver disease can be fulminant, acute, and chronic.

Fulminant hepatitis is a syndrome in which severe liver dysfunction is accompanied by hepatic encephalopathy, a clinical syndrome characterized by impaired mentation, neuromuscular disturbances, and altered consciousness. Fulminant liver disease is defined by the absence of preexisting liver disease and the rapid development of hepatic encephalopathy within 2 to 8 weeks of the onset of illness. The main cause of fulminant hepatitis is viral hepatitis; however, chemical toxicity (e.g., acetaminophen, drug reactions, poisonous mushrooms, industrial poisons), and other causes (e.g., Wilson's disease, fatty liver of pregnancy, Reye syndrome, hepatic ischemia, hepatic vein obstruction, and disseminated malignancies) are examples of other causes. Extrahepatic complications of fulminant hepatitis are cerebral edema, coagulopathy and bleeding, cardiovascular abnormalities, renal failure, pulmonary complications, acid-base disturbances, electrolyte imbalances, sepsis, and pancreatitis (inflammation of the pancreas).

Acute liver disease is identified typically as liver dysfunction that has been present for less than 6 months. Recovery is expected in a majority of patients who develop acute liver disease.

To be diagnosed with chronic hepatitis, a patient must have at least a 6-month course of hepatitis or biochemical and clinical evidence of liver disease with confirmatory biopsy findings of unresolving hepatic inflammation. Chronic hepatitis can be caused by autoimmune disease, viral infections, metabolic disorders, alcohol, drugs, or toxins. The most common causes of chronic hepatitis are hepatitis B, hepatitis C, and autoimmune hepatitis. Other causes are drug-induced liver disease, metabolic diseases, and NASH.

Clinical symptoms of chronic hepatitis are usually nonspecific, occur intermittently, and are mild. Common symptoms include fatigue, sleep disorders, difficulty concentrating, and mild upper quadrant pain. Severe advanced disease can lead to jaundice, muscle wasting, tea-colored urine, ascites (fluid accumulation in the abdomen), edema (fluid accumulation in the tissues), hepatic encephalopathy, gastrointestinal varices (abnormal enlarged veins often caused by portal hypertension) with resultant gastrointestinal bleeding, splenomegaly, palmar erythema (red palms), and spider angiomas (broken blood vessels).

In some instances, chronic hepatitis leads to cirrhosis and liver failure, also known as end-stage liver disease (ESLD). Cirrhosis, a build up of scar tissue and fibrosis of the liver, has many clinical manifestations, as illustrated in Fig. 28.4. There are several major complications of cirrhosis and ESLD.

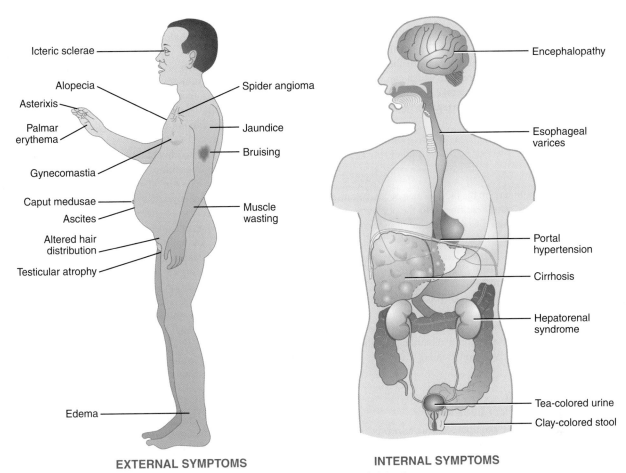

Icteric sclerae

Alopecia

Asterixis

Palmar
erythema

Gynecomastia

Caput medusae

Ascites

Altered hair
distribution

Testicular atrophy

Edema

Spider angioma

Jaundice

Bruising

Muscle
wasting

EXTERNAL SYMPTOMS

Encephalopathy

Esophageal
varices

Portal
hypertension

Cirrhosis

Hepatorenal
syndrome

Tea-colored urine

Clay-colored stool

INTERNAL SYMPTOMS

Fig. 28.4 Clinical manifestations of cirrhosis.

COMPLICATIONS OF ESLD: CAUSE AND NUTRITION TREATMENT

Decompensated ESLD can have several physical manifestations, including portal hypertension, ascites and edema, hyponatremia, and hepatic encephalopathy. It is important to understand the underlying cause of these complications as well as the medical and nutrition treatment options.

Portal Hypertension

Pathophysiology and Medical Treatment

Portal hypertension increases collateral blood flow and can result in swollen veins (varices) in the gastrointestinal tract (GIT). These varices often bleed, causing a medical emergency. Treatment includes administration of alpha-adrenergic blockers to decrease heart rate, endoscopic variceal banding, and radiologic placement of shunts. A transjugular intrahepatic portosystemic shunt (TIPS) involves a radiologically placed stent between the portal vein and the hepatic vein. During an acute bleeding episode, somatostatin or its analog may be administered to decrease bleeding, or a nasogastric tube equipped with an inflatable balloon is placed to alleviate bleeding from vessels.

Medical Nutrition Therapy

During acute bleeding episodes, nutrition cannot be administered enterally (using the gut); parenteral nutrition (PN) is indicated if a patient will be taking nothing enterally for at least 5 to 7 days (see Chapter 12). Repeated endoscopic therapies may cause esophageal

strictures or impair a patient's swallowing. Finally, placement of shunts may increase the incidence of encephalopathy and reduce nutrient metabolism because blood is shunted past the liver cells.

Ascites

Pathophysiology and Medical Treatment

Fluid retention is common, and ascites (accumulation of fluid in the abdominal cavity) is a serious consequence of liver disease. Portal hypertension, hypoalbuminemia, lymphatic obstruction, and renal retention of sodium and fluid contribute to fluid retention. Increased release of catecholamines, renin, angiotensin, aldosterone, and antidiuretic hormone secondary to peripheral arterial vasodilation causes renal retention of sodium and water.

Large-volume paracentesis (a procedure to drain the fluid) may be used to relieve ascites. Diuretic therapy often is used and frequently includes the medications spironolactone and furosemide. These drugs often are used in combination for best effect. Major side effects of loop diuretics such as furosemide include hyponatremia, hypokalemia, hypomagnesemia, hypocalcemia, and hypochloremic acidosis. Because spironolactone is potassium sparing, serum potassium levels must be monitored carefully and supplemented or restricted if necessary because deficiency or excess can contribute to metabolic abnormalities, including cardiac arrhythmias. Weight, abdominal girth (due to fluid accumulation), urinary sodium concentration, and serum levels of urea nitrogen, creatinine, albumin, uric acid, and electrolytes should be monitored during diuretic therapy.

Medical Nutrition Therapy

Dietary treatment for ascites includes restricting dietary sodium to 2 g/day (see Appendix 46). More severe limitations may be imposed; however, caution is warranted because of limited palatability and the risk of overrestricting sodium, which can lead to insufficient intake of sodium, or limited intake of calories and protein. Adequate protein intake is also important to replace losses from frequent paracentesis.

Hyponatremia

Pathophysiology

Hyponatremia (low sodium level in the blood) often occurs because of decreased ability to excrete water resulting from the persistent release of antidiuretic hormone, sodium losses via paracentesis, excessive diuretic use, or overly aggressive sodium restriction.

Medical Nutrition Therapy

Fluid intake is often restricted to 1 to 1.5 L/day, depending on the severity of the edema and ascites, although fluid restriction is utilized primarily if the sodium level is less than 125 mg/dL. Restricting sodium to about 2 g/day should be continued because excessive sodium intake results in worsened fluid retention and the further dilution of serum sodium levels (hyponatremia).

Hepatic Encephalopathy

Pathophysiology and Medical Treatment

Hepatic encephalopathy is a syndrome characterized by impaired mentation, neuromuscular disturbances, and altered consciousness. Gastrointestinal bleeding, fluid and electrolyte abnormalities, uremia, infection, use of sedatives, hyperglycemia or hypoglycemia, alcohol withdrawal, constipation, azotemia, dehydration, portosystemic shunts, and acidosis can precipitate hepatic encephalopathy. Subclinical or minimal hepatic encephalopathy also affects patients with chronic hepatic failure. Hepatic or portal systemic encephalopathy results in neuromuscular and behavioral alterations. Box 28.1 describes the four stages of hepatic encephalopathy.

Different theories exist regarding the mechanism by which hepatic encephalopathy occurs. However, one of the most common theories involves ammonia accumulation because it is considered to be an important causal factor in the development of encephalopathy. When the liver fails, it is unable to detoxify ammonia to urea. Ammonia levels are elevated in the brain and bloodstream, leading to impaired neural function through a complex system. The main source of ammonia is its endogenous production by the GIT from the metabolism of protein and from the degradation of bacteria and blood from gastrointestinal bleeding. Exogenous protein is also a source of ammonia. Some clinicians suggest that

dietary protein causes an increase in ammonia levels and subsequently hepatic encephalopathy, but this has not been proven in studies.

Drugs such as lactulose and rifaximin are given to treat hepatic encephalopathy. Lactulose is a nonabsorbable disaccharide. It acidifies the colonic contents, retaining ammonia as the ammonium ion. It also acts as an osmotic laxative to remove the ammonia. Rifaximin is a nonabsorbable antibiotic that helps decrease colonic ammonia production.

One nutrition-related hypothesis is the "altered neurotransmitter theory," which involves amino acid imbalance. A plasma amino acid imbalance exists in ESLD in which the branched-chain amino acids (BCAAs) valine, leucine, and isoleucine are decreased. The BCAAs furnish as much as 30% of energy requirements for skeletal muscle, heart, and brain when gluconeogenesis and ketogenesis are depressed, causing serum BCAA levels to fall. Aromatic amino acids (AAAs) tryptophan, phenylalanine, and tyrosine, plus methionine, glutamine, asparagine, and histidine are increased. Plasma AAAs and methionine are released into circulation by muscle proteolysis, but the synthesis into protein and liver clearance of AAAs is depressed. This changes the plasma molar ratio of BCAAs to AAAs and has been theorized to contribute to the development of hepatic encephalopathy. Conversely, high levels of AAAs have been theorized to limit the cerebral uptake of BCAAs because they compete for carrier-mediated transport at the blood-brain barrier. Convincing evidence to support this theory is lacking.

Medical Nutrition Therapy

The outdated practice of protein restriction in patients with low-grade hepatic encephalopathy is based on the premise that protein intolerance causes hepatic encephalopathy, but it has never been proven in a study. True dietary protein intolerance is rare except in fulminant hepatic failure, or in a rare patient with chronic endogenous hepatic encephalopathy. Unnecessary protein restriction may worsen body protein losses and must be avoided. In fact, patients with encephalopathy often do not receive adequate protein. Most patients with cirrhosis can tolerate mixed-protein diets up to 1.5 g/kg of body weight.

Studies evaluating the benefit of supplements enriched with BCAAs and restricted in AAAs have varied in study design, sample size, composition of formulas, level of encephalopathy, type of liver disease, duration of therapy, and control groups. When high-methodological quality studies are evaluated, no significant improvements or survival benefits are associated with giving extra BCAAs to patients.

Other theories postulate that vegetable proteins and casein may improve mental status compared with meat protein. Casein-based diets are lower in AAAs and higher in BCAAs than meat-based diets. Vegetable protein is low in methionine and ammoniagenic amino acids but BCAA rich. The high-fiber content of a vegetable-protein diet also may play a role in the excretion of nitrogenous compounds.

Finally, it has been proposed that probiotics and synbiotics (sources of gut-friendly bacteria and fermentable fibers) can be used to treat hepatic encephalopathy. Probiotics may improve hepatic encephalopathy by reducing ammonia and endotoxin levels. In a meta-analysis, probiotics were shown to reduce serum ammonia levels as effectively as lactulose (Cai et al, 2018) and improve minimal hepatic encephalopathy (Cao et al, 2018; Dalal et al, 2017). They decrease inflammation and oxidative stress in the hepatocyte (thus increasing hepatic clearance of toxins including ammonia), and minimize uptake of other toxins.

BOX 28.1	**Four Stages of Hepatic Encephalopathy**
Stage	**Symptoms**
I	Mild confusion, agitation, irritability, sleep disturbance, decreased attention
II	Lethargy, disorientation, inappropriate behavior, drowsiness
III	Somnolent but arousable, incomprehensible speech, confused, aggressive behavior when awake
IV	Coma

Glucose Alterations

Pathophysiology

Glucose intolerance occurs in almost two thirds of patients with cirrhosis, and as many as one third of patients develop diabetes mellitus. Glucose intolerance in patients with liver disease occurs because of insulin resistance in peripheral tissues. Hyperinsulinism also occurs in patients with cirrhosis, possibly because insulin production is increased, hepatic clearance is decreased, portal systemic shunting occurs, there is a defect in the insulin-binding action at the receptor site, or there is a postreceptor defect.

Fasting hypoglycemia, or low blood glucose, can occur because of the decreased availability of glucose from glycogen in addition to the failing gluconeogenic capacity of the liver when the patient has ESLD. Hypoglycemia occurs more often in acute or fulminant liver failure than in chronic liver disease. Hypoglycemia also may occur after alcohol consumption in patients whose glycogen stores are depleted by starvation because of the block of hepatic gluconeogenesis by ethanol.

Medical Nutrition Therapy

Patients with diabetes mellitus should receive standard medical and nutrition therapy to achieve normoglycemia (see Chapter 29). Patients with hypoglycemia need to eat frequently to prevent this condition (see *Clinical Insight:* Fasting Hypoglycemia). Evening snacks that contain low glycemic carbohydrates balanced with protein may help prevent morning hypoglycemia.

CLINICAL INSIGHT

Fasting Hypoglycemia

Two thirds of the glucose requirement in an adult is used by the central nervous system. During fasting, plasma glucose concentrations are maintained for use by the nervous system and the brain because liver glycogen is broken down, or new glucose is made from nonglucose amino acid precursors such as alanine. Fasting hypoglycemia occurs in liver and biliary disease when there is reduced synthesis of new glucose or reduced liver glycogen breakdown.

Causes of fasting hypoglycemia include cirrhosis, consumption of alcohol, extensive intrahepatic cancer, deficiency of cortisol and growth hormone, or non–beta-cell tumors of the pancreas (insulinomas). All patients with liver or pancreatic disease should be monitored for fasting hypoglycemia. Nutrition therapy involves balanced meals with small, frequent snacks to avoid periods of fasting. Monitoring of blood glucose and insulin levels is required.

Fat Malabsorption

Pathophysiology

Fat absorption may be impaired in liver disease. Possible causes include decreased bile salt secretion (as in PBC, sclerosing cholangitis, and biliary strictures), administration of medications such as cholestyramine, and pancreatic enzyme insufficiency. Stools may be greasy, floating, or light- or clay-colored, signifying malabsorption, which can be verified by a 72-hour fecal fat study (see Chapter 27).

Medical Nutrition Therapy

If significant steatorrhea (the presence of fat in the stool) is present, replacement of some of the long-chain triglycerides or dietary fat with medium-chain triglycerides (MCTs) can be useful. Because MCTs do not require bile salts and micelle formation for absorption, they are readily taken up via the portal route. Some nutrition supplements

contain MCTs, which can be used in addition to liquid MCT oil (see Chapter 12).

Significant stool fat losses may warrant a trial of a low-fat diet or evaluation of pancreatic insufficiency. If diarrhea does not resolve, fat restriction should be discontinued because it decreases the palatability of the diet and makes it difficult to take in adequate calories. Because of the degree of malabsorption and steatorrhea, it is important to consider that the patient may have deficiencies of multiple micronutrients, especially fat-soluble vitamins.

Renal Insufficiency and Hepatorenal Syndrome

Pathophysiology, Medical, and Nutrition Therapies

Hepatorenal syndrome is renal failure associated with severe liver disease without intrinsic kidney abnormalities. Hepatorenal syndrome is diagnosed when the urine sodium level is less than 10 mEq/L and oliguria persists in the absence of intravascular volume depletion. If conservative therapies, including discontinuation of nephrotoxic drugs, optimization of intravascular volume status, treatment of underlying infection, and monitoring of fluid intake and output fail, dialysis may be required. In any case, renal insufficiency and failure may necessitate alteration in fluid, sodium, potassium, and phosphorus intake (see Chapter 34).

Osteopenia

Pathophysiology

Osteopenia often exists in patients with PBC, sclerosing cholangitis, and alcoholic liver disease. Depressed osteoblastic function and osteoporosis also can occur in patients with hemochromatosis, and osteoporosis is prevalent in patients who have had long-term treatment with corticosteroids. Corticosteroids increase bone resorption; suppress osteoblastic function; and affect sex hormone secretion, intestinal absorption of dietary calcium, renal excretion of calcium and phosphorus, and vitamin D.

Medical Nutrition Therapy

Prevention or treatment options for osteopenia include prevention of excessive weight loss, ingestion of a well-balanced diet, adequate protein to maintain muscle mass, a minimum of the dietary reference intake (DRI) for calcium per day (1000 to 1300 mg depending on age), adequate vitamin D from the diet or supplements, avoidance of alcohol, and monitoring for steatorrhea, with diet adjustments as needed to minimize nutrient losses.

NUTRITION ISSUES RELATED TO END-STAGE LIVER DISEASE

Nutrition Assessment

Nutrition assessment must be performed to determine the extent and cause of malnutrition in patients with liver disease. However, many traditional markers of nutrition status are affected by liver disease, making traditional assessment difficult. Table 28.3 summarizes the factors that affect interpretation of nutrition assessment parameters in patients with liver dysfunction.

Objective nutrition assessment parameters that are helpful when monitored serially include anthropometric measurements and dietary intake evaluation (see Chapters 4 and 5). Caution should be taken when assessing biochemical markers in the advanced liver disease patient because the typical nutrition criteria will be affected due to the liver

TABLE 28.3   Factors That Affect Interpretation of Objective Nutrition Assessment Parameter in Patients With End-Stage Liver Disease

Parameter	Factors Affecting Interpretation
Body weight	Affected by edema, ascites, and diuretic use
Anthropometric measurements	Questionable sensitivity, specificity, and reliability
	Multiple sources of error
	Unknown if skinfold measurements reflect total body fat
	References do not account for variation in hydration status and skin compressibility
Nitrogen balance studies	Nitrogen is retained in the body in the form of ammonia
	Hepatorenal syndrome can affect the excretion of nitrogen
Single-frequency bioelectrical impedance	Invalid with ascites and edema

Modified from Hasse J: Nutritional aspects of adult liver transplantation. In Busuttil RW, Klintmalm GB, editors: *Transplantation of the liver*, ed 3, Philadelphia, 2015, Elsevier Saunders.

disease itself. The best way to perform a nutrition assessment may be to combine these parameters with the subjective global assessment (SGA) approach, which has demonstrated an acceptable level of reliability and validity. The SGA gives a broad perspective, but it is not sensitive to changes in nutrition status. Other available parameters should also be reviewed. The SGA approach is summarized in Box 28.2.

BOX 28.2   Subjective Global Assessment Parameters for Nutrition Evaluation of Liver Disease Patients

History
Weight change (consider fluctuations resulting from ascites and edema)
Appetite
Taste changes and early satiety
Dietary intake (calories, protein, sodium)
Persistent gastrointestinal problems (nausea, vomiting, diarrhea, constipation, difficulty chewing or swallowing)

Physical Findings
Muscle wasting
Fat stores
Ascites or edema

Existing Conditions
Disease state and other problems that could influence nutrition status such as hepatic encephalopathy, gastrointestinal bleeding, renal insufficiency, infection

Nutritional Rating Based on Results
Well nourished
Moderately (or suspected of being) malnourished
Severely malnourished

From Hasse J: Nutritional aspects of adult liver transplantation. In: Busuttil RW, Klintmalm GB, editors: *Transplantation of the liver*, ed 2, Philadelphia, 2005, Elsevier Saunders.

Malnutrition

Moderate to severe malnutrition is a common finding in patients with advanced liver disease (Fig. 28.5). This is extremely significant, considering that malnutrition plays a major role in the pathogenesis of liver injury and has a profound negative effect on prognosis. The prevalence of malnutrition depends on nutrition assessment parameters used, type and degree of liver disease, and socioeconomic status.

Numerous coexisting factors are involved in the development of malnutrition in liver disease (see *Pathophysiology and Care Management Algorithm: Malnutrition in Liver Disease*). Inadequate oral intake, a major contributor, is caused by anorexia, dysgeusia, early satiety, nausea, or vomiting associated with liver disease and the drugs used to treat it. Another cause of inadequate intake is dietary restriction.

Maldigestion and malabsorption also play a role. Steatorrhea is common in cirrhosis, especially if there is disease involving bile duct injury and obstruction. Medications also may cause specific malabsorptive losses. In addition, altered metabolism secondary to liver dysfunction causes malnutrition in various ways. Micronutrient function is affected by altered storage in the liver, decreased transport by liver-synthesized proteins, and renal losses associated with alcoholism and advanced liver disease. Abnormal macronutrient metabolism and increased energy expenditure also can contribute to malnutrition. Finally, protein losses can occur from large-volume paracentesis when several liters of fluid from the abdomen (ascites) are removed through a needle.

Route of Nutrition

Although oral diet is the preferred route of nutrition for patients with ESLD, anorexia, nausea, dysgeusia, and other gastrointestinal symptoms can make adequate nutrition intake difficult to achieve. Early satiety is also a frequent complaint such that smaller, more frequent meals are better tolerated than three large meals. In addition, frequent feedings

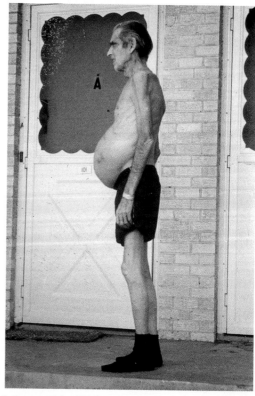

Fig. 28.5 Severe malnutrition and ascites in a man with end-stage liver disease.

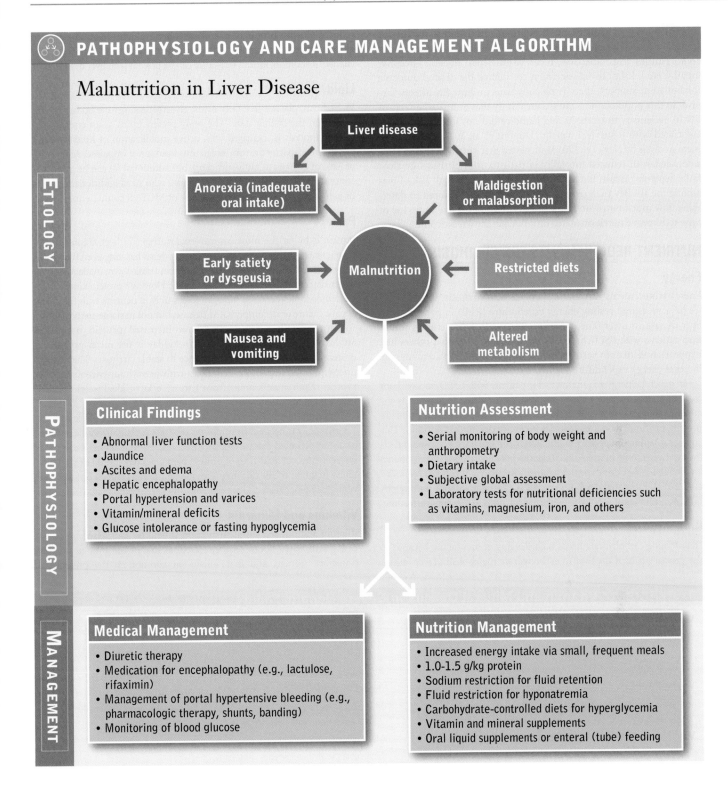

PATHOPHYSIOLOGY AND CARE MANAGEMENT ALGORITHM

Malnutrition in Liver Disease

ETIOLOGY

Liver disease

Anorexia (inadequate oral intake)

Maldigestion or malabsorption

Early satiety or dysgeusia

Malnutrition

Restricted diets

Nausea and vomiting

Altered metabolism

PATHOPHYSIOLOGY

Clinical Findings

- Abnormal liver function tests
- Jaundice
- Ascites and edema
- Hepatic encephalopathy
- Portal hypertension and varices
- Vitamin/mineral deficits
- Glucose intolerance or fasting hypoglycemia

Nutrition Assessment

- Serial monitoring of body weight and anthropometry
- Dietary intake
- Subjective global assessment
- Laboratory tests for nutritional deficiencies such as vitamins, magnesium, iron, and others

MANAGEMENT

Medical Management

- Diuretic therapy
- Medication for encephalopathy (e.g., lactulose, rifaximin)
- Management of portal hypertensive bleeding (e.g., pharmacologic therapy, shunts, banding)
- Monitoring of blood glucose

Nutrition Management

- Increased energy intake via small, frequent meals
- 1.0-1.5 g/kg protein
- Sodium restriction for fluid retention
- Fluid restriction for hyponatremia
- Carbohydrate-controlled diets for hyperglycemia
- Vitamin and mineral supplements
- Oral liquid supplements or enteral (tube) feeding

---

may also improve nitrogen balance and prevent hypoglycemia. Nutrient-dense snacks or supplements in the form of homemade or commercial oral drinks or foods should be encouraged, and, when necessary, use of enteral tube feedings should occur. Adjunctive nutrition support should be given to malnourished patients with liver disease if their intake is suboptimal and if they are at risk for fatal complications from the disease. Enteral nutrition (EN) is preferred over parenteral nutrition (PN) and history of varices are usually not a contraindication for tube feeding via a nasoenteric tube, provided there is no active bleeding (see Portal Hypertension Pathophysiology and Medical Treatment). Generally,

gastrostomy or jejunostomy tubes are not viable options in patients with liver disease given common complications of cirrhosis, including ascites and gastric varices. Instead, a nasoenteric tube (nasogastric, nasointestinal) tube is preferred although those could be contraindicated if the patient has severe epistaxis.

Treatment

EN support may be necessary in malnourished patients or patients with inadequate nutrient intake. The amount and duration of nutrition support depends on the goals of treatment (e.g., providing support during an acute event vs. improving nutrition to qualify for transplant), severity of the liver disease and malnutrition, and other comorbidities (e.g., infection, renal insufficiency, hepatic encephalopathy, etc.). If improved survival is considered the desired outcome for nutrition support, there is no consensus on how EN affects survival in this population. A multicenter study that evaluated effects of EN in patients with cirrhosis and jaundice did not find that EN was associated with a survival benefit (Dupont et al, 2012). However, a meta-analysis by Ney et al. (2013) suggested that nutrition therapy was associated with reduced mortality in patients with cirrhosis or alcoholic hepatitis disease, but a concern of the study was high risk of bias among the studies analyzed. Additional studies are required to determine how much nutrition support is needed and over what period of time to improve nutrition status or influence chosen outcomes.

NUTRIENT REQUIREMENTS FOR CIRRHOSIS

Energy

Energy requirements vary among patients with cirrhosis. Several studies have measured resting energy expenditure (REE) in patients with liver disease to determine energy requirements. Some studies found that patients with ESLD had normal metabolism and that others had hypometabolism or hypermetabolism. Ascites or shunt placement may increase energy expenditure slightly.

In general, energy requirements for patients with ESLD and without ascites are approximately 120% to 140% of the REE. Requirements increase to 150% to 175% of REE if ascites, infection, and malabsorption are present, or if nutritional repletion is necessary due to malnutrition. This equates to approximately 25 to 35 calories per kilogram body weight, although needs could be as low as 20 calories per kilogram for obese patients and as high as 40 calories per kilogram for underweight patients (Amodio et al, 2013). Estimated dry body weight (i.e., weight without fluid retention) or ideal weight should be used in calculations to prevent overfeeding.

Carbohydrate

Determining carbohydrate needs is challenging in liver failure because of the primary role of the liver in carbohydrate metabolism. Liver failure reduces glucose production and peripheral glucose use. The rate of gluconeogenesis is decreased, with preference for lipids and amino acids for energy. In addition, insulin resistance can be present with liver dysfunction.

Lipid

In cirrhosis, plasma-free fatty acids, glycerol, and ketone bodies are increased in the fasting state. The body prefers lipids as an energy substrate. Lipolysis is increased with active mobilization of lipid deposits, but the net capacity to store exogenous lipid is not impaired. An average of 30% of calories as fat is sufficient, but additional fat can be given as a concentrated source of calories for those who need additional calories. In patients with severe steatorrhea, use of MCT oil could be considered.

Protein

Protein is by far the most controversial nutrient in liver failure, and its management is also the most complex. Cirrhosis has long been thought of as a catabolic disease with increased protein breakdown, inadequate synthesis, depleted status, and muscle wasting. However, protein kinetic studies demonstrate increased nitrogen losses only in patients with fulminant hepatic failure or decompensated disease, but not in stable cirrhosis.

Patients with cirrhosis also have increased protein utilization. Studies suggest that 0.8 g of protein/kg/day is the mean protein requirement to achieve nitrogen balance in stable cirrhosis. Therefore in uncomplicated hepatitis or cirrhosis with or without encephalopathy, protein requirements range from 1 to 1.5 g/kg of ideal weight per day (Amodio et al, 2013).

To promote nitrogen accumulation or positive balance, at least 1.2 to 1.3 g/kg daily is needed. In situations of stress such as alcoholic hepatitis or decompensated disease (sepsis, infection, gastrointestinal bleeding, or severe ascites), at least 1.5 g of protein per kg per day should be provided. Small frequent meals not only provide additional calories but also prevent gluconeogenesis and wasting of muscle (Amodio et al, 2014).

Vitamins and Minerals

Vitamin and mineral supplementation should be considered for all patients with ESLD because of the essential role of the liver in nutrient transport, storage, and metabolism, in addition to the presence of

TABLE 28.4 Vitamin and Mineral Deficits in Severe Hepatic Failure

Vitamin or Mineral	Predisposing Factors	Signs of Deficiency (See Appendix 21)
Vitamin A	Steatorrhea, neomycin, cholestyramine, alcoholism	Night blindness, increased infection risk
Vitamin B_1 (thiamine)	Alcoholism, high-carbohydrate diet	Neuropathy, ascites, edema, central nervous system (CNS) dysfunction
Vitamin B_3 (niacin)	Alcoholism	Dermatitis, dementia, diarrhea, inflammation of mucous membranes
Vitamin B_6 (pyridoxine)	Alcoholism	Mucous membrane lesions, seborrheic dermatitis, glossitis, angular stomatitis, blepharitis, peripheral neuropathy, microcytic anemia, depression
Vitamin B_{12} (cyanocobalamin)	Alcoholism, cholestyramine	Megaloblastic anemia, glossitis, CNS dysfunction
Folate	Alcoholism	Megaloblastic anemia, glossitis, irritability
Vitamin D	Steatorrhea, glucocorticoids, cholestyramine	Osteomalacia, rickets (in children), possible link to cancer or autoimmune disorders
Vitamin E	Steatorrhea, cholestyramine	Peripheral neuropathy, ataxia, skeletal myopathy, retinopathy, immune system impairment
Vitamin K	Steatorrhea, antibiotics, cholestyramine	Excessive bleeding, bruising
Iron	Chronic bleeding	Stomatitis, microcytic anemia, malaise
Magnesium	Alcoholism, diuretics	Neuromuscular irritability, hypokalemia, hypocalcemia
Phosphorus	Anabolism, alcoholism	Anorexia, weakness, cardiac failure, glucose intolerance
Zinc	Diarrhea, diuretics, alcoholism	Immunodeficiency, impaired taste acuity, delayed wound healing, impaired protein synthesis

nutrient depletions due to drugs (Table 28.4). Vitamin deficiencies can contribute to complications. For example, folate and vitamin B_{12} deficiencies can lead to macrocytic anemia. Deficiency of pyridoxine, thiamin, or vitamin B_{12} can result in neuropathy. Confusion, ataxia, and ocular disturbances can result from a thiamin deficiency.

Deficiencies of fat-soluble vitamins have been found in all types of liver failure, especially in cholestatic diseases in which malabsorption and steatorrhea occur. Impaired dark adaptation can occur from vitamin A deficiency. Hepatic osteodystrophy or osteopenia can develop from vitamin D deficiency. Therefore supplementation is necessary, and may require using water-miscible forms of fat soluble vitamins. Intravenous or intramuscular vitamin K often is given for 3 days to rule out vitamin K deficiency as the cause of a prolonged prothrombin time. Water-soluble vitamin deficiencies associated with liver disease include thiamin (which can lead to Wernicke encephalopathy), pyridoxine (B_6), cyanocobalamin (B_{12}), folate, and niacin (B_3). Large doses (100 mg) of thiamin are given daily for a limited time if deficiency is suspected (see Appendices 12 and 13).

Mineral nutriture also is altered in liver disease. Iron stores may be depleted in patients experiencing gastrointestinal bleeding; however, iron supplementation should be avoided by persons with hemochromatosis or hemosiderosis (see Chapter 31). Manganese deposition has been noted to accumulate in brains of patients with cirrhosis, leading to impaired motor function and parkinsonism and increased occurrence of hepatic encephalopathy (Butterworth, 2013; Kobtan et al, 2016; Sureka et al, 2015). Elevated serum copper levels are found in cholestatic liver diseases (i.e., PBC and PSC).

In Wilson's disease, excess copper in various organs causes severe damage. Treatment typically includes administration of oral chelating agents such as D-penicillamine, trientine, or tetrathiomolybdate. Zinc acetate can block absorption of copper from food but typically is used with one of the chelating drugs. Dietary copper restriction can be useful during initial therapy. Copper also can be present in water where copper pipes are used. Running tap water for several seconds before using the water can reduce copper concentrations.

Zinc and magnesium levels are low in liver disease related to alcoholism and diuretic therapy. Calcium, as well as magnesium and zinc, may be malabsorbed with steatorrhea. Therefore the patient should take supplements of these minerals at least at the level of the DRI.

HERBAL AND DIETARY SUPPLEMENTS AND LIVER DISEASE

Hepatotoxicity is one of the greatest concerns associated with herbal and dietary supplementation. While most culinary herbs are safe, there are case reports of some herbal supplements resulting in liver failure (Box 28.3). One review lists more than 150 herbal products that have been reported as a cause of hepatotoxicity (Teschke et al, 2013). This extensive list emphasizes the gravity of the potential for harm to the liver from some herbal products, so practitioners should be vigilant in asking patients about supplement usage.

Other dietary products also have been implicated in hepatotoxicity. Among the most common products are garcinia cambogia, Herbalife products, Hydroxycut, and OxyElite Pro (Crescioli et al, 2018; Centers for Disease Control and Prevention [CDC], 2013; Fong et al, 2010; Jóhannsson et al, 2010; Schoepfer et al, 2007; Sharma et al, 2010). One of the most significant events occurred in 2013 when 56 individuals (43 in Hawaii) taking OxyElite Pro developed acute or fulminant liver failure. Several patients required liver transplantation and at least one patient died (CDC, 2013; Food and Drug Administration [FDA], 2014).

BOX 28.3 Selected Herbal Supplements Associated With Hepatotoxicity

Baikal skullcap (*Scutellaria*)
Chaparral (*Larrea tridentate*)
Pyrrolizidine alkaloids (found in herbs of the *Compositae, Leguminosae, Boraginaceae* family)
Comfrey (*Symphytum officinale*)
Heliotropium
Crotalaria
Germander (*Teucrium chamaedrys*)
Greater celandine (*Chelidonium majus*)
Saw palmetto (*Serenoa repens*)
Noni juice (*Morinda citrifolia*)
Margosa oil (*Antelaea azadirachta*)
Aloe vera (aloe latex)
Black cohosh (*Actea racemosa* or *Actea cimicifuga*)
LipoKinetix (*usnic acid*)
Atractylis gummifera
Impila (*Callilepis laureola*)
Mistletoe (*Viscum album*)
Valerian (*Valerian officinalis*)
Senna (*Cassia angustifolia*)
Pennyroyal (squaw mint oil)
Kava (*Piper methysticum*)
Liatris callilepis
Green tea extract (*Camellia sinensis*), although green tea in reasonable amounts appears safe
Cascara sagrada
OxyElite Pro
Jin Bu Huan (*Lycopodium serratum*)
Ma Huang (*Ephedra sinica*)
Dai-saiko-to (*Sho-saiko-to*)
Hydroxycut

LipoKinetix (Syntrax Innovations, Inc, Cape Girardeau, MO), OxyElite Pro (USP Labs, LLC, Dallas, TX), Hydroxycut (Iovate Health Sciences USA, Inc, Blasdell, NY).
Reprinted with permission from: Corey RL, Rakela J: Complementary and alternative medicine: risks and special considerations in pre- and post-transplant patients, *Nutr Clin Pract* 29:322, 2014.

Despite reports of hepatotoxicity with numerous herbal supplements, some supplements have been investigated for benefits on liver disease. *S*-adenosyl-*L*-methionine (SAMe) is sometimes suggested for use with liver disease. It is purported to act as a methyl donor for methylation reactions and participates in glutathione synthesis (an antioxidant). A recent systematic review and meta-analysis suggested SAMe may improve liver function but does not improve outcomes for chronic liver disease (Guo et al, 2015). Betaine has been proposed for treatment of NASH, alcoholic liver disease, and other conditions. Betaine functions in the liver as a methyl donor. Although there is theoretical promise, there is a lack of strong evidence for benefit (Day and Kempson, 2016; Abdelmalek et al, 2009; Mukherjee, 2011).

Milk thistle appears to be the most popular and extensively studied herbal supplement for liver disease. The active component in milk thistle is silymarin with silybin (constituting 50% to 70% of silymarin) believed to have the most biologic activity. Milk thistle is proposed to have antiinflammatory, antioxidant, and antifibrotic properties, which would be beneficial in liver disease (Abenavoli et al, 2010). Milk thistle has been evaluated for viral hepatitis, alcoholic liver disease, and toxin-induced liver disease. A recent meta-analysis evaluated the benefits of silymarin on NAFLD. The study showed that silymarin may reduce transaminases, but there was no evaluation of histologic changes in the liver (Zhong et al, 2017). Despite its popularity and widespread use, a clear consensus is lacking as to a beneficial effect of milk thistle on all forms of liver disease, so individual assessment is needed. However, data are not sufficient to suggest that it is unsafe or toxic for patients with liver disease.

LIVER RESECTION AND TRANSPLANTATION

As with any major surgery, protein and energy needs increase after liver resection. Needs also are increased for liver cell regeneration. EN can be beneficial by providing portal hepatotropic factors necessary for liver cell proliferation. Optimal nutrition is most important for patients with poor nutrition status before hepatectomy (e.g., patients with cholangiocarcinoma).

Liver transplantation has become an established treatment for ESLD. Malnutrition is common in liver transplant candidates. Dietary intake often can be enhanced if patients eat small, frequent, nutrient-dense meals, and oral nutritional supplements also may be well tolerated. EN is indicated when oral intake is inadequate or contraindicated.

Varices are not an absolute contraindication for placement of a feeding tube. Because PN can affect liver function adversely, EN is preferred. PN is reserved for patients without adequate gut function (see Chapter 12).

In the acute posttransplant phase, nutrient needs are increased to promote healing, deter infection, provide energy for recovery, and replenish depleted body stores. Nitrogen requirements are elevated in the acute posttransplant phase and can be met with early postoperative EN. Early postoperative EN has been associated with reduced infections in liver transplant recipients (Hasse et al, 1995; Ikegami et al, 2012; Masuda et al, 2014). Administration of probiotics and fiber with tube feeding may reduce postoperative infection rate better than tube feeding or fiber alone (Rayes et al, 2005).

Multiple medications used after transplant have nutritional side effects such as anorexia, gastrointestinal upset, hypercatabolism, diarrhea, hyperglycemia, hyperlipidemia, sodium retention, hypertension, hyperkalemia, and hypercalciuria. Therefore dietary modification is based on the specific side effects of drug therapy (Table 28.5). During the posttransplant phase, nutrient requirements are adjusted to prevent or treat problems of obesity, hyperlipidemia, hypertension, diabetes mellitus, and osteopenia. Table 28.6 summarizes nutrient needs after liver transplantation.

TABLE 28.5 Drugs Commonly Used After Liver Transplantation

Immunosuppressant Drug	Possible Nutritional Side Effects	Proposed Nutrition Therapy
Azathioprine	Macrocytic anemia	Give folate supplements.
	Mouth sores	Adjust food and meals as needed; monitor intake.
	Nausea, vomiting, diarrhea, anorexia, sore throat, stomach pain, decreased taste acuity	
Antithymocyte globulin (ATG), lymphocyte immune globulin	Nausea, vomiting	Adjust food and meals as needed; monitor intake.
Cyclosporine	Sodium retention	Decrease sodium intake.
	Hyperkalemia	Decrease potassium intake.
	Hyperlipidemia	Limit fat and simple carbohydrate intake.
	Hyperglycemia	Decrease simple carbohydrate intake.
	Decreased serum magnesium level	Increase magnesium intake; give supplements.
	Hypertension	Limit sodium intake.
	Nausea, vomiting	Adjust food and meals as needed; monitor intake.
Glucocorticoids	Sodium retention	Decrease sodium intake.
	Hyperglycemia	Decrease simple carbohydrate intake.
	Hyperlipidemia	Limit fat and simple carbohydrate intake.
	False hunger	Avoid overeating.
	Protein wasting with high doses	Increase protein intake.
	Decreased absorption of calcium and phosphorus	Increase calcium and phosphorus intake; give supplements as needed.
Mycophenolate mofetil, mycophenolic acid	Nausea, vomiting, diarrhea	Adjust food and meals as needed; monitor intake.
Sirolimus	Possible GI symptoms	Adjust food and meals as needed; monitor intake.
	Hyperlipidemia	Limit fat and simple carbohydrate intake.
	Inhibits wound healing	Ensure adequate macro- and micronutrients.
	Depressed appetite.	Consider appetite stimulants.
Tacrolimus	Hyperglycemia	Decrease simple carbohydrate intake.
	Hyperkalemia	Decrease potassium intake.
	Nausea, vomiting	Adjust food and meals as needed; monitor intake.

GI, Gastrointestinal.

TABLE 28.6 General Nutrient Requirements for Liver Transplant Patients

	Pretransplantation	Immediate Posttransplantation (First 2 Posttransplant Months)	Long-Term Posttransplantation
*Protein	Dependent on nutrition status and medical condition but usually 1-1.5 g/kg	Dependent on nutrition status, medical condition, and dialysis requirement but usually 1.2-2 g/kg	Maintenance – about 1 g/kg
*Calories	Dependent on nutrition status and losses; usually 20%-50% above basal	Dependent on nutrition status and metabolic stress but usually 20%-30% above basal	Dependent on activity and weight goals; usually 20% above basal for sedentary activity if at goal weight
Fat	As needed	Approximately 30% of calories	Moderate fat (30% of calories)
Carbohydrate	Reduced carbohydrate if diabetes or obesity present	Reduced carbohydrate if diabetes present	Reduced simple carbohydrate, especially if diabetes or obesity present
Sodium	2 g/day	2 g/day (as indicated)	2 g/day (as indicated)
Fluid	Restrict to 1000-1500 mL/day (if hyponatremic)	As needed	As needed
Calcium	800-1200 mg/day	800-1200 mg/day	1200-1500 mg/day
Vitamins	Multivitamin/mineral supplementation to DRI levels; additional water- and fat-soluble vitamins as indicated	Multivitamin/mineral supplementation to DRI levels; additional water- and fat-soluble vitamins as indicated	Multivitamin/mineral supplementation to DRI levels

*Use estimated dry or ideal weight.
DRI, Dietary reference intake.

PHYSIOLOGY AND FUNCTIONS OF THE GALLBLADDER

The gallbladder lies on the undersurface of the right lobe of the liver (Fig. 28.6). The main function of the gallbladder is to concentrate, store, and excrete bile, which is produced by the liver. During the concentration process, water and electrolytes are resorbed by the gallbladder mucosa. Bile is composed of bile salts and excretory endogenous and exogenous compounds. Other components include fatty acids, cholesterol, phospholipids, bilirubin, protein, and other compounds. Bile salts are made by liver cells from cholesterol and are essential for the digestion and absorption of fats, fat-soluble vitamins, and some minerals (see Chapter 1). Bilirubin, the main bile pigment, is derived

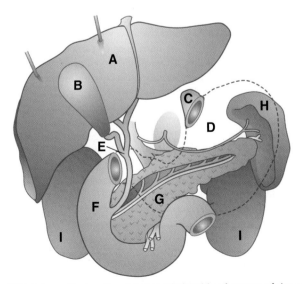

Fig. 28.6 Schematic drawing showing relationship of organs of the upper abdomen. **A,** Liver (retracted upward); **B,** gallbladder; **C,** esophageal opening of stomach; **D,** stomach (*shown in dotted outline*); **E,** common bile duct; **F,** duodenum; **G,** pancreas and pancreatic duct; **H,** spleen; **I,** kidneys. (Courtesy Cleveland Clinic, Cleveland, Ohio, 2002.)

from the release of hemoglobin from red blood cell destruction. It is transported to the liver, where it is conjugated and excreted via bile.

The primary transporter responsible for bile salt secretion is the bile salt export pump (BSEP). Overall, bile salts play a key role in a wide range of physiologic and pathophysiologic processes (Kubitz et al, 2012). Excreted into the small intestine via bile, bile salts are later resorbed into the portal system (enterohepatic circulation). This is the primary excretory pathway for the minerals copper and manganese.

Bile contains immunoglobulins that support the integrity of the intestinal mucosa. Fibroblast growth factor receptor (FGFR4) controls bile acid metabolism and protects the liver from fibrosis; FGFR1 and FGFR2 assist in regeneration of the liver (Böhm et al, 2010). Molecular crosstalk between bile acid–activated nuclear receptors and proinflammatory nuclear mediators provides new understanding of inflammation-induced cholestasis (Kosters and Karpen, 2010; Lam et al, 2010).

Bile is removed by the liver via bile canaliculi that drain into intrahepatic bile ducts. The ducts lead to the left and right hepatic ducts, which leave the liver and join to become the common hepatic duct. The bile is directed to the gallbladder via the cystic duct for concentration and storage. The cystic duct joins the common hepatic duct to form the common bile duct. The bile duct then joins the pancreatic duct, which carries digestive enzymes.

During the course of digestion, food reaches the duodenum, causing the release of intestinal hormones such as cholecystokinin (CCK) and secretin. This stimulates the gallbladder and pancreas and causes the sphincter of Oddi to relax, allowing pancreatic juice and bile to flow into the duodenum at the ampulla of Vater to assist in fat digestion. For this reason diseases of the gallbladder, liver, and pancreas often are interrelated.

DISEASES OF THE GALLBLADDER

Disorders of the biliary tract affect millions of people each year, causing significant suffering and even death by precipitating pancreatitis and sepsis. A diverse spectrum of disease affects the biliary system, often presenting with similar clinical signs and symptoms. Treatment may involve diet, medication, and/or surgery.

Cholestasis

Pathophysiology and Medical Management

Cholestasis is a condition in which little or no bile is secreted or the flow of bile into the digestive tract is obstructed. This can occur in patients without oral or enteral feeding for a prolonged period, such as those requiring PN, and can predispose to acalculous cholecystitis, an inflammatory disease of the gall bladder without evidence of gallstones or cystic duct obstruction. BSEP is the major transporter for the secretion of bile acids from the hepatocytes into bile. BSEP deficiency results in several different genetic forms of cholestasis and acquired forms of cholestasis such as drug-induced cholestasis and intrahepatic cholestasis of pregnancy (Lam et al, 2010). Prevention of cholestasis requires stimulation of biliary motility and secretions by at least minimum enteral feedings. If this is not possible, drug therapy is used.

Cholelithiasis

Pathophysiology

The formation of gallstones (calculi) is known as cholelithiasis. Virtually all gallstones form within the gallbladder. Gallstone disease affects millions of Americans each year and can cause significant health risks. In most cases gallstones are asymptomatic. Gallstones that pass from the gallbladder into the common bile duct may remain there indefinitely without causing symptoms, or they may pass into the duodenum with or without symptoms.

Choledocholithiasis develops when stones slip into the bile ducts, producing obstruction, pain, and cramps. If passage of bile into the duodenum is interrupted, cholecystitis, inflammation of the gallbladder, can develop. In the absence of bile in the intestine, lipid absorption is impaired, and without bile pigments, stools become light in color (acholic). If uncorrected, bile backup can result in jaundice and liver damage (secondary biliary cirrhosis). Obstruction of the distal common bile duct can lead to pancreatitis if the pancreatic duct is blocked.

Most gallstones are unpigmented cholesterol stones composed primarily of cholesterol, bilirubin, and calcium salts. Bacteria also play a role in gallstone formation. Low-grade chronic infections produce changes in the gallbladder mucosa, which affect its absorptive capabilities. Excess water or bile acid may be absorbed as a result. Cholesterol may then precipitate out and cause gallstones (Njeze, 2013).

There are numerous risk factors that may predispose an individual to gallstone formation (Stinton et al, 2010). Some of these are modifiable, others are not (Table 28.7) High dietary fat intake over a prolonged period may predispose a person to gallstone formation because of the constant stimulus to produce more cholesterol for bile

TABLE 28.7 Risk Factors for Gallstone Formation

Modifiable	Nonmodifiable
High-fat diet	Familial/genetics
Female sex hormone use	Ethnicity
Obesity/metabolic syndrome/diabetes	Female gender
Rapid weight loss	Increasing age
Physical inactivity	
Underlying disease: cirrhosis, Crohn's disease	
Drugs	
Parenteral nutrition	

Adapted from Stinton LM, Myers RP, Shaffer EA: Epidemiology of Gallstones, *Gastroenterol Clin North Am* 39:157–169, 2010; Shaffer EA: Gallstone disease: epidemiology of gallbladder stone disease, *Best Pract Res Clin Gastroenterol* 20(6):981–996, 2006.

synthesis required in fat digestion. Rapid weight loss (as with jejunoileal and gastric bypass surgery and fasting or severe calorie restriction) is associated with a high incidence of biliary sludge and gallstone formation. Indeed, cholelithiasis and fatty liver disease share risk factors, including central obesity, insulin resistance, and diabetes mellitus (Koller et al, 2012; Weikert et al, 2010).

Risk factors for cholesterol stone formation include female gender, pregnancy, older age, family history, obesity and truncal body fat distribution, diabetes mellitus, inflammatory bowel disease, and drugs (lipid-lowering medications, oral contraceptives, and estrogens). Certain ethnic groups are at greater risk of stone formation, including Native Americans, Scandinavians, and Mexican Americans. In addition, approximately 30% of individuals with cirrhosis have gallstones (Acalovschi, 2014).

Pigmented stones typically consist of bilirubin polymers or calcium salts. They are associated with chronic hemolysis. Risk factors associated with these stones include older age, sickle cell anemia, thalassemia, biliary tract infection, cirrhosis, alcoholism, and long-term PN.

Medical and Surgical Management

Cholecystectomy is surgical removal of the gallbladder, especially if the stones are numerous, large, or calcified. The cholecystectomy may be performed as a traditional open laparotomy or as a less invasive laparoscopic procedure.

Chemical dissolution with the administration of bile salts, chenodeoxycholic acid, and ursodeoxycholic acid (litholytic therapy), or dissolution by extracorporeal shockwave lithotripsy, may also be used less often than surgical techniques. Patients with gallstones that have migrated into the bile ducts may be candidates for a diagnostic procedure using X-ray called endoscopic retrograde cholangiopancreatography.

Medical Nutrition Therapy

The role of diet in the pathogenesis of gallstones and therefore treatment recommendations remains unclear. Obesity is a risk factor, but the exact composition of the diet that results in gallstones is less clear. Diets high in cholesterol and fat seem to increase the risk of cholelithiasis. In contrast, unsaturated fats, coffee, fiber, ascorbic acid (vitamin C), calcium, and moderate consumption of alcohol reduce the risk (Shaffer, 2006).

There also may be some benefit in replacing simple sugars and refined starches with high-fiber carbohydrates. Individuals consuming refined carbohydrates have a 60% greater risk for developing gallstones, compared with those who consumed the most fiber, in particular insoluble fiber (Mendez-Sanchez et al, 2007). Thus plant-based diets may reduce the risk of cholelithiasis. Vegetarian diets are high in fiber and low in fat, consisting primarily of unsaturated fat. Vitamin C, which is generally high in vegetarian diets, affects the rate-limiting step in the catabolism of cholesterol to bile acids and inversely is related to the risk of gallstones, especially in women.

Weight cycling (repeatedly losing and regaining weight), fasting, and very-low-calorie diets increase the likelihood of cholelithiasis. Along with weight reduction, some evidence indicates that physical activity reduces the risk of cholecystitis. In cholecystitis, MNT includes a high-fiber, low-fat, plant-based diet to prevent gallbladder contractions. Data are conflicting as to whether intravenous lipids stimulate gallbladder contraction.

After surgical removal of the gallbladder, oral feedings can be advanced to a regular diet as tolerated, although a lower fat diet with adequate soluble fiber may be important at first. In the absence of the gallbladder, bile is secreted directly by the liver into the intestine. The biliary tract dilates, forming a "simulated pouch" over time to allow bile to be held in a manner similar to the original gallbladder. Some patients may develop frequent loose, watery stools if they eat fatty meals during this adaptation time frame. In most cases, the diarrhea is temporary and self-limiting.

Cholecystitis

Pathophysiology

Inflammation of the gallbladder is known as cholecystitis, and it may be chronic or acute. It usually is caused by gallstones obstructing the bile ducts (calculous cholecystitis), leading to the backup of bile. Bilirubin, the main bile pigment, gives bile its greenish color. When biliary tract obstruction prevents bile from reaching the intestine, it backs up and returns to the circulation. Bilirubin has an affinity for elastic tissues (such as the eye and the skin); therefore when it overflows into the general circulation, it causes the yellow skin pigmentation and eye discoloration typical of jaundice.

Acute cholecystitis without stones (acalculous cholecystitis) may occur in critically ill patients or when the gallbladder and its bile are stagnant. Impaired gallbladder emptying in chronic acalculous cholecystitis appears to be due to diminished spontaneous contractile activity and decreased contractile responsiveness to CCK. The walls of the gallbladder become inflamed and distended, and infection can occur. During such episodes, the patient experiences upper-quadrant abdominal pain accompanied by nausea, vomiting, and flatulence.

Chronic cholecystitis is longstanding inflammation of the gallbladder. It is caused by repeated, mild attacks of acute cholecystitis. This leads to thickening of the walls of the gallbladder. The gallbladder begins to shrink and eventually loses the ability to perform its function: concentrating and storing bile. Eating foods that are high in fat may aggravate the symptoms of cholecystitis because bile is needed to digest such foods. Chronic cholecystitis occurs more often in women than in men, and the incidence increases after the age of 40. Risk factors include the presence of gallstones and a history of acute cholecystitis.

Surgical Management

Acute cholecystitis requires surgical intervention unless medically contraindicated. Without surgery, the condition may either subside or progress to gangrene.

Medical Nutrition Therapy

Acute cholecystitis. In an acute attack, oral feedings are temporarily discontinued. PN may be indicated if the patient is malnourished and it is anticipated that they will not be taking anything orally for a prolonged period. When feedings are resumed, a low-fat diet is recommended to decrease gallbladder stimulation. A hydrolyzed low-fat formula or an oral low-fat diet consisting of 30 to 45 g of fat per day can be given. Table 28.8 shows a fat-restricted diet.

TABLE 28.8 Fat-Restricted Diet

Food Allowed	Food to Limit or Exclude
Beverages Skim milk or buttermilk made with skim milk; coffee, tea, Postum, fruit juice, soft drinks, cocoa made with cocoa powder and skim milk	Whole milk, buttermilk made with whole milk, chocolate milk, cream in excess of amounts allowed under fats
Bread and Cereal Products Plain, nonfat cereals; spaghetti, noodles, rice, macaroni; plain whole grain or enriched breads, air-popped popcorn, bagels, English muffins	Biscuits, breads, egg or cheese bread, sweet rolls made with fat; pancakes, doughnuts, waffles, fritters, popcorn prepared with fat; muffins, natural cereals and breads to which extra fat is added
Cheese Fat-free or low-fat cottage cheese, ¼ c to be used as substitute for 1 oz of cheese, or low-fat cheeses containing less than 5% butterfat	Whole-milk cheeses
Desserts Sherbet made with skim milk; nonfat frozen yogurt; nonfat frozen nondairy desserts; fruit ice; sorbet; gelatin; rice, bread, cornstarch, tapioca, or pudding made with skim milk; fruit whips with gelatin, sugar, and egg white; fruit; angel food cake; graham crackers; vanilla wafers; meringues	Cake, pie, pastry, ice cream, or any dessert containing shortening, chocolate, or fats of any kind, unless especially prepared using part of fat allowance
Eggs Three per week prepared only with fat from fat allowance; egg whites as desired; low-fat egg substitutes	More than one/day unless substituted for part of the meat allowed
Fats Choose up to the limit allowed among the following (1 serving in the amount listed equals 1 fat choice): 1 tsp butter or margarine 1 tsp shortening or oil 1 tsp mayonnaise 2 tsp Italian or French dressing 1 Tbsp reduced-fat salad dressing 1 strip crisp bacon ⅛ avocado (4-inch diameter) 2 Tbsp light cream 1 Tbsp heavy cream 6 small nuts 5 small olives	Any in excess of amount prescribed on diet; all others

Continued

TABLE 28.8 Fat-Restricted Diet—cont'd

Food Allowed	Food to Limit or Exclude
Fruits	
As desired	Avocado in excess of amount allowed on fat list
Lean Meat, Fish, Poultry, and Meat Substitutes	
Choose up to the limit allowed among the following: poultry without skin, fish, veal (all cuts), liver, lean beef, pork, and lamb, all with visible fat removed—1 oz cooked weight equals 1 equivalent; ¼ c water-packed tuna or salmon equals 1 equivalent; tofu or tempeh—3 oz equals 1 equivalent	Fried or fatty meats, sausage, scrapple, frankfurters, poultry skins, stewing hens, spareribs, salt pork, beef unless lean, duck, goose, ham hocks, pig's feet, luncheon meats (unless reduced fat), gravies unless fat free, tuna and salmon packed in oil, peanut butter
Milk	
Skim, buttermilk, or yogurt made from skim milk	Whole, 2%, 1%, chocolate, buttermilk made with whole milk
Seasonings	
As desired	None
Soups	
Bouillon, clear broth, fat-free vegetable soup, cream soup made with skim milk, packaged dehydrated soups	All others
Sweets	
Jelly, jam, marmalade, honey, syrup, molasses, sugar, hard sugar candies, fondant, gumdrops, jelly beans, marshmallows, cocoa powder, fat-free chocolate sauce, red and black licorice	Any candy made with chocolate, nuts, butter, cream, or fat of any kind
Vegetables	
All plainly prepared vegetables	Potato chips; buttered, au gratin, creamed, or fried potatoes and other vegetables unless made with allowed fat; casseroles or frozen vegetables in butter sauce

Daily Food Allowances for 40-g Fat Diet

Food	Amount	Approximate Fat Content (g)
Skim milk	2 c or more	0
Lean meat, fish, poultry	6 oz or 6 equivalents	18
Whole egg or egg yolks	3 per week	2
Vegetables	3 servings or more, at least 1 or more dark green or deep yellow	0
Fruits	3 or more servings, at least 1 citrus	0
Breads, cereals	As desired, fat free	0
Fat exchanges*	4-5 exchanges daily	20-25
Desserts and sweets	As desired from permitted list	0
	Total Fat	38-43

*Fat content can be reduced further by reducing the fat exchanges. 1 fat exchange = 5 g of fat.

After cholecystectomy, patients may experience symptoms of gastritis secondary to duodenogastric reflux of bile acids. The reflux also may be responsible for symptoms in this postcholecystectomy syndrome. At present, there are no well-established pharmacologic approaches in the management of postcholecystectomy gastritis. The symptoms are not caused, but exacerbated, by the cholecystectomy. The use of ursodeoxycholic acid and various Chinese herbs have been suggested (Zhang et al, 2017). However, efficacy of their use is limited. The addition of soluble fiber to the diet may act as a sequestering agent and bind the bile in the stomach between meals to avoid gastritis.

Chronic cholecystitis. Patients with chronic conditions may require a long-term, low-fat diet that contains 25% to 30% of total kilocalories as fat (see Table 28.7). Stricter limitation is undesirable because fat in the intestine is important for some stimulation and drainage of the biliary tract. Additionally, saturated fats should be replaced with fish oil and polyunsaturated fats to reduce the risk of gallstone formation (Lee and Jang, 2012; Stinton et al, 2010; Berr et al, 1992). The degree of food intolerance varies widely among persons with gallbladder disorders; many complain of foods that cause flatulence and bloating. For this reason, it is best to determine with the patient which foods should be eliminated (see Chapter 27 for a discussion of potential gas-forming foods). Administration of water-soluble forms of fat-soluble vitamins may be of benefit in patients with chronic gallbladder conditions or in those in whom fat malabsorption is suspected.

Cholangitis

Pathophysiology and Medical Management

Inflammation of the bile ducts is known as cholangitis. Patients with acute cholangitis need resuscitation with fluids and broad-spectrum antibiotics. If the patient does not improve with conservative treatment, placement of a percutaneous biliary stent or cholecystectomy may be needed.

Sclerosing cholangitis can result in sepsis and liver failure. Most patients have multiple intrahepatic strictures, which makes surgical intervention difficult, if not impossible. Patients are generally on broad-spectrum antibiotics. Percutaneous ductal dilation may provide short-term bile duct patency in some patients. When sepsis is recurrent, patients may require chronic antibiotic therapy (see Primary Sclerosing Cholangitis).

COMPLEMENTARY AND INTEGRATIVE MEDICINE FOR GALLSTONES

Patients often seek complementary and integrative approaches to gallbladder disease, including various nutritional supplements, herbal medications, and gallbladder flushes. Vitamin C deficiency has been linked to gallstone formation in animal models (Jenkins, 1978). The data in humans are limited, but vitamin C supplementation has been associated with a decreased risk of gallstones in postmenopausal women who consume alcohol (Simon et al, 1998) and may protect against gallstones (Walcher et al, 2009). In a cross-sectional study of 582 elderly people, higher circulating levels of vitamin E was associated with a lower probability of gallstone disease (Waniek et al, 2018).

Choleretic (substances that increase the volume of secretion of bile from the liver) herbs such as milk thistle, dandelion root, artichoke, turmeric, greater celandine, and Oregon grape stimulate bile flow and reduce the amount of cholesterol in bile. Various herbs have been suggested as treatment options for cholestasis and other hepatobiliary disorders (Spiridonov, 2012). However, data from well-conducted randomized controlled trials is limited.

The use of acupuncture has been proposed for the treatment of gallstones (Moga, 2003). It is thought that acupuncture aids in the removal of stones. However, it may be that acupuncture aids in the relief of pain more so than the removal of stones.

PHYSIOLOGY AND FUNCTIONS OF THE EXOCRINE PANCREAS

The pancreas is an elongated, flattened gland that lies in the upper abdomen behind the stomach. The head of the pancreas is in the right upper quadrant below the liver within the curvature of the duodenum, and the tapering tail slants upward to the hilum of the spleen (see Fig. 28.6). This glandular organ has an endocrine and exocrine function. Pancreatic cells manufacture glucagon, insulin, and somatostatin for absorption into the bloodstream (endocrine function) for regulation of glucose homeostasis (see Chapter 29). Other cells secrete enzymes and other substances directly into the intestinal lumen, where they aid in digesting proteins, fats, and carbohydrates (exocrine function).

In most people, the pancreatic duct, which carries the exocrine pancreatic secretions, merges with the common bile duct into a unified opening through which bile and pancreatic juices drain into the duodenum at the ampulla of Vater. Many factors regulate exocrine secretion from the pancreas. Neural and hormonal responses play a role, with the presence and composition of ingested foods being a large contributor. The two primary hormonal stimuli for pancreatic secretion are secretin and CCK (see Chapter 1).

Factors that influence pancreatic secretions during a meal can be divided into three phases: (1) the cephalic phase, mediated through the vagus nerve and initiated by the sight, smell, taste, and anticipation of food that leads to the secretion of bicarbonate and pancreatic enzymes; (2) gastric distention with food initiates the gastric phase of pancreatic secretion, which stimulates enzyme secretion; and (3) the intestinal phase, mediated by the release of CCK, with the most potent effect.

DISEASES OF THE EXOCRINE PANCREAS

Pancreatitis

Pathophysiology and Medical Management

Pancreatitis is an inflammation of the pancreas and is characterized by edema, cellular exudate, and fat necrosis. The disease can range from mild and self-limiting to severe, with tissue autodigestion, necrosis, and hemorrhage of pancreatic tissue. Various prognostic scoring systems have been developed such as Ranson, acute physiology and chronic health evaluation (APACHE)-II, bedside index for severity in acute pancreatitis (BISAP) scores, and computed tomography severity index (CTSI) (Banks et al, 2013; Ranson, 1974; Larvin and McMahon, 1989; Balthazar et al, 1990; Wu et al, 2008; Petrov et al, 2009). These can help predict the mortality of acute pancreatitis (Cho et al, 2015). There may be differences in these scores but they help to predict the severity of the disease. Pancreatitis is classified as either acute or chronic, the latter with pancreatic destruction so extensive that exocrine and endocrine function are severely diminished, and maldigestion and diabetes mellitus may result.

The symptoms of pancreatitis can range from continuous or intermittent pain of varying intensity to severe upper abdominal pain, which may radiate to the back. Symptoms may worsen with the ingestion of food. Clinical presentation also may include nausea, vomiting, abdominal distention, and steatorrhea. Severe cases are complicated by hypotension, oliguria, and dyspnea. There is extensive destruction of pancreatic tissue with subsequent fibrosis, enzyme production is diminished, and serum amylase and lipase may appear normal. However, absence of enzymes to aid in the digestion of food leads to steatorrhea and malabsorption. Table 28.9 describes several tests used to determine the extent of pancreatic destruction.

TABLE 28.9	Some Tests of Pancreatic Function
Test	**Significance**
Secretin stimulation test	Measures pancreatic secretion, particularly bicarbonate, in response to secretin stimulation
Glucose tolerance test	Assesses endocrine function of the pancreas by measuring insulin response to a glucose load
72-hr stool fat test	Assesses exocrine function of the pancreas by measuring fat absorption that reflects pancreatic lipase secretion
Fecal elastase	Enzyme most commonly used to determine pancreatic function; indirect test. Levels >200 mcg/g are considered normal; concentration <15 mcg/g of feces consistent with pancreatic exocrine insufficiency

Medical Nutrition Therapy

Alcohol use, smoking, body weight, diet, genetic factors, and medications affect the risk of developing pancreatitis. Thus diet modification has an important role after diagnosis. Dietary recommendations differ, depending on whether the condition is acute or chronic. Obesity appears to be a risk factor for the development of pancreatitis and for increased severity (Martinez et al, 2004; Katuchova et al, 2014).

Depressed serum calcium levels are common. Hypoalbuminemia occurs, with subsequent edema (also known as third spacing of fluid). The calcium, which is bound to albumin, is thus affected and may appear artificially low. Another occurrence is "soap" formation in the gut by calcium and fatty acids, created by the fat necrosis that results in less calcium absorption. Checking an ionized calcium level is a method of determining available calcium.

Acute pancreatitis. Pain associated with acute pancreatitis (AP) is partially related to the secretory mechanisms of pancreatic enzymes and bile. Therefore, nutrition therapy is adjusted to provide minimum stimulation of these systems (International Association of Pancreatology, 2013) (see *Pathophysiology and Care Management Algorithm:* Pancreatitis). The basis for nutrition therapy is to put the pancreas "at rest." In patients with AP, early (within 24 hours) oral feeding as tolerated should be initiated rather than keeping the patient nil per os (NPO, nothing by mouth) (Crockett et al, 2018; Vege et al, 2018). Success of early feeding has been demonstrated using a variety of diets, including low fat, normal fat content, and soft or solid consistency, and thus starting with a clear liquid diet is not required (Lankisch et al, 2015). Early feeding is not successful in all AP due to pain, vomiting, or ileus (lack of peristalsis in the gut), and feeding may need to be delayed beyond 24 hours in some cases. Some patients who are intolerant of oral feeding may require placement of an enteral tube for nutritional support. The diet usually is progressed as tolerated to easily digested foods with a low-fat content with more fat added as tolerated. Foods may be better tolerated if they are divided into six small meals (see Table 28.8).

Severe acute pancreatitis (SAP) results in a hypermetabolic, catabolic state with immediate metabolic alterations in the pancreas and in remote organs. Metabolic demands are similar to those of sepsis. Amino acids are released from muscle and used for gluconeogenesis. These patients often exhibit signs of stress-induced malnutrition such as decreased serum levels of albumin, transferrin, and lymphocytes reflecting the inflammatory response (see Chapter 7). SAP is associated with significant morbidity and mortality. These patients often develop complications such as fluid collections, pseudocysts, pancreatic necrosis, and infection or multisystem organ failure.

The optimal route and timing of nutrition in SAP has been the subject of much controversy. PN and EN are equally effective in terms of days to normalization of serum amylase levels, days to resumption of oral feeding, days to clear nosocomial infections, and the clinical outcome in patients with mild to moderate pancreatitis (Wu et al, 2014). The favorable effect of either EN or PN on patient outcome may be enhanced by supplementation with modulators of inflammation such as arginine, glutamine, omega-3 fatty acids, or probiotics and systemic immunity (McClave et al, 2006; McClave et al, 2016) (see Chapter 7). However, failure to use the GIT in patients with SAP may exacerbate the stress response and disease severity, leading to more complications and prolonged hospitalization; thus EN is preferred for nutrition therapy (Al-Omran et al, 2010; McClave, 2013; Mirtallo et al, 2012; Crockett et al, 2018; Vege et al, 2018). Some data support the use of early EN in AP (Zou et al, 2014). In a meta-analysis of observational data from individuals with AP, starting EN within 24 hours after hospital admission, compared with after 24 hours, was associated with a reduction in complications (Bakker et al, 2014). Early EN in patients with AP may reduce length of hospital stay without adverse events for patients with mild to moderate pancreatitis (Vaughn et al, 2017). In

another meta-analysis, early EN was associated with a significant decrease in the incidence of multiple organ failure but was not significant for other complications and mortality compared with delayed EN (Feng et al, 2017).

Nasogastric EN has been shown to be efficacious in SAP (Nally et al, 2014). However, to minimize pancreatic stimulation it is best to place jejunal feeding tubes endoscopically as far down the intestine as possible, generally more than 40 cm past the ligament of Treitz (O'Keefe et al, 2001).

EN results in a substantial cost savings with fewer septic complications and overall reduction of morbidity and mortality (Petrov et al, 2008; Sun et al, 2013). The location of the feeding and the composition of the formula is thought to determine the degree of pancreatic stimulation. Infusion into the jejunum eliminates the cephalic and gastric phases of exocrine pancreatic stimulation which is optimal in AP. The use of jejunal feedings may be better tolerated and allow for an increase in the amount of nutrition that is delivered in the face of AP. However, no controlled trial has clearly demonstrated a significant improvement of feeding tolerance, mortality, or length of intensive care unit (ICU) stay with the use of jejunal feeding compared with gastric feedings (Zhang et al, 2013). Because the placement of a nasogastric feeding tube is easier than a jejunal tube, it is reasonable to consider gastric feedings for AP and reserve jejunal feedings for those who are intolerant to gastric feeding (Petrov, 2014). For those patients with SAP complicated by organ failure, pancreatic necrosis, or fluid collections, nasojejunal feeding is the preferred method of delivery (Seminerio and O'Keefe, 2014) to minimize pancreatic stimulation (see Chapter 12 for jejunal feeding details).

Although various formulations have been used in pancreatitis, no studies have determined the relative merits of standard, partially digested, elemental, or "immune-enhanced" formulations. Polymeric formulas infused at various sections of the gut stimulate the pancreas more than elemental and hydrolyzed formulas. Peptide-based formula can be used safely and standard formulas can be tried if the patient is tolerant (Mirtallo et al, 2012). Close observation for patient tolerance is important. Tolerance may be enhanced with the use of supplemental pancreatic enzymes during enteral feeding (Berry, 2014). These can be provided by mouth, mixed with water and delivered via the feeding tube, or added directly to the enteral formula. An enteral in-line lipase cartridge is also available which has been shown to hydrolyze a majority of the fat in EN formulas to monoglycerides and free fatty acids (Freedman, 2017). When the patient is allowed to eat, supplemental pancreatic enzymes may also be required to treat steatorrhea. In severe, prolonged cases, PN may be necessary.

Patients with mild to moderate stress can tolerate dextrose-based solutions, whereas patients with more severe stress require a mixed fuel system of dextrose and lipid to avoid complications of glucose intolerance. Lipid emulsion should not be included in a PN regimen if hypertriglyceridemia is the cause of the pancreatitis (Patel et al, 2014). A serum triglyceride level should be obtained before lipid-containing PN is initiated. Lipids may be should only given to patients with triglyceride values less than 400 mg/dL. Because of the possibility of pancreatic endocrine abnormalities and a relative insulin resistance, close glucose monitoring also is warranted. H_2-receptor antagonists may be prescribed to decrease hydrochloric acid production, which reduce stimulation of the pancreas. The hormone somatostatin is considered the best inhibitor of pancreatic secretion and may be used in conjunction with PN.

Chronic pancreatitis. In contrast to SAP, chronic pancreatitis (CP) evolves insidiously over many years. CP is characterized by recurrent attacks of epigastric pain of long duration that may radiate into the back. The pain can be precipitated by meals. Associated nausea, vomiting, or diarrhea make it difficult to maintain adequate nutrition status (Verhaeqh et al, 2013).

Patients with CP are at increased risk of developing protein-calorie malnutrition because of pancreatic insufficiency and inadequate oral

PATHOPHYSIOLOGY AND CARE MANAGEMENT ALGORITHM

Pancreatitis

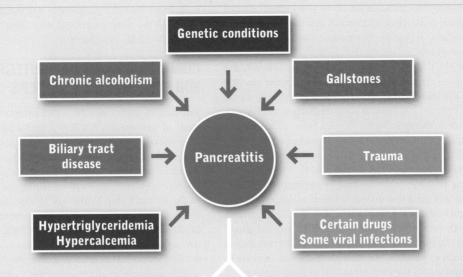

ETIOLOGY

- Genetic conditions
- Chronic alcoholism
- Gallstones
- Biliary tract disease
- Pancreatitis
- Trauma
- Hypertriglyceridemia Hypercalcemia
- Certain drugs Some viral infections

PATHOPHYSIOLOGY

Diagnosis

I: Apply Ranson's criteria
II: Tests of pancreatic function
   Secretin stimulation test
   Glucose tolerance test
   72-hour stool fat test
   Fecal elastase

Clinical Findings

Symptoms:
- Abdominal pain and distention
- Nausea
- Vomiting
- Steatorrhea

In severe form:
- Hypotension
- Oliguria
- Dyspnea

MANAGEMENT

Medical Management

Acute:
- Withhold oral feeding
- Give IV fluids
- Administer H_2-receptor antagonists, somatostatin

Chronic:
- Manage intestinal pH with:
  - Antacids
  - H_2-receptor antagonists
  - Proton pump inhibitors
- Administer insulin for glucose intolerance

Nutrition Management

Acute:
- Withhold oral and enteral feeding
- Support with IV fluids
- If oral nutrition cannot be initiated in 5 to 7 days, start tube feeding
- Once oral nutrition is started, provide
  - Easily digestible foods
  - Low-fat diet
  - 6 small meals
  - Adequate protein intake
  - Increased calories

Chronic:
- Provide oral diet as in acute phase
- Tube feeding (TF) can be used when oral diet is inadequate or as a treatment to reduce pain
- Prescription pancreatic enzymes
- Supplement fat-soluble vitamins and vitamin B_{12}

intake. Patients with CP admitted to a tertiary care center usually have malnutrition, increased energy requirements, weight loss, deficits of lean muscle and adipose tissue, visceral protein depletion, impaired immune function, and vitamin deficiencies (Duggan et al, 2014).

The objective of therapy for patients is to prevent further damage to the pancreas, decrease the number of attacks of acute inflammation, alleviate pain, decrease steatorrhea, and correct malnutrition. Dietary intake should be as liberal as possible, but modifications may be necessary to minimize symptoms.

The first goal of MNT is to provide optimal nutrition support, and the second is to decrease pain by minimizing stimulation of the exocrine pancreas. Because CCK stimulates secretion from the exocrine pancreas, one approach is to decrease CCK levels. If postprandial pain is a limiting factor, alternative enteral therapies, such as feeding beyond the ligament of Treitz, that minimally stimulate the pancreas are warranted. Nutrition counseling, antioxidants, and pancreatic enzymes may play a role in effective management of CP as well (Afghani et al, 2014).

When pancreatic function is diminished by approximately 90%, enzyme production and secretion are insufficient; maldigestion and malabsorption of protein and fat thus become a problem. In general, large meals with high-fat foods and alcohol should be avoided. However, there is a lot of variation among these patients and the diet should be liberalized as much as possible. For example, a gradual increase in the amount of fat and size of the meal is possible in some patients.

The patient may present with weight loss despite adequate energy intake and will complain of bulky, greasy stools. This is definitely the case with idiopathic CP associated with a cystic fibrosis gene mutation; therapies directed toward cystic fibrosis may benefit these patients (see Chapter 33). Of these therapies, pancreatic enzyme replacement has been shown to be efficacious (de la Iglesia-Garcia et al, 2016). Pancreatic enzyme replacements are given orally with meals; the dosage should be at least 30,000 units of lipase with each meal. To promote weight gain, the level of fat in the diet should be the maximum a patient can tolerate without increased steatorrhea or pain.

Additional therapies to maintain nutrition status and minimize symptoms in patients with maximum enzyme supplementation include a lower-fat diet (40 to 60 g/day) (see Table 28.7) or substitution of some dietary fat with MCT oil to improve fat absorption and weight gain (see Chapter 12). A lower-fat diet, primarily from vegetable-based oils such as olive oil may help reduce pain and ease nausea as well as eating small frequent meals. Trans fatty acids, found in commercially baked goods and other processed foods, can increase inflammation and are not recommended.

Malabsorption of the fat-soluble vitamins may occur in patients with significant steatorrhea. Also, deficiency of pancreatic protease, necessary to cleave vitamin B_{12} from its carrier protein, potentially could lead to vitamin B_{12} deficiency. Appropriate supplemental enzyme therapy will improve vitamin absorption; however, the patient should continue to be monitored periodically for vitamin deficiencies. Water-miscible forms of the fat-soluble vitamins or parenteral administration of vitamin B_{12} may be necessary. Some evidence indicates that increasing intake of antioxidants (found in fruits and vegetables) may help protect against pancreatitis or alleviate symptoms of the condition (Ahmed et al, 2014).

Because pancreatic bicarbonate secretion is frequently defective, medical management also may include maintenance of an optimal intestinal pH to facilitate enzyme activation. Antacids, H_2-receptor antagonists, or proton pump inhibitors that reduce gastric acid secretion may be used to achieve this effect.

In CP with extensive pancreatic destruction, the insulin-secreting capacity of the pancreas decreases, and glucose intolerance develops. Treatment with insulin and nutrition therapy is then required (see Chapter 29). Management is delicate and should focus on control of symptoms rather than normoglycemia.

Effort should be made to cater to the patient's tolerances and preferences for nutritional management; however, alcohol is discouraged because of the possibility of exacerbating the pancreatic disease. There is evidence that the progressive destruction of the pancreas will be slowed in the alcoholic patient who abstains from alcohol (Nordback et al, 2008; Yadav et al, 2009).

COMPLEMENTARY AND INTEGRATIVE MEDICINE FOR PANCREATIC DISORDERS

The role of complementary and integrative medicine in the treatment of pancreatic disorders remains unclear (Saxena et al, 2014). Over the counter digestive enzymes are sometimes used with pancreatic disease, but their use is not supported by evidenced-based research, the composition is often not guaranteed due to the way they are regulated, they can be costly, and they are often inactivated in the stomach due to the pH. The standard of care in pancreatic disease is prescription pancreatic enzymes such as Creon (Natural Medicines Database, 2019). There is little to no research on integrative approaches for pancreatic disease. In China, there are some studies involving herbal preparations, many of which are not readily available in other countries. Some of the studies are non-randomized and non-controlled. For traditional Chinese interventions, consider referring patients to a licensed Chinese medicine provider or licensed acupuncturist. Because chronic pancreatitis is an inflammatory condition, one of the most common integrative approaches is a nutritionally adequate anti-inflammatory diet (see Appendix 22 and chapter 7), although there is no direct scientific evidence supporting its use in the medical literature. Some studies suggest melatonin may have a protective effect and may alter the disease progression (Belyaev et al, 2011; Jaworek et al, 2012; Jin et al, 2013). See chapter 11 for more information about safely recommending dietary and herbal supplements.

PANCREATIC SURGERY

A surgical procedure often used for pancreatic carcinoma is a pancreaticoduodenectomy (Whipple procedure), in which distal segment (antrum) of the stomach, the first and second portions of the duodenum, the head of the pancreas, the common bile duct, and the gallbladder are removed. The basic concept behind the pancreaticoduodenectomy is that the head of the pancreas and the duodenum share the same arterial blood supply (the gastroduodenal artery). These arteries run through the head of the pancreas, so both organs must be removed if the single blood supply is severed. If only the head of the pancreas were removed, it would compromise blood flow to the duodenum, resulting in tissue necrosis. A cholecystectomy, vagotomy, or a partial gastrectomy also may be performed during the surgery. The pancreatic duct is reanastomosed (reattached) to the jejunum. Partial or complete pancreatic insufficiency can result, depending on the extent of the pancreatic resection. Most patients who have undergone pancreatic resection are at risk for vitamin and mineral deficiencies and will benefit from vitamin and mineral supplementation. Nutrition care is similar to that for CP.

Pancreatic and Islet Cell Transplantation

There have been significant improvements in the outcomes of patients undergoing pancreatic transplants or pancreatic transplants combined with a kidney transplant (Dean et al, 2017; Laftavi et al, 2017). In patients with unstable (brittle) diabetes mellitus who suffer from bouts of hyper- and hypoglycemia, transplantation can restore normal glucose homeostasis and prevent, halt, or reverse the progression of secondary complications (Dunn, 2014; Gruessner and Gruessner, 2013).

Pancreatic islet allotransplantation is a procedure in which islets from the pancreas of a deceased organ donor are purified, processed, and transferred into a recipient. It is performed in certain patients with type 1 diabetes mellitus whose blood glucose levels are extremely labile and difficult to control. Pancreatic islet autotransplantation is performed after total pancreatectomy in patients with severe and chronic, or long-lasting, pancreatitis that cannot be managed by other treatments. After pancreatectomy, islets are extracted and purified from the pancreas. The islets then are infused through a catheter into the liver. The goal is to give the body enough healthy islets to make insulin. A person who receives a pancreatic islet cell transplant should follow a meal plan designed for a person with diabetes mellitus if hyperglycemia is present. Some patients undergoing this procedure will achieve normoglycemia without exogenous insulin (see Chapter 29). Immunosuppressive medications are required for allo- but not autotransplantation; these medications can contribute to weight gain, hypertension, dyslipidemia, and labile blood glucose levels (Chhabra and Brayman, 2014).

Although pancreas transplantation has been favored for β-cell replacement, with improved outcomes following islet transplantation, the use of this minimally invasive therapy in carefully selected patients should be considered (Wisel et al, 2016; Hatipoglu, 2016; Markmann et al, 2016). Pancreas transplant remains the procedure of choice for β-cell replacement in uremic patients. Islet transplantation should be considered in nonuremic patients with low body mass index (BMI) and low insulin requirements, patients lacking the cardiovascular reserve to undergo open abdominal surgery, or patients who elect to forego the risks of a major operation in exchange for an increased risk of islet graft failure.

CLINICAL CASE STUDY 1

A 62-year-old white man is admitted to the hospital from the doctor's office with altered mental status. Past medical history reveals cirrhosis resulting from hepatitis C, esophageal varices, hepatic encephalopathy, and ascites. The patient reports missing his doses of lactulose the two previous days. Muscle wasting is noted in the form of squared shoulders, prominent clavicle, temporal wasting, and thin extremities. He has 3+ pitting edema in his lower extremities and a protuberant abdomen from ascites. His abnormal laboratory values on admission included elevated liver function enzymes and total bilirubin, sodium 127 mEq/L, glucose 68 mg/dL. Nutritional data include height, 177.8 cm; weight, 71.8 kg; dry weight, 75 kg; recent body weight range due to fluid fluctuations, 63.6 kg to 90.9 kg.

Nutrition Diagnostic Statements

- Involuntary weight loss related to cirrhosis as evidenced by 4.5% weight loss (based on dry weight) and physical signs of malnutrition.
- Altered laboratory values related to cirrhosis as evidenced by hyponatremia and hypoglycemia.

Interventions

- Initiate 2 g sodium diet with small, frequent meals.
- Ensure adequate kcals and protein.
- Fluid restriction (coordinate care with medical team).
- Initiate commercial beverage twice daily.

Monitoring and Evaluation

- Monitor food and beverage intake.
- Assess food and nutrition knowledge.
- Assess adherence to prescribed diet.

CLINICAL CASE STUDY 2

A 42-year-old Hispanic female presents with a history of chronic pancreatitis resulting from pancreatic divisum (a congenital abnormality in which there are two pancreatic ducts instead of one). The patient has had multiple hospitalizations for acute pancreatitis. Despite placement of pancreatic stents, she has developed chronic pancreatitis (confirmed by abnormal endoscopic ultrasound and low fecal elastase) and depends on chronic pain medications. She presents for evaluation of total pancreatectomy with islet autotransplantation. The patient is thin, with apparent muscle wasting, and reports that she is very fatigued and no longer able to work because of chronic pain. She describes chronic abdominal pain that worsens with eating so that she is only drinking clear soft drinks throughout the day and eating only one small meal per day. She often is constipated, but this can alternate with diarrhea with greasy, foul-smelling loose stools. Her nutritional data include height, 160 cm; weight, 40.5 kg; usual body weight, 54.5 kg (1 year ago). Her 25-hydroxy vitamin D level is <10 ng/mL.

Nutrition Diagnostic Statements

- Involuntary weight loss due to pain with eating as evidenced by 31-lb weight loss / 74% usual body weight (UBW).
- Altered nutrition-related laboratory values due to malabsorption as evidenced by vitamin D level less than 10 ng/mL.

Interventions

- Insert feeding tube (for supplemental nocturnal nutrition).
- Nutrition-related medication management (start pancreatic enzymes with meals).
- Initiate vitamin D supplement.
- Interview patient and family about culturally acceptable foods.

Monitoring and Evaluation

- Monitor total energy intake and body weight.
- Monitor enteral intake—formula/solution (for tolerance and adequacy).
- Monitor vitamin A, D, E levels.

USEFUL WEBSITES

American Liver Foundation
National Institute of Alcohol Abuse and Alcoholism
National Institute of Diabetes and Digestive and Kidney Disease

REFERENCES

Abdelmalek MF, Sanderson SO, Angulo P, et al: Betaine for nonalcoholic fatty liver disease: results of a randomized placebo-controlled trial, *Hepatology* 50:1818–1826, 2009.

Abenavoli L, Capasso R, Milic N, et al: Milk thistle in liver diseases: past, present, future, *Phytother Res* 24:1423–1432, 2010.

Acalovschi M: Gallstones in patients with liver cirrhosis: incidence, etiology, clinical and therapeutical aspects, *World J Gastroenterol* 20:7277–7285, 2014.

Afghani E, Sinha A, Singh VK: An overview of the diagnosis and management of nutrition in chronic pancreatitis, *Nutr Clin Pract* 29:295–311, 2014.

Ahmed Ali U, Jens S, Busch OR, et al: Antioxidants for pain in chronic pancreatitis, *Cochrane Database Syst Rev* 8:CD008945, 2014. doi:10.1002/14651858.CD008945.pub2.

Al-Omran M, Albalawi ZH, Tashkandi MF, et al: Enteral versus parenteral nutrition for acute pancreatitis, *Cochrane Database Syst Rev* CD002837, 2010.

Amodio P, Bemeur C, Butterworth R, et al: The nutritional management of hepatic encephalopathy in patients with cirrhosis: International Society for Hepatic Encephalopathy and Nitrogen Metabolism Consensus, *Hepatology* 58:325–326, 2013.

Amodio P, Canesso F, Montagnese S: Dietary management of hepatic encephalopathy revisited, *Curr Opin Clin Nutr Metab Care* 17:448–452, 2014.

Bacon BR: Iron overload (hemochromatosis). In Goldman L, Schafer AI, editors: *Goldman's cecil medicine*, ed 25, Philadelphia, 2015, Elsevier Saunders.

Bakker OJ, van Brunschot S, Farre A, et al: Timing of enteral nutrition in acute pancreatitis: meta-analysis of individuals using a single-arm of randomized trials, *Pancreatology* 14:340–346, 2014.

Balthazar EJ, Robinson DL, Megibow AJ, et al. Acute pancreatitis: value of CT in establishing prognosis, *Radiology* 174:331–336, 1990

Banks PA, Bollen TL, Dervenis C, et al. Classification of acute pancreatitis – 2012: revision of the Atlanta classification and definitions by international consensus, *Gut* 62:102–111, 2013.

Belyaev O, Herzog T, Munding J, et al: Protective role of endogenous melatonin in the early course of human acute pancreatitis, *J Pineal Res* 50:71–77, 2011.

Berr F, Holl J, Jüngst D, et al: Dietary N-3 polyunsaturated fatty acids decrease biliary cholesterol saturation in gallstone disease, *Hepatology* 16:960–967, 1992.

Berry AJ: Pancreatic enzyme replacement therapy during pancreatic insufficiency, *Nutr Clin Pract* 29:312–321, 2014.

Böhm F, Speicher T, Hellerbrand C, et al: FGF receptors 1 and 2 control chemically induced injury and compound detoxification in regenerating livers of mice, *Gastroenterology* 139:1385–1396, 2010.

Butterworth RF: Parkinsonism in cirrhosis: pathogenesis and current therapeutic options, *Metab Brain Dis* 28:261–267, 2013.

Cai XJ, Wang L, Hu CM: Efficacy of different drugs in the treatment of minimal hepatic encephalopathy: a network meta-analysis involving 826 patients based on 10 randomized controlled trials, *J Cell Biochem* 119:8336–8345, 2018.

Cao Q, Yu CB, Yang SG, et al: Effect of probiotic treatment on cirrhotic patients with minimal hepatic encephalopathy: a meta-analysis, *Hepatobiliary Pancreat Dis Int* 17:9–16, 2018.

Centers for Disease Control and Prevention (CDC): Notes from the field: acute hepatitis and liver failure following the use of a dietary supplement intended for weight loss or muscle building—May-October 2013, *MMWR Morb Mortal Wkly Rep* 62:817–819, 2013.

Chalasani N, Younossi Z, Lavine JE, et al: The diagnosis and management of non-alcoholic fatty liver disease: practice guidance from the American Association for the Study of Liver Diseases, American College of Gastroenterology, and the American Gastroenterological Association, *Hepatology* 67:328–357, 2018.

Chalasani NP: Alcoholic and nonalcoholic steatohepatitis. In Goldman L, Schafer AI, editors: *Goldman's cecil medicine*, ed 25, Philadelphia, 2016, Elsevier Saunders.

Chen S, Teoh NC, Chitturi S, et al: Coffee and non-alcoholic fatty liver disease: brewing evidence for hepatoprotection? *J Gastroenterol Hepatol* 29:435–441, 2014.

Chhabra P, Brayman KL: Overcoming barriers in clinical islet transplantation: current limitations and future prospects, *Curr Probl Surg* 51:49–86, 2014.

Cho JH, Kim TN, Chung HH, et al. Comparison of scoring systems in predicting the severity of acute pancreatitis, *World J Gastroenterol* 21:2387–2394, 2015.

Crescioli G, Lombardi N, Bettiol A, et al: Acute liver injury following Garcinia cambogea weight-loss supplementation: case series and literature review, *Intern Emerg Med* 13:857–872, 2018.

Crockett SD, Wani S, Gardner TB, et al: American Gastroenterological Association Institute Guideline on Initial Management of Acute Pancreatitis, *Gastroenterology*, 154:1096–1101, 2018

Dalal R, McGee RG, Riordan SM, et al: Probiotics for people with hepatic encephalopathy, *Cochrane Database Syst Rev* 2:CD008716, 2017.

Day CR, Kempson SA: Betaine chemistry, roles, and potential use in liver disease, *Biochim Biophys Acta*, 1860:1098–1106, 2016.

Dean PG, Kukla A, Stegall MD, et al. Pancreas transplantation, *BMJ* 357:j1321, 2017.

de la Iglesia-García D, Huang W, Szatmary P, et al. Efficacy of pancreatic enzyme replacement therapy in chronic pancreatitis: systematic review and meta-analysis, *Gut* 66:1354–1355, 2017.

Duggan SN, Smyth ND, O'Sullivan M, et al: The prevalence of malnutrition and fat-soluble vitamin deficiencies in chronic pancreatitis, *Nutr Clin Pract* 29:348–354, 2014.

Dunn TB: Life after pancreas transplantation: reversal of diabetic lesions, *Curr Opin Organ Transplant* 19:73–79, 2014.

Dupont B, Dao T, Joubert C, et al: Randomised clinical trial: enteral nutrition does not improve the long-term outcome of alcoholic cirrhotic patients with jaundice, *Aliment Pharmacol Ther* 35:1166–1174, 2012.

Feng P, He C, Liao G, et al: Early enteral nutrition versus delayed enteral nutrition in acute pancreatitis: A PRISMA-compliant systematic review and meta-analysis, *Medicine* 96(46):e8648, 2017.

Fogel EL, Sherman S: Diseases of the gallbladder and bile ducts. In Goldman L, Schafer AI, editors: *Goldman's cecil medicine*, ed 25, Philadelphia, 2016, Elsevier Saunders.

Food and Drug Administration (FDA): *FDA investigation summary: acute hepatitis illnesses linked to certain oxyelite pro products* (website), 2014. http://wayback.archive-it.org/7993/20171114154924/https://www.fda.gov/Food/RecallsOutbreaksEmergencies/Outbreaks/ucm370849.htm.

Fong TL, Klontz KC, Canas-Coto A, et al: Hepatotoxicity due to hydroxycut: a case series, *Am J Gastroenterol* 105:1561–1566, 2010.

Freedman SD: Options for addressing exocrine pancreatic insufficiency in patients receiving enteral nutrition supplementation, *Am J Manag Care* 23(Suppl. 12):S220–S228, 2017.

Gruessner RW, Gruessner AC: Pancreas transplant alone: a procedure coming of age, *Diabetes Care* 36:2440–2447, 2013.

Guo T, Chang L, Xiao Y, et al: S-adenosyl-L-methionine for the treatment of chronic liver disease: a systematic review and meta-analysis, *PLoS One* 10(3):e0122124, 2015.

Hasse JM, Blue LS, Liepa GU, et al: Early enteral nutrition support in patients undergoing liver transplantation, *JPEN J Parenter Enteral Nutr* 19:437–443, 1995.

Hatipoglu B: Islet cell transplantation and alternative therapies, *Endocrinol Metab Clin North Am* 45:923–931, 2016.

Ikegami T, Shirabe K, Yoshiya S, et al: Bacterial sepsis after living donor liver transplantation: the impact of early enteral nutrition, *J Am Coll Surg* 214:288–295, 2012.

International Association of Pancreatology (IAP), American Pancreatic Association (APA): IAP/APA evidence-based guidelines for the management of acute pancreatitis, *Pancreatology* 13(4 Suppl 2):e1–e15, 2013. doi:10.1016/j.pan.2013.07.063.

Jaworek J, Szklarczyk J, Jaworek AK, et al: Protective effect of melatonin on acute pancreatitis, *Int J Inflam*, 2012:173675, 2012.

Jenkins SA: Biliary lipids, bile acids and gallstone formation in the hypovitaminotic C guinea-pigs, *Br J Nutr* 40:317–322, 1978.

Jin Y, Lin CJ, Dong LM, et al: Clinical significance of melatonin concentrations in predicting the severity of acute pancreatitis, *World J Gastroeterol* 19:4066–4071, 2013.

Jóhannsson M, Ormarsdóttir S, Olafsson S: Hepatotoxicity associated with the use of Herbalife, *Laeknabladid* 96:167–172, 2010.

Kaler SG, Schilsky ML: Wilson disease. In Goldman L, Schafer AI, editors: *Goldman's cecil medicine*, ed 25, Philadelphia, 2015, Elsevier Saunders.

Katuchova J, Bober J, Harbulak P, et al: Obesity as a risk factor for severe acute pancreatitis patients, *Wien Kin Wochenschr* 127:223, 2014. Available at: https://doi.org/10.1007/s00508-014-0507-7.

Kelly RK, Venook AP: Liver and biliary tract cancers. In Goldman L, Schafer AI, editors: *Goldman's cecil medicine*, ed 25, Philadelphia, 2015, Elsevier Saunders.

Kobtan AA, El-Kalla FS, Soliman HH, et al: Higher grades and repeated recurrence of hepatic encephalopathy may be related to high serum manganese levels, *Biol Trace Elem Res* 169:153–158, 2016.

Koller T, Kollerova J, Hlavaty T, et al: Cholelithiasis and markers of non-alcoholic fatty liver disease in patients with metabolic risk factors, *Scand J Gastroenterol* 47:197–203, 2012.

Kosters A, Karpen SJ: The role of inflammation in cholestasis: clinical and basic aspects, *Semin Liver Dis* 30:186–194, 2010.

Kubitz R, Droge C, Stindt J et al: The bile salt export pump (BSEP) in health and disease, *Clin Res Hepatol Gastroenterol* 36:536–553, 2012.

Laftavi MR, Gruessner A, Gruessner R: Surgery of pancreas transplantation, *Curr Opin Organ Transplant* 22:389–397, 2017.

Lam P, Soroka CJ, Boyer JL: The bile salt export pump: clinical and experimental aspects of genetic and acquired cholestatic liver disease, *Semin Liver Dis* 30:125–133, 2010.

Lankisch PG, Apte M, Banks PA: Acute pancreatitis, *Lancet* 386:85–96, 2015.

Larvin M, McMahon MJ: APACHE-II score for assessment and monitoring of acute pancreatitis, *Lancet* 2:201–205, 1989.

Lee DK, Jang SI: Can fish oil dissolve gallstones? *J Gastroenterol Hepatol* 27;1649–1651, 2012.

Markmann JF, Barlett ST, Johnson P, et al: Executive summary of IPITA-TTS opinion leaders report on the future of β-cell replacement, *Transplantation* 100:e25–e31, 2016.

Martin P: Approach to the patient with liver disease. In Goldman L, Schafer AI, editors: *Goldman's cecil medicine*, ed 25, Philadelphia, 2015, Elsevier Saunders.

Martinez J, Sánchez-Payá J, Palazón JM, et al: Is obesity a risk factor in acute pancreatitis? A meta-analysis, *Pancreatology* 4:42–48, 2004.

Masuda T, Shirabe K, Ikegami T, et al: Sarcopenia is a prognostic factor in living donor liver transplantation, *Liver Transpl* 20:401–407, 2014.

McClave SA, Chang WK, Dhaliwal R, et al: Nutrition support in acute pancreatitis: a systematic review of the literature, *JPEN J Parenter Enteral Nutr* 30:143–156, 2006.

McClave SA, Taylor BE, Martindale RG et al. Guidelines for the provision and assessment of nutrition support therapy in the adult critically ill patient: Society of Critical Care Medicine (SCCM) and American Society for Parenteral and Enteral Nutrition (A.S.P.E.N.), *JPEN J Parenter Enteral Nutr* 40:159–2011, 2016.

McClave SA: Nutrition in pancreatitis, *World Rev Nutr Diet* 105:160–168, 2013.

Méndez-Sánchez N, Zamora-Valdés D, Chávez-Tapia NC, et al: Role of diet in cholesterol gallstone formation, *Clin Chim Acta* 376:1–8, 2007.

Mirtallo JM, Forbes A, McClave SA, et al: International consensus guidelines for nutrition therapy in pancreatitis, *JPEN J Parenter Enteral Nutr* 36:284–291, 2012.

Moga MM: Alternative treatment of gallbladder disease, *Med Hypotheses* 60:143–147, 2003.

Morisco F, Lembo V, Mazzone G, et al: Coffee and liver health, *J Clin Gastroenterol* 48(Suppl 1):S87–S90, 2014.

Mukherjee S: Betaine and nonalcoholic steatohepatitis: back to the future? *World J Gastroenterol* 17:3663–3664, 2011.

Nally DM, Kelly EG, Clarke M, et al: Nasogastric nutrition is efficacious in severe acute pancreatitis: a systematic review and meta-analysis, *Br J Nutr* 112:1769–1778, 2014.

Natural medicines database: pancreatic enzyme products professional monograph, stockton, CA, 2019, TRC Natural Medicines. Available at: https://naturalmedicines-therapeuticresearch-com.buproxy.bastyr.edu/databases/food,-herbs-supplements/professional.aspx?productid=254.

Ney M, Vandermeer B, van Zanten SJ, et al: Meta-analysis: Oral or enteral nutritional supplementation in cirrhosis, *Aliment Pharmacol Ther* 37:672–679, 2013.

Njeze GE: Gallstones, *Niger J Surg* 19(2):49–55, 2013.

Nordback I, Pelli H, Lappalainen-Lehto R, et al: The recurrence of acute alcohol-associated pancreatitis can be reduced: a randomized controlled trial, *Gastroenterology* 136:848–855, 2008.

O'Keefe SJ, Cariem AK, Levy M: The exacerbation of pancreatic endocrine dysfunction by potent pancreatic exocrine supplements in patients with chronic pancreatitis, *J Clin Gastroenterol* 32:319–323, 2001.

Patel KS, Noel P, Singh VP: Potential influence of intravenous lipids on the outcomes of acute pancreatitis, *Nutr Clin Pract* 29:291–294, 2014.

Pawlotsky JM: Acute viral hepatitis. In: Goldman L, Schafer AI, editors: *Goldman's cecil medicine*, ed 25, Philadelphia, 2016, Elsevier Saunders.

Petrov MS, Pylypchuk RD, Emelyanov NV: Systematic review: nutritional support in acute pancreatitis, *Aliment Pharmacol Ther* 28:704–712, 2008.

Petrov MS: Gastric feeding and "gut rousing" in acute pancreatitis, *Nutr Clin Pract* 29:287–290, 2014.

Petrov MS, Pylypchuk RD, Uchugina AF: A systematic review on the timing of artificial nutrition in acute pancreatitis, *Br J Nutr* 101:787–793, 2009.

Rayes N, Seehofer D, Theruvath T, et al: Supply of pre- and probiotics reduces bacterial infection rates after liver transplantation—a randomized, double-blind trial, *Am J Transplant* 5:125–130, 2005.

Saxena P, Chen JA, Mullin GE: The role of complementary and alternative medicine for pancreatic disorders, *Nutr Clin Pract* 29:409–411, 2014.

Schoepfer AM, Engel A, Fattinger K, et al: Herbal does not mean innocuous: ten cases of severe hepatotoxicity associated with dietary supplements from Herbalife products, *J Hepatol* 47:521–526, 2007.

Seminerio J, O'Keefe SJ: Jejunal feeding in patients with pancreatitis, *Nutr Clin Pract* 29:283–286, 2014.

Setiawan VW, Wilkens LR, Lu SC, et al: Association of coffee intake with reduced incidence of liver cancer and death from chronic liver disease in the US multiethnic cohort, *Gastroenterology* 148:118–125, 2015.

Shaffer EA: Gallstone disease: epidemiology of gallbladder stone disease, *Best Pract Res Clin Gastroenterol* 20(6):981–996, 2006.

Sharma T, Wong L, Tsai N, et al: Hydroxycut(®) (herbal weight loss supplement) induced hepatotoxicity: a case report and review of literature, *Hawaii Med J* 69:188–190, 2010.

Schilsky M: Wilson disease: treatment and prognosis. In Robson KM, ed. *UpToDate*. Waltham, MA, 2017. https://www.uptodate.com/contents/wilson-disease-treatment-and-prognosis#H19.

Simon JA, Grady D, Snabes MC, et al: Ascorbic acid supplement use and the prevalence of gallbladder disease. Heart & Estrogen-Progestin Replacement Study (HERS) Research Group, *J Clin Epidemiol* 51:257–265, 1998.

Spiridonov NA: Mechanisms of action of herbal cholagogues, *Med Aromat Plants* 1:5, 2012.

Stinton LM, Myers RP, Shaffer EA: Epidemiology of Gallstones, *Gastroenterol Clin North Am* 39:157–169, 2010.

Sun JK, Mu XW, Li WQ, et al: Effects of early enteral nutrition on immune function of severe acute pancreatitis patients, *World J Gastroenterol* 19:917–922, 2013.

Sureka B, Bansal K, Patidar Y, et al: Neurologic manifestations of chronic liver disease and liver cirrhosis, *Curr Probl Diagn Radiol* 44:449–461, 2015.

Teschke R, Schwarzenboeck A, Eickhoff A, et al: Clinical and causality assessment in herbal hepatotoxicity, *Expert Opin Drug Saf* 12:339–366, 2013.

Vaughn VM, Shuster D, Rogers MAM, et al: Early versus delayed feeding in patients with acute pancreatitis: a systematic review, *Ann Intern Med* 166;883–892, 2017.

Vege SS, DiMagno MJ, Forsmark CE, et al: Initial medical treatment of acute pancreatitis: American Gastroenterological Association institute technical review, *Gastroenterology* 154:1103–1139, 2018.

Verhaeqh BP, Reijven PL, Prins MH, et al: Nutritional status in patients with chronic pancreatitis, *Eur J Clin Nutr* 67:1271–1276, 2013.

Walcher T, Haenle MM, Kron M, et al: Vitamin C supplement use may protect against Gallstones: an observational study on a randomly selected population, *BMC Gastroenterol* 9:74, 2009.

Waniek S, di Giuseppe R, Esatbeyoglu T, et al: Association of circulating Vitamin E (α- and γ-Tocopherol) levels with Gallstone disease, *Nutrients* 10(2):pii: E133, 2018.

Weikert C, Weikert S, Schulze MB, et al: Presence of gallstones or kidney stones and risk of type 2 diabetes, *Am J Epidemiol* 171:447–454, 2010.

Wisel SA, Braun HJ, Stock PG: Current outcomes in islet versus solid organ pancreas transplant for β-cell replacement in type 1 diabetes, *Curr Opin Organ Transplant* 21:399–404, 2016.

Wu BU, Johannes RS, Sun X, et al: The early prediction of mortality in acute pancreatitis: a large population-based study, *Gut* 57:1698–1703, 2008.

Wu LM, Sankaran SJ, Plank LD, et al: Meta-analysis of gut barrier dysfunction in patients with acute pancreatitis, *Br J Surg* 101:1644–1656, 2014.

Yadav D, Hawes RH, Anderson MA, et al: Alcohol consumption, cigarette smoking, and the risk of recurrent acute and chronic pancreatitis, *Arch Intern Med* 169:1035–1045, 2009.

Zhang J, Lu Q, Ren YF, et al: Factors relevant to persistent upper abdominal pain after cholecystectomy, *HPB (Oxford)* 19:629–637, 2017.

Zhang Z, Xu X, Ding J, et al: Comparison of postpyloric tube feeding and gastric tube feeding in intensive care unit patients: a meta-analysis, *Nutr Clin Pract* 28:371–380, 2013.

Zhong S, Fan Y, Yan Q, et al: The therapeutic effect of silymarin in the treatment of nonalcoholic fatty disease: a meta-analysis (PRISMA) of randomized control trials, *Medicine (Baltimore)* 96(49):e9061, 2017.

Zou L, Ke L, Li W, et al: Enteral nutrition within 72 h after onset of acute pancreatitis vs delayed initiation, *Eur J Clin Nutr* 68:1288–1293, 2014.

Medical Nutrition Therapy for Diabetes Mellitus and Hypoglycemia of Nondiabetic Origin

Jessica Jones, MS, RDN, CDE

KEY TERMS

acanthosis nigricans
amylin
autonomic symptoms
basal or background insulin dose
C-peptide
carbohydrate counting
continuous glucose monitoring (CGM)
correction factor (CF)
counterregulatory (stress) hormones
dawn phenomenon
diabetic ketoacidosis (DKA)
fasting hypoglycemia
fasting plasma glucose (FPG)
gastroparesis
gestational diabetes mellitus (GDM)
glucagon
glucotoxicity
glycemic index (GI)
glycemic load (GL)
glycosylated hemoglobin (A1C)

honeymoon phase
hyperglycemia
hyperglycemic hyperosmolar state (HHS)
hypoglycemia (or insulin reaction)
hypoglycemia of nondiabetic origin
immune-mediated diabetes mellitus
impaired fasting glucose (IFG)
impaired glucose tolerance (IGT)
incretins
insulin
insulin deficiency
insulin resistance
insulin secretagogues
insulin to carbohydrate ratio
lag time
latent autoimmune diabetes of the adult
    (LADA)
lipotoxicity
macrosomia
macrovascular diseases

maturity onset diabetes of youth (MODY)
metabolic syndrome
microvascular diseases
neuroglycopenic symptoms
normoglycemia
polydipsia
polyphagia
polyuria
postprandial (after a meal) blood glucose
postprandial (reactive) hypoglycemia
prediabetes
preprandial (fasting/premeal) blood
    glucose
self-monitoring of blood glucose (SMBG)
Somogyi effect
type 1 diabetes mellitus (T1DM)
type 2 diabetes mellitus (T2DM)
Whipple's triad

For most people, eating carbohydrate foods will cause blood sugar levels to rise. However, the difference between people with diabetes and those without the disease is how high the blood sugar rises, and for how long.

Diabetes mellitus is a group of diseases characterized by prolonged high blood glucose concentrations. The cause of high blood glucose—also known as hyperglycemia—is the result of defects in insulin secretion, insulin action, or both. Insulin, a hormone produced by the beta-cells of the pancreas, is necessary for the use or storage of macronutrients (think carbohydrate, protein, and fat). Since people with diabetes do not produce adequate insulin—and/or have some degree of insulin resistance—hyperglycemia occurs.

Diabetes mellitus contributes to a considerable increase in morbidity and mortality, which can be reduced by early diagnosis and treatment. Direct medical expenditures such as inpatient care, outpatient services, and nursing home care are astronomical, and indirect costs such as disability, work loss, and premature mortality are equally high. Research estimates that the total costs of diagnosed diabetes have risen to $327 billion in 2017 from $245 billion in 2012 (Yang et al, 2018).

Thus providing medical nutrition therapy (MNT) for prevention and treatment of diabetes has tremendous potential to reduce these costs. Fortunately, people with diabetes can take steps to control the disease and lower the risk of complications or premature death.

INCIDENCE AND PREVALENCE

It is estimated that 9.4% of the U.S. population is living with diabetes. In 2017 total prevalence of diabetes in the United States in all ages was 30.3 million people (15.3 million adult men and 14.9 adult women), or 9.4% of the population. Of these, 23.1 million are diagnosed and 7.2 million are undiagnosed. In 2015 an estimated 1.5 million new cases of diabetes were diagnosed in people age 18 years or older (Centers for Disease Control and Prevention [CDC], 2017a). Diabetes prevalence also increases with age, affecting 12 million people age 65 years and older, or 39.7% of all people in this age group.

Much of the increase in prevalence is because the prevalence of type 2 diabetes is increasing dramatically in younger age groups in the last decade, especially in minority populations. Among youth with newly diagnosed diabetes, approximately 23% have type 2 diabetes (Mayer-Davis et al, 2017). The prevalence of type 2 diabetes is highest in ethnic groups in the United States. Data indicate in people aged 20 years or older, 15.1% of American Indians and Alaska Natives, 12.7% of non-Hispanic blacks,

Portions of this chapter were written by Marion J Franz, MS, RDN, LD, CDE and Alison B Evert, MS, RDN, CDE for the previous edition of this text.

12.1% of Hispanics, and 8.0% of Asian Americans had diagnosed diabetes. Among Hispanics, rates were 13.8% for Mexicans, 12% for Puerto Ricans, and 9% for Cubans. Of great concern are the 84.1 million people (34% of adults 18 years or older and 48.3% of adults 65 years or older) with prediabetes, which includes impaired glucose tolerance (IGT) and impaired fasting glucose (IFG) (CDC, 2017a). All are a high risk for conversion to type 2 diabetes and cardiovascular disease (CVD) if lifestyle prevention strategies are not implemented.

CATEGORIES OF GLUCOSE INTOLERANCE

Assigning a type of diabetes to an individual often depends on the circumstances present at the time of diagnosis, and many individuals do not easily fit into a single category. What is essential is the need to intercede early with lifestyle interventions, beginning with prediabetes and continuing through the disease process.

Prediabetes

Individuals with a stage of impaired glucose homeostasis that includes impaired fasting glucose (IFG) and impaired glucose tolerance (IGT) are referred to as having prediabetes, indicating their relatively high risk for the development of diabetes and CVD. Prediabetes is diagnosed with at least one of the following: IFG (fasting plasma glucose 100 to 125 mg/dL), IGT (2-hour postchallenge glucose of 140 to 199 mg/dL), both, or a hemoglobin A1C of 5.7% to 6.4%. Individuals diagnosed with prediabetes and should be counseled about effective diabetes prevention strategies, such as eating a balanced diet and increasing physical activity, to lower their risks (American Diabetes Association [ADA], 2018).

Type 1 Diabetes

The ADA estimates that about 1.25 million Americans have type 1 diabetes (ADA, 2018). At diagnosis, people with type 1 diabetes mellitus (T1DM) often experience excessive thirst, frequent urination, and significant weight loss. The primary defect is pancreatic beta-cell destruction, usually leading to absolute insulin deficiency and resulting in hyperglycemia, polyuria (excessive urination), polydipsia (excessive thirst), polyphagia (excessive hunger), unexpected weight loss, dehydration, electrolyte disturbance, and diabetic ketoacidosis (DKA)—a serious complication of diabetes characterized by extreme hyperglycemia and a buildup of ketones in the blood and urine. The rate of beta-cell destruction is variable, proceeding rapidly in infants and children and slowly in others (mainly adults.) The capacity of a healthy pancreas to secrete insulin is far in excess of what is needed normally. Therefore the clinical onset of diabetes may be preceded by an extensive asymptomatic period of months to years, during which beta-cells are undergoing gradual destruction.

T1DM accounts for 5% of all diagnosed cases of diabetes (CDC, 2017a). People with T1DM are dependent on exogenous insulin—meaning insulin produced outside of the body—to prevent ketoacidosis and death. T1DM can develop at any age. Although more cases are diagnosed in people before the age of 30 years, it also occurs in older individuals. Most individuals are lean but some are diagnosed without any (or with more subtle) symptoms and may be at a higher weight.

T1DM has two forms: immune-mediated and idiopathic (ADA, 2018). Immune-mediated diabetes mellitus results from an autoimmune destruction of the beta-cells of the pancreas, the only cells in the body that make the hormone insulin. Idiopathic T1DM refers to forms of the disease that have no known etiology. Although only a minority of individuals with T1DM fall into this category, of those who do, most are of African or Asian ancestry (ADA, 2018). At this time there is no known cure for T1DM.

Since autoimmune thyroid disease and celiac disease occur with increased frequency in people with T1DM, the ADA suggests screening for thyroid disease in people diagnosed with T1DM. Other autoimmune conditions, such as celiac disease, Addison's disease, autoimmune hepatitis, autoimmune gastritis, dermatomyositis, and myasthenia gravis, also occur more commonly in people with T1DM compared with the general pediatric population. Individuals with celiac disease that has been confirmed by a biopsy should be placed on a gluten-free diet by a registered dietitian nutritionist (RDN) experienced in managing diabetes and celiac disease (ADA, 2018).

Pathophysiology

As mentioned previously, people with T1DM experience destruction of the pancreatic beta cells, which results in decreased insulin production and prolonged elevation of blood glucose levels. Markers of the immune destruction of the beta-cells include islet cells autoantibodies; autoantibodies to insulin; autoantibodies to glutamic acid decarboxylase (GAD65) (a protein on the surface of the beta-cells); and autoantibodies to the tyrosine phosphatases IA-2, IA-2beta, and ZnT8. T1DM is defined by the presence of one or more of these autoimmune markers. It is important to note that T1DM also has strong genetic factors, which involve the association between T1DM and histocompatibility locus antigen (HLA) with linkage to the DQA and DQB and the DRB genes. These HLA-DR/DQ alleles can be either predisposing or protective (ADA, 2018). In T1DM, the rate of clinical beta-cell destruction is variable, being rapid in some individuals (mainly infants and children) and slow in others (mainly adults). Children and adolescents, for example, may present with DKA as the first manifestation of the disease. Adults can often retain sufficient b-cell function to prevent DKA for many years. Note that although T1DM commonly occurs in childhood and adolescence, it can occur at any age (ADA, 2018).

Frequently after diagnosis and the correction of hyperglycemia, metabolic acidosis, and ketoacidosis, endogenous insulin secretion—or insulin secreted inside the body—recovers. During this honeymoon phase, exogenous (outside the body) insulin requirements decrease dramatically for up to 1 year or longer, and good metabolic control may be easily achieved (Fonolleda et al, 2017). However, the need for increasing exogenous insulin replacement is inevitable and always should be anticipated. Intensive insulin therapy along with attention to MNT and self-monitoring of glucose from early diagnosis has been shown to prolong insulin secretion. One study found that children who were diagnosed with T1DM early in life—specifically before the age of 7 years—had a much greater loss of β-cells compared with those who are diagnosed with the illness in their teenage years or beyond (Leete et al, 2016).

Latent autoimmune diabetes of the adult (LADA)—also known as type 1.5 diabetes—is an autoimmune diabetes that occurs in adulthood. It is defined by adult-onset, presence of diabetes associated autoantibodies, and no insulin treatment requirement for a period after diagnosis. With genetic features of both type 1 and type 2 diabetes, LADA is the most prevalent form of adult-onset autoimmune diabetes (and possibly the most common form of autoimmune diabetes in general). LADA may be controlled initially with nutrition therapy, but within a relatively short period of time glucose-lowering medication and progression to insulin treatment are required (Laugesen et al, 2015).

Type 2 Diabetes

Type 2 diabetes mellitus (T2DM) accounts for 90% to 95% of all diagnosed cases of diabetes and is a progressive disease that, in many cases, is present long before it is diagnosed (ADA, 2018). Hyperglycemia develops gradually and is often not severe enough in the early stages for the person to notice any of the classic symptoms of diabetes. Although undiagnosed, these individuals are at increased risk of developing macrovascular and microvascular complications (CDC, 2017a).

PATHOPHYSIOLOGY AND CARE MANAGEMENT ALGORITHM

Type 1 Diabetes Mellitus

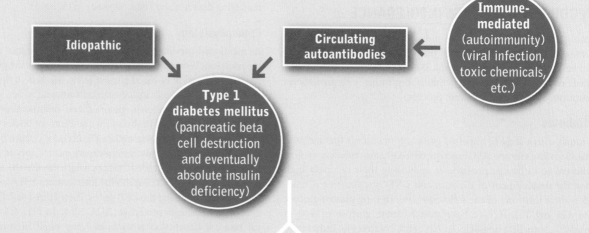

ETIOLOGY

Idiopathic

Circulating autoantibodies

Immune-mediated (autoimmunity) (viral infection, toxic chemicals, etc.)

Type 1 diabetes mellitus (pancreatic beta cell destruction and eventually absolute insulin deficiency)

PATHOPHYSIOLOGY

Symptoms

- Hyperglycemia
- Excessive thirst
- Frequent urination
- Significant weight loss
- Electrolyte disturbances

Complications

Ketoacidosis
Macrovascular diseases
- Coronary heart disease
- Peripheral vascular disease
- Cerebrovascular disease

Microvascular diseases
- Retinopathy
- Nephropathy

Neuropathy

MANAGEMENT

Medical Management

Medical nutrition therapy
Medications
- Insulin by injection or insulin infusion pumps

Monitoring
- Self-monitoring of blood glucose (SMBG)
- A1C testing
- Lipids
- Blood pressure
- Ketones
- Weight and growth in children

Self-management education

Medical Nutrition Therapy (MNT)

- Integrate insulin regimen into preferred eating and physical activity schedule; consistency in timing and amount of carbohydrate eaten if on fixed insulin doses
- Adjust premeal insulin dose based on insulin-to-carbohydrate ratios
- Adequate energy and nutrient intake to promote growth and development in children
- Cardioprotective nutrition interventions

Most people with T2DM are obese (defined as body mass index [BMI] >30 kg/m²), yet most obese individuals do not develop T2DM. Being at a higher weight may increase insulin resistance and can contribute to the destruction of the pancreatic beta-cells; however the exact mechanism of action remains unclear. Therefore obesity combined with a genetic predisposition may be necessary for T2DM to occur. Other risk factors include genetic and environmental factors, including a family history of diabetes, older age, physical inactivity, a prior history of gestational diabetes, prediabetes, hypertension or dyslipidemia, and race or ethnicity (Eckel et al, 2011).

Pathophysiology

T2DM is characterized by a combination of insulin resistance (decreased tissue sensitivity or responsiveness to insulin) and beta-cell failure. Endogenous insulin levels may be normal, depressed, or elevated, but they are inadequate to overcome concomitant insulin resistance. As a result, hyperglycemia ensues. At the time T2DM is diagnosed, there is an estimated 24% to 65% reduction in beta-cell function (Chen et al, 2017).

Insulin resistance is demonstrated first in target tissues, mainly muscle, liver, and adipose cells. Initially there is a compensatory increase in insulin secretion (hyperinsulinemia), which maintains glucose concentrations in the normal or prediabetic range. However, in many people, the pancreas is unable to continue to produce adequate insulin, which results in chronic hyperglycemia followed by a diabetes diagnosis.

Hyperglycemia is first exhibited as an elevation of postprandial (after a meal) blood glucose caused by insulin resistance at the cellular level and is followed by an elevation in fasting glucose concentrations. As insulin secretion decreases, hepatic glucose production increases, causing the increase in preprandial (fasting/premeal) blood glucose levels. The insulin response is also inadequate in suppressing alpha-cell glucagon secretion, resulting in glucagon hypersecretion and increased hepatic glucose production. Compounding the problem is glucotoxicity, the deleterious effect of hyperglycemia on insulin sensitivity and insulin secretion; hence the importance of achieving near-euglycemia in people with T2DM (Hædersdal et al, 2018).

Insulin resistance also is demonstrated at the adipocyte level, leading to lipolysis and an elevation in circulating free fatty acids. In particular, excess intraabdominal obesity, characterized by an excess accumulation of visceral fat around and inside abdominal organs, results in an increased flux of free fatty acids to the liver, leading to an increase in insulin resistance. Increased fatty acid levels (lipotoxicity) also cause a further decrease in insulin sensitivity at the cellular level, impair pancreatic insulin secretion, and disrupt hepatic glucose production. The above defects contribute to the development and progression of T2DM and are also primary targets for pharmacologic therapy.

People with T2DM may or may not experience the classic symptoms of uncontrolled diabetes (polydipsia, polyuria, polyphagia, weight loss) and they are not prone to develop ketoacidosis except during times of severe stress. The progressive loss of beta-cell secretory function means that people with T2DM require more medication(s) over time to maintain the same level of glycemic control; eventually exogenous insulin will be required. Insulin is also required sooner for control during periods of stress-induced hyperglycemia, such as during illness or surgery.

If at diagnosis it is not clear whether T1DM or T2DM is present, C-peptide may be measured. When the pancreas produces insulin, it begins as a large molecule—proinsulin. This molecule splits into two equal-sized pieces: insulin and C-peptide. A person with T1DM has a low level of C-peptide, whereas as a person with T2DM can have a normal or high level of C-peptide. As T2DM progresses, C-peptide also may be measured to see if endogenous insulin is still being produced by the pancreas. If it is not, exogenous insulin is needed (Leighton et al, 2017).

Gestational Diabetes Mellitus

Gestational diabetes mellitus (GDM) is a type of diabetes that occurs during pregnancy. About 2% to 10% of all pregnancies in the United States are affected by this condition (CDC, 2017b). Gestational diabetes increases a mother's risk of both hypertension during pregnancy and having a large baby requiring a cesarean section (C-section). Gestational diabetes also increases the baby's risk of premature labor (causing breathing and other problems), having low blood sugar, and developing diabetes later in life. Women of low socioeconomic status and those of Hispanic, Native American, Asian, and African American descent are more likely to experience GDM (Phelan, 2016).

For many women, blood sugar levels will revert back to normal after pregnancy. Others will end up developing diabetes. It is estimated that 15% to 25% of women with prior GDM will develop T2DM within 1 to 2 years after pregnancy, and that 35% to 70% will develop T2DM 10 to 15 years after pregnancy (Phelan, 2016).

Treatment for GDM includes checking blood sugar regularly (and making sure the numbers are within a healthy range), eating a balanced diet, being active (regular, moderate physical activity is recommended), and monitoring the baby's growth and development. Most women will be able to manage GDM with lifestyle changes, but some will require medications to achieve optimal blood glucose ranges (Kelley et al, 2015). Insulin is the preferred agent for management of both T1DM and T2DM in pregnancy because it does not cross the placenta. Furthermore, oral agents, such as metformin, are typically not sufficient in overcoming the insulin resistance in T2DM and are ineffective in T1DM (ADA, 2018). Previously GDM was defined as any degree of glucose intolerance with onset or first recognition during pregnancy. However, the number of pregnant women with undiagnosed diabetes has increased, and therefore it has now been recommended that women with risk factors for diabetes should be screened for undiagnosed T2DM at the first prenatal visit, using standard diagnostic criteria. Women found to have diabetes in the first trimester should receive a diagnosis of overt, not gestational, diabetes (ADA, 2018).

All women not previously known to have diabetes should be screened for GDM at 24 to 28 weeks of gestation. GDM is diagnosed most often during the second or third trimester of pregnancy because of the increase in insulin-antagonist hormone levels and insulin resistance that normally occurs at this time. Laboratory assessment of hemoglobin A1C, previously known as Hb A1C, at 24 to 28 weeks of gestation as a screening for GDM does not function as well as the glucose tolerance test (GTT). GDM screening can be accomplished with either of two strategies (for more details, see Table 14.5 in Chapter 14):

1. "One-step" 75-g oral glucose tolerance test (OGTT) or
2. "Two-step" approach with a 50-g (nonfasting) screen followed by a 100-g OGTT for those who screen positive.

For a comprehensive multisystem checklist for people with diabetes, please refer to the document *American Diabetes Association Standards of Medical Care in Diabetes*, which is published yearly online for free.

PATHOPHYSIOLOGY AND CARE MANAGEMENT ALGORITHM

Type 2 Diabetes Mellitus

ETIOLOGY

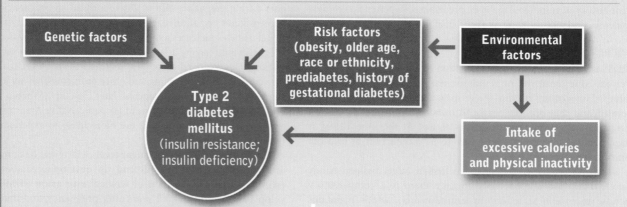

Genetic factors

Risk factors (obesity, older age, race or ethnicity, prediabetes, history of gestational diabetes)

Environmental factors

Type 2 diabetes mellitus (insulin resistance; insulin deficiency)

Intake of excessive calories and physical inactivity

PATHOPHYSIOLOGY

Symptoms (variable)

- Hyperglycemia
- Fatigue
- Excessive thirst
- Frequent urination

Clinical Findings

- Abnormal patterns of insulin secretion and action
- Decreased cellular uptake of glucose and increased postprandial glucose
- Increased release of glucose by liver (gluconeogenesis) resulting in fasting hyperglycemia
- Central obesity
- Hypertension
- Dyslipidemia

MANAGEMENT

Medical Management

Medical nutrition therapy
Physical activity
Medications
- Glucose-lowering medications
- Insulin

Monitoring
- Self-monitoring of blood glucose (SMBG)
- A1C testing
- Lipids
- Blood pressure
- Weight

Self-management education

Medical Nutrition Therapy (MNT)

- Lifestyle strategies (food/eating and physical activity) that improve glycemia, dyslipidemia, and blood pressure
- Nutrition education (regular balanced meal pattern, carbohydrate counting, fat modification) and counseling for health behavior change
- Blood glucose monitoring to determine adjustments in food or medications
- Cardioprotective nutrition interventions

During pregnancy, treatment to normalize maternal blood glucose levels reduces the risk of adverse maternal, fetal, and neonatal outcomes. Extra glucose from the mother crosses the fetal placenta and the fetus' pancreas responds by releasing extra insulin to cope with the excess glucose. The excess glucose is converted to fat, which results in macrosomia (a larger than normal baby). The fetus may become too large for a normal birth resulting in the need for C-section. Neonatal hypoglycemia at birth is another common problem. The above-normal levels of maternal glucose have caused the fetus to produce extra insulin. However, after birth the extra glucose is no longer available to the fetus, but until the pancreas can adjust, the neonate may require extra glucose through intravenous feedings for a day or two to keep blood glucose levels normal.

GDM does not cause congenital anomalies. Such malformations occur in women with diabetes before pregnancy who have uncontrolled blood glucose levels during the first 6 to 8 weeks of pregnancy when fetal organs are being formed. Because GDM does not appear until later in pregnancy, the fetal organs were formed before hyperglycemia became a problem.

When optimal blood glucose levels are not being maintained with MNT or the rate of fetal growth is excessive, pharmacologic therapy is needed (ADA, 2018). Research supports the use of insulin, insulin analogs, metformin, and glyburide during pregnancy. Women with GDM should be screened for diabetes 4 to 12 weeks postpartum and should have lifelong screening for the development of diabetes or prediabetes at least every 3 years (ADA, 2018). See Table 29.1 for a criteria for the diagnosis of diabetes and prediabetes.

Other Types of Diabetes

This category includes diabetes associated with specific genetic syndromes (such as neonatal diabetes and maturity onset diabetes of youth (MODY), genetic defects in insulin action, diseases of the exocrine pancreas (such as cystic fibrosis), endocrinopathies, (such as acromegaly or Cushing's syndrome), drug or chemical induced (such as in the treatment of HIV/AIDS or after organ transplantation), infections, and other illnesses. Monogenic defects that cause b-cell dysfunction, such as neonatal diabetes and MODY, represent a small fraction of patients with diabetes (<5%) (ADA, 2018).

SCREENING AND DIAGNOSTIC CRITERIA

Screening for Diabetes

1. Testing should be considered in overweight or obese (BMI greater than or equal to 25 kg/m² or greater than or equal to 23 kg/m² in Asian Americans) adults who have one or more of the following risk factors:
   - First-degree relative with diabetes
   - High-risk race/ethnicity (e.g., African American, Latino, Native American, Asian American, Pacific Islander)
   - History of CVD
   - Hypertension (greater than or equal to 140/90 mm Hg or on therapy for hypertension)
   - High-density lipoprotein (HDL) cholesterol level <35 mg/dL (0.90 mmol/L) and/or a triglyceride level >250 mg/dL (2.82 mmol/L)
   - Women with polycystic ovary syndrome (PCOS)
   - Physical inactivity
   - Other clinical conditions associated with insulin resistance (e.g., severe obesity; acanthosis nigricans, a condition in which dark raised areas appear on the sides of the neck and in body folds and creases).

TABLE 29.1	Criteria for the Diagnosis of Diabetes Mellitus and Increased Risk for Diabetes (Prediabetes)
Diagnosis	**Criteria**
Diabetes	A1C ≥6.5% (≥48 mmol/mol). The test should be performed in a laboratory using a method that is NGSP certified and standardized to the DCCT assay.*
	OR
	FPG ≥126 mg/dL (≥7.0 mmol/L). Fasting is defined as no caloric intake for at least 8 hr.*
	OR
	2-h PG ≥200 mg/dL (≥11.1 mmol/L) during an OGTT. The test should be performed as described by the WHO, using a glucose load containing the equivalent of 75-g anhydrous glucose dissolved in water.*
	OR
	In patients with classic symptoms of hyperglycemia or hyperglycemic crisis, a random PG ≥200 mg/dL (≥11.1 mmol/L)
Prediabetes*	FPG 100-125 mg/dL (5.6-6.9 mmol/L) (impaired fasting glucose)
	OR
	2-h PG during 75-g OGTT 140-199 mg/dL (7.8-11.0 mmol/L) (impaired glucose tolerance)
	OR
	A1C 5.7%-6.4% (39-47 mmol/mol)

*In the absence of unequivocal hyperglycemia, results should be confirmed by repeat testing.
*For all three tests, risk is continuous, extending below the lower limit of the range and becoming disproportionately greater at the higher end of the range.
DCCT, Diabetes Control and Complications Trial; *FPG*, fasting plasma glucose; *2-h PG*, 2-hour plasma glucose level (measured 2 hours after an oral glucose tolerance test [OGTT] with administration of 75 g of glucose); *NGSP*, National Glycohemoglobin Standardization Program; *WHO*, World Health Organization.
Modified from American Diabetes Association: Classification and of diabetes: standards of medical care in diabetes—2018, *Diabetes Care* 41(S1):S15-17, 2018.

2. Patients with prediabetes (A1C greater than or equal to 5.7% [39 mmol/mol], IGT, or IFG) should be tested yearly.
3. Women who were diagnosed with GDM should have lifelong testing at least every 3 years.
4. For all other patients, testing should begin at age 45 years.
5. If results are normal, testing should be repeated at a minimum of 3-year intervals, with consideration of more frequent testing depending on initial results and risk status.

Risk-based screening for T2DM or prediabetes in asymptomatic children and adolescents in a clinical setting (Persons aged <18 years):
   Criteria
   - Overweight (BMI >85th percentile for age and sex, weight for height >85th percentile, or weight >120% of ideal for height)

Plus one or more additional risk factors based on the strength of their association with diabetes as indicated by evidence grades:

- Maternal history of diabetes or GDM during the child's gestation
- Family history of T2DM in first- or second-degree relative
- Race/ethnicity (Native American, African American, Latino, Asian American, Pacific Islander)
- Signs of insulin resistance or conditions associated with insulin resistance (acanthosis nigricans, hypertension, dyslipidemia, PCOS, or small-for-gestational-age birth weight) (ADA, 2018)

Diagnostic Criteria

There are four methods used to diagnose diabetes. In the absence of unequivocal hyperglycemia, results should be confirmed by repeat testing (ADA, 2018). Diagnostic criteria for diabetes and prediabetes are summarized in Table 29.1.

1. Fasting plasma glucose (FPG) 126 mg/dL (7.0 mmol/L). Fasting is defined as no caloric intake for at least 8 hours. (In the absence of unequivocal hyperglycemia, results should be confirmed by repeat testing [ADA, 2018]).
2. OR 2-h plasma glucose 200 mg/dL (11.1 mmol/L) during OGTT. The test should be performed as described by the World Health Organization (WHO), using a glucose load containing the equivalent of 75-g anhydrous glucose dissolved in water.*
3. OR A1C 6.5% (48 mmol/mol). The test should be performed in a laboratory using a method that is National Glycohemoglobin Standardization Program (NGSP) certified and standardized to the Diabetes Control and Complications Trial (DCCT) assay.*
4. OR in a patient with classic symptoms of hyperglycemia or hyperglycemic crisis, a random plasma glucose <200 mg/dL (11.1 mmol/L).

Plasma glucose criteria, either the fasting plasma glucose (FPG) or the 2-hr plasma glucose after a 75-g OGTT, was the method usually used to diagnosis diabetes. However, the A1C assay now is highly standardized and is a reliable measure of chronic glucose levels. The A1C test reflects longer-term glucose concentrations and is assessed from the results of glycosylated hemoglobin (A1C) tests. When hemoglobin and other proteins are exposed to glucose, the glucose becomes attached to the protein in a slow, nonenzymatic, and concentration-dependent fashion (Fig. 29.1). Measurements of A1C therefore reflect a weighted average of plasma glucose concentration over the preceding weeks. In nondiabetic persons A1C values are 4% to 6%; these values correspond to mean blood glucose levels of about 70 to 126 mg/dL (3.9 to 7.0 mmol/L) (Table 29.2). A1C values vary less than FPG, and testing is more convenient because patients are not required to be fasting or to undergo an OGTT. However, A1C levels may vary with a person's race/ethnicity as glycation rates may differ by race (ADA, 2018). It is also unclear if the same A1C cutoff point should be used to diagnose children or adolescents with diabetes because studies used to recommend A1C to diagnose diabetes have all been performed in adult populations. For conditions with abnormal red cell turnover, such as hemolysis (blood loss), pregnancy, or iron deficiency, the diagnosis of diabetes must use glucose criteria exclusively (ADA, 2018). The A1C test should be performed using a method certified by the NGSP.

MANAGEMENT OF PREDIABETES

In no other disease does lifestyle—healthy food choices and physical activity—play a more important role in prevention and treatment than

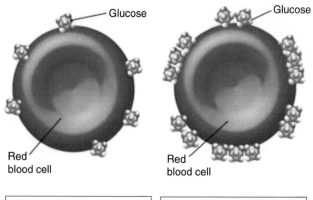

Fig. 29.1 Glycosylated Hemoglobin: Hemoglobin A1C. Glycosylated hemoglobin or A1C is the amount of glucose attached to the hemoglobin protein in a red blood cell. As blood sugar increases, the amount of glucose attached to hemoglobin increases. Because red blood cells last for 3 months in circulation, the A1C test is used to estimated average blood glucose over a 3-month time frame.

in diabetes. Studies comparing lifestyle modifications to medication have provided support for the benefit of weight loss (reduced energy intake) and physical activity as the first choice to prevent or delay diabetes. Clinical trials comparing lifestyle interventions to a control group have reported risk reduction for T2DM from lifestyle interventions ranging from 29% to 67% (Youssef, 2012). Two frequently cited

TABLE 29.2	**A1C and Estimated Average Glucose**
A1C (%)	**Estimated Average Glucose (mg/dL)**
4	68
4.5	82
5.0	97
5.5	111
6.0	126
6.5	140
7.0	154
7.5	169
8.0	183
8.5	197
9.0	212
9.5	226
10.0	240
10.5	255
11.0	269
11.5	283
12.0	298

The A1C test measures the percentage of red blood cells that have glucose bound to hemoglobin. This number correlates to blood glucose levels (mg/dL).
American Diabetes Association. *eAG / A1C Conversion Calculator* (website) https://professional.diabetes.org/diapro/glucose_calc.

studies are the Finnish Diabetes Prevention Study (FDPS) and the Diabetes Prevention Program (DPP), in which lifestyle interventions focused on a weight loss of 5% to 10%, physical activity of at least 150 min/week of moderate activity, and ongoing counseling and support. Both reported a 58% reduction in the incidence of T2DM in the intervention group compared with the control group and persistent reduction in the rate of conversion to T2DM within 3 to 14 years postintervention follow-up (DPP Research Group, 2009; Li et al, 2008; Lindström et al, 2006).

Medical Management

Use of the pharmacologic agents metformin, alpha-glucosidase inhibitors, orlistat, glucagon-like peptide-1 (GLP-1) receptor agonist, and thiazolidinediones has been shown to decrease incidence of diabetes by various degrees. However, none are approved by the U.S. Food and Drug Administration (FDA) specifically for diabetes prevention (ADA, 2018). Metformin has the strongest evidence base and has also demonstrated long-term safety as pharmacologic therapy for diabetes prevention. Keep in mind that diet and lifestyle modifications have been shown to be more effective than metformin when it comes to preventing and/or delaying diabetes (ADA, 2018).

Physical Activity

Physical activity helps to improve blood glucose control in T2DM, reduces cardiovascular risk factors, and may contribute to well-being. It is also important to note that physical activity, independent of weight loss, improves insulin sensitivity (ADA, 2018). Recommendations include moderate-intensity aerobic physical activity a minimum of 30 minutes 5 days per week (150 min/week) (i.e., walking 3 to 4 miles/hr) or vigorous-intensity aerobic physical activity a minimum of 20 minutes 3 days per week (90 min/week). Muscle-strengthening activities involving all major muscle groups two or more days per week are also recommended (U.S. Department of Health and Human Services and U.S. Department of Agriculture, 2015).

Medical Nutrition Therapy for Prediabetes

There is no one-size-fits-all meal plan for people living with prediabetes. One of the most important considerations for creating diabetes-centered goals around MNT is an emphasis on patient-centered care. This means the approach should be individualized and take into account a patient's health status, food preferences, food security, and housing situation (ADA, 2018). The ADA states that it is important to maintain the pleasure of eating by providing nonjudgmental messages about food choices. Adhering to a combination of healthy lifestyle habits (developing a healthy eating pattern, participating in regular physical activity, achieving and maintaining body weight goals, moderating alcohol intake, and being a nonsmoker) was shown to reduce the risk of developing T2DM by as much as 84% for women and 72% for men (Reis et al, 2011). More recently, moderate to high adherence to a Mediterranean-style eating pattern characterized by high levels of MUFAs such as olive oil, high intake of plant-based foods (vegetables, legumes, fruits, and nuts), moderate amounts of fish and wine, and a low intake of red and processed meat and whole-fat dairy products has been associated with a lower incidence of diabetes (Youssef, 2012; ADA, 2018).

In addition, whole grains and dietary fiber are associated with reduced risk of diabetes. Increased intake of whole grain–containing foods improves insulin sensitivity independent of body weight, and increased intake of dietary fiber has been associated with improved

insulin sensitivity and improved ability to secrete insulin adequately to overcome insulin resistance. Moderate consumption of alcohol (1 to 3 drinks per day [15 to 45 g alcohol]) is linked with decreased risk of T2DM, coronary heart disease, and stroke. But the data do not support recommending alcohol consumption to people at risk for diabetes who do not already drink alcoholic beverages.

High consumption of sugar-sweetened beverages, which includes soft drinks, fruit drinks, and energy and vitamin water-type drinks containing sucrose, high-fructose corn syrup, and/or fruit juice concentrates is associated with the development of T2DM (Malik et al, 2010). Studies also have reported that an eating pattern high in saturated fatty acids and trans fatty acids is associated with increased markers of insulin resistance and risk for T2DM, whereas unsaturated fatty acid intake is associated inversely with risk of diabetes (Youssef, 2012). Therefore individuals at increased risk for T2DM should be encouraged to limit their intake of sugar-sweetened beverages and decrease saturated fat intake (ADA, 2018).

MANAGEMENT OF DIABETES

Achieving glycemic control is the most important MNT goal in people with diabetes. Two classic clinical trials have demonstrated beyond a doubt the clear link between glycemic control and the development of complications in people with both T1DM and T2DM. The first is the DCCT, which studied approximately 1400 people with T1DM. Each individual involved in the study was treated with either intensive (multiple injections of insulin or use of insulin infusion pumps guided by blood glucose monitoring results) or conventional (one or two insulin injections per day) regimens. A 30-year follow-up of the DCCT demonstrated that an intervention that aimed to achieve normoglycemia, as close to the nondiabetic range as safely possible, reduced all of the microvascular and cardiovascular complications of diabetes and should be implemented as early as possible after diagnosis (Nathan, 2014). Another study, known as the United Kingdom Prospective Diabetes Study (UKPDS), demonstrated conclusively that glucose and blood pressure control decreased the risk of long-term complications in T2DM (Holman et al, 2008). Both of these trials emphasize importance of nutrition therapy in achieving continued glycemic control.

Medical Management

The management of all types of diabetes includes MNT, physical activity, blood glucose monitoring, medications, and self-management education and support. An important goal of medical treatment is to provide the individual with diabetes with the necessary tools to achieve the best possible control of glucose, lipids, and blood pressure to prevent, delay, or manage the microvascular (diabetic nephropathy, neuropathy, and retinopathy) and macrovascular complications (coronary artery disease, peripheral arterial disease, and stroke) while minimizing hypoglycemia and excess weight gain. Insulin, the primary hormone in glucose control is also anticatabolic and anabolic and facilitates cellular transport (Table 29.3). In general, the counterregulatory (stress) hormones (glucagon, growth hormone, cortisol, epinephrine, and norepinephrine) have the opposite effect of insulin.

The ADA's glycemic treatment goals for people with diabetes are listed in Table 29.4. Achieving goals requires open communication between the health care provider and the individual with diabetes and appropriate self-management education. Patients can assess day-to-day glycemic control by self-monitoring of blood glucose (SMBG) and measurement of urine or blood ketones. Longer-term glycemic

TABLE 29.3 Action of Insulin on Carbohydrate, Protein, and Fat Metabolism

Effect	Carbohydrates	Protein	Fat
Anticatabolic (prevents breakdown)	Decreases breakdown and release of glucose from glycogen in the liver	Inhibits protein degradation, diminishes gluconeogenesis	Inhibits lipolysis, prevents excessive production of ketones and ketoacidosis
Anabolic (promotes storage)	Facilitates conversion of glucose to glycogen for storage in liver and muscle	Stimulates protein synthesis	Facilitates conversion of pyruvate to free fatty acids, stimulating lipogenesis
Transport	Activates the transport system of glucose into muscle and adipose cells	Lowers blood amino acids in parallel with blood glucose levels	Activates lipoprotein lipase, facilitating transport of triglycerides into adipose tissue

TABLE 29.4 Recommendations for Glycemic Control for Many Nonpregnant Adults With Diabetes

Glycemic Control	Criteria
A1C	<7.0% (<53 mmol/mol)*
Preprandial capillary plasma glucose	80-130 mg/dL* (4.4-7.2 mmol/L)
Peak postprandial capillary plasma glucose†	<180 mg/dL* (<10.0 mmol/L)

*More or less stringent glycemic goals may be appropriate for individual patients. Goals should be individualized based on duration of diabetes, age/life expectancy, comorbid conditions, known CVD or advanced microvascular complications, hypoglycemia unawareness, and individual patient considerations.
†Postprandial glucose may be targeted if A1C goals are not met despite reaching preprandial glucose goals. Postprandial glucose measurements should be made 1 to 2 h after the beginning of the meal, generally peak levels in patients with diabetes.
Modified from American Diabetes Association: Glycemic Targets: Standards of medical care in diabetes—2018, *Diabetes Care* 41(S1):S60, 2018.

control (3-month average) is assessed by A1C testing. Cardiovascular risk factors should be assessed at least annually in all patients with diabetes. These risk factors include hypertension, dyslipidemia, smoking, a family history of premature coronary disease, chronic kidney disease, and the presence of albuminuria (ADA, 2018).

Patients with T1DM or T2DM who have hypertension should be treated to achieve blood pressure targets that are greater than or equal to 140/90 mm Hg (ADA, 2018). The ADA states that in adults with diabetes, it is reasonable to obtain a lipid profile (total cholesterol, low-density lipoprotein [LDL] cholesterol, HDL cholesterol, and triglycerides) at the time of diagnosis, at the initial medical evaluation, and at least every 5 years thereafter in patients under the age of 40 years. In patients who have had the disease for a longer period of time (typically younger patients with youth-onset T1DM), more frequent lipid profiles may be preferred (ADA, 2018). Providers should consider intensifying lifestyle therapy and optimizing glycemic control for patients with elevated triglyceride levels (>= 150 mg/dL [1.7 mmol/L]) and/or low HDL cholesterol (<40 mg/dL [1.0 mmol/L] for men, <50 mg/dL [1.3 mmol/L] for women) (ADA, 2018).

Optimal control of diabetes also requires the restoration of normal carbohydrate, protein, and fat metabolism. It is important that people with diabetes receive medical care from a team that ideally includes physicians, dietitians, nurses, pharmacists, and mental health professionals with expertise in diabetes. Individuals with diabetes also must assume an active role in their care. For T1DM a flexible, individualized management program using the principles of intensive insulin therapy is essential. T2DM is a progressive disease. In this instance it is not the diet that fails; rather, the pancreas is no longer able to secrete enough insulin to maintain adequate glucose control. As the disease progresses, MNT alone is not enough to keep A1C level at 7% or less. Therapy must intensify over time. Medications, and eventually insulin, need to be combined with nutrition therapy for optimal blood glucose control. Through the collaborative development of individualized nutrition interventions and ongoing support of behavior changes, health care professionals can facilitate the achievement of health goals for the person with diabetes.

Medical Nutrition Therapy for Diabetes

MNT is integral to total diabetes care and management. To integrate MNT effectively into the overall management of diabetes requires an RDN who is knowledgeable and skilled in implementing current nutrition therapy recommendations into the medical management of diabetes. Often times, RDNs acquire a specialized diabetes certification, known as a Certified Diabetes Educator (CDE) credential. CDEs are health professionals who possesses comprehensive knowledge of and experience in diabetes management and prevention.

MNT requires an individualized approach and effective nutrition, self-management education, counseling, and support. Monitoring glucose, A1C and lipid levels, blood pressure, weight, and quality-of-life issues is essential in evaluating the success of nutrition-related recommendations. Effective nutrition therapy interventions may be implemented in individualized sessions or in a comprehensive diabetes education program.

Since T2DM is a progressive disease, nutrition and physical activity interventions alone (i.e., without medications) are generally not adequate in maintaining glycemic control overtime. However, even after medications are initiated, nutrition therapy and proper education should continue to be an important component of the individualized treatment plan. For example, individuals with T1DM using multiple daily injections or continuous subcutaneous insulin infusion should focus on how to adjust insulin doses based on planned carbohydrate intake. For individuals using fixed daily insulin doses, carbohydrate intake on a day-to-day basis should be consistent with respect to time and amount. Retrospective studies reveal durable A1C reductions with these types of programs, with a significant improvement in quality of life over time. Finally, nutritional approaches for reducing CVD risk, including optimizing serum lipids and blood pressure, can effectively reduce CVD events and mortality (Evert et al, 2014).

The Academy of Nutrition and Dietetics (AND) published evidence-based nutrition practice guidelines (EBNPG) for T1DM and T2DM in adults in their Evidence Analysis Library and in print (AND, 2017; Franz et al, 2017). The ADA nutrition recommendations are published in a position statement and are summarized in their annual standards of care.

Goals and Desired Outcomes

The goals for MNT for diabetes emphasize the role of lifestyle in improving glucose control, lipid and lipoprotein profiles, and blood pressure. Goals of MNT are summarized in Box 29.1. Medicare reimburses qualified RDN providers for providing evidence-based MNT for diabetes management to eligible participants. Improving health through food choices and physical activity is the basis of all nutrition recommendations for the treatment of diabetes.

Besides being skilled and knowledgeable in assessing and implementing MNT, RDNs also must be aware of expected outcomes from MNT, when to assess outcomes, and what feedback (including recommendations) should be given to referral sources. Furthermore, the effect of MNT on A1C will be known by 6 weeks to 3 months, at which time the RDN must assess whether the goals of therapy have been met by changes in lifestyle or whether changes or additional medications are needed (Evert et al, 2014; AND, 2017).

Multiple research studies support MNT as an effective therapy in reaching diabetes treatment goals. MNT implemented by RDNs reduced A1C levels by 1.0% to 1.9% for people with T1DM and 0.3% to 2% for people with T2DM (ADA, 2018).

These outcomes are similar or greater to those from glucose-lowering medications. MNT also is reported to improve lipid profiles, decrease blood pressure, promote weight loss, decrease need for medications, and decrease risk of onset and progression to diabetes-related comorbidities. A variety of nutrition therapy interventions such as individualized MNT, portion control, sample menus, carbohydrate counting, exchange lists, simple meal plans, and low-fat vegan diets can be implemented (Franz and MacLeod, 2018). Individualized MNT, implemented in collaboration with the individual with diabetes, is essential because a variety of nutrition interventions are effective. A common focus of MNT for individuals with T2DM is reduced energy intake. Additionally, MNT may encourage the consumption of dietary fiber from fruit, vegetables, whole grains and legumes due to their overall health benefits. Sodium may also be a nutrient of focus. The recommendation for the general public to reduce sodium to <2300 mg/day is also appropriate for people with diabetes. However, if the individual has both diabetes and hypertension, additional reductions in sodium intake may be indicated (Franz and MacLeod, 2018). For individuals with T1DM, a common focus is using carbohydrate counting to determine premeal insulin boluses (Franz et al, 2017).

Energy Balance and Weight

Children/Adolescents

Historically, achieving and maintaining body weight goals has been a focus of MNT for diabetes. This is particularly true for children with T1DM. Provision of adequate calories for normal growth and development for children and adolescents with T1DM is a key component of MNT. Therefore height and weight should be measured at each visit and tracked via appropriate height and weight growth charts (Chiang et al, 2018) (See Appendix 4).

For youth with T2DM, traditional nutrition therapy goals included prevention of excessive weight gain while encouraging normal linear growth. However, the 2016 American Academy of Pediatrics (AAP) guidelines recommended shifting the focus from weight to healthy lifestyle behaviors. The guidelines state that while obesity may be a risk factor for T2DM in youth, obesity prevention efforts may lead to the development of an eating disorder (Golden et al, 2016). Furthermore, longitudinal research found that children whose parents used restrictive feeding have a higher likelihood of eating in the absence of hunger and an elevated BMI later in childhood (Birch et al, 2003).

Adults

Overweight and obesity are common in people both at risk for and with T2DM. Some research suggests that reduced calorie intake can lead to reductions in A1C of 0.3% to 2.0% in adults with T2DM. If appropriate for the individual, a reduction in caloric intake may also lead to improvements in medication doses and quality of life (ADA, 2018). Similarly, weight loss interventions implemented in people with prediabetes and newly diagnosed with T2DM have been shown to be effective in improving glycemic control, but the benefit of weight loss interventions in T2DM of longer duration is mixed (Franz et al, 2017). Substantial evidence suggests that weight loss diets are not sustainable. A review of over 30 long-term studies concluded that the more diets an individual has tried, the more weight they regain (Mann et al, 2007).

Furthermore, the AND EBNPG reported that approximately half of the weight loss intervention studies in people with T2DM improved A1C at 1 year and one-half did not (AND, 2008a). In the weight loss studies lasting 1 year or longer reviewed by the ADA, only 2 study groups achieved weight losses of 5% or greater. The first were people newly diagnosed with T2DM who followed a Mediterranean-style eating pattern (−6.2 kg) and the second were those who participated in an intensive lifestyle intervention as part of the Look AHEAD (Action for Health in Diabetes) study (−8.4 kg) (Esposito et al, 2009; Look AHEAD Research Group, 2010). Other weight loss interventions resulted in weight losses of less than 5% (4.8 kg or less) at 1 year (Evert et al, 2013). Weight losses greater than 5% resulted in consistent improvements in A1C, lipids, and blood pressure; however, weight losses less than 5% did not result in consistent 1-year improvements in A1C,

---

> ### BOX 29.1 Goals of Medical Nutrition Therapy That Apply to Adults With Diabetes
>
> 1. To promote and support healthful eating patterns, emphasizing a variety of nutrient-dense foods in appropriate portion sizes, to improve overall diet and specifically to:
>   - Attain individualized glucose, blood pressure, and lipids goals
>   - Achieve and maintain body weight goals
>   - Delay or prevent complications of diabetes
> 2. To address individual nutrition needs based on personal and cultural preferences, health literacy and numeracy, access to healthful food choices, willingness and ability to make behavioral changes.
> 3. To maintain the pleasure of eating by providing positive messages about food choices while limiting food choices only when indicated by scientific evidence.
> 4. To provide the individual with diabetes with practical tools for day-to-day meal planning rather than focusing on individual macronutrients, micronutrients, or single foods.

Adapted from Evert AB et al: Nutrition therapy recommendations for the management of adults with diabetes, *Diabetes Care* 36:3821, 2013.

lipids, or blood pressure (AND, 2008a; Franz, 2013). One approach that has recently gained popularity within the dietetics community is the Health at Every Size (HAES) weight neutral paradigm, which focuses on health gain/promotion rather than weight loss. A systematic review of 16 studies looking at the impact of nondiet approaches (such as HAES) on attitudes, behaviors, and health outcomes found that nondiet interventions resulted in statistically significant improvements in disordered eating patterns, self-esteem, and depression. Additionally, none of the interventions resulted in significant weight gain or worsening of blood glucose levels, cholesterol, or blood pressure. In two of the studies, biochemical measures improved significantly compared with the control or diet group. The researchers did note that there were limitations due to the inconsistent definitions of nondiet approaches and the use of various assessment instruments to measure outcomes. However, they concluded that "because of the long-term ineffectiveness of weight-focused interventions, the psychological improvements seen in weight-neutral, nondiet interventions warrant further investigation" (Clifford et al, 2015). It is important to keep in mind that potential weight discrimination may have an effect on health outcomes. One study found that weight discrimination, or negative weight-related attitudes toward individuals at higher weights or obesity, exacerbated the effects of waist-to-hip ratio on A1C, such that people who had higher waist-to-hip ratios and reported weight discrimination had the highest A1C levels (Tsenkova et al, 2011). Therefore the RDN should collaborate with individuals who have diabetes to integrate nutrient-dense eating patterns (which may or may not lead to weight loss) and regular physical activity and should not make assumptions on eating habits and lifestyle patterns based on weight.

Bariatric Surgery

Bariatric surgery can be an effective weight loss treatment for severely obese patients with T2DM and can result in marked improvements in glycemia (Schauer et al, 2014). The ADA states that metabolic surgery should be recommended as an option to treat T2DM in appropriate surgical candidates with BMI greater than or equal to 40 kg/m^2 (BMI greater than or equal to 37.5 kg/m^2 in Asian Americans), regardless of the level of glycemic control or complexity of glucose-lowering regimens, and in adults with BMI 35.0–39.9 kg/m^2 (32.5–37.4 kg/m^2 in Asian Americans) when hyperglycemia is inadequately controlled despite lifestyle and optimal medical therapy (ADA, 2018). In 4434 adults with T2DM, gastric bypass surgery resulted in 68.2% initial complete diabetes remission within 5 years after surgery (Arterburn et al, 2013). However, 35.1% had redeveloped diabetes within the next 5 years and the median duration of remission was 8.3 years. Predictors of relapse were poor preoperative glycemic control, insulin use, and longer diabetes duration.

Macronutrient Percentages and Eating Patterns

Although numerous studies have attempted to identify the optimal percentages of macronutrients for the eating plan of persons with diabetes, review of the evidence shows clearly that there is not an ideal percentage of calories from carbohydrate, protein, and fat for all persons with diabetes (Evert et al, 2014). Macronutrient distribution should be based on an individualized assessment of current eating patterns, preferences, and metabolic goals. In addition to metabolic goals, the RDN should consider personal preferences (including tradition, culture, religion, health beliefs and goals, economics) when working with individuals to determine the best eating pattern for them (ADA, 2018). Individualization of the macronutrient composition will depend on the metabolic status of the

individual (including lipid profile, renal function) and/or personal food preferences.

The ADA also reviewed research on eating patterns (Mediterranean-style, vegetarian and vegan, low-fat, low-carbohydrate, and Dietary Approaches to Stop Hypertension [DASH]) implemented for diabetes management and concluded that a variety of eating patterns are acceptable (ADA, 2018). The RDN must take into consideration personal preferences and metabolic goals when recommending one eating pattern over another.

Although numerous factors influence glycemic response to foods, monitoring total grams of carbohydrates, whether by use of carbohydrate counting or experienced based estimation, remains a key strategy in achieving glycemic control (Evert et al, 2013). While some evidence suggests that the type of carbohydrate eaten may influence blood glucose levels, the total amount of carbohydrate eaten is the primary predictor of glycemic response. Day-to-day consistency in the amount of carbohydrate eaten at meals and snacks is reported to improve glycemic control, especially in persons on either MNT alone, glucose-lowering medications, or fixed insulin regimens. In people with T1DM or T2DM who are on insulin pump therapy, insulin doses should be adjusted to match carbohydrate intake (Evert et al, 2013).

Carbohydrate counting is an eating plan method based on the principle that all types of carbohydrate (except fiber) are digested, and that the majority of carbohydrates are absorbed into the bloodstream as molecules of glucose. Carbohydrate foods include starches, such as breads, cereals, pasta, rice, beans and lentils, starchy vegetables, crackers, and snack chips; fruits and fruit juices; milk, milk substitutes, and yogurt; and sweets and desserts. One carbohydrate exchange (or serving) is a portion of food containing 15 grams of carbohydrate (see Appendix 18).

It is important for the RDN to ensure that the individual with diabetes has an understanding of which foods contain carbohydrates and the relationship between carbohydrate intake and blood glucose levels. It is equally important for the RDN to avoid vilifying carbohydrates, which unfortunately occurs too frequently in health care centers that work with patients who have diabetes. The RDN's role should include helping the individual understand that carbohydrates are part of a healthy diet, and collaboratively create an eating plan that lists the number of carbohydrate choices recommended for meals and, if desired, snacks. Individuals are encouraged to keep protein and fat food sources as consistent as possible because they do not greatly affect blood glucose levels even though they require insulin for metabolism.

There are two main eating plans using carbohydrate counting. The first uses insulin-to-carbohydrate ratios to adjust premeal insulin doses for variable carbohydrate intake (physiologic insulin regimens). Note that the insulin-to-carbohydrate ratio is typically calculated by dividing 500 by the total daily dose of insulin. For example, if a patient is taking 50 units of insulin per day, you would divide 500 by 50 to get 10. This means that 1 unit of rapid-acting insulin will cover the spike in blood glucose after the patient eats 10 grams of carbohydrate.

The second eating plan is following a consistent carbohydrate eating plan when using fixed insulin regimens. Testing premeal and postmeal glucose levels is important for making adjustments in either food intake or medication to achieve glucose goals.

Carbohydrate Intake

As noted earlier, blood glucose levels after eating are determined primarily by the speed of digestion and absorption of glucose into the bloodstream and the ability of insulin to clear glucose from the circulation. Low-carbohydrate diets may seem to be a logical approach to lowering postprandial glucose. However, foods that contain carbohydrates (whole grains, legumes, fruits, vegetables, and low-fat milk) are excellent sources of vitamins, minerals, dietary fiber, and energy and are encouraged over other sources of carbohydrates (namely highly processed carbohydrate with low fiber, added sugars and fats, or high sodium) to improve overall nutrient intake (ADA, 2018).

The long-held belief that sucrose—also known as common table sugar—must be restricted based on the assumption that sugars are more rapidly digested and absorbed than starches is not justified. The total amount of carbohydrate eaten at a meal, regardless of whether the source is starch or sucrose, is the primary determinant of postprandial glucose levels. The glycemic effect of carbohydrate foods cannot be predicted based on their structure (i.e., starch vs. sugar) owing to the efficiency of the human digestive tract in reducing starch polymers to glucose. Starches are rapidly metabolized into 100% glucose during digestion, in contrast to sucrose, which is metabolized into only approximately 50% glucose and approximately 50% fructose. Fructose has a lower glycemic response, which has been attributed to its slow rate of absorption and its storage in the liver as glycogen. Sucrose-containing foods can be substituted for isocaloric amounts of other carbohydrate foods. However, as for the general population, care should be taken to avoid excess energy intake and to avoid displacing nutrient-dense food choices (Ludwig et al, 2018). The ADA advises that people with or at risk for diabetes avoid sugar-sweetened beverages (soft drinks, fruit drinks, energy and vitamin-type water drinks containing sucrose, high-fructose corn syrup, and/or fruit juice concentrates) to reduce the risk of worsening the cardiometabolic risk profile and to prevent weight gain (ADA, 2018).

Glycemic Index and Glycemic Load

The glycemic index (GI) of food was developed to compare the physiologic effects of carbohydrates on glucose. The GI ranks carbohydrate foods according to how they affect blood glucose levels (for example, the GI of glucose = 100; the GI of white bread = 70).

The estimated glycemic load (GL) of foods, meals, and dietary patterns is calculated by multiplying the GI by the amount of available carbohydrate (divided by 100) in each food and then totaling the values for all foods in a meal or dietary pattern. For example, two slices of white bread with a GI of 75 and 30 g of carbohydrate has a GL of 22.5 ($75 \times 30/100 = 22.5$) (see Appendix 28 for GI and GL of foods).

The ADA conducted a systematic review of GI and GL diets in the management of diabetes and found that studies longer than 12 weeks report no significant impact of GI or GL, independent of weight loss, on A1C. However, mixed results were reported regarding fasting glucose levels and endogenous insulin levels. If GI or GL is proposed as a glycemia-lowering strategy, the RDN can advise adults with diabetes that lowering the GI or GL may or may not have a significant effect on glycemic control.

Fiber and Whole Grains

There is evidence to suggest that dietary fiber intake may lead to decreased all-cause mortality in individuals with diabetes (Evert et al, 2014). Additionally, a meta-analysis reviewing 15 studies that examined the relationship between fiber and diabetes found that an intervention involving fiber supplementation for T2DM can reduce fasting blood glucose (FBG) and A1C. Compared with the placebo, individuals who consumed dietary fiber as an intervention had an overall mean difference of a decrease in A1C of 0.26%. While this evidence is promising, one of the limitations is that the studies used a variety of grams of fiber per day in their interventions, from as low as an additional 4 g/day to 40 g/day (Post et al, 2012).

As with the general population, consuming 25 g fiber per day for adult women and 38 g per day for adult men is encouraged (Evert et al, 2014). It is also recommended that individuals with diabetes, along with the general population, consume at least half of all grains as whole grains.

Grams of fiber (and sugar alcohols) are included on food labels and are calculated as having about half the energy (2 kcal/g) of most other carbohydrates (4 kcal/g). However, for most people it is not necessary to subtract the amount of dietary fiber (or sugar alcohols) when carbohydrate counting (Evert et al, 2014). Adjustments in carbohydrate intake values is practical only if the amount per serving is more than 5 g. In that case, counting half of the carbohydrate grams from fiber (and sugar alcohols) would be useful in calculating food choices for food labels or recipes.

Nonnutritive and Hypocaloric Sweeteners

Reduced calorie sweeteners approved by the FDA include sugar alcohols (erythritol, sorbitol, mannitol, xylitol, isomalt, lactitol, and hydrogenated starch hydrolysates) and tagatose. All FDA-approved nonnutritive sweeteners, when consumed within the established daily intake levels, can be used by people with diabetes, including pregnant women. Furthermore, nonnutritive sweeteners could facilitate reductions in added sugars intake, thereby resulting in decreased total energy intake (ADA, 2018). However, although the use of nonnutritive sweeteners appears to be safe, some people report gastric discomfort after eating foods sweetened with these products, and consuming large quantities may cause diarrhea, especially in children.

Keep in mind that the intake of nutritive sweeteners, when substituted isocalorically for other carbohydrates, will not have a significant effect on A1C or insulin levels; however, they can reduce overall calorie and carbohydrate intake (ADA, 2018).

Protein Intake

According to the ADA, there is no evidence that adjusting the daily level of protein intake (typically 1 to 1.5 g/kg body weight/day or 15% to 20% total calories) will improve health in individuals without diabetic kidney disease. For people with diabetes, evidence is inconclusive to recommend an ideal amount of protein intake for optimizing glycemic control or improving CVD risk factors; therefore, goals should be individualized to reflect current eating patterns. Some research does suggest that slightly higher protein intake (20% to 30% of total calories) may lead to increased satiety in people with diabetes.

Although nonessential amino acids undergo gluconeogenesis, in well-controlled diabetes the glucose produced does not appear in the general circulation; the glucose produced is likely stored in the liver as glycogen. When glycolysis occurs, it is unknown if the original source of glucose was carbohydrate or protein. Although protein is just as potent a stimulant of acute insulin release as carbohydrate, it has no long-term effect on insulin needs. Adding protein to the treatment of hypoglycemia does not prevent subsequent hypoglycemia, due to the potential simultaneous rise in endogenous insulin (ADA, 2018).

Fat Intake

Evidence is also inconclusive for an ideal amount of total fat for people with diabetes and therefore goals should be individualized. The type of fat consumed appears to be more important than total fat in terms of metabolic and cardiovascular risk.

Monounsaturated fatty acid (MUFA)-rich foods as a component of the Mediterranean-style eating pattern are associated with improved glycemic control and improved CVD risk factors in persons with T2DM. Controversy exists on the best ratio of omega-6 to omega-3 fatty acids; however, polyunsaturated fatty acids (PUFAs) and MUFAs are recommended as substitutes for saturated fatty acids (SFAs) or trans fatty acids. The amount of SFAs, cholesterol, and trans fat recommended for people with diabetes is the same as for the general population.

There is evidence from the general population that foods containing omega-3 fatty acids have beneficial effects on lipoproteins and prevention of heart disease. Therefore the recommendations for the general public to eat fish (particularly fatty fish) at least two times (two servings) per week is also appropriate for people with diabetes. However, evidence from randomized controlled trial (RCTs) does not support recommending omega-3 supplements for people with diabetes for the prevention or treatment of CVD (ADA, 2018).

Alcohol

Small amounts of alcohol ingested with food have minimum, if any, acute effect on glucose and insulin levels. If individuals choose to drink alcohol, daily intake should be limited to one drink or less for adult women and two drinks or less for adult men (1 drink = 12 oz beer, 5 oz wine, or 1.5 oz distilled spirits). Each drink contains 15 grams of alcohol. The type of alcoholic beverage consumed does not make a difference. The same precautions that apply to alcohol consumption for the general population apply to persons with diabetes. Abstention from alcohol should be advised for people with a history of alcohol abuse or dependence; for women during pregnancy; and for people with medical problems such as liver disease, pancreatitis, advanced neuropathy, or severe hypertriglyceridemia (ADA, 2018).

Moderate to high alcohol consumption may place people with diabetes who take insulin or insulin secretagogues (medications that increase insulin production) at increased risk for delayed hypoglycemia (ADA, 2018). Consuming alcohol with food can minimize the risk of nocturnal hypoglycemia, or low blood sugar that occurs overnight when an individual is asleep. Education and awareness of delayed hypoglycemia after consuming alcoholic beverages is important. Alcoholic beverages should be considered an addition to the regular food and meal plan for all persons with diabetes. No food should be omitted, given the possibility of alcohol-induced hypoglycemia and because alcohol does not require insulin to be metabolized (ADA, 2018). Excessive amounts of alcohol (three or more drinks per day) on a consistent basis, contribute to hyperglycemia, which improves as soon as alcohol use is discontinued.

Small amounts of alcohol, in particular red wine, may be safe and potentially decrease cardiometabolic risk. One long-term RCT suggested that among well-controlled people with diabetes, initiating modest wine intake, especially red wine, as part of a healthy diet is probably safe and modestly decreases cardiometabolic risk (Blomster et al, 2014). However, chronic ingestion of alcohol does raise blood pressure and may be a risk factor for stroke (O'Keefe et al, 2018).

Micronutrients and Herbal Supplements

The evidence examining the effect of dietary supplements on blood glucose regulation are mixed; therefore the ADA does not endorse the use of routine vitamin or mineral supplementation in people with diabetes (compared with the general population) who do not have underlying deficiencies (ADA, 2018).

There is, however, some emerging evidence that suggests certain supplements may be helpful in lowering blood sugar levels. These include cinnamon, chromium, alpha-lipoic acid (ALA), and berberine.

A 2013 systematic review and meta-analysis found that cinnamon doses of 120 mg/day to 6 g/day for 4 to 18 weeks reduced levels of FPG, total cholesterol (−15.60 mg/dL), LDL cholesterol (−9.42 mg/dL), and triglycerides (−29.59 mg/dL) while increasing levels of HDL cholesterol (1.66 mg/dL). However, despite the reductions observed in FBG, no significant effect on hemoglobin A1C (HbA1C) levels (−0.16%) was seen (Allen et al, 2013).

A narrative review published in the *Journal of the Academy of Nutrition and Dietetics* had similar findings. The review analyzed 11 RCTs and found that all the studies reported some reductions in FPG during the cinnamon intervention. Of the studies measuring A1C, very modest decreases were also apparent with cinnamon, whereas changes in the placebo groups were minimal (Costello et al, 2016). It is important to use caution when combining cinnamon (in pill form) with other blood glucose-lowering herbs and supplements, as taking cinnamon with some antidiabetes drugs may cause hypoglycemic effects.

Chromium is an essential trace mineral required by the body in small amounts. Some research suggests that the mineral may be used to improve glycemic control for diabetes (types 1 and 2), prediabetes, PCOS, reactive hypoglycemia, metabolic syndrome, and other glucose regulation disorders (Natural Medicines Database, 2018). One study examined the effects of 42 µg Cr/day of chromium supplementation in a small number of people with newly diagnosed diabetes. After 3 months of chromium supplementation, the control group experienced a significant reduction in FBG. Additionally, A1C values improved significantly from 9.51% to 6.86%, indicating better glycemic control. In the experimental group, total cholesterol, triglycerides and LDL levels were also significantly reduced. These data demonstrate a possible beneficial effect of chromium supplementation on glycemic control and lipid variables in subjects with newly onset T2DM (Sharma et al, 2011). It should be noted that cell culture studies suggest a possibility of DNA damage with long-term chromium supplementation, however this has not been shown in living organisms (Linus Pauling Institute, 2018).

ALA is an essential cofactor in mitochondrial enzymes related to energy production that may improve glucose utilization in those with T2DM (Linus Pauling Institute, 2018b).

One trial randomized 105 people with diabetes to two groups. The first was instructed to take a supplement containing 600 mg of ALA (along with L-carnosine, zinc, and vitamins of group B). The second was given a placebo. The study found that after 3 months, there was a reduction of FPG, postprandial glucose, and A1C in the group that supplemented with ALA compared the placebo. The study also observed a reduction of LDL cholesterol, and triglycerides in the ALA group (Derosa et al, 2016).

Berberine is an alkaloid found in a variety of medicinal plants, including *Hydrastis canadensis* (goldenseal) and *Berberis aristata* (tree turmeric). It has been used for medicinal purposes in Chinese and Ayurvedic medicine and as a dye, thanks to its vibrant yellow color. In one clinical study, berberine significantly lowered FBG, A1C, triglyceride, and insulin levels in patients with T2DM. The FBG and A1C-lowering effects of berberine were similar to those of metformin and rosiglitazone. Liver function was improved greatly in these patients by showing reduction of liver enzymes (Ziegler et al, 2011). In another study, 36 adults with newly diagnosed T2DM were randomly assigned to treatment with berberine or metformin (0.5 g three times per day). After the 3 months, the hypoglycemic effect of berberine was similar to that of metformin. Significant decreases in A1C (9.5% to 7.5%), FBG (10.6 mmol/L to 6.9 mmol/L), postprandial blood glucose (19.8 mmol/L to 11.1 mmol/L), and triglycerides (1.13 mmol/L to 0.89 mmol/L) were observed in the berberine group (Yin et al, 2008).

Note that berberine may be contraindicated during lactation and pregnancy, and in children. Additionally, it can cause hypoglycemia in individuals on blood sugar-lowering medications (insulin, Amaryl, etc.) and may potentially lower blood pressure. Therefore it should be used with caution in people with low blood pressure or in people on blood sugar-lowering medications. Berberine can also inhibit activity of enzymes that break down certain drugs (Neoral, Sandimmune), which can lead to increased blood levels and increased risk of adverse effects. Other potential adverse effects include nausea, bloating, constipation, diarrhea, hypertension, respiratory failure, headache, bradycardia, jaundice, and paresthesias.

Even though there is some emerging evidence to suggest that herbal supplements may help with blood glucose regulation, it is important to remember that herbal products are not standardized and vary in their content of active ingredients (see Chapter 11). They have the potential to interact with and alter the effect of other medications. Therefore people with diabetes should always report the use of supplements and herbal products to their health care provider/RDN.

Metformin is associated with vitamin B_{12} deficiency. Because of this, a recent report from the Diabetes Prevention Program Outcomes Study (DPPOS) suggests that periodic testing of vitamin B_{12} levels should be considered in patients taking metformin, especially if the individual has a history of anemia or peripheral neuropathy.

Physical Activity/Exercise

Physical activity should be an integral part of the treatment plan for persons with diabetes. Exercise helps improve insulin sensitivity, reduce cardiovascular risk factors, control weight, and improve well-being. Given appropriate guidelines, the majority of people with diabetes can exercise safely. Individual activity plans will vary, depending on interest, age, general health, and level of physical fitness.

There are two types of exercise: aerobic and anaerobic. Both are important in people with diabetes. Aerobic exercise consists of rhythmic, repeated, and continuous movements of the same large muscle groups for at least 10 minutes at a time. Examples include walking, bicycling, jogging, swimming, and many sports. Anaerobic exercise, also known as resistance exercise, consists of activities that use muscular strength to move a weight or work against a resistive load. Examples include weight lifting and exercises using resistance-providing machines.

Despite the increase in glucose uptake by muscles during exercise, glucose levels change little in individuals without diabetes. Muscular work causes insulin levels to decline, while counterregulatory hormones (primarily glucagon) rise. As a result, the increased glucose use by the exercising muscles is matched with increased glucose production by the liver. This balance between insulin and counterregulatory hormones is the major determinant of hepatic glucose production, underscoring the need for insulin adjustments in addition to adequate carbohydrate intake during exercise for people with diabetes.

In people with T1DM, the glycemic response to exercise varies, depending on overall diabetes control, plasma glucose, and insulin levels at the start of exercise; timing, intensity, and duration of the exercise; previous food intake; and previous conditioning. An important variable is the level of plasma insulin during and after exercise. Hypoglycemia can occur because of insulin-enhanced muscle glucose uptake by the exercising muscle.

In people with T2DM, blood glucose control can improve with physical activity, largely because of decreased insulin resistance and increased insulin sensitivity, which results in increased peripheral use

of glucose not only during but also after the activity (Colberg et al, 2016). This exercise-induced enhanced insulin sensitivity occurs independent of any effect on body weight. Structured exercise interventions of at least 8 weeks in duration are reported to lower A1C. Exercise also decreases the effects of counterregulatory hormones, which reduces the hepatic glucose output, contributing to improved glucose control.

Potential Problems with Exercise

Hypoglycemia is a potential problem associated with exercise in people taking insulin or insulin secretagogues. Hypoglycemia can occur during, immediately after, or many hours after exercise, and is more common in people with T1DM (Colberg et al, 2016). Hypoglycemia has been reported to be more common after exercise—especially exercise of long duration. This can include strenuous activity, play, or sporadic exercise. Hypoglycemia in this instance is typically due to increased insulin sensitivity after exercise, requiring repletion of liver and muscle glycogen, which can take up to 24 to 30 hours (see Chapter 22).

Blood glucose levels before exercise reflect only the value at that time, and it is unknown if this is a stable blood glucose level or a blood glucose level that is dropping. If blood glucose levels are dropping before exercise, adding exercise can contribute to hypoglycemia during the activity.

Hyperglycemia also can result from exercise of high intensity, likely because the effects of counterregulatory hormones. When a person participates in a high level of exercise intensity, there is a greater-than-normal increase in counterregulatory hormones. As a result, hepatic glucose release exceeds the rise in glucose use. The elevated glucose levels also may extend into the postexercise state. Hyperglycemia and worsening ketosis also can result in people with T1DM who are deprived of insulin for 12 to 48 hours and are ketotic. Vigorous activity should be avoided in the presence of ketosis (ADA, 2018). It is not, however, necessary to postpone exercise based simply on hyperglycemia, provided the individual feels well and urine and/or blood ketones are negative.

Exercise Guidelines

The variability of glucose responses to exercise contributes to the difficulty in giving precise guidelines for exercising safely. Frequent blood glucose monitoring before, during, and after exercise helps individuals identify their response to physical activities. To meet their individual needs, it is important to modify general guidelines to reduce insulin doses before (or after) exercise. Additionally, an individual may choose to ingest carbohydrates before (or after) any physical activity. Similar to the general population without diabetes, it is also important for individuals with diabetes to stay hydrated when performing physical activities.

Carbohydrate recommendations for insulin or insulin secretagogue users. During moderate-intensity exercise, glucose uptake is increased by 8 to 13 g/hr; this is the basis for the recommendation to add 15 g carbohydrate for every 30 to 60 minutes of activity (depending on the intensity) over and above normal routines. Moderate exercise for less than 30 minutes usually does not require any additional carbohydrate or insulin adjustment, unless the individual is hypoglycemic before the start of exercise. Added carbohydrates should be ingested if preexercise glucose levels are less than 100 mg/dL (5.6 mmol/L). Supplementary carbohydrate is generally not needed in individuals with T2DM who are not treated with insulin or insulin secretagogues; it simply adds unnecessary calories (ADA, 2018).

In all people, blood glucose levels decline gradually during exercise, and ingesting carbohydrate during prolonged exercise can improve performance by maintaining the availability and oxidation of blood glucose. For the exerciser with diabetes whose blood glucose levels may drop sooner and lower than the exerciser without diabetes, ingesting carbohydrate after 40 to 60 minutes of exercise is important and also may assist in preventing hypoglycemia. Drinks containing 2% to 4% glucose empty from the stomach as quickly as water and have the advantage of providing both needed fluids and carbohydrates (Leiper, 2015). Consuming carbohydrates immediately after exercise optimizes repletion of muscle and liver glycogen stores. For the exerciser with diabetes, this takes on added importance because of increased risk for late-onset hypoglycemia.

Insulin Guidelines

It is often necessary to adjust the insulin dosage to prevent hypoglycemia. This occurs most often with moderate to strenuous activity lasting more than 45 to 60 minutes. For most persons a modest decrease (of about 1 to 2 units) in the rapid- (or short-) acting insulin during the period of exercise is a good starting point. For prolonged vigorous exercise, a larger decrease in the total daily insulin dosage may be necessary. After exercise, insulin dosing also may have to be decreased.

Precautions for Persons with Diabetes

Persons with T2DM may have a lower Vo$_2$max and therefore need a more gradual training program. Rest periods may be needed, but this does not impair the training effect from physical activity.

Exercise Recommendations

Adults with diabetes should be advised to perform at least 150 min/week of moderate-intensity aerobic physical activity spread over at least 3 days/week with no more than 2 consecutive days without physical activity. In the absence of contraindications, adults with T2DM should be encouraged to perform resistance exercise at least twice per week with each session consisting of at least one set of five or more different resistance exercises involving large muscle groups. There is an additive benefit of combined aerobic and resistance training in adults with T2DM. Children with diabetes or prediabetes should be encouraged to engage in at least 60 min/day of physical activity with vigorous muscle-strengthening and bone-strengthening activities at least 3 days/week (ADA, 2018).

Routine screening preexercise is not recommended. Providers should use clinical judgment in this area. High-risk patients should be encouraged to start with short periods of low-intensity exercise and increase the intensity and duration slowly (ADA, 2018).

Medications

A consensus statement on the approach to management of hyperglycemia in T2DM has been published by the ADA and the European Association for the Study of Diabetes (Inzucchi et al, 2015). Interventions at the time of diagnosis include healthy eating, weight control, physical activity, and diabetes education. Metformin is the preferred initial pharmacologic agent for T2DM, either in addition to lifestyle counseling and physical activity, or when lifestyle efforts alone have not achieved or maintained glycemic goals. If A1C target goals are not reached after approximately 3 months, a second oral agent, a GLP-1 receptor agent, or basal insulin is added. If A1C goals are not reached after 3 additional months, a three-drug intervention is implemented. If combination therapy that includes a long-acting insulin does not achieve A1C goals, a more complex insulin therapy involving multiple daily doses is started—usually in combination with one or more noninsulin agents. A patient-centered approach is always ideal, and should include patient preferences, cost, and potential side effects (ADA, 2018). The overall objective is to achieve and maintain glycemic control and to change interventions (including the use of insulin) when therapeutic goals are not being met.

All people with T1DM and many people with T2DM who no longer produce adequate endogenous insulin need replacement of insulin. Circumstances that require the use of insulin in T2DM include the failure to achieve adequate control with administration of glucose-lowering medications and periods of acute injury, infection, extreme heat exposure, surgery, or pregnancy.

Glucose-Lowering Medications for Type 2 Diabetes

Understanding that T2DM is a progressive disease is important for the understanding of treatment choices. Assisting individuals with diabetes to understand the disease process also helps them to understand and accept changes in medications that occur over time. Diabetes is first diagnosed when there is insufficient insulin available to maintain euglycemia, and as insulin deficiency progresses, medications and eventually insulin will be required to achieve glycemic goals.

Glucose-lowering medications target different aspects of the pathogenesis of T2DM—insulin resistance at the cellular level, incretin system defects, endogenous insulin deficiency, elevated levels of glucagon, and excessive hepatic glucose release. Because the mechanisms of action differ, the medications can be used alone or in combination. Table 29.5 lists the generic and brand names of glucose-lowering medications and their principal sites of action for persons with T2DM. Appendix 13 lists the nutrition implications of common drugs.

Biguanides

Metformin is the most widely used first-line type 2 medication. It suppresses hepatic glucose production, is not associated with hypoglycemia, may cause small weight losses when therapy begins, and is relatively inexpensive. The most common side effects are gastrointestinal (GI), which often disappear with time. To minimize these effects, the medication should be taken with food consumption and the smallest dose (500 mg) given twice a day for a week and gradually increased to maximum doses. If that does not help, Metformin XR (or extended release) is a good alternative that can help minimize GI side effects. This should also be taken with meals (Levy et al, 2010). A rare side effect of Metformin is severe lactic acidosis, which can be fatal. The acidosis usually occurs in patients who use alcohol excessively, have renal dysfunction, or have liver impairments. Metformin may also cause a decrease in B$_{12}$, so patients need to make sure to have adequate intake (ADA, 2018).

Sulfonylureas

The sulfonylureas (glyburide [DiaBeta], glipizide [Glucotrol], glimepiride [Amaryl]) are insulin secretagogues and promote insulin secretion by the beta-cells of the pancreas. First- and second-generation sulfonylurea drugs differ from one another in their potency, pharmacokinetics, and metabolism. Disadvantages of their use include weight gain, GI side effects—nausea, diarrhea, and constipation—and the potential to cause hypoglycemia. They also have the advantage of being inexpensive.

Thiazolidinediones (TZDs)

Thiazolidinediones (TZDs) or glitazones (pioglitazone [Actos] and rosiglitazone [Avandia]) decrease insulin resistance in peripheral tissues and thus enhance the ability of muscle and fat cells to take up glucose. TZDs also have a favorable effect on lipids and do not independently cause hypoglycemia. Adverse effects include weight gain, fluid retention leading to edema and/or heart failure, and increased risk of bone fractures.

Glucagon-like Peptide-1 (GLP-1) Receptor Agonists

Incretins are hormones made by the GI tract and include GLP-1. GLP-1 is released during nutrient absorption, which increases glucose-dependent

TABLE 29.5 Glucose-Lowering Medications for Type 2 Diabetes

Class	Compound(s)	Mechanism(s)	Effects/ Considerations
Biguanides	Metformin (Glucophage) Metformin Extended Release (Glucophage XR)	Decrease hepatic glucose production	Low cost, potential ASCVD benefit, contraindicated w/eGFR <30, gastrointestinal side effects common (nausea, diarrhea), potential for vitamin B_{12} and folate deficiency
Sulfonylureas (2nd generation)	Glipizide (Glucotrol) Glipizide (Glucotrol XL) Glyburide (Glynase PresTabs) Glimepiride (Amaryl)	Increase insulin secretion	Low cost, hypoglycemia, weight gain, glyburide not recommended with diabetic kidney disease, FDA special warning on increased risk of cardiovascular mortality
Meglitinides (Glinides)	Repaglinide (Prandin) Nateglinide (Starlix)	Increases insulin secretion	Hypoglycemia
Thiazolidinediones	Pioglitazone (Actos) Rosiglitazone (Avandia)	Increases insulin sensitivity	Low cost, weight gain, potential ASCVD benefit (pioglitazone), generally not recommended in renal impairment, fluid retention (edema, heart failure), FDA black box: May cause or worsen congestive heart failure, benefit in NASH, risk of bone fractures, bladder cancer (pioglitazone), raises LDL cholesterol (rosiglitazone)
Glucagon-like peptide-1 (GLP-1) receptor agonists	Exenatide (Byetta) Exenatide Extended Release (Bydureon) Liraglutide (Victoza) Albiglutide (Tanzeum) Dulaglutide (Trulicity)	Increases glucose-dependent insulin secretion Suppresses glucagon secretion (glucose dependent) Slows gastric emptying Increases satiety/activates GLP-1 receptors	High cost, weight loss, benefit ASCVD and progression of DKD (liraglutide), increased risk of side effect in patients with renal impairment, FDA black box: Risk of thyroid C-cell tumors, gastrointestinal side effects common (nausea, vomiting, diarrhea), injection site reactions, acute pancreatitis risk
Dipeptidyl peptidase-4 (DPP-4) inhibitors	Sitagliptin (Januvia) Saxagliptin (Onglyza) Linagliptin (Tradjenta) Alogliptin (Nesina)	Increases insulin secretion (glucose dependent) and decreases glucagon secretion (glucose dependent)/Inhibits DPP-4 activity, increasing postprandial incretin (GLP-1, GIP) concentrations	High cost, CHF potential risk (saxagliptin, alogliptin), can be used in renal impairment, potential risk of acute pancreatitis, joint pain
Bile acid sequestrants	Colesevelam (Welchol)	Decreases hepatic glucose and increases incretin levels/Binds bile acids in intestinal tract, increasing hepatic bile acid production	Do not use if history of bowel obstruction, triglycerides >500, or pancreatitis. Can decrease absorption of certain meds, soluble vitamins. Side effects GI in nature
Dopamine-2 agonists	Bromocriptine quick release QR (Cycloset)	Modulates hypothalamic regulation of metabolism, increases insulin sensitivity/activates dopaminergic receptors	Side effects: nausea, headache, fatigue, hypotension, syncope, somnolence
Alpha glucosidase inhibitors	Acarbose (Precose) Miglitol (Glyset)	Inhibits intestinal alpha glucosidase/slows intestinal carbohydrate digestion and absorption	Diarrhea, gas, and nausea If mild to moderate hypoglycemia occurs in combination with another antidiabetic drug such as a sulfonylurea or insulin, the hypoglycemia should be treated with oral glucose (dextrose) instead of sucrose (table sugar) because the drug blocks the digestion of sucrose to glucose.
Amylin mimetics	Pramlintide (Symlin)	Decreases glucagon secretion, slows gastric emptying, increases satiety/activates amylin receptors	FDA black box: severe hypoglycemic risk 3 hours post injection, consider decreasing insulin dose when starting. Side effects: nausea, weight loss

Continued

TABLE 29.5	Glucose-Lowering Medications for Type 2 Diabetes—cont'd		
Class	**Compound(s)**	**Mechanism(s)**	**Effects/ Considerations**
Sodium-glucose transport 2 inhibitors (SGLT2)	Canagliflozin (Invokana) Dapagliflozin (Farxiga) Empagliflozin (Jardiance)	Blocks reabsorption of glucose in the kidneys, increasing glucosuria/SGLT2 inhibition in the proximal nephron	High cost, weight loss, benefits ASCVD/CHF/ progression of DKD (canagliflozin not <45 eGFR, empagliflozin contraindicated with eGFR <30), FDA black box: risk of amputation (canagliflozin), risk of bone fractures (canagliflozin), DKA risk (rare in T2DM), risk of volume depletion/hypotension, raises LDL cholesterol, genitourinary infections
Insulins	See Table 29.6	Increases glucose disposal, decreases hepatic glucose production, suppresses ketogenesis/activates insulin receptors	Human insulin-low cost, analogs-high cost, hypoglycemia (higher risk with human insulin), weight gain, lower dose required with decreased eGFR, injection site reactions

Modified from American Diabetes Association: Pharmacologic approaches to glycemic treatment: Standards of medical care in diabetes—2018, *Diabetes Care* 41(S1):S77, S79-80, 2018.

insulin secretion, slows gastric emptying, decreases glucagon production, and enhances satiety. Exenatide (Byetta) and liraglutide (Victoza) are synthetic drugs that have many of the same glucose-lowering effects as the body's naturally occurring incretin, GLP-1. A primary benefit is weight loss (liraglutide has also been approved as a weight-loss drug). Typically exenatide is injected twice a day, at breakfast and at the evening meal, and liraglutide is injected once a day, at any time, independent of meals. There are three once-weekly injection GLP-1s: exenatide extended (Bydureon), dulaglutide (Trulicity), and semaglutide (Ozempic).

Dipeptidyl Peptidase 4 Inhibitors (DPP-4)

GLP-1 and glucose-dependent insulinotropic peptide (GIP), the main intestinal stimulants of insulin are rapidly degraded by the enzyme DPP-4. As a result, incretins have very short half-lives of 2 to 3 minutes. DPP-4 inhibitors prolong their half-lives. Oral DPP-4 inhibitors are sitagliptin (Januvia), saxagliptin (Onglyza), linagliptin (Tradjenta), and alogliptin (Nesina). They have a modest effect on A1C; however, advantages include being weight neutral and relatively well tolerated. Furthermore, they do not cause hypoglycemia when used as monotherapy.

Alpha Glucosidase Inhibitors

Acarbose (Precose) and miglitol (Glyset) are alpha-glucosidase inhibitors that work in the small intestine to inhibit enzymes that digest carbohydrates, thereby delaying carbohydrate absorption and lowering postprandial glycemia. They do not cause hypoglycemia or weight gain when used alone, but they can frequently cause flatulence, diarrhea, cramping, or abdominal pain. Symptoms may be alleviated by initiating therapy at a low dose and gradually increasing the dose to therapeutic levels.

Meglitinides (Glinides)

The meglitinides repaglinide (Prandin) and nateglinide (Starlix) differ from the sulfonylureas in that they have short metabolic half-lives, which result in brief episodic stimulation of insulin secretion. They are given before meals, decreasing postprandial glucose excursions and less risk of hypoglycemia. Nateglinide only works in the presence of glucose and is a somewhat less potent secretagogue. Possible weight gain is similar to sulfonylureas.

Sodium-Glucose Transporter 2 (SGLT-2) Inhibitors

Canagliflozin (Invokana), dapagliflozin (Farxiga), empagliflozin (Jardiance), and ertugliflozin (Steglatro) are drugs in a new class that target

blood glucose–lowering action in the kidneys. SGLT-2 inhibitors block a transporter protein that returns glucose to the bloodstream after it is filtered through the kidneys. Blocking this protein causes more glucose to be flushed out in the urine. Used independently it does not cause hypoglycemia or weight gain.

Amylin Agonists (Pramlintide)

Pramlintide (Symlin) is a synthetic analog of the hormone amylin, a hormone normally cosecreted with insulin by the beta-cell in response to food that is deficient in people with T1DM and T2DM. It is injected before meals, slowing gastric emptying and inhibiting glucagon production and resulting in a decrease in postprandial glucose excursions, which is related to a decrease in glucagon production from the pancreatic alpha cells. It must be injected separately from insulin.

Insulin

Insulin strategies for persons with T2DM may begin with basal insulin at bedtime to suppress nocturnal hepatic glucose production and to normalize fasting glucose levels. Glucose-lowering medications usually are continued during the day. The next step is to add one mealtime rapid-acting insulin with the basal insulin or use of premixed insulin, which is a combination of two insulins mixed together, twice daily. Premixed insulin is typically a combination of a short or rapid-acting insulin and an intermediate or long-acting insulin. If A1C goals are not achieved, mealtime rapid-acting insulin is used before each meal. Insulin secretagogues usually are stopped, but other glucose-lowering agents may be continued.

Insulin has three characteristics: onset, peak, and duration (Table 29.6). U-100 is the concentration of insulin used in the United States. This means it has 100 units of insulin per milliliter of fluid (100 units/mL). U-100 syringes deliver U-100 insulin; however, insulin pens are now being used more frequently as an alternative to the traditional syringe-needle units. Humulin R U-500 (500 units/mL) is useful in the treatment of insulin-resistant patients who require daily doses more than 200 units.

Rapid-acting insulins include lispro (Humalog), insulin aspart (Novolog), and insulin glulisine (Apidra) and are used as bolus (premeal or prandial) insulins. They are insulin analogs that differ from human insulin in amino acid sequence but bind to insulin receptors and thus function in a manner similar to human insulin. To determine

TABLE 29.6   Action Times of Human Insulin Preparations

Type of Insulin	Onset of Action	Peak Action	Usual Effective Duration	Monitor Effect In
Rapid-Acting				
Insulin lispro	<0.25-0.5 hr	0.5-2.5 hr	3-6.5 hr	1-2 hr
Insulin aspart	<0.25 hr	0.5-1.0 hr	3-5 hr	1-2 hr
Insulin glulisine	<0.25 hr	1-1.5 hr	3-5 hr	1-2 hr
Inhaled insulin				
Short-Acting				
Human Regular	0.5-1 hr	2-3 hr	3-6 hr	4 hr (next meal)
Intermediate-Acting Analogs				
Human neutral protamine hagedorn (NPH)	2-4 hr	4-10 hr	10-16 hr	8-12 hr
Basal Insulin Analogs				
Insulin glargine (Lantus)	2-4 hr	Peakless	20-24 hr	10-12 hr
Insulin detemir (Levemir)	0.8-2 hr (dose dependent)	Peakless	12-24 hr (dose dependent)	10-12 hr
Degludec				
Premixed Insulin Products				
70/30 (70% NPH, 30% regular)	0.5-1 hr	Dual	10-16 hr	
Humalog Mix (Lispro) 75/25 (75% neutral protamine lispro [NPL], 25% lispro)	<0.25 hr	Dual	10-16 hr	
Humalog Mix (Lispro) 50/50 (50% protamine lispro, 50% lispro)	<0.25 hr	Dual	10-16 hr	
NovoLog Mix 70/30 (70% neutral protamine aspart [NPA], 30% aspart)	<0.25 hr	Dual	15-18 hr	

Data from American Diabetes Association: Pharmacologic approaches to glycemic treatment: Standards of medical care in diabetes—2018, *Diabetes Care* 41(S1):S80, 2018.

the accuracy of the dose, blood glucose checking is done before meals and 2 hours after the start of the meals.

Regular insulin includes short-acting insulin with a slower onset of action and later activity peak. For best results the slow onset of regular insulin requires it to be taken 30 to 60 minutes before meals.

Neutral protamine hagedorn (NPH) is the only available intermediate-acting insulin and is cloudy in appearance. This type of insulin contains substrates that work over a long period of time, usually with an effective duration of 10 to 16 hours.

Long-acting insulins include insulin glargine (Lantus) and insulin detemir (Levemir). Insulin glargine is an insulin analog that, because of its slow dissolution at the injection site, results in a relatively constant and peakless delivery over 24 hours. Because of its acidic pH, it cannot be mixed with any other insulin in the same syringe before injection and usually is given at bedtime. However, glargine can be given before any meal. Keep in mind that consistency is key, as the dose must be administered consistently at whichever time is chosen. Basal insulin analogs decrease the chances of hypoglycemia, especially nocturnal hypoglycemia.

Premixed insulins include 70% NPH/30% regular, 75% lispro protamine (NPL [addition of neutral protamine to lispro to create an intermediate-acting insulin])/25% lispro, 50% lispro protamine and 50% lispro, and 70% protamine (addition of neutral protamine to aspart to create an immediate-acting insulin)/30% aspart (ADA, 2018). People using premixed insulins must eat at specific times and be consistent in carbohydrate intake to prevent hypoglycemia.

Insulin Regimens

All persons with T1DM and those with T2DM who no longer produce adequate endogenous insulin need replacement of insulin that mimics normal insulin action. After individuals without diabetes eat, their plasma glucose and insulin concentrations increase rapidly, peaking in 30 to 60 minutes, and return to basal concentrations within 2 to 3 hours. To mimic this, rapid-acting (or short-acting) insulin is given before meals, and this is referred to as bolus or mealtime insulin.

Mealtime insulin doses are adjusted based on the amount of carbohydrate in the meal. An insulin-to-carbohydrate ratio can be established for an individual that will guide decisions on the amount of mealtime insulin to inject based on grams of carbohydrate consumed. The basal or background insulin dose is that amount of insulin required in the postabsorptive state to restrain endogenous glucose output primarily from the liver, which helps maintain normal glucose levels between meals. Basal insulin also limits lipolysis and excess flux of free fatty acids to the liver. Long-acting insulins are used for basal insulin (Fig. 29.2).

These physiologic insulin regimens allow increased flexibility in the type and timing of meals. For nonobese persons with T1DM, the required insulin dosage is about 0.5 to 1 unit/kg of body weight per day. About 50% of the total daily insulin dose is used to provide for basal or background insulin needs. The remainder (rapid-acting insulin) is divided among the meals either proportionately to the carbohydrate content or by giving about 1 to 1.5 units of insulin per 10 to 15 g of carbohydrates consumed (insulin to carbohydrate ratio). As a result of the presence in the morning of higher levels of counterregulatory

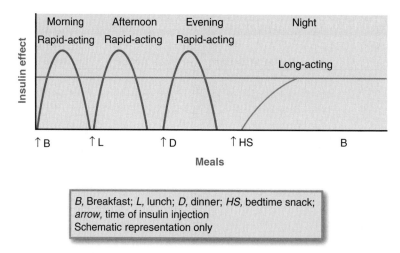

Fig. 29.2 Time actions of flexible insulin regimens. (Modified from Kaufman FR, editor: *Medical management of type 1 diabetes,* ed 6, Alexandria, VA, 2012, American Diabetes Association.)

hormones, many individuals may require larger doses of mealtime insulin for carbohydrates consumed at breakfast than meals later in the day. Persons with T2DM may require insulin doses in the range of 0.5 to 1.2 units/kg of body weight daily. Large doses, even more than 1.5 units/kg of body weight daily, may be required at least initially to overcome prevailing insulin resistance. The type and timing of insulin regimens should be individualized, based on eating and exercise habits and blood glucose concentrations.

Insulin Regimens: Continuous Sustained Insulin Infusion (CSII) or Insulin Pump Therapy

The insulin (usually a rapid-acting insulin) is pumped continuously by a mechanical device in micro amounts through a subcutaneous catheter (Fig. 29.3). The pump delivers insulin in two ways: in a steady, measured, and continuous dose (basal insulin) and as a surge (bolus) dose before meals.

The individual also should be educated about carbohydrate counting/estimation. Mealtime boluses are dependent on carbohydrate intake as well as circadian variation in insulin sensitivity, current blood glucose levels, and planned physical activity. Regularly scheduled

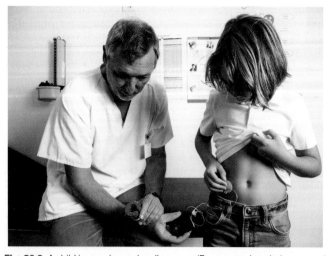

Fig. 29.3 A child is wearing an insulin pump. (From www.istockphoto.com.)

outpatient follow-up with diabetes care providers knowledgeable in the use of CSII is recommended to optimize glycemic control long term. Although there is an initial learning curve, insulin pump therapy provides many benefits, including eliminating the need for individual insulin injections. Using an insulin pump may also result in fewer large swings in blood glucose levels as well as allow users to be more flexible about when and what they eat.

Self-Management Education

Diabetes management is a team effort. Persons with diabetes must be at the center of the team because they have the responsibility for day-to-day management. RDNs, nurses, physicians, and other health care providers contribute their expertise to developing therapeutic regimens that help the person with diabetes achieve the best metabolic control possible. The goal is to provide patients with the knowledge, skills, and motivation to incorporate self-management into their daily lifestyles. The AND EBNPG recommends that individuals with diabetes be referred for MNT early after the diagnosis of diabetes. MNT is to be provided by an RDN in an initial series of three to four encounters, each lasting 45 to 90 minutes. This series should be completed within 3 to 6 months, and the RDN should determine whether additional encounters are needed after the initial series based on the nutrition assessment of learning needs and progress toward desired outcomes. At least one follow-up encounter is recommended annually to reinforce lifestyle changes and to evaluate and monitor outcomes that affect the need for changes in MNT or medication(s). The RDN should again determine whether additional MNT encounters are needed. Although glycemic control is the primary focus for diabetes management, cardioprotective nutrition interventions for the prevention and treatment of CVD also should be implemented in the initial series of encounters (AND, 2008a; Franz et al, 2010).

Dietitians can demonstrate their specialized diabetes knowledge by obtaining certification beyond the RDN credential. Two diabetes care certifications available to registered dietitians (RDs) are the CDE, a specialty certification, and board certified-advanced diabetes management (BC-ADM), an advanced practice certification.

Monitoring

The health care team, including the individual with diabetes, should work together to implement blood glucose monitoring and establish individual target blood glucose goals (see Table 29.4). Several methods are available to assess the effectiveness of the diabetes management plan on glycemic control: SMBG or continuous glucose monitoring (CGM) of interstitial glucose and A1C. SMBG is used on a day-to-day basis to manage diabetes effectively and safely; however, measurement of A1C levels provides the best available index of overall diabetes control.

Self-Monitoring of Blood Glucose (SMBG)

The ADA recommendations state that persons on multiple-dose insulin (MDI) or insulin pump therapy should do SMBG before meals and snacks, occasionally postprandially at bedtime, before exercise, when they suspect low blood glucose, after treating low blood glucose until they are normoglycemic, and before critical tasks such as driving. For people using less-frequent insulin injections or noninsulin therapies, SMBG results may be helpful to guide treatment decisions (ADA, 2018).

The AND EBNPG for diabetes reviewed the evidence on glucose monitoring and recommended that for persons with T1DM or T2DM on insulin therapy, at least three to four glucose tests per day are needed to determine the accuracy of the insulin dose(s) and to guide adjustments in insulin dose(s), food intake, and physical activity. Once established some insulin regimens require less-frequent SMBG. For persons on MNT alone or MNT in combination with glucose-lowering medications, frequency and timing are dependent on diabetes management goals and therapies.

Self-management education and training are necessary to use SMBG devices and data correctly (ADA, 2018). Individuals must be taught how to adjust their management program based on the results of SMBG. The first step in using such records is to learn how to identify patterns in blood glucose levels taken at the same time each day that are outside the target range—generally high readings for 3 or more days in a row or low readings 2 days in a row. The next step is to determine whether a lifestyle factor (meal times, carbohydrate intake, quantity and time of physical activity) or medication dose adjustment is needed.

If changes in medication doses such as insulin are needed, adjustments should be made to the insulin/mediations at the time of the problem glucose readings. After pattern management is mastered, algorithms for insulin dose changes to compensate for an elevated or low glucose value can be used. A commonly used formula determines the insulin sensitivity, or correction factor (CF), which defines how many milligrams per deciliter a unit of rapid-insulin (or short-acting) will lower blood glucose levels over a 2- to 4-hr period (Kaufman, 2012). The CF is determined by using the "1700 rule," in which 1700 is divided by the total daily dose (TDD) of insulin the individual typically takes. For example, if the TDD is 50 units of insulin, the CF = 1700/50 = 35. In this case 1 unit of rapid-acting insulin should lower the individual's blood glucose level by 35 mg/dL (2 mmol/L).

In using blood glucose monitoring records, remember that factors other than food affect blood glucose concentrations. An increase in blood glucose can be the result of insufficient insulin or insulin secretagogue; too much food; or increases in glucagon and other counter-regulatory hormones as a result of stress, illness, or infection. Factors that contribute to hypoglycemia include too much insulin or insulin secretagogue, not enough food, unusual amounts of exercise, and skipped or delayed meals. Urine glucose testing, which has been used in the past, has so many limitations that it should not be used.

Continuous Glucose Monitoring (CGM)

CGM systems include a tiny glucose-sensing device called a sensor that is inserted under the skin in the subcutaneous fat tissue for several days at a time. The sensor measures glucose in interstitial fluid and transmits readings every 5 minutes to a monitor that is worn or carried externally. CGM devices also provide information not just on current glucose level but also on the trend and rate of change in glucose levels (i.e., whether the glucose level is rising or falling and how quickly). Other features include alerts for glucose highs and lows and the ability to download data and track trends over time. The ADA recommends that CGM in conjunction with intensive insulin regimens can be a useful tool to lower A1C in selected adults with T1DM. Evidence is less strong for A1C lowering in children, teens, and younger adults; however, CGM may be also helpful in these groups (ADA, 2018).

A1C Monitoring

A1C tests should be done at least twice a year in persons who are meeting treatment goals and have stable glycemic control. They should be done quarterly in persons whose therapy has changed or who are not meeting glycemic goals. In persons without diabetes, A1C values are 4% to 6%. These values correspond to mean plasma glucose levels of approximately 70 to 126 mg/dL (3.9 to 7.0 mmol/L). Correlation between A1C levels and average glucose levels has recently been verified. An A1C of 6% reflects an average glucose level of 126 mg/dL (7.0 mmol/L) (See Table 29.2). Lowering A1C to below or around 7% is a reasonable goal for many nonpregnant adults with diabetes. An A1C less than 7% has been shown to reduce cardiovascular complications of diabetes and is associated with long-term reduction of macrovascular disease (ADA, 2018). Less stringent goals, such as less than 8%, may be appropriate for elderly individuals or individuals with advanced macrovascular and microvascular complications, history of severe hypoglycemia, or other extensive comorbid conditions (ADA, 2018).

Ketone, Lipid, and Blood Pressure Monitoring

Urine or blood testing can be used to detect ketones. Testing for ketonuria or ketonemia should be performed regularly during periods of illness and when blood glucose levels consistently exceed 240 mg/dL (13.3 mmol/L). The presence of persistent, moderate, or large amounts of ketones, along with elevated blood glucose levels, requires insulin adjustments. People with T2DM rarely have ketosis; however, ketone testing should be done when the person is seriously ill.

For most adults, lipids should be measured at least annually; however, in adults with low-risk lipid values (100 mg/dL [2.6mmol/L]), assessments may be repeated every 5 years. Blood pressure should be measured at every routine diabetes visit (ADA, 2018).

IMPLEMENTING THE NUTRITION CARE PROCESS

The nutrition care process (NCP) is a systematic and standardized approach to providing high-quality nutrition care. This system was adopted by the AND's House of Delegates in 2003 in an effort to provide dietetics professionals with a framework for critical thinking and decision making. The AND found that the use of the NCP can lead to more efficient and effective care and greater recognition of the role of dietetic professionals in all care settings.

There are two ways to deliver MNT using the NCP: individual or group sessions. While providing nutrition interventions in groups is becoming increasingly popular, it is important that group interventions allow for individualization of MNT and evaluation of outcomes. The NCP consists of four distinct, interrelated steps.

Nutrition Assessment

The AND EBNPG for diabetes recommends that the RDN assess the following domains in adults with T1DM and T2DM to formulate the nutrition care plan. The first is biomedical data, medical tests, and medication uses (including type of diabetes, glycemic control and targets, lipid profiles, blood pressure, renal function, and use of medications). The second is nutrition-focused physical findings (including height, weight, BMI and waist circumference, injection sites, and the relative importance of weight management). Third is the client history, which includes general health and demographic information, social history, cultural preferences, health literacy and numeracy, education and occupation, physical activity, patient or family nutrition-related medical and health history, and any other medical or surgical treatments. This section also includes knowledge, beliefs, attitudes, motivation, readiness to change, self-efficacy, and willingness and ability to make behavioral changes. Last but not least is the food and nutrition-related history. Here the RDN will gather information on food, beverage and nutrient, intake, including energy intake, serving sizes, meal-snack patterns, carbohydrate, fiber, types and amounts of fat, protein, micronutrient intake, and alcohol intake. It is also important to gather information on experience with food, previous and current food and nutrition history, eating environment, access to healthy foods, and eating out (Box 29.2).

Nutrition Diagnosis

The nutrition diagnosis identifies and describes a specific nutrition problem that can be resolved or improved through treatment/intervention by an RDN. Patients often have more than one nutrition diagnoses, in which case the RDN will need to prioritize them in the nutrition intervention step. Examples of diabetes-related nutrition diagnoses are listed in Box 29.3) .

Nutrition Interventions

Nutrition Therapy Interventions for All People with Diabetes

The first priority is to promote and support a healthful eating pattern, emphasizing a variety of nutrient-dense foods in appropriate portion sizes. However, monitoring carbohydrate intake also can be an important

---

> ### BOX 29.2 Nutrition Assessment
>
> **Nutrition Assessment Categories**
> - Biochemical data, medical tests, and procedures, which include laboratory data such as for A1C, glucose, lipids, kidney function, and blood pressure measurements
> - Anthropometric measurements, which include height, weight, body mass index (BMI), waist circumference, growth rate, and rate of weight change
> - Client history, which includes:
>   - General patient information, such as age, gender, race/ethnicity, language, literacy, and education
>   - Medical/health history and medical treatment, including goals of medical therapy and prescribed medications related to medical condition for which medical nutrition therapy (MNT) is being implemented
>   - Readiness to change nutrition-related behaviors
>   - Weight management goals
>   - Physical activity history and goals
>   - Social history, such as social and medical support, cultural and religious beliefs, and socioeconomic status
>   - Other medical or surgical treatments, therapy, and alternative medicine
> - Food/nutrition history
> - Food intake, nutrition and health knowledge and beliefs
> - Food availability
> - Supplement use
>
> Modified from Franz MJ et al: *ADA pocket guide to lipid disorders, hypertension, diabetes, and weight management*, Chicago, 2012, Academy of Nutrition and Dietetics.

> ### BOX 29.3 Examples of Problem, Etiology, and Signs and Symptoms (PES) Statements Related to Diabetes Mellitus
>
> **Nutrition Diagnosis: Inconsistent Carbohydrate Intake**
> - Inconsistent carbohydrate intake (P) related to incorrect application of carbohydrate counting (E) as evidenced by food records revealing 2 additional carbohydrate servings for many meals and wide fluctuations in blood glucose levels, most days of the week (S).
>
> **Nutrition Diagnosis: Inconsistent Carbohydrate Intake**
> - Inconsistent carbohydrate intake (P) related to inconsistent timing of meals (E) as evidenced by wide fluctuations in blood glucose levels (S).
>
> **Nutrition Diagnosis: Excessive Carbohydrate Intake**
> - Excessive carbohydrate intake (P) compared with insulin dosing related to inaccurate carbohydrate counting (E) as evidenced by the number of carbohydrate servings per meal noted in food record and postmeal glucose levels consistently greater than 200 mg/dL (S).
>
> **Nutrition Diagnosis: Inappropriate Intake of Food Fats**
> - Excessive saturated fat intake (P) related to lack of knowledge of saturated fat content of foods (E) as evidenced by self-report of high saturated fat intake (S).
>
> **Nutrition Diagnosis: Altered Laboratory Values**
> - Altered blood glucose values (P) related to insufficient insulin (E) as evidenced by hyperglycemia despite very good eating habits (S).
>
> **Nutrition Diagnosis: Food- and Nutrition-Related Knowledge Deficit**
> - Food- and nutrition-related knowledge deficit (P) related to lack of exposure to information (E) as evidenced by new diagnosis of diabetes (or prediabetes, lipid disorder, hypertension) (S).
>
> **Nutrition Diagnosis: Not Ready for Lifestyle Change**
> - Not ready for lifestyle change (P) related to denial of need to change in precontemplation (E) as evidenced by reluctance to begin participation in physical activity program (S).
>
> Modified from Franz MJ et al: *ADA pocket guide to lipid disorders, hypertension, diabetes, and weight management*, Chicago, 2012, Academy of Nutrition and Dietetics.

---

nutrition therapy strategy for persons with all types of diabetes. It is important that individuals with diabetes know which foods contain carbohydrates (starchy vegetables, grains, fruit, milk and milk products, vegetables, and sweets). They should also be educated on portion sizes and how many servings they should select for meals, and if they desire, snacks. When choosing carbohydrates, nutrient-dense, high-fiber foods are recommended whenever possible instead of processed foods with added sodium, fat, and sugars. Sugar-sweetened beverages and juice should also be minimized or avoided.

Nutrition Therapy Interventions for Specific Populations

For people with T1DM and insulin-requiring T2DM, the first priority is to integrate an insulin regimen into the usual eating habits and physical activity schedule. With the many insulin options now available (rapid- and long-acting insulins), an insulin regimen can be planned that will conform to an individual's preferred meal routines and food choices. While a medical doctor typically prescribes insulin, nurses and CDEs will often suggest modifications, depending on their scope of practice.

Physiologic insulin regimens that mimic natural insulin secretion involve multiple injections (three or more insulin injections per day) or use of insulin pump therapy. These types of insulin regimens allow increased flexibility in choosing when and what to eat. Mealtime insulin doses are adjusted to match carbohydrate intake (insulin-to-carbohydrate ratios). Therefore it is important that individuals learn how to count carbohydrates or use another meal planning approach to quantify carbohydrate intake. The insulin action times of the currently available rapid-acting insulin analogs are as follows: onset 5 to 15 minutes, a peak between 30 to 90 minutes, and a duration of approximately 4 to 6 hours. Lag time is defined as the amount of time that elapses between the injection of rapid-acting insulin and the meal; it is critical in control of postprandial hyperglycemia and in later risk of hypoglycemia. Given the pharmacodynamics of insulin analogs, a sufficient lag time of approximately 10 to 15 minutes before start of meal helps to decrease postprandial hyperglycemia.

Fixed insulin regimens are used for a variety of reasons, including age, cost, fewer required injections, lack of access to insulin analogs, personal preference, or prescribing habits of the health care provider. For people who receive fixed insulin regimens, such as premixed insulin formulas, day-to-day consistency in the timing and amount of carbohydrates eaten is key. This also applies to those who do not adjust their daily mealtime insulin doses. Carbohydrate intake can be individualized to meet the person's nutritional needs. The amount of mealtime insulin (rapid- or short-acting) that the person takes only changes based on the blood glucose level reading.

Persons with type 2 diabetes using mnt alone or with glucose-lowering medications. The first priority is to adopt lifestyle interventions that improve the metabolic abnormalities of glycemia, dyslipidemia, and hypertension. Lifestyle interventions independent of weight loss that can improve glycemia include reduced energy intake and increased energy expenditure through physical activity. Because many people with diabetes also have dyslipidemia and hypertension, a cardioprotective eating pattern also is recommended. These interventions should be implemented as soon as the diagnosis of diabetes is made.

MNT interventions for established T2DM differ from interventions for prevention. Some studies suggest that modest weight loss is beneficial in persons with insulin resistance; however, as the disease progresses to insulin deficiency, medications usually have to be combined with MNT. Emphasis should be on blood glucose control, improved food choices, increased physical activity, and moderate energy restriction rather than weight loss alone, as it is unclear whether weight loss alone may improve glycemic control. Additionally, reduction of caloric intake may result in nutritional inadequacies; therefore, special attention should be paid to maintaining adequate intake of vitamins and minerals.

The first step in food and meal planning is teaching which foods are sources of carbohydrate, what are appropriate portion sizes, and how many servings to select at meals (and snacks, if desired). Important components of successful MNT for T2DM include teaching that unsaturated fats should be substituted for foods high in saturated and trans fats, encouraging physical activity, and using blood glucose monitoring to adjust food and eating patterns. Medications are also important components of successful MNT for T2DM. Frequent follow-up with an RDN can provide the problem-solving techniques, encouragement, and support that lifestyle changes require.

Physical activity improves insulin sensitivity, acutely lowers blood glucose in people with diabetes, and also may improve cardiovascular status. By itself it has only a modest effect on weight; however, it is essential for long-term weight maintenance.

Youth with type 1 diabetes. Involvement of a multidisciplinary team, including a physician, RDN, nurse, and behavioral specialist, all trained in pediatric diabetes, is the best means of achieving optimal diabetes management in youth. However, the most important team members are the child or adolescent and the family members and caregivers.

A major nutrition goal for children and adolescents with T1DM is maintenance of normal growth and development. Possible causes of poor weight gain and linear growth include poor glycemic control, inadequate insulin, and overrestriction of calories. The last may be a consequence of the common erroneous belief that restricting food, rather than adjusting insulin, is the way to control blood glucose. Additional reasons for poor weight gain unrelated to diabetes management may include other autoimmune conditions such as thyroid abnormalities (Hashimoto's thyroiditis), malabsorption syndromes (celiac disease), or disordered eating behaviors. Some adolescents will even use less insulin in an effort to lose weight, an eating disorder known as diabulimia. Excessive weight gain can be caused by excessive caloric intake, overtreatment of hypoglycemia, or overinsulinization. Other causes include low physical activity levels and hypothyroidism, accompanied by poor linear growth (Corbin et al, 2018).

The nutrition prescription is based on the nutrition assessment. Newly diagnosed children often present with weight loss and hunger; as a result, the initial meal plan must be based on adequate calories to restore and maintain appropriate body weight. In about 4 to 6 weeks the initial caloric level may need to be modified to meet more usual caloric requirements. Nutrient requirements for children and adolescents with diabetes appear to be similar to those of children and adolescents without diabetes. The dietary reference intakes (DRIs) can be used to determine energy requirements (Institute of Medicine [IOM], 2011). However, it may be preferable to use a food and nutrition history of typical daily intake, providing that growth and development are normal, to determine an individual child's or adolescent's energy needs.

Consultation with an RDN to develop and discuss the eating plan is encouraged (Chiang et al, 2014). Because energy requirements change with age, physical activity, and growth rate, an evaluation of height, weight, BMI, and the eating plan must be updated at least every year. Height and weight should be recorded on a CDC pediatric growth charts every 3 months. Good metabolic control is essential for normal growth and development (for growth charts see Appendices 4–11). Linear growth can be affected by an insulin prescription that is not adjusted as the child grows. Chronic undertreatment with insulin along with longstanding poor diabetes control often leads to poor growth and weight loss. However, withholding food or having the child eat consistently without an appetite for food in an effort to control blood glucose should be discouraged.

Individualized eating plans, insulin regimens using basal (background) and bolus (mealtime) insulins, and insulin algorithms or insulin pumps can provide flexibility for children with T1DM as well as their families. This approach accommodates irregular meal times and schedules and varying appetites and activity levels. Blood glucose records are essential to assist in making appropriate changes in insulin regimens. Daily eating patterns in young children generally include three meals and two or three snacks, depending on the length of time between meals and the child's physical activity level. Children often prefer smaller meals and snacks. Snacks can prevent hypoglycemia between meals and provide adequate calories. Older children and teens may prefer only three meals. Blood glucose monitoring data are then used to integrate an insulin regimen into the meal, snack, and exercise schedules.

After the appropriate nutrition prescription has been determined, the meal planning approach can be selected. Keep in mind that a number of meal planning approaches can be used. Carbohydrate counting for food planning provides youth and their families with guidelines that facilitate glycemic control while still allowing the choice of many common foods that children and adolescents enjoy. However, whatever approach to food planning is used, the youth and family must find it understandable and applicable to their lifestyle.

Youth with type 2 diabetes. Childhood obesity has been accompanied by an increase in the prevalence of T2DM among children and adolescents. IGT has been shown to be highly prevalent in obese youth and is associated with insulin resistance. Once T2DM develops, beta-cell failure is also a factor. Thus T2DM in youth follows a progressive pattern similar to T2DM in adults. However, because of the increase in overweight and obesity in children and adolescents, it can be difficult to determine immediately whether a youth has T1DM or T2DM. Because of this, testing for islet antibodies is recommended, but it may take weeks to get the results of the test. Therefore guidelines for the management of T2DM in youth recommend starting the youth on insulin if it is unclear whether the youth has T1DM or T2DM (Springer et al, 2013). When the youth has been diagnosed with T2DM, metformin and lifestyle changes, including nutrition therapy and physical activity, are recommended (ADA, 2018).

Successful lifestyle treatment of T2DM in children and adolescents involves cessation of excessive weight gain, promotion of normal growth and development, and the achievement of blood glucose and A1C goals (ADA, 2018). Nutrition guidelines also should address comorbidities such as hypertension and dyslipidemia. Offer behavior modification strategies to decrease intake of high-caloric, high-fat, and high-carbohydrate foods and sugar-sweetened beverages, while encouraging healthy eating habits and regular physical activity for the entire family. Youth with T2DM should be encouraged to exercise at least 60 minutes a day and to limit their nonacademic "screen time" (video games, television) to less than 2 hours a day (Springer et al, 2013). The guidelines also emphasize the importance of a team effort using not only the physician but also the skills of an RDN, diabetes educator, and a psychologist or social worker to deal with the emotional and/or behavioral problems that may accompany T2DM.

Women with preexisting diabetes and pregnancy. Normalization of blood glucose levels during pregnancy is very important for women who have preexisting diabetes or who develop GDM. Table 29.7 lists glucose goals for pregnancy. The MNT goals are to assist in achieving and maintaining optimal blood glucose control and to provide adequate maternal and fetal nutrition throughout pregnancy, energy intake for appropriate maternal weight gain, and necessary vitamins and minerals (Reader, 2012). Nutrition recommendations during pregnancy and lactation appear to be similar for women with and without diabetes; therefore, the DRIs can be used to determine energy and nutrient requirements during pregnancy and for lactation (IOM, 2002) (see Chapter 14).

Preconception counseling and the ability to achieve near-normal blood glucose levels before pregnancy have been shown to be effective in reducing the incidence of anomalies in infants born to women with preexisting diabetes to nearly that of the general population. As a result of hormonal changes during the first trimester, blood glucose levels are often erratic. Although caloric needs do not differ from those preceding pregnancy, the eating plan may have to be adjusted to accommodate the metabolic changes. Women should be educated about the increased risk of hypoglycemia during pregnancy and cautioned against overtreatment.

TABLE 29.7 **Plasma Glucose Goals During Pregnancy**	
Gestational diabetes AND Pregnancy with preexisting type 1 or type 2 diabetes	Fasting: <95 mg/dL (5.3 mmol/L) and EITHER 1-h postmeal: <140 mg/dL (7.8 mmol/L) OR 2-h postmeal: <120 mg/dL (6.7 mmol/L) A1C: 6-6.5% (42-48 mmol/mol)

Data from American Diabetes Association, Management of Diabetes in Pregnancy: Standards of Medical Care in Diabetes—2018, *Diabetes Care* 41(S1):S138, 2018.

The need for insulin increases during the second and third trimesters of pregnancy. At 38 to 40 weeks' postconception, insulin needs and levels peak at two to three times prepregnancy levels. Pregnancy-associated hormones that are antagonistic to the action of insulin lead to elevated blood glucose levels. For women with preexisting diabetes, this increased insulin need must be met with increased exogenous insulin.

Eating plan adjustments are necessary to provide the additional calories required to support fetal growth, and weight should be monitored. During pregnancy the distribution of energy and carbohydrate intake should be based on the woman's food intake, eating habits, and blood glucose responses. Insulin regimens can be matched to food intake, but maintaining consistent eating times and intake is essential to avoid hypoglycemia caused by the continuous fetal draw of glucose from the mother. Smaller meals and more frequent snacks are often needed. Similarly, a late-evening snack is often necessary to decrease the likelihood of overnight hypoglycemia and fasting ketosis. Records of food intake and blood glucose values are essential for determining whether glycemic goals are being met and for preventing and correcting ketosis.

Regular follow-up visits during pregnancy are needed to monitor caloric and nutrient intake, blood glucose control, and whether starvation ketosis is present. Urine or blood ketones during pregnancy may signal ketosis that can be caused by inadequate energy or carbohydrate intake, omission of meals or snacks, or prolonged intervals between meals (e.g., more than 10 hours between the bedtime snack and breakfast). Ketonemia during pregnancy has been associated with fetal brain injury and may have long-term developmental impact, and women should be instructed to test for ketones periodically before breakfast (Mohan et al, 2017).

Women with gestational diabetes mellitus. MNT for GDM involves primarily a carbohydrate-controlled meal plan that promotes optimal nutrition for maternal and fetal health with adequate energy for appropriate gestational weight gain, achievement and maintenance of normoglycemia, and absence of ketosis. Specific nutrition and food recommendations are determined and modified based on individual assessment and blood glucose records. Monitoring blood glucose, fasting ketones, appetite, and weight gain can aid in developing an appropriate, individualized meal plan and in adjusting the meal plan throughout pregnancy.

Nutrition practice guidelines for gestational diabetes have been developed and tested (Academy of Nutrition and Dietetics Evidence Analysis Library, 2016). All women with GDM should receive MNT at diagnosis of GDM. Monitoring records guide nutrition therapy and are used to determine whether additional therapy is needed. Insulin, metformin, or glyburide therapy is added if glucose goals exceed target range (see Table 29.7) on two or more occasions in a 1- to 2-week period without some obvious explanation (Mohan et al, 2017). Inadequate weight gain and ketone testing can be useful in determining when women are undereating to keep glucose levels within target range in an effort to avoid insulin therapy.

Carbohydrates should be distributed throughout the day into three small-to-moderate size meals and two to four snacks. All pregnant women require a minimum of 175 g of carbohydrates daily (Academy of Nutrition and Dietetics Evidence Analysis Library, 2016). An evening snack usually is needed to prevent accelerated ketosis overnight. Carbohydrates are not as well tolerated at breakfast as they are at other meals because of increased levels of cortisol and growth hormones. To compensate for this, the initial eating plan may have approximately 30 g of carbohydrate at breakfast. To satisfy hunger, protein foods can be added because they do not affect blood glucose levels.

According to the EBNPG, the RDN should individualize the calorie prescription based on a thorough nutrition assessment with guidance from relevant references (DRIs, the IOM) and encourage adequate caloric intake to promote fetal/neonatal and maternal health, achieve glycemic goals, and promote appropriate gestational weight gain. Weight gain during pregnancy for women with GDM should be similar to that of women without diabetes.

Exercise assists in overcoming peripheral resistance to insulin and in controlling fasting and postprandial hyperglycemia and may be used as an adjunct to nutrition therapy to improve maternal glycemia. The ideal form of exercise is unknown, but a brisk walk after meals is often recommended.

Women with GDM (and women with preexisting diabetes) should be encouraged to breastfeed because breastfeeding is associated with a reduced incidence of future T2DM (ADA, 2018) (see Chapter 14). For women with GDM who are overweight/obese or with above-recommended weight gain during pregnancy, weight loss is advised after delivery. Weight loss may aid in reducing the risk of recurrent GDM or future development of T2DM (Reader, 2012).

Older adults. The prevalence of diabetes and IGT increases dramatically as people age. Many factors predispose older adults to diabetes: age-related decreases in insulin production, adiposity, decreased physical activity, multiple prescription medications, genetics, and coexisting illnesses. A major factor appears to be insulin resistance. Controversy persists as to whether the insulin resistance is a primary change or whether it is attributable to reduced physical activity, decreased lean body mass (sarcopenia), and increased adipose tissue, which are common in older adults. Furthermore, medications used to treat coexisting diseases may complicate diabetes therapy in older adults.

Despite the increase in glucose intolerance with age, aging should not be a reason for suboptimal control of blood glucose. Persistent hyperglycemia has deleterious effects on the body's defense mechanisms against infection. It also increases the pain threshold by exacerbating neuropathic pain, and it has a detrimental effect on the outcome of cerebrovascular accidents.

However, while it is important to control blood glucose levels in this population, the recommendations in blood glucose targets for older adults with diabetes have changed. Older adults who are otherwise healthy with few coexisting chronic illnesses and intact cognitive function and functional status should have lower glycemic goals (A1C <7.5% [58 mmol/mol]), while those with multiple coexisting chronic illnesses, cognitive impairment, or functional dependence should have less stringent glycemic goals (A1C <8.0% to 8.5% [64 to 69 mmol/mol]) (ADA, 2018).

Nutrition recommendations for older adults with diabetes should include meeting the DRI for age for nutrients, drinking adequate fluid, avoiding significant weight loss, and being sensitive to individual preferences and longstanding food habits while advocating good nutrition (Stanley, 2012) (see Chapter 19). Restrictive diets are contraindicated. Physical activity can reduce the decline in aerobic capacity significantly that occurs with age, improve risk factors for atherosclerosis, slow the decline in age-related lean body mass, decrease central adiposity, and improve insulin sensitivity; thus it should be encouraged. Flexibility training and balance training are recommended two to three times per week for older adults with diabetes. Yoga and tai chi may be included based on individual preferences to increase flexibility, muscular strength, and balance (ADA, 2018).

Malnutrition, not obesity, is the more prevalent nutrition-related problem in older adults. It often remains subclinical or unrecognized because the result of malnutrition—excessive loss of lean body mass—resembles the signs and symptoms of the aging process. Malnutrition and diabetes adversely affect wound healing and defense against infection, and malnutrition is associated with depression and cognitive deficits. The most reliable indicator of poor nutrition status in older adults is a change in body weight; involuntary weight gain or loss of more than 10 pounds or 10% of body weight in less than 6 months indicates a need to evaluate the reason.

It is essential that older adults, especially those in long-term care settings, focus on enjoyment of the meal experience in addition to meeting nutritional needs. Dietary restriction is not warranted for older residents in long-term health facilities. Residents should be served the regular, unrestricted menu. Strict carbohydrate control and use of sugar-free foods has not been shown beneficial in this population; however, routine meals with consistent portion sizes can assist with blood sugar control (Swift, 2012).

Hyperglycemia and dehydration can lead to a serious complication of diabetes in older adults: **hyperglycemic hyperosmolar state (HHS)**. Patients with HHS have a very high blood glucose level (>600 mg/dL [33.3 mmol/L]) without ketones (Pasquel and Umpierrez, 2014). Patients are markedly dehydrated, and mental alterations range from mild confusion to hallucinations or coma. Patients who have HHS have sufficient insulin to prevent lipolysis and ketosis. Treatment consists of hydration and small doses of insulin to control hyperglycemia.

The Nutrition Prescription

To develop, educate, and counsel individuals regarding the nutrition prescription, it is essential to learn about their lifestyle and eating habits. Food and eating histories can be done several ways, with the objective of determining a schedule and pattern of eating that will be the least disruptive to the lifestyle of the individual with diabetes and, at the same time, will facilitate improved metabolic control. With this objective in mind, asking the individual either to record or report what, how much, and when he or she typically eats during a 24-hour period may be the most useful. Another approach is to ask the individual to keep and bring a 3-day or 1-week food intake record (see Chapter 4 and Figs. 4.5 and 4.6). The request to complete a food record can be made when an appointment with the RDN is scheduled. It is also important to learn about daily routine and schedule. The following information is needed: (1) time of waking; (2) usual meal and eating times; (3) work schedule or school hours; (4) type, amount, and timing of exercise; (5) usual

Food Group	Meal/Snack/Time						Total servings/day	CHO (g)	Protein (g)	Fat (g)	Calories
	Breakfast	Snack	Lunch	Snack	Dinner	Snack					
Starches								15	3	1	80
Fruit								15			60
Milk								12	8	1	100
Vegetables								5	2		25
Meats/Substitutes									7	5(3)	75(55)
Fats										5	45
CHO Choices							Total grams				
							Calories/gram	X4=	X4=	X9=	Total calories
							Percent calories				

Calculations are based on medium-fat meats and skim/very low-fat milk. If diet consists predominantly of low-fat meats, use the factor 3 g instead of 5 g fat; if predominantly high-fat meats, use 8 g fat. If low-fat (2%) milk is used, use 5 g fat; if whole milk is used, use 8 g fat.

Fig. 29.4 Worksheet for assessment and design of a meal or food plan. *CHO,* Carbohydrate.

sleep habits; (6) type, dosage, and timing of diabetes medication; and (7) SMBG data.

Using the assessment data and food and nutrition history information, a preliminary eating plan can then be designed and, if the individual desires, sample menus provided. Developing an eating plan does not begin with a set calorie or macronutrient prescription; instead it is determined by modifying the individual's usual food intake as necessary. The worksheet in Fig. 29.4 can be used to record the usual foods eaten and to modify the usual food and nutrient intake as necessary. The macronutrient and caloric values for the food lists are listed on the form and in Table 29.8; see Appendix 18 for portion sizes of the foods on the food lists. These tools are useful in evaluating nutrition assessments.

Using the form in Fig. 29.4, the RDN begins by totaling the number of servings from each food list and multiplying this number by the grams of carbohydrate, protein, and fat contributed by each. Next, the grams of carbohydrate, protein, and fat are totaled from each column. Then the grams of carbohydrates and protein are multiplied by 4 (4 kcal/g of carbohydrates and protein), and the grams of fat are multiplied by 9 (9 kcal/g of fat). Total calories and percentage of calories from each macronutrient can then be determined. Numbers derived from these calculations are then rounded off. Fig. 29.5 provides an example of a preliminary eating plan. In this example the nutrition prescription would be the following: 1900 to 2000 calories, 230 g of carbohydrates (50%), 90 g of protein (20%), and 65 g of fat (30%). The number of carbohydrate choices for each meal and snack is the total of the starch, fruit, and milk

servings. Vegetables, unless starchy or eaten in very large amounts (three or more servings per meal), generally are considered "free foods." The carbohydrate choices are circled under each meal and snack column.

The next step is to evaluate the preliminary eating plan. First and foremost, is the eating plan feasible and will it fit into the individual's lifestyle? Second, is it appropriate for diabetes management? Third, does it encourage healthful eating? Fourth, if the individual is taking diabetes medicine, is the eating plan coordinated with the medication plan to reduce risk of hypoglycemia and/or minimize postprandial hyperglycemia?

To discuss feasibility, the eating plan is reviewed with the individual in terms of general food intake. Timing of meals and snacks and approximate portion sizes and types of foods are discussed. Calorie levels are only approximate, and adjustments in calories can be made during follow-up visits. A meal-planning approach can be selected later that will assist the patient in making food choices. At this point it must be determined whether this eating plan is reasonable.

To determine the appropriateness of the eating plan for diabetes management, distribution of the meals or snacks must be assessed along with the types of medications prescribed and treatment goals. Often the eating plan begins with three or four carbohydrate servings per meal for adult women and four or five for adult men and, if desired, one or two for a snack. Eating snacks when not hungry simply provides unnecessary calories. Adding protein to a snack may promote meal balance and optimize daily intake of macronutrients; however,

Food Group	Meal/Snack/Time						Total servings/day	CHO (g)	Protein (g)	Fat (g)	Calories
	Breakfast 7:30 AM	Snack 10:00	Lunch 12:00	Snack 3:00	Dinner 6:30	Snack 10:00					
Starches	2	1	2–3	1	2–3	1–2	10	15 / 150	3 / 30	1 / 10	80
Fruit	1		1		1	0–1	3	15 / 45			60
Milk	1				1		2	12 / 24	8 / 16	1 / 2	100
Vegetables			✓		✓			5 / 10	2 / 4		25
Meats/Substitutes			2–3		3–4		6		7 / 42	5(3) / 30	75(55)
Fats	1	0–1	1–2	0–1	1–2	0–1	5			5 / 25	45
CHO Choices	3–4 CHO	1 CHO	3–4 CHO	1 CHO	4–5 CHO	1–2 CHO	Total grams	229	92	67	
	1900–2000 calories 230 g CHO–50% 90 g protein–20% 65 g fat–30%						Calories/gram	X4= 916	X4= 368	X9= 603	Total calories
							Percent calories	50	19	30	1900–2000

Calculations are based on medium-fat meats and skim/very low-fat milk. If diet consists predominantly of low-fat meats, use the factor 3 g, instead of 5 g fat; if predominantly high-fat meats, use 8 g fat. If low-fat (2%) milk is used, use 5 g fat; if whole milk is used, use 8 g fat.

Fig. 29.5 An example of a completed worksheet from the assessment, the nutrition prescription, and a sample 1900- to 2000-calorie meal plan. *CHO,* Carbohydrate.

TABLE 29.8 Macronutrient and Caloric Values for Food Lists*

Food List	Carbohydrate (grams)	Protein (grams)	Fat (grams)	Calories
Carbohydrates				
Starch: breads, cereals and grains, starchy vegetables, crackers, snacks, and beans, peas, and lentils	15	3	1	80
Fruits	15	—	—	60
Milk and milk substitutes	12	8	0-3	100
Fat-free, low-fat, 1%	12	8	5	120
Reduced-fat, 2%	12	8	8	160
Whole				
Sweets, desserts, and other carbohydrates	15	Varies	Varies	Varies
Nonstarchy vegetables	5	2	—	25
Proteins				
Lean	—	7	2	45
Medium-fat	—	7	5	75
High-fat	—	7	8	100
Plant-based protein	—	7	Varies	Varies
Fats	—	—	5	45
Alcohol (1 alcohol equivalent)	Varies	—	—	100

*See Appendix 18.
From American Diabetes Association and Academy of Nutrition and Dietetics: *Choose your foods: Food lists for diabetes,* Alexandria, VA, Chicago, 2014 American Diabetes Association, Academy of Nutrition and Dietetics.

research does not support the need for protein for optimal glucose control (ADA, 2018). Results of blood glucose monitoring before the meal and 2 hours after the meal, plus feedback from the person with diabetes, are used to assess if these recommendations are feasible and realistic and to determine whether target glucose goals are being achieved.

Another strategy for meal planning is the U.S. Department of Agriculture (USDA) MyPlate method, which recommends making half your plate nonstarchy vegetables, one quarter protein, and one quarter carbohydrates. Many patients find this style of eating more flexible and user friendly.

For people who require insulin, the timing of eating is important, as insulin must be synchronized with food consumption (see Medications earlier in the chapter). If the eating plan is determined first, an insulin regimen can be selected that will fit with it. The best way to ensure that the eating plan promotes healthful eating is to encourage individuals to eat a variety of foods from all the food groups. The Dietary Guidelines for Americans, which includes a suggested number of servings from each food group, can be used to compare the individual's eating plan with the nutrition recommendations for all Americans (see Chapter 10).

Nutrition Education and Counseling

Implementation of MNT begins with the RDN selecting from a variety of interventions (reduced energy and fat intake, carbohydrate counting, simplified meal plans, healthy food choices, individualized meal planning strategies, insulin-to-carbohydrate ratios, physical activity, and behavioral strategies) (Pastors and Franz, 2012). All of the above interventions have been shown to lead to improved metabolic outcomes. Furthermore, nutrition education and counseling must be sensitive to the individual with diabetes, including personal needs, willingness to change, and ability to make changes (Fig. 29.6). Assessing the individual's health literacy and numeracy also may be beneficial. No single eating plan approach has been shown to be more effective than any other, and the eating plan approach selected should allow individuals with diabetes to select appropriate foods for meals and snacks.

A popular approach to meal planning is carbohydrate counting. Carbohydrate-counting educational tools are based on the concept that the carbohydrate in foods is the major predictor of postprandial

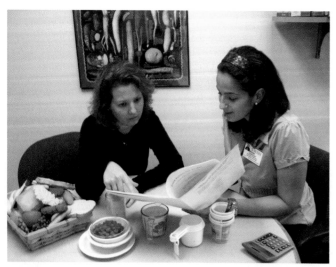

Fig. 29.6 A woman with type 1 diabetes mellitus is learning about carbohydrate counseling from her RDN counselor.

blood glucose levels. One carbohydrate serving contributes 15 g of carbohydrates. Basic carbohydrate counting emphasizes the following topics: basic facts about carbohydrates, primary food sources of carbohydrate, average portion sizes and the importance of consistency and accurate portions, amount of carbohydrates that should be eaten, and label reading. Advanced carbohydrate counting emphasizes the importance of record keeping, calculating insulin-to-carbohydrate ratios, and pattern management.

An important goal of nutrition counseling is to facilitate changes in existing food and nutrition-related behaviors and the adoption of new ones. The combined use of behavior change theories may potentially have a greater impact than any individual theory or technique used alone (Franz et al, 2012). The following five A's can guide the education/counseling sessions: step 1: ask; step 2: assess; step 3: advise; step 4: agree; and step 5: arrange. The "ask" step emphasizes the importance of questions as the RDN aims to develop a relationship with the client. Motivational interviewing techniques are used initially and throughout all of the encounters. In the "assess" step, the RDN evaluated the client's readiness to change. Different intervention strategies may be needed for individuals at different stages of the change process (see Chapter 13).

Nutrition Monitoring and Evaluation

Food intake, medication, metabolic control (glycemia, lipids, and blood pressure), anthropometric measurements, and physical activity should be monitored and evaluated. Medical and clinical outcomes should be monitored after the second or third visit to determine whether the individual is making progress toward established goals. If no progress is evident, the individual and RDN must reassess and perhaps revise nutrition interventions. Blood glucose monitoring results can be used to determine whether adjustments in foods and meals will be sufficient to achieve blood glucose goals or if medication additions or adjustments have to be combined with MNT. Nutrition care must be coordinated with an interdisciplinary team.

Documentation in the individual's medical record serves as a communication tool for members of the health care team. The medical record also serves as a legal document of what was done and not done and supports reimbursement of nutrition services billed to insurance carriers. There are many different formats available for medical record documentation. The appropriate format depends on where the RDN practices and whether electronic health records are used. Regardless of the specific format, the RDN can document using the assessment, diagnosis, interventions, monitoring, and evaluation (ADIME) content (Box 29.4).

Follow-Up Encounters

Successful nutrition therapy involves a process of assessment, problem solving, adjustment, and readjustment. Food records can be compared with the eating plan, which will help to determine whether the initial eating plan needs changing, and can be integrated with the blood glucose–monitoring records to determine changes that can lead to improved glycemic control.

Nutrition follow-up visits should provide encouragement and ensure realistic expectations for the individual with diabetes. A change in eating habits is not easy for most people, and they become discouraged without appropriate recognition of their efforts. Individuals should be encouraged to speak freely about problems they are having with their eating plan. Furthermore there may be major life changes that require changes in the eating plan. Job and schedule changes, travel, illness, and other factors all have an impact on the meal plan.

BOX 29.4 Nutrition Care Documentation

Nutrition Assessment
- Date and time of assessment
- Pertinent data collected and comparisons with standards (e.g., food and nutrition history, biochemical data, anthropometric measurements, client history, medical therapy, and supplement use)
- Patient's readiness to learn, food and nutrition-related knowledge, and potential for change
- Physical activity history and goals
- Reason for discontinuation of nutrition therapy, if appropriate

Nutrition Diagnoses
- Date and time
- Concise written statement of nutrition diagnosis (or nutrition diagnoses) written in the problem, etiology, signs and symptoms (PES) format. If there is no existing or predicted nutrition problem that requires a nutrition intervention, state "no nutrition diagnosis at this time"

Nutrition Interventions
- Date and time
- Specific treatment goals and expected outcomes
- Recommended nutrition prescription and nutrition interventions (individualized for the patient)
- Any adjustments to plan and justifications
- Patient's receptivity regarding recommendations
- Changes in patient's level of understanding and food-related behaviors
- Referrals made and resources used
- Any other information relevant to providing care and monitoring progress over time
- Plans for follow-up and frequency of care

Nutrition Monitoring and Evaluation
- Date and time
- Specific nutrition outcomes indicators and results relevant to the nutrition diagnosis (or diagnoses) and intervention plans and goals, compared with previous status or reference goals
- Progress toward nutrition intervention goals
- Factors facilitating or hindering progress
- Other positive or negative outcomes
- Future plans for nutrition care, monitoring, and follow-up or discharge

Adapted from Writing group of the nutrition care process/standardized language committee: Nutrition care process part II: Using the international dietetics and nutrition terminology to document the nutrition care process, *J Am Diet Assoc* 108:1287, 2008.

BOX 29.5 Common Causes of Hypoglycemia

Medication Errors
- Inadvertent or deliberate errors in medication (generally insulin) dosages
- Excessive insulin or oral secretagogue dosages
- Reversal of morning or evening insulin doses
- Improper timing of insulin in relation to food intake

Nutrition Therapy or Exercise
- Omitted or inadequate food intake
- Timing errors; delayed meals or snacks
- Unplanned or increased physical activities or exercise
- Prolonged duration or increased intensity of exercise

Alcohol and Drugs
- Alcohol intake without food
- Impaired mentation associated with alcohol, marijuana, or other illicit drugs

Adapted from Kaufman F: *Medical management of type 1 diabetes,* ed 6, Alexandria, VA, 2012, American Diabetes Association.

ACUTE COMPLICATIONS

Hypoglycemia and DKA are the two most common acute complications related to diabetes.

Hypoglycemia

A low blood glucose, or **hypoglycemia (or insulin reaction)**, is a common side effect of insulin therapy, although individuals taking insulin secretagogues also can be affected. **Autonomic symptoms** arise from the action of the autonomic nervous system and are often the first signs of mild hypoglycemia. Adrenergic symptoms include shakiness, sweating, palpitations, anxiety, and hunger. **Neuroglycopenic symptoms**, related to an insufficient supply of glucose to the brain, also can occur at similar glucose levels as autonomic symptoms but with different manifestations. The earliest signs of neuroglycopenia include a slowing down in performance and difficulty concentrating and reading. As blood glucose levels drop further, the following symptoms occur: confusion and disorientation, slurred or rambling speech, irrational or unusual behaviors, extreme fatigue and lethargy, seizures, and unconsciousness. While symptoms differ from person to person, they tend to be consistent from episode to episode for any one individual. Several common causes of hypoglycemia are listed in Box 29.5.

In T1DM and T2DM it has been demonstrated that counterregulatory responses to hypoglycemia steadily decline with frequent and repetitive episodes. It can become a vicious cycle as hypoglycemic episodes impair defenses against a subsequent hypoglycemic episode and thus can result in recurrent hypoglycemia. Hypoglycemia causes increased morbidity in most people with T1DM and many with long-duration T2DM.

In general, a blood glucose of 70 mg/dL (3.9 mmol/L) or lower should be treated immediately. Treatment of hypoglycemia requires ingestion of glucose or carbohydrate-containing food. Although any carbohydrate will raise glucose levels, glucose is the preferred treatment. The form of carbohydrates (i.e., liquid or solid) used to treat does not make a difference. Commercially available glucose tablets have the advantage of being premeasured to help prevent overtreatment. Ingestion of 15 to 20 g of glucose is an effective but temporary treatment. Note that pure glucose is the preferred treatment, but any form of carb that contains glucose will increase blood glucose levels. Initial response to treatment should be seen in about 10 to 20 minutes; however, blood glucose should be evaluated again in about 60 minutes as additional carbohydrate may be necessary (Box 29.6) (ADA, 2018).

Severely low blood glucose can cause loss of consciousness or seizures. If individuals are unable to swallow, administration of subcutaneous or intramuscular glucagon may be needed. Parents, siblings, friends, and spouses should be taught how to mix, draw up, and administer glucagon so that they are properly prepared for emergency situations. Kits that include a syringe prefilled with diluting fluid are available. After the injection, turn the patient on their side to prevent choking in case of vomiting. Nausea and vomiting are common side effects of glucagon. The patient should be given food or beverage containing carbohydrate as soon as they regain consciousness and can swallow.

SMBG is essential for prevention and treatment of hypoglycemia. Changes in insulin injections, eating, exercise schedules, and travel routines warrant increased frequency of monitoring. Some patients

---

BOX 29.6   Treatment of Hypoglycemia

- Immediate treatment with carbohydrates is essential.
  If the blood glucose level falls below 70 mg/dL (3.9 mmol/L), treat with 15 g of carbohydrates, which is equivalent to:
  - 15 g carbohydrate from glucose tablets (4) or glucose gel
  - 4-6 ounces of fruit juice or regular soft drinks
  - 6 ounces (1/2 can) of regular soda pop (not sugar-free)
  - 8 ounces (1 cup) of sports drink (not sugar-free)
  - 1 tablespoon of sugar, syrup or honey
- Retest in approximately 10-15 minutes. If the blood glucose level remains <70 mg/dL (<3.9 mmol/L), treat with an additional 15 g of carbohydrates.
- Repeat testing and treatment until the blood glucose level returns to within normal range.
- If it is more than 1 hour to the next meal, test again 60 minutes after treatment as additional carbohydrate may be needed.

Adapted from Kaufman F: *Medical management of Type 1 diabetes*, ed 6, Alexandria, VA, 2012, American Diabetes Association.

BOX 29.7   Sick-Day Guidelines for Persons With Diabetes

1. During acute illnesses, usual doses of insulin and other glucose-lowering medications are required. The need for insulin continues, or may even increase, during periods of illness. Fever, dehydration, infection, or the stress of illness can trigger the release of counterregulatory or "stress" hormones, causing blood glucose levels to become elevated.
2. Blood glucose levels and urine or blood testing for ketones should be monitored at least four times daily (before each meal and at bedtime). Blood glucose readings exceeding 250 mg/dL and the presence of ketones are danger signals indicating that additional insulin is needed.
3. Ample amounts of liquid need to be consumed every hour. If vomiting, diarrhea, or fever is present, small sips—1 or 2 tablespoons every 15-30 min—can usually be consumed. If vomiting continues and the individual is unable to take fluids for longer than 4 hr, the health care team should be notified.
4. If regular foods are not tolerated, liquid or soft carbohydrate-containing foods (such as regular soft drinks, soup, juices, and ice cream) should be eaten. Eating about 10-15 g of carbohydrate every 1-2 hr (or 50 g of carbohydrate every 3-4 hr) is usually sufficient.
5. The health care team should be called if illness continues for more than 1 day.

Adapted from Kaufman F: *Medical management of type 1 diabetes*, ed 6, Alexandria, VA, 2012, American Diabetes Association.

---

experience hypoglycemia unawareness, which means that they do not experience the usual symptoms of hypoglycemia. Patients must be reminded of the need to treat hypoglycemia, even in the absence of symptoms. Hypoglycemia unawareness, or one or more episodes of severe hypoglycemia, warrants reevaluation of the treatment regimen. A CGM may be a useful tool in those with hypoglycemia unawareness and/or frequent hypoglycemic episodes (ADA, 2018).

Hyperglycemia and Diabetic Ketoacidosis

Hyperglycemia can lead to DKA, a life-threatening but reversible complication, which occurs when the body produces high levels of blood acids called ketones. DKA is always the result of inadequate insulin for glucose use. As a result, the body depends on fat for energy, and ketones are formed. Acidosis results from increased production and decreased use of acetoacetic acid and 3-beta-hydroxybutyric acid from fatty acids. Ketones spill into the urine; hence the reliance on urine testing for ketones.

DKA is characterized by an elevated serum glucose level (greater than 250 mg/dL [13.88 mmol/L]), an elevated serum ketone level, a pH less than 7.3, and a serum bicarbonate level less than 18 mEq/L (18 mmol/L) (Westerberg, 2013). Symptoms include polyuria, polydipsia, hyperventilation, dehydration, the fruity odor of ketones, and fatigue. SMBG, testing for ketones, and medical intervention can help prevent DKA. If left untreated, DKA can lead to coma and death. Treatment includes supplemental insulin, fluid and electrolyte replacement, and medical monitoring. Acute illnesses such as flu, colds, vomiting, and diarrhea, if not managed appropriately, can lead to the development of DKA. Patients need to know the steps to take during acute illness to prevent DKA (Box 29.7). During acute illness, oral ingestion of about 150 to 200 g of carbohydrates per day (45 to 50 g every 3 to 4 hr) should be sufficient, along with medication adjustments, to keep glucose in the goal range and to prevent starvation ketosis.

Fasting hyperglycemia is a common finding in persons with diabetes. The amount of insulin required to normalize blood glucose levels during the night is less in the predawn period (from 1 AM to 3 AM) than at dawn (from 4 AM to 8 AM). The increased need for insulin at dawn causes a rise in FBG levels referred to as the dawn phenomenon. It results if insulin levels decline between predawn and dawn or if overnight hepatic glucose output becomes excessive as is common in T2DM. To identify the dawn phenomenon, blood glucose levels are monitored at bedtime and at 2 AM to 3 AM. With the dawn phenomenon, predawn blood glucose levels will be in the low range of normal but not in the hypoglycemic range. For patients with T2DM, metformin often is used because it decreases hepatic glucose output. For persons with T1DM, administering insulin that does not peak at 1 AM to 3 AM, such as a long-acting insulin, should be considered.

Hypoglycemia followed by rebound hyperglycemia is called the Somogyi effect. This phenomenon originates during hypoglycemia with the secretion of counterregulatory hormones (glucagon, epinephrine, growth hormone, and cortisol) and usually is caused by excessive exogenous insulin doses. Hepatic glucose production is stimulated, thus raising blood glucose levels. If rebound hyperglycemia goes unrecognized and insulin doses are increased, a cycle of overinsulinization may result. Decreasing evening insulin doses or, for the dawn phenomenon, taking a long-acting insulin should be considered.

LONG-TERM COMPLICATIONS

Long-term complications of diabetes include macrovascular diseases, microvascular diseases, and neuropathy. Macrovascular diseases involve diseases of large blood vessels. In contrast, microvascular diseases associated with diabetes involve the small blood vessels and include nephropathy and retinopathy.

Common consequences of diabetic neuropathy and/or peripheral arterial disease (PAD) include foot ulcers and amputation, and both represent major causes of morbidity and mortality in people with diabetes. Early detection is key in treatment of patients with diabetes and feet at risk for ulcers and amputations. Risk factors include poor glycemic control, peripheral neuropathy with loss of protective sensation (LOPS), cigarette smoking, foot deformities, preulcerative callus or corn, PAD, history of foot ulcer or amputation, visual impairment, and diabetic kidney disease (especially patients on dialysis) (ADA, 2018).

MNT is important in managing several long-term complications of diabetes. Nutrition therapy is also a major component in reducing risk factors for chronic complications, especially those related to macrovascular disease.

Macrovascular Diseases

Insulin resistance, which may precede the development of T2DM and macrovascular disease by many years, induces numerous metabolic changes known as the metabolic syndrome (see Chapter 20). It is characterized by intraabdominal obesity or the android distribution of adipose tissue (waist circumference greater than 102 cm [40 in] in men and greater than 88 cm [35 in] in women) and is associated with dyslipidemia, hypertension, glucose intolerance, and increased prevalence of macrovascular complications. Other risk factors include genetics, smoking, sedentary lifestyle, high-fat diet, renal failure, and microalbuminuria.

Macrovascular diseases including atherosclerotic cardiovascular disease (ASCVD), peripheral vascular disease (PVD), and cerebrovascular disease are more common, tend to occur at an earlier age, and are more extensive and severe in people with diabetes. People with diabetes have the CVD risk equivalent to persons with preexisting CVD and no diabetes (Low Wang et al, 2016). Furthermore, in women with diabetes the increased risk of mortality from heart disease is greater than in men, in contrast to the nondiabetic population, in which heart disease mortality is greater in men than in women (Recarti et al, 2015).

Dyslipidemia

Patients with diabetes have an increased prevalence of lipid abnormalities that contribute to higher rates of CVD. For example, in T2DM the prevalence of an elevated cholesterol level is about 28% to 34%. Similarly, about 5% to 14% of patients with T2DM have high triglyceride levels. Lower HDL cholesterol levels are common. People with T2DM typically have smaller, denser LDL particles, which increase atherogenicity even if the total LDL cholesterol level is not significantly elevated. Lifestyle intervention, including MNT, along with weight loss (if indicated) through reduced energy intake and increased physical activity and smoking cessation should be considered. Evidence is inconclusive for the ideal amount of total fat intake; fat quality may as important as quantity (Evert et al, 2013). Diet should be focused on reduction of saturated fat, trans fat, and cholesterol and increased intake of omega-3 fat (in food, not as supplements), viscous fiber, and plant stanols/sterols (ADA, 2018). In people with T2DM, a Mediterranean-style, MUFA-rich eating pattern may benefit glycemic control and CVD risk factors. Other CVD nutrition recommendations for people with diabetes are the same as for the general public. The most current American College of Cardiology (ACC)/American Heart Association (AHA) recommendations are for use of the DASH diet eating pattern (see Chapter 32). In addition to nutrition therapy, statin therapy is typically recommended, regardless of lipid levels, for all adults over 40 with diabetes (ADA, 2018) (Table 29.9).

Hypertension

Hypertension is a common comorbidity of diabetes, with about 74% of adults with diabetes having blood pressure of 140/90 mm Hg or higher or using prescription medications for hypertension (CDC, 2018). In order to reduce the risk of macrovascular and microvascular disease, treatment of hypertension in people with diabetes should be vigorous. Blood pressure should be measured at every routine visit, with a goal for blood pressure control of less than 140/80 mm Hg. MNT interventions for people with hypertension include weight loss (if overweight), DASH-style eating pattern (Appendix 17), reducing sodium intake and increasing potassium intake, moderation of alcohol intake, and increased physical activity (see Chapter 32). The recommendation for the general population to reduce sodium to less than 2300 mg/day is also appropriate for people with diabetes and hypertension (ADA, 2018). For individuals with both diabetes

and hypertension, further reduction in sodium intake should be individualized. Consideration must be given to issues such as the availability, palatability, and additional cost of low sodium food products. Pharmacologic therapy for hypertension includes either an angiotensin-converting enzyme (ACE) inhibitor, angiotensin receptor blockers, thiazide-like diuretics, and/or dihydropyridine calcium channel blockers (ADA, 2018). See Table 29.9.

Microvascular Diseases

Diabetic Kidney Disease

Diabetic kidney disease (DKD) or diabetic nephropathy occurs in 20% to 40% of patients with diabetes and is the single leading cause of end-stage renal disease (ESRD). Because of the much greater prevalence of T2DM, such patients constitute over half of the patients with diabetes currently starting on dialysis (see Chapter 34).

An annual screening to quantitate urine albumin excretion rate should be performed in patients who have had T1DM for more than 5 years, and in all patients with T2DM starting at diagnosis (ADA, 2014b). The serum creatinine is used to estimate glomerular filtration rate (GFR) and stage the level of chronic kidney disease (CKD), if present.

To reduce the risk and slow the progression of DKD, blood glucose and blood pressure control should be optimized. Although low protein diets (below 0.6 to 0.8 g/kg) have been shown to lower albuminuria, they do not alter the course of GFR decline or improve glycemic or CVD risk measures, and therefore are not recommended (Evert et al, 2013).

Retinopathy

Diabetic retinopathy is estimated to be the most frequent cause of new cases of blindness among adults 20 to 74 years of age. Glaucoma, cataracts, and other disorders of the eye also occur earlier and more frequently with diabetes (ADA, 2018). Laser photocoagulation surgery can reduce the risk of further vision loss but usually does not restore lost vision—thus the importance for a screening program to detect diabetic retinopathy.

Neuropathy

Chronic high levels of blood glucose also are associated with nerve damage, and an estimated 50% of people with diabetes have mild to severe forms of nervous system damage (CDC, 2018). Intensive treatment of hyperglycemia reduces the risk and slows progression of

---

TABLE 29.9 Recommendations for Lipid and Blood Pressure for Most Adults With Diabetes

Lipids/Blood Pressure	Criteria
LDL cholesterol	<100 mg/dL (<2.6 mmol/l)*
HDL cholesterol	Men: >40 mg/dL (>1.0 mmol/l)
	Women: >50 mg/d (>1.3 mmol/l)
Triglycerides	<150 mg/dL (<1.7 mmol/l)
Blood pressure	<140/90 mm Hg

*For patients with diabetes and atherosclerotic cardiovascular disease, if LDL cholesterol is greater than or equal to 70 mg/dL on maximally tolerated statin dose, consider adding additional LDL lowering therapy (such as ezetimibe or PCSK9 inhibitor).
HDL, High-density lipoprotein; *LDL*, low-density lipoprotein.
Data from American Diabetes Association: Cardiovascular disease and risk management: Standards of medical care in diabetes—2018, *Diabetes Care* 41(S1):S86-104, 2018.

diabetic neuropathy but does not reverse neuronal loss. Peripheral neuropathy usually affects the nerves that control sensation in the feet and hands. Autonomic neuropathy affects nerve function controlling various organ systems. Cardiovascular effects include postural hypotension and decreased responsiveness to cardiac nerve impulses, leading to painless or silent ischemic heart disease. Sexual function may be affected, with impotence the most common manifestation.

Damage to nerves innervating the gastrointestinal tract can cause a variety of problems. Neuropathy can be manifested in the esophagus as nausea and esophagitis, in the stomach as unpredictable emptying, in the small bowel as loss of nutrients, and in the large bowel as diarrhea or constipation.

Gastroparesis is characterized by delayed gastric emptying in the absence of mechanical obstruction of the stomach. Common symptoms include feelings of fullness, bloating, nausea, vomiting, diarrhea, or constipation. One study found that the prevalence of gastroparesis in patients with diabetes was 64%, which is higher than reported in some previous studies (Alipour et al, 2017). Therefore gastroparesis should be suspected in individuals with erratic glucose control.

The first step in management of patients with neuropathy should be to aim for stable and optimal glycemic control. MNT involves minimizing abdominal stress. Small, frequent meals may be better tolerated than three full meals a day, and these meals should be low in fiber and fat. If solid foods are not well tolerated, liquid meals may have to be recommended. For patients using insulin, the timing of insulin administration should be adjusted to match the usually delayed nutrient absorption. Insulin injections may even be required after eating. Frequent blood glucose monitoring is important to determine appropriate insulin therapy.

A prokinetic agent such as metoclopramide is used most commonly to treat gastroparesis. Antiemetic agents may be helpful for the relief of symptoms. In very severe cases, generally with unintentional weight loss, a feeding tube is placed in the small intestine to bypass the stomach. Gastric electric stimulation with electrodes surgically implanted in the stomach may be used when medications fail to control nausea and vomiting.

HYPOGLYCEMIA OF NONDIABETIC ORIGIN

Hypoglycemia of nondiabetic origin has been defined as a clinical syndrome with diverse causes in which low levels of plasma glucose eventually lead to neuroglycopenia. Hypoglycemia means low (hypo-) blood glucose (glycemia). Normally the body is remarkably adept at maintaining fairly steady blood glucose levels—usually between 60 and 100 mg/dL (3.3 to 5.6 mmol/L), despite the intermittent ingestion of food. Maintaining normal levels of glucose is important because body cells, especially the brain and central nervous system, must have a steady and consistent supply of glucose to function properly. Under physiologic conditions the brain depends almost exclusively on glucose for its energy needs. This is true even with the presence of hunger.

Pathophysiology

In a small number of people, blood glucose levels drop too low. Symptoms are often felt when blood glucose is below 65 mg/dL (3.6 mmol/L). If the brain and nervous system are deprived of the glucose they need to function, symptoms such as sweating, shaking, weakness, hunger, headaches, and irritability can develop. Symptoms of hypoglycemia have been recognized at plasma glucose levels of about 60 mg/dL, and impaired brain function has occurred at levels of about 50 mg/dL. A hypoglycemia alert value greater than or equal to 70 mg/dL (3.9 mmol/L) can help determine therapeutic dose adjustment of glucose-lowering drugs and is often related to symptomatic hypoglycemia (ADA, 2018).

Hypoglycemia can be difficult to diagnose because these typical symptoms can be caused by many different health problems. For example, adrenaline (epinephrine) released as a result of anxiety and stress can trigger the symptoms similar to those of hypoglycemia. The only way to determine whether hypoglycemia is causing these symptoms is to measure blood glucose levels while an individual is experiencing the symptoms. Hypoglycemia can best be defined by the presence of three features known as Whipple's triad: (1) a low plasma or blood glucose level, (2) symptoms of hypoglycemia at the same time, and (3) resolution of the symptoms once the blood glucose returns to normal.

A fairly steady blood glucose level is maintained by the interaction of several mechanisms. After eating, carbohydrates are broken down into glucose and enter the bloodstream. As blood glucose levels rise, the pancreas responds by releasing the hormone insulin, which allows glucose to leave the bloodstream and enter various body cells, where it fuels the body's activities. Glucose is also taken up by the liver and stored as glycogen for later use.

When glucose concentrations from the last meal decline, the body goes from a fed to a fasting state. Insulin levels decrease, which keeps the blood glucose levels from falling too low. Stored glucose is released from the liver back into the bloodstream with the help of glucagon from the pancreas. Normally the body's ability to balance glucose, insulin, and glucagon (and other counterregulatory hormones) keeps glucose levels within the normal range. Glucagon provides the primary defense against hypoglycemia; without it, full recovery does not occur. Epinephrine is not necessary for counterregulation when glucagon is present. However in the absence of glucagon, epinephrine has an important role.

Types of Hypoglycemia

Two types of hypoglycemia can occur in people who do not have diabetes. If blood glucose levels fall below normal limits within 2 to 5 hours after eating, this is postprandial (reactive) hypoglycemia. It can be caused by an exaggerated or late insulin response caused by either insulin resistance or elevated GLP-1, alimentary hyperinsulinism, renal glycosuria, defects in glucagon response, or high insulin sensitivity. Additionally it can be caused by rare syndromes such as hereditary fructose intolerance, galactosemia, leucine sensitivity or a rare beta-cell pancreatic tumor (insulinoma), causing blood glucose levels to drop too low. Alimentary hyperinsulinism is common after gastric surgery, associated with rapid delivery of food to the small intestine, rapid absorption of glucose, and exaggerated insulin response. These patients respond best to multiple, frequent feedings.

The ingestion of alcohol after a prolonged fast or the ingestion of large amounts of alcohol and carbohydrates on an empty stomach ("gin-and-tonic" syndrome) also may cause hypoglycemia within 3 to 4 hours in some healthy persons.

Idiopathic reactive hypoglycemia is characterized by normal insulin secretion but increased insulin sensitivity and, to some extent, reduced response of glucagon to acute hypoglycemia symptoms. The increase in insulin sensitivity associated with a deficiency of glucagon secretion leads to hypoglycemia late postprandially. Idiopathic reactive hypoglycemia has been inappropriately overdiagnosed by physicians and patients, to the point that some physicians doubt its existence. Although rare, it does exist but can be documented only in persons with hypoglycemia that occurs spontaneously and in persons who meet the criteria of Whipple's triad.

Fasting hypoglycemia, or postabsorptive hypoglycemia, often is related to an underlying disease. This food-deprived hypoglycemia may occur in response to having gone without food for 8 hours or longer and can be caused by conditions that upset the body's ability to balance blood glucose. These include eating disorders and other serious underlying medical conditions, including hormone deficiency states (e.g., hypopituitarism, adrenal insufficiency, catecholamine or glucagon deficiency), acquired liver disease, renal disease, certain drugs (e.g., alcohol, propranolol, salicylate), insulinoma (of which most are benign, but 6% to 10% can be malignant), and other nonpancreatic tumors. Taking high doses of aspirin also may lead to fasting hypoglycemia. Factitious hypoglycemia, or self-administration of insulin or sulfonylurea in people who do not have diabetes, is a cause as well. Symptoms related to fasting hypoglycemia tend to be particularly severe and can include a loss of mental acuity, seizures, and unconsciousness. If the underlying problem can be resolved, hypoglycemia is no longer a problem.

Diagnostic Criteria

One of the criteria used to confirm the presence of hypoglycemia is a blood glucose level of less than 70 mg/dL (3.9 mmol/L); however, clinically significant hypoglycemia (level 2), is 54 mg/dL (3.0 mmol/L) (ADA, 2018). Previously the OGTT test was the standard test for this condition; however, this test is no longer used. Recording finger stick blood glucose measurements during spontaneous, symptomatic episodes at home is used to establish the diagnosis. An alternative method is to perform a glucose test in a medical office setting, in which case the patient is given a typical meal that has been documented in the past to lead to symptomatic episodes. Whipple's triad can be confirmed if symptoms occur. If blood glucose levels are low during the symptomatic period and if the symptoms disappear on eating, hypoglycemia is probably responsible. It is essential to make a correct diagnosis in patients with fasting hypoglycemia because the implications are serious.

Management of Hypoglycemia

The management of hypoglycemic disorders involves two distinct components: (1) relief of neuroglycopenic symptoms by restoring blood glucose concentrations to the normal range and (2) correction of the underlying cause. The immediate treatment is to eat foods or beverages containing carbohydrates. As the glucose from the breakdown of carbohydrates is absorbed into the bloodstream, it increases the level of glucose in the blood and relieves the symptoms. If an underlying problem is causing hypoglycemia, appropriate treatment of this disease or disorder is essential.

The goal of treatment is to adopt eating habits that will keep blood glucose levels as stable as possible (International Diabetes Center, 2013).

BOX 29.9 Guidelines for Preventing Hypoglycemic Symptoms in People Who Do Not Have Diabetes

1. Eat small meals, with snacks interspersed between meals and at bedtime. This means eating five to six small meals rather than two to three large meals to steady the release of glucose into the bloodstream.
2. Spread the intake of carbohydrate foods throughout the day. Most individuals can eat two to four servings of carbohydrate foods at each meal and one to two servings at each snack. If carbohydrates are removed from the diet completely, the body loses its ability to handle carbohydrates properly, so this is not recommended. Carbohydrate foods include starches, fruits and fruit juices, milk and yogurt, and foods containing sugar.
3. Avoid or limit foods high in sugar and carbohydrate, especially on an empty stomach. Examples of these foods are regular soft drinks, syrups, candy, fruit juices, regular fruited yogurts, pies, and cakes.
4. Avoid beverages and foods containing caffeine. Caffeine can cause the same symptoms as hypoglycemia and make the individual feel worse.
5. Limit or avoid alcoholic beverages. Drinking alcohol on an empty stomach and without food can lower blood glucose levels by interfering with the liver's ability to release stored glucose (gluconeogenesis). If an individual chooses to drink alcohol, it should be done in moderation (one or two drinks no more than twice a week), and food always should be eaten along with the alcoholic beverage.

Modified from International Diabetes Center: *Reactive and fasting hypoglycemia*, Minneapolis, 2013, International Diabetes Center.

To stay symptom-free, it is important for individuals to eat five to six small meals or snacks per day, as this helps to provide manageable amounts of glucose to the body. Recommended guidelines are listed in Box 29.9.

Patients with hypoglycemia also may benefit from learning carbohydrate counting and, to prevent hypoglycemia, eating three to four carbohydrate servings (15 g of carbohydrate per serving) at meals and one to two for snacks (see Appendix 18). Foods containing protein can be eaten at meals or with snacks. These foods would be expected to have minimum effect on blood glucose levels and can add extra food for satiety and calories. However, because protein and carbohydrate stimulate insulin release, a moderate intake may be advisable.

CLINICAL CASE STUDY

MP is a 65-year-old, nonsmoking Hispanic female who is being seen for management of type 2 diabetes. Her blood glucose levels are uncontrolled as evidenced by an A1C > 10, and she complains of increasing numbness in her feet and occasionally in her fingers, and frequent urination during the day and overnight. From interviewing her and reviewing her health record, you learn the following about her:

Education: did not complete high school, attended through middle school.

Occupation: not employed outside the home, babysits infant grandchild on a daily basis.

Household Members: lives with her husband and with one of her four adult children.

Ethnic Background: Latin American, born in Mexico, emigrated to the United States in 1980.

Religious Affiliation: Catholic.

Language: Native Spanish, speaks English—has difficulty reading English.

Patient History: Weighed more than 9 lb at birth.

MP was diagnosed with T2DM 10 or 15 years ago and her diabetes management history is as follows:

Type of Treatment: Nutrition therapy plus oral diabetes medication and long-acting insulin at bedtime (HS)

Medications: glargine 80 units at HS, metformin XR 1000 mg BID, enalapril 10 mg daily, simvastatin 40 mg daily, levothyroxine 75 mcg daily

Family History: Mother had type 2 diabetes, 12-year-old grandson recently diagnosed with prediabetes

Medical History: type 2 diabetes, hypertension, hyperlipidemia, hypothyroidism, episodic migraines (last occurrence 2017)

Physical examination shows the following:

Weight: 201 lbs.

Height: 5'2".

Temperature: 98.6°F

Blood Pressure: 143/88 mm Hg

Continued

CLINICAL CASE STUDY—cont'd

Heart Rate: 80 bpm
Laboratories: A1C 10

Nutrition Diagnostic Statement

- Altered blood glucose levels related to difficulty match insulin to carbohydrate intake as evidenced by excessive mealtime carbohydrate intake and elevated postprandial self-monitoring of blood glucose (SMBG) download data report.

Interventions

- For each of the two problem, etiology, and signs and symptoms (PES) statements, write a goal based on signs and symptoms.

- For the two goals, write two to three nutrition interventions based on the etiology that would be appropriate for MP.

  NOTE: In a real face-to-face appointment between a registered dietitian nutritionist (RDN)/ Certified Diabetes Educator (CDE) and MP, they would collaboratively develop her goals together.

Evaluation and Monitoring

- When should the next nutrition counseling session be scheduled for MP?
- What would you assess at the follow-up visit based on the nutrition goals and interventions developed at the initial appointment?

USEFUL WEBSITES

Academy of Nutrition and Dietetics (AND)
Academy of Nutrition and Dietetics Evidence Analysis Library
American Association of Diabetes Educators (AADE)
American Diabetes Association (ADA)
Diabetes Care and Education Practice Group (DCE)
DCE Patient Education Handouts
International Diabetes Center (IDC)
IDC Publishing
Joslin Diabetes Center
National Diabetes Education Program (NDEP)
National Institute of Diabetes and Digestive Kidney Diseases (NIDDK)
Resources for Healthcare Professionals

REFERENCES

Academy of Nutrition and Dietetics Evidence Analysis Library: "*GDM: executive summary of recommendations* (2016)." https://www.andeal.org/topic.cfm?menu=5288&cat=5538. Accessed July 29, 2018.

Academy of Nutrition and Dietetics Evidence Analysis Library: "*In adults with type 1 and type 2 diabetes, what is the relationship of differing amounts of glycemic index on glycemia, insulin and CVD risk factors* (lipids and blood pressure)?" (2014). https://www.andeal.org/template.cfm?template=guide_summary&key=4348. Accessed July 29, 2018.

Academy of Nutrition and Dietetics Evidence Analysis Library: "*In women with GDM, what impact does the amount or type of carbohydrate consumed have on post-prandial breakfast glycemia?* (2016)" https://www.andeal.org/template.cfm?template=guide_summary&key=4429. Accessed July 29, 2018.

Academy of Nutrition and Dietetics Evidence Analysis Library: "*In women with GDM, what is the effect of caloric consumption on fetal/neonatal and maternal outcomes?* (2016)." https://www.andeal.org/template.cfm?template=guide_summary&key=4579. Accessed July 29, 2018.

Academy of Nutrition and Dietetics Evidence Analysis Library: https://www.andeal.org/vault/2440/web/files/20140527-ND%20Snapshot.pdf. Accessed July 29, 2018.

Alipour Z, Khatib F, Tabib SM, et al: Assessment of the prevalence of diabetic gastroparesis and validation of gastric emptying scintigraphy for diagnosis, *Mol Imaging Radionucl Ther* 26(1):17–23, 2017. doi:10.4274/mirt.61587.

Allen RW, Schwartzman E, Baker WL, et al: Cinnamon use in type 2 diabetes: an updated systematic review and meta-analysis, *Ann Fam Med* 11(5):452–459, 2013. doi:10.1370/afm.1517.

American Diabetes Association: Standards of Medical Care in Diabetes-2018, *Diabetes Care* 41(Suppl 1):S152–S153, 2018. doi:10.2337/dc18-S015.

Arterburn DE, Bogart A, Sherwood NE, et al: A multisite study of long-term remission and relapse of type 2 diabetes mellitus following gastric bypass, *Obes Surg* 23:93–102, 2013.

Birch LL, Fisher JO, Davison KK: Learning to overeat: maternal use of restrictive feeding practices promotes girls' eating in the absence of hunger, *Am J Clin Nutr* 78(2):215–220, 2003. doi:10.1093/ajcn/78.2.215.

Blomster JI, Zoungas S, Chalmers J, et al: The relationship between alcohol consumption and vascular complications and mortality in individuals with type 2 diabetes. *Diabetes Care* 37(5):1353–1359, 2014. doi:10.2337/dc13-2727.

Centers for Disease Control and Prevention (CDC): *Diabetes home: prevent complications.* https://www.cdc.gov/diabetes/managing/problems.html. Updated April 23, 2018.

Centers for Disease Control and Prevention (CDC): *National diabetes statistics report*, 2017a. https://www.cdc.gov/diabetes/pdfs/data/statistics/national-diabetes-statistics-report.pdf.

Centers for Disease Control and Prevention (CDC): *Gestational diabetes.* https://www.cdc.gov/diabetes/basics/gestational.html. Updated July 25, 2017b.

Chen C, Cohrs CM, Stertmann J, et al: Human beta cell mass and function in diabetes: recent advances in knowledge and technologies to understand disease pathogenesis, *Mol Metab* 6(9):943–957, 2017.

Chiang JL, Kirkman MS, Laffel LM, et al: Type 1 diabetes through the life span: a position statement of the American Diabetes Association, *Diabetes Care* 37:2034–2054, 2014.

Chiang JL, Maahs DM, Garvey KC, et al: Type 1 diabetes in children and adolescents: a position statement by the American Diabetes Association, *Diabetes Care* 41(9):2026–2044, 2018. doi:10.2337/dci18-0023.

Clifford D, Ozier A, Bundros J, et al: Impact of non-diet approaches on attitudes, behaviors, and health outcomes: a systematic review, *J Nutr Educ Behav* 47(2):143–155.e1, 2015.

Colberg SR, Sigal RJ, Yardley JE, et al: Physical activity/exercise and diabetes: a position Statement of the American Diabetes Association, *Diabetes Care* 39(11):2065–2079, 2016. doi:10.2337/dc16-1728.

Corbin KD, Driscoll KA, Pratley RE, et al: Advancing Care for Type 1 Diabetes and Obesity Network (ACT1ON): Obesity in Type 1 diabetes: pathophysiology, clinical impact, and mechanisms, *Endocr Rev* 39(5):629–663, 2018. doi:10.1210/er.2017-00191.

Costello RB, Dwyer JT, Saldanha L, et al: Do cinnamon supplements have a role in glycemic control in type 2 diabetes? A narrative review, *J Acad Nutr Diet* 116(11):1794–1802, 2016. doi:10.1016/j.jand.2016.07.015.

Derosa G, D'Angelo A, Romano D, et al: A clinical trial about a food supplement containing α-Lipoic acid on oxidative stress markers in Type 2 diabetic patients. Arráez-Román D, ed. *Int J Mol Sci* 17(11):1802, 2016. doi:10.3390/ijms17111802.

Diabetes Prevention Program Research Group: 10-year follow-up of diabetes incidence and weight loss in the Diabetes Prevention Program Outcome Study, *Lancet* 374:1677–1686, 2009.

Esposito K, Maiorino MI, Ciotola M, et al: Effects of a mediterranean-style diet on the need for antihyperglycemic drug therapy in patients with newly diagnosed type 2 diabetes: a randomized trial, *Ann Intern Med* 151:306–314, 2009.

Eckel RH, Kahn SE, Ferrannini E, et al: Obesity and type 2 diabetes: what can be unified and what needs to be individualized? *Diabetes Care* 34(6):1424–1430, 2011. doi:10.2337/dc11-0447.

Evert AB, Boucher JL, Cypress M, et al: Nutrition therapy recommendations for the management of adults with diabetes, *Diabetes Care* 36:3821–3842, 2013.

Evert AB, Boucher JL, Cypress M, et al: Nutrition therapy recommendations for the management of adults with diabetes, *Diabetes Care* 37(Suppl 1): S120–S143, 2014. doi:10.2337/dc14-S120.

Fonolleda M, Murillo M, Vázquez F, et al: Remission Phase in Paediatric Type 1 Diabetes: New Understanding and Emerging Biomarkers, *Horm Res Paediatr* 88(5):307–315, 2017. doi:10.1159/000479030.

Franz MJ, MacLeod J, Evert A, et al: Academy of Nutrition and Dietetics Nutrition Practice Guideline for Type 1 and Type 2 diabetes in adults: systematic review of evidence for medical nutrition therapy effectiveness and recommendations for integration into the nutrition care process, *J Acad Nutr Diet* 117(10):1659–1679, 2017. doi:10.1016/j.jand.2017.03.022.

Franz MJ, MacLeod J: Success of nutrition-therapy interventions in persons with type 2 diabetes: challenges and future directions, *Diabetes Metab Syndr Obes* 11:265–270, 2018. doi:10.2147/DMSO.S141952. eCollection 2018.

Franz MJ: The obesity paradox and diabetes, *Diabetes Spectr* 26:145–151, 2013.

Franz MJ, Boucher JL, Pereira RF: *ADA pocket guide to lipid disorders, hypertension, diabetes, and weight management*, Chicago, 2012, Academy of Nutrition and Dietetics.

Franz MJ, Powers MA, Leontos C, et al: The evidence for medical nutrition therapy for type 1 and type 2 diabetes in adults, *J Am Diet Assoc* 110: 1852–1889, 2010.

Gardner C, Wylie-Rosett J, Gidding SS, et al: Nonnutritive sweeteners: current use and health perspectives: a scientific statement from the American Heart Association and the American Diabetes Association, *Diabetes Care* 35:1798–1808, 2012.

Golden NH, Schneider M, Wood C: Preventing obesity and eating disorders in adolescents, *Pediatrics* 138(3):e20161649, 2016.

Gómez-Ríos MÁ, Gómez-Ríos D, Paech MJ, et al: Managing diabetic ketoacidosis in pregnancy, *Saudi J Anaesth* 10(2):238–239, 2016. doi:10.4103/1658-354X.168829.

Grembecka M: Sugar alcohols—their role in the modern world of sweeteners: a review, *Eur Food Res Technol* 241(1):1–14, 2015. doi:10.1007/s00217-015-2437-7.

Hædersdal S, Lund A, Knop FK, et al: The role of glucagon in the pathophysiology and treatment of Type 2 diabetes, *Mayo Clin Proc* 93(2):217–239, 2018. doi:10.1016/j.mayocp.2017.12.003.

Heidari-Beni M, Kelishadi R: *The role of dietary sugars and sweeteners in metabolic disorders and diabetes*, 2016, Springer, Cham, pp 1–19. doi:10.1007/978-3-319-26478-3_31-1.

Holman RR, Paul Sk, Bethel MA, et al: 10-year follow-up of intensive glucose control in type 2 diabetes, *N Eng J Med* 359:1577–1589, 2008.

Institute of Medicine: *Dietary reference intakes: energy, carbohydrate, fiber, fat, fatty acids, cholesterol, protein, and amino acids*, Washington, DC, 2002, National Academies Press.

International Diabetes Center: *Reactive and fasting hypoglycemia*, ed 4, Minneapolis, 2013, International Diabetes Center.

Inzucchi SE, Bergenstal RM, Buse JB, et al: Management of hyperglycemia in type 2 diabetes, 2015: a patient-centered approach. Update to a position statement of the American Diabetes Association (ADA) and the European Association for the Study of Diabetes (EASD), *Diabetes Care* 38:140–149, 2015.

Kaufman FR, editor: *Medical management of type 1 diabetes*, ed 6, Alexandria, Va, 2012, American Diabetes Association.

Kelley KW, Carroll DG, Meyer A: A review of current treatment strategies for gestational diabetes mellitus, *Drugs Context* 4:212282, 2015. doi:10.7573/dic.212282.

Laugesen E, Østergaard JA, Leslie RD: Latent autoimmune diabetes of the adult: current knowledge and uncertainty, *Diabet Med* 32(7):843–852, 2015. doi:10.1111/dme.12700.

Leete P, Willcox A, Krogvold L, et al: Differential insulitic profiles determine the extent of β-cell destruction and the age at onset of type 1 diabetes, *Diabetes* 65(5):1362–1369, 2016. doi:10.2337/db15-1615.

Leighton E, Sainsbury CA, Jones GC: A practical review of C-peptide testing in diabetes, *Diabetes Ther* 8(3):475–487, 2017. https://doi.org/10.1007/s13300-017-0265-4.

Leiper JB: Fate of ingested fluids: factors affecting gastric emptying and intestinal absorption of beverages in humans, *Nutr Rev* 73(Suppl 2):57–72, 2015.

Levy J, Cobas RA, Gomes MB: Assessment of efficacy and tolerability of once-daily extended release metformin in patients with type 2 diabetes mellitus, *Diabetol Metab Syndr* 2:16, 2010. doi:10.1186/1758-5996-2-16.

Li G, Zhang P, Wang J, et al: The long-term effect of lifestyle interventions to prevent diabetes in the China Da Qing Diabetes Prevention Study: a 20-year follow-up study, *Lancet* 371:1783–1789, 2008.

Lindström J, Ilanne-Parikka P, Peltonen M, et al: Sustained reduction in the incidence of type 2 diabetes by lifestyle intervention: follow-up of the Finnish Diabetes Prevention Study, *Lancet* 368:1673–1679, 2006.

Linus Pauling Institute: *Micronutrient Information Center: Chromium*. http://lpi.oregonstate.edu/mic/minerals/chromium. Published January 1, 2018.

Linus Pauling Institute Online: *Micronutrient Information Center: Lipoic Acid*. http://lpi.oregonstate.edu/mic/dietary-factors/lipoic-acid. Published 2002.

Look AHEAD Research Group: Long-term effects of a lifestyle intervention on weight and cardiovascular risk factors in individuals with type 2 diabetes mellitus: four-year results of the Look AHEAD trial, *Arch Intern Med* 170:1566–1575, 2010.

Low Wang CC, Hess CN, Hiatt WR, et al: Clinical update: cardiovascular disease in diabetes mellitus: atherosclerotic cardiovascular disease and heart failure in type 2 diabetes mellitus - mechanisms, management, and clinical considerations, *Circulation* 133(24):2459–2502, 2016. doi:10.1161/CIRCULATIONAHA.116.022194.

Ludwig DS, Hu FB, Tappy L, et al: Dietary carbohydrates: role of quality and quantity in chronic disease, *BMJ* 361:k2340, 2018. doi:10.1136/bmj.k2340.

Ma Y, Olendzki BC, Merriam PA, et al: A randomized clinical trial comparing low-glycemic index versus ADA dietary education among individuals with type 2 diabetes, *Nutrition* 24:45–56, 2008.

Malik VS, Popkin BM, Bray GA, et al: Sugar-sweetened beverages and risk of metabolic syndrome and type 2 diabetes: a meta-analysis, *Diabetes Care* 33:2477–2483, 2010.

Mann T, Tomiyama AJ, Westling E, et al: Medicare's search for effective obesity treatments: diets are not the answer, *Am Psychol* 62(3):220–233, 2007. doi:10.1037/0003-066X.62.3.220.

Mayer-Davis EJ, Lawrence JM, Dabelea D, et al: Incidence trends of type 1 and type 2 diabetes among youths, 2002–2012, *N Engl J Med* 376:1419–1429, 2017. doi:10.1056/NEJMoa1610187.

Mohan M, Baagar KAM, Lindow S: Management of diabetic ketoacidosis in pregnancy, *Obstet Gynaecol* 19(1):55-62, 2017. doi:10.1111/tog.12344.

Naik RG, Brooks-Worrell BM, Palmer JP: Latent autoimmune diabetes in adults, *J Clin Endocrinol Metab* 94:4635–4644, 2009.

Nathan DM: The diabetes control and complications trial/epidemiology of diabetes interventions and complications study at 30 years: overview, *Diabetes Care* 37:9–16, 2014.

Natural Medicines Database: *Chromium professional monograph*, Stockton, CA, 2019, TRC Natural Medicines. Available at: https://naturalmedicines.therapeuticresearch.com/databases/food-herbs-supplements/professional.aspx?productid=932.

O'Keefe EL, DiNicolantonio JJ, O'Keefe JH, et al: Alcohol and CV Health: Jekyll and Hyde J-Curves, *Prog Cardiovasc Dis* 61(1):68–75, 2018.

Pasquel FJ, Umpierrez GE: Hyperosmolar hyperglycemic state: a historic review of the clinical presentation, diagnosis, and treatment, *Diabetes Care* 37(11):3124-3131, 2014. doi:10.2337/dc14-0984.

Pastors JG, Franz MJ: Effectiveness of medical nutrition therapy in diabetes. In Franz MJ, Evert AB, editors: *American Diabetes Association guide to nutrition therapy for diabetes*, ed 2, Alexandria, VA, 2012, American Diabetes Association, p 1.

Phelan S: Windows of opportunity for lifestyle interventions to prevent gestational diabetes mellitus, *Am J Perinatol* 33(13):1291–1299, 2016. doi:10.1055/s-0036-1586504.

Post RE, Mainous AG, King DE, et al: Dietary fiber for the treatment of type 2 diabetes mellitus: a meta-analysis, *J Am Board Fam Med* 25(1):16–23, 2012. doi:10.3122/jabfm.2012.01.110148.

Reader D: Nutrition therapy for pregnancy, lactation, and diabetes. In Franz MJ, Evert AB, editors: *American Diabetes Association guide to nutrition therapy for diabetes*, ed 2, Alexandria, VA, 2012, American Diabetes Association, p 181.

Recarti C, Sep SJ, Stehouwer CD, et al: Excess cardiovascular risk in diabetic women: a case for intensive treatment, *Curr Hypertens Rep* 17(6):554, 2015. doi:10.1007/s11906-015-0554-0.

Reis JP, Loria CM, Sorlie PD, et al: Lifestyle factors and risk for new-onset diabetes: a population-based cohort study, *Ann Intern Med* 155:292–299, 2011.

Schauer PR, Bhatt DL, Kirwan JP, et al: Bariatric surgery versus intensive medical therapy for diabetes—3-year outcomes, *N Engl J Med* 370: 2002–2013, 2014.

Sharma S, Agrawal RP, Choudhary M, et al: Beneficial effect of chromium supplementation on glucose, HbA1C and lipid variables in individuals with newly onset type-2 diabetes, *J Trace Elem Med Biol* 25(3):149–153, 2011. doi:10.1016/j.jtemb.2011.03.003.

Springer SC, Silverstein J, Copeland K, et al: Management of type 2 diabetes mellitus in children and adolescents, *Pediatrics* 131:e648–e664, 2013.

Stanley K: Nutrition therapy for older adults with diabetes. In Franz MJ, Evert AB, editors: *American Diabetes Association guide to nutrition therapy for diabetes*, ed 2, Alexandria, VA, 2012, American Diabetes Association, p 169.

Swift CS: Nutrition therapy for the hospitalized and long-term care patient with diabetes. In Franz MJ, Evert AB, editors: *American Diabetes Association guide to nutrition therapy for diabetes*, ed 2, Alexandria, VA, 2012, American Diabetes Association, p 229.

Tsenkova VK, Carr D, Schoeller DA, et al: Perceived weight discrimination amplifies the link between central adiposity and nondiabetic glycemic control (HBA1C), *Ann Behav Med* 41(2):243–251, 2011. doi:10.1007/s12160-010-9238-9.

U.S. Department of Health and Human Services, U.S. Department of Agriculture: *Dietary guidelines for Americans 2015–2020*, ed 8, December 2015. https://health.gov/dietaryguidelines/2015/guidelines/.

U.S. Food & Drug Administration: *Additional information about high-intensity sweeteners permitted for use in food in the United States.* https://www.fda.gov/food/ingredientspackaginglabeling/foodadditivesingredients/ucm397725.htm#. Updated February 8, 2018.

Westerberg DP: Diabetic ketoacidosis: evaluation and treatment, *Am Fam Physician* 87(5):337–346, 2013.

Yang W, Dall TM, Beronjia K, et al: Economic costs of diabetes in the U.S. in 2017, *Diabetes Care* 41(5):917–928, 2018. doi:10.2337/dci18-0007.

Yin J, Xing H, Ye J: Efficacy of berberine in patients with type 2 diabetes mellitus, *Metabolism* 57(5):712–717, 2008. doi:10.1016/j.metabol.2008.01.013.

Youssef G: Nutrition therapy and prediabetes. In Franz MJ, Evert AB, editors: *American Diabetes Association guide to nutrition therapy for diabetes*, ed 2, Alexandria, VA, 2012, American Diabetes Association, pp 469–500.

Ziegler D, Low PA, Litchy WJ, et al: Efficacy and safety of antioxidant treatment with α-lipoic acid over 4 years in diabetic polyneuropathy: the NATHAN 1 trial, *Diabetes Care* 34(9):2054–2060, 2011. doi:10.2337/dc11-0503.

30

Medical Nutrition Therapy for Thyroid, Adrenal, and Other Endocrine Disorders

Sheila Dean, DSc, RDN, LDN, CCN, IFMCP

KEY TERMS

5-deiodinase
Addison's disease
adrenal fatigue
autoimmune thyroid disorders (AITDs)
calcitonin
cortisol
cretinism
euthyroid sick syndrome
free T$_4$
goitrin
Graves' disease

Hashimoto's thyroiditis
hyperthyroidism
hypothalamic-pituitary-thyroid axis (HPT axis)
hypothalamus
hypothyroidism
pituitary gland
polycystic ovary syndrome (PCOS)
reverse T$_3$ (rT$_3$)
Schmidt's syndrome
thyroglobulin antibodies (TGB Ab)

thyroid-binding globulin (TBG)
thyroid peroxidase (TPO)
thyroid peroxidase antibodies (TPO Ab)
thyroid-stimulating hormone (TSH)
thyrotoxicosis
thyrotropin-releasing hormone (TRH)
thyroxine (T$_4$)
triiodothyronine (T$_3$)
tyrosine

Diabetes mellitus is the most common endocrine-related chronic disease (Centers for Disease Control and Prevention [CDC], 2018; National Institutes of Health [NIH] MedlinePlus, 2018). However, according to a comprehensive review of the prevalence and incidence of endocrine and metabolic disorders in the United States (2009), about 5% of the U.S. population age 12 and older has hypothyroidism, and more than half remain undiagnosed. Furthermore, individuals with diabetes tend to have a higher prevalence of thyroid disorders. According to National Health and Nutrition Examination Survey (NHANES) data, the largest community-based study of thyroid function in the United States, the prevalence of high serum thyroid-stimulating hormone (a marker for underfunctioning thyroid) was 2% in people aged 60 to 69 years, 6% in those aged 70 to 79 years, and 10% in those aged 80 years and older (Hollowell et al, 2002).

In an analysis that examined thyroid disease risk among multiple ethnicities in the U.S. military, the incident rate for thyroid disease, specifically Graves' disease (autoimmune hyperthyroid), was significantly higher among blacks and Asian/Pacific Islanders. The incidence of autoimmune hypothyroid, Hashimoto's thyroiditis, was highest in whites and lowest in blacks and Asian/Pacific Islanders (McLeod et al, 2014).

In a study that examined gender, race, and socioeconomic influence on diagnosis and treatment of thyroid disorders in Brazilians, frequency of hypothyroidism treatment was higher in women and highly educated participants and those with high net family incomes. Frequency of hyperthyroidism treatment was higher in older than in younger individuals. Sociodemographic factors strongly influenced the diagnosis and treatment of thyroid disorders, including the use of levothyroxine (Olmos et al, 2015).

Thyroid-related diseases often are poorly diagnosed, and much about their treatment requires greater clarification and study. For example, radiation exposure of the thyroid at a young age is a risk factor for the development of thyroid cancer, lasting for a lifetime after exposure (Sinnott et al, 2010). Efforts to reduce exposure from medical x-ray examinations can protect the thyroid gland.

Genetic factors are implicated in endocrine autoimmune diseases. Recent genome-wide association studies (GWAS) have enabled identification of relevant immune response pathways; the same allele that predisposes someone to a certain autoimmune disease can be protective in another (Wiebolt et al, 2010). Thus endocrine GWAS are needed, especially for Graves' disease, Hashimoto's thyroiditis, and Addison's disease. Each of these disorders has stages beginning with genetic susceptibility, environmental triggers, and active autoimmunity, followed by metabolic derangements with overt symptoms of disease (Michels and Eisenbarth, 2010). Research is needed to clarify how nutrients interact with genetics, especially in these autoimmune thyroid disorders (AITDs).

THYROID PHYSIOLOGY

The thyroid gland is a small, butterfly-shaped gland found just below the Adam's apple. Although it weighs less than an ounce, it produces hormones that influence essentially every organ, tissue, and cell in the body, thus having an enormous effect on health. The thyroid gland responds to thyroid-stimulating hormone (TSH), a hormone secreted by the pituitary gland. When stimulated, the thyroid gland produces two main hormones: thyroxine (T$_4$), a thyroid hormone named for its four molecules of iodine, and triiodothyronine (T$_3$), a thyroid hormone named for its three molecules of iodine. T$_3$ is the most predominant and active form of thyroid hormone that the body can use. The thyroid gland regulates many processes in the body, including fat and carbohydrate metabolism, body temperature, and heart rate. The thyroid also produces calcitonin, a hormone that helps regulate the amount of blood calcium. Reverse T$_3$ (rT$_3$), an isomer of

T_3, is derived from T_4 through the action of deiodinase. Although the body cannot use rT_3, it is not simply an inactive metabolite with no physiologic effect on the body. This will be discussed more later in the chapter. Common reasons for elevated rT_3 include inadequate iron levels, chronic inflammation, elevated cortisol, and liver abnormalities (Gomes-Lima and Burman, 2018).

The synthesis of these hormones requires tyrosine, a key amino acid involved in the production of thyroid hormone, and the trace mineral iodine. Within the cells of the thyroid gland, iodide is oxidized to iodine by hydrogen peroxide, a reaction termed the *organification* of iodide. Two additional molecules of iodine bind to the tyrosyl ring in a reaction that involves thyroid peroxidase (TPO), an enzyme in the thyroid responsible for thyroid hormone production. Completed thyroid hormones are released into the circulation; however, metabolic effects of thyroid hormones result when the hormones ultimately occupy specific thyroid receptors. It is estimated that a cell needs five to seven times more T_4 to bind to the nuclear receptors to have a physiologic effect compared with the more biologically active T_3.

The biosynthetic processes resulting in the creation of thyroid hormones within the thyroid gland are controlled by feedback mechanisms within the hypothalamic-pituitary-thyroid axis (HPT axis). The HPT axis is part of the endocrine system responsible for the regulation of metabolism. As its name suggests, it depends on the hypothalamus (a tiny, cone-shaped structure located in the lower center of the brain that communicates between the nervous and endocrine systems), the pituitary gland (the master gland of the endocrine system located at the base of the brain), and the thyroid gland (Fig. 30.1).

The hypothalamus produces and secretes thyrotropin-releasing hormone (TRH), which travels to the pituitary gland, stimulating it to release TSH, which signals the thyroid gland to upregulate its synthetic machinery. Although T_4, T_3, and rT_3 are generated within the thyroid gland, T_4 is quantitatively the major secretory product. All T_4 found in circulation is generated in the thyroid unless exogenously administered via thyroid replacement medication (see Table 30.2). Production

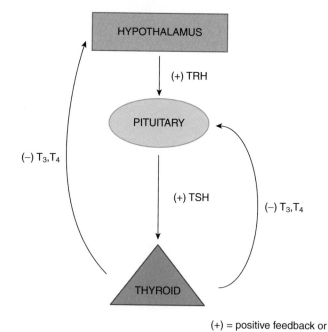

Fig. 30.1 The hypothalamus-pituitary-thyroid axis. *TRH*, Thyrotropin-releasing hormone; *TSH*, thyroid-stimulating hormone.

of T_3 and rT_3 within the thyroid is relegated to very small quantities and is not considered significant compared with peripheral production in other body tissues (Fig. 30.2).

When T_4 is released from the thyroid, it is primarily in a bound form with thyroid-binding globulin (TBG), a protein that transports thyroid hormones through the bloodstream, with lesser amounts bound

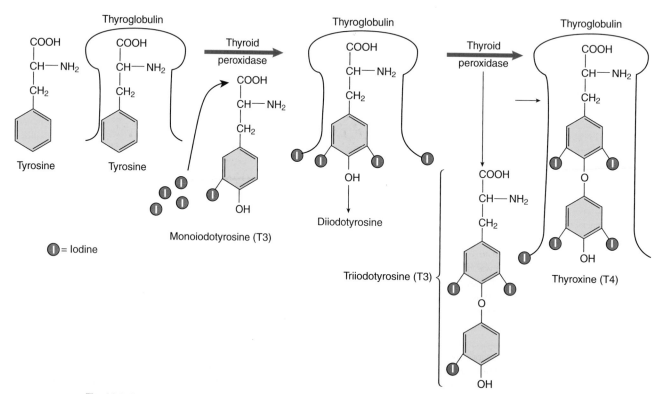

Fig. 30.2 Constructing thyroid hormones. (1) Accumulation of the raw materials tyrosine and iodide (I-), (2) fabrication or synthesis of the hormone, and (3) secretion of hormone into the blood either bound or as free T_4.

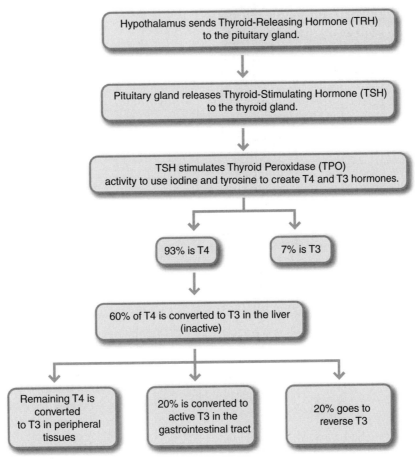

Fig. 30.3 Thyroid metabolism.

to T_4-binding prealbumin. It is estimated that only 0.03% to 0.05% of T_4 within the circulatory system is in a free or unbound form; this unbound T_4 is called free T_4. In peripheral tissues, approximately 70% of T_4 is converted to T_3 or rT_3 or eliminated. As mentioned, T_3 is considered to be the most metabolically active thyroid hormone. Although some T_3 is produced in the thyroid, approximately 80% to 85% is generated outside the thyroid gland, primarily by conversion via a deiodinase enzyme from T_4 to T_3 in the liver and kidneys. The pituitary and nervous system are also capable of converting T_4 to T_3, and so are not reliant on T_3 produced in the liver or kidney. Within the liver and kidney, the enzyme responsible for production of T_3 is a selenium-dependent enzyme called 5-deiodinase, an enzyme that removes one molecule of iodine from T_4 to form either T_3 or rT_3 (Fig. 30.3).

ASSESSMENT IN THYROID DISORDERS

Assessment begins with an evaluation of thyroid status based on laboratory data such as a full thyroid panel. In the absence of a full thyroid panel, a serum thyrotropin (also known as TSH) is the single best screening test for primary thyroid dysfunction for the vast majority of outpatient clinical situations (Garber et al, 2012). A TSH test does not screen for autoimmune disease. If autoimmune thyroid disease is suspected, additional tests must be done (described more below). Assessments also may include a diet history to evaluate micronutrients pertaining to thyroid health along with an evaluation of calorie and carbohydrate intake. In addition, an assessment of dietary intake of goitrogenic (thyroid-inhibiting) foods may be warranted.

Laboratory Norms: Functional versus Pathologic Ranges

A typical (statistical) reference range for TSH in many laboratories is approximately 0.2 to 5.5 mIU/L. Individuals with TSH values greater than 2 mIU/L have an increased risk of developing overt hypothyroidism during the next 20 years. Subclinical autoimmune thyroid disease is so common in the population that laboratory reference ranges derived from testing apparently healthy subjects easily could be misconstrued for those with disease. Importantly, several studies have detected an increase in thyroid antibody positivity with TSH concentrations outside the narrow range of 0.2 to 1.9 mIU/L (Fjaellagaard et al, 2015). This fact provides evidence that TSH in the upper reference range often is associated with abnormal pathologic findings (Hak et al, 2000; Khandelwal and Tandon, 2012; Saravanan et al, 2002), mitochondrial dysfunction, and morphologic skeletal muscle alterations including myalgia, muscle cramps, and weakness (Dunn et al, 2009). Additional evidence that thyroid function within the laboratory reference ranges can be associated with adverse outcomes is shown in Table 30.1. Conversely, decreased TSH levels combined with normal-to-high T_4 or T_3 levels may be suggestive of hyperthyroidism (see Thyroid Function Tests in Appendix 13).

Changes in 5-deiodination occur in a number of situations, such as stress, poor nutrition, illness, selenium deficiency, and certain drug therapies. Toxic metals such as cadmium, mercury, and lead have been associated with impaired hepatic 5-deiodination in animal models. (Soldin et al, 2008). Free radicals are also involved in inhibition of 5-deiodinase activity. In the course of chronic liver disease such as hepatic cirrhosis, alterations in hepatic deiodination resulting in

TABLE 30.1 Variation in Thyroid Function Within Reference Range and Adverse Outcomes

TSH >2 mIU/L*	Increased 20-year risk of hypothyroidism
TSH >2 mIU/L*	Increased frequency of thyroid autoantibodies
TSH >4 mIU/L*	Increased risk of heart disease
TSH 2-4 mIU/L*	Cholesterol values respond to thyroxine replacement
Free T$_4$ <10.4 pmol/L†	Impaired psychomotor development of infant if occurs in first trimester of pregnancy

T_3, Thyroxine; *TSH*, thyroid-stimulating hormone.
*Typical reference ranges: TSH 0.2-5.5 mIU/L
†Typical reference ranges: free T$_4$ 9.8-25 pmol/L

BOX 30.1 5-Deiodinase Inhibitors

Selenium deficiency
Inadequate protein, excess carbohydrates
High insulin
Chronic illness
Stress (cortisol)
Cd, Hg, Pb, and other heavy metal toxins
Compromised liver or kidney function

increased rT$_3$ and a simultaneous decrease in T$_3$ levels also have been observed (Box 30.1 and see Chapter 28).

HYPOTHYROIDISM

Of the detected cases of hypothyroidism (underactive thyroid) more than half are due to an autoimmune disorder called Hashimoto's thyroiditis, in which the immune system attacks and destroys thyroid gland tissue. A common clinical presentation of patients with functional changes of the endocrine system is altered thyroid function. Indeed *subclinical* hypothyroidism represents the first signs of thyroid hormone dysfunction for many individuals. Typical symptoms include low energy, cold hands and feet, fatigue, hypercholesterolemia, muscle pain, depression, and cognitive deficits (Box 30.2). Evaluation of thyroid hormone metabolism is needed before thyroid hormone replacement therapy.

BOX 30.2 Common Symptoms of Hypothyroidism and Hyperthyroidism

Hypothyroidism	Hyperthyroidism
Fatigue	Heat intolerance, sweating
Forgetfulness	Weight loss
Depression	Alterations in appetite
Heavy menses	Frequent bowel movements
Dry, coarse hair	Changes in vision
Mood swings	Fatigue and muscle weakness
Weight gain	Menstrual disturbance
Hoarse voice	Impaired fertility
Dry, coarse skin	Mental disturbances
Constipation	Sleep disturbances
	Tremors
	Thyroid enlargement

From Shomon M: *Thyroid Disease Symptoms—Hypothyroidism and Hyperthyroidism* (website): http://thyroid.about.com/cs/basics_starthere/a/symptoms.htm, 2008.

Women are five to eight times more likely than men to suffer from hypothyroidism. In addition, individuals who have celiac disease may be at risk (see *Clinical Insight: Was It Gluten That Caused Her Hypothyroidism?*)

CLINICAL INSIGHT

Gluten and Hypothyroidism

A case report described a 23-year-old woman with a diagnosis of hypothyroidism caused by Hashimoto's thyroiditis and autoimmune Addison's disease who was found in evaluation to have elevated antiendomysial antibody levels (a marker of celiac disease [CD]). During a 3-month period on a gluten-free diet, the patient demonstrated remarkable clinical improvement in her gastrointestinal (GI)-related symptoms and, more importantly, in her thyroid function. She required progressively less thyroid and adrenal replacement therapy. After 6 months, her endomysial antibody level became negative, her antithyroid antibody titer decreased significantly, and thyroid medication was discontinued. This case report points out the potential important effect of a gluten-free diet on thyroid function, especially in the presence of CD.

A number of studies show the importance of gluten in the induction of endocrine autoantibodies and organ system dysfunction in adolescent celiac patients (Cassio et al, 2010; Meloni et al, 2009). Furthermore, the genetic risk for CD is largely related to human leukocyte antigen genotypes, which in turn is linked to autoimmune thyroid disease (Barker and Liu, 2008). According to the international medical bibliography, autoimmune Hashimoto's thyroiditis and CD are clearly associated (Freeman, 2016). This might be explained partly by the increased immunosensitivity of CD patients, as part of an autoimmune polyglandular syndrome (APS), by the deficiency of key elements such as selenium and iodine due to malabsorption (Stazi and Trinti, 2010) or due to antibodies that affect both target-tissues (Naiyer et al, 2008). Based on recommendations from a recent meta-analysis, all patients with autoimmune Hashimoto's thyroiditis should be screened for CD, given the increased prevalence of the coexistence of these two disorders (Roy et al, 2016). This study advocates that patients with Hashimoto's thyroiditis undergo celiac serologic tests (serum IgA and IgG gliadin antibodies [AGA-IgA, AGA-IgG], IgA transglutaminase antibodies [TGA], and serum IgA endomysium antibodies [EMA]), and that if any of the celiac serologic tests is positive, the patients must be investigated with gastroduodenoscopy and duodenal biopsy. It must be considered that positive thyroid and celiac tests might represent an epiphenomenon because serum autoantibodies generally do not reflect a clinical autoimmune disease (Liontiris and Mazokopakis, 2017). It has been reported that gluten-dependent diabetes and thyroidal-related antibodies were found in patients with CD but were eliminated after the implementation of a gluten-free diet (Duntas, 2009). A gluten-free diet may be warranted in cases of Hashimoto's thyroiditis, as the mounting evidence shows that the avoidance of gluten may reduce inflammation and auto-antibody titers. See Chapter 27 for additional information about CD.

Pathophysiology

Hashimoto's thyroiditis is an autoimmune disorder in which the immune system attacks and destroys the thyroid gland. It is the most common form of hypothyroidism. The enlarged, chronically inflamed thyroid gland becomes nonfunctional, with reactive parts of the gland deteriorating after several years. Thyroid autoantibodies indicate the body's immune system is attacking itself and whether an autoimmune thyroid condition is present, be it hypothyroidism or hyperthyroidism, Epstein-Barr virus (EBV) has been implicated as a critical underlying factor in autoimmune thyroid disease. Janegova et al (2015) demonstrated a high prevalence of EBV infection in cases of Hashimoto's thyroiditis (80.7%) as well as in samples of Graves' disease (62.5%).

Specific antibody tests identify Hashimoto's thyroiditis. Thyroid peroxidase antibodies (TPO Ab) are immune cells that indicate the immune system is attacking TPO in the thyroid gland. The TPO Ab test is the most important because TPO is the enzyme responsible for the production of thyroid hormones, and the most frequent target of attack in Hashimoto's. Thyroglobulin antibodies (TGB Ab) are immune cells that indicate the immune system is attacking thyroglobulin in the thyroid gland. Sometimes this test is necessary as well because it is the second most common target for Hashimoto's disease.

Schmidt's syndrome refers to hypothyroidism with other endocrine disorders, including Addison's disease (adrenal insufficiency), hypoparathyroidism, and diabetes mellitus, all of which may be autoimmune in nature. Euthyroid sick syndrome is hypothyroidism associated with a severe systemic illness that causes decreased peripheral conversion of T_4 to T_3, an increased conversion of T_3 to the inactive rT_3, and decreased binding of thyroid hormones. Conditions commonly associated with this syndrome include protein-calorie malnutrition, surgical trauma, myocardial infarction, chronic renal failure, diabetic ketoacidosis, anorexia nervosa, cirrhosis, thermal injury, and sepsis. Once the underlying cause is treated, the condition usually is resolved (see *Pathophysiology and Care Management Algorithm: Thyroid Dysfunction*).

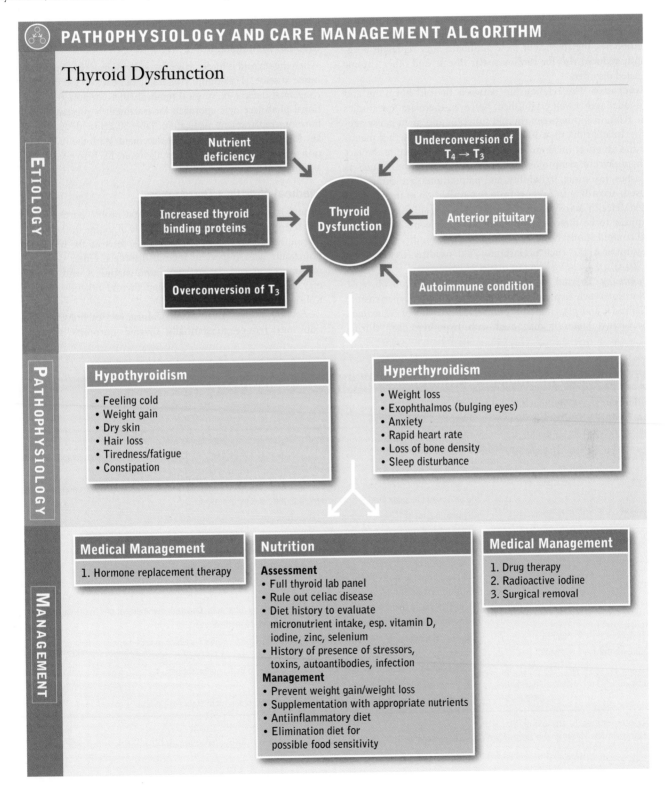

PATHOPHYSIOLOGY AND CARE MANAGEMENT ALGORITHM

Thyroid Dysfunction

ETIOLOGY

- Nutrient deficiency
- Underconversion of $T_4 \rightarrow T_3$
- Increased thyroid binding proteins
- Thyroid Dysfunction
- Anterior pituitary
- Overconversion of T_3
- Autoimmune condition

PATHOPHYSIOLOGY

Hypothyroidism
- Feeling cold
- Weight gain
- Dry skin
- Hair loss
- Tiredness/fatigue
- Constipation

Hyperthyroidism
- Weight loss
- Exophthalmos (bulging eyes)
- Anxiety
- Rapid heart rate
- Loss of bone density
- Sleep disturbance

MANAGEMENT

Medical Management
1. Hormone replacement therapy

Nutrition

Assessment
- Full thyroid lab panel
- Rule out celiac disease
- Diet history to evaluate micronutrient intake, esp. vitamin D, iodine, zinc, selenium
- History of presence of stressors, toxins, autoantibodies, infection

Management
- Prevent weight gain/weight loss
- Supplementation with appropriate nutrients
- Antiinflammatory diet
- Elimination diet for possible food sensitivity

Medical Management
1. Drug therapy
2. Radioactive iodine
3. Surgical removal

Triggers

Adrenal dysfunction and oxidative stress. Low thyroid function is almost always secondary to some other condition, often adrenal dysfunction (Kaltsas et al, 2010) (see Adrenal Disorders later in this chapter).

Aging. Maintaining thyroid hormone function throughout the aging process appears to be an important hallmark of healthy aging. The incidence of hypothyroidism (underactive thyroid) increases with age. By age 60, 9% to 17% of men and women have an underactive thyroid. The absence of circulating thyroid autoantibodies in healthy centenarians is noted. Because unhealthy aging is associated with a progressively increasing prevalence of organ-specific and non-organ-specific autoantibodies, the absence of these antibodies may represent a significantly reduced risk for cardiovascular disease and other chronic age-related disorders.

Menopause. The relationship between thyroid hormone and the gonadal axis is well established; however, there are few studies on the relationship between thyroid function and menopause specifically. In addition, they do not necessarily clarify whether menopause has an effect on thyroid regardless of aging, despite the fact that hypothyroid symptoms and menopause symptoms (such as hot flashes, insomnia, irritability, and palpitations) are commonly confused. According to a report from the evaluation of the Study of Women's Health Across the Nation (SWAN), thyroid function does not appear to be directly involved in the pathogenesis of menopausal complications; however, menopause may modify the clinical expression of AITDs such as Hashimoto's thyroiditis (Del Ghianda et al, 2014).

Pregnancy. Thyroid dysfunction has been related to obstetric complications such as premature delivery, gestational hypertension, preeclampsia, and placental abruption. Nearly 1 out of 50 women in the United States is diagnosed with hypothyroidism during pregnancy. Out of every 100 miscarriages, six are associated with thyroid hormone deficiency during pregnancy, up to 18% of women are diagnosed with postpartum thyroiditis, and approximately 25% of women develop permanent hypothyroidism (De Vivo et al, 2010; Yassa et al, 2010).

Global recommendations for iodine during pregnancy are 130-250 mcg/d depending on the country. In areas of severe iodine deficiency, maternal and fetal hypothyroxinemia can cause cretinism (condition of stunted physical growth and mental development). To prevent fetal damage, dietary iodine adequacy is essential during pregnancy (see Chapter 14 and Table 14.8) (Zimmermann, 2009).

Medical Management

When the thyroid is underactive (hypothyroidism) because of autoimmune disease (Hashimoto's disease), radioactive iodine treatment, congenital defects, or surgical removal (thyroidectomy), the conventional pharmacologic approach for treatment is prescription thyroid hormone replacement medication. Table 30.2 provides an overview of key forms of thyroid hormone replacement. With the further elucidation of the effects of genetics, new agents are likely to become available as adjunct therapy.

Medical Nutrition Therapy

Several nutrients are involved in thyroid health, particularly iodine and selenium. Because of the critical role of iodine in the synthesis of thyroid hormone, this trace mineral has received the most attention historically with respect to thyroid disorders. Other deficiencies of micronutrients such as iron, selenium, vitamin A, and possibly zinc may interact with iodine status and thyroid function (Hess, 2010; Köhrle, 2013).

Fasting or restrictive diets. Calorie and carbohydrate restriction may reduce substantially thyroid hormone activity. This

TABLE 30.2 Pharmacologic Treatments for Hypothyroidism

Medication Brand Name	Medication Generic Name	Use and Comments
Synthroid, Levoxyl	Levothyroxine—(synthetic T_4)	Most commonly prescribed synthetic form of thyroid hormone replacement drug (thyroxine) that provides a steady dose of T_4 for the body to convert to T_3. Available in a wide range of doses. Inactive ingredients include lactose and cornstarch.
Tirosint	Levothyroxine	A synthetic form of replacement hormone that includes only three inactive ingredients: gelatin, glycerin, and water. Is produced in a dedicated facility to eliminate the risk of cross-exposure.
Cytomel	Liothyronine—(synthetic T_3)	Synthetic form of T_3, which can also be compounded. Sometimes prescribed in addition to T_4. Only effective for approximately 10 hours and must be taken twice daily.
Armour Thyroid	Desiccated natural thyroid	Prepared from dried or powdered porcine (pig) or mixed beef and pork thyroid gland for therapeutic use. Available by prescription and frequently used as an alternative to synthetic thyroid drugs. All brands contain a mixture of approximately 80% T_4 and 20% T_3. Difficult to standardize. Compounded T_3 medication is available as a time-released formula. Compounded medications are frequently not insurance covered but are less expensive than standard medications.
WP Thyroid, Nature-Throid	Desiccated natural thyroid	Provides the full range of thyroid hormones, including T_4, T_3, T_2, and T_1, which may be beneficial for those who have difficulty with T_4-T_3 conversion. Available in 8-13 different strengths, ranging from low to high concentrations.
Thyrolar	Liotrix—(synthetic T_4-T_3 combination)	Synthetic combination of T_4 and T_3. Sometimes used in lieu of Armour Thyroid because of problem with standardization.

T_3, Triiodothyronine; T_4, thyroxine.
From Shomon M: *What is the best thyroid drug?* (website): http://thyroid.about.com/cs/thyroiddrugs/a/bestdrug.htm, 2014.

varies widely between individuals. Genetics, obesity, gender, and the macronutrient content of the hypocaloric diet influence the response. Nutritional status and energy expenditure influence thyroid function centrally at the level of TSH secretion, deiodination, and possibly elsewhere. Because an increase of rT_3 is found at the expense of T_3 during caloric restriction, it is possible that the hepatic pathways play a substantial role in metabolic control during energy balance. However, when caloric restriction is longer than 3 weeks, T_4 and rT_3 levels return to normal values (De Vries et al, 2015).

Fasting also exerts a powerful influence on the metabolism of thyroid hormones to save energy and limit catabolism. Mild elevations in endogenous cortisol levels may be partly responsible. Fasting decreases serum T_3 and T_4 concentrations, whereas intrahepatic thyroid hormone concentrations remain unchanged. However, ketones generated from calorie deprivation do not appear to suppress T_3 generation and hepatic 5-deiodinase activity. It appears that fasting-induced changes in liver thyroid hormone metabolism are not regulated via the hepatic autonomic input in a major way and more likely reflect a direct effect of humoral factors (factors that are transported by the circulatory system) on the hepatocyte. Overall during fasting, there is a down regulation of the HPT axis, which is assumed to represent an energy-saving mechanism, instrumental in times of food shortage (De Vries et al, 2015).

Goitrogens. Cyanogenic plant foods (cauliflower, broccoli, cabbage, Brussels sprouts, mustard seed, turnip, radish, bamboo shoot, and cassava) exert antithyroid activity through inhibition of the TPO enzyme. The hydrolysis of bioactive compounds called glucosinolates found in cruciferous vegetables may yield goitrin, a compound known to interfere with thyroid hormone synthesis. The hydrolysis of indole glucosinolates results in the release of thiocyanate ions, which can compete with iodine for uptake by the thyroid gland. Increased exposure to thiocyanate ions from cruciferous vegetable consumption, however, does not increase the risk of hypothyroidism unless accompanied by iodine deficiency. However, steaming, cooking, or fermenting may reduce the levels of goitrogens in goitrogenic foods (Jagminder et al, 2016).

Soybean, an important source of protein in many developing countries, also has goitrogenic properties when iodine intake is limited. The isoflavones, genistein and daidzein, inhibit the activity of TPO and can lower thyroid hormone synthesis. Furthermore, excessive intake of soybeans may interrupt the enterohepatic cycle of thyroid hormone metabolism. However, high intakes of soy isoflavones do not appear to increase the risk of hypothyroidism when iodine consumption is adequate.

Since the addition of iodine to soy-based formulas in the 1960s, there have been no further reports of hypothyroidism developing in soy formula–fed infants. Soybeans are by far the most concentrated source of isoflavones in the human diet. Small amounts are found in a number of legumes, grains, and vegetables. Average dietary isoflavone intakes in Asian countries, in particular in Japan and China, range from 11 to 47 mg/day because of intake of the traditional foods made from soybeans, including tofu, tempeh, miso, and matte, whereas intakes are considerably lower in Western countries (2 mg/day). Soy products (meat substitutes, soy milk, soy cheese, and soy yogurt), however, are gaining popularity in Western countries. Although research has not determined the exact effect of soy on the metabolic fate of thyroid hormones, excessive soy consumption is best approached cautiously in those with suspected impairment of thyroid metabolic pathways.

Iodine. As a trace element, iodine is present in the human body in amounts of 10 to 15 mg, and 70% to 80% of it is located in the thyroid gland. Ninety percent of it is organically bound to a protein produced in the thyroid gland called thyroglobulin (Tg). Iodide is actively absorbed in the thyroid gland to help produce the biochemically active thyroid hormones T_4 and T_3 (see Fig. 30.2). The thyroid gland must capture an estimated minimum of 60 mcg of iodide (the ionic form of iodine) daily to ensure an adequate supply for the production of thyroid hormone (Gropper and Smith, 2012). Inadequate intake of iodine impairs thyroid function and results in a spectrum of disorders. Randomized controlled intervention trials in iodine-deficient populations have shown that providing iron along with iodine results in greater improvements in thyroid function and volume than providing iodine alone (Hess, 2010). It is also vital to thyroid function, as it is a major cofactor and stimulator for the enzyme TPO.

In autoimmune Hashimoto's thyroiditis, supplementing with iodine may exacerbate the condition. Because iodine stimulates production of TPO, this in turn increases the levels of TPO Abs dramatically, indicating an autoimmune flare-up. Some people develop symptoms of an overactive thyroid, whereas others have no symptoms despite tests showing an elevated level of TPO Abs. Therefore one must be cautious regarding the use of high-dose iodine; however, a clinical evaluation and/or assessment (such as UI excretion laboratories) may help reveal whether iodine supplementation is warranted. Furthermore, although iodine deficiency is the most common cause of hypothyroidism for most of the world's population (Melse-Boonstra and Jaiswal, 2010), in the United States and other Westernized countries, Hashimoto's thyroiditis accounts for the majority of cases (Ebert, 2010).

Although the risk of iodine deficiency for populations living in iodine-deficient areas without adequate iodine fortification programs is well recognized, concerns have been raised that certain subpopulations may not consume adequate iodine in countries considered iodine sufficient. Vegetarian and nonvegetarian diets that exclude iodized salt, fish, and seaweed have been found to contain very little iodine.

Iron. Historically it has been thought that low thyroid function may contribute to anemia. Recent studies suggest that low thyroid function may be secondary to low iron status or anemia. The reason for this is because TPO is a glycosylated heme enzyme that is iron dependent. The insertion of heme iron into TPO is necessary for the enzyme to translocate to the apical cell surface of thyrocytes (or thyroid epithelial cells), thus assisting TPO to catalyze the two initial steps of thyroid hormone synthesis. A full assessment of iron status could likely help to identify the cause of many cases of thyroid malfunction. Treatment of anemic women with impaired thyroid function with iron improves thyroid-hormone concentrations, while T_4 (hormone replacement medication) and iron together are more effective in improving iron status (Hu and Rayman, 2017).

Selenium. Selenium, as selenocysteine, is a cofactor for 5-deiodinase. If selenium is deficient, the deiodinase activity is impaired, resulting in a decreased ability to deiodinate T_4 to T_3. In animals, deficiencies of selenium are associated with impaired 5-deiodinase activity in the liver and kidney, as well as reduced T_3 levels. Evidence suggests a strong linear association between lower T_3/T_4 ratios and reduced selenium status, even among individuals considered to be euthyroid based on standard laboratory parameters. This association is particularly strong in older adults, possibly as the result of impaired peripheral conversion. An inverse relationship between T_3 and breast cancer is associated with decreased selenium status, even when plasma T_4 and TSH concentrations may be similar. This combination of factors strongly suggests that low T_3 may be due to faulty conversion of T_4 to T_3 expected in selenium deficiency (De Sibio et al, 2014).

Selenium participates in the antioxidant network. It is a cofactor for glutathione peroxidase, an enzyme whose main biologic role is to protect the organism from oxidative damage. Several studies reported on the benefit of selenium treatment in Hashimoto's thyroiditis and Graves' disease. According to a systematic review and meta-analysis studies, selenium supplementation reduced serum TPO Ab levels in patients with chronic autoimmune thyroiditis (AIT) (Wichman et al, 2016).

Evidence also suggests that excessive intakes of selenium may exert a detrimental influence on thyroid hormone metabolism. Although individuals exposed to high dietary levels of selenium typically have normal levels of T_4, T_3, and TSH, a significant inverse correlation has been found between T_3 and selenium. Some researchers have hypothesized that the activity of 5-deiodinase may become depressed after a high dietary intake of selenium, suggesting a safe level of dietary selenium at or below 500 mcg daily. There is evidence from observational studies and randomized controlled trials that selenium/selenoproteins can reduce TPO-antibody titers, hypothyroidism, and postpartum thyroiditis (Hu and Rayman, 2017). In a 2016 study on selenium supplementation, authors conclude that selenium supplementation (83 mcg of selenomethionine per day orally for 4 months) could restore euthyroidism (healthy thyroid hormone balance) in one third of subclinical hypothyroidism patients with AIT (Pirola et al, 2016).

Magnesium. Magnesium is the fourth most abundant mineral in the body. It has been recognized as a cofactor for more than 300 enzymatic reactions, where it is crucial for adenosine triphosphate (ATP) metabolism and cellular energy production. Low serum magnesium is associated with several chronic diseases including thyroid disease. A cross-sectional study of over 1200 Chinese participants revealed that severely low serum magnesium was associated with increased risks of positive antithyroglobulin antibody and hypothyroidism. The risks of Hashimoto's thyroiditis diagnosed using ultrasonography in the lowest quartile group were higher than those in the adequate magnesium group (0.851 to 1.15mmol/L) ($p<0.01$, odds ratios [ORs] = 2.748 to 3.236). The risks of total and subclinical-only hypothyroidism in the lowest quartile group were higher than those in the adequate magnesium group (0.851 to 1.15mmol/L) ($p < 0.01$, ORs = 4.482 to 4.971) (Wang et al, 2018).

Ideal intake for magnesium should be based on the DRI. Magnesium supplements are available as magnesium oxide, magnesium chloride, magnesium citrate, magnesium taurate, magnesium orotate, as well as other amino acid chelates. In the treatment of magnesium deficiency, organic bound magnesium salts, such as magnesium citrate, gluconate, orotate, or aspartate recommendations were made due to their high bioavailability (Kisters, 2013).

Vitamin D. Lower vitamin D status has been found in Hashimoto's thyroiditis patients than in controls, and inverse relationships of serum vitamin D with TPO/TGB Ab have been reported. However, other data and the lack of trial evidence suggest that low vitamin D status is more likely the result of autoimmune disease processes that include vitamin D receptor dysfunction (Hu and Rayman, 2017).

Oral vitamin D supplementation was found to reduce titers of thyroid antibodies in levothyroxine-treated women with postpartum thyroiditis and low vitamin D status. Vitamin D increased serum levels of 25-hydroxy vitamin D, as well as reduced titers of thyroid antibodies. This effect was more pronounced for TPO than

for TGB Ab and correlated with their baseline titers. Authors concluded that vitamin D preparations may reduce thyroid autoimmunity in levothyroxine-treated women with Hashimoto's thyroiditis and normal vitamin D status (Krysiak et al, 2017). Taking into consideration the low cost and the minimal side effects of vitamin D supplementation, screening for vitamin D deficiency and careful vitamin D supplementation with monthly monitoring calcium and 25-hydroxy vitamin D levels, when required, may be recommended for patients with Hashimoto's thyroiditis (Liontiris and Mazokopakis, 2017).

Management of Thyroid Disorders During Pregnancy

The American Thyroid Association recommendations on diagnosis and management of thyroid disease during pregnancy and the postpartum period were reported in a review article in 2017 with the following guidelines (Kalra et al, 2017).

Hypothyroidism and Pregnancy
Laboratory Assessment
1. TSH assessment should be based on population-based trimester specific reference ranges, calculated from data of healthy pregnant women without history of thyroid disease, with optimal iodine intake, and negative TPO Ab status.
2. If pregnancy specific population-based data is not available, upper reference limit (URL) of 4.0 mU/L may be used.
3. A level 0.5mU/L lower than nonpregnant URL can also be taken as URL for TSH in pregnancy.
4. Serum T_4 (thyroxin) is a highly reliable marker for thyroid function in last trimester of pregnancy.

Preconception Investigations
1. Test TSH in all women presenting with infertility.
2. Test TSH either before, or 1 to 2 weeks after, controlled ovarian hyper stimulation (COHS).
3. Nonpregnant women with mild TSH elevation following COHS should undergo repeat testing after 2 to 4 weeks.
4. Test TSH at time of diagnosis of pregnancy, in euthyroid, antibody positive women.

Iodine Intake
1. Ensure iodine intake of 250 mg/day, at least 3 months before conception.
2. Such intake is not required in women who are on treatment for either hypo- or hyper-thyroidism.
3. Avoid iodine intake >500 mg/day.
4. Avoid iodine containing supplements in excess.

Additional Therapies
1. Selenium supplementation is not recommended for treatment of antibody positive pregnant women.
2. T_3 or desiccated thyroid is not recommended during pregnancy.

POLYCYSTIC OVARY SYNDROME

Polycystic ovary syndrome (PCOS) is a common endocrine disorder of unknown cause that affects an estimated 3% to 12% of women of reproductive age in Western societies (Moran et al, 2010; Velez and Motta, 2014). The condition is characterized by reproductive issues such as amenorrhea or other menstrual irregularities, anovulation, enlarged ovaries with multiple cysts, and infertility. More generalized symptoms include insulin resistance, acne, hirsutism (excessive or

TABLE 30.3 Nutrition Treatment for Polycystic Ovary Syndrome

Obesity	Institute weight management program of diet and exercise.
Insulin resistance	Restrict refined carbohydrates (low-glycemic index diet) and total calories. Increase high-fiber foods. Recommend small, frequent meals. Monitor carefully to ascertain benefit from high- versus low-carbohydrate diet. Consider supplementation with chromium picolinate.
Low serum 25 hydroxy vitamin D	Administer vitamin D_3 (cholecalciferol).
Clomiphene-citrate resistant infertility	Use short-term NAC as adjunct.
Laboratory or clinical evidence of hypothyroidism	Institute thyroid hormone replacement. Use foods or supplements with selenium and iodine.

NAC, N-acetylcysteine.

abnormal distribution of hair growth), male-pattern baldness, weight gain, and sleep apnea (Table 30.3).

Pathophysiology

Biochemical and endocrine abnormalities in women with PCOS include a hyperandrogenic state in which there is a higher concentration of free androgens (dehydroepiandrosterone, testosterone, and androstenedione) and decreased hepatic production of sex hormone binding globulin (Sirmans and Pate, 2013). In addition to the elevated levels of androgens, hyperinsulinemia (which results from insulin resistance), impaired glucose tolerance, and hyperlipidemia are seen. Hyperandrogenism is responsible for many of the symptoms of PCOS, such as reproductive and menstrual abnormalities, hirsutism, and acne. Elevated androgen levels, in turn, appear to be due in part to hyperinsulinemia, which triggers the increase in androgen production. Thus interventions that improve insulin resistance and hyperinsulinemia may reverse some of the manifestations of PCOS.

The insulin resistance seen in 50% to 70% of women with PCOS is unique in that it occurs independent of body weight to some extent and is not always corrected by weight loss. It appears to result from insulin receptor phosphorylation abnormalities in an insulin-mediated signaling pathway (Sirmans and Pate, 2013). Conventional treatment of PCOS includes diet and exercise to promote weight loss. In women who have gained an excessive amount of weight, weight loss may improve insulin resistance, decrease androgen levels and hirsutism, and restore ovulation in some cases. Low-glycemic load diets historically have been recommended with evidence of their clinical effectiveness. The capacity of dietary carbohydrates to increase postprandial blood sugar response may be an important consideration for optimizing metabolic and clinical outcomes in PCOS. Furthermore, independent of weight loss, a low-glycemic load diet appears to result in greater improvements in health, including improved insulin sensitivity, improved menstrual regularity, better emotion scores (on a questionnaire designed to detect changes in quality of life), and decreased markers of inflammation compared with a conventional low-fat diet when matched closely for macronutrient and fiber content (Marsh et al, 2010).

Medical Management

Hypothyroidism occurs in some cases of PCOS. Laboratory tests for thyroid function are frequently normal in patients with clinical evidence of hypothyroidism, and treatment with thyroid hormone results in clinical improvement in many patients. Therefore an empirical trial of thyroid hormone should be considered for patients with PCOS who have clinical evidence of hypothyroidism.

Thyroid antibody status should be taken into account when considering treatment with thyroid hormone in women with PCOS. Metformin frequently is prescribed to improve insulin resistance, and treatment with this drug may lead to resumption of ovulation. Other therapies include the drugs clomiphene citrate (to induce ovulation) and spironolactone (an antiandrogen), as well as oral contraceptives (to treat menstrual irregularities and hirsutism).

Medical Nutrition Therapy

Nutritional interventions that may be beneficial for women with PCOS include dietary modifications designed to enhance insulin sensitivity. This includes recommending a low-glycemic load diet, consuming high-fiber foods, and preventing excess weight gain via calorie awareness and promotion of physical activity. Eating a diet that keeps blood sugar balanced, including combining low-glycemic carbohydrates with protein and eating smaller meals may also be of benefit. It is important to ensure optimal nutrient status for vitamin D and to screen for sub optimal thyroid function (see Table 30.3).

Complementary and Integrative Approaches

A critical review of the 12 randomized controlled trials (RCTs) highlights that oral administration of myoinositol, alone or in combination with D-chiro-inositol, two stereoisomers of inositol (an intracellular messenger molecule), is capable of restoring insulin sensitivity and spontaneous ovulation and improving fertility in women with PCOS. These RCT studies support the hypothesis of a primary role of inositol phosphoglycans (IPGs) as second messengers of insulin signaling and demonstrate that myoinositol supplementation beneficially affects the hormonal milieu of PCOS patients. Indeed, these trials provide evidence that myoinositol reduces insulin levels, probably either by conversion to D-chiro-inositol (via the epimerase enzyme) or by serving as substrate for the formation of IPGs and D-chiro-inositol-containing IPGs, which would in turn amplify insulin signaling (Unfer et al, 2016).

N-Acetylcysteine (NAC) is an amino acid–derived supplement that may help improve insulin receptor activity, reduce testosterone, and increase spontaneous ovulation in PCOS. In a recent review of eight RCTs that compared metformin or placebo and NAC, women who took NAC were more likely to achieve pregnancy and to deliver a live baby, especially if resistant to the fertility drug clomiphene citrate. There was no benefit from NAC for improving menstrual regularity, acne, hirsutism, body mass index (BMI), fasting insulin, or fasting glucose. The typical dose of NAC was 1200 to 1800 mg/day (Thakker et al, 2015).

HYPERTHYROIDISM

Graves' disease is an autoimmune disease in which the thyroid is diffusely enlarged (goiter) and overactive, producing an excessive amount of thyroid hormones. It is the most common cause of hyperthyroidism (overactive thyroid) in the United States. Physical symptoms frequently include red, dry, swollen, puffy, and bulging eyes (exophthalmos), heat intolerance, difficulty sleeping, and anxiety (see Box 30.2). However,

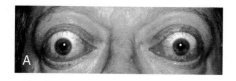

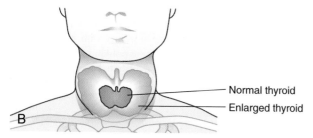

— Normal thyroid

— Enlarged thyroid

Fig. 30.4 A, Exophthalmos. (From SPL/Photo Researchers, Inc.) **B,** Thyroid enlargement. (From Buck C: *2011 ICD-9-CM, for Hospitals*, vols 1-3, St Louis, 2011, WB Saunders.)

the most common sign of Graves' disease is goiter or thyroid enlargement (Fig. 30.4). The excessive thyroid hormones may cause a serious metabolic imbalance called thyrotoxicosis. The prevalence of maternal thyrotoxicosis is approximately 1 case per 1500 persons, with maternal Graves' disease being the most common cause (80% to 85%) (American Thyroid Association, 2019).

Pathophysiology

Commonly, patients have a family history involving a wide spectrum of autoimmune thyroid diseases, such as Graves' disease, Hashimoto's thyroiditis, or postpartum thyroiditis. In Graves' disease, the TRH receptor itself is the primary autoantigen and is responsible for the manifestation of hyperthyroidism. The thyroid gland is under continuous stimulation by circulating autoantibodies against the TRH receptor, and pituitary TSH secretion is suppressed because of the increased production of thyroid hormones. These thyroid-stimulating antibodies cause release of thyroid hormone and Tg, and they also stimulate iodine uptake, protein synthesis, and thyroid gland growth.

The Tg and TPO Abs appear to have little role in Graves' disease. However, as mentioned earlier, they are markers of Hashimoto's thyroiditis autoimmune disease against the thyroid. A TSH antibody—typically referred to as thyroid-stimulating immunoglobulin—test is used to identify hyperthyroidism, or Graves' disease.

Triggers

Graves' disease is an autoimmune disorder, influenced by a combination of environmental and genetic factors. Genetic factors contribute to approximately 20% to 30% of overall susceptibility. Other factors include infection, excessive iodide intake, stress, female gender, steroids, and toxins. Smoking has been implicated in the worsening of Graves' ophthalmopathy (eye disease) (Wiersinga, 2016). Graves' disease also has been associated with infectious agents such as *Yersinia enterocolitica* and *Borrelia burgdorferi*, as these bacteria have been shown to contain high-affinity binding sites for the hormone TSH (Hargreaves et al, 2013).

Genetics. Several autoimmune thyroid disease susceptibility genes have been identified and appear to be specific to either Graves' disease or Hashimoto's thyroiditis, whereas others confer susceptibility to both conditions. The genetic predisposition to thyroid autoimmunity may interact with environmental factors or events to precipitate the onset of Graves' disease. HLA-DRB1 and HLA-DQB1 appear to be associated with Graves' disease susceptibility.

Stress. Stress can be a factor for thyroid autoimmunity. Acute stress-induced immunosuppression may be followed by immune system hyperactivity, which could precipitate autoimmune thyroid disease. This may occur during the postpartum period, in which Graves' disease may occur 3 to 9 months after delivery. Estrogen may influence the immune system, particularly the beta-cells. Trauma to the thyroid also has been reported to be associated with Graves' disease. This may include surgery of the thyroid gland, percutaneous injection of ethanol, and infarction of a thyroid adenoma.

Medical Management

For patients with sustained forms of hyperthyroidism, such as Graves' disease or toxic nodular goiter, antithyroid medications can be used. The goal with this form of drug therapy is to prevent the thyroid from producing hormones (Table 30.4).

The effects of immunotherapy drugs are also being evaluated (Salvi, 2014) (see *Pathophysiology and Care Management Algorithm: Thyroid Dysfunction*).

MANAGING IMBALANCES OF THE HYPOTHALAMUS-PITUITARY-THYROID AXIS

The thyroid has a relationship to hypothalamic, pituitary, immune, adrenal, and cardiovascular functions that affect clinical, cellular, and molecular outcomes. A checklist of considerations is found in Box 30.3 and is discussed here.

TABLE 30.4	**Treatments for Hyperthyroidism**	
Medication Brand Name	**Medication Generic Name**	**Use and Comments**
Tapazole	Methimazole (MMI)	Both drugs interfere with the thyroid gland's production of hormones. Both have side effects, which include rash, itching, joint pain, and fever.
Northyx	Propylthiouracil (PTU)	Liver inflammation or reduction in white blood cells may occur. Underlying hyperthyroidism can return when patient is no longer taking the medication.
Radioactive iodine		This is the most widely recommended permanent treatment of hyperthyroidism. Thyroid cells absorb radioactive iodine, which damages or kills them. If too many of the thyroid cells are damaged, remaining thyroid does not produce enough hormone, resulting in hypothyroidism, and supplemental thyroid hormone may be necessary.

Surgical Treatment
- Partial or complete removal of the thyroid
- Not as common as pharmacologic modes of treatment

BOX 30.3 Factors Promoting Thyroid Health in Adults

Consider

    Protein: 0.8 g/kg/day

    Iodine (once autoimmune disease has been ruled out): 150 mcg/day

    Selenium (as L-selenomethionine): 75-200 mcg/day

    Zinc (as zinc citrate): 10 mg/day

    Vitamin D (as D_3 or cholecalciferol): 1000 IU/day

    Vitamin E (as D-alpha tocopherol succinate): 100 IU/day

    Vitamin C (as ascorbic acid): 100-500 mg/day

    Guggulsterones (from guggul extract):100 mg/day

    Ashwaganda: 100 mg/day

Reduce or eliminate

    Gluten (found in wheat, rye, oats, and barley)

    Processed soy

    Excessive uncooked goitrogenic foods

    Stress

Provide adequate precursors for the formation of T_4. Iodide is a limiting nutrient in many individuals for the production of T_4. Adequate levels of organic iodide, which can come from sea vegetables, iodized salt, and seafood, are important in T_4 production. Adequate dietary protein intake is important in establishing proper protein calorie nutrition. Supplementation with tyrosine does not appear to have a beneficial effect on elevating thyroid hormones.

Reduce antithyroidal antibodies. A variety of food antigens could induce antibodies that cross-react with the thyroid gland. A food elimination diet using gluten-free grains and possible elimination of casein, the predominant milk protein, may be considered for hypothyroidism of unexplained origin. It also has been suggested that environmental toxins such as cadmium and lead may play a role in inducing AIT and thyroid dysfunction (Bajaj et al, 2016). Implementing nutritional support and providing adequate levels of vitamin D and selenium to support the immune system may be beneficial.

Improve the conversion of T_4 to T_3. Nutritional agents that help support proper deiodination by the type 1, 5-deiodinase enzyme include selenium (as L-selenomethionine) and zinc (as zinc glycinate or zinc citrate). Human studies repeatedly have demonstrated consequent reduced concentrations of thyroid hormones when a zinc deficiency is present (Blazewicz et al, 2010). In children with Down's syndrome, zinc sulfate may reduce thyroidal antibodies, improve thyroid function, and reduce the incidence of subclinical hypothyroidism (Mazurek and Wyka, 2016).

Zinc supplementation was also shown to ameliorate hazards of radiation on thyroid hormone indices (Al et al, 2016).

Enhance T_3 influence on mitochondrial function. A number of important nutritional relationships improve thyroid hormones' effects on the mitochondria, the organelles responsible for the majority of cellular energy production (Lanni et al, 2016). Selenium supplementation in animals can improve the production of T_3 and lower autoantibodies to thyroid hormones while improving energy production. Supplementation with selenomethionine results in improved deiodination of T_4, which may improve ATP formation by supporting improved mitochondrial activity. Food sources of selenium include the Brazil nut, snapper, cod, halibut, yellowfin tuna, salmon, sardines, shrimp, mushrooms, and barley.

Monitor use of botanical products. Based on animal studies, it appears that certain botanical preparations influence thyroid activity. The most significant products include *Commiphora mukul* (guggulsterones, from guggul extract) and *Withania somnifera* (ashwagandha). *C. mukul* demonstrates strong thyroid stimulatory action. Its administration (1 mg/100 g body weight) increases iodine uptake by the thyroid, increases TPO activity, and decreases lipid peroxidation, suggesting that increased peripheral generation of T_3 might be mediated by this plant's antioxidant effects. *W. somnifera* (ashwagandha) root extract (1.4 g/kg) may increase T_3 and T_4 concentrations without changing 5-deiodinase activity (Sharma et al, 2018).

Avoid disruption of thyroid hormone metabolism from flavonoids. Flavonoids, natural and synthetic, have the potential to disrupt thyroid hormone metabolism. Synthetic flavonoid derivatives can decrease serum T_4 concentrations and inhibit the conversion of T_4 to T_3 and the metabolic clearance of rT_3 by the selenium-dependent 5-deiodinase. Naturally occurring flavonoids appear to have a similar inhibitory effect. Of the naturally occurring flavonoids, luteolin (most often found in leaves, but also seen in celery, thyme, dandelion, green pepper, thyme, perilla, chamomile tea, carrots, olive oil, peppermint, rosemary, and oregano) is the most active inhibitor of 5-deiodinase activity. Because isolated or concentrated flavonoids are increasingly used as therapeutic interventions, more research on the potential influence of these substances on thyroid hormone metabolism is desirable (Gonçalves et al, 2013). However, in patients with thyroid cancer who have reduced ability to uptake iodide, flavonoids such as rutin and apigenin (found in asparagus, figs, and green and unpeeled apples) are able to increase iodide uptake and may be useful and adjuvant in radioiodine therapy since this flavonoid increased thyroid uptake without affecting adversely affecting thyroid function (Gonçalves et al, 2013; Gonçalves et al, 2017).

Use caution with supplements. Lipoic acid reduces the conversion of T_4 to T_3. Because it is usually not a therapeutic advantage to decrease peripheral activation of T_3 subsequent to T_4 therapy, use of lipoic acid supplements in hypothyroid patients receiving exogenous hormone therapy should be approached with caution. However, lipoic acid has been more recently shown to be a potential adjuvant therapy for advanced thyroid cancer because it could activate adenosine monophosphate activated protein kinase (AMPK) and inhibit transforming growth factor β-TGFβ pathway by reducing cancer cell migration and suppressing tumor growth (Jeon et al, 2016).

Maintain vitamin sufficiency. One nutrient that is critically important for establishing immune balance and preventing the production of autoantibodies is vitamin D. Vitamin D is considered a prohormone with antiproliferative, differentiating, and immunosuppressive activities. Vitamin D is an effective immune modulator and may suppress the development of autoimmune diseases, such as arthritis and multiple sclerosis (Baeke et al, 2010). Conversely, a vitamin D deficiency is associated with numerous autoimmune conditions, including Hashimoto's thyroiditis. More than 90% of people with autoimmune thyroid disease have a genetic defect affecting their ability to metabolize vitamin D (Feng et al, 2013; Kivity et al, 2011). Vitamin D also appears to work with other nutritional factors to help regulate immune sensitivity and may protect against development of autoantibodies. After exposure to heavy metals, decreases in a variety of hepatic antioxidant lipid peroxidation (the oxidative degradation of lipids) systems have been observed. Ascorbic acid has been shown to be effective in preventing lead-induced decreases in T_3 and hepatic 5-deiodination in an animal model (Ambali et al, 2011).

ADRENAL DISORDERS

Cushing's Syndrome

In Cushing's syndrome, too much cortisol remains in the bloodstream over a long period. The exogenous form occurs when individuals take steroids or other similar medications and ceases when the medication is stopped. Endogenous Cushing's syndrome is rare and occurs as the result of a tumor on the adrenal or pituitary gland. Weight gain, insulin resistance, high blood sugar, excessive thirst, easy bruising, depression, muscle loss, and weakness are common symptoms. Because cortisol causes bone loss over time, a diet rich in calcium and vitamin D may help prevent osteoporosis. Reducing sodium, optimal hydration, and caloric awareness can also assist with weight management and the prevention of fluid retention.

Addison's Disease

Primary adrenal insufficiency, also known as Addison's disease, is rare. In this condition, insufficient steroid hormones are produced in spite of adequate levels of the hormone adrenocorticotropic hormone (ACTH). People with Addison's disease lose the ability to appropriately regulate blood sugar and will have low levels of cortisol, aldosterone, epinephrine, and norepinephrine. This leads to loss of appetite, fatigue, low blood pressure, nausea and vomiting, and, for some, darkening of skin on the face and neck. Patients with Addison's disease have an increased need for salt and water and also need to eat regular balanced meals (with low-glycemic carbohydrate and protein) to regulate blood sugar.

Adrenal Insufficiency/Adrenal Fatigue

Adrenal fatigue has been identified as a collection of signs and symptoms caused by the decreased ability of the adrenal glands to respond adequately to stress. A variety of terms are found in the scientific literature that address adrenal fatigue, including subclinical adrenal insufficiency, adrenal stress, adrenal exhaustion, adrenal burnout, and adrenal imbalance (Allen Jr, 2013). The adrenals are the two triangular-shaped glands located at the top of each kidney and are responsible primarily for governing the body's adaptations to stress of any kind. Under the influence of stress, the adrenals will respond with increased hormone production, which can cause elevated blood sugar and blood pressure. Over time, the adrenal can become decompensated, where the hormone output may be diminished. This is often referred to as adrenal fatigue. This can occur whether the source of stress—physical, emotional, or psychological—is chronic and continues to persist causing a cumulative effect, or is a very intense single event stressor. In other words, the adrenal glands are unable to keep pace with the demands of perpetual fight-or-flight arousal, resulting in subclinical adrenal dysfunction. The most common symptoms of adrenal fatigue include, but are not limited to, excessive fatigue and exhaustion, hair loss, hypoglycemia, hormone imbalance, poor digestion, low immune function, slow recovery from illness, inability to concentrate, and inability to cope with stressors.

Chronic adrenal stress causes the following (Sun et al, 2016; Tsigos and Chrousos, 2002):

- Affects communication between the brain and hormone-secreting glands. The hypothalamus and pituitary gland direct hormone production, including that of the thyroid. When the hypothalamus and pituitary weaken because of chronic adrenal stress, they are not able to communicate well with the thyroid gland.
- Increases thyroid-binding protein activity, so that thyroid hormones cannot get into cells to do their job.
- Hampers the conversion of T_4 to active forms of T_3, which can lead to fatigue.
- Interferes with the biotransformation (detoxification) pathways through which thyroid hormones exit the body, leading to thyroid hormone imbalance.
- Causes cells to lose sensitivity to thyroid hormones.
- Weakens the immune barriers of the digestive tract, lungs, and brain; promotes poor immune regulation.

The impact of high stress on intestinal microflora has been examined as well. A significant decrease in the number of *Bifidobacteria* and *Lactobacilli* was reported. Conversely, an increase in the number of *Escherichia coli* and enterobacteria were also reported, suggesting that the increased chronic stress disrupts intestinal microflora ecology. The authors propose is that stress induces increased permeability of the gut, allowing bacteria and bacterial antigens to cross the epithelial barrier and activate a mucosal immune response, which in turn alters the composition of the microbiome and leads to enhanced hypothalamic-pituitary-adrenal (HPA) activation (Dinan and Cryan, 2012).

These are some of the ways adrenal stress directly affect thyroid function (Herman et al, 2016). Chronic adrenal stress affects other systems of the body, which in turn decreases thyroid function. For example, the adrenal hormone cortisol plays a large role in thyroid health. Cortisol is a life-sustaining hormone essential to the maintenance of homeostasis. It often is called the "stress hormone" because it influences, regulates, or modulates many of the changes that occur in the body in response to stress, including, but not limited to, the following:

- Antiinflammatory actions
- Blood glucose levels
- Blood pressure
- Central nervous system activation
- Fat, protein, and carbohydrate metabolism to maintain blood glucose
- Heart and blood vessel tone and contraction
- Immune responses

Cortisol levels follow a circadian rhythm and normally fluctuate throughout the day and night, peaking at about 8 a.m and reaching a low at about 4 p.m (Allen Jr, 2013). It is very important that bodily functions and cortisol levels return to normal after a stressful event. Adrenal fatigue appears to occur when the amount of stress or combined stresses overextends the capacity of the body to compensate for and recover from that stress. When this happens repeatedly, it exhausts the adrenal and thyroid glands, as well as the hypothalamus and the pituitary gland. Over time this exhaustion leads to functional hypothyroidism. In addition, constant cortisol production increases risk for obesity and weakens the gastrointestinal (GI) tract, making one more susceptible to inflammation, dysbiosis (poor gut health), and infection (Foster, 2017; van der Valk et al, 2018).

The following include common integrative interventions in the treatment of adrenal fatigue (Allolio et al, 2007; Charmandari, 2014):

- B-complex vitamins to provide cofactors for adrenal hormone production
- Exercise in moderation
- Low-glycemic load, nutrient-dense diet
- Antianxiolytic/sedative botanicals (i.e. chamomile and lavender) (Head and Kelly, 2009).
- Probiotics
- Optimizing sleep habits
- Relaxation and stress management

Overt stressors such as childhood emotional abuse and posttraumatic stress disorder (PTSD) may result in cortisol hyperactivity, thus leading to pituitary and adrenal hyperreactivity and adrenal fatigue and decompensation (Rasmusson et al, 2001). Increased cortisol signaling, however, has been shown to be neurocognitively beneficial in depressed women with a history of maltreatment (Abercrombie et al, 2018).

CLINICAL CASE STUDY

Frank is a 72-year-old black man from Jamaica who moved to the United States 2 years ago. He has been diagnosed with hypothyroidism this past year. He comes to your clinic taking Synthroid, garlic, and chamomile. His diet history indicates daily intake of chicken, rice, celery, green pepper, mango, and papaya. He states that he has been very tired lately, has little energy, and has constipation. His hormone levels on his last medical report were thyroxine (T_4): 1.7 ng/dL, triiodothyronine (T_3): 75 ng/dL, and thyroid-stimulating hormone (TSH): 6 U/mL, indicative that his hypothyroidism is still not well controlled.

Nutrition Diagnostic Statement
- Food-medication interaction related to mixing Synthroid with foods and herbs that aggravate thyroid dysfunction as evidenced by fatigue, constipation, high TSH, and low serum T_3 and T_4.

Nutrition Care Questions
1. What other information do you need for a more thorough assessment?
2. Taking into consideration his Jamaican heritage, advice would you offer Frank about his diet?
3. What foods and supplements conflict with Synthroid?
4. Because he is a recent immigrant, what potential stressors may he be experiencing?

USEFUL WEBSITES

American Association of Clinical Endocrinologists
American Thyroid Association
Endocrine Web
Thyroid Disease Information

REFERENCES

Abercrombie HC, Frost CP, Walsh EC, et al: Neural signaling of cortisol, childhood emotional abuse and depression-related memory bias, *Biol Psychiatry Cogn Neurosci Neuroimaging* 3:274–284, 2018.

Allen LV Jr: Adrenal fatigue, *Int J Pharm Compd* 17:39–44, 2013.

Allolio B, Arlt W, Hahner S: DHEA: why, when, and how much-DHEA replacement in adrenal insufficiency, *Ann Endocrinol (Paris)* 68:268–273, 2007.

Ambali SF, Orieji C, Abubakar WO, et al: Ameliorative effect of Vitamin C on alterations in thyroid hormone concentrations induced by sub-chronic Co-administration of Chloropyrifos and Lead in wistar rats, *J Thyroid Res* 214924, 2011.

American Thyroid Association: *Thyroid disease and pregnancy* (website). http://www.thyroid.org/thyroid-disease-and-pregnancy/.

Amin Al, Hegazy NM, Ibrahim KS, et al: Thyroid hormone indices in computer workers with emphasis on the role of Zinc supplementation, *Open Access Maced J Med Sci* 4:296–301, 2016.

Baeke F, Takiishi T, Korf H, et al: Vitamin D: modulator of the immune system, *Curr Opin Pharmacol* 10:482–496, 2010.

Bajaj JK, Salwan P, Salwan S: Various possible toxicants involved in thyroid dysfunction: a review, *J Clin Diagn Res* 10:FE01–FE03, 2016.

Barker JM, Liu E: Celiac disease: pathophysiology, clinical manifestations, and associated autoimmune conditions, *Adv Pediatr* 55:349–365, 2008.

Blazewicz A, Dolliver W, Sivsammye S, et al: Determination of cadmium, cobalt, copper, iron, manganese, and zinc in thyroid glands of patients with diagnosed nodular goitre using ion chromatography, *J Chromatogr B Analyt Technol Biomed Life Sci* 878:34–38, 2010.

Cassio A, Ricci G, Baronio F, et al: Long-term clinical significance of thyroid autoimmunity in children with celiac disease, *J Pediatr* 156:292–295, 2010.

Centers for Disease Control: *National diabetes statistics report*, 2018 (website). https://www.cdc.gov/diabetes/data/statistics/statistics-report.html.

Charmandari E: Adrenal Insufficiency, *Lancet* 383:2152–2167, 2014.

Chen ZP, Hetzel BS: Cretinism revisited, *Best Pract Res Clin Endocrinol Metab* 24:39–50, 2010.

De Sibio MT, de Oliveira M, Moretto FCF, et al: Triiodothyroinine and breast cancer, *World J Clin Oncol* 5:503–508, 2014.

De Vivo A, Mancuso A, Giacobbe A, et al: Thyroid function in women found to have early pregnancy loss, *Thyroid* 20:633–637, 2010.

de Vries EM, van Beeren HC, Ackermans MT, et al: Differential effects of fasting vs food restriction on liver thyroid hormone metabolism in male rats, *J Endocrinol* 224:25–35, 2015.

del Ghianda S, Tonacchera M, Vitti P: Thyroid and menopause, *Climacteric* 17:225–234, 2014.

Dinan TG, Cryan JF: Regulation of the stress response by the gut microbiota: implications for psychoneuroendocrinology, *Psychoneuroendocrinology* 37:1369–1378, 2012.

Dunn ME, Manfredi TG: Clinical Case Report: ultrastructural evidence of skeletal muscle mitochondrial dysfunction in patients with subclinical hypothyroidism, *Thyroid Sci* 4:1, 2009.

Duntas LH: Does celiac disease trigger autoimmune thyroiditis? *Nat Rev Endocrinol* 5:190–191, 2009.

Ebert EC: The thyroid and the gut, *J Clin Gastroenterol* 44:402–406, 2010.

Feng M, Li H, Chen SF, et al: Polymorphisms in the vitamin D receptor gene and risk of autoimmune thyroid diseases: a meta-analysis, *Endocrine* 43:318–326, 2013.

Fjaellegaard K, Kvetny J, Allerup PN, et al: Well-being and depression in individuals with subclinical hypothyroidism and thyroid autoimmunity – a general population study, *Nord J Psychiatry* 69:73–78, 2015.

Foster JA, Rinaman L, Cryan JF: Stress & the gut-brain axis: regulation by the microbiome, *Neurobiol Stress* 7:124–136, 2017.

Freeman HJ: Endocrine manifestations in celiac disease, *World J Gastroenterol* 22:8472–8479, 2016.

Garber JR, Cobin RH, Gharib H, et al: Clinical practice guidelines for hypothyroidism in adults: cosponsored by the American Association of Clinical Endocrinologists and the American Thyroid Association, *Endocr Pract* 18:988–1028, 2012.

Golden SH, Robinson KA, Saldanha I, et al: Clinical review: Prevalence and incidence of endocrine and metabolic disorders in the United States: a comprehensive review, *J Clin Endocrinol Metab* 94:1853–1878, 2009.

Gomes-Lima C, Burman KD: Reverse T3 or perverse T3? Still puzzling after 40 years, *Cleve Clin J Med* 85:450–455, 2018.

Gonçalves CF, Santos MC, Ginabreda MG, et al: Flavonoid rutin increases thyroid iodide uptake in rats, *PLoS One* 8:e73908, 2013, doi:10.1371/journal.pone.0073908. eCollection 2013.

Gonçalves CFL, de Freitas ML, Ferreira ACF: Flavonoids, thyroid iodide uptake and thyroid cancer – a review, *Int J Mol Sci* 18:1247, 2017.

Gropper S, Smith JL: *Advanced nutrition and human metabolism*, ed 6, Belmont, Calif, 2012, Wadsworth Cengage Learning.

Hak AE, Pols HA, Visser TJ, et al: Subclinical hypothyroidism is an independent risk factor for atherosclerosis and myocardial infarction in elderly women: the Rotterdam study, *Ann Intern Med* 132:270–278, 2000.

Hargreaves CE, Grasso M, Hampe CS, et al: Yersinia enterocolitica provides the link between thyroid-stimulating antibodies and their germline counterparts in graves' disease, *J Immunol* 190;5373–5381, 2013.

Head KA, Kelly GS: Nutrients and botanicals for treatment of stress: adrenal fatigue, neurotransmitter imbalance, anxiety, and restless sleep, *Altern Med Rev* 14(2):114–140, 2009.

Herman JP, McKlveen JM, Ghosal S, et al: Regulation of the hypothalamic-pituitary-adrenocortical stress response, *Compr Physiol* 6:603–621, 2016.

Hess SY: The impact of common micronutrient deficiencies on iodine and thyroid metabolism: the evidence from human studies, *Best Pract Res Clin Endocrinol Metab* 24:117–132, 2010.

Hollowell JG, Staehling NW, Flanders WD, et al: Serum TSH, T(4), and thyroid antibodies in the United States population (1988 to 1994): National Health and Nutrition Examination Survey (NHANES III), *J Clin Endocrinol Metab* 87:489–499, 2002.

Hu S, Rayman MP: Multiple nutritional factors and the risk of Hashimoto's thyroiditis, *Thyroid* 27:597–610, 2017.

Janegova A, Jenega P, Rychly B, et al: The role of Epstein-Barr virus infection in the development of autoimmune thyroid disease, *Endokrynol Pol* 66(2):132–136, 2015.

Jeon MJ, Kim WG, Lim S, et al: Alpha lipoic acid inhibits proliferation and epithelial mesenchymal transition of thyroid cancer cells, *Mol Cell Endocrinol* 419:113–123, 2016.

Kalra B, Sawhney K, Kalra S: Management of thyroid disorders in pregnancy: recommendations made simple, *J Pak Med Assoc* 67:1452–1455, 2017.

Kaltsas G, Vgontzas A, Chrousos G: Fatigue, endocrinopathies, and metabolic disorders, *PM R* 2:393–398, 2010.

Khandelwal D, Tandon N: Overt and subclinical hypothyroidism: who to treat and how, *Drugs* 72:17–33, 2012.

Kisters K: What is the correct magnesium supplement? *Magnes Res* 26:41–42, 2013.

Kivity S, Agmon-Levin N, Zisappl M, et al: Vitamin D and autoimmune thyroid diseases, *Cell Mol Immunol* 8:243–247, 2011.

Köhrle J: Selenium and the thyroid, *Curr Opin Endocrinol Diabetes Obes* 20:441–448, 2013.

Krysiak R, Szkróbka W, Okopień B: The effect of Vitamin D on thyroid autoimmunity in levothyroxine-treated women with hashimoto's thyroiditis and normal Vitamin D status, *Exp Clin Endocrinol Diabetes* 125: 229–233, 2017.

Lanni A, Moreno M, Goglia F: Mitochondrial actions of thyroid hormone, *Compr Physiol* 6:1591–1607, 2016.

Liontiris M, Mazokopakis EE: A concise review of Hashimoto's thyroiditis (HT) and the importance of iodine, selenium, vitamin D and gluten on the autoimmunity and dietary management of HT patients. Points that need more investigation, *Hell J Nucl Med* 20:51–56, 2017.

Marsh KA, Steinbeck KS, Atkinson FS, et al: Effect of a low glycemic index compared with a conventional healthy diet on polycystic ovary syndrome, *Am J Clin Nutr* 92:83–92, 2010.

Mazurek D, Wyka J: Down Syndrome – genetic and nutritional aspects of accompanying disorders, *Rocz Panstw Zakl Hig* 66:189–194, 2016.

McLeod DSA, Caturegli P, Cooper DS, et al: Variation in rates of autoimmune thyroid disease by race/ethnicity in US military personnel, *JAMA* 311: 1563–1565, 2014.

Meloni A, Mandas C, Jores RD, et al: Prevalence of autoimmune thyroiditis in children with celiac disease and effect of gluten withdrawal, *J Pediatr* 155: 51–55, 2009.

Melse-Boonstra A, Jaiswal N: Iodine deficiency in pregnancy, infancy and childhood and its consequences for brain development, *Best Pract Res Clin Endocrinol Metab* 24:29–38, 2010.

Michels AW, Eisenbarth GS: Immunologic endocrine disorders, *J Allergy Clin Immunol* 125:S226–S237, 2010.

Moran LJ, Lombard CB, Lim S, et al: Polycystic ovary syndrome and weight management, *Women's Health (Lond)* 6:271–283, 2010.

Naiyer AJ, Shah J, Hernandez L, et al: Tissue transglutaminase antibodies in individuals with celiac disease bind to thyroid follicles and extracellular matrix and may contribute to thyroid dysfunction, *Thyroid* 2008;18: 1171–1178.

National Institutes of Health, MedlinePlus: *Endocrine diseases* (website), 2018. http://www.nlm.nih.gov/medlineplus/endocrinediseases.html.

Nazarian S, St Peter JV, Boston RC, et al: Vitamin D3 supplementation improves insulin sensitivity in subjects with impaired fasting glucose, *Transl Res* 158:276–281, 2011.

Olmos RD, Figueiredo RC, Aquino EM, et al: Gender, race and socioeconomic Influence on diagnosis and treatment of thyroid disorders In the Brazilian Longitudinal Study of Adult Health (ELSA-Brasil), *Braz J Med Biol Res* 48:751–758, 2015.

Pirola I, Gandossi E, Agosti B, et al: Selenium supplementation could restore euthyroidism in subclinical hypothyroid patients with autoimmune thyroiditis, *Endokrynol Pol* 67:567–571, 2016.

Rasmusson A, Lipschitz DS, Wang S, et al: Increased pituitary and adrenal reactivity in premenopausal women with Posttraumatic stress disorder, *Biol Psychiatry* 50:965–977, 2001.

Roy A, Laszkowska M, Sundström J, et al: Prevalence of celiac disease in patients with autoimmune thyroid disease: a meta-analysis, *Thyroid* 26:880–890, 2016.

Salvi M: Immunotherapy for Graves' ophthalmopathy, *Curr Opin Endocrinol Diabetes Obes* 21:409–414, 2014.

Saravanan P, Chau WF, Roberts N, et al: Psychological well-being in patients on "adequate" doses of L-thyroxine: results of a large, controlled community based questionnaire study, *Clin Endocrinol (Oxf)* 57:577–585, 2002.

Sharma AK, Basu I, Singh S: Efficacy and safety of Ashwagandha root extract in subclinical hypothyroid patients: a double-blind, randomized placebo-controlled trial, *J Altern Complement Med* 24:243–248, 2018.

Sinnott B, Ron E, Schneider AB: Exposing the thyroid to radiation: a review of its current extent, risks, and implications, *Endocr Rev* 31: 756–773, 2010.

Sirmans SM, Pate KA: Epidemiology, diagnosis, and management of polycystic ovary syndrome, *Clin Epidemiol* 18(6):1–13, 2013.

Soldin OP, O'Mara DM, Aschner M: Thyroid hormones and methylmercury toxicity, Biol Trace Elem Res 126:1–12, 2008.

Stazi AV, Trinti B: Selenium status and over-expression of interleukin15 in celiac disease and autoimmune thyroid diseases, *Ann Ist Super Sanita* 46:389–399, 2010.

Sun HJ, Xiang P, Luo J, et al: Mechanisms of arsenic disruption on gonadal, adrenal and thyroid endocrine systems in humans: a review, *Environ Int* 95:61–68, 2016.

Thakker D, Raval A, Patel I, et al: N-acetylcysteine for polycystic ovary syndrome: a systemic review and meta-analysis of randomized controlled trials, *Obstet Gynecol Int* 2015:817849, 2015.

Tomer Y, Huber A: The etiology of autoimmune thyroid disease: a story of genes and environment, *J Autoimmun* 32:231–239, 2009.

Tsigos C, Chrousos GP: Hypothalamic-pituitary-adrenal axis, neuroendocrine factors and stress, *J Psychosom Res* 53:865–871, 2002.

Unfer V, Nestler JE, Kamenov ZA, et al: Effects of inositols in women with PCOS: a systematic review of randomized controlled trials, *Int J Endocrinol* 2016:1-12, 2016.

van der Valk ES, Savas M, van Rossum EFC: Stress and obesity: are there more susceptible individuals, *Curr Obes Rep* 7:193–203, 2018.

Vélez LM, Motta AB: Association between polycystic ovary syndrome and metabolic syndrome, *Curr Med Chem* 21:3999–4012, 2014.

Wang K, Wei H, Zhang W, et al: Severely low serum magnesium is associated with increased risks of positive anti-thyroglobulin antibody and hypothyroidism: a cross-sectional study, *Sci Rep* 8:9904, 2018.

Wichman J, Winther KH, Bonnema SJ, et al: Selenium supplementation significantly reduces thyroid autoantibody levels in patients with chronic Autoimmune thyroiditis: a systematic review and meta-analysis, *Thyroid* 26:1681–1692, 2016.

Wiebolt J, Koeleman BP, van Haeften TW: Endocrine autoimmune disease: genetics become complex, *Eur J Clin Invest* 40:1144–1155, 2010.

Wiersinga WM: Clinical relevance of environmental factors in the pathogenesis of Autoimmune thyroid disease, *Endocrinol Metab (Seoul)* 31:213–222, 2016.

Yassa L, Marqusee E, Fawcett R, et al: Thyroid hormone early adjustment in pregnancy (the THERAPY) trial, *J Clin Endocrinol Metab* 95:3234–3241, 2010.

Zimmermann MB: Iodine deficiency in pregnancy and the effects of maternal iodine supplementation on the offspring: a review, *Am J Clin Nutr* 89(2):S668– S678, 2009.

31

Medical Nutrition Therapy for Anemia

Michelle Loy, MPH, MS, RDN

KEY TERMS

anemia	intrinsic factor (IF)	polycythemia
aplastic anemia	iron deficiency anemia	protoporphyrin
ceruloplasmin	koilonychia	reticulocytosis
ferritin	macrocytic anemia	restless legs syndrome (RLS)
ferroprotein	meat-fish-poultry (MFP) factor	serum
glossitis	megaloblastic anemia	sickle cell disease (SCD)
hematocrit	microcytic anemia	sideroblastic (pyridoxine-responsive) anemia
heme iron	nonheme iron	soluble serum transferrin receptors (STFRs)
hemoglobin	normochromic	sports anemia
hemolytic anemia	nutritional anemias	thalassemia
hepcidin	pagophagia	total iron-binding capacity (TIBC)
hereditary hemochromatosis	pernicious anemia	transferrin
holotranscobalamin II (holo TCII)	pica	transferrin receptor
hypochromic	plasma	transferrin saturation

Anemia is the predominant hematologic disorder in the United States and is associated with medical consequences that influence morbidity and mortality. Anemia affects 5.6% of the nation's population with the prevalence being highest among women of reproductive age, adults 60 years or older, blacks, and Hispanics (Le, 2016). Anemia is also a serious global health burden affecting 2 billion people worldwide with the highest rates occurring in South Asia and central and west sub-Saharan Africa (Kassebaum, 2016). Globally, young children, women, and older adults are at highest risk of developing anemia. To best address this serious health problem, nutrition professionals need a solid understanding of the relevant terminology along with the etiology, pathophysiology, and medical and nutritional management of the most common types of anemia.

Hemoglobin is a conjugated protein containing four heme groups and globin; it is the oxygen-carrying pigment of the erythrocytes. The hematocrit is the volume percentage of erythrocytes in the blood. Plasma is the liquid portion of whole blood containing coagulation factors; serum is the liquid portion of whole blood without coagulation factors.

Anemia is a deficiency in the size or number of red blood cells (RBCs) or the amount of hemoglobin they contain. This deficiency limits the exchange of oxygen and carbon dioxide between the blood and the tissue cells. Anemia classification is based on cell size—macrocytic (large), normocytic (normal), and microcytic (small)—and on hemoglobin content: hypochromic (pale color from deficiency of hemoglobin) and normochromic (normal color) (Table 31.1).

Macrocytic anemia presents with larger-than-normal RBCs, plus increased mean corpuscular volume (MCV) and mean corpuscular hemoglobin concentration (MCHC). Microcytic anemia is characterized by smaller-than-normal erythrocytes and less circulating hemoglobin, as in iron deficiency anemia and thalassemia.

Most anemias are caused by a lack of nutrients required for normal erythrocyte synthesis, principally iron, vitamin B_{12}, and folate. These anemias that result from an inadequate intake of iron, protein, certain vitamins, copper, and other heavy metals are called nutritional anemias. Other anemias result from conditions such as hemorrhage, genetic abnormalities, chronic disease states, or drug toxicity and have varying degrees of nutritional consequence.

IRON-RELATED BLOOD DISORDERS

Iron status can range from overload to deficiency and anemia. Routine measurement of iron status is necessary because approximately 6% of Americans have a negative iron balance, approximately 10% have a gene for positive balance and increased storage of iron, and approximately 1% have iron overload. Anemia also affects some groups more than others. Non-Hispanic blacks and Hispanics have the highest prevalence of anemia followed by non-Hispanic whites. As shown in Fig. 31.1, stages of iron status range from iron overload to iron deficiency anemia and are summarized as follows (Herbert, 1992):

a. Stage I and stage II negative iron balance (i.e., iron depletion). In these stages iron stores are low and there is no dysfunction. In stage I negative iron balance, reduced iron absorption produces moderately depleted iron stores. Stage II negative iron balance is characterized by severely depleted iron stores.

b. Stage III and stage IV negative iron balance (i.e., iron deficiency). Iron deficiency is characterized by inadequate body

Portions of this chapter written by Tracy Stopler and Susan Weiner.

| TABLE 31.1 | **Morphologic Classification of Anemia** | | |

Morphologic Type of Anemia	Underlying Abnormality	Clinical Syndromes	Treatment
Macrocytic (MCV > 94; MCHC > 31)			
Megaloblastic	Vitamin B$_{12}$ deficiency	Pernicious anemia	Vitamin B$_{12}$
	Folate deficiency	Nutritional megaloblastic anemias, malabsorption syndromes	Folic acid
	Inherited disorders of DNA synthesis	Orotic aciduria Sickle cell disease	Treatment based on the nature of the disorder
	Drug-induced disorders of DNA synthesis	Side effects of chemotherapeutic agents, anticonvulsants, oral contraceptives	Discontinue offending drug and administer folic acid
Nonmegaloblastic	Accelerated erythropoiesis	Hemolytic anemia	Treatment of underlying disease
Hypochromic Microcytic (MCV < 80; MCHC < 31)			
	Iron deficiency	Chronic loss of blood, inadequate diet, impaired absorption, increased demands	Ferrous sulfate or ferrous bis glycinate and correction of underlying cause
	Disorders of globin synthesis	Thalassemia Hemoglobin E Hemoglobin C	Nonspecific Mild – does not require treatment; Severe – frequent blood transfusions to provide healthy RBCs with normal Hgb
	Disorders of porphyrin and heme synthesis	Pyridoxine-responsive anemia	Pyridoxine
	Other disorders of iron metabolism	Copper deficiency	Copper
Normochromic Normocytic (MCV 82-92; MCHC > 30)			
	Recent blood loss	Various	Transfusion, iron, correction of underlying condition
	Overexpansion of plasma volume	Edema of pregnancy	Restore homeostasis
	Hemolytic diseases	Overhydration	Treatment based on the nature of the disorder
	Hypoplastic bone marrow	Aplastic anemia Pure RBC aplasia	Transfusion Androgens
	Infiltrated bone marrow	Leukemia, multiple myeloma, myelofibrosis	Chemotherapy
	Endocrine abnormality	Hypothyroidism, adrenal insufficiency	Treatment of underlying disease
	Chronic disease		Treatment of underlying disease
	Renal disease	Renal disease	Treatment of underlying disease
	Liver disease	Cirrhosis	Treatment of underlying disease

DNA, Deoxyribonucleic acid; *MCHC,* mean corpuscular hemoglobin concentration: concentration of hemoglobin expressed in grams per deciliter (g/dL); *MCV,* mean corpuscular volume: volume of one red blood cell expressed in femtoliters (fl); *RBC,* red blood cell.
Modified from Wintrobe MM et al: *Clinical hematology,* ed 8, Philadelphia, 1981, Lea & Febiger.

iron, possibly causing dysfunction and disease. In stage III negative iron balance, dysfunction is not accompanied by anemia; anemia develops in stage IV negative iron balance.

c. Stage I and stage II positive iron balance. Stage I positive balance usually lasts for several years with no dysfunction. Supplements of iron and/or vitamin C promote progression to dysfunction or disease, whereas iron removal prevents progression to disease. Iron overload disease develops in persons with stage II positive balance after years of iron overload have caused progressive damage to tissues and organs.

Iron status has a variety of indicators. Serum ferritin is an iron apoferritin complex, one of the chief storage forms of iron. Serum ferritin levels are in equilibrium with body iron stores. Very early (stage I) positive iron balance may best be recognized by measuring total iron-binding capacity (TIBC), the capacity of transferrin to take on or become saturated with iron. Conversely, measurement of serum or plasma ferritin levels may best reveal early (stages I or II) negative iron balance, although serum TIBC may be as good an indicator (see Chapter 5). Transferrin saturation is the measure of the amount of iron bound to transferrin and is a gauge of iron supply to the tissues; the percent saturation = serum iron/TIBC × 100.

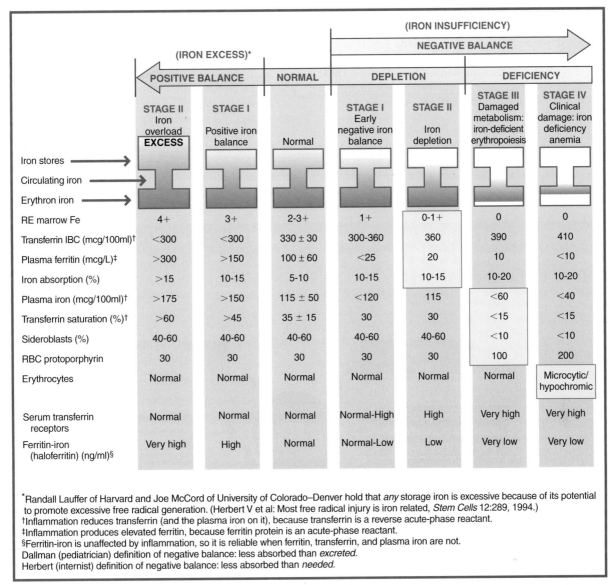

		(IRON EXCESS)*		NORMAL	(IRON INSUFFICIENCY) NEGATIVE BALANCE			
		POSITIVE BALANCE		NORMAL	DEPLETION		DEFICIENCY	
		STAGE II Iron overload **EXCESS**	STAGE I Positive iron balance	Normal	STAGE I Early negative iron balance	STAGE II Iron depletion	STAGE III Damaged metabolism: iron-deficient erythropoiesis	STAGE IV Clinical damage: iron deficiency anemia
Iron stores →								
Circulating iron →								
Erythron iron →								
RE marrow Fe		4+	3+	2-3+	1+	0-1+	0	0
Transferrin IBC (mcg/100ml)[†]		<300	<300	330 ± 30	300-360	360	390	410
Plasma ferritin (mcg/L)[‡]		>300	>150	100 ± 60	<25	20	10	<10
Iron absorption (%)		>15	10-15	5-10	10-15	10-15	10-20	10-20
Plasma iron (mcg/100ml)[†]		>175	>150	115 ± 50	<120	115	<60	<40
Transferrin saturation (%)[†]		>60	>45	35 ± 15	30	30	<15	<15
Sideroblasts (%)		40-60	40-60	40-60	40-60	40-60	<10	<10
RBC protoporphyrin		30	30	30	30	30	100	200
Erythrocytes		Normal	Normal	Normal	Normal	Normal	Normal	Microcytic/ hypochromic
Serum transferrin receptors		Normal	Normal	Normal	Normal-High	High	Very high	Very high
Ferritin-iron (haloferritin) (ng/ml)[§]		Very high	High	Normal	Normal-Low	Low	Very low	Very low

*Randall Lauffer of Harvard and Joe McCord of University of Colorado–Denver hold that *any* storage iron is excessive because of its potential to promote excessive free radical generation. (Herbert V et al: Most free radical injury is iron related, *Stem Cells* 12:289, 1994.)
[†]Inflammation reduces transferrin (and the plasma iron on it), because transferrin is a reverse acute-phase reactant.
[‡]Inflammation produces elevated ferritin, because ferritin protein is an acute-phase reactant.
[§]Ferritin-iron is unaffected by inflammation, so it is reliable when ferritin, transferrin, and plasma iron are not.
Dallman (pediatrician) definition of negative balance: less absorbed than *excreted.*
Herbert (internist) definition of negative balance: less absorbed than *needed.*

Fig. 31.1 Sequential stages of iron status. *IBC,* Iron-binding capacity; *RBC,* red blood cell; *RE,* reticuloendothelial cells. (Copyright Victor Herbert, 1995.)

Iron Deficiency Anemia

Pathophysiology

Iron deficiency anemia is characterized by the production of microcytic erythrocytes and a diminished level of circulating hemoglobin. This microcytic anemia is the last stage of iron deficiency, and it represents the end point of a long period of iron deprivation. There are many causes of iron deficiency anemia as discussed in Box 31.1.

A common cause of iron deficiency is blood loss, either chronic or acute, including heavy menstrual bleeding in women. It can also be caused by malabsorption, medications, and inadequate intake. Because anemia is the last manifestation of chronic, long-term iron deficiency, the symptoms reflect a malfunction of a variety of body systems. Inadequate muscle function is reflected in decreased work performance and exercise tolerance. Neurologic involvement is manifested by behavioral changes such as fatigue, anorexia, and pica (consumption of nonfood items), especially pagophagia (ice eating). Abnormal cognitive development in children may indicate iron deficiency before it has developed into overt anemia (Jáuregui-Lobera, 2014).

BOX 31.1	**Causes of Iron Deficiency Anemia**
Inadequate Ingestion	Poor diet without supplementation of iron
Inadequate Absorption	Diarrhea, achlorhydria, intestinal disease such as celiac disease, atrophic gastritis, partial or total gastrectomy, or drug interference
Inadequate Utilization	Chronic gastrointestinal disturbances
Increased Requirement	Increase of blood volume, which occurs during infancy, adolescence, pregnancy, and lactation and which is not being matched with intake
Increased Excretion	Excessive menstrual blood (in females); hemorrhage from injury; or chronic blood loss from a bleeding ulcer, bleeding hemorrhoids, esophageal varices, regional enteritis, celiac disease, Crohn's disease, ulcerative colitis, parasitic or malignant disease
Increased Destruction	Caused by a chronic inflammation or other chronic disorder leading to destruction of RBC's

Growth abnormalities, epithelial disorders, and a reduction in gastric acidity are also common. A possible sign of early iron deficiency is reduced immunocompetence, particularly defects in cell-mediated immunity and the phagocytic activity of neutrophils, which may lead to frequent infections. Restless legs syndrome (RLS) with leg pain or discomfort may result from a lack of iron in the brain; this alters dopamine production and movement (Connor et al, 2017).

As iron deficiency anemia becomes more severe, defects arise in the structure and function of the epithelial tissues, especially of the tongue, nails, mouth, and stomach. The skin may appear pale in people with lighter complexions, and the inside of the lower eyelid may be light pink instead of red regardless of skin tone. Mouth changes include atrophy of the lingual papillae, burning, redness, and in severe cases, glossitis, a completely smooth, waxy, and glistening appearance of the tongue. Angular stomatitis and a form of dysphagia may occur. Gastritis occurs frequently and may result in achlorhydria (low stomach acid). Fingernails can become thin and flat, and eventually koilonychia (spoon-shaped nails) may be noted (Fig. 31.2).

Progressive, untreated anemia results in cardiovascular and respiratory changes that can eventually lead to cardiac failure. Some social and emotional behavioral symptoms respond to iron therapy before the anemia is cured, suggesting they may be the result of tissue depletion of iron-containing enzymes rather than a decreased level of hemoglobin (see *Pathophysiology and Care Management Algorithm: Iron Deficiency Anemia*).

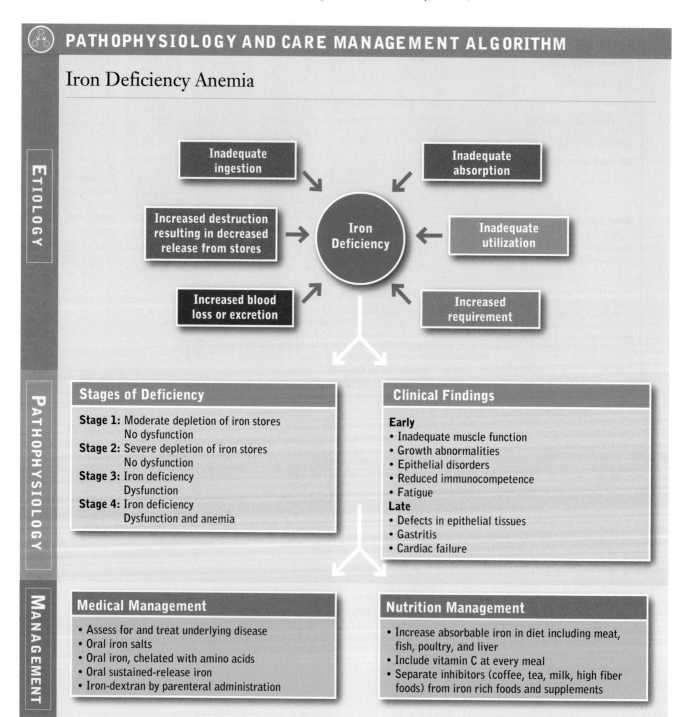

PATHOPHYSIOLOGY AND CARE MANAGEMENT ALGORITHM

Iron Deficiency Anemia

ETIOLOGY

- Inadequate ingestion
- Inadequate absorption
- Increased destruction resulting in decreased release from stores
- Inadequate utilization
- Increased blood loss or excretion
- Increased requirement

→ Iron Deficiency

PATHOPHYSIOLOGY

Stages of Deficiency

Stage 1: Moderate depletion of iron stores
No dysfunction
Stage 2: Severe depletion of iron stores
No dysfunction
Stage 3: Iron deficiency
Dysfunction
Stage 4: Iron deficiency
Dysfunction and anemia

Clinical Findings

Early
- Inadequate muscle function
- Growth abnormalities
- Epithelial disorders
- Reduced immunocompetence
- Fatigue

Late
- Defects in epithelial tissues
- Gastritis
- Cardiac failure

MANAGEMENT

Medical Management

- Assess for and treat underlying disease
- Oral iron salts
- Oral iron, chelated with amino acids
- Oral sustained-release iron
- Iron-dextran by parenteral administration

Nutrition Management

- Increase absorbable iron in diet including meat, fish, poultry, and liver
- Include vitamin C at every meal
- Separate inhibitors (coffee, tea, milk, high fiber foods) from iron rich foods and supplements

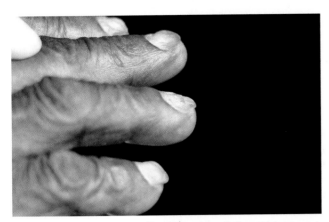

Fig. 31.2 Fingernails with cup-like depressions (koilonychia) are a sign of iron deficiency in adults. (From Heitz C. Koilonychia. In: Flickr [website]. https://www.flickr.com/photos/coreyheitzmd/15023020192. April 14, 2014.)

Assessment

A definitive diagnosis of iron deficiency anemia requires more than one method of iron evaluation; serum ferritin, iron, and transferrin are the most useful. The evaluation also should include an assessment of cell size and shape (morphology). By itself, hemoglobin concentration is unsuitable as a diagnostic tool in cases of suspected iron deficiency anemia for three reasons: (1) it is affected only late in the disease, (2) it cannot distinguish iron deficiency from other anemias, and (3) hemoglobin values may be within the normal range despite iron deficiency.

After absorption, iron is transported by plasma transferrin—a beta-1 globulin (protein) that binds iron derived from the gastrointestinal tract, iron storage sites, or hemoglobin breakdown—to the bone marrow (hemoglobin synthesis), endothelial cells (storage), or placenta (fetal needs). Transferrin molecules are generated on the surface of RBCs in response to the need for iron. With iron deficiency, so many transferrin receptors are on the cell surface unbound to iron that some of them break off and float in the serum. Their presence is an early sign of developing iron deficiency; a higher quantity of soluble serum transferrin receptors (STFRs) means greater deficiency of iron. Progressive stages of iron deficiency can be evaluated by measurements, as shown in Table 31.2.

Protoporphyrin is the iron-containing portion of the respiratory pigments that combines with protein to form hemoglobin or myoglobin. The zinc protoporphyrin (ZnPP)/heme ratio is measured to assess iron deficiency. However, both this ZnPP/heme ratio and hemoglobin levels are affected by chronic infection and other factors that can produce a condition that mimics iron deficiency anemia when, in fact, iron is adequate.

At higher altitudes, where there is a lower availability of oxygen, hematocrit and hemoglobin levels increase to adapt (Ryan et al, 2014). This must be considered when assessing anemia. High altitude is 4900 to 11,500 feet; very high altitude is 11,500 to 18,000 feet; extreme altitude is above 18,000 feet.

Medical Management

Treatment of iron deficiency anemia should focus primarily on the underlying cause, although this is often difficult to determine. The goal is repletion of iron stores.

Oral supplementation. The chief treatment for iron deficiency anemia involves oral administration of inorganic iron in the ferrous form. Although the body uses ferric and ferrous iron, the reduced ferrous is easier on the gut and better absorbed. At a dose of 30 mg, absorption of ferrous iron is three times greater than if the same amount were given in the ferric form.

Iron is best absorbed when the stomach is empty. However, under these conditions it tends to cause gastric irritation, which is a direct result of the high quantity of free ferrous iron in the stomach. Gastrointestinal side effects can include nausea, epigastric discomfort and distention, heartburn, diarrhea, or constipation. If these side effects occur, the patient is told to take the iron with meals instead of on an empty stomach; however, this sharply reduces the absorbability of the iron. Chelated forms of iron (combined with amino acids or Krebs cycle intermediaries) are more bioavailable than nonchelated iron. Chelated iron is less affected by inhibitors of iron absorption,

TABLE 31.2 Biochemical Evaluation of Iron Deficiency

Measure	Reference Range	Deficiency
Serum or plasma ferritin	Newborn 25-200 ng/mL; 25-200 mcg/dL Neonate – 5 mos 50-200 ng/mL; 50-200 mcg/dL 6 mos-15 yr 7-142 ng/mL; 7-142 mcg/dL F 15 yr + 10-150 ng/mL; 10-150 mcg/dL M 15 yr + 12-300 ng/mL; 12-300 mcg/dL	The most sensitive indicator of iron deficiency. Low levels of ferritin are also seen in severe protein depletion. Females – < 10 mcg/dL Males – < 12 mcg/dL
Serum or plasma iron	F 40-150 mcg/dL; 7.2-26.9 mmol/L M 50-160 mcg/dL; 8.9-28.7 mmol/L	A good measure of quantity of iron bound to transferrin. Females – < 40 mcg/dL Males – <50 mcg/dL
Total iron-binding capacity (TIBC)	250-460 mcg/dL; 45-82 mmol/L	TIBC primarily reflects liver function and is an indirect measurement of transferrin. Increases with iron-deficiency anemia.
Transferrin saturation	F 15%-50% M 20%-50%	Measures the iron supply to the tissues. Calculated by dividing serum iron by the TIBC multiplied by 100. Levels less than 16% are considered inadequate for erythropoiesis.
Soluble serum transferrin receptor (STFR)	F 1.9-4.4 mg/L M 2.2-5 mg/L	STFR reflects the rate of red blood cell (RBC) production in bone marrow. Ordered to differentiate between iron deficiency anemia and anemia of chronic disease. More sensitive than serum ferritin because it is elevated with iron deficiency, is within normal limits (WNL) in chronic disease or inflammation, and is low with iron overload.

Created with assistance by Mary Litchford, PhD, RDN, LDN.

TABLE 31.3 Forms of Iron Supplements

Iron Supplement	Advantages	Disadvantages
Ferrous sulfate	Most commonly studied Least expensive	Most constipating
Ferrous gluconate	Generally well tolerated with few gastrointestinal side effects	
Carbonyl iron (slow iron)	Generally well tolerated with few gastrointestinal side effects	Slow rate of solubilization, which slows the rate of absorption
Chelated iron (ferrous fumarate, succinate, aspartate, and bis glycinate)	Better absorbed Fewer side effects Least constipating	More expensive

including phytate, oxalate, phosphate, and calcium. Chelated iron, particularly ferrous bis glycinate, causes less gastrointestinal disturbances than elemental iron and it can be given in a lower dose (Ferrari et al, 2012; Milman et al, 2013). Micronutrient powders (MNPs) containing iron may be useful methods of home food fortification for children under age 2 (De-Regil et al, 2013). The MNPs can be added to semisolid foods without affecting the sensory appeal of the foods. Various forms of iron supplements are discussed in Table 31.3.

Health professionals usually prescribe oral iron three times daily for 3-6 months to treat iron deficiency. Depending on the severity of the anemia and the patient's tolerance, the daily dose of elemental iron recommended is 50 to 100 mg three times daily for adults and 2-6 mg/kg of body weight divided into three doses per day for children (Short and Domagalski, 2013; Wang, 2016). Vitamin C given with the iron greatly increases iron absorption, but at higher doses it may also increase gastric irritation by intensifying oxidative stress in the gastrointestinal tract. Taking it with a high vitamin C food such as orange juice may be better tolerated.

Absorption of 10 to 20 mg of iron per day permits RBC production to increase to approximately three times the normal rate and, in the absence of blood loss, hemoglobin concentration to rise at a rate of 0.2 g/dL daily. Increased reticulocytosis (an increase in the number of young RBCs) is seen within 2 to 3 days after iron administration, but affected persons may report subjective improvements in mood and appetite sooner. The hemoglobin level will begin to increase by day 4. Iron therapy should be continued for 4-6 months, even after restoration of normal hemoglobin levels, to allow for repletion of body iron reserves. Coordination of care with a physician is essential with therapeutic iron supplementation.

Parenteral iron administration. If iron supplementation fails to correct the anemia, (1) the patient may not be taking the supplemental iron as prescribed due to gastric distress, (2) bleeding may be continuing at a rate faster than the erythroid marrow can replace blood cells, or (3) the supplemental iron is not being absorbed, possibly as a result of malabsorption secondary to steatorrhea, celiac disease, or hemodialysis. Parenteral adminstration is also used for patients who are receiving erythropoietin, a hormone that stimulates blood cell production. It is most often given as iron dextran but can also be given as iron sucrose or ferric gluconate. Although replenishment of iron stores by this route is faster, it is more expensive and intravenous therapy carries additional risk.

Medical Nutrition Therapy

Nutrition assessments and interventions should consider the amount of absorbable dietary iron consumed. A good source of iron contains a substantial amount of iron in relation to its calorie content and contributes at least 10% of the recommended dietary allowance (RDA) for iron. Liver; kidney; beef; dried fruits; dried peas and beans; nuts; dark green leafy vegetables; and fortified whole-grain breads, muffins, cereals, and nutrition bars are among the foods that rank highest in iron content (see Appendix 42). It is estimated that 1.8 mg of iron must be absorbed daily to meet the needs of 80% to 90% of adult women and adolescent boys and girls.

Form of iron. Heme iron (approximately 15% of which is absorbable) is the organic form in meat, fish, and poultry, and is known as the meat-fish-poultry (MFP) factor. It is much better absorbed than nonheme iron. Nonheme iron can also be found in MFP, as well as in legumes, grains, vegetables, herbs and fruits, but it is not part of the heme molecule. The absorption rate of nonheme iron varies between 3% and 8% depending on the presence of dietary enhancing factors, specifically vitamin C and meat, fish, and poultry. Vitamin C not only is a powerful reducing agent, but also binds iron to form a readily absorbed complex. The mechanism by which the MFP factor potentiates the absorption of nonheme iron in other foodstuffs is unknown.

Inhibitors. Iron absorption can be inhibited to varying degrees by factors in foods that bind iron, including carbonates, oxalates, phosphates, and phytates (whole grain breads and cereals and legumes [beans]). Factors in vegetable fiber may inhibit nonheme iron absorption. If taken with meals, tea and coffee can reduce iron absorption by 50% through the formation of insoluble iron compounds with tannin. Iron in egg yolk is poorly absorbed because of the presence of phosvitin.

Bioavailability of dietary iron. Because typical Western diets generally contain 6 mg/1000 kcal of iron, the bioavailability of iron in the diet is more important in correcting or preventing iron deficiency than the total amount of dietary iron consumed. The rate of absorption depends on the iron status of the individual, as reflected in the level of iron stores. The lower the iron stores, the greater the rate of iron absorption. Individuals with iron deficiency anemia absorb approximately 20% to 30% of dietary iron compared with the 5% to 10% absorbed by those without iron deficiency.

IRON OVERLOAD

Excess iron is stored as ferritin and hemosiderin in the macrophages of the liver, spleen, and bone marrow. The body has a limited capacity to excrete iron and is efficient at recycling it. Approximately 1 mg of iron is excreted daily through the gastrointestinal tract, urinary tract, and skin. When red blood cells are no longer functional (after about 120 days), they are re-absorbed by the spleen. Iron from these cells can be recycled by the body. To maintain a normal iron balance, the daily obligatory loss must be replaced by the absorption of heme and nonheme food iron. Persons with iron overload excrete increased amounts of iron, especially in the feces, to compensate partially for the increased absorption and higher stores.

Excessive iron intake usually stems from accidental incorporation of iron into the diet from environmental sources. In the United States iron-containing supplements remain a common source of excessive iron ingestion, especially among children (Chang and Rangan, 2011). In other parts of the world, excessive iron intake may result from consumption of beverages or foods prepared in iron-containing cooking vessels (National Library of Medicine, 2019).

Uncommon disorders associated with iron overload include hemochromatosis, thalassemias, sideroblastic anemia, chronic hemolytic anemia, ineffective erythropoiesis, transfusional iron overload (secondary to multiple blood transfusions), porphyria cutanea tarda, aplastic anemia, and alcoholic cirrhosis. Aplastic anemia is a normochromic-normocytic anemia accompanied by a deficiency of all the formed elements in the blood; it can be caused by exposure to toxic chemicals, ionizing radiation, and medications, although the cause is often unknown.

Brain iron increases with age and is abnormally elevated in neurodegenerative diseases, including Alzheimer's disease and Parkinson's disease (Ward et al, 2014). Several gene variants affect iron metabolism and may contribute to early onset of these conditions.

Hemochromatosis

Hereditary hemochromatosis is a general term for a group of rare genetic disorders that are characterized by the accumulation of iron in body organs, typically the liver, pancreas, and heart. Over time this accumulation is associated with organ damage, organ failure, and sometimes premature death. The most common form of hemochromatosis goes by several names including hereditary iron overload (HFE-related) hemochromatosis, type I or classic hemochromatosis, or hereditary hemochromatosis. The disease generally does not become apparent until 20 to 40 years of age. Men are usually diagnosed earlier than women because they have no physiologic mechanisms for losing iron such as menstruation, pregnancy, or lactation. Symptoms include fatigue, joint pain, and enlarged liver and spleen. The exact prevalence of this disorder is unknown, but it is thought to be the most common autosomal recessive disorder in Caucasian populations. In individuals of Northern European descent, it is estimated to have an incidence of 1 in 227 people. People with this condition absorb three times more iron from their food than those without hemochromatosis. Those who have two affected genes (homozygous) will likely die of iron overload unless they donate blood frequently. Otherwise, the excessive iron absorption continues unabated.

The Hemochromatosis and Iron Overload Screening Study (HEIRS) notes that non-Hispanic whites have the highest prevalence of the C282Y mutation of the hereditary iron (HFE) gene and thus hemochromatosis, followed by Native Americans, Hispanics, African Americans, Pacific Islanders, and Asians (Adams, 2015). Asians and Pacific Islanders have the highest levels of iron in their blood of all racial and ethnic groups, but they have the lowest prevalence of the gene mutation found with the typical form of hemochromatosis. Results from the HEIRS study suggest that increased iron values in non-Caucasian populations may be associated with non-HFE hemochromatosis and secondary iron overload.

Pathophysiology

Hepcidin is a peptide synthesized in the liver that functions as the principal regulator of systemic iron homeostasis. It regulates iron transport from iron-exporting tissues into plasma. Hepcidin deficiency underlies most known forms of hereditary hemochromatosis. Hepcidin inhibits the cellular efflux of iron by binding to and inducing the degradation of ferroprotein, the sole iron exporter in iron-transporting cells. Hepcidin controls plasma iron concentration and tissue distribution of iron by inhibiting intestinal iron absorption, iron recycling by macrophages, and iron mobilization from hepatic stores (Ganz, 2011).

Hepcidin synthesis is increased by iron loading and decreased by anemia and hypoxia. Its synthesis is also greatly increased during inflammation, trapping iron in macrophages, decreasing plasma iron concentrations, and causing iron-restricted erythropoiesis that is characteristic of anemia of chronic disease. There is evidence that the mutation of the HFE gene leading to hemochromatosis is also associated with increased levels of gastrin in the stomach, leading to increased levels of gastric acid and thus increased absorption of iron (Ganz, 2011). In hemochromatosis iron absorption is enhanced, resulting in a gradual, progressive accumulation of iron. Most affected persons do not know they have it.

A progressive, positive iron balance may result in a variety of serious problems, including hepatomegaly, skin pigmentation, arthritis, heart disease, hypogonadism, diabetes mellitus, and cancer. Individuals with abnormally high iron levels are more likely to develop cancer of the colon. Iron is a prooxidant that can be used for tumor cell growth and proliferation. There also seems to be increased risk for age-related macular degeneration, Alzheimer's disease, and Parkinson's disease because of the oxidative damage associated with iron overload (Belaidi and Bush, 2016; Fleming and Ponka, 2012).

Assessment

If an iron overload is suspected, serum ferritin level (storage iron) and percent of transferrin saturation ([serum iron/TIBC] $\times$ 100) should be performed (Bacon et al, 2011). Iron overload may be present if the transferrin saturation is greater than or equal to 45% and if the serum ferritin level is elevated. If transferrin saturation and ferritin levels are elevated, HFE mutation analysis is recommended.

Medical Management

The patient with iron overload may simultaneously be anemic as a result of damage to the bone marrow, an inflammatory disorder, cancer, internal bleeding, or chronic infection. Iron supplements should not be taken until the cause is known.

For patients with significant iron overload, weekly phlebotomy for 2 to 3 years may be required to eliminate all excess iron (Bacon et al, 2011). Treatment for noninherited forms of secondary iron overload also may involve iron depletion with intravenous deferoxamine or oral deferasirox, chelating agents that are excreted by the kidneys, or with calcium disodium ethylenediaminetetraacetic acid (EDTA). Morbidity and mortality are reduced if excess body iron is removed by phlebotomy therapy before hepatic cirrhosis or diabetes develops.

Medical Nutrition Therapy

Individuals with iron overload should reduce meat, fish and poultry and consume more of a plant based or vegetarian diet. Reduced vitamin C is recommended as well as avoidance of vitamin C supplements, as this can increase absorption of iron.

Affected persons should avoid foods that are fortified with iron (i.e., breakfast cereals, energy or sports bars, and meal-replacement drinks or shakes). They should also avoid iron supplements or multiple vitamin and mineral supplements that contain iron. The RDA for iron should not be exceeded, and for some, lower intakes are recommended (see RDA tables at the beginning of the book).

MEGALOBLASTIC ANEMIAS

Megaloblastic anemia reflects a disturbed synthesis of DNA, which results in morphologic and functional changes in erythrocytes, leukocytes, and platelets and their precursors in the blood and bone marrow. This anemia is characterized by the presence of large, immature, abnormal, RBC progenitors in the bone marrow; 95% of cases are attributable to folate or vitamin B_{12} deficiency. Two disorders of cobalamin metabolism arise from mutations of the methionine synthase and methionine synthase reductase genes; these disorders feature megaloblastic anemia and neurologic manifestations (see Chapter 6).

Both vitamins are essential to the synthesis of nucleoproteins. Hematologic changes are the same for both; however, the folic acid deficiency is the first to appear. Normal body folate stores are depleted within 2 to 4 months in individuals consuming folate-deficient diets. By contrast, vitamin B_{12} stores are depleted only after several years of a vitamin B_{12}–deficient diet. In persons with vitamin B_{12} deficiency, folic acid supplementation can mask B_{12} deficiency (Fig. 31.3).

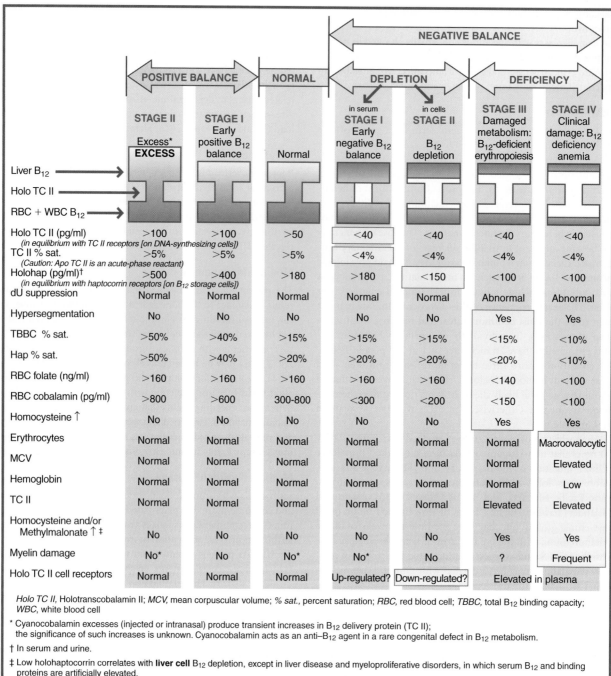

	NEGATIVE BALANCE			
	POSITIVE BALANCE		NORMAL	DEPLETION		DEFICIENCY	
	STAGE II	STAGE I Early positive B₁₂ balance	Normal	in serum STAGE I Early negative B₁₂ balance	in cells STAGE II B₁₂ depletion	STAGE III Damaged metabolism: B₁₂-deficient erythropoiesis	STAGE IV Clinical damage: B₁₂ deficiency anemia
	Excess* **EXCESS**						
Liver B₁₂ →							
Holo TC II →							
RBC + WBC B₁₂ →							
Holo TC II (pg/ml) *(in equilibrium with TC II receptors [on DNA-synthesizing cells])*	>100	>100	>50	<40	<40	<40	<40
TC II % sat. *(Caution: Apo TC II is an acute-phase reactant)*	>5%	>5%	>5%	<4%	<4%	<4%	<4%
Holohap (pg/ml)† *(in equilibrium with haptocorrin receptors [on B₁₂ storage cells])*	>500	>400	>180	>180	<150	<100	<100
dU suppression	Normal	Normal	Normal	Normal	Normal	Abnormal	Abnormal
Hypersegmentation	No	No	No	No	No	Yes	Yes
TBBC % sat.	>50%	>40%	>15%	>15%	>15%	<15%	<10%
Hap % sat.	>50%	>40%	>20%	>20%	>20%	<20%	<10%
RBC folate (ng/ml)	>160	>160	>160	>160	>160	<140	<100
RBC cobalamin (pg/ml)	>800	>600	300-800	<300	<200	<150	<100
Homocysteine ↑	No	No	No	No	No	Yes	Yes
Erythrocytes	Normal	Normal	Normal	Normal	Normal	Normal	Macroovalocytic
MCV	Normal	Normal	Normal	Normal	Normal	Normal	Elevated
Hemoglobin	Normal	Normal	Normal	Normal	Normal	Normal	Low
TC II	Normal	Normal	Normal	Normal	Normal	Elevated	Elevated
Homocysteine and/or Methylmalonate ↑ ‡	No	No	No	No	No	Yes	Yes
Myelin damage	No*	No	No*	No*	No	?	Frequent
Holo TC II cell receptors	Normal	Normal	Normal	Up-regulated?	Down-regulated?	Elevated in plasma	

Holo TC II, Holotranscobalamin II; *MCV,* mean corpuscular volume; *% sat.,* percent saturation; *RBC,* red blood cell; *TBBC,* total B₁₂ binding capacity;
WBC, white blood cell

* Cyanocobalamin excesses (injected or intranasal) produce transient increases in B₁₂ delivery protein (TC II);
the significance of such increases is unknown. Cyanocobalamin acts as an anti–B₁₂ agent in a rare congenital defect in B₁₂ metabolism.

† In serum and urine.

‡ Low holohaptocorrin correlates with **liver cell** B₁₂ depletion, except in liver disease and myeloproliferative disorders, in which serum B₁₂ and binding
proteins are artificially elevated.

There may be hematopoietic cell and glial cell B₁₂ depletion **prior to** liver cell depletion, and those cells may be in stage III or IV negative B₁₂ balance,
whereas liver cells are still in stage II.

Fig. 31.3 Sequential stages of vitamin B₁₂ status. (From Herbert V: Staging vitamin B₁₂. In Ziegler EE, Filer LJ,
editors: *Present knowledge in nutrition,* ed 7, Washington, DC, 1996, International Life Sciences Institute Press.)

In correcting the anemia, the vitamin B₁₂ deficiency may remain undetected, leading to the irreversible neuropsychiatric damage that is corrected only with B₁₂ supplementation (see Chapter 41).

Folate-Deficiency Anemia

Etiology

Folate is a naturally occurring B vitamin found in foods in the tetrahydrofolate (THF) form. Folic acid is the synthetic version of the vitamin found in the fully oxidized monoglutamate form, which may be found in fortified foods and supplements. Folate-deficiency anemia is associated with prolonged inadequate diets, inadequate absorption, inadequate use of folic acid caused by genetic aberrations, and increased requirements resulting from pregnancy or growth. Folate-deficiency anemia can affect pregnant women and occurs in infants born to mothers with folate deficiency. Folate deficiency in early pregnancy can result in an infant born with a neural tube defect (see Chapter 14). Other causes are intestinal disorders resulting in malabsorption (celiac

BOX 31.2 Causes of Folate Deficiency

Inadequate Ingestion	Poor diet (lack of or overcooked fruits and vegetables), vitamin B_{12} or vitamin C deficiency, chronic alcoholism
Inadequate Absorption	Celiac disease, tropical sprue, drug interactions, congenital defects
Inadequate Utilization	Antagonists, anticonvulsants, enzyme deficiency, vitamin B_{12} and vitamin C deficiency, chronic alcoholism, excess glycine and methionine
Increased Requirement	Extra tissue demand, infancy, increased hematopoiesis, increased metabolic activity, Lesch-Nyhan syndrome, drugs
Increased Excretion	Vitamin B_{12} deficiency, liver disease, kidney dialysis, chronic exfoliative dermatitis
Increased Destruction	Dietary oxidants

Modified from Herbert V, Das KC: Folic acid and vitamin B_{12}. In Shils ME et al, editors: *Modern nutrition in health and disease*, ed 8, vol 1, Philadelphia, 1994, Lea & Febiger.

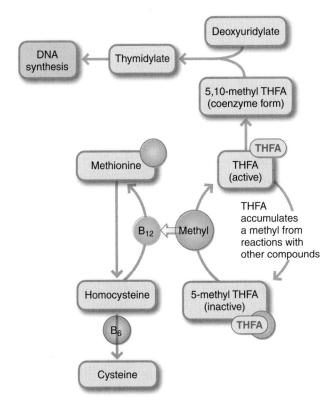

Fig. 31.4 Methylfolate trap. A deficiency of vitamin B_{12} can result in a deficiency of folic acid because folate is trapped in the form of 5-methyltetrahydrofolate (5-methyl THFA), which cannot be converted to THFA and methyl groups donated by the vitamin B_{12}–dependent pathway. *DNA*, Deoxyribonucleic acid; *THFA*, tetrahydrofolic acid.

disease, tropical sprue, and inflammatory bowel disease), use of certain drugs (anticonvulsants, barbiturates, cycloserine, sulfasalazine, cholestyramine, and metformin), amino acid excess (glycine and methionine), and alcohol.

Because alcohol interferes with the folate enterohepatic cycle, most people with alcoholism have a negative folate balance or a folate deficiency. Alcoholics constitute the only group that generally has all six causes of folate deficiency simultaneously: inadequate ingestion, absorption, and use, and increased excretion, requirement, and destruction of folate (see Chapter 28). Box 31.2 describes the causes of folate deficiency.

Folate absorption takes place in the small intestine. Enzyme conjugases (e.g., pteroylpolyglutamate hydrolase, the folate conjugase), found in the brush border of the small intestine, hydrolyze the polyglutamates to monoglutamates and reduce them to dihydrofolate and tetrahydrofolic acid (THFA) in the small intestinal epithelial cells (enterocytes). From the enterocytes these forms are transported to the circulation, where they are bound to protein and transported as methyl THFA into the cells of the body.

In the absence of vitamin B_{12}, 5-methyl THFA, the major circulating and storage form of folic acid, is metabolically inactive. To be activated the 5-methyl group is removed, and THFA is cycled back into the folate pool, where it functions as the main 1-carbon-unit acceptor in mammalian biochemical reactions. THFA may then be converted to the coenzyme form of folate required to convert deoxyuridylate to thymidylate, which is necessary for DNA synthesis.

MTHFR allele. A genetic defect found in 25% of Hispanics, 10% of Caucasians and Asians, and 1% of African Americans is the methylenetetrahydrofolate reductase (MTHFR) deficiency (National Institutes of Health, Office of Dietary Supplements, 2018) (see Chapter 6). The allele is problematic in pregnancy and may contribute to miscarriages, anencephaly, or neural defects (see Chapter 14). Because MTHFR irreversibly reduces 5,10-methylenetetrahydrofolate to 5-methyltetrahydrofolate, its deficiency may result in developmental delay, motor and gait dysfunction, seizures, neurologic impairment, extremely high levels of homocysteine, clotting disorders, and other conditions.

Methylfolate trap. Vitamin B_{12} deficiency can result in a folate deficiency by causing folate entrapment in the metabolically useless form of 5-methyl THFA (Fig. 31.4). The lack of vitamin B_{12} to remove the 5-methyl unit means that metabolically inactive methyl THFA is

trapped. It cannot release its 1-carbon methyl group to become THFA, the basic 1-carbon carrier that picks up 1-carbon units from one molecule and delivers them to another. Hence a functional folate deficiency results.

Pathophysiology

Folate deficiency develops in four stages: two that involve depletion, followed by two marked by deficiency (Fig. 31.5):

Stage 1: Characterized by early negative folate balance (serum depletion to less than 3 ng/mL)

Stage 2: Characterized by negative folate balance (cell depletion), with a decrease in erythrocyte folate levels to less than 160 ng/mL

Stage 3: Characterized by damaged folate metabolism, with folate-deficient erythropoiesis. This stage is characterized by slowed DNA synthesis, manifested by an abnormal diagnostic deoxyuridine (dU) suppression test correctable in vitro by folates, granulocyte nuclear hypersegmentation, and macroovalocytic red cells.

Stage 4: Characterized by clinical folate-deficiency anemia, with an elevated MCV and anemia.

Because of their interrelated roles in the synthesis of thymidylate in DNA formation, a deficiency of either vitamin B_{12} or folate results in a megaloblastic anemia. The immature nuclei do not mature properly in the deficient state; and large (macrocytic), immature (megaloblastic) RBCs are the result. The common clinical signs of folate deficiency include fatigue, dyspnea, sore tongue, diarrhea, irritability, forgetfulness, anorexia, glossitis, and weight loss.

Normal body folate stores are depleted within 2 to 4 months on a folate-deficient diet, resulting in a macrocytic, megaloblastic anemia

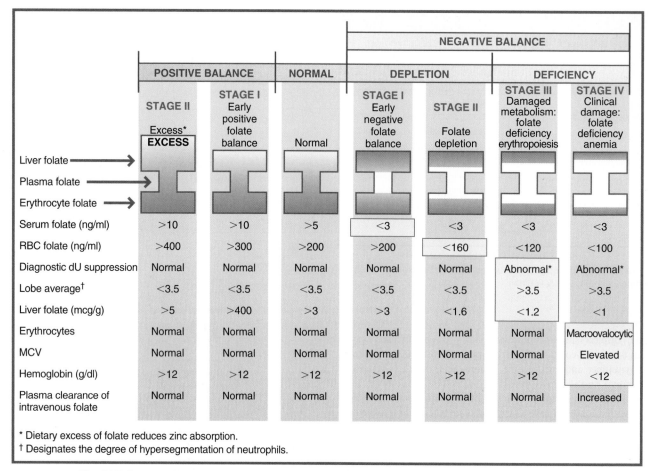

Fig. 31.5 Sequential stages of folate status. *dU*, Deoxyuridine; *MCV*, mean corpuscular volume; *RBC*, red blood cell. (From Herbert V: Folic acid. In Shils ME et al, editors: *Modern nutrition in health and disease*, ed 9, Philadelphia 1998, Lea & Febiger.)

with a decreased number of erythrocytes, leukocytes, and platelets. Folate-deficiency anemia is manifested by very low serum folate (<3 ng/mL) and RBC folate levels of less than 140 to 160 ng/mL. Whereas a low serum folate level merely diagnoses a negative balance at the time the blood is drawn, a red cell folate (RCF) level measures actual body folate stores, and thus is the superior measurement for determining folate nutriture. To differentiate folate deficiency from vitamin B_{12} deficiency, levels of serum folate, RCF, serum vitamin B_{12}, and vitamin B_{12} bound to transcobalamin II (TCII) can be measured simultaneously using a radioassay kit. Also diagnostic for folate deficiency is an elevated level of formiminoglutamic acid in the urine, as well as the dU suppression test in bone marrow cells or peripheral blood lymphocytes (see Chapter 5 and Appendix 12).

Medical Management

Before treatment is initiated, it is important to diagnose the cause of the megaloblastosis correctly. Administration of folate corrects megaloblastosis from either folate or vitamin B_{12} deficiency, but it can mask the neurologic damage of vitamin B_{12} deficiency, allowing the nerve damage to progress to the point of irreversibility.

A dosage of 1 mg of folate taken orally every day for 2 to 3 weeks replenishes folate stores. Maintaining repleted stores requires an absolute minimum oral intake of 50 to 100 micrograms of folate from food and or dietary supplements daily. When folate deficiency is complicated by alcoholism, genetic aberrations, or other conditions that suppress hematopoiesis, increase folate requirements, or reduce folate absorption, therapy should remain at 500 to 1000 micrograms daily.

Symptomatic improvement, as evidenced by increased alertness, and appetite, may be apparent within 24 to 48 hours, long before hematologic values revert to normal, a gradual process that takes approximately a month.

Medical Nutrition Therapy

After the anemia is corrected, the patient should be educated to eat multiple servings of folate-rich fresh fruit or dark green vegetables or to drink a glass of vegetable or fruit and vegetable juice daily (see Appendix 31 for a list of folate-containing foods). Fresh, uncooked fruits and vegetables are good sources of folate because folate can easily be destroyed by heat. In 1998 the Food and Drug Administration required that grains be fortified with folic acid. The RDAs for folate are summarized on the inside cover of this text. The RDA for adults is 400 mcg daily. The Dietary Guidelines for Americans recommend that women of childbearing age who may become pregnant and those in their first trimester of pregnancy consume adequate synthetic folic acid (400 mcg/day and 600 mcg/day, respectively) from fortified foods and supplements in addition to consuming a variety of foods containing folate (see Chapter 14 and Appendix 31).

Vitamin B_{12} Deficiency and Pernicious Anemias

Intrinsic factor (IF) is a glycoprotein secreted by parietal cells of the gastric mucosa in the gastric juice that is necessary for the absorption of dietary vitamin B_{12}. Ingested vitamin B_{12} is freed from protein by gastric acid and gastric and intestinal enzymes. The free vitamin B_{12} attaches to salivary R-binder, which has a higher affinity for the vitamin than does IF. An acid pH (2.3) is needed, such as that found in the healthy stomach.

Etiology

The release of pancreatic trypsin into the proximal small intestine destroys R-binder and releases vitamin B_{12} from its complex with R-protein. With an alkaline pH (6.8) in the intestine, IF binds the vitamin B_{12}. The vitamin B_{12}–IF complex is then carried to the ileum. In the ileum, with the presence of ionic calcium (Ca^{2+}) and a pH (>6), the complex attaches to the surface vitamin B_{12}–IF receptors on the ileal cell brush border. Here, the vitamin B_{12} is released and attaches to holotranscobalamin II (holo TCII). Holo TCII is vitamin B_{12} attached to the beta-globulin, the major circulating vitamin B_{12} delivery protein. Like IF, holo TCII plays an active role in binding and transporting vitamin B_{12}. The TCII–vitamin B_{12} complex then enters the portal venous blood.

Other binding proteins in the blood include haptocorrin, also known as transcobalamin I (TCI) and transcobalamin III (TCIII). These are alpha-globulins, larger macromolecular-weight glycoproteins that make up the R-binder component of the blood. Unlike IF, the R-proteins are capable of binding not only vitamin B_{12} but also many of its biologically inactive analogs. Although approximately 75% of the vitamin B_{12} in human serum is bound to haptocorrin and roughly 25% is bound to TCII, only TCII is important in delivering vitamin B_{12} to all the cells that need it. After transport through the bloodstream, TCII is recognized by receptors on cell surfaces. Patients with haptocorrin abnormalities have no symptoms of vitamin B_{12} deficiency. Those lacking TCII rapidly develop megaloblastic anemia. Vitamin B_{12} is excreted in urine.

Pathophysiology

Pernicious anemia is a megaloblastic, macrocytic anemia caused by a deficiency of vitamin B_{12}, most commonly from a lack of IF. Rarely, vitamin B_{12} deficiency anemia occurs in strict vegetarians whose diet contains no vitamin B_{12} except for traces found in plants contaminated by microorganisms capable of synthesizing vitamin B_{12}. Other causes include autoimmune disorders that destroy gastric parietal cells; antibody to IF; bariatric or intestinal surgery; bacterial overgrowth in the small intestine; malabsorption in the small intestine due to celiac disease, Crohn's disease, HIV, tropical sprue, and cancers involving the small intestine; drugs (paraaminosalicylic acid, colchicine, neomycin, metformin, antiretrovirals); and long-term ingestion of alcohol or calcium-chelating agents (Box 31.3).

Aging is associated with B_{12} deficiency for various reasons as discussed in Chapter 19. Approximately 1% to 2% of the U.S. population over the age of 51 years has clinical B_{12} deficiency, and it is thought that 10% to 20% have subclinical deficiency (Carmel, 2011). The incidence of B_{12} deficiency in older individuals may be related to medications commonly used in this population such as H_2 antagonists (see Appendix 13) and metformin used to treat type-2 diabetes (Herbert 2019).

Stages of Deficiency

As a result of normal enterohepatic circulation (i.e., excretion of vitamin B_{12} and analogs in bile and resorption of vitamin B_{12} in the ileum), it may take up to a year or two for strict vegetarians who are not receiving vitamin B_{12} supplementation to develop a vitamin B_{12} deficiency. Serum B_{12}, homocysteine, and methylmalonic acid levels are not as effective as predictors of B_{12}-responsive neurologic disorders; patients with unexplained leukoencephalopathy should be treated proactively because even long-standing deficits may be reversible (Graber et al, 2010).

Stage 1: Early negative vitamin B_{12} balance begins when vitamin B_{12} intake is low or absorption is poor, depleting the primary delivery protein, TCII. A low TCII (<40 pg/mL) may be the earliest detectable

---

BOX 31.3 Causes of Vitamin B_{12} Deficiency

Inadequate ingestion	Poor diet resulting from a vegan diet and lack of supplementation, chronic alcoholism, poverty
Inadequate absorption	Gastric disorders, small intestinal disorders, competition for absorption sites, pancreatic disease, HIV, or AIDS, gastritis, gastric surgery
Inadequate use	Vitamin B_{12} antagonists, congenital or acquired enzyme deficiency, abnormal binding proteins
Increased requirement	Hyperthyroidism, increased hematopoiesis
Increased excretion	Inadequate vitamin B_{12} binding protein, liver disease, renal disease
Increased destruction	Pharmacologic doses of ascorbic acid when it functions as a prooxidant
Medication induced	Drugs that suppress gastric acid and metformin have been associated with B_{12} deficiency

AIDS, Acquired immune deficiency syndrome; *HIV,* human immunodeficiency virus.

---

sign of a vitamin B_{12} deficiency (Nexo and Hoffmann-Lucke, 2011). This is a vitamin B_{12} predeficiency stage.

Stage 2: Vitamin B_{12} depletion shows a low B_{12} on TCII and a gradual lowering of B_{12} in haptocorrin (holohap <50 pg/mL), the storage protein.

Stage 3: Damaged metabolism and vitamin B_{12}–deficient erythropoiesis includes an abnormal dU suppression, hypersegmentation, a decreased TIBC and holohap percent saturation, a low RCF level (<140 ng/mL), and subtle neuropsychiatric damage (impaired short-term and recent memory).

Stage 4: Clinical damage occurs, including vitamin B_{12} deficiency anemia; it includes all preceding parameters, along with macroovalocytic erythrocytes, elevated MCV, elevated TCII levels, increased homocysteine and methylmalonic acid levels, and myelin damage. Leukoencephalopathy and autonomic dysfunction occur with very low serum B_{12} levels (<200 pg/mL); psychiatric changes, neuropathy, and dementia also may occur (Graber et al, 2010) (see Fig. 31.3).

Clinical Findings

Pernicious anemia affects not only the blood but also the gastrointestinal tract and the peripheral and central nervous systems. This distinguishes it from folate-deficiency anemia. The overt symptoms, which are caused by inadequate myelinization of the nerves, include paresthesia (especially numbness and tingling in the hands and feet), diminution of the senses of vibration and position, poor muscular coordination, poor memory, and hallucinations. If the deficiency is prolonged, the nervous system damage may be irreversible, even with initiation of vitamin B_{12} treatment.

Helicobacter pylori causes peptic ulcer disease and chronic gastritis (see Chapter 26). Both conditions are associated with hypochlorhydria, reduced production of IF by epithelial cells in the stomach, vitamin B_{12} malabsorption, and pernicious anemia. There is also a correlation between autoimmune gastritis and pernicious anemia. More than 90% of patients with pernicious anemia have parietal cell antibodies (PCAs), and 50% to 70% have elevated IF antibodies. Serum vitamin B_{12} levels of the *H. pylori*–infected patients are significantly lower than that of uninfected patients.

A study on *H. pylori* infection and autoimmune type atrophic gastritis examined serum markers for gastric atrophy (pepsinogen I, pepsinogen I/II, and gastrin) and autoimmunity. Positive serum autoimmune markers (IF antibodies and PCA) suggest that *H. pylori* contributes to autoimmune gastritis and pernicious anemia (Veijola et al, 2010).

Vitamin B_{12} deficiency is an important modifiable risk factor for osteoporosis in men and women. Adults with low vitamin B_{12} levels have a lower average bone mineral density and greater risk for osteoporosis (Karpouzos et al, 2017).

Reduced vitamin B_{12} status and elevated homocysteine concentrations are common. These alterations are problematic among vegans (Elmadfa and Singer, 2009). B_{12}-folate-homocysteine interactions aggravate heart disease and may lead to adverse pregnancy outcomes (Ganguly and Alam, 2015; Shahbazian et al, 2016) (see Chapters 14 and 32).

Assessment

Vitamin B_{12} stores are depleted after several years without vitamin B_{12} intake. A low holo TCII value (<40 pg/mL) is a sign of early B_{12} deficiency.

Other laboratory tests that may be helpful in diagnosing a vitamin B_{12} deficiency and determining its cause include measurements of serum B_{12}, IF antibody (IFAB), PCA, serum homocysteine and serum methylmalonic acid (MMA) levels (see Chapter 5 and Appendix 12). The IFAB and PCA tests can determine whether the deficiency is caused by a lack of IF.

Medical Management

Treatment usually consists of an intramuscular or subcutaneous injection of 100 mcg or more of vitamin B_{12} once per week. After an initial response is elicited, the frequency of administration is reduced until remission can be maintained indefinitely with monthly injections of 100 mcg. Very large oral doses of vitamin B_{12} (1000 mcg daily) are also effective, even in the absence of IF, because approximately 1% of vitamin B_{12} is absorbed by diffusion. Initial doses should be increased when vitamin B_{12} deficiency is complicated by debilitating illness such as infection, hepatic disease, uremia, coma, severe disorientation, or marked neurologic damage. A response to treatment is evidenced by improved appetite, alertness, and cooperation, followed by improved hematologic results, as manifested by marked reticulocytosis within hours of an injection.

Medical Nutrition Therapy

A high-protein diet (1.5 g/kg of body weight) is desirable for blood cell regeneration. Because green leafy vegetables contain iron and folate, the diet should contain increased amounts of these foods. Meats (especially beef and pork), eggs, milk, and milk products are particularly rich in vitamin B_{12} (see Appendix 31).

For those individuals prescribed metformin for treatment of diabetes, 10% to 30% have reduced vitamin B_{12} absorption. Metformin negatively affects the calcium-dependent membrane and the B_{12}-IF complex by decreasing the absorbability by the ileal cell surface receptors. Increased intake of calcium may reverse the vitamin B_{12} malabsorption. However a recent study found that supplementation with a multivitamin supplement was protective against B_{12} deficiency.

The Institute of Medicine recommends that people older than age 50 consume vitamin B_{12} in its crystalline form (i.e., in fortified cereals or supplements) to overcome the effects of atrophic gastritis. The RDAs for B_{12} are summarized in the front of the book. The RDA for adult men and women is 2.4 mcg daily.

OTHER NUTRITIONAL ANEMIAS

Anemia of Protein-Energy Malnutrition

Protein is essential for the proper production of hemoglobin and RBCs. Because of the reduction in cell mass and thus oxygen requirements in protein-energy malnutrition (PEM), fewer RBCs are required to oxygenate the tissue. Because blood volume remains the same, this reduced number of RBCs with a low hemoglobin level (hypochromic, normocytic anemia), which can mimic an iron deficiency anemia, is actually a physiologic (nonharmful) rather than harmful anemia. In acute PEM, the loss of active tissue mass may be greater than the reduction in the number of RBCs, leading to polycythemia (an increase in RBCs where they make up a larger proportion of the blood volume). The body responds to this RBC production, which is not a reflection of protein and amino acid deficiency but of an oversupply of RBCs. Iron released from normal RBC destruction is not reused in RBC production but is stored so that iron stores are often adequate. Iron deficiency anemia can reappear with rehabilitation when RBC mass expands rapidly.

The anemia of PEM may be complicated by deficiencies of iron and other nutrients and by associated infections, parasitic infestation, and malabsorption. A diet lacking in protein is usually deficient in iron, folic acid, and, less frequently, vitamin B_{12}. The nutrition counselor plays an important role in assessing recent and typical dietary intake of these nutrients.

Copper Deficiency Anemia

Copper and other heavy metals are essential for the proper formation of hemoglobin. Ceruloplasmin, a copper-containing protein, is required for normal mobilization of iron from its storage sites to the plasma. In a copper-deficient state, iron cannot be released; this leads to low serum iron and hemoglobin levels, even in the presence of normal iron stores. Other consequences of copper deficiency suggest that copper proteins are needed for use of iron by the developing erythrocyte and for optimal functions of the erythrocyte membrane. The amounts of copper needed for normal hemoglobin synthesis are so minute that they are usually amply supplied by an adequate diet; however, copper deficiency may occur in infants who are fed cow's milk or a copper-deficient infant formula. It also may be seen in children or adults who have a malabsorption syndrome or who are receiving long-term total parenteral nutrition that does not supply copper.

Sideroblastic (B_6-Responsive) Anemia

Sideroblastic (pyridoxine-responsive) anemia is characterized by a derangement in the final pathway of heme synthesis, leading to a buildup of immature RBCs. It has four primary characteristics: (1) microcytic and hypochromic RBCs; (2) high serum and tissue iron levels (causing increased transferrin saturation); (3) the presence of an inherited defect in the formation of δ-aminolevulinic acid synthetase, an enzyme involved in heme synthesis (pyridoxal-5-phosphate is necessary in this reaction); and (4) a buildup of iron-containing immature RBCs (sideroblasts, for which the anemia is named). The iron that cannot be used for heme synthesis is stored in the mitochondria of immature RBCs. These iron-laden mitochondria do not function normally, and the development and production of RBCs become ineffective. The symptoms are those of anemia and iron overload. Even though the anemia responds to the administration of pharmacologic doses of pyridoxine and thus is referred to as pyridoxine–responsive anemia, the neurologic and cutaneous manifestations of vitamin B_6 deficiency are not observed. This distinguishes it from anemia caused by a dietary vitamin B_6 deficiency.

Treatment consists of a therapeutic trial dose of 50 to 200 mg daily of pyridoxine or pyridoxal phosphate (PLP or pyridoxal-5-phosphate) which is 30 to 150 times the RDA. If the anemia responds to one or the other, pyridoxine therapy is continued for life. However, if the anemia is only partially corrected, a normal hematocrit value is never regained. Patients respond to this treatment to varying degrees, and some may only achieve near-normal hemoglobin levels.

Acquired sideroblastic anemias such as those attributable to drug therapy (isoniazid, chloramphenicol), copper deficiency, hypothermia, and alcoholism are not responsive to B_6 administration.

Vitamin E–Responsive Hemolytic Anemia

Hemolytic anemia occurs when defects in RBC membranes lead to oxidative damage and eventually to cell lysis. This anemia is caused by shortened survival of mature RBCs. Vitamin E, an antioxidant, is involved in protecting the membrane against oxidative damage, and one of the few signs noted in vitamin E deficiency is early hemolysis of RBCs.

NONNUTRITIONAL ANEMIAS

Anemia of Pregnancy

A physiologic anemia is the anemia of pregnancy, which is related to increased blood volume and usually resolves with the end of the pregnancy. However, demands for iron during pregnancy also are increased so that inadequate iron intake may also play a role in whether it develops (see Chapter 14 for further discussion).

Anemia of Chronic Disease

Anemia of chronic disease occurs from inflammation, infection, autoimmune disorders, chronic kidney and liver disease and malignancy because there is decreased RBC production, usually as a result of disordered iron metabolism. Ferritin levels are normal or increased, but serum iron levels and TIBC are low (see Chapter 5). It is important that this form of anemia, which is mild and normocytic, not be mistaken for iron deficiency anemia; iron supplements should not be given. Standard therapy involves treating the underlying disorder, which usually improves or corrects this anemia (Nemeth and Ganz, 2014). Erythrocyte transfusion and erythropoiesis-stimulating agents (ESAs) may be required in rare but severe cases.

Sickle Cell Disease

Pathophysiology

Sickle cell disease (SCD) describes a group of inherited blood disorders of RBCs. It is typically associated with African ancestry but affects millions of people worldwide including Central and South American, Mediterranean, and South Asian populations (Centers for Disease Control and Prevention [CDC], 2018). Those affected inherit two abnormal hemoglobin genes called hemoglobin S, one from each parent. This results in impaired hemoglobin synthesis, which produces sickle-shaped RBCs that get caught in capillaries and do not carry oxygen well (Fig. 31.6). The sickle-shaped RBCs die earlier than typical RBCs, usually in 10 to 20 days. The bone marrow cannot make new cells fast enough to replace them, which can result in anemia and enlargement of the spleen. The disease is usually diagnosed at birth and affects 100,000 in the United States, although 1 to 3 million Americans have the sickle cell trait, characterized by having only one copy of the sickle cell gene. (Centers for Disease Control and Prevention [CDC], 2018).

In addition to anemia, SCD is characterized by episodes of pain resulting from the occlusion of small blood vessels by the abnormally shaped erythrocytes. The occlusions frequently occur in the abdomen, causing acute, severe abdominal pain. The hemolytic anemia and vasoocclusive disease can result in impaired liver function, jaundice, gallstones, and deteriorating renal function. The constant hemolysis of erythrocytes increases iron stores in the liver; however, iron deficiency anemia and SCD can coexist. Iron overload is less common and is usually a problem only in those who have received multiple blood transfusions.

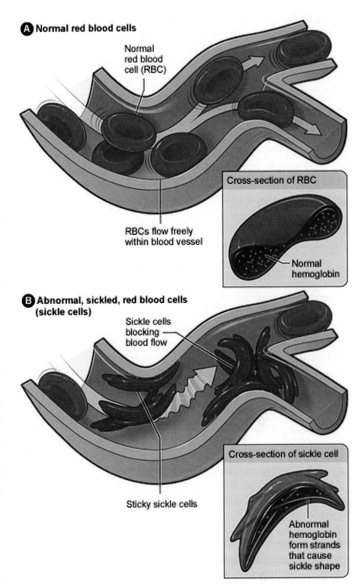

Fig. 31.6 A, Normal red blood cells and **B,** Abnormal, sickled red blood cells. (From National Institutes of Health (NIH), National Heart, Lung, and Blood Institute (NHLBI): *Sickle cell disease* (website). https://www.nhlbi.nih.gov/health-topics/sickle-cell-disease, 2018.)

Typically serum homocysteine levels are elevated, which may be due to low concentrations of vitamin B_6. Children with SCD were found to have these lower vitamin B_6 levels despite B_6 intakes comparable to those of unaffected children.

Medical Management

A new set of guidelines for managing SCD recommends using monthly blood transfusions and the drug hydroxyurea (Yawn et al, 2014). Consistent blood transfusions stop the body from producing sickle cells and attempts to normalize RBC count. Hydroxyurea increases the production of healthy fetal hemoglobin, reducing hospitalizations. Because hydroxyurea also lowers the number of white blood cells, patients must be monitored regularly with blood tests.

Other treatment for SCD focuses on relieving pain during a crisis, keeping the body oxygenated (using oxygen therapy if needed), and possibly administering an exchange transfusion. It is important that SCD not be mistaken for iron deficiency anemia, which can be treated with iron supplements, because iron stores in the patient with SCD secondary to transfusions are frequently excessive.

Zinc can increase the oxygen affinity of normal and sickle-shaped erythrocytes. Thus zinc supplements may be beneficial in managing SCD, especially because decreased plasma zinc is common in children with the SS genotype SCD and is associated with decreased linear and skeletal growth, muscle mass, and sexual maturation. Zinc supplementation also may prevent the deficit in growth that appears in these children (Hyacinth et al, 2010) Because zinc competes with copper for binding sites on proteins, the use of high doses of zinc may cause copper deficiency, so supplementation with at least the RDA of copper is recommended.

Medical Nutrition Therapy

Children with SCD and their families should receive instruction about how they can develop a well-balanced food plan providing enough calories and protein for growth and development. Their dietary intake may be low because of the abdominal pain characteristic of the disease. They also have increased metabolic rates, leading to a need for a higher caloric intake. This hypermetabolism probably is due to a constant inflammation and oxidative stress (Hyacinth et al, 2010; Yawn et al, 2014). Therefore their diets must be high enough in calories to meet these needs and must provide foods high in folate and the trace minerals zinc and copper (see Appendix 47 for sources of zinc).

In addition, these children may be low in vitamins A, C, D, and E; folate; calcium; and fiber. The diet should be high in folate (400 to 600 mcg daily) because the increased production of erythrocytes needed to replace the cells being continuously destroyed also increases folate requirements (see Appendix 31).

When assessing the nutrition status of patients with SCD, clinicians must pay attention to the questions related to the use of vitamin and mineral supplements, the consumption of alcohol (which increases iron absorption), and sources of protein (animal sources being high in zinc and iron) in the diet. A multivitamin and mineral supplement containing 50% to 150% of the RDA for folate, zinc, and copper (not iron) is recommended.

Dietary fluid and sodium intake influence the risk for vasoocclusive events in SCD; increasing fluid intake and limiting high-sodium foods should be discussed (Fowler et al, 2010) (see Chapter 32). Intake of 2 to 3 quarts of water daily is recommended. Finally, it is important to remember that patients with SCD may require higher than RDA amounts of protein.

If it is necessary for the diet to be low in absorbable iron, the diet should emphasize vegetable proteins. Iron-rich foods, such as liver, iron-fortified formula, iron-fortified cereals, and iron-fortified energy bars and iron-fortified sport drinks, should be excluded. Substances such as alcohol and vitamin C supplements, both of which enhance iron absorption, should be avoided. Rarely, iron deficiency may be present in some patients with SCD; iron deficiency should be confirmed and the diet adjusted appropriately.

Hypochromic Microcytic Transient Anemia (Sports Anemia)

Increased RBC destruction, along with decreased hemoglobin, serum iron, and ferritin concentrations, may occur at the initiation and early stages of a vigorous training program. Sports anemia is associated with a reduction in hemoglobin in the early stages of aerobic training due to hemodilution. The adaptations are considered advantageous and do not impair physical performance (see Chapter 22 for further discussion).

Athletes who have hemoglobin concentrations below those needed for optimal oxygen delivery may benefit from consuming nutrient and iron-rich foods; ensuring that their diets contain adequate protein; and

avoiding tea, coffee, antacids, H_2-blockers, and tetracycline, all of which inhibit iron absorption. No athlete should take iron supplements unless true iron deficiency is diagnosed based on a complete blood cell count with differential, serum ferritin level, serum iron level, TIBC, and percent saturation of iron-binding capacity. Athletes who are female, vegetarian, involved in endurance sports, or entering a growth spurt are at risk for iron deficiency anemia and therefore should undergo periodic monitoring (see Chapter 22).

Thalassemias

Thalassemias (alpha and beta) are inherited anemias characterized by microcytic, hypochromic, and short-lived RBCs resulting from defective hemoglobin synthesis, which primarily affect persons from the Mediterranean, Southern Asia, Africa, and the Middle East (National Heart, Lung, and Blood Institute, 2014). Severity of the disorder ranges from asymptomatic or mild anemia to more severe symptoms requiring routine blood transfusions. The ineffective erythropoiesis leads to an increase in plasma volume, progressive splenomegaly, and bone marrow expansion with the result of facial deformities, osteomalacia, and bone changes. Ultimately there is increased iron absorption and progressive iron deposition in tissues, resulting in oxidative damage. The accumulation of iron causes dysfunction of the heart, liver, and endocrine glands. Because patients with the more severe form require transfusions to stay alive, they also must have regular chelation therapy to prevent the damaging buildup of iron that can occur. Impaired growth in children accompanying thalassemia major can be partially corrected by increasing caloric intake.

Medical Nutrition Therapy

The diet should emphasize foods high in folate, vitamins A and C, and trace minerals, including zinc, copper, and selenium (Cunningham, 2016). Additionally, adequate intake of calcium and vitamin D is needed to support bone health. Patients not receiving blood transfusions should consume a moderately low-iron diet that limits iron-fortified foods and high red meat intakes. Multivitamin and mineral supplements that contain amounts of iron and vitamin C above the RDA should be also avoided. Patients receiving transfusions with chelation therapy do not need to follow a low-iron diet.

CLINICAL CASE STUDY

Marisa, a 27-year-old Hispanic female, reports increased symptoms of restless legs syndrome, fatigue, and heavy menses for the past year. A physical examination reveals inflammation and tenderness around her knee and ankle joints.

Her typical daily intake includes:

B: Coffee with milk, eggs and a white flour tortilla

L: Vegetable soup with chicken and water

S: sweet roll and another cup of coffee with milk.

D: Cheese enchiladas with red sauce and sour cream, pinto beans and hot tea.

Medications: None

Height: 5'5"

Weight: 164 lbs lb

Laboratory Values:

	Client	Normal Range	
WBC	8.3	3.8-10.5	K/uL
RBC	4.86	3.8-5.20	M/uL
HGB	10.8 L	12.0-16.0	g/dL
HCT	32.7 L	34.5-45.0	%
MCV	74.1 L	80.0-100.0	fl
MCH	24.3 L	27.0-34.0	pg

CLINICAL CASE STUDY—cont'd

	Client	Normal Range	
MCHC	30.4 L	32.0-36.0	gm/dL
IRON	28 L	40-160	ug/dL
UIBC	429 H	110-370	ug/dL
TIBC	508 H	220-430	ug/dL
% Saturation, Iron	12 L	14-50	%
Transferrin	435 H	200-400	mg/dL
Ferritin	12 L	15-150	ng/mL
C-Reactive Protein	0.96 H	0.00-0.40	mg/dL
Vitamin D	14.6 L	30.0-100.0	ng/mL

Nutrition Diagnostic Statements

- Increased nutrient needs (iron) related to heavy menses and suboptimal intake of dietary iron as evidenced by multiple low iron status labs including hematocrit (HCT), hemoglobin (HGB), and ferritin.
- Altered nutrition-related laboratory value related to predicted pro-inflammatory diet pattern as evidenced by low intake of omega-3 fatty acids and bioactive compounds, elevated C-reactive protein (CRP), and painful joints.

Nutrition Care Questions

1. Evaluate her laboratory test results. What type of anemia does she likely have? Are there any other concerning labs?
2. Assess Marisa's diet. Does it appear she is taking in adequate iron? What are her dietary inhibitors?
3. Considering her Mexican heritage, what nutrition recommendations would you have for Marisa?
4. What vitamin/mineral supplements, if any, should be part of her treatment plan?

USEFUL WEBSITES

American Society of Hematology
Centers for Disease Control and Prevention
Iron Disorders Institute
Linus Pauling Institute Micronutrient Information Center

REFERENCES

Adams PC: Epidemiology and diagnostic testing for hemochromatosis and iron overload, *Int J Lab Hematol* 37(Suppl 1):25–30, 2015.

Bacon BR, Adams PC, Kowdley KV, et al: Diagnosis and management of hemochromatosis: 2011 practice guideline by the American Association for the Study of Liver Diseases, *Hepatology* 54:328–343, 2011.

Belaidi AA, Bush AI: Iron neurochemistry in Alzheimer's disease and Parkinson's disease: targets for therapeutics, *J Neurochem* 139:179–197, 2016.

Carmel R: Biomarkers of cobalamin (vitamin B-12) status in the epidemiologic setting: a critical overview of context, applications, and performance characteristics of cobalamin, methylmalonic acid, and holotranscobalamin II, *Am J Clin Nutr* 94(Suppl 1):348S–358S, 2011.

Centers for Disease Control and Prevention: *Sickle Cell Disease (SCD)*, 2018. Available at: https://www.cdc.gov/ncbddd/sicklecell/index.html.

Chang TP, Rangan C: Iron poisoning: a literature-based review of epidemiology, diagnosis, and management, *Pediatr Emerg Care* 27:978–985, 2011.

Connor JR, Patton SM, Oexle K, et al: Iron and restless legs syndrome: treatment, genetics, and pathophysiology, *Sleep Med* 31:61–70, 2017.

Cunningham E: Is there a special diet for thalassemia? *J Acad Nutr Diet* 116:1360, 2016.

De-Regil LM, Suchdev PS, Vist GE, et al: Home fortification of foods with multiple micronutrient powders for health and nutrition in children under two years of age, *Evid Based Child Health* 8:112–201, 2013.

Elmadfa I, Singer I: Vitamin B-12 and homocysteine status among vegetarians: a global perspective, *Am J Clin Nutr* 89:1693S–1698S, 2009.

Ferrari P, Nicolini A, Manca ML, et al: Treatment of mild non-chemotherapy-induced iron deficiency anemia in cancer patients: comparison between oral ferrous bisglycinate chelate and ferrous sulfate, *Biomed Pharmacother* 66:414–418, 2012.

Fleming RE, Ponka P: Iron overload in human disease, *N Engl J Med* 366:348–359, 2012.

Fowler KT, Williams R, Mitchell CO, et al: Dietary water and sodium intake of children and adolescents with sickle cell anemia, *J Pediatr Hematol Oncol* 32:350–353, 2010.

Ganguly P, Alam SF. Role of homocysteine in the development of cardiovascular disease, *Nutr J* 14:6, 2015.

Ganz T: Hepcidin and iron regulation, 10 years later, *Blood* 117:4425–4433, 2011.

Graber JJ, Sherman FT, Kaufmann H, et al: Vitamin B12-responsive severe leukoencephalopathy and autonomic dysfunction in a patient with "normal" serum B12 levels, *J Neurol Neurosurg Psychiatry* 81:1369–1371, 2010.

Herbert V: Everyone should be tested for iron disorders. *J Am Diet Assoc* 92(12):1502–1509, 1992

Herbert l, Ribar A, Mitchell S, et al: Discovering metformin-induced vitamin B12 deficience in patients with type-2 diabetes in primary care, *J Am Assoc Nurse Pract.* 2019 Oct 18. doi:10.1097/JXX.0000000000000312. [Epub ahead of print]

Hyacinth HI, Gee BE, Hibbert JM: The role of nutrition in sickle cell disease, *Nutr Metab Insights* 3:57–67, 2010.

Jáuregui-Lobera I: Iron deficiency and cognitive functions, *Neuropsychiatr Dis Treat* 10:2087–2095, 2014.

Karpouzos A, Diamantis E, Farmaki P, et al: Nutritional aspects of bone health and fracture healing, *J Osteoporos* 2017:4218472, 2017.

Kassebaum NJ: The global burden of anemia, *Hematol Oncol Clin North Am* 30:247–308, 2016.

Kim, J; Ahn, C , Fang, et al: Association between metformin dose and B_{12} deficiency in patients with type-2 diabetes, Medicine 98:-Issue 46 - p e17918

Le CH: The prevalence of anemia and moderate-severe anemia in the US population (NHANES 2003-2012), *PLoS One* 11:e0166635, 2016.

Milman N, Jønsson L, Dyre P, et al: Ferrous bisglycinate 25 mg iron is as effective as ferrous sulfate 50 mg iron in the prophylaxis of iron deficiency and anemia during pregnancy in a randomized trial, *J Perinat Med* 42:197–206, 2013.

National Heart, Lung, and Blood Institute: *Thalassemias*, 2014. Available at: https://www.nhlbi.nih.gov/health-topics/thalassemias.

National Institutes of Health, Office of Dietary Supplements: *Folate fact sheet for health professionals*, 2018. Available at: https://ods.od.nih.gov/factsheets/Folate-HealthProfessional/.

National Library of Medicine: *African iron overload*, 2019. Available at: https://ghr.nlm.nih.gov/condition/african-iron-overload.

Nemeth E, Ganz T: Anemia of inflammation, *Hematol Oncol Clin North Am* 28:671–681, 2014.

Nexo E, Hoffmann-Lücke E: Holotranscobalamin, a marker of vitamin B-12 status: analytical aspects and clinical utility, *Am J Clin Nutr* 94:359S–365S, 2011.

Ryan BJ, Wachsmuth NB, Schmidt WF, et al: AltitudeOmics: rapid hemoglobin mass alterations with early acclimatization to and de-acclimatization from 5260 m in healthy humans, *PLoS One* 9:e108788, 2014.

Shahbazian N, Jafari RM, Haghnia S: The evaluation of serum homocysteine, folic acid, and vitamin B12 in patients complicated with preeclampsia, *Electron Physician* 8:3057–3061, 2016.

Short MW and Domagalski JE: Iron Deficiency anemia: evaluation and management, *Am Fam Physician*, 87:98–104, 2013.

Wang M: Iron deficiency and other types of anemia in infants and children, *Am Fam Physician*, 93:270–278, 2016.

Ward RJ, Zucca FA, Duyn JH, et al: The role of iron in brain ageing and neurodegenerative disorders, *Lancet Neurol* 13:1045–1060, 2014.

Veijola LI, Oksanen AM, Sipponen PI, et al: Association of autoimmune type atrophic corpus gastritis with Helicobacter pylori infection, *World J Gastroenterol* 16:83–88, 2010.

Yawn BP, Buchanan GR, Afenyi-Annan AN, et al: Management of sickle cell disease: summary of the 2014 evidence-based report by expert panel members, *JAMA* 312:1033–1048, 2014.

Medical Nutrition Therapy for Cardiovascular Disease

Janice L. Raymond, MS, RDN, CSG
Sarah C. Couch, PhD, RDN

KEY TERMS

3-hydroxy-3-methylglutaryl– coenzyme A (HMG-CoA)
angina
angiography
apolipoproteins
atherosclerotic cardiovascular disease (ASCVD)
atheroma
bile acid sequestrant
blood pressure
B-natriuretic peptide (BNP)
cardiac cachexia
cardiac catheterization
cardiovascular disease (CVD)
C-reactive protein (hs-CRP)
Cerebrovascular Accident (CVA)
chylomicron
coronary artery bypass graft (CABG)
diastolic blood pressure (DBP)
Dietary Approaches to Stop Hypertension (DASH)

dyslipidemia
dyspnea
edema
endothelial cell
essential hypertension
familial combined hyperlipidemia (FCHL)
familial dysbetalipoproteinemia
familial hypercholesterolemia (FH)
fatty streak
foam cells
heart failure (HF)
high-density lipoprotein (HDL)
homocysteine
hypertension
hypertriglyceridemia
intermediate-density lipoprotein (IDL)
ischemia
left ventricular hypertrophy (LVH)
lipoprotein

low-density lipoprotein (LDL)
Mediterranean diet (MeD)
metabolic syndrome
myocardial infarction (MI)
nitric oxide (NO)
plaque
prehypertension
renin-angiotensin system (RAS)
secondary hypertension
statins
stroke
syncope
systolic blood pressure (SBP)
thrombus
trans fatty acids
transient ischemic attack (TIA)
trimethylamine-N-oxide (TMAO)
very-low-density lipoprotein (VLDL)
xanthoma

Cardiovascular disease (CVD) is a group of interrelated diseases that includes atherosclerosis, hypertension, ischemic heart disease, peripheral vascular disease, and heart failure (HF). These diseases are interrelated and often coexist. An estimated 84,000,000 adult Americans (one in three) have one or more types of CVD (Box 32.1).

CVD remains the number one killer of men and women in the United States; one of every three deaths is attributed to CVD. CVD is the cause of more deaths than cancer, chronic lower respiratory diseases, and accidents combined. Every 25 seconds, an American suffers a coronary event and about every minute someone will die of one. On average, someone in the United States suffers a stroke every 40 seconds (American Heart Association [AHA], 2015). The lifetime risk for CVD in American men is two in three and for women is one in two (AHA, 2015). Worldwide, 18 million deaths per year are attributed to CVD (Yusuf et al, 2014).

Atherosclerotic cardiovascular disease (ASCVD) involves the narrowing of small blood vessels that oxygenate the heart muscle by the build-up of plaque (the lesion in the blood vessels). The plaque, known as atherosclerosis, can rupture, causing a blood clot to form that blocks the artery or travels somewhere else in the body, causing blockage at that site. The result can be a myocardial infarction (MI),

which is also called a heart attack or in the brain it is called an ischemic stroke, which is also known as a cerebrovascular accident (CVA). Heart disease and stroke cause the most deaths in both sexes of all ethnic groups, increasing with age. Until the age of 65 years, black men have the highest rates of ASCVD deaths; thereafter, white men have the highest rates. Black women have higher rates than white women at all ages. Among whites older than age 18, 12.1% have CVD. In the same age group, 10.2% of blacks have heart disease, and in Hispanics the incidence is 8.1%. The incidence in adult Native Americans is 12.1%, in Native Hawaiians or other Pacific Islanders it is 19.7 %, and in Asians it is 5.2% (AHA, 2015). This chapter discusses the incidence, pathophysiologic findings, prevention, and treatment of each of the CVDs.

ATHEROSCLEROSIS AND CORONARY HEART DISEASE

Anatomy and Physiology

Blood vessels are composed of three layers. The outer layer is mainly connective tissue that gives structure to the vessels. The middle layer is smooth muscle that contracts and dilates to control blood flow and

BOX 32.1 Types and Incidence of Cardiovascular Disease in the United States

Hypertension: 75,000,000
Coronary heart disease: 25,155,000
Myocardial infarction: 790,000
Heart failure: 6,500,000
Stroke: 7,950,000

Because of comorbidities, it is not possible to add these numbers together to reach a total (American Heart Association [AHA], 2010; https://www.ncbi.nlm.nih.gov/pmc/articles/PMC5408160/; https://www.cdc.gov/heartdisease/heart_attack.htm).

blood pressure. The inner lining is a thin layer of endothelial cells (the endothelium) that in a healthy state is smooth and responsive. The endothelium functions as a protective barrier between tissues and circulating blood. It facilitates bidirectional passage of macromolecules and blood gases to and from tissues and blood. Endothelial cells sense changes in blood flow and respond with the release of bioactive substances that maintain vascular homeostasis. One such substance is nitric oxide (NO). NO is a soluble gas continually synthesized from the amino acid L-arginine in endothelial cells. NO has a wide range of biologic properties that maintain vascular homeostasis. It appears to be involved in protection from injurious substances and plays a key role in vasodilation (Tousoulis et al, 2012). Decreased NO is a factor in the endothelial cell dysfunction that disrupts vascular balance and can result in vasoconstriction, platelet activation, leukocyte adherence, and vascular inflammation.

Pathophysiology

ASCVD involves the accumulation of plaque within the walls of the arteries. It starts with injury to the endothelial cells with an associated inflammatory response involving phagocytes and monocytes. Once in the tissue, monocytes evolve into a specialized type of macrophage called a foam cell that ingests oxidized cholesterol and becomes fatty streaks in these vessels. Intracellular microcalcification occurs, forming deposits within the vascular smooth muscle cells of the surrounding muscular layer (Fig. 32.1).

A protective fibrin layer or atheroma forms between the fatty deposits and the artery lining. Atheromas produce enzymes that cause the artery to enlarge over time, thus compensating for the narrowing

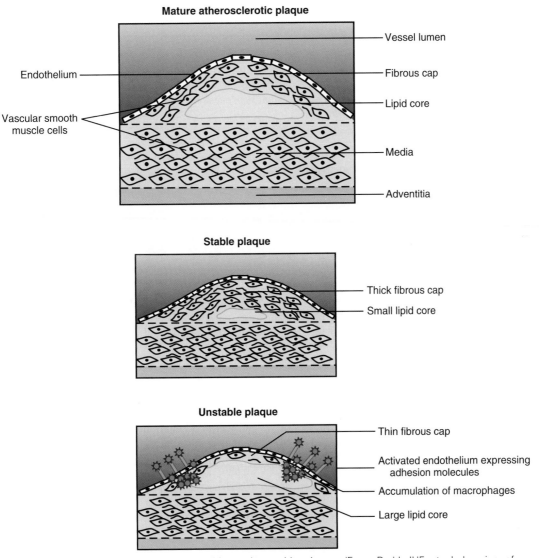

Fig. 32.1 The structure of mature, stable, and unstable plaque. (From Rudd JHF et al: Imaging of atherosclerosis—can we predict plaque rupture? *Trends Cardiovasc Med* 15:17, 2005.)

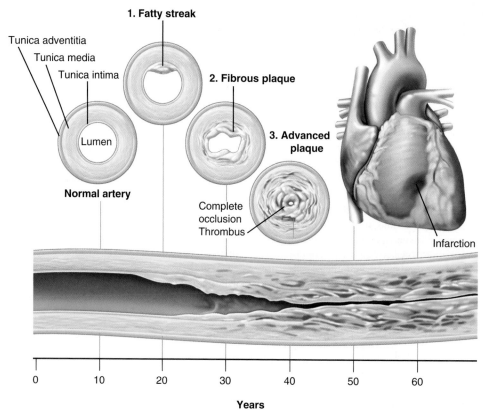

Fig. 32.2 Natural progression of atherosclerosis. (From Harkreader H: *Fundamentals of nursing: caring and clinical judgment,* Philadelphia, 2007, Saunders.)

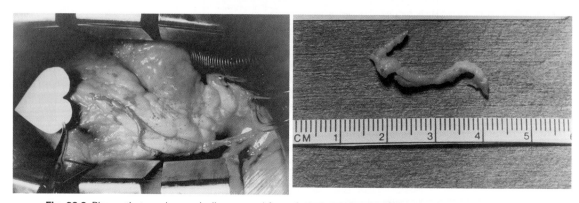

Fig. 32.3 Plaque that can be surgically removed from the coronary artery. (Photographs courtesy Ronald D. Gregory and John Riley, MD.)

caused by the plaque. This "remodeling" of the shape and size of the blood vessel may result in an aneurysm. Atheromas can rupture or break off, forming a **thrombus** (blood clot), where they attract blood platelets and activate the clotting system in the body. This response can result in a blockage and restricted blood flow.

Only high-risk or vulnerable plaque forms thrombi. Vulnerable plaques are lesions with a thin fibrous cap, few smooth muscle cells, many macrophages (inflammatory cells), and a large lipid core (Fig. 32.2). Arterial changes begin in infancy and progress asymptomatically throughout adulthood (Fig. 32.3).

The clinical outcome of impaired arterial function arising from atherosclerosis depends on the location of the impairment. In the coronary arteries atherosclerosis can cause **angina** (chest pain), MI, and sudden death; in the cerebral arteries it causes strokes and **transient ischemic attacks (TIAs)**; and in the peripheral circulation it causes intermittent claudication, limb **ischemia** (inadequate blood supply), and gangrene (Fig. 32.4). Thus atherosclerosis is the underlying cause of many forms of CVD.

Dyslipidemia refers to a blood lipid profile that increases the risk of developing atherosclerosis. Three important biochemical measurements in ASCVD include lipoproteins, total cholesterol, and triglycerides. Cholesterol is delivered into cell walls by **low-density lipoprotein (LDL)**, especially smaller particles. To attract and stimulate the macrophages, the cholesterol must be released from the LDL

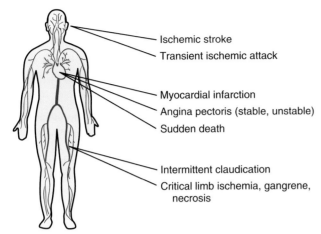

Fig. 32.4 Major clinical manifestations of atherothrombotic disease. (From Viles-Gonzalez JF, et al: Atherothrombosis: a widespread disease with unpredictable and life-threatening consequences, *Eur Heart J* 25:1197, 2004.)

Labels in figure:
- Ischemic stroke
- Transient ischemic attack
- Myocardial infarction
- Angina pectoris (stable, unstable)
- Sudden death
- Intermittent claudication
- Critical limb ischemia, gangrene, necrosis

particles and oxidized, a key step in the ongoing inflammatory process. Additionally, macrophages must move excess cholesterol quickly into high-density lipoprotein (HDL) particles to avoid becoming foam cells and dying. The typical dyslipidemic condition is one in which LDL levels are elevated (hyperlipidemia) and HDL levels are low.

Lipoproteins

Lipids are not water soluble, so they are carried in the blood bound to protein. These complex particles, called lipoproteins that are manufactured in the liver, vary in composition, size, and density. Lipoproteins measured in clinical practice—chylomicrons, very-low-density lipoprotein (VLDL), low-density lipoproteins (LDL), and high-density lipoproteins (HDL)—consist of varying amounts of triglyceride, cholesterol, phospholipid, and protein. Each class of lipoprotein actually represents a continuum of particles. The ratio of protein to fat determines the density; thus particles with higher levels of protein are the most dense (e.g., HDLs have more protein than LDLs). The physiologic role of lipoprotein includes transporting lipid to cells for energy, storage, or use as substrate for synthesis of other compounds such as prostaglandins, thromboxanes, and leukotrienes.

The largest particles, chylomicrons, transport dietary fat and cholesterol from the small intestine to the liver and periphery. Once in the bloodstream, the triglycerides within the chylomicrons are hydrolyzed by lipoprotein lipase (LPL), located on the endothelial cell surface in muscle and adipose tissue. Apolipoproteins carry lipids in the blood and also control the metabolism of the lipoprotein molecule. Apo C-II, one of the apolipoproteins, is a cofactor for LPL. When approximately 90% of the triglyceride is hydrolyzed, the particle is released back into the blood as a remnant. The liver metabolizes these chylomicron remnants, but some deliver cholesterol to the arterial wall and thus are considered atherogenic. Consumption of high-fat meals produces more chylomicrons and remnants. Plasma studies are done when fasting; chylomicrons are normally absent.

VLDL particles are synthesized in the liver to transport endogenous triglyceride and cholesterol. Triglyceride accounts for 60% of the VLDL particle. The large, buoyant VLDL particle is believed to be nonatherogenic. Vegetarian and low-fat diets increase the formation of large VLDL particles. Smaller VLDL particles (i.e., remnants) are formed from triglyceride hydrolysis by LPL. Normally these remnants, called intermediate-density lipoproteins (IDLs), are atherogenic and

are taken up by receptors on the liver or converted to LDLs. Some of the smaller LDL particles stay in the blood, are oxidized, and are then taken into the arterial wall. Clinically, a total triglyceride level is a measurement of the triglycerides carried on the VLDL and the IDL remnants.

LDL is the primary cholesterol carrier in blood, formed by the breakdown of VLDL. High LDL cholesterol is associated specifically with atherosclerosis (Stone et al, 2014). A recent change in recommendations from American College of Cardiology (ACC)/American Heart Association (AHA) was to drop the actual serum LDL ASCVD prevention target. LDL levels are used for dosing medication but are otherwise only considered part of a bigger picture of risk and should not be assessed in isolation. After LDL formation, 60% is taken up by LDL receptors on the liver, adrenals, and other tissues. The remainder is metabolized via nonreceptor pathways. The number and activity of these LDL receptors are major determinants of the LDL level in the blood. Apolipoprotein B is the structural protein for all of the atherogenic lipoproteins (VLDL, IDL, LDL) and modulates the transport of lipids from the gut and liver to the tissues. The two forms, apo B and apoB-100, are synthesized in the liver. ApoB-100 constitutes 95% of the apolipoproteins in LDL. ApoB-48 is synthesized in the intestines and is the structural component of chylomicrons.

HDL particles contain more protein than any of the other lipoproteins, which accounts for their metabolic role as a reservoir of the apolipoproteins that direct lipid metabolism. Apo A-I, the main apolipoprotein in HDL, is an antiinflammatory, antioxidant protein that also helps to remove cholesterol from the arterial wall to the liver for excretion or repackaging. This process prevents the build-up and oxidation of cholesterol in the arteries. Evaluation of apo A-I or the ratio of apo B to apo A-I has been proposed to assess risk and determine treatment (Navab et al, 2011). The lower the ratio, the lower the ASCVD risk. Both apo C and apo E on HDL are transferred to chylomicrons. Apo E helps receptors metabolize chylomicron remnants and also inhibits appetite. Therefore high HDL levels are associated with low levels of chylomicrons; VLDL remnants; and small, dense LDLs. Epidemiologic studies have shown an inverse correlation between HDL levels and risk of cardiovascular events. And generally a high HDL level is considered heart-protective. However there is recent evidence that very high levels of HDL cholesterol (greater than 97) are actually a risk factor (Madsen et al, 2017).

Total Cholesterol

A total cholesterol measurement captures cholesterol contained in all lipoprotein fractions: 60% to 70% is carried on LDL, 20% to 30% on HDL, and 10% to 15% on VLDL.

Triglycerides

The triglyceride-rich lipoproteins include chylomicrons, VLDLs, and any remnants or intermediary products formed in metabolism. Of these triglyceride-rich lipoproteins, chylomicrons and VLDL remnants are known to be atherogenic because they activate platelets, the coagulation cascade, and clot formation. All contain the apo B lipoprotein. Fasting triglyceride levels are classified as normal (<150 mg/dL), borderline high (150 to 199 mg/dL), high (200 to 499 mg/dL), and very high (<500 mg/dL) (Stone et al, 2014).

Patients with familial dyslipidemias have high triglyceride levels (hypertriglyceridemia). Triglycerides in the very high range place the patient at risk for pancreatitis. Triglyceride measurements are now considered along with glucose intolerance, hypertension, low HDL cholesterol, and high LDL cholesterol as part of the metabolic syndrome.

GENETIC HYPERLIPIDEMIAS

The study and identification of the genes responsible for the familial forms of hyperlipidemia have provided insight into the roles of enzymes, apolipoproteins, and receptors on cells involved in lipid metabolism. Several forms of hyperlipidemia have strong genetic components and are described here.

Familial Hypercholesterolemia

Familial hypercholesterolemia (FH) is a genetic disorder characterized by elevated LDL cholesterol and premature CVD, with a prevalence of approximately one in 200 to 500 for heterozygotes in North America and Europe (Brautbar, 2015).

In FH elevated cholesterol is already present at birth and results in early atherosclerotic disease. The optimal age range for screening is between 2 and 10 years. Currently, it is considered unreasonable to start a restricted diet before age 2, and there are no safety data on the use of statins before age 8 to 10 (Nordestgaard et al, 2013). Men with FH seem to develop CVD before women. Hypertension, smoking, diabetes, and high triglycerides and low HDL cholesterol are all well-established additional risk factors in FH.

The Familial Hypercholesterolemia Foundation recently convened a panel of international experts to "assess the utility of genetic testing." The rationale was (1) facilitation of definitive diagnosis; (2) pathogenic variants indicate higher cardiovascular risk, which indicates the potential need for more aggressive lipid lowering; (3) increase in initiation of and adherence to therapy; and (4) cascade testing of at-risk relatives. Their Expert Consensus Panel recommendations were to make FH genetic testing a standard of care for patients with definite or probable FH, as well as for their at-risk relatives. They recommended testing for the genes encoding the low-density lipoprotein receptor (LDLR), apolipoprotein B, and proprotein convertase subtilisin/kexin 9 (PCSK9) (Sturm et al, 2018). Treatment with statin drugs improves arterial function and structure (Masoura et al, 2011). Ultrasound of the Achilles tendon for xanthomas (cholesterol deposits from LDL) correctly identifies the majority of FH patients (Harada, 2017).

Polygenic Familial Hypercholesterolemia

Polygenic FH is the result of multiple gene defects. The *APOE-4* allele is common in this form. The diagnosis is based on two or more family members having LDL cholesterol levels above the 90th percentile without any tendon xanthomas. Usually these patients have lower LDL cholesterol levels than patients with the nonpolygenic form, but they remain at high risk for premature disease. The treatment is lifestyle change in conjunction with cholesterol-lowering drugs.

Familial Combined Hyperlipidemia

Familial combined hyperlipidemia (FCHL) is the most prevalent primary dyslipidemia, but its precise definition is controversial. FCHL is characterized by fluctuations in serum lipid concentrations and may present as mixed hyperlipidemia, isolated hypercholesterolemia, hypertriglyceridemia, or as a normal serum lipid profile in combination with abnormally elevated levels of apolipoprotein B. (Bello-Chavolla et al, 2018). Several lipoprotein patterns may be seen in patients with FCHL. These patients can have (1) elevated LDL levels with normal triglyceride levels (type IIa), (2) elevated LDL levels with elevated triglyceride levels (type IIb), or (3) elevated VLDL levels (type IV). Often these patients have the small, dense LDL associated with ASCVD. Consequently all forms of FCHL cause premature disease; approximately 15% of patients who have an MI before the age of 60 have FCHL. The defect in FCHL is hepatic overproduction of apo B-100 (VLDL) or a defect in the gene that produces hepatic lipase, the liver enzyme involved in triglyceride removal from the bloodstream. Patients with FCHL usually have other risk factors such as obesity, hypertension, diabetes, or metabolic syndrome. If lifestyle measures are ineffective, treatment includes medication. Patients with elevated triglyceride levels also need to avoid alcohol.

Familial Dysbetalipoproteinemia

Familial dysbetalipoproteinemia (type III hyperlipoproteinemia) is relatively uncommon. Catabolism of VLDL and chylomicron remnants is delayed because *APOE-2* replaces *APOE-3* and *APOE-4*. For dysbetalipoproteinemia to be seen, other risk factors such as older age, hypothyroidism, obesity, diabetes, or other dyslipidemias such as FCHL must be present. Total cholesterol levels range from 300 to 600 mg/dL, and triglyceride levels range from 400 to 800 mg/dL. This condition creates increased risk of premature ASCVD and peripheral vascular disease. Diagnosis is based on determining the isoforms of *APOE*. Treatment involves weight reduction, control of hyperglycemia and diabetes, and dietary restriction of saturated fat and cholesterol. If the dietary regimen is not effective, drug therapy is recommended.

Medical Diagnosis

Noninvasive tests such as electrocardiograms, treadmill stress tests, thallium scans, and echocardiography are used initially to establish a cardiovascular diagnosis. A more definitive, invasive test is angiography (cardiac catheterization), in which a dye is injected into the arteries, and radiographic images of the heart are obtained. Most narrowing and blockages from atherosclerosis are readily apparent on angiograms; however, neither smaller lesions nor lesions that have undergone remodeling are visible.

Magnetic resonance imaging (MRI) scans show the smaller lesions and can be used to follow atherosclerosis progression or regression after treatments. To predict MI or stroke, measuring the intimal thickness of the carotid artery may be used. Intracoronary thermography helps to determine the presence of vulnerable plaque.

Finally, the calcium in atherosclerotic lesions can be assessed. Electron beam computed tomography (ECT) measures calcium in the coronary arteries; persons with a positive scan are far more likely to have a future coronary event than those with a negative scan.

Approximately two thirds of cases of acute coronary syndromes (unstable angina and acute MI) happen in arteries that are minimally or mildly obstructed. This illustrates the role of thrombosis in clinical events. In the ischemia of an infarction, the myocardium or other tissue is deprived of oxygen and nourishment. Whether the heart is able to continue beating depends on the extent of the musculature involved, the presence of collateral circulation, and the oxygen requirement.

Prevention and Management of Risk Factors

The identification of risk factors for ASCVD and stroke has been a landmark achievement. The primary prevention of these disorders involves the assessment and management of the risk factors in the asymptomatic person. Persons with multiple risk factors are the target population, especially those with modifiable factors (Box 32.2).

Risk factor reduction has been shown to reduce CVD in persons of all ages. Many coronary events could be prevented with adoption of a healthy lifestyle (eating a heart-healthy diet, exercising regularly, managing weight, and not using tobacco) and adherence to lipid and hypertension drug therapy (Stone et al, 2014). The Framingham Heart Study, conducted over several decades, has provided a plethora of useful information to researchers (see *Focus On*: Framingham Heart Study).

BOX 32.2 Cardiovascular Disease Risk Factors

Major Risk Factors

Hypertension

Age (older than 45 years for men, 55 years for women)

Diabetes mellitus

Estimated glomerular filtration rate <60 mL/min

Microalbuminuria

Family history of premature cardiovascular disease (men <55 years of age, or women <65 years of age)

Modifiable Cardiovascular Risk Factors

Lipoprotein profile

Low-density lipoprotein (LDL) cholesterol, elevated

Total triglycerides, elevated

Elevated trimethylamine N-oxide (TMAO)

High-density lipoprotein (HDL) cholesterol, low

Inflammatory markers

Fibrinogen

C-reactive protein

Lifestyle Risk Factors

Tobacco use, particularly cigarettes

Physical inactivity

Poor diet

Stress

Insufficient sleep

Excessive alcohol consumption

Related Conditions

Hypertension

Obesity (body mass index >30)

Metabolic syndrome (including reduced HDL, elevated triglycerides, abdominal obesity)

Modified from National Institutes of Health, National Heart, Lung, and Blood Institute, National High Blood Pressure Education Program: The seventh report of the Joint National Committee on prevention, detection, evaluation, and treatment of high blood pressure, NIH Publication No. 04-5230, August 2004.

◎ FOCUS ON

Framingham Heart Study

The Framingham Heart Study (FHS) has conducted seminal research defining cardiovascular disease (CVD) risk factors and fundamentally shaping public health guidelines for CVD prevention over the past five decades. The success of the original cohort, initiated in 1948, paved the way for further epidemiologic research in preventive cardiology.

Since 1948 various leading investigators (Dr. Joseph Mountain, Dr. Thomas Dawber, Dr. William Kannel, and Dr. William Castelli) have been studying the population of Framingham, Massachusetts, to determine the prevalence and incidence of CVD and factors related to its development. This is the largest epidemiologic study of CVD in the world. Initial study participants (n = 5209) were healthy adults between 30 and 62 years of age. Because of the predominance of white individuals of European descent in the three original generations of FHS participants, the FHS enrolled the OMNI1 and OMNI2 cohorts in 1994 and 2003, respectively, aimed to reflect the current greater racial and ethnic diversity of the town of Framingham.

The study continues today, looking at the children and grandchildren of the original cohort. Through this cohort study, the concept of risk factors and thus prevention was born. Modifiable risk factors not only predict disease in healthy adults but also contribute to the disease process in those who have atherosclerotic disease. The seven major risk factors identified by the FHS are age, sex, blood pressure, total and high-density lipoprotein cholesterol, smoking, glucose intolerance, and left-ventricular hypertrophy (Opie et al, 2006). All FHS cohorts have been examined approximately every 2 to 4 years since the initiation of the study.

In addition to the contributions toward understanding CVD risk factors, the FHS has also been instrumental in establishing the epidemiology of specific CVD subtypes. The FHS demonstrated much of the characteristics and prognosis surrounding myocardial infarction (MI), including its frequent presentation as sudden cardiac death, and the high mortality associated with first MI, particularly in women. Heart failure has been and is a growing epidemic. The FHS was one of the first to describe the incidence, prevalence, and grim natural history of heart failure and also identified hypertension, valvular heart disease, and coronary disease as key etiologies for heart failure (Tsao and Vasan, 2015).

Milestones of the Framingham Heart Study

1960 Cigarette smoking found to increase the risk of heart disease.

1961 Cholesterol level, blood pressure, and electrocardiogram abnormalities found to increase the risk of heart disease.

1967 Physical activity found to reduce the risk of heart disease, and obesity found to increase the risk of heart disease.

1970 High blood pressure found to increase the risk of stroke.

1976 Menopause found to increase the risk of heart disease.

1978 Psychosocial factors found to affect heart disease.

1988 High levels of high-density lipoprotein cholesterol found to reduce risk of death.

1994 Enlarged left ventricle (one of two lower chambers of the heart) found to increase the risk of stroke.

1994 OMNI1 included changing racial and ethnic diversity.

1996 Progression from hypertension to heart failure described.

2003 OMNI2 included changing racial and ethnic diversity.

2006 Genetic Research Study begins to identify genes underlying CVDs in 9000 participants from three generations.

2008 Discovery and publication of four risk factors that raise probability of developing precursor of heart failure; new 30-year risk estimates developed for serious cardiac events.

2009 Researchers find parental dementia may be linked to poor memory in middle-aged adults.

2011 Blood lipids and the incidence of atrial fibrillation: The multiethnic study of atherosclerosis and the FHS.

In 1971 the offspring study was begun to measure the influence of heredity and environment on the offspring of the original cohort. The younger group appears to be more health conscious because they have lower rates of smoking, lower blood pressures, and lower cholesterol levels than their parents at the same age. The Generation III Cohort Study of the grandchildren is presently underway.

Data from Framingham Heart Study: *A timeline of milestones from the Framingham heart study* (website). http://www.framingham.com/heart/timeline.htm, 2015.

In the medical model, primary prevention of ASCVD and stroke involves altering similar risk factors toward a healthy patient profile. For ischemic stroke, atherosclerosis is the underlying disease. Therefore optimal lipid levels, as determined by the National Cholesterol Education Program (NCEP) for hypercholesterolemia, are also the target levels to prevent stroke.

Although the National Heart, Lung, and Blood Institute created the NCEP, the AHA has endorsed it. The AHA suggests that primary prevention of CVD should begin in children older than age 2 (Gidding et al, 2009). Dietary recommendations for children are a bit more liberal than those for adults. Activity is emphasized in maintaining ideal body weight. Early screening for dyslipidemia is recommended for children with a family history of hypercholesterolemia or ASCVD.

For adults, a total cholesterol level of 170 mg/dL or less is now considered optimal, including an HDL of at least 50 mg/dL. The new 2013 guidelines no longer rely strictly on cholesterol levels for advising patients or dosing medications. Instead the patient's overall health is evaluated for treatment decisions. The guidelines advise assessing factors such as age, gender, race, whether a patient smokes, blood pressure and whether it is being treated, whether a person has diabetes, and blood cholesterol levels in determining risk. They also suggest that health care providers should consider other factors, including family history. Only after that very personalized assessment is a decision made on what treatment would work best. The ASCVD Risk Calculator developed by the ACC/AHA expert panel is available at the ACC. org website.

Inflammatory Markers

Fifty percent of heart attacks occur in individuals with normal serum cholesterol, which has led to research on other risk markers. Increasing knowledge about the role of inflammation in ASCVD gives credence to the use of inflammatory markers to indicate the presence of atherosclerosis in asymptomatic individuals or the extent of atherosclerosis in patients with symptoms. Several markers have been suggested (Box 32.3), and research continues to look at the effects of diet on these biomarkers. Plasma levels of omega-3 fatty acids are inversely associated with the inflammatory markers C-reactive protein (hs-CRP), interleukin-6 (IL-6), fibrinogen, and homocysteine (Kalogeropoulos et al, 2010). An inflammatory marker specific to vascular inflammation has become available. The PLAC™ test measures Lp-PLA2 (Jellinger et al, 2012). Lp-PLA2 levels indicate ASCVD risk independent from other markers and provides information on the relationship between inflammation and atherosclerosis (see Chapters 5 and 7).

Fibrinogen. Most MIs are the result of an intracoronary thrombosis. Prospective studies have shown that plasma fibrinogen is an independent predictor of ASCVD risk. Factors associated with an elevated fibrinogen are smoking, diabetes, hypertension, obesity, sedentary lifestyle, elevated triglycerides, and genetic factors. More clinical trials are needed to determine whether fibrinogen is involved in atherogenesis or is just a marker of vascular damage. Blood thrombogenicity increases with high LDL cholesterol and in diabetes.

C-reactive protein. C-reactive protein (hs-CRP) is synthesized in the liver as the acute-phase response to inflammation. The *hs* refers to human serum. In a normal individual without infection or inflammation, hs-CRP levels are very low, less than 0.6 mg/dL. Because atherogenesis is an inflammatory process, hs-CRP has been shown to be elevated (>3 mg/dL) in people with angina, MI, stroke, and peripheral vascular disease; the elevated levels are independent of other risk factors (see Chapter 5). Despite a lack of specificity for the cause of the inflammation, data from more than 30 epidemiologic studies have shown significant association between elevated blood levels of hs-CRP and the prevalence of atherosclerosis (Morrow and Crea, 2014).

BOX 32.3 Inflammatory Markers for Cardiovascular Risk

Genetic markers: angiotensin II receptor type-1 polymorphism
Oxidized low-density lipoprotein cholesterol
Adhesion molecules
Selectins
Free fatty acids
Cytokines
    Interleukin-1
    Interleukin-6
    Tumor necrosis factor-alpha
Acute-phase reactants
    Fibrinogen
    C-reactive protein
    Serum amyloid A
White blood cell count
Erythrocyte sedimentation rate
Trimethylamine N-oxide (TMAO)

Derived from Fung MM, et al: Early inflammatory and metabolic changes in association with AGTR1 polymorphisms in prehypertensive subjects, *Am J Hypertens* 24:225, 2011; Pearson TA, et al: Markers of inflammation and cardiovascular disease: application to clinical and public health practice: a statement for healthcare professionals from the Centers for Disease Control and Prevention and the American Heart Association, *Circulation* 107:499, 2003.

Hs-CRP levels are categorized for risk as low (<1 mg/L), average (2 to 3 mg/L), and high (>3 mg/L) after the average of two measurements are taken at least 2 weeks apart. The Mediterranean diet pattern (Appendix 23) is most effective in inhibiting inflammation. The Dietary Approaches to Stop Hypertension model (described later in the chapter and in Appendix 17) and the plant nutrition model also have proven to be beneficial. The data on low-fat and low-carbohydrate diets are inconclusive (Lee et al, 2014; Smidowicz and Regula, 2015).

Homocysteine. Homocysteine is an amino acid metabolite of methionine. Elevated circulating total homocysteine (tHcy) concentrations have been regarded as an independent risk factor for CVD. However, several large clinical trials to correct hyperhomocysteinemia using B-vitamin supplements (particularly folic acid) have largely failed to reduce the risk of CVD (Baggot and Tamura, 2015).

Although some evidence suggests that homocysteine may promote atherosclerosis, no causal link has been established. And it appears more likely that increased homocysteine levels are markers rather than causes of CVD. Giving supplemental vitamins folate, B_6 and B_{12}, have been shown to lower homocysteine levels in some individuals and is being investigated actively as a treatment for CVD but as of now is not widely recommended.

Trimethylamine-N-oxide. Trimethylamine-N-oxide (TMAO) is a gut microbiota-dependent metabolite that contributes to heart disease (Tang et al, 2013). It is produced by the liver after intestinal bacteria have digested animal protein. TMAO has been shown to predict cardiac risk in individuals not identified by traditional risk factors and blood tests. This is speculated to be a factor in the emerging evidence that a plant-based diet is cardioprotective compared with one that includes animal sources (Tuso, 2015).

Lifestyle Guidelines

Lifestyle modification remains the backbone of CVD prevention and treatment. Adhering to a heart-healthy diet, regular exercising, avoidance of tobacco products, and maintenance of a healthy weight are

---

BOX 32.4 Summary of American College of Cardiology (ACC)/ American Heart Association (AHA) Recommendations for Lifestyle Management

DIET

LDL-C

Advise adults who would benefit from LDL-C lowering to

1. Consume a dietary pattern that emphasizes intake of vegetables, fruits, and whole grains; includes low-fat dairy products, poultry, fish, legumes, nontropical vegetable oils and nuts; and limits intake of sweets, sugar-sweetened beverages, and red meats.
   a. Adapt this dietary pattern to appropriate calorie requirements, personal and cultural food preferences, and nutrition therapy for other medical conditions (including diabetes mellitus).
   b. Achieve this pattern by following plans such as the DASH dietary pattern, the USDA Food Pattern, or the AHA Diet.
2. Aim for a dietary pattern that achieves 5%-6% of calories from saturated fat.
3. Reduce percent of calories from saturated fat.
4. Reduce percent of calories from trans fat.

Blood Pressure

Advise adults who would benefit from blood pressure lowering to

1. Consume a dietary pattern that emphasizes intake of vegetables, fruits, and whole grains; includes low-fat dairy products, poultry, fish, legumes, nontropical vegetable oils and nuts; and limits intake of sweets, sugar-sweetened beverages, and red meats.
   a. Adapt this dietary pattern to appropriate calorie requirements, personal and cultural food preferences, and nutrition therapy for other medical conditions (including diabetes mellitus).

b. Achieve this pattern by following plans such as the DASH dietary pattern, the USDA Food Pattern, or the AHA Diet.
2. Lower sodium intake.
3. a. Consume no more than 2400 mg of sodium/day.
   b. Further reduction of sodium intake to 1500 mg/day is desirable because it is associated with even greater reduction in blood pressure.
   c. Reduce intake by at least 1000 mg/day because that will lower blood pressure, even without meeting the desired daily sodium goal.
4. Combine the DASH dietary pattern with lower sodium intake.

PHYSICAL ACTIVITY

Lipids

In general, advise adults to engage in aerobic physical activity to reduce LDL–C and non-HDL–C: 3-4 sessions a week, lasting on average 40 minutes per session, and involving moderate-to-vigorous-intensity physical activity.

Blood Pressure

In general, advise adults to engage in aerobic physical activity to lower blood pressure: 3-4 sessions a week, lasting on average 40 minutes per session, and involving moderate-to-vigorous-intensity physical activity.

Eckel RH, Jakicic JM, Ard JD, et al. 2013 AHA/ACC guideline on lifestyle management to reduce cardiovascular risk: A report of the American College of Cardiology /American Heart Association Task Force on Practice Guidelines. Circulation 129: S76-S99, 2014.

---

known lifestyle factors that, along with genetics, determine CVD risk. Three critical questions (CQs) were addressed in the 2013 ACC/AHA lifestyle modification guidelines. CQ1 presents evidence on dietary patterns and macronutrients and their effect on blood pressure and lipids, CQ2 presents evidence on the effect of dietary sodium and potassium intake on blood pressure and CVD outcomes, and CQ3 presents the evidence on the effect of physical activity on lipids and blood pressure. The recommendations are summarized in Box 32.4.

Diet

The importance of diet and nutrition in modifying the risk of CVD has been known for some time. However, in general, individual dietary components have been the predominant focus. Because foods are consumed typically in combinations rather than individually and because of the possibility of synergist relationships between nutrients, there has been increasing attention to dietary patterns and their relationship to health outcomes such as CVD.

The Mediterranean Diet

There is no uniform definition of the Mediterranean diet (MeD) in the published studies, which makes it difficult to pool data. There are common features of the diet, such as greater number of servings of fruits and vegetables (mostly fresh) with an emphasis on root vegetables and greens, whole grains, fatty fish (rich in omega-3 fatty acids), lower amounts of red meat and with an emphasis on lean meats, lower fat dairy products, abundant nuts and legumes, and use of olive oil, canola oil, nut oil, or margarine blended with rapeseed oil or flaxseed oil (see Appendix 23). The MeD dietary patterns that have been studied were moderate in total fat (32% to 35%), relatively low in saturated fat (9% to 10%), high in polyunsaturated fatty acids (especially omega-3), and high in fiber (27 to 37 g per day). The Prevención con

Dieta Mediterránea (PREDIMED) trial was a randomized controlled trial (RCT) looking at the effect of a MeD on CVD outcomes. Those patients randomized to the MeD had a 30% reduced risk of CVD events (Estruch et al, 2013).

The Dietary Approaches to Stop Hypertension (DASH) Diet

The DASH dietary pattern is high in fruits and vegetables, low-fat dairy products, whole grains, fish, and nuts and low in animal protein and sugar. Two DASH variations were studied in the Optimal Macronutrient Intake Trial for Heart Health (OmniHeart) trial, one that replaced 10% of total daily energy from carbohydrate with protein; the other that replaced the same amount of carbohydrate with unsaturated fat. The former showed better results than the latter in lowering CVD risk (Swain et al, 2008; see Appendix 17). The 2013 ACC/AHA lifestyle guidelines recommend the DASH diet as best for prevention of CVD, but also suggest that a MeD pattern is cardioprotective.

Vegan Diet

A vegan diet is a strict vegetarian diet that includes no dietary sources from animal origins (see Appendix 30). There is ongoing research to suggest only this type of very restricted diet can actually reverse ASCVD (Esselstyn and Goulubić, 2014; Tuso, 2015).

Physical Inactivity

Physical inactivity and a low level of fitness are independent risk factors for ASCVD. Physical activity is associated with ASCVD, independent of the common cardiometabolic risk factors of obesity, serum lipids, serum glucose, and hypertension, in men and women. With the high prevalence of obesity, physical activity is a high priority. Physical activity lessens ASCVD risk by reducing atherogenesis, increasing vascularity of the myocardium, increasing fibrinolysis, increasing HDL cholesterol, improving glucose tolerance and insulin sensitivity, aiding in weight management, and reducing blood pressure.

The most recent AHA recommendations for exercise for adults are the following:

- Get at least 150 minutes per week of moderate-intensity aerobic activity or 75 minutes per week of vigorous aerobic activity, or a combination of both, preferably spread throughout the week.
- Add moderate- to high-intensity muscle-strengthening activity (such as resistance or weights) on at least 2 days per week.
- Spend less time sitting. Even light-intensity activity can offset some of the risks of being sedentary.
- Gain even more benefits by being active at least 300 minutes (5 hours) per week.
- Increase amount and intensity gradually over time.
  The AHA recommendations for children are the following:
- Children 3 to 5 years old should be physically active and have plenty of opportunities to move throughout the day.
- Kids 6 to 17 years old should get at least 60 minutes per day of moderate- to vigorous-intensity physical activity, mostly aerobic.
- Include vigorous-intensity activity on at least 3 days per week.
- Include muscle- and bone-strengthening (weight-bearing) activities on at least 3 days per week.
- Increase amount and intensity gradually over time.

Stress

Stress activates a neurohormonal response in the body that results in increased heart rate, blood pressure, and cardiac excitability. The stress hormone angiotensin II is released after stimulation of the sympathetic nervous system (SNS); exogenous infusion of angiotensin II accelerates the formation of plaque. The INTERHEART study found that the effect of stress on CVD risk is comparable to that of hypertension. Stress management was not part of the 2013 ACC/AHA lifestyle modification guidelines.

Diabetes

Diabetes is a disease that is an independent risk factor. The prevalence of diabetes mirrors that of obesity in the United States. Type 2 diabetes has continued to increase in incidence (see Chapter 29). Any form of diabetes increases the risk for ASCVD, with occurrence at younger ages. Most people with diabetes actually die of CVD. Some of the increased risk seen in patients with diabetes is attributable to the concurrent presence of other risk factors, such as dyslipidemia, hypertension, and obesity. Thus diabetes is now considered an ASCVD risk factor (see Chapter 29).

The Look AHEAD (Action for Health in Diabetes) study, conducted from 2001 to 2012, provided extensive longitudinal data on the effect of an intensive lifestyle intervention, targeting weight reduction through caloric restriction and increased physical activity, on CVD rates (the primary outcome) and CVD risk factors among adults with type 2 diabetes mellitus. Conclusions from the study were that increased physical activity and improvements in diet based on a MeD or DASH pattern can safely lead to weight loss and reduced requirement for medication to control CVD risk factors without a concomitant increase in the risk of cardiovascular events (Fox et al, 2015).

Metabolic Syndrome

Since the early findings of the Framingham Heart Study, it has been known that a clustering of risk factors markedly increases the risk of CVD (see Chapter 20 for an in-depth discussion of metabolic syndrome).

Obesity

Obesity has now reached epidemic levels in children and adults in many developed countries. Body mass index (BMI) and CVD are positively related; as BMI goes up, the risk of CVD also increases. The prevalence of overweight and obesity is the highest that it has ever been in the United States (see Chapter 20). Obesity rates vary by race and ethnicity in women. Non-Hispanic black women have the highest prevalence, followed by Mexican American women, American Indians, Alaskan natives, and non-Hispanic whites.

An obese-years metric was developed using more than 5000 participants of the Framingham Heart Study that captures the cumulative damage of obesity over years. The obese-years metric is calculated by multiplying the number of BMI units above 29 kg/m² by the number of years lived at that BMI. Higher obese years were associated with higher CVD risk in the study. The metric was found to provide a slightly more accurate measure of CVD risk than obesity alone (Abdullah et al, 2014).

Carrying excess adipose tissue greatly affects the heart through the many risk factors that are often present: hypertension, glucose intolerance, inflammatory markers (IL-6, tumor necrosis factor alpha [TNF-α], hs-CRP), obstructive sleep apnea, prothrombotic state, endothelial dysfunction, and dyslipidemia (small dense LDL, increased apo B, low HDL, high triglyceride levels). Many inflammatory proteins are now known to come from the adipocyte (see Chapters 7 and 20). These concurrent risk factors may help to explain the high morbidity and mortality rates observed in people who are obese.

Weight distribution (abdominal versus gynoid) is also predictive of CVD risk, glucose tolerance, and serum lipid levels. Central or abdominal length of adiposity also has been strongly related to markers of inflammation, especially hs-CRP. Therefore a waist circumference of less than 35 inches for women and 40 inches for men is recommended (see Chapter 20).

Small weight losses (10 to 20 lb) can improve LDL cholesterol, HDL cholesterol, triglycerides, high blood pressure, glucose tolerance, and hs-CRP levels, even if an ideal BMI is not achieved. Weight loss also has been correlated with lower hs-CRP levels. However, to restore vascular function, the amount of weight that must be lost, the time of weight maintenance, or the amount of improvement in endothelial function that lessens cardiovascular events is still unknown.

Nonmodifiable Risk Factors

Age and Sex

With increasing age, higher mortality rates from CVD are seen in both genders. However, gender is a factor for the assessment of risk. The incidence of premature disease in men 35 to 44 years of age is three times as high as the incidence in women of the same age. Therefore being older than 45 years of age is considered a risk factor for men. For women the increased risk comes after the age of 55 years, which is after menopause for most women. Overall the increased risk for CVD parallels age.

Family History and Genetics

A family history of premature disease is a strong risk factor, even when other risk factors are considered. A family history is considered to be positive when MI or sudden death occurs before the age of 55 years in a male first-degree relative or the age of 65 in a female first-degree relative (parents, siblings, or children). The presence of a positive family history, although not modifiable, influences the intensity of risk factor management.

Menopausal Status

Endogenous estrogen confers protection against ASCVD in premenopausal women, probably by preventing vascular injury. Loss of estrogen after natural or surgical menopause is associated with increased

ASCVD risk. Rates of ASCVD in premenopausal women are low except in women with multiple risk factors. During the menopausal period total cholesterol, LDL cholesterol, and triglyceride levels increase; HDL cholesterol level decreases, especially in women who gain weight.

Medical Nutrition Therapy

Medical nutrition therapy (MNT), which includes discussion of physical activity, is the primary intervention for patients with elevated LDL cholesterol (see Box 32.4). Physicians are encouraged to refer patients to registered dietitian nutritionists (RDNs) to help patients meet goals for therapy based on LDL cholesterol levels.

With diet, exercise, and weight reduction, patients can decrease LDL cholesterol and reduce body inflammation. The complexity of changes, number of changes, and motivation of the patient will dictate how many patient visits it will take for the adherent to be successful. An initial visit of 45 to 90 minutes followed by two to six visits of 30 to 60 minutes each with the RDN is recommended (Academy of Nutrition and Dietetics Evidence Analysis Library [EAL], 2011). Consequently these interventions are tried before drug therapy and also continue during pharmacologic treatment to enhance effectiveness of the medication (see *Pathophysiology and Care Management Algorithm: Atherosclerosis*).

Lifestyle Recommendations

The ACC/AHA recommends diet and lifestyle changes to reduce AS-CVD risk in all people older than the age of 2 (Eckel et al, 2014). The ACC/AHA recommendations are for a diet high in vegetables, fruits, whole grains, low-fat poultry, fish, nontropical vegetable oils, nuts, and low-fat dairy and low in sweets, sugar-sweetened beverages, and red meat. The DASH diet pattern or U.S. Department of Agriculture (USDA) food pattern (MyPlate) is recommended to achieve this diet. The MeD was not specifically recommended because in the evidence evaluated the diet was not specific or consistent enough to draw conclusions. In general, the MeD pattern (Fig. 32.5) fits the recommendations. A study recently presented at the ACC supports the MeD pattern for CVD risk reduction (ACC, 2015). The study included more than 2500 Greek adults over more than 10 years. Nearly 20% of men and 12% of women in the study developed or died from heart disease. People who closely followed the MeD were 47% less likely to develop heart disease than those who did not follow the diet. The MeD Score Tool was used (see Fig. 32.5) to validate the dietary pattern. A MeD may also reduce recurrent CVD by 50% to 70% and has been shown to affect lipoprotein levels positively in high-risk populations (Carter et al, 2010).

Saturated fatty acids. Currently in the United States the average intake of saturated fat is 11% of calories. The recommendation for decreasing LDL cholesterol is 5% to 6%. The guidelines have no specific recommendation for trans fatty acid intake but recommend it be decreased with the saturated fat. Saturated fat is generally found in animal proteins. It is recommended that intake of animal protein, especially red meat and high-fat dairy, be decreased.

Trans fatty acids. Trans fatty acids (stereoisomers of the naturally occurring cis-linoleic acid) are produced in the hydrogenation process used in the food industry to increase shelf life of foods and to make margarines, made from oil, firmer. Most trans fatty acids intake comes from these partially hydrogenated oils (PHOs). In 2013 the FDA made a decision to remove PHOs from the "generally recognized as safe" list. This was based on the mounting evidence that trans fats contributed to ASCVD and was associated with increased LDL cholesterol levels. Trans fat intake is inversely associated with HDL levels (Yanai et al, 2015).

Monounsaturated fatty acids. Oleic acid (C18:1) is the most prevalent monounsaturated fatty acid (MUFA) in the American diet. Substituting oleic acid for carbohydrate has almost no appreciable effect on blood lipids. However, replacing saturated fatty acids (SFAs) with MUFAs (as would happen when substituting olive oil for butter) lowers serum cholesterol levels, LDL cholesterol levels, and triglyceride levels. Oleic acid as part of the MeD (Fig. 32.6) has been shown to have antiinflammatory effects.

Polyunsaturated fatty acids. The essential fatty acid linoleic acid (LA) is the predominant PUFA consumed in the American diet; its effect depends on the total fatty acid profile of the diet. When added to study diets, large amounts of LA decrease HDL serum cholesterol levels. High intakes of omega-6 PUFAs may exert adverse effects on the function of vascular endothelium or stimulate production of proinflammatory cytokines (Harris et al, 2009). The AHA does not support concern for omega-6 PUFAs as proinflammatory. However, this position has been challenged by researchers in the field. A recent review of the evidence on the role of omega-6 PUFAS found limited conclusive evidence of an association between n-6 and CVD. Intervention trials were identified but they generally had a small sample size and varied in terms of the study subject characteristics and timing, duration, and dosage of the intervention (Khandelwal et al, 2013).

Omega-3 fatty acids. The main omega-3 fatty acids (eicosapentaenoic acid [EPA] and docosahexaenoic acid [DHA]) are high in fish oils, fish oil capsules, and ocean fish. Some studies have shown that eating fish is associated with a decreased ASCVD risk. The AHA recommendation for the general population is to increase fish consumption specifically of fish high in omega-3 fatty acids (salmon, tuna, mackerel, sardines) and eat a 3.5-ounce serving twice a week. Consumption of omega-3 fat in the form of fish oil has been associated with higher levels of HDL cholesterol and lower levels of serum triglycerides (Yanai et al, 2015; see Appendix 26). The AHA recommends a discussion with a physician before taking fish oil supplements.

An omega-3 fatty acid from vegetables, alpha-linolenic acid (ALA), has antiinflammatory effects (see Chapter 7). Omega-3 fatty acids are thought to be cardioprotective because they interfere with blood clotting and alter prostaglandin synthesis. Omega-3 fat stimulates production of NO, a substance that stimulates relaxation of the blood vessel wall (vasodilation). Unfortunately, high intakes (above 3 g EPA/DHA) prolong bleeding time, a common condition among Arctic Native populations with high omega-3 fat dietary intakes and low incidence of ASCVD.

Dietary cholesterol. Previous recommendations have been to decrease dietary cholesterol to decrease LDL cholesterol and reduce ASCVD risk. The ACC/AHA 2013 guidelines no longer make this recommendation, and they specifically state that dietary cholesterol does not raise LDLs (see Chapter 9). The 2015 U.S. Dietary Guidelines also eliminate the recommendation to restrict cholesterol. However it is important to remember that most high cholesterol foods are also high in saturated fats that do raise LDL cholesterol.

Fiber. High intake levels of dietary fiber are associated with significantly lower prevalence of ASCVD and stroke (Anderson et al, 2009). The USDA MyPlate, the DASH diet, and the MeD pattern emphasize fruits, vegetables, legumes, and whole grains, so they are innately high in fiber. This combination of foods provides a combination of soluble and insoluble fiber. Proposed mechanisms for the hypocholesterolemic effect of soluble fiber include the following: (1) the fiber binds bile acids, which lowers serum cholesterol and (2) bacteria in the colon ferment the fiber to produce acetate, propionate, and butyrate, which inhibit cholesterol synthesis. The role of fiber, if any, on inflammatory pathways is not well established. Minerals, vitamins,

PATHOPHYSIOLOGY AND CARE MANAGEMENT ALGORITHM

Atherosclerosis

ETIOLOGY

Smoking	Genes	Decreased HDL-cholesterol
Obesity	High saturated fat/cholesterol diet	Aging
Hypertension	Elevated serum triglycerides	Hyperhomocysteinemia
Elevated LDL-cholesterol	Inactivity	Endothelial dysfunction
	Diabetes	
	Stress	

Accumulation of plaque
Production of less nitric oxide
Oxidized LDL cholesterol taken up by macrophages
Formation of foam cells and fatty streaks

PATHOPHYSIOLOGY

Clinical Findings

- Elevated LDL cholesterol
- Elevated serum triglycerides
- Elevated C-reactive protein
- Low HDL-cholesterol

Nutrition Assessment

- BMI evaluation
- Waist circumference; waist to hip ratio (WHR)
- Dietary assessment for:
  SFA, *trans*-fatty acids, ω-3 fatty acids, fiber, sodium, alcohol, sugar, and phytonutrients

MANAGEMENT

Medical Management

- Lifestyle change (increase physical activity and lower stress)
- HMG CoA reductase inhibitors (statins)
- Triglyceride-lowering medication
- Blood pressure—lowering medication
- Medication for glucose management
- Percutaneous coronary intervention (PCI)
  - Balloon
  - Stent
- Coronary artery bypass graft (CABG)
- Antiplatelet therapy

Nutrition Management

- DASH dietary pattern
- Mediterranean diet pattern
- Weight reduction if needed
- Increase dietary fiber to 25–30 g/day or more
- Add ω-3 fats from food sources
- Add fruits and vegetables
- CoQ$_{10}$ for those on statin drugs

MEDITERRANEAN DIET SCORE TOOL

A Mediterranean dietary pattern ('Med diet') is typically one based on whole or minimally processed foods. It's rich in protective foods (fruits, vegetables, legumes, wholegrains, fish and olive oil) and low in adverse dietary factors (fast food, sugar-sweetened beverages, refined grain products and processed or energy-dense foods) with moderate red meat and alcohol intake.

Evidence shows **overall dietary pattern** (reflected in TOTAL SCORE) as well as **individual components** reflect risk; a higher score is associated with lower risk of CVD and all-cause mortality (BMJ 2008;337:a1344). During rehabilitation patient scores should ideally rise in response to dietary advice and support.

This tool can be used by health professionals with appropriate nutritional knowledge and competencies, such as Registered Dietitians (NICE, 2007, 2013). It can be used as both an *audit tool* and *as part of a dietary assessment* at baseline, end of programme and 1 year follow-up, along with assessment and advice for weight management, salt intake and eating behaviours. For information on complete requirements for dietary assessments and advice, please refer to the latest NICE/Joint British Societies guidelines (BACPR, 2012. The BACPR Standards and Core Components for Cardiovascular Disease Prevention and Rehabilitation, 2nd Ed.).

	Question	Yes	No	Nutritional issue to discuss in response
1.	Is olive oil the main culinary fat used?			**Choosing Healthier Fats** Olive oil is high in monounsaturated fat. Using unsaturated fats instead of saturated fats in cooking and preparing food is advisable.
2.	Are ≥ 4 tablespoons of olive oil used each day?			**Healthy fats are better than very low fat** Med diet is more beneficial than a very low fat diet in prevention of CVD. So replacing saturated with unsaturated fat is better than replacing it with carbohydrates or protein.
3.	Are ≥ 2 servings (of 200g each) of vegetables eaten each day?			**Eat plenty of fruits and vegetables** Eating a wide variety of fruit and vegetables every day helps ensure adequate intake of many vitamins, minerals, phytochemicals and fibre. Studies have shown that eating plenty of these foods is protective for CVD and cancer.
4.	Are ≥ 3 servings of fruit (of 80g each) eaten each day?			
5.	Is < 1 serving (100-150g) of red meat/ hamburgers/ other meat products eaten each day?			**Choose lean meats and consider cooking methods** Red and processed meats are high in saturated fat, can be high in salt and are best replaced with white meat or fish or vegetarian sources of protein. Grill or roast without fat, casserole or stir fry.
6.	Is < 1 serving (12g) of butter, margarine or cream eaten each day?			**Keep saturated fat low** These foods are high in saturated fat which can increase your blood cholesterol level. Choose plant-based or reduced-fat alternatives.
7.	Is < 1 serving (330ml) of sweet or sugar sweetened carbonated beverages consumed each day?			Excessive consumption of sugar-sweetened beverages can worsen many risk factors for CVD: keep consumption to < 1/day.
8.	Are ≥ 3 glasses (of 125ml) of wine consumed each week?			**Moderate alcohol intake with meals** While this does have some protective effect but **there is no evidence that non-drinkers should take up drinking alcohol.**
9.	Are ≥ 3 servings (of 150g) of legumes consumed each week?			**Include soluble fibre** These foods are high in soluble fibre and other useful nutrients. Regular consumption is advisable for raised cholesterol.
10.	Are ≥ 3 servings of fish (100-150g) or seafood (200g) eaten each week?			**Eat more oily and white fish** Oily fish is an excellent source of essential omega-3 fats. White fish is very low in saturated fat.
11.	Is < 3 servings of commercial sweets/pastries eaten each week?			**Eat less processed food** These foods are usually high in saturated fat, salt or sugar and often contain trans fats. Replacing these with healthy snacks such as fruit or unsalted nuts is beneficial.
12.	Is ≥ 1 serving (of 30g) of nuts consumed each week?			**Snack on modest servings of unsalted nuts** Nuts are rich in unsaturated fat, phytosterols, fibre, vitamin E and iron, **e.g. walnuts, almonds, hazelnuts**
13.	Is chicken, turkey or rabbit routinely eaten instead of veal, pork, hamburger or sausage?			'White meat' choices are lower in saturated fat. Remove the skin and consider your cooking method.
14.	Are pasta, vegetable or rice dishes flavoured with garlic, tomato, leek or onion eaten ≥ twice a week?			Using a tomato and garlic or onion or leek-based sauce regularly is a key feature of the Med diet.
	TOTAL SCORE (total no. of 'yes' answers)			

26.09.13
Version 1   Alison Hornby, Katherine Paterson

Fig. 32.5 Mediterranean Diet Score Tool. (Courtesy Alison Hornby and Katherine Paterson.)

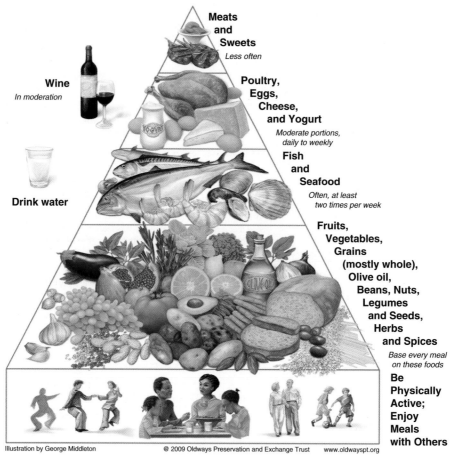

Fig. 32.6 The Traditional Healthy Mediterranean Diet Pyramid. (Courtesy Oldways Preservation and Exchange Trust, https://www.oldwayspt.org.) (http://www.cardiacrehabilitation.org.uk/docs/Mediterranean-Diet-Score.pdf.)

and antioxidants that are components of a high-fiber diet further enrich the diet.

Insoluble fibers such as cellulose and lignin have no effect on serum cholesterol levels. For the purpose of heart disease prevention, most of the recommended 25 to 30 g of fiber a day should be soluble fiber.

Antioxidants. Two dietary components that affect the oxidation potential of LDL cholesterol are the level of LA in the particle and the availability of antioxidants. Vitamins C, E, and beta-carotene at physiologic levels have antioxidant roles in the body. Vitamin E is the most concentrated antioxidant carried on LDLs, the amount being 20 to 300 times greater than any other antioxidant. A major function of vitamin E is to prevent oxidation of PUFAs in the cell membrane. The AHA does not recommend vitamin E supplementation for CVD prevention. A dietary pattern that includes increased amounts of whole grains, nuts, and seeds (especially sunflower seeds) has increased amounts of vitamin E. Foods with concentrated amounts of antioxidants are found in phytochemicals known as catechins and have been found to improve vascular reactivity. Red grapes, red wine, tea (especially green tea), berries, and broad beans (fava beans) are part of the MeD (see Figs. 32.5 and 32.6).

Stanols and sterols. Since the early 1950s, plant stanols and sterols isolated from soybean oils or pine tree oil have been known to lower blood cholesterol by inhibiting absorption of dietary cholesterol. Stanols and sterols have been shown to lower LDL cholesterol in adults (Yanai et al, 2015). Because these esters also can affect the absorption of and cause lower beta-carotene, alpha-tocopherol, and lycopene levels, further safety studies are needed for use in normocholesterolemic individuals, children, and pregnant women.

Weight loss. According to the Centers for Disease Control and Prevention (CDC), in 2015 to 2016 39.8% of adults and 18.5% of children in the United States were classified as obese. Obesity raises the risk of hypertension, dyslipidemia, type 2 diabetes, ASCVD, and stroke. Obesity is associated with increased risk in all-cause and CVD mortality (Stone et al, 2014). Recommendations of the panel are summarized in Box 32.5.

Medical Management

Pharmacologic Management

Determination of drug therapy depends on risk category and attainment of the LDL cholesterol goal. The 2013 ACC/AHA Guidelines for

BOX 32.5 Recommendations from The Obesity Society (TOS) Obesity Guideline

1. Patient/provider encounter for obesity prevention and management: A patient encounter is defined as an interaction with a primary care provider who assesses weight status to determine need for further assessment and treatment.
2. Measure weight and height and calculate body mass index (BMI).
3. BMI 25<30 (overweight) or BMI 30<35 (class I obese) or BMI 35<40 class II obese or BMI >40 (class III obese): these BMI cutpoints define overweight and obese individuals who are at increased risk of cardiovascular disease (CVD). Within these categories, additional personal risk assessment is needed.
4. Assess and treat CVD risk factors and obesity-related comorbidities: A waist circumference measurement is recommended for individuals with BMI 25-35 to provide additional information on risk. It is not necessary to measure waist circumference in patients with BMI >35 because the waist circumference will likely be elevated and it will add no additional information. Increased cardiometabolic risk is defined as >88 cm or >35 in for women and >102 cm or >40 in for men.
5. Assess weight and lifestyle histories: Ask questions about history of weight gain and loss over time, details of previous weight loss attempts, dietary habits, physical activity, family history of obesity, and other medical conditions and medications that may affect weight.
6. Assess need to lose weight: Weight loss treatment is indicated for (1) obese and (2) overweight with one or more indicators of increased CVD risk.
7. Advise to avoid weight gain and address other risk factors.

Jensen, et al: 2013 AHA/ACC/TOS guideline for the management of overweight and obesity in adults. *Circulation*, 129:S102, 2014.

Treatment of Blood Cholesterol have updated recommendations for prescribing statin drugs to be more focused on overall patient risk than on specific serum cholesterol targets. The primary treatment for those at risk of ASCVD are the 3-hydroxy-3-methylglutaryl–coenzyme A (HMG-CoA) reductase inhibitors, of which there are many (see Appendix 13). The classes of drugs include the following: (1) bile acid sequestrants such as cholestyramine (adsorbs bile acids); (2) nicotinic acid; (3) statins, or 3-hydroxy-3-methylglutaryl–coenzyme A (HMG-CoA) reductase inhibitors, which inhibit the rate-limiting enzyme in cholesterol synthesis; (4) fibric acid derivatives; and (5) probucol.

Medical Intervention

Medical interventions such as percutaneous coronary intervention (PCI) are now performed in patients with asymptomatic ischemia or angina. PCI, previously known as percutaneous transluminal coronary angioplasty, is a procedure that uses a catheter with a balloon that, once inflated, breaks up plaque deposits in an occluded artery. Coronary stenting involves a wire mesh tube inserted to hold an artery open; it can release medication that prevents clotting (Thom et al, 2006).

PCI is often possible because of earlier detection of blockages. The most common problem with PCI is restenosis of the artery. A recent study examined more than 2200 patients, half of whom received intervention of medication and lifestyle changes such as quitting smoking, exercise, and nutrition, and half of whom received lifestyle changes as well as angioplasty. After 5 years it was observed that the number who had heart attacks, were hospitalized, or died because of their heart problems was virtually identical in both groups. Angioplasty did not appear to provide an additional benefit versus lifestyle changes combined with medication (Boden et al, 2007).

Because PCI is performed with the patient under local anesthesia in a cardiac catheterization laboratory, recovery is quicker than with coronary artery bypass graft (CABG) surgery. In CABG surgery, an artery from the chest is used to redirect blood flow around a diseased vessel. Candidates for CABG usually have more than two occluded arteries. CABG surgeries have decreased since 1995 because more PCI procedures are being done. These surgeries improve survival time, relieve symptoms, and markedly improve the quality of life for patients with ASCVD. However, CABG does not cure atherosclerosis; the new grafts are also susceptible to atherogenesis. Consequently, restenosis is common within 10 years of surgery.

HYPERTENSION

Hypertension is persistently high arterial blood pressure, the force exerted per unit area on the walls of arteries. The systolic blood pressure (SBP), the upper reading in a blood pressure measurement, is the force exerted on the walls of blood vessels as the heart contracts and pushes blood out of its chambers. The lower reading, known as diastolic blood pressure (DBP), measures the force as the heart relaxes between contractions. Blood pressure is measured in millimeters (mm) of mercury (Hg). Adult blood pressure is considered normal at 120/80 mm Hg. The blood pressure cutoffs for elevated blood pressure (formerly prehypertension), stage 1 and stage 2 hypertension are found in Table 32.1.

The clinical practice guidelines from the ACC/AHA Task Force for the Prevention, Detection, Evaluation, and Management of High Blood Pressure in Adults (Whelton et al, 2018) state that the combination of diet and lifestyle therapy is especially useful in adults for the prevention of hypertension and for the management of elevated blood

TABLE 32.1 Categories of Blood Pressure in Adults

	SBP (mm Hg)*		DBP (mm Hg)*
Normal	<120 mm Hg	and	<80 mm Hg
Elevated	120-129 mm Hg	and	<80 mm Hg
Hypertension			
Stage 1	130-139 mm Hg	or	80-89 mm Hg
Stage 2	>130-139 mm Hg	or	>90 mm Hg

SBP, Systolic blood pressure; *DBP*, Diastolic blood pressure.

*Individuals with SBP and DBP in 2 categories should be designated to the higher blood pressure category. Blood pressure is based on an average of ≥2 careful readings obtained on ≥2 occasions.

Whelton PK, et al: 2017 ACC/AHA/AAPA/ABC/ACPM/APhA/ASH/ASPC/NMA/PCNA guideline for the prevention, detection, evaluation and management of high blood pressure in adults. *J Am Coll Cardiol* 71: e127-e240, 2018.

pressure and stage 1 hypertension without clinical ASCVD or estimated 10-year ASCVD risk of ≤10% (see http://tools.acc.org/ASCVD-Risk-Estimator-Plus/#!/calculate/estimate/). For adults with stage 1 hypertension with clinical ASCVD or estimated 10-year risk of ASCVD ≥10% or stage 2 hypertension, the ACC/AHA guidelines recommends blood pressure–lowering medication in combination with nonpharmacotherapy for primary prevention of CVD. The guidelines also call for individuals with diabetes, HF, and chronic kidney disease to be treated with blood pressure–lowering medication when their blood pressure exceeds 130/80 mm Hg. The recommendations are based on clinical evidence showing that stricter guidelines for these patients may prevent acceleration of target organ damage (kidney, heart, and pancreas) and related comorbidities. Importantly, the guidelines emphasize that people with high blood pressure should follow a healthy diet and lifestyle along with medication management. Diet and lifestyle modifications are important parts of primary prevention of hypertension.

Hypertension is a common public health problem in developed countries. In the United States one in three adults has high blood pressure (CDC, 2017). Untreated hypertension leads to many degenerative diseases, including HF, end-stage renal disease, and peripheral vascular disease. It is often called a "silent killer" because people with hypertension can be asymptomatic for years and then have a fatal stroke or heart attack. Although no cure is available, hypertension is easily detected and usually controllable. Some of the decline in CVD mortality during the last two decades has been attributed to the increased detection and control of hypertension. The emphasis on lifestyle modifications has given diet a prominent role in the primary prevention and management of hypertension.

Of those persons with high blood pressure, 90% to 95% have essential hypertension (hypertension of unknown cause) or primary hypertension. The cause involves a complex interaction between poor lifestyle choices and gene expression. Lifestyle factors that have been implicated include poor diet (i.e., high sodium, low fruit and vegetable intake), smoking, physical inactivity, stress, and obesity. Vascular inflammation has also been implicated (De Miguel et al, 2015). Many genes play a role in hypertension; most relate to the renal or neuroendocrine control of blood pressure. Genome-wide association studies have revealed more than 100 variants associated with blood pressure, although cumulatively these explain only a small percent of blood

pressure variability (Seidel and Scholl, 2017). The majority of the genetic contributors to blood pressure regulation are currently unknown (see Chapter 6). Hypertension that arises as the result of another disease, usually endocrine, is referred to as secondary hypertension. Depending on the extent of the underlying disease, secondary hypertension can be cured.

Prevalence and Incidence

Approximately 85.7 million American adults age 20 and older have hypertension or are taking antihypertensive medication (Benjamin et al, 2018). Projections show that by 2030, prevalence of hypertension will increase by 8.4% from 2013 estimates. Non-Hispanic black adults have a higher age-adjusted prevalence of hypertension (45.0% of men; 46.3% of women) than non-Hispanic whites (34.5% of men; 32.3% of women) and Mexican Americans (30.1% of men; 28.8% of women) (Benjamin et al, 2018). The prevalence of high blood pressure in blacks is one of the highest rates seen anywhere in the world. Because blacks develop hypertension earlier in life and maintain higher blood pressure levels, their risk of fatal stroke, heart disease, or end-stage kidney disease is higher than whites (Benjamin et al, 2018).

A person of any age can have hypertension. Approximately 12.9% of boys and 6.5% of girls have elevated blood pressure (Ma et al, 2016; Xi et al, 2016). With aging, the prevalence of high blood pressure increases (Fig. 32.7). Before the age of 45 more men than women have high blood pressure, and after age 65 the rates of high blood pressure among women in each racial group surpass those of the men in their group (Go et al, 2014). Because the prevalence of hypertension rises with increasing age, more than half the older adult population (more than 65 years of age) in any racial group has hypertension. Although lifestyle interventions targeted to older persons may reduce the prevalence of hypertension, early intervention programs provide the greatest long-term potential for reducing overall blood pressure-related complications (Whelton et al, 2018).

The relationship between blood pressure and risk of CVD events is continuous and independent of other risk factors. The higher the blood pressure, the greater is the chance of target organ damage, including left ventricular hypertrophy (LVH), HF, stroke, chronic kidney disease, and retinopathy (Benjamin et al, 2018). As many as 13% of adults with hypertension have treatment-resistant hypertension, which means that their blood pressure remains high despite the

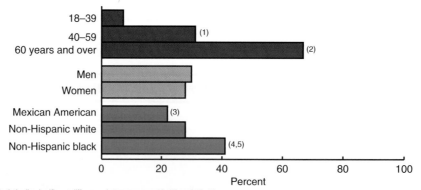

[1]Statistically significant difference between ages 18–39 and 40–59 years.
[2]Statistically significant difference between ages 40–59 and 60 years and over.
[3]Statistically significant difference between the non-Hispanic white and Mexican-American populations.
[4]Statistically significant difference between the non-Hispanic white and non-Hispanic black populations.
[5]Statistically significant difference between the non-Hispanic black and Mexican-American populations.
SOURCE: CDC/NCHS, National Health and Nutrition Examination Survey.

Fig. 32.7 Age-specific and age-adjusted prevalence of hypertension in adults: United States, 2005 to 2006. (Ostchega Y, et al: *Hypertension awareness, treatment, and control—continued disparities in adults: United States, 2005-2006.* NCHS data brief no. 3, Hyattsville, Md, 2008, National Center for Health Statistics.)

use of three or more antihypertensive drugs from different classes (Whelton et al, 2018). Treatment-resistant hypertension puts an individual at greater risk of target organ damage. Older age and obesity are two of the strongest risk factors associated with the condition. Identification and reversal of lifestyle factors contributing to treatment resistance, along with diagnosis and appropriate treatment of secondary causes and use of effective multidrug regimens, are essential treatment strategies.

The prevalence of hypertension among adults with diabetes is 80% and hypertension is at least twice as common among persons with type 2 diabetes as persons of the same age without diabetes (Whelton et al, 2018). Adults with diabetes have CVD death rates two to four times higher than adults without diabetes (Benjamin et al, 2018). Consequently, national health organizations, including the ACC/AHA, have set the target blood pressure goal for antihypertensive therapy for individuals with diabetes lower than that recommended for the general population, which is 140/90 mm Hg (Whelton et al, 2018). In adults with diabetes and hypertension, the ACC/AHA recommends antihypertensive drug treatment to be initiated at a blood pressure of 130/80 mm Hg or higher with a treatment goal of less than 130/80 mm Hg. Blood pressure control is often more difficult to achieve in patients with diabetes than in those without diabetes, necessitating use of a combination of blood pressure–lowering medications in the majority of patients (Whelton et al, 2018).

Although hypertensive patients are often asymptomatic, hypertension is not a benign disease. Cardiac, cerebrovascular, and renal systems are affected by chronically elevated blood pressure (Table 32.2). High blood pressure was the primary or a contributory cause in 427,631 of the 2.7 million U.S. deaths in 2009 (Benjamin et al, 2018). Between 2005 and 2015 the age-adjusted death rate from hypertension increased by 10.5%; overall deaths from hypertension increased by 37.5%. Death rates from hypertension are approximately three times higher in blacks than in whites (Benjamin et al, 2018). Hypertension is a major contributing factor to atherosclerosis, stroke, renal failure, and MI. Factors associated with a poor prognosis in hypertension are shown in Box 32.6.

Pathophysiology

Blood pressure is a function of cardiac output multiplied by peripheral resistance (the resistance in the blood vessels to the flow of blood). Thus the diameter of the blood vessel markedly affects blood flow. When the diameter is decreased (as in atherosclerosis) resistance and blood pressure increase. Conversely, when the diameter is increased (as with vasodilator drug therapy), resistance decreases and blood pressure is lowered.

Many systems maintain homeostatic control of blood pressure. The major regulators are the SNS for short-term control and the kidney for long-term control. In response to a fall in blood pressure, the SNS secretes norepinephrine, a vasoconstrictor, which acts on small arteries and arterioles to increase peripheral resistance and raise blood pressure. Conditions that result in overstimulation of the SNS (i.e., certain adrenal disorders or sleep apnea) result in increased blood pressure. The kidney regulates blood pressure by controlling the extracellular fluid volume and secreting renin, which activates the renin-angiotensin system (RAS) (Fig. 32.8). Abnormal blood pressure is usually multifactorial. In most cases of hypertension, peripheral resistance increases. This resistance forces the left ventricle of the heart to increase its effort in pumping blood through the system. With time, LVH and eventually HF can develop.

Common genetic variants of the RAS gene, including angiotensin-converting enzyme (ACE) and angiotensinogen, have shown relationships with hypertension (Heidari et al, 2017). An increased production

TABLE 32.2 Manifestations of Target Organ Disease from Hypertension

Organ System	Manifestations
Cardiac	Clinical, electrocardiographic, or radiologic evidence of arterial wall thickening left ventricular hypertrophy; left ventricular malfunction or cardiac failure
Cerebrovascular	Transient ischemic attack or stroke
Peripheral	Absence of one or more pulses in extremities (except for dorsalis pedis) Ankle-Brachial Index <0.9
Renal	Serum creatinine elevated: men 1.3-1.5 mg/dL, women 1.2-1.4 mg/dL Calculated GFR <60 mL/min/1.73 m² Elevated albumin excretion
Retinopathy	Hemorrhages or exudates, with or without papilledema

GFR, Glomerular filtration rate.
Adapted from Schmieder R: End organ damage in hypertension, *Dtsch Arztebl* 107:866, 2010.

BOX 32.6 Risk Factors and Adverse Prognosis in Hypertension

Risk Factors
Black race
Youth
Male gender
Persistent diastolic pressure >115 mm Hg
Smoking
Diabetes mellitus
Hypercholesterolemia
Obesity
Excessive alcohol intake
Evidence of end organ damage

Cardiac
Cardiac enlargement
Electrocardiographic signs of ischemia or left ventricular strain
Myocardial infarction
Heart failure

Eyes
Retinal exudates and hemorrhages
Papilledema

Renal
Impaired renal function

Nervous system
Cerebrovascular accident

From Fisher ND, Williams GH: Hypertensive vascular disease. In Kasper DL, et al, editors: *Harrison's principles of internal medicine*, ed 16, New York, 2005, McGraw-Hill.

of these proteins may increase production of angiotensin II, the primary mediator of the RAS, thus increasing blood pressure. Angiotensin II may also trigger low-grade inflammation within the blood vessel wall, a condition that predisposes to hypertension (McMaster et al, 2015).

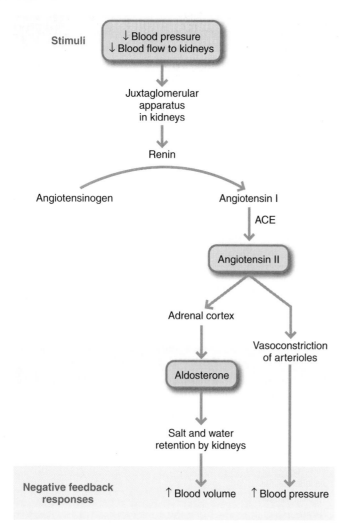

Stimuli — ↓ Blood pressure / ↓ Blood flow to kidneys

Juxtaglomerular apparatus in kidneys

Renin

Angiotensinogen

Angiotensin I

ACE

Angiotensin II

Adrenal cortex

Vasoconstriction of arterioles

Aldosterone

Salt and water retention by kidneys

Negative feedback responses — ↑ Blood volume   ↑ Blood pressure

Fig. 32.8 Renin-angiotensin cascade. *ACE,* Angiotensin-converting enzyme. (Reprinted with permission from Fox SI: *Human physiology,* ed 6, New York, 1999, McGraw-Hill.)

Hypertension often occurs with other risk factors for CVD, including visceral (intraabdominal) obesity, insulin resistance, high triglycerides, and low HDL cholesterol levels. The coexistence of three or more of these risk factors leads to metabolic syndrome. It is unclear whether one or more of these risk factors precede the others or whether they occur simultaneously. Accumulation of visceral fat synthesizes increased amounts of angiotensinogen, which activates the RAS and increases blood pressure (Zhou et al, 2012). Also, angiotensin II, the primary mediator of the RAS, promotes the development of large dysfunctional adipocytes, which produce increased amounts of leptin and reduced quantities of adiponectin. Higher levels of leptin and lower amounts of circulating adiponectin activate the SNS, a key component of the hypertensive response (DeMarco et al, 2014).

Primary Prevention

Positive changes in hypertension awareness, treatment, and control have occurred during the last several years. Based on analysis of National Health and Nutrition Examination Survey (NHANES) data from 2011 to 2014, 84.1% of people with hypertension are aware that they have it (Benjamin et al, 2018), up from 81% in 2007 to 2010. Although current hypertension treatment and control rates have increased from 48.4% to 53.3%, during this same time period, additional

efforts are needed to meet the *Healthy People 2020* objective of 61.2%. In 2015 women, younger adults (aged 18 to 39 years), and Hispanic individuals had lower rates of blood pressure control compared with men, younger individuals, and non-Hispanic whites. Improving hypertension treatment through targeted intervention programs should have a positive effect on CVD outcomes. Blood pressure treatment guidelines highlight the importance of evaluating patients for the presence of multiple CVD risk factors and individualizing lifestyle modification and drug therapies accordingly.

Changing lifestyle factors have documented efficacy in the primary prevention and control of hypertension. These factors were systematically reviewed and categorized by the Academy of Nutrition and Dietetics (AND) in 2015 (Lennon et al, 2017) and more recently by the ACC and AHA in 2018 (Whelton et al, 2018). These guidelines made a strong recommendation (i.e., high benefit/risk ratio with supporting evidence) for reducing intake of dietary sodium in adults with elevated blood pressure and hypertension and for weight loss in adults with elevated blood pressure or hypertension who are overweight or obese. A strong recommendation was also made for a heart-healthy dietary pattern such as the DASH diet rich in fruits, vegetables, whole grains, and low-fat dairy to lower blood pressure. Combining a low-sodium DASH diet with weight reduction was recommended as the most efficacious approach to substantially lowering blood pressure in adults at high CVD risk. Additional strong recommendations from both the ACC/AHA and the AND were made for increasing physical activity with a structured exercise program and for moderating alcohol consumption, particularly among heavy drinkers. The ACC/AHA also included a strong recommendation for supplementation with potassium to lower blood pressure. Increased potassium intake should preferably be in the form of diet modification and may be contraindicated for some patients with CKD. A summary of recommendations and ratings from the ACC/AHA and the AND can be found in Table 32.3.

Fats

Systematic reviews of RCTs that examined the effects of replacing calories from one fatty acid class with another have generally shown no or only a small effect on blood pressure (Al-Khudairy et al, 2015; Maki et al, 2018). Supplementation with n-3 PUFAs (EPA + DHA) in doses higher than 2 g/day showed modest reductions in SBP and DBP, especially in untreated hypertensive adults (Miller et al, 2014).

Protein

Evidence from observational studies and RCTs suggests replacement of protein for fat or carbohydrate in an isocaloric diet results in lowered blood pressure (Bazzano et al, 2013). Protein supplementation in doses of 60 g/day reduced SBP by 4.9 mm Hg and DBP by 2.7 mm Hg compared with 60 g/day of carbohydrate in overweight individuals with elevated blood pressure and untreated stage 1 hypertension (Teunissen-Beekman and van Baak, 2013).

Dietary Patterns Emphasizing Fruits and Vegetables

Several dietary patterns have been shown to lower blood pressure. Plant-based dietary patterns have been associated with lower SBP in observational studies and clinical trials (Alexander et al, 2017). Average SBP reductions of 5 to 6 mm Hg have been reported. Specifically, the Dietary Approaches to Stop Hypertension (DASH) controlled feeding study showed that a dietary pattern emphasizing fruits, vegetables, low-fat dairy products, whole grains, lean meats, and nuts significantly decreased SBP in hypertensive and normotensive adults. The DASH diet (see Appendix 17) was found to be more effective than just adding fruits and vegetables to a low-fat dietary pattern and was equally effective in men and women of diverse racial and ethnic backgrounds

TABLE 32.3 Recommendations on Blood Pressure in Hypertensive Adults from Evidence Analysis Library (2015) and American College of Cardiology/American Heart Association (2018)

Food or Nutrient	EAL Recommendation	Rating	ACC/AHA Recommendation	Rating
Sodium	The RDN should counsel on reducing sodium intake for blood pressure reduction in adults with HTN. Lowering dietary sodium intake to 1500-2000 mg/day reduced SBP and DBP up to 12 and 6 mm Hg, respectively.	Strong	Lower sodium intake Consume no more than 2400 mg of sodium/day; further reduction of sodium to 1500 mg/day is desirable because it is associated with even greater reduction in blood pressure; reduce intake by at least 1000 mg/day because that will lower blood pressure, even if the desired daily sodium intake is not achieved.	Strong Moderate
Dietary patterns emphasizing fruits and vegetables	The RDN should counsel on a DASH dietary pattern plus reduced sodium intake for blood pressure reduction.	Consensus	Consume a dietary pattern that emphasizes intake of vegetables, fruits, and whole grains; includes low-fat dairy products, poultry, fish, legumes, nontropical vegetable oils and nuts; and limits intake of sweets, sugar-sweetened beverages, and red meat; adapt the pattern to appropriate calorie requirements; achieve this pattern by following plans such as DASH, USDA food pattern, or the AHA Diet; combine the DASH dietary pattern with lower sodium intake.	Strong
Fruits and vegetables	Fruits and vegetables should be recommended at a level of 5 to 10 servings per day for significant blood pressure reduction.	Strong		Not evaluated
Weight management	Optimal body weight should be achieved and maintained (BMI 18.5-24.9) to reduce blood pressure.	Strong	Counsel overweight and obese adults with high blood pressure that lifestyle changes that produce even modest, sustained weight loss of 3% to 5% produce clinically meaningful benefits (e.g., reduce TG, blood sugar, Hb A1C); >5% will reduce blood pressure and reduce the need for medications to control blood pressure.*	Strong
Physical activity	Individuals should be encouraged to engage in aerobic physical activity for at least 30 minutes per day on most days of the week, because it reduces SBP.	Consensus	Advise adults to engage in aerobic physical activity to lower blood pressure: three to four sessions a week, lasting on average 40 minutes per session, and involving moderate-to-vigorous-intensity physical activity.	Moderate
Alcohol	For individuals who can safely consume alcohol, consumption should be limited to no more than two drinks (24 oz beer, 10 oz wine, or 3 oz of 80-proof liquor) per day in most men and to no more than one drink per day in women.	Consensus		Not evaluated
Potassium	Studies support a modest relationship between increasing intake of potassium and a lower sodium-potassium ratio with lowered blood pressure.	Fair	Insufficient evidence	Low
Calcium	The effect of increasing calcium intake with lowered blood pressure is unclear; although some research indicates minimal benefit.	Fair		Not evaluated
Magnesium	The effect of increasing magnesium intake with lowered blood pressure is unknown; although some research indicates minimal benefit.	Fair		Not evaluated
Omega-3 fatty acids	Studies investigating increased consumption of omega-3 fatty acids have not demonstrated a beneficial effect on blood pressure.	Fair		Not evaluated

ACC, American College of Cardiology; *AHA*, American Heart Association; *BMI*, body mass index; *DASH*, Dietary Approaches to Stop Hypertension; *DBP*, diastolic blood pressure; *Hb A1C*, hemoglobin A1C; *HTN*, hypertension; *RDN*, registered dietitian nutritionist; *SBP*, systolic blood pressure; *TG*, triglyceride; *USDA*, U.S. Department of Agriculture.

Recommendations listed are for those rated by the Academy of Nutrition and Dietetics and the American Academy of Cardiology (ACC)/American Heart Association (AHA) as strong, fair/moderate, and consensus; for those with weak ratings consult the American Dietetic Association Evidence Analysis Library for Hypertension (2009) http://www.adaevidencelibrary.com/topic.cfm?cat=3259 or the ACC/AHA data supplement at http://circ.ahajournals.org/lookup/suppl/doi:10.1161/01.cir.0000437740.48606.d1/-DC1

*Weight management guidelines are from Jensen MD, et al: 2013 AHA/ACC/TOS guideline for the management of overweight and obesity in adults: a report of the American College of Cardiology/American Heart Association Task Force on Practice Guidelines, and the Obesity Society, *J Am Coll Cardiol* 63:2985, 2014.

(Appel et al, 2006). This dietary pattern serves as the core for the ACC/AHA dietary recommendations for lowering blood pressure (Whelton et al, 2018). Although the DASH diet is safe and currently advocated for preventing and treating hypertension, the diet is high in potassium, phosphorus, and protein, depending on how it is planned. For this reason the DASH diet may not be advisable for individuals with end-stage renal disease with high-normal or elevated serum potassium and phosphorus levels (Tyson et al, 2012).

Several versions of the DASH diet have been examined in regard to blood pressure–lowering potential. The OmniHeart trial compared the original DASH diet to a high-protein version of the DASH diet (25% of energy from protein, approximately half from plant sources), and a DASH diet high in unsaturated fat (31% of calories from unsaturated fat, mostly monounsaturated). Although each diet lowered SBP, substituting some of the carbohydrate (approximately 10% of total calories) in the DASH diet with either protein or monounsaturated fat achieved the best reduction in blood pressure and blood cholesterol (Miller et al, 2006). This could be achieved by substituting nuts for some of the fruit, bread, or cereal servings.

Because many hypertensive patients are overweight, hypocaloric versions of the DASH diet also have been tested for efficacy in promoting weight loss and blood pressure reduction. A hypocaloric DASH diet versus a low-calorie, low-fat diet produced a greater reduction in SBP and DBP. More recently, the ENCORE study showed that the addition of exercise and weight loss to the DASH diet resulted in greater blood pressure reductions, greater improvements in vascular function, and reduction in left ventricular mass compared with the DASH diet alone (Lee et al, 2018).

The MeD dietary pattern has many similarities to the DASH diet but is generally higher in fat, primarily MUFA from olive oil, nuts, and seeds. A traditional MeD diet also contains fatty fish rich in omega-3 fatty acids. A systematic review of the MeD diet and CVD risk factors, found that although limited, evidence from RCTs was suggestive of a blood pressure–lowering effect of this style dietary pattern in adults with hypertension (Rees et al, 2013). According to the ACC/AHA, more studies on diverse populations are warranted before recommendations can be made related to the MeD diet for use in blood pressure management (Whelton et al, 2018).

Weight Reduction

There is a strong association between BMI and hypertension among men and women in all race or ethnic groups and in most age groups. It is estimated that at least 75% of the incidence of hypertension is related directly to obesity (Benjamin et al, 2018). Weight gain during adult life is responsible for much of the rise in blood pressure seen with aging.

Some of the physiologic changes proposed to explain the relationship between excess body fat and blood pressure are overactivation of the SNS and RAS and vascular inflammation (Hall et al, 2015). Visceral fat in particular promotes vascular inflammation by inducing cytokine release, proinflammatory transcription factors, and adhesion molecules (Hall et al, 2015). Low-grade inflammation occurs in the vasculature of individuals with elevated blood pressure; whether it precedes the onset of hypertension is unclear. Weight loss, exercise, and a MeD-style diet are beneficial (see Appendix 23).

Virtually all clinical trials on weight reduction and blood pressure support the efficacy of weight loss on lowering blood pressure. Reductions in blood pressure can occur without attainment of desirable body weight in most participants. Larger blood pressure reductions are achieved in participants who lost more weight and were also taking antihypertensive medications. This latter finding suggests a possible synergistic effect between weight loss and drug therapy. Although

weight reduction and maintenance of a healthy body weight is a major effort, interventions to prevent weight gain are needed before midlife. In addition, BMI is recommended as a screening tool in adolescence for future health risk (Flynn et al, 2017).

Sodium

Evidence from a variety of studies supports lowering blood pressure and CVD risk by reducing dietary sodium. For example, in the Trials of Hypertension Prevention more than 2400 individuals with moderately elevated blood pressure were assigned randomly to either cut their sodium by 750 to 1000 mg per day or to follow general guidelines for healthy eating for 18 months to 4 years. In 10 to 15 years after the studies ended, individuals who cut their sodium experienced a 32% lower risk of heart attacks, strokes, or other cardiovascular events compared with the group that did not (Cook et al, 2014). A meta-analysis of 37 RCTs further supports the positive effects of sodium reduction on blood pressure and cardiovascular outcomes for normotensive and hypertensive individuals (Aburto et al, 2013).

The DASH sodium trials tested the effects of three different levels of sodium intake (1500 mg, 2400 mg, and 3300 mg/day) combined with either a typical U.S. diet or the DASH diet in persons with prehypertension or stage 1 hypertension (Appel et al, 2006). The lowest blood pressures were achieved by those eating the 1500-mg sodium level in the DASH diet. In the DASH diet and the typical American diet groups, the lower the sodium, the lower the blood pressure. Such data provide the basis for the 2018 ACC/AHA (Whelton et al, 2018) sodium guideline for most adults to aim for at least 1000 mg/day reduction in sodium and for adults with elevated blood pressure to reduce sodium to an optimal goal of <1500 mg/day. For those with normal blood pressure, the Dietary Guidelines for Americans recommend an intake of less than 2300 mg of sodium, the equivalent of 6 g of salt, each day (USDA, 2015). This goal is supported by the AND Practice Guidelines (Lennon et al, 2017) and other organizations.

There is agreement that some persons with hypertension show a greater decrease in their blood pressures in response to reduced sodium intake than others. The term salt-sensitive hypertension has been used to identify these individuals. Salt-resistant hypertension refers to individuals with hypertension whose blood pressures do not change significantly with lowered salt intakes. Salt sensitivity varies, with individuals having greater or lesser degrees of blood pressure reduction. In general, individuals who are more sensitive to the effects of salt and sodium tend to be individuals who are black, obese, and middle-aged or older, especially if they have diabetes, chronic kidney disease, or hypertension. Currently, there are no clinical tests methods for identifying the salt-sensitive individual from the salt-resistant individual.

Calcium and Vitamin D

Calcium potentiates vascular contraction and relaxation through modification of 1,25-dihydroxy vitamin D_3 and parathyroid hormone levels (Brozovich et al, 2016). Peptides derived from milk proteins, especially fermented milk products, may also function as ACEs, thereby lowering blood pressure (Fekete et al, 2016). The DASH trial found that 8-week consumption of a diet high in fruits, vegetables, and fiber; three servings of low-fat dairy products/day; and lower total and saturated fat could lower SBP by 5.5 mm Hg and DBP by 3 mm Hg further than the control diet. The fruit and vegetable diet without dairy foods resulted in blood pressure reductions approximately half that of the DASH diet. The AND practice guidelines recommend a diet rich in fruits, vegetables, and low-fat dairy products for the prevention and management of elevated blood pressure (Lennon et al, 2017). The DASH serving recommendation of 2 to 3 low-fat dairy foods per day would provide the minimum calcium intake ($\sim$ 800 mg) necessary to achieve a SBP lowering of 4 mm Hg and DBP of 2 mm Hg in adults with hypertension (Lennon et al, 2017).

Cross-sectional studies suggest lower 25-hydroxy vitamin D (25[OH] D) levels are associated with higher blood pressure levels (Fraser et al, 2010) and higher rates of incident hypertension (Kunutsor et al, 2013). Mechanistically, vitamin D has been shown to improve endothelial function, reduce RAS activity, and lower parathyroid hormone (PTH) levels. However, recent evidence suggests that supplementation with vitamin D is not effective as a blood pressure–lowering agent on its own and therefore is not recommended as an antihypertension agent (Qi, 2017).

Magnesium

Magnesium is a potent inhibitor of vascular smooth-muscle contraction and may play a role in blood pressure regulation as a vasodilator. High dietary magnesium often is correlated with lower blood pressure (Schutten et al, 2018). Trials of magnesium supplementation have shown decreases in SBP of 3 to 4 mm Hg and DBP of 2 to 3 mm Hg with greater dose-dependent effects at supplementation of at least 370 mg/day (Zhang et al, 2016). The DASH dietary pattern emphasizes foods rich in magnesium, including green leafy vegetables, nuts, and whole-grain breads and cereals. Overall food sources of magnesium rather than supplemental doses of the nutrient are encouraged to prevent or control hypertension (Lennon et al, 2017).

Potassium

Supplemental doses of potassium in the range of 235 to 4700 mg/day lower blood pressure approximately 1 to 4 mm Hg DBP and 3 to 6 mm Hg SBP (Poorolajal et al, 2017). The effects of potassium are greater in those with higher initial blood pressure, in blacks compared with whites, and in those with higher intakes of sodium. Higher potassium intake also is associated with a lower risk of stroke (Aburto et al, 2013). Although the mechanism by which potassium lowers blood pressure is uncertain, several potential explanations have been offered, including decreased vascular smooth muscle contraction by altering membrane potential or restoring endothelium-dependent vasodilation (Bazzano et al, 2013). Failure of the kidney to adapt to a diet lower in potassium has been linked to sodium-sensitive hypertension.

The large number of fruits and vegetables recommended in the DASH diet makes it easy to meet the dietary potassium recommendations—approximately 4.7 g/day (Lennon et al, 2017). In individuals with medical conditions that could impair potassium excretion (e.g., chronic renal failure, diabetes, and congestive HF), a lower potassium intake (less than 4.7 g/day) is appropriate to prevent hyperkalemia (see Appendix 44).

Physical Activity

Less active persons are 30% to 50% more likely to develop hypertension than their active counterparts. Despite the benefits of activity and exercise in reducing disease, many Americans remain inactive. The prevalence of adults not meeting the Federal Physical Activity Guidelines for Americans (2008) is as follows: Hispanics (54.3% men, 59% women), blacks (49.7% men, 65% women), and whites (44.8% men, 49.1% women) all have a high prevalence of sedentary lifestyles (Benjamin et al, 2018). Exercise is beneficial to blood pressure. Increasing the amount of aerobic or dynamic resistance physical activity to a minimum of 90 to 150 minutes per week is an important adjunct to other blood pressure–lowering strategies (Whelton et al, 2018).

Alcohol Consumption

Excessive alcohol consumption is responsible for 5% to 7% of the hypertension in the population (Lennon et al, 2017). A three drink per day amount (a total of 3 oz of alcohol) is the threshold for raising blood pressure and is associated with a 3-mm Hg rise in SBP. For preventing high blood pressure, alcohol intake should be limited to no more than two drinks per day (24 oz of beer, 10 oz of wine, or 2 oz of 80-proof whiskey) in men, and no more than one drink a day is recommended for lighter-weight men and for women.

Medical Management

The goal of hypertension management is to reduce morbidity and mortality from stroke, hypertension-associated heart disease, and renal disease. The three objectives for evaluating patients with hypertension are to (1) identify the possible causes, (2) assess the presence or absence of target organ disease and clinical CVD, and (3) identify other CVD risk factors that help guide treatment. The presence of risk factors and target organ damage determines treatment priority.

Lifestyle modifications are definitive therapy for some and adjunctive therapy for all persons with hypertension. Several months of compliant lifestyle modifications should be tried before drug therapy is initiated. An algorithm for treatment of hypertension is shown in Fig. 32.9. Even if lifestyle modifications cannot completely correct blood pressure, these approaches help increase the efficacy of pharmacologic agents and improve other CVD risk factors. Management of hypertension requires a lifelong commitment.

Pharmacologic therapy is necessary for many individuals with hypertension, especially if blood pressure remains elevated after 6 to 12 months of lifestyle changes. The blood pressure target for initiating pharmacologic treatment is 130/80 mm Hg in adults with diabetes or kidney disease. For adults with stage 1 hypertension with clinical AS-CVD or estimated 10-year risk of ASCVD ≥10% or stage 2 hypertension, the ACC/AHA guidelines recommends blood pressure–lowering medication in combination with nonpharmacotherapy for primary prevention of CVD. Recommended pharmacologic treatment includes thiazide-type diuretics, calcium channel blockers (CCBs), angiotensin-converting enzyme inhibitors (ACEIs), or angiotensin receptor blockers (ARBs). Thiazide-type diuretics and CCBs are recommended in black populations, including those with diabetes, because they have been shown to be more effective in improving CVD outcomes compared to other classes of medications (Whelton et al, 2018). All these drugs can affect nutrition status (see Appendix 13).

Diuretics lower blood pressure in some patients by promoting volume depletion and sodium loss. At high doses other water-soluble nutrients are also lost and may have to be supplemented. Thiazide diuretics increase urinary potassium excretion, especially in the presence of a high salt intake, thus leading to potassium loss and possible hypokalemia. Except in the case of a potassium-sparing diuretic such as spironolactone or triamterene, additional potassium usually is required. Grapefruits and grapefruit juice can affect the action of many CCBs and should not be consumed while taking the medication.

A number of medications either raise blood pressure or interfere with the effectiveness of antihypertensive drugs. These include oral contraceptives, steroids, nonsteroidal antiinflammatory drugs, nasal decongestants and other cold remedies, appetite suppressants, cyclosporine, tricyclic antidepressants, and monoamine-oxidase inhibitors (see Appendix 13).

In addition to standard, conventional medical care, more than ½ of Americans also use complementary approaches and this includes treatment of hypertension and other cardiovascular diseases. Table 32.4 lists some that are most common.

Medical Nutrition Therapy

The appropriate course of nutrition therapy for managing hypertension should be guided by data from a detailed nutrition assessment.

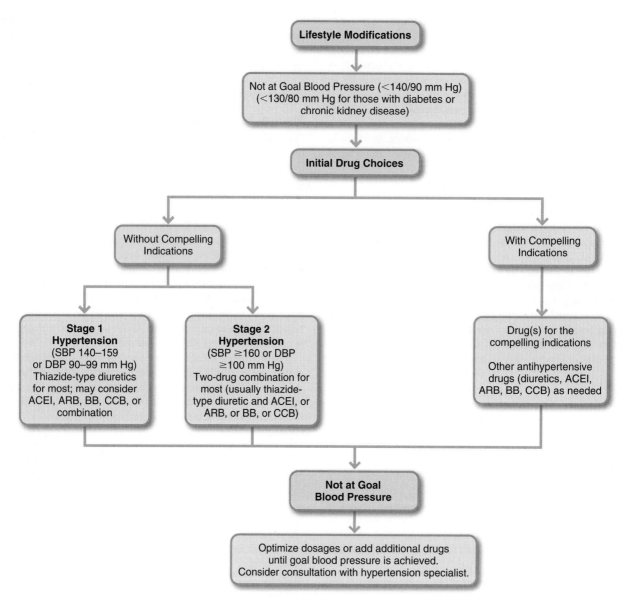

Fig. 32.9 Algorithm for treatment of hypertension. *ACEI*, Angiotensin-converting enzyme inhibitor; *ARB*, angiotensin-receptor blocker; *BB*, beta-blocker; *CCB*, calcium channel blocker; *DBP*, diastolic blood pressure; *SBP*, systolic blood pressure. (From National Institutes of Health, National Heart, Lung, and Blood Institute National High Blood Pressure Education Program: The seventh report of the Joint National Committee on prevention, detection, evaluation, and treatment of high blood pressure, NIH Publication No. 04-5230, August 2004.)

Weight history; leisure-time physical activity; and assessment of intake of sodium, alcohol, fat type (e.g., MUFA vs. SFA), and other dietary patterns (e.g., intake of fruits, vegetables, and low-fat dairy products) are essential components of the medical and diet history. Nutrition assessment should include evaluation of the individual in the following specific domains to determine nutrition problems and diagnoses: food and nutrient intake, knowledge, beliefs and attitudes, behavior, physical activity and function, and appropriate biochemical data. Following are the components of the current recommendations for managing elevated blood pressure.

Energy Intake

For each kilogram of weight lost, reductions in SBP and DBP of approximately 1 mm Hg are expected. Hypertensive patients who weigh more than 115% of ideal body weight should be placed on an individualized weight-reduction program that focuses on hypocaloric dietary intake and exercise (see Chapter 20). A modest caloric reduction is associated with a significant lowering of SBP and DBP, and LDL cholesterol levels. Hypocaloric diets that include a low-sodium DASH dietary pattern have produced more significant blood pressure reductions than low-calorie diets emphasizing only low-fat foods. Another benefit of weight loss on blood pressure is the synergistic effect with drug therapy. Weight loss should be an adjunct to drug therapy because it may decrease the dose or number of drugs necessary to control blood pressure.

DASH Diet

The DASH diet is used for preventing and controlling high blood pressure. Successful adoption of this diet requires many behavioral

TABLE 32.4 Complementary and Integrative Approaches for Cardiovascular Health

Common Name	Scientific Name	Effect on Cardiac Health	Side Effects and Risks
Coenzyme Q_{10}	Ubiquinone	Decreases SBP and DBP via a direct effect on the vascular endothelium and smooth muscle. May strengthen the heart muscle in heart failure.	May cause gastrointestinal discomfort, nausea, flatulence, and headaches
Vitamin C and vitamin E taken in combination as supplement	Ascorbic acid α-tocopherol	Decreases SBP and DBP, decreases arterial stiffness, and improves endothelial function by improving antioxidant status	Vitamin E may increase bleeding time with anticoagulants and reduce blood pressure. Vitamin C my cause diarrhea at high doses.
Vitamin D	1,25-dihydroxy vitamin D_3	Decreases SBP via suppression of renin expression and vascular smooth muscle cell proliferation	Hypercalcemia may occur depending on level of supplementation
Fish oil	Omega-3 polyunsaturated fatty acid	Therapeutic doses (2-3g EPA/DHA) lowers triglycerides. Lowers blood pressure by increasing endothelial vasodilatory response and may increase NO	May cause gastrointestinal discomfort, belching, bad breath, and increased bleeding time above 3g EPA/DHA
Garlic	*Allium sativum*	Reduces SBP and DBP in individuals with hypertension via vasodilation resulting from activation of potassium channels; may also be due to activation of NOS. Significantly lowers serum cholesterol.	May cause bad breath and body odor may increase bleeding time with anticoagulants
Resveratrol	Trans-3,4',5-trihydroxystilbene	Reduces systolic blood pressure in animals via enhanced NOS expression in the aorta	Unknown
Beet Extract	*Beta vulgaris*	Increases NO production and effective in reducing blood pressure	May have an additive effect when taken with antihypertensive medication
Hawthorn berry	*Crataegus oxycantha, Crataegus monogyna*	Exerts a mild, gradual blood pressure lowering effect; protective to the endothelium, antioxidant	May have an additive effect when taken with antihypertensive medication
Vitamin B3	Niacin	Lowers total cholesterol and raises HDL at doses above 1,000 mg/d	Causes flushing, itching and may raise liver enzymes. Coordination of care with a physician is necessary.
Hibiscus	*Hibiscus sabdariffa*	Lowers SBP in pre- and mildly hypertensive adults via calcium channel activation	May have an additive effect when taken with antihypertensive medication
Red Yeast Rice	*Monascus purpureus*	Contains a compound called Monakolin K that is identical to lovastatin. Lowers cholesterol.	Banned by the FDA in standardized quantities. May cause myalgias.
Plant sterols and stanols	β-sitosterol, campesterol, sitostanol and campestanol	Have been shown to lower cholesterol	none known

DBP, diastolic blood pressure; *NO*, nitric oxide; *NOS*, nitric oxide synthase; *SBP*, systolic blood pressure.
Data from Fragakis AS, Thomson C: *The health professional's guide to popular dietary supplements*, ed 3, Chicago, 2007, American Dietetic Association. © American Dietetic Association. Reprinted with permission. Natural Medicines [database on the Internet]. Somerville (MA): Therapeutic Research Center; publication year [December 10, 2019]. Available from: https://naturalmedicines.therapeuticresearch.com.

changes: eating twice the average number of daily servings of fruits, vegetables, and dairy products; limiting by one third the usual intake of beef, pork, and ham; eating half the typical amounts of fats, oils, and salad dressings; and eating one quarter the number of snacks and sweets. Lactose-intolerant persons may need to incorporate lactase enzyme or use other strategies to replace milk. Assessing patients' readiness to change and engaging patients in problem solving, decision making, and goal setting are behavioral strategies that may improve adherence.

The high number of fruits and vegetables consumed on the DASH diet is a marked change from typical patterns of Americans. To achieve the 8 to 10 servings, two to three fruits and vegetables should be consumed at each meal. Importantly, because the DASH diet is high in fiber, gradual increases in fruit, vegetables, and whole-grain foods should be made over time. Eight to 10 cups of fluids daily should be encouraged. Slow changes can reduce potential short-term gastrointestinal disturbances associated with a high-fiber diet, such as bloating and diarrhea. The DASH pattern is advocated in the 2017 ACC/AHA

nutrition guidelines on lifestyle management to reduce CVD risk (Whelton et al, 2018). Servings for different calorie levels are shown in Appendix 17.

Salt Restriction

The Dietary Guidelines for Americans recommend that young adults consume less than 2300 mg of sodium per day. This is also recommended for older people with hypertension (Whelton et al, 2018). Although further blood pressure improvements may be achieved by reducing sodium to 1500 mg/day (Appel et al, 2006), patients with HF should be cautioned against use of this dietary approach because adverse health effects of very-low-sodium diets in these patients have been reported (Institute of Medicine [IOM], 2013). Adherence to diets containing less than 2 g/day of sodium is very difficult to achieve.

In addition to advice on selection of minimally processed foods, dietary counseling should include instruction on reading food labels for sodium content, avoidance of discretionary salt in cooking or meal preparation (1 tsp salt = 2400 mg sodium), and use of alternative flavorings to satisfy individual taste. The DASH eating plan is rich in fruits and vegetables, which are naturally lower in sodium that many other foods.

Because most dietary salt comes from processed foods and eating out, changes in food preparation and processing can help patients reach the sodium goal. Sensory studies show that commercial processing could develop and revise recipes using lower sodium concentrations and reduce added sodium without affecting consumer acceptance. The food industry has made strides in reducing sodium in the American diet (see *Focus On:* Sodium and the Food Industry).

◎ FOCUS ON

Sodium and the Food Industry

Most foods sold in supermarkets and restaurants are high in salt. The dramatic differences in sodium from brand to brand suggest that many companies could easily achieve significant reductions without sacrificing taste. According to the Center for Science in the Public Interest (Liebman, 2014), processed foods and restaurant foods contribute approximately 80% of the sodium in Americans' diets: 10% comes from salt added during cooking at home or at the table and the remaining 10% is naturally occurring. Americans now consume approximately 3400 mg of sodium per day—1000 mg above the recommended amount. To help address this problem, in 2016, the Food and Drug Administration (FDA) issued draft guidance to the food industry on 2-year and 10-year voluntary sodium reduction targets for more than 150 foods, including snacks and frozen pizza. While not required, the proposed reduction targets would put significant public pressure on food manufacturers to reduce sodium in their products. The draft guidance triggered more than 200 written comments mostly from the leading food industry trade associations and food manufacturers. The majority of comments submitted to the FDA raised concerns about the challenges for the industry in reformulating food to lower sodium including consumer acceptance of reformulated products and concern with food safety and spoilage. In 2019 the FDA will issue the final guidance to food companies and restaurants on short-term sodium reduction targets. While some nutrition experts advocate for stronger action on the part of the FDA (mandatory sodium reduction), the guidelines still set a benchmark by which companies can be measured, something health advocates say is critical to lowering salt levels in the American diet.

Potassium-Calcium-Magnesium

Consuming a diet rich in potassium may lower blood pressure and blunt the effects of salt on blood pressure in some individuals (Appel et al, 2006). The recommended intake of potassium for adults is 4.7 g/day (IOM, 2004). Potassium-rich fruits and vegetables include leafy green vegetables, fruits, and root vegetables. Examples of such foods include oranges, beet greens, white beans, spinach, bananas, and sweet potatoes. Although meat, milk, and cereal products contain potassium, the potassium from these sources is not as well absorbed as that from fruits and vegetables (USDA, 2015).

Increased intakes of calcium and magnesium may have blood pressure benefits. Although there are not enough data to support a specific recommendation for increasing levels of magnesium intake, the AND EAL practice guidelines indicates that dietary calcium intakes of 800 mg or more may aid in blood pressure lowering (Lennon et al, 2017). The guidelines also recommend consideration of calcium supplementation of up to 1500 mg/day for adults with hypertension who are unable to achieve the dietary reference intake (DRI) of calcium with diet and

food alone. The DASH diet plan encourages foods that would be good sources of calcium and magnesium, including low-fat dairy products, dark green leafy vegetables, beans, and nuts (see Appendix 17).

Lipids

Current recommendations for lipid composition of the diet are recommended to help control weight and decrease the risk of CVD. Omega-3 fatty acids are not highlighted in blood pressure treatment guidelines (Lennon et al, 2017), although intakes of fish oils exceeding 2 g/day may have blood pressure benefits.

Alcohol

The diet history should contain information about alcohol consumption. Alcohol intake should be limited to no more than two drinks daily in men, which is equivalent to 2 oz of 80-proof whiskey, 10 oz of wine, or 24 oz of beer. Women or lighter-weight men should consume half this amount. Excessive alcohol consumption is associated with left ventricular function.

Exercise

Increasing the amount of aerobic or dynamic resistance physical activity to a minimum of 90 to 150 minutes per week is recommended as an adjunct therapy in hypertension management (Whelton et al, 2018). Because exercise is associated strongly with success in weight-reduction and weight-maintenance programs, any increase in activity level should be encouraged for those trying to lose weight. For substantial health benefits, the dietary guidelines recommends at least 150 minutes a week of moderate-intensity physical activity as well as muscle-strengthening activities that include all major muscle groups on 2 or more days for all Americans (USDA, 2015).

Treatment of Hypertension in Children and Adolescents

The prevalence of primary hypertension among children in the United States is increasing in concert with rising obesity rates and increased intakes of high-calorie, high-salt foods (Flynn et al, 2017). Hypertension tracks into adulthood and has been linked with carotid intimal-medial thickness, LVH, and fibrotic plaque formation. Secondary hypertension is more common in preadolescent children, mostly from renal disease; primary hypertension caused by obesity or a family history of hypertension is more common in adolescents (Miller and Joye Woodward, 2014). In addition, intrauterine growth retardation leads to hypertension in childhood (Longo et al, 2013).

High blood pressure in youth is based on a normative distribution of blood pressure in healthy children. Hypertension is defined as an SBP or DBP of greater than the 95th percentile for age, sex, and height. The designation for prehypertension in children is SBP or DBP of greater than the 90th percentile. Therapeutic lifestyle changes are recommended as an initial treatment strategy for children and adolescents with prehypertension or hypertension. These lifestyle modifications include regular physical activity, avoiding excess weight gain, limiting sodium, and consuming a DASH-type diet.

Weight reduction is considered the primary therapy for obesity-related hypertension in children and adolescents. Unfortunately, sustained weight loss is difficult to achieve in this age group. The Framingham Children's Study showed that children with higher intakes of fruits, vegetables (a combination of four or more servings per day), and dairy products (two or more servings per day) had lower SBP compared with those with lower intakes of these foods. Couch and colleagues (2008) showed that adolescents with prehypertension and hypertension could achieve a significant reduction in SBP in response to a behaviorally oriented nutrition intervention emphasizing the DASH diet. Because adherence to dietary interventions may be particularly challenging among children and teenagers, innovative nutrition intervention approaches that address the unique needs and circumstances of this age group are important considerations in intervention design (see Chapters 16 and 17).

Treatment of Blood Pressure in Older Adults

More than half of the older population has hypertension; this is not a normal consequence of aging. The lifestyle modifications discussed previously are the first step in treatment of older adults, as with younger populations. The Trial of Nonpharmacologic Interventions in the Elderly study found that losing weight (8 to 10 lb) and reducing sodium intake (to 1.8 g/day) can lessen or eliminate the need for drugs in obese, hypertensive older adults. Although losing weight and decreasing sodium in older adults are very effective in lowering blood pressure, knowing how to facilitate these changes and promote adherence remains a challenge for health professionals.

Blood pressure should be controlled regardless of age, initial blood pressure level, or duration of hypertension. Severe sodium restrictions

are not adopted because these could lead to volume depletion in older patients with renal damage. Drug treatment in the older adult is supported by very strong data. Additionally, the benefits of treating hypertensive persons age 65 years and older to reach a blood pressure goal of less than 130/80 mm Hg are well supported in the literature. For older adults with hypertension and a high burden of comorbidity and limited life expectancy, a team-based approach is recommended to assess risk/benefit for decisions regarding intensity of blood pressure–lowering and choice of pharmacotherapy (Whelton et al, 2018).

HEART FAILURE

Normally the heart pumps adequate blood to perfuse tissues and meet metabolic needs (Fig. 32.10). In heart failure (HF), formerly called congestive HF, the heart cannot provide adequate blood flow to the rest of the body, causing symptoms of fatigue, dyspnea (shortness of breath), and fluid retention. Diseases of the heart (valves, muscle,

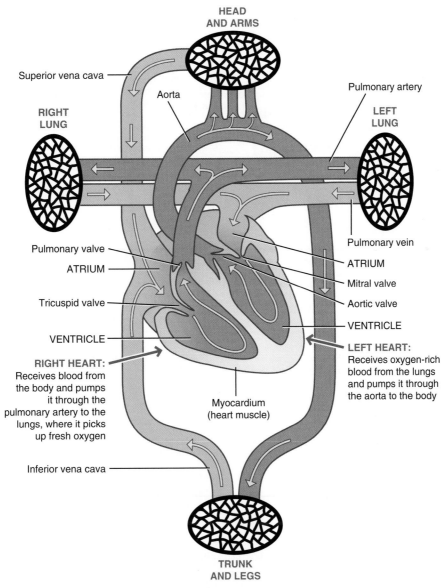

Fig. 32.10 Structure of the heart pump.

blood vessels) and vasculature can lead to HF (see *Pathophysiology and Care Management Algorithm: Heart Failure*). HF can be right-sided or left-sided or can affect both sides of the heart. It is further categorized as systolic failure when the heart cannot pump or eject blood efficiently out of the heart or diastolic failure, meaning the heart cannot fill with blood as it should.

The lifetime risk of developing HF is 20% for Americans age 40 or older. Approximately 5.1 million in the United States have HF. The incidence increases with age, rising from approximately 20 per 1000 individuals 65 to 69 years to greater than 80 per 1000 in those individuals 85 and older (Stone et al, 2014). Black men have been shown to be at the highest risk of HF; white women have the lowest. HF in non-Hispanic black males and females has a prevalence of 4.5% and 3.8% respectively, versus 2.7% and 1.8% in non-Hispanic white males and females, respectively (Stone et al, 2014).

Pathophysiology

The progression of HF is similar to that of atherosclerosis because there is an asymptomatic phase when damage is silently occurring (stages A and B) (Fig. 32.11). HF is initiated by damage or stress to the heart muscle either of acute MI or insidious (hemodynamic pressure or volume overloading) onset (see Table 32.5 for classifications of HF).

The progressive insult alters the function and shape of the left ventricle such that it hypertrophies in an effort to sustain blood flow, a process known as cardiac remodeling. Symptoms do not usually arise until months or years after cardiac remodeling begins. Many compensatory mechanisms from the SNS, RAS, and cytokine system are activated to restore homeostatic function. Proinflammatory cytokines, such as TNF-α, IL-1, and IL-6, are increased in blood and the myocardium and have been found to regulate cardiac remodeling.

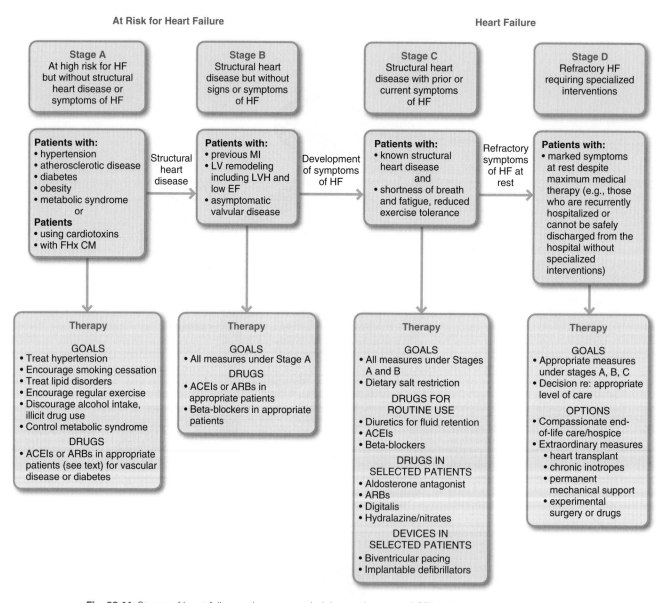

Fig. 32.11 Stages of heart failure and recommended therapy by stage. *ACEI,* Angiotensin-converting enzyme inhibitor; *ARB,* angiotensin receptor blocker; *CM,* cardiomyopathy; *EF,* ejection fraction; *FHx,* family history; *HF,* heart failure; *IV,* intravenous; *LV,* left ventricular; *LVH,* left ventricular hypertrophy; *MI,* myocardial infarction. (From Hunt SA, et al: ACC/AHA 2005 guideline update for the diagnosis and management of chronic heart failure in the adult: a report of the American College of Cardiology/American Heart Association Task Force, *J Am Coll Cardiol* 46:e1, 2005.)

PATHOPHYSIOLOGY AND CARE MANAGEMENT ALGORITHM

Heart Failure

ETIOLOGY

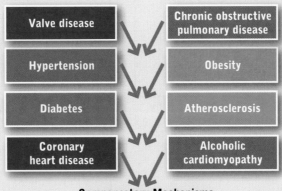

Valve disease	Chronic obstructive pulmonary disease
Hypertension	Obesity
Diabetes	Atherosclerosis
Coronary heart disease	Alcoholic cardiomyopathy

Compensatory Mechanisms
Sympathetic nervous system
Renin-angiotensin system
Cytokine system

Left Ventricular Hypertrophy or Hemodynamic Stress on a Diseased Heart

Dietary sodium excess
Medication noncompliance
Arrhythmias
Pulmonary embolism
Infection
Anemia

Heart Failure

PATHOPHYSIOLOGY

Clinical Findings

- Shortness of breath
- Fatigue
- Fluid retention
- Peripheral vasoconstriciton
- Elevated B-natriuretic peptide
- Mental confusion
- Memory loss
- Anxiety
- Insomnia
- Syncope and headache
- Dry cough

Nutrition Assessment

- Anorexia
- Nausea, abdominal pain, and feeling of fullness
- Constipation
- Malabsorption
- Malnutrition
- Cardiac cachexia
- Hypomagnesemia
- Hyponatremia

MANAGEMENT

Medical Management

- ACE inhibitors
- Angiotensin receptor blockers
- Aldosterone blockers
- β-blockers
- Digoxin
- Vasodilators
- Implantable defibrillator
- Heart transplant

Nutrition Management

- DASH diet
- Diet low in saturated fat, *trans* fat
- Restricted sodium diet—<3 gm/day
- Increased use of whole grains, fruits, vegetables
- Limit fluid to 2 L per day
- Lose to or maintain appropriate weight
- Magnesium supplementation
- Thiamin supplementation
- Increase physical activity as tolerated
- Avoid alcohol and tobacco

TABLE 32.5	**Classifications of Heart Failure**
Class I	No undue symptoms associated with ordinary activity and no limitation of physical activity
Class II	Slight limitation of physical activity; patient comfortable at rest
Class III	Marked limitation of physical activity; patient comfortable at rest
Class IV	Inability to carry out physical activity without discomfort; symptoms of cardiac insufficiency or chest pain at rest

Modified from Hunt SA, et al: ACC, AHA, 2005 guideline update for the diagnosis and management of chronic heart failure in the adult: a report of the American College of Cardiology/American Heart Association Task Force on practice guidelines, *J Am Coll Cardiol* 46:e1, 2005.

TABLE 32.6	**Skeletal Muscle Changes in Heart Failure**
Function loss	Weakness
	Fatigability
Structural	Loss of muscle mass
	Atrophy, fibrosis, no ≠ apoptosis
	Fiber type switch type I–type IIb
	Loss of mitochondria
	Endothelial damage
Blood flow	Capillary density ↓
	Vasodilation
	Peak leg blood flow ↓
Metabolism	Proteolysis
	Oxidative metabolism ↓ Acidosis glycolysis ≠
Inflammation	Cytokine and oxidative markers
Neuroendocrine	GH, IGF-1, epinephrine, norepinephrine, cortisol
Inactivity	TNF-α ≠ ≠
Genetic factors	Myostatin, IGF

GH, Growth hormone; *IGF*, insulin-like growth factor; *TNF-α*, tumor necrosis factor alpha.
From Strassburg S, et al: Muscle wasting in cardiac cachexia, *Int J Biochem Cell Biol* 37:1938, 2005.

Another substance, B-natriuretic peptide (BNP), is secreted by the ventricles in response to pressure and is predictive of the severity of HF and mortality at any level of BMI. BNP is often highly elevated in patients with HF (greater than 100 pg/mL is abnormal, and some patients have levels more than 3000 pg/mL). For every 100 pg/mL rise in BNP concentration, there is a corresponding 35% increase in the relative risk of death (Desai, 2013).

Eventually overuse of compensatory systems leads to further ventricle damage, remodeling, and worsening of symptoms (stage C). HF patients have elevated levels of norepinephrine, angiotensin II, aldosterone, endothelin, and vasopressin; all of these are neurohormonal factors that increase the hemodynamic stress on the ventricle by causing sodium retention and peripheral vasoconstriction. These neurohormones and the proinflammatory cytokines contribute to disease progression; hence, current studies focus on inhibition of these undesirable pathways and promotion of desirable ones.

For the final stages of HF, there is a subjective scale used to classify symptoms based on the degree of limitation in daily activities (Table 32.5). The severity of symptoms in this classification system is weakly related to the severity of left ventricular dysfunction; therefore treatment encompasses improving functional capacity and lessening progression of the underlying disease.

In HF the heart can compensate for poor cardiac output by (1) increasing the force of contraction, (2) increasing in size, (3) pumping more often, and (4) stimulating the kidneys to conserve sodium and water. For a time this compensation maintains near-normal circulation, but eventually the heart can no longer maintain a normal output (decompensation). Advanced symptoms can develop in weeks or months, and sudden death can occur at any time.

Three symptoms—fatigue, shortness of breath, and fluid retention—are the hallmarks of HF. Shortness of breath on exertion, or effort intolerance, is the earliest symptom. The shortness of breath known as orthopnea is breathlessness while lying down. Fluid retention can manifest as pulmonary congestion or peripheral edema. Evidence of hypoperfusion includes cool forearms and legs, sleepiness, declining serum sodium level caused by fluid overload, and worsening renal function.

Decreased cranial blood supply can lead to mental confusion, memory loss, anxiety, insomnia, syncope (loss of oxygen to the brain causing brief loss of consciousness), and headache. The latter symptoms are more common in older patients and often are the only symptoms; this can lead to a delay in diagnosis. Often the first symptom in older adults is a dry cough with generalized weakness and anorexia.

Cardiac cachexia is the end result of HF in 10% to 15% of patients. It is defined as involuntary weight loss of at least 6% of nonedematous body weight during a 6-month period (Springer et al, 2006). Unlike normal starvation, which is characterized by adipose tissue loss, this cachexia is characterized by a significant loss of lean body mass. This decrease in lean body mass further exacerbates HF because of the loss of cardiac muscle and the development of a heart that is soft and flabby. In addition, there are structural, circulatory, metabolic, inflammatory, and neuroendocrine changes in the skeletal muscle of patients with HF (Delano and Moldawer, 2006) (Table 32.6). Some changes in cardiac function can be attributed to aging and are listed in Box 32.7.

Cardiac cachexia is a serious complication of HF with a poor prognosis and mortality rate of 50% in 18 months (Carlson and

BOX 32.7	**Principal Effects of Aging on Cardiovascular Structure and Function**

Increased vascular stiffness
Increased myocardial stiffness
Decreased beta-adrenergic responsiveness
Impaired mitochondrial ATP production
Decreased baroreceptor responsiveness
Impaired sinus node function
Impaired endothelial function
Net effect: Marked reduction in cardiovascular reserve

ATP, Adenosine triphosphate.
From Rich MW: Office management of heart failure in the elderly, *Am Med* 118:342, 2005.

Dahlin, 2014). Symptoms that reflect inadequate blood supply to the abdominal organs include anorexia, nausea, a feeling of fullness, constipation, abdominal pain, malabsorption, hepatomegaly, and liver tenderness. All of these contribute to the high prevalence of malnutrition observed in hospitalized patients with HF. Lack of blood flow to the gut leads to loss of bowel integrity; bacteria and other endotoxins may enter the bloodstream and cause cytokine activation. Proinflammatory cytokines such as TNF-α and adiponectin are highest in patients with cardiac cachexia. An increased level of TNF-α is associated with a lower BMI, smaller skinfold measurements, and decreased plasma total protein levels, indicative of a catabolic state.

Adiponectin levels are high in HF and are a marker for wasting and a predictor of mortality. As with TNF-α, adiponectin levels also are correlated inversely with BMI. Pharmacologic treatments for muscle wasting are being explored.

Risk Factors

The Framingham Heart Study (see *Focus On:* Framingham Heart Study) showed the risk factors for HF were hypertension, diabetes, ASCVD, and left ventricular hypertrophy (LVH) (enlargement of the left ventricle of the heart). Antecedent hypertension is present in about three fourths of HF patients. Individuals who have diabetes mellitus and ischemic heart disease more frequently develop HF compared with patients without diabetes (Rosano et al, 2006). Left ventricular dysfunction without ischemia is often related to excessive alcohol intake. Diabetes is an especially strong risk factor for HF in women. The prevalence of hypertension and diabetes increases with age, making the elderly particularly vulnerable to HF. Another large cohort study of older adults (70 to 79 years old) showed that waist circumference and percentage of body fat were the strongest predictors of who would develop HF (Nicklas et al, 2006). A recent study of elderly individuals with HF found a strong association between vitamin D deficiency and HF risk (Porto, 2018). Data from the Multi-ethnic Study of Atherosclerosis (also known as MESA) concluded that high EPA blood levels were significantly inversely correlated with risk of HF (Block, 2019). Numerous changes in cardiovascular structure and function also place the elderly at high risk for developing HF (see Box 32.7).

Prevention

Because long-term survival rates for persons with HF are low, prevention is critical. HF is categorized into four stages ranging from persons with risk factors (stage A—primary prevention) to persons with advanced HF (stage D—severe disease). For stages A and B the aggressive treatment of underlying risk factors and diseases such as dyslipidemia, hypertension, and diabetes is critical to prevent structural damage to the myocardium and the appearance of HF symptoms. Such prevention has been very effective. Even patients who experience an MI can reduce the risk of HF with antihypertensive therapy. Patients are often asymptomatic during these two stages.

For stages C and D, secondary prevention strategies to prevent further cardiac dysfunction are warranted. These strategies include the use of ACE inhibitors (first line of therapy), ARBs, aldosterone blockers, beta-blockers, and digoxin. Early detection, correction of asymptomatic left ventricular dysfunction, and aggressive management of risk factors are needed to lower the incidence and mortality of HF.

Medical Management

Therapy recommendations correspond to the stage of HF. For patients at high risk of developing HF (stage A), treatment of the underlying conditions (hypertension, dyslipidemia, thyroid disorders, arrhythmias), avoidance of high-risk behaviors (tobacco, excessive alcohol, illicit drug use), and lifestyle changes (weight reduction, exercise, reduction of sodium intake, heart-healthy diet) are recommended. All these recommendations are carried through the other stages. In addition, an implantable defibrillator, which shocks the heart when it stops, can be placed in patients at risk of sudden death. Pharmacologic treatment of HF is the hallmark of therapy with progressive stages. The last stage also includes surgically implanted ventricular-assist devices, heart transplantation, and continual intravenous therapy.

The short-term goals for the treatment of HF are to relieve symptoms, improve the quality of life, and reduce depression if it is present. The long-term goal of treatment is to prolong life by lessening, stopping, or reversing left ventricular dysfunction. Medical management is tailored to clinical and hemodynamic profiles with evidence of hypoperfusion and congestion. In some cases, surgical procedures are needed to alleviate the HF caused by valvular disease; medical management is limited in these instances.

Standard fluid restrictions are to limit total fluid intake to 2 L (2000 mL) daily. When patients are severely decompensated, a more restrictive fluid intake (1000 to 1500 mL daily) may be warranted for adequate diuresis. A sodium-restricted diet should be maintained despite low-sodium blood levels because in this case the sodium has shifted from the blood to the tissues. Serum sodium appears low in a patient who is fluid overloaded because of dilution; diuresis improves the levels by decreasing the amount of water in the vascular space.

An ACE inhibitor is the first line of pharmacologic treatment for HF. As the stages progress, a beta-blocker or angiotensin receptor blocker may be added. In stages C and D selected patients also may take a diuretic, aldosterone antagonists, digitalis, and vasodilators (e.g., hydralazine). Basically these medications reduce excess fluid, dilate blood vessels, and increase the strength of the heart's contraction. Several of these medications have neurohormonal benefits along with their primary mechanism of action. For example, ACE inhibitors (e.g., captopril, enalapril) not only inhibit the RAS but also improve symptoms, quality of life, exercise tolerance, and survival. Similarly, spironolactone has diuretic and aldosterone-blocking functions that result in reduced morbidity and mortality in patients. Most of these medications can affect nutrition status (see Chapter 8).

Medical Nutrition Therapy

The RDN provides MNT, which includes assessment, a nutrition diagnosis, and interventions (education, counseling). As part of a multidisciplinary team (physician, pharmacist, psychologist, nurse, and social worker), the RDN positively affects patient outcomes. Reduced readmission to the hospital, fewer days in the hospital, improved compliance with restricted sodium and fluid intakes, and improved quality of life scores are the goals in HF patients.

Nutrition screening for HF in older adults can help prevent disease progression and improve disease management, overall health, and quality-of-life outcomes. The first step in screening is determination of body weight. Altered fluid balance complicates assessment of body weight in the patient with HF. Weights should be taken before eating and after voiding at the same time each day. A dry weight (weight without edema) should be determined on the scale at home. Patients should record daily weights and advise their care providers if weight gain exceeds more than 1 lb a day for patients with severe HF, more than 2 lb a day for patients with moderate HF, and more than 3 to 5 lb with mild HF. Restricting sodium and fluids along with diuretic therapy is recommended to restore fluid balance.

Dietary assessments in HF patients reveal that more than half have malnutrition, usually related to the cardiac cachexia mentioned earlier. Negative energy balance and negative nitrogen balances can be noted. In overweight patients, caloric reduction must be monitored carefully to avoid excessive and rapid body protein catabolism. Nutrition education to promote behavior change is a critical component of MNT. The benefits of MNT should be communicated to patients.

The total diet must be addressed in patients with HF because underlying risk factors are often present; dietary changes to modify these risk factors are an important component of MNT. For dyslipidemia or atherosclerosis, a heart-healthy diet low in SFAs, trans fatty acids, and cholesterol and high in fiber, whole grains, fruits, and vegetables is recommended. For persons with hypertension, the DASH diet is recommended. Both of these dietary patterns emphasize lower-sodium foods and higher intake of potassium. Total energy expenditure is higher in HF patients because of the catabolic state; adequate protein and energy should be provided (Academy of Nutrition and Dietetics, Evidence Analysis Library, 2017).

Salt Restriction

Excessive sodium intake is associated with fluid retention and edema. A 2-g sodium restriction is regularly prescribed for patients with HF. The AND (2012) EAL recommends a 2-g sodium restriction but notes

that the evidence for this recommendation is only "fair." The Heart Failure Society of America recommends 2 to 3 g of sodium daily unless severe symptoms are present, then the recommendation is for 2 g (Gupta et al, 2012). The updated AHA recommendation is for "moderate" sodium restriction. Table 32.7 summarizes the recommendations from multiple organizations. The inconsistencies in the different organizations are due to the weak database of studies. Many have small sample sizes and many were not randomized trials. Three of the larger studies that were randomized had consistent results but showed that sodium restriction was associated with worse outcome (Gupta et al, 2012). It is hypothesized that this effect may be related to neurohormones including aldosterone, norepinephrine, and angiotensin II, all of which increased with dietary restriction. These hormones act to conserve fluid, thus trying to restore blood flow. Aldosterone promotes sodium reabsorption, and vasopressin promotes water conservation in the distal tubules of the nephron. This complex balance is further complicated by the medications used for HF.

Patient compliance with sodium restriction of 2 g/day has been shown to be poor. This can lead to generally inadequate nutritional intake that may be a contributing factor to poor outcomes associated with sodium restriction. A one-size-fits-all sodium restriction is not possible. The HF stage, amount of edema present, overall nutritional status, and medications must be taken into consideration. There is consensus that high sodium intake (above 3 g/day) is contraindicated for HF.

The degree of restriction depends on the individual (see *Focus On: Sodium and Salt Measurement Equivalents*).

TABLE 32.7 Dietary Sodium Intake in Heart Failure

Guideline	Year	Sodium/Fluid Restriction Recommendations	Level of Evidence
National Heart Foundation of Australia/Cardiac Society of Australia and New Zealand	2006	<3 g/day for NYHA class II without peripheral edema/ <2 g/day for NYHA class III and IV	C
		<2 L/day for all patients and <1.5 L/day during fluid retention episodes	
Heart Failure Society, India	2007	<2 g/day	Not stated
		<2 L/day	
European Society of Cardiology	2008	Moderate restriction 1.5-2 L/day in patients with severe symptoms and especially with hyponatremia	C
Canadian Cardiovascular Society	2008	<2 g/day	Not stated
		2 L/day	
American College of Cardiology/ American Heart Association	2009	Moderate restriction (≤2 g/day if volume overload, followed by fluid intake restriction to 2 L/day if fluid retention persists)	C
Royal College of Physicians	2010	Salt reduction Fluid restriction	Limited; further research required
Heart Failure Society of America	2010	2-3 g/day; <2 g/day may be considered in moderate to severe heart failure	C
		<2 L/day, if fluid retention persists and if severe hyponatremia (serum Na <130 mEq/L) is present	
Scottish Intercollegiate Guidelines Network	2010	<2.4 g/day tailored fluid restriction	1+
American Dietetic Association	2011	<2 g/day 1.4-1.9 L/day depending on clinical symptoms	Fair

Level of Evidence: *C,* Limited populations evaluated. Only consensus opinion of experts, case studies, or standard of care; *Fair,* Benefits exceed the harms but quality of evidence is not as strong; *1+,* well-conducted meta-analysis, systemic reviews, or randomized controlled trials with low risk of bias.
NYHA, New York Heart Association.
From American Heart Association: *Contemporary reviews in cardiovascular medicine* (website). http://circ.ahajournals.org/content/126/4/479/T1.expansion.html, 2015.

⊚ FOCUS ON

Sodium and Salt Measurement Equivalents

Sodium chloride is approximately 40% (39.3%) sodium and 60% chloride. To convert a specified weight of sodium chloride to its sodium equivalent, multiply the weight by 0.393. Sodium also is measured in milliequivalents (mEq). To convert milligrams of sodium to mEq, divide by the atomic weight of 23. To convert sodium to sodium chloride (salt), multiply by 2.54. Millimoles (mmol) and milliequivalents (mEq) of sodium are the same. For example:

1 tsp of salt = approximately 6 g NaCl = 6096 mg NaCl
6096 mg NaCl × 0.393 = 2396 mg Na (approximately 2400 mg)
2396 mg Na/23 = 104 mEq Na
1 g Na = 1000 mg/23 = 43 mEq or mmol
1 tsp of salt = 2400 mg or 104 mEq Na

BOX 32.9 Food Labeling Guide for Sodium

Sodium-free	Less than 5 mg per standard serving; cannot contain any sodium chloride
Very low sodium	35 mg or less per standard serving
Low sodium	140 mg or less per standard serving
Reduced sodium	At least 25% less sodium per standard serving than in the regular food
Light in sodium	50% less sodium per standard serving than in the regular food
Unsalted, without added salt, or no salt added	No salt added during processing; the product it resembles is normally processed with salt
Lightly salted	50% less added sodium than is normally added; product must state "not a low-sodium food" if that criterion is not met

https://www.labelcalc.com/nutrient-content-claims/low-sodium-nutrition-label-guidelines-for-your-food-product/.

Adherence to sodium restrictions can be problematic for many individuals, and individualized instruction is recommended. Ethnic differences in sodium consumption must be considered. Some cultures have traditional diets that are very high in sodium such as Kosher and Asian diets. In some cases regional cooking, like in some areas in the southern United States, depends heavily on salt.

Positive outcomes (i.e., decreased urinary sodium excretion, less fatigue, less frequent edema) have been observed in HF patients receiving MNT. The type of sodium restriction prescribed should be the least restrictive diet that will achieve the desired results. The first step is to minimize or eliminate the use of table salt and high-sodium foods (Box 32.8) (see Appendix 46 for sodium content of foods).

Poor adherence to low-sodium diets occurs in part as a result of lack of knowledge about sodium and lower-sodium food choices by the patient, and perception that the diet interferes with the social aspects of eating. Lack of cooking skills or adequate cooking facilities is another obstacle because it leads patients to eat premade foods that tend to be high in salt. Memory loss, severe fatigue, and economic issues are all challenges to following a low-sodium diet. In addition, food labels, although informative, may be hard for many patients or their caregivers to comprehend (Box 32.9).

BOX 32.8 Top Ten Categories of High-Sodium Foods

1. Smoked, processed, or cured meats and fish (e.g., ham, bacon, corned beef, cold cuts, hot dogs, sausage, salt pork, chipped beef, pickled herring, anchovies, tuna, and sardines)
2. Tomato juices and tomato sauce, unless labeled otherwise
3. Meat extracts, bouillon cubes, meat sauces, MSG, and taco seasoning and other packaged seasonings
4. Salted snacks (potato chips, tortilla chips, corn chips, pretzels, salted nuts, popcorn, and crackers)
5. Prepared salad dressings, condiments, relishes, ketchup, Worcestershire sauce, barbecue sauce, cocktail sauce, teriyaki sauce, soy sauce, commercial salad dressings, salsa, pickles, olives, and sauerkraut
6. Packaged mixes for sauces, gravies, casseroles, and noodle, rice, or potato dishes; macaroni and cheese; stuffing mix
7. Cheeses (processed and cheese spreads)
8. Frozen entrees and pot pies
9. Canned soup
10. Foods eaten away from home

Note: Reading labels is most important; some brands are lower in sodium than others.
MSG, Monosodium glutamate.

Alcohol

In excess, alcohol contributes to fluid intake and raises blood pressure. Many cardiologists recommend avoiding alcohol. Chronic alcohol ingestion may lead to cardiomyopathy and HF (Mirijello, 2017). Although heavy drinking should be discouraged, there is no evidence to support total abstinence from alcohol (AND, 2012). Quantity, drinking patterns, and genetic factors influence the relationship between alcohol consumption and HF (Djoussé and Gaziano, 2008). If alcohol is consumed, intake should not exceed one drink per day for women and two drinks per day for men. A drink is equivalent to 1 oz of alcohol (1 oz of distilled liquor), 5 oz of wine, or 12 oz of beer.

Caffeine

Until recently caffeine has been considered detrimental to patients with HF because it contributes to irregular heartbeats. However, a study in the Netherlands suggests that moderate intake of either tea or coffee reduces ASCVD risk; tea actually reduces ASCVD deaths (de Koning Gans et al, 2010). Researchers in the United States followed 130,054 men and women and found that those who reported drinking four or more cups of coffee each day had an 18% lower risk of hospitalization for heart rhythm disturbances. Those who reported drinking one to three cups each day had a 7% reduction in risk (Klatsky, 2010). The antioxidant effects of coffee and tea may be beneficial. A recently published randomized trial concluded that a high dose of caffeine did not induce arrhythmias in patients with systolic HF (Zuchinali, 2016).

Calcium

Patients with HF are at increased risk of developing osteoporosis because of low activity levels, impaired renal function, and prescription drugs that alter calcium metabolism (Zittermann et al, 2006). Cachectic HF patients have lower bone mineral density and lower calcium levels than HF patients without cachexia (Anker et al, 2006). Caution must be used with calcium supplements because they have been shown to be associated with adverse outcomes (Drozd et al, 2014).

L-Arginine

In patients with HF, decreased exercise capacity may be in part due to reduced peripheral blood flow related to impairment of endothelium-dependent vasodilation. L-Arginine is converted to NO, an endothelium-derived relaxing factor. At least four studies have shown some benefit with supplementation. The studies were small, and more research is needed to establish clear recommendations.

Coenzyme Q₁₀

Some studies on the use of coenzyme Q_{10} (CoQ_{10}) supplementation in HF patients showed positive outcome. Outcomes included significantly improved exercise tolerance, decreased symptoms, and improved quality of life. CoQ_{10} levels are generally low in HF patients; it is postulated that repletion can prevent oxidative stress and further myocardial damage. A systematic review of 7 studies and over 900 patients on the use of CoQ_{10} in HF patients concluded that the studies were too small and too diverse in study design to draw any useful conclusions (Madmani et al, 2014). Patients on statins (HMG-CoA reductase inhibitors) may have a different reason to consider supplementation. HMG-CoA reductase inhibitors are a class of cholesterol-lowering drugs that are known to interfere with synthesis of CoQ_{10}.

D-Ribose

D-ribose is a component of adenosine triphosphate (ATP) for cellular metabolism and energy production. Myocardial ischemia lowers cellular energy levels, integrity, and function. The failing heart is energy starved. D-ribose is being tested to correct this deficient cellular energy as a naturally occurring carbohydrate (Shecterle et al, 2010). A recent prospective study that gave 6 weeks of D-ribose supplement was inconclusive in determining benefit (Bayram et al, 2015).

Energy

The energy needs of patients with HF depend on their current dry weight, activity restrictions, and the severity of the HF. Overweight patients with limited activity should be encouraged to maintain an appropriate weight that will not stress the myocardium. However, the nutrition status of the obese patient must be assessed to ensure that the patient is not malnourished. In patients with HF, energy needs are unclear. At least two studies found that standard energy equations used to determine calorie needs underestimated the needs of HF patients. Another study found lower calorie needs compared with healthy controls (AND, 2012). This area requires more research. Standard nutritional assessment should be employed with careful monitoring.

Fats

Fish consumption and fish oils rich in omega-3 fatty acids can lower elevated triglyceride levels and may prevent atrial fibrillation in HF patients (Roth and Harris, 2010). Intake of at least 1 g daily of omega-3 fatty acids from either oily fish or fish-oil supplements was used in the study. However, further studies are needed. Some evidence suggests that high saturated fat feeding in mild to moderate HF preserves contractile function and prevents the switch from fatty acid to glucose metabolism, thus serving a cardioprotective role (Chess et al, 2009; Christopher et al, 2010).

Meal Strategies

Patients with HF often tolerate small, frequent meals better than larger, infrequent meals because the latter are more tiring to consume, can contribute to abdominal distention, and markedly increase oxygen consumption. All these factors tax the already stressed heart. Caloric supplements can help to increase energy intake; however, this intervention may not reverse this form of malnutrition (Anker et al, 2006).

Folate, Vitamin B₆, and Vitamin B₁₂

High dietary intakes of folate and vitamin B_6 have been associated with reduced risk of mortality from HF and stroke in some populations (Cui et al, 2010). However, deficiencies of vitamin B_{12} and folate have been studied and found to be relatively rare in HF patients (van der Wal et al, 2015).

Magnesium

Magnesium deficiency is common in patients with HF as a result of poor dietary intake and the use of diuretics, including furosemide. As with potassium, the diuretics used to treat HF increase magnesium excretion. Magnesium deficiency aggravates changes in electrolyte concentration by causing a positive sodium and negative potassium balance. Because deficient magnesium status is associated with poorer prognosis, blood magnesium levels should be measured in HF patients and treated accordingly. Poor dietary intake of magnesium has been associated with elevated hs-CRP, a product of inflammation. Hypermagnesemia may be found in some cases of renal failure, HF, and high doses of furosemide.

Thiamin

Patients with HF are at risk for thiamin deficiency because of poor food intake; use of loop diuretics, which increases excretion; and advanced age. Thiamin is a required coenzyme in the energy-producing reactions that fuel myocardial contraction. Therefore thiamin deficiency can cause decreased energy and weaker heart contractions. Studies have shown thiamin deficiency to be associated with HF, in great part due to the effect of commonly used medications. Loop diuretics (e.g., furosemide) can deplete body thiamin and cause metabolic acidosis. Supplementation with thiamin has been shown to improve cardiac function, urine output, weight loss, and signs and symptoms of HF (DiNicolantonio et al, 2013). Thiamin deficiency is diagnosed using erythrocyte thiamin pyrophosphate. Thiamin status should be assessed in HF patients on loop diuretics and appropriate supplementation recommended if necessary. Thiamin supplementation (e.g., 100 mg/day) can improve left ventricular ejection fraction (fraction of blood pumped out of the ventricles with each heartbeat) and symptoms.

Vitamin D

Patients with a polymorphism of the vitamin D receptor gene have higher rates of bone loss than HF patients without this genotype. Vitamin D may improve inflammation in HF patients (Vieth and Kimball, 2006). In a double-blind, randomized, placebo-controlled trial, supplementation with vitamin D (50 mcg or 2000 international units of vitamin D_3 per day) for 9 months increased the antiinflammatory cytokine IL-10 and decreased the proinflammatory factors in HF patients (Schleithoff et al, 2006). As a steroid hormone, vitamin D regulates gene expression and inversely regulates renin secretion (Meems et al, 2011). With the recent study showing a relationship between vitamin D deficiency and the development of HF (Porto, 2018), the case for supplementation of vitamin D is now stronger.

CARDIAC TRANSPLANTATION

Cardiomyopathies represent a heterogeneous group of diseases that often lead to progressive HF; types include dilated cardiomyopathy, hypertrophic cardiomyopathy, restrictive cardiomyopathy, and arrhythmogenic right ventricular cardiomyopathy (Wexler et al, 2009). Cardiac transplantation is the only cure for refractory, end-stage HF. Because the number of donor hearts is limited, careful selection of recipients with consideration of the likelihood for adherence to lifelong therapeutic regimen and their quality of life is imperative. Nutrition support before and after transplantation is crucial to decrease morbidity and mortality. Thus the nutrition care of the heart transplant patient can be divided into three phases: pretransplant, immediate posttransplant, and long-term posttransplant.

Pretransplant Medical Nutrition Therapy

A comprehensive nutrition assessment of the pretransplant patient should include a history, physical and anthropometric assessment, and biochemical testing. Recommended lifestyle changes before transplantation include restricting alcohol consumption, losing weight, exercising, quitting smoking, and eating a low-sodium diet (Wexler et al, 2009). Extremes in body weight (less than 80% or more than 140% of ideal body weight) increase the patient's risk for infection, diabetes, morbidity, and higher mortality. Pretransplant comorbidities such as hyperlipidemia and hypertension also reduce survival rates. If oral intake is inadequate, an enteral feeding should be tailored to the nutritional and comorbid conditions of the patient.

Immediate Posttransplant Nutrition Support

Nutrition guidelines are consistent for all types of organ transplants and not specific just to heart transplants (Table 32.8). The nutritional goals in the acute posttransplant patient are to (1) provide adequate protein and calories to treat catabolism and promote healing, (2) monitor and correct electrolyte abnormalities, and (3) achieve optimal blood glucose control (Hasse, 2015). In the immediate posttransplant period nutrient needs are increased, as is the case after any major surgery. Protein needs are increased because of steroid-induced catabolism, surgical stress, anabolism, and wound healing.

Patients progress from clear liquids to a soft diet given in small, frequent feedings. Enteral feeding may be appropriate in the short term, especially if complications arise. Nutrient intake is often maintained by using liquid supplements and foods of high caloric density, especially in patients with poor appetite. Weight gain to an ideal weight is the nutritional goal for patients who were cachectic before transplant. The increase in cardiac function helps to halt the presurgical cachectic state. Hyperglycemia can be exacerbated by the stress of the surgery and the immunosuppressive drug regimen. Dietary adjustments can be made to aid in glucose control (see Table 32.8).

Long-Term Posttransplant Nutrition Support

Comorbid conditions that often occur after transplantation include hypertension, excessive weight gain, hyperlipidemia, osteoporosis, and infection. Hypertension is managed by diet, exercise, and medications. Minimizing excessive weight gain is important because patients who become obese after transplantation are at higher risk for rejection and lower rates of survival.

Increases in total LDL cholesterol and triglycerides are a consequence of immunosuppressive drug therapy and increase the risk of HF after transplantation. Along with a heart-healthy diet, patients also need a lipid-lowering drug regimen to normalize blood lipids. Statins are recommended in the early and long-term postoperative periods. Because of their LDL-lowering effect, stanols or sterols may be helpful to reduce statin dosages (Goldberg et al, 2006).

Before transplantation, patients are likely to have osteopenia because of their lack of activity and cardiac cachexia. After transplantation, patients are susceptible to steroid-induced osteoporosis. Patients require optimal calcium and vitamin D intake to slow bone loss; weight-bearing exercise and antiresorptive drug therapy are often necessary. Infection must be avoided because of the necessity of lifelong use of immunosuppressive drugs. Food safety should be discussed.

TABLE 32.8 Posttransplant Nutrient Recommendations

Nutrient	Short-Term Recommendations	Long-Term Recommendations
Calories	120%-140% of BEE (30-35 kcal/kg) or measure REE	Maintenance: 120%-130% BEE (20-30 kcal/kg) depending on activity level
Protein	1.3-2 g/kg/day	1 g/kg/day
Carbohydrate	~50% of calories Restrict simple sugars if glucose level elevated	~50% of calories Restrict simple sugars and encourage high-fiber complex carbohydrate choices
Fat	30% of calories (or higher with severe hyperglycemia)	≤30% of total calories <10% of calories as saturated fat
Calcium	1200 mg/day	1200-1500 mg/day (consider the need for estrogen or vitamin D supplements)
Sodium	2 g/day	2 g/day
Magnesium and phosphorus	Encourage intake of foods high in these nutrients Supplement as needed	Encourage intake of foods high in these nutrients Supplement as needed
Potassium	Supplement or restrict based on serum potassium levels	Supplement or restrict based on serum potassium levels
Other vitamins and minerals	Multivitamin/mineral—supplement to RDI levels May need additional supplements to replete suspected or confirmed deficiencies	Multivitamin/mineral—supplement to RDI levels May need additional supplements to replete suspected or confirmed deficiencies
Other	Avoid complementary or alternative products without proven safety and effectiveness in transplant patients	Avoid complementary or alternative products without proven safety and effectiveness in transplant patients

BEE, Basal energy expenditure; *RDI*, reference daily intake; *REE*, resting energy expenditure.

CLINICAL CASE STUDY

Tom is a 55-year-old single white man with hypertension (blood pressure 145/92 mmHg), high low-density lipoprotein cholesterol (241 mg/dL), and low high-density lipoprotein cholesterol (38 mg/dL) and a C-reactive protein (CRP) of 4mg/L. He has a strong family history of heart disease. He reports that he often eats in his car, so he frequents fast-food restaurants. He works long hours and, other than gardening on the weekends, he does not exercise. He is 5′10″ and 220 lb with a BMI of 31.6. His breakfast is usually a cheese-egg biscuit, bacon, and coffee with milk or cream. Lunch is often a bean and cheese burrito and ice cream. His favorite dinner is fried chicken, mashed potatoes with gravy, collards sautéed with bacon fat, and pie.

Nutrition Diagnostic Statements

- Intake of types of fats inconsistent with needs (saturated fat) (NI-5.5.3) related to eating fast food on the run and busy schedule as evidenced by unfavorable cholesterol profile (elevated LDL and low HDL) and regular consumption of fried foods, bacon and full fat dairy.
- Excessive mineral intake (sodium) (NI-5.10.7) related to frequent fast food consumption as evidenced by elevated blood pressure of 145.92 mmHg.
- Overweight/Obesity (NC-3.3) related to physical inactivity and consuming large portions of kcal dense foods as evidenced by BMI of 31.6 and frequent eating in fast food restaurants.

Nutrition Care Questions

1. What additional nutrition diagnoses would be appropriate for Tom?
2. What more would you want to know about Tom's diet and lifestyle to help him with health behavior change?
3. What is the significance of a CRP level of 4 mg/dL?
4. What nutrition and lifestyle interventions would be most helpful for Tom?

USEFUL WEBSITES

Academy of Nutrition and Dietetics, Evidence Analysis Library
American Association of Cardiovascular and Pulmonary Rehabilitation
American Heart Association
DASH Eating Plan (NIH)
Framingham Heart Study
National Heart, Lung, and Blood Institute (NIH)
Old Ways Foundation (Mediterranean Diet)

REFERENCES

Abdullah A, Amin FA, Stoelwinder J, et al: Estimating the risk of cardiovascular disease using an obese-years metric, *BMJ Open* 4:e005629, 2014.

Aburto NJ, Ziolkovska A, Hooper L, et al: Effect of lower sodium intake on health: systematic review and meta-analyses, *BMJ* 346:f1326, 2013.

Academy of Nutrition and Dietetics: *Evidence Analysis Library,* Heart Failure 2017 Guideline. Accessed at: https://www.andeal.org/topic.cfm?menu=5289 on 11-3-2019.

Academy of Nutrition and Dietetics Evidence Analysis Library (EAL): *Disorders of Lipid Metabolism: Executive Summary of Recommendations,* 2011. Available at: https://www.andeal.org/topic.cfm?menu=5300&cat=4528. Accessed November 3, 2019.

Alexander S, Ostfeld RJ, Allen K, et al: A plant-based diet and hypertension, *J Geriatr Cardiol* 14:327–330, 2017

Al-Khudairy L, Hartley L, Clar C, et al: Omega 6 fatty acids for the primary prevention of cardiovascular disease, *Cochrane Database Syst Rev* 16:CD011094, 2015

American College of Cardiology: *Mediterranean diet cuts heart disease risk by nearly half,* March 4, 2015. Available at: http://www.acc.org/about-acc/press-releases/2015/03/04/16/36/mediterranean-diet-cuts-heart-disease-risk-by-nearly-half.

American Heart Association: *Heart and stroke statistics,* 2015. Available at: http://www.heart.org/HEARTORG/General/Heart-and-Stroke-Association-Statistics_UCM_319064_SubHomePage.jsp.

Anderson JW, Baird P, Davis RH, et al: Health benefits of dietary fiber, *Nutr Rev* 67:188–205, 2009.

Anker SD, John M, Pedersen PU, et al: ESPEN guidelines on enteral nutrition: cardiology and pulmonology, *Clin Nutr* 25:311–318, 2006.

Appel LJ, Brands MW, Daniels SR, et al: Dietary approaches to prevent and treat hypertension: a scientific statement from the American Heart Association, *Hypertension* 47:296–308, 2006.

Baggott JE, Tamura T: Homocysteine, iron and cardiovascular disease: a hypothesis, *Nutrients* 7:1108–1118, 2015.

Bayram M, St Cyr JA, Abraham WT: D-Ribose aids heart failure patients with preserved ejection fraction and diastolic dysfunction: a pilot study, *Ther Adv Cardiovasc Dis* 9:56–65, 2015.

Bazzano LA, Green T, Harrison TN, et al: Dietary approaches to prevent hypertension, *Curr Hypertens Rep* 15:694–702, 2013.

Bello-Chavolla OY, Kuri-García A, Ríos-Ríos M, et al: Familial Combined Hyperlipidemia: current knowledge, perspectives, and controversies, *Rev Invest Clin* 70:224–236, 2018.

Benjamin EJ, Virani SS, Callaway CW, et al: Heart disease and stroke statistics-2018 update: A report from the American Heart Association, *Circulation* 137:e67–e492, 2018

Boden WE, O'Rourke RA, Teo KK, et al: Optimal medical therapy with or without PCI for stable coronary disease, *N Engl J Med* 356:1503–1516, 2007.

Block CB, Liu L, Herrington DM, et al: Predicting risk for incident heart failure with omega-3 fatty acids: From MESA, *JACC: Heart Failure* 7:651–661, 2019.

Brautbar A, Leary E, Rasmussen K, et al: Genetics of familial hypercholesterolemia, *Curr Atheroscler Rep* 17:491–498, 2015.

Brozovich FV, Nicholson CJ, Degen CV, et al: Mechanisms of vascular smooth muscle contraction and the basis for pharmacologic treatment of smooth muscle disorders, *Pharmacol Rev* 68:476–532, 2016.

Carlson H, Dahlin CM: Managing the effects of cardiac cachexia, *J Hosp Palliat Nurs* 16:15–20, 2014.

Carter SJ, Roberts MB, Salter J, et al: Relationship between Mediterranean diet score and atherothrombotic risk: findings from the Third National Health and Nutrition Examination Survey (NHANES-III), 1988-1994, *Atherosclerosis* 210:630–636, 2010.

Centers for Disease Control and Prevention: *Hypertension,* 2017. Available at: https://www.cdc.gov/nchs/fastats/hypertension.htm.

Chess DJ, Khairallah RJ, O'Shea KM, et al: A high-fat diet increases adiposity but maintains mitochondrial oxidative enzymes without affecting development of heart failure with pressure overload, *Am J Physiol Heart Circ Physiol* 297:H1585–H1593, 2009.

Christopher BA, Huang HM, Berthiaume JM, et al: Myocardial insulin resistance induced by high fat feeding in heart failure is associated with preserved contractile function, *Am J Physiol Heart Circ Physiol* 299:H1917–H1927, 2010.

Cook NR, Appel LJ, Whelton PK. Lower levels of sodium intake and reduced cardiovascular risk, *Circulation* 129:981–989, 2014.

Couch SC, Saelens BE, Levin L, et al: The efficacy of a clinic-based behavioral nutrition intervention emphasizing a DASH-type diet for adolescents with elevated blood pressure, *J Pediatr* 152:494–501, 2008.

Cui R, Iso H, Date C, et al: Dietary folate and vitamin B6 and B12 intake in relation to mortality from cardiovascular diseases: Japan collaborative cohort study, *Stroke* 41:1285–1289, 2010.

de Koning Gans JM, Uiterwaal CS, van der Schouw YT, et al: Tea and coffee consumption and cardiovascular morbidity and mortality, *Arterioscler Thromb Vasc Biol* 30:1665–1671, 2010.

Delano MJ, Moldawer LL: The origins of cachexia in acute and chronic inflammatory diseases, *Nutr Clin Pract* 21:68–81, 2006.

DeMarco VG, Aroor AR, Sowers JR: The pathophysiology of hypertension in patients with obesity, *Nat Rev Endocrinol* 10:364–376, 2014.

De Miguel C, Rudemiller NP, Abais JM, et al: Inflammation and hypertension: new understandings and potential therapeutic targets, *Curr Hypertens Rep* 17:507, 2015.

Desai AS: Controversies in cardiovascular medicine. Are serial BNP measurements useful in heart failure management? *Circulation* 127:509, 2013.

DiNicolantonio JJ, Niazi AK, Lavie CJ, et al: Thiamine supplementation for the treatment of heart failure: a review of the literature, *Congest Heart Fail* 19:214–222, 2013.

Djoussé L, Gaziano JM: Alcohol consumption and heart failure: a systematic review, *Curr Atheroscler Rep* 10:117–120, 2008.

Drozd M, Cubbon R, Gierula J, et al: 54 calcium supplementation in patients with chronic heart failure: Is it Safe? *Heart* 100:A31, 2014.

Eckel RH, Jakicic JM, Ard JD, et al: 2013 AHA/ACC guideline on lifestyle management to reduce cardiovascular risk: A report of the American College of Cardiology/American Heart Association Task Force on Practice Guidelines, *Circulation* 129:S76–S99, 2014.

Esselstyn CB, Golubić M: The nutritional reversal of cardiovascular disease – Fact or fiction? Three case reports, *Cardiology* 20:1901–1908, 2014.

Estruch R, Ros E, Salas-Salvadó J, et al: Primary prevention of cardiovascular disease with a Mediterranean diet, *N Engl J Med* 368:1279–1290, 2013.

Fekete ÁA, Giromini C, Chatzidiakou Y, et al: Whey protein lowers blood pressure and improves endothelial function and lipid biomarkers in adults with prehypertension and mild hypertension: results from the chronic Whey2Go randomized controlled trial, *Am J Clin Nutr* 104:1534–1544, 2016.

Flynn JT, Kaelber DC, Baker-Smith CM, et al: Clinical practice guideline for screening and management of high blood pressure in children and adolescents, *Pediatrics* 140:e20171904, 2017.

Fox CS, Golden SH, Anderson C, et al: Update on prevention of cardiovascular disease in adults with type 2 diabetes mellitus in light of recent evidence: a scientific statement from the American Heart Association and the American Diabetes Association, *Circulation* 132:691–718, 2015.

Fraser A, Williams D, Lawlor DA: Associations of serum 25-hydroxyvitamin D, parathyroid hormone and calcium with cardiovascular risk factors: analysis of 3 NHANES cycles (2001-2006), *PLoS One* 5:e13882, 2010.

Gidding SS, Lichtenstein AH, Faith MS, et al: Implementing American Heart Association pediatric and adult nutrition guidelines: a scientific statement from the American Heart Association Nutrition Committee of the Council on Nutrition, Physical Activity and Metabolism, Council on Cardiovascular Disease in the Young, Council on Arteriosclerosis, Thrombosis and Vascular Biology, Council on Cardiovascular Nursing, Council on Epidemiology and Prevention, and Council for High Blood Pressure Research, *Circulation* 119:1161–1175, 2009.

Go AS, Mozaffarian D, Roger VL, et al: Heart disease and stroke statistics—2014 update: a report from the American Heart Association, *Circulation* 129:e28–e292, 2014.

Goldberg AC, Ostlund RE, Bateman JH, et al: Effect of plant stanol tablets on low-density lipoprotein cholesterol lowering in patients on statin drugs, *Am J Cardiol* 97:376–379, 2006.

Gupta D, Georgiopoulou VV, Kalogeropoulos AP, et al: Dietary sodium intake in heart failure, Circulation 126:479–485, 2012.

Hall JE, do Carmo JM, da Silva AA, et al: Obesity-induced hypertension: Interaction of neurohumoral and renal mechanisms, *Circ Res* 116:991–1006, 2015.

Harada T, Inagaki-Tanimura K, Nagao M, et al: Frequency of achilles tendon xanthoma in patients with acute coronary syndrome, *J Atheroscler Thromb* 24:949–953, 2017.

Harris WS, Mozaffarian D, Rimm E, et al: Omega-6 fatty acids and risk for cardiovascular disease: a science advisory from the American Heart Association Nutrition Subcommittee of the Council on Nutrition, Physical Activity, and Metabolism; Council on Cardiovascular Nursing; and Council on Epidemiology and Prevention, *Circulation* 119:902–907, 2009.

Hasse JM: Nutritional aspects of transplantation in adults. In Busuttil RW, Klintmalm GB, editors: *Transplantation of the liver*, ed 3, St Louis, MO, 2015, Elsevier Saunders, pp 4994–4509.

Heidari F, Vasudevan R, Mohd Ali SZ, et al: RAS genetic variants in interaction with ACE inhibitors drugs influences essential hypertension control, *Arch Med Res* 48:88–95, 2017.

Institute of Medicine: *Dietary reference intakes: water, potassium, sodium chloride, and sulfate*, ed 1, Washington, DC, 2004, National Academies Press.

Institute of Medicine: *Sodium intake in populations: assessment of evidence*, Washington, DC, 2013, National Academies Press.

Jellinger PS, Smith DA, Mehta AE, et al: American Association of Clinical Endocrinologists' guidelines for management of dyslipidemia and prevention of atherosclerosis, *Endocr Pract* 18(Suppl 1):1–78, 2012.

Kalogeropoulos N, Panagiotakos DB, Pitsavos C, et al: Unsaturated fatty acids are inversely associated and n-6/n-3 ratios are positively related to inflammation and coagulation markers in plasma of apparently healthy adults, *Clin Chim Acta* 411:584–591, 2010.

Khandelwal S, Kelly L, Malik R, et al: Impact of omega-6 fatty acids on cardiovascular outcomes: a review, *J Preventive Cardiol* 2:325–336, 2013.

Klatsky AL: *Coffee drinking and caffeine associated with reduced risk of hospitalization for heart rhythm disturbances*. AHA 50th Annual Conference on Cardiovascular Disease, Epidemiology and Prevention, San Francisco, CA, 2010.

Kunutsor SK, Apekey TA, Steur M: Vitamin D and risk of future hypertension: meta-analysis of 283,537 participants, *Eur J Epidemiol* 28:205–221, 2013.

Lee CJ, Kim JY, Shim E, et al: The effects of diet alone or in combination with exercise in patients with prehypertension and hypertension: a randomized controlled trial, *Korean Circ J* 48:637–651, 2018

Lee Y, Kang D, Lee SA: Effect of dietary patterns on serum C-reactive protein level, *Nutr Metab Cardiovasc Dis* 24:1004–1011, 2014.

Lennon SL, DellaValle DM, Rodder SG, et al: 2015 Evidence analysis library evidence-based nutrition practice guideline for the management of hypertension in adults, *J Acad Nutr Diet* 117:1445–1458.e17, 2017.

Liebman B. *Is a low salt diet plan healthy?* 2016. Available at: https://www.nutritionaction.com/daily/salt-in-food/salt/. Accessed November 2, 2019.

Longo S, Bollani L, Decembrino L, et al: Short-term and long-term sequelae in intrauterine growth retardation (IUGR), *J Matern Fetal Neonatal Med* 26:222–225, 2013.

Ma C, Zhang T, Xi B: Prevalence of elevated blood pressure among US Children, 2013-2014. *J Clin Hypertens (Greenwich)* 18:1071–1072, 2016.

Madmani ME, Yusuf Solaiman A, Tamr Agha K, et al: Coenzyme Q10 for heart failure, *Cochrane Database Syst Rev* 6:CD008684, 2014.

Madsen CM, Varbo A, Nordestgaard BG: Extreme high high-density lipoprotein cholesterol is paradoxically associated with high mortality in men and women: two prospective cohort studies, *Eur Heart J* 28(32):2478–2486, 2017.

Maki KC, Eren F, Cassens ME, et al: Omega-6 polyunsaturated fatty acids and cardiometabolic health: current evidence, controversies, and research gaps, *Adv Nutr* 9:688–700, 2018.

Masoura C, Pitsavos C, Aznaouridis K, et al: Arterial endothelial function and wall thickness in familial hypercholesterolemia and familial combined hyperlipidemia and the effect of statins. A systematic review and meta-analysis, *Atherosclerosis* 214:129–138, 2011.

McMaster WG, Kirabo A, Madhur MS, et al: Inflammation, immunity, and hypertensive end-organ damage, *Circ Res* 116:1022–1033, 2015.

Meems LM, van der Harst P, van Gilst WH, et al: Vitamin D biology in heart failure: molecular mechanisms and systematic review, *Curr Drug Targets* 12:29–41, 2011.

Miller D, Joye Woodward N: Clinical inquiries. Whom should you test for secondary causes of hypertension? *J Fam Pract* 63:41–42, 2014.

Miller ER III, Erlinger TP, Appel LJ: The effects of macronutrients on blood pressure and lipids: an overview of the DASH and OmniHeart trials, *Curr Atheroscler Rep* 8:460–465, 2006.

Miller PE, Van Elswyk M, Alexander DD: Long-chain omega-3 fatty acids eicosapentaenoic acid and docosahexaenoic acid and blood pressure: a meta-analysis of randomized controlled trials, *Am J Hypertens* 27: 885–896, 2014.

Mirijello A, Tarli C, Vassallo GA, et al: Alcoholic cardiomyopathy: What is known and what is not known, *Eur J Int Med* 43:1–5, 2017.

Morrow DA, Crea F: *C-reactive protein in cardiovascular disease, UpToDate,* 2014, Wolters Kluwer, Alphen aan den Rijn, Netherlands Available at: http://www.uptodate.com/ contents/c-reactive-protein-in-cardiovascular-disease.

Navab M, Reddy ST, Van Lenten BJ, et al: HDL and cardiovascular disease: atherogenic and atheroprotective mechanisms, *Nat Rev Cardiol* 8:222–232, 2011.

Nicklas BJ, Cesari M, Penninx BW, et al: Abdominal obesity is an independent risk factor for chronic heart failure in older people, *J Am Geriatr Soc* 54:413–420, 2006.

Nordestgaard BG, Chapman MJ, Humphries SE, et al: Familial hypercholesterol-aemia is underdiagnosed and undertreated in the general population: guidance for clinicians to prevent coronary heart disease: consensus statement of the European Atherosclerosis Society, *Eur Heart J* 34:3478–3490a, 2013.

Opie LH, Commerford PJ, Gersh BJ: Controversies in stable coronary artery disease, *Lancet* 367:69–78, 2006.

Poorolajal J, Zeraati F, Soltanian AR, et al: Oral potassium supplementation for management of essential hypertension: a meta-analysis of randomized controlled trials, *PLoS One* 12:e0174967, 2017.

Porto CM, Silva VL, da Luz JSB, Filho BM, da Silveira VM: Association between vitamin D deficiency and heart failure risk in the elderly, *ESC Heart Fail* 5:63–74, 2018.

Priccila Zuchinali, ScD, Gabriela C, Souza, ScD, et al: Short-term Effects of High-Dose Caffeine on Cardiac Arrhythmias in Patients With Heart Failure: a randomized clinical trial, *JAMA Intern Med* 176(12):1752–1759, 2016. doi:10.1001/jamainternmed.2016.6374.

Qi D, Nie X, Cai J: The effect of vitamin D supplementation on hypertension in non-CKD populations: A systematic review and meta-analysis, *Int J Cardiol* 227:177–186, 2017.

Rees K, Hartley L, Flowers N, et al: 'Mediterranean' dietary pattern for the primary prevention of cardiovascular disease, *Cochrane Database Syst Rev* 8:CD009825, 2013.

Rosano GM, Vitale C, Fragasso G: Metabolic therapy for patients with diabetes mellitus and coronary artery disease, *Am J Cardiol* 98:14J–18J, 2006.

Roth EM, Harris WS: Fish oil for primary and secondary prevention of coronary heart disease, *Curr Atheroscler Rep* 12:66–72, 2010.

Schleithoff SS, Zittermann A, Tenderich G, et al: Vitamin D supplementation improves cytokine profiles in patients with congestive heart failure: a double-blind, randomized, placebo-controlled trial, *Am J Clin Nutr* 83:754–759, 2006.

Schutten JC, Joosten MM, de Borst MH, et al: Magnesium and blood pressure: a physiology-based approach, *Adv Chronic Kidney Dis* 25:244–250, 2018.

Seidel E, Scholl UI. Genetic mechanisms of human hypertension and their implications for blood pressure physiology, *Physiol Genomics* 49:630–652, 2017.

Shecterle LM, Terry KR, St Cyr JA: The patented uses of D-ribose in cardiovascular diseases, *Recent Pat Cardiovasc Drug Discov* 5:138–142, 2010.

Smidowicz A, Regula J: Effect of nutritional status and dietary patterns on human serum C-reactive protein and interleukin-6 concentrations, *Adv Nutr* 6:738–747, 2015.

Springer J, von Haehling S, Anker SD: The need for a standardized definition for cachexia in chronic illness, *Nat Clin Prac Endocrinol Metab* 2:416–417, 2006.

Stone NJ, Robinson JG, Lichtenstein AH, et al: 2013 ACC/AHA guideline on the treatment of blood cholesterol to reduce atherosclerotic cardiovascular risk in adults: a report of the American College of Cardiology/American Heart Association Task Force on Practice Guidelines, *Circulation* 129(Suppl 2):S1–S45, 2014.

Sturm AC, Knowles JW, Gidding SS, et al: Clinical genetic testing for familial hypercholesterolemia: JACC scientific expert panel, *J Am Coll Cardiol* 72(6):660–680, 2018.

Swain JF, McCarron PB, Hamilton EF, et al: Characteristics of the diet patterns tested in the optimal macronutrient intake trial to prevent heart disease (OmniHeart): options for a heart-healthy diet, *J Am Diet Assoc* 108: 257–265, 2008.

Tang WH, Wang Z, Levison BS, et al: Intestinal microbial metabolism of phosphatidylcholine and cardiovascular risk, *N Engl J Med* 368: 1575–1584, 2013.

Teunissen-Beekman KF, van Baak MA: The role of dietary protein in blood pressure regulation, *Curr Opin Lipidol* 24:65–70, 2013.

Thom T, Haase N, Rosamond W, et al: Heart disease and stroke statistics—2006 update: a report from the American Heart Association Statistics Committee and Stroke Statistics Subcommittee, *Circulation* 113:e85–e151, 2006.

Tousoulis D, Kampoli AM, Tentolouris C, et al: The role of nitric oxide on endothelial function, *Curr Vasc Pharmacol* 10:4–18, 2012.

Tsao CW, Vasan RS: Cohort Profile: The Framingham Heart Study (FHS): overview of milestones in cardiovascular epidemiology, *Int J Epidemiol* 44:1800–1813, 2015.

Tuso P, Stoll SR, Li WW: A plant-based diet, atherogenesis, and coronary artery disease prevention, *Perm J* 19:62–67, 2015.

Tyson CC, Nwankwo C, Lin PH, et al: The Dietary Approaches to Stop Hypertension eating pattern in special populations, *Curr Hypertens Rep* 14:388–396, 2012.

US Department of Agriculture (USDA), United States Department of Health and Human Services (USDHHS): *Dietary guidelines for Americans 2015-2020,* 2015. Available at: https://www.cnpp.usda.gov/2015-2020-dietary-guidelines-americans.

van der Wal HH, Comin-Colet J, Klip IT, et al: Vitamin B12 and folate deficiency in chronic heart failure, *Heart* 101:302–310, 2015.

Vieth R, Kimball S: Vitamin D in congestive heart failure, *Am J Clin Nutr* 83:731–732, 2006.

Wexler RK, Elton T, Pleister A, et al: Cardiomyopathy: an overview, *Am Fam Physician* 79:778–784, 2009.

Whelton PK, Carey RM, Aronow WS, et al: 2017 ACC/AHA/AAPA/ABC/ ACPM/AGS/APHA/ASH/ASPC/NMA/PCNA Guideline for the Prevention, Detection, Evaluation, and Management of High Blood Pressure in Adults, *J Am Coll Cardiol* 71:e127, 2018.

Xi B, Zhang T, Zhang M, et al: Trends in elevated blood pressure among US children and adolescents: 1999-2012, *Am J Hypertens* 29:217–225, 2016.

Yanai H, Katsuyama H, Hamasaki H, et al: Effects of dietary fat intake on HDL metabolism, *J Clin Med Res* 7:145–149, 2015.

Yusuf S, Rangarajan S, Teo K, et al: Cardiovascular risk and events in 17 low-, middle-, and high-income countries, *N Engl J Med* 371:818–827, 2014.

Zhang X, Li Y, Del Gobbo LC, et al: Effects of magnesium supplementation on blood pressure: a meta-analysis of randomized double-blind placebo-controlled trials, *Hypertension* 68:324–333, 2016.

Zhou MS, Schulman IH, Zeng Q: Link between the renin-angiotensin system and insulin resistance: implications for cardiovascular disease, *Vasc Med* 17:330–341, 2012.

Zittermann A, Schleithoff SS, Koerfer R: Markers of bone metabolism in congestive heart failure, *Clin Chim Acta* 366:27–36, 2006.

33

Medical Nutrition Therapy for Pulmonary Disease

Laith Ghazala, MD, FRCP
A. Christine Hummell, MS, RDN, LD, CNSC
Bette Klein, MS, RDN, CSP, LD

KEY TERMS

acinar
acinus
acute respiratory distress syndrome (ARDS)
adiponectin
asthma
aspiration pneumonia
bronchiectasis
bronchogenic carcinomas
bronchopulmonary dysplasia (BPD)
cancer cachexia syndrome
chronic bronchitis
chronic obstructive pulmonary
    disease (COPD)
cilia
chylothorax
clubbing
continuous positive airway pressure
    (CPAP)

cor pulmonale
cyanosis
cystic fibrosis (CF)
cystic fibrosis related diabetes (CFRD)
distal intestinal obstruction syndrome
    (DIOS)
dyspnea
elastase
emphysema
ghrelin
hypercapnia
hypopnea
idiopathic pulmonary fibrosis
interstitial lung disease (ILD)
interstitial pulmonary fibrosis
kyphosis
leptin
obesity hypoventilation syndrome (OHS)

obstructive sleep apnea (OSA)
osteopenia
pancreatic enzyme replacement
    therapy (PERT)
pancreatic insufficiency (PI)
pleural effusion
pneumonia
pulmonary cachexia
pulmonary function tests
pulmonary hypertension (PH)
pulse oximetry
resistin
resolvin
spirometry
steatorrhea
surfactant
tachypnea
tuberculosis (TB)

Optimal nutrition supports the development, growth, and maintenance of the respiratory organs, supporting structures of the skeleton and muscles and related nervous, circulatory, and immunologic systems. A well-functioning pulmonary system enables the body to obtain the oxygen needed to meet its cellular demands for energy from macronutrients and to remove carbon dioxide as a byproduct of metabolism.

THE PULMONARY SYSTEM

The respiratory structures include the nose, pharynx, larynx, trachea, bronchi, bronchioles, alveolar ducts, and alveoli. Supporting structures include the skeleton and the muscles (e.g., the intercostal, abdominal, and diaphragm muscles). Within a month after conception, pulmonary structures are recognizable. The pulmonary system grows and matures during gestation and childhooduntil it reaches full maturity and aveoli density at about 20 years of age. As aging occurs, the lungs lose elasticity and functional capacity declines.

The primary function of the respiratory system is gas exchange, and the anatomy and physiology is geared to fulfill this function (Fig. 33.1). The lungs enable the body to obtain the oxygen needed to meet its cellular metabolic demands and to remove the carbon dioxide (CO_2) produced. Healthy nerves, and efficient blood and lymph circulation are needed to supply oxygen and nutrients to all tissues. The lungs also filter, warm, and humidify inspired air.

The respiratory center is the name for structures involved in the generation of rhythmic respiratory movements and reflexes and is located in the medulla and pons (see Fig. 39.2 in Chapter 39). The electrical impulses generated by the respiratory center are carried by the phrenic nerves to the diaphragm and other respiratory muscles. Contraction of diaphragm and other muscles increases the intrathoracic volume, which creates negative intrathoracic pressure and allows air to be sucked in. The air traverses through the upper airways into the lower airways (see Fig. 33.1, A) and reaches the alveoli (see Fig. 33.1, B). The alveoli are surrounded by capillaries where gas exchange takes

---

Portions of this chapter were written by Sameera H. Kahn and Ashok M. Karnik.

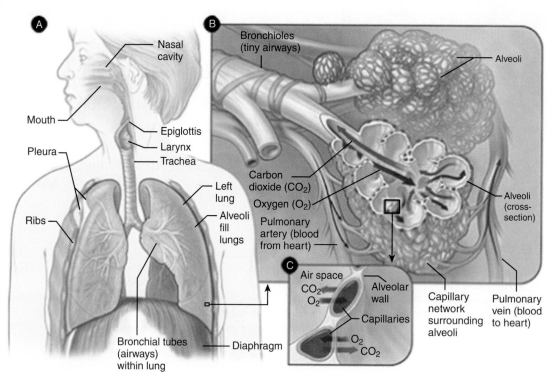

Fig. 33.1 Functional anatomy and physiology of the respiratory system. **A,** Various parts of respiratory system. **B,** Gas exchange unit. **C,** Alveolar-capillary interface. *National Heart, Lung, and Blood Institute; National Institutes of Health; U.S. Department of Health and Human Services.*

place (see Fig. 33.1, *C*). The pulmonary artery carries blood from the right ventricle of the heart into the small capillaries where gas exchange takes place with the alveoli; oxygenated blood returns back through the pulmonary veins into the left atrium of the heart to be delivered into the rest of the body. The large pulmonary blood vessels and the conducting airways are located in a well-defined connective tissue compartment—the pleural cavity.

The lungs are an important part of the body's immune system, because inspired air is laden with particles and microorganisms. Mucus keeps the airways moist and traps the particles and microorganisms from inspired air. The airways have 12 types of epithelial cells, and most cells that line the trachea, bronchi, and bronchioles have cilia. The cilia are "hair-like" structures that move the superficial liquid lining layer from deep within the lungs toward the pharynx to enter the gastrointestinal tract, thereby playing an important role as a lung defense mechanism by clearing bacteria and other foreign bodies. Each time a person swallows, microorganism-containing mucus passes into the digestive tract, in addition to the food. When inhaled bacteria or food particles are not cleared effectively, the patient is prone to develop recurrent chest infections that may eventually lead to bronchiectasis. The epithelial surface of the alveoli contains macrophages. By the process of phagocytosis, these alveolar macrophages engulf inhaled inert materials and microorganisms and digest them. The alveolar cells also secrete surfactant, a compound synthesized from proteins and phospholipids that maintains the stability of pulmonary tissue by reducing the surface tension of fluids that coat the lung.

The lungs have several metabolic functions. For example, they help regulate the body's acid-base balance (see Chapter 3). The body's pH is maintained partially by the proper balance of CO_2 and oxygen (O_2). The lungs also synthesize arachidonic acid that ultimately may be converted to prostaglandins or leukotrienes. These appear to play a role in

bronchoconstriction seen in asthma. The lungs convert angiotensin I to angiotensin II by the angiotensin-converting enzyme (ACE) found mainly in the numerous capillary beds of the lungs. Angiotensin II increases blood pressure. Because of the ultrastructure and the fact that they receive the total cardiac output, lungs are well suited to function as a chemical filter. They protect the systemic circulation from exposure to high levels of circulating vasoactive substances. Although serotonin, 5-hydroxytryptamine (5-HT), and norepinephrine are totally or partially eliminated or inactivated in the pulmonary circulation, epinephrine and histamines pass through the lungs unchanged.

Effect of Malnutrition on the Pulmonary System

The relationship between malnutrition and respiratory disease has long been recognized. Malnutrition adversely affects lung structure, elasticity, and function; respiratory muscle mass, strength, and endurance; lung immune defense mechanisms; and control of breathing. For example protein and iron deficiencies result in low hemoglobin levels that diminish the oxygen-carrying capacity of the blood. Low levels of calcium, magnesium, phosphorus, and potassium compromise respiratory muscle function at the cellular level. Hypoalbuminemia, as measured by serum albumin, contributes to the development of pulmonary edema by decreasing colloid osmotic pressure, allowing body fluids to move into the interstitial space. Decreased levels of surfactant contribute to the collapse of alveoli, thereby increasing the work of breathing. The supporting connective tissue of the lungs is composed of collagen, which requires ascorbic acid for its synthesis. Normal airway mucus is a substance consisting of water, glycoproteins, and electrolytes, and thus requires adequate nutritional intake.

Effect of Pulmonary Disease on Nutritional Status

Pulmonary disease substantially increases energy requirements. This factor explains the rationale for including body composition and

BOX 33.1 Adverse Effects of Lung Disease on Nutrition Status

Increased Energy Expenditure
Increased work of breathing
Chronic infection
Medical treatments (e.g., bronchodilators, chest physical therapy)

Reduced Intake
Fluid restriction
Shortness of breath
Decreased oxygen saturation while eating
Anorexia resulting from chronic disease
Gastrointestinal distress and vomiting

Additional Limitations
Difficulty preparing food because of fatigue
Impaired feeding skills (for infants and children)
Altered metabolism
Food-drug interactions

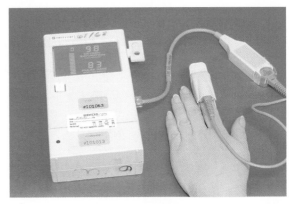

Fig. 33.2 Pulse oximeter.

weight parameters in nutrition assessment. Weight loss from inadequate energy intake is significantly correlated with a poor prognosis in persons with pulmonary diseases. Malnutrition leading to impaired immunity places any patient at high risk for developing respiratory infections. Malnourished patients with pulmonary disease who are hospitalized are likely to have lengthy stays and are susceptible to increased morbidity and mortality compared with well-nourished patients.

The complications of pulmonary diseases or their treatments can make adequate food intake and digestion difficult. For example, patients who are unable to breathe well will find it tiring to prepare food or to eat. Absorption and metabolism of most nutrients are affected. As pulmonary disease progresses, several conditions may interfere with food intake and overall nutrition status. For example, abnormal production of sputum, vomiting, tachypnea (rapid breathing), hemoptysis, thoracic pain, nasal polyps, anemia, depression, and altered taste secondary to medications are often present. Weight loss, low body mass index (BMI), and other adverse effects are listed in Box 33.1.

Medical Management

Pulmonary system disorders may be categorized as primary, such as tuberculosis (TB), asthma, and lung cancer; or secondary when associated with cardiovascular disease, obesity, infection, sickle cell disease, or scoliosis. Conditions also may be acute or chronic. Examples of acute conditions include aspiration pneumonia, airway obstruction from foods such as peanuts, and allergic anaphylaxis from consumption of shellfish. Examples of chronic conditions include cystic fibrosis (CF) and chronic obstructive pulmonary disease (COPD).

The assessment of the pulmonary status starts with obtaining a thorough history with a focus on the social history such as smoking and other inhalational toxins as well as exposure history. Typical symptoms of pulmonary disorders include dyspnea (shortness of breath), cough, sputum production, chest discomfort, fatigue, early satiety, and weight loss. The pulmonary assessment continues with percussion and auscultation. These bedside techniques provide important information on the patient's breathing.

Numerous diagnostic and monitoring tests such as imaging procedures, arterial blood gas determinations, sputum cultures, and biopsies also can be employed. Pulmonary function tests are used to diagnose or monitor the status of lung disease; they are designed to measure the ability of the respiratory system to exchange O_2 and CO_2. Pulse oximetry is one such test. A small device called a pulse oximeter, which uses light waves to measure the O_2 saturation of arterial blood, is placed on the end of the finger (Fig. 33.2). Normal for a young, healthy person is 95% to 99%. Spirometry is another common pulmonary function test. This involves breathing into a spirometer that gives information on lung volume and the rate at which air can be inhaled and exhaled.

CHRONIC PULMONARY DISEASE

Cystic Fibrosis

Cystic fibrosis (CF) is a life-threatening autosomal recessive inherited disorder that is most commonly seen in white populations with a CF incidence of 1 out of 3000 babies born in the United States (Cystic Fibrosis Foundation, 2016). According to the Cystic Fibrosis Foundation 2016 Patient Registry, 29,497 persons have CF. CF is caused by mutations in the cystic fibrosis transmembrane conductance regulator (CFTR) protein, a complex chloride channel and regulatory protein found in all exocrine tissues. The function of CFTR is to regulate the passage of chloride, sodium, and bicarbonate in the epithelial cells. Due to absent or abnormal CFTR in CF, the decreased secretion of chloride and water and increased reabsorption of sodium result in the production of thick, viscous secretions in the lungs, pancreas, liver, intestines, and reproductive tract, and lead to increased salt content in the sweat gland secretions. Most of the clinical manifestations are related to the thick, viscous secretions (Fig. 33.3). Lung disease and malnutrition are predominant consequences of the disease.

In the past, most patients were diagnosed with CF because of symptoms related to various organ systems. All 50 states now provide newborn screening for CF in the first 2 to 3 days of life, with the majority of cases diagnosed by 1 month of age. Screening consists of using a neonatal blood spot to determine the concentration of immunoreactive trypsinogen; if it is elevated, then genetic analysis and sweat chloride tests are completed to confirm the diagnosis. The diagnosis of CF in persons other than neonates who have a clinical history consistent with the disease or have a sibling with CF, is determined by an abnormal sweat chloride test (chloride level in sweat >60 mmol/L). If the chloride sweat test is abnormal, genetic analysis is used to confirm the diagnosis and the CFTR mutation (Katkin, 2014). Abnormal sweat chloride tests can occur with malnutrition and adrenal insufficiency.

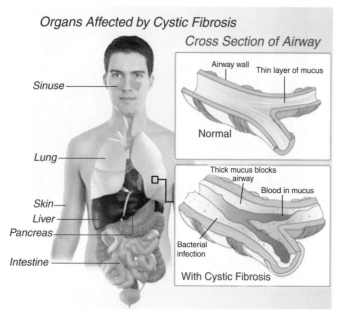

Fig. 33.3 Illustration showing multisystem involvement in cystic fibrosis (CF) and tenacious secretions.

Pathophysiology

Pulmonary and Sinus Disease

Due to the difficulty of expelling thick and viscous mucus in the respiratory tract, CF patients present with chronic persistent cough, dyspnea, and wheezing. Thick and viscous mucus is considered a rich environment for bacteria to grow, leading to a form of obstructive airway disease, bronchiectasis, a chronic condition of dilatation of the bronchi that develops as a result of recurrent lung infections. Examination of a patient with bronchiectasis may show presence of clubbing. Digital clubbing is characterized by increased digital tip mass and increased longitudinal and transverse nail plate curvature (Fig. 33.4), and lung auscultation reveals diffuse coarse crackles in the lungs and decreased breath sounds. Chest radiograph may show hyperinflation in advanced disease, and a computed tomography (CT) scan may show cystic and nodular densities, the classical picture of cystic bronchiectasis (Fig. 33.5). Pulmonary function testing shows

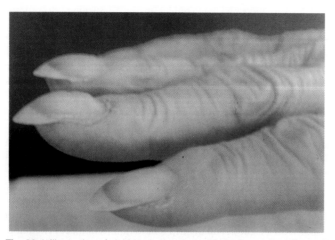

Fig. 33.4 Illustration of clubbing in a patient with "yellow nail syndrome."

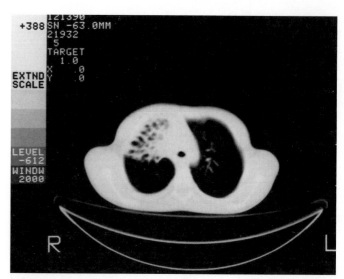

Fig. 33.5 Computed tomography (CT) scan of a patient showing cystic changes of bronchiectasis in right upper lobe.

airway obstruction. The spirogram shows reduced forced vital capacity (FVC), known as "restrictive pattern." The reduced forced expiratory volume (FEV$_1$) and the reduced FEV$_1$/FVC ratio are suggestive of airway obstruction.

Sputum cultures are used to identify bacteria growing in the respiratory tract in CF patients. Most common bacteria in CF patients are *Staphylococcus aureus* and *Pseudomonas aeruginosa*, which colonize the airways frequently. Evidence exists that these bacteria play an important role in disease progression. Many children with CF develop chronic rhinosinusitis with nasal polyposis. Some questions remain unanswered as to the origin of polyps in CF patients.

Pancreatic Disease in Cystic Fibrosis

Several different types of pancreatic disease occur in CF patients.

Pancreatic insufficiency. Pancreatic insufficiency (PI), in which the pancreas fails to make adequate enzymes to digest food in the small intestine, is the most common gastrointestinal complication of CF, affecting approximately 90% of patients at some time in their lives (Rogers, 2013).

Up to 90% of patients exhibit fat malabsorption by 1 year of age. The production of pancreatic enzymes is decreased, which leads to the malabsorption of fats and steatorrhea. Steatorrhea is characterized by foul smelling, bulky, oily stools and failure to thrive or poor weight gain. Such patients may also present with clinical features of deficiency of the fat-soluble vitamins A, D, E, and K. The CF population frequently presents with suboptimal vitamin D status. CF patients also suffer from vitamin K deficiencies and need routine supplementation.

Pancreatitis. The abnormal pancreatic secretions cause progressive pancreatic damage, so these patients can present with acute or recurrent pancreatitis.

CF-related diabetes. Patients with exocrine PI also may develop impaired function of the endocrine pancreas, leading to the development of cystic fibrosis related diabetes (CFRD). It is the most common comorbidity in the CF population, occurring in 20% of the adolescents and 40% to 50% of the adults with CF. CFRD is associated with poor growth, clinical and nutritional deterioration, and early death. The American Diabetes Association and the Cystic Fibrosis Foundation recommend yearly CFRD screenings, starting at age 10 (see Chapter 29 for discussion of diabetes management), to be performed using a 2-hour 75 mg oral glucose tolerance test during a period of stable health. The use of hemoglobin A1C is not recommended for screening because it has low sensitivity in CFRD (Moran et al, 2010). Hemoglobin A1C is often normal in patients with CFRD regardless of the degree of hyperglycemia. However, if it is already measured and the value is >6.5, this is still consistent with a diagnosis of CFRD.

Bone Disease

Due to vitamin D deficiency, bone disease is common in CF patients and is characterized by increased fracture rates, low bone density, and kyphosis, which is increased curvature of the upper back. Multiple risk factors contribute to developing bone disease—chronic corticosteroid use; multiple courses of antibiotics; failure to thrive; malabsorption of calcium, vitamin D, vitamin K, and magnesium; inadequate overall intake; and reduced weight-bearing activities. Obtaining and monitoring serum 25-hydroxy vitamin D level should be done yearly.

Other Conditions

Meconium ileus, rectal prolapse, biliary disease, infertility, musculoskeletal disorders, and recurrent venous thrombosis are other less common conditions that occur in patients with CF. Meconium ileus is an obstruction of the small intestine caused by thickened meconium (first feces) that can occur in neonates with CF. CF patients are susceptible to small intestine bacterial overgrowth due to decreased motility. This disorder interferes with fat absorption and appetite and can lead to multiple food intolerances and digestive disturbances (Baker et al, 2013) (see Chapter 27).

Medical Management

CF is a multisystem disease that requires a multidisciplinary approach to manage symptoms, correct deficiencies, and prevent complications and progression of the disease. The CF team usually includes medical and nursing staff; respiratory therapists, physical therapists, registered dietitian nutritionists; social workers; and genetic counselors. Impairment of the respiratory and gastrointestinal systems is responsible for significant mortality and morbidity. Sinus infection, glucose control, nutritional status, and psychosocial issues must be assessed and managed at regular intervals (Fig. 33.6).

CF management is usually separated into chronic maintenance therapy and acute exacerbation of the disease. Chronic therapy focuses on prevention and treatment of airway infections and obstructions as CF patients are prone to recurrent chest infections. Medical management consists of chest physiotherapy, nebulizer therapy, antiinflammatory agents, pulmonary hygiene, pneumococcal and influenza vaccinations, and, frequently, chronic prophylactic antibiotic use. A major step forward in the treatment of CF came in 2011 with the invention of a medication that targets the correction of the mutant CFTR function, Ivacaftor (VX-770). It is a small molecular weight oral drug that is designed specifically to treat patients who have a G551D mutation in at least one of their CFTR genes. Ivacaftor is the first approved CF therapy that restores the functioning of a mutant CF protein rather than trying to target one or more of its downstream consequences (Davis, 2011). In clinical trials, it was found to improve respiratory status, reduce pulmonary exacerbations, enhance quality of life, and promote weight gain. Currently, other drugs are coming onto the market that target the mutant CFTR function. If the CF patient continues to decline despite medical therapy, bilateral lung transplantation may be needed. The acute management of CF sometimes requires

hospitalization, usually to treat an infection with intravenous antibiotics and more frequent pulmonary hygiene.

Because of the PI, pancreatic enzyme replacement therapy (PERT) is an important component of the management for CF patients to adequately absorb carbohydrates, protein, and fat. The pancreatic ducts are obstructed in approximately 85% to 90% of CF individuals, and this prevents pancreatic enzymes such as lipase, amylase, and protease from secreting into the small intestine. The build-up of these enzymes in the pancreas leads to auto digestion of the pancreas and destruction of acinus. Pancreatic acinus is the secretory unit of exocrine pancreas, where pancreatic juice is produced. Destruction of pancreatic acinus, or acinar destruction, results in impaired secretion of pancreatic juice, which results in loose, oily, frequent stools and malabsorption. These individuals need PERT to combat the PI and maintain adequate absorption and digestion of nutrients (see Focus On: PERT).

◎ FOCUS ON

PERT

Pancreatic enzyme replacement therapy (PERT) is the first step taken to correct maldigestion and malabsorption. The microspheres, designed to withstand the acidic environment of the stomach, release enzymes in the duodenum, where they digest protein, fat, and carbohydrate. Pharmaceutical advancements have improved the medications. The quantity of enzymes to be taken with food depends on the degree of pancreatic insufficiency; the quantity of food eaten; the fat, protein, and carbohydrate content of food consumed; and the type of enzymes used.

Enzyme dosage per meal or snack is adjusted empirically to control gastrointestinal symptoms, including steatorrhea, and to promote growth appropriate for age. Following the manufacturer's directions about storage and administration of a particular brand of enzyme is important to emphasize. If gastrointestinal symptoms cannot be controlled, enzyme dosage, patient adherence, and enzyme type should be reevaluated. Fecal elastase (protein-digesting enzyme secreted by the pancreas and involved in hydrolysis of peptide bonds), fecal fat, or nitrogen balance studies may help to evaluate the adequacy of enzyme supplementation.

The acidic environment of the stomach does not allow the enzymes of the enteric coated PERT to be degraded. This normally occurs once the pH is above 5.5, usually when the PERT reaches the duodenal jejunum. A common practice is placing cystic fibrosis (CF) patients on proton pump inhibitors in order to increase the duodenal pH by decreasing gastric acid secretion (Rogers, 2013).

Intestinal abnormalities such as gastroesophageal reflux disease (GERD), meconium ileus (MI), and **distal intestinal obstruction syndrome (DIOS)**, which is the blockage of intestines resulting from stool and intussusceptions (obstructions), are some of the complications seen in patients (Katkin, 2014).

Hepatobiliary problems are seen more commonly now in this population because of an increased survival rate. In the liver, the cystic fibrosis transmembrane conductance regulator (CFTR) is located in the biliary epithelium. Bile produced in patients with CF is thick and tenacious, causing blockage of the intrahepatic bile ducts. Blockage of these ducts eventually leads to cirrhosis. Use of ursodeoxycholic acid (UDCA) may delay the progression of liver disease (Kappler et al, 2012) (see Chapter 28); however, a recent Cochrane Review found little evidence to support routine use of UDCA, citing the small number of trials assessing its effectiveness (Cheng et al, 2017). At this time, there is little evidence-based research for the prevention and management of liver disease in persons with CF (Palanippan et al, 2017).

PATHOPHYSIOLOGY AND CARE MANAGEMENT ALGORITHM

Cystic Fibrosis

ETIOLOGY

Autosomal recessive inheritance

↓

Cystic Fibrosis Gene
Cystic fibrosis transmembrane receptor (CFTR)

↓

Cystic Fibrosis (CF)

PATHOPHYSIOLOGY

Obstruction of Glands and Ducts

- Secretion of abnormally thick, tenacious mucus by exocrine glands

Affected Organs

- Respiratory organs
- Pancreas; gallbladder, liver
- Reproductive organs
- Sweat glands
- Salivary glands
- Intestines

Physical Growth

- Short stature
- Low body weight (children and adults)
- Low muscle mass
- Malabsorption

MANAGEMENT

Medical Management

- Genotyping
- Oral or IV antibiotics
- Aerosol antibiotics
- Inhaled medications
- Chest and physical therapy

Nutrition Management

- Monitor ongoing nutrition status and support maintenance of lean body mass
- Supply pancreatic enzyme replacement therapy (PERT)
- Meet increased energy requirements
- Provide vitamin and mineral supplementation due to malabsorption

Fig. 33.6 Algorithm for diagnosis and management of cystic fibrosis.

Medical Nutrition Therapy

Medical nutrition therapy (MNT), critical to management of CF and all of its comorbidities, is vital in promoting longevity and positive outcomes. MNT begins with evaluation of the nutritional status of the patient (Baker et al, 2013) (see Chapters 4 and 5). CF patients frequently have growth failure, the cause of which is multifactorial: malabsorption, increased energy needs, and reduced appetite. Nutritional status is closely correlated to pulmonary function and survival in CF. As a result, close attention to growth status in children should be monitored; clinical care guidelines for infants and preschoolers have been published (Borowitz et al, 2009; Lahiri et al, 2016). All patients with CF should have regular nutritional assessments for early detection of nutritional status deterioration (see *Pathophysiology and Care Management Algorithm: Cystic Fibrosis*). Older children should be evaluated for bone density, using the dual-energy x-ray absorptiometry (DEXA) (see Chapter 23).

CF is typically associated with malnutrition; however, the number of overweight and obese patients has also increased in this population, raising concern for the effect of excess energy intake on lung function. Dietary recommendations should emphasize a balanced healthy diet with good exercise habits.

Major goals of nutritional therapy are increasing muscle strength, promoting optimal growth and weight maintenance, and enhancing the quality of life. To achieve these goals, the objectives of treatment are to correct maldigestion and malabsorption and to provide nutrients that are commonly deficient.

Energy. Evidenced-based nutrition goals for individuals with CF are based on the Cystic Fibrosis Foundation registry data analysis for age and sex:

- Newborn to 24 months: weight/length ≥50th percentile, using Centers for Disease Control and Prevention (CDC) growth charts
- 2 to 20 years old: BMI 50th to 85th percentile, using CDC growth charts
- Adult females: BMI 22 to 27 kg/m^2
- Adult males: BMI 23 to 27 mg/km^2

These weight goals are associated with a desirable pulmonary function.

A broad range of energy requirements are reported in patients with CF, ranging from 120% to 150% of recommendations for the general population, depending on the CF mutation, the patient's age, degree of malabsorption, presence of pulmonary exacerbation, pulmonary function, sex, pubertal status, presence of additional medical complications (CFRD, CF liver disease), and the current state of health (Schindler et al, 2015).

A challenging issue is attaining an adequate energy intake with an energy dense diet. The determination to initiate enteral feedings is individualized for those who are unable to consume adequate calories and protein to meet growth/weight maintenance goals or those with moderate or severe malnutrition (Schwarzenberg, 2016). Tube feeding options include gastrostomy tube, nasogastric tube, and jejunostomy tube. The most common delivery option is the percutaneous endoscopic gastrostomy (PEG) tube (see Chapter 12). Appropriate PERT management should be maintained with general guidelines based on fat grams provided. If the patient is eating, PERT can be administered orally. For those who are not taking anything by mouth, PERT may be crushed (depending on the type of PERT), dissolved in a sodium bicarbonate solution, and then administered as an enteral medication. Recently a digestive enzyme cartridge became available that attaches to feeding tube sets, which simplifies PERT administration.

Vitamins and minerals. In CF patients, liver disease and pancreatic dysfunction lead to fat malabsorption, which predisposes these patients to deficiencies of fat-soluble vitamins A, D, E, and K and some minerals even with PERT use. Vitamin levels should be assessed at diagnosis (except the newborn) and supplemented as indicated. CF-specific vitamins contain fat and water-soluble vitamins as well as zinc to enhance absorption. Deficiencies of vitamins A, D, E, and K, which significantly affect CF patients, reduce their response to pulmonary infections.

Because bone disease is common in patients with CF and progresses with age (Rana et al, 2014), the Cystic Fibrosis foundation recommends patients be treated with cholecalciferol (D$_3$). A daily vitamin D dosage of 1500 to 2000 IU is suggested by the Endocrine Society with dosages increasing to 10,000 IU daily for CF patients 18 or older (Rogers, 2013).

It is also recommended that the CF patient be supplemented with vitamin K. Taking at least 1000 mcg/day was found to achieve an optimal status of vitamin K (Rogers, 2013).

Fat-soluble vitamin testing is important in the identification of deficiencies in CF patients with PI. Fat-soluble vitamins are supplemented routinely and annually monitored. Patients may be noncompliant with vitamin supplementation or require higher dosages (Rana et al, 2014).

Salt. Excessive sodium loss in perspiration in patients with CF predisposes them to hyponatremic dehydration under conditions of heat stress. Most patients need supplementation of sodium chloride starting in infancy. The amount of salt supplementation should be increased under circumstances such as high temperature and humidity; a dry, desert climate; strenuous exercise in hot weather; excessive sweating; fever; and presence of diarrhea or vomiting.

Zinc. Additional zinc is recommended if a deficiency is suspected in patients with an unexplained decline in growth or appetite or those with prolonged diarrhea (Schindler et al, 2015).

ASTHMA

Asthma is a chronic disorder that affects the airways and is characterized by bronchial hyper-reactivity, reversible airflow obstruction, and airway remodeling. Asthmatic symptoms include periodic episodes of chest tightness, breathlessness, and wheezing. Asthma has become more prevalent and has been increasing at the rate of 25% to 75% every decade since 1960 in westernized countries (Allan and Devereux, 2011). It affects all age groups.

Pathophysiology

Asthma is the result of a complex interaction between environmental exposures and genetics. When people are genetically susceptible, environmental factors exacerbate airway hyper-responsiveness, airway inflammation, and atopy (tendency to develop allergic reaction), which eventually leads to asthma.

Environmental factors that are linked to the development of asthma include indoor allergies (dust mites, animal allergies) and outdoor allergies (pollen and fungi), exposure to tobacco smoke, air pollution, recurring respiratory infections, gastrointestinal esophageal reflux, sulfites in foods, and medication sensitivities (Fanta, 2017). A younger gestational age and a higher infant weight gain are associated with the development of asthma (Sonnenschein-van der Voort et al, 2014). Lower socioeconomic status may also be correlated with the incidence of asthma (Chen et al, 2016).

Clinicians identify three key areas when diagnosing asthma:

1. Airflow obstruction that is at least partially reversible
2. Airflow obstruction that recurs in response to a trigger
3. Symptoms consistent with asthma

Symptoms such as wheezing, coughing, shortness of breath, and chest tightness occur in most patients, and symptoms that worsen at night is a common feature. Although allergic asthma or "extrinsic asthma" is due to chronic allergic inflammation of the airways, "intrinsic asthma" is triggered by nonallergic factors such as exercise, certain chemicals, and extreme emotions (Chih–Hung Guo et al, 2012).

A life-threatening situation with markedly narrow airways, known as status asthmaticus, can result when asthma has not been treated properly. Corticosteroid therapy is often prescribed, but chronic use may place the individual at risk for osteopenia (precursor to osteoporosis), bone fractures, or steroid-induced hyperglycemia (see Appendix 13). Some evidence supports the effectiveness of sublingual immunotherapy in the treatment of asthma and rhinitis, but more studies are needed on optimal dosages (Lin et al, 2013).

Medical Management

The essential components of asthma therapy are routine monitoring of symptoms and lung function, patient education, control of environmental triggers, and pharmacotherapy.

Pharmacologic treatment must be tailored to the individual patient and is used in a stepwise manner. The medications and the regime chosen depend on the severity of the asthma, which can be classified as an acute attack, intermittent, mild persistent, moderate persistent, or severe persistent.

Quick-relief and long-term controller medications are used as therapy for asthma. Although quick-relief medications include short-acting beta agonists (bronchodilators) and steroid pills, long-term controller medications include inhaled corticosteroid, long-acting beta agonists, and leukotriene modifiers. Long-acting anticholinergics are now considered as additional therapy in those not controlled with inhaled corticosteroids (Sobieraj et al, 2018).

Inhaled corticosteroids are the cornerstone of pharmacologic management with persistent asthma. Some patients with refractory asthma need maintenance doses of systemic steroids. Because steroids change bone metabolism and the development of osteoporosis, these patients benefit from increased calcium intake. Therapies developed over the past decade for severe asthmatics focus on immunotherapy: anti-immunoglobulin E (anti-IgE), antiinterleukin-5 (anti-IL-5) antibodies, tumor necrosis factor-alpha (TNF-α) inhibitors, and macrolide antibiotics.

Antibiotics for exacerbation of asthma are not recommended by current clinical practice guidelines, because respiratory infection triggering asthma attacks are more often viral rather than bacterial.

Medical Nutrition Therapy

When treating asthma, the dietitian nutritionist addresses dietary triggers, corrects energy and nutrient deficiencies and excesses in the diet, educates the patient on a personalized diet that provides optimal levels of nutrients, monitors growth in children, and watches for food-drug interactions.

Modulation of antioxidant intake with nutritional supplementation has a beneficial effect on the severity and progression of asthma (Fabian et al, 2013). Although a slight inverse association was seen between a low vitamin E intake and wheezing symptoms, no association was found between vitamin E and asthma. Further studies are required to understand the mechanism of vitamin E on the inflammation of the immune system (Fabian et al, 2013). Low blood carotenoid levels also have been linked with asthma. A diet rich in

antioxidants and monounsaturated fats seems to have a protective effect on childhood asthma by counteracting oxidative stress (Garcia-Marcos et al, 2013). The relationship between selenium status and the incidence and severity of asthma has been inconsistent in humans so selenium supplementation is not recommended (Norton et al, 2012).

In the childhood asthma prevention study omega-3 polyunsaturated fatty acid (PUFA) fish oil was supplemented throughout childhood, and wheezing was reduced. This effect did not continue into later childhood. Supplementation of vitamin C and zinc also have been reported to improve asthma symptoms and lung function (Allan and Devereux, 2011).

Conflicting results on the efficacy of vitamin D supplementation have been reported. In one study an insufficient serum level of less than 30 ng/dL of vitamin D was associated with an increase in asthma exacerbation in the form of emergency room (ER) visits and hospitalizations (Brehm et al, 2010). In another, high doses of vitamin D supplementation were not shown to have any protective effect (Litonjua et al, 2014). Due to the conflicting results of these studies, it can be concluded that vitamin D supplementation should not be recommended at this time as therapy for asthma (Jiao and Castro, 2015).

Other nutritional interventions could potentially include use of probiotics, oral magnesium, and the Mediterranean diet. Reduced diversity or aberrant composition of the infant gut microbiota may be associated with the development of asthma in later life, so breastfeeding is recommended to ensure growth of healthy microbiota (Milani et al, 2017; Hendaus et al, 2016). A nutritionally healthy diet such as the Mediterranean diet may help prevent asthma during childhood (Hendaus et al, 2016). In a small study of 55 males and females with mild to moderate asthma, supplementing with 340 mg magnesium/ day (in two divided doses of 170 mg) for 6 months reduced bronchial reactivity and improved pulmonary function tests (Kazaks et al, 2010).

A higher than desirable BMI during childhood is associated with a significant increase in the development of asthma. Institution of diets that help with weight loss in asthmatic obese children seem to show improvements with the control of asthma, static lung function, and improved quality of life (Gibson et al, 2013). However, a large study of adult obese asthmatics found that the degree of weight loss needed to improve cardiometabolic risk factors was not enough to enhance asthma control (Ma et al, 2015).

Gastroesophageal reflux disease (GERD) and food allergens are the two most common dietary triggers for asthma. GERD is highly prevalent in asthmatic patients. A critical component of MNT for asthmatic patients is a diet free of known irritants such as spicy foods, caffeine, chocolate, and acidic foods (see Chapter 26). Limiting the intake of high fat foods and portion control can prevent gastric secretions, which exacerbate GERD.

Food allergens and food additives are other potential dietary triggers for asthma. An IgE-mediated reaction to a food protein can lead to bronchoconstriction. Completely avoiding the allergenic food protein is the only dietary treatment currently available for food allergies. Some sulfites, such as potassium metabisulfite and sodium sulfide, used in the processing of foods have been found to be a trigger for asthmatics (Gaur et al, 2013)

Some asthma patients need maintenance oral steroids, and these patients are prone to develop drug-nutrient interaction problems. Due to risk of developing osteoporosis while on long-term steroids, intakes of 1000 mg calcium/day and 600 IU Vitamin D is suggested for children ages 4-17 (Buckley, 2017).

CHRONIC OBSTRUCTIVE PULMONARY DISEASE

Chronic obstructive pulmonary disease (COPD) is now the third most common cause of death in the world and is predicted to be the fifth most common cause of disability by 2020 (Burney et al, 2014). Smoke from cigarettes is a major risk factor, along with that from biomass fuel used for cooking and heating in rural areas of developing countries. Occupational smoke or dust, air pollution, and genetic factors are also factors in the development of COPD (Table 33.1). Patients with COPD suffer from decreased food intake and malnutrition that causes respiratory muscle weakness, increased disability, increased susceptibility to infections, and hormonal alterations.

Pathophysiology

COPD is a term that encompasses chronic bronchitis (a long-term condition of COPD in which inflamed bronchi lead to mucus, cough, and difficulty breathing) and emphysema (a form of long-term lung disease characterized by the destruction of lung parenchyma with lack of elastic recoil). These conditions may coexist in varying degrees and are generally not reversible. Fig. 33.7 shows the overlap between these three conditions: asthma, chronic bronchitis, and emphysema. Asthma-COPD overlap syndrome (ACOS) is a new entity that entails those who have features of both COPD and asthma. ACOS was recognized in 2015 by the Global Initiative for Chronic Obstructive Lung Disease (GOLD) and Global Initiative for Asthma (GINA).

Patients with primary emphysema suffer from greater dyspnea and cachexia. On the other hand patients with bronchitis have hypoxia, hypercapnia (increased amount of CO_2), and complications such as pulmonary hypertension and right heart failure (Papaioannou et al, 2013).

Alpha-1 antitrypsin deficiency is present in 1% to 2% of COPD patients and is likely underrecognized. COPD exacerbations can be caused by *Haemophilus influenzae*, *Moraxella catarrhalis*, *Streptococcus pneumonia*, rhinovirus, coronavirus, and to a lesser degree, organisms such as *P. aeruginosa*, *S. aureus*, Mycoplasma spp., and *Chlamydia pneumoniae*. Allergies, smoking, congestive heart failure, pulmonary embolism, pneumonia, and systemic infections are the reason for 20% to 40% of COPD exacerbations (Nakawah et al, 2013).

Prolonged tobacco use is associated with an increased risk of having COPD besides other respiratory disorders (Liu et al, 2015). Osteoporosis in COPD patients not only predisposes patients to painful vertebral fractures but also affects lung function by altering the configuration of the chest wall. Frequent acute exacerbations in COPD patients increase the severity of chronic system inflammation. This leads to bone loss by inhibiting bone metabolism. Lack of sun

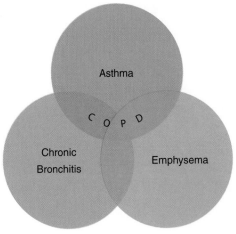

Fig. 33.7 The overlap of asthma, chronic bronchitis, and emphysema making up chronic obstructive pulmonary disease (COPD).

exposure and physical activity with COPD leads to a lack of 25-hydroxy vitamin D (25[OH]D), which regulates bone metabolism by promoting the absorption of calcium (Xiaomei et al, 2014).

Factors that influence the prognosis of COPD are the severity of disease, genetic predisposition, nutritional status, environmental exposures, and acute exacerbations.

Medical Management

In general, COPD therapies have a limited effect compared with therapies for asthma. With the exception of smoking cessation, no disease-modifying medications exist that can change the progression of airway obstruction in COPD. The airflow obstruction in COPD is irreversible.

Inhaled bronchodilators remain the mainstay of treatment for COPD patients. Usually these are given by metered dose inhalers (MDI), but for severe dyspnea or those unable to use inhalers (i.e., arthritis, cognitive dysfunction), they may be administered in a nebulized form. Anticholinergic medications such as ipratropium bromide or Spiriva (tiotropium bromide), a long-acting anticholinergic agent with specificity for muscarinic receptors, can be added to the treatment. Theophylline continues to be used but less often due to associated toxicity. Inhaled steroids and a trial of oral steroids may be required for some patients. Antibiotics often are prescribed when an exacerbation is considered to be due to bacterial infection.

Acute exacerbation of COPD is associated with adverse effects such as declining lung function, reduced quality of life, and increased mortality. In many institutions, reducing early (≤30 days) readmission for COPD has become a health care policy goal. Identifying reasons for readmissions are important. Some of these reasons include depression, smoking, anxiety, GERD, reduced functional status, unwillingness to use oxygen, and malnutrition.

Pulmonary hypertension is a risk factor that shortens life expectancy and is common in advanced COPD. The first step in treating pulmonary hypertension in patients with COPD is appropriate medical management of their obstructive lung disease, as mentioned earlier.

Patients with low oxygen levels (hypoxemic) need supplemental oxygen. Pulmonary rehabilitation may be helpful in advanced COPD. Patients with severe COPD may suffer respiratory failure related to complications such as pneumothorax, pneumonia, and congestive

TABLE 33.1 Risk Factors for Chronic Obstructive Pulmonary Disease (COPD)

Definite	Probable
Tobacco smoking	Pulmonary tuberculosis
Occupational exposure	Repeated lower respiratory infection during childhood
Exposure to biomass fuel smoke	
Environmental tobacco smoke	Poorly treated asthma

Adapted from Gupta D, et al: Guidelines for diagnosis and management of chronic obstructive pulmonary disease: Joint ICS/NCCP (I) recommendations, *Lung India* 30:228, 2013.

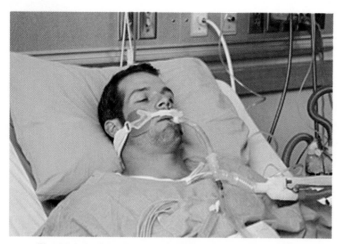

Fig. 33.8 An intensive care unit (ICU) patient on ventilator.

heart failure, or due to uncontrolled administration of high-dose oxygen or narcotic sedatives. The patients in respiratory failure need mechanical ventilation (Fig. 33.8).

In addition to facing major physical impairment and chronic dyspnea, COPD patients are at an increased risk of developing depression that should be identified and treated.

Medical Nutrition Therapy

Malnutrition is a common problem associated with COPD, with prevalence rates of 30% to 60% due to the extra energy required by the work of breathing and frequent and recurrent respiratory infections. Breathing with normal lungs expends 36 to 72 kcal/day; it increases 10-fold in patients with COPD (Hill et al, 2013). Infection with fever increases metabolic rate even further (see Chapter 2). Malnourished patients, identified as those having decreased body weight, reduced fat-free body mass, or a BMI ≤20 kg/m², are likely to have more COPD exacerbations and a shorter survival time than those who are well-nourished (Itoh et al, 2013). Increasing energy intake can maintain or improve muscle strength and exercise tolerance in these patients (Itoh et al, 2013).

Low body weight is due to poor nutritional intake, an increased metabolic rate, or both. Inadequate food intake and poor appetite are the primary targets for intervention in patients with COPD. These two issues are the reasons COPD patients struggle to meet their nutritional needs. Depletion of protein and vital minerals such as calcium, magnesium, potassium, and phosphorus contribute to respiratory muscle function impairment. In severe malnutrition inadequate electrolyte repletion during aggressive nutrition repletion can lead to severe metabolic consequences related to refeeding syndrome (see Chapter 12).

There are two main goals in managing the hypermetabolism seen in stable COPD: (1) the prevention of weight loss and (2) the prevention of the loss of lean body mass (LBM). These goals can be achieved by ensuring the following:

- Small frequent meals that are nutritionally dense
- The patient eats the main meal when energy level is at its highest
- Adequate calories, protein, vitamins, and minerals to maintain a desirable weight—a BMI of 20 to 24 kg/m²
- Availability of foods that require less preparation and can be heated easily in a microwave oven if patients prepare their own food

- Limitation of alcohol to fewer than 2 drinks/day (30 g alcohol)
- A period of rest before mealtimes

People with COPD suffer a poor prognosis when they have malnutrition that predisposes them to infections. The ability to produce lung surfactant, exercise tolerance, and respiratory muscle force are reduced in the presence of infection. Weight loss leads to an increased load on the respiratory muscles, contributing to the onset of acute respiratory failure (Hill et al, 2013).

Many factors affect nutritional status during the progression of COPD. Although body weight and BMI should be followed because they are easily obtained markers of nutritional status in patients, they can underestimate the extent of nutritional impairment (Hill et al, 2013).

Current evidence suggests that a healthy diet pattern helps in protecting smokers against malnutrition. A combination of nutritional counseling and nicotine replacement seems to optimize success (Hill et al, 2013).

Studies have shown an inverse relationship between dietary iron and calcium intake and COPD risk. Iron deficiency anemia is seen in 10% to 30% of patients with COPD (Silverberg et al, 2014). It has been seen that correcting the anemia and iron deficiency by either blood transfusions or intravenous iron therapy improves dyspnea (shortness of breath) in COPD patients (Silverberg et al, 2014). COPD patients are also at higher risk of developing osteoporosis resulting from steroid usage, smoking, and vitamin D depletion. Maintaining adequate levels of 25(OH)D is important for COPD patients (Lee et al, 2013; see Appendix 38).

The primary goals of nutrition care for patients with COPD are to facilitate nutritional well-being, maintain an appropriate ratio of LBM to adipose tissue, correct fluid imbalance, manage drug-nutrient interactions (see Appendix 13), and prevent osteoporosis.

Nutritional depletion may be evidenced clinically by low body weight for height and decreased grip strength. Calculation of BMI may be insufficient to detect changes in fat and muscle mass. Instead, determination of body composition helps to differentiate lean muscle mass from adipose tissue and overhydration from dehydration. In patients with cor pulmonale (increased blood pressure that leads to enlargement and failure of the right ventricle of the heart) and the resultant fluid retention, weight maintenance, or gain from fluid may camouflage actual wasting of LBM. Thus for patients retaining fluids, careful interpretation of anthropometric measurements, biochemical indicators, and functional measures of nutrition status are necessary (see Chapter 5 and Appendices 11 and 12).

A combination of protein rich supplements and anabolic steroids can increase muscle mass and reverse any negative effects of weight loss. Exercise tolerance has been shown to improve with a dietary supplement that contains omega-3 PUFA, which has antiinflammatory effects (Berman, 2011) (see Chapter 7).

Adipokines is a generic term for the bioactive proteins that are secreted by adipocytes. They include adiponectin, leptin, IL-6, and TNF-α. They play a vital role in influencing the nutritional status and regulating the appetite. Leptin (satiety hormone) is secreted promptly in response to food intake and plays a role in suppressing appetite and enhancing energy expenditure. It has been suggested that measuring levels of leptin in the sputum can be useful in determining the severity of lung disease because it has been shown to increase during acute exacerbations (Itoh et al, 2013). Adiponectin (a protein involved in fatty acid breakdown and glucose regulation), like leptin, is secreted from adipocytes, but has an opposite effect. Adiponectin enhances appetite and has an antiinflammatory, antidiabetic, and antiatherosclerotic effect and is considered beneficial.

TABLE 33.2 Blood Levels of Hormones and Adipokines in Patients with Chronic Obstructive Pulmonary Disease (COPD)

Hormone	Function	Changes in Blood Levels with COPD
Leptin	• Suppresses appetite • Promotes inflammation • Regulates hematopoiesis, angiogenesis, and wound healing	Decreased in patients with a low BMI compared with patients with a normal and high BMI
Ghrelin	Stimulates appetite and release of growth hormone	Increased in underweight patients compared with normal weight patients
Adiponectin	• Stimulates fatty acid oxidation • Increases insulin sensitivity and inhibits inflammatory process	Increased during acute exacerbation Decreased levels in current smokers
Resistin	Promotes inflammation and insulin resistance by the production of IL-6 and TNF-α	Inversely correlated with predicted FEV_1 %
TNF-α	Antagonizes insulin signaling and promotes inflammation	Increased compared with healthy individuals
IL-6	• Loss of appetite • Promotes inflammation	Increased compared with healthy individuals

BMI, Body mass index; *FEV₁,* forced expiratory volume; *IL-6,* interleukin-6; *TNF-α,* tumor necrosis factor alpha.
Adapted from Itoh M, et al: Undernutrition in patients with COPD and its treatment, *Nutrients* 5:1316, 2013.

Resistin, another adipokine, induces inflammation and insulin resistance. In addition to being an appetite stimulant, **ghrelin** also stimulates growth hormone secretion, with antagonistic effects to leptin. Table 33.2 summarizes the functions and change in the blood levels of these adipokines in COPD patients, and how they can influence management and recovery (Itoh et al, 2013).

Macronutrients

In stable COPD, requirements for water, protein, fat, and carbohydrate are determined by the underlying lung disease, oxygen therapy, medications, weight status, and any acute fluid fluctuations. Attention to the metabolic side effects of malnutrition and the role of individual amino acids is necessary. Determination of a specific patient's macronutrient needs is made on an individual basis, with close monitoring of outcomes.

Energy

Meeting energy needs can be difficult. For patients participating in pulmonary rehabilitation programs, energy requirements depend on the intensity and frequency of exercise therapy and can be increased or decreased. It is crucial to remember that energy balance and nitrogen balance are intertwined. Consequently, maintaining optimal energy balance is essential to preserving visceral and somatic proteins. Preferably, indirect calorimetry should be used to determine energy needs and to prescribe and monitor the provision of sufficient, but not excessive calories. When energy equations are used for prediction of needs, increases for physiologic stress must be included. Caloric needs may vary significantly from one person to the next and even in the same individual over time (see Chapter 2).

Fat

Omega-3 and omega-6 are PUFAs that are essential fatty acids. The simplest forms of these fatty acids are the omega-6 linoleic acid (LA) and alpha-linolenic acid (ALA). The body is unable to synthesize them, and they must be consumed in the human diet. These fatty acids are desaturated to form long-chain omega-3 PUFAs or omega-6 PUFAs. Docosahexaenoic acid (DHA), eicosapentaenoic acid (EPA), and ALA are the major omega-3 PUFAs, and the major long-chain omega-6 fatty acids are LA and arachidonic acid (AA). See Appendix 26 for the sources of these fatty acids in the diet. In theory, intake of long-chain omega-3 PUFAs, which reduces inflammation,

should improve the efficacy of COPD treatments. PUFA supplementation is beneficial in COPD, but various factors such as supplement adherence, comorbidities, and duration of the supplementation play vital roles (Fulton et al, 2013).

Dietary supplementation of DHA and AA has been shown to delay and reduce risk of upper respiratory infections and asthma, with lowering the incidence of bronchiolitis during the first year of life (Shek et al, 2012). Data from various studies have shown the positive impact of long-chain PUFAs in initiating and providing resolution of inflammation in respiratory diseases (Shek et al, 2012). It has been shown that aspirin helps to trigger resolvin, a molecule naturally made by the body from omega-3 fatty acids. **Resolvin** resolves or turns off the inflammation in underlying destructive conditions such as inflammatory lung diseases (Dalli et al, 2013). At this time, there are ongoing large studies evaluating the effectiveness of omega-3 PUFAs in the treatment of COPD.

Protein

Sufficient protein of 1.2 to 1.5 g/kg of dry body weight is necessary to maintain or restore lung and muscle strength, as well as to promote immune function. Other concurrent disease processes such as cardiovascular or renal disease, cancer, or diabetes affect the total amounts, ratios, and kinds of protein, fat, and carbohydrate prescribed.

Vitamins and Minerals

As with macronutrients, vitamin and mineral requirements for individuals with stable COPD depend on the underlying pathologic conditions of the lung, other concurrent diseases, medical treatments, weight status, and bone mineral density. For people continuing to smoke tobacco, additional vitamin C is necessary (see Appendix 35). One study indicated that vitamin C's role as an antioxidant improved plasma glutathione levels (Pirabbasi et al, 2016).

The role of minerals such as magnesium and calcium in muscle contraction and relaxation may be important for people with COPD. Intakes at least equivalent to the dietary reference intake (DRI) should be provided. Depending on bone mineral density test results, coupled with food intake history and glucocorticoid medications use, additional vitamins D and K also may be necessary (see Chapter 23).

Patients with cor pulmonale and subsequent fluid retention require sodium and fluid restriction. Depending on the diuretics prescribed, increased potassium supplementation may be required (Appendix 13).

BOX 33.2 Planning the Diet for the Patient with Pulmonary Cachexia

Energy requirements during healing = 30 kcal/kg of usual body weight or 13.7 cal/usual body weight (pounds)

Protein (g)/day during healing = [(1.2 g − 1.4 g) × body weight (kg) or 0.55 × usual body weight (pounds)

Fluid requirements = body weight (lb)/2 = ounces per day or body weight (lb) × 9/16 = cups per day

Fluid requirements are increased because of fever, chemotherapy regimen, oxygen use, and presence of chronic obstructive pulmonary disease (COPD). Lack of energy or dehydration increases fatigue and constipation. Fluid deficits of 1% body weight lower metabolic function by 5%.

Levin RM: *Nutrition in the patient with lung cancer, caring ambassadors lung cancer choices* (website). http://lungcancercap.org/wp-content/uploads/2014/10/Chapter_8_2014.pdf, 2012.

And other water-soluble vitamins, particularly thiamin, may need to be supplemented.

Patients are recommended to drink adequate fluids and stay hydrated to help sputum consistency and easier expectoration. The Parenteral and Enteral Nutrition Group (PENG) recommends a fluid intake of 35 mL/kg body weight daily for adults 18 to 60 years and 30 mL of fluid/kg body daily for adults over 60 years (PENG, 2011).

COPD patients report difficulties with eating because of low appetite, increased breathlessness when eating, difficulty shopping and preparing meals, dry mouth, early satiety and bloating, anxiety and depression, and fatigue. In addition to the above, inefficient and overworking respiratory muscles lead to increased nutritional requirements (Evans, 2012).

Patients in the Advanced Stage of COPD

Patients with advanced COPD are undernourished and in a state of pulmonary cachexia, which is defined as a BMI of less than 17 in men and less than 14 in women (Allen et al, 2017). The cause of cachexia in advanced COPD is poorly understood. The role for myostatin has been suggested. Myostatin is a member of the transforming growth factor-beta superfamily that functions as a negative regulator of muscle growth. This has been suggested by the significantly high levels of myostatin in patients with stable COPD compared with healthy individuals (Benedik et al, 2011).

These cachectic patients have anorexia as a typical symptom. Pulmonary cachexia is an independent risk factor and is common in the advanced stage of COPD. Pharmacotherapy and nonpharmacotherapeutic treatments such as respiratory rehabilitation and nutrition counseling are the mainstays of COPD treatment in such patients (Itoh et al, 2013). Sarcopenia and cachexia result from the accelerated loss of lean tissue (Raguso and Luthy, 2011). This muscle wasting has a detrimental effect on the respiratory function (Collins et al, 2012).

Osteoporosis exists as a significant problem in 24% to 69% of patients with advanced COPD (Evans and Morgan, 2014). Any sudden drop in height is a mark of developing osteoporosis. As COPD progresses, osteoporosis results because of immobility, which also leads to deconditioning and dyspnea. Smoking, low BMI, low skeletal muscle mass, and corticosteroid usage can lead to bone loss along with low serum vitamin D levels (Evans and Morgan, 2014) (Box 33.2).

PULMONARY HYPERTENSION

Pulmonary hypertension (PH) is defined as elevated pressure within the pulmonary circulation that includes the pulmonary artery,

capillaries, and pulmonary veins. The pulmonary artery takes deoxygenated blood from the right ventricle into the small capillaries, where gas exchange takes place, and oxygenated blood returns via the pulmonary vein into the left atrium.

Patients with PH usually complain of shortness of breath, mainly on exertion. As the disease advances, the shortness of breath becomes more prominent even at rest, and patients have symptoms related to hypoxia such as headache, dizziness, and chest pain. Upon evaluation by a pulmonologist or cardiologist, some of the important signs to look for would include cardiac murmur, right-sided ventricular heave (the heel of hand lifts off the chest with every beat, indicating an enlarged right ventricle), loud heart sound, and an elevated jugular vein pressure. Cyanosis can be evident with worsening hypoxia. Cyanosis occurs when hemoglobin is inadequately saturated with oxygen, and it is characterized by a bluish discoloration of the skin, nails, lips, or around the eyes.

An echocardiogram (ECHO) is usually the screening tool for PH. ECHO is used to measure the right ventricle function and to measure the right ventricle systolic pressure (RVSP), which can be used to estimate pulmonary artery systolic pressure. A RVSP >50 mm Hg suggests an elevated pulmonary systolic pressure and will need confirmation by direct measurements of the pulmonary artery pressure, using right heart catheterization.

Elevated pulmonary circulation pressure can occur due to primary pulmonary artery disease (primary PH) or secondary to pulmonary or extrapulmonary diseases. In 2013 the World Health Organization (WHO) classified PH into five categories (Hopkins and Rubin, 2018).

Category 1: Pulmonary arterial hypertension; PH due to autoimmune disorders, human immunodeficiency virus (HIV), toxins, drugs, sickle cell disease; porto-PH

Category 2: PH due to left heart disease

Category 3: PH due to underlying lung disease such as COPD, interstitial pulmonary fibrosis (scar tissue in the lungs)

Category 4: chronic thromboembolic PH

Category 5: multifactorial and unclear mechanisms leading to PH. Examples include sarcoidosis (a condition that can lead to inflammation primarily in the lung and the lymph nodes)

Medical Management

Treatment of PH largely depends on the cause of the elevated pulmonary pressure. Those with category 1 can benefit from keeping oxygen above 90% and with medical therapy to reduce the pressure by acting directly on pulmonary circulation. Those with categories 2 and 3 will need to treat the underlying cause. Patients with category 4 require anticoagulation therapy and may benefit from mechanical or medical thrombolysis of their clots. Treatment for patients in category 5 depends on the underlying disorder.

Medical Nutrition Therapy

There is no evidence-based guidelines or research in this area. Nutrition interventions should be directed at the underlying cause of PH such as sodium and fluid restriction for those with left-sided heart failure or improving oral intake in persons with COPD. Persons with PH can have nutritional statuses ranging from malnutrition to overnutrition, so nutrition interventions should be designed to diagnose and correct these issues accordingly.

DIFFUSE PARENCHYMAL LUNG DISEASE

Diffuse parenchymal lung disease (DPLD) (also known as interstitial lung diseases [ILD]) is common and more recognized now with advances that have been made in imaging. DPLD comprises a long list of diseases and can be primary or secondary due to other systemic disorders or medications. Patients typically complain of chronic shortness of breath, nonproductive cough, and fatigue. If the disease advances, patients become hypoxic, requiring oxygen, and are limited in their physical activity. The prognosis for these diseases vary due to the underlying cause and the response to treatment.

Idiopathic pulmonary fibrosis (IPF) is the most common ILD and is associated with the worst prognosis. IPF is a chronic progressive disease characterized by progressive lung scarring. The incidence of IPF is 0.22 to 8.8/100,000 in the United States. Men are affected more than women. Patients with IPF commonly present in the sixth and seventh decades of life. Typical symptoms are chronic shortness of breath that progresses and nonproductive cough. Pulmonary function tests show restrictive pattern with reduced volumes. The diagnosis of IPF includes the following:

1. Exclusion of known causes of ILD such as medication, environmental exposure, or systemic disorders
2. Symptoms that are consistent with IPF such as chronic progressive shortness of breath, nonproductive cough, and hypoxia
3. CT scan consistent with IPF pattern
4. If diagnosis remains uncertain, then open lung biopsy and histologic confirmation are necessary

Pathophysiology

Most cases of IPF are sporadic although some genetic component has been described. Risk factors for IPF include smoking and exposures to metals and some organic dusts. Gastroesophageal reflux may contribute to the progression of the disease (Lederer and Martinez, 2018).

Medical Management

The evaluation and management of IPF requires a pulmonologist, radiologist, and pathologist. Investigations need to rule out other diseases that could mimic IPF and to assess the severity of the disease. Lung biopsy is not always required if secondary causes were excluded and CT scan is consistent with all the radiographic features of IPF.

The medical management of IPF can be divided into acute and chronic courses. IPF slowly progresses over time without clear understanding. Patients are usually recommended to start treatment with antifibrotic medications early in the course with the goal to slow down progression of the disease. Currently, two antifibrotic medications are used in the United States (pirfenidone, nintedanib). Pirfenidone is associated with rash, photosensitivity, and possible gastrointestinal disturbances such as diarrhea, nausea, vomiting, or abdominal discomfort. Dose adjustment may help relieve some of these symptoms. Nintedanib is associated with more gastrointestinal side effects with diarrhea occurring in up to 60% of the patients; consequently, antidiarrheal agents are usually prescribed at the same time. Other less common adverse effects include nausea, vomiting, and elevated liver enzymes.

Those with acute presentation usually are admitted to the intensive care unit (ICU) due to increased oxygen requirements. Their management is most often supportive care. High doses of steroids were used in the past with conflicting results and therefore are not always recommended. Patients who become more symptomatic and worsen quickly might benefit from an early referral to a lung transplant center.

Pulmonary Diagnostic Tests

Pulmonary Function Tests (PFT): includes spirometry, measuring lung volumes, and diffusion capacity. Used to diagnose asthma and COPD and to assess severity of lung disease such as ILD.

Chest Radiograph (chest x-ray)

Computed Tomography (CT) Scan: scans cross-section of chest. More accurate and higher sensitivity and specificity compared with chest x-ray. Greater radiation exposure than chest x-ray.

Bronchoscopy: Scope with a camera is inserted in the mouth or nose and goes through the upper airways and trachea. Used for airway examination, sampling fluid for infection workup, and biopsies to rule out malignancies or sarcoidosis.

Lung Biopsy: either by bronchoscopy or more invasive approach in the operating room by using video-assisted thoracoscopic surgery (VATS) and requiring general anesthesia.

Medical Nutrition Management

At this time, there are neither evidenced-based guidelines nor research studies specifically for patients with IPF. Patients with IPF can have weights varying from being underweight to obese, so nutrition interventions should be designed to diagnose and correct nutritional abnormalities. Pulmonary cachexia syndrome can occur similar to that seen in persons with COPD and is due to hypoxemia, low-grade inflammation, and corticosteroid use (Allen et al, 2017). As shortness of breath worsens, oral intake begins to decline so the suggestions for improving intake for persons with COPD may be appropriate for patients with IPF:

- small frequent meals
- consumption of main meal when energy level is at its highest
- adequate calories, protein, vitamins, and minerals to achieve appropriate weight
- use of foods that are easily prepared (i.e., microwave)
- use of protein and calorie dense liquid nutritional supplements, homemade or premade, if oral intake is poor

Sometimes, chewing becomes tiring for patients who are short of breath. Changing the diet to softer foods or relying more on nutritionally adequate liquid supplements to ensure adequate nutrition may be necessary nutrition interventions.

TUBERCULOSIS

Mycobacterium tuberculosis, the causative organism of tuberculosis (TB), is an intracellular bacterial parasite, has a slow rate of growth, is an obligate aerobe, and induces a granulomatous response in the tissues of a normal host.

Even though TB is not as common in the United States as in some other countries, there has been a resurgence associated with HIV and drug-resistant forms of TB (see Chapter 36). In 2017 the WHO estimated approximately 10.4 million individuals became ill with TB and 1.7 million died. According to the WHO, multidrug resistant TB accounted for approximately 600,000 cases of TB worldwide.

Pathophysiology

When an infectious TB patient coughs, the cough droplets contain tuberculous bacilli. Small particles penetrate deep into the lungs. Each of these tiny droplets may carry 1 to 5 bacilli, which are enough to establish infection. This is the reason why cases of active TB must be isolated in an airborne infection isolation room (a room with a ventilation system that creates negative pressure by allowing air to enter the room but not leave it). This form of isolation should continue until patients become noninfectious. In about 5% of cases, the infection progresses and produces active TB. In 95% of cases when a host has an effective cell-mediated immune response, the infection is contained. When patients with active TB are left untreated, they can die as a result of progression and complications (Hood, 2013).

Although there may be minimal symptoms and the diagnosis is suspected because of an abnormal chest radiograph, most patients with pulmonary TB present with chronic cough, prolonged fever, night sweats, anorexia, and weight loss.

Medical Management

An important component of management is to place these patients in respiratory isolation to prevent spread of infection until the smear for sputum acid fast bacillus (AFB) comes back negative. As soon as the diagnosis is established, treatment with four anti-TB medications—INH, rifampin, pyrazinamide, and ethambutol—is started. Each drug has food-nutrient interactions (see Appendix 13). These medications are continued for 2 months, and then only rifampin and INH are continued for an additional 4 months. Duration of treatment may be longer in some patients.

Medical Nutrition Therapy

Malnutrition is common in patients with pulmonary TB, and nutritional supplementation is necessary. Protein status can be assessed by looking at blood levels of acute phase reactants (inflammatory proteins) (see Table 5.4 in Chapter 5), anthropometric indices, and the micronutrient status of TB patients (Miyata et al, 2013).

TB leads to or worsens any preexisting condition of malnutrition and increases catabolism. The WHO guidelines suggest hospitalization of patients who are severely undernourished due to increased risk of death. Dietary supplementation is recommended until the patient achieves a BMI of 18.5 (Bhargava et al, 2013).

Active TB is associated with weight loss, cachexia, and low serum concentration of leptin. There is a synergistic interaction between malnutrition and infection. Recurrent infection leads to worsening nutritional status and loss of body nitrogen. The resulting malnutrition, in turn, creates a higher susceptibility to infection (Miyata et al, 2013).

In the short term, malnutrition increases the risk of infection and early progression of infection to produce active TB. In the long term, malnutrition increases the risk of reactivation of the TB disease. Malnutrition also can lower the effectiveness of the anti-TB drug regime, which patients have to be on for several months. The efficacy of Bacillus Calmette-Guerin (BCG) vaccine can also be impaired by malnutrition.

Upon correction of nutritional deficiencies, malnutrition-induced loss of certain immune processes can be reversed rapidly. Nutritional intervention in combination with appropriate medications does improve the outcome of malnourished TB patients.

Energy

Current energy recommendations are those for undernourished and catabolic patients, 35 to 40 kcal/kg of ideal body weight. For patients with any concomitant infections such as HIV, energy requirements increase by 20% to 30% to maintain body weight.

Protein

Protein is vital in preventing muscle wasting, and an intake of 15% of energy needs or 1.2 to 1.5 g/kg ideal body weight, approximately 75 to 100 g per day, is recommended.

Vitamins and Minerals

Poor nutritional intake associated with TB will likely promote micronutrient deficiencies (Kant et al, 2015). Providing supplemental zinc, vitamin D, vitamin E, and selenium will probably increase serum levels of these nutrients but the evidence has not demonstrated significant clinical benefit (Grobler et al, 2016). Supplementing these nutrients above the recommended daily amounts seems to be unnecessary due to the unreliable evidence (Grobler et al, 2016).

Isoniazid is an antagonist of vitamin B_6 (pyridoxine) and is frequently used in TB treatment. It may cause rare instances of peripheral neuropathy resulting from the nutritional depletion of vitamin B_6. A standard procedure is to supplement adults with 25 mg of vitamin B_6 per day to overcome this drug-nutrient interaction. Vitamin B_6 supplementation will be needed for exclusively breastfed infants, malnourished children, and HIV-infected children and adolescents (Rodà et al, 2016). Research indicates some healthy children could develop mild symptom-free pyridoxine deficiency (Rodà et al, 2016).

Studies have documented an increased prevalence of anemia in TB patients, which is associated with increased risk of death. To guide clinical decision making and provide treatment recommendations, factors that contribute to the TB-associated anemia have to be determined. Although other causes do coexist, iron deficiency anemia is the most important contributor in the development of anemia in TB patients (Isanaka et al, 2012).

Iron is an essential micronutrient not only for humans but also for bacteria such as *M. tuberculosis*; TB is dependent on the host's iron supply (Carver, 2018). Providing iron either as a supplement or blood transfusion could increase risk of infection but at this time this is controversial (Carver, 2018). The use of iron therapy is not universally recommended. However, if iron studies show iron deficiency, iron therapy is then initiated (see Chapter 31 for management of iron deficiency anemia).

LUNG CANCER

Lung cancer remains the leading cause of cancer deaths for males and females in the United States. In 2012 1.8 million patients worldwide were diagnosed with lung cancer (Mannino, 2014).

Neoplasms of the lower respiratory tract are a heterogeneous group of tumors. The group commonly called bronchogenic carcinomas comprises squamous cell carcinoma, adenocarcinoma, small cell undifferentiated carcinoma, and large cell undifferentiated carcinoma and account for 90% of all the neoplasms of the lower respiratory tract. Mortality is more common in males than females, although this difference is diminishing. While the female incidence rate is stabilizing, the male incidence rate seems to be decreasing (Baldini, 2014).

Pathophysiology

Often lung cancer is detected on a routine chest radiograph in an asymptomatic smoker. Other patients may present with symptoms related to the tumor itself, symptoms related to the local extension of the tumor or widespread metastases, or systemic symptoms such as anorexia, weight loss, weakness, and paraneoplastic syndromes.

Dyspnea is the most burdensome cancer symptom and occurs in 25% to 40% of lung cancer patients at diagnosis. In addition to the tumor, other factors contribute to the symptom of dyspnea—factors such as pericardial effusion, anemia, fatigue, depression, anxiety, metastatic involvement of other organs, aspiration, anorexia-cachexia syndrome, and pleural effusion.

Patients with lung cancer suffer from progressive weight loss with changes in body composition. Malnutrition impairs the contractility of the respiratory muscles, affecting endurance and respiratory mechanics.

Cough is present in 50% to 75% of lung cancer patients at presentation and occurs most frequently in squamous cell and small cell carcinoma because of their tendency to involve central airways (Kocher et al, 2015).

Pain and fatigue are common symptoms associated with lung cancer. The tumor may produce pleuritic pain because of tumor extension into the pleura, or musculoskeletal type pain because of extension into the chest wall. Bone pain may occur as a result of metastases to the bones. Bone metastases in patients with lung cancer account for 30% to 40% of the pain. About 50% of early stage cancer and 75% to 100% of advanced stage cancer patients report fatigue (Kocher et al, 2015).

Pulmonary cachexia syndrome affects patients with advanced lung disease. In lung cancer, weight loss is associated with increasing mortality, and weight loss of even 5% indicates a poor prognosis. Although anorexia and cachexia are two different entities, they often are used interchangeably (Kocher et al, 2015) (see Chapter 35).

Medical Management

The choice of definitive management for a particular patient is determined by numerous factors, such as the tumor cell type, tumor stage, resectability of the tumor, and suitability of the patient for general anesthesia and surgery. Some patients need general palliative care in terms of psychological support, control of distressing symptoms, and palliative radiation. Nutritional support plays a very important role in the management of advanced lung cancer.

Medical Nutrition Therapy

The National Comprehensive Cancer Network (NCCN) guidelines include nutritional assessments, medications, and nonpharmacologic approaches to achieve the following:

1. Treat the reversible causes of anorexia such as early satiety
2. Evaluate the rate and severity of weight loss
3. Treat the symptoms interfering with food intake: nausea and vomiting, dyspnea, mucositis, constipation, and pain
4. Assess the use of appetite stimulants like megestrol acetate and Decadron (corticosteroids)
5. Provide nutritional support (enteral or parenteral) (Del Ferraro et al, 2012)

Cancer cachexia syndrome (CCS) is the presence of a metabolic state that leads to energy and muscle store depletion in lung cancer patients. When patients experience CCS, they lose adipose and skeletal muscle mass. Changes in hormone and cytokine levels, along with tumor byproducts, cause CCS. Weight loss seen with CCS, unlike starvation, is irreversible and continues to worsen despite increased nutritional intake (Huhmann and Camporeale, 2012) (see Chapter 35).

However, despite these findings, reversible causes of anorexia should be sought and treated. Although nutritional support does not improve spirometric values and arterial blood gas and does not stop weight loss, it does modestly improve clinical outcomes such as the 6-minute walk test, quality of life, and inspiratory and expiratory muscle strength (Bellini, 2013).

Nutrition repletion is problematic in advanced lung disease because fatigue and dyspnea tend to interfere with the preparation and consumption of food. Alterations in the taste of food because of chronic sputum production, early satiety resulting from flattening of the diaphragm, nausea and indigestion resulting from side effects of medications, and lack of motivation to eat because of depression make it difficult for the patient to take adequate nutrition by the oral route. However, accepted components of oral nutrition therapy are the following:

1. Small frequent meals that are calorie and protein dense
2. Provide calorie level that meets or exceeds the resting energy expenditure (REE)
3. Rest before meals
4. Meals that require minimal preparation
5. Oral nutritional supplements (homemade or preprepared)

With pulmonary CCS, patients are unable to gain weight with nutritional interventions alone. Prokinetic agents for delayed gastric emptying can be used with careful consideration of side effects. Megestrol acetate, an appetite stimulant, may result in increasing appetite and caloric intake. Ghrelin (a growth hormone releasing peptide) lowers fat use and stimulates feeding through growth hormone independent mechanisms, thereby inducing a positive energy balance. Studies have shown that repeated intravenous (IV) administration of ghrelin improves body composition, lowers muscle wasting, and increases functional capacity (Bellini, 2013).

One study suggests that whole body protein metabolism in pulmonary patients may benefit from branched-chain amino acid (BCAA) supplementation. This study was the first of its kind in assessing the clinical benefits of supplementing BCAA in a preoperative pulmonary rehabilitation center; 6.2 g of BCAA supplementation was the recommended daily dosage. However the effect of BCAA supplementation for lung cancer patients has not been clarified and requires further study before specific recommendations can be made. A comprehensive pulmonary rehabilitation protocol includes nutritional support and physical exercise (Harada et al, 2013).

OBESITY HYPOVENTILATION SYNDROME

Obesity hypoventilation syndrome (OHS) is defined as a BMI of more than 30 kg/m^2 and alveolar hypoventilation defined by arterial CO$_2$ (Paco$_2$) level of more than 45 mm Hg during wakefulness, which occurs in the absence of other conditions that cause hypoventilation (Piper and Grunstein, 2011).

Alveolar hypoventilation in OHS is related to the multiple physiologic abnormalities associated with obesity: obstructive sleep apnea (OSA), increased work of breathing, respiratory muscle impairment, a depressed central ventilator drive, and reduced effects of neurohumoral modulators (e.g., leptin) (Koenig, 2011; Piper and Grunstein, 2011).

Obstructive sleep apnea (OSA) is a common chronic disorder, which is characterized by loud snoring, excessive daytime sleepiness, and witnessed breathing interruptions or awakenings because of gasping or choking. The presence or absence of OSA and its severity usually is confirmed by a sleep study (polysomnography) before initiating treatment (Kapur et al, 2017). The polysomnography also serves as a baseline to establish the effectiveness of the subsequent treatment (Epstein et al, 2009).

Medical Management

Depending on the number of episodes of apnea or hypopnea (overly shallow breathing) per hour, OSA is graded as mild, moderate, or severe. Patients with OSA commonly are treated with a continuous positive airway pressure (CPAP) machine, which includes a mask worn over the nose, or nose and mouth that provides oxygen under pressure to aid in breathing. These primary treatment modalities for OSA must be used in addition to weight loss because of the low success and low cure rates by dietary approach alone.

Medical Nutrition Therapy

Weight reduction by MNT or by bariatric surgery remains an important component of management of these cases (see Chapter 20). A guideline from the American Thoracic Society recommends a lifestyle intervention consisting of reduced calorie intake, exercise or increased physical activity, and behavioral guidance, stating that weight loss is associated with improvements in respiratory function, cardiometabolic comorbidities, and quality of life (Hudgel et al, 2018). In a multicenter study of patients with OSA undergoing Roux-en-Y gastric bypass surgery, OSA was reduced from 71% to 44% one year later in these patients; however, moderate to severe OSA remained in 20% of the patients (Peromaa-Haavisto et al, 2017).

PLEURAL EFFUSION

Pleural effusion is the accumulation of the fluid in the pleural space. The pleura, which is the layer that surrounds the lung, is divided into visceral and parietal layers and in between is a small space that contains about 10 to 20 mL fluid. If there is increased production or decreased drainage in the pleural space, fluid can accumulate. Pleural effusion can be either transudate or exudate (Feller-Kopman and Light, 2018). Transudate effusion is usually due to congestive heart failure, liver disease, or kidney disease, while exudate effusion may occur due to infection, malignancy, and autoimmune disorders.

Pleural effusion can be found incidentally on chest imaging in patients who are asymptomatic or can present with shortness of breath, chest pain, or symptoms related to the underlying cause such as pneumonia or congestive heart failure. Effusions can be unilateral or bilateral. Fig. 33.9 is a CT scan of a patient with bilateral pleural effusion.

Medical Management

The management of pleural effusion depends on numerous factors and usually involves drainage of the fluid either to make a diagnosis or to relieve symptoms in those with large effusions. Fluid can be drained by a procedure called thoracentesis, which can be done as an outpatient or inpatient at the bedside. Those who have recurrent effusion might benefit from a long-term therapy such as placement of an indwelling pleural catheter to drain the fluid as needed or through more invasive procedures such as injection of chemicals (talc or doxycycline) to achieve pleurodesis, which is an obliteration of the pleural space to prevent accumulation of fluid or recurrent pneumothorax.

Medical Nutrition Therapy

Neither evidence-based guidelines nor research exists for appropriate MNT for the patient with a pleural effusion. However, MNT

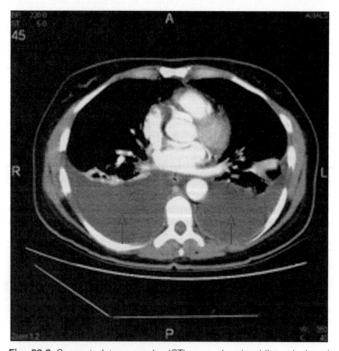

Fig. 33.9 Computed tomography (CT) scan showing bilateral pleural effusions.

interventions should be directed toward the underlying disorder causing the pleural effusion; for example, sodium and fluid restriction for the patient with congestive heart failure. Malnutrition may exist due to the primary disorder and should be appropriately diagnosed and treated.

CHYLOTHORAX

Chylothorax is a rare cause of pleural effusion. It is caused by the disruption or obstruction of the thoracic duct, which results in the leakage of chyle (lymphatic fluid of intestinal origin) into the pleural space. The fluid typically has a milky appearance. A pleural fluid triglyceride concentration of more than 110 mg/dL strongly supports the diagnosis of a chylothorax (Heffner, 2018).

Chylothorax can result from nontraumatic causes such as sarcoidosis or benign idiopathic chylothorax. It can occur because of surgical trauma such as postoperative chylothorax or postpneumonectomy chylothorax.

Medical Management

The principles of management of chylothorax are (1) treatment of the underlying condition such as sarcoidosis, infection, lymphoma, or metastatic carcinoma and (2) pleural drainage to relieve dyspnea. Those patients who do not improve by thoracentesis and dietary control measures may have to be treated by pleurodesis or thoracic duct ligation (Heffner, 2018).

Medical Nutrition Therapy

The goal of MNT is to reduce the flow of chyle, particularly in patients with low volume chylous drainage (less than one liter daily), by consuming a high-protein, low-fat (less than 10 grams) diet (Heffner, 2018). Decreasing fat intake will result in less fat to be absorbed in the gastrointestinal tract and therefore reduces chyle production. Long-chain triglycerides should be avoided. The restrictive very-low-fat diets may promote vitamin, particularly fat-soluble vitamin, and essential fatty acid deficiencies so intravenous vitamins and lipid emulsions may be needed. Very-low-fat enteral formulas are also available. If the pleural drainage decreases, medium-chain triglycerides (MCTs) could be added to the diet or enteral formula because MCTs, after absorption in the gastrointestinal tract, bypass the lymphatic system and are directly transported to the liver via the portal vein. MCTs are not very palatable and they have side effects such as gastrointestinal upset, steatorrhea, and hyperlipidemia. As the chylous drainage declines, fat intake can be gradually increased. It may take 7 to 10 days for the chylous drainage to clear. Patients with high volume chylous drainage (greater than one liter) will likely need surgery for correction. Parenteral nutrition may be needed for patients with high volume drainage and for those who do not respond to a very-low-fat intake.

ACUTE RESPIRATORY DISTRESS SYNDROME

Acute respiratory distress syndrome (ARDS) is a clinical state in which patients develop diffuse pulmonary infiltrates, severe hypoxia, and respiratory failure. Underlying clinical events such as sepsis or trauma that lead to the development of ARDS also result in a hypermetabolic state that markedly increases nutritional requirements (ARDS Definition Task Force et al, 2012).

Pathophysiology

For normal gas exchange, it is essential that dry, patent alveoli be in close proximity to capillaries. When an injury produces diffuse alveolar

TABLE 33.3 Common Clinical Conditions Associated with Acute Respiratory Distress Syndrome (ARDS)

Most Common	Less Common
Pneumonia	Drug toxicity
Sepsis	Aspiration
	Inhalation injury
	Near drowning
	Respiratory syncytial virus
	Transfusion related acute lung injury
	Trauma

Adapted from Saguil A, Fargo M: Acute respiratory distress syndrome: diagnosis and management, *Am Fam Phys* 85:352, 2012.

TABLE 33.4 Complications Resulting from Overfeeding and Underfeeding in Acute Respiratory Distress Syndrome (ARDS) Patients

Overfeeding	Underfeeding
Nosocomial infections	Nosocomial infections
Hypercapnia	Immunosuppression
Immunosuppression	Depressed respiratory muscle strength
Failure in weaning from mechanical ventilator	Failure in weaning from mechanical ventilator
Poor wound healing	Low ventilatory drive
Electrolyte imbalance	
Azotemia	

Adapted from Krzak A, et al: Nutrition therapy for ALI and ARDS, *Crit Care Clin* 27:647, 2011.

damage, proinflammatory cytokines are released. These cytokines promote migration of neutrophils to the lungs, where they become activated and release toxic mediators, which produce further damage to the alveolar epithelium and capillary endothelium. This damage allows protein to escape into the interstitium. Alveoli get filled with bloody, proteinaceous fluid which interferes with gas exchange, and severe, refractory hypoxemia results. Various clinical conditions can lead to the development of ARDS (Table 33.3).

Patients with ARDS present with acute onset of shortness of breath, tachypnea, and hypoxemia, which is refractory to oxygen supplementation.

Medical Management

The principles of ARDS management are the following (Siegel, 2013):
- Treatment of underlying cause such as sepsis, aspiration, or bacterial pneumonia
- Mechanical ventilatory support
- ICU including sedation with or without paralytic drug
- Ensuring hemodynamic stability
- Prevention of complications such as stress ulcers (gastrointestinal prophylaxis), hyperglycemia, deep venous thrombosis, and aspiration pneumonia
- Nutritional support
- Therapies with corticosteroids, exogenous surfactant, antioxidants, and inhaled nitric oxide have been used but have not shown consistent benefit.

Medical Nutrition Therapy

Malnutrition is common in these patients who require mechanical ventilation. Patients with severe respiratory disease have increased metabolic needs and require prompt initiation of supplemental nutrition. It is important to consider issues related to energy and protein use.

Nutrition support in ARDS patients is necessary for preventing cumulative caloric deficits, loss of LBM, malnutrition, and deterioration of respiratory muscle strength (Krzak et al, 2011). According to the 2016 Society of Critical Care Medicine and American Society for Parenteral and Enteral Nutrition (SCCM/ASPEN) guidelines, a standard enteral formula can be administered and a concentrated formula may be needed for those who are fluid-overloaded or have pulmonary edema (McClave et al, 2016).

Patients with ARDS are at high risk for complications as a result of underfeeding or overfeeding (Table 33.4). Reduction in respiratory

muscle strength is a negative consequence of underfeeding, which leads to problems in weaning from mechanical ventilation. In addition, poor wound healing, immunosuppression, and risk of nosocomial (hospital acquired) infections increase related to inadequate calories and protein. Overfeeding leads to undesirable outcomes such as stress hyperglycemia, delayed weaning from mechanical ventilation, and delayed wound healing (Krzak et al, 2011). Effective MNT requires careful assessment and monitoring. See Chapter 37 for further discussion on MNT for metabolically stressed patients.

PNEUMONIA

An inflammatory condition of the lungs that causes chest pain, fever, cough, and dyspnea is called pneumonia. In the clinical setting there are various kinds of pneumonias, such as community-acquired pneumonia, which may be viral or bacterial; hospital-acquired pneumonia; pneumonia in an immune compromised host; ventilator-associated pneumonia (VAP); and aspiration pneumonia, which will be discussed here. Aspiration is a common event even in healthy adults and usually causes no deleterious effects. At least one half of healthy adults aspirate during sleep. However, when this aspirate results in pulmonary infection, it results in aspiration pneumonia (Box 33.3).

Box 33.3 Conditions That Predispose a Patient to Aspiration Pneumonia

- Impaired level of consciousness, with compromised closure of glottis and impaired cough reflex
- Dysphagia from neurologic conditions (i.e., stroke)
- Gastric reflux, disorders of or surgery on the upper gastrointestinal tract
- Mechanical disruption of the glottis closure because of endotracheal tube, tracheostomy, bronchoscopy, and interference with the cardiac sphincter by gastroduodenal endoscopy or placement of a nasogastric tube
- Miscellaneous conditions such as protracted vomiting, feeding via gastrostomy at less than a 45-degree angle, and persistent recumbent position

Bartlett JG: Aspiration pneumonia in adults. In Baslow DS, editor: Wolters Kluwer: *UpToDate*, Waltham, Mass, 2012. Retrieved from http://www.uptodate.com/contents/aspiration-pneumonia-in-adults.

Pathophysiology

Two conditions must exist for aspiration pneumonia to develop. First, there is a breach in the normal defense mechanisms, such as failure of glottis closure or impaired cough reflex, and second, a large enough inoculum enters the lungs. The aspirate contains gastric acid, which has a direct toxic effect on the lungs, particulate matter that may cause airway obstruction and atelectasis, and oral bacteria, which can result in infection and pneumonia. Pathogens such as *S. pneumonia, Haemophilus influenzae*, gram-negative bacilli, and *S. aureus* are virulent, and only a small inoculum is needed to cause pneumonia. By convention, aspiration pneumonia is caused by less-virulent organisms such as anaerobes, which are part of the normal oral flora, with predisposing situations.

Medical Management

Three clinical syndromes exist within the category of aspiration pneumonia: (1) chemical pneumonitis resulting from aspiration of acid, (2) bacterial infection, and (3) airway obstruction. The clinical features depend on which of these predominates, but often there is an overlap. The details of the management of these syndromes is beyond the scope of this chapter but an understanding of pathophysiology and predisposing conditions helps in the effective treatment and prevention of aspiration pneumonia.

Patients who are observed to have aspirated should be cleared of the fluids or food with immediate tracheal suction. However, this maneuver will not necessarily protect the lungs from chemical injury, which occurs instantly (Bartlett, 2012). The main treatment in this situation is antibiotics and to support the pulmonary function. Use of glucocorticoids in chemical pneumonitis is controversial and not usually recommended.

Aspiration pneumonia usually presents with indolent symptoms. Many patients present with complications such as lung abscess, emphysema, and necrotizing pneumonia. Once a patient has been diagnosed with aspiration pneumonia, antibiotic therapy should include coverage for anaerobic pathogens because they may cause significant disease when present (Allen et al, 2013).

Medical Nutrition Therapy

Patients with aspiration pneumonia may have dysphagia so a swallow evaluation by a speech pathologist will be needed before allowing oral intake. Diet textures and liquid viscosities may need modification to prevent further aspiration. Dysphagia diets are described in Chapter 39 and Appendix 20.

If the patient has dysphagia and must have nothing by mouth, then enteral nutrition will be the preferred route of feeding. As per the 2016 SCCM/ASPEN and the American College of Gastroenterology guidelines (McClave et al, 2016), nutritional interventions for preventing aspiration pneumonia and managing it when it exists in the patient in the acute care setting are the following:

- Direct tube feedings into the small bowel rather than the stomach for those who are at high risk for aspiration
- Implement continuous feedings rather than bolus feedings
- Elevate the head of the patient's bed to 30 to 45 degrees
- Use prokinetic agents
- Minimize use of sedatives
- Optimize oral hygiene using chlorhexidine mouthwash

Gastric residuals volumes have been found not to correlate with incidences of aspiration. Also coloring agents, including blue food coloring, should not be used as markers of aspiration due to their potential toxicity.

LUNG TRANSPLANTATION

Lung transplantation was done for the first time in 1963 with good pulmonary results but the patient died 18 days after transplant due to comorbidities and malnutrition. Subsequently, multiple lung transplants were done without evaluating outcomes compared with other solid organ transplants. In the past, one of the main obstacles associated with lung transplantation was the type of immunosuppression required with the high dose of steroids that can affect airway anastomosis healing. Over the last 20 years, the number of lung transplants performed increased rapidly with 4122 lung transplants done in 2015. Outcomes have improved with better donor and recipient selection, surgical techniques, and medical therapy. The current median survival for lung transplant patients is about 5.5 years with chronic rejection being the most common complication.

Major indications for lung transplant are the following:
- COPD
- Idiopathic interstitial pneumonia (most commonly IPF)
- CF
- Pulmonary arterial hypertension
- Alpha-1 antitrypsin deficiency

Multiple factors are considered when a patient is being evaluated for lung transplantation; nutritional status is an important factor. Patients usually get referred to a registered dietitian nutritionist (RDN) before being listed for transplant. Nutritional status can adversely impact posttransplant outcomes. Patients with class I obesity (BMI: 30 to 34.9 kg/m^2) are relatively contraindicated while those with class II obesity (BMI: >35 kg/m^2) are absolutely contraindicated. A low BMI has not been a risk factor for mortality after lung transplantation (Weill et al, 2015). However, multiple studies have shown that malnutrition or a low BMI <18 kg/m^2 can be associated with worse outcomes (Christie et al, 2012; Lederer et al, 2009).

Medical Nutrition Therapy

As stated above, nutritional status plays a crucial role in a patient's hospital course and survival after lung transplantation. The pretransplant assessment by the RDN will determine the presence of malnutrition, and the nutrition interventions should include plans to correct the nutritional status. Postoperatively, the immediate concern is adequate nutrition for wound healing and recovery. Immunosuppressant medications have multiple adverse effects, some of which have nutritional implications that will need attention, including the need for education abut food safety.

BRONCHOPULMONARY DYSPLASIA

Bronchopulmonary dysplasia (BPD) is a chronic lung disease most commonly seen in premature infants who require mechanical ventilation and oxygen therapy for acute respiratory distress. BPD occurs in 40% of preterm neonates less than or equal to 28 weeks gestational age (Davidson et al, 2017). BPD is a lung development disorder characterized by impairment of alveolarization. This leads to pulmonary and vascular hypoplasia with less interstitial cellularity and fibrosis (Jobe, 2011).

Common interventions have little impact on long-term outcomes, with respiratory care remaining supportive. Decreased lung compliance and increased need for respiratory support exists in these patients (Dani and Poggi, 2012).

Medical Management

Management should minimize any further injuries, while providing an optimal environment for growth and recovery (Adams and Stark, 2014).

Ongoing pulse oximetry is used to monitor oxygenation, whereas intermittent blood gas sampling monitors pH and Paco$_2$. Periodic attempts are made to progressively wean infants from ventilator support. Prolonged ventilation is associated with laryngeal injury and subglottic stenosis, especially with infants who require multiple intubations. Suctioning should be limited to only when needed because it is associated with tracheal and bronchial injury (Adams and Stark, 2014).

The use of supplemental oxygen is challenging in patients with BPD because of the need to treat hypoxemia on one hand, and on the other, to avoid exposure to excess oxygen. Increasing the inhaled oxygen concentrations could have a negative affect by increasing the risk of retinopathy, pulmonary edema, or inflammation.

Most infants are managed with a modest fluid restriction of 140 to 150 mL/kg per day. Although diuretic therapy may improve short-term pulmonary status, there is no evidence that it improves clinical outcomes. Use of diuretics leads to serum electrolyte abnormalities such as hyponatremia and hypokalemia (Adams and Stark, 2014).

Medical Nutrition Therapy

Using the criteria in Box 33.4, assessment of the infant with BPD begins with MNT. Energy needs of infants with BPD are 15% to 20% higher than those of healthy infants, and they benefit from 140 to 150 kcal/kg/day during active stages of the disease (Dani and Poggi, 2012). Inadequate caloric intake leads to a catabolic state and muscle fatigue of the diaphragm. Adequate nutrition is essential for lung growth, alveolar development, surfactant production, and protection against infections.

Infants with BPD have decreased LBM, indicating an inadequate protein intake. Treatment with corticosteroids also increases body fat and lowers protein, thereby altering the composition of weight gain. Protein intakes of 3.5 to 4.0 g/kg body weight in infants with BPD help in meeting the growth and anabolic needs (Dani and Poggi, 2012). Amino acids are administered within the first 26 hours of life because they are well tolerated, improve glucose tolerance, and create positive nitrogen balance. An amino acid requirement of 1.5 to 2 g/kg/day is suggested for term infants, 2 to 3 g/kg/day for infants at 30 to 36 weeks, and 3.6 to 4.8 g/kg/day for infants at 24 to 30 weeks (Dani and Poggi, 2012) (see Chapter 41).

Although lipids remain a vital component in providing essential fatty acids and meeting energy goals, the role of lipid administration remains controversial. Lipids are held or administered in small quantities because they can cause hyperbilirubinemia and increase the risk of kernicterus (brain dysfunction due to hyperbilirubinemia) in these infants. Lipids result in less CO$_2$ production compared with carbohydrate, and although high-fat formulas do not show a significant change in respiration in adults, infants who receive high-fat formulas exhibit decreased CO$_2$ production and improved respiration (Dani and Poggi, 2012). Further investigation is required to determine the optimal lipid intake for infants with BPD. The European Society of Pediatric Gastroenterology, Hepatology and Nutrition (ESPGHAN) recommends a reasonable range of 4.4 to 6.0 g of fat/100 kcal or 40% to 55% of caloric intake.

Sodium and potassium depletion are seen in infants with BPD who are treated with diuretics. Because sodium administration counteracts the action of diuretics, mild deficiencies in sodium and chloride are anticipated (Dani and Poggi, 2012).

Decreased bone mineralization is seen in infants with BPD. Urinary loss of calcium is increased with the administration of corticosteroids and diuretics. Osteopenia of prematurity is common in infants with BPD resulting from nutritional deficiencies of calcium and phosphorus. Enteral feeds are not useful in providing adequate amounts of calcium and phosphorus, whereas parenteral feeds restrict the intake because of limited solubility of calcium and phosphorus.

BOX 33.4 Components of Nutrition Assessment for Infants with Bronchopulmonary Dysplasia

History
Birthweight
Gestational age
Medical history
Nutrition history
Previous growth pattern

Medical Status
Respiratory status
Oxygen saturation
Use of medications
Emesis
Stool pattern
Urine output
Urine specific gravity
Ventilator dependency

Nutrition-Biochemical Measures
Anthropometrics
Weight
Length
Growth percentiles
Head circumference

Hemoglobin
Hematocrit
Serum electrolytes
C-reactive protein

Feeding History
Volume of intake
Frequency of feedings
Behavior during feedings
Formula composition
Use of solid foods
Developmental feeding milestones
Swallowing difficulty
Gastroesophageal reflux

Environmental Concerns
Parent-child interaction
Home facilities
Access to safe food supply
Community resources
Economic resources
Access to adequate food and nutrients

Infants with BPD are monitored every 1 to 2 weeks for calcium and phosphorus and it is recommended to supplement with vitamin D (Dani and Poggi, 2012) and milk fortifiers (see Chapter 41).

The use of vitamin A, corticosteroids, and caffeine have been shown to reduce BPD at 36 weeks of age. 5000 IU of vitamin A was administered intramuscularly three times a week for a month to show a significant reduction in BPD and death in those infants receiving the supplementation (Ehrenkranz, 2014).

Parenteral nutrition is continued along with enteral feeds till the feeding volume reaches 100 mL/kg/day. Starting enteral feeds earlier induces gastric motility and promotes progression to full enteral feedings. Better neurologic development in preterm infants with BPD can be accomplished with early nutrition support, appropriate enteral feeds, and parenteral feed selection (Dani and Poggi, 2012). See Chapter 41 for further discussion on feeding the low birth weight infant.

Complementary and Integrative Approaches for Pulmonary Disease

Complementary and integrative approaches for pulmonary disease usually focus on providing support for the underlying pathology, whether it is inflammation and fibrosis or excess mucous production. It also focuses on exacerbating factors such as stress and environmental exposures (such as chemicals and pollution). Chapter 7 and appendix 22 provide a review of nutrition support for inflammation. Vitamin D and Omega-3 fatty acids have shown benefit for reducing inflammation, fibrosis and exacerbations in asthma and COPD and further study is underway on the long term benefit of these supplements (Gold, 2016). A recent review on diet and asthma concluded that study results are contradictory for single nutrient interventions and the authors recommend a whole diet approach (Han, 2015). Mind body therapies such meditation, yoga, tai chi, and mindfulness based stress reduction may be helpful for reducing stress and may reduce incidence of exacerbations in patients who are able and motivated to participate (McClafferty, 2014). N-acetyl cysteine (NAC), a derivative of the amino acid cysteine, has been used as a mucolytic for airway diseases such as COPD and chronic bronchitis. A recent Cochrane review concluded that while there is a small reduction in acute exacerbations and hospitalizations, there is not a significant improvement in overall lung function or reduction in mortality with the use of NAC. The authors stated that there was a high degree of heterogenicity in study participants and design, thus making the conclusions less certain (Poole, 2019). Contradictions in research on integrative approaches may come from the need for individualized assessment. For example, people who are not nutrient deficient will not respond to supplementation or dietary interventions to boost intake of that nutrient. Additionally, single nutrient interventions, including antioxidant vitamins, are typically inadequate for treating complex conditions. For this reason, integrative interventions are usually multi-modal, including whole diet, specific nutrient and mind body therapies, and work best when the patient is a willing and active participant.

CLINICAL CASE STUDY

Ray is a 75-year-old single white male who started smoking when he was in high school and quit several years ago because his breathing was becoming more difficult. His medical history includes chronic obstructive pulmonary disease (COPD), hypertension, hyperlipidemia, and coronary artery disease requiring a stent. He was admitted to the medical intensive care unit for a COPD exacerbation, his third exacerbation in the past 6 months. Significant findings are weight 120 lb, height 5'10", blood pressure 1357/90 mm Hg, heart rate 82/minute, respiratory rate 28/minute, temperature 98.6° F, oxygen saturation 90% on 6L of O_2. Prescribed medications include an inhaled bronchodilator, antihypertensives, and a statin. Upon interviewing the patient, the registered dietitian nutritionist (RDN) learns the patient has not been eating well due to early satiety and shortness of breath, eating about 50% of usual intake in 2 meals, lost 50 lb in the past 6 months, and spends most of his day in a recliner as any physical activity leaves him breathless. His adult children bring in meals several times weekly, which he will reheat if he has the energy. Due to his limited income, he consumes no nutritional supplement, including herbal, vitamin, and mineral supplements.

Nutrition Diagnosis Statement
- Unintended weight loss related to decreased food intake due to COPD as evidenced by 50% of usual intake and weight loss of 50 lb/30% of body weight in 6 months.

Nutrition Care Questions
1. What are the interrelationships between COPD, food intake, and nutrient metabolism?
2. What are the goals of nutrition care for this patient? Keep in mind the frequency of the COPD exacerbations and their effect on the patient's prognosis.
3. What nutrition interventions can you suggest to increase intake of calories and protein? Why?
4. Due to his history of heart disease, the medical team ordered a low-fat, low-cholesterol, restricted-sodium diet for the patient. Is this diet appropriate? Why?
5. While hospitalized, what do you want to monitor to ensure the patient is making progress toward the agreed-upon nutrition goals?
6. The patient has a limited income and lives alone. Are there any food programs that may be beneficial? Also, if nutritional supplements are recommended, who will pay for them? Are there programs that will pay for them? If not, are there alternatives that are free or at a much lower price?

USEFUL WEBSITES

American Academy of Allergy, Asthma, and Immunology
American Association for Respiratory Care
American Lung Association
American Thoracic Society
Cystic Fibrosis Foundation
Cystic Fibrosis Genetic Analysis Consortium (Cystic Fibrosis Mutation Database)
National Cancer Institute (Lung Cancer)
National Institute of Diabetes and Digestive and Kidney Diseases— Cystic Fibrosis Research

REFERENCES

Adams JM, Stark AR: Management of bronchopulmonary dysplasia. In Basow DS, editor: *UpToDate*, Waltham, 2014, Mass. Available at: http://www. uptodate.com/contents/management-of-bronchopulmonary-dysplasia.

Allan K, Devereux G: Diet and asthma: nutritional implications from prevention to treatment, *J Amer Diet Assoc* 111:258–268, 2011.

Allen KS, Mehta I, Cavallazzi R: When does nutrition impact respiratory function? *Curr Gastroenterol Rep* 15:327, 2013.

Allen KS, Hoffman L, Jones K, et al: Pulmonary disease. In: Mueller CM, editor: *The ASPEN adult nutrition support core curriculum*, 3rd ed, American Society for Parenteral and Enteral Nutrition, 2017, Silver Spring, MD pp 489.

The ARDS Definition Task Force, Ranieri VM, Rubenfeld GD, et al: Acute respiratory distress syndrome: the Berlin definition, *JAMA* 307:2526–2533, 2012.

Baker RD, Coburn-Miller C, Baker SS, et al: Cystic fibrosis: nutritional issues. In Basow DS, editor: *UpToDate*, Waltham, 2013, Mass.

Baldini EH: Women and lung cancer. In Basow DS, editor: *UpToDate*, Waltham, 2014, Mass. Available at: http://www.uptodate.com/contents/women-and-lung-cancer.

Bartlett JG: Aspiration pneumonia in adults. In Baslow DS, editor: *UpToDate*, Waltham, Mass, 2012, Wolters Kluwer. Available at: http://www.uptodate.com/contents/aspiration-pneumonia-in-adults.

Bellini L: Nutritional support in advanced lung disease. In Baslow DS, editor: *UpToDate*, Waltham, 2013, Mass. Available at: http://www.uptodate.com/contents/nutritional-support-in-advanced-lung-disease.

Benedik B, Farkas J, Kosnik M, et al: Mini nutritional assessment, body composition, and hospitalizations in patients with chronic obstructive pulmonary disease, *Respir Med* 105(Suppl 1):S38–S43, 2011.

Berman AR: Management of patients with end stage chronic obstructive pulmonary disease, *Prim Care* 38:277–297, 2011.

Bhargava A, Chatterjee M, Jain Y, et al: Nutritional status of adult patients with pulmonary tuberculosis in rural central India and its association with mortality, *PLos One* 8:e77979, 2013.

Borowitz D, Robinson KA, Rosenfeld M, et al: Cystic Fibrosis Foundation evidence-based guidelines for management of infants with cystic fibrosis, *J Pediatr* 115(Suppl 6):S73–S93, 2009.

Brehm JM, Schuemann B, Fuhlbrigge AL, et al: Serum vitamin D levels and severe asthma exacerbations in the Childhood Asthma Management Program Study, *J Allergy Clin Immunol* 126:52–58.e5, 2010.

Buckley L, Guyatt G, Fink HA, et al: 2017 American College of Rheumatology guideline for the prevention and treatment of glucocorticoid-induced osteoporosis, *Arthritis Care Res* 69:1095–1110, 2017.

Burney P, Jithoo A, Kato B, et al: Chronic obstructive pulmonary disease mortality and prevalence: the associations with smoking and poverty—a BOLD analysis, *Thorax* 69:465–473, 2014.

Carver PL: The battle for iron between humans and microbes, *Curr Med Chem* 25(1):85–96, 2018.

Chen E, Shalowitz MU, Story RE, et al: Dimensions of socioeconomic status and childhood asthma outcomes: evidence for distinct behaviorial and biological associations, *Psychosom Med* 78(9):1043–1052, 2016.

Cheng K, Ashby D, Smyth RL: Ursodeoxycholic acid for cystic fibrosis-related liver disease, *Cochran Database Syst Rev* 9:CD000222, 2017.

Guo CH, Liu PJ, Lin KP, et al: Nutritional supplement therapy improves oxidative stress, immune response, pulmonary function, and quality of life in allergic asthma patients: an open label pilot study, *Altern Med Rev* 17:42–56, 2012.

Christie JD, Stehlik J, Edwards LB, et al: The registry of the International Society for Heart and Lung Transplantation: 29th adult lung and heart-lung transplant report-2012, *J Heart Lung Transplant* 31(10):1052–1064, 2012.

Collins PF, Stratton RJ, Elia M: Nutritional support in chronic obstructive pulmonary disease: a systemic review and meta-analysis, *Am J Clin Nutr* 95:1385–1395, 2012.

Cystic Fibrosis Foundation: *Patient Registry: 2016 Annual Data Report,* Bethesda, MD, 2016, Cystic Fibrosis Foundation.

Dalli J, Winkler JW, Colas RA, et al: Resolvin D3 and aspirin-triggered Resolvin D3 are potent immune resolvents, *Chem Biol* 20:188–201, 2013.

Dani C, Poggi C: Nutrition and bronchopulmonary dysplasia, *J Matern Fetal Neonatal Med* 25(Suppl 3):37–40, 2012.

Davidson LM, Berkelhamer SK: Bronchopulmonary dysplasia: chronic lung disease of infancy and long-term pulmonary outcomes, *J Clin Med* 6(1):E4, 2017.

Davis PB: Therapy for cystic fibrosis—the end of the beginning, *New Engl J Med* 365:1734–1735, 2011.

Del Ferraro C, Grant M, Koczywas M, et al: Management of anorexia-cachexia in late-stage lung cancer patients, *J Hosp Palliat Nurs* 14(6), 2012. doi:10.1097/NJH.0b013e31825f3470.

Ehrenkranz RA: Ongoing issues in the intensive care for the periviable infant-nutritional management and prevention of bronchopulmonary dysplasia and nosocomial infections, *Semin Perinatol* 38:25–30, 2014.

Epstein LJ, Kristo D, Friedman N, et al: Clinical guidelines for the evaluation, management and long-term care of obstructive sleep apnea in adults, *J Clin Sleep Med* 5:263–276, 2009.

Evans A: Nutrition screening in patients with COPD, *Nurs Times* 108:12–14, 2012.

Evans RA, Morgan MD: The systemic nature of chronic lung disease, *Clin Chest Med* 35:283–293, 2014.

Fabian E, Pölöskey P, Kósa L, et al: Nutritional supplements and plasma anti-oxidants in childhood asthma, *Wien Klin Wochenschr* 125:309–315, 2013.

Fanta CH: An overview of asthma management. In Hollingsworth H, editor: *UpToDate,* Waltham, 2017, Mass.

Feller-Kopman D, Light R: Pleural effusion, *N Engl J Med* 378:740–751, 2018.

Fulton AS, Hill AM, Williams MT, et al: Feasibility of omega-3 fatty acid supplementation as an adjunct therapy for people with chronic obstructive pulmonary disease: study protocol for a randomized controlled trial, *Trials* 14:107, 2013.

Garcia-Marcos L, Castro-Rodriguez JA, Weinmayr G, et al: Influence of Mediterranean diet on asthma in children: a systematic review and meta-analysis, *Pediatr Allergy Immunol* 24:330–338, 2013.

Gaur P, Kumar C, Shukla RK, et al: Nutritional scenario in bronchial asthma, *Int J Curr Microbiol Appl Sci* 2:119–124, 2013.

Gibson PG, Jensen ME, Collins CE, et al: Diet induced weight loss in obese children with asthma: a randomized control trial, *Clin Exp Allergy* 43:775–784, 2013.

2019 GINA Report: *Global Strategy for Asthma Management and Prevention.* 2019. Available at: https://ginasthma.org/wp-content/uploads/2019/06/GINA-2019-main-report-June-2019-wms.pdf.

Global Initiative for Chronic Obstructive Lung Disease: *GOLD report;* 2019: 1–155. Available at: https://goldcopd.org/wp-content/uploads/2018/11/GOLD-2019-POCKET-GUIDE-DRAFT. Accessed August 2019.

Gold DR, Litonjua AA, Carey VJ, et al: Lung VITAL: Rationale, design, and baseline characteristics of an ancillary study evaluating the effects of vita-min D and/or marine omega-3 fatty acid supplements on acute exacerba-tions of chronic respiratory disease, asthma control, pneumonia and lung function in adults. *Contemp Clin Trials* 47:185–195, 2016.

Grobler L, Nagpal C, Sudarsanam TD, et al: Nutritional supplements for people being treated for active tuberculosis, *Cochrane Database Syst Rev* (6):CD006086, 2016.

Han YY, Forno E, Holguin F, et al: Diet and asthma: an update, *Curr Opin Allergy Clin Immunol* 15(4):369–374.

Harada H, Yamashita Y, Misumi K, et al: Multidisciplinary team–based approach for comprehensive preoperative pulmonary rehabilitation including intensive nutritional support for lung cancer patients, *PLoS One* 8:e59566, 2013.

Heffner JE: Management of chylothorax. In Basow DS, editor: *UpToDate,* Waltham, 2018, Mass. Available at: http://www.uptodate.com/contents/management-of-chylothorax.

Hendaus MA, Jomha FA, Ehlayel M: Allergic disease among children: nutritional prevention and intervention, *Ther Clin Risk Manag* 12:361–372, 2016.

Hill K, Vogiatzis I, Burtin C: The importance of components of pulmonary rehabilitation, other than exercise training in COPD, *Eur Respir Rev* 22:405–413, 2013.

Hood ML: A narrative review of recent progress in understanding the relationship between tuberculosis and protein energy malnutrition, *Eur J Clin Nutr* 67:1122–1128, 2013.

Hopkins W, Rubin LJ: Treatment of pulmonary hypertension in adults. In Baso DS, editor: *UpToDate,* Wolters Kluwer, Waltham, 2018.

Hudgel DW, Patel SR, Ahasic AM, et al: The role of weight management in the treatment of adult obstructive sleep apnea. An official American Thoracic Society clinical practice guideline, *Am J Respir Crit Care Med* 198(6):e70–e87, 2018.

Huhmann M, Camporeale J: Supportive care in lung cancer: clinical update, *Semin Oncol Nurs* 28(2):e1–e10, 2012.

Isanaka S, Mugusi F, Urassa W, et al: Iron deficiency and anemia predict mortality in patients with tuberculosis, *J Nutr* 142:350–357, 2012.

Itoh M, Tsuji T, Nemoto K, et al: Undernutrition in patients with COPD and its treatment, *Nutrients* 5:1316–1335, 2013.

Jiao J, Castro M: Vitamin D and asthma: current perspectives, *Curr Opin Allergy Clin Immunol* 15:375–382, 2015.

Jobe AH: The new bronchopulmonary dysplasia, *Curr Opin Pediatr* 23(2):167–172, 2011.

Kant S, Gupta H, Ahluwalia S: Significance of nutrition in pulmonary tuberculosis, *Crit Rev Food Sci Nutr* 55(7):955–963, 2015.

Kappler M, Espach C, Schweiger-Kabesch A, et al: Ursodeoxycholic acid therapy in cystic fibrosis liver disease-a retrospective long-term follow-up case control study, *Aliment Pharmacol Ther* 36:266–273, 2012.

Kapur VK, Auckley DH, Chowdhuri S, et al: Clinical practice guideline for diagnostic testing for adult obstructive sleep apnea: an American Academy of Sleep Medicine clinical practice guideline, *J Clin Sleep Med* 13(3):479–504, 2017.

Katkin JP: Cystic fibrosis: clinical manifestations and diagnosis. In Baslow DS, editor: *UpToDate,* Waltham, 2014, Mass. Available at: http://www.uptodate.com/contents/cystic-fibrosis-clinical-manifestations-and-diagnosis?source=search_result&search=cystic+fibrosis&selectedTitle=1~150.

Kazaks AG, Uriu-Adams JY, Albertson TE, et al: Effect of oral magnesium sup-plementation on measures of airway resistance and subjective assessment of asthma control and quality of life in men and women with mild to moderate asthma: a randomized placebo controlled trial, *J Asthma* 47(1):87–92, 2010.

Kocher F, Hilbe W, Seeber A, et al: Longitudinal analysis of 2293 NSCLC patients: a comprehensive study from the TYROL registry, *Lung Cancer* 87:193–200, 2015.

Koenig SM: Pulmonary complications of obesity, *Am J Med Sci* 321:249–279, 2011.

Krzak A, Pleva M, Napolitano LM: Nutrition therapy for ALI and ARDS, *Crit Care Clin* 27:647–659, 2011.

Lahiri T, Hempstead SE, Brady C, et al: Clinical practice guidelines from the Cystic Fibrosis Foundation for preschoolers with cystic fibrosis, *Pediatrics* 137(4):e20151784, 2016.

Lederer DJ, Martinez FJ: Idiopathic pulmonary fibrosis, *N Engl J Med* 378:1811–1823, 2018.

Lederer DJ, Wilt JS, D'Ovidio F, et al: Obesity and underweight are associated with an increased risk of death after lung transplantation, *Am J Respir Crit Care Med* 180(9):887–895, 2009.

Lee H, Kim S, Lim Y, et al: Nutritional status and disease severity in patients with chronic obstructive pulmonary disease (COPD), *Arch Gerontol Geriatr* 56(3):518–523, 2013.

Lin SY, Erekosima N, Kim JM, et al: Sublingual immunotherapy for the treatment of allergic rhinoconjunctivitis and asthma, a systematic review, *JAMA* 309:1278–1288, 2013.

Litonjua AA, Lange NE, Carey VJ, et al: The Vitamin D Antenatal Asthma Reduction Trial (VDAART): rationale, design, and methods of a randomized, controlled trial of vitamin D supplementation in pregnancy for the primary prevention of asthma and allergies in children, *Contemp Clin Trials* 38:37–50, 2014.

Liu Y, Pleasants RA, Croft JB, et al: Smoking duration, respiratory symptoms, and COPD in adults aged ≥45 years with a smoking history, *Int J Chron Obstruct Pulmon Dis* 10:1409–1416, 2015.

Ma J, Strub P, Xiao L, et al: Behavioral weight loss and physical activity intervention in obese adults with asthma. A randomized trial, *Ann Am Thorac Soc* 12:1–11, 2015.

Mannino DM: Cigarette smoking and other risk factors for lung cancer. In Baslow DS, editor: *UpToDate*, Waltham, 2014, Mass. Available at: http://www.uptodate.com/contents/cigarette-smoking-and-other-risk-factors-for-lung-cancer?source=search_result&search=cigarette+smoking+and+other+risks+for+lung+cancer&selected.

McClafferty H: An Overview of integrative therapies in asthma treatment, *Current Allergy Asthma Rep* 14(10):464, 2014. doi:10.1007/s11882-014-0464-2.

McClave SA, Taylor BE, Martindale RG, et al: Guidelines for the provision and assessment of nutrition support therapy in the adult critically ill patient: Society of Critical Care Medicine (SCCM) and American Society for Parenteral and Enteral Nutrition (A.S.P.E.N.), *J Parenter Enteral Nutr* 40:159–211, 2016.

McClave SA, DiBaise JK, Mullin GE, et al: ACG clinical guideline: nutrition therapy in the adult hospitalized patient, *Am J Gastroenterol* 111(3):315–334, 2016.

Milani C, Duranti S, Bottacini F, et al: The first microbial human colonizers of the human gut: composition, activities, and health implications of the infant gut microbiota, *Microbiol Mol Biol Rev* 81(4):e00036-17, 2017.

Miyata S, Tanaka M, Ihaku D: The prognostic significance of nutritional status using malnutrition universal screening tool in patients with pulmonary tuberculosis, *Nutr J* 12:42, 2013.

Moran A, Brunzell C, Cohen RC, et al: Clinical care guidelines for cystic fibrosis-related diabetes, *Diabetes* 33(12):2697–2708, 2010.

Nakawah MO, Hawkins C, Barbandi F: Asthma, chronic obstructive pulmonary disease (COPD) and the overlap syndrome, *J Am Board Fam Med* 26:470–477, 2013.

Norton RL, Hoffmann PR: Selenium and asthma, *Mol Aspects Med* 33(1):98–106, 2012.

Papaioannou AI, Loukides S, Gourgoulianis KI, et al: Global assessment of the COPD patient: time to look beyond FEV1? *Respir Med* 103:650–660, 2013.

Palanippan SK, Than NN, Thein AW, et al: Interventions for preventing and management advanced liver disease in cystic fibrosis, *Cochrane Database Syst Rev* 8:CD012056, 2017.

Parenteral and Enteral Nutrition Group (PENG): *A pocket guide to clinical nutrition*, ed 4, Birmingham, 2011, British Dietetic Association.

Peromaa-Haavisto P, Tuomilehto H, Kössi J, et al: Obstructive sleep apnea: the effect of bariatric surgery after 12 months. A prospective trial, *Sleep Med* 35:85–90, 2017.

Piper AJ, Grunstein RR: Current perspectives on the obesity hypoventilation syndrome, *Curr Opin Pulm Med* 13:490–496, 2007.

Piper AJ, Grunstein RR: Obesity hypoventilation syndrome: mechanisms and management, *Am J Respir Crit Care Med* 183:292–298, 2011.

Pirabbasi E, Shahar S, Manaf ZA, et al: Efficacy of ascorbic acid (Vitamin C) and/N-acetylcysteine (NAC) supplementation on nutritional and antioxidant status of male chronic obstructive pulmonary disease (COPD) patients, *J Nutr Sci Vitaminol* 62(1):54–61, 2016.

Poole P, Sathananthan K, Fortescue R: Mucolytic agents vs placebo for chronic bronchitis or chronic obstructive pulmonary disease. *Cochrane Database Syst Rev* 20(5):CD001287, 2019.

Raguso CA, Luthy C: Nutritional status in chronic obstructive pulmonary disease: role of hypoxia, *Nutrition* 27:138–143, 2011.

Rana M, Wong-See D, Katz T, et al: Fat soluble vitamin deficiency in children and adolescents with cystic fibrosis, *J Clin Pathol* 67:605–608, 2014.

Rodà D, Rozas L, Fortuny C, et al: Impact of the increased recommended dosage of isoniazid on pyridoxine levels in children and adolescents, *Pediatr Infect Dis J* 35(5):586–589, 2016.

Rogers CL: Nutritional management of the adult with cystic fibrosis – Part 1, *Practical Gastroenterology Series* 113:10, 2013.

Saguil A, Fargo M: Acute respiratory distress syndrome: diagnosis and management, *Am Fam Physician* 85:352–358, 2012.

Schindler T, Michel S, Wilson AW: Nutrition management of cystic fibrosis in the 21st century, *Nutr Clin Pract* 30(4):488–500, 2015.

Schwarzenberg SJ, Hempstead SE, McDonald CM, et al: Enteral tube feeding for individuals with cystic fibrosis: Cystic Fibrosis Foundation evidence-informed guidelines, *J Cyst Fibros* 15(6):724–735, 2016.

Siegel MD: Acute Respiratory Distress Syndrome: Supportive care and oxygenation in adults. In: Basow DS, editor: *UpToDate*, Wolters Kluwer, Waltham MA, 2013.

Shek LP, Chong MF, Lim JY, et al: Role of dietary long-chain polyunsaturated fatty acids in infant allergies and respiratory diseases, *Clin Dev Immunol*, 2012(12):730568, 2012. doi:10.1155/2012/730568.

Silverberg DS, Mor R, Weu MT, et al: Anemia and iron deficiency in COPD patients: prevalence and the effects of correction of the anemia with erythropoiesis stimulating agents and intravenous iron, *BMC Pulm Med* 14:24, 2014.

Sobieraj DM, Baker WL, Nguyen E, et al: Association of inhaled corticosteroids and long acting muscarinic antagonists with asthma control in patients with uncontrolled, persistent asthma: a systemic review and meta-analysis, *JAMA* 319:1473–1484, 2018.

Sonnenschein-van der Voort AM, Arends LR, de Jongste JC, et al: Preterm birth, infant weight gain, and childhood asthma risk: a meta-analysis of 147,000 European children, *J Allergy Clin Immunol* 133(5):1317–1329, 2014.

Weill D, Benden C, Corris PA, et al: A consensus document for the selection of lung transplant candidates: 2014-an update from the Pulmonary Transplantation Council for the International Society for Heart and Lung Transplantation, *J Heart Lung Transplant* 34(1):1–15, 2015.

World Health Organization (WHO): *Global tuberculosis report 2017*, Geneva, Switzerland, 2017, World Health Organization.

Xiaomei W, Hang X, Lingling L, et al: Bone metabolism status and associated risk factors in elderly patients with chronic obstructive pulmonary disease (COPD), *Cell Biochem Biophys* 70:129–134, 2014.

34

Medical Therapy for Renal Disorders

Katy G. Wilkens, MS, RDN
Veena Juneja, MSc, RDN
Elizabeth Shanaman, RDN

KEY TERMS

angiotensin-converting enzyme (ACE)
acute glomerulonephritis
acute kidney injury (AKI)
adynamic (low turnover) bone disease
antidiuretic hormone (ADH)
angiotensin II receptor blocker (ARB)
azotemia
blood urea nitrogen (BUN)
calciphylaxis
chronic kidney disease (CKD)
continuous renal replacement therapy (CRRT)
continuous venovenous hemodialysis (CVVHD)
continuous venovenous hemofiltration (CVVH)
creatinine
dialysate
end-stage renal disease (ESRD)

estimated glomerular filtration rate (eGFR)
erythropoietin (EPO)
fistula
glomerular filtration rate (GFR)
graft
hemodialysis (HD)
hypercalciuria
hyperoxaluria
idiopathic hypercalciuria (IH)
intradialytic parenteral nutrition (IDPN)
intraperitoneal nutrition (IPN)
Kidney Dialysis Outcome Quality Initiative (KDOQI)
Kidney Disease Improving Global Outcomes (KDIGO)
kinetic modeling
Kt/V
metastatic calcification

nephrolithiasis
nephrotic syndrome
oliguria
osteitis fibrosa cystica
osteomalacia
peritoneal dialysis (PD)
phosphate binders
protein-nitrogen appearance (PNA) rate
recombinant human EPO (rHuEPO)
renal failure
renal osteodystrophy
renal replacement therapy (RRT)
renal tubular acidosis (RTA)
renin-angiotensin mechanism
ultrafiltrate
urea reduction ratio (URR)
uremia
vasopressin

PHYSIOLOGY AND FUNCTION OF THE KIDNEYS

The main function of the kidney is to maintain the balance of fluids, electrolytes, and organic solutes. The normal kidney performs this function over a wide range of fluctuations in sodium, water, and solutes. This task is accomplished by the continuous filtration of blood with alterations in secretion and reabsorption of this filtered fluid. The kidney receives 20% of cardiac output, filtering approximately 1600 L/day of blood and producing 180 L of fluid called ultrafiltrate. Through active processes of reabsorbing certain components and secreting others, composition of this ultrafiltrate is changed into the 1.5 L of urine excreted in an average day.

Each kidney consists of approximately 1 million functioning nephrons (Fig. 34.1), consisting of a glomerulus connected to a series of tubules. Tubules consist of different segments: the proximal convoluted tubule, loop of Henle, distal tubule, and collecting duct. Each nephron functions independently and contributes to the final urine, although all are under similar control and coordination. If one segment of a nephron is destroyed, that complete nephron is no longer functional.

The glomerulus is a spheric mass of capillaries surrounded by a membrane, Bowman's capsule. The glomerulus produces the ultrafiltrate, which then is modified by the next segments of the nephron.

Production of ultrafiltrate is mainly passive and relies on the perfusion pressure generated by the heart and supplied by the renal artery.

The tubules reabsorb the vast majority of components that compose the ultrafiltrate. Much of this process is active and requires a large expenditure of energy in the form of adenosine triphosphate (ATP). The tubule is a unique structure; differences in permeability between the various segments and hormonal responses allow the tubule to produce the final urine, which can vary widely in concentration of electrolytes, osmolality, pH, and volume. Ultimately, this urine is funneled into common collecting tubules and into the renal pelvis. The renal pelvis narrows into a single ureter per kidney, and each ureter carries urine into the bladder, where it accumulates before elimination.

The kidney has almost unlimited ability to regulate water homeostasis. Its ability to form a large concentration gradient between its inner medulla and outer cortex allows the kidney to excrete urine as dilute as 50 mOsm or as concentrated as 1200 mOsm. Given a daily fixed solute load of approximately 600 mOsm, the kidney can get rid of as little as 500 mL of concentrated urine or as much as 12 L of dilute urine. Control of water excretion is regulated by vasopressin, a small peptide hormone secreted by the posterior pituitary, which is also called antidiuretic hormone (ADH). An excess of relative body water, indicated by a low osmolality, leads to prompt shut-off of all vasopressin secretion. Likewise, a small rise in osmolality brings about

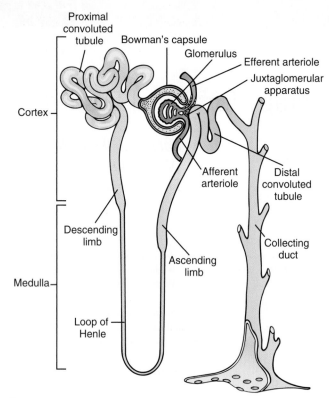

Fig. 34.1 The nephron. (Modified from Patton KT, Thibodeau GA: *The human body in health and disease*, ed 6, Maryland Heights, Mo, 2013, Mosby.)

marked vasopressin secretion and water retention. However, the need to conserve sodium sometimes leads to a sacrifice of the homeostatic control of water for the sake of volume.

The minimum urinary volume capable of eliminating a relatively fixed 600 mOsm of solute is 500 mL, assuming that the kidney is capable of maximum concentration. Urinary volume of less than 500 mL/day is called oliguria; it is impossible for such a small urine volume to eliminate all of the daily waste.

The majority of the solute load consists of nitrogenous wastes, primarily the end products of protein metabolism. Urea predominates in amount, depending on the protein content of the diet. Uric acid, creatinine (Cr), and ammonia are present in small amounts. If normal waste products are not eliminated appropriately, they collect in abnormal quantities in the blood, known as azotemia. The ability of the kidney to adequately eliminate nitrogenous waste products is defined as renal function. Thus renal failure is the inability to excrete the daily load of wastes.

The kidney also performs functions unrelated to excretion. One of these involves the renin-angiotensin mechanism, a major control of blood pressure. Decreased blood volume causes cells of the glomerulus (the juxtaglomerular apparatus) to react by secreting renin, a proteolytic enzyme. Renin acts on angiotensinogen in the plasma to form angiotensin I, which is converted to angiotensin II, a powerful vasoconstrictor and a potent stimulus of aldosterone secretion by the adrenal gland. As a consequence, sodium and fluid are reabsorbed, and blood pressure is returned to normal.

The kidney also produces the hormone erythropoietin (EPO), a critical determinant of erythroid activity in the bone marrow. Deficiency of EPO is the primary cause of the severe anemia present in chronic renal disease.

Maintenance of calcium-phosphorus homeostasis involves the complex interactions of parathyroid hormone (PTH); calcitonin; active vitamin D; and three effector organs: the gut, kidney, and bone. The role of the kidney includes production of the active form of vitamin D—1,25-dihydroxycholecalciferol ($1,25[OH]_2D_3$)—as well as elimination of calcium and phosphorus. Active vitamin D promotes efficient absorption of calcium by the gut and is one of the substances necessary for bone remodeling and maintenance. Active vitamin D also suppresses PTH production, which is responsible for mobilization of calcium from bone (see Chapter 23).

RENAL DISEASES

The manifestations of renal disease are significant. They can be ordered by degree of severity: (1) kidney stones, (2) acute kidney injury (AKI), (3) chronic kidney disease (CKD), and (4) end-stage renal disease (ESRD) (National Kidney Foundation, 2018). Objectives of nutritional care depend on the abnormality being treated.

Kidney Stones (Nephrolithiasis)

Nephrolithiasis is a highly prevalent disease worldwide with rates ranging from 7% to 13% in North America, 5% to 9% in Europe, and 1% to 5% in Asia (Sorokin et al, 2017). National Health and Nutrition Examination Survey (NHANES) reveals a lower occurrence rate in black non-Hispanic and Hispanic individuals compared with white non-Hispanic individuals (Scales et al, 2012).

About one in 11 people has a kidney stone in their lifetime and more than 50% of these will have a recurrence within 5 to 10 years. A positive family history influences the clinical course of idiopathic calcium stones with significant gender related differences:

-Earlier onset in females and higher rate of recurrence.

-Men are one and a half times more likely than women to develop stones overall. (Guerra et al, 2016). Increased incidence of obesity, diabetes, hypertension, and metabolic syndrome have been linked to increasing rates of nephrolithiasis.

Health care cost of evaluation, hospitalization, and treatment of kidney stone disease in the United States exceeds 4.5 billion dollars per year. Preventing recurrence can have a significant cost-saving potential as a result of reduced stone burden. Medical nutrition therapy can play an important role in prevention and is economical compared with management with drugs. Medical evaluation and drug and diet therapy are underused. Only 7.4% of patients with visits to the emergency room (ER) with a stone submitted 24-hour urine collection for evaluation within 6 months (Morgan and Pearle, 2016). A low urine volume is the single most important risk factor for all types of nephrolithiasis. Body mass index (BMI), fluid intake, Dietary Approaches to Stop Hypertension (DASH)-style diet, dietary calcium intake, and sugar-sweetened beverage intake are the five modifiable risk factors that account for more than 50% of incident kidney stones (Ferraro et al, 2017a).

Pathophysiology

Kidney stone formation is a complex process that consists of saturation; supersaturation; nucleation; crystal growth or aggregation; crystal retention; and stone formation in the presence of substances that promote, inhibit, and precipitate stones in urine. A typical metabolic evaluation is described in Table 34.1.

Calcium stones are the most common: 60% of stones are calcium oxalate, 10% calcium oxalate and calcium phosphate, and 10% calcium phosphate. Other stones are 5% to 10% uric acid, 5% to 10% struvite, and 1% cystine.

TABLE 34.1 Baseline Information and Metabolic Evaluation of Urolithiasis

Information	Description and Data
History of urolithiasis	History of onset, frequency Family history Spontaneous passage or removal Retrieval, analysis of stone Current status with radiologic examination
Medical history, investigation	Hyperparathyroidism Renal tubular acidosis Urinary tract infection Sarcoidosis Hypertension Osteoporosis Inflammatory bowel disease, malabsorption syndrome, intestinal bypass surgery for obesity (Roux-en-Y or gastric banding/sleeve gastrectomy) Metabolic syndrome or insulin resistance Diabetes mellitus Obesity
Blood tests	Serum—calcium, phosphorus, creatinine, uric acid, CO_2, albumin, parathyroid hormone, Hgb A1C
Urinalysis	Urine analysis with pH Urine culture
24-hr urine collection	Volume, calcium, oxalate, uric acid, sodium, citrate, magnesium, phosphorus Urea Creatinine Qualitative cystine
Medications and vitamins	Thiazide, allopurinol, vitamin C, vitamin B_6, vitamin D, cod liver oil, calcium carbonate, glucocorticoid therapy, potassium citrate, antacids
Occupation history and strenuous exercise	Dermal water losses Dehydration Low urine volume Type of job and activity level
Environment	Hard water area
Dietary evaluation	Intake of calcium, oxalate, animal protein, salt, purines, fructose, potassium Fruits and vegetables (related to urine pH) Herbal products, probiotics, fish oils Volume of fluid intake Type of fluids containing citrate, malate, caffeine, fructose, phosphoric acid; mineral water; sports drinks

CO_2, Carbon dioxide; *Hgb A1C*, hemoglobin A1C.

Stone formers with obesity excrete increased amounts of sodium, calcium, uric acid, and citrate, and have lower urine pH. Obesity is the strongest predictor of stone recurrence in first-time stone formers. As body weight increases, the excretion of calcium, oxalate, and uric acid also increases. Patients with a higher BMI have a decrease in ammonia excretion and impaired hydrogen ion buffering. With increasing BMI, uric acid stones become more dominant than calcium oxalate stones, especially in men.

Uric acid stones are common in the presence of type 2 diabetes. Hyperinsulinemia also may contribute to the development of calcium stones by increasing urinary calcium excretion. Uric acid stones are also associated with higher prevalence of CKD (Li et al, 2018).

TABLE 34.2 Causes and Composition of Renal Stones

Pathogenetic Causes	Composition of Stone
Hypercalciuria, hyperoxaluria, hyperuricosuria, or hypocitraturia	Calcium oxalate
Primary hyperparathyroidism	Calcium oxalate
Cystinuria	Cystine
Infection	Struvite
Acid urine pH	Uric acid
Hyperuricosuria	Uric acid
Renal tubular acidosis	Calcium phosphate
Alkaline urine pH	Calcium phosphate

Weight control may be considered one of the preventive modalities, and in stone formers a BMI of 18 to 25 kg/m² is recommended.

With malabsorptive bariatric procedures such as Roux-en-Y gastric bypass (RYGB), urolithiasis is higher than in obese controls, probably because of the increased prevalence of hyperoxaluria and hypocitraturia in RYGB patients. However, restrictive gastric surgery (i.e., gastric banding or sleeve gastrectomy) is not associated with increased risk of kidney stones (Semins et al, 2010).

Some oral antibiotics such as sulfa and broad-spectrum penicillins play a role in increasing stone risk in adults and children given the latter are prescribed antibiotics at a higher rate than adults (Tasian et al, 2018). Antibiotics alter the composition of human microbiome, and disruptions in the intestinal and urinary microbiome have been linked to the occurrence of kidney stones.

Agents added intentionally or unintentionally to food or drug products have led to the appearance of new types of stones containing melamine and indinavir (Zilberman et al, 2010) (Table 34.2).

Calcium Stones. Hypercalciuria is the most common abnormality identified in stone formers, occurring in 30% to 60% of patients. Ninety percent of patients with idiopathic hypercalciuria never form a stone. Hypercalciuria describes a value of calcium in excess of 300 mg (7.5 mmol) per day in men, 250 mg (6.25 mmol) per day in women, or 4 mg (0.1 mmol)/kg/day for either in random urine collections of outpatients on unrestricted diets.

Idiopathic hypercalciuria (IH) is a familial disorder characterized by abnormal serum calcium in the absence of known causes of hypercalciuria, such as primary hyperparathyroidism, sarcoidosis, excess vitamin D intake, hyperthyroidism, glucocorticoid use, or renal tubular acidosis (RTA).

The relationship between calcium intake and the risk of calcium stone formation is complex. Besides increased calcium intake raising urine calcium, other factors impact the risk of calcium stones. Higher calcium intake is associated with reduced risk of incident stone formation in all except men older than 60 years of age. The protective effect of dietary calcium has been attributed to the interaction between calcium and oxalate in the intestinal lumen to form an insoluble complex that is excreted in the stool. When calcium intake is low the formation of calcium oxalate complex declines and more oxalate is absorbed.

Low calcium intake in patients with IH increases bone loss associated with higher net acid excretion and greater risk of fractures. The loss of more calcium in urine than is in the diet indicates a total net loss of body calcium, its source being the skeleton. For decades low-calcium diets were recommended to reduce the hypercalciuria in stone formers. However, chronic prolonged calcium restriction, deficient calcium intake, and increased losses from hypercalciuria decrease bone mineral density (BMD). The decreased BMD also correlates with an increase in markers of bone turnover as well as increased fractures (Krieger and Bushinsky, 2013). Vertebral fracture risk is four times higher in patients with urolithiasis than in the general population.

Negative calcium balance appears to be greater in stone formers than in non–stone formers. Patients with IH may also tend toward negative phosphorus balance even on normal intakes. The defective phosphate metabolism may lead to increased $1,25(OH)_2D_3$ levels and increased intestinal calcium absorption. A high protein intake of nondairy origin may enhance undesirable bone resorption. An inadequate calcium intake along with high protein intake induces metabolic acidosis, increases calcium excretion by inhibiting renal reabsorption of calcium secondary to the acid load, and lowers urinary pH. A reduction in nondairy animal protein, as well as potentially alkaline foods such as vegetables and fruit, is recommended (see *Clinical Insight:* Acid and Alkaline Diets).

Calcium supplementation is associated with an increased risk of stone formation compared with no supplementation as calcium supplements do not have the same protective effect against stone formation as dietary calcium. Widespread use of calcium supplements to prevent osteoporosis corresponds to an increase in kidney stones in women. A trial of combined calcium–vitamin D supplementation to prevent bone loss and fractures led to a 17% increase in new stone formation in women who increased their calcium intake to 2000 mg a day by adding a 1000 mg calcium supplement to their baseline diet (Wallace et al, 2011).

If calcium is taken as a supplement, timing is important. Calcium supplements taken with meals increase urinary calcium and citrate but decrease urinary oxalate; thus the increase in citrate and decrease in oxalate counterbalance the effects of elevated urinary calcium. Therefore, if used by patients who cannot tolerate dairy products because of lactose intolerance, allergies, or preference, calcium supplements should be taken with meals. Urine calcium should be measured before starting the supplement and afterward to see the effect; if urine calcium increases, patients should increase fluid intake to dilute the urine concentration of calcium.

Higher dietary calcium from either nondairy or dairy foods is independently associated with a lower kidney stone risk (Taylor and Curhan, 2013). Therefore based on dietary reference intake (DRI) recommendations for age (1000 to 1200 mg/day) patients may select calcium from dairy or nondairy choices. Given recent concerns for increased risk for cardiovascular disease and kidney stones with increased use of calcium supplements, women should aim to meet DRI recommendations from a calcium-rich diet, taking calcium supplements only if needed to reach DRI goals. Calcium should be taken in divided doses, choosing a source with each meal to maximize oxalate

---

CLINICAL INSIGHT

Acid and Alkaline Diets

Dietary intake can influence the acidity or alkalinity of the urine (Berardi et al, 2008). It has been shown that excessive dietary protein (particularly high in sulfur-containing amino acids such as methionine and cysteine), and chloride, phosphorous, and organic acids are the main sources of dietary acid load. When these animal proteins, such as meat and cheese, are eaten with other acid-producing foods and not balanced with alkaline-producing foods, such as fruit and vegetables, there is an increased risk of chronic acidosis. Acidosis (which is not to be confused with acidemia) has been linked to inflammatory-related chronic diseases such as urolithiasis, hypertension, insulin resistance, low immune function, and osteoporosis (Adeva and Souto, 2011; Minich and Bland, 2007).

Consequently, when working with higher protein intakes it is important to provide a diet balanced with high alkaline foods. The most abundant alkaline foods are plant-based foods; particularly vegetables and fruit abundant in alkalinizing micronutrients such as magnesium, calcium, sodium, and potassium. A more alkaline diet consisting of a higher fruit and vegetable intake and lower meat and refined carbohydrate intake is associated with a low potential renal acid load (PRAL) (Remer and Manz, 1995). Although acute acid loading may only temporarily disrupt acidbase equilibrium, a chronic perturbation occurs when metabolism of the diet repeatedly releases acids into the systemic circulation in amounts that exceed the amount of base released at the same time. To overcome the imbalance, the skeleton, which serves as the major reservoir of base, provides the buffer needed to main blood pH (Pizzorno et al, 2010).

Remer and Manz developed a physiologically based model to calculate the PRAL of selected, frequently consumed foods. By means of these PRAL data, the daily net acid excretion can be calculated, allowing for an accurate prediction of the effects of diet on acid load. This has been a reason to recommend animal protein limited diets, to control the dietary source of acids (Kiwull-Schone et al, 2008). The following food lists serve as a guide to influencing potential renal acid load (PRAL).

Potentially Acid Foods

Protein: meat, fish, fowl, shellfish, eggs, all types of cheese, peanut butter, peanuts

Fat: bacon, butternuts, walnuts, pumpkin seeds, sesame seeds, sunflower seeds, creamy salad dressings

Carbohydrate: all types of bread including cornbran, oats, macaroni, ricebran, rye, wheat, and especially wheat gluten, sugar (white)

Potentially Basic or Alkaline Foods

Fat: dried beechnuts, dried chestnuts, acorn

Vegetables: all types including legumes but especially beets, beet greens, Swiss chard, dandelion greens, kale, leeks, mustard greens, spinach, turnip greens

Fruit: all types, especially currants, dates, figs, bananas, dried apricots, apples, prunes, raisins

Spices/Herbs: all types, especially fresh dill weed and dried spices/herbs such as spearmint, basil, coriander, curry powder, oregano, parsley

Sweets: sorghum syrup, sugar (brown), molasses, cocoa (dry powder)

Beverages: coffee

Neutral Foods

Fats: butter, margarine, oils

Dairy: milk

Vegetables: corn

Sweets: sugar, maple syrup, honey

Beverages: water, tea

by Sheila Dean, DSc, RDN, LDN, CCN, IFMCP

binding. Calcium carbonate may be the best option. Low-fat dairy choices are good options for their lower saturated fat content.

Oxalate Stones. Hyperoxaluria (more than 40 mg of oxalate in urine per day) plays an important role in calcium stone formation and is observed in 10% to 50% of recurrent stone formers. Hyperoxaluria increases urinary saturation of calcium oxalate. Urinary oxalate levels are determined by calcium and oxalate in diet, functional integrity of gastrointestinal (GI) tract, presence of oxalate degrading bacteria in the gut, and genetic disorders. Primary hyperoxaluria is a feature of an autosomal-recessive genetic defect of a hepatic enzyme that results in overproduction of oxalate and a urinary oxalate concentration three to eight times normal. Multiple stones occur in these children, causing renal failure and early death.

GI malabsorptive conditions including inflammatory bowel diseases and gastric bypass often develop hyperoxaluria related to fat malabsorption. The bile acids produced during the digestive process normally are reabsorbed in the proximal GI tract, but when this fails to occur, bile salts and fatty acids increase colonic permeability to oxalate (see Chapter 27). The unabsorbed fatty acids also bind calcium to form soaps, decreasing availability of calcium in a soluble form. With less calcium available to bind oxalate in the gut and prevent its absorption, serum oxalate and thus urinary oxalate levels increase.

Urinary oxalate also comes from endogenous synthesis. Oxalate is generated in the liver from the metabolism of the amino acids hydroxyproline, glycine, phenylalanine, and tryptophan, and the dialdehyde glyoxal. GI oxalate absorption is not subject to regulation and its absorption is low and less than 15%. The oxalate absorbed is practically all excreted in the urine. Ascorbic acid accounts for 35% to 55%, and glyoxylic acid accounts for 50% to 70% of urinary oxalate. Pyridoxine acts as cofactor in the conversion of glyoxylate to glycine, and its deficiency could increase endogenous oxalate production (Holmes et al, 2016). In patients with CKD, excessive vitamin C intake may lead to stone formation. Dietary hyperoxaluria in patients on intensive, short time weight loss programs (Khneizer et al, 2017) or on high oxalate vegan diets (Hermann and Suarez, 2017) has been identified in case studies as a cause of acute or chronic kidney failure (oxalate nephropathy) due to oxalate crystal deposition in the tubules of the kidney.

The bioavailability of food oxalate and thus urine oxalate are affected by salt forms of oxalate, food processing and cooking methods, meal composition, and the presence of *Oxalobacter formigenes* in the GI tract. *O. formigenes* is part of the normal intestinal flora that degrades oxalate. Stone-forming patients who lack this bacterium have significantly higher urinary oxalate excretion secondary to reduced degradation and stone episodes compared with patients colonized with the bacteria. There is a strong inverse relationship between colonization and risk of recurrent calcium oxalate stone formation. In Western society 30% to 40% of the general population is colonized with *O. formigenes*. Stone formers are colonized at half this rate. Those not colonized are 70% more likely to develop a kidney stone (Holmes et al, 2016). Fecal samples from stone formers exhibit significantly lower bacterial representation of genes involved in oxalate degradation with inverse correlation with 24-hour urinary oxalate excretion (Ticinesi et al, 2018).

Administration of *O. formigenes* as enteric-coated capsules significantly reduces urine oxalate in patients with primary hyperoxaluria. Dietary advice for reducing urinary oxalate should include use of this probiotic and reduction of dietary oxalate, if needed, and simultaneous consumption of calcium-rich food or supplement to reduce oxalate absorption (Holmes et al, 2016; Box 34.1).

Uric Acid Stones. Uric acid is an end product of purine metabolism from food, de novo synthesis, and tissue catabolism. Approximately half

---

> **BOX 34.1 Foods to Avoid for a Low-Oxalate Diet**
>
> Rhubarb
> Spinach
> Strawberries
> Chocolate
> Wheat bran and whole-grain wheat products
> Nuts (almonds, peanuts, or pecans)
> Beets
> Tea (green, black, iced, or instant)
> High doses of the spice turmeric

Data from Siener R, et al: Oxalate content of cereals and cereal products, *J Agric Food Chem* 54:3008, 2006.

---

of the purine load is from endogenous sources and is constant. Exogenous dietary sources provide the other half, accounting for the variation in urinary uric acid. The solubility of uric acid depends on urine volume, the amount excreted, and urine pH (Table 34.3). Uric acid stones form when urine is supersaturated with undissociated uric acid, which occurs at urinary pH less than 5.5.

The most important feature in uric acid stone formers is low urine pH resulting from increased net acid excretion (NAE) and impaired buffering caused by reduced urinary ammonium excretion. The former can be a result of low intake of alkali-producing foods or increased consumption of acid-producing foods. Fruits, vegetables, and grains are alkai-producing foods while meat and dairy foods are acid-producing.

Inflammatory bowel disease results in chronically acidic urine, usually from dehydration. GI bicarbonate loss from diarrhea may predispose these patients to uric acid stones. Uric acid stones also are associated with lymphoproliferative and myeloproliferative disorders, with increased cellular breakdown that releases purines and thus increases uric acid load. Diabetes, obesity, and hypertension appear to be associated with nephrolithiasis; diabetes is a common factor in uric acid stone development (Scales et al, 2012). Besides diabetes management for patients with uric acid lithiasis and hyperuricosuric calcium oxalate stones, dietary purines also should be restricted (Morgan and Pearle, 2016).

Meat, fish, and poultry are rich in purines and acid ash and thus should be used in moderation to meet DRI for protein. Purines and metabolism of sulfur-rich amino acids, cystine, and methionine in animal protein confer an acid load to the kidney, thus lowering urine pH. Potential renal acid load (PRAL) value is assigned to groups of foods in terms of their positive or negative effect on acidic load (Trinchieri, 2012). Dietary factors that increase purines including fructose, excess animal protein, and alcohol should be minimized (see Chapter 38). Dietary noncompliance or persistence of hyperuricosuria warrants use of medication. Uric acid stones are the only stones amenable to dissolution therapy by urine alkalinization to a pH of 6 to 6.5. An alkali load can raise urine pH, prevent uric acid stone, and dissolve

---

TABLE 34.3 Effect of Urine pH on Stone Formation

pH	State of Urate	Likely Stone Development
<5.5	Undissociated urate	Uric acid stones
5.5-7.5	Dissociated urate	Calcium oxalate stones
>7.5	Dissociated urate	Calcium phosphate stones

them. Potassium citrate has been used as the first line of treatment. If this is not attainable or alkalization is not effective, allopurinol can be added. Sodium bicarbonate increases urinary monosodium urate and calcium and should not be used as a supplement.

Cystine Stones. Cystine stones represent 1% to 2% of urinary calculi and are caused by homozygous cystinuria. Cystine stones affect approximately 1 in 15,000 persons in the United States. Whereas normal individuals daily excrete 20 mg or less of cystine in their urine, stone-forming cystinuric patients excrete more than 250 mg/day. Cystine solubility increases when urine pH exceeds 7; therefore an alkaline urine pH must be maintained 24 hours per day, even while the patient sleeps. The primary goal of treatment is to reduce urinary cystine concentration to a level below the solubility limit of 250 mg/L. This is achieved almost always with the use of medication. Fluid intake of more than 4 L daily is recommended to prevent cystine crystallization and aim for urine volume of at least 3 to 4 L. Lower sodium intake (less than 100 mEq/day) may be useful in reducing cystine in the urine. Restriction of animal protein is associated with lower intake of cystine and methionine, a precursor of cystine. Ingestion of vegetables and fruit high in citrate and malate, such as melons, limes, oranges, and fresh tomato juice, may help alkalinize the urine (Heilberg and Goldfarb, 2013). Potassium citrate can be used to raise urine pH of 7 to 7.5 (this may increase risk of calcium phosphate stones). Severe cystinuria requires the thiol drugs tiopronin, D-Penicillamine, and captopril, which form a complex with cysteine that is highly soluble. These drugs have significant side effects (Morgan and Pearle, 2016).

Melamine and Indinavir Stones. Kidney stones, acute renal failure (ARF), and death have been reported in young children who received melamine-contaminated infant formula. Melamine is an organic base synthesized from urea. When added as an adulterant to liquid milk or milk powder, it deceptively increases the protein content. Melamine precipitates in the distal renal tubules, forming crystals and sand-like stones. Hydration and urine alkalinization help with stone passage.

The treatment of human immunodeficiency virus infection with protease inhibitors, such as indinavir, has led to the appearance of another previously unknown urinary calculus. Hypocitraturia is universal in all patients with indinavir stones as well as decreased solubility in a low urine volume with a low pH. These stones are soft, gelatinous, and radiolucent and are not amenable to basket removal or ureteroscopy. Intravenous (IV) hydration and temporary cessation of indinavir should be the first choice of treatment (Zilberman et al, 2010).

Struvite Stones. Struvite stones are composed of magnesium ammonium phosphate and carbonate apatite. They are also known as triple-phosphate or infection stones. Unlike most urinary stones, they occur more commonly in women than in men, at a ratio of 2:1. They form only in the presence of bacteria such as *Pseudomonas, Klebsiella, Proteus mirabilis,* and *Urealyticum,* which carry urease, a urea-splitting enzyme. Urea breakdown results in ammonia and carbon dioxide (CO_2) production, thus raising urine pH and the level of carbonate. Struvite stones grow rapidly to large staghorn calculi in the renal pelvic area. The mainstay of treatment is extracorporeal shockwave lithotripsy (ECSWL) with adjunctive culture-specific antimicrobial therapy that uses urease inhibitors. The goal is to eliminate or prevent urinary tract infections by regularly screening and monitoring urine cultures. Because of their infectious origin, diet has no definitive role except avoidance of urine alkalinization. Acetohydroxamic acid is a potent urease inhibitor that prevents bacterial induced urease to alter the urinary milieu.

Medical Management

Uric acid stones are the only type amenable to dissolution therapy or dissolving of the stone by alkalinization of the urine. This is done with consumption of a more vegetarian diet that is also lower in purines or

by the use of medication. Shockwave lithotripsy and endourologic techniques almost have replaced the open surgical procedures of stone removal of 20 years ago. Struvite stones also are treated with adjunctive culture-specific antimicrobial therapy that uses urease inhibitors. Management strategies are now aimed at kidney stone prevention.

Medical Nutrition Therapy

After corrective treatment, nutrition assessment is needed to determine risk factors for stone recurrence. The risk in men and women rises with increasing urine calcium and oxalate and decreases with increasing citrate and urine volume. There is a continuum of risk related to increasing urinary calcium and urinary oxalate. For patients with no metabolic abnormality there is a graded increase in stone risk that begins when the rate of urinary excretion of calcium, oxalate, and citrate is still within the normal range (Curhan and Taylor, 2008). Because urine chemistries change from day to day based on changes in the environment and diet, two 24-hour urine specimens are needed based on a usual diet, one during a weekday and one on the weekend. Specific medical nutrition therapy (MNT) is then based on comprehensive metabolic evaluations consisting of radiologic studies to assess stone burden, crystallographic stone analysis, and laboratory studies with standard serum chemistries and 24-hour urine collections. Nutrition counseling and metabolic monitoring can be effective (Table 34.4). Evaluation and management should be personalized according to risk

TABLE 34.4 Recommendations for Diet and 24-Hour Urine Monitoring in Kidney Stone Disease

Diet Component	Intake Recommendation	24-Hour Urine
Protein	Normal intake: avoid excess	Monitor urinary urea
Calcium	Normal intake:1000 mg if age <50 years; 1200 mg if age >50 years Divide intake between three or more eating sessions. Choose from dairy or nondairy sources	Calcium <150 mg/L (<3.75 mmol/L)
Oxalate	Avoid moderate- to high-oxalate foods if urinary oxalate is high	Oxalate <20 mg/L (<220 µmol/L)
Fluid	2.5 L or more; assess type of fluids consumed; provide guidelines	Volume > 2 L/day
Purines	Avoid excessive protein intake; avoid specific high-purine foods	Uric acid <2 mmol/L (<336 mg/L)
Vitamin C	Avoid supplementation	Monitor urinary oxalate
Vitamin D	Meet DRI for vitamin D intake; use supplements to reach DRI	Serum 25(OH)D_3 in acceptable range
Vitamin B_6	No risk associated; no recommendation made except for primary hyperoxaluria	
Sodium	<100 mmol/day	Monitor urinary sodium

DRI, Dietary reference intake.

of recurrence, severity of stone disease, and presence of associated medical conditions (Shah and Calle, 2016).

When a patient passes a stone, it should be determined whether it is a new stone or a preexisting one and advisement given accordingly. The effectiveness of any MNT should be monitored with evaluation of subsequent 24-hour urine collections. This gives the dietitian and patient a measure of the effect of dietary changes. Once diet therapy is initiated, the goal is to prevent new stones from forming and preexisting stones from growing (see *Pathophysiology and Care Management Algorithm:* Kidney Stones).

Fluid and Urine Volume. A low urine volume is by far the most common abnormality noted in the metabolic evaluation of stone formers, and its correction with a high fluid intake should be the focus with all types of kidney stones. The objective is to maintain urinary solutes in the undersaturated zone to inhibit nucleation; this is accomplished by an increase in urine volume and reduction of solute load. The goal is the amount of urine flow rather than a specified fluid intake. High urine flow rate tends to wash out any formed crystals, and a urine volume of 2 to 2.5 L/day should prevent stone recurrence (Shah and Calle, 2016). Fluid intake should change based on different rates of extrarenal fluid loss that affect rate of urine flow. The concentration of urinary risk factors is important, not the absolute amount excreted, as the former will be high when the urine volume is low. The goal should be to maintain appropriate concentration of solutes per liter of urine.

Achieving a urine volume of 2 to 2.5 L/day usually requires an intake of 250 mL of fluid at each meal, between meals, at bedtime, and when arising to void at night. Hydration during sleep hours is important to break the cycle of the "most-concentrated" morning urine. Half of this daily 2.5 L should be taken as water. Even higher fluid intake, perhaps as much as 3 L/day, may be necessary to compensate for any GI fluid loss, excessive sweating from strenuous exercise, or an excessively hot or dry environment. Barriers to fluid intake success include lack of knowledge about the benefits of fluid or not remembering to drink, disliking the taste of water, lack of thirst, lack of availability of water, needing to void frequently, and not wanting workplace disruptions. Fluid intake behavior can be improved by specifically addressing barriers relevant to the individual patient.

Not all fluids are equally beneficial for reducing the risk of kidney stones. Cranberry juice acidifies urine and is useful in the treatment of struvite stones. Black currant juice increases urinary citrate and oxalate and, because of its urine alkalinizing effect, may prevent the occurrence of uric acid stones. Orange juice has citrate that delivers an alkali load.

Tea, coffee, decaffeinated coffee, orange juice, beer, and wine have been associated with reduced risk of stone formation. Coffee and tea induce moderate diuresis because of their caffeine content. Because decaffeinated coffee has no caffeine, it is suggested that other mechanisms may be involved, such as phytochemicals with antioxidant properties. Alcohol also helps because of diuresis. In a dose response meta-analysis each 500 mL increase in water intake was associated with a significantly reduced risk of kidney stone formation. Protective associations were found for an increasing intake of tea, coffee, and alcohol but no significant risk associated with an intake of juice, soda, or milk (Xu et al, 2015). Sugar-sweetened noncola soda and punch are associated with a 33% higher risk of kidney stones versus cola sodas with a 23% higher risk (Ferraro et al, 2013).

The oxalate content of tea brewed from regular black or green tea is 300 to 1500 μmol/L. Because of this high oxalate content of black tea, it should be taken with generous amounts of added milk; milk appears to reduce oxalate absorption by binding it in the gut lumen as calcium oxalate, making it less absorbable. Herbal teas have much lower oxalate content of 31 to 75 μmol/L and are an acceptable alternative.

Animal Protein. Epidemiologic studies find a correlation between improved standard of living, high animal protein intake, and the rising incidence of kidney stones. Meat, fish, poultry, eggs, cheese, and grains are the primary contributors of acid; a load of acid to kidney evaluation (LAKE) score can be a simple and useful tool to evaluate dietary PRAL. Dietary modifications can be made to achieve LAKE reduction for the prevention of kidney stones. Fruits, juices, vegetables, potatoes, and legumes have negative PRAL values (Trinchieri, 2012) (see *Clinical Insight:* Acid and Alkaline Diets). An adequate-calcium (1200 mg/day), low-animal protein (52 g/day), low-salt diet (50 mmol/day) was associated with a lower incidence of stone recurrence compared with low calcium (400 mg/day) diet. Several multicomponent dietary interventions to study the effect of restricting animal protein have taken place but an independent evaluation of the effect of animal protein restriction has not been done. A protein moderation with a recommended intake of 0.8-1.0 g/kg/day is recommended (Shah and Calle, 2016; Morgan and Pearle, 2016) in calcium oxalate and uric acid stone formers who have relatively high levels of uric acid. Long-term consumption of protein supplements (whey protein and albumin) to increase muscle mass and improve performance may cause variable increase in urinary calcium, lower pH, and increase in urinary sodium (albumin). Caution and monitoring are warranted (Hattori et al, 2017).

Oxalate. Because much less oxalate than calcium exists in urine (the ratio is 1:5), changes in oxalate concentration have a greater effect than changes in urinary calcium. However, oxalate absorption, which is 3% to 8% of the amount in food, is affected by the amount of dietary calcium. Dietary calcium reduces oxalate absorption and appears to have more impact on urinary oxalate than the amount of dietary oxalate. The impact of dietary oxalate on urinary oxalate appears to be small. Absorption of soluble oxalate with varying amounts of daily calcium intake from 200 to 1800 mg/day showed a linear inverse relationship between daily calcium intake and oxalate absorption. Normal healthy people who consume oxalate at 100 to 750 mg/day can have an increase of 2 mg urinary oxalate per 100 mg of oxalate consumed. A difference of 5 mg increase in urinary oxalate can be associated with a 70% to 100% increase in stone risk in some groups (Holmes et al, 2016). Age is associated independently and inversely with urinary oxalate.

Dietary counseling to reduce oxalate absorption is beneficial for stone-forming individuals who have large intakes of high-oxalate foods and who excrete more than 30 mg (350 μmol) of oxalate per day. Based on the available evidence, severe oxalate restriction is not necessary. A low oxalate intake is considered at 80 to 100 mg/day (Holmes et al, 2016). Strategies to reduce urine oxalate excretion should be dually controlled with a reasonable reduction in oxalate intake (see Box 34.1 for foods high in oxalate) and maintenance of normal calcium consumption. The growth of kidney stones is not likely to be a constant process; it responds to transient sharp increases in oxalate concentration. It should be emphasized to patients that deviations in any meal or snack could potentially result in significant stone growth. Infrequent ingestion of high-oxalate and low-calcium foods (e.g., spinach) could risk rapid stone growth (Holmes et al, 2016). The patient is advised to add calcium to each meal to bind oxalate. The total calcium intake for the day can be divided between at least three meals or as many eating occasions as possible. Patients should include approximately 150 mg calcium in each meal, such as that found in ½ cup milk, ice cream, pudding, yogurt, or ¾ oz cheese. In recurrent stone formers the DASH diet, which includes foods rich in oxalate compared with a low-oxalate diet, showed lower urinary saturation of calcium-oxalate, higher urine pH, and increased urinary magnesium and citrate excretion. A modified DASH diet with a reduced oxalate content may be more effective (Noori et al, 2014; Morgan and Pearle, 2016). Probiotics, specifically *Lactobacillus acidophilus*, have been shown to prevent

PATHOPHYSIOLOGY AND CARE MANAGEMENT ALGORITHM

Kidney Stones

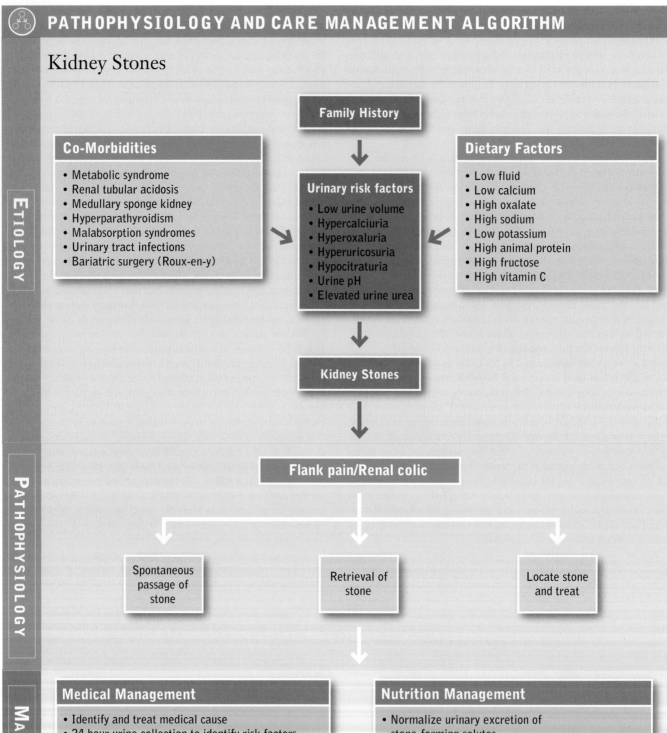

Family History

↓

Co-Morbidities

- Metabolic syndrome
- Renal tubular acidosis
- Medullary sponge kidney
- Hyperparathyroidism
- Malabsorption syndromes
- Urinary tract infections
- Bariatric surgery (Roux-en-y)

Urinary risk factors

- Low urine volume
- Hypercalciuria
- Hyperoxaluria
- Hyperuricosuria
- Hypocitraturia
- Urine pH
- Elevated urine urea

Dietary Factors

- Low fluid
- Low calcium
- High oxalate
- High sodium
- Low potassium
- High animal protein
- High fructose
- High vitamin C

↓

Kidney Stones

↓

Flank pain/Renal colic

| Spontaneous passage of stone | Retrieval of stone | Locate stone and treat |

Medical Management

- Identify and treat medical cause
- 24 hour urine collection to identify risk factors
- Stone analysis
- Shockwave lithotripsy
- Surgical, endourologic stone removal
- Antimicrobial therapy
- Pharmacologic treatment

Nutrition Management

- Normalize urinary excretion of stone-forming solutes
- Increase fluids to achieve daily urine volume >2 L
- Dietary calcium based on DRI
- Avoid high oxalate foods
- Lower salt intake
- Moderate animal protein
- Vitamin C not >500 mg/day

ETIOLOGY

PATHOPHYSIOLOGY

MANAGEMENT

intestinal oxalate absorption and therefore decrease its urinary excretion (Hermann and Suarez, 2017). New therapies include an oral formulation of the recombinant form of microbial enzyme that degrades dietary oxalate in the gut and decreases urinary oxalate excretion but needs more trials before it is accepted for use (Langman et al, 2016).

Potassium. Potassium intake is related inversely to the risk of kidney stones. Stone formers often have a low to normal potassium intake and high sodium intake that results in an adversely raised Na:K ratio. Estimation of fruit and vegetable intake should be included in the metabolic evaluation. Stone formers should be encouraged to consume diets high in potassium by choosing low-oxalate fruit and vegetables many times throughout the day (see Appendix 44 and Box 34.1). Foods high in potassium are replete with alkali, which stimulates urinary citrate excretion, raises pH and urine volume as shown in the study of dietary protein type (dairy, nondairy animal, and vegetable) and potassium, and animal protein to potassium ratio (an estimate of net acid load). Potassium intake is associated with lower risk of incident kidney stones. Greater risk is associated with higher animal protein to potassium ratio. Dairy protein was a better option compared with nondairy protein (Ferraro et al, 2016b).

Magnesium. Magnesium is a low-molecular-weight inhibitor that forms soluble complexes with oxalate. Like calcium, it inhibits oxalate absorption and may have a role to play in hyperoxaluric patients.

Phosphate. Excess urine phosphate contributes to calcium phosphate stone risk, but it is not as important a risk factor as urinary pH, which determines how much phosphate will be in the form of hydrogen phosphate (HPO_4). Calcium phosphate stones tend to occur in pregnant women in the second and third trimesters of pregnancy.

Sodium. The daily amount of sodium in modern diets reaches excessive levels that average 3500 mg/day in the United States. The amount of sodium in the urine and hypercalciuria are correlated directly because sodium and calcium are reabsorbed at common sites in the renal tubule. The risk for nephrolithiasis is significantly higher in hypertensive individuals compared with normotensive individuals. A low-sodium diet and water therapy lowered urine sodium, calcium, and oxalate in idiopathic hypercalciuric stone formers compared with controls on water therapy alone (Taylor et al, 2009). Urine sodium is associated positively with urine calcium and urine volume and negatively with urine calcium-oxalate supersaturation. Increased volume may confer a protective effect.

Sodium intake should be lowered to less than 2300 mg/day in patients with hypercalciuria. Consumption of a diet modeled on the DASH diet reduces the risk for kidney stones. Higher DASH scores are associated with higher intakes of calcium, potassium, magnesium, oxalate, and vitamin C and lower intakes of sodium as the diet is moderately high in low-fat dairy products, fruits and vegetables, and nuts and low in animal proteins (see Appendix 17).

Citrate. Citrate inhibits urinary stones by forming a complex with calcium in urine. Thus less calcium is available to bind urinary oxalate, which helps prevent the formation of calcium oxalate or calcium phosphate stones. Distal renal tubular acidosis (RTA) is an acidosis accompanied by hypokalemia. RTA, malabsorption syndrome with enteric hyperoxaluria, and excessive meat intake (lower urine pH) are associated with decreased urinary citrate levels.

Many citrate-containing beverages have been tested for their effect on urine. Several diet sodas contain moderate amounts of citrate and malate, bicarbonate precursors; malate increases the total alkali load delivered, which augments citraturia. One commercial sports drink tested in non–stone formers increased urine citrate as much as 170 mg/day, but many sports drinks also contain too much fructose and do not increase urinary citrate. Melon juice has citrate and malate and a PRAL value more negative than orange juice. Fresh tomato juice has citrate and malate and is low in sodium and oxalate.

Hypocitraturia is most commonly idiopathic but also may be caused by acidosis accompanied by hypokalemia, malabsorption syndrome with enteric hyperoxaluria, excessive meat intake, and acid ash. Half of recurrent calcium stone formers have hypocitraturia (urinary citrate of less than 300 mg/day). Normal daily urinary citrate level should be more than 640 mg/day. Long-term lemonade or lime or lemon juice therapy in hypocitraturic stone formers results in increased urinary citrate levels and decreased stone formation rate. Mineral water, with its magnesium and bicarbonate content, raises urine pH and stone inhibition.

Fructose. Fructose intake has increased approximately 2000% during the past 30 years from the widespread use of high-fructose corn syrup in foods. Fructose may increase urinary excretion of calcium and oxalate. It is the only carbohydrate known to increase the production of uric acid and its urinary excretion. Fructose also may increase insulin resistance, which is associated with low urine pH. Fructose intake has been positively associated with risk for all types of kidney stones. Increased fruit and vegetable consumption is recommended to increase potassium intake, but because of the fructose content of fruit, there should be more emphasis on vegetables.

Vitamins. Vitamin C can break down to oxalate in tissues as it performs its antioxidant function. Studies support vitamin C intake as a significant risk factor for the development of kidney stones. Men with an intake >218 mg/day had a 31% higher risk of forming stones than those consuming <105 mg/day. Supplemental vitamin C at 1000 mg/day was associated with twofold increased risk of kidney stones in men compared with less than 90 mg/day. Greater than 1000 mg/day results in 6.8 mg more oxalate in urine (Holmes et al, 2016). In another study, which included women, total vitamin C intake and supplemental vitamin C intake correlated with risk for stone formation in men but not women. In another study dietary vitamin C intake was not associated with stones among men or women although few participants had dietary intakes >700 mg/day (Ferraro et al, 2016a). Thus individuals with calcium oxalate stone disease and high levels of urine oxalate should avoid vitamin C supplementation and watch their intake of vitamin C–rich foods (Holmes et al, 2016).

Vitamin B_6 in the form of pyridoxal phosphate is a required cofactor in oxalate metabolism in promoting the activity of alanine glyoxylate aminotransferase, which diverts glyoxylate away from oxalate synthesis and may reduce urinary oxalate excretion. Conflicting results were found between intake of vitamin B_6 and risk of kidney stones in previous studies. Based on the result of a large cohort, no association was found between intake of vitamin B_6 and incident stones (Ferraro et al, 2018). Marginal B_6 status should be avoided. Pyridoxine supplementation, incrementally up to a dosage of 20 mg/kg/day in primary hyperoxaluria, has shown a 25% relative reduction in urinary oxalate, with benefit seen in 50% of patients (Morgan and Pearle, 2016; Holmes, et al 2016).

Patients with kidney stones have significantly higher vitamin D levels compared with controls (Wang et al, 2016). There is no statistically significant association between total vitamin D intake (<100 to = > 1000 IU/day) and supplemental vitamin D intake (0 to = > 1000 IU/day) and risk of incident stones (Ferraro et al, 2017b). Use of vitamin D in typical amounts used appears safe (Ferraro et al, 2017b). Long-term vitamin D supplementation did not increase the risk of kidney stones (Malihi, 2016).

Omega-3 Fatty Acids. Elevated levels of arachidonic acid (AA) in cell membranes may promote hypercalciuria and hyperoxaluria. The intake of omega-3 fatty acids such as eicosapentaenoic acid (EPA) and docosahexaenoic acid (DHA) may decrease the AA content of cell membranes and reduce urinary excretion of calcium and oxalate. EPA is an inhibitor of AA metabolism resulting in decreased synthesis of prostaglandin E2 (PGE2), a substance known to potentiate urine calcium excretion. The use of fish oil (omega-3 fatty acids at 1200 mg/day) in the treatment of hypercalciuric stone formers combined with diet counseling resulted in a measurable decrease in urine calcium (24% became normocalciuric) and oxalate excretion, and an increase in urinary citrate. Calcium-oxalate supersaturation decreased in 38% of subjects. EPA at 1800 mg/day showed significant reduction in stone episodes (Yasui et al, 2008). Fish oil administration needs further exploration to confirm its effects and mode of action.

EDUCATION, ADHERENCE, AND COMPLIANCE

Based on current practice patterns more than half of the urologists provide dietary recommendations for greater than 75% of patients, time spent varying from less than 4 minutes to greater than or equal to 10 minutes. Although greater than 76% would like another provider to give recommendations, only 23% partner with a registered dietitian nutritionist (RDN) to do so (Wertheim et al, 2014). Multiple patient factors account for compliance and adherence with diet recommendations. Less than three recommendations are associated with higher patient recall. Most important dietary strategies to reduce stone risk should be prioritized, reserving those less important for follow-up (Penniston et al, 2016).

ACUTE KIDNEY INJURY (ACUTE RENAL FAILURE)

Pathophysiology

Acute kidney injury (AKI) is characterized by a sudden reduction in glomerular filtration rate (GFR), the amount of filtrate per unit in the nephrons, and altered ability of the kidney to excrete the daily production of metabolic waste. AKI can occur in association with oliguria (decreased output of urine) or normal urine flow, but it typically occurs in previously healthy kidneys. Duration varies from a few days to several weeks. The causes of AKI are numerous and can occur simultaneously (Table 34.5). These causes are generally classified into three categories: (1) inadequate renal perfusion (prerenal), (2) diseases within the renal parenchyma (intrinsic), and (3) urinary tract obstruction (postrenal).

A technique to help clinicians assess the severity and progression of AKI uses the acronym RIFLE (Risk, Injury, Failure, Loss, and ESRD), indicating the likelihood of a patient recovering or progressing to chronic renal failure. This, in turn, helps dietitians know whether to increase protein intake goals or be more moderate to preserve kidney function.

Medical Management

The ratio of blood urea nitrogen (BUN) to Cr can be used diagnostically to assess the location of damage to the kidney. Depending on where the insult occurs, BUN is increased because of poor filtration and is more actively reabsorbed. In this situation, with a BUN/Cr ratio greater than 20:1, damage is prerenal (before the kidney). Generally, if careful attention is directed at diagnosing and correcting the prerenal or obstructive causes, AKI is short lived and requires no particular nutritional intervention.

When damage is intrinsic (within the kidney), the BUN/Cr ratio decreases to less than 10:1. Intrinsic AKI can result from causes listed in Table 34.5; of these, a prolonged episode of ischemia leading to ischemic acute tubular necrosis is the most devastating. Typically patients develop this illness as a complication of an overwhelming infection, severe trauma, surgical accident, or cardiogenic shock. The clinical course and outcome depend mainly on the underlying cause. Patients with AKI caused by drug toxicity generally recover fully after they stop taking the drug. On the other hand, the mortality rate associated with ischemic acute tubular necrosis caused by shock is approximately 70%. Typically these patients are highly catabolic, and extensive tissue destruction occurs in the early stages. Hemodialysis (HD), which is discussed later, is used to reduce the acidosis, correct the uremia, and control hyperkalemia.

If recovery is to occur, it generally takes place within 2 to 3 weeks after the insult is corrected. The recovery (diuretic) phase is characterized first by an increase in urine output and later by a return of waste elimination. During this period dialysis may still be required, and careful attention must be paid to fluid and electrolyte balance and appropriate replacement.

Medical Nutrition Therapy

Nutritional care in AKI is particularly important because the patient not only has uremia, metabolic acidosis, and fluid and electrolyte imbalance but also usually suffers from physiologic stress (e.g., infection or tissue destruction) that increases protein needs. The problem of balancing protein and energy needs with treatment of acidosis and excessive nitrogenous waste is complicated and delicate. In the early stages of AKI the patient is often unable to eat. Early attention to nutritional support and early dialysis improves patient survival.

At the onset of AKI, depending on severity, some patients can be treated with medical management, and other patients require renal replacement therapy (RRT) with standard hemodialysis (HD) or peritoneal dialysis (PD) to remove wastes and fluids until kidney function returns. In significant AKI, a patient in the intensive care unit (ICU) may require continuous treatments, rather than periodic dialysis. Continuous renal replacement therapy (CRRT) is the broad category term that includes a whole host of modalities. Most often used are continuous venovenous hemofiltration (CVVH) and continuous venovenous hemodialysis (CVVHD), which use a small ultrafiltration membrane to produce an ultrafiltrate that can be replaced by parenteral nutrition (PN) fluids. This treatment allows parenteral feeding without fluid overload.

Protein. The amount of protein recommended is influenced by the underlying cause of AKI and the presence of other conditions. A

TABLE 34.5	Some Causes of Acute Kidney Injury
Causes	**Condition**
Prerenal inadequate renal perfusion	Severe dehydration Circulatory collapse
Intrinsic diseases within the renal parenchyma	Acute tubular necrosis • Trauma, surgery • Septicemia Ischemic acute tubular necrosis Nephrotoxicity • Antibiotics, contrast agents, and other drugs Local reaction to drugs Vascular disorders • Bilateral renal infarction **Acute glomerulonephritis** of any cause • Poststreptococcal infection • Systemic lupus erythematosus
Postrenal urinary tract obstruction	Benign prostatic hypertrophy with urinary retention Carcinoma of the bladder or prostate Retroperitoneal or pelvic cancer Bilateral ureteral stones and obstruction Rhabdomyolysis

range of recommended levels can be found in the literature, from 0.5 to 0.8 g/kg for nondialysis patients to 1 to 2 g/kg for patients receiving dialysis. With CRRT protein losses are high, and estimated protein needs increase to 1.5 to 2.5 g/kg. As the patient's overall medical status stabilizes and improves, metabolic requirements decrease. During this stable period before renal function returns, a minimum protein intake of 0.8 to 1 g/kg of body weight should be given. This remains dependent on the patient's overall status and comorbidities and should be evaluated individually. In the past AKI patients were maintained in the hospital. Recent changes in Centers for Medicare and Medicaid Services (CMS) regulations have stable AKI patients moving to outpatient dialysis units. Questions may be posed to the nephrologist to clarify if the goal is lower protein for preserving or regaining kidney function versus a higher protein goal to address needs for healing and immune function.

Energy. Energy requirements are determined by the underlying cause of AKI and comorbidity. Energy needs can be measured at the bedside by indirect calorimetry in most ICUs (see Chapter 2). If this equipment is not available, calorie needs should be estimated at 25 to 40 kcal/kg/day of upper end ideal body weight (IBW). Excessive calorie intake can lead to excess CO_2 production, depressing respiration (see Chapter 33). With newer solutions available, glucose can be either absorbed or lost, depending on the concentration or type of solution used, and can be a source of calorie loss or gain. Large intakes of carbohydrate and fat are needed to prevent the use of protein for energy production. For patients who receive PN, high concentrations of carbohydrate and lipid can be administered to fulfill these needs as long as respiratory status is monitored.

A high-calorie, low-protein diet may be used in cases in which dialysis or hemofiltration is unavailable. In addition to the usual dietary sources of refined sweets and fats, special high-calorie, low-protein, and low-electrolyte formulas have been developed to augment the diet. However, care must be taken with these products because hyperglycemia is not uncommon as a result of glucose intolerance, and additional insulin often is needed.

Fluid and Sodium. During the early (often oliguric) phase of AKI, meticulous attention to fluid status is essential. Ideally fluid and electrolyte intake should balance the net output. With negligible urine output, significant contributions to total body water output include emesis and diarrhea, body cavity drains, and skin and respiratory losses. If fever is present, skin losses can be excessive, whereas if the patient is on humidified air, almost no losses occur. Because of the numerous IV drugs, blood, and blood products necessitated by the underlying disease, the challenge in managing patients at this point becomes how to cut fluid intake as much as possible while providing adequate protein and energy.

Sodium is restricted based on decreased urinary production. In the oliguric phase when the sodium output is very low, intake should be low as well, perhaps as low as 20 to 40 mEq/day. However, limiting sodium is often impossible because of the requirement for many IV solutions (including IV antibiotics, medications for blood pressure, and PN). The administration of these solutions in electrolyte-free water in the face of oliguria quickly leads to water intoxication (hyponatremia). For this reason, all fluid above the daily calculated water loss should be given in a balanced salt solution. Furthermore, aggressive fluid removal in AKI is generally discouraged. The risk of myocardial stunning, meaning damaging the heart by reducing left ventricular function from removing fluid too quickly, goes against the goals of returning the patient to prior stable health (Mahmoud, 2017).

Potassium. Most of the excretion of potassium and the control of potassium balance are normal functions of the kidney. When renal function is impaired, potassium balance should be scrutinized

TABLE 34.6 Summary of Medical Nutrition Therapy for Acute Kidney Injury

Nutrient	Amount
Protein	Adjust per MD. For goal of regain of function 0.8-1 g/kg IBW increasing as GFR returns to normal, but if the cause of AKI requires protein for healing, the goal should be closer to 1-1.2 g/kg IBW
Energy	30-40 kcal/kg of body weight
Potassium	30-50 mEq/day in oliguric phase (depending on urinary output, dialysis, and serum K^+ level); replace losses in diuretic phase
Sodium	20-40 mEq/day in oliguric phase (depending on urinary output, edema, dialysis, and serum Na^+ level); replace losses in diuretic phase
Fluid	Replace output from the previous day (vomitus, diarrhea, urine) plus 500 mL
Phosphorus	Limit as necessary

AKI, Acute kidney injury; *GFR,* glomerular filtration rate; *IBW,* ideal body weight; K^+, potassium; *MD,* medical doctor; Na^+, sodium.

carefully. In addition to dietary sources, all body tissues contain large amounts of potassium; thus tissue destruction can lead to potassium overload. Potassium levels can shift abruptly and have to be monitored frequently. Potassium intake must be individualized according to serum levels (see Appendix 44). The primary mechanism of potassium removal during AKI is dialysis. Control of serum potassium levels between dialysis administrations relies mainly on IV infusions of glucose, insulin, and bicarbonate, all of which drive potassium into cells. Exchange resins, such as sodium polystyrene sulfonate (Kayexalate), which exchange potassium for sodium in the GI tract, can be used to treat high potassium concentrations; however, for many reasons these resins are less than ideal. Table 34.6 summarizes MNT for AKI.

CHRONIC KIDNEY DISEASE

Many forms of kidney disease, two of which are described earlier, are characterized by a slow, steady decline in renal function and lead to renal failure in some patients, whereas other patients have a benign course without loss of renal function. It is unclear why some patients remain stable with chronic kidney disease (CKD) for many months to years, whereas others progress rapidly to renal failure and dialysis. The nature of this progressive loss of function has been the subject of an enormous amount of basic and clinical research during the past several decades and the subject of several excellent reviews (National Kidney Foundation, 2018; Yang et al, 2014). MNT begins when the patient is diagnosed, with the goal of preventing the progression of the disease as well as mitigating symptoms.

Pathophysiology

Diabetes is the leading risk factor for CKD followed by hypertension and glomerulonephritis. The National Kidney Foundation divides CKD into five stages related to the estimated glomerular filtration rate (eGFR), the rate at which the kidneys are filtering wastes (Table 34.7). Stages 1 and 2 are early stages with markers such as proteinuria, hematuria, or anatomic issues. Stages 3 and 4 are considered advanced stages. Stage 5 results in death unless dialysis or transplantation is initiated. See Box 34.2 for additional causes of CKD.

TABLE 34.7   Stages of Chronic Kidney Disease

				Albuminuria Categories		
				A1	**A2**	**A3**
				Normal to mildly increased	Moderately increased	Severely increased
				<30 mg/g <3 mg/mmol	30–299 mg/g 3-29 mg/mmol	≥300 mg/g ≥30 mg/mmol
GFR stages	**G1**	Normal or high	≥90			
	G2	Mildly decreased	60–90			
	G3a	Mildly to moderately decreased	45–59			
	G3b	Moderately to severely decreased	30–44			
	G4	Severely decreased	15–29			
	G5	Kidney failure	<15			

Key to Figure:
Colors: Represents the risk for progression, morbidity and mortality by color from best to worst.

Green: Low risk (if no other markers of kidney disease, no CKD)
Yellow: Moderately increased risk
Orange: High risk
Red: Very high risk
Deep red: Highest risk

From National Kidney Foundation. *Estimated Glomerular Filtration Rate* (website). https://www.kidney.org/atoz/content/gfr.

BOX 34.2   Causes of Chronic Kidney Disease (CKD)

	Examples of systemic diseases affecting the kidney	Examples of primary kidney diseases (absence of systemic diseases affecting the kidney)
Glomerular diseases	Diabetes, systemic autoimmune diseases, systemic infections, drugs, neoplasia (including amyloidosis)	Diffuse, focal or crescentic proliferative glomerulonephritis; focal and segmental glomerulosclerosis; membranous nephropathy, minimal change disease
Tubulointerstitial diseases	Systemic infections, autoimmune, sarcoidosis, drugs, urate, environmental toxins (lead, aristolochic acid), neoplasia (myeloma)	Urinary-tract infections, stones, obstruction
Vascular diseases	Atherosclerosis, hypertension, ischemia, cholesterol emboli, systemic vasculitis, thrombotic microangiopathy, systemic sclerosis	ANCA-associated renal limited vasculitis; fibromuscular dysplasia
Cystic and congenital diseases	Polycystic kidney disease, Alport's syndrome, Fabry's disease	Renal dysplasia, medullary cystic disease, podocytopathies

Genetic diseases are not considered separately because some diseases in each category are now recognized as having genetic determinants.

National Kidney Foundation. *How to Classify CKD* (website). https://www.kidney.org/professionals/explore-your-knowledge/how-to-classify-ckd.

Medical Management

The prevalence of CKD is now estimated at approximately 15% of adults in the United States, or greater than 30 million Americans. This estimated prevalence of CKD shows that 1 in 3 people with diabetes and 1 in 5 people with hypertension have CKD (Centers for Disease Control and Prevention [CDC], 2019). Many states have legislated clinical laboratories reporting serum Cr also to report the patient's eGFR. Patients with a low calculated eGFR do not necessarily have CKD. They must have several blood samples drawn 3 months apart that are consistently low (showing eGFR of less than 60) (see Table 34.7). The National Kidney Foundation and the American Society for Clinical Pathology and many other laboratories have standardized testing, so that doctors can easily identify and diagnose patients. Evidenced-based clinical practice guidelines recommend two tests for CKD assessment: eGFR and urine albumin-Cr ratio. These tests come paired on most laboratory profiles. This streamlining of tests helps doctors easily monitor all patients for the presence of kidney disease.

An online eGFR calculator can be found at the National Kidney Foundation website. With screening tools such as the calculated eGFR and a greater awareness of the progressive nature of CKD, more attention has focused on its social, medical, and financial effects. For example, CKD is strongly linked with cardiovascular disease (see *Clinical Insight:* Chronic Kidney Disease and Heart Disease—A Deadly Union).

CLINICAL INSIGHT

Chronic Kidney Disease and Heart Disease—A Deadly Union

The presence of chronic kidney disease (CKD) increases the risk category for those with cardiovascular disease (CVD), and exacerbates existing CVD. An alarming fact is that most patients with CKD die of heart disease before they develop end-stage renal disease. Recommendations are that CKD patients should decrease their cardiovascular risks: quit smoking, increase exercise, choose healthy fats, increase intake of fruits and vegetables, and reach and maintain a healthy body weight. Fortunately, intervention makes a difference. The United States Renal Data System Dialysis M/M Study included 2264 patients with CKD. More than half had not seen a nephrologist in the year before needing dialysis, and a third had their first nephrologist encounter less than 4 months before starting dialysis. This late referral to nephrologists resulted in low serum albumin and hematocrit levels. Patients who had seen a nephrologist at least 2 years before dialysis had a decrease in mortality. Thus patients who have CKD and receive early nutrition counseling may postpone the need for dialysis, or come to dialysis better nourished. The expertise of the renal dietitian has been recognized by the Center for Medicare Services, allowing for physician-ordered medical nutrition therapy by registered dietitian nutritionist (RDN) providers for Americans with CKD who are not on dialysis.

Medical Nutrition Therapy

With each level of CKD, a different nutritional therapy may be proposed. The primary objectives of MNT are to manage the symptoms associated with the syndrome by treating the primary cause of the disease and then the secondary symptoms (edema, hypoalbuminemia, and metabolic acidosis), decrease the risk of progression to renal failure, decrease inflammation, and maintain nutritional stores. Patients are treated primarily with sodium bicarbonate, blood pressure medicines such as angiotensin-converting enzyme (ACE) inhibitors and angiotensin II receptor blockers (ARBs), low-sodium diets, and diuretics. Research has shown that starting with diet modification, specifically increasing fruits and vegetables, can be as effective alone or paired with these treatments (Goraya et al, 2013). Research further shows that use of ACEs and ARBs work poorly when not in the setting of a low-sodium diet (Garofalo et al, 2018). The DASH and Mediterranean diet are being utilized more and more for MNT in CKD to support patients (Gallieni and Cupisti, 2016).

Protein. Patients with an established severe protein deficiency who continue to lose protein may require an extended time of carefully supervised nutritional care. The diet should attempt to provide sufficient protein and energy to maintain a positive nitrogen balance and to support tissue synthesis while not overtaxing the kidneys. In most cases, sufficient intake from carbohydrate and fats is needed to spare protein for anabolism. Providing adequate protein remains the same goal with Nephrotic Syndrome. With this diagnosis, giving excess protein tends to cause more protein to spill into the urine further damaging the kidneys, with little impact on improving nutritional status.

The recommended dietary protein level for CKD patients has changed over time. Historically, these patients received diets low in protein to prevent symptoms of uremia prior to the development of dialysis. Studies have shown that a reduction of protein intake to 0.8 g/kg/day may decrease proteinuria without adversely affecting serum albumin. Multiple studies comparing protein intake in this population have had inconsistent results. It seems prudent to encourage adequate protein targeted to their overall nutrition needs.

A large multicenter trial, Modification of Diet in Renal Disease (MDRD), attempted to determine the role of protein, phosphorus restriction, and blood pressure control in the progression of renal disease. Thus the National Institute of Diabetes and Digestive and Kidney Diseases (NIDDKD) developed recommendations for the management of patients with progressive renal disease or pre-ESRD. Those recommendations for dietary protein intake in progressive renal failure are 0.8 g/kg/day with 60% high biologic value (HBV) for patients whose GFR is greater than 55 mL/min, and 0.6 g/kg/day with 60% HBV for patients whose GFR is 25 to 55 mL/min.

The National Kidney Foundation's Kidney Dialysis Outcome Quality Initiative (KDOQI) panel who establish national renal guidelines and Kidney Disease Improving Global Outcomes (KDIGO) who establish international guidelines, suggests that patients whose GFR is less than 25 mL/min and who have not yet begun dialysis should be maintained on 0.6 g/kg/day of protein and 35 kcal/kg/day. If patients cannot maintain an adequate caloric intake on this protein recommendation, their protein intake should be increased to 0.75 g/kg/day. In both cases approximately 50% of the protein should be of HBV.

The potential benefits of protein restriction in the patient with moderate renal insufficiency must be weighed against the potential hazards of such treatment (i.e., protein malnutrition). If protein is restricted, careful monitoring and anthropometric studies should be carried out periodically as directed by the KDOQI guidelines.

Systemic hypertension, which aggravates the progressive loss of renal function, must be well controlled to produce benefits from protein restriction. Also important in the control of the progression of renal failure in people with diabetes is good blood glucose control. In a national multicenter trial, the Diabetes Control and Complications Trial (DCCT) showed that blood glucose control was more important than protein restriction in delaying the onset of renal failure in individuals who have diabetes (see Chapter 29).

Research continues about the use of more plant-based proteins in CKD, including tofu and legumes. Some benefits can be assessed looking at inflammation and improvement in mortality rates, but it is not yet conclusive that this is related to the plant-based proteins, or a result of the nutrition and lifestyle changes associated with a more plant-based diet (Sparks, 2018).

Energy. Energy intake should be approximately 35 kcal/kg/day for adults to spare protein for tissue repair and maintenance. In patients who are significantly overweight, some adjustment should be made to normalize requirements (see Box 2.1 in Chapter 2).

Sodium. Edema, the most clinically apparent manifestation, indicates total body sodium overload. In addition, because of low oncotic pressure from hypoalbuminemia, the volume of circulating blood may be reduced because of migration of fluid to interstitial space. Attempts to severely limit sodium intake or to use diuretics may cause marked hypotension, exacerbation of coagulopathy, and deterioration of renal function. Therefore control of edema in this group of diseases should be with dietary intake of 1500mg of sodium daily (Whelton et al, 2012).

Potassium. Potassium management is possible through use of medications such as diuretics, individualized diet prescription, and rate of progression of CKD. Many patients in early-stage CKD take potassium-wasting diuretics (e.g., furosemide) that require supplementation of potassium. When urine output drops below 1 L/day, these same patients may require a change to potassium restriction as the kidney is no longer able to excrete all the potassium ingested. This typically occurs rather late in stage 4 CKD.

Phosphorus. The importance of controlling phosphate in patients with early-stage disease often is overlooked. Serum phosphorous levels elevate at the same rate as eGFR decreases. Early initiation of phosphate reduction therapies is advantageous for delaying hyperparathyroidism and bone disease. Unfortunately, patients are often asymptomatic during the early phase of hyperparathyroidism and hyperphosphatemia; they may not attend to their modified diets or understand the need to take phosphate binders with meals.

Those with an eGFR of less than 60 should be evaluated for renal bone disease and benefit from phosphorus restriction. Ongoing monitoring of a patient's phosphorus and use of phosphate binders is recommended. The diet typically is modified to allow no more than 1000 mg of phosphates daily, a limit that allows approximately one to two dairy foods per day. Because of the recommended decrease in protein intake, the control of phosphorus is somewhat easier to manage. Patients who are in later stages of CKD and intolerant of red meats because of uremic taste alterations often are able to substitute milk foods for meat and still maintain a limited phosphate intake.

Lipids. The important consequence of dyslipidemia is cardiovascular disease. Pediatric patients with frequently relapsing or resistant nephrotic syndrome are at particular risk for premature atherosclerosis. Certain lipid-lowering agents in combination with a cholesterol-lowering diet can reduce total cholesterol, low-density lipoprotein cholesterol, and triglycerides in these patients (see Chapter 32). KDIGO, a global nonprofit organization that develops guidelines for the treatment of CKD, recently made the recommendation not to use statins in CKD patients as they do not improve cardiovascular outcomes despite lowering cholesterol (KDIGO, 2013). Standard diet recommendations for lowering cholesterol remain appropriate, with the understanding of protein goals.

Vitamins and Probiotics. CKD patients routinely are recommended a water-soluble renal customized vitamin supplement, because restrictions of fruits, vegetables, and dairy foods may cause the diet to be inadequate. Significant research is being done at this time linking the gut microbiome to progression of CKD paired with research to see if probiotics are both safe and effective in the treatment of this dysbiosis (Lau, 2017; Borges et al, 2018). Further research will continue to try to unlock the answers to the balance of gut repair paired with safety and efficacy of probiotics use in this immunocompromised population.

END-STAGE RENAL DISEASE

End-stage renal disease (ESRD) reflects the kidney's inability to excrete waste products, maintain fluid and electrolyte balance, and produce certain hormones. As renal failure slowly progresses, the level of circulating waste products eventually leads to symptoms of uremia (see *Pathophysiology and Care Management Algorithm:* Chronic Kidney Disease and End-Stage Renal Disease). Uremia is a clinical syndrome of malaise, weakness, nausea and vomiting, muscle cramps, itching, metallic taste in the mouth, and neurologic impairment that is brought about by an unacceptable level of nitrogenous wastes in the body.

Pathophysiology

ESRD can result from a wide variety of different kidney diseases. Currently 90% of patients reaching ESRD have chronic (1) diabetes mellitus, (2) hypertension, or (3) glomerulonephritis. The manifestations are somewhat nonspecific and vary by patient. No reliable laboratory parameter corresponds directly with the beginning of symptoms. However, as a rule of thumb, BUN of more than 100 mg/dL and Cr of 10 to 12 mg/dL are usually close to this threshold.

Medical Treatment

Once the patient progresses from stage 4 to stage 5 CKD, options for treatment for ESRD include dialysis, transplantation, or medical management progressing to death.

Dialysis

Patients may choose to dialyze in an outpatient dialysis facility, or they may prefer hemodialysis (HD) at home using either conventional daily or nocturnal dialysis. They may choose peritoneal dialysis (PD) and have a choice of continuous ambulatory peritoneal dialysis (CAPD) or automated peritoneal dialysis (APD, formerly called continuous cyclic peritoneal dialysis, or CCPD), or combinations of the two. Patients, families, and their physicians together evaluate the therapy that best meets the patient's needs (Table 34.8).

HD requires permanent access to the bloodstream through a fistula created by surgery to connect an artery and a vein (Fig. 34.2). If the patient's blood vessels are fragile, an artificial vessel called a graft may be implanted surgically. Large needles are inserted into the fistula or graft before each dialysis and removed when dialysis is complete. Temporary access through subclavian catheter is common until the patient's permanent access can be created or can mature; however, problems with infection make these catheters undesirable. In 2003 the CMS paired with the national oversight groups called the Renal Network to establish a quality improvement project called Fistulas First to encourage fistula placement and catheter removal to work toward better patient outcomes.

The HD dialysate fluid and electrolyte content is similar to that of normal plasma. Waste products and electrolytes move by diffusion, ultrafiltration, and osmosis from the blood into the dialysate and are removed (Fig. 34.3). Outpatient HD usually requires treatment of 3 to 5 hours three times per week in a dialysis unit (Fig. 34.4). Newer therapies can shorten the duration of treatment by increasing its frequency. Patients on these more frequent dialysis therapies have lower mortality rates, approaching that of transplantation. Patients on daily dialysis at home typically have treatments lasting from 2 to 3.5 hours 5 to 6 days a week, whereas some home dialysis patients receive nocturnal dialysis three to six times a week for 8 hours, while they sleep.

PD makes use of the body's own semipermeable membrane, the peritoneum. A catheter is implanted surgically through the abdomen

PATHOPHYSIOLOGY AND CARE MANAGEMENT ALGORITHM

Chronic Kidney Disease and End-Stage Renal Disease

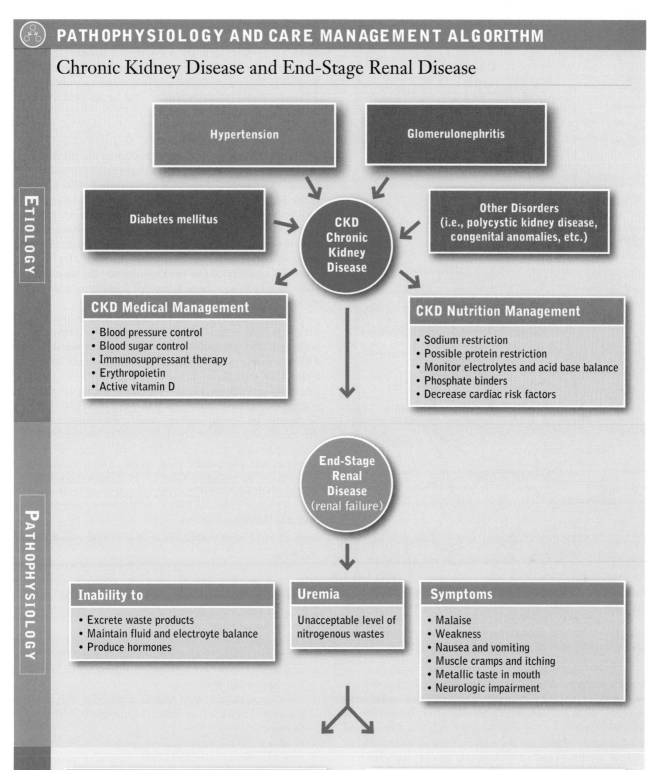

ETIOLOGY

Hypertension

Glomerulonephritis

Diabetes mellitus

CKD Chronic Kidney Disease

Other Disorders (i.e., polycystic kidney disease, congenital anomalies, etc.)

CKD Medical Management
- Blood pressure control
- Blood sugar control
- Immunosuppressant therapy
- Erythropoietin
- Active vitamin D

CKD Nutrition Management
- Sodium restriction
- Possible protein restriction
- Monitor electrolytes and acid base balance
- Phosphate binders
- Decrease cardiac risk factors

PATHOPHYSIOLOGY

End-Stage Renal Disease (renal failure)

Inability to
- Excrete waste products
- Maintain fluid and electroyte balance
- Produce hormones

Uremia
Unacceptable level of nitrogenous wastes

Symptoms
- Malaise
- Weakness
- Nausea and vomiting
- Muscle cramps and itching
- Metallic taste in mouth
- Neurologic impairment

MANAGEMENT

ESRD Medical Management
- Dialysis
- Kidney transplantation
- Immunosuppressant therapy
- Psychologic support
- Conservative treatment and preparation for death
- Erythropoietin
- Active vitamin D

ESRD Nutrition Management

Goals
- Prevent nutrient deficiencies
- Control edema and serum electrolytes
  - Sodium and potassium restriction
- Prevent renal osteodystrophy
  - Use of phosphate binders, low phosphorus diet, and calcium supplementation
- Provide a palatable and attractive diet

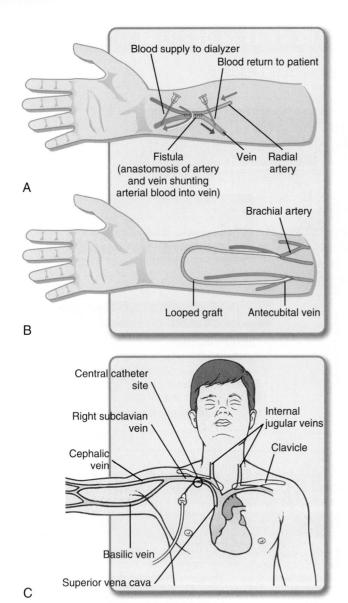

Fig. 34.2 Types of access for hemodialysis. **A,** Arteriovenous fistula. **B,** Artificial loop graft. **C,** Subclavian catheter (usually temporary). (From Lewis SL, et al: *Medical-surgical nursing: assessment and management of clinical problems,* ed 9, St Louis, 2013, Elsevier Mosby.)

and into the peritoneal cavity. **Dialysate** containing a dextrose concentration is instilled into the peritoneum, where diffusion carries waste products from the blood through the peritoneal membrane and into the dialysate; water moves by osmosis. This fluid then is withdrawn and discarded, and new solution is added multiple times each day providing 24 hours per day dialysis and is more similar to normal kidney function.

Several types of PD exist. In CAPD, the dialysate is left in the peritoneum and exchanged manually by gravity. Exchanges of dialysis fluid are done four to five times daily (Fig. 34.5). In APD, patient treatments are done at night by a machine that mechanically performs the exchanges. During the day these patients sometimes keep a single dialysate exchange in the peritoneal cavity for extended periods of time, perhaps the entire day. Different combinations of CAPD and APD are possible and are referred to here as PD.

Advantages of PD are avoidance of large fluctuations in blood chemistry, maintaining residual renal function, and achievement of a more normal lifestyle. Complications include peritonitis, challenges

managing blood sugars, and weight gain. Tissue weight gain is experienced by most patients as a result of absorbing 400 to 800 calories per day from the dextrose in the dialysate. The amount depends on the concentration of the dialysate solution and how many exchanges are done daily. This may be desirable in patients who are underweight, but eventually dietary intake or activity must be modified to account for the calories absorbed from dialysate.

Evaluation of Dialysis Efficacy

Kinetic modeling is a method for evaluating the efficacy of dialysis that measures the removal of urea from the patient's blood over a given period. This formula, often called **Kt/V** (where K is the urea clearance of the dialyzer, t is the length of time of dialysis, and V is the patient's total body water volume), should ideally produce a result higher than 1.4 per HD, or 3.2 per week. These calculations are somewhat complex and are typically calculated using a computer program. A more accurate method for determining adequacy of HD is eKt/V, in which e stands for equilibrated and takes into account the amount of time it takes for urea to equilibrate across cell membranes after dialysis has stopped. An acceptable eKt/V is 1.2 or greater.

Another method to determine effective dialysis treatment is the **urea reduction ratio (URR)**, which looks at the reduction in urea before and after dialysis. The patient is considered well dialyzed when a 65% or greater reduction in the serum urea occurs during dialysis. Unlike Kt/V, this calculation can be done quickly at the patient's bedside by the practitioner. The method for calculating the efficacy of PD is somewhat different, but a weekly Kt/V of 2 is the goal. The Kt/V can be altered by several patient- and dialysis-associated variables. The calculations for Kt/V can also be used to determine the patient's **protein-nitrogen appearance (PNA) rate**, which compares to a simplified nitrogen balance study in the dialysis patient. The PNA values should be between 0.8 and 1.4. Patients on short daily HD and nocturnal HD require different calculations to estimate their Kt/V.

Medical Nutrition Therapy

Goals of MNT in the management of ESRD are intended to do the following:

1. Prevent deficiency and maintain good nutrition status (and, in the case of children, growth) through adequate protein, energy, vitamin, and mineral intake (Table 34.9).
2. Control edema and electrolyte imbalance by controlling sodium, potassium, and fluid intake.
3. Prevent or slow the development of renal osteodystrophy by balancing calcium, phosphorus, vitamin D, and PTH.
4. Enable patients to eat a palatable, attractive diet that fits their lifestyle as much as possible.
5. Coordinate patient care with families, dietitian nutritionists, nurses, and physicians in acute care, outpatient, or skilled nursing facilities.
6. Provide initial nutrition education, periodic counseling, and long-term monitoring of patients, with the goal of patients receiving enough education to direct their own care and diet.

Table 34.10 presents a guide for teaching patients about their blood values and control of their disease. Because dialysis is done at home or in an outpatient unit, most patients with ESRD assume responsibility for their own diets. Most long-term patients know their diets very well (Fig. 34.6), having been instructed many times by renal dietitian nutritionists at their dialysis units.

Protein

Dialysis is a drain on body protein, so protein intake must be increased. In addition, exposure of patients' blood to an artificial membrane three

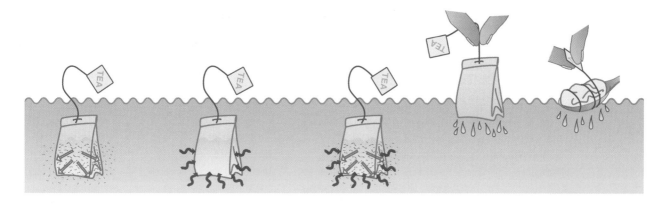

Diffusion
is the passage of particles through a semipermeable membrane. Tea, for example, diffuses from a tea bag into the surrounding water.

Osmosis
is the movement of fluid across a semipermeable membrane from a lower concentration of solutes to a higher concentration of solutes. (The water moves into the teabag.)

Diffusion and Osmosis
can occur at the same time. (Particles move out and fluid moves in at the same time.)

Filtration
is the passage of fluids through a membrane.

Ultrafiltration
provides additional pressure to squeeze extra fluid through the membrane.

Fig. 34.3 Dialysis: how it works. (Modified from Core curriculum for the dialysis technician: a comprehensive review of hemodialysis, 2001, AMGEN, Inc.)

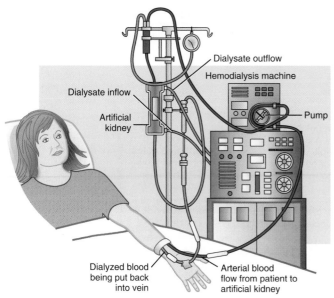

Fig. 34.4 Hemodialysis. Treatment is usually for 3 to 5 hours, three times per week.

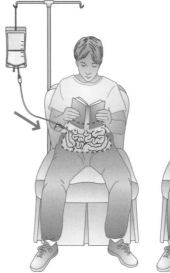
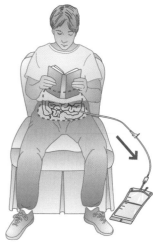

The peritoneal cavity is filled with dialysate, using gravity.

At the end of the exchange, the dialysate is drained into the bag, again using gravity.

Fig. 34.5 Continuous ambulatory peritoneal dialysis; 20-minute exchanges are given four to five times daily every day.

or more times a week induces a state of chronic inflammation and distorts protein metabolism. Patients who receive HD three times per week can lose about 15 g of protein per dialysis treatment and require a daily protein intake of 1.2 g/kg of body weight. Protein losses of 20 to 30 g can occur during a 24-hour PD, with an average of 1 g/hr. Those receiving PD need a daily protein intake of 1.2 to 1.5 g/kg of body weight. At least 50% should be HBV protein. Serum BUN and serum Cr levels, uremic symptoms, and weight should be monitored, and the diet should be adjusted accordingly.

In renal failure, prealbumin, which is metabolized by the kidney, is not a good nutritional marker, because values are routinely elevated. Albumin is not recommended by the Academy of Nutrition and Dietetics

to be used as an indicator of protein but continues to be routinely used in evaluating ESRD patients based on KDQOI goals. However, because of the complexity of either acute or chronic inflammation, albumin remains predictive more of poor survival in ESRD and less of nutritional status. Current international research cites Subjective Global Assessment as being even more predictive of clinical outcomes (Lu et al, 2017). Hypoalbuminemia is multifactorial and may be related to fluid status, inflammation, or comorbid disease. When interpreting albumin values, it is important to know the laboratory's methodology for measuring serum albumin, because different laboratory techniques give

TABLE 34.8   Options for Treatment in ESRD

	Hemodialysis	Peritoneal Dialysis	Short Daily Hemodialysis or Nocturnal Dialysis	Transplant
Primary treatment responsibility	Health care personnel	Patient and/or family member	Patient and/or family member	Patient
Diet	Low K, low PO_4, low Na, moderate protein, fluid restriction	High K, low PO_4, low Na, high protein, moderate fluid restriction	High K, low PO_4, low Na, high protein, moderate fluid restriction	High and moderate protein, no K or PO_4 restrictions, no fluid restriction.
Location	Clinical dialysis unit	Home, office, vacation	Home, vacation	No limitations
Risks	Bleeding, sepsis, infection	Peritonitis, hernia, constipation, exit site infections, poorly controlled diabetes, weight gain, early satiety	Unattended dialysis, rare user error bleeding	Immuno-compromised, diabetes, cancer
Contraindications	Poor cardiac status, poor blood vessels for access creation	Multiple abdominal surgeries, lack of a clean home, altered mental status	Dementia, illiteracy, inability to communicate, lack of a clean home	High body mass index, noncompliance with medications, less than 5-year hx of cancer

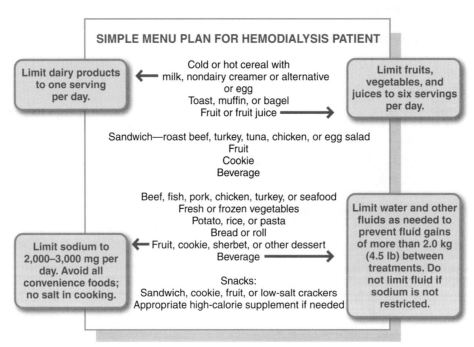

Fig. 34.6 A simple menu plan for a patient on hemodialysis. The diet should allow for less than 4% fluid weight gain between dialyses.

different results in renal failure (see Table 34.10). Federal mandates require some nutrition intervention at levels below 4 g/dL to attempt to improve albumin to this level despite the evidence that low albumin is not a function of nutritional intake.

Most patients find it challenging to consume adequate protein because uremia itself causes taste aberrations, notably to red meats. Some patients cannot tolerate even the smell of meat cooking. Often this protein aversion makes it difficult to achieve recommended HBV protein intake. Patients may prefer eggs, tofu, and "white" meats. Spices can be used to alter the taste of meats, and serving animal proteins cold, minimizes the urea taste. Nutritional supplements may be helpful in some patients, and occasionally the phosphate restriction may have to be lifted to allow the consumption of dairy products to meet protein needs. Vegetarian protein sources are able to meet protein goals for HD, and the diet can be safely recommended (Sparks, 2018). As with all the nutritional parameters, meeting patient needs must be individualized.

Energy

Energy intake should be adequate to spare protein for tissue protein synthesis and to prevent its metabolism for energy. Depending on the patient's nutrition status and degree of stress, between 25 and 40 kcal/kg of body weight should be provided, with the lower amount for transplantation and PD patients and the higher level for the nutritionally depleted patient (see Chapter 5 and Appendix 8 for determining BMI and appropriate body weight). Tools have been developed to allow the renal

TABLE 34.9 Nutrient Requirements of Adults with Renal Disease Based on Type of Therapy

Therapy	Energy	Protein	Fluid	Sodium	Potassium	Phosphorus
Impaired renal function	30-35 kcal/kg IBW	0.6-1.0 g/kg IBW	Ad libitum	Variable, 1.5-2 g/day	Variable, usually ad libitum or increased to cover losses from diuretics	0.8-1.2 g/day or 8-12 mg/kg IBW
Hemodialysis	35 kcal/kg IBW	1.2 g/kg IBW	750-1000 mL/day plus urine output	1.5-2 g/day	2-3 g/day or 40 mg/kg IBW	0.8-1.2 g/day or <17 mg/kg IBW
Peritoneal dialysis (CAPD)(CCPD)	30-35 kcal/kg IBW	1.2-1.5 g/kg IBW	Ad libitum (minimum of 1000 mL/day from urine plus output)	1.5-4 g/day	3-4 g/day	0.8-1.2 g/day
Transplant, 4-6 weeks after transplant	30-35 kcal/kg IBW	1.3-2 g/kg IBW	Ad libitum	1.5-2 g/day	Variable; may require restriction with cyclosporine-induced hyperkalemia	Calcium 1.2 g/day No need to limit phosphorus
6 weeks or longer after transplant	Kcal/kg to achieve/ maintain IBW Limit simple CHO Fat <35% cal CHO <400 mg/day PUFA/SFA ratio >1	1 g/kg IBW	Ad libitum	1.5-2 g/day	Variable	Calcium 1.2 g/day No need to limit phosphorus

CAPD, Continuous ambulatory peritoneal dialysis; *CCPD*, continuous cyclical peritoneal dialysis; CHO, cholesterol; *IBW*, ideal body weight; *PUFA*, polyunsaturated fat; *SFA*, saturated fat.
Modified from National Kidney Foundation: KDOQI clinical practice guidelines for nutrition in chronic renal failure, *Am J Kidney Dis* 35(suppl 2):S1, 2000; Wiggins K: Guidelines for nutrition care of renal patients, ed 3, Chicago, 2002, American Dietetic Association.

TABLE 34.10 Guide to Blood Values in End-Stage Renal Disease Patients

This guide is to help in understanding laboratory reports. In the following table, the normal values are for people with good kidney function. Acceptable values for dialysis patients are also given. Many things affect blood values. Diet is only one of these. Underlying disease, adequacy of treatment, medications, and complications all may affect laboratory values.

Substance	Normal Values	Normal for People on Dialysis	Function	Diet Changes
Sodium	135-145 mEq/L	135-145 mEq/L	Found in salt and many preserved foods. A diet high in sodium causes thirst. When patients drink too much fluid, it may actually dilute their sodium, and serum levels will appear low. If patients eat too much sodium and do not drink water, sodium may be high. Too much sodium and water raise blood pressure and can cause fluid overload, pulmonary edema, and congestive heart failure.	High: Check fluid status. If high fluid gains, tell patient to eat fewer salty foods. If low fluid gains, make sure patient is gaining about 1.5 kg between dialyses (or <4% body weight) and is not dehydrated (this is rare). Low: If high fluid gains, tell patient to eat less salt and fluid. Check fluid status—patient is probably drinking too much fluid. Limit weight gains to less than 4% of body weight between runs and ask patient to eat fewer salty foods and limit fluid to 3 C plus urine output.
Potassium	3.5-5.5 mEq/L	3.5-5.5 mEq/L	Found in most high-protein foods, milk, fruits, and vegetables. Affects muscle action, especially the heart. High levels can cause the heart to stop. Low levels can cause symptoms such as muscle weakness and atrial fibrillation.	High: Ascertain that no other causes, such as gastrointestinal bleeding, trauma, or medications are creating high potassium values. Tell patient to avoid foods with more than 250 mg/serving and limit daily intake to 2000 mg. Consider lowering potassium in dialysate bath. Recheck blood level next treatment. Low: Add one high-potassium food/day and recheck blood level. Use salt substitutes or potassium supplements. Consider raising potassium in dialysate bath if diet changes are not working.
Urea nitrogen (BUN)	7-23 mg/dL	50-100 mg/dL	Waste product of protein breakdown. Unlike creatinine, this is affected by the amount of protein in the diet. Dialysis removes urea nitrogen.	High: Patient is probably underdialyzed. Check eKt/V. Check nPNA. Low: Underdialysis is also a cause. BUN may decrease if patient is not eating because of uremic symptoms. Also decreases with loss of muscle.

Continued

TABLE 34.10   Guide to Blood Values in End-Stage Renal Disease Patients—cont'd

Substance	Normal Values	Normal for People on Dialysis	Function	Diet Changes
Creatinine	0.6-1.5 mg/dL	Less than 15 mg/dL	A normal waste product of muscle breakdown. This value is controlled by dialysis. Patients have a higher amount because they are not dialyzing 24 hours a day, 7 days a week, as they would with normal kidney function.	Dialysis normally controls creatinine. Low creatinine may indicate good dialysis or low body muscle. Check the clearance of urea during dialysis (Kt/V) to assess dialysis adequacy. If patient is losing weight, will break down more muscle, so creatinine may be higher. Patient may need to eat more protein and calories to stop weight loss.
URR	N/A	Above 65% (or 0.65)	A measure of reduction of urea that occurs during a dialysis treatment. Postdialysis BUN is subtracted and divided by predialysis BUN to give a percentage.	No diet changes, but catabolism or anabolism will affect values, as with Kt/V and equilibrated clearance of urea during dialysis (eKt/V).
eKt/V	N/A	Above 1.2	A mathematic formula that attempts to quantify how well a patient is dialyzed. Represents the clearance of urea by the dialyzer, multiplied by the minutes of treatment, and divided by the volume of water the patient's body holds.	No diet changes. Low: Values below 1.2 are associated with increased morbidity and mortality. High: Higher values are associated with better outcomes.
Kt/V		Above 1.2 for hemodialysis Above 2 for peritoneal dialysis	Not adjusted for urea equilibration. See above.	No diet changes. See above.
nPNA	N/A	0.8-1.4	A calculation used to look at the rate of protein turnover in the body. Assumes patient is not catabolic because of infection, fever, surgery, or trauma. A good indicator of stable patient's protein intake, when combined with dietary history and albumin. The term *normalized* means that values have been adjusted to the patient's normal or ideal weight.	High: Patient may need to decrease protein intake. Patient may be catabolic or may be eating large amounts of protein. Low: Patient may need to increase protein intake. If patient is putting out urine, a small urine volume can make a big difference in results. Have patient keep a 48-hour urine collection.
Albumin	3.5-5 g/dL (bromcresol green) 3-4.5 g/dL (bromcresol purple)	3.5-5 g/dL Above 4 g/dL	Protein is lost with all dialysis. If albumin is below 2.9, fluid will leak from blood vessels into the tissue, thus causing edema. When fluid is in the tissue, it is more difficult to remove with dialysis. Low albumin is closely associated with increased risk of death in dialysis patients.	Low: Increase intake of protein-rich foods: meat, fish, chicken, eggs. A protein supplement may be needed. Intravenous albumin corrects short-term problems with oncotic pressure but does not change serum albumin levels.
Calcium	8.5-10.2 mg/dL	8.5-10.2 mg/dL	Found in dairy products. Dialysis patients' intakes are usually low. Active vitamin D is needed for absorption. The calcium value multiplied by the phosphorus value should not exceed 59, or patient will get calcium deposits in soft tissue. Because it is bound to albumin, calcium can be falsely lower if albumin is low. Ionized calcium is a more accurate test in this case.	High: Check if patient is taking calcium supplement or a form of active vitamin D. These should be temporarily stopped. Low: If albumin is low, suggest an ionized calcium be drawn. Patient may need a calcium supplement between meals and active vitamin D. Check with physician.
Phosphorus	2.5-4.8 mg/dL	3-6 mg/dL	Found in milk products, dried beans, nuts, and meats. Used to build bones and helps the body produce energy. Acceptable levels depend on variety of factors, including calcium, PTH levels, and the level of phosphorus in diet. If calcium and PTH levels are normal, a slightly higher-than-normal level of phosphorus is acceptable.	High: Limit milk and milk products to 1 serving/day. Remind patient to take phosphate binders as ordered with meals and snacks. Noncompliance with binders is the most common cause of high phosphorus. Low: Add 1 serving milk product or other high-phosphorus food per day or decrease phosphate binders.

TABLE 34.10 Guide to Blood Values in End-Stage Renal Disease Patients—cont'd

Substance	Normal Values	Normal for People on Dialysis	Function	Diet Changes
PTH intact (I-PTH)	10-65 pg/mL	150-600 pg/mL	A high level of PTH indicates that calcium is being pulled out of bone to maintain serum calcium levels. This syndrome is called secondary hyperparathyroidism. Leads to osteodystrophy. Pulsed doses of oral or IV vitamin D usually lower PTH.	High: Check whether patient taking oral or IV active vitamin D. Contact patient's physician regarding therapy. If patient has no symptoms (high phosphorus, bone pain, fractures), treat less aggressively. Low: No treatment available.
Aluminum	0-10 mcg/L	Less than 40 mcg/L	Patients taking aluminum hydroxide phosphate binders may develop aluminum toxicity, which can cause bone disease and dementia. Value should be checked every 6 months.	High: Discontinue aluminum hydroxide treatment.
Magnesium	1.5-2.4 mg/dL	1.5-2.4 mg/dL	Magnesium normally is excreted in the urine and can become toxic to dialysis patient. High levels may be caused by antacids or laxatives that contain magnesium such as Milk of Magnesia or Maalox.	No dietary changes, except to use nontoxic methods such as fiber to aid in relief of constipation. If magnesium is used as a phosphate binder, levels will have to be checked more often.
Ferritin	Male: 20-350 mcg/L Female: 6-350 mcg/L	300-800 mcg/L with EPO; 50 mcg/L without EPO	This is the way iron is stored in the liver. If iron stores are low, red blood cell production is decreased.	Low: Iron in food is not well absorbed. Most patients need an IV iron supplement. Patients should not take oral iron at same time as phosphate binders.
CO_2	22-25 mEq/L	22-25 mEq/L	Dialysis patients are often acidotic because they do not excrete metabolic acids in their urine. Acidosis may increase the rate of muscle and bone catabolism.	Low: Review eKt/V, BUN, nPNA. Oral sodium bicarbonate may be given to raise CO_2, but it presents a significant sodium load to patient.
Glucose	65-114 mg/dL	Same for nondiabetic patients Less than 300 mg/dL (patients with diabetes)	Because the kidney metabolizes insulin, low blood sugar levels caused by a longer half-life of insulin are possible. For patients with diabetes: a high blood sugar may increase thirst.	Most people need 6-11 servings of breads and starches or cereals per day and 2-4 servings of fruit per day to provide energy. Patients with diabetes should avoid concentrated sweets, unless blood sugar level is low.

BUN, Blood urea nitrogen; *CO₂*, carbon dioxide; *DHT*, dihydrotachysterol; *EPO*, erythropoietin; *IV*, intravenous; *N/A*, not applicable; *nPNA*, normalized protein nitrogen appearance; *PTH*, parathyroid hormone; *URR*, urea reduction ratio.
Developed by Katy G. Wilkens, MS, RDN, Northwest Kidney Centers, Seattle, Washington.

dietitian to assess the quality of the patient's nutrition status (see Chapter 5 and Appendices 12 and 21). Indirect calorimetry remains a valid tool (Morrow et al, 2017) but is rarely available in outpatient practices.

Fluid and Sodium Balance

The kidney's ability to handle sodium and water in ESRD must be assessed frequently through measurement of blood pressure, edema, fluid weight gain, serum sodium level, and dietary intake. The vast majority of dialysis patients need to restrict sodium and fluid intakes. Excessive sodium intake is responsible for increased thirst, increased fluid gain, and resultant hypertension. Even those patients who do not experience these symptoms but produce minimal amounts of urine benefit from a reduced sodium intake to limit their thirst and prevent large intradialytic fluid gains.

In the patient who is maintained on HD, sodium and fluid intake are regulated to allow for a weight gain of 4 to 5 lb (2 to 3 kg) from increased fluid in the vasculature between dialyses. The goal is a fluid gain of less than 4% of body weight. A sodium intake of 65 to 87 mEq

(1500 to 2000 mg) daily and a limit on fluid intake (usually about 750 mL/day plus the amount equal to the urine output) is usually sufficient to meet these guidelines. Only fluids that are liquid at room temperature are included in this calculation. The fluid contained in solid foods is not included in the 750 mL limit. Solid foods in the average diet contribute approximately 500 to 800 mL/day of fluid. This fluid in solid food is calculated to approximately replace the 500 mL/day net insensible water loss.

A 65 to 87 mEq (1500 to 2000 mg) sodium diet requires no salt in cooking; no salt at the table; no salted, smoked, enhanced, or cured meat or fish; no cheese except Swiss or cream cheese; and no salted snack foods, canned soups, packaged bread products, or high-sodium convenience foods. In today's marketplace, increased intake of convenience foods is the norm and it is estimated that 75% to 90% of sodium intake is consumed in convenience foods, with only 10% to 25% added to foods in cooking or at the table.

The most effective way to reduce the renal patient's thirst and fluid intake is to decrease sodium intake. It is salt intake that drives fluid consumption. Appendix 21 gives the details of a low-sodium meal plan. Attempts to restrict fluid in patients who are not on a restricted sodium diet are futile, because feelings of thirst become overwhelming to the patient with a high sodium intake.

When educating about fluid balance, the health care provider must teach the patient how to deal with thirst without drinking. Sucking on a few ice chips, cold sliced fruit, or sour candies or using artificial saliva are good suggestions. In approximately 15% to 20% of patients, hypertension is not alleviated even after meticulous attention to fluid and water balance. In these patients hypertension usually is perpetuated by a high level of renin secretion and requires medication for control.

Although the majority of patients with ESRD retain sodium, a small number may lose it. Examples of conditions with a salt-losing tendency are polycystic disease of the kidney, medullary kidney disease, chronic obstructive uropathy, chronic pyelonephritis, ostomy losses, and analgesic nephropathy. To prevent hypotension, hypovolemia, cramps, and further deterioration of renal function, extra sodium may be required. A diet for these types of patients may contain 130 mEq (3 g) or more of sodium per day. Not limiting sodium in the diet can satisfy the need for extra sodium. The number of patients who require this level of sodium intake is small, but these patients exemplify the need for individual consideration of the diet prescription and a thorough understanding of the patient's underlying disease and present diet.

Potassium

Potassium usually requires restriction, depending on the serum potassium level, urine output, medications, and the frequency of HD. The daily intake of potassium for most Americans is 75 to 100 mEq (3 to 4 g). This usually is reduced in ESRD to 60 to 80 mEq (2.3 to 3.1 g) per day and is reduced for the anuric patient on dialysis to 51 mEq (2 g) per day. Some patients (i.e., those on high-flux dialysis or with increased dialysis times or frequencies such as PD, short daily or nocturnal) require higher intakes. Again, a close monitoring of the patient's laboratory values, potassium content of the dialysate, and dietary intake is essential.

The potassium content of foods is listed in Appendix 44. When counseling HD patients on a low-potassium diet, clinicians should take care to point out that some low-sodium foods contain potassium chloride as a salt substitute rather than sodium chloride. Nutrition labels for products such as salt substitutes and low-sodium herb mixtures must be checked carefully to be sure they do not contain dangerous levels of potassium. Low-sodium soy sauces, low-sodium soups, and other low-sodium products may require particular review by a trained professional (see Chapter 10 for labeling definitions). Reviewing food preparation techniques should include anyone who may be cooking for the patient, such as restaurants, family members, friends, or neighbors.

When a thorough diet history does not reveal the reason for elevated serum potassium, other nondietetic sources for the elevated potassium should be researched. Examples include incomplete dialysis or missed dialysis treatments, too high a concentration of potassium in the dialysate bath, defective HD access or recirculation of blood within the access, very elevated blood sugar, acidosis, constipation, significant GI bleeding, some medications, blood transfusions, major trauma, chemotherapy, or radiation therapy. Occasionally blood samples are handled improperly, resulting in hemolysis and falsely elevated potassium levels.

Phosphorus

More than 99% of excess phosphate is excreted in the urine. However, as GFR decreases, phosphorus is retained in the plasma. Phosphorus is not easily removed by dialysis, and patients experience net gain of about one half of the phosphate they consume daily. Phosphate intake is lowered by restricting dietary sources to 1200 mg/day or less. The difficulty in implementing the phosphorus restriction comes from the necessity for a high-protein diet. High-protein foods, such as meats and dairy, contain high levels of phosphorus in the form of ATP. In addition, other sources of protein—nuts and legumes (including soy)—are also high in phosphorus. Thus high-phosphorus foods cannot be eliminated without restricting protein, creating a challenge to balance intake with dietary intervention alone.

The American diet, which contains highly processed foods, has resulted in increases in the types and amounts of phosphorus available for absorption, making compliance with a phosphorus restriction more difficult. Naturally occurring phosphate in food is only approximately 60% absorbed. Commonly used phosphate additives such as trisodium phosphate, disodium phosphate, and dicalcium phosphate are nearly 100% absorbed, making the processed diet a contributor to elevated phosphorus levels (Chang and Anderson, 2017). Dietary intervention should focus on a balance of limiting dairy, nuts, beans, and processed foods while still encouraging enough proteins of HBV to meet dietary needs. Phosphorus management through diet has the added challenge of not being included in the values on the standard nutrition label. Phosphate additives are becoming more prevalent throughout our food system (León et al, 2013) and dietitian nutritionists are crucial to helping patient find foods that are better choices.

Because dietary restrictions alone are not adequate to control serum phosphorus, nearly all patients who undergo dialysis require phosphate-binding medications. Phosphate binders such as calcium carbonate, calcium acetate, sevelamer carbonate, sucroferric oxyhydroxide, ferric citrate, and lanthanum carbonate are used routinely with each meal and snack to bind to phosphorus. These medications bind excess dietary phosphate and transport it through the GI tract for elimination, thus preventing its absorption into the blood. Side effects of taking these medications over long periods are common. Some may cause GI distress, diarrhea, or gas. Severe constipation, leading to intestinal impaction, is a potential risk of excessive use of some types of phosphate binders; occasionally this may lead to perforation of the intestine resulting in peritonitis or death. Common medications are listed in Table 34.11 (see *Clinical Insight:* Why Don't Clients Take Their Phosphate Binders?).

CLINICAL INSIGHT

Why Don't Clients Take Their Phosphate Binders?

Phosphate binders are prescribed to be taken with all meals and snacks, whether the client eats at home, at work, or in a restaurant. Reasons clients give for not taking their phosphate binders are that they:
- cause gastrointestinal discomfort and acid reflux
- cause severe constipation and can lead to bowel impaction
- may be difficult to chew or swallow
- may need to take an average of 2 to 5 pills each meal
- forget to take them
- do not like to be reminded of being "sick"
- cannot feel a difference when taking them
- may be expensive and not always covered by insurance

Calcium and Parathyroid Hormone

In ESRD, the body's ability to maintain phosphorus-calcium balance is complicated by calcium and PTH controls. As GFR decreases, the

TABLE 34.11 Common Medications and Nutritional Supplements for Patients with End-Stage Renal Disease

Phosphate Binders
Taken with meals and snacks to prevent dietary phosphorus absorption

Calcium carbonate	TUMS, Os-Cal, Calci-Chew, Calci-Mix
Calcium acetate	PhosLo
Mg/Ca^{++} carbonate	MagneBind
Sevelamer carbonate	Renvela
Lanthanum carbonate	Fosrenol
Aluminum hydroxide	AlternaGEL
Iron-based binders	Velphoro, Auryxia

Vitamins
Increased need for water-soluble vitamins because of losses during dialysis

Fat-soluble vitamins A, E, and K are not supplemented

Dialysis Recommendations

Vitamin C	60 mg (not to exceed 200 mg daily)
Folic acid	1 mg
Thiamin	1.5 mg
Riboflavin	1.7 mg
Niacin	20 mg
Vitamin B$_6$	10 mg
Vitamin B$_{12}$	6 mcg
Pantothenic acid	10 mg
Biotin	0.3 mg

Brand names include Nephrocap, Nephron FA, Nephplex, Nephro-Vites, and Dia-tx

Iron
Iron needs are increased because of EPO therapy and oral iron is not adequate

IV iron	Iron dextran (Infed), Iron gluconate (Ferrlecit), Iron sucrose (Venofer)

EPO
Stimulates bone marrow to produce red blood cells

IV or IM	Erythropoietin Stimulating Agents

Activated Vitamin D
Used for the management of hyperparathyroidism

Oral	Calcitriol (Rocaltrol), doxercalciferol (Hectorol)
IV	Calcitriol (Calcijex), paricalcitol (Zemplar)

Bisphosphonates
Inhibit bone resorption by blocking osteoclast activity

Oral	Alendronate (Fosamax)
IV	Pamidronate (Aredia)

Calcium Supplements
TUMS, Os-Cal, Calci-Chew

Phosphorus Supplements

	Kphos neutral, NutraPhos, NutraPhos K

Calcimimetics

Mimic calcium and bind to parathyroid gland	Cinacalcet (Sensipar) and Etelcalcetide (Parsabiv)

Potassium Lowering Agents
For the treatment of hyperkalemia

Oral or rectal	SPS (Kayexalate)
	Patiromer (Veltassa)
	Sodium Zirconium Cyclocilicate (Lokelma)

Ca^{++}, Calcium; *CHO*, cholesterol; *EPO*, epoetin; *ESRD*, end-stage renal disease; *IV*, intravenous; *IM*, intramuscular; *MVI*; multiple vitamin injection; *SPS*, sodium polystyrene sulfonate.

Developed by Fiona Wolf, RDN, and Thomas Montemayor, RPh, Northwest Kidney Centers, Seattle, Washington, 2015.

serum calcium level declines for several reasons. First, decreased ability of the kidney to convert inactive vitamin D to its active form, $1,25(OH)_2D_3$, leads to poor GI absorption of calcium. Second, the need for serum calcium increases as serum phosphate levels increase. Both of these causes lead to hypertrophy of the parathyroid gland, which is responsible for calcium homeostasis. The resultant oversecretion of PTH increases resorption of bone to provide a calcium source. Because calcium is bound to albumin in the blood serum calcium will appear low when albumin is low (see Chapter 3).

The resulting metabolic bone disease, renal osteodystrophy, is essentially one of four types: (1) osteomalacia, (2) osteitis fibrosa cystica, (3) metastatic calcification, or (4) adynamic (low turnover) bone disease. With a deficit of calcium available from dietary absorption due to lack of vitamin D, the low calcium level triggers the release of PTH from the parathyroid glands. PTH acts to increase release of calcium from the bones by stimulating osteoclast activity. This can lead to osteomalacia or bone demineralization, as a result of lack of osteoblast stimulation to replace lost calcium in the bones.

Ongoing low calcium causes the parathyroid glands to continue producing PTH in an attempt to elevate serum calcium levels. In time this leads to secondary hyperparathyroidism, in which even the baseline production of PTH by these enlarged glands is enough to cause severe bone demineralization (osteitis fibrosa cystica), which is characterized by dull, aching bone pain.

Even though the serum calcium level is elevated in response to PTH, serum phosphate concentration remains high as the GFR falls lower. If the product of serum calcium multiplied by the serum phosphate level is greater than 70, metastatic calcification is imminent. Metastatic calcification occurs when calcium phosphate is deposited in nonbone cells. This extraskeletal calcification may develop in joints, soft tissue, and vessels.

Calciphylaxis occurs when calcium phosphate is deposited in wound tissues with resultant vascular calcification, thrombosis, nonhealing wounds, and gangrene. It is closely linked with use of blood thinners, so bone mineral management paired with coagulation management are the primary treatments. It is frequently fatal. Newer treatments pair calcium and phosphorus control with increased dialysis, antibiotic therapy, sodium thiosulfate, and hyperbaric chamber treatments (Nigwekar et al, 2015).

Many patients on dialysis suffer from hypocalcemia, despite calcium supplementation. Because of this, the routine drug of choice is active vitamin D, $1,25(OH)_2D_3$, available as calcitriol (Rocaltrol and Calcijex). Analogs such as doxercalciferol (Hectorol) and paricalcitol (Zemplar) are also effective in lowering PTH and raising calcium levels, but with less enhancement of gut absorption of calcium than the 1,25 forms.

Other mechanisms for controlling PTH include the oral medication cinacalcet (Sensipar) or IV medication etelcalcetide (Parsabiv), and calcimimetic or calcium-imitating drugs. They bind to sites on the parathyroid gland, simulating acceptable calcium levels. The drugs are effective in suppressing PTH production and also may lower calcium levels dramatically, with significant benefit. Known complications of low calcium means that overall, close monitoring is essential.

In more extreme cases of hyperparathyroidism, use of surgical excision of portions of the parathyroid glands can be used in an attempt to restore balance. This creates the risk of low PTH and can lead to adynamic (low turnover) bone disease, characterized by decreased levels of bone turnover and suppression of both osteoclasts and osteoblasts. This condition is unique to ESRD, in which oversuppression of the parathyroid gland and too much active vitamin D lead to decreased bone formation and fragile bones with very little matrix. Usually diagnosed by a low PTH level, this disease results in a high risk of nonhealing fractures. Oversuppression of the parathyroid gland by use of vitamin D or its analogs can mimic this as well.

Overall the dietary balance of phosphorus, the use of phosphate binders, vitamin D analogs, calcium memetics (drugs that mimics the action of calcium on tissue), the removal of phosphate by dialysis, and intense monitoring of laboratory values contribute to complex bone management in ESRD.

Lipid

Atherosclerotic cardiovascular disease (AHD) is a common cause of death among patients maintained on long-term dialysis (Sarnak M et al. 2019). This appears to be a function of underlying disease (e.g., diabetes mellitus, hypertension, nephrotic syndrome) and a lipid abnormality common among patients with ESRD. As stated earlier in the chapter the use of statins is no longer recommended in CKD based on KDIGO 2013 guidelines. Low-fat diet recommendations for AHD have been replaced with recommendations to replace unhealthy fats with healthier ones (see Chapter 32). General diet education for cardiac health is advised, with consideration for the higher protein recommendations and the need to limit potassium.

Iron and Erythropoietin

The anemia of chronic renal disease is caused by an inability of the kidney to produce erythropoietin (EPO), the hormone that stimulates the bone marrow to produce red blood cells; an increased destruction of red blood cells secondary to circulating uremic waste products; and blood loss with dialysis or blood sampling. A synthetic form of EPO, recombinant human EPO (rHuEPO), is used to treat this form of anemia. Clinical trials have demonstrated a dramatic improvement in correcting anemia and restoring a general sense of well-being. Recent studies have indicated that higher dosages of EPO pose increased risk of stroke, adverse cardiac events, and death, so close monitoring and balancing the needs of the patient are essential.

Use of EPO increases red blood cell production 2.5-fold. Almost always accompanying the rise in hematocrit is an increased need for iron that requires IV supplementation. While many things can be managed by diet, the increased need for iron to increase red blood cells formed with use of EPO outweighs what can be accomplished from food. Oral supplementation of iron is also not effective in maintaining

adequate iron stores in patients on EPO. Unless a documented allergic reaction exists, almost all patients taking EPO require periodic IV or intramuscular iron. For patients who are allergic to IV iron, several better-tolerated forms are now available as iron dextran (Infed), iron gluconate (Ferrlecit), and iron sucrose (Venofer).

Serum ferritin is an accurate indicator of iron status in renal failure. Patients who have received several transfusions and who are storing extra iron may have high serum ferritin levels of 800 to 5000 ng/mL (a normal level is 68 ng/mL for women and 150 ng/mL for men; see Appendix 12). In patients who are receiving EPO, ferritin should be kept above 300 ng/mL but below 800 ng/mL. When ferritin values fall below 100 ng/mL, IV iron is usually given. The percent of transferrin saturation is another useful indicator of iron status in these patients and should be between 25% to 30%.

Vitamins

Water-soluble vitamins are rapidly lost during dialysis. In general, ascorbic acid and most B vitamins are lost through dialysate at approximately the same rate they would have been lost in the urine (depending on the type and duration of treatment), with the exception of folate, which is highly dialyzable. Patients who still produce urine may be at increased risk of loss of water-soluble vitamins. Folate is recommended to be supplemented at 1 mg/day based on extra losses. Because vitamin B_{12} is protein-bound, losses of this B vitamin during dialysis are minimal. Altered metabolism and excretory function, as well as drug administration, also may affect vitamin levels. Little is known about GI absorption of vitamins in uremia, but it may be significantly decreased. Uremic toxins may interfere with the activity of some vitamins, such as inhibition of phosphorylation of pyridoxine and its analogs.

Another cause of decreased vitamin intake in uremia is the restriction of dietary phosphorus and potassium. Water-soluble vitamins are usually abundant in high-potassium foods such as citrus fruits, vegetables, and high-phosphorus foods such as milk. Diets for patients on dialysis tend to be low in folate, niacin, riboflavin, and vitamin B_6. With frequent episodes of anorexia or illness, vitamin intake is decreased further. Whereas levels of water-soluble vitamins decrease as a result of dialysis, replacement of fat-soluble vitamins usually is not required in renal disease.

Several vitamin supplements that fit the needs of the uremic patient or the dialysis patient are now available by prescription: Nephrocaps, Renavite, Dialyvite, Folbee Plus, and Renal Caps or Virt-Caps. An over-the-counter supplement containing the vitamin B complex and vitamin C often is used and can be less expensive than a prescription, but additional supplements of folic acid and pyridoxine may be needed.

Niacin has been found to be helpful in lowering phosphate levels in ESRD patients. It interferes with the sodium-phosphate pump in the GI lumen, causing decreased transport of phosphate, and thus works with a different mechanism than phosphate binders (Cheng et al, 2008; Edalat-Nejad et al, 2012). It has shown benefit in improving outcomes in patients that struggle with a serum phosphorus of more than 6.0 when used in conjunction with phosphate binders as a once-daily pill. Potential side effects such as GI bleeding, liver disease, and flushing must be carefully considered.

Nutrition Support in End-Stage Renal Disease
Enteral Tube Feeding

Patients with ESRD who require enteral tube feeding generally can use standard formulas used for most tube-fed patients (see Chapter 12) and do not require a specialty or renal formula. Formulas marketed as renal products are more calorie-dense, higher in protein, and lower in specific nutrients such as potassium and phosphorus. If patients are receiving renal products only, they may develop problems with low phosphorus or potassium levels as these products are designed to be used in conjunction with oral intake.

Oral Protein Supplementation During Dialysis

Recent research has focused on use of oral protein supplements while a patient is receiving dialysis treatments. The theory is that muscle protein will be replaced, offsetting catabolism, which occurs during dialysis. This is thought to be similar to what an athlete might experience using a protein supplement immediately after exercise. Study results show possible links to reduction in mortality from use during dialysis treatments, not related to serum albumin levels (Lacson et al, 2012). Another study by Beddhu et al (2015) measured midarm muscle circumference, albumin and C-reactive protein (hs-CRP) in response to intradialytic protein supplementation and found no change.

Parenteral Nutrition

PN in ESRD is similar to PN used for other malnourished patients with respect to protein, carbohydrates, and fat, but differs in use of vitamins and minerals. Most researchers agree that vitamin needs for ESRD during PN differ from normal requirements; however, they do not agree on recommendations for individual nutrients. Folate, pyridoxine, and biotin should be supplemented. Vitamin A should not be provided parenterally unless retinol-binding protein is monitored during each HD treatment because it is elevated in patients with ESRD. Because there is currently no parenteral vitamin that is specifically designed for patients with renal failure, a standard vitamin preparation usually is administered. Little information related to parenteral trace mineral supplementation is available. Because most trace minerals, including zinc, chromium, and magnesium, are excreted in the urine, a close monitoring of these minerals in the serum seems to be appropriate.

Intradialytic Parenteral Nutrition

Malnourished patients with chronic renal failure who are on HD have easy access to PN because of the direct blood access required by the dialysis therapy itself. Intradialytic parenteral nutrition (IDPN) can be administered to support a patient's nutritional status. IDPN is administered typically through a connection to the venous side of the extracorporeal circuit during dialysis. Because of the high blood flow rate achieved through use of the surgically created fistula and the high blood pump speeds that are attained, glucose protein and lipids can be administered without requiring a separate port.

Another method of nutrition support in PD patients is called intraperitoneal nutrition (IPN) using a peritoneal dialysate solution that contains amino acids instead of dextrose. Typically one bag of this solution is used per day.

End-Stage Renal Disease in Patients with Diabetes

Because renal failure is a complication of diabetes, approximately 45% of all new patients starting dialysis have diabetes (United States Renal Data System, 2017). The need to control blood sugar in these patients requires specialized diet therapy. The diet for diabetes management (see Chapter 29) can be modified for the patient on dialysis. In addition, the diabetic patient on dialysis often has other complications such as retinopathy, neuropathy, gastroparesis, and amputation, all of which can place this patient at high nutritional risk.

Chronic Kidney Disease and End-Stage Renal Disease in Children

Although CKD may occur in children at any age, from the newborn infant to the adolescent, it is a relatively uncommon diagnosis. Causal factors in children include congenital defects, anatomic defects (urologic malformations or dysplastic kidneys), inherited disease (autosomal-recessive polycystic kidney disease), metabolic disorders that eventually result in renal failure (cystinosis or methylmalonic aciduria), or acquired conditions or illnesses (untreated kidney infections, physical trauma to kidneys, exposure to nephrotoxic chemicals or medications, hemolytic anemia resulting from *Escherichia coli* 0157 ingestion, or glomerular nephritis).

As with all children, the major concern is to promote normal growth and development. Without aggressive monitoring and encouragement, children with renal failure rarely meet their nutritional requirements. If the renal disease is present from birth, nutrition support needs to begin immediately to avoid losing the growth potential of the first few months of life. Growth in children with CKD usually is delayed. Although no specific therapy ensures normal growth, factors capable of responding to therapy include metabolic acidosis, electrolyte depletion, osteodystrophy, chronic infection, and protein-calorie malnutrition. Energy and protein needs for children with chronic renal disease are at least equivalent to the DRIs for normal children of the same height and age. If nutrition status is poor, energy needs may be even higher to promote weight gain and linear growth.

Feeding by tube is required in the presence of poor intake, particularly in the critical growth period of the first 2 years of life. Gastrostomy tubes almost always are placed in these children to enhance nutritional intake and facilitate growth. PN rarely is initiated unless the GI tract is nonfunctional. For the nutritional requirements of children with renal failure see the National Kidney Foundation website.

Control of calcium and phosphorus balance is especially important for maintaining good growth. The goal is to restrict phosphorus intake while promoting calcium absorption with the aid of $1,25(OH)_2D_3$. This helps prevent renal osteodystrophy, which can cause severe growth retardation. Use of calcium carbonate formulations to supplement the dietary intake enhances calcium intake while binding excess phosphorus. Persistent metabolic acidosis is often associated with growth failure in infancy. In chronic acidosis the titration of acid by the bone causes calcium loss and contributes to bone demineralization. Bicarbonate may be added to the infant formula to counteract this effect.

Restriction of protein in pediatric diets is controversial. The so-called protective effect on kidney function must be weighed against the clearly negative effect of possible protein malnutrition on growth. The recommended dietary allowance for protein for age is usually the minimum amount given.

Each child's diet should be adjusted for individual food preferences, family eating patterns, and biochemical needs. This is often not an easy task. In addition, care must be taken not to place too much emphasis on the diet to avoid food becoming a manipulative tool and an attention-getting device. Special encouragement, creativity, and attention are required to help the child with CKD consume the necessary energy. When possible, PD is given intermittently during the day and continuously at night because it allows liberalization of the diet. The child is more likely to meet nutritional requirements with fewer dietary restrictions and therefore experience better growth.

Other treatments that help renal disease in children include the use of rHuEPO and recombinant deoxyribonucleic acid–produced human growth hormone. EPO usually is started when the child's serum hemoglobin falls below 10 g/dL, with a goal of maintaining hemoglobin between 11 and 12 g/dL. Correction of anemia with the use of rHuEPO may increase appetite, intake, and feeling of well-being, but it has not been found to affect growth, even with seemingly adequate nutrition support.

Medical Nutrition Therapy for Transplantation

The nutritional care of the adult patient who has received a transplanted kidney is based mainly on the metabolic effects of the required immunosuppressive therapy. Medications typically used for the long term include azathioprine (Imuran), corticosteroids (e.g., prednisone), calcineurin inhibitors (cyclosporine A, Gengraf, SangCya, Sandimmune, tacrolimus [Prograf, F506]), sirolimus (Rapamune), everolimus (Zortress), mycophenolate mofetil (CellCept), and mycophenolic acid (Myfortic). Corticosteroids are associated with accelerated protein catabolism, hyperlipidemia, sodium retention, weight gain, hyperglycemia, osteoporosis, and electrolyte disturbances. Calcineurin inhibitors are associated with hyperkalemia, hypertension, hyperglycemia, and hyperlipidemia. The doses of these medications used after transplantation are decreased over time until a maintenance level is reached.

During the first 6 weeks after surgery, a high-protein diet is often recommended (1.2 to 1.5 g/kg IBW), with an energy intake of 30 to 35 kcal/kg IBW, to prevent negative nitrogen balance. A moderate sodium restriction of 2 to 3 g/day during this period minimizes fluid retention and helps to control blood pressure. After recovery, protein intake should be decreased to 1 to 1.5. g/kg IBW, with calorie intake providing sufficient energy to maintain or achieve an appropriate weight for height. A balanced low-fat diet aids in lowering cardiac complications, whereas sodium intakes are individualized based on fluid retention and blood pressure.

Hyperkalemia warrants a temporary dietary potassium restriction. After transplantation, many patients exhibit hypophosphatemia and mild hypercalcemia caused by bone resorption; this is associated with persistent hyperparathyroidism and the effects of steroids on calcium, phosphorus, and vitamin D metabolism. The diet should contain adequate amounts of calcium and phosphorus (1200 mg of each daily) and cholecalciferol (vitamin D_3, 2000 IU daily). Supplemental phosphorus also may be necessary to correct hypophosphatemia.

Hydration must also be monitored closely after transplantation. Because most kidney recipients required a fluid restriction while on dialysis, they must be reminded of the importance of maintaining fluid intake after transplant. Typically, patients are encouraged to drink 2 L/day, but their overall needs depend on their urine output.

The majority of transplant recipients have elevated serum triglycerides or cholesterol for a variety of reasons. Intervention consists of medications, calorie restriction for those who are overweight, cholesterol intake limited to less than 300 mg/day, and limited total fat (see Chapter 32). In patients with glucose intolerance, limiting carbohydrates and a regular exercise regimen are appropriate. Tissue weight gain with resultant obesity is common after transplantation. Medication side effects, fewer dietary restrictions, and the lack of physical exercise can contribute to posttransplant weight gain.

Because of immunosuppression, care must be taken with food safety similar to other significantly at-risk groups. Handwashing, food temperature monitoring, and avoidance of uncooked foods remain appropriate infection control behaviors.

Referral to bariatric surgery is being seen in patients needing weight loss to qualify for a transplant. Much coordination and collaboration is needed between the bariatric RDN and the renal RDN to be sure that the patient's very specific diet needs are met based on their treatment modality and progression of kidney disease (see Chapter 20).

Counseling and Education of Patients with End-Stage Renal Disease

For effective intervention, it is important to look at the long-range goals for educating patients with ESRD about their nutritional needs.

The average patient survives on dialysis 7 to 10 years, the average mortality is approximately 20% per year, equal to that of serious cancers such as ovarian cancer. However, some patients with a relatively benign diagnosis may look forward to life spans of 20 to 40 years, particularly if they receive kidney transplants as a part of their treatment. The challenge for the dietitian nutritionist is educating patients with a chronic disease who will be primarily responsible for implementing nutritional recommendations for the rest of their life. Thus intervention for ESRD and that for diabetes share many similarities.

It is incumbent on the renal dietitian nutritionist to develop a long-standing rapport with patients and their families, and to serve as an ally to help them make the best nutritional choices over an extended period. Understanding the burdens of a complex, challenging, ever-changing diet suggests the transfer of information to the renal patient and family in a workable, flexible, and easily understood manner. Skills for this task are just as challenging, if not more so, than maintaining a patient's iron status or keeping the patient at a good body weight. Empathy and use of techniques such as motivational interviewing or cognitive behavioral therapy are essential tools (see Chapter 13).

Coordination of Care in End-Stage Renal Disease

The position of the registered dietitian nutritionist (RDN) in the care of dialysis patients is unique because it is a federally mandated position. So, too, is the RDN's place on the mandated interdisciplinary health care team that exists within each dialysis unit. The team approach is an important aspect of all health care; however, its importance is magnified in the dialysis team, which consists of the patient, renal nurse, renal social worker, nephrologist, and renal dietitian nutritionist. Care of these complex, long-term ESRD patients requires the skill and compassion of each member of the health care team working together. Advanced levels of practice are available for dietitians who wish to be certified as renal RDNs; they can be certified through examination by the Academy of Nutrition and Dietetics and become a Board Certified Specialist in Renal Nutrition.

Emergency Diets for Dialysis Patients

When power outages, flooding, storms, hurricanes, or earthquakes threaten a community, they threaten the most vulnerable people in that community. Patients on HD require power and water sources to do their own treatments at home. PD patients need a clean environment and access to their supplies. If they travel to a dialysis unit, they need access to transportation. Because of poor outcomes in recent natural disasters, the federal government's ESRD program has specified that patients and caregivers must be familiar with alternative nutritional therapies when dialysis is not available because of a natural or manmade emergency. Box 34.3 demonstrates the type of nutrient and practical information that must be considered when patients may be without dialysis for days, or because they must be evacuated to a site that cannot meet their urgent nutritional needs.

Medical Management (Conservative Treatment) or Palliative Care

The decision to forego or discontinue dialysis and opt for end-of-life care is a difficult and emotional one. Factors such as religious practices, age, quality of life, and comorbid disease play a role. Patients who are poor candidates for dialysis or transplantation may benefit from a low-protein, low-sodium diet to minimize physical symptoms, such as shortness of breath and uremia. Palliative care can be offered with the goal of balancing patient wishes for food choice with these complex side effects (Rak et al, 2017).

BOX 34.3 Emergency Dialysis Diet Plan

This plan will work for short periods (5 days or less) when patients cannot dialyze.

The Emergency Diet Plan does not replace dialysis; it should be used only in case of an emergency.

Guidelines

1. Limit meat to 3-4 oz/day.
2. Avoid all high-potassium fruits and vegetables.
3. Consume only one to two 8-oz cups of fluid per day.
4. Choose low-salt foods.
5. Do not use salt or salt substitute.
6. Use fats and sugars for extra calories.
7. If the power is off for a day, foods in refrigerator should be eaten first.
8. Patients should eat food from the freezer while they still have ice crystals in the center.
9. Patients should have a portable emergency kit they can take with them to a disaster relief center. Sample foods are listed in the following diet plan.

Emergency Diet Plan

If a food is not on this list, dialysis patients should not eat it.

Meat and Protein Foods (three to four 1-oz choices/day)

1 egg
1 oz meat, fish, tofu, or poultry
¼ cup unsalted or rinsed canned fish or poultry
2 tablespoons unsalted peanut butter
¼ cup cottage cheese
½ can commercial liquid nutritional supplement

Starch (six to ten choices/day)

1 slice white bread
½ English muffin or bagel
5 unsalted crackers
2 graham crackers
6 shortbread cookies, vanilla wafers
1 cup unsalted rice, noodles, pasta
1 cup puffed wheat, rice, shredded wheat
1 cup of rice or pasta

Vegetables (one choice/day)

½-cup serving of green beans, summer squash, corn, beets, carrots, or peas
Should be fresh or frozen, not canned

Fruits (three to four choices/day)

1 small apple
15 grapes
½ cup serving of berries, cherries, applesauce, canned pears, or canned pineapple

Fats and Oil (six or more choices/day)

1 tsp butter, margarine, oil, or mayonnaise

Fluids (one to two choices/day)

1 cup water, coffee, tea, soda
½ cup Ensure Plus, Boost Plus, or Nepro
½ cup serving of milk, half and half, soy, or rice milk
Cranberry, apple, or grape juice; or Kool-Aid

Emergency Kit

Have the following things stored in a box or bag easily accessible:
Foods listed in the Emergency Diet Plan
Can opener
Two-gallon jugs of distilled water
Bleach, 1 Tbsp/gallon of water to sterilize
Flashlight and extra batteries
Sharp knife
Aluminum foil
Plastic mixing containers and lids
Measuring cup
Fork, knife, spoon
Battery-operated transistor radio
One-week supply of personal medicines kept in a handy place, including blood pressure medications and phosphate binders (insulin and some other medications must be kept refrigerated or cold)

Storage Tips

1. Store things in a clean, dry place such as a new garbage can or rubber tub.
2. Label and date when food is put in storage.
3. Change all food and water once a year. Eat unused food or donate to a food bank.

Dialysis Emergency Diet information from Katy Wilkens, MS, RDN. Copyright Northwest Kidney Centers, 2019. For more emergency diet info see https://www.nwkidney.org or your local Network Coordinating Council website.

CLINICAL CASE STUDY

HC is a 67-year-old Japanese American male.

Serum creatinine 3.3 mg/dL, BUN 72 mg/dL, albumin 2.9 mg/dL, potassium 3.3 mEq/L, phosphorus 6.7 mg/dL, calcium 8.5 mg/dL

Hx: Type 2 diabetes mellitus (DM), heart attack, A-Fib

Pt seen re: 5 kg wt loss/1mo. Pt reports a poor appetite x 3mo.

c/o "I just don't enjoy eating like I used to…food tastes funny."

c/o being too weak to do anything but read or watch TV.

Diet hx reveals pt eats 0% to 10% of meals. Declines enteral supplements.

DW: 48.0 kg, % IBW: 91, BMI: 17.6, moderate fat and muscle wasting.

Pt is reported to have a stage III pressure injury on his coccyx.

Nutrition Care Questions

1. What is HC's calculated eGFR?
2. What is his stage of chronic kidney disease (CKD)?
3. What is the first goal for education?
4. What dietary factors would you address based on these laboratory values?
5. What is the goal for protein intake?
6. How would you assess for improvement or stability of his CKD?
7. What would you expect for him during the next few years if no diet intervention is followed?

REFERENCES

Adeva MM, Souto G: Diet-induced metabolic acidosis, *Clin Nutr* 30:416–421, 2011.

Beddhu S, Filipowicz R, Chen X, et al: Supervised oral protein supplementation during dialysis in patients with elevated C-reactive protein levels: a two phase, longitudinal, single center, open labeled study, *BMC Nephrol* 16:87, 2015.

Borges NA, Carmo FL, Stockler-Pinto MB, et al: Probiotic supplementation in chronic kidney disease: a double blind randomized placebo controlled trial, *J Ren Nutr* 28(1):28–36, 2018.

Centers for Disease Control and Prevention: *Chronic kidney disease in the United States, 2019*, Atlanta, GA, 2019, US Department of Health and Human Services, Centers for Disease Control and Prevention.

Chang AR, Anderson C: Dietary phosphorus intake and the kidney, *Annu Rev Nutr* 37:321–346, 2017.

Cheng SC, Young DO, Huang Y, et al: A randomized, double-blind, placebo-controlled trial of niacinamide for reduction of phosphorus in hemodialysis patients, *Clin J Am Soc Nephrol* 3(4):1131–1138, 2008. doi:10.2215/CJN.04211007

Collins AJ, Foley RN, Gilbertson DT, et al: United States Renal Data System public health surveillance of chronic kidney disease and end-stage renal disease, *Kidney Int Suppl* 5(1):2–7, 2015.

Curhan GC, Taylor EN: 24-h uric acid excretion and the risk of kidney stones, *Kidney Int* 73:489–496, 2008.

Edalat-Nejad M, Zameni F, Talaiei A: The effect of niacin on serum phosphorus levels in dialysis patients, *Indian J Nephrol* 22(3):174–178, 2012.

Ferraro PM, Taylor EN, Gambaro G, et al: Soda and other beverages and the risk of kidney stones, *Clin J Am Soc Nephrol* 8:1389–1395, 2013.

Ferraro PM, Curhan GC, Gambaro G, et al: Total, dietary and supplemental vitamin C intake and risk of incident kidney stones, *Am J Kidney Dis* 67:400–407, 2016a.

Ferraro PM, Mandel EI, Curhan GC, et al: Dietary protein and potassium, diet- dependent net acid load, and risk of incident kidney stones, *Clin J Am Soc Nephrol* 11(10):1834–1844, 2016b.

Ferraro PM, Taylor EN, Gambaro G, et al: Dietary and lifestyle risk factors associated with incident kidney stones in men and women, *J Urol* 198(4):858–863, 2017a.

Ferraro PM, Taylor EN, Gambaro G, et al: Vitamin D intake and the risk of incident kidney stones, *J Urol* 197(2):405–410, 2017b.

Ferraro PM, Taylor EN, Gambaro G, et al: Vitamin B6 intake and the risk of incident stones, *Urolithiasis* 46(3):265–270, 2018. doi:10.1007/s00240-017-0999-5.

Goraya N, Simoni J, Jo CH, et al: A comparison of treating metabolic acidosis in CKD stage 4 hypertensive kidney disease with fruits and vegetables or sodium bicarbonate, *Clin J Am Soc Neprhol* 8(3):371–381, 2013.

Garofalo C, Borrelli S, Provenzano M, et al: Dietary salt restriction in chronic kidney diseas: a meta-analysis of randomized clinical trials, *Nutrients* 10:732, 2018.

Gallieni M, Cupisti A: DASH and mediterranean diets as nutritional interventions for CKD Patients, *Am J Kidney Dis* 68(6):828–830; 2016.

Guerra A, Folesani G, Nouvenne A, et al: Family history influences clinical course of idiopathic calcium nephrolithiasis: case control study of a large cohort of Italian patients, *J Nephrol* 29(5):645–651, 2016.

Hattori CM, Tiselius HG, Heilberg IP: Whey protein and albumin effects upon urinary risk factors for stone formation, *Urolithisis* 45(5):421–428, 2017.

Heilberg IP, Goldfarb DS: Optimum nutrition for kidney stone disease, *Adv Chronic Kidney Dis* 20:165–174, 2013.

Hermann SM, Suarez LG: Oxalate nephropathy due to high oxalate vegan diet, Renal, *Nutrition Forum* 36(3):1, 2017.

Holmes RP, Knight J, Assimos DG: Lowering urinary oxalate excretion to decrease calcium oxalate stone disease, *Urolithiasis* 44(1):27–32, 2016.

Khneizer G, Al-Taee A, Mallick MS, et al: Chronic dietary oxalate nephropathy after intensive dietary weight loss regimen, *J Nephropathol* 6(3):126–129, 2017.

KDIGO 2013: *Kidney International Supplements.* 3(3):271–279, 2013. doi:10.1038/kisup.2013.34.

Kiwull-Schöne H, Kiwull P, Manz F, et al: Food composition and acid-base balance: alimentary alkali depletion and acid load in herbivores, *J Nutr* 138:431S–434S, 2008.

Krieger NS, Bushinsky DA: The relation between bone and stone formation, *Calcif Tissue Int* 93:374–381, 2013.

Lacson E, Wang W, Zebrowski B, et al: Outcomes associated with intradialytic oral nutritional supplements in patients undergoing maintenance hemodialysis: a quality improvement report, *Am J Kidney Dis* 60(4):591–600, 2012.

Langman CB, Grujic D, Pease RM et al. A Double-Blind, Placebo Controlled, Randomized Phase 1 Cross-Over Study with ALLN-177, an Orally Administered Oxalate Degrading Enzyme. Am Jour Nephrol, 44(2):150-8, 2016

Lau WL, Vaziri ND: The leaky gut and altered microbiome in chronic kidney disease, *J Ren Nutr* 27(6), 458–461, 2017. doi:10.1053/j.jrn.2017.02.010.

León JB, Sullivan CM, Sehgal AR: The prevalence of phosphorus containing food additives in top-selling foods in grocery stores, *J Ren Nutr* 23(4):265-270.e2, 2013.

Li CC, Chien TM, Wu WJ, et al: Uric acid stones increase the risk of chronic kidney disease, *Urolithiasis* 46(6):543–547, 2018.

Lu D, Mukai H, Lindholm B, et al: Clinical global assessment of nutritional status as predictor of mortality in chronic kidney disease patients, *PLoS One* 12(12):e0186659, 2017.

Mahmoud H, Forni LG, McIntyre CW, et al: Myocardial Stunning occurs during intermittent haemodialysis for acute kidney injury, *Intensive Care Med* 43(6):942–944, 2017.

Malihi Z: Hypercalcemia, hypercalciuria, and kidney stones in long-term studies of vitamin D supplementation: a systematic review and meta-analysis, *Am J Clin Nutr* 104(4):1039–1051, 2016.

Minich DM, Bland JS: Acid-alkaline balance: role in chronic disease and detoxification, *Altern Ther Health Med* 13:62–65, 2007.

Morrow E, Marcus A, Byham-Gray L: Comparison of handheld indirect calorimetry device and. predictive energy equations among individuals on maintenance hemodialysis, *J Ren Nutr* 27(6):402–411, 2017.

Morgan MS, Pearle MS: Medical management of kidney stones, *BMJ* 352:i52, 2016.

National Kidney Foundation: *How to classify CKD,* Website: 2018.

National Kidney Foundation: *Know your kidney number: two simple tests,* 2017.

Nigwekar SU, Kroshinsky D, Nazarian RM, et al: Calciphylaxis: risk factors, diagnosis and treatment, *Am J Kidney Dis* 66(1):133–146, 2015.

Noori N, Honarkar E, Goldfarb DS, et al: Urinary lithogenic profile in recurrent stone formers with hyperoxaluria: a randomized controlled trial comparing DASH style and low oxalate diets, *Am J Kidney Dis* 63:456–463, 2014.

Penniston KL, Wertheim ML, Nakada SY, et al: Factors associated with patient recall of individualized dietary recommendations for kidney stone prevention, *Eur J Clin Nutr* 70(9):1062–1067, 2016.

Pizzorno J, Frassetto LA, Katzinger J: Diet induced acidosis: is it real and clinically relevant? *Br J Nutr* 103:1185–1194, 2010.

Rak A, Raina R, Suh T, et al: Palliative care for patients with end-stage renal disease: approach to treatment that aims to improve quality of life and relieve suffering for patients (and families) with chronic illnesses, *Clin Kidney J* 10(1):68–73, 2017.

Remer T, Manz F: Potential renal acid load of foods and its influence on urine pH, *J Am Diet Assoc* 95:791–797, 1995.

Sarnak MJ, Amann K, Bangalore S, et al: Chronic kidney disease and coronary artery disease, *J Am Coll Cardiol* 74(14):1823–1838, 2019.

Scales CD, Smith AC, Hanley JM, et al: Prevalence of kidney stones in the United States, *Eur Urol* 62(1):160–165, 2012.

Semins MJ, Asplin JR, Steele K, et al: The effect of restrictive bariatric surgery on urinary stone risk factors, *Urology* 76:826–829, 2010.

Shah S, Calle JC: Dietary and medical management of recurrent nephrolithiasis, *Cleve Clin J Med* 83(6):463–471, 2016.

Sorokin I, Mamoulakis C, Miyazawa K, et al: Epidemiology of stone disease across the world, *World J Urol* 35(9):1301–1320, 2017.

Sparks B: Nutritional considerations for dialysis vegetarian patients, part one, *J Ren Nutr* 28(2) e11–e14, 2018.

Tasian GE, Jemielita T, Goldfarb DS, et al: Oral antibiotics may raise risk of kidney stones Disease, *J Am Soc Nephrol* 29(6):1731–1740, 2018. doi:10.1681/ASN.2017111213

Taylor EN, Curhan GC: Dietary calcium from dairy and nondairy sources, and risk of symptomatic kidney stones, *J Urol* 190:1255–1259, 2013.

Taylor EN, Fung TT, Curhan GC: DASH-style diet associates with reduced risk of kidney stones, *J Am Soc Nephrol* 20:2253–2259, 2009.

Ticinesi A, Milani C, Guerra A, et al: Understanding the gut-kidney axis in nephrolithiasis: an analysis of the gut microbiota composition and functionality of stone formers, *Gut* 67(12):2097–2106, 2018.

Trinchieri A: Development of a rapid food screener to assess the potential renal acid load of diet in renal stone formers (LAKE score), *Arch Ital Urol Adrol* 84:36–38, 2012.

United States Renal Data System (USRDS): *2017 USRDS annual data report: epidemiology of kidney disease in the United States*, Bethesda, MD, 2016, US Department of Health and Human Services, National Institutes of Health, National Institute of Diabetes and Digestive and Kidney Diseases. Available at: https://www.usrds.org/adr.aspx.

Wallace RB, Wactawski-Wende J, O'Sullivan MJ, et al: Urinary tract stone occurrence in the Women's Health Initiative randomized clinical trial of calcium and vitamin D supplements, *Am J Clin Nutr* 94:270–277, 2011.

Wang H, Man L, Li G, et al: Association between serum vitamin D levels and the risk of kidney stone: evidence from a meta-analysis, *Nutr J* 15:32, 2016.

Wertheim ML, Nakada SY, Penniston KL: Current practice patterns of urologists providing nutrition recommendations to aptients with kidney stones, *J Endourol* 28(9):1127–1131, 2014.

Whelton PK, Appel LJ, Sacco RL, et al: Sodium, blood pressure, and cardiovascular disease: further evidence supporting the American Heart Association sodium reduction recommendations, *Circulation* 126:2880–2889, 2012.

Xu W, Zhang C, Wang XL, et al: Self-fluid management in prevention of kidney stones: a PRISMA-compliant systematic review and dose-response meat-analysis of observational studies, *Medicine (Baltimore)* 94(27):e1042, 2015.

Yang W, Xie W, Anderson AH, et al: Association of Kidney Disease Outcomes with risk factors for CKD: Findings from the Chronic Renal Insufficiency Cohort (CRIS) study, *Am J Kidney Dis* 63:236–243, 2014.

Yasui T, Suzuki S, Itoh Y, et al: Eicosapentanoic acid has protective effect on the recurrence of nephrolithissis, *Urol Int* 81:135–138, 2008.

Zilberman DE, Yong D, Albala DM, et al: The impact of societal changes on patterns of urolithiasis, *Curr Opin Urol* 20:148–153, 2010.

35

Medical Nutrition Therapy for Cancer Prevention, Treatment, and Survivorship

Ginger Hultin, MS, RDN, CSO

KEY TERMS

antiangiogenic agents
antineoplastic therapy
antioxidants
apoptosis
benign
biotherapy
bisphenol A (BPA)
cancer cachexia
carcinogen
carcinogenesis
certified specialist in oncology nutrition
   (CSO)
chemoprevention
chemotherapy
cytokines
dumping syndrome
emetogenic
graft-versus-host disease (GVHD)
hematopoietic cell transplantation (HCT)

hematopoietic growth factors
hormonal therapy
hospice
initiation
insulin-like growth factor-1 (IGF-1)
isotonic
malignant neoplasm
metastasis
mitogen
mucositis
mutations
myelosuppression
neoplasm
neutropenia
nutrigenomics
nutrition impact symptoms
oncogenes
oncology
osteoradionecrosis

palliative care
pancytopenia
peripheral neuropathy
phytochemicals
polycyclic aromatic hydrocarbons (PAHs)
progression
promotion
radiation enteritis
radiation therapy
thrombocytopenia
trismus
tumor
tumor angiogenesis
tumor necrosis factor-α (cachectin)
tumor-node-metastasis (TNM) staging
   system
tumor suppressor genes
xerostomia

Cancer is a group of diseases that involves the abnormal and uncontrolled division and reproduction of cells that can spread throughout the body. Some cancers can be monitored over time and treated like a chronic disease while others are harder to treat and lead to early death. The etiology of cancer is not clearly understood but is likely multifactorial with genetic, environmental, medical, and lifestyle factors interfacing to produce a given malignancy (American Cancer Society [ACS], 2019b; National Institutes of Health [NIH, 2019] and National Cancer Institute [NCI], 2019b). The ACS predicts the lifetime risk for developing cancer in the United States is slightly less than half of men and a little more than one third of women (ACS, 2019b). Annually in the United States, cancer is responsible for almost one in four deaths and is the second most common cause of death after heart disease (ACS, 2019b). It is estimated that one third of the more than 580,000 anticipated cancer deaths can be attributed to nutrition and lifestyle behaviors such as poor diet, physical inactivity, alcohol use, and overweight and obesity. Tobacco use contributes significantly to death from cancer with more than 15 million lives lost since the surgeon general released the warning in 1964. Today, nearly one in five deaths from cancer and other diseases in the United States are caused by tobacco use (ACS, 2019b).

Overall, fewer Americans are dying from cancer, a trend that began more than 20 years ago. For many, cancer is now a chronic disease, like heart disease and diabetes. According to the ACS, there are 15.5 million American cancer survivors living with a history of cancer; this means they are cancer free, are living with evidence of disease, or are undergoing cancer treatment (ACS, 2019b). As a result of progress in early detection of cancer and the development of new anticancer therapies, survivorship for all cancers is now 70% among whites and 63% among blacks, up from 39% and 27% respectively in the 1960's (ACS, 2019b). The Annual Report to the Nation on the Status of Cancer 1999 to 2015 found that cancer incidence rates decreased among men but were stable among women. Overall, cancer death rates are significantly declining in men and women yet differences in rates and trends by race and ethnicity do remain (Cronin et al, 2018).

The cost of cancer care in the United States is a burden to patients, their families, and society, estimated to be more than $216.6 billion annually—$80.2 billion for direct medical costs and $130 billion for loss of productivity resulting from lost income and premature death (ACS, 2019b; Inoue-Choi and Robien, 2013) (Fig. 35.1).

The ACS has created guidelines for the prevention and early detection of cancer (Box 35.1). These prevention guidelines, for those who do not use tobacco, include weight control, dietary choices, and levels

---

Portions of this chapter were written by Barbara Grant and Kathryn Hamilton.

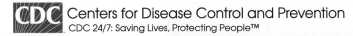

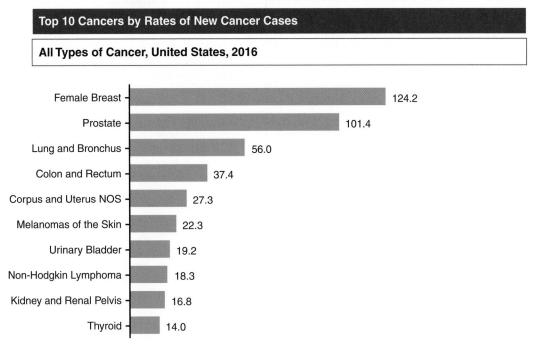

A   Rate per 100,000 people, male and female

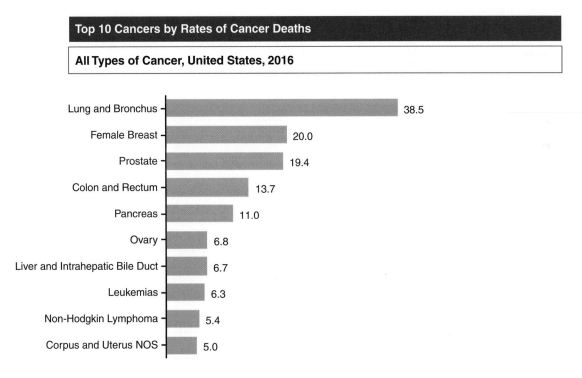

B   Rate per 100,000 people, male and female

Fig. 35.1 U.S. Cancer Statistics Working Group. U.S. Cancer Statistics Data Visualizations Tool, based on November 2018 submission data (1999-2016): U.S. Department of Health and Human Services, Centers for Disease Control and Prevention and National Cancer Institute; www.cdc.gov/cancer/dataviz, June 2019.

of physical activity as the most important modifiable determinants of cancer risk (ACS, 2018b).

PATHOPHYSIOLOGY

Carcinogenesis is the origin or development of cancer. Oncology is the branch of medicine that specializes in the prevention, diagnosis, and treatment of cancer. Researchers believe changes in gene function cause normal cells to transform into cancerous cells.

Oncogenes are altered genes that promote tumor growth and inhibit apoptosis (programmed cell death). The inhibition of cell death pathways allows for survival of the genetically damaged cancer cells. Tumor suppressor genes are the opposite of oncogenes; these genes become deactivated in cancer cells. This loss in function can lead to unregulated cell growth and, ultimately, cancer. Examples of tumor suppressor genes include adenomatosis polyposis coli (APC), breast cancer types BRCA1 and BCRA2, and tumor suppressor, a protein that

is involved in preventing cancer. Only approximately 5% to 10% of all cancers occur as result of inherited genetic alterations, also called mutations (ACS, 2018b). Factors observed in families with hereditary cancers include the following:

- Many cases of an uncommon or rare type of cancer
- A cancer diagnosis at an earlier age than normal for certain kinds of cancer
- Individuals with one type of cancer being diagnosed with a second type of cancer
- More than one childhood cancer diagnosed in a set of siblings
- Cancers occurring in a pair of organs like both eyes, both kidneys, or both breasts
- Cancers occurring in the gender not usually affected (e.g., breast cancer in men)
- Cancers occurring in many generations
- Certain types of cancers observed in specific ethnic populations (e.g., individuals of Ashkenazi Jewish ancestry with breast and ovarian cancer)
- Recognized cancer syndromes, such as hereditary nonpolyposis colorectal cancer or Lynch syndrome, which cause individuals to be at greater risk for developing gastrointestinal (GI), ovarian, uterine, brain, or skin cancer (NIH, 2019a; NCI, 2018a)

Genetic counselors assist individuals and their families to evaluate their risk of hereditary predisposition, such as testing positive for gene mutations and assessing risk.

Phases of Carcinogenesis

A carcinogen is a physical, chemical, or viral agent that induces cancer. Carcinogenesis is a biologic, multistage process that proceeds on a continuum in three distinct phases: initiation, promotion, and progression. Initiation involves transformation of cells produced by the interaction of chemicals, radiation, or viruses with cellular deoxyribonucleic acid (DNA). This transformation occurs rapidly, but cells can remain dormant for a variable period until they are activated by a promoting agent. After the initial cellular damage has occurred, transformation from normal cells to a detectable cancer can take many years or even decades. During promotion, initiated cells multiply and escape the mechanisms set in place to protect the body from uncontrolled growth and spread. A neoplasm, new and abnormal tissue with no useful function, is established. In the third phase, progression, tumor cells aggregate and grow into a fully malignant neoplasm or a tumor.

In the process known as metastasis, the neoplasm has the capacity for invasion that can spread to distant tissues and organs. For a cancer to metastasize, it must develop its own blood supply to sustain its growth of rapidly dividing abnormal cells. In normal cells, angiogenesis promotes the formation of new blood vessels, which are essential to supply the body's tissues with oxygen and nutrients. In cancer cells, tumor angiogenesis occurs when tumors are able to develop new blood vessels needed for their growth and metastasis.

NUTRITION AND CARCINOGENESIS

Nutrition may modify the carcinogenic process at any stage, including carcinogen metabolism, cellular and host defense, cell differentiation, and tumor growth. Estimates produced by the World Cancer Research Fund indicate one quarter to one third of all of the cancers that occur in higher-income countries such as the United States, Canada, and Australia are due to poor nutrition, physical inactivity, and excess weight (ACS, 2019b).

Studies looking at the role of nutrition and diet as causal factors of cancer seek to identify relationships between the diets of population

TABLE 35.1	Phytochemicals in Vegetables and Fruits that May Have Cancer Protective Properties		
Color	**Phytochemical**	**Vegetables and Fruits**	**Potential Benefits**
Red	Lycopene	Tomatoes and tomato products, papaya, pink grapefruit, watermelon	Protect against prostate cancer
Red and purple	Anthocyanins, polyphenols	Berries, grapes, red wine, plums, purple cabbage, peanuts	Prevent cancer formation, decrease inflammation and provide antioxidant support
Orange	Alpha- and beta-carotene	Carrots, mangos, pumpkin, sweet potato	Protect against oral, esophageal, pharynx, larynx, and lung cancers. Improve immune response
Yellow and green	Lutein, zeaxanthin	Kale, spinach, collard, dandelion, mustard and turnip greens, asparagus, cooked winter squash	Protect DNA from damage
Green	Sulforaphanes, indoles	Arugula, Bok choy, cabbage, broccoli, Brussels sprouts, cauliflower, watercress	Change DNA methylation that directly and indirectly regulates cancer progression
White and green	Allyl sulfides	Leeks, onion, garlic, chives	Protect against stomach and colorectal cancer

American Institute for Cancer Research/World Cancer Research Fund: *Diet – what to eat to lower cancer risk*, 2018b; Bender A, Collins K, Higginbotham S: Nutrition and cancer prevention. In Leser M, Ledesma N, Bergerson S, et al, editors: *Oncology nutrition for clinical practice*, Chicago, 2013, Oncology Dietetic Practice Group.

groups and categories of individuals and the incidence of specific cancers (Thomson et al, 2014). Sets of individuals are compared in case control, cohort, or cross-sectional studies. In cancer research, epidemiologists look at human populations and evaluate how many people are diagnosed with cancer, what types of cancer occur in different populations and cultures, and what factors (such as diet and lifestyle) play a role in the development of the cancers.

The sheer complexity of diverse diet patterns presents a difficult challenge for research. Thousands of compounds are found in a normal diet; some are well studied and some are less known and unmeasured. Some dietary carcinogens are naturally occurring pesticides or herbicides produced by plants for protection against fungi, insects, animal predators, or mycotoxins, which are secondary metabolites produced by molds present in foods (e.g., aflatoxins, fumonisins, or ochratoxins). Food preparation and preservation methods also may contribute to dietary carcinogen ingestion. Examples of dietary enhancers of carcinogenesis may be the saturated fat in red meat or the polycyclic aromatic hydrocarbons (PAHs) that form on the surface of meat when grilling at high temperatures. Fortunately, diets also contain inhibitors of carcinogenesis. Dietary carcinogen inhibitors include antioxidants (e.g., vitamin C, carotenoids, vitamin E, selenium, zinc) and phytochemicals (biologically active components of plants) (Table 35.1). Dietary antioxidants scavenge and neutralize free radicals, preventing them from causing damage in the body (NCI, 2017).

Complicating the study of nutrition, diet, and cancer is the fact that an alteration of one major component of the diet can precipitate a change in other facets of the diet. For example, decreasing animal protein also decreases saturated fat. This cascade makes the interpretation of research findings difficult because the effects cannot be associated clearly with one single factor. Additional complications in interpretation can result from the fact that cancer cells can either be fast growing or have a long latent or dormant period. The slow-growing, latent, or dormant aspect of the disease progression makes pinpointing dietary patterns at the time of cancer cell initiation or promotion, and not at time of diagnosis, difficult. Epidemiologic research, together with animal studies, provides a viable method for discovering the links between nutrition and cancer in humans.

Alcohol

Alcohol consumption was responsible for 3 million deaths each year globally, in 2018, and is a modifiable risk factor for cancer-related deaths in the United States (Bender et al, 2013; World Health Organization

[WHO], 2018). It is associated with increased cancer risk for cancers of the oral cavity, pharynx, larynx, esophagus, colon, rectum, stomach, pancreas, gallbladder, liver, and breast (pre- and postmenopausal women). For colorectal, stomach, liver, and kidney cancers, daily consumption of two or more drinks increases risk significantly compared with non-drinkers. (Bagnardi et al, 2015; World Cancer Research Fund/American Institute for Cancer, 2018).

Alcohol can also negatively affect health outcomes for some cancer survivors. Alcohol consumption was associated with an increased risk of overall mortality in cancer survivors particularly in head and neck cancer leading to lower survival rates. Alcohol intake recommendations should be tailored to the individual given the type of cancer, dietary history, and health goals (Rock et al, 2012). An increased risk for cancer recurrence was also found when data for pre- and postdiagnosis levels of alcohol were combined. Alcohol is associated with an increased risk of breast cancer recurrence and increased mortality rates among survivors of hepatocellular carcinoma, non-Hodgkin's lymphoma, laryngeal and pharyngeal, and head and neck cancer (Schwedhelm et al, 2016).

Concurrent tobacco and alcohol use greatly increases cancer risk, particularly for cancers of the upper digestive area and respiratory tract (WCRF/AICR, 2018). In addition, malnutrition associated with alcoholism is likely to be important in the increased risk for certain cancers. In the United States if individuals choose to drink, men are recommended to limit alcohol intake to no more than two drinks per day and women to one drink per day. Serving sizes of alcoholic drinks include beer (12 oz), wine (5 oz), and liquors (1.5 oz of 80-proof liquors) though the WCRF/AICR recommends that it is best to not drink alcohol at all (Dietary Guidelines for Americans, 2018; Kushi et al, 2012; WCRF/AICR, 2018). (Fig. 35.2).

Energy Intake and Body Weight

Obesity is a risk factor for some cancers and may account for up to 20% of all cancer-related mortality (Arnold et al, 2016; Arnold et al, 2017; Bender et al, 2013; Kushi et al, 2012). This makes maintaining a healthy body weight status the second most important lifestyle factor to reduce cancer risk after not using tobacco (Bender et al, 2013). Currently 70.2% of American adults are overweight or obese (Centers for Disease Control and Prevention [CDC], 2018). The relationship between body weight, body mass index (BMI), or relative body weight and site-specific cancer has been widely investigated; a positive association has been seen with cancers of the mouth/larynx/pharynx,

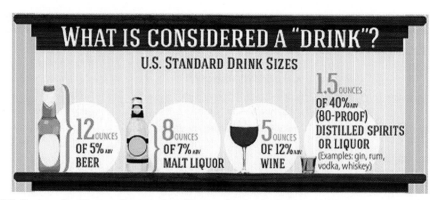

Fig. 35.2 Centers for Disease Control. Fact Sheet – Moderate Drinking (website). https://www.cdc.gov/alcohol/fact-sheets/moderate-drinking.htm.

TABLE 35.2	American Cancer Society: Moderate and Vigorous Physical Activity	
	Moderate Activities (moving fast enough that you can speak but cannot sing)	**Vigorous Activities (moving fast enough that you can speak a few words but not in complete sentences)**
Exercise and leisure	Walking, dancing, leisurely bicycling, ice and roller skating, horseback riding, canoeing, yoga	Jogging or running, fast bicycling, circuit weight training, aerobic dance, martial arts, jumping rope, swimming
Sports	Volleyball, golfing, softball, baseball, badminton, doubles tennis, downhill skiing	Soccer, field or ice hockey, lacrosse, singles tennis, racquetball, basketball, cross-country skiing
Home activities	Mowing the lawn, general yard and garden maintenance	Digging, carrying and hauling, masonry, carpentry
Workplace activity	Walking and lifting as part of the job (custodial work, farming, auto or machine repair)	Heavy manual labor (forestry, construction, firefighting)

American Cancer Society (ACS): https://www.cancer.org; Kushi LH, et al: American Cancer Society guidelines on nutrition and physical activity for cancer prevention: reducing the risk of cancer with healthy food choices and physical activity, *CA Cancer J Clin* 62:30, 2012.

esophagus, pancreas, gallbladder, breast (postmenopausal), endometrium, kidney, colon, rectum, gastric cardia, liver, ovary, thyroid, multiple myeloma, and meningioma (Arnold et al, 2016; Arnold et al, 2017). Body fat is a metabolically active tissue that produces estrogen and proteins that cause high levels of insulin and other hormones including insulin-like growth factor-1 (IGF-1) and leptin that can lead to inflammation. The longer a person is overweight, the more significant the association with the incidence of all obesity-related cancers. For example, in postmenopausal breast and endometrial cancer, every 10-year increase in adulthood overweight status is associated with a 5% and 17% increase in risk, respectively (Arnold et al, 2016; Arnold et al, 2017; AICR, 2018a; Bender et al, 2013).

Obesity, age, hyperglycemia, and the incidence of metabolic syndrome play a role in the circulating levels of insulin-like growth factor-1 (IGF-1). IGF-1 is a polypeptide secreted primarily by the liver and plays a key role in normal growth and development, acting as a mitogen, a chemical substance that encourages cells to divide, that may promote growth and reproduction of cancer cells while inhibiting apoptosis. High circulating levels have been associated with the development and progression of prostate, breast, lung, and colon cancer (Adachi et al, 2016; Bender et al, 2013). IGF-1 secretion is increased when insulin levels are elevated. Obesity and high simple carbohydrate intakes potentially increase insulin resistance and raise circulating insulin levels. This area of research connects several known risk factors between nutrition, diet, and cancer (Park et al, 2014).

Physical activity is a critical component of weight management, optimal lean body mass, and energy balance. The ACS Nutrition and Physical Activity Guidelines for Cancer Prevention and the Guidelines for Cancer Survivors encourage individuals to strive for a minimum of 150 minutes per week of moderate activity or a minimum of 75 minutes per week of vigorous activity (Kushi et al, 2012; Rock et al, 2012) (Table 35.2).

Achieving and maintaining energy balance and a reasonable weight should be a primary health goal for all individuals, including cancer survivors, because being overweight or obese appears to increase risk of developing cancer, cancer recurrence, and decreased survival (Kushi et al, 2012; Rock et al, 2012) (Box 35.2).

BOX 35.2   Does Eating Less Reduce the Risk for Cancer?

Animal studies have demonstrated that both chronic restriction of calories and intermittent calorie restriction have shown anticancer effects. Both forms of restriction may decrease insulin-like growth factor-1 (IGF-1) and leptin while increasing adiponectin and improving insulin sensitivity. There have been population-based studies on breast cancer and chronic caloric restriction though compliance has been low in some studies due to the challenges of constant restriction. For this reason, intermittent fasting (IF) may be better suited to some individuals and has been linked to weight loss and significantly lower serum IGF-1 in some participants. IF can be done several ways including alternate day fasting, fasting 2 days per week, or fasting for 12 to 16 hours out of 24 hours. This is also referred to as time restricted feeding. Caloric restriction, without malnutrition, appears to have a positive effect on cancer prevention in animals; it is unclear whether that effect translates to humans and if chronic restriction or IF may be more desirable for compliance and cancer outcomes (Chen et al, 2016; Fontana et al, 2016; Harvie and Howell, 2016).

Fat

Dietary fat has been studied in relationship to cancer risk and recurrence. There appears to be an inconsistent link between certain types of cancer and the amount of fat in the diet. Of note, diets that contain a significant amount of fat often contain more meat and more calories, which can contribute to overweight and obese conditions and increased cancer risk.

To further complicate the picture, an additional link a fat, meat, and cancer risk results from meat preparation and processing, such as the presence of heterocyclic amines (HCAs) and/or PAHs from cooking, formation of carcinogenic N-nitroso compounds (NOCs) from processing, and the potential cancer-promoting influence of heme-iron (Bender et al, 2013; WCRF/AICR, 2018).

Because dietary fat intake is correlated with the intake of other nutrients and dietary components, it is difficult to distinguish between the effects of dietary fat, protein, total calories, and carcinogenic compounds in cancer prevention. So the current ACS recommendation is to limit consumption of processed meats and red meats (Kushi et al, 2012).

A large prospective randomized trial examined dietary fat consumption as part of the diet composition, and all cancer mortality showed mixed results. The Women's Health Initiative (WHI) found that adoption of a low-fat dietary pattern led to a lower incidence of deaths after breast cancer but no reduction in mortality from other cancer sites (Chlebowski et al, 2018). Current recommendations focus on limiting highly processed foods high in fat and added sugar as well as limiting red meat. Doing so naturally reduces the amount of trans and saturated fat in the diet (WCRF/AICR, 2018).

Eating more omega-3 fatty acids (foods such as fatty fish, flaxseed oil, walnuts, and certain algae) in relation to omega-6 fatty acids (polyunsaturated fats such as safflower oil and sunflower oil) potentially reduces risk of cancer by acting to decrease inflammation, cell proliferation, and angiogenesis while increasing apoptosis (Bender et al, 2013). However, there have been contradictory results in human studies so the benefit remains unclear (Weylandt et al, 2015). The differences seen are possibly due to the difference in response to omega-3 in food versus taking omega-3 as a supplement.

Sugar and Nonnutritive Sweeteners

Studies suggest that high glycemic diets that raise postprandial blood glucose may increase cancer risk by creating higher levels of IGF-1 in the body. A large prospective study (EPIC-Italy) found that a high glycemic diet was associated with an increased risk of colon and bladder cancer (Sieri et al, 2017). The 2015–2020 Dietary Guidelines for Americans recommends limiting calories from added sugars in the diet, specifically consuming less than 10% of calories per day from added sugars (Dietary Guidelines for Americans, 2018). Sugary drinks, energy-dense foods, and highly processed foods can promote weight gain so consumption should be limited for cancer prevention (Bender et al, 2013).

The Food and Drug Administration (FDA) has approved eight nonnutritive sweeteners (acesulfame-potassium, aspartame, luo han guo fruit extract [monk fruit], neotame, saccharin, stevia, advantame, and sucralose) for use in the food supply and regulates them as food additives; they are generally recognized as safe (GRAS) when used in moderation (Academy of Nutrition and Dietetics [AND], 2012 ; FDA, 2018). Described as "high-intensity" sweeteners, nonnutritive sweeteners provide little or no energy because they sweeten in minute amounts. Nonnutritive sweeteners have been investigated primarily in relation to potential adverse health concerns, including long-term safety and

carcinogenicity, but multiple studies during the past 20 or more years have indicated that when consumed in reasonable amounts, they are safe (NCI, 2016a). Additional sugar substitutes on the market include sugar alcohols (e.g., mannitol, sorbitol, xylitol). Sugar alcohols are not considered nonnutritive sweeteners even though they are used in a similar way (AND, 2012).

Protein

Most diets that contain significant amounts of protein also contain significant amounts of meat and fat and lower amounts of fiber. The effect of protein on carcinogenesis depends on origin and type of tumor as well as the type of protein consumed and the overall calorie content of the diet as it relates to body weight regulation. Some studies suggest that restricting protein intake can lower IGF-1 levels and be cancer protective, even slowing tumor progression in animal models. Note that human studies state protein restriction is not appropriate for older adults age 65+ and people undergoing cancer treatment at any age also have increased needs. Because of the link between red and processed meat consumption and cancer, the American Cancer Society and the American Institute for Cancer Research recommend limiting these foods and eating more plant based proteins such as legumes, nuts, and seeds. (Levine et al, 2014; Melina 2016; WCRF/AICR, 2018).

Smoked, Grilled, and Preserved Foods and Processed Meats

Processed meats are treated in some way to preserve flavor generally by smoking, curing, salting, or adding chemical preservatives. Processed meats include beef jerky, bologna, pepperoni, ham, bacon, hot dogs and frankfurters, pastrami, salami, and sausages. Nitrates are added as preservatives to processed meats. Nitrates can be readily reduced to form nitrites, which can interact with dietary substrates such as amines and amides to produce NOCs nitrosamines and nitrosamides, which are known mutagens and carcinogens. Nitrates or nitrites are used in smoked, salted, and pickled foods. They are linked especially to colorectal cancer (WCRF/AICR, 2018). Twenty-two experts from 10 countries reviewed more than 800 studies and found that eating 50 grams of processed meat every day increased the risk of colorectal cancer by 18%. That is the equivalent of about four strips of bacon or one hot dog. For those eating any red meat, there was evidence of increased risk of colorectal, pancreatic, and prostate cancer (WHO, 2015).

Charring or cooking meat at high temperatures over an open flame (400° F/204.4° C or more) can cause the formation of PAHs and HCAs. Polycyclic aromatic hydrocarbons (PAHs) have shown clear indications of mutagenicity and carcinogenicity. Normal roasting or frying food does not produce large amounts of PAHs compared with the amount produced when cooking over open flames. Animal proteins that produce the greatest dripping of fat on to the flames register the highest PAH formation. For example, grilled beef produces larger amounts of PAHs than grilled chicken, which produces higher amounts than oven-grilled chicken. The source of the flame can also influence PAH production; charcoal grilling promotes the most, followed by flame gas, and finally oven grilling (Ewa and Danuta, 2017).

Organic and Genetically Modified (GM) Foods

Food growing techniques and modifications made to food leave some patients fearing that conventionally grown or GM foods can be cancer promoting. Though studies have shown that organically produced foods are less likely than conventionally grown foods to contain pesticide residues, a large study presented in the *British Journal of Cancer* found that consumption of organic food was not associated with a reduction in the incidence of all cancer, soft tissue sarcoma, or breast cancer (Bradbury et al, 2014). While some studies have suggested that organic foods are higher in certain nutrients, others have found that not to be true to a notable degree. At this time, risk of cancer or a decreased nutritional value are not reasons to avoid conventionally grown produce (Bradbury et al, 2014; Brantsæter et al, 2017). For patients who are concerned about limiting their pesticide exposure or who have environmental concerns, purchasing organic foods is an option. See Chapter 8 for further discussion of organic versus conventional agriculture.

Biotechnology in agriculture includes genetically modified organisms (GMOs) such as corn and soybean crops among others in the United States. Some people fear that there is a link between cancer and GMOs though studies do not show that the process of genetic modification is a risk. Some studies have suggested a link between tumors in animals and non-Hodgkin's lymphoma in humans due to the use of herbicide glyphosate used on GM crops. It was previously deemed a probable human carcinogen by the International Agency for Research on Cancer (IARC). One benefit to GMOs can be to decrease the number of herbicides used directly on crops. However, some GMO crops have been developed to be resistant to herbicides, so while GMO crops decrease the amount of pesticide needed, the amount of herbicide is actually increased. The National Academy of Sciences has reviewed the safety of GM crops and found that they pose no unique hazards to human health, including cancer incidence. Ongoing evaluation of GMO safety is important to understanding the long-term effects of GMOs on human health and the environment (Kushi et al, 2012; Landrigan and Benbrook, 2015).

Chemical Exposures

The Environmental Protection Agency (EPA) was established in 1970 to oversee the acute and long-term health threats caused by substances in the environment. As part of this protection, the Toxic Substances Control Act passed in 1976 requires manufacturers to submit health and safety information on all new chemicals. However, many were grandfathered in with the passage of this law and are still untested. To date, 248 compounds have been identified by the NIH as carcinogenic (NIH/National Institute of Environmental Health Services [NIEHS], 2016).

Everyday activities expose people to a myriad of chemicals through air, water, food, and beverages. In fact, an estimated 12% of cancers diagnosed each year are likely caused by these very common exposures (Israel, 2010; NIH/NIEHS, 2016). Studies of people with high exposures to pesticides such as agricultural workers including farmers and crop duster pilots, have higher rates of overall cancer incidence as well as increased risk of lymphohematopoietic cancers; leukemia; non-Hodgkin's lymphoma; multiple myeloma; breast, bladder, prostate, brain, lung, pancreatic, and colorectal cancers; and melanoma. There are specific types of cancer associated with specific types of pesticide application and exposure (Alavanja, 2009; Weichenthal et al, 2010).

A good environmental history can be performed at clinical visits and then quickly reviewed for outdoor air pollutants such as nitrogen dioxide, ozone, and carbon monoxide, which pose health risks. Exposure to heavy metals, pesticides, herbicides, and occupational exposures also may be noted. Oxidative stress caused by these environmental exposures can be reduced by changes in lifestyle, including eliminating smoking and implementing dietary changes such as the consumption of phytonutrient-rich foods and a nutrient-rich diet (Kushi et al, 2012).

> ### BOX 35.3   Tips from the FDA to Minimize Exposure to Bisphenol A (BPA)
>
> - Check plastic container recycle codes on the bottom of container. Some, but not all, plastics that are marked with recycle codes 3 or 7 may be made with BPA.
> - Avoid putting very hot or boiling liquids in plastic containers made with BPA. BPA levels rise in food when containers and products made with the chemical are heated and come in contact with the food. Don't microwave polycarbonate plastic food containers.
> - Reduce your use of canned foods or choose BPA-free products. Opt instead for glass, porcelain, or stainless-steel containers.

Food and Drug Administration: *Bisphenol A (BPA): for use in food content application*, 2014; Environmental Protection Agency: *Risk management for bisphenol A (BPA)*, 2017; National Institutes of Health: *Bisphenol A (BPA)*, 2017.

Bisphenol A (BPA)

Bisphenol A (BPA) is an industrial chemical used since the 1960s in the manufacturing of many hard, plastic bottles and the epoxy linings of metal-based food and beverage cans. It is also an ingredient in the production of epoxy resin used in paints and adhesives. Studies done when the product was developed indicated it was safe to use in food and beverage containers. However, multiple studies have demonstrated that BPA may disrupt the function of some hormones, including sex hormones, leptin, insulin, and thyroxin causing hepatotoxic, immunologic, and carcinogenic effects (Michałowicz, 2014).

Other findings from the combined efforts of the NIEHS, the National Toxicology Program, and FDA scientists at the National Center for Toxicologic Research Program conclude that the health threat from BPA is less than previously estimated and safe at the levels occurring in foods. Health damage from BPA may not be as likely because based on mathematical models, BPA rapidly metabolizes in the body, rather than accumulating (FDA, 2014).

Until more is known, the current goal is to reduce the use and exposure to BPA through several actions: restricting the use of BPA in plastic bottles, using alternatives to the glue resins used in food containers, and increasing the oversight on the use of BPA in manufacturing and testing. The U.S. Department of Health and Human Services (USDHHS) supports eliminating BPA from all food-related product production. Originally it was thought to leech from the plastic only when exposed to heat; now it is believed to leech even at cold temperatures (FDA, 2014). Note that BPA-free products are now easy to find. Consumers can read labels and choose BPA-free cans or foods packaged in BPA-free boxes or glass (Box 35.3).

CHEMOPREVENTION

Eating behaviors play an important role in health promotion and disease prevention. Chemoprevention is defined as the use of drugs, vitamins, or other agents to reduce the risk of, or delay the development or recurrence of cancer (NIH and NCI, 2015). Examples include nonsteroidal antiinflammatory drugs that may protect against colon cancer, and metformin, a commonly used medication to treat diabetes; these are currently being explored as cancer prevention and treatment agents (Guppy et al, 2011; Quinn et al, 2013). Other natural products or molecules currently being investigated include the hundreds of polyphenols in fruits and vegetables, green tea, curcumin (turmeric), and resveratrol from red grapes and berries. Phenolic acid, flavonoids, terpenes, and lignans are the most abundant polyphenols; the chemopreventive potential of these compounds comes from their ability to modulate epigenetic alterations in cancer cells (Choi and Friso, 2010). Many of these substances likely have complementary and overlapping mechanisms including antioxidant, antiangiogenesis, immune modulating, detox enzyme enhancing, antiproliferative, and nitrosamine formation inhibiting properties in addition to diluting and binding carcinogens in the digestive tract and altering hormone metabolism, all relevant to cancer prevention (see Table 35.1).

The epigenetic modification step occurs early in the development of a cancer cell, at a time when it is potentially reversible. Scientists do not fully understand how this process works, yet it is reasonable to recommend a health-promoting and possibly cancer-preventing diet rich in fruits, vegetables, soy, therapeutic culinary herbs such as turmeric and cinnamon, green tea, and coffee (Link et al, 2010). The overall evidence of association between these and other dietary factors enable health organizations to draft diet and lifestyle recommendations for the purpose of reducing cancer risk (see the ACS website https://www.cancer.org and Box 35.1).

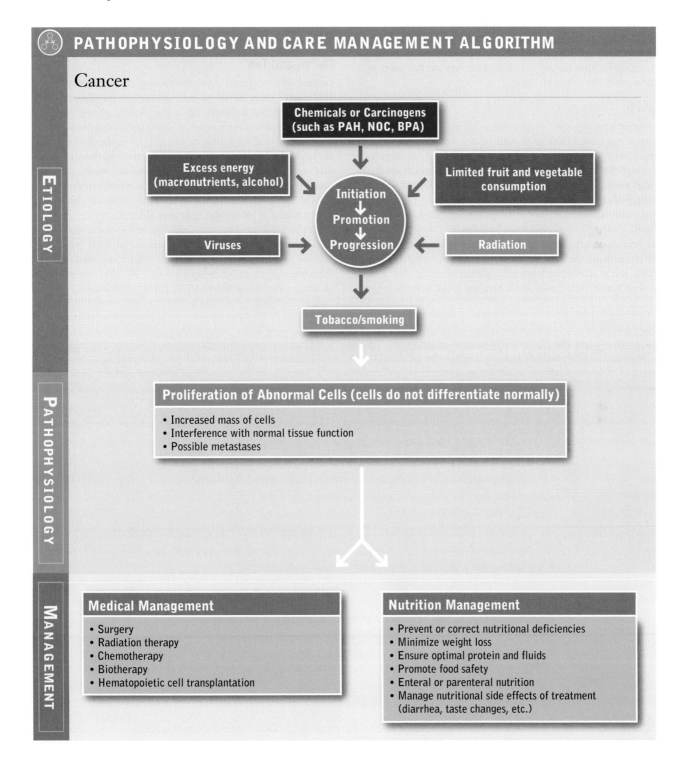

PATHOPHYSIOLOGY AND CARE MANAGEMENT ALGORITHM

Cancer

ETIOLOGY

Chemicals or Carcinogens (such as PAH, NOC, BPA)

Excess energy (macronutrients, alcohol)

Limited fruit and vegetable consumption

Initiation → Promotion → Progression

Viruses

Radiation

Tobacco/smoking

PATHOPHYSIOLOGY

Proliferation of Abnormal Cells (cells do not differentiate normally)
- Increased mass of cells
- Interference with normal tissue function
- Possible metastases

MANAGEMENT

Medical Management
- Surgery
- Radiation therapy
- Chemotherapy
- Biotherapy
- Hematopoietic cell transplantation

Nutrition Management
- Prevent or correct nutritional deficiencies
- Minimize weight loss
- Ensure optimal protein and fluids
- Promote food safety
- Enteral or parenteral nutrition
- Manage nutritional side effects of treatment (diarrhea, taste changes, etc.)

Antioxidants and Bioactive Compounds

The American Institute for Cancer Research (AICR) lists 19 foods that fight cancer based on bioactive compounds that inhibit the reproduction of cancer cells, slow the growth of tumors, inhibit division of cancer cells, and decrease risk of developing cancer. Bioactive compounds including saponins, protease inhibitors, phytic acid, quercetin, resveratrol, glucosinolates, chlorogenic acid, and many more can act as chemoprotective agents (AICR, 2018c). (Table 35.3).

Studies have shown promise that diets higher in antioxidants including vitamins C and E, selenium, flavonoids, and carotenoids may prevent certain types of cancer including breast cancer. A large prospective cohort study, the Rotterdam Study, found that high overall dietary antioxidant capacity was associated with a lower risk of developing breast cancer (Pantavos et al, 2015). Research supports potential chemoprotection from dietary antioxidant sources but not from supplement sources (Bender et al, 2013).

Vitamin D

Some studies have reported an association of poor vitamin D status and greater incidence of cancer though other studies do not support this hypothesis. Vitamin D is the precursor to steroid hormone calcitriol—1,25-dihydroxyvitamin D_3 (1,25[OH]$_2$ D_3), which mediates numerous actions in many tissues of the body. It is known that calcitriol regulates multiple signaling pathways involved in proliferation, apoptosis, differentiation, inflammation, invasion, angiogenesis, and metastasis, creating a potential to affect cancer development and growth. Studies on what blood levels of serum 25-hydroxy vitamin D (25[OH]D) provide the most protection but concentrations of 45 to 50 ng/mL levels experienced lower incidence of colon and breast cancer than those with lower levels ranging from 8 to 12 ng/mL

(American Academy of Dermatology [AAD], 2018; Baggerly et al, 2015; Feldman et al, 2014).

More work must be done in this area to determine whether supplementation with vitamin D can prevent cancer, or if low levels of the vitamin simply increases an individual's cancer risk. Until more is learned about the interaction between vitamin D_3 and cancer prevention, taking 600 IU of vitamin D per day to maintain normal serum 25(OH)D levels is considered safe for males and females ages 1-70 years at which time recommendations increase to 800 IU (Kushi et al, 2012). Individuals with abnormal serum levels should consult their medical team for supplement suggestions, monitoring, and evaluation. Correcting a deficiency in vitamin D may be important for its health promotion benefits as well as its effect on calcium absorption and bone health.

Coffee and Tea

Coffee contains various antioxidant and phenolic compounds, some of which have been shown to have anticancer properties. Coffee also contains caffeine, a compound in the alkaloid phytochemical family. Coffee as a major source of antioxidants in the American diet may offer a protective effect against cancer. Though coffee does contain acrylamide, created during high temperature roasting, there is no evidence that regular consumption of coffee is associated with increased risk of cancer. It has shown to be potentially carcinogenic when given to animals at high levels but is not a concern for humans at this time (AICR, 2018c; NIH and NCI, 2010; Wilson et al, 2010).

Tea is also a good source of phenols and antioxidants. Green tea is made from leaves that have been pressed and dried but not roasted. Because of this, green tea, more so than black tea, contains catechins, including epigallocatechin-3-gallate (EGCG) that possess potentially anticancer biologic activity (AICR, 2018c; NIH and NCI, 2010).

TABLE 35.3	Foods that Fight Cancer
Food	**Bioactive Compound**
Apples	Fiber, vitamin C, quercetin, flavonoids, triterpenoids
Blueberries	Fiber, vitamins C and K, manganese, anthocyanins, catechins, quercetin, kaempferol, ellagitannins, pterostilbene, resveratrol
Cruciferous Vegetables	Vitamins C, K, and manganese, glucosinolates that form isothiocyanates and indoles
Carrots	Fiber, vitamins A and K, beta-carotene and alpha-carotene, luteolin, falcarinol
Cherries	Fiber, vitamin C, potassium, anthocyanins, hydroxycinnamic acid, perillyl alcohol
Coffee	Riboflavin, chlorogenic acid, quinic acid, cafestol and kahweol, N-methylpyridinium (NBM)
Cranberries	Fiber, vitamin c, flavonoids, ursolic acid, benzoic and hydroxycinnamic acid
Dark Leafy Greens	Fiber, folate, carotenoids (lutein and zeaxanthin), saponins and flavonoids
Legumes	Fiber, lignans, saponins, triterpenoids, inositol, sterols, protease inhibitors, resistant starch that produce short-chain fatty acids (SCFA)
Flaxseed	Fiber, magnesium, manganese, thiamin, selenium, lignans, alpha-linolenic acid (ALA), gamma-tocopherol: a form of vitamin E
Garlic	Allicin, S-allyl cysteine, flavonoids (kaempferol and quercetin), inulin, saponins
Grapefruit	Vitamin C, naringenin, limonin, beta-carotene, lycopene
Grapes	Resveratrol
Soy	Isoflavones (genistein, daidzein and glycitein), saponins, phenolic acids, phytic acid, sphingolipids
Squash	Fiber, vitamins A and C, potassium, beta-carotene and alpha-carotene, lutein, zeaxanthin
Tea	Theophylline and theobromine, catechins (epigallocatechin gallate [EGCG], epicatechin, epigallocatechin [EGC], epicatechin-3-gallate [ECG], thearubigins and theaflavins (black tea), theasinensins (oolong tea), flavonols quercetin, kaempferol and myricetin, L-theanine
Tomatoes	Vitamins A and C, potassium, lycopene, phytoene and phytofluene
Walnuts	Ellagitannins, gamma-tocopherol, ALA, polyphenols including (flavonoids and phenolic acids), phytosterols, melatonin
Whole Grains	Fiber, polyphenols (phenolic acids and flavonoids), lignans, saponins alkylresorcinols, phytic acid, protease inhibitors, tocotrienols

American Institute for Cancer Research: *Foods that fight cancer,* 2018c. http://www.aicr.org/foods-that-fight-cancer/

Fruits and Vegetables

Fruit intake is protective against cancers of the esophagus, lung, and stomach (WCRF/AICR, 2018). Nonstarchy vegetables, such as spinach, tomatoes, and peppers, probably provide protection against mouth, pharynx, larynx, esophageal, lung, and breast cancers. All vegetables, but particularly green and yellow ones, probably protect against stomach cancer (WCRF/AICR, 2018). The Dietary Guidelines for Americans suggests 2 cups per day of fruit and 2 ½ cups per day of vegetables including dark green and red and orange colored varieties (Dietary Guidelines for Americans, 2018).

Anticarcinogenic agents found in fruits and vegetables include antioxidants such as vitamins C and E, selenium, and phytochemicals. Phytochemicals include carotenoids, flavonoids, isoflavones, lignans, organosulfides, phenolic compounds, and monoterpenes. It is still unclear which specific substances of fruits and vegetables are the most protective against cancer (Kushi et al, 2012). It appears extremely unlikely that any one substance is responsible for all the observed associations. See Table 35.1 for a discussion of chemoprotective agents in fruits and vegetables.

Soy and Phytoestrogens

Soy is a plant-based protein that contains isoflavones such as genistein and daidzein, plant based estrogens (phystoestrogens). Diets containing modest amounts of soy protect against breast cancer (ACS, 2019a), especially if the soy foods have been consumed early in life (ACS, 2019a). Confusion regarding soy abounds because soy isoflavones have been shown to promote in vitro growth of breast cancer cells and mammary tumor growth in rodent models, creating some concern about the potential adverse effect of soy consumption on prognosis in women who have been diagnosed with breast cancer. Soy is metabolized differently in humans and recent large epidemiologic studies have found no adverse effects of soy food intake on breast cancer recurrence or total mortality, alone or in combination with tamoxifen. The ACS and other researchers state that there is the potential for these foods to exert a beneficial synergistic effect with tamoxifen (ACS, 2019a; Rock et al, 2012).

Commercially prepared soy supplement powders and foods made from soy products can but may not always contain isoflavones at much higher concentrations than traditional whole soy foods such as edamame beans, tofu, tempeh, miso, or soy milk (U.S. Department of Agriculture [USDA], 2016). According to the ACS current evidence does not support that consuming soy foods will have an adverse effect on recurrence or survival of breast cancer patients. (Rock et al, 2012). Men with hormone-sensitive cancer such as prostate cancer may also benefit from regular consumption of soy foods. Prostate cancer is a testosterone-driven cancer and phytoestrogens are antagonists. Tofu and other soy foods are also linked to lower rates of heart disease and may help to lower cholesterol (ACS, 2019a).

Vegetarian and Vegan Plant-Based Diets

Plant foods may aid in cancer prevention by functioning as cancer inhibitors through antiinflammatory mechanisms and changes in gene expression and hormone activity (Bender et al, 2013). Diets primarily composed of plant foods including vegetarian and vegan dietary patterns may provide anticancer properties. Results from the Adventists Health Study 2 found an association between vegetarian diets and lower overall cancer risk, especially a lower risk of GI cancer (Melina et al, 2016). In fact, a vegan diet appeared to protect against cancer more than any other dietary pattern (Melina et al, 2016). Fruits, vegetables, and whole grains contain biologically active phytochemicals,

---

BOX 35.4 **Nutrigenomics: The Future of Personalized Cancer Prevention?**

Nutrigenomics, is the interaction between nutrients and the genome as they impact host health and disease risk. Because the progression of cancer is enhanced by the genetic instability of cells due to defective DNA repair processes, damage to the genome and what could be done to prevent it is an area of interest for further study. It is known that nutrients and other environmental factors interact with the genome and could either further DNA damage or perhaps help prevent it. Human nutrigenomic and cancer research is an area of exciting possibility as nutrition professionals position themselves as experts in the field and are involved in discussing genetic concepts with patients (Sharma and Dwivedi, 2017; Camp and Trujillo, 2014; Spees and Grainger, 2013).

vitamins, minerals, and dietary fiber that have demonstrated functions in preventing and treating disease. In fact, vegetarian and vegans are at reduced risk of ischemic heart disease, type 2 diabetes, hypertension, and obesity (Melina et al, 2016). Vegetarians typically consume higher levels of fiber compared with other diets which may target a reduction in colorectal cancer risk (Melina et al, 2016). In addition, the ACS Prevention Guidelines suggest that individuals who eat more vegetables and fruits further benefit by experiencing less weight gain and greater satiety and are at a lower risk of developing obesity, thereby reducing overall cancer risk (Kushi et al, 2012).

Physical Activity

Physical activity is an important part of cancer prevention, treatment, and survival. Studies clearly show that increasing physical activity reduces cancer risk. Engaging in moderate to vigorous levels of activity reduces the risk of developing breast, colon, and endometrial cancers as well as advanced prostate cancer and pancreatic cancer (Kushi et al, 2012). Physical activity helps regain and maintain muscle; regain strength, energy, and flexibility; and relieve symptoms of stress, anxiety, and even depression. Physical activity may reduce risk of cancer by strengthening the immune system and regulating sex hormones, insulin, and prostaglandins (Kushi et al, 2012) Evidence reflects that exercising during and after treatment is safe and even associated with improved quality of life and positive outcomes due to reduced risk of other chronic diseases including heart disease, diabetes, osteoporosis, and hypertension (Kushi et al, 2012). Research is particularly strong for breast and colorectal cancer survivors undergoing treatment. With medical clearance for safety, cancer survivors in all phases of the cancer-care spectrum should be as physically active as possible (Marian, 2013) (see Table 35.2 and Box 35.4).

MEDICAL DIAGNOSIS AND STAGING OF CANCER

Despite the progress made in understanding possible prevention strategies, cancer remains a significant health threat. Assessing symptoms of cancer at the earliest stage is critical for treatment effectiveness and survival. Many symptoms of early or metastatic cancer affect an individual's ability to eat, digest, or absorb. According to the ACS, the following early warning signs and symptoms of cancer are described using the acronym CAUTION:

Change in bowel or bladder habits
A sore that does not heal
Unusual bleeding or discharge
Thickening or lump in breast or elsewhere
Indigestion or difficulty in swallowing or chewing

TABLE 35.4	Imaging Studies for Cancer Diagnosis and Disease Monitoring
Type of Imaging	**Description and Use in Cancer Diagnosis and Treatment**
Computed tomography (CT) scan	**Description:** A CT scan is a radiographic procedure in which a series of detailed pictures of areas inside the body are taken from different angles. Images are created by a computer and are linked to an x-ray machine. **Use:** A CT scan is used to evaluate for abnormalities of possible cancer in a general anatomic area such as the head, chest, abdomen, or pelvis. Radiologists use CT scans to visualize suspicious lesions, internal organs, and lymph nodes.
Magnetic resonance imaging (MRI) scan	**Description:** An MRI scan is an imaging procedure that uses radio waves and a powerful magnet linked to a computer to create detailed pictures of areas inside the body. This type of scanning often creates better images of body organs and soft tissue than other type of scanning methods. **Use:** Images produced show differences between normal and cancerous tissue. An MRI scan is commonly used to evaluate suspicious areas of the brain, spinal cord, and liver.
Positron emission tomography (PET) scan	**Description:** A PET scan is a procedure in which a small amount of radioactive glucose is injected into a vein and a scanner is used to make detailed, computerized pictures of areas where glucose is used in the body. **Use:** Cancerous cells have an enhanced rate of glycolysis, using more glucose than normal cells. Areas of glucose metabolism with high activity or "hot spots" appearing on the PET scan generally correlate to findings of cancer.

Data from American Cancer Society (ACS): *Cancer Glossary* (website). http://www.cancer.org/cancer/cancerglossary/index; National Institutes of Health (NIH), National Cancer Institute (NCI): *NCI Dictionary of Cancer Terms.* http://www.cancer.gov/publications/dictionaries/cancer-terms?expand.

Obvious change in a wart or mole

Nagging cough or hoarseness

When symptoms or screening tests suggest cancer, physicians use the following to establish a definitive diagnosis: evaluation of an individual's medical, social, and family histories; physical examination; laboratory tests; imaging procedures; and tissue biopsy. Laboratory evaluation is composed of analysis of blood, urine, and other body fluids. Oncologists evaluate tumor markers (e.g., α-fetoprotein [AFP], cancer antigen [CA] 125, CA 19-9, carcinoembryonic antigen [CEA], prostate-specific antigen [PSA]) and other substances in blood or body fluids that can be elevated when someone has cancer. Imaging procedures help determine a diagnosis (Table 35.4). Pathologists perform cytologic examinations by analyzing body fluids, sputum, urine, or tissue under a microscope. To detect malignant cells, they use a histopathologic examination to review specially stained tissue flow cytometry to count and examine cells and chromosomes, immunohistochemistry to review antibodies for specific cell proteins, and cytogenetics to visualize genetic defects.

Staging is used to identify how much a cancer has spread throughout the body. The stage of the cancer at the time of diagnosis is a strong predictor of survival, and it directs oncologists to the most effective treatment plan. Cancer staging is most frequently described as stage I, II, III, or IV—stage I being the least amount of disease and stage IV being the most advanced. The tumor-node-metastasis (TNM) staging system is also commonly used by oncologists. *T* stands for the size of the tumor, *N* stands for nodes or whether it has spread into lymph nodes, and *M* stands for metastasis, or whether the cancer has spread to distant organs (Fig. 35.3) (American Joint Committee on Cancer, 2018).

Classification and Common Types of Cancer

For classification, solid cancers are often referred to as tumors and hematologic-related cancers are frequently called blood cancers. The classification of tumors is based on their tissue of origin, their growth properties, and their invasion of other tissues. Tumors that are not malignant typically are described as benign.

Because cancer occurs in cells that are replicating, patterns are different in children and adults. In early life the brain, nervous system, bones, muscles, and connective tissues are still growing; therefore, cancers involving these tissues are more prevalent in children. Common childhood cancers include neuroblastoma; medulloblastoma; osteosarcoma; and soft tissue sarcomas such as rhabdomyosarcoma,

schwannoma, and germ cell tumors. Conversely, adult cancers frequently involve epithelial tissues that cover and line the body's internal and external surfaces. Cancers of the epithelial tissues include cancers of the skin, and circulatory, digestive, endocrine, reproductive, respiratory, and urinary systems. Cancers arising from these tissues are referred to as carcinomas, and common types are classified as adenocarcinomas, basal cell carcinomas, papillomas, and squamous cell carcinomas.

Leukemias, lymphomas, and myelomas are cancers of the immune system and can occur in children or adults. Leukemias arise most frequently from white blood cells of the bone marrow. Lymphomas are cancers that develop in the lymphatic system—in nodes, glands, and organs. Myeloma is cancer that originates in the plasma cells of the bone marrow and most frequently occurs in older adults. These cancers are diagnosed using blood tests and bone marrow biopsies.

Other types of cancer are related to infectious causes and cancer experts recommend antibiotics, vaccines, and changes in behavior for their prevention (ACS, 2018a). Examples include hepatocellular carcinoma linked to hepatitis B virus (HBV) exposure and alcoholic-related cirrhosis leading to liver cancer, oropharyngeal and cervical cancers linked to human papillomavirus infection (HPV), and stomach cancer caused by chronic inflammation by *Helicobacter pylori* (see Chapter 26).

MEDICAL TREATMENT

In the United States and many other countries around the world, cancer treatment is guided by oncologists, medical doctors specializing in the prevention, treatment, and palliation of cancer, and by evidence-based standards known as the National Comprehensive Cancer Network (NCCN) Clinical Practice Guidelines in Oncology (NCCN, 2018). The NCCN Guidelines encompass evidence-based care for 97% of all cancers treated in oncology practice. Also listed with these guidelines are evidence-based recommendations for providing supportive care (e.g., survivorship, palliative care, cancer-related pain, fatigue, and antiemesis).

Conventional modalities include antineoplastic therapy (e.g., chemotherapy, biotherapy, or hormonal therapy), radiation therapy, and surgery used alone or in combination with other cancer therapies. Solid tumors and hematologic malignant diseases such as leukemias, lymphomas, and multiple myelomas may be treated with hematopoietic cell transplantation (HCT).

THE STAGING OF CANCER

In the Tumor-Node-Metastasis (TNM) system:

- The T refers to the size and extent of the main tumor. The main tumor is usually called the primary tumor.
- The N refers to the number of nearby lymph nodes that have cancer.
- The M refers to whether the cancer has metastasized. This means that the cancer has spread from the primary tumor to other parts of the body.

Primary tumor (T)

- TX: Main tumor cannot be measured.
- T0: Main tumor cannot be found.
- T1, T2, T3, T4: Refers to the size and/or extent of the main tumor. The higher the number after the T, the larger the tumor or the more it has grown into nearby tissues. T's may be further divided to provide more detail, such as T3a and T3b.

Regional lymph nodes (N)

- NX: Cancer in nearby lymph nodes cannot be measured.
- N0: There is no cancer in nearby lymph nodes.
- N1, N2, N3: Refers to the number and location of lymph nodes that contain cancer. The higher the number after the N, the more lymph nodes that contain cancer.

Distant metastasis (M)

- MX: Metastasis cannot be measured.
- M0: Cancer has not spread to other parts of the body.
- M1: Cancer has spread to other parts of the body.

Stage	What it means
Stage 0	Abnormal cells are present but have not spread to nearby tissue. Also called carcinoma in situ, or CIS. CIS is not cancer, but it may become cancer.
Stage I, Stage II, and Stage III	Cancer is present. The higher the number, the larger the cancer tumor and the more it has spread into nearby tissues.
Stage IV	The cancer has spread to distant parts of the body.

Fig. 35.3 The tumor-node-metastasis (TNM) system of grading cancer tumors and the staging of cancer. Adapted from the National Cancer Institute (website). https://www.cancer.gov/about-cancer/diagnosis-staging/staging.

Chemotherapy is the use of chemical agents or medications to systematically treat cancer. These agents interfere with the steps or phases of the cell cycle, specifically with the synthesis of DNA and replication of cancer cells. Treatment regimens often involve the use of more than one type of chemotherapy to maximally interrupt the cancer cell growth cycle. The basic five phases of cell reproduction in normal and malignant cells are the following (Polovich et al, 2014):

- G0—resting phase
- G1—postmitotic phase; ribonucleic acid (RNA) and protein are synthesized
- S—DNA is synthesized
- G2—premeiotic phase; the second phase where RNA and protein are synthesized
- M—mitosis; cell division

Most chemotherapy agents are categorized by their biochemical activity and their mechanism of action such as alkylating agents (cell-cycle nonspecific), antimetabolites (cell-cycle specific, usually S-phase), and taxanes (M-phase specific). **Biotherapy** is the use of biologic agents to produce anticancer effects indirectly by inducing, enhancing, or suppressing an individual's own immune response. **Antiangiogenic agents** are used to inhibit the development of new blood vessels needed by cancers (tumor vasculature) and thus prevent their growth, invasion, and spread. **Hormonal therapy** is systemic therapy used for the treatment of hormone-sensitive cancers (e.g., breast, ovarian, prostate) by blocking or reducing the source of a hormone or its receptor site.

Radiation oncologists use **radiation therapy**, high-energy (ionizing radiation) in multiple fractionated doses, or radioactive chemicals to treat cancer. Cancerous tissue can also be removed using surgery.

Response to cancer treatment is defined as complete or partial response, stable disease, or disease progression. Factors that affect an individual's response to treatment include tumor burden because the larger the tumor the greater risk of metastatic disease, rate of tumor growth because rapidly growing tumors are usually more responsive to therapy, and drug resistance. Tumors mutate as they grow, and with successive mutations new cancer cells can become resistant to therapy. Other factors contributing to an individual's response to cancer treatment include comorbid diseases (e.g., diabetes, renal disease, cardiopulmonary disease), age, performance status, psychosocial support systems, bone marrow reserve, and overall general health (NIH and NCI, 2018c; Polovich et al, 2014).

Goals of Treatment

The goal of cancer treatment may be to cure, control, or palliate (remove symptoms without curing). A cure is a complete response to treatment. Even when treatment does not cure the cancer, it can diminish its effects and extend life. Cancer treatment can last for years, even decades. When the treatment is no longer working or the side effects cause a patient to reject further treatment, palliative care is offered. Palliative care helps individuals be as comfortable as possible and promotes quality of life. Palliation is designed to relieve pain and manage symptoms of illness; lessen isolation, anxiety, and fear; and help maintain independence as long as possible (National Hospice and Palliative Care Organization [NHPCO], 2018). Hospice is care for individuals with a life expectancy of 6 months or less. It focuses on relieving symptoms, controlling pain, and providing emotional and spiritual support to patients and their families. Patients are made as comfortable as possible through the end of their lives.

Cultural Considerations

Cultural competency in health care providers is a critical piece of cancer treatment. Aside from existing racial and health disparities in racial and ethnic minority populations in the United States regarding screening, diagnosis, and treatment of cancer, there is some evidence that interventions to improve cultural competency can improve patient/client health outcomes (Truong et al, 2014). Cultural and linguistic barriers can negatively affect health care delivery. Treatment preferences, end-of-life values, health literacy, and dietary patterns should all be assessed when working with a diverse population in cancer care (see Chapter 10).

MEDICAL NUTRITION THERAPY

Medical nutrition therapy (MNT) improves treatment tolerance, reduces the need for breaks in treatment, decreases unintentional weight and lean body mass loss, and can improve quality of life. Nutrition therapy has been shown to decrease unplanned hospitalizations by >50%, reduce length of hospital stays, and improve overall survival for patients undergoing cancer treatment (Trujillo et al, 2018). The Commission on Dietetic Registration has developed a board certification in oncology nutrition: certified specialist in oncology nutrition (CSO). To further assist clinicians working in the cancer care setting, the AND has developed the Oncology Toolkit with MNT protocols for breast, colorectal, esophageal, gastric, head and neck, hematologic, lung, and pancreatic cancers (AND, 2010). Another AND resource for clinicians when providing MNT in the cancer care setting is the Pocket Guide to the Nutrition Care Process in Cancer (Grant, 2015).

Nutrition Screening and Assessment
Validated Screening Tools
With the continued shift of cancer care from the hospital setting to outpatient settings, nutrition screening and assessment should continue throughout the continuum of care. Ideally, nutrition screening and assessment for risk of nutrition problems should be interdisciplinary, instituted at the time of diagnosis, and reevaluated and monitored throughout treatment and recovery. See Chapter 4 for screening tools validated for use with individuals diagnosed with cancer (AND Evidence Analysis Library [EAL], 2013) including the Patient Generated-Subjective Global Assessment (PG-SGA) for inpatient and outpatient settings, Malnutrition Screening Tool (MST) for inpatient and outpatient settings, and Malnutrition Universal Screening Tool (MUST) for inpatient and outpatient settings. (AND EAL, 2013; PG-SGA©, 2014).

Other assessment tools specific to patients with cancer are the Activities of Daily Living (ADLs) Tool, the Common Toxicity Criteria for Adverse Events (CTCAE), and the Karnofsky Performance Scale (KPS) Index. CTCAE is an outcome measure used in anticancer therapy that compares acute toxicities of cancer treatment, and KPS is a scoring index that associates an individual's functional status with disease status and survival (Polovich et al, 2014).

In-depth assessment including a nutrition-focused physical examination is used to obtain more information and to identify nutrition problems and assess degree of risk (see Chapter 5 and Appendix 11). Careful review of the individual's appetite and oral intake is required, with an assessment of symptoms (e.g., nausea, vomiting, and diarrhea), weight status, comorbidities, and laboratory studies. Components of this type of assessment include a general survey of the body, review of vital organs and anthropometrics, and an evaluation of the subcutaneous fat stores, muscle mass, and fluid status (see Chapter 5).

General Assessment

When working with patients in active treatment for cancer, it is important to first assess where each patient is in their journey without assumption or bias. For example, during treatment, some people have a range of classic side effects including pain, nausea, and vomiting while others experience few if any of these. As treatment options expand and improve, patients are thriving during treatment and are often able to carry on with their normal life activities. Recommendations should be prioritized with input from the patient. Whether the focus is on food safety due to neutropenia (reduced white blood cells), hydration status, undesired weight loss or gain, individual nutrient needs, or emotional well-being, patient safety is the first concern for a dietetic practitioner. Use critical assessment to treat each patient as an individual, meeting their unique needs that prioritize challenges in each stage of treatment.

Patients have highly variable side effects with cancer treatment that can effect their energy level, mood, and tolerance of foods. Each patient should be approached in an individualized manner based on their unique needs and treatment plan.

During nutrition screening, assess factors that may affect intake and well-being. Discuss gastrointestinal function with each patient to assess for diarrhea, constipation or other factors related to digestion and absorption of nutrients. Inquire about energy levels, sleep, and fatigue, considering how this may affect food acquisition or preparation. Cancer treatment can be highly stressful and potentially traumatic for patients. Cancer-related posttraumatic stress disorder (PTSD) has been documented in patients and family members. Studies show that cancer-related fatigue, sleep disturbances, stressful life events, and psychological distress do contribute to higher levels of breast cancer-mortality (Haller et al, 2017). As part of the medical team, the dietitian can help advocate for psychological support and counseling for the patient (Chasen and Dippenaar, 2008; Cordova et al, 2017) (Box 35.5).

Energy

Determining individualized energy needs is vital to helping people maintain energy balance during treatment and prevent unintentional weight gain or loss. Not every person who undergoes cancer treatment will lose weight. In fact, some may gain, so energy adjustments should be made to support a healthy weight depending on the unique needs of each individual. Methods used to estimate energy requirements for adults include using standardized equations or measuring resting metabolic rate using indirect calorimetry (Hamilton, 2013; see Chapter 2 for methods for determining energy requirements). To ensure that adequate energy is being provided, the individual's diagnosis, presence of other diseases, intent of treatment (e.g., curative, control, or palliation), therapies (e.g., surgery, chemotherapy, biotherapy, or radiation therapy), presence of fever or infection, and other metabolic complications such as refeeding syndrome must be considered. Evidence-based guidelines from the American Society for Parenteral and Enteral Nutrition (ASPEN) for quickly estimating energy and fluid needs of people with cancer based on body weight are shown in Table 35.5.

Protein

An individual's need for protein is increased during times of illness and stress. Additional protein is required by the body to repair and rebuild tissues affected by cancer treatments and to maintain a healthy immune system (Hamilton, 2013). Adequate energy should be provided as a fuel source and to prevent lean tissue loss. The degree of malnutrition, extent of disease, degree of stress, and ability to metabolize and use protein are factors in determining protein requirements (Hamilton, 2013). For example, though the dietary reference intake (DRI) for protein for healthy individuals is 0.8 g/kg/day, protein needs for a catabolic patient may be 1.2 to 2.0 g/kg/day or more, and protein needs for an individual undergoing a hematopoietic cell transplant are estimated at 1.5 g/kg/day. Daily protein requirements generally are calculated using actual body weight rather than ideal body weight unless the patient is obese and not at risk for malnutrition during treatment. If appropriate based on individualized assessment, adjusted body weight may be used (see Table 35.5).

Fluid

Dietitians managing cancer patients must ensure adequate hydration and electrolyte balance to prevent dehydration and hypovolemia. Altered fluid balance may occur with fever, ascites, edema, fistulas, profuse vomiting or diarrhea, multiple concurrent intravenous (IV) therapies, impaired renal function, or medications such as diuretics. Individuals need close monitoring for dehydration (e.g., intracellular fluid losses caused by inadequate intake of fluid because of mucositis or anorexia), hypovolemia (e.g., extracellular fluid losses from fever or GI fluids such as vomiting, diarrhea, or malabsorption), and nephrotoxic effects from anticancer treatments.

Signs and symptoms of dehydration include fatigue, acute weight loss, hypernatremia, poor skin turgor, dry oral mucosa, dark or strong-smelling urine, and decreased urine output. To carefully assess for hypovolemia, levels of serum electrolytes, blood urea nitrogen, and creatinine also should be evaluated. A general guideline for estimating fluid needs for all adults without renal concerns is 20 to 40 mL/kg though some patients may experience increased needs (30 to 40 mL/kg) due to chemotherapy (Hamilton, 2013). Other methods including mL per kcal and using Body Surface Area (BSA) are listed in Table 35.5. IV hydration may be recommended for individuals struggling to achieve adequate hydration, but infusion frequency and volume must be determined on an individual basis, considering fluid intake and output (see Table 35.5).

Micronutrients

For patients undergoing cancer treatment, micronutrient status may be affected by the severity of illness, type of treatment, location type of tumor, and ability to consume a normal diet. If individuals are experiencing difficulty with eating and treatment-related side effects, a standard multivitamin and mineral supplement that provides no more than 100% of the DRIs is considered safe (Rock et al, 2012). People who are ill can experience deficiencies in zinc, iron, selenium, and vitamins A, B, and C. Inflammation can increase demands for selenium, copper, iron, and zinc (Hamilton, 2013).

To date, vitamin and mineral supplements have not proven effective for cancer prevention. The AICR encourages all people including cancer survivors not to use dietary supplements for cancer prevention because evidence is insufficient to assess the potential benefits versus harm of doing so (WCRF/AICR, 2018). There are some emerging exceptions. In the most recent WCRF/AICR report, calcium supplements showed a probable decreased risk for colorectal cancer (WCRF/AICR, 2018). In the Physicians Health Study II, a daily multivitamin modestly but significantly reduced risk of total cancer in male physicians (Gaziano et al, 2012). Purified eicosapentaenoic acid (EPA)/docosahexaenoic acid (DHA) omega-3 supplements up to 2 grams/day

TABLE 35.5 Estimating Energy and Fluid Needs of People with Cancer

Condition	Energy Needs	Protein Needs
Cancer, nutritional repletion, weight gain	30-35 kcal/kg/day	1.0-1.5 g/kg/day
Cancer, inactive, nonstressed	25-30 kcal/kg/day	0.8-1.0 g/kg/day
Cancer, hypermetabolic, stressed	35 kcal/kg/day	1.5-2.5 g/kg/day
Hematopoietic cell transplant	30-35 kcal/kg/day	1.5 g/kg/day
Sepsis	25-30 kcal/kg/day	1.5-2.0 g/kg/day

Fluid needs:

Typical fluid requirements for adults 20 to 40 mL/kg/day or 1 to 1.5 mL/kcal energy expended

RDA Method: 1 mL per 1 kcal consumed

Body Surface Area (BSA) Method: 1500 mL/m2 or BSA x 1500 mL

Data from Gottschlich MM, editor: *The A.S.P.E.N. nutrition support core curriculum: a case-based approach—the adult patient,* Silver Spring, Md, 2007, American Society for Parenteral and Enteral Nutrition; Hamilton KK: Nutrition needs of the adult oncology patient. In Leser M et al, editors: *Oncology nutrition for clinical practice,* Chicago, 2013, Oncology Nutrition Dietetic Practice Group of the Academy of Nutrition and Dietetics.

have shown antitumor activity and reduced neuropathy in patients treated for neuropathy (Vernieri et al, 2018).

In some instances, during and after a cancer diagnosis, supplementation or restriction of specific micronutrients may be required above or below DRI levels, depending on medical diagnosis and laboratory analysis (e.g., iron supplementation for iron-deficiency anemia, B_{12} injections, and folic acid supplementation during treatment with the chemotherapy agent pemetrexed ([Alimta]). There is evidence that some supplements may be harmful before or during treatment. Food sources of antioxidants are safe, but some supplemental forms of antioxidants have proven ill effects. For example, high-dose beta-carotene supplements in people who smoke have been shown to increase the risk of lung cancer while dietary derived beta-carotene has been shown to decrease lung cancer risk (WCRF/AICR, 2018). Curcumin, a phytochemical in turmeric, provides some proven anti-inflammatory and anti-cancer benefits and is generally well tolerated in supplement forms. Patients treated with irinotecan or cyclophosphamide should avoid taking curcumin until more data can clear potential antagonistic interactions shown in a laboratory setting. Although drinking green tea is safe, studies on green tea extracts are mixed and carry the risk of potential liver damage at very high doses. Vitamin C can cause GI distress and is still under investigation for efficacy and potential for reducing chemotherapy cytotoxicity (Vernieri et al, 2018). Until more research is available, best practices are for patients to focus on food sources of nutrients and antioxidants.

Nutrition Diagnosis

Nutrition diagnosis identifies the specific nutrition problems that can be resolved or improved through nutrition intervention (AND, 2018; Box 35.6).

Nutrition Intervention

The Oncology Toolkit (https://www.eatright.org) includes the recommendation for careful appraisal if the planned nutrition intervention will negatively affect patient safety or possibly interfere with the cancer treatment (AND, 2010). The Toolkit also advises evaluation of the nutrition intervention's likely effectiveness for improving nutrition status, possible financial burden, and patient acceptance.

Intervention goals should be specific, achievable, and individualized to maximize benefit. Goals must be directed toward an objective measure such as body weight or some other meaningful index. Another goal is to minimize the effects of nutrition impact symptoms and to maximize the individual's nutritional parameters. Nutrition impact symptoms can be defined as symptoms and side effects of cancer and cancer treatment that directly affect the nutrition status resulting in a depletion of nutrient stores and deterioration in nutrition status. Consultation with the individual, caregivers, or family members regarding expected problems and their possible solutions should be initiated early in the course of cancer therapy and should continue in conjunction with follow-up nutrition assessment and care. Malnutrition, anorexia (loss of appetite), and weight loss are significant issues in cancer care and are often present in many individuals at the time of diagnosis, even in children.

The incidence of malnutrition among individuals with cancer has been estimated to be between 15% and 80% depending on the type of cancer and intensity of treatment (Santarpia et al, 2011). Studies consistently show that even small amounts of weight loss (less than 5% of body weight) before treatment is associated with a poorer prognosis and decreased quality of life, thus reinforcing the importance of early MNT (Arends et al, 2017).

Oral Nutrition Management Strategies

Oral feeding is the goal though individuals often experience symptoms that make it difficult. The causes of impaired oral intake are multifactorial and include oral ulceration, xerostomia (dryness of the mouth from decreased saliva), poor dentition, intestinal obstruction, malabsorption, constipation, diarrhea, nausea, vomiting, reduced intestinal motility, chemosensory alteration, uncontrolled pain, and medication side effects (Arends et al, 2017). Strategies for

---

BOX 35.6 Common Nutrition Diagnoses for Patients with Cancer Using the Problem, Etiology, and Signs and Symptoms Format

Intake Domain

- Inadequate protein-energy intake related to decreased ability to consume sufficient protein and/or energy as evidenced by >5% weight loss in 1 month, estimated energy intake from diet less than estimated, and conditions associated with a diagnosis (colon cancer).
- Excessive energy intake related to food- and nutrition-related knowledge deficit concerning energy intake as evidenced by body mass index (BMI) of 37, intake of energy in excess of estimated energy needs, and reports of higher consumption of nutritional supplements than recommended.
- Inadequate oral intake related to conditions associated with head and neck cancer treatment as evidenced by 5% weight loss in past week, decreased appetite, estimates of insufficient intake of energy and high-quality protein from diet compared with requirements.

Clinical Domain

- Swallowing difficulty related to mechanical causes (tongue cancer) as evidenced by decreased estimated food intake, avoidance of foods, and pain while swallowing.
- Biting/chewing (masticatory) difficulty related to xerostomia after chemotherapy as evidenced by dry mouth, and eating ~30% of meals.

- Altered gastrointestinal (GI) function related to side effect from chemotherapy as evidenced by patient reports of cramping, pain, and diarrhea.
- Malnutrition (undernutrition) related to alteration in GI tract function as evidenced by evidence of temporomandibular wasting, and intake <50% of estimated energy requirement.

Behavioral-Environmental Domain

- Food- and nutrition-related knowledge deficit related to new breast cancer diagnosis and lack or prior dietary education as evidenced by pt report and multiple questions about foods to eat or avoid during chemotherapy.
- Inability to manage self-care related to lack of permanent housing and financial stress as evidenced by skipping one or more meals each day while under treatment for cancer.
- Limited access to food related to lack of financial resources to purchase a sufficient quantity of appropriate healthful foods as evidenced by BMI <18.5, estimated inadequate intake of energy, and patient reports of lack of resources for food.

Academy of Nutrition and Dietetics. Nutrition Terminology Reference Manual (eNCPT): Dietetics Language for Nutrition Care, 2019.

modifying dietary intake may be necessary and depend on the specific eating problem and the individual's nutritional status. Food choices, preparation, and presentation may need modification. Liquid medical food supplements may be recommended for those unable to consume enough energy and protein to maintain weight and nutrition status (see Chapter 13). Education materials with suggestions for improving oral intake and managing treatment-related side effects are at the end of the chapter and include Eating Hints,

Chemotherapy and You, and Radiation Therapy and You (NIH and NCI, 2011, 2018a, 2016a). Table 35.6 outlines examples of nutrition intervention strategies.

Managing Anorexia and Alterations in Taste and Smell

Sometimes even before diagnosis, and throughout cancer treatment, individuals may report anorexia, early satiety, and decreased food intake. Alterations in taste and smell are common problems. Taste

---

TABLE 35.6 Nutrition Intervention Strategies for Patients with Cancer

Side Effect or Symptom	Strategies
Anorexia, poor appetite	• Encourage small, more frequent nutrient-dense meals and snacks. • Add protein and fats to favorite foods. • Use protein and calorie-containing supplements (e.g., whey or soy powder, nutritional supplements). • Keep nutrient-dense foods close at hand and snack frequently. • Maximize intake at times when feeling best. • Eat meals and snacks in a pleasant atmosphere. • View eating as part of treatment. • Have high protein and calorie liquid supplements and smoothies • Eat by the clock instead of waiting for hunger cues (set a timer). • Consume liquids between meals rather than with meals. • Engage in light physical activity as able.
Nausea and vomiting	• Eat small, more frequent meals and snacks. • Sip on cool or room temperature clear liquids in small amounts. • Avoid high-fat, greasy, spicy, or overly sweet foods. • Avoid foods with strong odors such as fish or eggs. • Consume bland, soft, easy-to-digest foods on scheduled treatment days. • Encourage compliance with medications that are prescribed to control nausea. • Rest with head elevated for 30 minutes after eating. • Consider complementary therapies including ginger tea, relaxation techniques, or acupressure bracelets.
Diarrhea	• Encourage the intake of hydrating liquids such as water, clear juices, broth, gelatin, popsicles, and commercially prepared hydration fluids (see Chapter 27). • Avoid high-fiber foods, such as nuts, raw fruits and vegetables, and whole-grain breads and cereals and avoidance of dairy foods is sometimes helpful. • Avoid sugar alcohol–containing foods such as sugar-free candies and gums (e.g., mannitol, xylitol, sorbitol). • Choose high-soluble fiber such as applesauce, bananas, canned peaches, and oatmeal. • Encourage compliance with medications prescribed to control diarrhea.
Constipation	• Increase the intake of high-fiber foods such as whole grains, fresh or cooked fruits and vegetables, especially those with skins and seeds, dried fruits, beans, and nuts. • Consume at least 64 ounces of fluid each day. • Use probiotic-containing foods or supplements. • Include activities of daily living and physical activity as able. • Encourage compliance with fiber supplements and/or medications that affect bowel function and are prescribed to manage constipation. • Schedule adequate bathroom time to facilitate bowel movements without psychological stress and pressure.
Sore throat, esophagitis Sore mouth, mucositis, or thrush	• Recommend the intake of soft, moist foods with extra sauce, dressing or gravy. • Avoid dry, coarse, or rough foods. • Avoid alcohol, citrus, caffeine, tomatoes, vinegar, and hot peppers or other spicy food. • Experiment with food temperatures (e.g., warm, cool, or icy) to find which temperatures are most soothing. • Prepare smoothies with low acid fruits like melon, banana, peaches and add yogurt, milk, or silken tofu. • Encourage compliance with medications prescribed to manage esophagitis, painful swallowing, oral pain, and/or infection.
Fatigue	• Recommend the intake of small, frequent meals and snacks. • Choose easy-to-prepare, easy-to-eat foods. • Advise keeping nutrient-dense snacks close at hand and snack frequently. • Suggest eating when appetite is best. • Encourage activities of daily living and physical activity as able. • Consider physical therapy consult for strengthening.

Continued

TABLE 35.6 Nutrition Intervention Strategies for Patients with Cancer—cont'd

Side Effect or Symptom	Strategies
Neutropenia	• Advise frequent hand washing and keep kitchen surfaces and utensils clean. • Advise the avoidance of raw or undercooked animal products, including meat, pork, game, poultry, eggs, and fish. • Wash all fresh fruits and vegetables well before eating. • Ensure proper temperatures for cooking, cooling and reheating. • Check expirations dates on all foods. • Avoid bulk bins, salad bars and buffets. • Prevent cross contamination between raw meat and ready to eat foods. • "When in doubt, throw out" and "No oldy or moldy."
Altered taste or smell	• Recommend good oral hygiene practices (e.g., rinse mouth frequently, keep mouth clean). • Use marinades and spices to mask altered tastes. • Use plastic utensils if metallic tastes are a problem. • Eat cooler foods, rather than warmer foods. • Flavor water with lemon or other fruit or herbs. • Choose nonmeat protein sources such as tofu, dairy, or beans.
Thickened saliva/or dry mouth (xerostomia)	• Suggest sipping on liquids throughout the day to keep the oral cavity moist. Aim for 8-10 cups per day. • Thin oral secretions with club soda or seltzer water. • Chew on carrots or celery. • Suck on frozen grapes or melon balls. • Recommend using a cool mist humidifier while sleeping. • Suggest trying tart foods to stimulate saliva, if open sores are not present. • Recommend alternating bites of food with sips of liquids at meals. • Recommend eating soft, moist foods with extra sauces, dressings, or gravies. • Advise avoidance of alcoholic beverages and alcohol-containing mouthwash as these will dry the mouth.

Data from Grant BL et al, editors: *American Cancer Society's complete guide to nutrition for cancer survivors*, ed 2, Atlanta, 2010, American Cancer Society; National Cancer Institute (NCI): *Eating Hints* (website). http://www.cancer.gov/publications/patient-education/eatinghints.pdf, 2018; Elliot L: Symptom management of cancer therapies. In Leser M et al, editors: *Oncology nutrition for clinical practice*, Chicago, 2013, Oncology Nutrition Dietetic Practice Group of the Academy of Nutrition and Dietetics.

alterations can be associated with the disease itself, certain chemotherapy agents, radiation therapy, or surgery to the head and neck. Chemotherapy-induced, learned taste aversions have been reported in adults and children. Individuals also may develop a heightened sense of smell that results in sensitivity to food preparation odors and aversions to nonfood items such as soaps or perfumes. These sensation abnormalities do not consistently correlate with the tumor site, extent of tumor involvement, tumor response to therapy, or food preferences and intake. Nutrition interventions that decrease the aroma of foods, such as serving foods cold instead of hot, may be helpful (See Table 35.6).

Alterations in Energy Metabolism Resulting from Cancer

Energy metabolism is related intimately to carbohydrate, protein, and lipid metabolism, all of which are altered by tumor growth. Tumors exert a consistent demand for glucose, exhibit a characteristically high rate of anaerobic metabolism, and yield lactate as the end product. This expanded lactic acid pool requires an increased rate of host gluconeogenesis via Cori cycle activity, which is increased in some people with cancer but not in others. Protein breakdown and lipolysis take place at increasing rates to maintain high rates of glucose synthesis. There is glucose intolerance and insulin resistance, characterized by excess fatty acid oxidation and decreased uptake and use of glucose by muscle.

Because cancer patients lose muscle tissue and have decreased energy utilization, they have an increased need for protein and calories. Most notable is the loss of skeletal muscle protein caused by increased protein breakdown, as well as decreased protein synthesis. Additional protein is especially critical when undergoing treatment or experiencing malnutrition or cachexia (Hamilton, 2013).

Managing Cancer Cachexia

A common secondary diagnosis in people with advanced cancer is a variant of protein-energy malnutrition. This syndrome is termed cancer cachexia and is characterized by progressive weight loss, anorexia, generalized wasting and weakness, immunosuppression, altered basal metabolic rate, and abnormalities in fluid and energy metabolism. There is also increased loss of adipose tissue, which is related to an increased rate of lipolysis, rather than a decrease in lipogenesis. Increased levels of lipid-mobilizing factor and proteolysis-inducing factor secreted by tumor cells will lead to increased loss of fat and muscle mass. Individuals at the time of diagnosis with breast or hematologic cancers rarely present with significant weight loss, whereas individuals with lung, esophageal, or head and neck cancers often exhibit substantial weight loss.

Cancer cachexia is caused in part by cytokines (immune-modulating agents), produced by the cancer itself or by the immune system in response to the cancer. Cytokines can cause metabolic changes and wasting that is similar to changes seen in inflammation (see Chapter 3). Proinflammatory cytokines include tumor necrosis factor (TNF)-α (cachectin) and TNF-β, interleukin (IL)-1, IL-6, and interferon-α. These cytokines have overlapping physiologic activities, which makes it likely that no single substance is the sole cause. Many people undergoing cancer treatment will be treated with steroids as part of their protocol, partially to address the inflammatory process. Resting energy expenditure (REE) is elevated, which is in contrast to the REE in chronic starvation, wherein the body adapts to conserve energy and preserve body tissue. Cancer cachexia and the associated wasting often increase closer to the time of death and are also indicated as a factor in the cause of death of 30% to 50% of all patients with cancer, which is why increased protein and calorie needs are indicated (Levin, 2013).

Pharmacotherapy

The pharmacologic management of cachexia and anorexia requires careful evaluation based on the individual's treatment goals and prognosis and on close monitoring of symptoms. Cancer cachexia cannot be reversed without medical management of the underlying inflammation and hypermetabolism. Anorexia, a common cancer-related condition, is amenable to treatment with nutrition counseling, diet modification, and pharmacotherapy. A number of pharmacologic agents are utilized when treating anorexia and cachexia, including antihistamines (Periactin), corticosteroids (Decadron, Solu-Medrol), progestational agents (Provera, Megace), prokinetic agents (Reglan), and antidepressants (Remeron) (Elliot, 2013).

Medical marijuana, or cannabis, is a controlled substance in the United States, though over 50% of states have now enacted laws to legalize its use. According to the NCI Physician Data Query (PDQ), cannabinoids, which are the active chemicals in cannabis, can provide relief from side effects including pain, nausea and vomiting, anxiety, and anorexia from cancer and cancer treatment (NIH, 2019b; NCI, 2017). The FDA has not approved medical marijuana for cancer or cancer treatment application; however, it has approved two cannabinoids, Marinol and Cesamet, for individuals experiencing chemotherapy-related nausea and vomiting (NIH, 2019b; NCI, 2017).

Managing Other Cancer-Related Metabolic Abnormalities

Metabolic alterations vary by tumor type. An individual's immunologic function can be impaired, as the result of the disease, cancer treatment, or progressive malnutrition. In addition to the cancer-induced metabolic effects, the mass of the tumor may anatomically alter the physiology of specific organ systems. The activity of several enzyme systems involved with digestion and absorption can be affected, as can certain endocrine functions.

Critical imbalances in fluid and electrolyte status can occur in people who have cancers or are undergoing cancer treatments that promote excessive diarrhea, vomiting, or malabsorption. Profuse and often severe diarrhea can result from partial bowel obstructions and endocrine-secreting tumors such as those secreting serotonin (carcinoid tumors), calcitonin, or gastrin (Zollinger-Ellison's syndrome). The use of antimetabolites, alkylating agents, and antibiotics may also lead to the development of severe diarrhea. In some instances, people who are immunocompromised or have undergone GI surgery may experience profuse diarrhea that is caused by intestinal pathogens such as *Clostridium difficile* (see Chapter 27).

Persistent vomiting is associated with intestinal obstruction, radiation therapy to the stomach and abdomen or brain, highly emetogenic (nausea-causing) chemotherapy agents, intracranial tumors, and advanced cancer (Iwamoto et al, 2012). Careful assessment and evaluation of the cause of diarrhea or vomiting is critical for effective management. Malabsorption may be caused by treatment-related pancreatic dysfunction, postsurgical short gut syndrome, acute or chronic radiation enteritis (inflammation of the GI tract tissues secondary to radiation), excess serotonin, steatorrhea, or chronic diarrhea.

Hypercalcemia may occur in individuals with bone metastases, caused by the osteolytic activity of tumor cells releasing calcium into the extracellular fluid causing nausea, weakness, fatigue, lethargy, and confusion. Hypercalcemia is potentially fatal and is associated most commonly with multiple myeloma, lung cancer, and advanced breast and prostate cancer. Medical management of hypercalcemia includes rehydration and use of antihypercalcemic agents. Calcium supplementation from dietary supplements and antacids should be avoided. Restricting the intake of foods containing calcium is not indicated because the consumption of these foods has little effect in the overall management of hypercalcemia.

INTEGRATIVE, COMPLEMENTARY, AND FUNCTIONAL ONCOLOGY

Research shows that 40% to 50% of cancer patients use complementary and integrative medicine during and after treatment though over 80% of health care providers report limited knowledge about the role of complementary therapies in the cancer care setting (King et al, 2015).

The health care team working in oncology must be informed on the different therapies and should be knowledgeable regarding resources used to evaluate and educate the individuals in their care. Increasing consumer demand has encouraged health care institutions to create integrative medicine departments with onsite complementary services. Cancer survivors look for open, honest discussions or recommendations from their health care teams. Nondisclosure with the care team regarding complementary therapies such as special dietary patterns or supplements is common because patients fear healthcare providers will suggest they stop or because they believe physicians have limited knowledge on the topic of supplements (Huebner et al, 2014). Medical, nursing, and nutrition assessments should include open-ended questions on dietary supplement use and questions regarding the additional integrative or complementary therapies or diets they are following at the time. The core components to discuss integrative or alternative therapies involve understanding and respecting the need for personal empowerment. Having a willingness to listen, explore, and respond frankly to questions; taking the time to discuss the options and offer advice; summarizing the discussion; documenting the dialog; and monitoring the progress of the therapy are critical to supporting patients going through cancer treatment (Abrams, 2013). The NIH established the National Center for Complementary and Integrative Health (NCCIH), which works to create a framework in which to evaluate and research these therapies. See Chapter 11 on Dietary Supplements and Integrative Medicine for more information.

Dietary Supplements

Nondisclosure of use is a common occurrence, with a reported 53% of individuals receiving chemotherapy not discussing use of dietary supplements with their health care team (Abrams, 2013; Davis et al, 2014). Data from the Intergroup Phase III Breast Cancer Chemotherapy Trial found that over half of all study participants received no advice on dietary supplements (Gröber et al, 2016). People may view dietary supplements as a more natural alternative to prescription medications or a quick, easy remedy to an underlying medical problem.

It is the position of the Academy of Nutrition and Dietetics that micronutrient supplements are warranted when requirements are not being met through the diet alone. This is a population that may greatly benefit from certain forms of supplementation. According to the European Society for Clinical Nutrition and Metabolism (ESPEN) guidelines on enteral nutrition, it can be assumed that any patient with cancer who is able to consume <60% of their daily energy requirements for a period of 7 to 10 days has an inadequate supply of micronutrients (Gröber et al, 2016). Consumers are often not comfortable interpreting labels, understanding needs, and assessing safety when choosing supplements. When working with patients undergoing cancer treatment, assess the safety and efficacy of supplements they report taking, paying special attention to those that may interact with medications or cause increased risk of bleeding. For more information, refer to Appendix 13 and Chapter 11. (Marra and Bailey, 2018).

Some supplements show promise for malignancies including omega-3 fatty acids, vitamin D, curcumin, selenium, and medicinal mushrooms such as maitake, reishi, and turkey tail (Abrams, 2013; Baggerly et al, 2015; Blagodatski et al, 2018; Gröber et al, 2016;

TABLE 35.7 Popular Anticancer Dietary Plan

Diet	Description	Potential Benefit or Harm
Alkaline Diet	Attempts to create a more alkaline environment in the body by eliminating acidic foods (red meat, sugar, refined flours, alcohol, coffee).	While there is no evidence that supports the efficacy of this diet currently available because the body regulates its own pH balance, it does reduce or eliminate some foods that increase cancer risk (red meat, high glycemic foods, alcohol) and increases legumes and vegetables which could be helpful. Ensure adequate calorie and protein intake.
Budwig Diet	Flaxseed oil and cottage cheese preparation is consumed twice per day. Emphasis on natural, unprocessed foods low in added sugar or fat/oils; no dairy or animal fats, pork, seafood, soy. or corn.	No clinical trials available at this time. No evidence that flaxseed oil and cottage cheese are specifically anticancer though this mixture can be supportive in adding calories to a patient experiencing weight loss.
Essiac	An herbal mixture often taken as a tea, consumed three times per day designed to shrink tumors and strengthen the immune system.	No published clinical trials, no proven efficacy in animal studies, though some of the herbs do exhibit antitumor effects on their own in vitro. May have a laxative effect and cause nausea or vomiting.
Gerson Therapy	Vegetarian diet, raw juices, and coffee enemas. 15-20 pounds of organic fruit and vegetables are consumed, juiced, each day. Avoids fat. Nutritional and biological supplements are used including pancreatic enzymes.	The National Cancer Institute suggests avoiding this diet due to risk for protein energy malnutrition, dehydration, and concerns for food safety with neutropenic patients. Available studies are limited at this time regarding safety and efficacy.
Intermittent Fasting (IF)	Abstaining from food for various periods of time including before and during chemotherapy, alternate day, or for a number of hours each day in an effort to limit fuel to cancer cells. Preliminary studies have shown reduced tumor development in mouse studies.	Malnutrition and weight loss are serious consequences of fasting during treatment when calorie and protein needs are increased. Human studies are limited at this time though some short-term data ($\leq$6 months) in overweight and obese participants have suggested IF improves insulin sensitivity and reduces inflammatory markers.
Ketogenic	High fat (>80%), low carbohydrate (<10%) diets used to treat childhood epilepsy, neurodegenerative diseases, and also as alternative therapy for some cancer treatment, often glioma and other brain cancers.	Though there is some promising preliminary research in rodent studies and the best efficacy currently for humans is likely for brain cancers, more research is needed to understand if ketogenic is a supportive diet for people undergoing cancer treatment. Ketogenic diets should be closely medically managed. They can cause fatigue, kidney damage, constipation, weight loss, and nutritional deficiencies.
Macrobiotic	A diet and lifestyle philosophy brought to the United States from Japan in the 1950s with an emphasis on organic, vegetarian foods high in grains and low in fat. Chewing food and special cooking techniques required.	This diet does focus on many potentially beneficial foods within a vegetarian dietary pattern. However, there is a potential for nutrient deficiencies given the exclusion of some foods. May be challenging to adhere to because of special cooking and preparation requirements.
Raw Food Diet	Allows only raw foods heated to 105° F or less. Usually avoids meat, dairy, and eggs unless raw which is dangerous (food safety issue).	May be deficient in protein, calories, and certain nutrients. Can irritate the gut, especially if diarrhea is a side effect. May be a food safety concern. A potential beneficial emphasis on unprocessed foods and high in fruit and vegetables.

Melina V, Craig W, Levin S: Position of the Academy of Nutrition and Dietetics: vegetarian diets, *J Acad Nut Diet* 116(12):1970–1980, 2016; Schwalfenberg GK: The alkaline diet: is there evidence that an alkaline pH diet benefits health? *J Environ Pub Health* 2012:727630, 2012; O'Brien S, Leser M, Ledesma N: Diets, functional foods and dietary supplements for cancer prevention and survival. In Leser M, Ledesma N, Bergerson S, et al, editors: *Oncology nutrition for clinical practice*, Chicago, 2013, Oncology Nutrition Dietetic Practice Group; National Cancer Institute: Gerson therapy, 2016b, NCI; Harvie MN, Howell T: Could intermittent energy restriction and intermittent fasting reduce rates of cancer in obese, overweight, and normal-weight subjects? A summary of evidence, *Adv Nutr* 7(4):690–705, 2016; Weber DD, Aminazdeh-Gohari S, Kofler B: Ketogenic diet in cancer therapy, *Aging* 10(2):164–165, 2018; Allen BG, Bhatia SK, Anderson CM, et al: Ketogenic diets as an adjuvant cancer therapy: history and potential mechanism, *Redox Biol* 2:963–970, 2014; National Institutes of Health, National Cancer Institute: Gerson therapy PDQ, 2016b.

LeMay-Nedjelski et al, 2018, Zhou et al, 2017). Others may cause damage in a variety of ways. For example, common supplements like garlic and vitamin E can increase bleeding risk and thin the blood (Marra and Bailey, 2018; Alsanad et al, 2014). Some interact negatively with common cancer medications. Garlic, green tea, mistletoe, Chinese herbs, iron, St. John's Wort, and ginger have been shown to interact with drugs including cyclophosphamide, nonsteroidal antiinflammatory drugs, irinotecan, vinorelbine, warfarin, and paclitaxel (Alsanad et al, 2014). Others are in fact toxic to the body. Anticancer supplement B_{17}/laetrile/amygdalin is a source of cyanide and is associated with toxicity and poisoning (Dang et al, 2017). Educating patients about the safety of supplements while maintaining an open mind is key for relationship building and safety when it comes to integrative, complementary, and functional oncology nutrition (Alsanad et al, 2014; Gröber et al, 2016; Table 35.7).

NUTRITIONAL IMPACT OF CANCER TREATMENTS

Chemotherapy

Chemotherapy uses chemical agents or medications to treat cancer. Classifications of chemotherapy cytotoxic agents are listed in Table 35.8. Once in the bloodstream, these agents are carried through the body to reach as many cancer cells as possible. Routes of administration for chemotherapy include the following:

- Oral: capsule, pill, or liquid
- IV: delivery of medication via an injection or an indwelling catheter into a vein
- Intraperitoneal: delivery of medication via a catheter directly into the abdominal cavity
- Intravesicular: delivery of medication via a Foley catheter directly into the bladder

- Intrathecal: delivery of medication via an injection into the central nervous system using an Ommaya reservoir or a lumbar puncture (Polovich et al, 2014)

Whereas surgery and radiation therapy are used to treat localized tumors, chemotherapy is a systemic therapy that affects the malignant tissue and normal cells as well. Cells of the body with a rapid turnover such as bone marrow, hair follicles, and the mucosa of the digestive tract are the most affected. As a result, nutrition intake and nutrition status can be adversely affected. Nutrition-related symptoms include myelosuppression, also called pancytopenia, (suppression of bone marrow production of neutrophils, platelets, and red blood cells), anemia, fatigue, nausea and vomiting, loss of appetite, mucositis, changes in taste and smell, xerostomia (mouth dryness), dysphagia, and altered bowel function such as diarrhea or constipation (Table 35.8).

The severity of the side effects depends on the specific agents used, dosage, duration of treatment, number of treatment cycles, accompanying drugs, individual response, and current health status. The timely and appropriate use of supportive therapies such as antiemetics, antidiarrheals, corticosteroids, hematopoietic agents, and antibiotics, as well as dietary changes, is important. Many people experience significant side effects, especially in "dose-intensive" multiple-agent chemotherapy regimens; neutropenia (reduced white blood cells or neutrophils), thrombocytopenia (low blood platelet counts), and

TABLE 35.8 Nutrition-Related Effects of Antineoplastic Agents: Chemotherapy, Biotherapy, and Hormone Therapy

Agent Classification	Common Side Effects and Nutrition Implications
Chemotherapy	
Alkylating Agents	
• Altretamine (Hexalen), Busulfan (Buselfex), Bendamustine (Treanda), carboplatin (Paraplatin), cisplatin (Platinol), cyclophosphamide (Cytoxan), oxaliplatin (Eloxatin), temozolomide (Temodar)	• Myelosuppression, anorexia, nausea, vomiting, fatigue, renal toxicity • Treat lung, breast, ovary cancers, leukemia, lymphoma, Hodgkin's disease, multiple myeloma, and sarcoma by stopping cells from reproducing by damaging their DNA. They work in all phases of the cell cycle.
Antitumor Antibiotics	
• Bleomycin (Blenoxane), doxorubicin (Adriamycin), Mitomycin (Mutamycin), Epirubicin, Idarubicin, Daunorubicin	• Myelosuppression, anorexia, nausea, vomiting, fatigue, diarrhea, mucositis, can damage the heart • Treat a wide variety of cancers because they change the DNA inside cancer cells to stop them from growing and multiplying.
Antimetabolites	
• Capecitabine (Xeloda), Pemetrexed (Alimta®), cytarabine (ARA-C), 5-fluorouracil (5-FU), Floxuridine, Fludarabine, 6-mercaptopurine (6-MP), gemcitabine (Gemzar), methotrexate	• Myelosuppression, anorexia, nausea, vomiting, fatigue, diarrhea, mucositis • Treat leukemias and cancers of the breast, ovary, and intestinal tract by interfering with DNA and RNA, damaging the cells during the phase when chromosomes are being copied.
Topoisomerase Inhibitors	
• Topotecan (Hycamtin), irinotecan (CPT-11, Camptosar), etoposide (VP-16, Etopopos), teniposide, mitoxantrone • Treat leukemias, lung, ovarian, testicular, and gastrointestinal cancers by interfering with enzymes that help separate strands of DNA so it can be copied.	• Anorexia, nausea, vomiting, diarrhea, constipation, muscle cramps, risk of infection
Mitotic Inhibitors	
• Docetaxel (Taxotere), estramustine (Emcyt), ixabepilone (Ixempra), paclitaxel (Abraxane), vinblastine, vincristine (Marqibo), vinorelbine (Navelbine) • Treat breast and lung cancers, myelomas, lymphomas, and leukemias by stopping cell division.	• Anorexia, nausea, vomiting, fatigue, muscle and joint aches, mouth sores, hair loss, and peripheral neuropathy (tingling and nerve irritation in the hands and feet)
Miscellaneous	
• Procarbazine (Matulane)	• Myelosuppression, nausea, vomiting, diarrhea, monoamine oxidase (MAO) inhibitor/avoid foods high in tyramine. • Treats non-Hodgkin's lymphoma, brain tumors, melanoma, lung cancer.
Biotherapy	
Cytokines	
• Interferon-alfa (Intron A, Roferon), interleukin (IL-2, Aldesleukin)	• Myelosuppression, anorexia, fatigue, nausea, flu-like symptoms, chills
Monoclonal Antibodies	
• Cetuximab (Erbitux), rituximab (Rituxan), trastuzumab (Herceptin), tositumomab (Bexxar)	• Infusion reaction of chills, fever, headache, hypotension; myelosuppression; nausea; vomiting; rash

Continued

TABLE 35.8   Nutrition-Related Effects of Antineoplastic Agents: Chemotherapy, Biotherapy, and Hormone Therapy—cont'd

Agent Classification	Common Side Effects and Nutrition Implications
Protein-Targeted Therapies: Small Molecule Inhibitors • Tyrosine kinase inhibitors: erlotinib (Tarceva), imatinib mesylate (Gleevec), gefitinib (Iressa), sorafenib (Nexavar), sunitinib (Sutent) • mTOR inhibitors: everolimus (Afinitor), temsirolimus (Torisel) • Proteasome inhibitor: bortezomib (Velcade)	• Fever, chills, rash, diarrhea, fatigue, anorexia
Angiogenesis Inhibitors • Bevacizumab (Avastin), lenalidomide (Revlimid), thalidomide	• Hypertension, arterial thromboembolic events, gastrointestinal perforation, hemorrhage, proteinuria, hypothyroidism
Cancer Vaccines • Sipuleucel-T (Provenge)	• Fever, chills, back pain, loss of appetite, fatigue, nausea, flu-like symptoms
Hormone Therapy **Antiandrogens** • Bicalutamide (Casodex); flutamide (Eulexin)	• Hot flashes, weight gain, fatigue, bone pain, decreased libido/impotence
Luteinizing Hormone-Releasing Hormone (LHRH) Antagonist • Leuprolide (Lupron), goserelin (Zoladex)	• Hot flashes, fatigue, edema, nausea, bone pain, muscle weakness, headache, gynecomastia, decreased libido/impotence
Selective Estrogen Receptor Modulators (SERMs) • Raloxifene (Evista), tamoxifen (Nolvadex), toremifene (Fareston)	• Thromboembolic events, fluid retention, hot flashes, nausea, joint discomfort, diarrhea, weight gain, skin changes/rash
Aromatase Inhibitors (AIs) • Anastrozole (Arimidex), letrozole (Femara), exemestane (Aromasin)	• Hot flashes, nausea, vomiting, thromboembolic events, high cholesterol, fever, joint aches and pains
Progesterones • Megestrol acetate (Megace)	• Increased appetite, weight gain, fluid retention, hyperglycemia, thromboembolic events

Data from Polovich M, et al: *Chemotherapy and biotherapy guidelines and recommendations for practice*, ed 4, Pittsburgh, 2014, Oncology Nursing Society; Wilkes GM, Barton-Burke M: 2014 *Oncology nursing drug handbook*, Burlington, 2013, Jones and Bartlett; Chu E, Devita VT: *Physician's cancer chemotherapy drug manual*, Boston, 2014, Jones and Bartlet, http://www.chemocare.com; American Cancer Society: How chemotherapy drugs work, 2016; Grant BL: Nutritional effects of cancer treatment: chemotherapy, biotherapy, hormone therapy and radiation therapy. In Leser M, Ledesma N, Bergerson S, et al, editors: Oncology nutrition for clinical practice, Chicago, 2013, Oncology Nutrition Dietetic Practice Group.

myelosuppression are the primary factors limiting chemotherapy administration. Commonly experienced chemotherapy induced toxicities affecting the gastrointestinal system include mucositis, nausea, vomiting, diarrhea, and constipation. Chemotherapy related taste abnormalities can lead to anorexia and decreased oral intake.

Anemia of Chronic Disease

Certain chemotherapies are more likely to cause anemia including platinum-based chemotherapy such as cisplatin, carboplatin, and oxaliplatin. Certain tumor types such as lung or ovarian, may also increase the likelihood for anemia (ACS, 2017). Hallmark symptoms of anemia that can compound other side effects include severe fatigue, weakness, swelling in the hands and feet, and dizziness. Patients may inquire about what they can do nutritionally to aid in supporting healthy red blood cell counts but not all anemia during cancer treatment has a nutrition-based etiology. Anemia of chronic disease is different than iron deficiency anemia in that it is caused by myelosuppression from chemotherapy and other cancer treatments. Cancer patients can also become iron deficient due to malnutrition and blood

loss, which can also lead to anemia. It is important understand the difference in order to correctly assess patient needs. Severe anemia may need to be treated with blood transfusions or medications (ACS, 2017). Dietetic practitioners should ensure that nutrition status is adequate including adequate protein and calories plus vitamin A and dietary folate. See Chapter 31 on anemia.

Diarrhea

Diarrhea is a common side effect of certain chemotherapy agents, radiation therapy that covers the intestines and surgery. Left unmanaged, it can lead to depletion of fluids, electrolytes, malnutrition, and even hospitalization. The intestinal mucosa and digestive processes can be affected, thus altering digestion and absorption to some degree. Protein, energy, and vitamin metabolism may be impaired. It is essential to maintain hydration status and replace electrolytes if three or more stools per day compared with usual or an increase in liquidity of bowel movements occurs. Institute a low-fat, low-fiber, and possibly low-lactose diet that avoids gas producing foods, caffeine, and alcohol. Suggest foods such as applesauce, banana, oatmeal, potatoes, and rice as soluble fiber bulking agents with diarrhea (Elliott, 2013).

Nausea and Vomiting

Chemotherapy induced nausea and vomiting are commonly classified as anticipatory (occurs before receiving treatment), acute (occurs within the first 24 hours after receiving treatment), or delayed (occurs 1 to 4 days after treatment), each of which is characterized by distinct pathophysiologic events and requires different therapeutic interventions. Effective agents for treatment-related nausea and vomiting are the serotonin antagonists (e.g., ondansetron, granisetron, and dolasetron), neurokinin-1 (NK-1) receptor antagonists (e.g., aprepitant), dopamine antagonists (e.g., metoclopramide, prochlorperazine), and corticosteroids such as dexamethasone (Polovich et al, 2014). Other antiemetic agents include cannabinoids (e.g., dronabinol, nabilone), benzodiazepines (e.g., lorazepam, diazepam), and ginger tea or extract (Elliott, 2013). To support patients with nausea and vomiting, suggest five to six small meals per day, cool and light foods without strong odors, resting with head elevated after eating, and consuming liquids between meals rather than with meals (Elliott, 2013) (see Table 36.6).

Food-Drug Interactions

Nutrition professionals can gain valuable insights regarding possible drug-nutrient interactions and contraindications by reviewing product medication inserts, pharmacy resource books, and medication databases or by consulting with pharmacy personnel (see Appendix 13). Some chemotherapy agents can cause potentially severe adverse events (Grant, 2013), for example:

- Individuals with certain types of lung cancer who are being treated with pemetrexed (Alimta) require vitamin B_{12} (often by injection) and folic acid supplementation throughout the duration of their therapy to avoid significant anemia associated with this chemotherapy agent.
- A severe hypertensive event is possible when tyramine-rich foods and beverages are consumed while taking procarbazine (Matulane), a chemotherapy agent commonly used to treat brain cancer.
- Individuals with colon cancer receiving oxaliplatin (Eloxatin) should not drink, eat, or handle cold drinks or foods for up to 5 days because of treatment-related neuropathy or transient paresthesias of the hands, feet, and throat.
- To prevent unnecessary gastric upset, individuals taking the medication capecitabine (Xeloda) must take the medication within 30 minutes of eating food or a meal. Conversely, medications such as erlotinib (Tarceva) should not be taken with food; it can cause a rash and profound diarrhea unless taken on an empty stomach.
- Individuals with certain types of cancer or rheumatoid arthritis who are being treated with methotrexate (Trexall) may benefit from supplemental folate which can reduce the toxicity of treatment similar or better than a common medication given for the same effect, leucovorin. (Merzel, 2017). Always coordinate care with a physician to ensure appropriateness of supplementation with folate in cancer therapy.

Oral Changes

People with altered taste acuity (dysgeusia, hypogeusia, ageusia) may benefit from increased use of flavorings and seasonings during food preparation. Meat aversions may require the elimination of red meats and the substitution of alternative protein sources including soy foods, beans, dairy, or eggs. Herpes simplex virus and *Candida albicans* (thrush) account for most oral infections. In addition to causing oral infections, some agents, especially corticosteroids, can cause hyperglycemia and can lead to excessive losses of urinary protein, potassium, and calcium. Support patients with oral changes by trialing fruity and salty flavors. Fruit marinades on meat and other foods including lemon, herbs, and spices can help. Prepare foods without strong smells including foods that are not cooked or are covered with a lid. Suggest patients follow good oral hygiene and brush teeth before eating (Elliott, 2013) (see Chapter 24).

Mucositis

The rapidly dividing epithelial cells of the mouth are vulnerable to the side effects of therapy and oral mucositis can be a serious consequence. An inflammation of the mucous membranes lining the oropharynx and esophagus, mucositis is among the most common debilitating complication of chemotherapy and radiation. It can result in pain, inability to eat, and increased susceptibility to infection due to open sores. It is known that a good oral care regimen can help prevent or decrease the severity of mucositis and, just as important, help prevent the development of infection through open mouth sores. The mainstay of an effective oral care regimen is mouth rinses, and numerous studies have determined that a rinse with ¾ teaspoon salt and 1 teaspoon of baking soda in 4 cups of water is one of the best and most cost-effective mouth rinses available (Elliott, 2013). A mouth rinse aides in removing debris and keeping the oral tissue moist and clean.

General care guidelines include avoidance of tobacco, alcohol, and irritating foods such as spicy or acidic including citrus, tomato, chilies, and hot sauce. Bland liquids and soft solids are usually better tolerated in individuals with oral or esophageal mucositis and strong-flavored, acidic, or spicy foods also should be avoided. Chewing on ice can sometimes help (Elliott, 2013) (see Chapter 24).

The amino acid L-glutamine, often taken in a powder mixed into water, has been shown to decrease the severity of mucositis at 5 grams three times daily (Elliott, 2013; Tsuimoto et al, 2015).

Biotherapy

Biotherapy is immunotherapy in which a group of cancer treatment drugs prescribed to stimulate the body's own immune system and natural defenses are used to treat cancer. Biotherapy is sometimes used by itself, but it is given most often in combination with chemotherapy drugs. Different kinds of biotherapy drugs used to help the immune system recognize cancer cells and strengthen its ability to destroy them include the following:

- Cytokines such as interferon and IL-2 for treatment of malignant melanoma and metastatic melanoma.
- Monoclonal antibodies such as trastuzumab (Herceptin) for treatment of specific types of breast cancer, and rituximab (Rituxan) for treatment of non-Hodgkin's lymphoma.
- Antiangiogenesis inhibitors prevent and reduce the growth of new blood vessels and prevent tumor invasion. These agents are most frequently used in combination with other chemotherapy agents to maximize their effectiveness. An example of an antiangiogenic agent used to treat colon or brain cancer is bevacizumab (Avastin).
- Cancer vaccines such as sipuleucel-T (Provenge) made from an individual's own cancer or substances from tumor cells are currently under investigation in clinical cancer trials (Grant, 2013; Wilkes and Barton-Burke, 2013).

Other types of biotherapy drugs are groups of proteins that cause blood cells to grow and mature (NIH and NCI, 2015). These drugs are called hematopoietic growth factors. They include supportive care medications such as darbepoetin (Aranesp) or epoetin alfa (Procrit) to stimulate red blood cell production, and filgrastim (Neupogen) or pegfilgrastim (Neulasta) to stimulate the production of neutrophils in the bone marrow. Individuals receiving these agents may experience fatigue, chills, fever, and flu-like symptoms.

Hormone Therapy

Hormone therapy adds, blocks, or removes hormones to slow or stop the growth of hormone-sensitive breast or prostate cancer (NIH and NCI, 2015). Examples of these agents include tamoxifen (Nolvadex) and anastrozole (Arimidex) for breast cancer and leuprolide (Lupron) or bicalutamide (Casodex) for prostate cancer. Side effects commonly include hot flashes, decreased libido and sexual function, and bone pain (Wilkes and Barton-Burke, 2013).

Radiation Therapy

Radiation therapy, ionizing radiation used in multiple fractionated doses, is used to cure, control, or palliate cancer. Radiation therapy can be delivered externally into the body from a megavoltage machine or with brachytherapy by placing a radioactive source (implant) in or near the tumor to deliver a highly localized dose. Advances in technology to deliver radiation therapy with precise accuracy include radiation surgery (e.g., stereotactic radiosurgery) and intensity-modulated radiation therapy (IMRT). Whereas chemotherapy is a systemic therapy, radiation therapy affects only the tumor and the surrounding area. The side effects of radiation therapy are usually limited to the specific site being irradiated. Chemotherapy agents may also be given in combination with radiation therapy to produce a radiation-enhancing effect. People receiving multimodality therapy often experience side effects sooner and with greater intensity.

The acute side effects of radiation therapy when used alone generally occur around the second or third week of treatment and usually resolve within 2 to 4 weeks after the radiation therapy has been completed. Late effects of radiation therapy may happen several weeks, months, or even years after treatment. Commonly experienced nutrition-related symptoms include fatigue, loss of appetite, skin changes, and hair loss in the area being treated (Table 35.9).

Radiation to the Head and Neck

Treatment for head and neck cancer usually includes a multimodal approach with aggressive chemotherapy, radiation therapy, and often surgery. Radiation therapy to the head and neck can cause acute nutrition-related symptoms: sore mouth, altered taste and smell, dysphagia and odynophagia, mucositis, xerostomia, anorexia, fatigue, and weight loss (Havrila et al, 2010). Diminished oral intake, weight loss, and dehydration are a serious risk due to impaired chewing and swallowing during treatment. In fact, patients with head and neck cancers experience among the highest rates of malnutrition of any cancer diagnosis (25% to 50%) (Nguyen and Nadler, 2013). Prophylactic placement of percutaneous endoscopic gastrostomy (PEG) feeding tubes can help to reduce treatment-associated weight loss and malnutrition particularly for patients who have experienced undesired preoperative weight loss of 10 or more pounds, advanced (stage IV) tumors, pharyngeal tumors, or a planned combined surgery and radiotherapy treatment plan (Nguyen and Nadler, 2013).

Salivary stimulants and substitutes or oral lubricants are beneficial for temporary relief of xerostomia (diminished salivation or loss of salivation) caused by head and neck radiation therapy or certain types of medications (e.g., pain medications). In addition, liquids and foods with sauces and gravies are usually well tolerated. Late effects of radiation therapy may include dental caries, permanent xerostomia, trismus (an inability to fully open the mouth), and osteoradionecrosis of the jaw (necrosis of the bone caused by exposure to radiation therapy).

Radiation to the Thorax

Nutrition-related symptoms of radiation therapy to the thorax (chest) can include heartburn and acute esophagitis, accompanied by dysphagia and odynophagia. Late effects include possible esophageal fibrosis and stenosis. When this occurs, individuals are generally able to

TABLE 35.9	Nutrition-Related Effects of Radiation Therapy
Site of Radiation Therapy	**Common Nutrition-Related Symptom**
Central nervous system (brain and spinal cord)	**Acute Effects** Nausea, vomiting Fatigue Loss of appetite Hyperglycemia associated with corticosteroids **Late Effects (>90 days after treatment)** Headache, lethargy
Head and neck (tongue, larynx, pharynx, oropharynx, nasopharynx, tonsils, salivary glands)	**Acute Effects** Xerostomia Mucositis Sore mouth and throat Thick saliva/oral secretions Dysphagia, odynophagia Alterations in taste and smell Fatigue Loss of appetite **Late Effects (>90 days after treatment)** Mucosal atrophy and dryness Salivary glands—xerostomia, fibrosis Trismus Osteoradionecrosis Alterations in taste and smell
Thorax (esophagus, lung, breast)	**Acute Effects** Esophagitis Dysphagia, odynophagia Heartburn Fatigue Loss of appetite **Late Effects (>90 days after treatment)** Esophageal—fibrosis, stenosis, stricture, ulceration Cardiac—angina on effort, pericarditis, cardiac enlargement Pulmonary—dry cough, fibrosis, pneumonitis
Abdomen and pelvis (stomach, ovaries, uterus, colon, rectum)	**Acute Effects** Nausea, vomiting Changes in bowel function—diarrhea, cramping, bloating, gas Changes in urinary function—increased frequency, burning sensation with urination Acute colitis or enteritis Lactose intolerance Fatigue Loss of appetite **Late Effects (>90 days after treatment)** Diarrhea, malabsorption, maldigestion Chronic colitis or enteritis Intestinal—stricture, ulceration, obstruction, perforation, fistula Urinary—hematuria, cystitis

Data from Iwamoto RR, et al: *Manual for radiation oncology and nursing practice and education*, ed 4, Pittsburgh, 2012, Oncology Nursing Society; Grant B: Nutritional effects of cancer treatment: chemotherapy, biotherapy, hormone therapy and radiation therapy. In Leser M et al, editors: *Oncology nutrition for clinical practice*, Chicago, 2013, Oncology Nutrition Dietetic Practice Group of the Academy of Nutrition and Dietetics.

swallow only liquids, and the use of medical food supplements and enteral nutrition (EN) support may be necessary to meet nutritional needs (see Chapter 12). Often individuals undergo esophageal dilations or swallowing therapy and rehabilitation to improve swallowing function.

Radiation to the Abdomen or Pelvis

Radiation therapy to the abdomen or pelvis may cause gastritis or enteritis that can be accompanied by nausea, vomiting, diarrhea, and anorexia. Late effects can include lasting GI damage such as malabsorption of disaccharides (e.g., lactose), fats, vitamins, minerals, and electrolytes. Proactive management includes encouraging affected individuals to consume soluble fiber, to increase intake of hydrating liquids, and to avoid eating high nonsoluble fiber or lactose-containing foods. To alleviate symptoms, medications such as antidiarrheals like loperamide may be given to reduce intestinal motility.

Chronic radiation enteritis can develop with diarrhea, ulceration, or obstruction, intensifying the risk of malnutrition. Chronic radiation enteritis combined with or without significant bowel resection can result in bowel dysfunction and short bowel syndrome (SBS). The severity of this condition depends on the length and location of the nonfunctional or resected bowel and generally is diagnosed when the individual has less than 150 cm of small intestine remaining. The sequelae of SBS include malabsorption, malnutrition, dehydration, weight loss, fatigue, and lactose intolerance (Havrila et al, 2010) (see Chapter 27).

Initially parenteral nutrition (PN) may be required, and frequent monitoring of fluids and electrolytes may be necessary for weeks or months. Individuals with SBS may require an oral diet restricted to defined formula tube feedings or to frequent small meals high in protein, low in fat and fiber, and lactose-free. Dietary supplements that contain vitamin B_{12}, folic acid, thiamin, calcium, and vitamins A, E, and K often are indicated to prevent deficiencies. Serum concentrations of various minerals also should be monitored and adjusted as needed.

Total-Body Irradiation

Total-body irradiation (TBI) is a technique of radiation therapy that is used in HCT to eliminate malignant cells, to ablate the bone marrow and make room for the engraftment of the infused hematopoietic cells, and to suppress the immune system to decrease the risk of rejection. Commonly encountered side effects are fever, nausea, vomiting, headache, mucositis, parotitis (inflammation of the parotid glands), xerostomia, diarrhea, anorexia, fatigue, and associated weight loss.

Surgery

The surgical resection or removal of any part of the alimentary tract (mouth to anus), as well as the malignant disease process, can potentially impair normal digestion and absorption. Surgery may be used as a single mode of cancer treatment, or it may be combined with preoperative or postoperative adjuvant chemotherapy or radiation therapy. After surgery, individuals commonly experience fatigue, temporary changes in appetite and bowel function caused by anesthesia, and pain. They often require additional energy and protein for wound healing and recovery. Most side effects are temporary and dissipate a few days after surgery. However, some surgical interventions have long-lasting nutritional implications (Table 35.10). When performing a nutrition assessment, it is important to understand which part of the alimentary tract has been affected or surgically removed so that the appropriate nutrition intervention can be recommended (see Chapter 1 for a review in GI physiology).

Head and Neck Cancer

Individuals with head and neck cancer often have difficulty with chewing and swallowing caused by the cancer itself, the specific surgical intervention required to remove cancerous tissues, and/or radiation therapy. There can be additional problems due to history of smoking and alcohol abuse, illicit drug use, and subsequent poor nutrition intake, which place these individuals at high risk for malnutrition and postoperative complications. Surgery often necessitates temporary or long-term reliance on EN support (e.g., PEG tube feedings) (see Chapter 12). Individuals who resume oral intake often have prolonged dysphagia and require modifications of food consistency and extensive training in chewing and swallowing. Referrals to a speech therapist can yield dramatic positive results through evaluation and individualized instruction in swallowing and positioning techniques, as well as evaluation for aspiration risk (see Chapter 39).

Esophageal Cancer

Surgical intervention for treatment of esophageal cancer often requires partial or total removal of the esophagus. The stomach is commonly used for esophageal reconstruction. A feeding jejunostomy tube, which allows for early postoperative tube feedings, can be placed before an individual undergoes surgery or at the time of surgery. Usually the individual is able to progress to oral intake with specific dietary recommendations to minimize nutrition-related symptoms, which include reflux, dumping syndrome (discussed later in this chapter), dysmotility, gastroparesis, early satiety, vomiting, and fluid and electrolyte imbalances (Huhmann and August, 2010). Postsurgical recommendations include a low-fat diet with small, frequent feedings of energy-dense foods and avoidance of large amounts of fluids at any one time (see Chapter 26).

Gastric Cancer

Surgery is the most common treatment for cancer of the stomach, although chemotherapy and radiation therapy can be used before or after surgery to improve survival. Surgical interventions include partial, subtotal, or total gastrectomy. Placement of a jejunostomy feeding tube at surgery is advisable, and EN support using a jejunal feeding tube is generally feasible within a few days after surgery.

Postgastrectomy syndrome encompasses a myriad of symptoms, including dumping syndrome, general and fat malabsorption, gastric stasis, lactose intolerance, anemias, and metabolic bone disease (osteoporosis, osteopenia, osteomalacia). Dumping syndrome is a common complication of gastric surgery, manifested by the rapid transit of foods or liquids, and the dilutional response of the small remaining stomach to highly osmotic bolus feedings. Individuals may experience GI and vasomotor symptoms such as abdominal cramps, diarrhea, nausea, vomiting, flushing, faintness, diaphoresis, and tachycardia (Huhmann and August, 2010). Individuals experiencing malabsorption may have deficiencies in iron, folic acid, and vitamin B_{12}, which can lead to anemia. Micronutrient deficiencies of calcium and fat-soluble vitamins are also common (Gill, 2013; Huhmann and August, 2010).

Pancreatic Cancer

Cancer of the pancreas, with or without surgical resection, can have significant nutritional consequences. The Whipple procedure and the pylorus-sparing pancreatic duodenectomy are the most common pancreatic cancer surgeries. Postsurgical complications include delayed gastric emptying, early satiety, glucose intolerance, bile acid insufficiency, diarrhea, and fat malabsorption. Pancreatic enzyme replacement, the use of small, more frequent low-fat meals and snacks, and avoidance of simple carbohydrates aid digestion and absorption (see Chapter 28).

TABLE 35.10	Nutrition-Related Effects of Surgery in Cancer Treatment
Anatomic Site	**Nutrition Impact Symptoms**
Oral cavity	Difficulty with chewing and swallowing Aspiration potential Sore mouth and throat Xerostomia Alteration in taste and smell
Larynx	Alterations in normal swallowing, dysphagia Aspiration
Esophagus	Gastroparesis Indigestion, acid reflux Alterations in normal swallowing, dysphagia Decreased motility Anastomotic leak
Lung	Shortness of breath Early satiety
Stomach	Dumping syndrome Dehydration Early satiety Gastroparesis Fat malabsorption Vitamin and mineral malabsorption (vitamin B_{12} and D; calcium, iron)
Gallbladder and bile duct	Gastroparesis Hyperglycemia Fluid and electrolyte imbalance Vitamin and mineral malabsorption (vitamin A, D, E, and K; magnesium, calcium, zinc, iron)
Liver	Hyperglycemia Hypertriglyceridemia Fluid and electrolyte malabsorption Vitamin and mineral malabsorption (vitamin A, D, E, K, B_{12} and folic acid, magnesium, zinc)
Pancreas	Gastroparesis Fluid and electrolyte imbalance Hyperglycemia Fat malabsorption (vitamin A, D, E, K, B_{12}; calcium, zinc, iron)
Small bowel	Chyle leak Lactose intolerance Bile acid depletion Diarrhea Fluid and electrolyte imbalance Vitamin and mineral malabsorption (vitamin A, D, E, K, B_{12}; calcium, zinc, iron)
Colon and rectum	Increased transit time Diarrhea Dehydration Bloating, cramping, gas Fluid and electrolyte imbalance Vitamin and mineral malabsorption (vitamin B_{12}, sodium, potassium, magnesium, calcium)
Ovaries and uterus	Early satiety Bloating, cramping, and gas
Brain	Nausea, vomiting Hyperglycemia associated with corticosteroids

Data from Leser M et al, editors: *Oncology nutrition for clinical practice,* Chicago, 2013, Oncology Nutrition Dietetic Practice Group of Nutrition of the Academy of Nutrition and Dietetics; Huhmann MB, August D: Surgical oncology. In Marian M, Roberts S, editors: *Clinical nutrition for oncology patients,* Sudbury, Mass, 2010, Jones and Bartlett.

Cancers of the Intestinal Tract

Partial or total resections of the intestinal tract because of colorectal cancer or carcinoid syndrome may induce profound losses of fluid and electrolytes secondary to decreased transit time and diarrhea, the severity of which are related to the length and site of the resection. Resections of as little as 15 cm of the terminal ileum can result in bile salt losses that exceed the liver's capacity for resynthesis, and vitamin B_{12} absorption is affected. With depletion of the bile salt pool, steatorrhea develops. Nutrition intervention strategies consist of a diet low in fat, osmolality, lactose, and oxalates (see Chapters 27 and 37).

Hematopoietic Cell Transplantation (HCT)

Hematopoietic cell transplantation (HCT), commonly referred to as a "stem cell transplant," is performed for the treatment of certain hematologic cancers such as leukemia, lymphoma, and multiple myeloma. The stem cells used for HCT arise from bone marrow, peripheral blood, or umbilical cord blood. The preparative regimen includes cytotoxic chemotherapy, with or without TBI, followed by IV infusion of hematopoietic cells from the individual (autologous), or from a histocompatible related or unrelated donor (allogeneic), or from an identical twin (syngeneic) (National Marrow Donor Program, 2018). Autologous transplants often have a shortened period of pancytopenia (reduction in the cellular components of the blood), when individuals are at risk for bleeding, serious infections, or sepsis.

The HCT procedure is associated with severe nutritional consequences that require prompt, proactive intervention. The patient should have a thorough nutrition assessment before the initiation of therapy, ongoing reassessments, and monitoring throughout the entire transplant course. The acute toxicities of immunosuppression can last for 2 to 4 weeks after the transplant and include nausea, vomiting, anorexia, dysgeusia, stomatitis, oral and esophageal mucositis, fatigue, and diarrhea. In addition, immunosuppressive medications can also adversely affect nutrition status. Complications of delayed-onset nutrition-related symptoms include varying degrees of mucositis, xerostomia, and dysgeusia. Mucositis, which is often severe and extremely painful, develops in more than 75% of transplant patients (Macris Charuhas, 2013).

Depending on the transplant regimen, individuals may have little or no oral intake, and the GI tract can be significantly compromised in the early posttransplant period. For many patients, PN is a standard component of care and is indicated for those who are unable to tolerate oral or enteral feeding (AND EAL, 2013; Macris Charuhas, 2013). In addition, administration of optimal levels of PN often is complicated by the frequent need to interrupt it for the infusion of antibiotics, blood products, and IV medications. Careful monitoring and the use of more concentrated nutrient solutions, increased flow rates and volumes, and double- or triple-lumen catheters often are needed to achieve optimal nutrition intakes.

Graft-Versus-Host Disease (GVHD)

Graft-versus-host disease (GVHD) is a major complication seen primarily after allogeneic transplants, in which the donated "donor" stem cells react against the tissues of the transplant recipient "host." The functions of several target organs (skin, liver, gut, lymphoid cells) are disrupted and are susceptible to infection. Acute GVHD can occur within the first 100 days after the transplant (Macris Charuhas, 2013). It may resolve, or it may develop into a chronic form that requires long-term treatment and dietary management. Chronic GVHD can develop up to 3 months after transplant and is observed with increased frequency in nonidentical related donors and unrelated donors. Chronic GVHD can affect the skin, oral mucosa (ulcerations, stomatitis, xerostomia), and the GI tract (anorexia, reflux symptoms, diarrhea) and can cause changes in body weight. Skin GVHD is characterized by a maculopapular rash. GVHD of the liver, evidenced by jaundice and abnormal liver function tests, often accompanies GI GVHD and further complicates nutrition management. Other acute or chronic complications of HCT include osteoporosis, pulmonary disease, impaired renal function, rejection of the graft, growth abnormalities in children, sepsis, and infection (Flowers et al, 2018; Macris Charuhas, 2013) Nutrition-related symptoms associated with HCT may persist; individuals receiving outpatient marrow transplantation require frequent monitoring and intervention (Macris Charuhas, 2013).

The symptoms of acute GI GVHD can be severe; individuals may experience gastroenteritis, abdominal pain, nausea, vomiting, and large volumes of secretory diarrhea. Immunosuppressive medications and a phased dietary regimen should be instituted (Flowers et al, 2018; Macris Charuhas, 2013). The first phase consists of total bowel rest and the use of PN until diarrhea subsides. The second phase reintroduces oral feedings of beverages that are isotonic (mimic the balance of water, salt, and sugar that can be as easily taken up by the body as water), low residue, and lactose-free so as to compensate for the loss of intestinal enzymes secondary to alterations in the intestinal villi and mucosa (Flowers et al, 2018). If these beverages are tolerated, phase three includes the reintroduction of solids that contain low levels of lactose, fiber, fat, and total acidity, and no gastric irritants. In phase four dietary restrictions are progressively reduced as foods are gradually introduced and tolerance is established. Phase five is the resumption of the individual's regular diet (Flowers et al, 2018).

Nutrition Precautions with Neutropenia

Individuals receiving HCT become immunocompromised and require supportive therapy, including medications and dietary changes to prevent infection. Some cancer centers and hospitals continue to prescribe a low-microbial, low-bacteria, "neutropenic" diet for people with neutropenia. However, there is no clear evidence that a restrictive diet of only cooked foods reduces overall rates of infection or death (Wolfe et al, 2018). Current recommendations are for nutrition education to include dietary counseling on safe food handling and avoidance of foods that pose a risk of infection while patients are neutropenic and until immunosuppressive therapy has been completed (Macris Charuhas, 2013; Wolfe et al, 2018). These patients should avoid foods that contain unsafe levels of bacteria (raw meats, spoiled or moldy foods including some artisanal and soft cheeses, and unpasteurized beverages) and use special handling of raw meats, game, poultry, eggs, utensils, cutting boards, and countertops. Thorough hand washing is critical to food safety as is the avoidance of untested well water. Store foods at appropriate temperatures (below 40° F and above 140° F) (Macris Charuhas, 2013) (see Table 35.6).

NUTRITION MONITORING AND EVALUATION

Dietetic professionals must determine and quantify their patients' nutrition care goals by monitoring progress, measuring and evaluating outcomes and changes, and documenting this information throughout the process. Symptoms can evolve throughout treatment so monitoring and evaluation needs to be tailored to each person's therapeutic needs based on the severity of disease and intensity of treatment. Monitoring and evaluation of these factors is needed to effectively diagnose nutrition problems that should be the focus of future nutrition interventions (AND EAL, 2013) (see Chapter 9; Box 35.7.)

PEDIATRIC CANCER

Like adults, children with cancer can experience malnutrition and nutrition-related symptoms as a result of their cancer and its treatment.

Malnutrition can have long-term side effects with childhood cancer treatment such as slow or stunted growth and development, compromised bone health, eating disorders, and decreased quality of life (Fatemi and Sheridan-Neumann, 2013). Children with advanced cancer are at greater risk of severe nutritional depletion than adults are due to the frequent use of more aggressive, multimodality treatment. Deficiencies in energy and protein can affect growth adversely, although the effects may be temporary, and catch-up growth depends on how much energy children are able to consistently consume (Fatemi and Sheridan-Neumann, 2013). Some cancer treatment regimens may have an effect on growth and development that is independent of nutritional deprivation. HCT is now an accepted and increasingly successful intensive therapy for a wide range of disorders in children.

Psychogenic food refusal in children requires interventions that address underlying psychological issues. Families and caregivers often express their fears through a preoccupation with eating and maintaining weight. Creative efforts are required to minimize the psychological effects of fear, unpleasant hospital routines, unfamiliar foods, learned food aversions, and pain. Nutrition intervention strategies that use oral intake should stress the maximum use of favorite, nutrient-dense foods during times when intake is likely to be best, and food aversions are least likely to occur. Oral medical foods can be useful, but their acceptance is often a problem.

EN support by nasogastric tube (up to 3 months) or gastrostomy tube (more than 3 months) may be indicated for some children who are able to cooperate and who have functional GI tracts. PN is indicated for children who are receiving intense treatment associated with severe GI toxicity (intractable vomiting and severe diarrhea) and for children with favorable prognoses who are malnourished or have a high risk of developing malnutrition. PN is seldom indicated for children with advanced cancer associated with significant deterioration or with diseases that are unresponsive to therapy.

American Society for Parenteral and Enteral Nutrition has established standards for the nutrition screening and specialized nutrition support for all hospitalized pediatric patients. The nutritional requirements of pediatric patients with cancer are similar, with an adjustment for activity, to those of normal growing children. Often pediatric patients with cancer are not bedridden but are as active as their healthy peers. Factors that may alter nutrient requirements in cancer include the effect of the disease on host metabolism, the catabolic effects of cancer therapy, and physiologic stress from surgery, fever, malabsorption, and infection. Fluid requirements are increased during anticancer therapy or in the presence of fever, diarrhea, or renal failure. Micronutrients may require supplementation during periods of poor intake, stress, or malabsorption. The best long-term indicator of adequate nutrient intake is growth. Children have increased nutritional requirements for growth and development that must be met despite extended periods of cancer treatment (see Chapters 15 through 17). A special vulnerability exists during the adolescent growth spurt.

Advanced Cancer and Palliative Care

Palliative care is the care of an individual when curative measures are no longer considered an option by either the medical team or the individual. Hospice care focuses on relieving symptoms and supporting individuals with a life expectancy of months, not years (NHPCO, 2018c). The objectives are to provide for optimal quality of life; relieve physical symptoms; alleviate isolation, anxiety, and fear associated with advanced disease; and to help patients maintain independence as long as possible. The goals of nutrition intervention should focus on managing nutrition-related symptoms such as pain, weakness, loss of appetite, early satiety, constipation, weakness, dry mouth, and dyspnea (Trentham, 2013). Another important goal is maintaining strength and energy to enhance quality of life, independence, and the ability to perform activities of daily living. Nutrition should be provided as tolerated, according to patient preference or as desired along with emotional support and awareness of and respect for individual needs and wishes. The pleasurable aspects of eating should be emphasized.

The use of nutrition support and hydration in individuals with advanced, incurable cancer is a difficult and often controversial issue and should be determined on a case-by-case basis. Providing hydration to a terminal patient may cause pain, is intrusive, and may cause symptoms including vomiting, ascites, edema, and pulmonary congestion (Trentham, 2013). Dehydration can be part of the natural transition process. Advance directives are legal documents that guide health care providers regarding the specific wishes of individuals, outlining the extent of their desired medical care, including the provision of artificial nutrition and hydration.

NUTRITION RECOMMENDATIONS FOR CANCER SURVIVORS

Recommendations for survivors are very similar to the recommendations for cancer prevention already discussed. The ACS defines anyone living with a cancer diagnosis as a cancer survivor from the time of diagnosis through the balance of life (Rock et al, 2012). The ACS guidelines as well as the WCRF and AICR recommendations provide sound diet, nutrition, and physical activity advice for primary cancer prevention and health for all individuals, including cancer survivors. See the recommendations on cancer prevention (Rock et al, 2012; WCRF/AICR, 2018).

Cancer survivorship encompasses three phases: active treatment and recovery, living after recovery (including living disease-free or with stable disease), and advance cancer and end of life (Rock et al, 2012). Cancer survivors represent one of the largest groups of people living with a chronic disease. It is estimated that there will be 15.5 million survivors in the United States in 2018 (ACS, 2019b). The majority of individuals with cancer are able to return to full function and regain quality of life. This trend is expected to continue because of recent awareness in cancer prevention, advances in cancer detection, development of more effective cancer treatments, and advancements in determining the genetic causes of cancer. Long-term cancer survivors should now focus on healthy weight management, healthy diets, and physical activity geared toward secondary cancer and chronic disease prevention (Box 35.8).

Box 35.8 Physical Activity for Survivors

Before participating in any type of physical activity and exercise program, individuals should be advised to undergo evaluation by qualified professional to first assess for cardiovascular fitness post cancer treatment and design an individualized physical assessment and activity plan if safe and appropriate.

- The Survivorship Training and Rehab (STAR) certified specialists are available around the country in large and small cancer centers; the program's goal is the health care professionals seeking certification how rehab can help cancer patients and about the unique needs of cancer survivors after cancer treatment (Oncology Rehab Partners [ORP], 2018).

- The American College of Sports Medicine (ACSM) offers a certification program for trainers working with people diagnosed with cancer (a certified cancer exercise trainer) (ACSM, 2018).

- The YMCA's Livestrong (http://www.ymca.net/livestrong-at-the-ymca) is available across the United States and offers physical activity and exercise opportunities to support cancer survivors.

CLINICAL CASE STUDY

Daniel is a 54-year-old white man with a recent diagnosis of colon cancer. He has experienced some blood in the stool over time but never followed up on his doctor's referral. He lost 20 pounds in the 3 months before his diagnosis because of lack of appetite and lower intestinal discomfort. Prediagnosis, his diet consisted of drinking protein shakes his son purchased at the local gym. He has been very pleased with his weight loss as he has struggled with obesity over time but knew something was wrong. His medical history also includes hypertension and elevated cholesterol levels.

Daniel underwent surgery to remove the tumor and 2 rounds of chemotherapy. He recalls that he received some nutrition information from the inpatient registered dietitian nutritionist right before he was discharged but was anxious to go home, did not pay attention to the diet instruction, and could not find the paperwork once he got home. He has lost an additional 15 pounds in the past month and has been admitted once for dehydration caused by lack of fluid intake and because of symptoms related to ongoing episodes of diarrhea after eating. He states he is not sleeping well and doesn't feel rested.

His current food and nutrition history includes small meals with a usual intake of approximately 1500 calories daily. He eats three times a day and reports he does not have the energy to prepare food, so while his wife is at work, he has started drinking the prepared protein shakes again and is warming canned soup in the microwave. He is also drinking sports drinks because he has been encouraged to increase his fluid intake. He has a sweet tooth, and because his appetite is low, he rewards himself with ice cream or sherbet. His beverages include whole milk, apple juice, and an occasional "finger" of scotch each night. He has been referred to see the outpatient registered dietitian nutritionist.

Biochemical Data
WBC count: 4.2 th/mm3 (low end WNL)
Hematocrit: 32% (L)
Fasting Blood Glucose: 93 mg/dL (WNL)
Hematocrit: 31 mg/dL (L)
Ferritin 21 ng/mL (L)
Serum sodium: 147 mmol/L (H)

Anthropometric Data
Height: 70"
Weight history: Usual body weight: 220 lb, preoperative weight: 200 lb, 1-month postoperative weight: 185 lb
Current body mass index (BMI): 28

Medications
Metoclopramide (Reglan) 30 minutes before each meal
Metoprolol (Toprol)

Hydrochlorothiazide
FOLFOX (Folinic Acid, 5-Fluorouracil (5-FU) and Oxaliplatin)

Dietary Supplements
One-A-Day for Men
Lycopene

Nutrition Diagnostic Statements
- Inadequate fluid intake related to increased needs from chemotherapy and surgery induced diarrhea as evidenced by typical day intake and high serum sodium level.
- Inadequate protein and energy intake related to poor appetite and diarrhea as evidenced by decreased food and beverage and unintended weight loss.

Nutrition Care Questions
1. Assess Daniel's labs and medical history. What kind of a daily eating plan would you design with Daniel so that he can meet his nutritional requirements with food and fluid?
2. After reviewing Daniel's medical, social, and physical activity history, what other factors could be contributing to his difficulty with eating and his inability to regain weight?
3. Would you include Daniel's family members in your counseling sessions? If so, why? If not, why?
4. As Daniel continues to be seen for survivorship care at your clinic, what late-occurring side effects of cancer treatment should you anticipate and continue to monitor? Could any of these side effects affect his ongoing nutritional status? If so, should any laboratory tests be ordered or evaluated? What other factors should be monitored as a part of your nutritional care?
5. What type of integrative strategies would you deploy with Daniel to support his healing and survivorship?

Nutrition Interventions
Nutrition prescription: Small, frequent meals consisting of energy-dense, well cooked, low residue and moderate fat foods and limited simple carbohydrates. Monitor white blood cell count and educate on principles of food safety.

Nutrition education: Update Daniel's knowledge of appropriate nutrition therapy after a colon resection. Discuss tolerance of different food groups; sources of protein; energy-dense, easy-to-prepare menu options; and healthy beverage selections, including advising him to discontinue consumption of daily alcoholic beverage; and goal caloric intake needed for slow, steady weight gain. Suggest he consider eating every 2 hours to create an external reminder to eat. Recommend he review his hypertension and cholesterol lowering medications and doses with his physicians because his need for medication may have changed with his significant weight loss.

Continued

CLINICAL CASE STUDY—cont'd

At follow-up visits address weight stabilization, bowel function, food and beverage intake and tolerance; encourage physical activity (physician approved) starting with short walks to regain muscle strength. Daniel should be accompanied by a friend or family member on these walks. Encourage Daniel to follow-up with his primary care physician to discuss his problems sleeping.

Nutrition counseling: Coordinate with patient and family members to ensure appropriate foods and beverages are available for consumption. Discuss expected acute and long-term side effects from surgery. Establish physical activity goals for next 3 months.

Nutrition Monitoring and Evaluation

1. Body weight trends
2. Hydration status
3. Serum prealbumin levels and creatinine levels (over 3 months)
4. Physical activity
5. Schedule follow-up session in 2 weeks, with optional phone call between visits

USEFUL WEBSITES

Academy of Nutrition and Dietetics Oncology Tool Kit
Academy of Nutrition and Dietetics (AND) Standards of Practice and Standards of Professional Performance for Oncology Nutrition Practice
American Cancer Society (ACS)
American Institute for Cancer Research (AICR)
National Cancer Institute (NCI)
National Center for Complementary and Integrative Health (NCCIH)
Oncology Nutrition Dietetic Practice Group (ONDPG)
World Cancer Research Fund (WCRF)

REFERENCES

Abrams D: Integrative Oncology: The Role of Nutrition. In Leser M, Ledesma N, Bergerson S, et al, editors: *Oncology nutrition for clinical practice*, Chicago, 2013, Oncology Nutrition Dietetic Practice Group.

Academy of Nutrition and Dietetics (AND), Evidence Analysis Library (EAL): *Oncology nutrition evidence-based nutrition practice guidelines*, Chicago, 2013, Academy of Nutrition and Dietetics.

Academy of Nutrition and Dietetics: *Nutrition Terminology Reference Manual (eNCPT): Dietetics Language for Nutrition Care*. Available at: http://www.ncpro.org.

Academy of Nutrition and Dietetics: *Oncology tool kit*, Chicago, 2010, Academy of Nutrition and Dietetics.

Academy of Nutrition and Dietetics: Position of the Academy of Nutrition and Dietetics: use of nutritive and nonnutritive sweeteners, *J Acad Nutr Diet* 112(5):739–758, 2012.

Adachi Y, Nojima M, Mori M, et al: For JACC Study Insulin-like growth factor-related components and the risk of liver cancer in a nested case-control study, *Tumour Biol* 37(11):15125–15132, 2016.

Alavanja MC: Introduction: pesticides use and exposure, extensive worldwide, *Rev Environ Health* 24(4):303–309, 2009.

Allen BG, Bhatia SK, Anderson CM, et al: Ketogenic diets as an adjuvant cancer therapy: history and potential mechanism, *Redox Biol* 2:963–970, 2014.

Alsanad SM, Williamson EM, Howard RL: Cancer patients at risk of herb/food supplement–drug interactions: a systematic review, *Phytother Res* 28(12):1749–1755, 2014.

American Academy of Dermatology: *Vitamin D*. Available at: https://www.aad.org/media/stats-vitamin-d. 2018.

American Cancer Society: *Anemia in people with cancer*, 2017.

American Cancer Society: *Soy and Cancer: Our Expert's Advice*. Retrieved from https://www.cancer.org/latest-news/soy-and-cancer-risk-our-experts-advice.html. 2019a.

American Cancer Society: *Cancer facts and figures 2018*, Atlanta, GA, 2019b, American Cancer Society.

American Cancer Society: *Prevention and early detection guidelines*. Available at: https://www.cancer.org/health-care-professionals/american-cancer-society-prevention-early-detection-guidelines.html. 2018a.

American Cancer Society: *Family cancer syndromes* 2018b.

American Cancer Society: *How chemotherapy drugs work*, 2016.

American College of Sports Medicine: *ACSM/ACS certified cancer exercise trainer*. Available at: https://www.acsm.org/get-stay-certified/get-certified/specialization/cet. 2018.

American Institute for Cancer Research: *Continuous Update projects 2018*, 2018a.

American Institute for Cancer Research/World Cancer Research Fund: *Diet – what to eat to lower cancer risk*. Available at: https://www.aicr.org/reduce-your-cancer-risk/recommendations-for-cancer-prevention/2018b.

American Institute for Cancer Research: *Foods that fight cancer*, 2018c.

American Joint Committee on Cancer: *Cancer staging system*, 2018.

Applebaum AJ, Stein EM, Lordebaum A J, et al: Optimism, social support, and mental health outcomes in patients with advanced cancer, *Psychooncology* 23(3):299–306, 2014.

Arends J, Bachmann P, Baracos V, et al: ESPEN guidelines on nutrition in cancer patient, *Clin Nut* 35(1):11–48, 2017.

Arnold M, Renehan AG, Colditz GA: Excess weight as a risk factor common to many cancer sites: words of caution when interpreting meta-analytic evidence, *Cancer Epidemiol Biomarkers Prev* 26(5):663–665, 2017.

Arnold M, Jiang L, Stefanick ML, et al: Duration of adulthood overweight, obesity, and cancer risk in the women's health initiative: a longitudinal study from the United States, *PLoS Med* 13(8):e1002081, 2016.

Baggerly CA, Cuomo RE, French CB, et al: Sunlight and vitamin D: necessary for public health, *J Am Coll Nutr* 34(4):359–365, 2015.

Bagnardi V, Rota M, Botteri E, et al: Alcohol consumption and site-specific cancer risk: a comprehensive dose–response meta-analysis, *Brit J Cancer* 112(3):580–593, 2015.

Bender A, Collins K, Higginbotham S: Nutrition and cancer prevention. In Leser M, Ledesma N, Bergerson S, et al, editors: *Oncology nutrition for clinical practice*, Chicago, 2013, Oncology Dietetic Practice Group.

Blagodatski A, Yatsunskaya M, Mikhailova V, et al: Medicinal mushrooms as an attractive new source of natural compounds for future cancer therapy, *Oncotarget* 9(49):29259–29274, 2018.

Bradbury KE, Balkwill A, Spencer EA, et al: Organic food consumption and the incidence of cancer in a large prospective study of women in the United Kingdom, *Brit J Cancer* 110(9):2321–2326, 2014.

Brantsæter AL, Ydersbond TA, Hoppin JA, et al: Organic food in the diet: exposure and health implications, *Ann Rev Pub Health* 38:295–313, 2017.

Camp KM, Trujillo E: Position of the Academy of Nutrition and Dietetics: nutritional genomics, *J Acad Nut Diet* 114(2):299–312, 2014.

Centers for Disease Control and Prevention: *Health, United States, 2018: adult obesity facts*, Hyattsville, MD, 2018, US Department of Health and Human Services.

Chasen MR, Dippenaar AP: Cancer nutrition and rehabilitation—its time has come! *Curr Oncol* 15(3):117–122, 2008.

Chlebowski RT, Anderson GL, Manson JE, et al: Low-fat dietary pattern and all cancer mortality in the Women's Health Initiative (WHI) randomized controlled trial, *J Clin Oncol* 35(25):2919–2926, 2018.

Chen Y, Ling L, Su G, et al: Effect of intermittent versus chronic calorie restriction on tumor incidence: a systematic review and meta-analysis of animal studies, *Sci Rep* 6:33739, 2016.

Choi SW, Friso S: Epigenetics: a new bridge between nutrition and health, *Adv Nutr* 1(1):8–16, 2010.

Cordova MJ, Riba MB, Spiegel D: Post-traumatic stress disorder and cancer, *Lancet Psychiatry* 4(4):330–338, 2017.

Cronin KA, Lake AJ, Scott S, et al: Annual Report to the Nation on the Status of Cancer, part I: National cancer statistics, *Cancer* 124(13): 2785–2800, 2018.

Dang T, Nguyen C, Tran PN: Physician beware: severe cyanide toxicity from amygdalin tablets ingestion, *Case Rep Emerg Med* 2017:4289527, 2017.

Davis EL, Oh B, Butow PN, et al: Cancer patient disclosure and patient-doctor communication of complementary and alternative medicine use: a systematic review, *Oncologist* 21(1)58–59, 2014.

Elliott L: Symptom management of cancer therapies. In Leser M, Ledesma N, Bergerson S, et al, editors: *Oncology nutrition for clinical practice*, Chicago, 2013, Oncology Nutrition Dietetic Practice.

Environmental Protection Agency: *Risk management for bisphenol A (BPA).* Available at: https://www.epa.gov/assessing-and-managing-chemicals-under-tsca/risk-management-bisphenol-bpa 2017.

Ewa B, Danuta MŠ: Polycyclic aromatic hydrocarbons and PAH-related DNA adducts, *J Appl Genet* 58(3):321–330, 2017.

Fatemi D, Sheridan-Neumann. Nutritional management of the pediatric oncology patient. In Leser M, Ledesma N, Bergerson S, et al, editors: *Oncology nutrition in clinical practice*, Chicago, 2013, Oncology Nutrition Dietetic Practice Group.

Feldman D, Krishnan AV, Swami S, et al: The role of vitamin D in reducing cancer risk and progression, *Nat Rev Cancer* 14(5):342–357, 2014.

Flowers ME, McDonald G, Carpenter P, et al: *Long-term follow-up after hematopoietic stem cell transplant; general guidelines for referring physicians,* Fred Hutchinson Cancer Research Center/Seattle Cancer Care Alliance, Version June 2018, pp 1–108.

Fontana L, Villareal DT, Das SK, et al: Effects of 2-year calorie restriction on circulating levels of IGF-1, IGF-binding proteins and cortisol in nonobese men and women: a randomized clinical trial. *Aging Cell* 15(1):22–27, 2016.

Food and Drug Administration: *Additional information about high-intensity sweeteners permitted for use in food in the United States.* Retrieved from https://www.fda.gov/food/food-additives-petitions/additional-information-about-high-intensity-sweeteners-permitted-use-food-united-states. 2018.

Food and Drug Administration: *Bisphenol A (BPA): for use in food content application.* Available at: https://www.fda.gov/food/food-additives-petitions/bisphenol-bpa-use-food-contact-application. 2014.

Gaziano JM, Sesso HD, Christen WG, et al: Multivitamins in the prevention of cancer in men: the Physicians' Health Study II randomized controlled trial, *JAMA* 308(18):1871–1880, 2012.

Gill C: Nutrition Management for Cancers of the Gastrointestinal Tract. In Leser M, Ledesma N, Bergerson S, et al, editors: *Oncology nutrition for clinical practice*, Chicago, 2013, Oncology Nutrition Dietetic Practice Group.

Grant BL: Nutritional effects of cancer treatment: chemotherapy, biotherapy, hormone therapy and radiation therapy. In Leser M, Ledesma N, Bergerson S, et al, editors: *Oncology nutrition for clinical practice*, Chicago, 2013, Oncology Nutrition Dietetic Practice Group.

Grant BL: *Academy of Nutrition and Dietetics pocket guide to the nutrition care process and cancer*, Chicago, 2015, Academy of Nutrition and Dietetics.

Gröber U, Holzhauer P, Kisters K, et al: Micronutrients in oncological intervention, *Nutrients* 8(3):163, 2016.

Guppy A, Jamal-Hanjani M, Pickering L: Anticancer effects of metformin and its potential as a therapeutic agent for breast cancer, *Future Oncol* 7(6):727–736, 2011.

Haller H, Winkler MM, Klose P, et al: Mindfulness-based interventions for women with breast cancer: an updated systematic review and meta-analysis, *Acta Oncol* 56(12):1665–1676, 2017.

Hamilton KK: Nutritional needs of the adult oncology patient. In Leser M, Ledesma N, Bergerson S, et al, editors: *Oncology nutrition for clinical practice*, Chicago, 2013, Oncology Nutrition Dietetic Practice Group.

Harvie MN, Howell T: Could intermittent energy restriction and intermittent fasting reduce rates of cancer in obese, overweight, and normal-weight subjects? A summary of evidence, *Adv Nutr* 7(4):690–705, 2016.

Havrila C, Read CP, Mack D: Medical and radiation oncology. In Marian M, Roberts S, editors: *Clinical nutrition for oncology patients*, Sudbury, Mass, 2010, Jones and Bartlett.

Huebner J, Marienfeld S, Abbenhardt C, et al: Counseling patients on cancer diets: a review of the literature and recommendations for clinical practice, *Anticancer Res* 34(1):39–48, 2014.

Huhmann MB, August D: Surgical oncology. In Marian M, Roberts S, editors: *Clinical nutrition for oncology patients*, Sudbury, Mass, 2010, Jones and Bartlett.

Inoue-Choi M, Robien K: Cancer and Nutrition: Significance and Background. In Leser M, Ledesma N, Bergerson S, et al, editors: *Oncology nutrition for clinical practice*, Chicago, 2013, Oncology Dietetic Practice Group.

Israel B: *How many cancers are caused by the environment?* Scientific American. 2010.

Iwamoto RR, Haas ML, Gosselin TK: *Manual for radiation oncology and nursing practice and education*, ed 4, Pittsburgh, 2012, Oncology Nursing Society.

King N, Balneaves LG, Levin GT, et al: Surveys of cancer patients and cancer health care providers regarding complementary therapy use, communication, and information needs, *Integr Cancer Ther* 14(6): 515–524, 2015.

Kushi LH, Doyle C, McCullough M, et al: American Cancer Society guidelines on nutrition and physical activity for cancer prevention: reducing the risk of cancer with healthy food choices and physical activity, *CA Cancer J Clin* 62(1):30–67, 2012.

Landrigan PJ, Benbrook C: GMOs, herbicides, and public health, *New Eng J Med* 373(8):693–695, 2015.

LeMay-Nedjelski L, Mason-Ennis JK, Taibi A: Omega-3 Polyunsaturated Fatty Acids Time-Dependently Reduce Cell Viability and Oncogenic MicroRNA-21 Expression in Estrogen Receptor-Positive Breast Cancer Cells (MCF-7), *Int J Mol Sci* 19(1):E244, 2018.

Levin R: Nutrition Risk Screening and Assessment of the Oncology Patient. In Leser M, Ledesma N, Bergerson S, et al, editors: *Oncology nutrition for clinical practice*, Chicago, 2013, Oncology Nutrition Dietetic Practice Group.

Levine ME, Suarez JA, Brandhorst S, et al: Low protein intake is associated with a major reduction in IGF-1, cancer, and overall mortality in the 65 and younger but not older population, *Cell Metab* 19(3):407–417, 2014.

Link A, Balaguer F, Goel A: Cancer chemoprevention by dietary polyphenols: promising role for epigenetics, *Biochem Pharmacol* 80(12):1771–1792, 2010.

Park J, Morley TS, Kim M, et al: Obesity and cancer—mechanisms underlying tumour progression and recurrence, *Nat Rev Endocrinol* 10(8):455–465, 2014.

Macris Charuhas PM: Medical nutrition therapy for hematopoietic cell transplantation. In Leser M, Ledesma N, Bergerson S, et al, editors: *Oncology nutrition for clinical practice*, Chicago, 2013, Oncology Nutrition Dietetic Group.

Marian M: Energetics, exercise and cancer: In Leser M, Ledesma N, Bergerson S, et al, editors: *Oncology nutrition for clinical practice*, Chicago, 2013, Oncology Nutrition Dietetic Practice Group.

Marra MV, Bailey RL: Position of the Academy of Nutrition and Dietetics: Micronutrient supplementation, *J Acad Nut Diet* 118(11):2162–2173, 2018.

Melina V, Craig W, Levin S: Position of the Academy of Nutrition and Dietetics: vegetarian diets, *J Acad Nut Diet* 116(12):1970–1980, 2016.

Merzel RL, Boutom SM, Chen J: Folate binding protein: therapeutic natural nanotechnology for folic acid, methotrexate, and leucovorin, *Nanoscale* 9(7):2603–2615, 2017.

Michałowicz J: Bisphenol A—sources, toxicity and biotransformation, *Environ Toxicol Pharmacol* 37(2):738–758, 2014.

National Cancer Institute: *Artificial sweeteners and cancer,* 2016a.

National Cancer Institute: *Gerson therapy*, 2016b.

National Cancer Institute: *Antioxidants and cancer prevention*, 2017.

National Center for Complementary and Integrative Health: *The use of complementary and alternative medicine in the United States: cost data*, 2018.

National Comprehensive Cancer Network: *NCCN clinical practice guidelines in. Oncology* (NCCN Guidelines). Available at: https://www.nccn.org/professionals/. 2019.

National Hospice and Palliative Care Organization: *How can palliative care help?* Available at: https://www.nhpco.org/palliative-care-overview/explanation-of-palliative-care/, 2019.

National Institutes of Health, National Cancer Institute: *Cancer genetics overview PDQ*, 2018a.

National Institutes of Health, National Cancer Institute: *Cannabis and cannabinoids PDQ*, 2019b.

National Institutes of Health, National Cancer Institute: *Chemotherapy and you*, 2018a.

National Institutes of Health, National Cancer Institute: *Eating hints before, during, and after treatment*, 2018b.

National Institutes of Health, National Cancer Institute: *Radiation therapy and you*, 2016a.

National Institutes of Health, National Cancer Institute: *Gerson therapy PDQ*, 2016b.

National Institutes of Health, National Cancer Institute: *NCI dictionary of cancer terms*, 2015.

National Institutes of Health, National Cancer Institute: *SEER Stat fact sheet: all cancer sites*, 2018c.

National Institutes of Health, National Cancer Institute: *Tea and cancer prevention*, 2010.

National Institutes of Health, National Institute of Environmental Health Services: *14th Report on Carcinogens*, 2016.

National Institutes of Environmental Health Services: *Bisphenol A (BPA)*, 2017.

National Marrow Donor Program: *Transplant basics*, 2018.

Nguyen A, Nadler E: Integrative oncology: medical nutrition therapy for head and neck cancer. In Leser M, Ledesma N, Bergerson S, et al, editors: *Oncology nutrition for clinical practice*, Chicago, 2013, Oncology Nutrition Dietetic Practice Group.

O'Brien S, Leser M, Ledesma N: Diets, functional foods and dietary supplements for cancer prevention and survival. In Leser M, Ledesma N, Bergerson S, et al, editors: *Oncology nutrition for clinical practice*, Chicago, 2013, Oncology Nutrition Dietetic Practice Group.

Oncology Rehab Partners: *STAR Program Information*, 2018.

Pantavos A, Ruiter R, Feskens EF, et al: Total dietary antioxidant capacity, individual antioxidant intake and breast cancer risk: the Rotterdam study, *Int J Cancer* 136(9):2178–2186, 2015.

Park J, Morley TS, Kim M, et al: Obesity and cancer—mechanisms underlying tumour progression and recurrence, *Nat Rev Endocrinol* 10(8):455–465, 2014.

Polovich M, Whitford JM, Olsen MM: *Chemotherapy and biotherapy guidelines and recommendations for practice*, ed 4, Pittsburgh, 2014, Onc Nurs Soc.

Quinn BJ, Kitagawa H, Memmott RM, et al: Repositioning metformin for cancer prevention and treatment, *Trends Endocrinol Metab* 24(9):469–480, 2013.

Rock CL, Doyle C, Demark-Wahnefried W, et al: Nutrition and physical activity guidelines for cancer survivors, *CA Cancer J Clin* 62(4):243–274, 2012.

Santarpia L, Contaldo F, Pasanisi F: Nutritional screening and early treatment of malnutrition in cancer patients, *J Cachexia Sarcopenia Muscle* 2(1): 27–35, 2011.

Schwalfenberg GK: The alkaline diet: is there evidence that an alkaline pH diet benefits health? *J Environ Pub Health* 2012:727630, 2012.

Schwedhelm C, Boeing H, Hoffmann G, et al: Effect of diet on mortality and cancer recurrence among cancer survivors: a systematic review and meta-analysis of cohort studies, *Nut Rev* 74(12):737–748, 2016.

Sharma P, Dwivedi S: Nutrigenomics and nutrigenetics: new insight in disease prevention and cure, *Indian J Clin Biochem* 32(4):371–373, 2017.

Sieri S, Agnoli C, Pala V, et al: Dietary glycemic index, glycemic load, and cancer risk: results from the EPIC-Italy study, *Sci Rep* 7(1):9757, 2017.

Spees CK and Grainger EM. Nutrigenomics and Cancer. In Leser M, Ledesma N, Bergerson S, et al, editors: *Oncology nutrition for clinical practice*, Chicago, 2013, Oncology Dietetic Practice Group.

The Scored Patient-Generated Subjective Global Assessment (PG-SGA©): Website. Available at: http://pt-global.org/wp-content/uploads/2014/09/PG-SGA-Sep-2014-teaching-document-140914.pdf. 2014.

Thomson CA, McCullough ML, Wertheim BC, et al: Nutrition and physical activity cancer prevention guidelines, cancer risk and mortality in the women's health initiative, *Cancer Prev Res* 7(1):42–53, 2014.

Trentham K. Nutritional management of oncology patients in palliative and hospice settings. In Leser M, Ledesma N, Bergerson S, et al, editors: *Oncology nutrition for clinical practice*, Chicago, 2013, Oncology Nutrition Dietetic Practice Group.

Trujillo EB, Dixon SW, Claghorn K, et al: Closing the gap in nutrition care at outpatient cancer centers: ongoing initiatives of the oncology nutrition dietetic practice group, *J Acad Nut Diet* 118(4):749–760, 2018.

Truong M, Paradies Y, Priest N: Interventions to improve cultural competency in healthcare: a systematic review of reviews, *BMC Health Serv Res* 14(1):99, 2014.

Tsuimoto T, Yamamoto Y, Wasa M, et al: L-glutamine decreases the severity of mucositis induced by chemoradiotherapy in patients with locally advanced head and neck cancer: a double-blind, randomized, placebo-controlled trial, *Oncol Rep* 33(1):33–39, 2015.

U.S. Department of Agriculture: *USDA Database for the isoflavone content of selected foods, release 2.0* . Available at: http://www.ars.usda.gov/nutrientdata/isoflav. 2016.

U.S. Department of Health and Human Services and U.S. Department of Agriculture: *2015–2020 Dietary Guidelines for Americans*, ed 8, December 2015.

Vernieri C, Nichetti F, Raimondi A, et al: Diet and supplements in cancer prevention and treatment: Clinical evidences and future perspectives, *Crit Rev Oncol Hematol* 123:57–73, 2018.

Weber DD, Aminazdeh-Gohari S, Kofler B: Ketogenic diet in cancer therapy, *Aging* 10(2):164–165, 2018.

Weichenthal S, Moase C, Chan P: A review of pesticide exposure and cancer incidence in the Agricultural Health Study cohort, *Environ Health Perspec* 118(8):1117–1125, 2010.

Weylandt KH, Serini S, Chen YO, et al: Omega-3 Polyunsaturated fatty acids: the way forward in times of mixed evidence, *BioMed Res Int* Volume 2015, Article ID 143109. doi:10.1155/2015/143109.

Wilkes GM, Barton-Burke M: *2013 Oncology nursing drug handbook*, Burlington, 2013, Jones and Bartlett.

Wilson KM, Mucci LA, Rosner BA, et al: A prospective study of dietary acrylamide intake and the risk of breast, endometrial, and ovarian cancers, *Cancer Epidemiol Biomarkers Prev* 19(10):2503–2515, 2010.

Wolfe HR, Sadeghi N, Agrawal D, et al: Things we do for no reason: neutropenic diet, *J Hosp Med* 13(8):573-576. 2018.

World Cancer Research Fund/American Institute for Cancer Research: *Diet, nutrition, physical activity, cancer: a global perspective*. Continuous Update Project Expert Report, 2018.

World Health Organization: *Global status report on alcohol and health 2018*. World Health Organization, 2019.

World Health Organization: *Carcinogenicity of the consumption of red and processed meat*, 2015.

Zhou S, Zhang S, Shen H, et al: Curcumin inhibits cancer progression through regulating expression of microRNAs, *Tumor Biol* 39(2): 1010428317691680, 2017.

36

Medical Nutrition Therapy for HIV and AIDS

Maureen Lilly, MS, RDN
Solenne Vanne, MS, RDN

KEY TERMS

acquired immune deficiency syndrome (AIDS)
acute HIV infection
antiretroviral therapy (ART)
asymptomatic HIV infection
Bioelectrical Impedance Analysis (BIA)
CD4+ cells
CD4 count

clinical latency
drug resistance
HIV-associated lipodystrophy syndrome (HALS)
HIV ribonucleic acid (RNA)
human immunodeficiency virus (HIV)
lipoatrophy
lipohypertrophy

long-term nonprogression
opportunistic infections (OIs)
people living with HIV/AIDS (PLWHA)
preexposure prophylaxis or PrEP
seroconversion
symptomatic HIV infection
T-helper lymphocyte cells
viral load

Acquired immune deficiency syndrome (AIDS) is caused by the human immunodeficiency virus (HIV). HIV affects the body's ability to fight off infection and disease, which if left untreated, can ultimately lead to AIDS and death. Medications used to treat HIV have enhanced the quality of life and increased life expectancy of people living with HIV/AIDS (PLWHA). These antiretroviral therapy (ART) medications slow the replication of the virus but do not eliminate HIV infection. With increased access and improvements to ART, people are living longer with HIV.

THE CHANGING FACE OF HIV IN THE UNITED STATES

During the start of the HIV epidemic in the 1980s much of the nutrition therapy focused on symptoms such as anorexia, catabolism and wasting syndrome, chronic infection, fever, poor nutrient intake, nausea, vomiting, diarrhea, malabsorption, metabolic disturbances, lack of access to food, depression, and side effects of drugs and treatment (Young, 1997). Life expectancy before treatment became available was around 12 years from time of infection. Since the release of the first antiretroviral therapy AZT (azidothymidine) in 1996 to the release of the newest single tablet regimens starting in 2006, the face of HIV has changed dramatically. In a recent study on life expectancy in PLWHA, researchers found that the average life expectancy of a 20-year-old patient who started ART after 2008 and had a low viral load was 78 years, similar to the general population (Trickery, 2017). With these new advancements in treatment much of the nutrition therapy focus has shifted. Unfortunately, health issues such as cardiovascular disease and insulin resistance are increasingly prevalent, and

PLWHA are at a greater risk of the same chronic diseases as the general population.

Special consideration should be taken into account when working with the aging population of PLWHA who are more likely to have experienced trauma during the beginning of the HIV epidemic. Many have a long history of loss of close friends and partners, isolation and criminalization, and years of poor health due to drug side effects and opportunistic infections (OIs).

A New Era in HIV Prevention

Even though antiretroviral therapy (ART) has been a revolutionary advance in keeping HIV positive individuals from progressing to AIDS, it is estimated that globally an average of about 5000 new HIV infections occur daily (UNAIDS, 2018).

The primary route of HIV transmission remains sexual contact. Although prevention efforts have reduced sexual transmission significantly, the rate of new infection demonstrates the need for better tools. In 2012 the Food and Drug Administration approved an antiretroviral drug combination for preexposure prophylaxis, or PrEP. In a study of heterosexual partners in which one partner was HIV positive and one partner HIV negative, consistent use of the drug Truvada (emtricitabine/tenofovir) reduced infections by at least 90% (Baeten et al, 2012). Similarly, in a study of 2500 HIV-negative men and transgender women who have sex with men, participants were randomly assigned to receive either Truvada or a placebo once daily. Participants with detectable levels of the antiretrovirals in their blood showed a 92% to 99% greater protection against HIV (Grant et al, 2010).

Short-term side effects of Truvada for PrEP have been reported to be gastric distress, diarrhea, headaches, and weight loss. The long-term side effects of PrEP in HIV-negative individuals are still unknown. However, the same possible long-term effects observed in HIV-positive individuals using Truvada should be monitored in this patient population. Monitoring for lactic acidosis, liver damage, renal issues, and bone density are important (Gilead Sciences, 2017).

Portions of this chapter were written by Kimberly R. Dong MS, RDN, and Cindy Mari Imai, PhD, RDN.

Furthermore in the advancement of HIV prevention and ending stigmatization, there is now strong evidence showing that a PLWHA who is on ART medication with an undetectable viral load, cannot sexually transmit the virus to an HIV-negative individual. The public health campaign that has launched from two long-term PARTNER studies starting in 2009 is called U=U (Undetectable=Untransmittable). This messaging is key to public health and provider understanding of HIV. (Eisinger et al, 2019).

Other prevention efforts being researched have focused on HIV vaccines, microbicides, and antibodies. Development of a prophylactic HIV vaccine has been difficult as HIV's ability to elude the immune system makes traditional vaccines like those used for smallpox and measles ineffective. However, two potential vaccines, Imbokodo and HVTN 702, show some promise. Two vaccine efficacy trials are currently underway in Africa for Imbokodo, and trials for HVTN 702 are set to begin in 2020 (National Institutes of Health [NIH], 2017). A microbicide vaginal ring, dapivirine, has been shown to partially reduce risk of HIV infection in clinical trials. Additional trials are underway while waiting for regulatory approval (Microbicide Trials Network, 2016). Antibody-mediated prevention has shown great potential in laboratory studies; the antibody VRC01 prevented over 90% of nearly 200 sample HIV strains from infecting human cells. Two multinational placebo-controlled trials using intravenous infusion of VRC01 have also recently begun (National Institute of Allergy and Infectious Diseases [NIAID], 2016). These efforts give hope to greatly reducing the transmission of HIV, especially in areas where there is poor access to medication.

Nutritional status plays an important role in maintaining a healthy immune system and preventing the progression of HIV to AIDS. To develop appropriate nutrition recommendations, the nutrition professional should be familiar with the pathophysiology of HIV infection, the medication and nutrient interactions, and the barriers to adequate nutrition.

EPIDEMIOLOGY AND TRENDS

Global Status of HIV and AIDS

The first cases of AIDS related to HIV were described in 1981. In 1983 HIV was isolated and identified as the core agent leading to AIDS. Since then, the number of people with HIV has increased gradually, leading to a global pandemic affecting socioeconomic development worldwide. The continuing rise in the population of people living with HIV is reflective of new HIV infections and the widespread use of ART, which has delayed the progression of HIV infection to death. Globally, an estimated 36.9 million people were living with HIV or AIDS in 2017. The number of new HIV infections and related deaths has fallen in the last decade. In 2017 there were 1.8 million new HIV infections and 960,000 AIDS-related deaths reported (UNAIDS, 2018).

Despite increased prevention efforts and availability of ART, geographic variation in HIV infection is evident. The majority of infections continue to occur in the developing world (Fig. 36.1). Sub-Saharan Africa remains the region most heavily affected by HIV, accounting for 66% of new HIV infections and 61% of AIDS-related deaths (UNAIDS, 2018). Within sub-Saharan Africa, heterosexual transmission is the most prevalent mode of HIV transmission. Other populations particularly at risk of HIV infection include injection drug users, men who have sex with men, sex workers, and clients of sex workers (Fig. 36.2).

The United States

Within the United States, more than 1.1 million people are living with HIV infection and 14% may be unaware of their HIV status (Dailey

et al, 2017). Although more people are living with a diagnosis of HIV or AIDS, incidence has remained relatively stable since the 1990s. In 2016 men accounted for 70% of all diagnoses of HIV infection, and the most common route of transmission was male-to-male sexual contact (Centers for Disease Control and Prevention [CDC], 2017a). The rate of new infections among women, primarily through heterosexual contact, has decreased since 2011 (CDC, 2017a). The largest percentage of persons living with HIV infection is among those aged 50 to 54. However, in 2016, people aged 25 to 29 accounted for the highest rate of new HIV infections. Ethnic populations disproportionately affected by HIV include African Americans and Latinos, who accounted for 44% and 25% of new HIV diagnoses, respectively, in 2016 (CDC, 2017a). The most common route of transmission among men is male-to-male sexual contact and among women is heterosexual contact (see Fig. 36.2).

While there is limited research on transgender PLWHA (those with a differing gender identity than the sex assigned at birth), growing evidence indicates a disproportionately high rate of HIV infection within the transgender (also referred to as trans) community. According to the Report of the 2015 Transgender Survey, the rate of HIV among transgender respondents is 1.4%, among trans women (male-to-female) the rate is 3.4%, and an estimated 19% of black trans women are living with HIV (James et al, 2016). Additionally, the 2009–2014 National HIV Surveillance System reported that 2351 of U.S. transgender people were newly diagnosed with HIV. Of those diagnosed, 84% were transgender women, 15.4% were transgender men (female-to-male), and 0.7% were an additional gender identity. Moreover, more than half of those diagnosed lived in the South and 52% identified as African American (Clark et al, 2017).

PATHOPHYSIOLOGY AND CLASSIFICATION

Primary infection with HIV is the underlying cause of AIDS. HIV invades the genetic core of the CD4+ cells, which are T-helper lymphocyte cells, and which are the principal agents involved in protection against infection. HIV infection causes a progressive depletion of CD4+ cells, which eventually leads to immunodeficiency.

HIV infection progresses through four clinical stages: acute HIV infection, clinical latency, symptomatic HIV infection, and progression of HIV to AIDS. The two main biomarkers used to assess disease progression are HIV ribonucleic acid (RNA) (also known as the viral load) and CD4+ T-cell count (CD4 count).

Acute HIV infection is the time from transmission of HIV to the host until seroconversion, the production of detectable antibodies against the virus, occurs. Half of individuals experience physical symptoms such as fever, malaise, myalgia, pharyngitis, or swollen lymph glands at 2 to 4 weeks after infection, but these generally subside after 1 to 2 weeks. Because of the nonspecific clinical features and short diagnostic window, acute HIV infection is rarely diagnosed. HIV seroconversion occurs within 3 weeks to 3 months after exposure. If HIV testing is done before seroconversion occurs, a false negative may result despite HIV being present. During the acute stage, the virus replicates rapidly and causes a significant decline in CD4+ cell counts. Eventually, the immune response reaches a viral set point, when the viral load stabilizes and CD4+ cell counts return closer to normal.

A period of clinical latency, or asymptomatic HIV infection, then follows. Further evidence of illness may not be exhibited for as long as 10 years postinfection. The virus is still active and replicating, although at a decreased rate compared with the acute stage, and CD4+ cell counts continue to steadily decline. In 3% to 5% of HIV-infected individuals, long-term nonprogression occurs, in which CD4+ cell

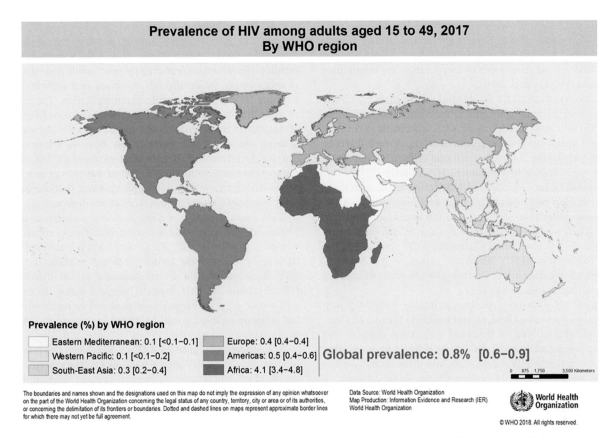

Fig. 36.1 Global prevalence of HIV/AIDS among adults aged 15 to 49. (World Health Organization [website]. https://www.who.int/gho/hiv/epidemic_status/prevalence/en/.)

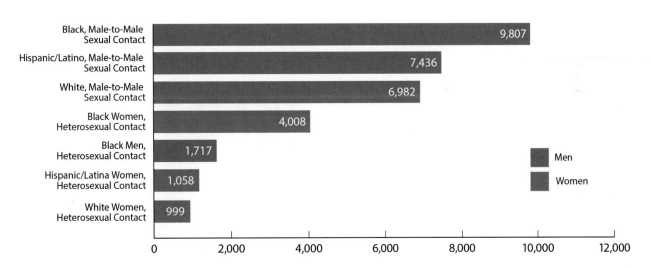

Note: Subpopulations representing 2% or less of all people who received an HIV diagnosis in 2017 are not represented in this chart.

Fig. 36.2 Estimated percentage of HIV diagnoses by route of transmission in the United States, 2013. (Centers for Disease Control and Prevention [CDC]: *HIV Surveillance Report* [website]. https://www.cdc.gov/hiv/library/reports/surveillance, 2015.)

counts remain normal and viral loads can be undetectable for years without medical intervention (Department of Health and Human Services [DHHS], 2017). It has been suggested that this unique population has different and fewer receptor sites for the virus to penetrate cell membranes (Wanke et al, 2009).

In the majority of cases, HIV slowly breaks down the immune system, making it incapable of fighting the virus. When CD4+ cell counts fall below 500 cells/mm³ individuals are more susceptible to developing signs and symptoms such as persistent fevers, chronic diarrhea, unexplained weight loss, and recurrent fungal or bacterial infections, all of which are indicative of symptomatic HIV infection.

As immunodeficiency worsens and CD4 counts fall to even lower levels, the infection becomes symptomatic and progresses to AIDS. The progression of HIV to AIDS increases the risk of opportunistic infections (OIs), which generally do not occur in individuals with healthy immune systems. The CDC classifies AIDS cases as positive laboratory confirmation of HIV infection in persons with a CD4+ cell count less than 200 cells/mm³ (or less than 14%) or documentation of an AIDS-defining condition (Box 36.1).

HIV is transmitted via direct contact with infected body fluids such as blood, semen, preseminal fluid, vaginal fluid, and breastmilk. Cerebrospinal fluid surrounding the brain and spinal cord, synovial fluid surrounding joints, and amniotic fluid surrounding a fetus are other fluids that can transmit HIV. Saliva, tears, and urine do not contain enough HIV for transmission. In the United States sexual transmission is the most common way HIV is transmitted, and injection drug use is the second most prevalent method of transmission (see Fig. 36.2).

Most HIV positive people have HIV-1 infection, which, unless specified, is the type discussed in this chapter. HIV-1 mutates readily and has become distributed unevenly throughout the world in different strains, subtypes, and groups. HIV-2, first isolated in Western Africa, is less easily transmitted, and the time between infection and illness takes longer.

MEDICAL MANAGEMENT

HIV-related morbidity and mortality stem from the HIV virus weakening the immune system as well as the virus's effects on organs (such as the brain and kidneys). If untreated, the HIV virion (virus particle) can replicate at millions of particles per day and rapidly progress through the stages of HIV disease. Due to the ability of the virus to rapidly replicate and become drug resistant, taking more than one class of drugs allows for significantly decreased viral replication through targeting HIV on different pathways of replication. The introduction of three-drug combination ART in 1996 transformed the treatment of patients living with HIV and has significantly decreased AIDS-defining conditions and mortality (see Box 36.1). Previously, most drugs were formulated as individual medications, but increasingly many are available as fixed-dose (two or more drugs in a single pill) combinations to simplify treatment regimens, decrease pill burden, and potentially improve patient medication adherence.

CD4 count is used as a major indicator of immune function in people with HIV infection. CD4 counts generally are monitored every 3 to 4 months. In addition, HIV RNA (viral load) is monitored on a regular basis because it is the primary indicator to gauge the efficacy of ART. Initiation of ART is recommended for all individuals with HIV regardless of CD4 levels. There are a few occasions when ART would be deferred due to clinical and or psychosocial factors, but initiation of therapy is to be started as soon as possible (Roberts et al, 2016).

The fundamental goals of ART are to achieve and maintain viral suppression, reduce HIV-related morbidity and mortality, improve the quality of life, and restore and preserve immune function. This generally can be achieved within 10 to 24 weeks if there are no complications with adherence or resistance to medications (DHHS, 2017). Because the guidelines for HIV management evolve rapidly, it is beneficial to frequently check for updated recommendations.

Classes of Antiretroviral Therapy Drugs

Currently ART includes more than 25 antiretroviral agents from six mechanistic classes of drugs:

- Nucleoside and nucleotide reverse transcriptase inhibitors (NRTIs)
- Nonnucleoside reverse transcriptase inhibitors (NNRTIs)
- Protease inhibitors (PIs)
- Integrase inhibitors (INSTIs)

BOX 36.1   CDC Case Definition AIDS-Defining Clinical Conditions/Opportunistic Infections (OIs)

Bacterial infections, multiple or recurrent (among children <13 years)
Candidiasis (bronchi, trachea, or lungs)
Candidiasis (esophagus)
Cervical cancer (invasive)
Coccidioidomycosis (disseminated or extrapulmonary)
Cryptococcosis (extrapulmonary)
Cryptosporidiosis (intestinal, >1-month duration)
Cytomegalovirus disease (other than liver, spleen, or nodes)
Cytomegalovirus retinitis (with loss of vision)
Encephalopathy (HIV related)
Herpes simplex: chronic ulcers (>1-month duration)
Herpes simplex: bronchitis, pneumonitis, or esophagitis
Histoplasmosis (disseminated or extrapulmonary)
Isosporiasis (intestinal, >1-month duration)
Kaposi sarcoma
Lymphoid interstitial pneumonia or pulmonary lymphoid hyperplasia complex
Lymphoma, Burkitt (or equivalent term)

Lymphoma, immunoblastic (or equivalent term)
Lymphoma, primary (brain)
Mycobacterium avium complex (disseminated or extrapulmonary)
Mycobacterium kansasii (disseminated or extrapulmonary)
Mycobacterium tuberculosis (any site, pulmonary, disseminated, or extrapulmonary)
Pneumocystis jiroveci pneumonia
Pneumonia (recurrent)
Progressive multifocal leukoencephalopathy
Salmonella septicemia (recurrent)
Toxoplasmosis (brain)
  Wasting syndrome attributed to HIV: >10% involuntary weight loss of baseline body weight plus (1) diarrhea (two loose stools per day for ≥30 days) or (2) chronic weakness and documented fever (≥30 days, intermittent or constant) in the absence of concurrent illness or condition other than HIV infection that could explain the findings (e.g., cancer, tuberculosis).

Schneider E et al: Revised surveillance case definitions for HIV infection among adults, adolescents, and children aged <18 months and for HIV infection and AIDS among children aged 18 months to <13 years—United States, 2008, *MMWR Recomm Rep* 57(RR-10):1, 2008.
AIDS, Acquired immune deficiency syndrome; *CDC,* Centers for Disease Control and Prevention; *HIV,* human immunodeficiency virus.

- Fusion inhibitors
- Chemokine receptor 5 (CCR5) antagonists

Advances in HIV ART treatments have been moving rapidly. The focus of medication development includes continuing to create single tablet regimens, decreasing metabolic complications, decreasing overall toxicities, and better prevention of drug resistance. Nonadherence to ART can lead to drug resistance due to HIV's tendency to rapidly mutate.

Predictors of Adherence

When initiating ART, patients must be willing and able to commit to lifelong treatment, and they should understand the benefits and risks of therapy and the importance of adherence. The patient's understanding about HIV disease and the specific regimen prescribed is critical. A number of factors have been associated with poor adherence, including low levels of health literacy, neurocognitive impairment, psychosocial issues (e.g., mental illness, housing instability, low social support, stressful life events, dementia, or psychosis), active substance use, stigma, denial, difficulty with taking medication (e.g., trouble swallowing pills, daily schedule issues), complex regimens (e.g., pill burden, dosing frequency, food requirements), adverse drug effects, treatment fatigue, and inconsistent access to medication (DHHS, 2017).

Food insecurity has been associated with increased behaviors that can transmit HIV and decreased access to HIV treatment and care; it also can be a predictor of poor adherence (Singer et al, 2015; Young et al, 2014) because medications are costly and they often compete with food for available resources. Continued encouragement is needed to help patients adhere as closely as possible to the prescribed doses for all ART regimens.

Illicit Drug Use

In the United States injection drug use is the second most common mode of HIV transmission after sexual contact. The most commonly used illicit drugs associated with HIV infection are heroin, cocaine, and methamphetamine. The chaotic lifestyle associated with drug use is associated with poor or inadequate nutrition, food insecurity, homelessness, and mental health concerns. This complicates treatment of HIV if the individual is using drugs and potentially can lead to poor adherence with ART medications.

Injection drug use is linked strongly to transmission of blood-borne infections such as HIV, hepatitis B virus, and hepatitis C virus (HCV), especially if needles are reused or shared (see *Focus On: HIV and Hepatitis C Virus Coinfection*). Coinfection of HIV and HCV increases the risk of cirrhosis. Chronic HCV infection also complicates HIV treatment because of ART-associated hepatotoxicity. Special medical and nutrition treatment considerations should be taken into account if the liver is damaged from drug use, if there is coinfection with hepatitis, or if there is increased nutrient excretion from diuresis and diarrhea (Hendricks and Gorbach, 2009; Tang et al, 2010).

Food-Drug Interactions

Some ART medications require attention to dietary intake. It is important to ask individuals with HIV to report all medications, including vitamins, minerals, other supplements, and recreational substances that they consume in order to assess their needs fully and prevent drug interactions and nutrient deficiencies. Some nutrients can affect how drugs are absorbed or metabolized. Interactions between food and drugs can influence the efficacy of the drug or may cause additional or worsening adverse effects. For example, grapefruit juice and

◎ FOCUS ON

HIV and Hepatitis C Virus Coinfection

About one quarter of people in the United States who have human immunodeficiency virus (HIV) also are coinfected with hepatitis C virus (HCV). According to the Centers for Disease Control and Prevention (CDC), 70% of HIV-infected injection drug users also have HCV (CDC, 2017b). Although it is unknown if HCV accelerates HIV disease progression, it has been shown to damage the liver more quickly in HIV-infected persons. In the presence of hepatic impairment, the metabolism and excretion of antiretroviral medications may be impaired, affecting the efficacy of HIV treatment. In addition, three classes of anti-HIV medications (nucleoside and nucleotide reverse transcriptase inhibitors, nonnucleoside reverse transcriptase inhibitors, and protease inhibitors) are associated with hepatotoxicity. Therefore it is important for HIV-infected patients to be tested for HCV, preferably before starting ART, to appropriately manage treatment and prolong healthy liver function.

HCV is viewed as an opportunistic infection (OI) (not an acquired immune deficiency syndrome–defining illness) in HIV-infected persons because there are higher titers of HCV, more rapid progression to liver disease, and increased risk of cirrhosis (DHHS, 2017). Nutrition recommendations and dosing and choice of HIV medications must be adjusted for those with liver failure (see Chapter 29).

In 2014 the Food and Drug Administration (FDA) approved Harvoni, a simple one-pill-a-day regimen taken for 12 weeks.

Clinical studies show a 96% to 99% cure rate in individuals with HCV genotype 1 (Gritsenko and Hughes, 2015). The most common side effects of treatment are slow heart rate, weakness, fatigue, and headaches (Gilead Sciences, 2018).

PIs compete for the cytochrome P450 enzymes; thus individuals taking PIs who also drink grapefruit juice may have either increased or decreased blood levels of the drug. Table 36.1 provides potential nutrient interactions with ART medications (see Appendix 13).

Some ART medications can cause diarrhea, fatigue, gastroesophageal reflux, nausea, vomiting, dyslipidemia, and insulin resistance. Timing is also important for ART efficacy, so patients with HIV must take medications on a schedule. Some medications indicate that they must be taken with food or on an empty stomach. Sometimes food must be taken within a specific time frame of administering a medication. Refer to Table 36.1 for timing considerations with ART.

Medical Management

HIV infection should be confirmed by laboratory testing and not based on patient report (CDC, 2019). The presence of comorbidities such as heart disease, diabetes, hepatitis, and OIs may complicate the patient's treatment profile. Important assessment information includes the patient's past medical history and pertinent immediate family history for heart disease, diabetes, cancers, or other disorders. Metabolic issues such as dyslipidemia and insulin resistance are common in people with HIV due to inflammation from the viral infection and medication side effects, and are important to monitor. Biochemical measurements should be documented to determine the course of HIV treatment, efficacy of ART, and underlying malnutrition and nutrient deficiencies. Some common biochemical measurements include CD4 count, viral load, albumin, hemoglobin, iron status, lipid profile, liver function tests, renal function tests, glucose, insulin, and vitamin levels. Table 36.2 discusses conditions associated with HIV and their nutritional implications.

TABLE 36.1   Medication Interactions and Common Adverse Effects

	Take with Meal or Snack	Take on Empty Stomach	Take Without Regard to Food	Nausea	Vomiting	Diarrhea	Hyperlipidemia	Hyperglycemia	Fat Maldistribution	Pancreatitis	Taste Alterations	Loss of Appetite	Anemia	Vitamin or Mineral Deficiencies	Liver Toxicity
NRTIs															
emtricitabine and tenofovir disoproxil fumarate (Truvada) made by Gilead			X	X		X									X
zidovudine, lamivudine (Combivir) made by ViiV Healthcare			X	X		X			X	X		X	X		X
abacavir and lamivudine (Epzicom) made by ViiV Healthcare			X	X		X			X						X
Protease Inhibitors															
atazanavir and cobicistat (Evotaz) made by Bristol-Myers Squibb	X			X			X	X	X						
darunavir and cobicistat (Prezcobix) made by Janssen Therapeutics	X			X	X	X	X	X							
Integrase Inhibitors															
elvitegravir (Vitekta) made by Gilead	X			X		X									
Monoclonal Antibodies															
ibalizumab (Trogarzo) made by TaiMed Biologics and Theratechnologies				X		X									
Pharmacokinetic Enhancers															
cobicistat (Tybost) made by Gilead	X			X		X									
Combinations															
emtricitabine and tenofovir alafenamide (Descovy) made by Gilead			X	X		X									
emtricitabine, rilpivirine, and tenofovir alafenamide (Odefsey) made by Gilead	X														X
elvitegravir, cobicistat, emtricitabine, and tenofovir alafenamide (Genvoya) made by Gilead	X			X		X	X								X
bictegravir, emtricitabine, and tenofovir disoproxil fumarate (Biktarvy) made by Gilead			X	X		X									

HIV Drug Chart. POZ. (https://www.poz.com/drug_charts/hiv-drug-chart)
Medicines: HIV/AIDS. Gilead Sciences. (http://www.gilead.com/medicines)
Our Medicines. ViiV Healthcare (https://www.viivhealthcare.com/our-medicines.aspx)
Our Medicines. Bristol-Myers Squibb (https://www.bms.com/patient-and-caregivers/our-medicines.html)
Prezcobix. Janssen Therapeutics (https://www.prezcobix.com/home)
Ibalizumab. AIDS Info (https://aidsinfo.nih.gov/drugs/511/ibalizumab/0/patient)

TABLE 36.2 HIV-Related Conditions with Specific Nutrition Implications

Condition	Brief Description	Nutrition Implications
Pneumocystis pneumonia (PCP)	Potentially fatal fungal infection	Difficulty chewing and swallowing caused by shortness of breath
Tuberculosis (TB)	Bacterial infection that attacks the lungs	Prolonged fatigue, anorexia, nutrient malabsorption, altered metabolism, weight loss
Cryptosporidiosis	Infection of small intestine caused by parasite	Watery diarrhea, abdominal cramping, malnutrition and weight loss, electrolyte imbalance
Kaposi sarcoma	Type of cancer-causing abnormal tissue growth under the skin	Difficulty chewing and swallowing caused by lesions in oral cavity or esophagus Diarrhea or intestinal obstruction caused by lesions in intestine
Lymphomas	Abnormal, malignant growth of lymph tissue	Side effects from chemotherapy and cancer treatment - diarrhea, poor appetite, difficulty eating, neutropenia (see Chapter 35)
Brain abnormalities	Changes in motor and cognitive abilities	Inability to prepare food and coordinate movement
Small bowel abnormalities	Malabsorption	Weight loss, diarrhea, loss of appetite
Cytomegalovirus (disseminated)	Infection caused by herpes virus	Loss of appetite, weight loss, fatigue, enteritis, colitis
Candidiasis	Infection caused by fungi or yeast	Oral sores in mouth, difficulty chewing and swallowing, change in taste
HIV-induced enteropathy	Idiopathic, direct or indirect effect of HIV on enteric mucosa	Chronic diarrhea, weight loss, malabsorption, changes in cognition and behavior
HIV encephalopathy (AIDS dementia)	Degenerative disease of brain caused by HIV infection	Loss of coordination and cognitive function, inability to prepare food
Pneumocystis jiroveci pneumonia	Infection caused by fungi	Fever, chills, shortness of breath, weight loss, fatigue
Mycobacterium avium complex (disseminated)	Bacterial infection in lungs or intestine, spreads quickly through bloodstream	Fever, cachexia, abdominal pain, diarrhea, malabsorption

Coyne-Meyers K, Trombley LE: A review of nutrition in human immunodeficiency virus infection in the era of highly active antiretroviral therapy, *Nutr Clin Prac* 19:340, 2004; Falcone EL et al: Micronutrient concentrations and subclinical atherosclerosis in adults with HIV, *Am J Clin Nutr* 91:1213, 2010; McDermid JM et al: Mortality in HIV infection is independently predicted by host iron status and SLC11A1 and HP genotypes, with new evidence of a gene-nutrient interaction, *Am J Clin Nutr* 90:225, 2009; Pitney CL et al: Selenium supplementation in HIV-infected patients: is there any potential clinical benefit? *J Assoc Nurses AIDS Care* 20:326, 2009; Rodriguez M et al: High frequency of vitamin D deficiency in ambulatory HIV-positive patients, *AIDS Res Hum Retroviruses* 25:9, 2009.
AIDS, Acquired immune deficiency syndrome; *HIV,* human immunodeficiency virus; *PCP, Pneumocystis pneumonia; TB,* tuberculosis.

MEDICAL NUTRITION THERAPY

For people living with HIV, adequate and balanced nutrition intake is essential to maintain a healthy immune system, delay disease progression, and prolong life. As ART medications have evolved the overall risk for AIDS-related wasting has decreased and a shift to an increase in prevalence of obesity and cardiometabolic disease has occurred. Proper nutrition may help maintain lean body mass, reduce the severity of HIV-related symptoms (including cardiometabolic and digestive), improve quality of life, and enhance adherence to and effectiveness of ART. Therefore medical nutrition therapy (MNT) is integral to successfully manage HIV (see *Pathophysiology and Care Management Algorithm:* Human Immunodeficiency Virus Disease).

A registered dietitian nutritionist (RDN) can help patients mitigate potential adverse effects from medications or disease states and address nutritional concerns. Some common nutrition diagnoses in this population include the following:

- Inadequate oral food intake NI-2.1
- Inadequate energy intake NI-1.2
- Increased nutrient needs NI-5.1
- Swallowing difficulty NC-1.1
- Biting and chewing difficulty NC-1.2
- Altered gastrointestinal (GI) function NC-1.4
- Food-medication interaction NC-2.3
- Involuntary weight loss NC-3.2
- Overweight and obesity NC-3.3
- Food- and nutrition-related knowledge deficit NB-1.1
- Impaired ability to prepare foods or meals NB-2.4
- Poor nutrition quality of life NB-2.5

- Limited access to food NB-3.2
- Intake of unsafe foods NB-3.1

Having regular access to an RDN or other qualified nutrition professional can help PLWHA maintain a better quality of life. Patients are recommended to undergo a baseline nutrition assessment upon diagnoses with HIV (see Chapters 4 and 5). Because patients with HIV can have multifactorial complications, those who receive ongoing nutrition assessments have lower risk of complications from treatment. The Academy of Nutrition and Dietetics (AND) recommends that an RDN provide at least one to two MNT encounters per year for individuals with asymptomatic HIV infection and at least two to six MNT encounters per year for those with symptomatic but stable HIV infection (Willig, 2018). Individuals diagnosed with AIDS usually need to be seen more often because they may require nutrition support (see Chapter 12).

Ultimately, RDNs need to individualize MNT and determine frequency of nutrition counseling based upon the patient's needs. The major goals of MNT for persons living with HIV infection are to optimize nutritional status, immunity, and well-being; to maintain a healthy weight and lean body mass; to prevent nutrient deficiencies and reduce the risk of comorbidities; and to maximize the effectiveness of medical and pharmacologic treatments. Thus screening should be performed on all patients medically diagnosed with HIV to identify those at risk for nutritional deficiencies or in need of MNT. Due to the effects of HIV on the immune system, education around food safety concerns is important to discuss with clients, especially for individuals with low CD4 counts.

Patients who exhibit the various HIV-related symptoms or conditions listed in Table 36.3 would benefit from a referral to an RDN with

PATHOPHYSIOLOGY AND CARE MANAGEMENT ALGORITHM

Human Immunodeficiency Virus Disease

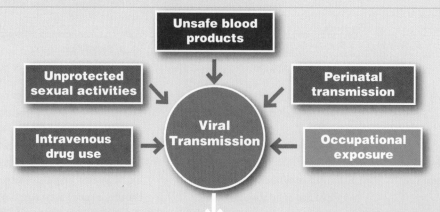

Clinical Findings

Acute HIV infection (Acute retroviral syndrome) Fever, fatigue, rash, headache, generalized lymphadenopathy, pharyngitis, myalgia, nausea/vomiting, diarrhea, night sweats, adenopathy, oral ulcers, genital ulcers, neurological symptoms, malaise, anorexia, weight loss, wasting syndrome
Seroconversion
HIV Positive Test HIV rapid tests; ELISA test, Western blot; PCR test
Asymptomatic HIV infection Abnormal metabolism, change of body composition (body cell mass loss with/without weight loss, lipoatrophy, lipohypertrophy), vitamin B_{12} deficiency, susceptibility to pathogens
Symptomatic HIV infection Weight loss, thrush, fever, loss of LBM with/without weight loss, diarrhea, oral hairy leukoplakia, herpes zoster, peripheral neuropathy, idiopathic thrombocytopenic purpura, pelvic inflammatory disease
Asymptomatic AIDS
Symptomatic AIDS (AIDS defined conditions) CD4 cell count <200/mm³, opportunistic infectious diseases (pneumocystitis jirovecii, pneumonia, others), Kaposi's sarcoma, lymphoma, HIV-associated dementia, HIV-associated wasting, vitamins/minerals deficiencies

Medical Management

Treat possible co-morbidities
Hyperglycemia, hyperlipidemia, hypertension, body composition changes, pancreatitis, kidney and liver diseases, hypothyroidism, hypogonadism, osteopenia, hepatitis-C
Monitoring
Fasting blood lipid, fasting glucose/insulin level, protein status, blood pressure, TSH/testosterone level, CD4 cell count, and viral load
Medication
Antiretroviral therapy, lipid lowering agents, antidiabetic agents, antihypertensive agents, appetite stimulants, hormone replacement therapy, treatment for coinfection diseases (i.e. hepatitis), prophylaxis and treatment for opportunistic infectious diseases

Nutrition Management

Considerations for generally healthy individuals with a well controlled viral load.
- Complete nutrition assessment 2-6 times/year
- Emphasize importance of early/ongoing nutritional intervention
- Promote adequate intake of nutrients and fluids, including vitamins A, B12, C, D, selenium, and zinc
- Emphasize regular exercise and physical activity
- Assess for psychosocial and economic barriers to food and provide resources
- Assess need for dietary supplementation, emphasizing food first when possible
- Inform patient of possible side effects, symptoms, and/or complications
- Monitor/manage metabolic and cardiovascular abnormalities (fasting glucose, blood lipids) and digestive complaints

Special considerations for symptomatic individuals with a high viral load and low CD4.
- Emphasize importance of food safety and sanitation
- Small, frequent, nutrient dense meals if necessary
- Monitor/manage gastrointestinal symptoms
- Appetite stimulants if necessary
- Parenteral nutrition if necessary
- Anabolic therapies

Management of drug side effects

TABLE 36.3 Nutrition Recommendations for Typical Adverse Effects

Adverse Effect	Nutrition Recommendations
Nausea, vomiting	Eat small, frequent meals. Avoid drinking liquids with meals. Drink cool, clear liquids. Try dry crackers, rice cakes, or toast. Try bland foods such as potatoes, noodles, rice, or canned fruits. Try adding ginger to meals and sipping on ginger tea between meals. Limit high-fat, greasy foods or foods that have strong odors such as ripe cheese or fish. Eat foods at room temperature or cooler. Wear loose-fitting clothes. Rest sitting up after meals. Keep a log of when nausea and vomiting occur and which foods seem to trigger it. Try eating ready-to-eat foods to eliminate smells from cooking. Incorporate mindful eating techniques into meal and snack times.
Diarrhea	Eat low residue, well-cooked foods Try plain carbohydrates such as white rice, rice congee, noodles, crackers, or white toast. Try low-fiber fruits like bananas and applesauce. Drink fluids that will replace electrolytes such as broths and oral hydration drinks. Try small, frequent meals. Avoid fatty, greasy foods. Avoid highly spiced foods. Avoid sugary items such as soda and fruit juice. Avoid milk and milk products or choose lactose free. Limit caffeine. Try gentle probiotic and prebiotic foods such as Greek yogurt and bananas. Try supplementing with glutamine (5-10 grams 2-3 times per day).
Loss of appetite	Eat small, frequent meals. Avoid drinking too many liquids that contain no calories. Focus on nutrient-dense foods such as yogurt smoothies and high callorie meal replacement drinks and bars, eggs, avocado, Greek yogurt, nut butters, cheese and whole grain breads. Add extra oils and fats to foods. Try to eat in a pleasant environment or eating with friends and family. Assess for signs of depression or changes in mental health that could be factoring into appetite changes.
Taste alterations	Add spices and herbs to foods. Avoid canned foods or canned oral supplements as these can have a metallic taste. Keep mouth clean by frequently brushing teeth and rinsing mouth before and after eating. Use plastic utensils if metal ones taste bad.
Hyperlipidemia	NCEP diet (see Chapter 32).
Hyperglycemia	Diet for patients with elevated blood sugar and diabetes (see Chapter 29).
Mouth and esophageal ulcers and sore throat	Try soft foods such as oatmeal, rice, applesauce, scrambled eggs, refried beans, shredded lean meat or fish, avocado, pureed soups, smoothies, or yogurt. Avoid acidic foods such as citrus, vinegar, spicy, salty, or hot foods. Moisten foods with gravy or sauces. Drink liquids with meals. Avoid acidic beverages. Try foods and beverages at room temperature. Use a food processor or blender to create desired consistency
Pancreatitis	Focus on low-fat foods and limit fat at each meal (see Chapter 28). May need pancreatic enzymes to aid in digestion.
Weight loss	Eat small, frequent meals. Focus on nutrient-dense foods such as protein and calorie rich smoothies and meal replacement beverages, eggs, nut butters, avocado, Greek yogurt, trail mixes, and tofu. Add rice, barley, avocado, and legumes to soups. Add dry milk powder, Greek yogurt, or protein powder to casseroles, hot cereals, and smoothies. Add a little olive oil, avocado, or nuts to meals.
Weight gain	Balanced Mediterranean, anti-inflammatory or DASH dietary pattern. Identify triggers for overeating. Increase physical activity and strength training.

NCEP, National Cholesterol Education Program.

TABLE 36.4	Factors to Consider in Nutrition Assessment
Medical	Stage of HIV disease Comorbidities Opportunistic infections Metabolic complications Biochemical measurements
Physical	Changes in body shape Weight or growth concerns Oral or gastrointestinal symptoms Functional status (i.e., cognitive function, mobility) Anthropometrics
Social	Living environment (support from family and friends) Behavioral concerns or unusual eating behaviors Mental health (i.e., depression)
Economical	Barriers to nutrition (i.e., access to food, financial resources)
Nutritional	Typical intake Food shopping and preparation Food allergies and intolerances Vitamin, mineral, and other supplements Alcohol and drug use

HIV, Human immunodeficiency virus.

TABLE 36.5	HIV-Associated Lipohypertrophy and Lipoatrophy	
Lipohypertrophy: Fat buildup		**Lipoatrophy: Fat loss**
Can occur: • Around the organs in the abdomen • On the back of the neck between the shoulders (buffalo hump) • In the breasts • Just under the skin, causes fatty bumps called lipomas		Can occur: • In the arms and legs • In the buttocks • In the face
Primary interventions: • Diet and exercise • Metformin (in patients with diabetes mellitus)		Primary interventions: • Switch HIV medications that contain a thymidine analog (stavudine or zidovudine to abacavir or tenofovir)

Guzman N, Al Aboud AM: HIV-associated lipodystrophy. In: *StatPearls [Internet]. Treasure Island (FL)*, StatPearls Publishing, 2019. Available from: https://www.ncbi.nlm.nih.gov/books/NBK493183/. Updated October, 27 2018.
HIV, Human immunodeficiency virus.

expertise in managing this disease. A comprehensive nutrition assessment should be performed at the initial visit. In addition, regular monitoring and evaluation are essential to detect and manage any undesirable nutritional consequences of medical treatments or the disease process. Strategies for managing the adverse effects are given in Table 36.3. Key factors to assess are listed in Table 36.4.

Anthropometry and Body Composition Measurements

Historically, the prevalence of undernutrition, AIDS-related wasting syndrome, and HIV-associated lipodystrophy syndrome (HALS) were much higher, but with advancements in HIV care and treatments these conditions occur less frequently (Table 36.5). Even though rates are lower, it is still important to assess patients early and evaluate for both undernutrition and overnutrition. Taking anthropometric measurements during the initial assessment provides a baseline for understanding the patients' nutritional status. Patients with HIV are aware of changes in their body shape and are instrumental in identifying these changes. Asking patients about body shape changes every 3 to 6 months helps practitioners catch any changes early on. Changes in body shape and fat redistribution can be monitored by anthropometric measurements. Commonly these are taken as circumferences around the waist, hip, midupper arm, and thigh, and as skinfold measurements of the triceps, subscapular, suprailiac, thigh, and abdomen. The use of Bioelectric Impedance Analysis (BIA) (see Chapter 5) can be a helpful tool for monitoring changes in both lean body mass and fat mass. Due to the decreased reliability of BIA in the presence of dehydration, which commonly can occur in individuals experiencing wasting and chronic diarrhea, the use of Bioelectric Impedance Vector Analysis (BIVA) can be a more useful aid in assessing nutritional status.

Wasting

Wasting implies unintentional weight loss and loss of lean body mass that is equal to or greater than 10% of a person's body weight and may be seen along with diarrhea and fever that is not associated with an infection (U.S. Department of Veterans Affairs, 2018). Wasting is strongly associated with an increased risk of disease progression and mortality.

The populations most at risk of experiencing wasting are individuals not receiving ART. Although wasting may be caused by a combination of factors, including inadequate dietary intake, malabsorption, and increased metabolic rates from viral replication or complications from the disease. Inadequate dietary intake can be caused by several issues related to conditions that affect the ability to chew or swallow food, gastrointestinal motility, neurologic diseases that affect perceptions of hunger or ability to eat, food insecurity related to psychosocial or economic factors, and anorexia from medications, malabsorption, systemic infections, or tumors (Mankal and Kotler, 2014). Until the underlying cause of weight loss is discovered, it will remain difficult to target effective nutrition therapy. It is important to closely monitor patients for unintentional weight loss because it can indicate progression of HIV disease.

HIV-associated Lipodystrophy Syndrome (HALS)

There is no consensus on the clinical definition of HALS, and the manifestations vary greatly from patient to patient. The syndrome encompasses both the metabolic abnormalities and body shape changes seen in some, but not all patients with HIV, similar to metabolic syndrome found in the general population. The lipodystrophy body shape changes that can occur include a buildup of body fat (lipohypertrophy) or loss of body fat (lipoatrophy). Individuals typically present with one or the other, but some present with a mixed picture of both (Figs. 36.3 and 36.4). Metabolic abnormalities have been associated with both lipohypertrophy and lipoatrophy and can also develop separately with no body composition changes (Currier, 2018). The most common metabolic abnormalities include hyperlipidemia (particularly high triglycerides and low-density lipoprotein [LDL] cholesterol and low high-density lipoprotein [HDL] cholesterol) and insulin resistance. These factors raise concern for increased risk of cardiovascular disease.

Cardiometabolic Risk

Individuals living with HIV are at a 1.5 to 2.0 increased risk for cardiovascular disease (CVD), compared with the general population (Glesby, 2017). Increasing evidence shows that this elevated risk is in

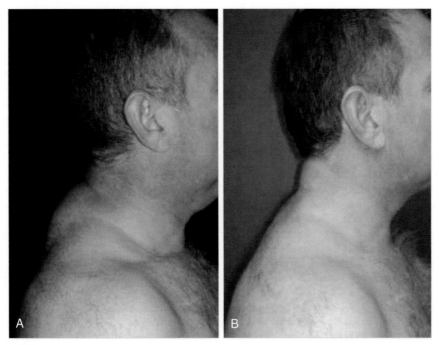

Fig. 36.3 A, Preoperative view of a 48-year-old man with cervicodorsal lipodystrophy that developed 7 years before his initial consultation. He also complained of anterior neck lipodystrophy and facial lipoatrophy. **B,** Postoperative view 21 months after excisional lipectomy, SAL of the cervicodorsal fat pad, rhytidectomy, anterior neck lift with submental fat excision, and autologous fat transfer from the abdomen to the nasolabial folds bilaterally.

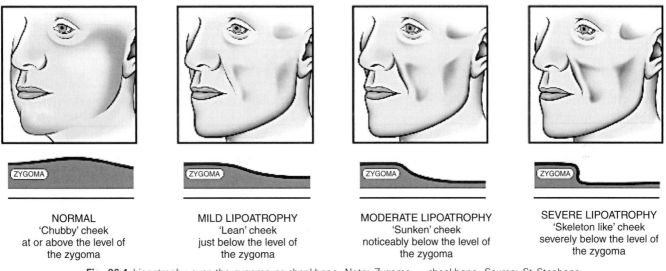

NORMAL	MILD LIPOATROPHY	MODERATE LIPOATROPHY	SEVERE LIPOATROPHY
'Chubby' cheek at or above the level of the zygoma	'Lean' cheek just below the level of the zygoma	'Sunken' cheek noticeably below the level of the zygoma	'Skeleton like' cheek severely below the level of the zygoma

Fig. 36.4 Lipoatrophy over the zygoma or cheekbone. Note: Zygoma = cheekbone. Source: St Stephens AIDS Trust, Chelsea and Westminster Hospital

part due to chronic immune activation and inflammation from the HIV virus itself, as well as the effects of ART on lipid profiles.

Inflammation plays a role in the general development of atherosclerosis, and HIV has been linked to an increase in several markers of inflammation including C-reactive protein (CRP) and interleukin (IL)-6. This low-level chronic activation of the immune system may adversely affect endothelial cells and promote a prothrombotic environment leading to atherosclerosis and plaque rupture (Currier, 2019).

Additionally, various medications have been shown to elicit a greater effect on lipid profiles than others (see Table 36.1). Even though receiving ART has been shown to increase risk of cardiovascular events,

not starting or being on ART increases risk of CVD to a greater extent (Currier, 2018).

Other general risk factors of CVD must also be taken into account when assessing an individual's CVD risk such as hypertension, diabetes mellitus, dyslipidemia, and cigarette smoking.

The cause of HALS is multifactorial and includes duration of HIV infection, duration and type of ART medications, age, gender, race and ethnicity, increased viral load, and increased body mass index (BMI). It is important to monitor individual anthropometric measurements along with blood lipid profile, A1C, and blood glucose.

For nutrition recommendations regarding lipohypertrophy and metabolic abnormalities, the guidelines set by the American Heart Association (AHA), the American College of Cardiology (ACC), and the American Diabetes Association are followed (see Chapters 29 and 32). Patients who complement a cardio-protective diet (see Chapter 32) with regular physical activity, such as aerobic exercise and resistance training, are likely to see further improvements in their health.

For patients who have high triglycerides, omega-3 fatty acids may be useful. Studies focusing on the impact of omega-3 fatty acids in individuals with HIV are limited. Some studies have shown 2 to 4 g of fish oil supplements per day lower serum triglyceride levels in patients with HIV (Paranandi et al, 2014). In a meta-analysis, which included four studies, omega-3 fatty acids intake lowered serum triglyceride concentrations in PLWHA on ART (Oliveira and Rondó, 2011). However, because the studies were not homogenous with regards to dose, population, and length of intervention, it is challenging to determine the amount of omega-3 fatty acids needed to see positive benefits. Nevertheless, supplementing with omega-3 fatty acids tends to be low risk and potentially beneficial. Coordination of care is advised for supplementation above 3 grams eicosapentaenoic acid (EPA)/ docosahexaenoic acid (DHA). This can help to mitigate potential side effects from supplementation including GI distress, hyperglycemia, and increased LDL cholesterol levels. It is important to discuss and monitor use of dietary supplements with each patient's health care team.

Obesity

Obesity in people with HIV also has been noted. Unintentional weight loss in HIV infection has been associated with mortality, but more careful review of individuals with a BMI greater than 25 kg/m^2 is needed. Recently a lower risk of developing a noncommunicable disease was observed among HIV-positive adults initiating ART who had a BMI of 25 to 29.9 kg/m^2 compared with HIV-positive adults initiating ART with a BMI of less than 25 kg/m^2 (Koethe et al, 2015). However, excess adiposity is associated with cardiovascular risk factors and inflammation. In the era of ART, it is no longer believed that continuously gaining body weight is a protective cushion against HIV-related wasting and progression to AIDS.

Some of the ART medications increase the risk of hyperlipidemia, insulin resistance, and diabetes. It is important to monitor these risk factors and provide nutrition recommendations to maintain a healthy weight. Physical activity, aerobic exercise, and resistance training are recommended to work synergistically with optimal nutrition intake to achieve a healthy weight and maintain lean body mass.

Social and Economic Factors

Depending on a patient's mental status, psychosocial issues may take precedence over nutrition counseling. Mental health conditions such as depression, bipolar disorder, anxiety, and posttraumatic stress disorder (PTSD) are common. Monitoring for mental health issues is important in order to provide referrals or engage in coordination of care with the patient's health care providers.

When individuals are unable to care for themselves, discussion with caretakers may be necessary to understand the patient's nutrition history. Particular habits, food aversions, timing of meals with medications, and related concerns should be documented.

Evaluation of access to safe, affordable, and nutritious food is a priority as this information will guide appropriate interventions. Common barriers include cost, location of supermarkets, lack of transportation, and lack of knowledge of healthier choices. Furthermore, stigma not only is a predictor of ART adherence, but also may prevent individuals with HIV from using nutrition programs and seeking support systems. HIV-related stigma is hypothesized to be a strong deterrent from seeking medical care, treatment, or support.

Marginalized populations, such as racial/ethnic minorities and those in the lesbian, gay, bisexual, transgender, queer (LGBTQ) community, often face increased discrimination and stigma, making them less likely to engage in health care. Additionally, some PLWHA, such as young gay African American males and transgender women, may be more likely to be experiencing multiple layers of marginalization and decreased community support (Arnold et al, 2014, Mayer et al, 2016). Providers who are mindful of individual considerations, such as preferred gender pronouns (e.g., he, she, they) and cultural food preferences, help to reduce stigmatization (see Chapter 10).

Nutrient Recommendations

When collecting the diet history, include a review of current intake, changes in intake, limitations with food access or preparation, food intolerances or allergies, supplement use, current medications, and alcohol and recreational drug use to help determine the potential for any nutrient deficiencies and assist in making individualized recommendations (see Chapter 4).

Adequate nutrition intake can help patients with HIV with symptom management and improve the efficacy of medications, disease complications, and overall quality of life (see Fig. 36.5 for a sample nutrition screening form). Note that a one-size-fits-all approach does not address the complexity of HIV. Recommendations in Box 36.2 to improve nutritional status, immunity, and quality of life; address drug-nutrient interactions or side effects; and identify barriers to desirable food intake should be personalized for the patient.

Energy and Fluid

When determining energy needs, take into consideration factors such as weight loss or gain, altered metabolism, nutrient deficiencies, severity of disease, comorbidities, and OIs, which can impact energy needs. Calculating energy and protein needs for this population is difficult because of other issues with wasting, obesity, HALS, and lack of accurate prediction equations. Some research suggests that resting energy expenditure is increased by approximately 10% in adults with asymptomatic HIV (Kosmiski, 2011). Limited research suggests that energy expenditure may increase by a similar amount in virally immune suppressed individuals on antiretrovirals. After an OI, nutritional requirements may increase up to 20% to 50% in adults and children (World Health Organization [WHO], 2005a). Continuous medical and nutrition assessment is necessary to make adjustments as needed. Individuals with well-controlled HIV are encouraged to follow the same principles of healthy eating and fluid intake recommended for the general population (see Chapter 10).

Generalized nutrient recommendations for transgender HIV patients are not yet established so clinicians need to determine which comparative standards to use when calculating energy needs. Gender-neutral kcal/kg calculations may be preferred. Notable metabolic changes following hormone therapy include the potential for transgender women on antiandrogens and estrogen therapy to exhibit a decrease in lean body mass and an increase in body fat. In turn, transgender men who receive androgen therapy may exhibit an increase in lean body mass and a decrease in body fat (World Professional Association for Transgender Health [WPATH], 2012; Wellington et al, 2012).

Protein

Currently, limited evidence-based research exists around ideal protein intake for PLWHA. When determining protein needs the clinician must take into account an individual's weight, activity level, other comorbidities, and complications related to HIV. The Association of Nutrition Services Agency (ANSA) proposed protein recommendations between 1.0 g/kg to 1.4 g/kg for weight maintenance and 1.5 g/kg

HIV/AIDS Screening Form

DATE: _____

Patient Name: _____ MR#: _____

DOB: _____ Age: ____Yrs. ____ Mos. Gender: ☐ Male ☐ Female

Medical Provider: _____

Ensure that all people with HIV infection are screened for nutrition-related problems, based on referral criteria regardless of setting, at each primary care provider visit. **Review and check all that apply:**

High Risk (HR) To Be Seen by RDN Within One Week	Moderate Risk (MR) To Be Seen by RDN Within One Month	Low Risk (LR) To Be Seen by RDN at Least Annually
A. HIV Diagnosis and Nutrition Assessment		
	☐ 1. HIV or AIDS newly diagnosed ☐ 2. No nutrition assessment by a registered dietitian or not seen by a registered dietitian in 12 months ☐ 3. Patient requests RDN consult	
B. Body Composition and Weight Concerns		
☐ 1. New wasting diagnosis ☐ 2. Poor growth, lack of weight gain or failure to thrive in pediatric patients ☐ 3. Five (5%) or more unintentional weight loss within four weeks ☐ 4. Ten (10%) or more unintentional weight loss over four to six months, (% weight change = last body wt − current body weight / last body weight x 100)	☐ 1. Underweight (< 20 BMI) ☐ 2. Evidence or suspected muscle loss ☐ 3. Obesity (>30 BMI) ☐ 4. Client or provider initiated weight management ☐ 5. Evidence for body fat change: ☐ a. Central fat adiposity ☐ b. Fat accumulation: ☐ 1. Neck ☐ 2. Upper back ☐ 3. Breasts ☐ 4. Other: _____	☐ 1. Stable desirable weight ☐ 2. In pediatrics, appropriate: ☐ a. Weight gain ☐ Growth and weight-for-height
C. Oral/GI Symptoms and Side Effects		
☐ 1. Severe dysphagia (swallowing difficulty) ☐ 2. Enteral or parenteral feedings ☐ 3. Complicated food-drug interactions	☐ 1. Possible food-drug-nutrient interactions ☐ 2. Food allergies or food intolerances: _____ ☐ 3. Oral or esophageal thrush ☐ 4. Dental problems interfering with intake ☐ 5. Persistent: ☐ a. Nausea or vomiting ☐ b. Diarrhea ☐ c. Heartburn ☐ d. Gas ☐ e. Bloating ☐ f. Poor appetite ☐ g. Other: _____	☐ 1. No oral symptoms or side effects ☐ 2. No GI symptoms or side effects
D. Metabolic and Other Medical Conditions and Labs		
☐ 1. Poorly controlled diabetes mellitus ☐ 2. Pregnancy ☐ 3. Infancy ☐ 4. Current illness or opportunistic infection ☐ 5. Dialysis	Abnormal, trending abnormal or taking medications to control: ☐1. Cholesterol, LDL-cholesterol, HDL-cholesterol or triglycerides ☐ 2. Blood glucose ☐ 3. Blood pressure ☐ 4. Creatinine, BUN, LFT, GFR ☐ 5. Potassium, phosphorous, sodium, or calcium, other_____ ☐ 6. Vitamin blood levels ☐ 7. Other nutrition-related labs: ___ ☐ 8. Osteopenia or osteoporosis ☐ 9. Liver disease ☐ 10. Kidney disease ☐ 11. Anemia, type: _____ ☐ 12. Cancer ☐ 13. Tuberculosis ☐ 14. CNS disease resulting in a decrease in functional capacity ☐ 15. Other: _____	☐ 1. Stable HIV disease and with no active infections ☐ 2. Normal blood levels of: ☐ a. Cholesterol ☐ b. Triglycerides ☐ c. Albumin ☐ d. Glucose ☐ 3. Normal: ☐ a. Hepatic function ☐ b. Renal function

Fig. 36.5 Nutrition screen and referral criteria for adults with HIV and AIDS. (From ADA MNT Evidence Based Guides for Practice. Copyright 2005, American Dietetic Association, now Academy of Nutrition and Dietetics, March 2005. For interim revisions see https://andevidencelibrary.com/topic.cfm?cat=4458.

High Risk (HR) To Be Seen by RDN Within One Week	Moderate Risk (MR) To Be Seen by RDN Within One Month	Low Risk (LR) To Be Seen by RDN at Least Annually
E. Psychosocial Barriers, Eating and Other Behaviors		
☐ Severely dysfunctional psychosocial situation (especially in children)	☐ 1. Suspected poor composition or adequacy of diet ☐ 2. Evidence of inappropriate or excessive vitamin, mineral or other dietary or herbal supplement intake ☐ 3. Inappropriate use of diet pills, laxatives or other over-the-counter medications ☐ 4. Substance abuse: Current or in the recovery process ☐ 5. Disordered eating: 　　☐ a. Anorexia 　　☐ b. Binging 　　☐ c. Purging 　　☐ d. Purposely skips meals 　　☐ e. Other: _____ ☐ 6. Follows diet for religious, vegetarian or other reasons ☐ 7. Evidence for: 　　☐ a. Sedentary lifestyle 　　☐ b. Excessive exercise regimen ☐ 8. Unstable psychosocial situation (especially in children): 　　☐ a. Homelessness 　　☐ b. Homebound 　　☐ c. Difficulty securing food 　　☐ d. Other: _____	☐ 1. Adequate and balanced diet ☐ 2. Regular exercise regimen ☐ 3. Psychosocial issues stable (especially in children)
_____ Total number of checks	_____ Total number of checks	_____ Total number of checks
≥1 check: ☐ **High Risk**	**≥1 + Ø high risk checks:** ☐ **Moderate Risk**	**Ø high risk + Ø moderate risk checks:** ☐ **Low Risk**
Action needed		
☐ To be seen by RDN within one week	☐ To be seen by RDN within one month	☐ To be seen by RDN at least annually

_____   _____   _____
Authorized Provider's Name, Printed   Authorized Provider's Name, Signed   Date

Medical Nutrition Therapy (MNT) by an RDN is indicated for at least one to two MNT encounters per year for people with HIV infection who are asymptomatic, and at least two to six or more MNT encounters per year for people with HIV infection who are symptomatic but stable, acute or palliative.

* Based upon the Screening and Referral recommendations in the *HIV/AIDS Evidence-Based Nutrition Practice Guideline*, Academy of Nutrition and
Dietetics Evidence Analysis Library (2010) www.andeal.org © 2015. Academy of Nutrition and Dietetics.

Fig. 36.5, cont'd

BOX 36.2   Nutrition Education and MNT for the HIV Infected

Pregnancy, Lactation, Infancy, and Childhood
Nutrition and food choices for healthy pregnancy and lactation
Transmission risk in breastfeeding and replacement feeding alternatives
Growth failure and developmental delay in children
Support for normal growth trends in children

Adolescents and Adults
Basic nutrition concepts and healthy habits, cardio-protective diet
Physical activity recommendations
Body image and altered body weight and shape
Attention to cultural or ethnic practices

Nutrition Interactions
Prevention, restoration, and maintenance of optimal body composition with an emphasis on lean tissues

Food medication interactions
Management of barriers to nutritional wellness, nutrition-related side effects of treatments, and symptoms requiring attention
Review of beverage or nutrient supplements
Review of potential interactions with nonprescription medications and herbal supplements
Evaluation of alcohol and recreational drug use

Life Skills and Socioeconomic Issues
Safe food handling and water sources
Access to adequate food choices
Food preparation skills and abilities

Adapted from Willig A, Wright L, and Galvin TA. Practice paper of the Academy of Nutrition and Dietetics: nutrition intervention and human immunodeficiency virus infection. *J Acad Nutr Diet* 118:486-498, 2018.

to 2.0 g/kg for increasing lean body mass. Recognize that these recommendations are educated guesses, not based on experimental studies; however, evidence suggests that protein needs tend to increase as CD4 counts drop below 500, particularly when HIV progresses to AIDS (Cervero and Watson, 2015). It is important for dietitians to individualize protein needs and consider weight changes and OIs (AND, 2010). With an OI, an additional 10% increase in protein intake may be recommended because of increased protein turnover (WHO, 2005b).

Fat

Currently PLWHA without other risk factors for CVD are recommended to follow the dietary reference intake (DRI) for dietary fat intake, 20% to 35% total calories as fat and <10% saturated fat (Richmond et al, 2010). If individuals have hyperlipidemia, tailor fat intake to help reduce risk of CVD (AND, 2010) (see Chapter 32). Additionally, promising research suggests that increasing the intake of omega-3 fatty acids may decrease serum triglycerides, reduce inflammation, and improve depression (Paranandi et al, 2014; Ravi et al, 2016).

Micronutrients

Vitamins and minerals are important for optimal immune function. Nutrient deficiencies can affect immune function and lead to disease progression. Micronutrient deficiencies are common in people with HIV infection as a result of malabsorption, drug-nutrient interactions, altered metabolism, gut infection, and altered gut barrier function. Vitamin A, zinc, and selenium serum levels are often low during a response to infection, so it is important to assess dietary intake to determine whether correction of serum micronutrients is warranted (Coyne-Meyers and Trombley, 2004).

There are benefits to correcting some depleted serum levels of micronutrients. Low levels of vitamins A, B_{12}, and zinc are associated with faster disease progression. Higher intakes of vitamins C and B have been associated with increased CD4 counts and slower disease progression to AIDS (Visser et al, 2017).

Studies on micronutrients are difficult to interpret because there are a variety of study designs and outcomes. Serum micronutrient levels reflect conditions such as acute infection, liver disease, technical parameters, and recent intake. Adequate micronutrient intake can be achieved through consumption of a balanced, healthy diet. However, diet alone may not be sufficient for some people living with HIV. A multivitamin and mineral supplement that provides 100% of the DRI also may be recommended for PLWHA who are unable to consistently meet daily micronutrient recommendations solely through dietary intake (Forrester and Sztam, 2011; Visser et al, 2017).

Research has been increasing in the area of micronutrient supplementation in people with HIV. It is important to consider the populations in which these studies have been conducted, and the findings need to be individualized to the client's needs. Factors to consider are underlying nutritional status, the stage of HIV infection or AIDS, use of ART medications, the presence of coinfections, and indication of an actual micronutrient deficiency (preferably from laboratory documentation), as well as intended length of supplement use. Caution should be used when recommending micronutrient supplementation for all people with HIV, because megadosing on some micronutrients such as vitamin A and zinc can have adverse outcomes (Coyne-Meyers and Trombley, 2004; Forrester and Sztam, 2011).

Studies have suggested that selenium supplementation may slow HIV progression (Baum et al, 2013). However low serum 25-hydroxy vitamin D levels may hasten HIV disease progression and increase disease progression and all-cause mortality, alluding to a possible benefit of vitamin D supplementation in people with HIV with a vitamin D deficiency (Shepherd et al, 2014; Eckard and McComsey, 2014). Certain medications, such as Efavirenz, have also been found to interfere with the metabolism of Vitamin D, making individuals on these medications at greater risk for deficiency. Vitamin D_3 supplementation has been effective at correcting these deficiencies (Eckard and McComsey, 2014). Recent studies also suggest that Vitamin D_3 and calcium supplementation may slow bone loss following initiation of ART (Overton et al, 2015).

The challenging question is whether a low serum micronutrient laboratory value is indicative of a true deficiency or an acute phase response to the virus (Forrester and Sztam, 2011). Because of these uncertainties, micronutrient supplementation should be thoroughly evaluated before being prescribed and, if indicated, be monitored to determine the optimal dosage and duration for supplementation.

The most beneficial levels of micronutrient supplementation have yet to be determined. At this time, there is not enough evidence to support micronutrient supplementation in adults with HIV infection above the recommended levels of the DRI (Kawai et al, 2010; AND, 2010) (Table 36.6).

Gastrointestinal Health

While PLWHA are experiencing less side effects overall, gastrointestinal symptoms are some of the most commonly reported side effects from use of ART (see Table 36.1). Additionally, emerging research indicates that HIV-positive individuals have significantly altered intestinal microbiota composition compared with HIV-negative individuals, regardless of medical management. This appears to be more prevalent among those with lower CD4 count, as CD4 T cells are involved in the regulation and promotion of beneficial microbes (Lozupone et al, 2013; Bandera et al, 2018). Dietitians play an important role in helping patients mitigate symptoms such as nausea, poor appetite, or diarrhea. Recommendations may range from suggesting more easily digestible foods for someone with diarrhea or helping a patient with nausea figure out the most tolerable foods to eat before taking medications. Nutrition recommendations are listed in Table 36.3.

Dietary supplements such as protein powder and protein-rich smoothies or soups may be helpful for patients who have difficulty meeting protein needs. Probiotics, yogurt, and glutamine may help those with gastrointestinal side effects. Although the evidence is conflicting whether glutamine may reduce antiviral (ARV) drug-related diarrhea, more promising research suggests it may improve intestinal permeability. The best results came from clinical trials where glutamine was combined with other amino acids, such as alanyl-glutamine, or glutamine in combination with arginine and beta-hydroxy-beta-methylbutyrate (Cervero and Watson, 2015; Clark et al, 2000; Leite et al, 2013). The recommended dosage of glutamine has yet to be determined; however, studies have demonstrated enhanced intestinal absorption with well-tolerated doses ranging from 3 g to 40 g and improved nelfinavir-associated diarrhea with doses of 10 g taken three times daily (Cervero and Watson, 2015; Huffman and Walgren, 2003).

Probiotics are beneficial microorganisms that may be consumed in the form of cultured or fermented foods, or as a dietary supplement. Probiotics are used clinically to help support intestinal barrier function. Certain strains, such as *Lactobacillus rhamnosus GG*, have been beneficial in helping to prevent diarrhea and inflammatory bowel diseases (Rao and Samak, 2013). Studies illustrate mixed results with the use of probiotics for antiretroviral-associated diarrhea, with most studies showing some benefit (Carter et al, 2016; D'Angelo et al, 2017). It is important to note that supplements vary in concentration, absorption, and product integrity. Products with the *live and active cultures* seal are preferential as these products should contain at least 100 million (10^8) cultures per gram at the time of manufacture (Sanders, 2003). The best food sources of probiotics include lactic acid fermented foods such as yogurt, sauerkraut, and olives (Hakansson and Molin, 2011). In order to get the most benefits from probiotics, in any form, it is best for individuals to regularly consume probiotics along with prebiotics which feed probiotics. Good food sources of prebiotics include chicory root, dandelion greens, garlic, onion, oats, barley, and bananas.

TABLE 36.6 Common Micronutrient Deficiencies and Indications for Supplementation

Vitamin or Mineral	Potential Cause for Deficiency	Results of Vitamin Deficiency	Supplementation Indications
B₁₂	Malabsorption Inadequate intake	Increased risk of progression to AIDS Dementia Peripheral neuropathy Myelopathy Diminished performance (information processing and problem-solving skills)	Little evidence for benefits of supplementation beyond correcting low serum levels
A	Inadequate intake Fat malabsorption	Increased risk of progression to AIDS	Necessary to correct low levels Should not exceed DRI when serum levels are normal High intakes beyond correcting low levels can be detrimental to health and potentially increase risk of mortality from AIDS (Coyne-Meyers and Trombley, 2004) Needs more research
Beta-carotene	Inadequate intake Fat malabsorption	Potential relationship with oxidative stress Potentially weakens immune function	May increase lung cancer risk in smokers, avoid mega-doses Needs more research
E	Inadequate intake Fat malabsorption	Potential increased progression to AIDS Oxidative stress Impaired immune response	High intake: may be associated with increased surrogate markers of atherosclerosis Needs more research
D	Inadequate intake Inadequate exposure to sunshine Fat malabsorption Kidney disease Medications	Immune suppression Poor calcium absorption Low bone mineral density	Correct low levels Needs more research
Selenium	Inadequate intake	Potential increased progression to AIDS Weakened immune function Oxidative stress	Multivitamin/mineral providing DRI Higher doses not recommended at this time until further research
Zinc	Inadequate intake Diarrhea	Increased risk for HIV-related mortality Weakened immune system Impaired healing processes Lower CD4 counts	Recommend supplementing to intakes of DRI High levels above DRI may lead to faster disease progression Needs more research
Iron	Low levels during initial asymptomatic HIV infection caused by inadequate absorption Inadequate intake	Anemia Progression and mortality in HIV infection Increased susceptibility to and severity from other infections such as TB	Correct low levels as needed Recommend intakes at DRI High levels potentially lead to increased viral load Needs more research

Academy of Nutrition and Dietetics Evidence Analysis Library *HIV/AIDS: Executive Summary of Recommendations (2010)*, 2010. https://www.andeal.org/topic.cfm?menu=5312&cat=4458. Accessed June 6, 2018. Cervero M, Watson RR: *Health of HIV Infected People: Food, Nutrition and Lifestyle with Antiretroviral Drugs* (vol 1), London, UK, 2015, Elsevier Inc. Coyne-Meyers K, Trombley LE: A review of nutrition in human immunodeficiency virus infection in the era of highly active antiretroviral therapy, *Nutr Clin Prac* 19:340, 2004; Eckard AR, McComsey GA: Vitamin D deficiency and altered bone mineral metabolism in HIV-infected individuals. *Curr HIV/AIDS Rep.* 2014;11(3):263-270; Falcone EL et al: Micronutrient concentrations and subclinical atherosclerosis in adults with HIV, *Am J Clin Nutr* 91:1213, 2010; McDermid JM et al: Mortality in HIV infection is independently predicted by host iron status and SLC11A1 and HP genotypes, with new evidence of a gene-nutrient interaction, *Am J Clin Nutr* 90:225, 2009; Pitney CL et al: Selenium supplementation in HIV-infected patients: is there any potential clinical benefit? *J Assoc Nurses AIDS Care* 20:326, 2009; Rodriguez M et al: High frequency of vitamin D deficiency in ambulatory HIV-positive patients, *AIDS Res Hum Retroviruses* 25:9, 2009.

AIDS, Acquired immune deficiency syndrome; *DRI,* dietary reference intake; *HIV,* human immunodeficiency virus; *TB,* tuberculosis.

HIV IN WOMEN

Around the world, women represent about half the people who are living with HIV or AIDS. In the United States women accounted for 7529 (19%) of the estimated number of new HIV infections in 2017 (CDC, 2017a). The highest rate of new HIV infection was seen in African American women, representing 61% of new diagnosis, more than 3 times higher than white or Latina women, although the rate has decreased by 20% since 2013 (CDC, 2017a).

Women contract HIV less than men in the United States, but several factors put them at higher risk. Biologically, women are more likely to get HIV during unprotected vaginal sex because the lining of the vagina provides a larger area that can be exposed to HIV-infected semen. Barriers to receiving appropriate medical care also exist. Social and cultural stigma, lack of financial resources, responsibility of caring for others, and fear of disclosure may prevent women from seeking proper care. Stigma and discrimination is thought to be particularly high among African American women living with HIV in the Southern states (Fletcher et al, 2016).

Preconception and Prenatal Considerations

Receiving counseling before conception can help HIV-positive women of childbearing age decrease the risk of perinatal transmission. Current recommendations include prenatal screening for HIV, hepatitis C virus, and tuberculosis infection; initiation of ART during pregnancy; and ART for the child once they are born. In the United States these interventions have reduced the risk of perinatal transmission to less than 2% (DHHS, 2012). Monitoring HIV-positive pregnant women during pregnancy can help prevent nutritional deficiencies.

Postpartum and Other Considerations

In the United States breastfeeding is not recommended for HIV-infected women, including those on ART, or where safe, affordable, and feasible alternatives are available and culturally appropriate (Kemp, 2017; CDC, 2018). Banked milk from human milk banks is an option (see *Focus On: What Is a Human Milk Bank?* in Chapter 41). In developing countries, recommendations may differ depending on safety and availability of formula and access to clean drinking water and availability of human milk banks.

HIV IN CHILDREN

An estimated 180,000 new HIV infections occurred globally among children younger than the age of 15 in 2017. In 2016 in the United States, 99 children under the age of 13 received a diagnosis of perinatally acquired HIV. The majority of these infections stem from perinatal transmission in utero, during delivery, or through consumption of HIV-infected breastmilk (UNAIDS, 2017). Premastication (chewing foods or medicine before administering to a child) also has been reported as a route of transmission through blood in saliva (CDC, 2011).

Growth is the most valuable indicator of nutritional status in childhood. Poor growth may be an early indicator for progression of HIV disease. Growth failure can result from HIV infection itself and HIV-associated OIs (Vreeman et al, 2015; WHO, 2010) (see Appendices 4 through 11).

HIV treatment has improved the clinical outcomes for children, with ART initiation resulting in significant catch-up in weight and height, but not to the level of uninfected children. The presence of HALS seen in adults is also seen in children (Miller et al, 2012). Multivitamin and micronutrient supplementation may be beneficial at the DRI levels for children who are malnourished. Research does not currently support any supplementation at higher doses.

INTEGRATIVE AND FUNCTIONAL NUTRITION (IFN)

The use of IFN is prevalent in patients with HIV infection. The Natural Medicines Database suggests that IFN use in people living with HIV and AIDS is about 53% (Natural Medicines Clinical Management Series, 2019). Vitamins, herbs, and supplements are the most common followed by prayer and other spiritual approaches (Lorenc and Robinson, 2013). People experiencing greater HIV symptom severity and longer disease duration are more likely to use complementary and integrative medicine (CIM) (Lorenc and Robinson, 2013).

Despite the high percentage of IFN use, less than one third of patients disclose IFN use to their health care providers (Reed and Lagunas, 2012). Some patients with HIV have noted benefits with taking dietary supplements; however, patients need to be made aware of any potential interactions with ART medications. In addition, caution with anecdote-based remedies should be monitored regarding credibility for a vulnerable population such as PLWHA (Kalichman et al, 2012). It is important to gather a detailed list of all dietary supplements in order to screen for potential drug-nutrient interactions and side effects.

Several popular dietary supplements have a significant potential drug-nutrient interactions with ART medication. For example concentrated garlic supplements and St. John's wort (*Hypericum perforatum*) decrease blood levels of ART medications, decreasing the efficacy of ART and potentially leading to drug resistance. Additionally, while some studies have shown potential antiretroviral properties of spirulina blue-green algae, supplemental use is not advised as there is potential for it to be contaminated with pathogenic microorganisms (Ngo-Matip et al, 2015; Winter et al, 2014).

Probiotic supplements, with or without prebiotics, are commonly used for reducing HIV/AIDS -related infectious diarrhea and general dysbiosis (see Gastrointestinal Health). Current research is also examining how altering microbiota may impact immune health. Probiotics are hypothesized to support immune health by supporting healthy intestinal microbiota, improving barrier function, and helping to regulate immune supportive natural killer cells, lymphocytes, and antibodies (Carter et al, 2016; Sanders et al, 2013). A 2016 meta-analysis analyzed the impact of probiotics and prebiotics on CD4 count. While overall results were inconclusive, most of fifteen experimental studies analyzing the impact of probiotics and prebiotics on CD4 count illustrated an increase in CD4 count (nine with significant improvements). More promising results came from using probiotics and synbiotics with *Bifidus* or *Lactobacilli* probiotic strains, in pill, or in food form (yogurt) (Carter et al, 2016). While probiotics tended to be well tolerated in these studies, there have been rare cases of pathogenic infection from probiotics (Riquelme et al, 2003). Because of the way dietary supplements are regulated, it is prudent to recommend brands that carry 3rd party certification, thus assuring their potency and quality (see Chapter 11 for more details on dietary supplement regulation). Taking probiotics and prebiotics in food form may be a safer and more economical choice for PLWHA, especially those with limited income.

Recreational and medical cannabis use is common among PLWHA to help improve appetite, reduce pain and neuropathy, enhance mood, and reduce nausea. While current research is investigating the effectiveness of cannabis on these symptoms, more specific research is needed within the HIV-positive population. Evidence on the specific benefits in the population is increasing. According to the Natural Medicine Database smoking marijuana is possibly effective in stimulating appetite, increasing calorie intake, and increasing weight gain in PLWHA experiencing poor appetite. Furthermore, it may possibly be effective in reducing the intensity of pain associated with neuropathy (Natural Medicines Clinical Management Series, 2019).

While some dietary supplements and integrative therapies may help support immune function, reduce side effects, and improve nutrient status and quality of life, a food-first strategy should be primary. This is particularly relevant when working with clients that have limited resources. Making specific IFN recommendations might be more costly as this can lead to individuals losing funds that would otherwise be spent on basic healthy food.

CLINICAL CASE STUDY

Edwin is a 42-year-old white male who has been human immunodeficiency virus (HIV) positive for 20 years. His viral load is undetectable and his CD4+ count is 643. Edwin's medical history also includes depression, gastroesophageal reflux disease (GERD), high blood pressure, and hyperlipidemia. His current HIV antiretroviral regimen was recently changed to Genvoya; he also takes atorvastatin (Lipitor), and ranitidine (Zantac). His height is 5'9" and his current weight is 188 lb, up from 175 lb. His fasting lipid profile shows a total cholesterol 235 mg/dL, triglycerides 304 mg/dL, high-density lipoprotein 25 mg/dL, and low-density lipoprotein 96 mg/dL. Since his last visit 3 months ago, he has been having moderate diarrhea with general gastrointestinal (GI) upset that he states is "left over" from when he had the flu and took 2 rounds of antibiotics a few months ago. Edwin lives by himself and doesn't like to cook. He also receives one meal per day from a community program and gets groceries once per week from a food bank. He walks his dog for 30 minutes daily. Upon taking a 24-hour recall, you find his caloric intake to be 2700 kcal/day coming primarily from ready-to-eat items. He also expresses that ice cream is his emotional comfort food, which he eats 5 to 7 days per week.

Nutrition Diagnostic Statements

- Excessive dietary intake (NB-1.7) related to frequent intake of highly processed foods and limited food access as evidenced by 24-hour recall reflecting intake of 2700 kcal per day and weight gain of 13 lb (7.4%) in the past 3 months.
- Altered GI function (NC-1.4) related to history of antibiotic use and high intake of lactose as evidenced by patient report of moderate diarrhea since taking 2 rounds of antibiotics in past few months and diet recall revealing eating ice cream 5 to 7 days a week.

Nutrition Care Questions

1. What factors may be contributing to the GI symptoms that Edwin is experiencing? What recommendations do you suggest for these symptoms? Are there any drug-nutrient interactions of which you need to be aware?
2. What nutrition and lifestyle interventions would you recommend to address his nutrition diagnoses?
3. What are some biochemical and nutritional parameters you would monitor to determine whether the nutrition interventions are effective?
4. How would you evaluate the desired nutrition outcomes to determine whether they have been met?
5. Are there any integrative therapies that may help Edwin? Any potential drug nutrient interactions you would need to consider?

USEFUL WEBSITES

Academy of Nutrition and Dietetics Infectious Diseases Nutrition Dietetic Practice Group

Centers for Disease Control and Prevention HIV Research, Prevention, and Surveillance

Centers for Disease Control and Prevention Website: Resources for Persons Living with HIV

Joint United Nations Program on HIV/AIDS

National Center for Complementary Integrative Health (NCCIH)

Preexposure Prophylaxis and ART in Uninfected Individuals

REFERENCES

Academy of Nutrition and Dietetics Evidence Analysis Library HIV/AIDS: *Executive Summary of Recommendations,* 2010. Available at: https://www.andeal.org/topic.cfm?menu=5312&cat=4458. Accessed June 6, 2018.

Arnold EA, Rebchook GM, Kegeles SM: "Triply cursed": Racism, homophobia and HIV-related stigma are barriers to regular HIV testing, treatment adherence and disclosure among young Black gay men, *Cult Health Sex* 16(6): 710–722, 2014.

Baeten JM, Donnell D, Ndase P, et al: Antiretroviral prophylaxis for HIV prevention in heterosexual men and women, *N Engl J Med* 367:399–410, 2012.

Bandera A, De Benedetto I, Bozzi G, et al: Altered gut microbiome composition in HIV infection: causes, effects and potential intervention, *Curr Opin HIV AIDS* 13(1):73–80, 2018.

Baum MK, Campa A, Lai S, et al: Effect of micronutrient supplementation on disease progression in asymptomatic, antiretroviral-naive, HIV-infected adults in Botswana: a randomized clinical trial, *JAMA* 310:2154–2163, 2013.

Carter GM, Esmaeili A, Shah H, et al: Probiotics in human immunodeficiency virus infection: a systematic review and evidence synthesis of benefits and risks, *Open Forum Infect Dis* 3(4):1–10, 2016.

Centers for Disease Control and Prevention (CDC): Diagnoses of HIV infection in the United States and dependent areas, 2016, *HIV Surveill Rep* 28:6–8, 2017a.

Centers for Disease Control and Prevention (CDC): *HIV and Viral Hepatitis,* 2017b. Available at: https://www.cdc.gov/hiv/pdf/library/factsheets/hiv-viral-hepatitis.pdf. Accessed October 23, 2019.

Centers for Disease Control and Presentation (CDC): *Human Immunodeficiency Virus (HIV)-Breastfeeding,* 2018. Available at: https://www.cdc.gov/breastfeeding/breastfeeding-special-circumstances/maternal-or-infant-illnesses/hiv.html. Accessed November 3, 2019.

Centers for Disease Control and Prevention (CDC): *HIV Testing,* 2019. Available at: https://www.cdc.gov/hiv/testing/index.html. Accessed October 28, 2019.

Centers for Disease Control and Prevention (CDC): Premastication of food by caregivers of HIV-exposed children—nine U.S. sites, 2009-2010, *MMWR Morb Mortal Wkly Rep* 60(9):273–275, 2011.

Cervero M, Watson RR: *Health of HIV Infected People: Food, Nutrition and Lifestyle with Antiretroviral Drugs* (vol 1), London, UK, 2015, Elsevier Inc.

Clark H, Babu AS, Wiewel EW, et al: Diagnosed HIV infection in transgender adults and adolescents: results from the National HIV Surveillance System, 2009-2014, *AIDS Behav* 21(9):2774–2783, 2017.

Clark RH, Feleke G, Din M, et al: Nutritional treatment for acquired immunodeficiency virus-associated wasting using beta-hydroxy beta-methylbutyrate, glutamine, and arginine: a randomized, double-blind, placebo-controlled study, *JPEN* 24:133–139, 2000.

Coyne-Meyers K, Trombley LE: A review of nutrition in human immunodeficiency virus infection in the era of highly active antiretroviral therapy, *Nutr Clin Prac* 19:340, 2004.

Currier JS: Epidemiology of cardiovascular disease and risk factors in HIV infected patients, *Up to Date,* 2018. Available at: https://www.uptodate.com/contents/epidemiology-of-cardiovascular-disease-and-risk-factors-in-hiv-infected-patients. Accessed November 5, 2019.

Currier JS: *Pathogenesis and biomarkers of cardiovascular disease in HIV-infected patients,* 2019. Available at: https://www.uptodate.com/contents/pathogenesis-and-biomarkers-of-cardiovascular-disease-in-hiv-infected-patients. Updated October 15, 2019. Accessed November 5, 2019.

Dailey AF, Hoots BE, Hall HI, et al: Vital signs: human immunodeficiency virus testing and diagnosis delays — United States, *MMWR Morb Mortal Wkly Rep* 66:1300–1306, 2017.

D'Angelo C, Reale M, Costantini E, et al: Microbiota and probiotics in health and HIV infection, *Nutrients* 9(6):E615, 2017.

Department of Health and Human Services (DHHS): *Panel on Antiretroviral Guidelines for Adults and Adolescents. Guidelines for the Use of Antiretroviral Agents in Adults and Adolescents Living with HIV*, 2017. Available at: https://aidsinfo.nih.gov/contentfiles/AdultandAdolescentGL003510.pdf. Updated October 17, 2017. Accessed October 28, 2019.

Department of Health and Human Services (DHHS): *Panel on Treatment of HIV Infected Pregnant Women and Prevention of Perinatal Transmission. Recommendations for Use of Antiretroviral Drugs in Pregnant HIV-1-Infected Women for Maternal Health and Interventions to Reduce Perinatal HIV Transmission in the U.S*, 2012. Available at: https://aidsinfo.nih.gov/contentfiles/PerinatalGL003381.pdf. Accessed March 2, 2014.

Eckard AR, McComsey GA: Vitamin D deficiency and altered bone mineral metabolism in HIV-infected individuals, *Curr HIV/AIDS Rep* 11(3): 263–270, 2014.

Eisinger RW, Dieffenbach CW, Fauci AS: HIV viral load and transmissibility of HIV infection: undetectable equals untransmittable, *JAMA* 321(5): 451–452, 2019.

Fletcher F, Ingram LA, Kerr J, et al: "She told them, oh that bitch got AIDS": experiences of multilevel HIV/AIDS-related stigma among African American women living with HIV/AIDS in the South, *AIDS Patient Care STDS* 30(7):349–356, 2016.

Forrester JE, Sztam KA: Micronutrients in HIV/AIDS: Is there evidence to change the WHO 2003 recommendations? *Am J Clin Nutr* 94(6): 1683S–1689S, 2011.

Glesby D: Cardiovascular complications of HIV, *Top Antivir Med* 24(4): 127–131, 2017.

Grant RM, Lama JR, Anderson PL, et al: Preexposure chemoprophylaxis for HIV prevention in men who have sex with men, *N Engl J Med* 363: 2587–2599, 2010.

Gilead Sciences HCP: *Truvada for Pre-Exposure Prophylaxis (PrEP)™ Side Effects,* 2019. https://www.truvada.com/what-is-truvada/side-effects. Published July 2019. Accessed October 31, 2019.

Gilead Sciences HCP: *HARVONI® (ledipasvir 90 mg/sofosbuvir 400 mg) tablets,* 2018. Available at: https://hcp.harvoni.com. Accessed October 31, 2019.

Gritsenko D, Hughes G: Ledipasvir/Sofosbuvir (harvoni): improving options for hepatitis C virus infection, *P T* 40(4):256–276, 2015.

Hakansson A, Molin G: Gut microbiota and inflammation, *Nutrients.* 3: 637–682, 2011.

Hendricks K, Gorbach S: Nutrition issues in chronic drug users living with HIV infection, *Addict Sci Clin Prac* 5(1):16–23, 2009.

Huffman FG, Walgren ME: L-glutamine supplementation improves nelfinavir-associated diarrhea in HIV-infected individuals, *HIV Clin Trials* 4(5): 324–329, 2003.

James SE, Herman JL, Rankin S, et al: *The report of the 2015 U.S. transgender survey,* Washington, DC, 2016, National center for Transgender Equality.

Joint United Nations Programme on HIV/AIDS, World Health Organization: *UNAIDS 2018.* September 20, 2018.

Kalichman SC, Cherry C, White D, et al: Use of dietary supplements among people living with HIV/AIDS is associated with vulnerability to medical misinformation on the internet, *AIDS Res Ther* 9:1, 2012.

Kawai K, Kupka R, Mugusi F, et al: A randomized trial to determine the optimal dosage of multivitamin supplements to reduce adverse pregnancy outcomes among HIV- infected women in Tanzania, *Am J Clin Nutr* 91:391–397, 2010.

Kemp C: *Debate to focus on pros, cons of breastfeeding by HIV-positive mothers, American Academy of Pediatrics,* 2017. Available at: https://www.aappublications.org/news/2017/09/15/NECBreastfeeding091917. Accessed November 4, 2019.

Koethe JR, Jenkins CA, Turner M: et al: Body mass index and the risk of incident noncommunicable diseases after starting antiretroviral therapy, *HIV Med* 16:67–72, 2015.

Kosmiski L: Energy expenditure in HIV infection, *Am J Clin Nutr* 94(6):1677S–1682S, 2011.

Leite RD, Lima NL, Leite CA, et al: Improvement of intestinal permeability with alanyl-glutamine in HIV patients: a randomized, double blinded, placebo-controlled clinical trial, *Arq Gastroenterol* 50(1):56–63, 2013.

Lorenc A, Robinson N: A review of the use of complementary and alternative medicine and HIV: issues for patient care, *AIDS Patient Care STDS* 27:503–510, 2013.

Lozupone CA, Li M, Campbell TB, et al: Alterations in the gut microbiota associated with HIV-1 infection, *Cell Host Microbe* 14(3):329–339, 2013.

Mankal PK, Kotler DP: From wasting to obesity, changes in nutritional concerns in HIV/AIDS, *Endocrinol Metab Clin North Am* 43:647–663, 2014.

Mayer KH, Grinsztejn B, El-Sadr WM: Transgender people and HIV prevention: what we know and what we need. to know, a call to action, *J Acquir Immune Defic Syndr* 72(Suppl 3):S207–S209, 2016.

Microbicide Trials Network: *MTN Trials Fact Sheet,* 2016. Available at: https://mtnstopshiv.org/news/mtn-trials-fact-sheet. Accessed November 1, 2019.

Miller TI, Borkowsky W, DiMeglio LA, et al: Metabolic abnormalities and viral replication are associated with biomarkers of vascular dysfunction in HIV-infected children, *HIV Med* 13(5):264–275, 2012.

Natural Medicines Clinical Management Series: *Natural medicines in the clinical management of HIV/AIDS,* 2019. Available at: http://naturaldatabase.therapeuticresearch.com/ce/CECourse.aspx?cs=naturalstandard&s=ND&pm=5&pc=17-107. Accessed November 5, 2019.

Ngo-Matip ME, Pieme CA, Azabji-Kenfack M, et al: Impact of daily supplementation of Spirulina platensis on the immune system of naïve HIV-1 patients in Cameroon: a 12-months single blind, randomized, multicenter trial, *Nutr J* 14:70, 2015.

National Institutes of Health: *NIH and partners launch HIV vaccine efficacy study.* Updated November 30, 2017.

National Institute of Allergy and Infectious Diseases (NIAID): *NIH launches large clinical trials of antibody-based HIV prevention,* Bethesda, Maryland, 2016, U.S. Department of Health and Human Service. Accessed November 1, 2018.

National Institutes of Health (NIH): *NIH and partners launch HIV vaccine efficacy Study,* Bethesda, Maryland, 2017, U.S. Department of Health and Human Service. Available at: https://www.nih.gov/news-events/news-releases/nih-partners-launch-hiv-vaccine-efficacy-study. Accessed November 1, 2019.

Novella, S: *HIV Treatment Extends Life Expectancy.* Science-Based Medicine, 2008. Available at: https://sciencebasedmedicine.org/hiv-treatment-extends-life-expectancy. Accessed November 4, 2019

Oliveira JM, Rondó PH: Omega-3 fatty acids and hypertriglyceridemia in HIV-infected subjects on antiretroviral therapy: systematic review and meta-analysis, *HIV Clin Trials* 12:268–274, 2011.

Overton E, Chan ES, Brown TT, et al: High-dose vitamin D and calcium attenuates bone loss with antiretroviral therapy initiation: a prospective, randomized placebo-controlled trial for bone health in HIV-infected individuals, *Ann Intern Med* 162(12):815–824, 2015.

Paranandi A, Asztalos BF, Mangili A, et al: Short communication: effects of omega-3 fatty acids on triglycerides and high-density lipoprotein subprofiles in HIV-infected persons with hypertriglyceridemia, *AIDS Res Hum Retroviruses* 30(8):800–805, 2014.

Rao RK, Samak G: Protection and restitution of Gut Barrier by probiotics: nutritional and clinical implications, *Curr Nutr Food Sci* 9(2):99–107, 2013.

Ravi S, Khalili H, Abbasian L, et al: Effect of omega-3 fatty acids on depressive symptoms in HIV-positive individuals: a randomized, placebo-controlled clinical trial, *Ann Pharmacother* 50(10):797–807, 2016.

Reed R, Lagunas LF: Complementary and alternative medicine use among people living with hiv or aids el uso de medicina complementaria y alternativa en personas viviendo con vih o sida, *Horiz Enferm* 23(1):81–88, 2012.

Richmond SR, Carper MJ, Lei X, et al: HIV-protease inhibitors suppress skeletal muscle fatty acid oxidation by reducing CD36 and CPT1 fatty acid transporters, *Biochim Biophys Acta* 1801(5):559–566, 2010.

Riquelme AJ, Calvo MA, Guzmán AM, et al: Saccharomyces cerevisiae fungemia after Saccharomyces boulardii treatment in immunocompromised patients, *J Clin.Gastroenterol* 36(1):41–43, 2003.

Roberts T, Cohn J, Bonner K, et al: Scale-up of routine viral load testing in resource-poor settings: current and future implementation challenges, *Clin Infect Dis* 62(8):1043–1048, 2016.

Sanders ME: Probiotics: considerations for human health, *Nutr Rev* 61(3): 91–99, 2003.

Sanders ME, Guarner F, Guerrant R, et al: An update on the use and investigation of probiotics in health and disease, *Gut* 62(5):787–796, 2013.

Shepherd L, Souberbielle JC, Bastard JP, et al: Prognostic value of vitamin D level for all-cause mortality, and association with inflammatory markers, in HIV-infected persons, *J Infect Dis* 210(2):234–243, 2014.

Singer AW, Weiser SD, McCoy SI: Does food insecurity undermine adherence to antiretroviral therapy? A systematic review, *AIDS Behav* 19(8): 1510–1526, 2015.

Tang AM, Forrester JE, Spiegelman D, et al: Heavy injection drug use is associated with lower percent body fat in a multi-ethnic cohort of HIV-positive and HIV-negative drug users from three US cities, *Am J Drug Alcohol Abuse* 36:78–86, 2010.

Trickery A, May MT, Vehreschild JJ, et al. Survival of HIV-positive patients starting antiretroviral therapy between 1996 and 2013: a collaborative analysis of cohort studies, *Lancet HIV* 4:e349–356, 2017.

Joint United Nations Programme on HIV/AIDS (UNAIDS): *UNAIDS DATA 2018,* 2018:5–19. Available at: https://www.unaids.org/sites/default/files/media_asset/unaids-data-2018_en.pdf. Accessed October 31, 2019.

United States Department of Veterans Affairs: *HIV wasting syndrome,* 2018. Available at: https://www.hiv.va.gov/patient/diagnosis/OI-wasting-syndrome.asp. Accessed July 9, 2018.

Visser ME, Durao S, Sinclair D, et al: Micronutrient supplementation in adults with HIV infection, *Cochrane Database Syst Rev* 5:CD003650, 2017.

Vreeman RC, Scanlon ML, McHenry MS, et al: The physical and psychological effects of HIV infection and its treatment on perinatally HIV-infected children, *J Int AIDS Soc* 18(Suppl 6):20258, 2015.

Wanke C, et al: Overview of HIV/AIDS today. In Hendricks KM, Dong KR, Gerrior JL, eds. *Nutrition management of HIV and AIDS,* Chicago, 2009, American Dietetic Association.

Wellington C, Bilyk H: Gender identity: a culture with unique nutrition concerns, *J Acad Nutr Diet* 112:A21, 2012.

Willig A, Wright L, Galvin TA: Practice paper of the academy of nutrition and dietetics: nutrition intervention and human immunodeficiency virus infection, *J Acad Nutr Diet* 118:486–498, 2018.

Winter FS, Emakam F, Kfutwah A, et al: The effect of Arthrospira platensis capsules on CD4 T-cells and antioxidative capacity in a randomized pilot study of adult women infected with human immunodeficiency virus not under HAART in Yaoundé, Cameroon, *Nutrients* 6(7):2973–2986, 2014.

World Health Organization (WHO): *Antiretroviral therapy for HIV infection in infants and children: towards universal access: recommendations for a public health approach,* 2010 revision, 2010. Geneva, Switzerland, World Health Organization. Available at: https://apps.who.int/iris/bitstream/handle/10665/164255/9789241599801_eng.pdf;jsessionid=888AF2CD3C44958FA2C8CA160AA4BB76?sequence=1. Accessed November 1, 2019.

World Health Organization (WHO): *Executive summary of a scientific review: consultation on nutrition and HIV/AIDS in Africa: evidence, lessons and recommendations for action,* Durban, South Africa, 2005a, World Health Organization, Department of Nutrition for Health and Development. Available at: https://www.who.int/nutrition/topics/Executive_Summary_Durban.pdf. Accessed November 1, 2019.

World Health Organization (WHO): *Macronutrients and HIV/AIDS: a review of current evidence: consultation on nutrition and HIV/AIDS in Africa: evidence, lessons, and recommendations for action,* Durban, South Africa, 2005b, World Health Organization, Department of Nutrition for Health and Development. Available at: https://www.who.int/nutrition/topics/Paper_1_Macronutrients_bangkok.pdf?ua=1. Accessed November 1, 2019.

World Professional Association for Transgender Health: *Standards of care for the health of transsexual, transgender, and gender nonconforming people the world professional association for transgender health,* 2012.

Young JS: HIV and Medical Nutrition Therapy, *J Am Diet Assoc* 97(10): S161–166, 1997.

Young, S, Wheeler AC, McCoy SI, et al: A review of the role of food insecurity in adherence to care and treatment among adult and pediatric populations living with HIV and AIDS, *AIDS Behav* 18(Suppl 5):S505–S515, 2014.

37

Medical Nutrition Therapy in Critical Care

Britta Brown, MS, RD, LD, CNSC
Katherine Hall, RD, LD, CNSC

KEY TERMS

abdominal compartment syndrome
acute-phase proteins
adrenocorticotropic hormone
catecholamines
cortisol
counterregulatory hormones
cytokines
ebb phase
epithelial barrier function (EBF)
flow phase

hemodynamic
ileus
interleukin-1 (IL-1)
interleukin-6 (IL-6)
multiple organ dysfunction syndrome
 (MODS)
nutrition support therapy
quick sequential organ failure
 assessment criteria (qSOFA)
sepsis

shock
systemic inflammatory response
 syndrome (SIRS)
tight junction
total body surface area (TBSA) burned
tumor necrosis factor (TNF)

Critical care is the complex medical management of a seriously ill or injured person. This level of illness or injury involves acute impairment of one or more vital organ systems with a high probability of life-threatening deterioration of the patient's condition. Critical care requires complex decision making and support of vital organ systems to prevent failure involving one or more of the following: the central nervous system, the circulatory system, the renal and hepatic systems, the metabolic and respiratory systems, and shock. Critical care patients are treated in an intensive care unit (ICU) that contains specialized equipment and highly trained staff. The presence of multiple monitors, tubes, catheters, and infusions makes these patients difficult to assess nutritionally (Fig. 37.1). Critical illness and injury results in profound metabolic alterations, beginning at the time of injury and persisting until wound healing and recovery are complete. Whether the event involves sepsis (infection), trauma, burns, or surgery, the systemic response is activated. The physiologic and metabolic changes that follow may lead to shock and other negative outcomes (Fig. 37.2). Disorders that frequently are treated in an ICU include, but are not limited to, acute respiratory distress syndrome (ARDS), asthma, burn, chronic obstructive pulmonary disease (COPD), pneumonia, respiratory distress syndrome, sepsis, and trauma.

METABOLIC RESPONSE TO STRESS

The metabolic response to critical illness, traumatic injury, sepsis, burns, or major surgery is complex and involves most metabolic pathways. Accelerated catabolism of lean body or skeletal mass

Portions of this chapter were written by Marion Winkler and Ainsley Malone.

occurs, which clinically results in net negative nitrogen balance and muscle wasting. The response to critical illness, injury, and sepsis characteristically involves ebb and flow phases. The ebb phase, occurring immediately after injury, is associated with hypovolemia (decreased blood volume circulating in the body), shock, and tissue hypoxia. Typically, decreased cardiac output, oxygen consumption, and body temperature occur in this phase. Insulin levels fall in direct response to the increase in glucagon, most likely as a signal to increase hepatic glucose production. Increased cardiac output, oxygen consumption, body temperature, energy expenditure, and total body protein catabolism characterize the flow phase that follows fluid resuscitation (the replacement of bodily fluids typically using crystalloids [intravenous fluid solutions], colloids [i.e., albumin or blood]) and restoration of oxygen transport. Physiologically, in this phase is a marked increase in glucose production, free fatty acid release, circulating levels of insulin, catecholamines (epinephrine and norepinephrine released by the adrenal medulla), glucagon, and cortisol. The magnitude of the hormonal response appears to be associated with the severity of injury.

HORMONAL AND CELL-MEDIATED RESPONSE

Metabolic stress is associated with an altered hormonal state that results in an increased flow of substrate but poor use of carbohydrate, protein, fat, and oxygen. Counterregulatory hormones, which are elevated after injury and sepsis, play a role in the accelerated proteolysis (muscle and tissue breakdown). Glucagon promotes gluconeogenesis, amino acid uptake by the liver, ureagenesis, and protein catabolism. Cortisol, which is released from the adrenal cortex in response to stimulation by adrenocorticotropic hormone secreted by the anterior pituitary gland, enhances skeletal muscle catabolism and promotes

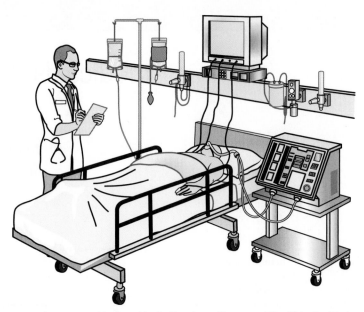

Fig. 37.1 Common equipment used in the critically ill patient. (Courtesy Afford Medical Technologies Pvt Ltd.)

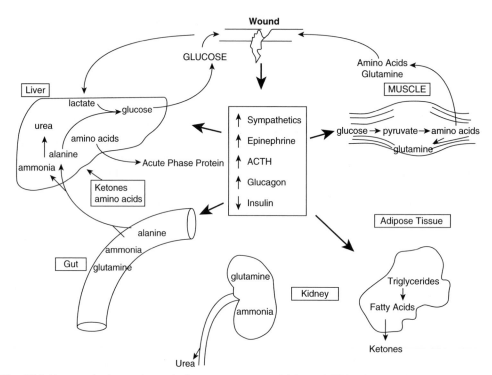

Fig. 37.2 Neuroendocrine and metabolic consequences of injury. *ACTH*, adrenocorticotropic hormone. (Reprinted from Lowry SF, Perez JM: *Modern nutrition in health and disease*, Philadelphia, 2006, Lippincott Williams & Wilkins, pp 1381–1400.)

hepatic use of amino acids for gluconeogenesis, glycogenolysis, and acute-phase protein synthesis (Table 37.1).

After injury or sepsis, energy production increasingly depends on protein. Branched-chain amino acids (BCAAs leucine, isoleucine, and valine) are oxidized from skeletal muscle as a source of energy for the muscle; carbon skeletons are made available for the glucose-alanine cycle and muscle glutamine synthesis. The mobilization of acute-phase proteins (secretory proteins produced by the liver) are altered in response to injury or infection, resulting in rapid loss of lean body

mass and an increased net negative nitrogen balance, which continues until the inflammatory response resolves. Breakdown of protein tissue also causes increased urinary losses of potassium, phosphorus, and magnesium. Lipid metabolism also is altered in stress and sepsis. Increased circulation of free fatty acids is thought to result from increased lipolysis caused by elevated catecholamines and cortisol, as well as a marked elevation in the ratio of glucagon to insulin.

Most notable is the hyperglycemia observed during stress. This initially results from a marked increase in glucose production and

TABLE 37.1 The Metabolic Response to Injury

Physiologic Changes in Catabolism	
Carbohydrate metabolism	↑ Glycogenolysis
	↑ Gluconeogenesis
	Insulin resistance of tissues
	Hyperglycemia
Fat metabolism	↑ Lipolysis
	Free fatty acids used as energy substrate by tissues (except brain)
	Some conversion of free fatty acids to ketones in liver (used by brain)
	Glycerol converted to glucose in the liver
Protein metabolism	↑ Skeletal muscle breakdown
	Amino acids converted to glucose in liver and used as substrate for acute-phase proteins
	Negative nitrogen balance
Total energy expenditure is increased in proportion to injury severity and other modifying factors	
Progressive reduction in fat and muscle mass until stimulus for catabolism ends	

From Forsythe JLR, Parks RW: *The metabolic response to injury: principles and practice of surgery*, ed 6, 2012, Elsevier, Churchill Livingstone.

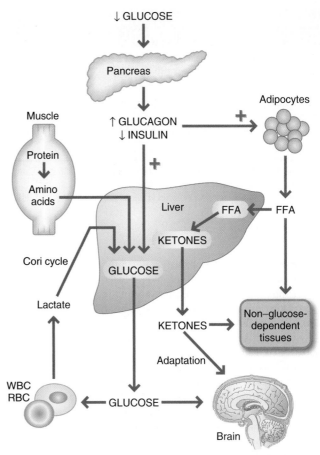

Fig. 37.3 Metabolic changes in starvation. *FFA*, Free fatty acid; *RBC*, red blood cell; *WBC*, white blood cell. (From Simmons RL, Steed DL: *Basic science review for surgeons*, Philadelphia, 1992, Saunders.)

uptake secondary to gluconeogenesis and elevated levels of hormones, including epinephrine, that diminish insulin release. Stress also initiates the release of aldosterone, a corticosteroid that causes renal sodium retention, and vasopressin (antidiuretic hormone), which stimulates renal tubular water resorption. The action of these hormones results in conservation of water and salt to support the circulating blood volume.

The response to injury also is regulated by metabolically active cytokines (proinflammatory proteins) such as interleukin-1 (IL-1), interleukin-6 (IL-6), and tumor necrosis factor (TNF), which are released by phagocytic cells in response to tissue damage, infection, inflammation, and some medications. IL-6 is secreted by T cells and macrophages to stimulate the immune response to trauma or other tissue damage leading to inflammation; it has proinflammatory and antiinflammatory actions (see Chapter 7). Cytokines are thought to stimulate hepatic amino acid uptake and protein synthesis, accelerate muscle breakdown, and induce gluconeogenesis. IL-1 appears to have a major role in stimulating the acute-phase response. The vagus nerve helps to regulate cytokine production through a cholinergic antiinflammatory pathway, releasing nicotinic acetylcholine receptor alpha-7 to reduce excessive cytokine activity.

As part of the acute-phase response, serum iron and zinc levels decrease, and levels of ceruloplasmin increase, primarily because of sequestration and, in the case of zinc, increased urinary zinc excretion. The net effect of the hormonally and cell-mediated response is an increase in oxygen supply and a greater availability of substrates for metabolically active tissues.

STARVATION VERSUS STRESS

The metabolic response to critical illness is very different from simple or uncomplicated starvation in which loss of muscle is much slower in an adaptive response to preserve lean body mass. Stored glycogen, the primary fuel source in early starvation, is depleted in approximately 24 hours. After the depletion of glycogen, glucose is available from the breakdown of protein to amino acids, depicted in Fig. 37.3. The depressed glucose levels lead to decreased insulin secretion and increased glucagon secretion. During the adaptive state of starvation, protein catabolism is reduced, and hepatic gluconeogenesis decreases.

Lipolytic activity is also different in starvation and in stress. After approximately 1 week of fasting or food deprivation, a state of ketosis develops, in which ketone bodies supply the bulk of energy needs, thus reducing the need for gluconeogenesis and conserving body protein to the greatest possible extent. In late starvation, as in stress, ketone body production is increased, and fatty acids serve as a major energy source for all tissues. Starvation is characterized by decreased energy expenditure, diminished gluconeogenesis, increased ketone body production, and decreased ureagenesis. Conversely, energy expenditure in stress is increased markedly, as are gluconeogenesis, proteolysis, and ureagenesis. As discussed, the stress response is activated by hormonal and cell mediators—counterregulatory hormones such as catecholamines, cortisol, and growth hormone. This mediator activation does not occur in starvation.

SYSTEMIC INFLAMMATORY RESPONSE SYNDROME, SEPSIS, AND ORGAN DYSFUNCTION OR FAILURE

Pathophysiology

Sepsis and the systemic inflammatory response syndrome (SIRS) often complicate the course of a critically ill patient. The term sepsis is used

BOX 37.1 Systemic Inflammatory Response Syndrome (SIRS)

Two or more of the following are present:
- Body temperature >38° C or <36° C
- Heart rate >90 beats/minute
- Respiratory rate >20 breaths/minute (tachypnea)
- White blood cell count >12,000/mm³ or <4000/mm³ or >10% immature bands (immature neutrophils in the absence of chemotherapy-induced neutropenia and leukopenia)

From Bone RC, et al: American College of Chest Physicians/Society of Critical Care Medicine Consensus Conference: definitions for sepsis and organ failure and guidelines for the use of innovative therapies in sepsis, *Crit Care Med.* 20:864, 1992.

when a patient has a life-threatening organ dysfunction caused by a dysregulated host response to infection (Singer et al, 2016). Bacteria and their toxins lead to a strong inflammatory response during critical illness. Other microorganisms that lead to an inflammatory response include viruses, fungi, and parasites.

Systemic inflammatory response syndrome (SIRS) describes the widespread inflammation that can occur in infection, pancreatitis, ischemia, burns, multiple trauma, hemorrhagic shock, or immunologically mediated organ injury. The inflammation is usually present in areas remote from the primary site of injury, affecting otherwise healthy tissue. Each condition leads to release of cytokines, proteolytic enzymes, or toxic oxygen species (free radicals) and activation of the complement cascade. Currently used SIRS criteria were published by Bone et al in 1992. Patients are classified with SIRS if they demonstrate any two of the following: heart rate >90 beats per minute, respiratory rate >20 beats per minute, body temperature >38° C or <36° C, or white blood cell count >12,000/mm³ or <4000/mm³ or >10% immature bands (Bone et al, 1992) and are shown in Box 37.1. The authors of the Third International Consensus Definitions for Sepsis and Septic Shock (Sepsis-3) also recommend using the quick sequential organ failure assessment (qSOFA) tool as a practical scoring system to define organ dysfunction of a potentially septic patient (Table 37.2).

A common complication of SIRS is the development of organ dysfunction or failure, often referred to as multiple organ dysfunction syndrome (MODS). The syndrome generally begins with lung failure and is followed by failure of the liver, intestines, and kidney in no particular order. Hematologic and myocardial failures usually manifest later; however, central nervous system changes can occur at any time. MODS may occur as the direct result of injury to an organ from trauma, major surgery, burns, sepsis, acute kidney injury, or acute

TABLE 37.2 Quick Sequential Organ Failure Assessment (qSOFA) Criteria

Criteria	Points*
Respiratory rate ≥22/minute	1
Change in mental status	1
Systolic blood pressure ≤100 mm Hg	1

*qSOFA score ≥2 indicates organ dysfunction
From Singer M, et al: The third international consensus definitions for sepsis and septic shock (sepsis-3), *JAMA* 315:801, 2016.

pancreatitis. Secondary MODS occurs in the presence of inflammation or infection in organs remote from the initial injury.

Patients with SIRS and MODS are clinically hypermetabolic and exhibit high cardiac output, low oxygen consumption, high venous oxygen saturation, and lactic acidemia. Patients generally have a strong positive fluid balance associated with massive edema and a decrease in plasma protein concentrations.

Multiple hypotheses have been proposed to explain the development of SIRS or MODS. In some studies, SIRS leading to MODS appears to be mediated by excessive production of proinflammatory cytokines and other mediators of inflammation. The gut hypothesis suggests that the trigger is injury or disruption of the gut barrier function, with corresponding translocation of enteric bacteria into the mesentery lymph nodes, liver, and other organs. Unique gut-derived factors carried in the intestinal lymph but not the portal vein usually lead to acute injury- and shock-induced SIRS and MODS. Shock results in gut hypoperfusion; the hypoperfused gut is a source of proinflammatory mediators. Early gut hypoperfusion causes an ileus or lack of peristalsis in the stomach and small bowel, and late infections cause further worsening of this gut dysfunction. Early enteral feeding is thought to restore gut function and influence the clinical course. The mechanism for this effect is due to the enhanced functional and structural integrity of the gut.

Enteral nutrition (EN) may have a role in maintaining tight junctions between the intraepithelial cells, stimulating blood flow and inducing the release of trophic factors (Fig. 37.4). Maintenance of villous height supports the secretory immunocytes that make up the gut-associated lymphoid tissue. With central parenteral nutrition (PN), mucosal atrophy and a loss of epithelial barrier function (EBF) may occur. Clinical trials evaluating the use of parenteral and enteral glutamine supplementation have demonstrated mixed results without clear clinical benefit, such as reduction in mortality, infectious complications, and faster recovery of organ dysfunction (Rhodes et al, 2017). Both the Surviving Sepsis Campaign Guidelines and the Society for Critical Care Medicine (SCCM) and American Society for Parenteral and Enteral Nutrition (ASPEN) Guidelines for the Provision and Assessment of Nutrition Support Therapy in the Critically Ill Patient recommend against exogenous glutamine supplementation (Rhodes et al, 2017; McClave et al, 2016).

MALNUTRITION: THE ETIOLOGY-BASED DEFINITION

The historical approach to defining malnutrition in the patient undergoing the stress response has recently been reevaluated. In an effort to provide consistency in its definition, in 2009 an international group of nutrition support leaders developed an etiology basis for the definition of malnutrition for hospitalized adult patients (see Appendix 11). This approach focuses on the following three causes: starvation-related malnutrition, chronic disease–related malnutrition, and acute disease–related malnutrition (Fig. 37.5). Using this framework, a collaborative workgroup of ASPEN and the Academy of Nutrition and Dietetics (AND) published a consensus document outlining specific criteria for diagnosing severe and nonsevere malnutrition. Each malnutrition cause is defined by specific criteria and thresholds (Box 37.2 for criteria specific to the acute illness and injury malnutrition cause). This specific category includes those patients experiencing SIRS and MODS and is characterized by a heightened cytokine response, which in turn leads to profound losses in fat-free mass. In this setting, multiple factors impede the body's ability to maintain or replete lean body mass despite provision of nutrition support therapy (Looijaard et al, 2018; Jensen et al, 2009, 2010).

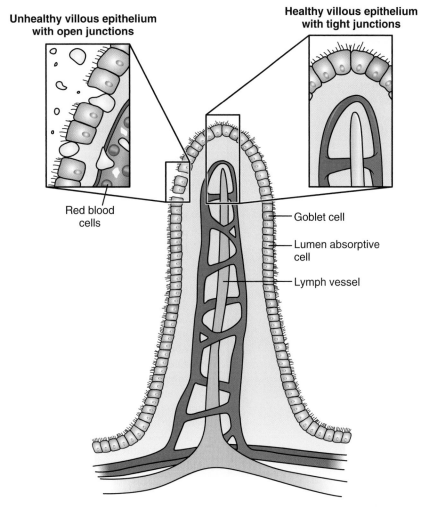

Fig. 37.4 Tight junction in the intestinal villus, supporting gut membrane integrity.

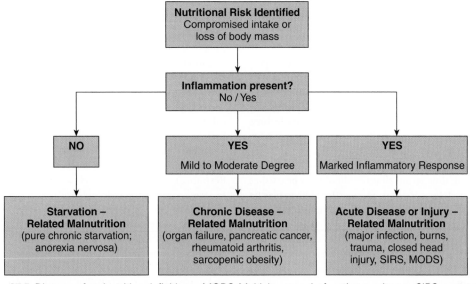

Fig. 37.5 Diagram of malnutrition definitions. *MODS*, Multiple organ dysfunction syndrome; *SIRS*, systemic inflammatory response syndrome. (Adapted from Jensen GL, et al: Malnutrition syndromes: a conundrum versus continuum, *J Parenter Enteral Nutr* 33:710, 2009; Jensen G, et al: Adult starvation and disease-related malnutrition: a proposal for etiology-based diagnosis in the clinical practice setting from the International Consensus Guideline Committee, *J Parenter Enteral Nutr* 34:156, 2010.)

BOX 37.2 Consensus Malnutrition Criteria for Acute Illness and Injury Cause

Severe Malnutrition
- Energy intake
  - ≤50% of estimated energy requirement for ≥5 days
- Weight loss (percentage of usual body weight over time period)
  - >2% over 1 week
  - >5% over 1 month
  - >7.5% over 3 months
- Loss of body fat
  - Moderate
- Loss of muscle mass
  - Moderate
- Fluid accumulation
  - Moderate to severe
- Hand grip strength
  - Measurably reduced

Nonsevere Malnutrition
- Energy intake
  - <75% of estimated energy requirement for >7 days
  - Weight loss (percentage of usual body weight over time period)
  - 1% to 2% over 1 week
  - 5% over 1 month
  - 7.5% over 3 months
- Loss of body fat
  - Mild
- Loss of muscle mass
  - Mild
- Fluid accumulation
  - Mild
- Hand grip strength
  - Not applicable

From Consensus statement: Academy of Nutrition and Dietetics and American Society for Parenteral and Enteral Nutrition: characteristics recommended for the identification and documentation of adult malnutrition (undernutrition). From White JA, et al: *J Parent Enteral Nutr* 36:275, 2012.

Medical Nutrition Therapy

The critically ill patient typically enters an ICU because of a cardiopulmonary diagnosis, intraoperative or postoperative complication, multiple trauma, burn injury, or sepsis. Traditional methods of assessing nutritional status are often of limited value in the ICU setting. The severely injured patient is usually unable to provide a dietary history. Values for weight may be erroneous after fluid resuscitation, and anthropometric measurements are not easily attainable, nor are they sensitive to acute changes. Hypoalbuminemia reflects severe illness, injury, and inflammation; thus serum albumin should not be used as a marker of nutritional status (McClave et al, 2016). Other plasma proteins such as prealbumin and transferrin often drop precipitously, related not to nutrition status but to an inflammation-induced decrease in hepatic synthesis and changes caused by compartmental shifts in body fluid. This is part of the acute-phase response in which secretory and circulating proteins are altered in response to inflammation or injury (see Chapters 5 and 7).

The critical role of physical assessment cannot be overlooked. Loss of lean body mass and accumulation of fluid are common among ICU patients, and the ability to recognize these changes, as well as other important physical parameters, is essential. In addition to conducting a nutrition-focused physical examination, researchers are evaluating body composition technologies including computed tomography (CT), dual-energy x-ray absorptiometry (DEXA), bioelectrical impedance analysis (BIA), and ultrasound (US) to evaluate their efficacy in characterizing nutritional status in an ICU setting (Teigen et al, 2017). In general, assessment and care planning focus on the preadmission, preoperative, or preinjury nutrition status; presence of any organ system dysfunction; the need for early nutrition support therapy; and options that exist for enteral or parenteral access.

Because the patient is so ill, oral intake of food or fluid may be severely limited. Some common nutrition diagnoses used in critical illness include the following:

- Inadequate oral food and beverage intake (requiring another mode of nutrient or fluid administration)
- Inadequate or excessive intake from EN or PN infusion
- Inappropriate infusion of EN or PN (e.g., using PN when EN is possible)
- Inadequate or excessive fluid intake (e.g., intravenous [IV] infusions, nutrient solutions, tube flushes)
- Increased nutrient needs (e.g., protein requirements for wound healing)
- Excessive carbohydrate intake (e.g., dextrose-containing [IV] infusions or PN, especially among patients who are malnourished or at risk for refeeding)
- Abnormal nutrition-related laboratory values
- Altered gastrointestinal (GI) function (e.g., vomiting, diarrhea, constipation, ileus)

If malnutrition or an inflammatory response is present, the nutrition diagnosis should be framed around those conditions. The rationale for focusing on malnutrition and the inflammatory response is that these conditions increase the risk of complications related to nutritional status. An example of such a problem, etiology, and signs and symptoms (PES) statement would be the following: Increased nutrient needs (energy and protein) related to an inflammatory response to injury as evidenced by elevated body temperature and minute ventilation.

Nutrition Support Therapy

Nutrition support therapy incorporates early EN (within 48 hours of ICU admission) when feasible, appropriate macro- and micronutrient delivery, and glycemic control. Favorable expected outcomes from these practices include reduced disease severity, decreased length of time in the ICU, and decreased infectious disease morbidity and overall mortality.

The traditional goals of nutrition support therapy during sepsis and after injury include minimization of starvation, prevention or correction of specific nutrient deficiencies, provision of adequate calories to meet energy needs while minimizing associated metabolic complications, and fluid and electrolyte management to maintain adequate urine output and normal homeostasis (see *Pathophysiology and Care Management Algorithm:* Hypermetabolic Response). Clinicians focus on attenuating the metabolic response to stress, preventing oxidative cellular injury, and modulating the immune response. The first emphasis of care in the ICU is establishing hemodynamic stability (maintenance of airway and breathing, adequate circulating fluid volume and tissue oxygenation, and acid-base neutrality). It is important to follow the patient's heart rate, blood pressure, cardiac output, mean arterial pressure (MAP), and oxygen saturation to assess hemodynamic stability because this determines when nutrition support therapy can commence. It is common practice to withhold EN if a patient's MAP is <50 mm Hg (McClave et al, 2016).

Glycemic control and its relationship to improved outcomes has been the focus of extensive study. It is now recognized that more moderate (blood glucose 140 to 180 mg/dL), rather than tight (blood glucose 80 to 110 mg/dL), control is associated with positive outcomes in critically ill patients (AND, 2018a). Dietitians must recognize the significant contribution of dextrose in PN formulas or IV fluids and its influence on glycemic control.

Nutritional Requirements

Energy. Ideally, indirect calorimetry (IC) should be used to determine energy requirements for critically ill patients (see Chapter 2). Oxygen consumption is an essential component in the determination of energy expenditure. Septic and trauma patients have substantial increases in energy expenditure associated with the magnitude of injury. IC can be performed serially as a patient's clinical status changes (AND, 2018b); this allows for a more accurate assessment of energy requirements during a patient's stay in the ICU. IC is not appropriate for all patients, however, and should be performed and interpreted by experienced clinicians (AND, 2018b). High oxygen requirements, the presence of a chest tube, acidosis, and the use of supplemental oxygen are factors that may lead to invalid results. In these situations measurement of energy expenditure by IC is not recommended (AND, 2018b).

In the absence of a metabolic cart for IC, energy requirements may be calculated as 25 to 30 kcal/kg/day (McClave et al, 2016) or by using one of the many published predictive equations (see Chapter 2). Avoidance of overfeeding in the critically ill patient is important. Although adequate energy is essential for metabolically stressed patients, excess calories can result in complications such as hyperglycemia, hepatic steatosis, and excess carbon dioxide production, which can exacerbate respiratory insufficiency or prolong weaning from mechanical ventilation.

There has been long-standing controversy about the value of increased energy intake for critically ill patients. Newer research may differentiate the conflicting outcomes observed in prior studies by stratifying patient populations by the degree of malnutrition or nutritional risk. For example, the Nutrition Risk in the Critically Ill (NUTRIC) score (Heyland et al, 2011) (Table 37.3) has been used to distinguish between low- and high-risk patients. Using this tool, greater energy and protein intake has been associated with lower mortality and faster time to discharge alive among high-risk (NUTRIC score ≥5) patients, but not among nutritionally low-risk patients (Compher et al, 2017).

Some debate also exists in practice regarding what value should be used for body weight in predictive equations. Actual body weight is a better predictor of energy expenditure than ideal body weight in obese individuals (Breen and Ireton-Jones, 2004). The 2012 Critical Illness Update recommends that when IC is unavailable, the Penn State University (PSU [2003b]) equation, using actual body weight, should be used in obese and nonobese patients who are younger than 60 years of age. For obese patients 60 years or older, the PSU (2010) equation should be used. Research indicates that these equations have the best prediction accuracy (AND, 2018b).

Available research suggests that hypocaloric, high-protein nutrition support therapy or "permissive underfeeding" in critically ill obese patients results in achievement of net protein anabolism and minimizes complications resulting from overfeeding. The SCCM and ASPEN guidelines suggest that clinical outcomes in patients supported with high-protein hypocaloric feeding are at least equivalent to those supported with high-protein eucaloric feeding (McClave et al, 2016). Furthermore, the guidelines recommend that for all classes of obesity, goal EN should not exceed 60% to 70% of target energy requirements as measured by IC. If IC is unavailable, 11 to 14 kcal/kg actual body weight (body mass index [BMI] 30 to 50) and 22 to 25 kcal/kg ideal body weight (BMI >50) can be used to estimate energy needs. Protein can be provided in a range from 2.0 grams/kg ideal body weight (BMI 30 to 40), up to 2.5 grams/kg ideal body weight

TABLE 37.3 Nutrition Risk in the Critically Ill (NUTRIC) Score

Variable	Range	Points
Age	<50	0
	50 to <75	1
	≥75	2
APACHE II	<15	0
	15 to <20	1
	20 to 28	2
	≥28	3
SOFA	<6	0
	6 to <10	1
	≥10	2
Number of comorbidities	0 to 1	0
	≥2	1
Days from hospital to ICU admission	0 to <1	0
	≥1	1
IL-6	0 to <400	0
	≥400	1

NUTRIC SCORE SCORING SYSTEM: IF IL-6 AVAILABLE

Sum of points	Category	Explanation
6-10	High score	• Associated with worse clinical outcomes (mortality, ventilation). • These patients are the most likely to benefit from aggressive nutrition therapy.
0-5	Low score	• These patients have a low malnutrition risk.

NUTRIC SCORE SCORING SYSTEM: IF NO IL-6 AVAILABLE

Sum of points	Category	Explanation
5-9	High score	• Associated with worse clinical outcomes (mortality, ventilation). • These patients are most likely to benefit from aggressive nutrition therapy.
0-4	Low score	• These patients have a low malnutrition risk.

APACHE, Acute physiologic assessment and chronic health evaluation; *ICU*, intensive care unit; *IL-6*, interleukin-6; *SOFA*, sequential organ failure assessment.
From Heyland DK, et al: Identifying critically ill patients who benefit the most from nutrition therapy: the development and initial validation of a novel risk assessment tool, *Crit Care* 15:R268, 2011.

(BMI >40) (McClave et al, 2016). Hypocaloric low protein feedings are associated with unfavorable outcomes and should be avoided. Clinical vigilance for adequate protein provision is important, and nitrogen balance studies may help guide in the establishment of protein goals. More research is needed to validate hypocaloric feeding as the standurd approach to nutrition support in obese patients, especially because of the wide variability in body composition (Choban and Dickerson, 2005; Port and Apovian, 2010).

PATHOPHYSIOLOGY AND CARE MANAGEMENT ALGORITHM

Hypermetabolic Response

ETIOLOGY

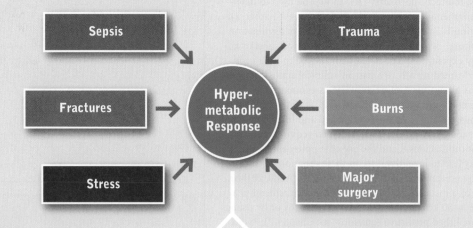

PATHOPHYSIOLOGY

EBB Phase

Hypovolemia
Shock
Tissue hypoxia
Decreased:
- Cardiac output
- O_2 consumption
- Body temperature

Flow Phase

Acute-phase proteins
Hormonal responses
Immune responses (cell-mediated and antibody)
Increased:
- Cardiac output
- O_2 consumption
- Body temperature
- Energy expenditure
- Protein catabolism

MANAGEMENT

Medical Management

- Treat cause of hypermetabolism
- Hemodynamic stability

Nutrition Management

- Minimize catabolism
- Meet energy requirements, but do not overfeed
  - Use indirect calorimetry if possible
  - Non-obese: 25-30 kcal/kg/day
  - Obese: 14-18 kcal/kg/day of actual body weight
- Meet protein, vitamin, and mineral needs
- Establish and maintain fluid and electrolyte balance
- Plan nutrition therapy (oral, enteral, and/or parenteral nutrition)
- Need for individualized therapeutic nutrient repletion
- Physical therapy
- Exercise as tolerated

Protein. Determination of protein requirements is difficult for critically ill patients. Patients typically require 1.2 to 2 g/kg/day depending on their baseline nutritional status, degree of injury and metabolic demand, and abnormal losses (e.g., through open abdominal wounds or burned skin) (Hoffer and Bistrian, 2012). Patients with acute kidney injury undergoing continuous renal replacement therapy (CRRT) may have a higher protein requirement because of the increased loss via the filtration process (see Chapter 34). A systematic review of protein requirements in critical illness concluded that protein delivery of 2.0 to 2.5 g/kg/day is safe and may be optimal for most critically ill patients except for those with refractory hypotension, overwhelming sepsis, or severe liver disease (Hoffer and Bistrian, 2012). A multicenter, registration-based randomized control trial is currently underway to better define optimal protein requirements in critical illness. Administration of excessive amounts of protein does not decrease the characteristic net negative nitrogen balance seen among hypermetabolic patients.

Vitamins, minerals, and trace elements. No specific guidelines exist for the provision of vitamins, minerals, and trace elements in metabolically stressed individuals. Conditions such as wounds, burns, malnutrition, chemical dependency (i.e., alcohol), and refeeding syndrome can all affect a patient's micronutrient requirements. Supplementation with antioxidant vitamins E and C, and trace minerals (selenium, zinc, copper) may improve outcomes among burn, trauma, and mechanically ventilated critically ill patients, but dosing, frequency, and route of administration have not been standardized (McClave et al, 2016). Micronutrient needs are elevated during acute illness because of increased urinary and cutaneous losses and diminished GI absorption, altered distribution, and altered serum carrier protein concentrations. With increased caloric intake there may be an increased need for B vitamins, particularly thiamin and niacin. Catabolism and loss of lean body tissue increase the loss of potassium, magnesium, phosphorus, and zinc. GI and urinary losses, organ dysfunction, and acid-base imbalance necessitate that mineral and electrolyte requirements be determined and adjusted individually. Fluid and electrolytes should be provided to maintain adequate urine output and normal serum electrolytes.

Feeding strategies. The preferred route for nutrient delivery is an orally consumed diet of whole foods. However, critically ill patients are often unable to eat because of endotracheal intubation and ventilator dependence. Furthermore, oral feeding may be delayed by impairment of chewing, swallowing, anorexia induced by pain-relieving medications, or posttraumatic shock and depression. Patients who are able to eat may not be able to meet the increased energy and nutrient requirements associated with metabolic stress and recovery. They often require combinations of oral nutritional supplements, EN, and PN. When EN fails to meet nutritional requirements or when GI feeding is contraindicated, PN support should be initiated.

Timing and route of feeding. Tools including the Nutritional Risk Screening (NRS 2002) and the NUTRIC score (see Table 37.3) have been used to identify critically ill patients who are most likely to benefit from nutrition support therapy (Kondrup et al, 2003; Heyland et al, 2011). The NRS 2002 is a simpler tool that includes the patient's BMI, weight loss in the past 3 months, reduced dietary intake in the last week, and presence of severe illness (Table 37.4), while the

---

TABLE 37.4 Nutrition Risk Screening [NRS 2002]

INITIAL SCREENING

		Yes	No
1	Is BMI <20.5?		
2	Has the patient lost weight within the last 3 months?		
3	Has the patient had a reduced dietary intake in the last week?		
4	Is the patient severely ill? (e.g., intensive care)		

Yes: If the answer is "yes" to any question, further screening is performed (see below).

No: Is the answer is "no" to all questions, the patient is rescreened weekly. If the patient is scheduled for major operation, a preventative nutritional care plan is considered to avoid the associated risk status.

FINAL SCREENING

Impaired nutritional status		Severity of disease (increase in requirements)	
Absent **Score 0**	Normal nutritional status	Absent **Score 0**	Normal nutritional requirements
Mild **Score 1**	Weight loss >5% in 3 months or food intake <50%-75% of normal requirement in preceding week	Mild **Score 1**	Hip fracture, chronic patients with acute complications: cirrhosis, COPD, chronic hemodialysis, diabetes, oncology
Moderate **Score 2**	Weight loss >5% in 2 months or BMI 18.5-20.5 + impaired general condition or food intake 25%-60% of normal requirement in preceding week	Moderate **Score 2**	Major abdominal surgery, stroke, severe hematologic malignancy
Severe **Score 3**	Weight loss >5% in 1 month (>15% in 3 months) or BMI <18.5 + impaired general condition or food intake 0%-25% of normal requirement in preceding week	Severe **Score 3**	Head injury, bone marrow transplantation, intensive care patients (APACHE >10)
Score:	+	**Score:**	= Total score
Age	If ≥70 years, add 1 to total score above = age − adjusted total score		

Score ≥3: The patient is nutritionally at risk and a nutritional care plan is initiated.

Score <3: Weekly rescreening of the patient. If the patient is scheduled for a major operation, a preventative nutritional care plan is considered to avoid the associated risk status.

APACHE, Acute physiologic assessment and chronic health evaluation; *BMI,* body mass index; *COPD,* chronic obstructive pulmonary disease.
From Kondrup J, et al: ESPEN guidelines for nutrition screening 2002, *Clin Nutr,* 22:415, 2003.

NUTRIC score uses a rubric composed of the patient's age, acute physiologic assessment and chronic health evaluation (APACHE II), SOFA, number of comorbidities, days from hospital to ICU admission, and IL-6 (if available) (see Table 37.3).

EN is the preferred route of feeding for the critically ill patient who cannot eat food and yet has good intestinal function. Feedings should be initiated early within the first 24 to 48 hours of ICU admission and advanced toward goal calories during the next 48 to 72 hours. Intake of 50% to 65% of goal calories during the first week of hospitalization is thought to be sufficient to achieve the clinical benefit of EN. This practice is intended for patients who are hemodynamically stable. In the setting of hemodynamic instability (large fluid volume requirements or use of high-dose catecholamine agents), tube feeding should be withheld until the patient is resuscitated fully or stable to minimize risk of ischemic or reperfusion injury.

Either gastric or small-bowel feedings can be used. Small-bowel feedings are indicated for patients who do not tolerate gastric feeding or who are deemed high risk for aspiration (McClave et al, 2016). Nasoenteric or surgically placed feeding tubes can be placed intraoperatively for patients with severe head, major thoracic, or spinal injury; facial injury requiring jaw wiring; proximal gastric or esophageal injuries; major pancreatic or duodenal injury; and severe trauma with plans for repeated surgeries.

Enteral tolerance should be monitored by assessing the level of pain, presence of abdominal distention, passage of flatus and stool, physical examination, and, if appropriate, abdominal x-ray examination. Elevating the head of the bed and using promotility medication can reduce aspiration risk. The cause of diarrhea, when present, should be determined, including assessment for infectious diarrhea. Patients should be evaluated for intake of hyperosmolar medications and broad-spectrum antibiotics. PN is indicated for patients in whom EN is unsuccessful or contraindicated.

Formula selection and fluid, energy, and nutrient requirements, as well as GI function, determine the choice of an enteral product. Most standard polymeric enteral formulas can be used to feed the critically ill patient. However, intolerance to standard formulas sometimes occurs because of their fat content, and the patient may temporarily require a lower-fat formula or a product containing a higher ratio of medium-chain triglycerides. Several commercially available products (see Appendix 15) are marketed specifically for patients with trauma and metabolic stress. These products typically have higher protein content and a higher ratio of BCAAs and/or additional glutamine, arginine, or antioxidant vitamins and minerals.

Immune modulating enteral formulations that contain arginine, glutamine, nucleic acids, antioxidants, and omega-3 fatty acids potentially have beneficial effects and favorable outcomes for critically ill patients who have undergone GI surgery, as well as for trauma and burn patients. However, these formulations should not be used routinely for ICU patients with sepsis because they may worsen the inflammatory response (McClave et al, 2016). Insoluble fiber should be avoided in critically ill patients; however, soluble fiber may be beneficial for the hemodynamically stable, critically ill patient who develops diarrhea (McClave et al, 2016). Patients at high risk for bowel ischemia initially should not receive fiber-containing formulas or diets.

TRAUMA AND THE OPEN ABDOMEN

After major abdominal trauma, bowel distention, and states of shock, some patients experience increased intraabdominal pressure leading to hypoperfusion and ischemia of the intestines and other peritoneal and retroperitoneal structures. Abdominal compartment syndrome

occurs with increased intraabdominal pressure, often after major abdominal trauma or sepsis. This condition has profound consequences, including hemodynamic instability and respiratory, renal, and neurologic abnormalities. Because the abdominal cavity has become too small, management consists of emergent decompressive laparotomy (surgical incision through the abdominal wall) to release intraabdominal pressure. Closure of the abdomen is not performed, either because the visceral edema is too great to close or to help with future reexploration. Temporary abdominal closure (TAC) is applied. Negative pressure wound therapy with continuous fascial traction is the recommended method for managing TAC. Fascial closure should be done as soon as the patient can tolerate it (Coccolini et al, 2018).

Patients with an open abdomen have severe metabolic alterations, increased loss of fluids, and elevated nutritional requirements. The open abdomen also may be a significant source of protein loss depending on the amount of drainage. It is recommended that an extra 15 to 30 grams of protein per liter of exudate be added to the nutrition prescription (McClave et al, 2016). There has been some controversy as to whether patients with an open abdomen can be fed enterally. As long as the patient is hemodynamically stable and does not require large-volume fluid resuscitation or increasing doses of pressor agents, enteral feeding should be possible (McClave et al, 2016). Ideally, a nasojejunal feeding tube should be positioned at the time of surgery to facilitate early EN support therapy.

Management of patients with intestinal fistulas and large draining wounds is also challenging surgically and nutritionally because these patients have metabolic abnormalities associated with losses of fluid, electrolytes, and nutrients (Friese, 2012; Majercik et al, 2012). The priorities for management of intestinal fistulas are to restore blood volume, replace fluid and electrolyte losses, treat sepsis, control fistula drainage, protect the surrounding skin, and provide optimal nutrition support therapy. ASPEN-La Federación Latinoamericana de Terapia Nutricional (FELANPE) guidelines were created to help guide the clinician when caring for the adult patient with enterocutaneous fistula (Kumpf et al, 2017). EN is the preferred route of feeding if the fistula output is less than 500 mL/day and access can be gained through or distal to the fistula site. If output is >500 mL/day or if the output impairs skin integrity or electrolyte and fluid balance, PN may be needed. Recommended protein needs are 1.5 to 2.0 grams/kg or up to 2.5 grams/kg if the patient has a high output enteroatmospheric fistula. No specific calorie goals have been established, but needs are likely similar to that of other critically ill patients. Somatostatin or somatostatin analogs can decrease drainage and assist with spontaneous closure (see Chapters 12 and 27).

MAJOR BURNS

Pathophysiology

Major burns result in severe trauma, and this response can be more pronounced and prolonged than any other injury. The release of inflammatory mediators results in a multitude of metabolic challenges. Hypermetabolism, muscle protein catabolism, MODS, insulin resistance, and infection are all common. Energy requirements can increase as much as 100% above resting energy expenditure (REE), depending on the extent and depth of the injury (Fig. 37.6). Exaggerated protein catabolism and increased urinary nitrogen excretion accompany this hypermetabolism, and protein is also lost through the burn wound exudate. Mechanical ventilation is usually required, especially in

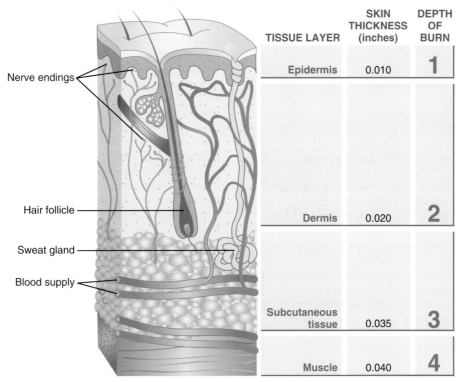

TISSUE LAYER	SKIN THICKNESS (inches)	DEPTH OF BURN
Epidermis	0.010	1
Dermis	0.020	2
Subcutaneous tissue	0.035	3
Muscle	0.040	4

Fig. 37.6 Interpretation of burn classification based on damage to the integument.

patients who have been in a smoke environment for prolonged periods of time, resulting in an inhalation injury. Side effects such as ileus, nausea, anorexia, and dysphagia are common following injury and can further complicate a patient's ability to meet their nutritional needs. In children, healing after burn and trauma requires not only restoration of oxygen delivery and adequate calories to support metabolism and repair but also awareness of how children differ from adults in metabolic rate, growth requirements, and physiologic response (Cook and Blinman, 2010).

Medical Management
Fluid and Electrolyte Repletion

The first 24 to 48 hours of treatment for thermally injured patients are devoted to fluid resuscitation. The volume of resuscitation fluid is approximately 2 to 4 mL/kg body weight per percentage of burn depending on the patient's physiologic demands or response. Generally, half of the calculated volume for the first 24 hours is given during the first 8 hours after burn injury and the remaining half in the next 16 hours. Urine output is used to titrate the rate of IV fluid replacement.

The volume of fluid needed is based on the age and weight of the patient and the extent of the injury designated by percentage of total body surface area (TBSA) burned. Once resuscitation is complete, ample fluids must be given to cover maintenance requirements and evaporative losses that continue through open wounds. Evaporative water loss can be estimated at 2 to 3.1 mL/kg of body weight per 24 hours per percent of TBSA burn. Serum sodium, osmolar concentrations, and body weight are used to monitor fluid status. Providing adequate fluids and electrolytes as soon as possible after injury is paramount for maintaining circulatory volume and preventing ischemia.

Wound Management

Wound management depends on the depth and extent of the burn. Current surgical management promotes use of topical antimicrobial agents and biologic and synthetic dressings, early debridement, excision, and grafting. Energy expenditure may be reduced slightly by the practice of covering wounds as early as possible to reduce evaporative heat and nitrogen losses and prevent infection.

Ancillary Measures

Passive and active range of motion exercises should be started early in the hospital to prevent contracture formation. Physical and occupational therapy helps maintain function and prevents muscle wasting and atrophy. A warm environment minimizes heat loss and the expenditure of energy to maintain body temperature. Thermal blankets, heat lamps, and individual heat shields often are used to maintain environmental temperature near 86° F. Minimizing fear and pain with reassurance from the staff and adequate pain medication also can reduce catecholamine stimulation and help avoid increases in energy expenditure. Treatments such as biofeedback, guided imagery, and good sleep hygiene are helpful. A number of pharmacologic strategies have been used to attenuate the hypermetabolic state and net protein loss sustained by burn patients (Abdullahi and Jeschke, 2014). These anabolic agents including insulin, oxandrolone, and propranolol improve lean body mass through metabolic effects on skeletal muscle or fat tissue. Insulin decreases protein breakdown, oxandrolone decreases protein breakdown and fat oxidation, and propranolol decreases fat oxidation and promotes glucose homeostasis. These pharmacologic agents are used now in conjunction with nutrition support in the care of burn patients.

Medical Nutrition Therapy

A burn patient has greatly accelerated metabolism and needs increased energy, carbohydrates, proteins, fats, vitamins, minerals, and antioxidants to heal and prevent detrimental sequelae.

BOX 37.3 Medical Nutrition Therapy Goals for Burn Patients

1. Minimize metabolic stress response by
   - Controlling environmental temperature
   - Maintaining fluid and electrolyte balance
   - Controlling pain and anxiety
   - Excising and covering wounds early
   - Considering pharmacologic agents to attenuate metabolic demands
2. Meet nutritional needs by
   - Providing adequate calories to prevent weight loss of greater than 10% of usual body weight
   - Providing adequate protein to promote wound healing, improve immune function, and limit loss of lean body mass
   - Providing vitamin and mineral supplementation if indicated
3. Continue to reassess nutritional requirements
   - Repeat indirect calorimetry (IC) weekly in the early stages of burn injury and as needed thereafter
   - Compare enteral nutrition (EN) volumes received to volumes ordered and adjust rates when needed
   - Repeat physical assessment and monitor weight trends compared with admission (preresuscitation) weight

The goals of nutrition support therapy after major burn injury include provision of adequate calories to meet energy needs while minimizing associated metabolic complications, prevention or correction of specific nutrient deficiencies, and fluid and electrolyte management for adequate urine output and normal homeostasis (see Box 37.3 for the nutritional goals for the burned person). Adequate surgical care, infection control, and nutrition should be implemented as soon as possible after burn resuscitation. Delays in admission to an organized burn unit can be detrimental, especially for children, because malnutrition is a common concern. Nutritional assessment of the adult burn patient should include evaluation of any preexisting substance abuse, psychiatric illness, or chronic disease that may be associated with malnutrition and could influence energy and nutrient requirements.

Many burn patients are able to eat food, and nutrition counseling should focus on selection of high protein and calorically dense food and fluids. It is not uncommon that patients require supplemental nutrition support, and EN should be considered for those patients who are unable to eat or cannot achieve adequate intake by food alone. With major burns, placement of enteral tubes should occur as soon as possible after the injury. Early initiation of EN support has been shown to blunt the hypermetabolic response and lessen the degree of protein catabolism. Postpyloric trophic feeds have been safely initiated 4 to 6 hours post burn and titrated to goal volumes following the resuscitation period. Feeding tube placement into the duodenum or jejunum also allows for uninterrupted delivery of nutrition during frequent surgical procedures (Varon et al, 2017). In contrast, many patients with gastric tubes must be made nothing by mouth (NPO) for wound excisions and skin grafting, thus limiting their ability to receive adequate nutrition.

Energy

Increased energy needs of the burn patient vary according to the size of the burn, with severely burned patients often approaching twice their predicted energy expenditure. Burn size makes the largest contribution to measured energy expenditure, followed by age (Shields et al, 2013). Most predictive equations used to calculate energy expenditure in severely burned adults do not correlate strongly with measured energy expenditure (Shields et al, 2013). Therefore measuring energy expenditure via IC is the most reliable method for assessing energy expenditure in burn patients. It is believed that increasing energy requirements by 10% to 30% above measured REE may be necessary to limit weight loss in burn patients and account for energy expenditure associated with wound care and physical therapy. If IC is not an option, there is debate as to which predictive equation is optimal. Dickerson compared 46 predictive equations to the IC results of 24 adult patients and found Xie (1993), Zawacki (1970), and Milner (1994) to be the most precise, unbiased predictive equations (Dickerson et al, 2002), whereas Shields compared nine predictive equations to the IC results of 31 adult burn patients and found Milner (1994), Carlson (1992), and Harris-Bennedict equations with an injury factor of 1.5 were the only equations that were not statistically different from measured energy expenditure (Shields et al, 2013). European Society for Clinical Nutrition and Metabolism (ESPEN) guidelines suggest the Toronto equation for adult burn patients and the Schofield equation for burn children (Rousseau et al, 2013).

Additional calories may be required because of fever, sepsis, multiple traumas, or the stress of surgery. Although weight gain may be desirable for the severely underweight patient, this is generally not feasible until acute illness has resolved. Overfeeding can lead to difficulty weaning from mechanical ventilation, fatty liver, azotemia, and hyperglycemia. When a factor of 1.4 was added to measured REE, patients gained weight but it was an increase in fat mass without improvements in lean body mass (Hart et al, 2002). Adjustments in caloric goals may be required when patients receive a large amount of IV dextrose solutions and propofol (an anesthetic in a lipid-delivery system).

Weight maintenance should be the goal for overweight patients until the healing process is complete. Obese individuals may be at higher risk of wound infection and graft disruption. There is limited data on energy requirements for the obese burned patient, and while the PSU equation has been recommended for obese, critically ill patients, this has not been validated with the burn population. A small study including obese trauma as well as nine obese burn patients found that 21 kcal/kg/day was more similar to the average measured REE than the studied equations (Stucky et al, 2008).

Protein

The protein needs of burn patients are elevated because of losses through urine and wounds, increased use in gluconeogenesis, and wound healing. Recent evidence promotes the feeding of high amounts of protein. Providing 1.5 to 2.0 grams/kg in adults and 2.4 to 4.0 grams/kg in children is recommended (McClave et al, 2016).

The adequacy of energy and protein intake is best evaluated by monitoring wound healing, graft take, and basic nutrition assessment parameters. Wound healing or graft take may be delayed if weight loss exceeds 10% of the usual weight. An exact evaluation of weight loss may be difficult to obtain because of fluid shifts or edema, or because of differences in the weights of dressings or splints. The coordination of weight measurement with dressing changes or hydrotherapy may allow recording of a weight without dressings and splints. Monitoring weight trends compared with admission, preresuscitation weight, and ongoing physical assessment is necessary.

Nitrogen balance often is used to evaluate the efficacy of a nutritional regimen, but it cannot be considered accurate without accounting for wound losses, which is difficult to accomplish in a clinical setting. Nitrogen excretion should begin to decrease as wounds heal, are grafted, or are covered. Unfortunately, serum proteins such as albumin and prealbumin are more representative of the acute phase response than nutritional status. Using these laboratory tests to monitor nutritional status is not recommended (SCCM and ASPEN, 2016).

Micronutrients and Antioxidants

Vitamin and trace elements are required for many stages of the burn healing process, and circulating levels of these nutrients have been shown to be lower than normal either due to the inflammatory process or due to losses in wound exudate. Although it is known that levels of many vitamins and minerals are low in this population after injury, exact supplementation guidelines have not been determined and practice among facilities is varied. The ASPEN and ESPEN guidelines both recommend supplementation but do not give dosing recommendations (McClave et al, 2016; Rousseau et al, 2013). A recent systematic review and meta-analysis evaluated supplementation of selenium, copper, and zinc either alone or combined. Results showed no effect on length of stay (LOS) nor mortality but a significant decrease in infectious episodes was found (Kurmis et al, 2016).

Vitamin C is involved in collagen synthesis, fibroblast and capillary formation, and immune system maintenance; it also acts as a powerful antioxidant (Nordlund et al, 2014). Furthermore, vitamin C levels decrease after burn injury and may be a result of cutaneous losses (Vinha et al, 2013). Vitamin C frequently is supplemented to promote wound healing (0.5 to 1.0 grams/day), and some centers are using high-dose vitamin C (0.66 mg/kg/h for 24 h) during the resuscitation period to minimize the amount of fluid resuscitation requirements (Rousseau et al, 2013).

Vitamin A is also an important nutrient for immune function and epithelialization. Vitamin A deficiency impairs collagen synthesis and may affect wound healing negatively. Toxicity is also possible, however, and vitamin A supplementation should be limited in patients with kidney and liver disease. Few clinical data suggest routine supplementation of vitamin A in burns, and vitamin A levels have been shown to return to normal 2 weeks after injury without supplementation (Nordlund et al, 2014).

Vitamin D deficiency has been reported in pediatric and adult burn patients. It is still unknown how to interpret vitamin D levels in critical illness, and optimal dosing levels for supplementation have not been established. Vitamin D is an area of ongoing research, especially in the burn population, as burn survivors have a long-term increased risk of vitamin D deficiency because the major source of vitamin D synthesis is in the skin (Al-Tarrah et al, 2018).

Electrolyte imbalances that involve serum sodium or potassium usually are corrected by adjusting fluid therapy. Hyponatremia may be seen in patients whose evaporative losses are reduced drastically by the application of dressings or grafts; who have had changes in maintenance fluids; or who have been treated with silver nitrate soaks, which tend to draw sodium from the wound. Restricting the oral consumption of free water and sodium-free fluids may help correct hyponatremia. Hypokalemia often occurs after the initial fluid resuscitation and during protein synthesis. Slightly elevated serum potassium may indicate inadequate hydration.

Depression of serum calcium levels may be seen in patients with burns that involve more than 30% TBSA. Hypocalcemia accompanies hypoalbuminemia. Calcium losses may be exaggerated if the patient is immobile or being treated with silver nitrate soaks. Early ambulation and exercise should help minimize these losses.

Hypophosphatemia also has been identified in patients with major burns. This occurs most commonly in patients who receive large volumes of resuscitation fluid along with parenteral infusion of glucose solutions and large amounts of antacids for stress ulcer prophylaxis. Serum levels must be monitored and appropriate phosphate supplementation provided. Magnesium levels also may require

attention because a significant amount of magnesium can be lost from the burn wound. Supplemental phosphorus and magnesium often are given parenterally to prevent GI irritation.

A depressed serum zinc level has been reported in burn patients, but whether this represents total body zinc status or is an artifact of hypoalbuminemia is unclear, because zinc is bound to serum albumin. Zinc is a cofactor in energy metabolism and protein synthesis. Supplementation with 220 mg of zinc sulfate (50 mg elemental zinc) is common (Nordlund et al, 2014). However, zinc content of enteral tube feedings and other multivitamins should be monitored to prevent long-term over-supplementation of zinc, which can result in copper deficiency. The anemia initially seen after a burn usually is unrelated to iron deficiency and is treated with packed red blood cells.

Methods of Nutrition Support Therapy

Methods of nutrition support therapy must be implemented on an individual basis. Most patients with burns of less than 20% TBSA are able to meet their needs with a regular high-calorie, high-protein oral diet. Often the use of concealed nutrients such as protein added to puddings, milks, and gelatins is helpful because consuming large volumes of foods can be overwhelming to the patient. Patients should have immediate access to food and fluids at the bedside. They should be encouraged to consume calorically dense, high-protein drinks. Involving family and caregivers during mealtimes helps to promote good oral intake.

Patients with major burns, elevated energy expenditure, or poor appetites may require tube feeding or PN. Enteral feeding is the preferred method of nutrition support therapy for burn patients, but PN may be necessary if unable to use the enteral route. Because ileus is often present only in the stomach, severely burned patients can be fed successfully by tube into the small bowel. PN may be needed for patients who do not tolerate tube feeds or do not have enteral access. Soybean oil–based parenteral lipid infusions may inhibit immune function. Alternative mixed oil lipid emulsions are now available, but they have not been specifically studied in the burn population. With careful monitoring, central lines for PN can be maintained through burn wounds (see Chapter 12).

SURGERY

The delivery of correctly formulated and safely administered nutritional and metabolic support is a matter of life or death in surgical and critical care units; obese patients have a higher surgical risk (Blackburn et al, 2010). Although surgical morbidity correlates best with the extent of the primary disease and the nature of the operation performed, malnutrition also may compound the severity of complications. A well-nourished patient usually tolerates major surgery better than a severely malnourished patient. Malnutrition is associated with a high incidence of operative complications, morbidity, and death. If a malnourished patient is expected to undergo major upper GI surgery and EN is not feasible, PN should be initiated 7 to 10 days preoperatively and continued into the postoperative period if the duration of therapy is anticipated to be longer than 7 days. For a patient who is not malnourished at the time of admission and EN is not feasible, PN should be delayed for 5 to 7 days following surgery (McClave et al, 2016; see Chapter 12).

Medical Nutrition Therapy
Preoperative Nutrition Care

The routine practice of requiring a patient take NPO at midnight before surgery has been discontinued in many settings. The American Society of Anesthesiologists historically recommended withholding solids for 6 hours preoperatively and clear liquids for 2 hours before induction of anesthesia. This practice was intended to minimize aspiration and regurgitation. The use of a carbohydrate-rich beverage in the preoperative period has been shown to enhance glycemic control and decrease losses of nitrogen, lean body mass, and muscle strength after abdominal and colorectal surgery (Bilku et al, 2014).

Postoperative Nutrition Care

Postoperative patients who are critically ill and receiving care in the ICU should receive early EN unless there is an absolute contraindication (McClave et al, 2016). This practice after major GI surgery is associated with reduced infection and decreased hospitalization. If the patient is malnourished (severe or nonsevere), however, the use of PN is indicated to provide perioperative support until patients are able to tolerate goal enteral feeding regimens (McClave et al, 2016). The use of arginine-containing immune-enhanced enteral formulas is associated with a decrease in wound complications and a reduced hospital LOS in patients who have undergone GI surgery (Drover et al, 2011; Marik and Zaloga, 2010).

If oral feeding is not possible or an extended NPO period is anticipated, an access device for enteral feeding should be inserted at the time of surgery. Combined gastrostomy-jejunostomy tubes offer significant advantages over standard gastrostomies because they allow for simultaneous gastric drainage from the gastrostomy tube and enteral feeding via the jejunal tube.

The timing of introduction of solid food after surgery depends on the patient's degree of alertness and condition of the GI tract. A general practice has been to progress over a period of several meals from clear liquids to full liquids and finally to solid foods. However, no physiologic reason exists for solid foods not to be introduced as soon as the GI tract is functioning and a few liquids are tolerated. Surgical patients can be fed a regular solid-food diet rather than a clear liquid diet.

CLINICAL CASE STUDY

Chronologic Clinical Case Study with Suggested Answers

First Assessment

A 44-year-old Native American man was admitted to a hospital with an incarcerated ventral hernia and probable bowel compromise. He underwent hernia repair and was found to have dusky areas of small bowel (clinical sign of lack of oxygenation). He was left in temporary abdominal closure and remained mechanically ventilated and sedated. On hospital day 5, 30 cm of jejunum was resected and the patient was left in discontinuity (the jejunum had not been reconnected yet) with a plan to return to the operating room in the next 24 hours.

Screening and Assessment Data

Height = 72" (183 cm)
Weight = 364 lb (165 kg)
Body mass index = 49 kg/m^2
Ideal body weight = 178 lb (81 kg)
Weight change in the 1 month before admission: none
Decreased intake in the previous month: no
Physical examination: bilateral severe pitting edema of ankles and upper extremities.
Abdominal examination: distended with absent bowel sounds
Currently receiving 0.45% normal saline at 120 mL/h
Intake/Output = 3305/3725 mL

Laboratory Values

Sodium: 138 mmol/dL
Potassium: 3 mmol/dL
Chloride: 105 mmol/dL
Carbon dioxide: 27 mmol/dL
Blood urea nitrogen: 13 mg/dL
Creatinine: 1.28 mg/dL
Glucose: 185 mg/dL
Ionized calcium: 1.12 mm/L
Magnesium: 1.6 mg/dL
Phosphorus: 2.1 mg/dL
Albumin: 1.9 g/dL

1. Write pertinent nutrition diagnosis statements (problem, cause, and signs and symptoms [PES] format) in order of priority for this patient.
   Malnutrition in the context of acute illness as evidenced by energy intake <50% of requirements (≥5 days) and severe fluid accumulation.
   Altered nutrition-related laboratory values related to the metabolic response to stress and a lack of electrolyte intake in diet and intravenous fluids as evidenced by low serum sodium, potassium, and phosphorus.

2. Should the patient be started on parenteral nutrition (PN)? Explain.
   By the information presented in the case, the patient should be started on PN because he is malnourished, has been NPO for 6 days, and cannot begin enteral nutrition (EN).

3. Calculate the patient's nutritional needs.
   His caloric requirement should be estimated using the hypocaloric, high-protein approach because he is morbidly obese (grade III) and renal function is normal. Ideal body weight should be used.
   Hypocaloric regimen for this patient is 11 to 14 kcal/kg actual body weight: 1815 to 2310 kcal/day.
   Protein requirement may be set at 2 to 2.5 g/kg ideal body weight or 162 to 203 g/day.

First Change of Status with Reassessment

Patient returned to the operating room (OR) on hospital day 6 where remaining small bowel appeared viable. He was placed back in continuity (the jejunum was reconnected at the site of the prior resection) and the abdomen was closed. On hospital day 7 the patient's body temperature spiked to 39° C, and he was found to have multiple infected abdominal abscesses. He goes to the operating room for abscess drainage. During this time his blood pressure (BP) and urine output dropped considerably, requiring initiation of fluid resuscitation and vasopressor agents for BP stabilization. His kidney function is noted to worsen. There is no plan for renal replacement therapy at the present.

Current status is noted:
T$_{max}$ 39.3° C
VE = 15.6 L/min (minute ventilation)
PN continues
Intravenous fluids: 0.45% normal saline solution at 150 mL/h + additional fluid boluses
Sodium: 131 mmol/dL
Potassium: 5.1 mmol/dL
Chloride: 96 mmol/dL
Carbon dioxide: 15 mmol/dL
Blood glucose: 225 mg/dL
Ionized calcium: 1.01 mm/L
Magnesium: 2.8 mg/dL
Phosphorus: 4.8 mg/dL
Albumin: 1.2 gm/dL
Arterial blood gas: 7.31/24/115/11

CLINICAL CASE STUDY—cont'd

Chronologic Clinical Case Study with Suggested Answers

4. Upon monitoring, what is the patient's metabolic state?

He has become hypermetabolic and hypercatabolic, and he has worsening kidney function.

Hyperglycemia has worsened.

Electrolyte excess (potassium, phosphorus, magnesium).

5. What is the patient's acid-base status?

He has a metabolic acidosis resulting from an impaired renal excretion of acid, and reabsorption and regeneration of bicarbonate.

6. Write updated PES statements:

Increased nutrient needs (energy and protein) related to a systemic inflammatory response as evidenced by fever and elevated minute ventilation.

Altered nutrition-related laboratory values (hyperglycemia) related to stress metabolism and glucose intake as evidenced by blood glucose of 225 mg/dL.

Altered nutrition-related laboratory values related to acute kidney injury as evidenced by elevated potassium, phosphorus, and magnesium.

7. Is the patient's blood glucose control adequate? If not, why and what should be done?

His blood glucose is not adequately controlled. There is evidence that when glucose levels are controlled between 140 to 180 mg/dL, survival is better.

The dextrose load in his PN should be reduced or a standardized insulin protocol should be instituted, or both. In addition, energy intake should be assessed to confirm absence of overfeeding because this could result in hyperglycemia.

8. Why is the patient's serum albumin level falling?

Decreased acute-phase proteins are a response to the inflammatory process his body has mounted to try to reestablish homeostasis.

Second Change of Status with Reassessment

On hospital day 10, the patient has not yet stooled, but his abdomen is soft. His acute kidney injury continues, although hemodialysis has been initiated and electrolyte levels have normalized. On rounds, the dietitian asks whether the patient is stable enough to start tube feeding through a postpyloric feeding tube. The surgical and critical care teams believe that the patient's gastrointestinal status has improved sufficiently to initiate an enteral feeding.

9. What feeding formula should be used? Is an immune-enhancing tube feeding formula indicated?

Commercial immune-enhancing formulas that combine several nutrients thought to enhance immune function are not indicated for routine use, and may be contraindicated in the severely critically ill, such as this patient.

A polymeric enteral feeding was initiated via postpyloric access and gradually advanced to goal rate during the next 2 to 3 days. Tolerance was demonstrated via no change in abdominal distention, pain, or nausea and vomiting. As the feeding advanced, the PN was gradually weaned, then discontinued when > 60% of goal (EN) was achieved.

CLINICAL INSIGHT

Factors to consider when interpreting the literature with respect to conflicting data among nutrition support outcomes studies:

- Study designs may differ
- Sample size may be too small
- Patient sample may be heterogeneous; subjects may differ by underlying illness or injury, acuity level, mortality risk
- Inclusion of well-nourished patients who would likely not show an effect of nutrition intervention
- Preexisting malnutrition may or may not be present and may or may not be diagnosed with similar criteria

- Length of intensive care unit (ICU) stay may vary
- Short interval time of nutrition therapy in the ICU
- Differences may be present with respect to timing of initiation of enteral nutrition (EN) or parenteral nutrition (PN)
- Contribution of nonnutritional calorie sources such as D5W (5% dextrose in water) and medications in lipid delivery systems (i.e., propofol, clevidipine)
- Differences in techniques to establish target energy goals (i.e., indirect calorimetry, predictive equations, kcal/kg)

CLINICAL INSIGHT

Enhanced Recovery After Surgery (ERAS)

First presented in the late 1990s, this multimodal pathway for care of the surgical patient has become a standard of care for many conditions including colon, rectal, liver, and esophageal resections; pancreatoduodenectomy; bariatric surgery; major gynecologic procedures; and head and neck cancer surgery (Ljungqvist et al, 2017). This management approach involves aspects of the patient's care preoperatively, during the surgical procedure, and postoperatively (Fig. 37.7). The central elements of the ERAS pathway address key factors including pain control, gut dysfunction, the need for intravenous fluids, and ambulation. The ERAS components help clarify how these areas interact to affect patient recovery, and mounting evidence demonstrates that use of the ERAS pathway results in positive outcomes compared with standard surgical care.

In a meta-analysis, Varadhan and colleagues reported the ERAS pathway was shown to reduce surgical care time by more than 30% and reduce postoperative complications by up to 50% (Varadhan et al, 2010). An international ERAS society was formed in 2010 with its mission to "develop perioperative care and to improve recovery through research, audit education and implementation of evidence-based practice" (Gustafsson et al, 2012).

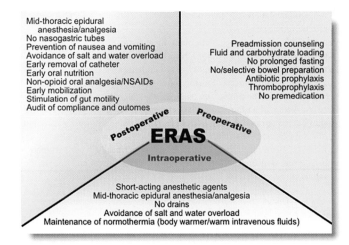

Fig. 37.7 The enhanced recovery after surgery (ERAS) Protocol. *NSAIDs,* Nonsteroidal antiinflammatory drugs. From Short HL, Taylor N, Thakore M et al, *J Ped Surg,* 53(March), pp 418–430, 2018.

USEFUL WEBSITES

American Burn Association
American Society for Parenteral and Enteral Nutrition (ASPEN)
ERAS® Society
Society of Critical Care Medicine (SCCM)

REFERENCES

Abdullahi A, Jeschke MG: Nutrition and anabolic pharmacotherapies in the care of burn patients, *Nutr Clin Pract* 29:621–630, 2014.

Academy of Nutrition and Dietetics: *Critical illness: glucose control. Evidence-analysis library*, 2012. Available at: https://www.andeal.org/template.cfm?template=guide_summary&key=3204.

Academy of Nutrition and Dietetics: *Critical illness: determination of resting metabolic rate*, 2012. Available at: https://www.andeal.org/template.cfm?template=guide_summary&key=3200.

Al-Tarrah K, Hewison M, Moiemen N, et al: Vitamin D status and its influence on outcomes following major burn injury and critical illness, *Burns Trauma* 6:11, 2018.

Bilku DK, Dennison AR, Hall TC, et al: Role of preoperative carbohydrate loading: a systematic review, *Ann R Coll Surg Engl* 96:15–22, 2014.

Blackburn GL, Wollner S, Bistrian BR: Nutrition support in the intensive care unit: an evolving science, *Arch Surg* 145:533–338, 2010.

Bone RC, Balk RA, Cerra FB, et al: American Society of Chest Physicians/Society of Critical Care Medicine consensus conference: definitions for sepsis and organ failure and guidelines for the use of innovative therapies in sepsis, *Crit Care Med* 20:864–874, 1992.

Breen HB, Ireton-Jones CS: Predicting energy needs in obese patients, *Nutr Clin Pract* 19:284–289, 2004.

Choban PS, Dickerson RN: Morbid obesity and nutrition support: is bigger different? *Nutr Clin Pract* 20:480–487, 2005.

Coccolini F, Roberts D, Ansaloni L, et al: The open abdomen in trauma and non-trauma patients: WSES guidelines, *World J Emerg Surg* 13:7, 2018.

Compher C, Chittams J, Sammarco T, et al: Greater protein and energy intake may be associated with improved mortality in higher risk critically ill patients: a multicenter, multinational observational study, *Crit Care Med* 45:156–163, 2017.

Cook RC, Blinman TA: Nutritional support of the pediatric trauma patient, *Semin Pediatr Surg* 19:242–251, 2010.

Dickerson RN, Gervasio JM, Riley ML, et al: Accuracy of predictive methods to estimate resting energy expenditure of thermally-injured patients, *JPEN J Parenter Enteral Nutr* 26:17–29, 2002.

Drover JW, Dhaliwal R, Weitzel L, et al: Perioperative use of arginine-supplemented diets: a systematic review of the evidence, *J Am Coll Surg* 212:385–399, 2011.

Friese RS: The open abdomen: definitions, management principles, and nutrition support considerations, *Nutr Clin Pract* 27:492–498, 2012.

Gustafsson UO, Scott MJ, Schwenk W, et al: Guidelines for perioperative care in elective colonic surgery: Enhanced Recovery After Surgery (ERAS) Society recommendations, *Clin Nutr* 31:783–800, 2012.

Hart DW, Wolf SE, Herdon DN, et al: Energy expenditure and caloric balance after burn: increased feeding leads to fat rather than lean muscle accretion, *Ann Surg* 235:152–161, 2002.

Heyland DK, Dhaliwal R, Jiang X, et al: Identifying critically ill patients who benefit the most from nutrition therapy: the development and initial validation of a novel risk assessment tool, *Crit Care* 15:R268, 2011.

Hoffer LJ, Bistrian BR: Appropriate protein provision in critical illness: a systematic and narrative review, *Am J Clin Nutr* 96:591–600, 2012.

Jensen GL, Bistrian B, Roubenoff R, et al: Malnutrition syndromes: a conundrum versus continuum, *JPEN J Parenter Enteral Nutr* 33:710–716, 2009.

Jensen GL, Mirtallo J, Compher C, et al: Adult starvation and disease-related malnutrition: a proposal for etiology-based diagnosis in the clinical practice setting from the International Consensus Guideline Committee, *J Parenter Enteral Nutr* 34:156–159, 2010.

Kondrup J, Allison SP, Elia M, et al: ESPEN guidelines for nutrition screening 2002, *Clin Nutr* 22:415–421, 2003.

Kumpf VJ, de Aguilar-Nascimento JE, Diaz-Pizarro Graf JI, et al: ASPEN-FELANPE clinical guidelines, *J Parenter Enteral Nutr* 41:104–112, 2017.

Kurmis R, Greenwood J, Aromataris E, et al: Trace element supplementation following severe burn injury: a systematic review and meta-analysis, *J Burn Care Res* 37:143–159, 2016.

Looijaard WGPM, Molinger J, Weijs PJM: Measuring and monitoring lean body mass in critical illness, *Curr Opin Crit Care* 24:241–247, 2018.

Ljungqvist O, Scott M, Fearon KC, et al: Enhanced recovery after surgery: a review. *JAMA Surg* 152:292–298, 2017.

Majercik S, Kinikini M, White T: Enteroatmospheric fistula: from soup to nuts, *Nutr Clin Pract* 27:507–512, 2012.

Marik PE, Zaloga GP: Immunonutrition in high-risk surgical patients: a systematic review and analysis of the literature, *J Parenter Enteral Nutr* 34:378–386, 2010.

McClave SA, Taylor BE, Martindale RG, et al: Guidelines for the provision and assessment of nutrition support therapy in the adult critically ill patient: Society of Critical Care Medicine (SCCM) and American Society for Parenteral and Enteral Nutrition (ASPEN), *J Parenter Enteral Nutr* 40:159–211, 2016.

Nordlund MJ, Pham TN, Gibran NS, et al: Micronutrients after burn injury: a review, *J Burn Care Res* 35:121–133, 2014.

Port AM, Apovian C: Metabolic support of the obese intensive care unit patient: a current perspective, *Curr Opin Clin Nutr Metab Care* 13:184–191, 2010.

Rhodes A, Evans LE, Alhazzani W, et al: Surviving sepsis campaign: international guidelines for management of sepsis and septic shock 2016, *Crit Care Med* 45:486–552, 2017.

Rousseau AF, Losser MR, Ichai C, et al: ESPEN endorsed recommendations: Nutritional therapy in major burns, *Clin Nutr* 32:497–502, 2013.

Shields BA, Doty KA, Chung KK, et al: Determination of resting energy expenditure after severe burn, *J Burn Care Res* 34:e22–e28, 2013.

Short HL, Taylor N, Thakore, M et al: A survey of pediatric surgeons' practices with enhanced recovery after children's surgery, *J Ped Surg*, 53:418–430, 2018.

Singer M, Deutschman CS, Seymour CW, et al: The third international consensus definitions for sepsis and septic shock (sepsis-3), *JAMA* 23:801–810, 2016.

Stucky CC, Moncure M, Hise M, et al: How accurate are resting energy expenditure prediction equations in obese trauma and burn patients? *J Parenter Enteral Nutr* 32:420–426, 2008.

Teigen LM, Kuchnia AJ, Mourtzakis M, et al: The use of technology for estimating body composition: strengths and weaknesses of common modalities in a clinical setting, *Nutr Clin Pract* 32:20–29, 2017.

Varadhan KK, Neal KR, Dejong CH, et al: The enhanced recover after surgery (ERAS) pathway for patients undergoing major elective open colorectal surgery: a meta-analysis of randomized trials, *Clin Nutr* 29:434–440, 2010.

Varon DE, Freitas G, Goel N, et al: Intraoperative feeding improves calorie and protein delivery in acute burn patients, *J Burn Care Res* 38:299–303, 2017.

Vinha PP, Martinez EZ, Vannucchi H, et al: Effect of acute thermal injury in status of serum vitamins, inflammatory markers, and oxidative stress markers: preliminary data, *J Burn Care Res* 34:e87–e91, 2013.

38

Medical Nutrition Therapy for Rheumatic and Musculoskeletal Disease

F. Enrique Gómez, MSc, PhD
Gabriela E. Mancera-Chávez, MSc, NC
Martha Kaufer-Horwitz, MSc, DSc, NC, FTOS

KEY TERMS

ankylosing spondylitis (AS)
antiinflammatory diet
antinuclear antibodies (ANA)
arachidonic acid (ARA)
arthritis
autoimmune arthritis
biologic response modifiers (BRMs)
cyclooxygenase (COX)
C-reactive protein (CRP)
cytokines
dihomo-γ-linolenic acid (DGLA)
disease-modifying antirheumatic drugs
    (DMARDs)
docosahexaenoic acid (DHA)
eicosanoids
eicosapentaenoic acid (EPA)
gamma-linolenic acid (GLA)
gout

hyperuricemia
leukotrienes (LT)
lipoxygenase (LOX)
maresins
monosodium urate (MSU) crystals
nonsteroidal antiinflammatory drug
    (NSAIDs)
osteoarthritis (OA)
polymyalgia rheumatica (PMR)
polymyositis (PM)
polyunsaturated fatty acids (PUFAs)
prostaglandins (PG)
prostanoids
protectins
purines
Raynaud's syndrome
resolvins

rheumatic fever
rheumatoid arthritis (RA)
rheumatic and musculoskeletal diseases
    (RMDs)
rheumatoid factor (RF)
scleroderma
Sjögren's syndrome (SS)
specialized proresolving mediators (SPMs)
spondylarthritides
systemic lupus erythematosus (SLE)
systemic sclerosis (SSc)
temporomandibular disorders (TMDs)
thromboxanes (Tx)
tophi
uric acid
uricostatic
uricosuric

Rheumatic and musculoskeletal diseases (RMDs) are a diverse group of inflammatory diseases that commonly affect the connective tissue and joints but can affect any organ of the body. There are more than 200 different RMDs, affecting both children and adults. They are usually caused by immune dysregulation, infections, or gradual deterioration of joints, muscles, ligaments, and bones. Some of them have an autoimmune component while the origin of others is unknown. They are typically progressive, painful, and limit function. In severe cases, RMDs can result in significant disability, having a major impact on both quality of life and life expectancy (van der Heijde et al, 2018).

Medical nutrition therapy (MNT), pharmacotherapy, and physical and occupational therapies must be tailored and designed to treat each disease and its symptoms. A diet with adequate protein and energy content, rich in vitamins, minerals, and omega-3 polyunsaturated fatty acids (PUFAs) can promote a beneficial protective effect against tissue damage and suppression of inflammatory activity. Table 38.1 provides an overview of these disorders and their nutritional management.

RMDs are among the most prevalent chronic disease conditions in the United States. The annual cost for medical care to treat all forms of arthritis and joint pain is estimated to be $303.5 billion (Murphy et al, 2018). Rheumatic disease affects all population groups. Data from the 2015 National Health Interview Survey estimated that arthritis affects 91.2 million adults in the United States, equivalent to 36.8% of the total 247.7 million Americans (Jafarzadeh and Felson, 2018). Among persons with heart disease, diabetes, and obesity, the prevalence of doctor-diagnosed arthritis was 49.3%, 47.1%, and 30.6%, respectively (Barbour et al, 2017).

The National Arthritis Data Workgroup reviewed data to estimate national prevalence rates of various rheumatic diseases based on 2005 U.S. census data, finding that in the United States rheumatoid arthritis (RA) affects 1.3 million adults; juvenile arthritis 294,000 people; spondylarthritides (the current name of spondyloarthropathies) 0.64 to 2.4 million adults ages 25 and older; systemic lupus erythematosus (SLE) 161,000 to 322,000 adults; systemic sclerosis (SSc) 49,000 adults; Sjögren's syndrome (SS) 0.4 to 3.1 million adults; clinical osteoarthritis 27 million people aged 25 and older; polymyalgia rheumatica 711,000 people; gout 8 million adults; and fibromyalgia 5 million people (Helmick and Watkins-Castillo, 2014)

Arthritis is a generic term that comes from the Greek word arthro, which means "joint," and the suffix -itis, which means "inflammation." There are two distinct categories of disease: systemic, autoimmune arthritis and nonsystemic osteoarthritis (OA). The more debilitating autoimmune arthritis group includes RA, psoriatic arthritis, juvenile RA, gout, SS, fibromyalgia, SLE, and scleroderma. The OA group includes OA, bursitis, and tendonitis. Other rheumatic diseases include spondylarthritides, polymyalgia rheumatica, and polymyositis.

TABLE 38.1 Summary of Medical Nutrition Therapy for Rheumatic Diseases

Disease	Medical Nutrition Therapy	Complementary and Integrative Medicine (CIM)	Supplements or Herbs that Can Be Safely Considered
Rheumatoid arthritis	Vegan, Mediterranean diet; antiinflammatory diet; appropriate calories for maintenance of normal body weight; RDA for protein unless malnutrition present; moderate-fat diet with emphasis on omega-3 PUFAs and fish 1-2 times per week and monounsaturated fats; modifications as needed for jaw pain, anorexia	Exercise, meditation, tai chi, spiritual practice, relaxation techniques; topical rubbing gels based on capsaicin. A gluten-free diet may be helpful to reduce inflammation.	Supplement diet as needed to meet DRI for antioxidant nutrients and calcium, folate, vitamins B_6, B_{12}, D; GLA from evening primrose oil, black currant oil, and borage oil; fish oils; bromelain, rosemary, turmeric, curry, ginger, and other culinary herbs. Probiotic supplementation may be helpful.
Osteoarthritis	Weight management; diet adequate in calcium, folate, vitamins B_6, D, K; magnesium; antiinflammatory diet (see Box 38.2)	Exercise, acupuncture; SAM-e; topical rubbing gels based on capsaicin, turmeric (curcumin), ginger	Supplement diet as needed to meet DRI for antioxidant nutrients and calcium, folate, vitamins B_6, B_{12}, and D; glucosamine and chondroitin (mixed results); fish oils; bromelain, type 2 collagen
Gout	Weight management; adequate fluid consumption; alcohol, particularly beer, restricted or eliminated; limit or eliminate fructose intake from sweetended beverages and fruit juice. Limit animal foods except dairy and moderate amounts of cold water, oily fish, eggs, and poultry; coffee is protective.	Exercise; alkaline-ash foods; see *Clinical Insight* on Acid and Alkaline Diets in Chapter 34.	Cherry juice, vitamin C
Lupus	Tailor diet to individual needs based on organ involvement; calories to maintain IBW; restriction of protein, fluid, and sodium if renal involvement; check for gluten intolerance.	Antiinflammatory diet, meditation, and stress reduction	Supplement diet as needed to meet DRI for antioxidant nutrients, omega-3 fatty acids, turmeric (curcumin)
Scleroderma	Adequate fluid; high-energy, high-protein supplements as needed to prevent or correct weight loss; moist foods; modifications for GERD if needed.		
Sjögren's syndrome	Balanced diet with adequate B_6 or vitamin supplementation; restrict sugary foods and beverages; modify food portions to smaller size and soft consistency to improve chewing and swallowing processes.		GLA improves eye discomfort and tear production
TMD	Balanced diet with soft foods in small pieces to improve chewing and reduce pain.		

DRI, Dietary reference intake; *GERD*, gastroesophageal reflux disease; *GLA*, gamma-linolenic acid; *IBW*, ideal body weight; *RDA*, recommended dietary allowance; *SAM-e*, S-adenosyl-L-methionine; *TMD*, temporomandibular disorder.

ETIOLOGY

Body changes associated with aging—including decreased somatic protein, body fluids, and bone density—and obesity may contribute to the onset and progression of arthritis. The aging body mass causes changes in neuroendocrine regulators, immune regulators, and metabolism, which affect the inflammatory process. Therefore recent increases in the frequency of these conditions may be the result of aging of the U.S. population. It is estimated that by 2030 approximately 67 million Americans will be at risk for rheumatic disease (Barbour et al, 2017).

Rheumatic conditions are usually chronic and have no known cure but may present as acute episodes with short or intermittent duration. Chronic arthritic conditions are associated with alternating periods of remission without symptoms and flares with worsening symptoms that occur without any identifiable cause. Risk factors include repetitive joint injury, genetic susceptibility, and environmental factors, particularly smoking. Gender is a risk factor because women are more susceptible than men for most rheumatic diseases; the female to male ratio varies from 3:1 for RA, to 9:1 for SLE and SS. Only in gout is there a clear dominance of male over female patients. Recently a transcriptome analysis of RNA levels showed that healthy women carry a proinflammatory profile, particularly to develop RA (Jansen et al, 2014).

Patients with RMDs also have higher risk of developing other conditions such as cardiovascular disease (CVD) (Arida et al, 2018), metabolic syndrome (Medina et al, 2018), and psychiatric disorders such as depression (Marrie et al, 2018).

PATHOPHYSIOLOGY AND INFLAMMATION

Inflammation plays an important role in health and disease. The inflammatory process normally occurs to protect and repair tissue damaged by infections, injuries, toxicity, or wounds via accumulation of fluid and cells. Once the cause is resolved, the inflammation usually subsides. Whether inflammation is due to stress on the joints as in OA, or to an autoimmune response as in RA, an uncontrolled and long-lasting inflammatory reaction causes more damage than repair (see Chapter 7 for discussion of the inflammation and the pathophysiology of chronic disease) (see *Focus On:* The Biochemistry of Inflammation).

PUFAs play an important role in inflammation as precursors of a potent group of modulators of inflammation termed eicosanoids (*eicos* means "20" in Greek), which include the prostanoids and the leukotrienes (LT). The prostanoids are the products of the enzyme cyclooxygenase (COX) and include the prostaglandins (PG) and thromboxanes (Tx), whereas LTs are produced by the enzyme lipoxygenase (LOX) (Box 38.1).

The Biochemistry of Inflammation

Cyclooxygenase (COX, officially known as prostaglandin-endoperoxide synthase [PTGS]), has three isoforms: COX-1, COX-2, and COX-3 (the latter is a splice variant of COX-1, so it is sometimes called COX-1b or COX-1var). COX-1 is widely distributed and constitutively expressed in most tissues, whereas COX-2 is induced by inflammatory and proliferative stimuli. The difference in tissue distribution of COX expression may explain the existence of the two COX isoforms: COX-1 providing prostaglandin (PG) that is required for homeostatic functions (including gastric cytoprotection), and COX-2 playing the predominant role in PG formation during pathophysiologic states, such as in inflammation (Seo and Oh, 2017).

In the synthesis of prostanoids, COX consumes two double bonds from the original polyunsaturated fatty acid (PUFA), whereas lipoxygenase (LOX) consumes none; therefore, depending on the PUFA used as substrate, different eicosanoids are produced. For instance, arachidonic acid (ARA) (20:4, omega-6) has four double bonds and is the precursor of the series 2 of PG and thromboxanes (Tx), and of the series 4 of leukotrienes (LT), which are the most potent inflammatory eicosanoids (Calder, 2017). The series 2 of prostanoids (PG_2 and Tx_2) are abundant because ARA is the most abundant in plasma membranes of cells involved in inflammation (macrophages, neutrophils, fibroblasts). If the substrate is eicosapentaenoic acid (EPA) (20:5, omega-3)

that has five double bonds, series 3 of PG and Tx, and series 5 of LT are produced. Dihomo-γ-linolenic acid (DGLA) (20:3, omega-6) has three double bonds and is the precursor of series 1 of PG and Tx, and of series 3 of LT that have antiinflammatory activities (Food and Agricultural Organization [FAO] of the United Nations [UN], 2010). Finally, docosahexaenoic acid (DHA) (22:6, omega-3) and EPA are converted to novel bioactive lipid mediators termed specialized proresolving mediators (SPMs), which include three families: resolvins (Rv), protectins, and maresins, which promote the resolution of inflammation. Rv of the E series (RvE1-2) derived from EPA, and Rv of the D series (RvD1-6) derived from DHA, are produced by the sequential actions of the enzymes 15-lipoxygenase (15-LO) and 5-lipoxygenase (5-LO). Recent studies have shown that PUFAs also may regulate the expression of genes associated with the inflammatory response (Serhan and Levy, 2018). Based on this information, it is desirable to increase the omega-3/omega-6 ratio by increasing the consumption of antiinflammatory EPA, DGLA, and DHA (oily fish), while reducing the intake of ARA (vegetable oils and meat). Similarly, the increase in vegetables and fruits consumption also results in reduced risk of rheumatic diseases by contributing phytonutrients that have antiinflammatory effects (van Breda and de Kok, 2018).

BOX 38.1 Production of Bioactive Lipid Mediators from Omega-3 and Omega-6 PUFAs

Eicosapentaenoic acid (EPA) (20:5, omega-3)

Thromboxane A_3: weak vasoconstrictor and weak platelet aggregator

Prostacyclin PGI_3: vasodilator and platelet antiaggregator

Leukotriene B_5: weak inflammation inducer and weak chemotactic agent

E-series resolvins (RvE1 and 2): promote resolution of inflammation

Arachidonic Acid (ARA) (20:4, omega-6)

Thromboxane A_2: vasoconstrictor and potent platelet aggregator

Prostaglandin E_2: vasodilator and platelet antiaggregator

Leukotriene B_4: inflammation inducer and potent leukocyte chemotaxis and adherence inducer

Dihomo-γ-linoleic acid (DGLA) (20:3, omega-6)

Thromboxane A_1: antiinflammatory and pain reducer

Prostaglandin E_1: vasodilator, inhibits monocyte and neutrophil function, platelet antiaggregator

Leukotriene B_3: very weak proinflammatory effects

Eicosapentaenoic acid (EPA) (20:5, omega-3)

E-series resolvins (RvE 1-3): inhibit neutrophil recruitment, promote lymphatic removal of phagocytes, reduce PMN infiltration

Docosahexaenoic acid (DHA) (22:6, omega-3)

D-series resolvins (RvD 1-6): promote resolution of inflammation, analgesics, reduce leukocyte recruitment and activation, reduce interleukin (IL)-1 and tumor necrosis factor (TNF) production

Protectins (PD1) and maresins 1 (MaR 1 and 2): promote resolution of inflammation

Calder PC: Omega-3 fatty acids and inflammatory processes: from molecules to man, *Biochem Soc Trans* 45: 1105, 2017; Food and Agricultural Organization (FAO) of the United Nations: Fat and fatty acid intake and inflammatory and immune response. In *Fats and fatty acids in human nutrition. Report of an expert consultation*, Rome, 2010, Food and Agricultural Organization of the United Nations; Serhan CN and Levy BD: Resolvins in inflammation: emergence of the pro-resolving superfamily of mediators, *J Clin Invest* doi: 10.1172/JCI97943. [Epub ahead of print], 2018.

MEDICAL DIAGNOSIS AND TREATMENT

A thorough history of symptoms and a detailed physical examination are the cornerstones for an accurate diagnosis. However, laboratory testing can help to further refine the diagnosis and identify appropriate treatment.

Biochemical Assessment

Acute-phase proteins are plasma proteins whose concentrations increase more than 25% during inflammatory states. Two acute-phase proteins traditionally used to screen for and monitor rheumatic disease are rheumatoid factor (RF) and C-reactive protein (CRP), although they are nonspecific and, in the case of CRP, also may indicate an infection or even a recent cardiac event. The term RF is used to refer to a group of self-reacting antibodies (an abnormal IgM against normal IgG) found in the sera of rheumatic patients. The American College of Rheumatology (ACR) recommends periodic measurements of RF and CRP in addition to a detailed assessment of symptoms and functional status and radiographic examination to determine the current level of disease activity.

The detection of autoantibodies to a variety of antigens is important in the diagnosis of several rheumatic diseases (Jog and James, 2017). These antibodies can be directed against the nucleus (antinuclear antibodies [ANA]) either to double-stranded DNA (dsDNA), ribonucleoproteins (RNPs), or other nuclear structures. Some autoantibodies recognize intracellular structures, or proteins that constitute extracellular matrices. Very often, the presence of a particular set of autoantibodies is a distinct characteristic of a rheumatic disease such as anti-dsDNA and anti-Sm for SLE, anticitrullinated protein antigens (ACPAs) for RA, and anti-Ro/SSA, and anti-La/SSB for SS. Routine blood testing also should include complement levels, a complete blood count, serum creatinine, and hematocrit; urine or synovial fluid may be tested as well (Jog and James, 2017).

PHARMACOTHERAPY

Many of the drugs used in treating RMDs provide relief from pain and inflammation, with hopes of controlling symptoms and slowing disease progress rather than providing a cure. Table 38.2 describes the

TABLE 38.2 Nutritional Side Effects of Medications Used in the Treatment of Rheumatic and Musculoskeletal Diseases*

Drug Category	Nutritional Side Effects*
Analgesics	
Acetaminophen with codeine, hydrocodone with acetaminophen, hydrocodone with ibuprofen, methadone hydrochloride, morphine sulfate, morphine sulfate with naltrexone, oxycodone, oxycodone hydrochloride with acetaminophen, oxycodone with aspirin, tramadol	Constipation, nausea, vomiting, urinary retention, abdominal pain, diarrhea, dry mouth, flatulence, infection, insomnia, abdominal or stomach cramps, heartburn or indigestion
Acetaminophen and tapentadol	No gastrointestinal side effects
Biologics	
Belimumab, rituximab, canakinumab, ustekinumab, brodalumab, secukinumab, ixekizumab, brodalumab	Nausea, vomiting, abdominal pain, diarrhea, stomach ache
Adalimumab, certolizumab pegol, etanercept, golimumab, infliximab, abatacept, anakinra, tocilizumab	No nutritional side effects
NSAIDs	
Diclofenac potassium, diclofenac sodium, diclofenac sodium with misoprostol, diflunisal, etodolac, fenoprofen calcium, ibuprofen, indomethacin, ketoprofen, meloxicam, naproxen, naproxen sodium, piroxicam, sulindac, celecoxib, acetylsalicylic acid, choline and magnesium trisalicylates	Abdominal cramps, pain or discomfort, peptic ulcer, constipation, diarrhea, gastrointestinal bleeding, heartburn or indigestion, acid reflux, nausea or vomiting
Corticosteroids	
Betamethasone, cortisone acetate, dexamethasone, hydrocortisone, methylprednisolone, prednisolone, prednisone	Elevated blood fats (cholesterol, triglycerides), elevated blood sugar, hardening of arteries (atherosclerosis), hypertension, increased appetite, indigestion, weight gain, ulcers
DMARDs	
Azathioprine	Liver problems, loss of appetite, nausea or vomiting
Cyclophosphamide	Loss of appetite, nausea or vomiting
Cyclosporine	Abdominal pain, gingivitis, high blood pressure, kidney problems, loss of appetite, nausea
Gold sodium thiomalate	Irritation and soreness of tongue, irritated or bleeding gums, metallic taste, ulcers or white spots on lips or in mouth or throat
Hydroxychloroquine	Abdominal cramps, diarrhea, loss of appetite, nausea or vomiting
Leflunomide	Gastrointestinal problems, heartburn, high blood pressure, liver problems, stomach pain
Methotrexate	Folic acid antagonist, abdominal pain, liver problems, mouth sores, nausea
Minocycline, Mycophenolate mofetil	Diarrhea, gastrointestinal ulcers or bleeding, nausea, vomiting
Sulfasalazine	Abdominal discomfort, diarrhea, headache, loss of appetite, nausea and vomiting
Tofacitinib	Diarrhea, hypertension, increased lipid level

*Some of these side effects are usually short term and go away gradually after treatment stops.
Arthritis Foundation: Arthritis today, Drug Guide. https://www.arthritis.org/living-with-arthritis/treatments/medication/drug-guide/search-alphabetical.php.

commonly used drugs and their nutritional side effects (also see Appendix 13).

Analgesics

Analgesics are drugs designed specifically to relieve pain. There are several types of analgesics: acetaminophen (Tylenol) and a variety of opioid analgesics (also called narcotics). Some products combine acetaminophen with an opioid analgesic for added relief. Opioid analgesics work by binding to receptors on cells mainly in the brain, spinal cord, and gastrointestinal system.

Nonsteroidal Antiinflammatory Drugs

Nonsteroidal antiinflammatory drugs (NSAIDs) are used to relieve pain and inflammation associated with arthritis and related conditions. All NSAIDs work by blocking the synthesis of PG, which are involved in pain and inflammation, as well as many other bodily functions including protecting the stomach lining.

Traditional NSAIDs include more than 20 different drugs. They work by blocking PG synthesis by inhibiting COX-1 and COX-2, making the lining of the stomach vulnerable to ulcers and bleeding. Aspirin (acetylsalicylic acid) is the only NSAID that inhibits all COX proteins by covalent modification; all other NSAIDs act noncovalently.

Ibuprofen and naproxen slow down the body's production of PG by inhibiting COX-1. They are considered useful tools in the management of most rheumatic disorders; however, long-term use of NSAIDs may cause gastrointestinal problems (see Table 38.2).

Because of the damage to the gastric mucosa caused by COX-1 inhibitors, a drug was developed to block only COX-2: celecoxib (Celebrex). Because it only inhibits COX-2 without affecting COX-1, this drug does not harm the stomach and is well tolerated by patients requiring long-term antiinflammatory therapy. However, celecoxib is not exempt of side effects, like increased thrombotic events, skin reactions, and cardiotoxicity, so continuous medical monitoring is advised. Calcitriol (1,25-dihydroxy-D_3, the active form of vitamin D), flavonoids, and BDMC33 (a curcumin derivative) are also specific blockers of COX-2, they inhibit inflammation by interfering with *COX-2* gene expression (Lee et al, 2015). In addition, calcitriol also blocks PG receptor expression in their target cells PG production and secretion of proinflammatory cytokines in macrophages (Wang et al, 2014).

Disease-Modifying Antirheumatic Drugs

Disease-modifying antirheumatic drugs (DMARDs) is a category of otherwise unrelated drugs defined by their use in RA and other diseases such as SLE and SS, to slow down disease progression. Each DMARD works in different ways to slow or stop the inflammatory process that damages the joints and internal organs.

Of particular interest is the drug methotrexate (MTX), originally used to treat certain types of cancer, which is widely used to treat RA alone, or in combination with other DMARDs. MTX works by competitively inhibiting dihydrofolate reductase (DHFR), an enzyme that converts folic acid to its active metabolite tetrahydrofolate (THF), which is required for nucleic acid (DNA and RNA) synthesis. Therefore patients taking MTX must consume supplemental folate to reduce the adverse effects caused by MTX such as anemia, abdominal pain, nausea, and mouth sores. Supplemental folate can be in the form of folic acid, folinic acid, or 5-methyltetrahydrofolate (5-MTHF) (see Appendix 31). Folinic acid (Leucovorin) is a folate derivative that is easily converted to THF and is unaffected by the inhibition of DHFR by MTX, while relieving some of the side effects of MTX (Shea et al, 2014). 5-MTHF (Metafolin) is the active form of folic acid used at the cellular level for DNA synthesis and also is not affected by MTX (Scaglione and Panzavolta, 2014). MTX should not be taken by pregnant and lactating women (Gerosa et al, 2016).

Biologic Response Modifiers or Biologics

Biologic response modifiers (BRMs), or biologics, are medications genetically engineered from a living organism, such as a virus, gene, or protein, to simulate the body's natural response to infection and disease. BRMs target proteins, cells, and pathways responsible for the symptoms and damage of RA and other types of inflammatory arthritis.

The biologics used for treating RMDs work in one of several ways: (1) by blocking proteins that are produced in response to injury such as interleukin-1 (IL-1), IL-6, IL-17, tumor necrosis factor alpha (TNF-α); (2) by blocking B cells, which produce antibodies that are produced excessively in some forms of arthritis and SLE; and (3) by inhibiting the activation of T cells, thereby preventing the chain reactions that result in inflammation. These molecules are administered by injection (intravenously or subcutaneously) because they are proteins and oral administration would destroy their biologic activities. Patients taking these drugs should be monitored for chronic infections or malignancies (Ramiro et al, 2017). The main drawback is their high cost, which varies depending on the information source, from $43,000 dollars per patient per year to over $110,000 (Popp et al, 2018).

Corticosteroids

Corticosteroids, sometimes called glucocorticoids, are medications that mimic the effects of the hormone cortisol, which is produced naturally by the adrenal glands. Cortisol affects many parts of the body, including the immune system. Corticosteroids are prescribed for patients who need quick relief from severe inflammation by lowering the levels of PG. In some cases of RA, corticosteroids pills are taken while waiting for other DMARDs to start to take effect. Low-dose corticosteroids also may be prescribed long term for some patients with RA. However, the use of corticosteroids in RA is debated, because some doctors believe the long-term benefits do not outweigh the risk of side effects. If used alone, the immediate relief corticosteroids provide may defer the start of treatment, which could make a difference in the course of the disease.

As the most potent of the antiinflammatory drugs used to treat RA, steroids have extensive catabolic effects that can result in negative nitrogen balance and blood sugar imbalance. Hypercalciuria and reduced calcium absorption can increase the risk of osteoporosis (see Chapters 8 and 24). Concomitant calcium and vitamin D supplementation and monitoring of bone status should be considered to minimize osteopenia. Many drugs used for treating RMDs can cause one or more nutritional side effects (see Table 38.2).

Vitamin D (cholecalciferol)

Vitamin D is a fat-soluble vitamin obtainable from the diet, as well as a prohormone produced in the skin by ultraviolet B from sunlight (see Appendix 38). The active form of vitamin D (1,25-dihydroxy vitamin D_3, termed calcitriol) binds to the vitamin D receptor (VDR), a protein that acts as a transcriptional factor and regulates the expression of several genes. The VDR forms a heterodimer with the retinoid-X receptor (RXR), and the VDR-RXR complex binds to vitamin D response element (VDRE) in the promoter region of its target genes to regulate mRNA expression.

The classical role of vitamin D is to regulate metabolism of calcium and phosphate. However, several nonclassical effects of vitamin D, such as regulation of cell proliferation and differentiation, have been recognized. Of particular interest is the regulatory effect of vitamin D on immune cells because virtually all immune cell types (macrophages/monocytes, neutrophils, T and B cells and dendritic cells) express VDR, making them susceptible to calcitriol-mediated modulation. Most of the immune cells (monocytes, dendritic cells, macrophages, B cells, and T cells) also have the capability to convert vitamin D into calcitriol, which allows for local regulation of its concentration at sites of inflammation and illustrates an important role for these cells in the systemic effects of vitamin D (Kongsbak et al, 2014).

Dendritic cells (DC) could be considered as the primary immune cell target of vitamin D. It inhibits DC maturation and differentiation and consequently impairs antigen processing and presentation to immune cells, resulting in a decline in proinflammatory cytokines (IL-6, IL-23, IL-1, IL-8, IL-12, TNF-α, and interferon [IFN]-α) along with an increase in tolerogenic molecules such as IL-10. Furthermore, through the DC modulation, vitamin D suppresses the activity of Th17, a T cell subset widely engaged in inflammatory responses, and enhances regulatory T (Treg) cell expansion (Vasile et al, 2017).

Extensive research over the past decades has suggested that low sunlight exposure and vitamin D deficiency are also associated with signs and symptoms of autoimmune diseases (Holick, 2016; Dankers et al, 2017). Body levels of vitamin D are documented to fluctuate with changing seasons, due to the influence of ultraviolet (UV) radiation exposure during different times of the year and to location. Seasonal relapses of autoimmune diseases could also be explained by low UV exposure, and, therefore, low levels of vitamin D. Vitamin D levels, which reach a nadir during late winter and early spring, are correlated with increased disease activity and clinical severity, as well as relapse rates in several disease entities noncutaneous flares of SLE, psoriasis, and RA (Watad et al, 2017). As most studies indicate that vitamin D insufficiency is associated with high disease activity of RA, it would be logical to supplement these patients with vitamin D (Jeffery et al, 2016; Pludowski et al, 2018). Most clinicians agree that with the increasing adverse health outcomes associated with hypovitaminosis D, screening and supplementation should be performed routinely in RA patients.

Vitamin A (retinol)

Vitamin A (retinol [ROL]) is essential for multiple functions, including the maintenance of the immune system. Vitamin A can be obtained preformed from animal products, or as its precursor (carotenes) from vegetables in the diet. Inside the cells, ROL is converted to retinaldehyde

(RAL) which is oxidized to form retinoic acid, the active form of vitamin A. Two isoforms of retinoic acid are produced, all-trans RA (at-RA) and 9-cis RA (9cis-RA), which are ligands for the nuclear retinoic acid receptors (RAR alpha, beta, and gamma) whereas the retinoid X receptors (RXR alpha, beta, and gamma) only bind to 9cis-RA. Therefore vitamin A regulates gene expression via RAR and RXR, which bind to specific sequences in the DNA known as RARE (retinoic acid response elements), as homodimers (RAR/RAR), or as heterodimers (RAR/RXR) (Kim, 2018).

Vitamin A plays an essential role in the proliferation and differentiation of immune cells via RAR and RXR interactions. T cells can be divided in to two main subsets: proinflammatory and antiinflammatory, which are defined by the cytokines they produce. Th1 and Th17 are proinflammatory whereas Th2 and Treg are antiinflammatory. Vitamin A metabolites modulate specific functional aspects of the immune response, such as the Th1/Th2 cell balance and the differentiation of Treg cells and Th17 cells. In vitamin A deficiency there is an increase in the Th1 type response and an increase in the Th1/Th2 ratio. The addition of at-RA reestablishes the Th1/Th2 balance due to an increase in Th2 cells (Miyabe et al, 2015). Dietary retinoids have regulatory effects on immune cells and have been shown to improve rheumatic diseases in animal models. These findings suggest a possible role for dietary retinoids in the therapy for of rheumatic disease.

ANTIINFLAMMATORY DIET

The antiinflammatory diet, a diet resembling the Mediterranean diet, has been useful for the treatment of inflammatory diseases, including RMDs. The diet aims for the inclusion of as much fresh food as possible, the least amount of processed foods and fast food, minimal amounts of sugar (particularly fructose and sucrose), and an abundance of fruits (especially berries) and vegetables, lean proteins from animal sources such as chicken and fish, and vegetarian sources such as legumes and nuts, plus essential fatty acids and dietary fiber. If weight loss is a desired outcome to reduce inflammation, people may lose weight with these dietary changes (Arthritis Foundation [AF], 2014a) (Box 38.2; see Appendix 22). There is plenty of evidence for a relationship between a Mediterranean diet and lower levels of inflammation both in observational and intervention studies. A recent systematic review and meta analysis of randomized controlled trials showed that a Mediterranean dietary pattern decreases inflammation (Bonaccio et al, 2017). The antiinflammatory diet works by reducing the expression of genes involved in the inflammatory process such as IL-1, IL-6, and TNF-α.

One of the main components of the Mediterranean diet is extra virgin olive oil (EVOO). Diverse studies show evidence that EVOO and its components may have potential positive properties on the modulation of immune-inflammatory processes. The trend toward the use of natural compounds and diet, due to fewer side effects compared with classical pharmacotherapy, has given rise to EVOO and EVOO compounds consumption as an alternative therapy for the prevention and management of different immune-inflammatory diseases such as RA, SLE, and multiple sclerosis, because of the beneficial fatty acid profile of EVOO and the presence of a high content of phenolic compounds (Aparicio-Soto et al, 2016).

COMPLEMENTARY AND INTEGRATIVE HEALTH APPROACHES

Because of the chronic nature of arthritic diseases, their effects on quality of life, and the fact that most treatments result only in modest improvement in symptoms and function, patients commonly try complementary and integrative medicine (CIM). Rheumatologists

---

BOX 38.2 General Principles of the Antiinflammatory Diet

Aims for variety, with a whole foods, plant-based diet with minimal processed foods.

Consume a variety of fruits and vegetables; some people may need to avoid potatoes and other nightshade vegetables, which contain the alkaloid solanine

Low in saturated fat and devoid of trans fats

Low in omega-6 fats, such as vegetable oils and animal fat

High in Monounsaturated fatty acids (MUFAs) such as those found in olive oil, walnuts, pumpkin seeds, and those high in omega-3 fats found in flax and chia seeds and fatty cold-water oily fish such as salmon, sardines, mackerel, and herring.

Low in refined carbohydrates such as white pasta, white bread, white rice, other refined grains, sucrose (table sugar), and sucrose-containing products such as pastries, cookies, cakes, energy bars, and candy

Increase whole grains such as brown rice, bulgur wheat, and other unrefined grains such as amaranth, quinoa, and spelt

Includes lean protein sources such as chicken and fish

Limits eggs, red meat, butter, and other full-fat dairy products

Includes spices such as ginger, curry, turmeric, and rosemary, which have antiinflammatory effects

Includes good sources of phytonutrients: fruits and vegetables of all bright and dark colors, especially berries, orange and yellow fruits, and dark leafy greens; cruciferous vegetables (cabbage, broccoli, Brussels sprouts, cauliflower); soy foods; tea (especially white, green, or oolong), dark plain chocolate in moderation

Additionally, weight should be maintained within healthy parameters, and exercise should be included.

Note: Please refer to Appendix 22 for a thorough description of the antiinflammatory diet.
Arthritis Foundation. https://www.arthritis.org/living-with-arthritis/arthritis-diet/anti-inflammatory/anti-inflammatory-diet.php; Van Breda SGJ and de Kok TMCM: Smart combinations of bioactive compounds in fruits and vegetables may guide new strategies for personalized prevention of chronic diseases, *Mol Nutr Food Res* 62: 1700597, 2018.

---

show moderate acceptance toward some types of CIM. A substantial proportion of rheumatologists perceive some integrative therapies, including bodywork, meditation, and acupuncture, to be beneficial for their patients (Grainger and Walker, 2014). CIM use is popular among patients with rheumatological diseases. An estimated 60% to 90% of arthritis patients have reported using CIM (Seca et al, 2016). A recent systematic review identified good quality randomized clinical trials using CIM as intervention in patients with different rheumatic diseases including acupuncture, Ayurvedic treatment, homeopathic treatment, natural products, megavitamin therapies, chiropractic and osteopathic manipulation. It is clear from this review that there is no particular type of CIM that proves effective for all types for rheumatic diseases, although some CIM interventions appear to be more effective than others. For example, acupuncture appears to be beneficial for OA but not RA. The review could not show evidence for all diseases because of scarcity of trials or contradictory findings. CIM interventions were associated, if at all, with minor adverse reactions (Phang et al, 2018). Some of the main categories in which CIM can be grouped are presented below (National Institutes of Health [NIH], National Center for Complementary and Integrative Health [NCCIH], 2018).

Mind and body practices include a large and diverse group of procedures or techniques administered or taught by a trained practitioner or teacher. These include acupuncture, massage therapies, meditation, movement therapies (Feldenkrais method, Alexander technique, Pilates), relaxation techniques (breathing exercises, guided imagery, progressive muscle relaxation), spinal manipulation, tai chi, qi gong, and yoga.

Natural products encompass herbs (botanicals), vitamins and minerals, and probiotics. The most common dietary supplements used for AORD include glucosamine, chondroitin, S-adenosyl-L-methionine (SAM-e), fish oil, EVOO, curcumin, turmeric, boswellia, and methylsulfonylmethane (MSM). Capsaicin, the compound responsible for the burning sensation produced by chili peppers, is used as a rubbing topical gel to relieve pain, particularly in joints of OA and RA patients (see Chapter 11 for further discussion of botanicals).

Patients decisions to try any CIM should be discussed with their physician. The main drawback for some patients is the additional costs of CIM, which are often not covered by insurance, and the potential for drug-nutrient interactions.

Elimination Diets and Other Therapeutic Diets

Adverse reactions to food can contribute to inflammatory symptoms in some people with rheumatic conditions, including trial elimination of gluten, animal products (vegan), and nightshade elimination (see Chapter 25 for strategies for testing for food allergies or sensitivities and implementing an elimination diet). Gluten-free diet has been associated with benefits in patients with RA though the existing evidence is inconclusive (Badsha, 2018). Eliminating any animal product or byproducts has been reported to be clinically beneficial for disease remission in RA patients. Studies conclude that the improvements in disease activity might have been a result of reduction in immune-reactivity to certain food antigens in the gastrointestinal tract that were eliminated by changing the diet (Khanna et al, 2017). One dietary compound that has been suspected to increase painful swelling in the joints is nightshade plants. Nightshades are a diverse group of foods, herbs, shrubs, and trees that include more than 2800 species of plants of the *Solanaceae* family, such as potatoes, tomatoes, sweet and hot peppers, and eggplants. They contain a group of chemicals termed alkaloids, like solanine and chaconine, which are believed to cause damage to the joints and increase the loss of calcium from the bones. The nightshade elimination diet is believed to be safe, but there is always the risk that when eliminating certain foods from their diet, arthritis patients may not get enough of the necessary nutrients (vitamins, minerals, antioxidants; see Chapter 25). Although there are anecdotal claims of its effectiveness, the nightshade elimination diet has not been studied in depth, and no formal research has ever confirmed its beneficial effects.

Fasting has been actively studied as an alternative therapy for RA, and a number of clinical trials have been conducted to test its efficacy since the 1970s. Either periodic fasting or a fasting-mimicking diet followed by vegan diets have the potential to treat RA, although larger randomized studies are necessary to test this possibility (Choi et al, 2018).

MICROBIOTA AND ARTHRITIS

Increased levels of antibodies directed against antigens of certain species of gut bacteria point to the relationship between bacteria and arthritis (De Luca and Shoenfeld, 2018). Three sites have been associated particularly with it, mainly the lungs, oral mucosa, and gastrointestinal tract. The idea that intestinal microorganisms are associated with the development of RA is not new: alterations of microbiota (dysbiosis) are related to risk and severity of the disease. Mechanisms through which the microbiota may be involved in the pathogenesis of rheumatic diseases include altered epithelial and mucosal permeability, loss of immune tolerance to components of the indigenous microbiota, and trafficking of activated immune cells and antigenic material to the joints.

A previously unrecognized bacterium termed *Prevotella copri* was recovered from human feces. *P. copri* is an obligate anaerobic, nonmotile, gram-negative rod. The importance of this discovery is that *P. copri* has been recovered in 75% of patients with new-onset untreated RA (NORA) and only in 21.4% of healthy individuals (Bernard, 2014).

Studies on the effect of diet on the microbiota, particularly with regard to the proinflammatory effects of the Western diet, are needed to gain insight into the treatment of rheumatic diseases. Given that alterations in the intestinal microbiota are associated with arthritis, modifying the microbiota might be a valuable therapeutic strategy. The main approaches that have been used to modify the microbiota in disease are probiotics, the administration of single or multiple strains of beneficial bacteria or yeasts; dietary modification to increase fiber and prebiotics; and fecal microbial transplantation (Bravo-Blas et al, 2016), although currently fecal transplantation is undertaken only in the case of intractable diarrhea, not for the purpose of influencing inflammation.

Some bacterial infections have been related to the development of reactive arthritis, the most widely documented from infection with *Streptococcus pyogenes*, a Group A beta-hemolytic bacteria that is the cause of streptococcal pharyngeal infection. Rheumatic fever is a systemic disease affecting the peri-arteriolar connective tissue and can occur after an untreated *S. pyogenes* infection. Acute rheumatic fever commonly appears in children between the ages of 6 and 15, with only 20% of first-time attacks occurring in adults. The illness is so named because of its similarity in presentation to RA.

Diagnosis of acute rheumatic fever is based on the presence of documented Group A streptococcal infection. The most common symptoms include arthritis (most of the time unilateral, instead of the common bilateral presentation in RA), carditis (inflammation of the heart tissue), and Sydenham chorea (involuntary movements of the face, hands, and feet, also known as Saint Vitus' dance) (Rhodes et al, 2018). Heart complications may be long term and severe, particularly if valves are involved.

Molecular mimicry accounts for the tissue injury that occurs in rheumatic fever. In this process, the patient's immune responses are unable to distinguish between *S. pyogenes* structures and certain host tissues, attacking both. The resultant inflammation may persist well beyond the acute infection and produces the manifestations of rheumatic fever. The recurrence of rheumatic fever is relatively common in the absence of maintenance of low-dose antibiotics, especially during the first 3 to 5 years after the first episode. Survivors of rheumatic fever often have to take penicillin to prevent streptococcal infection, which could possibly lead to another case of rheumatic fever that could prove fatal.

OSTEOARTHRITIS

Osteoarthritis (OA), formally known as degenerative arthritis or degenerative joint disease, is the most prevalent form of arthritis. Obesity, aging, female gender, white ethnicity, greater bone density, and repetitive-use injury associated with athletics have been identified as risk factors. OA is not systemic or autoimmune in origin but involves cartilage destruction with asymmetric inflammation. It is caused by joint overuse, whereas RA is a systemic autoimmune disorder that results in symmetric joint inflammation.

Pathophysiology

OA is a chronic joint disease that involves the loss of habitually weight-bearing articular (joint) cartilage. This cartilage normally allows bones to glide smoothly over one another. The loss can result in stiffness, pain, swelling, loss of motion, and changes in joint shape, in addition to abnormal bone growth, which can result in osteophytes (bone spurs) (Fig. 38.1; see *Pathophysiology and Care Management Algorithm: Osteoarthritis*).

A Healthy Joint

A Joint with Osteoarthritis

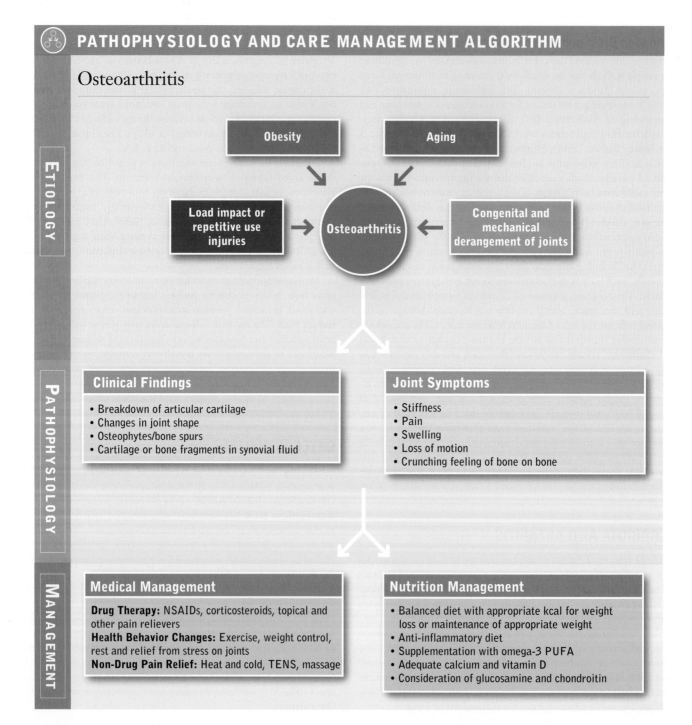

Fig. 38.1 A healthy joint and a joint with severe osteoarthritis. From National Institutes of Health, National Institute of Arthritis and Musculoskeletal and Skin Diseases. https://www.niams.nih.gov/file/823.

PATHOPHYSIOLOGY AND CARE MANAGEMENT ALGORITHM

Osteoarthritis

ETIOLOGY

- Obesity
- Aging
- Load impact or repetitive use injuries
- Osteoarthritis
- Congenital and mechanical derangement of joints

PATHOPHYSIOLOGY

Clinical Findings

- Breakdown of articular cartilage
- Changes in joint shape
- Osteophytes/bone spurs
- Cartilage or bone fragments in synovial fluid

Joint Symptoms

- Stiffness
- Pain
- Swelling
- Loss of motion
- Crunching feeling of bone on bone

MANAGEMENT

Medical Management

Drug Therapy: NSAIDs, corticosteroids, topical and other pain relievers
Health Behavior Changes: Exercise, weight control, rest and relief from stress on joints
Non-Drug Pain Relief: Heat and cold, TENS, massage

Nutrition Management

- Balanced diet with appropriate kcal for weight loss or maintenance of appropriate weight
- Anti-inflammatory diet
- Supplementation with omega-3 PUFA
- Adequate calcium and vitamin D
- Consideration of glucosamine and chondroitin

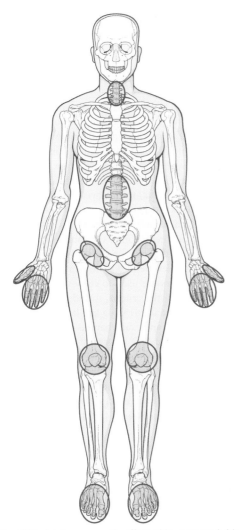

Fig. 38.2 Joints commonly affected by osteoarthritis.

The joints most often affected in OA are the distal interphalangeal joints, the thumb joint, and, in particular, the joints of the knees, hips, ankles, and spine, which bear the bulk of the body's weight (Fig. 38.2). The elbows, wrists, and ankles are less often affected. OA generally presents as pain that worsens with weight bearing and activity and improves with rest, and patients often report morning stiffness or "gelling" of the affected joint after periods of inactivity. Diseases of the joints influenced by congenital and mechanical derangements may contribute to OA as well. Inflammation occurs at times but is generally mild and localized.

Medical and Surgical Management

The patient's medical history and level of pain should determine the most appropriate treatment. This should include nonpharmacologic modalities (patient education, massage therapy, physical and occupational therapy), pharmacologic agents, and surgical procedures with the goals of pain control, improved function and health-related quality of life, and avoidance of toxic effects from treatment. Weight loss and/or achievement of ideal body weight (body mass index [BMI] of 18.5 to 24.9 kg/m^2) should be part of the medical treatment because it improves OA dramatically (see Chapter 20).

Patients with severe symptomatic OA pain who have not responded adequately to medical treatment and who have been progressively limited in their activities of daily living (ADLs), such as walking, bathing, dressing, and toileting, should be evaluated by an orthopedic surgeon. Surgical options include arthroscopic debridement (with or without arthroplasty), total joint arthroplasty, and osteotomy. Surgical reconstruction has been successful but should not be viewed as a replacement for overall good nutrition, maintenance of healthy body weight, and exercise (Smink et al, 2014).

Exercise

OA limits the ability to increase energy expenditure through exercise. It is critical that the exercise be done with correct form so as not to cause damage or exacerbate an existing problem. Physical and occupational therapists can provide unique expertise for OA patients by making individualized assessments and recommending appropriate exercise programs and assistive devices, in addition to offering guidance regarding joint protection and energy conservation. Nonloading aerobic (swimming), range-of-motion, and weight-bearing exercises have been shown to reduce symptoms, increase mobility, and lessen continuing damage from OA. Non–weight-bearing exercise also may serve as an adjunct to NSAID use.

Sports or strenuous activities that subject joints to repetitive high impact and loading increase the risk of joint cartilage degeneration. Therefore increased muscle tone and strength, correct form, general flexibility, and conditioning help protect these joints in the habitual exerciser. A walking program and lower-extremity strength training are beneficial for individuals with knee OA.

Medical Nutrition Therapy

Weight and Adiposity Management

Excess weight puts an added burden on the weight-bearing joints. Epidemiologic studies have shown that obesity and injury are the two greatest risk factors for OA. The risk for knee OA increases as BMI increases. Controlling obesity can reduce the burden of inflammation on OA and thus delay disease progression and improve symptoms. A well-balanced diet that is consistent with established dietary guidelines and promotes attainment and maintenance of a desirable body weight is an important part of MNT for OA (Bliddal et al, 2014).

An antiinflammatory diet combined with moderate exercise and diet-induced weight loss has been shown to be an effective intervention for knee OA. There is also an antiinflammatory effect from weight loss in OA management because the reduced fat mass results in the presence of less inflammatory mediators from adipose tissue (see Chapters 7 and 20).

Vitamins and Minerals

Cumulative damage to tissues mediated by reactive oxygen species has been implicated as a pathway that leads to many of the degenerative changes seen with aging.

At present, there are insufficient data to show benefit from antioxidant supplementation in OA. However, for general health, patients should be encouraged to eat a healthy diet that includes adequate amounts of dietary antioxidants (Thomas et al, 2018)

Many patients with OA consume deficient levels of calcium and vitamin D. Low serum levels of 25-OH-vitamin D are frequent and there is an inverse association between serum 25-OH-vitamin D and clinical findings (cartilage loss in the joint space) and joint pain. Calcitriol (1,25-dihydroxy vitamin D$_3$) binds to the VDR followed by their interaction with specific sequences in the DNA. However, the VDR gene also presents polymorphisms, and some of these have been associated with OA and another condition called intervertebral disc degeneration. Given the role of vitamin D in the cartilaginous tissue, the very common low levels of serum vitamin D, and the genetic polymorphism of the VDR, more studies are necessary to determine the role of vitamin D in the pathogenesis of OA (Liu et al, 2014; Thomas et al, 2018).

Complementary Integrative Therapies

A meta-analysis has found that capsaicin gel and SAM-e are useful in treating OA; articulin F (an ayurvedic mixture of Withania, Boswellia, curcuma, and zinc) improved pain and function (Phang et al, 2018).

Glucosamine and Chondroitin

Glucosamine and chondroitin are involved in cartilage production, but their mechanism for eliminating pain has not been identified. The Glucosamine/Chondroitin Arthritis Intervention Trial (GAIT) was a large, randomized, placebo-controlled trial conducted at several sites across the United States (NIH, 2017). The GAIT team, funded by the NCCIH of the NIH and the National Institute of Arthritis and Musculoskeletal and Skin Diseases (NIAMS), actually conducted two studies: a primary, or original, study that investigated whether glucosamine and/or chondroitin could treat the pain of knee OA, and an ancillary, or additional, study that investigated whether the dietary supplements could diminish the structural damage of knee OA.

The results of the primary GAIT study showed that the popular dietary supplement combination of glucosamine plus chondroitin sulfate did not provide significant relief from OA pain among all participants. However, a smaller subgroup of study participants with moderate-to-severe pain showed significant relief with the combined supplements.

The results of the ancillary GAIT study showed that glucosamine and chondroitin sulfate, together or alone, appeared to fare no better than placebo in slowing loss of cartilage in knee OA (Sawitzke et al, 2010).

In a meta-analysis review of 43 studies with 9110 patients it was found that chondroitin may improve pain slightly in the short term (less than 6 months); chondroitin improves knee pain by 20% in slightly more people and probably improves quality of life slightly as measured by Lequesne's index (combined measure of pain, function, and disability). Chondroitin has little or no difference in adverse and serious adverse events versus other agents and slightly slows down the narrowing of joint space on x-rays of the affected joint. The combination of some

efficacy and low risk associated with chondroitin may explain its popularity among patients as an over-the-counter supplement (Singh et al, 2016).

RHEUMATOID ARTHRITIS

Rheumatoid arthritis (RA) is a debilitating and frequently crippling autoimmune disease with overwhelming personal, social, and economic effects. Although less common than OA, RA is usually more severe and occurs more frequently in women than in men, with a peak onset commonly between 20 and 45 years of age.

RA affects the interstitial tissues, blood vessels, cartilage, bone, tendons, and ligaments, as well as the synovial membranes that line joint surfaces. Measurements of RF, and antinuclear antibodies (ANA) and antibodies to citrullinated protein antigens (ACPAs), are useful in the diagnosis as well as the prediction of the course and outcomes of RA. For RA patients, one of the most important type of biomarkers at the moment is autoantibodies. Besides joint pain and inflammation, several serologic biomarkers are used to classify RA patients. Serologic biomarkers, described in the criteria, include autoantibodies such as RF and ACPA (Verheul et al, 2015; Jog and James, 2017).

Numerous remissions and exacerbations generally follow the onset of RA, although for some people it lasts just a few months or years and then goes away completely. Although any joint may be affected by RA, involvement of the small joints of the extremities—typically the proximal interphalangeal joints of the hands and feet—is most common (Fig. 38.3). Although the exact cause of RA is still unknown, certain genes have been discovered that play a role (Nigrovic et al, 2018).

Pathophysiology

RA is a chronic, autoimmune, systemic disorder in which cytokines and the inflammatory process play a role. RA has articular manifestations that involve chronic inflammation that begins in the synovial membrane and progresses to subsequent damage in the joint cartilage (see *Pathophysiology and Care Management Algorithm:* Rheumatoid

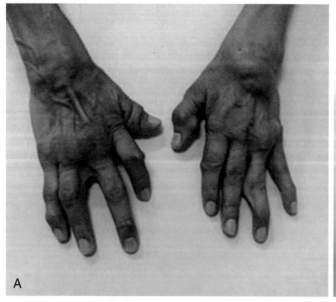
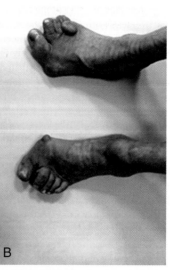

Fig. 38.3 A female patient with advanced rheumatoid arthritis. The twisted hands (**A**) and feet (**B**), and the puffiness of the metacarpal joints are typical of the disease. (Photos courtesy Dr. F. Enrique Gómez. Instituto Nacional de Ciencias Médicas y Nutrición Salvador Zubirán. Mexico City, México, 2015.)

Normal Joint

Joint Affected by Rheumatoid Arthritis

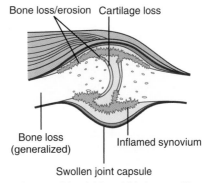

Fig. 38.4 Comparison of a normal joint and one affected by rheumatoid arthritis, which has swelling of the synovium. From National Institute of Arthritis and Musculoskeletal and Skin Diseases. https://www.niams.nih.gov/file/813.

Arthritis). Citrullination, also termed deimination, is a modification of arginine side chains catalyzed by peptidylarginine deiminase (PAD) enzymes. This posttranslational modification has the potential to alter the structure, antigenicity, and function of proteins. Four citrullinated antigens, fibrinogen, vimentin, collagen type II, and alpha-enolase, are expressed in the joints.

The appearance of RF may precede symptoms of RA. Pain, stiffness, swelling, loss of function, and anemia are common. The swelling or puffiness is caused by the accumulation of synovial fluid in the membrane lining the joints and inflammation of the surrounding tissues (Fig. 38.4).

Some controversy exists regarding green tea: It has been suggested that drinking large amounts of tea may increase the risk of developing RA, whereas other studies suggest a protective role (Lee et al, 2014). Smoking is the environmental risk factor that is most associated with RA. The association of smoking and the development of RA has been demonstrated through epidemiologic studies, as well as through in vivo and animal models of RA. With increased use of biological agents in addition to standard DMARDs, there has been interest in how smoking affects drug response in RA treatment. Recent evidence suggests the response and drug survival in people treated with anti-TNF therapy is less effective in heavy smokers (Chang et al, 2014). In a recent meta-analysis, lifelong cigarette smoking was positively associated with the risk of RA even among smokers with a low lifelong exposure. The risk of RA did not further increase with an exposure higher than 20 pack-years (Di Giuseppe et al, 2014). Coffee consumption also represents a risk factor for RA (Lee et al, 2014), whereas dietary antioxidants and breastfeeding may be protective (Chen et al, 2015).

Medical Management

RA patients are at increased risk for CVD, explained by the systemic inflammatory response. This is especially significant considering findings regarding COX-2 selective NSAIDs. In fact, many of the drugs used to treat RA (see Appendix 13) can result in hyperhomocysteinemia, hypertension, and hyperglycemia, all risk factors for CVD. Conveniently, treatment aimed at reducing inflammation may benefit both diseases.

Pharmacologic Therapy

Medications to control pain and inflammation are the mainstay of treatment for RA. Salicylates and NSAIDs are often the first line of treatment. MTX commonly is prescribed as well, but these drugs may cause significant side effects. The choice of drug class and type is based on patient response to the medication, incidence and severity of adverse reactions, and patient compliance. Drug-nutrient side effects can occur with any of the drugs (see Chapter 5 and Appendix 13).

Salicylates are used commonly. However, chronic aspirin ingestion is associated with gastric mucosal injury and bleeding, increased bleeding time, and increased urinary excretion of vitamin C. Taking aspirin with milk, food, or an antacid often alleviates the gastrointestinal symptoms. Vitamin C supplementation is prescribed when serum levels of ascorbic acid are abnormally low. Statins have a significant antiinflammatory effect in RA patients by reduction of disease activity and several blood parameters like erythrocyte sedimentation rate (ESR), CRP, and lipid profile (Li et al, 2018).

DMARDs may be prescribed because of their unique ability to slow or prevent further joint damage caused by arthritis. These include MTX, sulfasalazine (Azulfidine), hydroxychloroquine (Plaquenil), azathioprine (Imuran), and leflunomide (Arava). In fact, the ACR recommends that the majority of patients with newly diagnosed RA be prescribed a DMARD within 3 months of diagnosis. Depending on which drug is selected, side effects can include myelosuppression or macular or liver damage. A main adverse effect of the DMARD MTX treatment is folate antagonism. Treatment with MTX induces a significant rise in serum homocysteine, which is corrected by folic acid supplementation and a properly balanced diet. Folate supplementation is advised to offset the toxicity of this drug, for protection against gastrointestinal disturbances, and for maintenance of red blood cell production without reducing the efficacy of MTX therapy. Long-term folate supplementation in patients on MTX is also important to prevent neutropenia, mouth ulcers, nausea, and vomiting.

D-penicillamine acts as an immunosuppressor by reducing the number of T cells, inhibiting macrophage function, and decreasing IL-1 and RF production. Additional DMARDs include gold salt therapy and antimalarials and may lead to a remission in RA symptoms. Proteinuria may occur with administration of gold and D-penicillamine; therefore, toxicity must be monitored continually.

Surgery

Surgical treatment for RA may be considered if pharmacologic and nonpharmacologic treatment cannot adequately control the pain or maintain acceptable levels of functioning. Common surgical options include synovectomy, joint replacement, and tendon reconstruction.

After substantial weight loss from bariatric surgery, obese patients with RA showed lower disease activity, decreased inflammatory markers (CRP, ESR, total leukocytes) and less RA-related medication use.

PATHOPHYSIOLOGY AND CARE MANAGEMENT ALGORITHM

Rheumatoid Arthritis

Inflammation

Autoimmune disorder

Genetic susceptibility

Rheumatoid Arthritis

Viral or bacterial infection

Hormonal factors

ETIOLOGY

PATHOPHYSIOLOGY

Joint Symptoms

- Warmth
- Redness
- Swelling
- Pain
- Stiffness
- Loss of function

Articular

- Chronic inflammation in synovial membranes
- Damage to joint cartilage and bone
- Weakening of surrounding muscles, ligaments, and tendons

Extra-Articular

- Generalized bone loss
- Rheumatoid cachexia
- Changes in GI mucosa
- Anemia
- Sjögren's syndrome
- Cardiovascular disease

MANAGEMENT

Medical Management

Routine Monitoring and Ongoing Care Doctor visits, blood, urine and lab tests, x-rays
Drug Therapy DMARDS, biological response modifiers, analgesics, NSAIDs, corticosteroids
Health Behavior Changes
- Rest and exercise
- Joint care
- Stress reduction
Surgery Joint replacement, tendon reconstruction, synovectomy

Nutrition Management

- Whole foods, balanced diet
- Avoidance of possible food allergens
- Adequate B vitamins
- Adequate calcium and vitamin D
- Supplementation with ω-3 PUFA
- Anti-inflammatory diet
- Intermittent fasting and a vegetarian diet may be helpful during an acute phase

These findings show that weight loss is important to reduce RA disease activity and should be encouraged by nutrition professionals (Sparks et al, 2015; Hassan and Hassan, 2016).

Exercise

Physical and occupational therapy are often part of the initial therapy for newly diagnosed RA but also may be integrated into the treatment plan as the disease progresses and ADLs are affected. To maintain joint function, recommendations may be given for energy conservation, along with range-of-motion and strengthening exercises. Although the patient may be reluctant at first, individuals with RA can participate in conditioning exercise programs without increasing fatigue or joint symptoms while improving joint mobility, muscle strength, aerobic fitness, and psychological well-being.

Medical Nutrition Therapy

The nutrition care process and model serve as a guide for implementing MNT with RA patients. A comprehensive nutrition assessment of individuals with RA is essential to determine the systemic effects of the disease process. A physical examination provides diagnostic signs and symptoms of nutrient deficiencies (see Appendix 11). Weight change is an important measure of RA severity. In cases where a person is overweight, weight loss (5 kg or more) can bring improvement in RA disease activity (Kreps et al, 2018). In some cases, patients with RA will present as underweight due to the progression of their disease. The characteristic progression of malnutrition in RA is attributed to excessive protein catabolism evoked by inflammatory cytokines and by muscle disuse atrophy resulting from functional impairment.

The diet history should review the usual diet, the effect of the physical impairment and impact on ADLs, types of food consumed, and changes in food tolerance. The effect of the disease on food shopping and preparation, self-feeding ability, appetite, and intake also must be assessed.

Articular and extraarticular manifestations of RA affect the nutrition status of individuals in several ways. Articular involvement of the small and large joints may limit the ability to perform nutrition-related ADLs, including shopping for, preparing, and eating food. Involvement of the temporomandibular joint can affect the ability to chew and swallow and may necessitate changes in diet consistency including a soft diet. Extraarticular manifestations include increased metabolic rate secondary to the inflammatory process, SS, and changes in the gastrointestinal mucosa.

Increased metabolic rate secondary to the inflammatory process leads to increased nutrient needs, often in the face of a diminishing nutrient intake. Taste alterations secondary to xerostomia and dryness of the nasal mucosa; dysphagia secondary to pharyngeal and esophageal dryness; and anorexia secondary to medications, fatigue, and pain may reduce dietary intake. Changes in the gastrointestinal mucosa affect intake, digestion, and absorption. The effect of RA and the medications used may be evident throughout the gastrointestinal tract. Based on the patient's unique profile, a registered dietitian nutritionist can determine the most appropriate nutrition intervention, followed by monitoring and evaluation.

The association of foods with disease flares should be discussed. Whether food intake can modify the course of RA is an issue of continued scientific debate and interest. Dietary manipulation by either modifying food composition or reducing body weight may give some clinical benefit in improving RA symptoms. A vegan, gluten-free diet causes improvement in some patients, possibly because of the reduction of immunoreactivity to food antigens (Badsha, 2018). Identification of possible food allergies and use of an elimination diet may be useful (Khanna et al, 2017) (see Chapter 25).

Fasting has been practiced for millennia but, only recently, studies have shed light on its role in adaptive cellular responses that reduce oxidative damage and inflammation. In humans, it helps reduce hypertension, asthma, and symptoms of RA. Thus findings from well-controlled studies in animal models, and emerging findings from human studies, indicate that different forms of fasting may provide effective strategies to minimize age-related debility, optimize health, and help prevent and treat diseases while minimizing the side effects caused by medications (Choi et al, 2017). Intermittent fasting during the acute phase of RA may provide some pain relief; however, after the normal diet is resumed, inflammation returns unless the fasting period is followed by a vegetarian diet. Thus the combination of fasting and a vegetarian diet may be beneficial for the treatment of RA (Longo and Mattson, 2014).

An antiinflammatory diet described in Box 38.2 should be considered. The similar Mediterranean-style eating plan includes foods that almost everyone should aim to consume on a daily basis, such as moderate amounts of lean meat, unsaturated fats instead of saturated fats, plenty of fruits and vegetables, and fish (AF, 2018; van Breda and de Kok, 2018). These diets are also nutritionally adequate and cover all of the food groups (see Appendix 22 for additional description of the antiinflammatory diet).

Preliminary studies demonstrate the beneficial effects of probiotic supplementation in RA patients on their clinical and metabolic status, although it is still early to generalize recommendation of probiotics for RA patients (Zamani et al, 2016).

Energy

There are three unique aspects of energy metabolism in RA. The first is elevated resting energy expenditure. RA causes cachexia, a metabolic response characterized by loss of muscle mass and elevated resting energy expenditure. The second is elevated whole-body protein catabolism, a destructive form of muscle metabolism that translates to muscle wasting. The third is low body cell mass, which leads to increased fat mass. People with RA tend to be less active than people without it; the stiffness and swelling caused by inflammation naturally prompt them to pursue less physical, more sedentary lifestyles. Such habits lead to overall gains in fat mass. Being overweight puts an extra burden on weight-bearing joints when they are already damaged or under strain.

Total energy expenditure is significantly lower in RA patients, mainly because of less moderate-intensity physical activity performance. Disease activity and fatigue are important contributing factors. Energy requirements should be adjusted according to the weight and activity level of the individual as well as nutritional complications, for example metabolic syndrome, if present (Hugo et al, 2016).

People with RA should consume nutrient-rich diets and incorporate physical activity throughout the day to boost their total energy expenditure. This helps them improve their physical function and quality of life and maintain a healthy weight.

Protein

Protein requirements for individuals who are poorly nourished or who are in the inflammatory phase of the disease are 1.2 to 1.5 g protein/kg body weight. Well-nourished individuals do not have increased requirements.

Fat

Fat should contribute less than 30% of the total energy intake for the purposes of healthy eating and weight management. The type of fat included in the diet is important: An increase in the amount of omega-3 fatty acids primarily from fish and alpha-linolenic acid (found in flaxseed, soybean oils, and green leaves) has been shown to reduce inflammation in RA. There is evidence of the efficacy of marine omega-3 PUFAs on improvement in joint swelling and pain and duration of morning stiffness (Calder, 2015; Calder, 2017; Veselinovic et al, 2017). Fish oil at a high dose (3.5 g/day) has been shown to have additional benefits to those achieved by combination DMARD with similar MTX use, including reduced triple DMARD failure and a higher rate of remission (Proudman et al, 2015). Recently it was reported that the consumption of whole fish (tuna, salmon, sardines, trout, sole, halibut, poke, and grouper) more than two times/week by RA patients had a significant impact on their disease activity, but this effect was not observed in those patients who consumed whole fish with lesser frequency (less than one time/week) or ever (Tedeschi et al, 2018). Although these benefits along with improved dietary habits are known, they usually cannot replace conventional drug therapies.

CLINICAL INSIGHT

Fatty Acids in Foodstuffs and the Inflammatory Process

Inflammation is the body's attempt at self-protection to remove harmful stimuli, including damaged cells, irritants, or pathogens, and begin the healing process. When the offending stimuli are removed, inflammation subsides. The resolving phase of inflammation is not a passive process but actively "switches off" via the biosynthesis of endogenous antiinflammatory mediators. It could therefore be considered that chronic, nonresolving inflammation not only is associated with excessive production of proinflammatory mediators but also is attributed to a defect in the synthesis of antiinflammatory compounds.

Two classes of polyunsaturated omega-6 and omega-3 fatty acids are metabolized competitively, including conversion to their corresponding prostanoids (prostaglandins [PG] and thromboxanes [Tx]) and leukotrienes (LT). Eicosapentaenoic acid (EPA, 20:5) and docosahexaenoic acid (DHA, 22:6) are omega-3 polyunsaturated fatty acids (PUFA) that are abundant in cold-water fish such as salmon, sardines, mackerel, herring, tuna, fish oils, and some algae. Alpha-linolenic acid (ALA, 18:3) is also an omega-3 PUFA found in abundance in flaxseed, walnuts, and soy and canola (rapeseed) oils. EPA, DHA, and ALA have all been shown to replace the synthesis of inflammatory eicosanoids by competing with the conversion of arachidonic acid (ARA, 20:4 omega-6) to the series 2 of PG and Tx. Also, EPA and DHA are enzymatically converted to novel specialized proresolving mediators (SPMs) that involve three separate families termed resolvins, protectins, and maresins, which promote the resolution of inflammation (Serhan and Levy, 2018). ARA comes exclusively from animal foods. Linoleic acid (LA, 18:2), an omega-6 PUFA found in safflower and other vegetable oils, is a precursor of ARA; therefore its consumption should be limited in rheumatic patients.

The type of mediator that is produced is determined by the type of PUFAs present in the phospholipids of the cell membrane, which in turn is influenced by the type of PUFAs in the diet. Theoretically, a person can replace omega-6 PUFAs with omega-3 PUFAs by increasing omega-3 PUFA consumption. This, in turn, will result in the synthesis of prostanoids (PG and Tx) with antiinflammatory effects. Similarly, reducing the amount of ARA minimizes inflammation and can enhance the benefits of fish oil supplementation.

Studies during the last 20 years clearly show beneficial changes in eicosanoid metabolism with fish oil supplementation in patients with RA, even when administered parenterally (Calder, 2017). Although fish oil seems to exert an antiinflammatory effect in short-term studies, these effects may vanish during long-term treatment because of decreased numbers of autoreactive T cells via apoptosis.

These oils should be used in conjunction with improved eating that includes more omega-3 PUFA. This means a diet that includes baked or broiled fish one to two times per week. However, the Food and Drug Administration (FDA) has identified shark, swordfish, king mackerel, and tilefish as high-mercury fish that should be avoided (see *Focus On:* Childhood Methylmercury Exposure and Toxicity: Media Messaging in Chapter 16).

A daily consumption of omega-3 PUFA (mainly EPA and DHA) for an RA patient varies from 2.7 g to 4.6 g (Akbar et al, 2017; Calder, 2017). Nowadays the quality of fish oil supplements is higher and with fewer side effects (mostly fishy odor, mild diarrheas, abdominal cramps).

The combination of fish oils with olive oil results in greater clinical improvements in RA patients than those consuming fish oils alone. These results are attributed to oleocanthal, a naturally occurring phenolic compound found in extra virgin olive oil. Oleocanthal exerts its antiinflammatory activity by inhibiting cyclooxygenase (COX)-1 and COX-2 in a similar way as ibuprofen does (Casas et al, 2018) as well as iNOS, interleukin (IL)-1, IL-6, and tumor necrosis factor (TNF) among others (Pang and Chin, 2018).

Minerals, Vitamins, and Antioxidants

Several vitamins and minerals function as antioxidants and therefore affect inflammation. Vitamin E is just such a vitamin, and along with omega-3 fatty acids may decrease proinflammatory cytokines and lipid mediators. Synovial fluid and plasma trace element concentrations, including zinc, change in inflammatory RA. Altered trace element concentrations in inflammatory RA may result from changes of the immunoregulatory cytokines. Degradation of collagen and eicosanoid stimulation are associated with oxidative damage.

RA patients often have nutritional intakes below the dietary reference intakes (DRIs) for folic acid, calcium, vitamin D, vitamin E, zinc, vitamin B, and selenium. In addition, the commonly used drug MTX is known to decrease serum folate levels with the result of elevated homocysteine levels (Kawami et al, 2018). Low serum level of pyridoxal-5-phosphate correlates with increased markers of inflammation (Ueland et al, 2017), and continuous use of NSAID (Naproxen) also impairs pyridoxine metabolism by a mechanism related to COX inhibition (Chang et al, 2013). Thus in these patients, adequate intakes of folate and vitamins B_6 and B_{12} should be encouraged.

Calcium and vitamin D malabsorption and bone demineralization are characteristic of advanced stages of the disease, leading to osteoporosis or fractures. Prolonged use of glucocorticoids also can lead to osteoporosis. Therefore supplementation with calcium and vitamin D should be considered. Vitamin D status should be assessed and supplementation started if below normal. Indeed, vitamin D is a selective immunosuppressant and greater intakes of vitamin D may be beneficial. Because of drug-induced alterations in specific vitamin or mineral levels, mounting evidence supports supplementation beyond the minimum levels for vitamins D, E, folic acid, and vitamins B_6 and B_{12}.

In RA patients, inflammatory Th17 cells producing IL-17 are inversely associated with antiinflammatory Treg cells. Flavonoids found in many fruits, vegetables, cocoa, tea, and some herbs and spices have been used as therapeutic agents in autoimmune inflammatory diseases. The antiinflammatory properties of flavonoids are increasingly elucidated in vitro and in animal models of arthritis, as flavonoids have been shown to inhibit COX, to reduce the production of inflammatory cytokines, to suppress p38 MAPK, to inhibit Th17 cells, and to increase Tregs (Kelepouri et al, 2018). Elevated levels of copper and ceruloplasmin in serum and joint fluid are seen in RA. Plasma copper levels correlate with the degree of joint inflammation, decreasing as the inflammation is diminished. Elevated plasma levels of ceruloplasmin, the carrier protein for copper, may have a protective role because of ceruloplasmin's antioxidant activity.

Complementary and Integrative Therapies

The increasing popularity of the use of complementary treatments appears to be particularly evident with people afflicted with RA. Herbal therapy such as the use of turmeric and ginger have shown benefits in RA with very low risk of adverse events. As with all herbal therapies, it is important to fully assess the potential for drug nutrient interactions (Dragos et al, 2017).

Gamma-linolenic acid (GLA) is an omega-6 fatty acid found in the oils of black currant, borage, and evening primrose that can be converted into the antiinflammatory prostaglandin E (PGE)$_1$ or into ARA, a precursor of the inflammatory PGE$_2$. Because of competition between omega-3 and omega-6 fatty acids for the same enzymes, the relative dietary contribution of these fats appears to affect which pathways are favored. The enzyme delta-5 desaturase converts GLA into ARA, but a diet high in omega-3 fats pulls more of this enzyme to the omega-3 pathway, allowing the body to use GLA to produce PGE_1 (see *Clinical Insight: Fatty Acids and the Inflammatory Process*). This antiinflammatory PGE_1 may relieve pain, morning stiffness, and joint tenderness with no serious side effects. Further studies are required to establish optimum dosage and duration.

SJÖGREN'S SYNDROME

Sjögren's syndrome (SS) is a chronic autoimmune inflammatory disease that affects the exocrine glands, particularly the salivary and the lacrimal glands, leading to dryness of the mouth (xerostomia) and of the eyes (xerophthalmia). SS can present alone (primary SS) or secondary as a result of a previous rheumatic disorder (commonly RA or SLE). It mainly affects middle-aged women, with a female to male ratio of 9:1 (Mariette and Criswell, 2018).

Common oral signs include thirst, burning sensation in the oral mucosa, inflammation of the tongue (glossitis) and lips (cheilitis), cracking of the corners of the lips (cheilosis), difficulties in chewing and swallowing (dysphagia), severe dental caries, oral infections (candidiasis), progressive dental decay, and nocturnal oral discomfort. Patients may also suffer from extraglandular disorders affecting the skin, lung, kidney, nerve, connective tissue, and digestive systems (Mariette and Criswell, 2018). SS patients also may develop disturbances in smell perception (dysosmia) and in taste acuity (dysgeusia) (Gomez et al, 2004; Al-Ezzi et al, 2017).

Pathophysiology

Although the pathogenesis of SS remains elusive, environmental, genetic, and hormonal contributors seem to be involved. The majority of lymphocytes infiltrating the salivary glands are mostly CD4 T cells. Increased levels of IL-1 and IL-6 in the saliva of SS patients suggest that a Th1 response participates in the pathogenesis of the disease. A recent meta-analysis reported an increase in IL-17 in serum and saliva of primary SS (pSS) patients (Zhang et al, 2018), which also was associated with the severity of the symptoms. Furthermore, patients with pSS without immunosuppressive treatment show markedly higher IL-17 levels.

Although T cells were originally considered to play the initiating role in SS, whereas B cells were restricted to autoantibody production, it has been shown that B cells play a central role in the development of the disease (Nocturne and Mariette, 2018). A distinctive hallmark of SS is the presence of anti-Ro/SSA and anti-La/SSB autoantibodies. Interestingly, anti-Ro/SSA may be found either solely or concomitantly with anti-La/SSB antibodies, whereas exclusive anti-La/SSB positivity is rare (Jog and James, 2017).

Recent studies indicate that dysbiosis may play a role in SS pathogenesis. The cause-effect direction is not clear yet because the dysfunction of salivary glands induces alterations in the microbiome, which is linked to worsening of symptoms and disease severity. Although this information is preliminary, dietary patterns that support a healthy microbiome including a plant-based, fiber-rich diet may be reasonable (Tsigalou et al, 2018).

Medical Management

The therapeutic management of SS is based on symptomatic treatment of glandular manifestations and on the use of DMARD for systemic involvement (van der Heijden et al, 2018). Symptomatic treatment has beneficial effects on oral and ocular dryness and prevents further complications such as oral candidiasis, periodontal disease, and corneal ulceration and perforation.

Topical treatment of xerostomia begins by avoiding irritants such as caffeine, alcohol, and tobacco, followed by appropriate hydration (small sips of water) and the use of saliva substitutes, lubricating gels, mouth rinses, chewing gum, lozenges, or oils. Any of these treatments is effective in the short term, but none improves saliva production. After consumption of sugary foods or beverages, the teeth should be brushed and rinsed with water immediately to prevent dental caries. Topical treatment for xerophthalmia starts by avoiding dry, smoky, or windy environments and prolonged reading or computer use. Artificial tears can be used. The muscarinic receptor agonists pilocarpine (Salagen) and cevimeline (Evoxac) may be used for the treatment of dry mouth and dry eyes only in patients with residual gland function (Mariette and Criswell, 2018).

B-cell depletion therapy with rituximab (anti-CD20) improves the stimulated whole saliva flow rate and lacrimal gland function, as well as other variables including RF levels, extraglandular manifestations (arthritis, skin vasculitis), fatigue, and quality of life, indicating a major role of B cells in the pathogenesis of SS (Mariette and Criswell, 2018).

IL-1 and TNF-α play a major role in the development of SS. Blocking IL-1 (anakinra) is beneficial in the treatment of SS, whereas blocking TNF-α (etanercept) is ineffective in controlling SS symptoms (Nocturne and Mariette, 2018). The management of extraglandular features must be tailored to the specific organs involved. Antimalarials (hydroxychloroquine), besides improving salivary flow, can help SS patients with arthromyalgia. The use of corticosteroids may be used in patients with extraglandular manifestations, although they have no effect in salivary or lacrimal flow rates.

Medical Nutrition Therapy

The first goal of dietary management for patients with SS is to help them relieve their oral symptoms and reduce the eating discomfort derived from the difficulty with chewing and swallowing (Sjögren's Syndrome Foundation, 2018). Very often SS patients modify their dietary habits on a trial and error basis to cope with their oral symptoms, particularly to improve biting (cutting fruits, vegetables, and meats in small pieces), chewing (making foods softer by preparing them as soups, broths, casseroles, or as tender cooked vegetables and meats), and swallowing (moistening foods with sauces, gravies, yogurts, or salad dressings). Foods that worsen oral symptoms should be limited, such as citrus fruits, as well as irritating, hot, or spicy foods and alcohol (Sjögren's Syndrome Foundation, 2018).

Malnutrition or weight loss are not common in SS patients, although deficiencies of several nutrients are common. These include vitamin D (Garcia-Carrasco et al, 2017), vitamin B_6, vitamin B_{12}, folate, and iron, which can be corrected easily by proper nutritional counseling or supplementation (Erten et al, 2015). More importantly single nutrient deficiencies in SS have been associated with other diseases, such as low levels of vitamin D with neuropathy and lymphoma, suggesting a possible role of vitamin D deficiency in the development of other symptoms, and the plausible beneficial effect for vitamin D supplementation (Garcia-Carrasco et al, 2017).

Preliminary studies demonstrate that the beneficial effects of probiotic supplementation in RA patients might also benefit patients with SS and other autoimmune conditions, to shift their microbiome away from a disease promoting and proinflammatory pattern (Zamani et al, 2016).

TEMPOROMANDIBULAR DISORDERS

Temporomandibular disorders (TMDs) affect the temporomandibular joint, which connects the lower jaw (mandible) to the temporal bone. TMDs can be classified as myofascial pain, internal derangement of the joint, or degenerative joint disease. One or more of these conditions may be present at the same time, causing pain or discomfort in the muscles or joint that control jaw function.

Pathophysiology

Besides experiencing a severe jaw injury, little scientific evidence suggests a cause for TMD. It is generally agreed that physical or mental stress may aggravate this condition.

Medical Nutrition Therapy

The goal of dietary management is to alter food consistency to reduce pain while chewing. According to the National Institute of Dental and Craniofacial Research (NIDCR), diet should be soft in consistency; all foods should be cut into bite-size pieces to minimize the need to chew or open the jaw widely; chewing gum, sticky foods, and hard foods such as raw vegetables, candy, and nuts should be avoided (NIH, NIDCR, 2018). It is recommended to cut all foods into small pieces, select moist foods or use gravies or sauces to moisten foods to a comfortable consistency, peel fruits (with the exception of berries) and vegetables that have skin, chop whole foods to consistencies that can be comfortably tolerated, limit jaw opening to the extent that is comfortable, take small bites of food, and chew slowly. Although mechanically altering the patient's diet to enable pain-free eating is the goal, in some instances, patients may benefit from taking liquid oral supplements to meet their energy, protein, and micronutrient needs (Nasri-Heir et al, 2016). Nutrient intake of TMD patients appears to be the same as for the general population with regard to total calories, protein, fat, carbohydrates, vitamins, and minerals. However, during times of acute pain, intake of fiber is often reduced.

GOUT

Gout is one of the oldest diseases in recorded medical history. It is a disorder of purine metabolism in which abnormally high levels of uric acid accumulate in the blood (hyperuricemia). Contrary to what is observed in most rheumatic diseases, gout predominantly affects men. Gout is common in most countries in North America and Western Europe, with prevalence in the range 1% to 4%. By contrast, gout is reportedly rare in former Soviet Union regions, Guatemala, Iran, Malaysia, Philippines, Saudi Arabia, rural Turkey, and African countries. In all countries, men have a significantly higher prevalence of gout than women. The male to female ratio is generally in the order of 3:1 to 4:1 (Kuo et al, 2015)

Gout is associated with cardiovascular and renal diseases and is an independent predictor of premature death. The frequencies of obesity, chronic kidney disease (CKD), hypertension, type 2 diabetes, dyslipidemias, cardiac diseases (including coronary heart disease, heart failure, and atrial fibrillation), stroke, and peripheral arterial disease have been repeatedly shown to be increased in gout. Therefore the screening and care of these comorbidities as well as of cardiovascular risk factors are of utmost importance in patients with gout (Bardin and Richette, 2017).

Pathophysiology

Gout is a crystal deposition disease in which the clinical symptoms are caused by the formation of monosodium urate (MSU) crystals in the joints and soft tissues, and the elimination of these crystals "cures" the disease. Uric acid is the end-product of purine metabolism in humans, but it is an intermediary product in most other mammals. It is produced primarily in the liver by the action of the enzyme xanthine-oxidase, a molybdenum-dependent enzyme. In most mammals, uric acid is further degraded by the enzyme urate oxidase (uricase), to allantoin, which is more soluble than uric acid, and hence more readily excreted by kidneys. In humans and higher primates, the gene encoding for uricase is nonfunctional and due to this evolutionary event, uric acid levels are higher in humans than in many other mammals. Endogenous production of uric acid from degradation of purines accounts for two thirds of the body urate pool, the remainder being of dietary origin. Because most uric acid is excreted via the kidney (approximately 70%), hyperuricemia results from reduced efficiency of renal urate clearance.

Two proteins have been well characterized in urate clearance: the urate transporter 1 (URAT1) and the glucose and fructose transporter (GLUT9). URAT1 localizes in the brush border membrane of the proximal tubule kidney and is responsible mainly for renal reabsorption of uric acid, whereas GLUT9 is located in the apical and basolateral membrane of the distal tubule where it functions as the main exit of urate from the body (Mandal and Mount, 2015).

In the vast majority of people with gout, hyperuricemia results from reduced renal urate clearance. MSU crystals preferentially form within cartilage and fibrous tissues; however if shed from these sites, they are highly immunogenic particles that are quickly phagocytosed by monocytes and macrophages, activating the NALP3 inflammasome and triggering the release of IL-1 and other cytokines, thus initiating an inflammatory response that affects the joint. MSU crystals act as a danger signal that can be recognized by pattern recognition receptors at the cell surface and in the cytoplasm, indicating the importance of innate immunity in gout (Benn et al, 2018). Persistent accumulation of MSU crystals causes joint damage through mechanical effects (pressure erosion) leading to chronic symptoms of arthritis (Fig. 38.5). MSU crystals can deposit in the small joints and surrounding tissues, producing recurrent episodes of extremely painful and debilitating joint and soft tissue inflammation (acute gout). In chronic gout, classic sites are the big toe, wrists and finger joints, elbow (Fig. 38.6), ankle, knee, and the helix of the ear. Occasionally, uric acid crystals called tophi can be seen as white patches on the skin and in cartilage such as the ear.

Pseudogout, also called CPPD (calcium pyrophosphate deposition) disease has a prevalence of around 0.5% of the general population (for the U.S. and Europe). The average age of onset is over 68 years and is more common in men. There is no reported treatment (pharmacological or nutritional) that can lower the production and deposition of CPP in these patients. Although the treatment for the symptoms of CPPD (inflammation and pain) is identical to that of "classical" gout (due to monosodium urate crystals), there is no dietary intervention known to prevent or treat this condition (Zamora & Kaik 2019).

Medical Management

Colchicine is a medication used to treat the pain associated with acute flares of gout (within 12 to 24 hours) by reducing the inflammation caused by MSU crystals; it has no effect on serum urate levels. Colchicine may be used with other NSAIDs and only for a limited time because of its toxicity.

Because monocytes and macrophages produce IL-1 in response to MSU crystals, treatment with IL-1 antagonists (Anakinra) or with soluble IL-1 receptor (rilonacept) results in rapid and complete pain relief (Pascart and Richette, 2017).

Two classes of drugs have been used to lower serum urate: uricostatic drugs, which reduce the synthesis of uric acid by inhibiting xanthine oxidase, and uricosuric drugs, which increase the excretion of uric acid by blocking its renal tubular reabsorption. Allopurinol (Zyloprim) and febuxostat are uricostatic drugs; they are the drugs of choice for long-term treatment of hyperuricemia. On the other hand, sulfinpyrazone, probenecid, and benzbromarone are uricosuric drugs that act by inhibiting URAT1, therefore increasing the urinary excretion of uric acid (Mandal and Mount, 2015; Pascart and Richette, 2017).

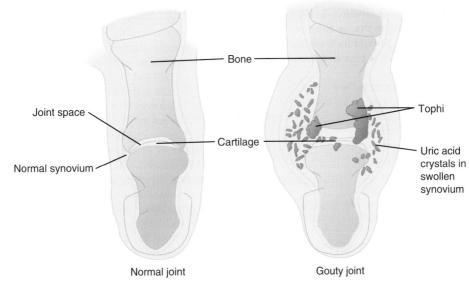

Fig. 38.5 Comparison of a gouty joint and a normal joint in the toe. (From Black JM, et al: *Medical surgical nursing*, ed 7, Philadelphia, 2005, Saunders.)

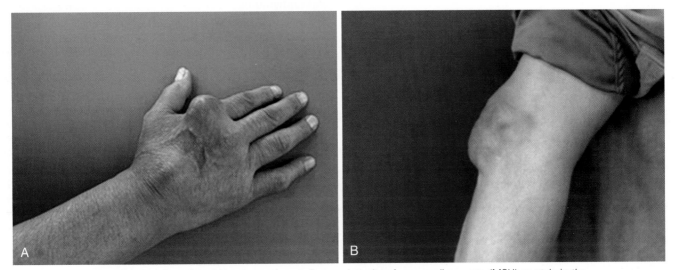

Fig. 38.6 A male patient with advanced gout. Severe deposits of monosodium urate (MSU) crystals in the hand (**A,** wrist and fingers) and in the elbow (**B**). (Photos courtesy Dr. F. Enrique Gómez. Instituto Nacional de Ciencias Médicas y Nutrición Salvador Zubirán. Mexico City, México, 2015.)

Pegloticase, a recombinant uricase, reduces serum urate levels by converting uric acid to allantoin, which is excreted rapidly in the urine (Guttmann et al, 2017). Pegloticase is used for rapid debulking of tophi, and together with colchicine it reduces the impact of acute gout flares.

Medical Nutrition Therapy

Purine-containing foods (such as meats, organ meat, seafood, legumes, yeast, mushrooms, and gravies) have been the target of many early gout diets, mainly on the basis of the concept that the biochemical degradation end product of purines is urate. More recent studies have found that this is not necessarily true. National Health and Nutrition Examination Survey data show that the age-adjusted differences in serum urate between the lowest and highest intake of meat was 0.48 mg/dL (95% CI 0.34-0.61 mg/dL, p<0.001) and 0.16 mg/dL for

seafood (95% CI 0.06-0.27 mg/dL, p = 0.005). Total protein intake was not found to be related to increasing urate levels.

In a similar prospective study, the relative risk for gout in men with the highest meat intake compared with the lowest was 1.41 (95% CI 1.07-1.80), whereas seafood was 1.51 (95% CI 1.17-1.95). Each additional serving of meat per day increased the risk of gout by 21%, whereas each additional weekly seafood serving increased risk by 7%. The intake of dried beans and greens is not associated with gouty flares, as shown by a relative risk of 0.73 (95% CI 0.56-0.96).

Fructose is the only carbohydrate known to increase urate. Fructose and sugar intake also predispose to insulin resistance and metabolic syndrome, which further increase the risk of hyperuricemia (Beyl et al, 2016).

On the other hand, diets that contain low-fat dairy products and supplemental vitamin C have been associated with reduced

BOX 38.3 Purine Content of Foods

High Purine Content (100-1000 mg of Purine Nitrogen per 100 g of Food): Foods in This List Should be Omitted from the Diet of Patients Who have Gout (Acute and Remission Stages).

Anchovies	Meat extracts
Bouillon	Mincemeat
Brains	Mussels
Broth	Partridge
Consommé	Roe
Goose	Sardines
Gravy	Scallops
Heart	Sweetbreads
Herring	Yeast (baker's and brewer's), taken as
Kidney	supplement
Mackerel	

Moderate Purine Content (9-100 mg of Purine Nitrogen per 100 g of Food): One Serving (2-3 oz) of Meat, Fish, or Poultry Daily

Meat, fish and shellfish not listed above
Poultry

risk of gout. Consumption of black coffee (without sugar) is associated with low levels of serum urate, and therefore may be protective for gout.

Alcohol consumption, particularly beer (which is rich in purines), increases the risk of gout. Consumption of fructose, mainly as soft drinks sweetened with high fructose corn syrup, is associated with higher risk for gout. It is unclear whether this is a particular effect of fructose derived from high-fructose corn syrup, or whether it extends to sucrose (Beyl et al, 2016). Excess consumption of naturally occurring fructose such as in fruit juices also may increase risk of gout.

It is prudent to advise patients to consume a balanced meal plan with limited intake of animal foods and beer, avoidance of high-purine foods (Box 38.3), limited consumption of fructose and refined carbohydrates (sweetened soft drinks and juices, candies, and sweet pastries). If a patient is overweight, weight loss may also help reduce risk of gout. Liberal intake of plant proteins, nuts, vegetables, legumes, whole grains, lower sugar fruits, and plant oils is supported, and up to two servings daily of low-fat dairy products is recommended. Although fish intake can increase serum urate, there may be greater overall cardiovascular benefit from the addition of moderate amounts of cold water, oily fish such as tuna, salmon, and trout, which are high in omega-3 fatty acids. Eggs and poultry are lower risk protein sources when used in moderation. One or fewer servings of red meat or shellfish per week may be recommended. Wine in moderation is acceptable. Up to 6 cups of coffee daily has been shown beneficial but new initiation of coffee may exacerbate gout flares. Supplementation with vitamin C may be useful, but a dosing range and long-term safety recommendations have not been made. Cherry products may be beneficial, but better data are needed before making this a recommendation to patients. During an acute flare it is recommended to increase water intake to at least 8 cups per day and avoid alcohol or meat (Beyl et al, 2016).

Dairy products (milk or cheese), eggs, vegetable protein, and coffee appear to be protective, possibly because of the alkaline ash effect of these foods (see *Clinical Insight:* Acid and Alkaline Diet in Chapter 34). Cherry juice has also been studied for its ability to lower uric acid levels and gout flares.

SCLERODERMA (SYSTEMIC SCLEROSIS OR SSc)

Scleroderma (currently known as systemic sclerosis or SSc) is a chronic disease characterized by three features: early microvascular obliterative changes, early activation of the immune system with activation of T cells and B cells, and widespread fibrosis of skin and internal organs. SSc is characterized by multisystem involvement, mainly the skin, respiratory tract (lung parenchyma and pulmonary arteries), kidneys, skeletal muscles, the gastrointestinal tract and cardiovascular system (Eldoma and Pope, 2018). As with other RMDs, women are more prone to develop SSc but the incidence is very low (between 10 and 20/100,000).

Based on the extent of skin involvement, SSc is classified into two subtypes: limited cutaneous scleroderma (lcSSc), defined by thickened skin distal to elbows and knees, face, and neck, and diffuse cutaneous scleroderma (dcSSc) which involves the trunk and the proximal part of upper and lower limbs. It is important to identify the patient's subtype due to differences in prognosis and organ involvement. LcSSc is more likely to be associated with anticentromere autoantibodies (ACA) and Raynaud's syndrome before disease onset and a better prognosis. DcSSc is more likely to have internal organ involvement and a worse prognosis.

Pathophysiology

Systemic sclerosis (SSc) is characterized by vascular abnormalities, followed by hypoxia and coldness of the hands and feet (Raynaud's syndrome) as well as excessive production of extracellular matrix and collagen. The pathogenesis of SSc is incompletely understood, but immune activation and microvasculopathy could lead to the development of fibrosis. The activation of B cells results in the presence of autoantibodies, whereas activation of proinflammatory Th1 and Th17 cells is enhanced by a reduction in IL-10. Other cytokines such as IL-4, IL-13, IL-6, and TGFβ, are among the profibrotic mediators implicated in SSc pathogenesis.

Scleroderma renal crisis (SRC) is a rare complication of SSc characterized by hypertension and oliguric or anuric acute renal failure. Intestinal involvement is frequent in SSc and represents a significant cause of morbidity. The pathogenesis of intestinal involvement includes vascular damage, nerve dysfunction, smooth muscle atrophy, and fibrosis, causing hypomotility, which may lead to small intestinal bacterial overgrowth (SIBO), malabsorption, malnutrition, diarrhea, pseudoobstruction, constipation, and fecal incontinence (Sakkas et al, 2018; Eldoma and Pope, 2018). Manifestations are often troublesome and reduce quality of life and life expectancy (Smirani et al, 2018; Sakkas et al, 2018).

Medical Management

SSc is a serious, sometimes life-threatening connective tissue disease with treatment options that have been shown to provide only mild to modest benefit. The limited efficacy of available therapies can be explained by several factors including heterogeneity of the disease, lack of complete understanding of pathophysiology, and limited use of combination or maintenance therapy. Treatment guidelines for SSc provide therapy options for disease manifestations based on the affected organs or systems. However, the current therapy available shows mild improvement in disease with mostly loss of benefit after discontinuation of treatment.

Several immunosuppressive treatments (MTX, cyclophosphamide, and mycophenolate mofetil) have been used to reduce the deposition of collagen in skin in early dcSSc. Immunomodulation should be considered early in intestinal involvement. Since the advent of angiotensin-converting enzyme (ACE) inhibitors, mortality associated with SRC decreased from 76% to <10%. Some patients may progress to end-stage renal disease and need dialysis. SSc has been treated with biologicals (Abatacept, Tocilizumab) with some promising results (Eldoma and Pope, 2018).

Medical Nutrition Therapy

Management of concomitant digestive complaints is a primary focus of MNT for SSc. Patients with diarrhea are managed with a low-residue and low-fat diet, medium-chain triglycerides, avoidance of lactulose and fructose, and/or a low-FODMAP diet if SIBO is present. In diarrhea/malabsorption, bile acid sequestrant and pancreatic enzyme supplementation may help. General measures are applied for constipation (fiber, fluids, physical activity, and fermented foods or probiotics supplements), and intestine rest plus antibiotics for pseudoobstruction. Fecal incontinence is managed with measures for associated SIBO or constipation, and with behavioral therapies. A multidisciplinary approach to management of intestinal manifestations in SSc by gastroenterologists, rheumatologists, and dietitians is required for optimum management (Sakkas et al, 2018; Smirani et al, 2018).

Patients with SSc often experience dry mouth and dysphagia (see Chapter 39 and Appendix 20). Dry mouth with resultant tooth decay, loose teeth, and tightening facial skin make eating difficult. Consuming adequate fluids, choosing moist foods, chewing sugarless gum, and using saliva substitutes help moisten the mouth and offer temporary relief.

If gastroesophageal reflux is a concern, small, frequent meals are recommended along with avoidance of late-night eating, alcohol, caffeine, and spicy or fatty foods (see Chapter 26).

Malabsorption of lactose, vitamins, fatty acids, and minerals can cause further malnutrition and supplementation may be required. A high-energy, high-protein supplement or enteral feeding may prevent or correct weight loss. Home enteral or parenteral nutrition often is required when problems such as chronic diarrhea and malabsorption persist (see Chapter 12).

SYSTEMIC LUPUS ERYTHEMATOSUS

Systemic lupus erythematosus (SLE) is known commonly as lupus. SLE is a chronic autoimmune disease characterized by production of autoantibodies directed against nuclear (anti-dsDNA, anti-Sm, anti-RNP) and cytoplasmic antigens affecting several organs and tissues (Jog and James, 2017). SLE is most prevalent in women of childbearing age with a female to male ratio of 9:1, suggesting that sex-related factors are important in its development. It has also been shown that SLE is more common in African Americans and women of Hispanic, Asian, and Native American descent than in Caucasians. In the United States, SLE is among the top 20 leading causes of death in females between 5 and 64 years of age (Yen and Singh, 2018).

Pathophysiology

The cause of SLE is multifactorial and involves multiple genes and environmental factors such as infections, hormones, and drugs. In SLE, circulating ANA (anti-dsDNA, anti-Sm, anti-RNP) and others (anticardiolipin) can deposit in several tissues (Jog and James, 2017). The production of cytokines such as type 1 IFN activates B and T cells and propagates the signal to produce more IFN by DC. This upregulation of the type 1-IFN pathway is critical in the severity and progression of SLE (Connelly et al, 2018).

Common symptoms include extreme fatigue, painful or swollen joints, muscle pain, sensitivity to the sun, unexplained fever, skin rashes most commonly on the face, mouth ulcers, pale or purple fingers or toes from cold or stress (Raynaud's syndrome), and kidney insufficiency (NIH, NIAMS, 2018). SLE is characterized by periods of remission and relapse and may present with various constitutional and organ-specific symptoms.

Medical Management

General treatment of SLE includes sun protection, diet and nutrition, smoking cessation, and exercise, whereas organ-specific treatments include use of steroids, NSAIDs, DMARDs, and biologics. Pharmacologic treatment includes the cytotoxic agents cyclophosphamide and azathioprine; their combination with corticosteroids must be employed early if there is major organ involvement in order to prevent or minimize irreversible damage.

The hallmark of SLE is B-cell activation and the production of harmful autoantibodies. Therefore B-cell depletion and cytokine or Treg cells targeted therapies, alone or combined with cytotoxic drugs, have been used to treat SLE. There are more than 20 biologic therapies used for SLE. They have different immune targets, such as B cells, T cells, and myeloid cells and their cytokines, known to contribute to lupus pathogenesis (Davis and Reimold, 2017).

Hydroxychloroquine (Plaquenil, an antimalarial drug) has potential benefits for dermatologic manifestations, arthritis, preventing lupus flares, reducing thrombosis in APS, atherosclerotic risk, and type 2 diabetes risk. Steroid hormones, azathioprine and MTX and mycophenolate mofetil, are some of the DMARDs used to control SLE manifestations (Davis and Reimold, 2017).

Medical Nutrition Therapy

Because kidney insufficiency is common in SLE, total protein intake may need to be reduced (see Chapter 34). SLE patients tend to have higher consumption of carbohydrates and low intake of dietary fiber and omega-3 (EPA and DHA) and omega-6 fatty acids. The latter has been negatively associated with increased disease activity, altered serum lipid profiles, and increased carotid plaque presence (Lourdudoss et al, 2016). In addition, SLE patients often have inadequate intakes of calcium, fruits, and vegetables and high consumption of oils and fats (Aparicio-Soto et al, 2017).

Photosensitivity, sunlight avoidance, the use of sun protection, and low dietary intake, in combination with medications prescribed to treat the symptoms of the disease, may be responsible for the observed low levels of vitamin D (Dall'Ara et al, 2018). Decreased conversion of 25-hydroxy vitamin D to its active form, calcitriol (1,25-dihydroxy vitamin D_3), is possible because of renal impairment common in SLE, putting additional stress on vitamin D metabolism.

Vitamin D deficiency has been associated with higher ANA levels in healthy subjects and in treatment-naive SLE patients, suggesting it might be a trigger for autoantibody production. Vitamin D supplementation may be beneficial to patients with high anti-dsDNA positivity, possibly reducing clinical flares (Aparicio-Soto et al, 2017; Franco et al, 2017).

Vitamin D supplementation in patients with SLE is recommended because increased vitamin D levels seem to ameliorate inflammatory and blood markers and show a tendency toward subsequent clinical improvement. General international recommendations have established that vitamin D supplementation with 800 to 1000 IU/day or 50000 IU/month is safe for most individuals and can ensure levels of vitamin D within the optimal range (Aparicio-Soto et al, 2017; Dall'Ara et al, 2018).

Vitamin A has also shown beneficial effects, alone or in combination with low-dose immunosuppressive drugs, in lupus nephritis and cytokine modulation in both mouse models and patients with SLE (Aparicio-Soto et al, 2017). The most likely mechanism of action for vitamin A in SLE is via IL-17 and transforming growth factor (TGFβ), cytokine regulation, and possibly others like IL-6 (Handono et al, 2016).

An adequate intake of dietary fiber is recommended in SLE because of the beneficial effects of fiber in decreasing cardiovascular risk, promoting gut mobility, and reducing serum levels of inflammation markers such as CRP, cytokines, and homocysteine (Aparicio-Soto et al, 2017).

Complementary Integrative Therapies

More than an estimated 50% of patients with SLE have used CIM to reduce symptoms and manage their health. Supplements of N-acetyl cysteine and turmeric reduce SLE activity and, together with mind-body methods (cognitive-behavioral therapy and other counseling interventions), improve mood and quality of life of SLE patients (Greco et al, 2013). A small study showed short-term turmeric supplementation can decrease proteinuria, hematuria, and systolic blood pressure in patients suffering from relapsing or refractory lupus nephritis (Khajehdehi et al, 2012). No systematic reviews have been performed for the application of integrative medicine for lupus nephritis on patients with SLE (Choi et al, 2018).

SPONDYLARTHRITIDES

The most important clinical features of this group of diseases are inflammatory back pain, asymmetric peripheral oligoarthritis (predominantly of the lower limbs), and enthesitis (inflammation at the site where the tendon attaches to the bone). Conventional medical treatment is based mainly on the use of NSAIDs (ibuprofen, COX-2 inhibitors) and DMARDs (sulfasalazine); patients with persistently active disease are also treated with blocking agents (TNF, IL-6). Physiotherapy is of major importance in the general approach to patients with any of these spondylarthritides. Nutritional therapy must emphasize keeping a healthy body weight, as well as increasing the consumption of foods rich in antioxidants and with antiinflammatory activities (see Box 38.2 and Appendix 22).

Ankylosing spondylitis (AS) is the major subtype of the spondylarthritides. AS (from Greek *ankylos*, fused; *spondylos*, vertebra; *-itis*, inflammation) affects joints in the spine and the sacroiliac joint in the pelvis and can cause eventual fusion of the spine. AS most often develops in young adult men and it lasts a lifetime. Enthesitis, inflammation of the site where ligaments and tendons insert into the bone, accounts for much of the pain and stiffness of AS. This inflammation eventually can lead to bony fusion of the joints, where the fibrous ligaments transform to bone, and the joint permanently grows together. Other joints also can develop synovitis, with lower limb joints more commonly involved than upper-limb joints. Pain in the low back and buttocks are usually the first symptoms of AS. In contrast to mechanical low back pain, low back pain and stiffness in AS patients are worse after a period of rest or on waking up in the morning and improve after exercise, a hot bath, or a shower. Progressive stiffening of the spine is usual, with ankylosis occurring after some years of disease in many, but not all, patients. A majority of patients have mild or moderate disease with intermittent exacerbations and remissions and maintain some mobility and independence throughout life. Complete fusion results in a complete rigidity of the spine, a condition known as bamboo spine.

Polymyalgia rheumatica (PMR) means "pain in many muscles," and is a syndrome with pain or stiffness, usually in the neck, shoulders, and hips. It may be caused by an inflammatory condition of blood vessels such as temporal arteritis (inflammation of blood vessels in the face, which can cause blindness if not treated quickly). Most PMR sufferers wake up in the morning with pain in their muscles; however, there have been cases in which the patient has developed the pain during the evenings. Treatment for PMR includes the use of corticosteroids (prednisone) alone or with an NSAID (ibuprofen) to relieve pain, exercises to strengthen the weak muscles, and a healthy diet (antiinflammatory diet) (see Appendix 22).

Polymyositis (PM), which means "inflammation of many muscles," is a type of chronic inflammation of the muscles (inflammatory myopathy) and is more common in adult women. Symptoms include pain with marked weakness or loss of muscle mass in the muscles of the head, neck, torso, and upper arms and legs. The hip extensors are often severely affected, leading to particular difficulty in ascending stairs and rising from a seated position. Early fatigue while walking is caused by weakness in the upper leg muscles. Sometimes the weakness presents itself as an inability to raise from a seated position without help or an inability to raise one's arms above one's head. Dysphagia or other problems with esophageal motility occur in as many as one third of patients; foot drop in one or both feet can be a symptom of advanced PM.

Treatment for PM includes corticosteroids, specialized exercise therapy, and a whole-foods antiinflammatory diet tailored to individual needs. Patients with dysphagia may benefit by changing the consistency of foods (softened, increased moisture) and a referral to a speech language therapist for further assessment.

CLINICAL CASE STUDY

Linda is a 33-year-old Mexican female, team manager at a service company and mother of two. She is an active smoker with periodontal disease. Six months ago, she presented with chronic additive symmetric polyarthritis, involving the wrists, hands, knees, and toes. Linda has morning stiffness for about an hour, her symptoms improve with movement and worsen with rest. She has taken several NSAIDs with no major improvement. At examination, the doctor noted inflammation in the joints.

Laboratory tests showed mild normocytic normochromic anemia, elevated erythrocyte sedimentation rate, and high C-reactive protein. She was positive for rheumatoid factor and antibodies to cyclic citrullinated peptide (ACPAs).

Marginal erosions in the metacarpophalangeal joints were found by x-ray imaging.

Linda was diagnosed with rheumatoid arthritis. Based on polyarthritis, positivity of antibodies and erosions, it was determined to be a severe case, and she was started on disease-modifying antirheumatic drugs (DMARDs) methotrexate (MTX) and corticosteroids.

Nutrition Assessment

Patient is 33-year-old Mexican woman with a recent diagnosis of rheumatoid arthritis. Anthropometric Data

CLINICAL CASE STUDY—cont'd

Ht 5'8" (1.73 m); Wt 152 lb (69 kg) (lost 6 lb [4%] over past 2 months)
Body mass index (BMI) = 23
Biochemical data: Hb 10.5 g/dL

Food and Nutrition History

Diet reflects reliance on convenience foods and highly processed take-out fast foods with inadequate intake of antiinflammatory fruits, vegetables, whole grains, and omega 3 fatty acids.

Decline in food preparation due to difficulty in shopping and cooking. Pt reports having a lower than normal appetite due to stress and pain.

Caloric intake: 1600 kcal/day (80% of estimated need)

Estimated energy requirement (EER): 2070 kcal (30 kcal/kg) and 82 g protein (1.2 g/kg body weight [BW] for acute phase).

Nutrition Diagnostic Statements

- Inadequate energy intake related to reduced appetite from stress and pain as evidenced by consuming an estimated 80% of caloric needs and involuntary weight loss of 4% in 2 months (NI-1.4) (NC-3.2).
- Impaired ability to prepare foods/meals related with pain and swelling in hands and wrist joints as evidenced by patient's report.
- Undesirable food choices related to food and nutrition knowledge deficit about the relationship between whole foods antiinflammatory diet and the progression of autoimmune disease as evidenced by a reliance on highly processed convenience foods and low intake of omega-3 fatty acids, fruits, vegetables, and whole grains.

- Altered nutrition-related laboratory values (Hemoglobin) related to drug-nutrient interaction with MTX and inadequate iron intake, as evidenced by anemia diagnosis.

Interventions

- Ensure adequate energy, protein, and iron intake (2000 kcals, 80 g protein)
- Whole foods, iron-rich diet with an emphasis on vegetables, whole grains, oily fish, and antiinflammatory herbs and spices (turmeric)
- Education about whole foods based on convenience foods and adaptive utensils that may make food preparation easier
- Omega-3 fatty acid supplementation (2,000 to 3000 mg daily). Folinic acid (due to MTX) and iron supplementation as prescribed by her physician
- Advice to cease smoking and perform moderate intensity physical activity

Monitoring and Evaluation

- Monthly weight measurements; although Linda's BMI is currently adequate in spite of her weight loss, it is important to stop weight loss due to her autoimmune condition.
- Repeat iron laboratories in 3 months
- Evaluate energy, protein, and iron intake. If arthritis is not active, adjust protein to 1 g/kg BW.

USEFUL WEBSITES

American Autoimmune Related Diseases Association, Inc.
American College of Rheumatology
Arthritis Foundation
Arthritis Research UK
Arthritis Society
European League Against Rheumatism (EULAR)
Lupus Foundation of America
National Center for Complementary and Integrative Health
National Institute of Arthritis and Musculoskeletal and Skin Diseases
Scleroderma Foundation
Sjögren's Syndrome Foundation

REFERENCES

Akbar U, Yang M, Kurian D, et al: Omega-3 fatty acids in rheumatic diseases. A critical review, *J Clin Rheumatol* 23:330–339, 2017.

Al-Ezzi MY, Pathak N, Tappuni AR, et al: Primary Sjögren's syndrome impact on smell, taste, sexuality and quality of life in female patients: a systematic review and meta-analysis, *Mod Rheumatol* 27:623–629, 2017.

Arida A, Protogerou AD, Kitas GD, et al: Systemic inflammatory response and atherosclerosis: the paradigm of chronic inflammatory rheumatic diseases, *Int J Mol Sci* 19:1890, 2018.

Aparicio-Soto M, Sánchez-Hidalgo M, Rosillo MÁ, et al: Extra virgin olive oil: a key functional food for prevention of immune-inflammatory diseases, *Food Funct* 9:4492–4505, 2016.

Aparicio-Soto M, Sánchez-Hidalgo M, Alarcón-de-la-Lastra C: An update on diet and nutritional factors in systemic lupus erythematosus management, *Nutr Res Rev* 30:118–137, 2017.

Arthritis Foundation: https://www.arthritis.org/living-with-arthritis/arthritis-diet/anti-inflammatory/anti-inflammatory-diet.php.

Arthritis Foundation: *Arthritis today, Drug Guide.* Available at: www.arthritis.org/living-with-arthritis/treatments/medication/drug-guide/search-alphabetical.php.

Badsha H: Role of diet in influencing rheumatoid arthritis disease activity, *Open Rheumatol J* 12:19–28, 2018.

Barbour KE, Helmick CG, Boring M, et al: Vital signs: prevalence of doctor-diagnosed arthritis and arthritis-attributable activity limitation-United States, 2013-2015, *MMWR Morb Mortal Wkly Rep* 66:246–253, 2017.

Bardin T, Richette P: Impact of comorbidities on gout and hyperuricaemia: an update on prevalence and treatment options, *BMC Med* 15:123, 2017.

Bernard NJ: Rheumatoid arthritis: prevotella copri associated with new-onset untreated RA, *Nat Rev Rheumatol* 10:2, 2014.

Benn CL, Dua P, Gurrell R, et al: Physiology of hyperuricemia and urate-lowering treatments, *Front Med (Lausanne)* 5:160, 2018.

Beyl RN Jr, Hughes L, Morgan S: Update on importance of diet in gout, *Am J Med* 129:1153–1158, 2016.

Bliddal H, Leeds AR, Christensen R: Osteoarthritis, obesity and weight loss: evidence, hypotheses and horizons - a scoping review, *Obes Rev* 15:578–586, 2014.

Bonaccio M, Pounis G, Cerletti C, et al: Mediterranean diet, dietary polyphenols and low grade inflammation: results from the MOLI-SANI study, *Br J Clin Pharmacol* 83:107–113, 2017.

Bravo-Blas A, Wessel H, Milling S: Microbiota and arthritis: correlations or cause? *Curr Opin Rheumatol* 28:161–167, 2016.

Calder PC: Marine omega-3 fatty acids and inflammatory processes: effects, mechanisms and clinical relevance, *Biochim Biophys Acta* 1851:469–484, 2015.

Calder PC: Omega-3 fatty acids and inflammatory processes: from molecules to man, *Biochem Soc Trans* 45:1105–1115, 2017.

Casas R, Estruch R, Sacanella E: The protective effects of extra virgin olive oil on immune-mediated inflammatory responses, *Endocr Metab Immune Disord Drug Targets* 18:23–35, 2018.

Chang HY, Tang FY, Chen DY, et al: Clinical use of cyclooxygenase inhibitors impairs vitamin B-6 metabolism, *Am J Clin Nutr* 98:1440–1449, 2013.

Chang K, Yang SM, Kim SH, et al: Smoking and rheumatoid arthritis, *Int J Mol Sci* 15:22279–22295, 2014.

Chen H, Wang J, Zhou W, et al: Breastfeeding and risk of rheumatoid arthritis: a systematic review and metaanalysis, *J Rheumatol* 42:1563–1569, 2015.

Choi IY, Lee C, Longo VD: Nutrition and fasting mimicking diets in the prevention and treatment of autoimmune diseases and immunosenescence, *Mol Cell Endocrinol* 455:4–12, 2017.

Choi TY, Jun JH, Lee MS: Integrative medicine for managing the symptoms of lupus nephritis: a protocol for systematic review and meta-analysis, *Medicine (Baltimore)* 97:e0224, 2018.

Connelly KL, Kandane-Rathnayake R, Huq M, et al: Longitudinal association of type 1 interferon-induced chemokines with disease activity in systemic lupus erythematosus, *Sci Rep* 19:3268, 2018.

Dall'Ara F, Cutolo M, Andreoli L, et al: Vitamin D and systemic lupus erythematous: a review of immunological and clinical aspects, *Clin Exp Rheumatol* 36:153–162, 2018.

Dankers W, Colin Em, van Hamburg JP, et al: Vitamin D in autoimmunity: molecular mechanisms and therapeutic potential, *Front Immunol* 7:697, 2017.

Davis LS, Reimold AM: Research and therapeutics—traditional and emerging therapies in systemic lupus erythematosus, *Rheumatology (Oxford)* 56:i100–i113, 2017.

De Luca F, Shoenfeld Y: The microbiome in autoimmune diseases, *Clin Exp Immunol* 195(1):74–85, 2019. doi:10.1111/cei.13158.

Di Giuseppe D, Discacciati A, Orsini N, et al: Cigarette smoking and risk of rheumatoid arthritis: a dose-response meta-analysis, *Arthritis Res Ther* 16:R61, 2014.

Eldoma M, Pope J: The contemporary management of systemic sclerosis, *Expert Rev Clin Immunol*, 14:573–582, 2018. doi:10.1080/17446 66X.2018.1485490.

Erten S, Şahin A, Altunoğlu A, et al: Comparison of plasma vitamin D levels in patients with Sjögren's syndrome and healthy subjects, *Int J Rheum Dis* 18:70–75, 2015.

Food and Agricultural Organization (FAO) of the United Nations: *Fat and fatty acid intake and inflammatory and immune response. In Fats and fatty acids in human nutrition. Report of an expert consultation*, Rome, 2010, Food and Agricultural Organization of the United Nations.

Franco AS, Freitas TQ, Bernardo WM, et al: Vitamin D supplementation and disease activity in patients with immune-mediated rheumatic diseases: a systematic review and meta-analysis, *Medicine (Baltimore)* 96:e7024, 2017.

Garcia-Carrasco M, Jiménez-Herrera EA, Gálvez-Romero JL, et al: Vitamin D and Sjögren syndrome, *Autoimmun Rev* 16:587–593, 2017.

Gerosa M, Schioppo T, Meroni PL: Challenges and treatment options for rheumatoid arthritis during pregnancy, *Expert Opin Pharmacother* 17:1539–1547, 2016.

Gomez FE, Cassís-Nosthas L, Morales-de-León JC, et al: Detection and recognition thresholds to the 4 basic tastes in Mexican patients with primary Sjögren's syndrome, *Eur J Clin Nutr* 58:629–636, 2004.

Greco CM, Nakajima C, Manzi S: Updated review of complementary and alternative medicine treatments for systemic lupus erythematosus, *Curr Rheumatol Rep* 15:378, 2013.

Grainger R, Walker J: Rheumatologists' opinions towards complementary and alternative medicine: a systematic review, *Clin Rheumatol* 33:3–9, 2014.

Guttmann A, Krasnokutsky S, Pillinger MH, et al: Pegloticase in gout treatment-safety issues, latest evidence and clinical considerations, *Ther Adv Drug Saf* 8:379–388, 2017.

Handono K, Firdausi SN, Pratama MZ, et al: Vitamin A improve Th17 and Treg regulation in systemic lupus erythematosus, *Clin Rheumatol* 35:631–638, 2016.

Hassan S, Hassan C: Bariatric surgery: what the rheumatologist needs to know, *J Rheumatol* 43:1001–1007, 2016.

Helmick CG, Watkins-Castillo SI: Prevalence of AORC. in *United States bone and joint initiative: the burden of musculoskeletal diseases in the United States (BMUS)*, ed 3, Rosemont, IL, 2014. http://www.boneandjointburden.org.

Holick MF: Biological effects of sunlight, ultraviolet radiation, visible light, infrared radiation and vitamin D for health, *Anticancer Res* 36:1345–1356, 2016.

Hugo M, Mehsen-Cetre N, Pierreisnard A, et al: Energy expenditure and nutritional complications of metabolic syndrome and rheumatoid cachexia in rheumatoid arthritis: an observational study using calorimetry and actimetry, *Rheumatology (Oxford)* 55:1202–1209, 2016.

Jansen R, Batista S, Brooks AI, et al: Sex differences in the human peripheral blood transcriptome, *BMC Genomics* 15:33, 2014.

Jafarzadeh SR, Felson DT: Updated estimates suggest a much higher prevalence of arthritis in United States adults than previous ones, *Arthritis Rheumatol* 70:185–192, 2018.

Jeffery LE, Raza K, Hewison M: Vitamin D in rheumatoid arthritis-towards clinical application, *Nat Rev Rheumatol* 12:201–210, 2016.

Jog NR, James JA: Biomarkers in connective tissue diseases, *J Allergy Clin Immunol* 140:1473–1483, 2017.

Kawami M, Harabayashi R, Harada R, et al: Folic acid prevents methotrexate-induced epithelial-mesenchymal transition via suppression of secreted factors from the human alveolar epithelial cell line A549, *Biochem Biophys Res Commun* 497:457–463, 2018.

Kelepouri D, Mavropoulos A, Bogdanos DP, et al: The role of flavonoids in inhibiting Th17 responses in inflammatory arthritis, *J Immunol Res* 5:9324357, 2018.

Khajehdehi P, Zanjaninejad B, Aflaki E, et al: Oral supplementation of turmeric decreases proteinuria, hematuria, and systolic blood pressure in patients suffering from relapsing or refractory lupus nephritis: a randomized and placebo-controlled study, *J Ren Nutr* 22:50–57, 2012.

Khanna S, Jaiswal KS, Gupta B: Managing rheumatoid arthritis with dietary interventions, *Front Nutr* 4:52, 2017.

Kim CH: Control of innate and adaptive lymphocytes by the RAR-retinoic acid axis, *Immune Netw* 18:e1, 2018.

Kongsbak M, von Essen MR, Levring TB, et al: Vitamin D-binding protein controls T cell responses to vitamin D, *BMC Immunol* 15:35, 2014.

Kreps DJ, Halperin F, Desai SP, et al: Association of weight loss with improved disease activity in patients with rheumatoid arthritis: a retrospective analysis using electronic medical record data, *Int J Clin Rheumtol* 13:1–10, 2018.

Kuo CF, Grainge MJ, Zhang W, et al: Global epidemiology of gout: prevalence, incidence and risk factors, *Nat Rev Rheumatol* 11:649–662, 2015.

Lee KH, Abas F, Mohamed Alitheen NB, et al: Chemopreventive effects of a curcumin-like diarylpentanoid [2,6-bis(2,5-dimethoxybenzylidene) cyclohexanone] in cellular targets of rheumatoid arthritis in vitro, *Int J Rheum Dis* 18:616–627, 2015.

Lee YH, Bae SC, Song GG: Coffee or tea consumption and the risk of rheumatoid arthritis: a meta-analysis, *Clin Rheumatol* 33:1575–1583, 2014.

Li GM, Zhao J, Li B, et al: The anti-inflammatory effects of statins on patients with rheumatoid arthritis: a systemic review and meta-analysis of 15 randomized controlled trials, *Autoimmun Rev* 17:215–225, 2018.

Liu H, He H, Li S, et al: Vitamin D receptor gene polymorphisms and risk of osteoarthritis: a meta-analysis, *Exp Biol Med (Maywood)* 239:559–567, 2014.

Longo VD, Mattson MP: Fasting: molecular mechanisms and clinical applications, *Cell Metab* 19:181–192, 2014.

Lourdudoss C, Elkan AC, Hafström I, et al: Dietary micronutrient intake and atherosclerosis in systemic lupus erythematosus, *Lupus* 25:1602–1609, 2016.

Mandal AK, Mount DB: The molecular physiology of uric acid homeostasis, *Annu Rev Physiol* 77:323–345, 2015.

Mariette X, Criswell LA: Primary Sjögren's syndrome, *N Engl J Med* 378:931–939, 2018.

Marrie RA, Hitchon CA, Walld R, et al: Increased burden of psychiatric disorders in Rheumatoid Arthrititis, *Arthritis Care Res (Hoboken)* 70:970–978, 2018.

Medina G, Vera-Lastra O, Peralta-Amaro AL, et al: Metabolic syndrome, autoimmunity and rheumatic diseases, *Pharmacol Res* 133:277–288, 2018. doi:10.1016/j.phrs.2018.01.009.

Miyabe Y, Miyabe C, Nanki T: Could retinoids be a potential treatment for rheumatic disease? *Rheumatol Int* 35:35–41, 2015.

Murphy LB, Cisternas MG, Pasta DJ, et al: Medical expenditures and earning losses among US adults with arthritis in 2013, *Arthritis Care Res (Hoboken)* 70:869–876, 2018.

Nasri-Heir C, Epstein JB, Touger-Decker R, et al: What should we tell patients with painful temporomandibular disorders about what to eat? *J Am Dent Assoc* 147:667–671, 2016.

National Center for Complementary and Integrative Health: *Complementary, alternative, or integrative health: what's in a name?* 2018. https://nccih.nih.gov/health/integrative-health.

National Institute of Arthritis and Musculoskeletal and Skin Diseases: *Systemic lupus erythematosus (Lupus)*, 2018. https://www.niams.nih.gov/health-topics/lupus.

National Institutes of Health (NIH), National Institute of Dental and Craniofacial Research: *TMJ (Temporomandibular joint and muscle disorders)*, 2018. https://www.nidcr.nih.gov/health-info/tmj.

Nigrovic PA, Raychaudhuri S, Thompson SD: Review: genetics and the classification of arthritis in adults and children, *Arthritis Rheumatol* 70: 7–17, 2018.

Nocturne G, Mariette X: B cells in the pathogenesis of primary Sjögren syndrome, *Nat Rev Rheumatol* 14:133–145, 2018.

Pascart T, Richette P: Current and future therapies for gout, *Expert Opin Pharmacother* 18:1201–1211, 2017.

Pang KL, Chin KY: The biological activities of oleocanthal from a molecular perspective, *Nutrients* 10:E570, 2018.

Phang JK, Kwan YH, Goh H, et al: Complementary and alternative medicine for rheumatic diseases: a systematic review of randomized controlled trials, *Complement Ther Med* 37:143–157, 2018.

Pludowski P, Holick MF, Grant WB, et al: Vitamin D supplementation guidelines, *J Steroid Biochem Mol Biol* 175:125–135, 2018.

Popp RA, Rascati K, Davis M, et al: Refining a claims-based algorithm to estimate biologic medication effectiveness and cost per effectively treated patient with rheumatoid arthritis, *Pharmacotherapy* 38:172–180, 2018.

Proudman SM, James MJ, Spargo LD, et al: Fish oil in recent onset rheumatoid arthritis: a randomized, double-blind controlled trial within algorithm-based drug use, *Ann Rheum Dis* 74:89–95, 2015.

Ramiro S, Sepriano A, Chatzidionysiou K, et al: Safety of synthetic and biological DMARDs: a systematic literature review informing the 2016 update of the EULAR recommendations for management of rheumatoid arthritis, *Ann Rheum Dis* 76:1101–1136, 2017.

Rhodes KL, Rasa MM, Yamamoto LG: Acute rheumatic fever: revised diagnostic criteria, *Pediatr Emerg Care* 34:436–440, 2018.

Sakkas LI, Simopoulou T, Daoussis D, et al: Intestinal involvement in systemic sclerosis: a clinical review, *Dig Dis Sci* 63:834–844, 2018.

Sawitzke AD, Shi H, Finco MF, et al: Clinical efficacy and safety of glucosamine, chondroitin sulphate, their combination, celecoxib or placebo taken to treat osteoarthritis of the knee: 2-year results from GAIT, *Ann Rheum Dis* 69:1459–1464, 2010.

Scaglione F, Panzavolta G: Folate, folic acid and 5-methyltetrahydrofolate are not the same thing, *Xenobiotica* 44:480–488, 2014.

Seca S, Miranda D, Cardoso D, et al: The effectiveness of acupuncture on pain, physical function and health-related quality of life in patients with rheumatoid arthritis: a systematic review protocol, *JBI Database System Rev Implement Rep* 14:18–26, 2016.

Seo MJ, Oh DK: Prostaglandin synthases: molecular characterization and involvement in prostaglandin biosynthesis, *Prog Lipid Res* 66:50–68, 2017.

Serhan CN, Levy BD: Resolvins in inflammation: emergence of the pro-resolving superfamily of mediators, *J Clin Invest* 128:2657–2669, 2018. doi:10.1172/JCI97943.

Shea B, Swinden MV, Ghogomu ET, et al: Folic acid and folinic acid for reducing side effects in patients receiving methotrexate for rheumatoid arthritis, *J Rheumatol* 41:1049–1060, 2014.

Singh JA, Noorbaloochi S, MacDonald R, et al: Chondroitin for osteoarthritis, *Cochrane Database Syst Rev* 1:CD005614, 2016.

Sjögren's Syndrome Foundation: *Diet & food tips*, 2018. www.sjogrens.org/home/about-sjogrens/living-with-sjogrens/diet-a-food-tips.

Smink AJ, Bierma-Zeinstra SM, Schers HJ, et al: Non-surgical care in patients with hip or knee osteoarthritis is modestly consistent with a stepped care strategy after its implementation, *Int J Qual Health Care* 26:490–498, 2014.

Smirani R, Truchetet ME, Poursac N, et al: Impact of systemic sclerosis oral manifestations on patients' health-related quality of life: a systematic review, *J Oral Pathol Med*, 47:808–815, 2018. doi:10.1111/jop.12739.

Sparks JA, Halperin F, Karlson JC, et al: Impact of bariatric surgery on patients with rheumatoid arthritis, *Arthritis Care Res (Hoboken)* 67:1619–1626, 2015.

Tedeschi SK, Bathon JM, Giles JT, et al: Relationship between fish consumption and disease activity in rheumatoid arthritis, *Arthritis Care Res (Hoboken)* 70:327–332, 2018.

Thomas S, Browne H, Mobasheri A, et al: What is the evidence for a role for diet and nutrition in osteoarthritis? *Rheumatology (Oxford)* 57:iv61–iv74, 2018.

Tsigalou C, Stavropoulou E, Bezirtzoglou E: Current insights in microbiome shifts in Sjogren's syndrome and possible therapeutic interventions, *Front Immunol* 9:1106, 2018.

Ueland PM, McCann A, Midttun Ø, et al: Inflammation, vitamin B6 and related pathways, *Mol Aspects Med* 53:10–27, 2017.

van Breda SGJ, de Kok TMCM: Smart combinations of bioactive compounds in fruits and vegetables may guide new strategies for personalized prevention of chronic diseases, *Mol Nutr Food Res* 62:1700597, 2018.

van der Heijde D, Daikh DL, Betteridge N, et al: Common language description of the term rheumatic and musculoskeletal diseases (RMDs) for use in communication with the lay public, healthcare providers, and other stakeholders endorsed by the European League Against Rheumatism (EULAR) and the American College of Rheumatology (ACR), *Arthritis Rheumatol* 70:826–831, 2018.

van der Heijden EHM, Kruize AA, Radstake TRDJ, et al: Optimizing conventional DMARD therapy for Sjögren's syndrome, *Autoimmun Rev* 17:480–492, 2018.

Vasile M, Corinaldesi C, Antinozzi C, et al: Vitamin D in autoimmune rheumatic diseases, *Pharmacol Res* 117:228–241, 2017.

Verheul MK, Fearon U, Trouw LA, et al: Biomarkers for rheumatoid and psoriatic arthritis, *Clin Immunol* 161:2–10, 2015.

Veselinovic M, Vasiljevic D, Vucic V, et al: Clinical benefits of n-3 PUFA and ɣ-linolenic acid in patients with rheumatoid arthritis, *Nutrients* 9:325, 2017.

Wang Q, He Y, Shen Y, et al: Vitamin D inhibits COX-2 expression and inflammatory response by targeting thioesterase superfamily member 4, *J Biol Chem* 289:11681–11694, 2014.

Watad A, Azrielant S, Bragazzi NL, et al: Seasonality and autoimmune diseases: the contribution of the four seasons to the mosaic of autoimmunity, *J Autoimmun* 82:13–30, 2017.

Yen EY, Singh RR: Lupus—An unrecognized leading cause of death in young females: a population-based study using nationwide death certificates, 2000–2015, *Arthritis Rheumatol* 70:1251–1255, 2018.

Zamani B, Golkar HR, Farshbaf S, et al: Clinical and metabolic response to probiotic supplementation in patients with rheumatoid arthritis: a randomized, double-blind, placebo-controlled trial, *Int J Rheum Dis* 16:869–879, 2016.

Zhang LW, Zhou PR, Wei P, et al: Expression of interleukin-17 in primary Sjögren's syndrome and the correlation with disease severity: a systematic review and meta-analysis, *Scand J Immunol* 87(4):e12649, 2018. doi:10.1111/sji.12649.

Zamora EA, Naik R: Calcium phosphate deposition disease (pseudogout), [Updated 2019 Aug 26]. In: *StatPearls [Internet]*, Treasure Island FL, 2019, StatPearls Publishing. Available at: https://www.ncbi.nlm.nih.gov/books/NBK540151/.

39

Medical Nutrition Therapy for Neurologic Disorders

Maggie Moon, MS, RDN
Ashley Contreras-France, MA, MS, CCC-SLP

KEY TERMS

absence seizure (petit mal)
adrenomyeloleukodystrophy (ALD)
adrenomyeloneuropathy
Alzheimer's disease (AD)
amyotrophic lateral sclerosis (ALS)
anosmia
aphasia
apraxia
areflexia
aspiration
aspiration pneumonia
basilar skull fractures
central nervous system (CNS)
chronic inflammatory demyelinating
    polyneuropathy (CIDP)
concussion
contusion
cortical blindness
deglutory dysfunction
diffuse axonal injury
Disability Adjusted Life Year (DALY)
dysarthria
dysosmia
dysphagia

embolic stroke
epidural hematoma
epilepsy
Frazier Free Water Protocol
Glasgow Coma Scale
Guillain-Barré syndrome (GBS)
hemianopsia
hemiparesis
hydrocephalus
hyperosmia
intracranial pressure (ICP)
intraparenchymal hemorrhage
International Diet Standardisation
    Initiative (IDDSI)
ketogenic diet
Lewy bodies
medium-chain triglyceride (MCT) oil
motor strips
multiple sclerosis (MS)
myasthenia gravis (MG)
myelin
myelopathy
neglect
neuromuscular junction

otorrhea
paraplegia
paresthesia
Parkinson's disease (PD)
partial seizures
peripheral nervous system (PNS)
peripheral neuropathy
refractory epilepsy
rhinorrhea
seizure
speech-language pathologist (SLP)
spinal cord injury (SCI)
stroke (cerebrovascular accident)
subarachnoid hemorrhage (SAH)
subdural hematoma
syndrome of inappropriate antidiuretic
    hormone secretion (SIADH)
tetraplegia
thromboembolic event
thrombotic stroke
tonic-clonic (grand mal) seizure
transient ischemic attack (TIA)
traumatic brain injury (TBI)
Wernicke-Korsakoff syndrome (WKS)

The nervous system is essential to daily existence, health, and well-being: from breathing to how we perceive the world around us, to how we think and store memories, to movement and coordination. It is also involved in sleep, healing, stress responses, hunger, thirst, digestion, and more. That is why this chapter starts with the basic anatomy and physiology of the central nervous system (CNS) and how good nutrition supports its health.

Conversely, poor nutrition can also have an impact on the brain (Table 39.1). In addition, medical nutrition therapy supports the medical management of neurologic disorders from trauma (e.g., sports injury, surgery), as well as other diseases and conditions (e.g., Alzheimer's, epilepsy, Parkinson's) (Table 39.2).

Though relatively rare, neurologic disorders affect hundreds of millions of people globally (World Health Organization [WHO], 2016a). Neurologic disorders, when combined, make up the world's number one cause of years lost to disability, also known as Disability Adjusted Life Years (DALY) (GBD 2015 Neurological Disorders Collaborator Group, 2017). The measure of DALY includes the years people live with a disability as well as their shortened lifespan. Grouped together, neurologic disorders are the second leading cause of death, and the

number of those deaths has risen by 36.7% in just 25 years (1990–2015). This number is expected to grow as the aging population grows.

To meet this growing demand, dietetics professionals need to understand the fundamental nutrition required for a healthy nervous system, and be equipped with current evidence and best practices for the neurologic conditions in which nutrition has the most potential impact. Many elements of nutrition care for neurologic diseases and conditions are similar regardless of the origin of the disease process. For example, it is important to know how to develop a diet appropriate for varying degrees of dysphagia, as it is the most common issue complicating nutrition therapy for neurologic disorders and international guidelines have recently been updated. For an overview, see Box 39.1.

THE NERVOUS SYSTEM

There are two main components of the nervous system: the central nervous system (CNS), which includes the brain and spinal cord, and the peripheral nervous system (PNS), which includes the nerves that extend from the spinal cord to the rest of the body (i.e., neck, chest, abdomen, arms, legs, muscles, and internal organs). The CNS and PNS

TABLE 39.1 Neurologic Diseases of Nutritional Origin

Disease	Deficient Nutrient	Physiologic Effect	Treatment
Protein-calorie deprivation	Protein and calories	Impaired cognitive and intellectual function	Protein foods, adequate calories
Wet beriberi	B_1 Thiamin	Peripheral or central neurologic dysfunction	Thiamin, food and/or supplement as needed
Pellagra	B_3 Niacin	Memory loss, hallucinations, dementia	Niacin, food and/or supplement as needed
Pernicious anemia	Vitamin B_{12} cobalamin	Lesions occur in myelin sheaths of optic nerves, cerebral white matter, peripheral nerves	Monthly vitamin B_{12} injections, oral vitamin B_{12} supplements
Wernicke-Korsakoff syndrome	B_1 Thiamin	Encephalopathy, involuntary eye movements, impaired movement, amnesia	Eliminate alcohol; thiamin food or supplement, adequate hydration
Magnesium deficiency	Magnesium	Muscle spasms, anxiety, headache, insomnia, cramps	Magnesium in food/supplements
Zinc deficiency	Zinc	Taste and smell loss, hallucinations, depression, brain defects during pregnancy	Zinc in food/supplements
B_2 deficiency	B_2 Riboflavin	Burning, itching of eyes, sensitivity to light, burning sensations around mouth, peripheral nerve damage	Riboflavin, food and/or supplement as needed. Keep food sources away from heat and light.
B_5 deficiency	B_5 Pantothenic acid	Rare but can lead to fatigue, burning sensations on hands and feet, and headaches	Pantothenic acid, food and/or supplement as needed
B_6 deficiency	B_6 Pyridoxine	Abnormal touch sensations, mania, convulsions, abnormal EEG readings	Pyridoxine, food and/or supplement as needed. Eliminate alcohol
B_9 deficiency	B_9 Folic acid	Peripheral nerve problems, memory disorder, convulsions; neural tube defects	Folate in food and supplements/Folic Acid in supplements
Hypocalcemia and tetany seizures	Vitamin D	When combined with low calcium can lead to seizures	Vitamin D, food and/or supplement as needed. Sensible sun exposure.
Cretinism	Iodine	Stunted physical and mental growth	Seafood, fortified salt, supplement
Wilson's disease	Excessive copper	Mental and movement problems; genetic disorder	Low copper diet, including supplements

EEG, Electroencephalography.

TABLE 39.2 Nutritional Considerations for Neurologic Conditions

Medical Condition	Relevant Nutrition Therapy
Adrenoleukodystrophy	Lorenzo's oil may lower VLCFA levels.
Dementia	Recommend antiinflammatory diet such as MIND diet or Mediterranean diet.
	Minimize distractions at mealtime.
	Initiate smell or touch of food.
	Guide hand to initiate eating. May require verbal cueing for sequential bites.
	Provide nutrient-dense foods, omega-3 fatty acids.
Amyotrophic lateral sclerosis	Intervene to prevent malnutrition and dehydration. Possibly ketogenic diet. Monitor dysphagia progression.
	Antioxidant use (vitamins C, E, selenium, methionine) is well tolerated, but not proven.
Epilepsy	Provide ketogenic diet (see Appendix 19, Ketogenic Diets)
Guillain-Barré syndrome	Attain positive energy balance with high-energy, high-protein tube feedings.
	Assess dysphagia.
	Discuss safe food handling to prevent recurrence.
Migraine headache	Coffee is therapeutic. Coenzyme Q_{10}, riboflavin, feverfew, butter bur, and chiropractic services may possibly be effective. B_6, B_{12}, and folic acid are potentially prophylactic.
	Possibly avoid tyramine-containing foods (e.g., aged cheese, wine), which can be trigger foods.
	Possibly avoid tomatoes, citrus, chocolate, spinach, aged meats and cheeses (histamine in or released by these foods may trigger, maintain, or aggravate headache).
	Consider a supervised elimination diet to identify individualized food triggers.
	Maintain adequate dietary and fluid intake.
	Keep extensive records of symptoms and foods.

Continued

TABLE 39.2 Nutritional Considerations for Neurologic Conditions—cont'd

Medical Condition	Relevant Nutrition Therapy
Myasthenia gravis	Provide nutritionally dense foods at beginning of meal.
	Small, frequent meals are recommended.
	Limit physical activity before meals.
	Place temporary feeding tube in advanced disease.
Multiple sclerosis	Recommend antiinflammatory diet.
	Increase omega-3 intake, especially from marine sources. Decrease saturated fat intake.
	Evaluate health and especially vitamin D status of patient.
	Nutrition support may be needed in advanced stages.
	Distribute fluids throughout waking hours; limit before bed.
Parkinson's disease (see Appendix 19, Ketogenic Diets)	Focus on drug-nutrient interactions with dietary protein and vitamin B_6.
	Minimize dietary protein at breakfast and lunch.
	Recommend antiinflammatory diet.
Pernicious anemia	Patient will need B_{12} injections through medical management.
	Provide diet liberal in HBV protein.
	Provide diet supplemented with Fe^+, vitamin C, and B complex vitamins (especially B_{12} and folate).
Spinal trauma	Assess site of trauma and degree of impairment Possibly provide enteral or parenteral nutrition support.
	Provide high-fiber diet, adequate hydration to minimize constipation.
	Provide healthful diet to meet nutrient needs (e.g., Mediterranean diet, DASH diet, MIND diet).
Stroke	Mediterranean, DASH, or MIND diet.
	Assess possible dysphagia.
	Enteral nutrition via tube feeding may be needed if motor functions are poor.
Wernicke-Korsakoff syndrome	Provide thiamin-rich foods and supplementation.
	Provide adequate hydration.
	Eliminate alcohol.
	Dietary protein may have to be restricted.

DASH, Dietary Approaches to Stop Hypertension; *Fe⁺,* iron; *HBV,* high biologic value; *MIND,* Mediterranean-DASH intervention for neurodegenerative delay; *VLCFA,* very-long-chain fatty acid.

BOX 39.1 Issues Complicating Nutrition Therapy

Nutrition assessment requires taking a detailed patient history. The diet history and mealtime observations are used to assess patterns of normal chewing, swallowing, and rate of ingestion. Weight loss history establishes a baseline weight; a weight loss of 10% or more is indicative of nutritional risk. Assessment for nutrients involved in neurotransmitter synthesis is particularly important in these patients. It is important to ask about all supplements and medications to determine food-drug interactions or side effects that will impact adequate nourishment. Nutrition diagnoses common in the neurologic patient population include the following:

- Chewing difficulty
- Increased energy expenditure
- Inadequate energy intake
- Inadequate fluid intake
- Physical inactivity
- Poor nutritional quality
- Difficulty with independent eating
- Swallowing difficulty
- Underweight
- Elimination problems
- Inadequate access to food or fluid

Meal Preparation

Confusion, dementia, impaired vision, or poor ambulation may contribute to difficulty with meal preparation, thus hindering oral food and beverage intake. Assistance with shopping and meal planning are frequently necessary. Food manufacturers are facilitating the management of modified textures through use of the International Dysphagia Diet Standardisation Initiative (IDDSI) framework for easy identification. Further, the growing use of food delivery decreases the cognitive burdens associated with grocery shopping and meal planning.

Eating Difficulties and Inadequate Access to Food or Fluid

With chronic neurologic diseases, a decline in function may hinder the ability for self-care and nourishment. Access to food and satisfying basic needs may depend on the involvement of family, friends, or professionals. With acute neurologic situations such as seizures, trauma, stroke, or Guillain-Barré syndrome (GBS), the entire process of eating can be interrupted abruptly. The patient may require enteral nutrition for a time until overall function improves, and adequate oral intake is resumed (see Chapter 13).

Eating Issues: Presentation of Food to the Mouth

The patient with neurologic disease may be unable to eat independently because of limb weakness, poor body positioning, hemianopsia, limb apraxia,

BOX 39.1 Issues Complicating Nutrition Therapy—cont'd

confusion, or neglect. Tremors in Parkinson's disease (PD), spastic movements, or involuntary movements that occur with cerebral palsy, Huntington's disease, or tardive dyskinesia may further restrict dietary intake. The affected region of the central nervous system (CNS) determines the resulting disability (see Table 39.3).

If limb weakness or paralysis occurs on the dominant side of the body, poor coordination resulting from a new reliance on the nondominant side may make eating difficult and unpleasant. The patient may have to adjust to eating with one hand or using the nondominant hand. An occupational therapist can facilitate strategies and provide adaptive equipment to support self-feeding. **Hemiparesis** is weakness on one side of the body, usually both limbs and sometimes the face, that causes the body to slump toward the affected side; it may increase a patient's risk of aspiration.

Hemianopsia is blindness for one half of the field of vision. Patients must learn to recognize that they no longer have a normal field of vision and must

compensate by turning the head. **Neglect** is a failure to respond to stimuli on the weakened or paralyzed side of the body; this occurs when the right parietal side of the brain suffers an insult. The patient ignores the affected body part, and the perception of the body's midline is shifted. This phenomenon may occur after insult to the left side of the brain, resulting in right-sided neglect. However, right-sided neglect is less frequent, less severe, and more likely to resolve than left-sided neglect (Myers, 2009). Hemianopsia and neglect can occur together and severely impair the patient's function. Patients may eat only half of the contents of a meal because they recognize only half of it (Fig. 39.1).

Another potential deterrent to independent eating is apraxia because the person is unable to carry out an action and follow directions. Demonstration may make it possible for the action to occur; however, judgment may be affected as well and can result in the performance of dangerous tasks. This makes it unsafe to leave the patient alone.

---

work together to control voluntary actions (e.g., muscle movement) and involuntary activity (e.g., breathing, temperature regulation, heart beat).

A careful history of the patient's signs and symptoms can help determine where CNS lesions may originate. Through this process, the lesion can be localized to muscle, nerve, spinal cord, or brain as part of the medical diagnosis. Nerve tracts coming to and from the brain cross to opposite sides in the CNS (Fig. 39.2). Therefore a lesion on the

cortex that affects the right arm is found on the left side of the brain. Fig. 39.3 shows the segments of the brain.

Symptoms of muscle weakness, loss of coordination, and impaired range of motion are the most quantifiable clinical signs of nervous system disease. The neurons in the motor strip (upper motor neurons) receive input from all parts of the brain and project their axons all the way to their destinations in the spinal cord. Axons connect to the spinal cord motor neurons (lower motor neurons). These neurons extend from the spinal cord to muscles without interruption. The location of a lesion in the nervous system often can be deduced clinically by observing stereotypical abnormalities and function of either upper or lower motor neurons (Table 39.3).

TABLE 39.3 Basic Functions of Cranial Nerves

Number	Nerve Function
Olfactory (I)	Smell
Optic (II)	Vision
Oculomotor (III)	1. Eye movement 2. Pupil constriction
Trochlear (IV)	Eye movement
Trigeminal (V)	1. Mastication 2. Facial heat, cold, touch 3. Noxious odors 4. Input for corneal reflex
Abducens (VI)	Eye movement
Facial (VII)	1. All muscles of facial expression 2. Corneal reflex 3. Facial pain 4. Taste on anterior two thirds of tongue
Vestibulocochlear (VIII)	Hearing and head acceleration and input for oculocephalic reflex
Glossopharyngeal (IX)	1. Swallowing 2. Gag reflex 3. Palatal, glossal, and oral sensation
Vagus (X)	1. Heart rate, gastrointestinal activity, sexual function 2. Cough reflex 3. Taste on posterior third of tongue
Spinal accessory (XI)	1. Trapezius 2. Sternocleidomastoid muscle
Hypoglossal (XII)	Tongue movement

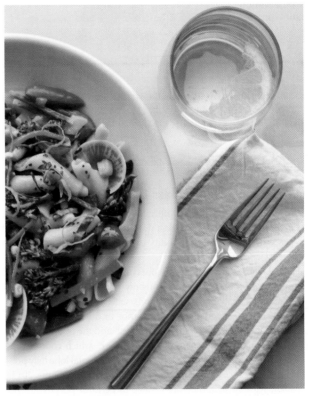

Fig. 39.1 A, Vision with hemianopsia (half of the visual field is absent). Food photography credit: Courtesy Maggie Moon, MS, RDN.

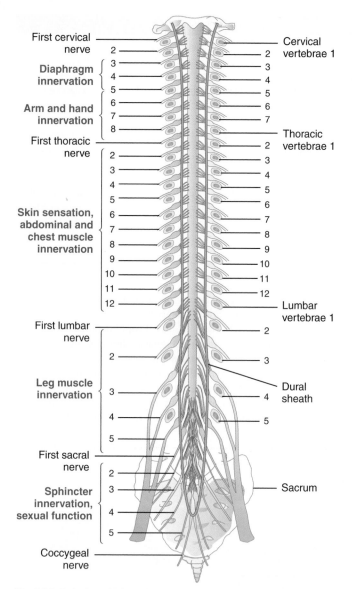

Fig. 39.2 Spinal cord lying within the vertebral canal. Spinal nerves are numbered on the left side; vertebrae are numbered on the right side; body areas supplied by various levels are in blue.

First cervical nerve
Diaphragm innervation
Arm and hand innervation
First thoracic nerve
Skin sensation, abdominal and chest muscle innervation
First lumbar nerve
Leg muscle innervation
First sacral nerve
Sphincter innervation, sexual function
Coccygeal nerve

Cervical vertebrae 1
Thoracic vertebrae 1
Lumbar vertebrae 1
Dural sheath
Sacrum

Locations and Signs of Mass Lesions

Eating and drinking require complex coordination within many parts of the nervous system. Therefore a problem at any location within the nervous system can affect the ability to meet nutritional requirements (Table 39.4).

- Frontal lobe lesions: The frontal lobes in the brain are the source of the most complex activities and commonly offer the most complex presentations. Psychiatric manifestations such as depression, mania, or personality change may indicate a tumor or other frontal lobe mass, either right or left. Frontal lobes are larger, and the posterior portions of the frontal lobes contain the motor strips, which control muscle movement. Lesions that develop in the central frontal lobe may present as motor apraxia, an impairment of motor planning (Duffy, 2013). A person with apraxia may not be able to perform purposeful movements such as independent eating despite a willingness to do so.
- Skull base lesions: Lesions or tumors near the skull base can lead to changes in smell and vision because olfactory and

optic nerves track along the bottom of these frontal lobes. Changes to sense of smell include anosmia (absence of smell), hyperosmia (increased sensitivity of smell), or dysosmia (distortion of normal smell).

- Temporal lobe lesions: Temporal lobes control memory and speech, and lesions in this part of the brain are seen in Alzheimer's dementia, stroke, and seizures. A right parietal lobe mass or insult may result in chronic inability to focus attention to the body's left side, a condition known as neglect. Because language centers are located near the junction of the left temporal, parietal, and frontal lobes, pathologic conditions in this region may cause aphasia, the inability to process language.
- Occipital lobe lesions: The occipital lobes are reserved for vision, and dysfunction here may bring about cortical blindness of varying degrees. In this condition the people are unaware that they cannot see.
- Cerebellum and brainstem lesions: Lesions of the cerebellum and brainstem may obstruct the ventricular system where it is the narrowest. This obstruction may precipitate life-threatening hydrocephalus, a condition of increased intracranial pressure (ICP) that may quickly result in death due to increased accumulation of fluid in the brain. Other signs of hydrocephalus include trouble with balance, walking and coordination, marked sleepiness, and complaints of a headache that is worse on awakening. Lesions in the brainstem may infiltrate any of the cranial nerves that innervate structures of the face and head, including the eyes, ears, jaw, tongue, pharynx, and facial muscles. These lesions have consequences for nutrition, because the patient is often unable to eat without risk of aspiration of food or liquids into the lungs. Tumors or other lesions in the medulla oblongata (the lower half of the brainstem) may infiltrate respiratory and cardiac centers with grim consequences.
- Spinal cord lesions: Lesions in the spinal cord are much less common than brain tumors and ordinarily cause lower motor neuron signs at the level of the lesion and upper motor signs in segments below the level of the lesion. Spinal cord injury (SCI) is the most common pathologic condition in this region. Other examples of spinal cord abnormalities are multiple sclerosis (MS), amyotrophic lateral sclerosis (ALS), tumor, syrinx (fluid-filled neurologic cavity), chronic meningitis, vascular insufficiency, and mass lesions of the epidural space. Injuries to the cervical and thoracic regions of the spinal cord may result in respiratory dysfunction requiring assisted ventilation which presents challenges for intake.
- Pituitary gland and hypothalamus lesions: Lesions of the pituitary gland and hypothalamus often manifest systemically; for example, electrolyte and metabolic abnormalities secondary to adrenocortical, thyroid, and antidiuretic hormone dysregulation. Because of the proximity to the visual pathways, changes may occur in visual field or acuity. The syndrome of inappropriate antidiuretic hormone secretion (SIADH) is often a complication; volume status and hyponatremia are part of the medical diagnosis (see Chapter 5). Because the hypothalamus is the regulatory center for hunger and satiety, lesions here may present as anorexia or overeating.
- Peripheral nerve and neuromuscular junction lesions: Disorders of peripheral nerves and the neuromuscular junction affect one's ability to maintain proper nutrition from fluctuating weakness and easy fatigability in voluntary muscle movements. Disorders such as Guillain-Barré syndrome (GBS) or myasthenia gravis (MG) may counteract the efforts to maintain nutritional balance. While respiratory and limb muscles are obviously affected, the impact of weakness on oral, pharyngeal, and laryngeal muscles presents challenges for safe intake of food and drink.

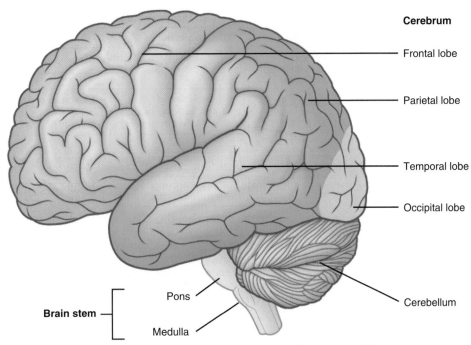

Fig. 39.3 Parts of the brain. Trauma or disease in one area may affect speech, vision, movement, or eating ability. (From Scully C: *Medical problems in dentistry*, ed 6, 2010, Churchill Livingstone.)

TABLE 39.4 Common Impairments with Neurologic Diseases

Site in the Brain	Impairment	Results
Cortical lesions of the parietal lobe (perception of sensory stimuli)	Sensory deficits	Fine regulation of muscle activities impossible if the patient is unable to perceive joint position and motion and tension of contracting muscles
Lesions of the nondominant hemisphere	Hemi inattention syndrome (neglect)	Patient neglects the affected side of the body
Optic tract lesions (usually of the middle cerebral artery or the artery near the internal capsule)	Visual field cuts	Patient reads one half of a page, eats from only half of the plate, etc. (see Fig. 39.1)
Loss of subcortically stored pattern of motor skills	Apraxia	Inability to perform a previously learned task (e.g., walking, rising from a chair), but paralysis, sensory loss, spasticity, and incoordination are not present
No identification with a particular brain disorder or a specifically located lesion	Language apraxia	Inability to produce meaningful speech, even though oral muscle function is intact and language production has not been affected; may produce groping oral movements in attempts at production
Lesion of Broca area	Nonfluent aphasia	Thought and language formulation are intact, but the patient is unable to connect them into fluent speech production; word-finding deficits (anomia) are common
Lesion of Wernicke area	Fluent aphasia	Flow of speech and articulation seem normal, but language output makes little or no sense; characterized by deficits in auditory comprehension and the presence of jargon, or nonwords that follow the language conventions
Extensive brain damage	Global aphasia	Language expression and reception are severely impaired
Brainstem lesions, bilateral hemispheric lesions, cerebellar disorders, cranial nerve lesions, and diffuse neurologic diseases	Dysarthria	Inability to produce intelligible words due to impairments in respiration, phonation, articulation, resonance, and prosodic systems

Duffy JR: Motor speech disorders: Substrates, differential diagnosis, and management, ed 3, St. Louis, MO, 2013, Elsevier Mosby; Greenberg DA, Aminoff MJ, Simon RP: Clinical neurology, 8th ed, New York, NY, 2012, McGraw-Hill Companies, Inc; Steinberg FU: Rehabilitating the older stroke patient: what's possible? *Geriatrics* 41:85, 1986.

Nutrition and Lifestyle Factors for a Healthy Nervous System

The healthy nervous system, like the body it is housed in, requires optimal consumption of the right macronutrients, micronutrients, and phytonutrients, as well as adequate water intake. There is no specialized diet for maintaining a healthy CNS, and an eating pattern that has appropriate portions of a variety and balance of healthful foods applies as it does to the general population. However, certain compounds are of active interest in the research community, including curcumin, choline, polyphenols, and omega-3 fatty acids (Fig. 39.4).

The brain consumes up to 20% of the energy needed to maintain the body's resting metabolic rate, far outpacing it being only 2% of total body weight. About 75% of the brain is water, and 60% of the remaining brain matter is made of lipids. The brain is especially sensitive to oxidative stress and inflammation, and does not have access to

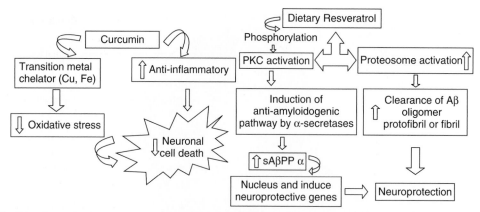

Fig. 39.4 The role of curcumin and resveratrol in neuroprotection. Left: Curcumin has multiple biologic effects: it chelates transition metals (iron and copper) and acts as an antioxidant and antiinflammatory molecule, protecting from oxidative stress. Right: Resveratrol favors phosphorylation in protein kinase C, activating the nonamyloidogenic pathway of AβPP cleavage, and this leads to reduction in Aβ formation. sAβPPβ, a product of AβPP cleavage, gets translocated to the nucleus and modulates the genes. All these events favor neuronal cell survival. *Aβ*, Amyloid beta; *PKC*, protein kinase C; *sAPPβ*, secreted fragment of amyloid protein precursor beta. (From Ramesh BN, et al: Neuronutrition and Alzheimer's disease, *J Alzheimer's Dis* 19:1123, 2010. With permission from IOS Press.)

as many endogenous antioxidant enzymes as other areas of the body, which is why dietary antioxidants are important for brain health, even in small amounts (Morris, 2012).

Nonnutritive lifestyle factors that improve nervous system health include adequate sleep for rest and repair, exercise for maintaining neural connections related to memory and learning, social engagement, and a constant supply of oxygen.

DYSPHAGIA

The nutritional management of patients with neurologic disease is complex. Severe neurologic impairments often compromise the mechanisms and cognitive abilities needed for adequate nourishment. A common result is dysphagia (difficulty swallowing), and the ability to obtain, prepare, and present food to the mouth can be compromised. Modified food textures are often required for the individual with swallowing problems. The International Dysphagia Diet Standardisation Initiative (IDDSI) has created a system for naming, describing, and testing various texture modifications for liquids and solids (Steele et al, 2015). However, not all institutions have adopted the new system and are still operating under the National Dysphagia Diet system (Box 39.2).

Early recognition of signs and symptoms, implementation of an appropriate care plan to meet the nutritional requirements of the individual, and counseling for the patient and family members on dietary choices are essential. Regular evaluation of the patient's nutrition status and disease management are priorities, with the ultimate goal of improving outcomes and the patient's nutritional quality of life. Active coordination with swallowing professionals, including speech-language pathologists (SLP) and occupational therapists (OT), aids in achieving this outcome.

Dysphagia often leads to malnutrition because of inadequate intake. Symptoms of dysphagia include drooling, choking, or coughing during or following meals; inability to suck from a straw; a "gurgly," or wet, voice quality; holding pockets of food in the buccal recesses or sublingual cavity (of which the patient may be unaware); absent gag reflex; and chronic respiratory infections. Patients with intermediate

or late-stage Parkinson's disease, MS, ALS, dementia, or stroke are likely to have dysphagia.

A swallowing evaluation by an SLP is important in assessing and treating swallowing disorders. The SLP is often consulted for individual patients following traumatic brain injury (TBI), stroke, or cancers of the head and neck, and for those at risk of aspiration, or the inhalation of foreign material, such as food and liquid, into the lungs. Aspiration pneumonia may result from the bacteria in saliva that is carried into the lungs; a common misconception is that pneumonia results from the food and liquid (Coyle, 2018). Coordination with an SLP for the management of other conditions that result in poor swallowing coordination may also be necessary for incorporating compensatory strategies or diet texture modifications. Many registered dietitian nutritionists (RDNs) have acquired additional training in swallowing therapies to help coordinate this evaluation process.

Phases of Swallowing

Proper positioning for effective swallowing should be encouraged (i.e., sitting upright, and in some cases, a chin down position). Concentrating on the swallowing process can also help reduce choking. Initiation of the swallow begins voluntarily but is completed reflexively. Normal swallowing allows for safe and easy passage of food from the oral cavity through the pharynx and esophagus into the stomach by propulsive muscular force, with some benefit from gravity. The process of swallowing can be organized into three phases, as shown in Fig. 39.5.

Oral Phase

During the preparatory and oral phases of swallowing, food is placed in the mouth, where it is combined with saliva, chewed if necessary, and formed into a bolus by the tongue. The tongue pushes the food to the rear of the oral cavity by gradually squeezing it backward against the hard and soft palate in a stripping action and creating negative pressure in the anterior oral cavity. Adequate muscle bulk in the buccal muscles supports fixing the lateral portion of the tongue, the movement of the soft palate to seal off the nasopharynx, and the allowance for respiration during the oral phase of the swallow. Increased ICP or

BOX 39.2 Development of Dysphagia Diets

Transitional Phasing Out of National Dysphagia Diet (NDD)

Not all facilities have transitioned to the new International Dysphagia Diet Standardisation Initiative (IDDSI) system, and some still use NDD. As such, it is important to be aware of both during this transition period. Below, find an overview of the NDD system.

Texture Modifications

Level 3: Dysphagia Advanced (Previously: Mechanical Soft)
- Soft-solid foods. Include easy-to-cut whole meats, soft fruits and vegetables (i.e., bananas, peaches, melon without seeds, tender meat cut into small pieces and well moistened with extra gravy or sauce).
- Crusts should be cut off bread.
- Chopped or cut into small pieces.
  EXCLUDES hard, crunchy fruits and vegetables, sticky foods, and very dry foods. NO nuts, seeds, popcorn, potato chips, coconut, hard rolls, raw vegetables, potato skins, corn, etc.

Level 2: Dysphagia Mechanically Altered (Previously: Ground)
- Cohesive, moist, semisolid foods that require some chewing ability.
- Includes fork-mashable fruits and vegetables (i.e., soft canned or cooked fruits with vegetables in pieces smaller than ½ inch).
- Meat should be ground and moist. Extra sauce and gravy should be served.

EXCLUDES most bread products, crackers, and other dry foods. No whole grain cereal with nuts, seeds, and coconut. No food with large chunks. Most food should be ground texture.

Level 1: Dysphagia Puree
- Smooth, pureed, homogenous, very cohesive, pudding-like foods that require little or no chewing ability.
- No whole foods.
- Includes mashed potatoes with gravy, yogurt with no fruit added, pudding, soups pureed smooth, pureed fruits and vegetables, pureed meat/poultry/fish served with sauces/gravies, and pureed desserts without nuts, seeds, or coconut. AVOID scrambled, fried, or hard-boiled eggs.

Fluid Modifications

Thin liquids: includes water, soda, juice, broth, coffee, and tea. This also includes foods like Jello, ice cream, and sherbet that melt and become thin in the mouth.

Nectar-thick liquids: are pourable and the consistency of apricot nectar.

Honey-thick liquids: slightly thicker than nectar and can be drizzled; consistency of honey.

Pudding-thick liquids: should hold their shape, and a spoon should stand up in them; they are not pourable and are eaten with a spoon.

Adapted from National Dysphagia Diet Task Force: *National Dysphagia Diet: standardization for optimal care,* Chicago, IL, 2002, American Dietetic Association.

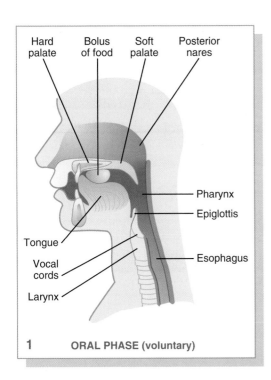

ORAL PHASE (voluntary)

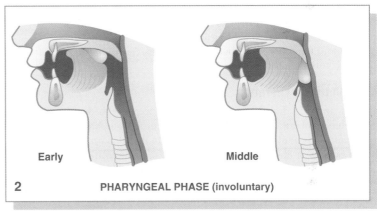

PHARYNGEAL PHASE (involuntary)

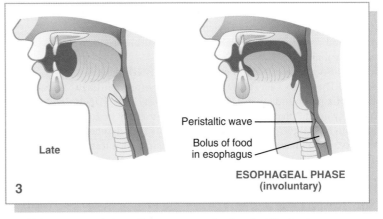

ESOPHAGEAL PHASE (involuntary)

Fig. 39.5 Swallowing occurs in three phases: Voluntary or oral phase: Tongue presses food against the hard palate, forcing it toward the pharynx. Involuntary, pharyngeal phase: Early: wave of peristalsis forces a bolus between the tonsillar pillars. Middle: soft palate draws upward to close posterior nares, and respirations cease momentarily. Late: vocal cords approximate, and the larynx pulls upward, covering the airway and stretching the esophagus open. Involuntary, esophageal phase: Relaxation of the upper esophageal (hypopharyngeal) sphincter allows the peristaltic wave to move the bolus down the esophagus.

intracranial nerve damage may result in weakened or poorly coordinated tongue movements. Weakened lip muscles result in the inability to completely seal the lips, form a seal around a cup, or suck through a straw. Patients are often embarrassed by drooling and may not want to eat in front of others. The patient may have difficulty forming a cohesive bolus and moving it through the oral cavity. Food can become pocketed in the buccal recesses, especially if sensation in the cheek is lost or facial weakness exists.

Pharyngeal Phase

The pharyngeal phase is initiated when the bolus is propelled past the faucial arches. Four events must occur in rapid succession during this phase. The soft palate elevates to close off the nasopharynx and prevent oropharyngeal regurgitation. The hyoid bone and larynx elevate, causing the epiglottis to flip downward while the vocal cords adduct to protect the airway. The pharynx sequentially contracts while the cricopharyngeal sphincter relaxes, allowing the food to pass into the esophagus. Breathing resumes with exhalation at the end of the pharyngeal phase. Symptoms of poor coordination during this phase include gagging, choking, and nasopharyngeal regurgitation. Individuals with dysphagia may initiate swallow during inhalation, increasing the risk for aspiration.

Esophageal Phase

The final or esophageal phase, during which the bolus continues through the esophagus into the stomach, is completed involuntarily. Normal esophageal transit takes 8 to 20 seconds for the peristaltic wave to push the bolus through the lower esophageal sphincter. Difficulties that occur during this phase are generally the result of a mechanical obstruction, but neurologic disease cannot be ruled out. For example, impaired peristalsis can arise from a brainstem infarct.

Medical Nutrition Therapy

Weight loss, anorexia, and dehydration are key concerns with dysphagia. Observation during meals allows the nurse or RDN to screen informally for signs of dysphagia and bring them to the attention of the health care team. Environmental distractions and conversations during mealtime increase the risk for aspiration and should be curtailed. Reports of coughing and unusually long mealtimes are associated with tongue, facial, and masticator muscle weakness. Changing the consistency of foods served may be beneficial while simultaneously keeping the diet palatable and nutritionally adequate. A soft, blended, or pureed consistency may reduce the need for oral manipulation and conserve energy while eating though this may compromise palatability.

In 2002 the Academy of Nutrition and Dietetics (AND) published the National Dysphagia Diet (NDD), which was developed through consensus of a panel of dietitians, SLPs, and scientists. The NDD is prescribed by an SLP that evaluates the individual's ability to safely swallow both food textures and liquids. Standard levels of dysphagia from severe to mild were designated with assigned diet texture modifications for each level to promote the safety of swallow (Fig. 39.6). The traditional levels of dysphagia severity range from mild to severe (see Box 39.2).

More recently, a collaborative group of dietitians, SLPs, food scientists, physicians, OTs, engineers, nurses, and food service professionals recognized a professional deficiency in the language and implementation of modified diet textures for the management of dysphagia. These individuals created a nonprofit international organization known as the IDDSI which tested and created norms for each dysphagia diet texture modification. The findings of this organization are supported by both the AND and the American

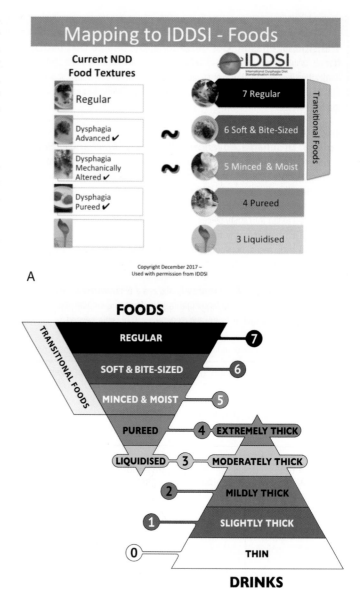

B

Fig. 39.6 Levels of National Dysphagia Diet (NDD) and updated framework as created by the International Dysphagia Diet Standardisation Initiative (IDDSI).

Speech-Language-Hearing Association. As such, international implementation standards are in process to support the medical necessity of implementation.

In November 2015 IDDSI created a new framework which utilizes current evidence to create diet texture specifications that are cross-cultural, through the lifespan, and applicable in all care settings (Steele et al, 2015). The framework consists of eight levels. Solids are defined across levels three through seven: liquidized, pureed, minced and moist, soft and bite-sized, and regular (Cichero et al, 2013) (see Table 39.5).

TABLE 39.5	International Dysphagia Diet Standardisation Initiative (IDDSI) Framework	
Level	Name & Description	Testing Methods
0	**Thin** • Flows like water • Can drink through nipple, cup, or straw	Flows through a 10 mL slip tip syringe completely within 10 seconds without any residue
1	**Slightly Thick** • Thicker than water, requiring more effort • Flows through a straw, syringe, or nipple • Found in infant formula	Flows through a 10 mL slip tip syringe leaving 1-4 mL in the syringe after 10 seconds
2	**Mildly Thick** • Flows off a spoon • Sippable, but requires effort to drink through a straw	Flows through a 10 mL slip tip syringe leaving 4-8 mL in the syringe after 10 seconds
3	**Liquidized/Moderately Thick** • Can be drunk from a cup • Effort is required for using a straw • Cannot be molded on a plate, nor eaten with a fork • No chewing required • No lumps, fibers, or particles present	• Flows through a 10 mL slip tip syringe leaving >8 mL in the syringe after 10 seconds • Easily pours from a spoon when tilted; does not stick to spoon • Fork prongs do not leave a clear pattern on the surface
4	**Pureed/Extremely Thick** • Eaten with a spoon though a fork is possible • Cannot be drunk from a cup • Will maintain molding on a plate • Falls off a spoon when tilted and holds shape • No lumps • Not sticky	• Fork tines make a clear pattern on the surface • Will not flow through the fork tines though may form a small tail • Will hold shape on a spoon

5	**Minced & Moist**
	• Eaten with a fork or spoon
	• Can be scooped or shaped
	• No separate thin liquid
	• Small lumps visible
	  • 2 mm for pediatrics
	  • 4 mm for adults
	• Lumps mash with tongue pressure only
		• When pressed with a fork, particles easily separated
		• Scooped sample sits in a pile and does not flow through fork tines
		• Holds shape on a spoon

6	**Soft & Bite-Sized**
	• Can be mashed down with pressure from a fork
	• A knife is not required to cut this food
	• Chewing is required before swallowing
	• No separate thin liquid
	• Bite-sized pieces
	  • 8 mm for pediatric
	  • 15 mm for adults
		• Pressure from a fork on side can cut pieces
		• When pressed down, the bite will squash and change shape; it does not return to original shape

7	**Regular** • Normal, everyday foods • Sample size is not restricted • Hard, tough, chewy, fibrous, stringy, dry, crispy, crunchy, or crumbly textures permitted • Mixed consistency foods and liquids	No testing
Transitional Foods	Foods that start as one texture but change into another when moisture is applied, or temperature changes occur • Cheetos ™ puffs • Ice cream	After moisture or temperature introduced, the bite becomes deformed with fork pressure and cannot recover its shape

Table created by Ashley Contreras-France, MA, MS, CCC, SLP, adapted from IDDSI, 2017.

It is important to be aware of both the NDD and IDDSI standards while health care facilities transition fully to IDDSI.

Liquids

Swallowing liquids of thin consistency such as juice or water is the most difficult swallowing task because of the timely coordination and control required. Liquids are easily aspirated into the lungs and may pose a life-threatening event because aspiration pneumonia may ensue. Aspiration occurs when any material, including saliva, goes below the level of the vocal folds. The development of aspiration pneumonia is contingent on the condition of the individual's pulmonary system, the volume and pH of the aspirated bolus, and the potential pathogens present. Of greatest concern is the bacteria present within the oral cavity as this creates the greatest risk for aspiration pneumonia (Coyle, 2018). Therefore oral care is often prescribed as a primary component of aspiration precautions and pneumonia prevention.

If a patient has difficulty consuming thin liquids, meeting fluid needs can become a challenge. Dry milk powder as a thickener alters the taste and might raise protein content too high for children, especially with limited free water. Commercial thickeners now have xanthan gum or modified food starches as ingredients. Benefits of xanthan gum include the following: it is tasteless, holds its thickening level over time, is easy to mix, and can be used on the ketogenic diet as it does not contain any carbohydrate or calories. Xanthan gum is not recommended for children less than 1 year of age because it has been implicated in the development of necrotizing enterocolitis (NEC) (Beal et al, 2012). Modified food starches add calories and continue to thicken over time, so it is more difficult to be accurate in the level of thickening.

The thickening of fluids should be prescribed with careful assessment of risk. Risks associated with thickening fluids include dehydration, drink aversion, and difficulty clearing aspirated fluids. Clinical studies suggest that patients with dysphagia have more difficulty clearing a thickened liquid from the respiratory system than a thinner liquid (Carlaw et al, 2012). Modifications in fluids were addressed in the NDD report, and the four terms used to identify the viscosity level of fluids are thin, nectar-thick, honey-thick, and spoon-thick (McCullough et al, 2003). These levels of thickness have since been redefined within the IDDSI framework under levels zero through four: thin, slightly thick, mildly thick, moderately thick, and extremely thick (Cichero et al, 2013) (see Table 39.5).

Infant cereals, pudding, or yogurt blend well into fluids, provide calories and protein, and are less expensive than commercial thickeners. Stage 2 baby fruits or applesauce can be added to juice to create a nectar or honey consistency, maintain a good flavor, and add calories, and they are less expensive than commercial supplements.

It is difficult to maintain adequate fluid intake with thickened liquids, especially if drinking skills are poor. Mild chronic dehydration resulting from limited water intake can cause fatigue and malaise. Encouraging soft or blended fruits and vegetables provides, a good source of free water. A systematic assessment, such as the Dehydration Risk Appraisal Checklist, may be beneficial to alert providers of the patient's elevated risk for dehydration, especially for those with modified diets (Bulgarelli, 2015). Determination of dehydration risk facilitates coordination with all professionals as to the considerations of downgrade in liquid textures for reduction of aspiration risk versus complex medical risks associated with dehydration resulting from thickened liquids. The decision, therefore, should be made as a team with documented risk levels.

The Frazier Free Water Protocol, which allows for drinking water in those who otherwise require thickened liquids, is being increasingly used in long-term care. This protocol is based on the following assumptions:
1. Aspiration of water poses little risk to the patient if oral bacteria associated with the development of aspiration pneumonia can be minimized.
2. Allowing free water decreases the risk of dehydration.
3. Allowing free water increases patient compliance with swallowing precautions and improves quality of life.
4. Good oral hygiene is a key ingredient of the water protocol and offers other benefits to swallow function.

A key component for implementation of the Frazier Free Water Protocol is based on the understanding that aspiration does not always lead to pneumonia. Therefore the prescribed oral care regimen serves to decrease overall risk as it serves to reduce oral bacteria, a likely cause for the development of pneumonia (Carlaw et al, 2012).

Liquid intake is a concern in those with neurogenic bladder and urinary retention, a common management issue in patients with a myelopathy (a pathologic condition of the spinal cord) or an SCI. This predisposes the individual to urinary tract infections (UTIs). Alternately, myelopathy and SCI may result in urinary urgency, frequency, or incontinence. To minimize these problems, distributing fluids evenly throughout the waking hours and limiting them before bedtime may help. Some patients limit fluid intake severely to decrease urgency or frequent urination. This practice increases the risk of UTI and is not recommended.

One nontraumatic cause of myelopathy and neurogenic bladder is MS, an unpredictable and severe progressive disease of the CNS. Individuals with MS have a higher incidence of UTIs.

Milk is considered a liquid with unique properties. Some people associate consumption of milk with symptoms of excess mucus production; however, research evidence does not support this belief. When the dysphagic patient reports increased phlegm after milk consumption, it may actually be a consequence of poor swallowing ability rather than mucus production.

Textures

As chronic neurologic disease progresses, cranial nerves become damaged, leading to neurologic deficits often manifested by dysphagia or elimination of entire food groups. Nutrition intervention should be individualized according to the type and extent of dysfunction. Vitamin and mineral supplementation may be necessary. If chewable supplements are not handled safely, liquid forms may be added to acceptable foods.

Presented with small, frequent meals, the patient may eat more. Swallowing can also be improved by carefully selecting various tastes, textures, and temperatures of foods. Juices can be substituted for water and provide flavor, nutrients, and calories. Thermal and gustatory stimulation may aid in triggering a swallow response; therefore cold food items may be better tolerated. Carbonation combined with citrus helps with the sensory issues by "awakening" the mouth. Sauces and gravies lubricate foods for ease in swallowing and can help prevent fragmentation of foods in the oral cavity. Moist pastas, casseroles, and egg dishes are generally well tolerated. Avoid foods that crumble easily in the mouth, because they can increase choking risk. Alcoholic beverages and alcohol-containing mouth washes should be avoided because they dry out the oral membranes.

Enteral Tube Nutrition

Patients with acute and chronic neurologic diseases may benefit from nutrition support. Enteral tube nutrition does not minimize the risk for aspiration pneumonia. In fact, in individuals post stroke, aspiration pneumonia was the most common complication. Aspiration precautions should be maintained in the patient with dysphagia even in the presence of enteral tube nutrition and no oral intake.

In most instances the gastrointestinal tract function remains intact, and enteral nutrition is the preferred method of administering nutrition support. One noted exception occurs after SCI, in which ileus, an obstruction in the ileum, is common for 7 to 10 days after the insult, and parenteral nutrition may be necessary. Although a nasogastric (NG) tube can be a short-term option, a percutaneous endoscopic gastrostomy (PEG) tube, commonly known as a G-tube, or gastrostomy-jejunostomy (PEG/J) tube, commonly known as a GJ-tube, is preferred for long-term management. These should be considered for patients whose swallowing is inadequate (see Chapter 12). A benefit of the PEG or PEG/J is in the reversibility should swallow function return.

Malnutrition itself can produce neuromuscular weakness that negatively affects quality of life; it is a prognostic factor for poor survival. In the acutely ill but previously well-nourished individual who is unable to resume oral nourishment within 7 days, nutrition support is used to prevent decline in nutritional health and aid in recovery until oral intake can be resumed. Conversely, in the chronically ill, nutrition support is an issue that each patient must eventually address because it may result in prolonged therapy. However, adequate nutrition can promote health and may be a welcome relief to an overburdened patient.

NEUROLOGIC DISEASES OF NUTRITIONAL ORIGIN

Most neurologic symptoms arising from primary nutritional deficiency or excess can be corrected with increased or decreased food or supplement intake (see Table 39.1). For example, dietary deficiencies of vitamin B_{12}, folate, thiamin, and niacin—or excessive long-term intake (12 months or more) of vitamin B_6 supplements (but not food)—can directly result in neurologic symptoms that can be reversed through dietary changes and supplements when addressed early. Though, with Wernicke-Korsakoff syndrome (WKS), the severe and acute thiamin deficiency and its neurologic effect occur secondary to alcoholism. In this case the primary cause of alcoholism should be addressed, as well as repletion of thiamin.

Emerging neurologic disorders that may have nutritional origins stem from gluten sensitivity. Numerous reports of patients with neurologic dysfunction related to gluten sensitivity have been reported since 1966 including ataxia, headache, and seizures (Hadjivassiliou et al, 2010), with up to 60% of patients with gluten ataxia showing evidence of cerebellar atrophy (Hadjivassiliou et al, 2015). Symptoms of gluten sensitivity typically are focused on gut function; however, most patients who present with neurologic manifestations of gluten sensitivity have no gastrointestinal symptoms. Celiac disease is common in people with autism with and without gastrointestinal symptoms.

NEUROLOGIC DISORDERS FROM TRAUMA

Cerebrovascular Accident (Stroke)

Stroke (cerebrovascular accident) occurs either when the brain's blood supply is suddenly interrupted (i.e., ischemic stroke, which accounts for 87% of all strokes [American Heart Association [AHA], 2017]), or when a blood vessel in the brain bursts (hemorrhagic stroke). Both of these situations cause brain cells to die within minutes, either due to loss of oxygen and nutrients or bleeding around the brain, respectively.

Severe strokes are often preceded by transient ischemic attacks (TIAs), brief attacks of cerebral dysfunction of vascular origin with no persistent neurologic defect. Stroke is responsible for about one in every 20 deaths in the United States (Centers for Disease Control and Prevention [CDC], 2017a), and stroke is a leading cause of death and a common cause of serious, long-term disability in the United States (AHA, 2017). Advanced age is the most significant risk factor for stroke. Among modifiable risk factors, hypertension and smoking are the major contributors (see Chapter 32). Other factors include poor diet, obesity, coronary heart disease, diabetes, physical inactivity, excessive alcohol intake, and genetics. About 80% of strokes are preventable (CDC, 2018a). The high costs of stroke in the United States, estimated at $34 billion a year, include the disability-related costs of health care services, medicines, and missed days at work (AHA, 2017).

Pathophysiology

Embolic stroke occurs when a cholesterol plaque is dislodged from a proximal vessel, travels to the brain, and blocks an artery, most commonly the middle cerebral artery (MCA). In patients with

dysfunctional cardiac atria, clots may be dislodged from there and embolize. In thrombotic stroke a cholesterol plaque within an artery ruptures, and platelets subsequently aggregate to clog an already narrowed artery. Most strokes are incited by a thromboembolic event, which may be aggravated by atherosclerosis, hypertension, diabetes, and gout (see *Pathophysiology and Care Management Algorithm: Neurological Diseases*).

Intracranial hemorrhage occurs in only 13% of strokes but is often fatal immediately. Intracranial hemorrhage occurs more commonly in individuals with hypertension. In intraparenchymal hemorrhage, a vessel inside the brain ruptures. A variation of intraparenchymal hemorrhage is a lacunar (deep pool) infarct. These smaller infarcts occur in the deep structures of the brain such as the internal capsule, basal ganglia, pons, thalamus, and cerebellum. Even a small lacunar infarct can produce significant disability because the brain tissue in the deep structures is so densely functional. A second type of intracranial hemorrhage is subarachnoid hemorrhage (SAH). SAH occurs commonly as a result of head trauma but more often as a result of a ruptured aneurysm of a vessel in the subarachnoid space.

Medical Management

A thromboembolic stroke is more likely to occur when the patient is fully conscious, but the onset of motor or sensory changes occurs suddenly. Hemorrhage is suspected when the patient presents with headache, decreased level of consciousness, and vomiting, all of which occur within minutes to hours. As with all neurologic disease, the clinical presentation depends on the location of the abnormality. An infarct of a particular cerebrovascular territory can be suspected by seeking out various neurologic deficits. An MCA occlusion produces paresis, with sensory deficits of limbs on the opposite side of the body because this artery supplies the motor and sensory strips. If the left MCA is occluded, aphasia, or loss of language or expression, may be present. Individuals often receive rehabilitative services, such as physical therapy, occupational therapy, and speech-language pathology, in a skilled nursing facility for short-term daily intervention with transition to intermittent long-term periodic management.

In the past, treatment for embolic stroke was supportive; it focused on prevention of further brain infarction and rehabilitation. Use of thrombolytic, "clot-busting" drugs reverses brain ischemia by lysing the clots. Initiation of therapy needs to occur within 6 hours of the onset of symptoms. Use of aspirin may be of some value in preventing further cerebrovascular events, but its effectiveness varies from one patient to another.

Controlling ICP while maintaining sufficient perfusion of the brain is the treatment for intracranial hemorrhage. This may include surgical evacuation of large volumes of intracranial blood and severe functional consequences, and therefore intracranial hemorrhage has a longer period of convalescence than ischemic stroke.

Postevent, more than two out of three stroke survivors use rehabilitation services, including physical and occupational therapy, for which updated guidelines from the AHA and American Stroke Association were issued in 2016 (AHA, 2016). Survivors may be admitted to a long-term care facility if their activities of daily living are severely impaired.

Medical Nutrition Therapy

Lifestyle and behavior changes that include diet are key components to primary prevention of stroke (Meschia et al, 2014). The landmark PREDIMED randomized controlled trial (RCT) showed how a Mediterranean diet supplemented with tree nuts or extra virgin olive oil reduced cardiac events, including stroke (Estruch et al, 2018). See Appendix 23 on the Mediterranean diet.

Efforts should be directed toward maintaining the overall health of the patient. For example, foods that support cellular repair and improved inflammatory markers include nuts, low-fat dairy, whole grains, and antioxidant-rich fruits and vegetables. In particular, a diet high in omega-3 fatty acids has been shown in some studies to provide a protective benefit against stroke, and current dietary recommendations to eat seafood twice per week helps meet omega-3 intake goals. Keep in mind that omega-3 fatty acid supplements have not shown the same benefit, and are contraindicated for anyone taking a blood thinner such as warfarin or aspirin (National Institutes of Health [NIH], National Center for Complimentary and Integrative Health [NCCIH], 2013). See Table 39.6 for additional information on nutrition and stroke (Iacoviello et al, 2018).

Eating difficulties and resulting behavioral problems are determined by the extent of the stroke and the area of the brain affected. Dysphagia, an independent predictor of mortality, commonly

TABLE 39.6	Nutrition Guidance to Reduce Stroke Risk
	Guidance and Rationale
Recommended	
Mediterranean-type diet	• Antiinflammatory, antioxidant, antiatherogenic, and antithrombotic • Diet pattern associated with lower morbidity and mortality from stroke
DASH diet	• Largely plant-based plus dairy products with low salt Intake • Associated with reduced risk of stroke
Plant-based diets	• Large amounts of vegetable dietary sources compared with animal sources • Pattern overlaps with other patterns that lower stroke risk
Fruits and vegetables	• 5-9 servings a day • Ensures adequate intake of dietary fibers, minerals (potassium, magnesium), vitamins (e.g., folic acid), and other nutrients • Reduction of blood pressure and improvement of microvascular function • Dose-dependent inverse association with reduced risk of total, ischemic, and hemorrhagic stroke
Nuts	• 20-30 g/day for heart health and reduced risk of stroke • Improves markers of oxidation, inflammation, and endothelial function
Whole-grain cereals	• Adequate intake for heart health recommended • Improvement of blood pressure, body weight, insulin resistance, lipid profile, and subclinical inflammation (limited evidence for a reduced risk of stroke at higher intakes)
Legumes	• Intake needed to support heart health recommended • No association between legumes intake and stroke risk
Olive oil	• Use extra virgin olive oil as main fat • Polyphenols, tocopherols, and monounsaturated fatty acids • Reduced risk of stroke with higher intakes of extra virgin olive oil
Chocolate	• Moderate intake of dark chocolate is associated with reduced risk of total stroke • Increased high-density lipoprotein (HDL), decreased low-density lipoprotein (LDL) oxidation, improved endothelial function, and reduced blood pressure
Fish	• Fatty and semifatty fish twice a week for heart health • PUFA, vitamins D and B, potassium, calcium, and magnesium contained in fish may have favorable vascular effects • Reduced risk of total and ischemic stroke with higher fish consumption; no consistent association with hemorrhagic stroke
Milk and dairy products	• Regular intake of low-fat milk and dairy products recommended • Possibly mediated by high content of calcium, magnesium, potassium, and bioactive peptides • Lower risk of ischemic and hemorrhagic stroke observed with regular moderate consumption of low-fat milk and dairy products
Coffee	• Moderate regular intake recommended and associated with lower risk of total and ischemic stroke • Contains polyphenols, chlorogenic acid, caffeine, niacin, and lignans
Tea	• Moderate intake recommended, especially green tea • Favorable health effects of antioxidants, catechins, L-theanine • Higher tea consumption is associated with reduced risk of total, ischemic, and hemorrhagic strokes
Alcohol	• Moderate intake of 1 drink/day for women; 2 drinks/day for men may reduce risk • Evidence of a J-shaped relationship between ethanol intake and stroke risk • Moderate consumption is associated with improved lipid profile, reduction in platelet aggregation, beneficial effects on inflammation, antiatherogenic and antithrombotic effects, and regulation of endothelial function and blood pressure • Alcohol abuse associated with increased risk of total, ischemic, and hemorrhagic stroke
Dietary calcium	• Adequate dietary intake recommended • Possible beneficial effects of low-fat dairy products on blood pressure and systemic inflammation, particularly in overweight individuals
Magnesium	• Adequate dietary intake recommended • Beneficial effects on blood pressure, insulin resistance, and blood lipids

TABLE 39.6 Nutrition Guidance for Stroke Risk—cont'd

	Guidance and Rationale
Potassium	• Meet DRI recommendations • Blood pressure–lowering effect • Evidence of an inverse association between potassium intake and risk of stroke, likely more favorable for ischemic rather than hemorrhagic stroke
Folates	• Adequate dietary intake recommended as it has been associated with lower risk of stroke, especially ischemic • Beneficial effect likely independent of homocysteine
Vitamin C	• Adequate dietary intake recommended • Prevention of endothelial dysfunction, antiinflammatory and antihypertensive role • Both higher dietary and blood levels of vitamin C have been associated with reduced risk of stroke
Vitamin D	• Correct for deficiency, indicated by a plasma concentration of 25-hydroxycholecalciferol below 50 nmoL/L (20 ng/mL) • Favorable role on blood pressure, insulin sensitivity, renin-angiotensin system, endothelial function, proliferation of vascular smooth muscle cells, regulation of parathyroid hormone levels • Low blood levels of vitamin D are associated with increased stroke incidence
Dietary fiber	• Adequate dietary intake of at least 25 g/day through plant foods recommended to reduce blood pressure levels, improve insulin resistance, lipid profile fibrinolysis, inflammation, and endothelial function • Dietary fiber intake is associated with reduced risk of stroke: effect more pronounced for ischemic stroke and for women
Low-glycemic load carbohydrates	• A low-glycemic load diet is recommended • Vascular injury induced by a chronic increase in blood glucose and postprandial insulinemia, oxidative stress, and a subclinical systemic inflammation with production of oxidized lipoproteins and AGEs • A high dietary GL is associated with the risk of stroke while total CHO intake and GI are not
Dietary fats	• Intake of MUFA-rich and PUFA-rich foods recommended, especially to replace saturated fats and refined carbohydrates
Protein	• Adequate dietary intake recommended without specific sufficient evidence in support of any association between dietary protein intake and stroke
Eggs	• No recommendation available as no association with either ischemic or hemorrhagic stroke was documented
Avoid	
Western diet	• A typical Western diet that is high in meat, saturated fats, and refined carbohydrates and low in whole grains, fruits, vegetables, legumes, nuts, seeds, and fiber is associated with multiple chronic diseases including stroke
Meat and processed meat	• Limit meat to 1-2 times per week; limit processed meat as much as possible • Likely linked to the unfavorable effects of SFA content, high heme, lipid peroxidation, and high salt content of processed meat on blood pressure • High intake of meat and processed meat is associated with a higher risk of total and ischemic stroke
Calcium supplement	• Extreme caution when prescribing calcium supplements, unless needed to correct proven deficits. Calcium supplements may increase the risk of myocardial infarction and stroke especially in post menopausal women
Sodium	• Reduce to 2 g/day or below (5 g of salt) • Strong relationship between higher salt intake and risk of elevated blood pressure and stroke
Supplements of folates, B₆, B₁₂, Vitamin A, Vitamin E	• The use of antioxidant vitamin supplements for the prevention of stroke is not indicated • Association between dietary or plasma levels of vitamin B_6/vitamin B_{12} with stroke risk is uncertain • Vitamin B_6/vitamin B_{12}/folate supplements are not beneficial for the prevention of stroke • No association between vitamin A intake and stroke risk • Both higher dietary and supplemented vitamin E intakes are associated with increased risk of hemorrhagic stroke
Dietary fats	• Foods rich in SFA should be limited and trans fatty acids (TFA) should be avoided • Reduction or substitution of SFAs with PUFAs or MUFAs is associated with reduced stroke risk.
PUFA supplements	• Evidence from intervention studies of primary and secondary prevention of stroke failed to find any association between omega-3 fatty acid supplementation and either ischemic or hemorrhagic stroke
Sweetened beverages	• Limit due to unfavorable effect on LDL-cholesterol, VLDL, blood glucose, and insulin associated with increased risk of total and ischemic stroke

AGEs, Advanced glycation end products; *CHO*, cholesterol; *DASH*, Dietary Approaches to Stop Hypertension; *GI*, gastrointestinal; *GL*, glycemic load; *MUFA*, monounsaturated fatty acid; *PUFA*, polyunsaturated fatty acids; *SFA*, saturated fatty acid; *VLDL*, very-low-density lipoprotein.
Iacoviello L, Bonaccio M, Cairella G, et al: Diet and primary prevention of stroke: Systematic review and dietary recommendations by the ad hoc Working Group of the Italian Society of Human Nutrition, *Nutr Metab Cardiovasc Dis* 28:309–334, 2018.

accompanies stroke and contributes to complications and poor outcomes from malnutrition, pulmonary infections, disability, increased length of hospital stay, and institutional care. In some instances, enteral nutrition via a tube feeding is required to maintain nutritional health until oral alimentation can be resumed. As motor functions improve, eating and other activities of daily living are part of the patient's rehabilitation process and necessary for resuming independence. Malnutrition predicts a poor outcome and should be prevented.

HEAD TRAUMA OR NEUROTRAUMA

Traumatic brain injury (TBI) refers to any of the following, alone or in combination: brain injury, skull fractures, extraparenchymal hemorrhage—epidural, subdural, subarachnoid—or hemorrhage into the brain tissue itself, including intraparenchymal or intraventricular hemorrhage. In the United States TBI is a major cause of death and disability, affiliated with 30% of all injury-related deaths, or 153 people each day (Taylor et al, 2017). For people ages 65 and older, the leading cause of TBI-related death was falls; for those 64 years of age and younger, preventable causes ranged from assault to car accidents to intentional self-harm.

Morbidity is high, and headache is one of the most common complaints. It is difficult to accurately predict neurologic recovery. Despite intensive intervention, long-term disability occurs in a large portion of severe head injury survivors.

Pathophysiology

Brain injury can be categorized as three types: concussion, contusion, and diffuse axonal injury. A concussion is a brief loss of consciousness, less than 6 hours, with no damage found on computed tomography (CT) or magnetic resonance imaging (MRI) scans. Microscopic studies have failed to find any evidence of structural damage in areas of known concussion, although evidence of change in cellular metabolism exists. A contusion is characterized by damaged capillaries and swelling, followed by resolution of the damage. Large contusions may dramatically increase ICP and may lead to ischemia or herniation. Contusions can be detected by CT or MRI scans. Diffuse axonal injury results from the shearing of axons by a rotational acceleration of the brain inside the skull. Damaged areas are often found in the corpus callosum (the bridge between the two hemispheres) and the upper, outer portion of the brainstem. The variation in cognitive changes present with TBI reflect the physical trauma to the brain. However, mild TBI will not show any physical trauma to neurologic structures but manifest complex cognitive presentations in behavior and processing (Hovda, 2017).

Skull fractures of the calvarium and the base are described in the same manner as other fractures. Displacement refers to a condition in which bones are displaced from their original positions. Open or closed describes whether a fracture is exposed to air. Open fractures dramatically increase the risk of infection (osteomyelitis), and open skull fractures carry an increased risk for meningitis because the dura mater is often violated.

Epidural and subdural hematomas are often corrected by surgical intervention. The volume of these lesions often displaces the brain tissue and may cause diffuse axonal injury and swelling. When the lesion becomes large enough, it may cause herniation of brain contents through various openings of the skull base. Consequent compression and ischemia of vital brain structures often rapidly lead to death.

Medical Management

The body's response to stress from TBI results in production of cytokines (interleukin-1, interleukin-6, interleukin-8, and tumor necrosis factor) and inflammation (see Chapter 7). These are elevated in the body after head injury and are associated with the hormonal changes

that negatively affect metabolism and organ function (see Chapter 37). Inflammatory cytokines tend to cause organ demise; tissue damage has been observed in the gut, liver, lung, and brain. Overall, the molecular basis of functional recovery is poorly understood.

Clinical findings of brain injury often include a transient decrease in level of consciousness. Headache and dizziness are relatively common and not worrisome unless they become more intense or are accompanied by vomiting. Focal neurologic deficits, progressively decreasing level of consciousness, and penetrating brain injury demand prompt neurosurgical evaluation.

Skull fractures underneath lacerations often can be felt as a "drop off" or discontinuity on the surface of the skull and are readily identifiable by CT scan. Basilar skull fractures, bone breaks at the skull base, are manifested by otorrhea (fluid leaking from the ear) or rhinorrhea (salty fluid dripping from the nose or down the pharynx). Other signs include raccoon eyes and Battle's sign—blood behind the mastoid process. Basilar skull fractures may precipitate injuries to cranial nerves, which are essential for chewing, swallowing, taste, and smell.

Hematomas are neurosurgical emergencies because they may rapidly progress to herniation of brain contents through the skull base and to subsequent death. These lesions may present similarly, with decreased level of consciousness, contralateral hemiparesis, and pupillary dilation. These lesions damage brain tissue by gross displacement and traction. Classically the epidural hematoma presents with progressively decreasing consciousness after an interval of several hours during which the patient had only a brief loss of consciousness. Subdural hematoma usually features progressively decreasing consciousness from the time of injury.

Sequelae most often include epilepsy and postconcussive syndrome, a constellation of headache, vertigo, fatigue, and memory difficulties. Treatment for these patients can be highly complex, but the two goals of any therapeutic intervention are to maintain cerebral perfusion and to regulate ICP. Perfusion and pressure control have implications for nutrition therapy.

Medical Nutrition Therapy

The intersection of nutrition and TBI is complex, and in some cases adequate evidence does not exist to answer questions about best nutritional support. However, the updated Brain Trauma Foundation guidelines (Carney et al, 2017) provide two key nutrition-related recommendations for improved clinical outcomes:

- Feed patients to replace basal caloric needs within 5 to 7 days postinjury to decrease mortality.
- Use transgastric jejunal feeding to reduce the incidence of ventilator-associated pneumonia.

Hypermetabolism contributes to increased energy expenditure. Correlations between the severity of brain injury as measured by the Glasgow Coma Scale (Fig. 39.7) and energy requirements have been shown. The Glasgow Coma Scale is based on a 15-point scale for estimating and categorizing the outcomes of brain injury based on overall social capability or dependence on others.

The previous edition of the guidelines (Brain Trauma Foundation, 2007) indicate that nitrogen needs are higher at 14 to 25 g/day for a fasting patient with severe head injury, compared with just 3 to 5 g/day in a normal fasting person. This is due to protein degradation caused by inflammation-associated hypercatabolism, and evidenced by profound urinary urea nitrogen excretion. If a patient continues to fast, they can lose up to 10% of lean mass in a week. For context, 30% weight loss increases mortality rate.

In patients medicated with barbiturates, metabolic expenditure may be decreased to 100% to 120% of basal metabolic rate. This

GLASGOW COMA SCALE : Do it this way

Institute of Neurological Sciences NHS Greater Glasgow and Clyde

CHECK

For factors Interfering with communication,
ability to respond and other injuries

OBSERVE

Eye opening , content of speech and movements of right and left sides

STIMULATE

Sound: spoken or shouted request
Physical: Pressure on finger tip, trapezius or supraorbital notch

RATE

Assign according to highest response observed

Eye opening

Criterion	Observed	Rating	Score
Open before stimulus	✔	Spontaneous	4
After spoken or shouted request	✔	To sound	3
After finger tip stimulus	✔	To pressure	2
No opening at any time, no interfering factor	✔	None	1
Closed by local factor	✔	Non testable	NT

Verbal response

Criterion	Observed	Rating	Score
Correctly gives name, place and date	✔	Orientated	5
Not orientated but communication coherently	✔	Confused	4
Intelligible single words	✔	Words	3
Only moans / groans	✔	Sounds	2
No audible response, no interfering factor	✔	None	1
Factor interferring with communication	✔	Non testable	NT

Best motor response

Criterion	Observed	Rating	Score
Obey 2-part request	✔	Obeys commands	6
Brings hand above clavicle to stimulus on head neck	✔	Localising	5
Bends arm at elbow rapidly but features not predominantly abnormal	✔	Normal flexion	4
Bends arm at elbow, features clearly predominantly abnormal	✔	Abnormal flexion	3
Extends arm at elbow	✔	Extension	2
No movement in arms / legs, no interfering factor	✔	None	1
Paralysed or other limiting factor	✔	Non testable	NT

Sites For Physical Stimulation

Finger tip pressure   Trapezius Pinch   Supraorbital notch

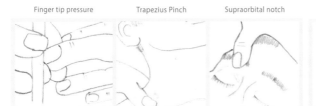

Features of Flexion Responses

Modified with permission from Van Der Naalt 2004
Ned Tijdschr Geneeskd

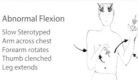

Abnormal Flexion

Slow Sterotyped
Arm across chest
Forearm rotates
Thumb clenched
Leg extends

Normal flexion

Rapid
Variable
Arm away from body

For further information and video demonstration visit www.glasgowcomascale.org

Graphic design by Margaret Frej based on layout and illustrations from Medical Illustration M I • 268093
(c) Sir Graham Teasdale 2015

Fig. 39.7 Glasgow Coma Scale (GCS) Aid. A summary of the structured assessment of each component in the GCS. (From https://www.glasgowcomascale.org and the Institute of Neurological Sciences NHS Greater Glasgow and Clyde.)

decreased metabolic rate in pharmacologically paralyzed patients suggests that maintaining muscle tone is an important part of metabolic expenditure. See Chapter 37 for guidelines on care of the critically ill patient with head trauma.

Choline and its derivative citicoline support cell membrane integrity, the impairment of which is a suggested part of the pathophysiology of TBI. Recent research found citicoline significantly improves the recovery of patients with TBI (Secades, 2016). Therefore supplementation with citicoline and increasing dietary intake of choline may be supportive. Common supplementation of citicoline in the literature is 500 to 1000 mg/day. Good dietary sources of choline ($>/= 10\%$ daily value [DV]) include eggs, beef, soybeans, chicken, cod, shiitake mushrooms, and red potatoes (skin on). Foods with a smaller but still significant amount of choline ($>/= 5\%$ DV) include wheat germ, kidney beans, quinoa, low-fat milk, nonfat yogurt, cooked Brussels sprouts, cooked broccoli, nonfat cottage cheese, and white tuna fish.

Experimental dietary interventions of natural plant compounds exist in animal models of young mice and rats in blunt force trauma models. Of these, the most studied with common food sources and a promising trend of positive results include allicin, baicalein, crocin, curcumin, ellagic acid, epigallocatechin gallate, formononetin, gallic acid, ginseng, luteolin, quercetin, resveratrol, and rutin (Table 39.7; see Fig. 39.6).

TABLE 39.7 Role of Dietary Compounds in Traumatic Brain Injury (TBI)

# Studies	Compound	Impact	Food Sources
1	Allicin Compound that gives garlic its aroma	In mild TBI, 50 mg/kg 2-4 hrs posttrauma was the therapeutic window and most effective dose for improving oxidative stress, neuroinflammation, apoptosis, and TBI-related declines in neuroscores. Possible mechanism is by activating nitric oxide synthase (NOS).	Garlic, onions, shallots, green onions, chives, leeks
1	Crocin Bioactive compound in saffron	In moderate cortical impact TBI, a 20 mg/kg dose 30 minutes preinjury decreased the severity of motor skills damage, brain edema 24-hours post injury, and modest reduction in neuroinflammatory markers.	Saffron (*Crocus sativus L.*)
7	Curcumin polyphenol	In a lateral fluid percussion (LFP) injury model, a diet with 500 ppm curcumin was provided for either 4 weeks prior (moderate improvement in spatial learning and memory, as measured by Morris Water Maze [MWM], reduced oxidative stress, increased brain-derived neurotrophic factor [BDNF], and protected mitochondria and synaptic proteins); or 2 weeks postinjury (greater impact on improved oxidative stress, mitochondrial homeostasis, and MWM performance). In a secondary injury cascade (SIC) of cortical contusion model, both 50 or 100 mg/kg injection pretreatment led to improved locomotor behavior. Posttreatment was not measured. In moderate to severe injury, dosing immediately before (75 or 150 mg/kg) or 30-minutes postinjury (300 mg/kg) significantly reversed some of the SIC, neuroinflammation, and edema. However, the cortical lesion size was not affected, so there was no neuroprotection. In another severe cortical injury model, 100 mg/kg curcumin postinjury improved neuroscores at 24 hours postinjury with small but significant reductions in edema, inflammation, and indicators of damaged and dying neuronal cells.	Turmeric (*Curcuma longa L.*); strong antiinflammatory and antioxidant potential
1	Ellagic acid Polyphenol antioxidant	In a mild to moderate diffuse injury model, 100 mg/kg for 7 days before injury led to improved learning and memory, as measured by a passive avoidance task, reduced blood-brain barrier (BBB) permeability and inflammatory cytokines, and improved signs of long-term synaptic strengthening in the hippocampus. The mechanism is unknown, but ellagic acid is generally known to have antiinflammatory, antioxidant, and immunomodulatory characteristics.	Found in various fruits and nuts including black raspberry (38 mg/100 g), blackberry (44 mg/100 g), cloudberry (15 mg/100 g), pomegranate juice (17 mg/100 mL), raw chestnut (735 mg/100 g), walnut (29 mg/100 g), Japanese walnut (16 mg/100 g)
3	Epigallocatechin gallate (EGCG) polyphenol	In three studies of very mild TBI, a 4-week pretreatment with 0.1% solution of EGCG in the drinking water improved neuronal survival and cognitive performance in MWM postinjury, supported by significantly reduced lipid peroxidation, DNA damage, and a proapoptotic protein. Pretreatment had stronger benefits than limited postinjury treatment. The proposed mechanism is the antioxidant properties of EGCG.	Freshly brewed green tea (27 mg/100 mL), oolong tea (18 mg/100 mL), black tea (9 mg/100 mL). For an alternate source, pecans offer 2 mg/100 g. Bottled teas offer 2-9 mg/100 mL.

TABLE 39.7 Role of Dietary Compounds in Traumatic Brain Injury (TBI)—cont'd

# Studies	Compound	Impact	Food Sources
1	Formononetin Phytoestrogen isoflavone	In one mild to moderate closed-head TBI model, 10 or 20 mg/kg was injected 5 days postinjury and improved neuroscores and reduced brain edema, supported by increased antioxidant enzyme levels and reduced lipid peroxidation.	Roasted soybeans (6 mg/100 g)
1	Gallic acid Phenolic acid	In severe TBI, 100 mg/kg by mouth for 7 days prior and 2 days post injury significantly improved neuroscore and learning and memory behaviors as measured by passive avoidance tests.	Found in various fruits, vegetables, seeds, and nuts: Raw chestnuts (480 mg/100 g) and cloves (458 mg/100 g) are among the highest sources. Green chicory leaf (26 mg/100 g), red chicory leaf (15 mg/100 g), dried sage and oregano (5 mg/100 g), black tea (5 mg/100 mL), black-berry and cloudberry (4-5 mg/100 g), vinegar (3 mg/100 mL), and dried dates (2 mg/100 g)
4	Ginseng	In moderate TBI models, a component of ginseng, ginseng total saponins (GTS), was tested at varying doses twice a day for 14 days postinjury, and the best benefit was at 20 mg/100 g for improving neuroscores starting within 6 hours of injury, hippocampal CA3 region neuron protection and reduced cortical neuron death, supported by signs of reduced oxidation and inflammation. However there was no change in brain edema or lesion volume at 24 hours. Another ginseng-derived compound, ginsenoside Rb1 (GS-Rb1), reduced brain infarction and edema and improved neuroscores when given at 20-40 mg/kg immediately postinjury. For severe TBI, oral intake of total ginseng at 100 or 200 mg/kg eliminated oxidative stress and neuroinflammation when provided daily starting at 14 days postinjury. After 9 days, animals performed better in spatial learning and memory, as measured by MWM.	Root of *Panax ginseng*
4	Luteolin Flavone in a variety of vegetables such as broccoli and celery, and aromatic plants such as mint	In moderate to severe TBI, 10, 30, and 50 mg/kg given 30-minutes postinjury all decreased edema, and the 10 and 30 mg/kg dose improved grip strength and reduced oxidative stress and apoptosis. With 30 mg/kg there was a significant reduction in BBB opening, cell damage, and inflammation. With a 15-day pretreatment of 20 mg/kg reduced TBI-induced Alzheimer's disease.	Dried Mexican oregano (56 mg/100 g), fresh common thyme (40 mg/100 g), fresh common sage (33 mg/100 g), raw globe artichoke (42 mg/100 g), dried lemon verbena (5 mg/100 g). Black olives and dried rosemary (3 mg/100 g)
2	Quercetin Bioflavonoid found in many vegetables and fruits	In severe TBI, 30 mg/kg was given immediately posttrauma and for 3 following days, resulting in improved MWM scores at 4-weeks postinjury.	Black elderberry (42 mg/100 g), dried Mexican oregano (42 mg/100 g), capers (33 mg/100 g), cloves (28 mg/100 g), dark chocolate (25 mg/100 g), raw shallots (2 mg/100 g)
6	Resveratrol Polyphenol with high levels in grapes, nuts, and red wine	In moderate TBI, 100 mg/kg immediately postinjury significantly reduced oxidative stress and edema at 24-hours posttrauma, decreased lesion size at 14 days. In moderate to severe TBI, 100 mg/kg immediately after injury and for 2 following days resulted in improved balance and learned memory behavior as measured by beam balance and MWM at 5 days posttrauma. Another study using the same treatment found resveratrol significantly reduced edema, enhanced motor coordination, and MWM navigation. These findings were supported by reduced inflammation and neuron protection.	Raw lingonberry (3 mg/100 g), muscadine red wine (3 mg/100 mL), European cranberry (2 mg/100 g), raw redcurrant (2 mg/100 g)
2	Rutin A flavonol glycoside of quercetin found widely in plants	In severe TBI, 20, 40, or 80 mg/kg doses were given 14 days post-trauma for an additional 2 weeks, resulting in near-preinjury cognition levels and decreased inflammation, lipid peroxidation, and increases in markers for antioxidants.	Buckwheat, citrus fruit, but found widely in plants, apples, other fruits and vegetables

Chart created by Maggie Moon, MS, RDN, adapted from data in Scheff and Ansari, 2017.

The omega-3 fatty acids docosahexaenoic acid (DHA) and eicosapentaenoic acid (EPA) have antioxidant, antiinflammatory, and antiapoptosis properties, leading to neuron protection in the damaged brain (Dyall, 2015). Studies have shown that short-term implementation of a ketogenic diet acutely postinjury improves structural and functional outcome in TBI in animals and shows potential in humans (McDougall et al, 2018) (see Appendix 19).

Immune-enhancing nutrition formulas are available for critically ill head-injured patients; the formulas are enhanced with glutamine, arginine, and omega-3 fatty acids. Data to support their use has not been consistent. One recent human clinical trial did show increased markers of antioxidants and decreased inflammatory markers (Rai et al, 2017); an earlier preliminary human study found increased prealbumin levels and some benefit of decreased infection in those patients using the immune-enhanced formula (Painter et al, 2015).

SPINE TRAUMA AND SPINAL CORD INJURY

Spine trauma encompasses many types of injuries, ranging from stable fractures of the spinal column to catastrophic transection of the spinal cord. A complete spinal cord injury (SCI) is defined as a lesion in which there is no preservation of motor or sensory function more than three segments below the level of the injury. With an incomplete injury there is some degree of residual motor or sensory function more than three segments below the lesion.

Pathophysiology

The spinal cord responds to insult similarly to the brain. Bleeding, contusion, and shorn axons appear first, followed by a multiyear remodeling process consisting of gliosis and fibrosis.

The location of the SCI and the disruption of the descending axons determine the extent of paralysis. Tetraplegia (formerly known as quadriplegia) exists when the injury to the spinal cord affects all four extremities. When the SCI location results in only lower extremity involvement, it is called paraplegia.

Medical Management

SCIs have numerous clinical manifestations, depending on the level of the injury. Complete transection results in complete loss of function below the level of the lesion, including the bladder and sphincters. After the patient is stabilized hemodynamically, the doctor evaluates the degree of neurologic deficit. Patients with suspected SCI are usually immobilized promptly in the field. Complete radiographic evaluation of the spinal column is obligatory in multitrauma and unconscious patients.

In the awake patient, clinical evidence of spine compromise is usually sufficient to determine the need for further workup. CT and MRI are used to more accurately delineate bony damage and spinal cord compromise. A dismal 3% of patients with complete spinal cord insults recover some function after 24 hours. Failure to regain function after 24 hours predicts a poor prognosis for reestablishment of function in the future. Incomplete spinal cord syndromes may have somewhat better outcomes.

Morbidity and mortality rates associated with SCI have improved dramatically, particularly in the last two decades. Advances in acute-phase care have reduced early mortality and prevented complications frequently associated with early death, such as respiratory failure and pulmonary emboli. Today, fewer than 10% of patients with SCI die of the acute injury.

Medical Nutrition Therapy

Technologic advances in enteral and parenteral feeding techniques and formulas have played a role in maintaining the nutrition status of these patients (see Chapter 12). Although the metabolic response to neurotrauma has been studied extensively, the acute metabolic response to SCI has not, but it is similar to other forms of neurotrauma during the acute phase. Initially paralytic ileus may occur but often resolves within 72 hours postinjury.

In the acute phase, calorie estimates should be based on energy expenditure measured by indirect calorimetry. Metabolic activity is decreased due to muscle enervation. Actual energy needs are at least 10% lower than predicted levels. If indirect calorimetry is unavailable, consider the Harris-Benedict formula, using admission weight, injury factor of 1.2, and activity factor of 1.1. Acute protein needs are 2 g/kg of ideal body weight (Academy of Nutrition and Dietetics, 2009) (see Chapter 2).

Because DHA and EPA have antioxidant, antiinflammatory, and antiapoptosis properties, patients may benefit from fish oil supplementation (Dyall, 2015).

For those who survive the injury but are disabled for life, there are significant alterations in lifestyle, as well as the possibility of secondary complications. In general, the number and frequency of complications, such as the impaired ability to prepare food and self-feed, and the presence of constipation, pressure ulcers, changes in weight status, and pain vary but will involve nutrition management (Box 39.3). Evidence-based practice guidelines for SCI were released in 2010 by the Academy of Nutrition and Dietetics. While updated guidelines do not exist as of 2018, opportunities for future research to improve the guidelines have been proposed (DiTucci, 2014). Individuals with SCI have significantly higher fat mass and lower lean mass. Loss of muscle tone caused by skeletal muscle paralysis below the level of injury contributes to decreased metabolic activity, initial weight loss, and predisposition to osteoporosis. The higher the injury, the lower the metabolic rate, which results in lower energy requirements. Guidelines for accepted weights adjusted for paraplegia and tetraplegia are as follows:

	Weight adjustment from ideal body mass index (BMI)
Paraplegic	Reduce by 10 to 15 lb
Tetraplegic	Reduce by 15 to 20 lb

Tetraplegic patients have lower metabolic rates than paraplegic patients, proportional to the amount of denervated muscle in their arms and legs, caused in part by the loss of residual motor function. In the rehabilitation phase, tetraplegics may require approximately 25% to 50% fewer calories than conventional equations predict. Thus these patients have the potential to become overweight. It has been proposed that obesity may slow the eventual rehabilitation process by limiting functional outcome. In the rehabilitation phase, estimated energy needs are approximately 22.7 kcalories per kg body weight (quadriplegia), and 27.9 kcalories per kg body weight (paraplegia). Protein needs range from 0.8 to 1 g/kg body weight as long as there are no pressure ulcers or infections (Academy of Nutrition and Dietetics, 2009).

SCI is associated with osteopenia and osteoporosis as a result of bone mineralization losses secondary to immobilization, and the prevalence of long-bone fractures increases. Adequate intake of vitamin D and calcium should be planned without excessive daily intakes.

NEUROLOGIC DISEASES

Neurologic diseases are relatively rare, and their exact causes are largely unknown. Many are being actively studied, and the science that informs our understanding will continue to rapidly evolve in the next

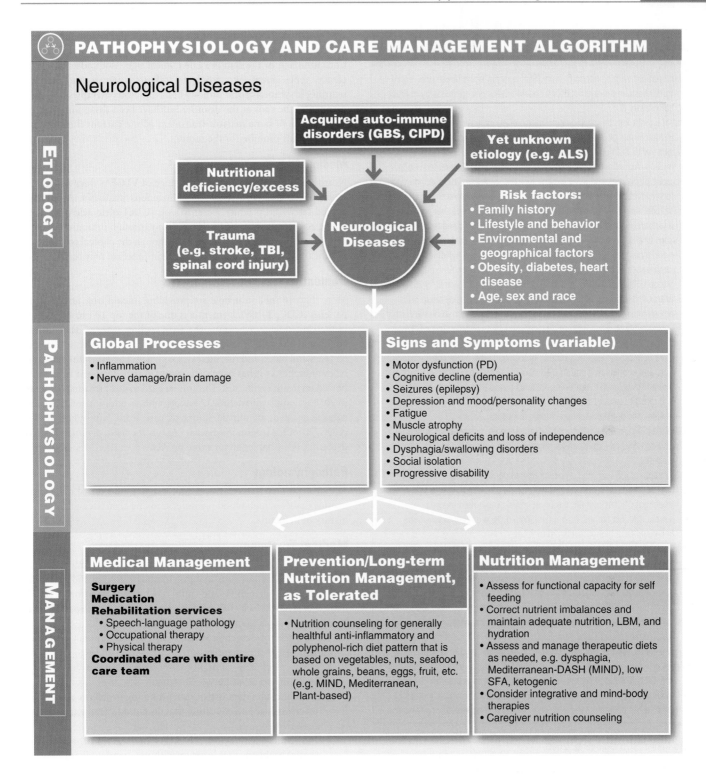

PATHOPHYSIOLOGY AND CARE MANAGEMENT ALGORITHM

Neurological Diseases

ETIOLOGY

Acquired auto-immune disorders (GBS, CIPD)

Yet unknown etiology (e.g. ALS)

Nutritional deficiency/excess

Neurological Diseases

Trauma (e.g. stroke, TBI, spinal cord injury)

Risk factors:
- Family history
- Lifestyle and behavior
- Environmental and geographical factors
- Obesity, diabetes, heart disease
- Age, sex and race

PATHOPHYSIOLOGY

Global Processes
- Inflammation
- Nerve damage/brain damage

Signs and Symptoms (variable)
- Motor dysfunction (PD)
- Cognitive decline (dementia)
- Seizures (epilepsy)
- Depression and mood/personality changes
- Fatigue
- Muscle atrophy
- Neurological deficits and loss of independence
- Dysphagia/swallowing disorders
- Social isolation
- Progressive disability

MANAGEMENT

Medical Management

Surgery
Medication
Rehabilitation services
- Speech-language pathology
- Occupational therapy
- Physical therapy

Coordinated care with entire care team

Prevention/Long-term Nutrition Management, as Tolerated
- Nutrition counseling for generally healthful anti-inflammatory and polyphenol-rich diet pattern that is based on vegetables, nuts, seafood, whole grains, beans, eggs, fruit, etc. (e.g. MIND, Mediterranean, Plant-based)

Nutrition Management
- Assess for functional capacity for self feeding
- Correct nutrient imbalances and maintain adequate nutrition, LBM, and hydration
- Assess and manage therapeutic diets as needed, e.g. dysphagia, Mediterranean-DASH (MIND), low SFA, ketogenic
- Consider integrative and mind-body therapies
- Caregiver nutrition counseling

---

several decades. What we do know is that neurologic diseases can significantly impact nutritional status.

Adrenomyeloleukodystrophy

Pathophysiology

Adrenomyeloleukodystrophy (ALD) is a rare congenital enzyme deficiency that affects the metabolism of very-long-chain fatty acids (VLCFAs). This leads to accumulation of VLCFAs, particularly hexacosanoic acid (C26:0) and tetracosanoic acid (C24:0) in the brain and adrenal glands. The incidence is 1 in 21,000 male births and 1 in 14,000 female births (Hung et al, 2013). While ALD more commonly presents in young males, it should be considered in women with chronic myelopathy or peripheral neuropathy, especially with early fecal incontinence (Engelen et al, 2014); there have also been cases of men presenting with ALD as late as their mid-30s (Chen et al, 2018).

ALD is an X-linked recessive disorder characterized by myelopathy, peripheral neuropathy, and cerebral demyelination. The adult variant, adrenomyeloneuropathy, has chronic distal axonopathy of spinal

BOX 39.3 Key Guidelines for Managing Spinal Cord Injury

If the patient with spinal cord injury (SCI) is in the acute phase, the registered dietitian nutritionist (RDN) should assess energy needs by indirect calorimetry (IC).

Initial weight loss during the acute phase of injury may lead to weight gain in the chronic phase because of body mass redistribution.

Patients with SCI have reduced metabolic activity because of denervated muscle. Actual energy needs are at least 10% below predicted needs.

Because of decreased energy expenditure and caloric needs, secondary to lower levels of spontaneous physical activity and a lower thermic effect of food, adults in the chronic phase of SCI are often overweight or obese and therefore at risk for diabetes and cardiovascular disease.

Persons of all ages with SCI appear to be at high risk for cardiovascular disease, atherogenesis, and undesirable blood lipid values. Modifiable risk factors such as obesity, inactivity, dietary factors, and smoking must be addressed. Physical activity, including sports, swimming, electrically stimulated exercise, and body-weight supported treadmill training, may result in improvements in blood lipid parameters. Dietary intervention using the current evidence-based guide for lipid disorders should be provided by an RDN.

Nutrition care provided by the RDN as part of a multidisciplinary team results in improved nutrition-related outcomes in the acute care, rehabilitation, and community settings. SCI patients experience improvements in nutrient deficiencies, nutrition problems associated with social isolation and mobility issues, overweight and obesity, bowel management, swallowing, and nutrition-related chronic diseases.

Cranberry juice may be beneficial for prevention of urinary tract infections. One cup (250 mL) daily can be recommended, unless the patient has diabetes.

A minimum of 1.5 L of fluid is recommended per day. Therapeutic diets of high fiber and adequate water intake alone often do not suffice for treatment of constipation; a routine bowel preparation program may be required. For chronic bowel dysfunction, 15 g of fiber seems more beneficial than higher levels (20 to 30 g).

Maintenance of nutritional health is important because poor nutrition is a risk factor for infection and pressure ulcer development. Regular assessment of nutritional status, the provision of adequate nutritional intake, and the implementation of aggressive nutritional support measures are indicated. Reduced pressure ulcer development occurs in patients who maintain a normal weight, higher activity levels, and better serum levels of total protein, albumin, prealbumin, zinc, vitamin D, and vitamin A. Thus sufficient intake of calories, protein, zinc, and vitamins C, A, and B-complex is warranted.

When pressure ulcers are present, use 30 to 40 kcal/kg of body weight/day and 1.2 g to 1.5 g of protein/kg body weight/day (see Chapter 20). Fluid requirements should be at least 1 mL fluid per kcal provided; increase if air-fluidized beds are used and when losses are increased for any reason.

Academy of Nutrition and Dietetics Evidence Analysis Library: Spinal Cord Injury (SCI) Guideline, 2009.

cord and peripheral nerves marked by cerebral inflammatory demyelination; head trauma is an environmental factor that is detrimental in those people genetically at risk. The mental and physical deterioration progresses to dementia, aphasia, apraxia, dysarthria, and blindness.

Medical Management

Clinical manifestations usually occur before age 7, with average age of onset between 5 and 12 years, and may manifest as adrenal insufficiency or cerebral decompensation.

Dysarthria (impairment of the neuromuscular system for the production of speech) and dysphagia may interfere with oral alimentation. Bronzing of the skin is a late clinical sign. With adrenal insufficiency, replacement of steroids is indicated, which may improve neurologic symptoms and prolong life. Numerous therapies have been directed at the root of the disorder but have been disappointing. The selective use of bone marrow transplant is one current therapy; gene therapy holds promise for the future.

Medical Nutrition Therapy

Nutritional therapy by dietary avoidance of VLCFAs does not lead to biochemical change because of endogenous synthesis. A specialty altered fatty acid product, Lorenzo's oil (C18:1 oleic acid and C22:1 erucic acid), lowers the VLCFA level, likely through inhibition of elongation activities (Morita et al, 2018). Although the clinical course is not significantly improved, a slower decline in function may result.

Dementia

More than 16 million people are providing unpaid care for dementia patients (CDC, 2018b). Dementia is one of the top 10 causes of death in the United States where it is the sixth leading cause of death among adults and the fifth leading cause of death among older adults aged 65 years and older, and risk increases with age. The mortality rates may be even higher as it has been demonstrated that dementia is underreported on death certificates. The annual hard costs of treating dementia in 2018 was approximately $277 billion, with an additional $232 billion equivalent spent in unpaid hours of care from family and friends (CDC, 2018c). Alzheimer's disease (AD) is the most common form of dementia. See Chapter 40 for more on AD.

Pathophysiology

The primary risk factor for dementia is aging. Additional risk factors include diabetes, high blood pressure, smoking cigarettes, and a family history of dementia.

Medical Treatment

Expert international groups collaborated with the Alzheimer's Association and National Institute on Aging to update criteria and guidelines for diagnosing dementia and mild cognitive impairment (MCI) (Albert et al, 2011; Jack et al, 2011; McKhann et al, 2011; Sperling et al, 2011). Key updates to the prior 1984 guidelines include:

- Three stages of dementia where it had previously only identified the final stage of dementia:
  1. Early preclinical asymptomatic stage: marked by amyloid buildup and other nerve cell changes
  2. MCI: includes memory or other thinking problems unusual for a person's age and education that do not interfere with independent living
  3. Dementia: memory loss, difficulty finding words, and visual/spatial problems that interfere with independent living
- Definition of AD expanded beyond memory loss to include other aspects of cognition such as word-finding ability and judgment, which may be impaired earlier
- Better differentiation between AD and other dementias and disorders that may increase risk for AD, such as vascular disease, that were not previously recognized or understood
- Identification of potential biomarkers of underlying brain disease that can be used for research purposes (not clinical); these simply did not exist in 1984 when confirmation of diagnosis was only possible by autopsy

Most medical management is targeted to improving the quality of life for those with the condition and their caregivers, including maintaining mental function, managing behavioral issues, and delaying symptoms. Preliminary and observational evidence suggests that the risk of developing dementia can be reduced through lifestyle factors (see Chapter 40).

A review paper on the pros and cons of medical marijuana suggest that cannabis may diminish adverse effects of conditions such as ALS, MS, AD, and Parkinson's disease, but that chronic cannabis may lead to cognitive impairments (Suryadevara et al, 2017).

Medical Nutrition Treatment

Potential Risk Reduction

Preliminary research suggests an eating pattern called the Mediterranean-DASH intervention for neurodegenerative delay (MIND) diet may help slow cognitive decline and reduce the risk of developing AD (see Chapter 40). It is based on established heart-healthy eating patterns and enhanced with foods specifically for brain health. Two large prospective studies suggest that this diet may slow cognitive decline by 7.5 years and reduce the risk of AD by up to 53% (Morris et al, 2015a, 2015b).

A literature review on nutrition in cognitive function and brain aging in the elderly determined that the MIND diet substantially slowed cognitive decline over and above the Mediterranean and DASH diets individually, though all are healthy eating patterns (Gardener and Rainey-Smith, 2018). A phase 3 RCT began in 2017 to test the effects of a 3-year MIND diet intervention, with an estimated completion date in April 2021. One of the underlying mechanisms may be related to polyphenol content (Figueira et al, 2017) (Table 39.8).

Public Health Approaches to Promoting Health and Independence for an Aging Population

Clinicians can participate in public health efforts and improve patient outcomes by training caregivers through the REACH OUT program, which trains caregivers of people with dementia, including AD. Participants had improved health and less depression, and those in their care were less likely to be left unsupervised, wander, or have access to dangerous objects. Information on how to implement a community-based program for dementia caregivers with examples, tips, resources, websites, and references in a step-by-step guide is available (National Association of Chronic Disease Directors, 2009).

Clinical Approaches

In early stages, the goal of nutrition therapy is maintenance of membrane integrity and correction of existing nutritional deficiencies. A person with preclinical or early dementia may have olfactory and taste dysfunction that may reduce appetite. RDNs can guide caregivers to make meal times simple and social, and to encourage eating.

In the MCI phase, the goal of nutrition therapy is to manage nutrition in the context of behavioral changes, monitor for weight loss and signs of dysphagia, and consider the need for oral nutritional supplements to fill deficiencies. When dementia progresses to a severe stage, the goal is to provide appropriate therapy for dysphagia as needed, correct weight loss, monitor for signs of pulmonary aspiration risk, and consider finger foods and high calorie drinks when intake at meals decreases (Pivi et al, 2017).

TABLE 39.8 The Mediterranean-DASH Intervention for Neurodegenerative Delay (MIND) Diet

Food	Frequency	Food Sources
Olive oil	Daily, main fat	Extra virgin olive oil
Wine	Daily, 5 oz glass only	Red wine
Whole grains	3x/day	Amaranth, barley, brown rice, buckwheat, bulgur, corn, farro, oatmeal, sorghum, quinoa, wheat berry, whole wheat, wild rice
Vegetables	Daily	Asparagus, cauliflower, carrot, onions, bell peppers, celery, cucumber, sweet potato, garlic, mushrooms, green beans
Leafy green vegetables	Near daily, 6x/week	Arugula, broccoli, lettuces, spinach, cabbage, kale, Swiss chard, collard greens, mustard greens, watercress, bok choy
Nuts	5x/wk	Almonds, cashews, pecans, pistachios, walnuts
Beans	3-4x/wk, every other day	Black beans, black-eyed peas, cannellini beans, chickpeas, great northern beans, kidney beans, lima beans, pinto beans
Berries	2x/wk	Wild blueberries, highbush blueberries, strawberries, raspberries, pomegranate, blackberry, gooseberry, cranberry, cloudberry, lingonberry, boysenberry, huckleberry, bilberry, goji berry, currants, mulberry, acai
Poultry	2x/wk	Chicken, turkey
Seafood	1x/wk	Salmon, arctic char, sardines, rainbow trout, mussels, oysters, barramundi, crab, squid
Red meat	Less than 4x/week	Beef, bison, pork, lamb
Cheese	Less than once a week	Cheddar, mozzarella, parmigiano-reggiano, feta, brie, Camembert, provolone, Swiss cheese, Gouda, Gorgonzola, manchego, Emmental
Butter and stick margarine	Less than 1 tablespoon per day	Inclusive of fats with a large percentage of saturated fat or trans fats: butter, margarine, ghee, and coconut oil (would include trans fatty acids if they were not already banned)
Pastries and sweets	Less than 5 times a week	Éclair, croissant, pie, baklava, donut, bear claw, cannoli, cinnamon roll, samosa, empanada, cronut, danish, dutch baby pancake, macaron, mooncake, pain au chocolat, pan dulce, candy, chocolate, gummies, fudge, jelly beans, sour candy
Fried/fast foods	Less than one serving per week	French fries, fried chicken, mozzarella sticks, hushpuppy, fried shrimp, fried green tomatoes, fried clams, arancini, churro, jalapeno poppers, onion rings, bacon, fried calamari rings, chicken fingers

Severe dementia causes complications of immobility, swallowing disorders, and accompanying risk of malnutrition that raises the risk of acute problems that can lead to death (e.g., pneumonia). However, note that there is a lack of evidence for using a feeding tube for people with advanced dementia, and the practice is declining.

European Society for Clinical Nutrition and Metabolism (ESPEN) guidelines for nutrition in dementia provide 26 recommendations (Volkert et al, 2015). Screening for malnutrition and closely monitoring body weight are recommended. For patients with inadequate intake who are in crisis caused by a potentially reversible condition, artificial nutrition may be appropriate for mild to moderate—but not severe or terminal stage—dementia. Supplements of single nutrients are not recommended unless there is a deficiency, and supplements in general would only be to improve nutrition status, not to treat or prevent cognitive decline. However, the clinician should use best judgment when compounds, such as curcumin, are generally safe and possibly effective (Table 39.9).

There is preliminary research regarding the antioxidant and antiin-flammatory properties of the polyphenol curcumin, found naturally in turmeric or in supplement form. High-dose animal and in vitro studies suggest a therapeutic role through improved glucose homeostasis, lipid metabolism, endothelial function, insulin immunosupport and inhibiting amyloid plaque aggregation. While it shows promise, adequate human studies have been less convincing to date, and more research is needed. However, in amounts normally found in food, this is a safe and possibly helpful compound to include in a therapeutic diet. Note that bioavailability tends to be low, but is improved 2000 times in the presence of piperine (naturally found in black pepper), which suppresses rapid processing in the liver and urinary extraction of curcumin (Kim and Clifton, 2018).

In addition to nutrition care, integrative patient-centered approaches to care are low-cost, low-risk, and helpful to people with dementia (Anderson et al, 2017), including:

- Support groups for social engagement and relieving social isolation
- Aerobic exercise, which has been shown to improve spatial memory, executive functioning and brain connectivity, as well as improve activities of daily living (ADL) and cognition, through reducing inflammation and supporting neurogenesis
- Cognitive training and stimulation for improved word associations (e.g., names of things) and money tasks (e.g., making change)
- Stress-reducing mind-body interventions such as meditation and mindfulness, which have been shown to improve logical memory, working memory, verbal fluency, attention, sleep, mood, cerebral blood flow, and agitation. Reflective exercise such as yoga and tai chi may help improve cognitive function through similar mechanisms as aerobic exercise. Guided imagery has been shown to improve cognitive function and mood. These activities promote relaxation through psychoneuroimmunological pathways that can be dysregulated in people with dementia.

Amyotrophic Lateral Sclerosis

Etiology

Amyotrophic lateral sclerosis (ALS), also known as Lou Gehrig's disease, is a progressive and fatal neurodegenerative disorder affecting the motor neurons in the CNS. ALS involves a progressive denervation, atrophy, and weakness of muscles; hence the name amyotrophy. ALS affects about 5 in 100,000 people in the United States (Mehta et al, 2018), with 1.9 new cases each year per 100,000 people. Global cases are projected to increase by 69% by 2040 primarily due to aging (Arthur et al, 2016). The hereditary form accounts for 5% to 10% of cases, but the remaining 90% to 95% of cases have no clear cause. Whites, males, non-Hispanics, people aged 60 years and older, and

TABLE 39.9 ESPEN Guidelines on Nutrition in Dementia: Interventions to Support Adequate Food Intake

Potential Cause of Malnutrition	Reasonable Intervention
Mastication problems	Oral care Dental treatment Texture modification
Swallowing problems	Swallowing evaluation Swallowing training Texture modification
Xerostomia	Check medication for adverse side effects, remove or change medication if possible Ensure adequate fluid intake Use mouth rinse and gel
Restricted mobility, immobility	Physiotherapy Group exercise Resistance training Help with shopping and cooking Meals on wheels
Psychiatric disorders (e.g., depressive mood, depression, anxiety)	Adequate medical treatment Eating with others/shared meals Pleasant meal ambience/eating environment Group activities, occupational therapy
Acute disease, (chronic) pain	Adequate medical treatment
Adverse effects of medications (e.g., xerostomia, nausea, apathy)	Coordinate care regarding medications, manage side effects (i.e., moist foods, easy to digest, and enjoyable foods)
Social problems (e.g., lacking support, family conflict)	Help with shopping, cooking, and eating Meals on wheels, shared meals Resolve conflicts
Difficulties in shopping, preparing meals, and/or eating regularly	Help with shopping Domestic help Meals on wheels Person who is present at mealtimes
Forgetting to eat	Supervision during meals Verbal prompting, encouragement
Decreasing ability to remember eating, to recognize food, and to eat independently	Feeding assistance Increased time spent by nurses during feeding Energy-dense meals
Behavioral problems, wandering	Emotional support Specific behavioral and communication strategies
Dysphagia	Texture modification in coordination with SLP

ESPEN, European Society for Clinical Nutrition and Metabolism; *SLP*, speech-language pathologist.
Adapted from data presented in Volkert D, Chourdakis M, Faxen-Irving G, et al: ESPEN guidelines on nutrition in dementia, *Clin Nutr* 34:1052–1073, 2015.

those with a family history are more likely to develop ALS. One study found obesity (BMI >30) was a significant predictor for younger-age onset of ALS (Hollinger et al, 2016).

The cause of ALS is not clear. Thus there is no cure, and survival is typically 3 to 5 years after disease onset. However, in a very unique case, renowned physicist Stephen Hawking (1942–2018) lived with ALS for 55 years. Risk factors related to occupation, trauma, diet, or socioeconomic status are not consistent, although environmental toxins have been suspected to play a role (Su et al, 2016). One of the first clues that ALS may involve an environmental factor was obtained on the island of Guam, where an unusually high proportion of people over the past century have developed symptoms similar to ALS as they age. Studies are ongoing but thus far without proof of cause.

Pathophysiology

The pathologic basis of weakness in ALS is the selective death of motor neurons in the ventral gray matter of the spinal cord, brainstem, and in the motor cortex. Clinical manifestations are characterized by generalized skeletal muscular weakness, atrophy, and hyperreflexia (NIH, GARD, 2018). The typical presentation is:

- Signs of lower motor neuron deficits: weakness, wasting, fasciculation (muscle twitching)
- Signs of upper motor neuron deficits: hyperactive tendon reflexes, Hoffman signs, Babinski signs, or clonus (muscle contractions)

Muscle weakness begins in the legs and hands and progresses to the proximal arms and oropharynx. As these motor nerves deteriorate, almost all of the voluntary skeletal muscles are at risk for atrophy and complete loss of function. The loss of spinal motor neurons causes the denervation of voluntary skeletal muscles of the neck, trunk, and limbs, resulting in muscle wasting, flaccid weakness, involuntary twitching (fasciculations), and loss of mobility.

Progressive loss of function in cortical motor neurons can lead to spasticity of jaw muscles, resulting in strained speech and dysphagia. The onset of dysphagia is usually insidious. Swallowing difficulties usually follow speech difficulties. Discussions regarding eventual need for enteral nutrition often coincide with the introduction of augmentative and alternative communication systems as the speech and swallow function decline (Coyle, 2018). Although some weight loss is inevitable given the muscle atrophy, consistent or dramatic loss may be an indicator of chewing difficulties or dysphagia. Eye movement and eye blink are spared, as are the sphincter muscles of the bowel and bladder; thus incontinence is rare. Sensation remains intact and mental acuity is maintained.

Medical Management

No currently known therapy cures the disease. In 2017 the Food and Drug Administration (FDA) approved a second drug for ALS called edaravone. Both riluzole and edaravone help slow the progression of ALS (Mehta et al, 2018). Edaravone's documented benefit is among early ALS patients with rapid disease progression, though it is approved in the United States for all ALS patients (Dorst et al, 2018). It was initially developed and approved in Japan, and is being considered for approval in Europe as of mid-2018. Treatment with a high dose of methylcobalamin (B_{12}) is being studied to preserve muscle integrity (NIH, 2014). The ketogenic diet has shown positive results in disease amelioration in mouse models (Yang and Fan, 2017). Although mechanical ventilation can extend the life of patients, most decline this option. Quality of life is poor in advanced ALS and supportive comfort measures are primarily used.

Medical Nutrition Therapy

There are decreases in body fat, lean body mass, muscle power, and nitrogen balance and an increase in resting energy expenditure as death approaches. Hypermetabolic status and increased resting energy expenditure measurements have been noted. Hypercaloric enteral diets were demonstrated to be safe and well tolerated in a small phase 2 RCT (Wills et al, 2014). A study of 148 ALS patients found survival time was associated with early intake of a higher fat and protein diet (Kim et al, 2018).

The relationship between dysphagia and respiratory status is important. As ALS progresses, a progressive loss of function in bulbar and respiratory muscles contributes to oral and pharyngeal dysphagia. This results in the need for nutrition support, generally via gastrostomy tube. In late stages, when respiratory muscles are impaired, feeding tube placement is associated with more risk. For that reason, early feeding tube placement is recommended.

The clinician should become familiar with common clinical findings in ALS to prevent secondary complications of malnutrition and dehydration. The functional status of each patient should be monitored closely so that timely intervention with the appropriate management techniques can be started. Oropharyngeal weakness affects survival in ALS by placing the patient at continuous risk of aspiration, pneumonia, and sepsis and by curtailing the adequate intake of energy and protein. These problems can compound the deteriorating effects of the disease. The Amyotrophic Lateral Sclerosis Severity Scale often is used to assess the functional level of swallowing, speech, and upper and lower extremities. Once the severity of deficits has been identified, appropriate interventions can be implemented (see *Focus On:* Dysphagia Intervention for Amyotrophic Lateral Sclerosis [ALS]).

⊚ **FOCUS ON**

Dysphagia Intervention for Amyotrophic Lateral Sclerosis (ALS)

Strand and colleagues (1996) outlined dysphagia intervention on a continuum of five stages that correlate to the amyotrophic lateral sclerosis (ALS) severity scale. They include the following:

Normal Eating Habits (ALS Severity Scale Rating 10-9)

Early assessment and intervention are critical for maintaining nutritional health in ALS. This is the appropriate time to begin educating the patient, before the development of speech or swallowing symptoms. Hydration and maintenance of nutritional health are critical at this stage. Fluid intake of at least 2 qt/day is important. Dehydration contributes to fatigue and thickens saliva. For patients with spinal ALS, emphasis on fluids is important because they may intentionally limit fluid intake because of difficulties with toileting. The diet history is helpful to assess patterns of normal chewing, swallowing, and the rate of ingestion. Weight loss history establishes a baseline weight. A weight loss of 10% or more is indicative of nutritional risk.

Early Eating Problems (Severity Scale Rating 8-7)

At this point patients begin to report difficulties eating; reports of coughing and unusually long mealtimes are associated with tongue, facial, and masticator muscle weakness. Dietary intervention begins to focus on modification of consistency, avoidance of thin liquids, and use of foods that are easier to chew and swallow.

Dietary Consistency Changes (Severity Scale Rating 6-5)

As symptoms progress, the oral transport of food becomes difficult as dry, crumbly foods tend to break apart and cause choking. Foods that require more chewing (e.g., raw vegetables or steak) are typically avoided. As dysphagia progresses, ingestion of thin liquids, especially water, may become more problematic. Often the patient has fatigue and malaise, which may be associated with a mild chronic dehydration resulting from a decreased fluid intake. Dietary intervention should change food consistency (see Appendix 20) to reduce the need for oral manipulation and to conserve energy. Small, frequent meals

Continued

also may increase intake. Thick liquids that contain a high percentage of water, as well as attempts to increase fluid intake, must be emphasized to maintain fluid balance. Popsicles, gelatin, ice, and fresh fruit are additional sources of free water. Liquids can be thickened with a modified cornstarch thickener. Swallowing can be improved by emphasizing taste, texture, and temperature. Juices can be substituted for water to provide taste, nutrients, and calories. A cool temperature facilitates the swallowing mechanism; therefore cold food items may be better tolerated; heat does not provide the same advantage. Carbonation also may be better tolerated because of the beneficial effect of texture. Instructions for preventing aspiration should be addressed: Safe swallowing includes sitting upright with the head in a chin-down position. Concentrating on the swallowing process can also help reduce choking. Avoid environmental distractions and conversation during mealtime; however, families should be encouraged to maintain a normal mealtime routine. As dysphagia progresses, the limitation of food consistencies may result in the exclusion of entire food groups. Vitamin and mineral supplementation may be necessary. If chewable supplements are not handled safely, liquid forms may be added to acceptable foods. Fiber also may have to be added along with fluids for constipation problems.

Tube Feeding (Severity Scale Rating 4-3)
Dehydration will occur acutely before malnutrition, which is a more chronic state. This may be an early indication of the need for nutrition support. Weight

loss from muscle wasting and dysphagia eventually leads to placement of a percutaneous endoscopic gastrostomy (PEG) tube for nutrition and protection against aspiration caused by dysphagia. Enteral nutrition support is preferred because the gastrointestinal tract should be functioning properly. Given the progressive nature of ALS, placing feeding tubes when there are signs of dysphagia and dehydration is better than initiating this therapy later, after the patient has become overtly malnourished or when respiratory status is marginal. The decision of whether to place a feeding tube for nutrition support is part of the decision-making process each patient must face. Adequate nourishment can maintain health of the individual longer and may be a welcome relief for the patient. The purpose of nutrition support should be to enhance the quality of life. Long-term access should be considered via a PEG or percutaneous endoscope jejunostomy tube (see Chapter 12).

Nothing by Mouth (Severity Scale Rating 2-1)
The final level of dysphagia is reached when patients can neither eat orally nor manage their own oral secretions. Although saliva production is not increased, it tends to pool in the front of the mouth as a result of a declining swallow response. Once the swallowing mechanism is absent, mechanical ventilation is required to manage saliva flow. Tube feeding is permanent at this stage.

Epilepsy

Epilepsy is a chronic condition characterized by unprovoked, recurring seizures. Seizures are caused by abnormal electrical activity of a group of neurons. According the latest available estimates from 2015 data, an estimated 1.2% of the total U.S. population has active epilepsy, which translates to 3.4 million people including 3 million adults and 470,000 children (CDC, 2017b).

Pathophysiology

Most seizures begin in early life, but a resurgence occurs after age 60. The first occurrence of a seizure should prompt investigation into a cause. A clinical workup usually reveals no anatomic abnormalities, and the cause of the seizure may remain unknown (idiopathic). Seizures before age 2 are usually caused by fever, developmental defects, birth injuries, or a metabolic disease (see Chapters 42 and 43). The medical history is the key component for suggesting further avenues of diagnostic investigation and potential treatments, especially in children. An electroencephalogram can help delineate seizure activity. It is most helpful in localizing partial complex seizures.

Medical Management

The dramatic tonic-clonic (grand mal) seizure is the most common image of a convulsive seizure, yet numerous classifications of seizures, each with a different and often less dramatic clinical presentation, exist. A generalized tonic-clonic seizure typically involves the entire brain cortex from its beginning phases. After such a seizure the patient wakes up slowly and will be groggy and disoriented for minutes to hours. This is termed the postictal phase and is characterized by deep sleep, headache, confusion, and muscle soreness.

The absence seizure (petit mal) is also generalized in nature. Patients with absence seizures may appear to be daydreaming during an episode, they recover consciousness within a few seconds and have no postictal fatigue or disorientation.

Partial seizures occur when there is a discrete focus of epileptogenic brain tissue. A simple partial seizure involves no loss of consciousness, whereas a complex partial seizure is characterized by a

change in consciousness. Failure of partial seizure control may prompt consideration of seizure surgery. A localized focus resected from nonessential brain renders a patient seizure free in 75% of cases.

Determining the seizure type is key to implementing effective therapy. Antiepileptic drugs control seizures in 70% of people; however, these drugs can have undesirable side effects. Use of just one antiseizure medication is recommended initially, resorting to combination therapies only when needed. If seizures are not well controlled after a trial of two antiseizure drugs, the likelihood of control from an additional medication or combination of medications is minimal.

Medications used in anticonvulsant therapy may alter the nutrition status of the patient (see Appendix 13). For example, phenobarbital has been associated with decreased cognitive function (memory and attention) in children, perhaps because it depletes folate; further, an animal study showed widespread apoptosis in the developing brain after phenobarbital exposure (Kim and Ko, 2016). It occasionally is considered for use after failure of other antiepileptic drugs. Phenobarbital, phenytoin, and valproates interfere with intestinal absorption of calcium by interfering with vitamin D metabolism in the kidneys. Long-term therapy with these drugs may lead to osteomalacia in adults or rickets in children, and vitamin D supplementation is recommended. Folic acid supplementation interferes with phenytoin metabolism; thus it contributes to difficulties in achieving therapeutic levels.

Phenytoin, valproates, and phenobarbital are bound primarily to albumin in the bloodstream. Decreased serum albumin levels limit the amount of drug that can be bound. This results in an increased free drug concentration and possible drug toxicity even with a standard dose.

Absorption of phenobarbital is delayed by the consumption of food; therefore administration of the drug must be staggered around mealtimes if it is used. Continuous enteral feeding slows the absorption of phenytoin, thus necessitating an increase in the dose to achieve a therapeutic level. Stopping the tube feeding 1 hour before and 1 hour after the phenytoin dose was common practice in the past but is no longer recommended. The phenytoin dose should be adjusted based on the tube feeding.

Marijuana is being explored for its anticonvulsant properties, especially for treatment-resistant epilepsy (O'Connell et al, 2017; Reddy, 2017), though a number of neurologic adverse effects have been reported, highlighting the need to weigh risks and benefits (Solimini et al, 2017).

Medical Nutrition Therapy

The classic ketogenic diet, which has been in existence since the 1920s, is a well-established nonpharmacologic treatment for epilepsy. A 2018 consensus statement advocates for implementing a ketogenic diet in hard-to-manage epilepsy even before medical intractability, defined as failure of two or more antiseizure medications (see Appendix 19 on the ketogenic diet).

While the exact mechanisms are not clearly understood, therapeutic benefits may be due to neuronal metabolism, neurotransmitter function, neuronal membrane potential, and neuron protection against reactive oxygen species (Zhang et al, 2018). Two mouse models suggest the way the gut microbiota is altered by ketogenic diet therapy correlates to seizure protection (Olson et al, 2018) (Box 39.4).

It is absolutely contraindicated when a patient has a metabolic disorder that limits fat metabolism or carnitine production, and may be relatively contraindicated when there are certain issues that need to be addressed before initiating a ketogenic diet.

Originally designed using ratios of 4:1 or 3:1 (grams of fat to non-fat) to achieve strong and consistent ketosis, less restrictive versions are now available that can also be effective. The modified ketogenic diet uses lower ratios (e.g., 1:1 and 2:1), and modified Atkins and the low glycemic index treatment (LGIT) are also available for those who may benefit from a less restricted approach (Roehl and Sewak, 2017).

Glucose Transporter Type I Deficiency Syndrome (Glut-1 DS) and pyruvate dehydrogenase deficiency (PDHD) are two genetically inherited disorders that typically include seizures and are treatable with ketogenic diet therapy. The diet also has been effective for other inherited disorders in which seizures are also typical: glycogen storage diseases, nonketotic hyperglycinemia, and respiratory chain defects. The common feature of each of these conditions is the failure of the brain to derive adequate fuel from glucose. Ketones provided by ketogenic diet therapy offer an alternative fuel source which improves symptoms, preserves neurons, and can prevent further decline.

Short-term side effects include fatigue, headaches, nausea, emesis, constipation, hypoglycemia, or acidosis, especially in the first few weeks on the diet (Kossoff et al, 2018; Roehl and Sewak, 2017). An oral citrate or sodium bicarbonate can help buffer acidosis, or the dietary fat ratio can be decreased to improve tolerability and palatability. Ensuring adequate fiber and fluid can help manage gastrointestinal distress and improve compliance with the ketogenic diet.

Although the diet is restrictive and requires continued effort, ketogenic diets are effective in reducing seizure frequency by 50% or more in about half of patients who are otherwise resistant to drug therapy and considered to have refractory epilepsy.

Improvement in seizure control can take up to 3 months after diet has been implemented. Antiepileptic drugs are not stopped but may be reduced before initiation, if medication toxicity occurs, or after it has been established that the diet therapy is effective.

The majority of the diet is composed of fresh meats, eggs, cheese, fish, heavy whipping cream, butter, oils, nuts, and seeds. Vegetables and fruits are added in small amounts, within the current diet prescription. A carbohydrate-free multiple vitamin and mineral supplement is necessary to ensure that the diet is nutritionally complete. However, additional vitamins and minerals are often necessary, including calcium, vitamin D, and selenium. All prescription and over-the-counter medications (e.g., pain relievers, cold remedies, mouthwash, toothpaste, and lotions) must be scrutinized for sugar content to minimize carbohydrate. It is important that the diet be strictly followed; the smallest amount of extra carbohydrate can cause a breakthrough seizure. Weight and height should be monitored, because a rapid rate of weight gain can decrease ketosis and reduce effectiveness. The RDN should work closely with the patient throughout the course of therapy to ensure nutritional adequacy and optimal seizure control.

Attention to the patient's health status, growth, and development is required during the course of therapy. For the child whose epilepsy is controlled by diet, complying with the diet is much easier than dealing with devastating seizures and injuries.

As clinical and scientific research evolves, improvements in which diet to use, how long to use it, and specific guidelines for certain epilepsies will emerge. Some patients may benefit from a simple diet initially then graduate to the more restrictive ketogenic therapy based on their seizure outcome results. Others may start off with the most restrictive ketogenic therapy and transition to a less restrictive one for long-term maintenance (see Fig. 39.8 and Appendix 19).

Guillain-Barré Syndrome (GBS) and Chronic Inflammatory Demyelinating Polyneuropathy (CIDP)

GBS and chronic inflammatory demyelinating polyneuropathy (CIDP) are acute and chronic, respectively, acquired immune-mediated inflammatory disorders of the PNS. They are rare autoimmune disorders that damage the nerves, causing muscle weakness, and in severe cases, paralysis. The incidence of GBS is approximately 1 in 100,000, or about 3000 to 6000 people each year in the United States (CDC, 2017c). It is also called acute inflammatory demyelinating polyneuropathy and Landry's ascending paralysis. Similarly, there are 1 to 2 new cases of CIDP per 100,000 people in the United States each year (GBS-CIDP Foundation International, 2018). CIDP is sometimes called chronic relapsing polyneuropathy and is considered the chronic form of GBS.

Etiology

In 60% of GBS cases the disorder follows an infection, surgery, or an immunization. Some of the more common organisms are *Campylobacter jejuni* (responsible for up to 40% of cases in the United States) and *Mycoplasma* spp. It can also develop after flu, cytomegalovirus, Epstein-Barr virus, and Zika virus infection. In very rare cases, it can develop in the days and weeks following a vaccination. Despite an association with infections, GBS and CIDP are not contagious.

BOX 39.4 Gut Microbiota In Neurologic Conditions

The gut microbiota communicates with the central nervous system through the gut-brain axis. Gut microbiota dysbiosis is seen in neurologic diseases. Exactly how these are connected is not yet fully understood, but emerging science on the gut microbiome suggests a role in neurologic diseases. The gut and brain communicate via three basic mechanisms: direct neuronal communication, endocrine signaling mediators, and the immune system. Dietary habits can affect intestinal microbial composition, and microbiome dysbiosis may be one factor in the development of multiple sclerosis (MS) (Chu et al, 2018). People with Parkinson's disease and Alzheimer's disease also suffer from gut microbiota dysbiosis, though whether it is a cause or effect of the condition is not clearly understood (Parashar and Udayabanu, 2017; Westfall et al, 2017). Dietary factors can theoretically modulate chronic activation of inflammatory response in aging, a risk factor for many neurologic conditions (Erro et al, 2018). There is not enough evidence to support clinical recommendations at this time, but this is an active area of research. In the meantime, greater intake of fermented foods, polyphenols, and dietary fiber are generally safe ways to support a healthy microbiome.

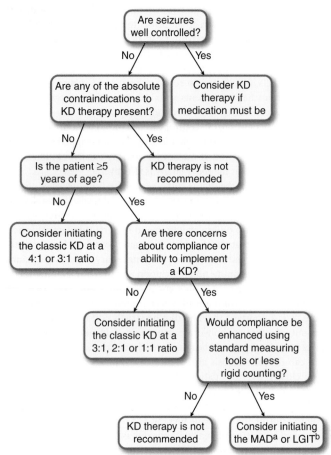

Fig. 39.8 Ketogenic diet (KD) therapy initiation decision tree. [a]*MAD*, Modified Atkins diet. [b]*LGIT,* low glycemic index treatment. (From *Journal of the Academy of Nutrition and Dietetics* 2017 117, 1279–1292. With permission from Elsevier).

Several pathologic varieties exist related to which segment of the immune system is inflicting nerve damage. The clinical course of GBS is similar regardless of subtype, although GBS after a *Campylobacter* infection tends to be more severe. Gluten sensitivity has been reported in some cases as a cause of GBS. The cause of CIDP is similar to GBS; however, the illness follows a longer course (Eldar and Chapman, 2014).

Pathophysiology

Relatively symmetric weakness with **paresthesia** (numbness and tingling) usually begins in the legs and progresses to the arms and face, potentially leading to paralysis. Chest muscles are affected in 20% to 30% of people with GBS, making it difficult to breathe (WHO, 2016b). In severe cases, the ability to speak and swallow is compromised, which is life-threatening and requires hospitalization. Most people fully recover within a few months of diagnosis and treatment, even from severe cases, though about 30% continue to experience some muscle weakness years after the first GBS symptom (NIH, Genetic and Rare Diseases [GARD] Information Center, 2017).

The loss of function in affected nerves occurs because of demyelination. **Myelin** is the specialized fatty insulation that envelops the conducting part of the nerve, the axon. In GBS, the immune system mounts an attack against the body's own myelin. Presumably myelin shares a common characteristic with the pathogen from the antecedent infection; thus the immune system cannot differentiate what is foreign (pathogen) from what is native (myelin). When the nerve is demyelinated, its ability to conduct signals is severely impaired, resulting in neuropathy.

Medical Management

GBS reveals itself in a matter of days. The most common sequence of symptoms is **areflexia** (absence of reflexes), followed by proximal limb weakness, cranial nerve weakness, and respiratory insufficiency. These symptoms normally peak by 2 weeks but may progress up to 1 month. Medical diagnosis is ordinarily made on clinical grounds, but nerve conduction studies are also beneficial. Before the clinical course is apparent, myelopathic disorders must be considered.

Because of the precipitous progression, vital capacity and swallowing function may rapidly deteriorate such that intensive care is sometimes necessary. Intubation and respiratory support should be instituted early in respiratory decline to avoid the need for resuscitation. Any endotracheal tube intubation lasting longer than 7 to 10 days increases the risk for laryngeal injury; this factor increases the risk of dysphagia. A systematic review of documented incidence of dysphagia following endotracheal intubation found that the highest rates of dysphagia (62%, 56%, and 51%) were in patients intubated for more than 24 hours (Skoretz et al, 2010).

Plasmapheresis, the exchange of the patient's plasma for albumin, is often helpful to reduce the load of circulating antibodies. Intravenous immunoglobulin or steroids have been shown to help.

Medical Nutrition Therapy

GBS progresses quickly. During the acute stage, the metabolic response of GBS is similar to the stress response that occurs in neurotrauma. Energy needs assessed by indirect calorimetry may be as high as 40 to 45 kcal/kg and protein needs are twice the usual amount. Supportive nutritional care should be offered to attenuate muscle wasting.

For a small percentage of patients, oropharyngeal muscles may be affected, leading to dysphagia and dysarthria. In this situation, a visit by the RDN at mealtime can be a valuable way to observe difficulties the patient may have with chewing or swallowing. Specific difficulties warrant evaluation by a swallowing specialist. The SLP can evaluate the degree of dysphagia and make appropriate dietary recommendations pertaining to texture. As the patient recovers, it is important to discuss safe food handling and future prevention of *C. jejuni* infection.

Myasthenia Gravis

Myasthenia gravis (MG) is the most well-known auto-immune disorder of the neuromuscular junction. The **neuromuscular junction** is the site on the striated muscle membrane where a spinal motor neuron connects. Here the signal from the nerve is carried to the muscle via a submicron-size gap: a synapse. The molecule that carries the signal from the nerve ending to the muscle membrane is acetylcholine (Ach), and acetylcholine receptors (AchRs) populate the muscle membrane. These receptors translate the chemical signal of Ach into an electrical signal that is required for contraction of muscle fibers. MG is one of the most well-characterized autoimmune diseases, a class of disorders in which the body's immune system raises a response to AchRs.

The prevalence of MG is approximately 14 to 20 per 100,000 people in the United States, or about 36,000 to 60,000 cases (Myasthenia Gravis Foundation of America, 2015). It is underdiagnosed and true prevalence is likely higher. Males are more affected than females, with symptoms appearing most commonly after age 50.

Pathophysiology

In MG the body unwittingly makes antibodies to AchR. These antibodies are the same that fight off colds. The AchR antibodies bind to

AchR and make them unresponsive to Ach. There is no disorder of nerve conduction and no intrinsic disorder of muscle. The characteristic weakness in MG occurs because the signal of the nervous system to the muscle is garbled at the neuromuscular junction. Patients with MG commonly have an overactive thymus gland. This gland resides in the anterior thorax and plays a role in the maturation of B-lymphocytes, the cells that are charged with synthesizing antibodies.

Relapsing and remitting weakness and fatigue, varying from minutes to days, characterize MG. The most common presentation is diplopia (double vision) caused by extraocular muscle weakness, followed by dysarthria, facial muscle weakness, and dysphagia. Dysphagia or swallowing disorders (resulting from fatigue after mastication) may cause malnutrition. Less commonly, proximal limb weakness in the hips and shoulders may be present. Severe diaphragmatic weakness can result in respiratory difficulty. Sensory nerves are not involved.

Medical Management

Anticholinesterases are medicines that inhibit acetylcholinesterase, thus serving to increase the amount of Ach in the neuromuscular junction. Removal of the thymus results in symptomatic improvement in most patients. Corticosteroids are immunosuppressive. Additional immunosuppressant drugs can reverse symptoms while in use, though each comes with side effects: azathioprine, cyclosporine, cyclophosphamide, mycophenolate mofetil, methotrexate, and eculizumab—a first-in-its-kind therapy for patients unresponsive to at least two immunotherapies for at least a year; it was approved by the FDA in October 2017. Plasma exchange is a short-term strategy for rapidly declining patients, to quickly strengthen patients before surgery and as intermittent therapy for those who are unresponsive to all other treatments. Intravenous immune globulin improves 50% to 100% of patients within a week and lasting several weeks or months; the mechanism is unknown (Myasthenia Gravis Foundation of America, 2015).

Medical Nutrition Therapy

Chewing and swallowing often are compromised in MG. Because this compromise is due to fatigue, it is important to provide nutritionally dense foods at the beginning of meals before the patient fatigues. Small, frequent meals that are easy to chew and swallow are helpful. Difficulties holding a bolus on the tongue have been observed, suggesting that foods that do not fall apart easily may be better tolerated, for example IDDSI level 5, minced and moist. For patients treated with anticholinesterase drugs, it is crucial to time medication with feeding to facilitate optimal swallowing.

Physical activity should be limited before mealtime to ensure maximum strength to eat a meal. It is also important not to encourage food consumption once the patient begins to fatigue because this may contribute to aspiration. If and when respiratory crisis occurs, it is usually temporary. Nutrition support via tube feeding may be implemented in the interim to assist in maintaining vital functions of the patient until the crisis subsides. Once extubated, a swallow evaluation using a videofluoroscopic swallow study (VFSS) is appropriate to assess the degree of deglutory dysfunction (swallowing irregularity) or risk of aspiration associated with an oral diet.

Multiple Sclerosis

Multiple sclerosis (MS) is a chronic inflammatory disorder of the CNS and is one of the most common causes of nontraumatic disability among young and middle-aged adults, more women than men and more common among people of Northern European ancestry (National Multiple Sclerosis Society, 2018a).

MS affects approximately 2.5 million worldwide. In the United States the National Multiple Sclerosis Society estimates that nearly 403

per 100,000 people are affected, representing nearly a million people, which is more than double previous estimates. This is according to preliminary results presented in October 2017 (National Multiple Sclerosis Society, 2017). MS symptoms can start anywhere between 10 and 80 years of age, but onset is usually between 20 and 40 years, with a mean of 32 years. Although MS is more frequently seen in European Americans than African Americans, the latter group appears to accumulate disability more quickly, suggesting more destructive tissue injury in this population. The prevalence of MS varies by geographic location and generally increases the further one travels from the equator in either hemisphere. It remains unclear whether this altered incidence represents an environmental influence, genetic difference, or variable surveillance (Hersh and Fox, 2018).

MS affects the CNS and is characterized by destruction of the myelin sheath, which protects nerve axons, which transmit electrical nerve impulses. Multiple areas of optic nerves, spinal cord, and brain undergo sclerosis, whereby myelin is replaced with sclera or scar tissue. No single test can ascertain whether a patient has MS; however, diagnostic criteria (revised McDonald criteria) were developed for use by practicing clinicians (Thompson et al, 2018).

The signs and symptoms of MS are easily distinguished, and they recur over the natural history of this disease. In the worst scenario, MS can render a person unable to write, speak, or walk. Fortunately, the majority of patients are only mildly affected.

Pathophysiology

The precise cause of MS remains undetermined. A familial predisposition to MS has been noted in a minority of cases. Geographic latitude and diet are implicated. Epidemiologic studies have linked the incidence of MS to geographic location and sunshine exposure. Studies have shown that people born in an area with a high risk of MS who then migrate to an area with a lower risk before the age of 15 assume the risk of their new area. Such data suggest that exposure to some environmental agent before puberty may predispose a person to develop MS.

There is growing evidence that higher sunlight exposure—and therefore vitamin D production—reduces the risk of MS, and poor levels of vitamin D have been linked to increased risk, suggesting a protective effect for vitamin D. The degree of sunlight exposure catalyzes the production of vitamin D in the skin. Vitamin D produced by the skin is eventually metabolized to vitamin D_3, which is a selective immune system regulator and may inhibit MS progression (Zahoor and Haq, 2017).

Given the current evidence of the potential benefits of vitamin D, it appears to be reasonable and safe to consider vitamin D supplementation adequate to achieve optimal levels in patients with MS, though the mechanism is not yet clearly understood (Rosen et al, 2016).

The evidence is also growing that smoking plays an important role in MS. Studies have shown that smoking increases a person's risk of developing MS and is associated with more severe and rapid disease progression. Fortunately, the evidence also suggests that stopping smoking—whether before or after the onset of MS—is associated with a slower progression of disability (National Multiple Sclerosis Society, 2015).

Obesity in childhood and adolescence, especially among females, has been shown to increase risk of developing MS later in life. There is some data of early adulthood obesity and increased risk as well, and obesity in the already diagnosed may exacerbate inflammation (Novo and Batista, 2017).

Various viruses and bacteria are being studied for their role in developing MS. For example, previous infection with Epstein-Barr virus (EBV) appears to increase the risk of developing MS. Human herpes virus 6 (HHV-6) is being studied related to triggering relapses. This is an area of active research. The theories that have been disproven include living with a dog or other small pet, having allergies, exposure to heavy metals, experiencing physical trauma, and exposure to aspartame (National Multiple Sclerosis Society, 2018b).

Four disease courses have been identified by the National Multiple Sclerosis Society:

1. Clinically isolated syndrome (CIS): an isolated episode lasting at least 24 hours that looks like MS but does not yet meet full criteria of diagnosis. People may or may not go on to develop MS.
2. Relapsing-remitting MS (RRMS): the most common type of MS (about 85% of new cases), RRMS is characterized by intermittent neurologic symptoms during attacks (relapses) followed by periods of remission during which the disease does not appear to progress (remissions).
3. Secondary progressive MS (SPMS): most people with RRMS eventually develop SPMS, in which disability progresses over time.
4. Primary progressive MS (PPMS): accounts for about 15% of people with MS, in which neurologic function declines from the onset of symptoms.

Medical Management

Fluctuating symptoms and spontaneous remissions make MS treatments difficult to evaluate. Medical intervention attempts to reduce exacerbation of symptoms, also called flares, manage daily manifestations of disease process, and slow, possibly halt, disease course (National Multiple Sclerosis Society, 2018). Initially, recovery from relapses is nearly complete, but over time, neurologic deficits remain. Therefore measures to maximize recovery from initial attacks or exacerbations, prevent fatigue and infection, and use all available rehabilitative measures to postpone the bedridden stage of disease are imperative. Rehabilitative services are standard practice for the management of weakness, spasticity, tremor, incoordination, and other symptoms.

Drugs for spasticity can be initiated at a low dose and cautiously increased until the patient responds. Physical therapy for gait training and range-of-motion exercises may be implemented. Steroid therapy is used in treating exacerbations; adrenocorticotropic hormone (ACTH) and prednisolone are the drugs of choice. However, treatment is not consistently effective and tends to be more useful in cases of less than 5 years' duration. Side effects of short-term steroid treatment include increased appetite, weight gain, fluid retention, nervousness, and insomnia. Reduced cerebrospinal fluid and serum levels of vitamin B_{12} and folate have been noted in MS patients who receive high-dose steroids. Methotrexate also may be used with ACTH, causing anorexia and nausea.

A 2014 guideline from the American Academy of Neurology provides a summary of evidence-based guidance on complementary and integrative medicine in MS including conclusions related to marijuana use for pain, spasticity, and reduced urinary frequency (American Academy of Neurology, 2014).

Medical Nutrition Therapy

The role of diet in MS requires continued prospective and clinical trials to fully illuminate. To date, there are preclinical models, epidemiologic studies, and a limited number of prospective studies that provide early direction on which specific dietary components and dietary patterns may have an impact.

In two epidemiologic studies of about 9000 total patients with MS, healthier eating habits were associated with lower levels of disability, and better mental health–related quality of life (Sand, 2018). While there are mixed data on high-fat (ketogenic) versus low-fat (Swank or McDougall) diets, longer terms studies seem to favor a diet lower in saturated fat.

- A pilot short-term trial of 60 RRMS patients suggests ketogenic and fasting-mimicking diet (FMD) of 3 days a week on a very-low-calorie diet had higher health-related quality of life at 3 months compared with controls.
- In the 1950s Dr. Swank started to follow a small group of 144 MS patients for more than 3 decades, and those who complied with a low-saturated-fat diet (<20 g/day) experienced significantly less disability and had lower mortality rates than those who did not. However, this study lacked randomization or controls for potential confounders, so it is more directional.
- A small study found the very-low-fat vegan McDougall diet (10% calories from fat) had neutral results (no differences in clinical relapses), but was only powered to find a much bigger shift and so there is now a larger trial underway to test its impact on fatigue.
- A prospective 2-year study in more than 200 pediatric MS patients found that saturated fat tripled the risk of relapse for every 10% increase in energy intake from saturated fat.
- A very small study of 10 subjects found that a Paleolithic diet in combination with dietary supplements, exercise program, electrical stimulation, and meditation significantly improved fatigue in PPMS patients.

Observational data suggest that the specific dietary components that may reduce the risk of MS include fish, marine sources of omega-3 fatty acids, vitamin D, fruits and vegetables, and whole grains. Preclinical studies suggest a high-salt diet may worsen disease progression, but human studies have found both positive and neutral associations, making sodium and MS a topic to watch in the scientific literature (Sand, 2018).

Though very little work has been done to date on the Mediterranean diet and MS, the preliminary evidence on foods and nutrients that may positively impact MS suggests it is worth studying. A pilot clinical trial of a modified Mediterranean diet in MS is in progress.

The National Multiple Sclerosis Society published a guide to vitamins, minerals, and herbs in 2015 that can be useful when working with an MS patient (National Multiple Sclerosis Society, 2015) (Table 39.10).

The RDN's evaluation of the patient to maximize nutritional intake is imperative. Vitamin D status should be assessed by measuring 25-hydroxy vitamin D. Evidence suggests high serum vitamin D may decrease the risk of MS and risk of relapse and new lesions, and supplementation may be warranted (Bagur et al, 2017). There is now some evidence that an antiinflammatory diet (see Chapter 7 and Appendix 22) can be of use in treating MS. This is an active area of research.

As the disease progresses, neurologic deficits and dysphagia may occur as the result of damaged cranial nerves. Thus, diet consistency may have to be modified along the IDDSI continuum of regular (level 7) to pureed (level 4) foods, even progressing to thickened liquids (levels 2 or 3) to prevent aspiration (IDDSI, 2017). Impaired vision, dysarthria, and poor ambulation make meal preparation difficult. In this situation, reliance on meal delivery services, prepackaged, single-serving, or convenience foods often permits independent preparation of meals. Given the chronic nature of this debilitating disease, patients may require enteral nutrition support.

Neurogenic bladder is common, causing urinary incontinence, urgency, and frequency. To minimize these problems, distributing fluids evenly throughout the waking hours and limiting them before bed is helpful. Some patients severely limit fluid intake to decrease urination frequency, which unintentionally increases the risk of UTIs. UTIs and recurrent falls are common in patients with MS and are associated with MS relapse (Zelaya et al, 2017).

Neurogenic bowel can cause either constipation or diarrhea, and incidence of fecal impaction is increased in MS. A diet that is high in

TABLE 39.10	**Supplemental Vitamins, Minerals, and Herbs Used in MS**			
Vit/Min/Herb	**Relation to MS**	**Risks**	**Food Sources**	**Role of RDN**
Vitamin D Evidence suggestive not conclusive	Higher blood levels associated with lower risk of developing MS For those with MS, low levels associated with increased risk of MS relapses and developing new MRI lesions and increased levels of disability	High doses may increase risk of kidney stones in some people	Fish, fortified dairy and plant-based alternatives, breakfast cereals. Also produced in the skin in response to sunlight.	Guide patients to choose food first and sensible sun exposure; for supplements, D3 supplement form preferred over D2; and stay under UL
AOX vitamins A, C, E	Preliminary evidence suggests damage caused by free radicals may be involved in the disease process	Safety of supplement AOX in MS not clearly established; theoretical risk of stimulating the immune system and MS has an overactive immune system part of the disease process, not good to stimulate. Given the theoretical benefits and risks, food sources are safest and supplements can be tested in moderation under care.	A wide variety of fruits and vegetables. A: eggs, fish, carrots, sweet potato, spinach, mangos, broccoli, salmon, pistachios. C: citrus, tomatoes, broccoli, kiwi, bell peppers, strawberries, cauliflower, peas, brussels sprouts, cantaloupe, spinach. E: almonds, hazelnuts, peanut butter, spinach, broccoli, sunflower seeds, safflower oil, sunflower oil, peanuts, corn oil, soybean oil.	Encourage food sources over supplements
B_6	No clear link, but patients reportedly take for help with energy	High doses can cause numbness, tingling or pain at doses as low as 50–100 mg/d	B_6: chickpeas, yellowfin tuna, salmon, chicken breast, fortified cereals, turkey, banana, bulgur, cottage cheese, winter squash, rice, nuts, onions, spinach, tofu, watermelon.	DRI level from food and dietary supplements. Do not exceed the UL
B_{12}	People with MS have low B_{12} more than general population; no evidence that normal B_{12} levels in MS patient and then supplementation does anything to improve MS	N/A	Eggs, meat, poultry, shellfish, dairy products	Supplement if necessary, especially if serum B_{12} is low or methylmalonic acid (MMA) level is elevated.
Selenium	Observational data that selenium levels are lower in people with MS than general population; but in animal study selenium supplementation worsened an MS-like disease	Theoretically may increase the immune response	Seafood, beans, whole grains, low-fat meats, dairy	Get selenium from foods; if using supplements, avoid exceeding the UL
Calcium	Old hypothesis with very little evidence supporting it that MS was linked to high intake of milk in childhood with sudden drop off in teen years Could help generally with bone health and this population tends to be at risk for osteoporosis		Dairy, eggs, green leafy vegetables, bone-in anchovies, calcium-made tofu	Encourage food sources at the DRI level or supplementation if dietary adequacy is not achieved.
Zinc	Data is equivocal; may activate immune system; may worsen an animal model of MS	High dose can cause copper deficiency leading to copper-deficiency myelopathy, which causes symptoms that mimic MS	Zinc Oysters, beef, crab, fortified cereal, beans, chicken, yogurt, cashews, chickpeas, oatmeal, milk, almonds, kidney beans, peas, flounder	Food and supplemental forms not exceeding the RDA

Continued

TABLE 39.10	Supplemental Vitamins, Minerals, and Herbs Used in MS—cont'd			
Vit/Min/Herb	**Relation to MS**	**Risks**	**Food Sources**	**Role of RDN**
Ginkgo Biloba	One small study shows it may help improve MS fatigue; inhibits platelet activating factor to decrease activity of certain immune cells, theoretically could help MS; two human studies: one suggested benefit, the larger showed no benefit to prevent relapses or cognitive dysfunction	May inhibit blood clotting so avoid on bleeding disorder or blood-thinning, or surgery; may interact with medications	Ginkgo	Discuss with health care team
St. John's Wort	No published data on effects on immune system that could concern MS patients. Typically used for depression.	Interactions with medications for MS	St. John's wort	Check for drug nutrient interactions and consult care team about interventions for depression
Valerian	Not studied in MS population; used to help with sleep as MS patients may have difficulty sleeping and fatigue; valerian could decrease time to sleep	May increase effects of sedating drugs prescription	Valerian root	Check for drug nutrient interactions
Asian ginseng Panax ginseng	One small MS study reports improvement in fatigue; inconsistent results in general population studies	May stimulate immune system		Too little evidence to gauge effectiveness
Cranberry	May help prevent UTI, a common issue in MS	May interact with warfarin/ Coumadin	Cranberry juice, sauce, fresh	Monitor blood glucose with diabetes, check for drug nutrient interactions
Marijuana, most specifically cannabidiol (CBD)	Acts on CNS in ways that may reduce MS symptoms and slow disease activity		Recomendation from AAN summary of evidence: https://www.nationalmssociety.org/Treating-MS/Complementary-Alternative-Medicines/Marijuana	Work in accordance with legal regulations, but consider for medicinal use

AAN, American Academy of Neurology; *CNS,* central nervous system; *MRI,* magnetic resonance imaging; *MS,* multiple sclerosis; *RDA,* recommended dietary allowance; *UL,* tolerable upper intake level; *UTI,* urinary tract infection.
Table created by Maggie Moon, MS, RDN, based on information presented at National Multiple Sclerosis Society, 2015

fiber with additional prunes and adequate fluid can moderate both problems.

Parkinson's Disease

Parkinson's disease (PD) is a progressive, disabling, neurodegenerative disease, first described by James Parkinson in 1817. PD is characterized by motor system dysfunction, seen as trembling in the hands, arms, legs, jaw, and face; rigid or stiff limbs and trunk; bradykinesia or slow movement; and impaired balance and coordination. These signs are due to the loss of dopamine-producing brain cells (NIH, National Institute of Neurological Disorders and Stroke [NINDS], 2018).

Although the natural history of this disease can be remarkably benign in some cases, approximately 66% of patients are disabled within 5 years and 80% are disabled after 10 years (Yao et al, 2013). MCI or dementia may affect up to 80% of people with PD (Goldman et al, 2018).

PD is one of the most common neurologic diseases in North America, costing an estimated $25 billion a year in the United States (Parkinson's Foundation, 2018). About 1 million people in the United States live with PD, and about 60,000 will be diagnosed each year. Prevalence by state is available at Parkinson's Foundation. The incidence is similar across socioeconomic groups, although PD is less common in African Americans and Asians compared with European Americans. It most commonly occurs between the ages of 40 and 70, and affects men 1.5 times more than women. Risk increases slightly if there is family history of PD or ongoing exposure to herbicides and pesticides.

Pathophysiology

PD is caused by the progressive impairment or deterioration of dopaminergic neurons in an area of the brain known as the substantia nigra, which sits within the midbrain, beneath the cerebral cortex, functionally part of the basal ganglia. When functioning normally, these neurons produce the vital neurotransmitter dopamine. The cause of PD is unknown, but several factors appear to play a role. The presence of Lewy bodies, which are clumps of specific substances within brain cells, are microscopic markers of PD. Researchers believe these Lewy bodies hold an important clue to the cause of PD. Lewy bodies are proteins found in abundance in the brainstem area that deplete the neurotransmitter dopamine.

The role of endogenous toxins from cellular oxidative reactions has emerged because aging has been associated with a loss of dopamine-containing neurons and an increase in monoamine oxidase, an enzyme that removes dopamine from the brain (Gaweska and Fitzpatrick, 2011). When metabolized (enzymatic oxidation and autoxidation), dopamine produces endogenous toxins (hydrogen peroxide and free radicals), causing peroxidation of membrane lipids and cell death. In the presence of an inherited or acquired predisposition, severe oxidative injury can lead to substantial loss of dopaminergic neurons similar to that observed in PD.

Several other environmental factors also have been implicated as causal factors of PD. The connection between smoking and a lowered risk for PD has been evaluated for therapeutic potential in epidemiologic and basic research studies, but clinical results remain inconsistent (Ma et al, 2017). In older patients, drug-induced PD may occur as a side effect of neuroleptics or metoclopramide (see Appendix 13).

Recent epidemiologic studies have shown a link between PD and environmental factors including drinking well water, rural living, farming, diet, and exposure to agricultural chemicals (Pan-Montojo and Reichmann, 2014). PD has also been linked to exposure to different metals and industrial compounds. Many studies performed in the 1990s identified manganese, lead, copper, iron, zinc, aluminium, or amalgam. Higher incidence of PD has been reported in manganese miners. It was shown that manganese, a component of various pesticides, also reproduces PD symptoms after long and chronic exposure (between 6 months and 16 years). Remarkably, some populations have witnessed a decreasing prevalence of certain types of neurodegenerative diseases that coincide with the disappearance of an environmental factor unique to these populations (Pan-Montojo and Reichmann, 2014). A meta-analysis of observational studies found that 5 and 10 years of pesticide exposure were associated with 5% and 11% increased risk of developing PD (Yan et al, 2018).

Nutrient-related findings are biologically plausible and support the hypothesis that oxidative stress may contribute to the pathogenesis of PD (Członkowska and Kurkowska-Jastrzębska, 2011). The relationships of folate, elevated plasma homocysteine levels, and caloric deficits are being evaluated.

Medical Management

The five clinical signs—resting tremor (e.g., limbs, head, and presence of pill rolling), rigidity (e.g., resistance to passive range of motion), bradykinesia (e.g., slow initiation of movement), akinesia (e.g., festinating gait, masked face, reduced limb movement), and postural abnormalities (e.g., stooped and poor adjustment to tilting or falling)—remain the criteria for medical diagnosis. In the 1960s, L-dopa (a precursor to dopamine) was introduced for controlling PD symptoms of bradykinesia, rigidity, and tremor, and it remains the most effective pharmacologic agent to treat PD today (Lees at al, 2015). Sinemet is a combination of levodopa and carbidopa, which enhances levodopa, helping to lower the effective dosage and reduce side effects. Safinamide is sometimes added to the regimen when new symptoms appear. Types of medications include dopamine precursors, inhibitors of levodopa breakdown, dopamine agonists, inhibitors of dopamine breakdown (monoamine oxidase [MAO]-B inhibitors), and anticholinergic. A full list of Parkinson's medications approved in the United States and common side effects are available at the website for the American Parkinson Disease Association.

Pharmacotherapy agents, surgical interventions, and physical therapy are the best adjunctive therapies.

Medical Nutrition Therapy

The primary focus of nutrition intervention is to optimize dietary intake, particularly to maintain muscle mass for strength and mobility. One cross-sectional study of more than 1000 individuals suggests a diet pattern rich in vegetables, fruits, nuts, fish, and olive oil was associated with a slower rate of PD progression (Mischley et al, 2017).

Nutrition intervention should also focus on drug-nutrient interactions, especially between dietary protein and L-dopa. Side effects of medications for PD include anorexia, nausea, reduced sense of smell, constipation, and dry mouth. To diminish the gastrointestinal side effects of L-dopa, it should be taken with meals. Foods that contain natural L-dopa such as broad beans (fava beans) should be avoided. For some patients, dyskinesia may be reduced by limiting dietary protein at breakfast and lunch and including it in the evening meal. Table 39.11 presents a sample menu for this diet.

TABLE 39.11 Dietary Protein Redistribution with L-Dopa Therapy

	Amount of Protein (g)
Breakfast	
½ C oatmeal	2
1 orange	0.5
1 C Rice Dream beverage	0.5
Egg replacer (unlimited)	0
Low-protein bread toast	0
Olive oil (unlimited)	0
Fruit (unlimited)	0
Coffee or tea (unlimited)	0
Lunch	
½ C vegetable soup	2
1 C tossed salad	1
Salad dressing (unlimited)	0
1 banana	1
Low-protein pasta (unlimited)	0
Olive oil (unlimited)	0
Juice, coffee, tea, or water	0
Afternoon Snack	
Fruit-only smoothies (unlimited)	0
100% juice (up to half of total daily fruit)	0
Total	7
Dinner	
4 oz (at least) fish, chicken, pork, beef	28 or more
1 C stuffing	4
Gravy	0
½ C peas	2
¾ C yogurt	8
1 C milk	8
Evening Snack	
1 oz cheese or deli meat	7
4 crackers	2
Water, herbal tea, or 100% juice	0
Daily total	73 or more

Fiber and fluid adequacy lessen constipation, a common concern for people with PD. Pyridoxine (vitamin B_6) has a possible efficacy-lowering interaction with L-dopa. Decarboxylase, the enzyme required to convert L-dopa to dopamine, depends on pyridoxine. The nutrient-drug interaction does not occur when carbidopa is used in combination with levodopa (Sinemet), which it commonly is, so likelihood of occurrence is low (Hansten and Horn, 1997). Interactions between pyridoxine and aspartame should be considered as well. In addition, manganese should be carefully monitored to avoid excesses above dietary reference intake (DRI) levels. The high demand for molecular oxygen, the enrichment of polyunsaturated fatty acids in membrane phospholipids, and the relatively low abundance of antioxidant defense enzymes are all relevant factors (Sun et al, 2008). Antiinflammatory and neuroprotective effects come from phenolic compounds, such as resveratrol from grapes and red wine, curcumin from turmeric, and epigallocatechin from green tea (Sun et al, 2008). Sufficient intake of vitamin D_3 and omega-3 fatty acids should be recommended.

In a small clinical study seven volunteers with PD agreed to maintain a ketogenic diet for 1 month. Five had improvement in their postdiet test scores (Hashim and VanItallie, 2014). An 8-week pilot RCT of 38 PD patients tested a low-fat versus ketogenic diet (Phillips et al, 2018), and both groups significantly improved motor symptoms. However, at least in the short term of 8 weeks, the ketogenic group had greater improvements in nonmotor symptoms. Although these studies are preliminary in nature, they raise awareness for the potential role of ketogenic diet therapy in this disease

A yearlong study of 257 patients with PD and 198 controls found that those who were more compliant with a Mediterranean diet had later age-at-onset of PD (Alcalay et al, 2012); these findings match large epidemiologic studies (Gao et al, 2007).

As the disease progresses, rigidity of the extremities can interfere with the patient's ability to eat independently. Rigidity interferes with the ability to control the position of the head and trunk, necessary for eating. Eating is slowed; mealtimes can take up to an hour. Simultaneous movements such as those required to handle a knife and fork become difficult. Tremors in the arms and hands may make consuming liquids independently impossible without spilling. Perception and spatial organization can become impaired. Dysphagia is often a late complication. Patients may be silent aspirators, that is the individual will aspirate without a cough response, a change to voicing, or a latent protective behavior such as a throat clear, which affects nutrition status and increases the risk for aspiration pneumonia.

Experimental treatment procedures are an active area of study. Deep brain stimulation, other surgical interventions, and efforts with stem cell research continue in hope of a cure. Over the counter and complementary therapies are also common, and the Parkinson's Foundation maintains a summary of these, including two of the most common: coenzyme Q_{10} and St. John's Wort. A common supplement is coenzyme Q_{10}, which has been used safely in studies lasting up to 5 years (Natural Medicines Database, 2018a). Data are mixed on coenzyme Q_{10} and PD, but appear to either neutralize or improve activities of daily living and slow functional decline for early Parkinson's. A large clinical trial was stopped midstudy in 2011 due to lack of improvement in delaying early PD progression (Parkinson Study Group QE3 Investigators, 2014). St. John's Wort is another popular supplement that may be effective for mild to moderate depression (Natural Medicines Database, 2018b).

CLINICAL CASE STUDY

Michael is a 67-year-old white man who is a lifelong resident of Sherman Oaks, CA, a suburb of Los Angeles. He was a high school football star and now runs a small landscaping business and volunteers as a local football coach. He enjoys taking walks in a park that is next to a large freeway. Sometimes he will go on an easy hike in the nearby hills with his wife, Lisa. They are happily married and both love Mexican food (especially chips and salsa, tacos, and margaritas) and music by the Beatles.

Michael was diagnosed with Parkinson's disease 3 years ago, after Lisa noticed that his hands were shaking at rest. She noted that he had been complaining about having to move more slowly at work and at football practices, too.

Michael is coming in for a regular check-up appointment. He has been taking Sinemet (mix of levodopa and carbidopa) and Neupro (rotigotine) to control his symptoms. His symptoms are well managed, but he's experienced some nausea and dizziness on these medications that he just lives with because they keep him functional. He also takes coenzyme Q_{10}, St. John's Wort, and a high potency multivitamin with 75 mg pyridoxine.

He is 6'0" and currently weighs 160 lb. He was 180 lb at his last visit 3 months ago. Lisa thinks he's lost a little weight, but isn't sure. He's always been fit and lean. What she has noticed is that they don't talk as much during meals anymore and that it takes him a long time to finish his food. After speaking with the couple for a while, Lisa remembers one time recently when she'd made his favorite banana bread and the whole house smelled amazing, but he didn't notice. Her feelings had been hurt. She admits that sometimes he loses interest and doesn't seem to have the energy to finish his meals. When she encourages him to eat, he can be either apathetic or irritable.

Nutrition Diagnostic Statements

- Inadequate energy intake related to PD progression, hyposmia, and decreased appetite, as evidenced by recent weight loss of 12% in 3 months (severe), decreased food intake, and fatigue.
- Difficulty swallowing related to PD progression as evidenced by slow eating pace.
- Environmental factors to consider are long-term exposure to car pollution and herbicides from his landscaping work.

Nutrition Care Questions

1. What dietary advice do you have for Michael and his caregiver?
2. What changes in Michael's diet and lifestyle would you recommend?
3. What other evaluations does Michael need?
4. What possible food-drug interactions could be occurring?
5. What strategies can Michael use to decrease his exposure to car pollution and herbicides?

USEFUL WEBSITES

Alzheimer's Association
American Academy of Neurology
American Parkinson Disease Association
American Stroke Association
Centers for Disease Control and Prevention (CDC): Stroke Education Materials for Health Professionals
The Charlie Foundation for Ketogenic Therapies
Clinical Trials
Epilepsy Foundation
GBS-CIDP Foundation International
International Dysphagia Diet Standardisation Initiative (IDDSI)
KetoDietCalculator
The Michael J. Fox Foundation for Parkinson's Research
Migraine Awareness Group

Myasthenia Gravis Foundation of America, Inc

National Headache Foundation

National Human Genome Research Institute

National Institutes of Health: Genetic and Rare Disease Information Center (NIH, GARD)

National Institutes of Health: National Institute on Aging (NIH, NIA)

National Institutes of Health: National Institute of Neurological Disorders and Stroke (NIH, NINDS)

National Multiple Sclerosis Society

Parkinson's Foundation

Phenol Explorer

USDA Database for the Flavonoid Content of Selected Foods

REFERENCES

Academy of Nutrition and Dietetics Evidence Analysis Library: *Spinal Cord Injury (SCI) guideline*, 2009. Available at: https://www.andeal.org/topic.cfm?menu=5292&cat=3485.

Albert MS, et al: The diagnosis of mild cognitive impairment due to Alzheimer's disease: Recommendations from the National Institute on Aging – Alzheimer's Association workgroups on diagnostic guidelines for Alzheimer's disease, *Alzheimers Dement* 7(3):270–279, 2011.

Alcalay RN, et al: The association between Mediterranean diet adherence and Parkinson's disease, *Mov Disord* 27(6):771–774, 2012.

American Academy of Neurology Guideline Subcommittee: Summary of evidence-based guideline: Complementary and alternative medicine in multiple sclerosis, *Neurology* 82(12):1083–1092, 2014.

American Heart Association Statistics Committee and Stroke Statistics Subcommittee: Heart disease and stroke statistics—2017 update: a report from the American Heart Association, *Circulation* 135:e229–e445, 2017.

American Heart Association Stroke Council, Council on Cardiovascular and Stroke Nursing, Council on Clinical Cardiology, et al: Guidelines for adult stroke rehabilitation and recovery: a guideline for healthcare professionals from the American Heart Association/American Stroke Association, *Stroke* 47:e98–e169, 2016.

Anderson JG, Lopez RP, Rose KM, et al: Nonpharmacological strategies for patients with early-stage dementia or mild cognitive impairment: a 10-year update, *Res Gerontol Nurs* 10(1):5–11, 2017.

Arthur KC, Calvo A, Price TR, et al: Projected increase in amyotrophic lateral sclerosis from 2015 to 2040, *Nat Commun* 7:12408, 2016.

Bagur MJ, Murcia MA, Jiménez-Monreal AM, et al: Influence of diet in multiple sclerosis: a systematic review, *Adv Nutr* 8(3):463–472, 2017.

Beal J, Silverman B, Bellant J, et al: Late onset necrotizing enterocolitis in infants following use of xanthan gum-containing thickening agent, *J Pediatr* 161(2):354–6, 2012.

Brain Trauma Foundation: *Guidelines for the management of severe traumatic brain injury*, ed 3, New York, NY, 2007, Brain Trauma Foundation. Available at: https://www.braintrauma.org/uploads/11/14/Guidelines_Management_2007w_bookmarks_2.pdf.

Bulgarelli K: Proposal for the testing of a tool for assessing the risk of dehydration in the elderly patient, *Acta Biomed* 86(2):134–141, 2015.

Carlaw C, Finlayson H, Beggs K, et al: Outcomes of a pilot water protocol project in a rehabilitation setting, *Dysphagia* 27:297–306, 2012. doi:10.1007/s00455-011-9366-9.

Carney N, Totten AM, O'Reilly C, et al: Guidelines for the management of severe traumatic brain injury, 4th edition, *Neurosurgery* 80(1):6–15, 2017.

Centers for Disease Control and Prevention: *Stroke statistics*, 2017a. Available at: https://www.cdc.gov/stroke/facts.htm.

Centers for Disease Control and Prevention: *Epilepsy fast facts*, 2017b. Available at: https://www.cdc.gov/epilepsy/about/fast-facts.htm.

Centers for Disease Control and Prevention: *Guillain-Barré syndrome: How common is GBS?* 2017c. Available at: https://www.cdc.gov/campylobacter/guillain-barre.html.

Centers for Disease Control and Prevention: *Preventing stroke: healthy living*, 2018a. Available at: https://www.cdc.gov/stroke/healthy_living.htm.

Centers for Disease Control and Prevention: *Alzheimer's disease*, 2018b. Available at: https://www.cdc.gov/dotw/alzheimers/index.html.

Centers for Disease Control and Prevention: *Promoting health and independence for an aging population at a glance*, 2018c. Available at: https://www.cdc.gov/chronicdisease/resources/publications/aag/alzheimers.htm.

Chen Y, Polara F, Pillai A: Rare variability in adrenoleukodystrophy: a case report, *J Med Case Rep* 12(1):182, 2018.

Chu F, Shi M, Lang Y, et al: Gut microbiota in multiple sclerosis and experimental autoimmune encephalomyelitis: current applications and future perspectives, *Mediators Inflamm* 2018:8168717, 2018.

Cichero JA, Steele C, Duivestein J, et al. The need for international terminology and definitions for texture-modified foods and thickened liquids used in dysphagia management: foundations of a global initiative, *Curr Phys Med Rehabil Rep* 1:280–291, 2013.

Coyle JL: Medical speech pathology: *Managing dysphagia in complex adult patients with pulmonary, digestive, and airway disorders*, Seattle, WA, June 2018, Northern Speech Services, Inc.

Członkowska A, Kurkowska-Jastrzębska I: Inflammation and gliosis in neurological diseases—clinical implications, *J Neuroimmunol* 231:78–85, 2011.

DiTucci A: Academy of Nutrition and Dietetics evidence based spinal cord injury nutrition practice guidelines and research opportunities, *J Acad Nutr Diet* 114(9):A34, 2014.

Dorst J, Ludolph AC, Huebers A: Disease-modifying and symptomatic treatment of amyotrophic lateral sclerosis, *Ther Adv Neurol Disord* 11:1–16, 2018.

Duffy JR: *Motor speech disorders: Substrates, differential diagnosis, and management*, ed 3, St. Louis, MO, 2013, Elsevier Mosby.

Dyall SC: Long-chain omega-3 fatty acids and the brain: a review of the independent and shared effects of EPA, DPA and DHA, *Front Aging Neurosci* 7:52, 2015.

Eldar AH, Chapman J: Guillain Barré syndrome and other immune mediated neuropathies: diagnosis and classification, *Autoimmun Rev* 13:525–530, 2014.

Engelen M, Barbier M, Dijkstra IM, et al: X-linked adrenoleukodystrophy in women: a cross-sectional cohort study, *Brain* 137(Pt 3):693–706, 2014.

Erro R, Brigo F, Tamburin S, et al: Nutritional habits, risk, and progression of Parkinson disease, *J Neurol* 265(1):12–23, 2018.

Estruch R, Ros E, Salas-Salvadó J, et al: Primary prevention of cardiovascular disease with a Mediterranean diet supplemented with extra-virgin olive oil or nuts, *N Engl J Med* 378(25):e34, 2018.

Figueira I, Menezes R, Macedo D, et al: Polyphenols beyond barriers: a glimpse into the brain, *Curr Neuropharmacol* 15(4):562–594, 2017.

Gao X, Chen H, Fung TT, et al: Prospective study of dietary pattern and risk of Parkinson disease, *Am J Clin Nutr* 86:1486–1494, 2007.

Gardener SL, Rainey-Smith SR: The role of nutrition in cognitive function and brain ageing in the elderly, *Curr Nutr Rep* 7(3):139–149, 2018. https://www.ncbi.nlm.nih.gov/pubmed/29974344.

Gaweska H, Fitzpatrick PF: Structures and mechanism of the monoamine oxidase family, *Biomol Concepts* 2(5):365–377, 2011.

GBD 2015 Neurological Disorders Collaborator Group: Global, regional, and national burden of neurological disorders during 1990-2015: a systematic analysis for the Global Burden of Disease Study 2015, *Lancet Neurol* 16(11):877–897, 2017.

GBS-CIDP Foundation International: *What is chronic inflammatory demyelinating polyneuropathy (CIPD)?* 2018. Available at: https://www.gbs-cidp.org/cidp/.

Goldman JG, Vernaleo BA, Camicioli R, et al: Cognitive impairment in Parkinson's disease: A report from a multidisciplinary symposium on unmet needs and future directions to maintain cognitive health, *NPJ Parkinsons Dis* 4:19, 2018.

Greenberg DA, Aminoff MJ, Simon RP: *Clinical neurology*, 8th ed, New York, NY, 2012, McGraw-Hill Companies, Inc.

Hadjivassiliou M, Sanders DS, Grünewald RA, et al: Gluten sensitivity: from gut to brain, *Lancet Neurol* 9:318–330, 2010.

Hadjivassiliou M, Sanders DD, Aeschlimann DP: Gluten-related disorders: gluten ataxia, *Dig Dis* 33(2):264–8, 2015.

Hansten PD, Horn JR: *Drug interactions analysis and management*, Vancouver, WA, 1997, Applied Therapeutics Inc. Accessed through Natural Medicines Database monograph on pyridoxine. Available with subscription at: https://

naturalmedicines.therapeuticresearch.com/databases/food,-herbs-supplements/professional.aspx?productid=934#interactionsWithDrugs.

Hashim SA, VanItallie TB: Ketone body therapy: from the ketogenic diet to the oral administration of ketone ester, *J Lipid Res* 55:1818–1826, 2014.

Hersh CM, Fox RJ: *Multiple sclerosis*, 2018. Available at: http://www.clevelandclinicmeded.com/medicalpubs/diseasemanagement/neurology/multiple_sclerosis/Default.htm#top.

Hollinger SK, Okosun IS, Mitchell CS: Antecedent disease and amyotrophic lateral sclerosis: What is protecting whom? *Front Neurol* 7:47, 2016.

Hovda DA: *The translation of the science of traumatic brain injury from bench to bedside and back.* Academy of Neurologic Communication Disorders and Sciences: 2017 Annual Meeting, Los Angeles, CA, November, 2017.

Hung KL, Wang JS, Keng WT, et al: Mutational analyses on X-linked adrenoleukodystrophy reveal a novel cryptic splicing and three missense mutations in the ABCD1 gene, *Pediatr Neurol* 49:185–190, 2013.

Iacoviello L, Bonaccio M, Cairella G, et al: Diet and primary prevention of stroke: Systematic review and dietary recommendations by the ad hoc Working Group of the Italian Society of Human Nutrition, *Nutr Metab Cardiovasc Dis* 28:309–334, 2018.

International Dysphagia Diet Standardisation Initiative: *Complete IDDSI framework: detailed definitions*, March 4, 2017. Available at: http://iddsi.org/framework/.

Jack CR, Albert MS, Knopman DS, et al: Introduction to the recommendations from the National Institute on Aging-Alzheimer's Association workgroups on diagnostic guidelines for Alzheimer's disease, *Alzheimers Dement* 7(3):257–262, 2011.

Kim B, Jin Y, Kim SH, et al: Association between macronutrient intake and amyotrophic lateral sclerosis prognosis, *Nutr Neurosci*, 1–8, 2018.

Kim EH, Ko TS: Cognitive impairment in childhood onset epilepsy: up-to-date information about its causes, *Korean J Pediatr* 59(4):155–164, 2016.

Kim Y, Clifton P: Curcumin, cardiometabolic health and dementia, *Int J Environ Res Public Health* 15:E2093, 2018.

Kossoff EH, Zupec-Kania BA, Auvin S, et al: Optimal clinical management of children receiving dietary therapies for epilepsy: updated recommendations of the International Ketogenic Diet Study Group, *Epilepsia Open* 3(2): 175–192, 2018.

Lees AJ, Tolosa E, Olanow CW: Four pioneers of L-dopa treatment: Arvid Carlsson, Oleh Hornykiewicz, George Cotzias, and Melvin Yahr, *Mov Disord* 30(1):19–36, 2015.

Ma C, Liu Y, Neumann S, et al: Nicotine from cigarette smoking and diet and Parkinson disease: a review, *Transl Neurodegener* 6:18, 2017.

McCullough G, Pelletier C, Steele C: National Dysphagia Diet: What to swallow? *The ASHA Leader*, November 2003.

McDougall A, Bayley M, Munce SE: The ketogenic diet as a treatment for traumatic brain injury: a scoping review, *Brain Inj* 32(4):416–422, 2018.

McKhann GM, Knopman DS, Chertkow H, et al: The diagnosis of dementia due to Alzheimer's disease: Recommendations from the National Institute on Aging-Alzheimer's Association workgroups on diagnostic guidelines for Alzheimer's disease, *Alzheimers Dement* 7(3):263–269, 2011.

Mehta P, Kaye W, Raymond J, et al: Prevalence of amyotrophic lateral sclerosis – United States, 2014, *MMWR Morb Mortal Wkly Rep* 67: 216–218, 2018.

Meschia JF, Bushnell C, Boden-Albala B, et al: Guidelines for the primary prevention of stroke: a statement for healthcare professionals from the American Heart Association/American Stroke Association, *Stroke* 45: 3754–3832, 2014.

Mischley LK, Lau RC, Bennett RD: Role of diet and nutritional supplements in Parkinson's disease progression, *Oxid Med Cell Longev* 2017:6405278, 2017.

Morita M, Honda A, Kobayashi A, et al: Effect of Lorenzo's oil on hepatic gene expression and the serum fatty acid level in abcd1-deficient mice, *JIMD Rep* 38:67–74, 2018.

Morris MC, Tangney CC, Wang Y, et al: MIND diet slows cognitive decline with aging, *Alzheimers Dement* 11(9):1015–1022, 2015a.

Morris MC, Tangney CC, Wang Y, et al: MIND diet associated with reduced incidence of Alzheimer's disease, *Alzheimers Dement* 11(9):1007–1014, 2015b.

Morris MC. Nutritional determinants of cognitive aging and dementia, *Proc Nutr Soc* 71(1):1–13, 2012.

Myasthenia Gravis Foundation of America: *Clinical overview of MG*, 2015. Available at: https://cdn.ymaws.com/www.chronicdisease.org/resource/resmgrHealthy_Aging_Critical_Issues_Brief/ReachOutActionGuide.pdf.

Myers PS: *Right hemisphere damage: disorders of communication and cognition*, Clifton Park, NY, 2009, Delmar Cengage Learning.

National Association of Chronic Disease Directors: *Implementing a community-based program for dementia caregivers: an action guide using REACH OUT*, 2009. Available at: https://cdn.ymaws.com/www.chronicdisease.org/resource/resmgrHealthy_Aging_Critical_Issues_Brief/ReachOutActionGuide.pdf.

National Dysphagia Diet Task Force: *National Dysphagia Diet: standardization for optimal care*, Chicago, IL, 2002, American Dietetic Association.

National Institutes of Health: *Genetic and Rare Diseases (GARD) Information Center: Amyotrophic lateral sclerosis*, 2018. Available at: https://rarediseases.info.nih.gov/diseases/5786/amyotrophic-lateral-sclerosis.

National Institutes of Health: *Genetic and Rare Diseases (GARD) Information Center: Guillain-Barre syndrome*, 2017. Available at: https://rarediseases.info.nih.gov/diseases/6554/guillain-barre-syndrome#ref_1747.

National Institutes of Health: *National Center for Complimentary and Integrative Health (NCCIH): Omega-3 supplements: an introduction*, 2013. Available at: https://nccih.nih.gov/health/omega3/introduction.htm.

National Institutes of Health: *National Institute of Neurological Disorders and Stroke: Parkinson's disease information page*, 2018. Available at: https://www.ninds.nih.gov/Disorders/All-Disorders/Parkinsons-Disease-Information-Page.

National Multiple Sclerosis Society: *Preliminary results of MS prevalence study estimate nearly 1 million living with MS in the U.S.*, presented at ECTRIMS, October 26, 2017. Available at: https://www.nationalmssociety.org/About-the-Society/News/Preliminary-Results-of-MS-Prevalence-Study.

National Multiple Sclerosis Society: *Smoking*, 2015. Available at: https://www.nationalmssociety.org/NationalMSSociety/media/MSNationalFiles/Research/Stroup_T_Smoking_and_MS_20151110.pdf.

National Multiple Sclerosis Society: *Treating MS: Medications*, 2018. Available at: https://www.nationalmssociety.org/Treating-MS/Medications.

National Multiple Sclerosis Society: *Vitamins, minerals & herbs in MS: an introduction*, 2015. Available at: https://www.nationalmssociety.org/NationalMSSociety/media/MSNationalFiles/Brochures/Brochure-Vitamins,-Minerals,-and-Herbs-in-MS_-An-Introduction.pdf.

National Multiple Sclerosis Society: *Who gets MS?* 2018a. Available at: https://www.nationalmssociety.org/What-is-MS/Who-Gets-MS.

National Multiple Sclerosis Society: *Disproved theories*, 2018b. Available at: https://www.nationalmssociety.org/What-is-MS/What-Causes-MS#section-5.

Natural Medicines Database: *CoEnzyme Q10 professional monograph*, 2018a. Available at: https://naturalmedicines.therapeuticresearch.com/databases/food,-herbs-supplements/professional.aspx?productid=938#effectiveness.

Natural Medicines Database. *St. John's Wort professional monograph*, 2018b. Available at: https://naturalmedicines.therapeuticresearch.com/databases/food,-herbs-supplements/professional.aspx?productid=329#effectiveness.

Novo AM, Batista S: Multiple sclerosis: implications of obesity in neuroinflammation, *Adv Neurobiol* 19:191–210, 2017.

O'Connell BK, Gloss D, Devinsky O: Cannabinoids in treatment-resistant epilepsy: a review, *Epilepsy Behav* 70(Pt B):341–348, 2017.

Olson CA, Vuong HE, Yano JM, et al: The gut microbiota mediates the anti-seizure effects of the ketogenic diet, *Cell* 173(7):1728–1741.e13, 2018.

Pan-Montojo F, Reichmann H: Considerations on the role of environmental toxins in idiopathic Parkinson's disease pathophysiology, *Transl Neurodegener* 3:10, 2014.

Painter TJ, Rickerds J, Alban RF: Immune enhancing nutrition in traumatic brain injury – a preliminary study, *Int J Surg* 21:70–74, 2015.

Parashar A, Udayabanu M: Gut microbiota: Implications in Parkinson's disease, *Parkinsonism Relat Disord* 38:1–7, 2017.

Parkinson study group QE3 Investigators: A randomized clinical trial of high-dosage coenzyme Q10 in early Parkinson disease: no evidence of benefit, *JAMA Neurol* 71(5):543–552, 2014.

Parkinson's Foundation: *Understanding Parkinson's: statistics,* 2018. Available at: Available at: http://www.parkinson.org/Understanding-Parkinsons/Causes-and-Statistics/Statistics.

Phillips MCL, Murtagh DKJ, Gilbertson LJ, et al: Low-fat versus ketogenic diet in Parkinson's disease: a pilot randomized controlled trial, *Mov Disord* 33(8):1306–1314, 2018.

Pivi GAK, de Andrade Vieira NM, et al: Nutritional management for Alzheimer's disease in all stages: mild, moderate, and severe, *BMC Nutrire* 42:1, 2017.

Rai VRH, Phang LF, Sia SF, et al: Effects of immunonutrition on biomarkers in traumatic brain injury patients in Malaysia: a prospective randomized controlled trial, *BMC Anesthesiol* 17(1):81, 2017.

Reddy DS: The utility of cannabidiol in the treatment of refractory epilepsy, *Clin Pharmacol Ther* 101(2):182–184, 2017.

Roehl K, Sewak SL: Practice paper of the Academy of Nutrition and Dietetics: classic and modified ketogenic diets for treatment of epilepsy, *J Acad Nutr Diet* 117(8):1279–1292, 2017.

Rosen Y, Daich J, Soliman I, et al: Vitamin D and autoimmunity, *Scand J Rheumatol* 45(6):439–447, 2016.

Sand IK: The role of diet in multiple sclerosis: mechanistic connections and current evidence, *Curr Nutr Rep* 7:150–160, 2018.

Scheff SW, Ansari MA: Natural compounds as a therapeutic intervention following traumatic brain injury: the role of phytochemicals, *J Neurotrauma* 34(8):1491–1510, 2017.

Secades JJ: Citicoline: pharmacological and clinical review, 2016 update, *Rev Neurol* 63(S03):S1–S73, 2016.

Skoretz SA, Flowers HL, Martino R: The incidence of dysphagia following endotracheal intubation: a systematic review, *Chest* 137:665–673, 2010.

Solimini R, Rotolo MC, Pichini S, et al: Neurological disorders in medical use of cannabis: an update, *CNS Neurol Disord Drug Targets* 16(5):527-533, 2017.

Sperling RA, Aisen PS, Beckett LA, et al: Toward defining the preclinical stages of Alzheimer's disease: recommendations from the National Institute on Aging-Alzheimer's Association workgroups on diagnostic guidelines for Alzheimer's disease, *Alzheimers Dement* 7(3):280–292, 2011.

Steele CM, Alsanei WA, Ayanikalath S, et al: The influence of food texture and liquid consistency modification on swallowing physiology and function: a systematic review, *Dysphagia* 30(1):2–26, 2015.

Steinberg FU: Rehabilitating the older stroke patient: what's possible? *Geriatrics* 41:85, 1986.

Strand EA, Miller RM, Yorkston KM, et al: Management of oral-pharyngeal dysphagia symptoms in amyotrophic lateral sclerosis, *Dysphagia* 11:129–139, 1996.

Su FC, Goutman SA, Chernyak S, et al: Association of environmental toxins with amyotrophic lateral sclerosis, *JAMA Neurol* 73(7):803–811, 2016.

Sun AY, Wang Q, Simonyi A, et al: Botanical phenolics and brain health, *Neuromolecular Med* 10:259–274, 2008.

Suryadevara U, Bruijnzeel DM, Nuthi M, et al: Pros and cons of medical cannabis use by people with chronic brain disorders, *Curr Neuropharmacol* 15(6):800–814, 2017.

Taylor CA, Bell JM, Breiding MJ, et al: Traumatic brain injury-related emergency department visits, hospitalizations, and deaths – United States, 2007 and 2013, *MMWR Surveill Summ* 66(9):1–16, 2017.

Thompson AJ, Banwell BL, Barkhof F, et al: Diagnosis of multiple sclerosis: 2017 revisions of the McDonald criteria, *Lancet Neurol* 17(2):162–173, 2018.

Volkert D, Chourdakis M, Faxen-Irving G, et al: ESPEN guidelines on nutrition in dementia, *Clin Nutr* 34:1052–1073, 2015.

Westfall S, Lomis N, Kahouli I, et al: Microbiome, probiotics and neurodegenerative diseases: deciphering the gut brain axis, *Cell Mol Life Sci* 74(20):3769–3787, 2017.

Wills AM, Hubbard J, Macklin EA, et al: Hypercaloric enteral nutrition in patients with amyotrophic lateral sclerosis: a randomised, double-blind, placebo-controlled phase 2 trial, *Lancet* 383(9934):2065–2072, 2014.

World Health Organization: *What are neurological disorders?* 2016a. Available at: http://www.who.int/features/qa/55/en/.

World Health Organization: *Guillain-Barré syndrome: key facts,* 2016b. Available at: http://www.who.int/news-room/fact-sheets/detail/guillain-barré-syndrome.

Yan D, Zhang Y, Liu L, et al: Pesticide exposure and risk of Parkinson's disease: dose-response meta-analysis of observational studies, *Regul Toxicol Pharmacol* 96:57–63, 2018.

Yang LP, Fan DS: Diets for patients with amyotrophic lateral sclerosis: pay attention to nutritional intervention, *Chin Med J (Engl)* 130(15):1765–1767, 2017.

Yao SC, Hart AD, Terzella M: An evidence-based osteopathic approach to Parkinson disease, *Osteopath Fam Phys* 5:96–101, 2013.

Zahoor I, Haq E: Vitamin D and multiple sclerosis: an update. In Zagon IS, McLaughlin PJ, editors. *Multiple sclerosis: perspectives in treatment and pathogenesis*, Brisbane, AU, 2017, Codon Publications.

Zelaya JE, Murchison C, Cameron M: Associations between bladder dysfunction and falls in people with relapsing-remitting multiple sclerosis, *Int J MS Care* 19(4):184–190, 2017.

Zhang Y, Xu J, Zhang K, et al: The anticonvulsant effects of ketogenic diet on epileptic seizures and potential mechanism, *Curr Neuropharmacol* 16(1):66–70, 2018.

40

Medical Nutrition Therapy in Psychiatric and Cognitive Disorders

Christina Troutner, MS, RDN

KEY TERMS

addiction
advanced glycation end products (AGEs)
adverse childhood experience (ACE)
alpha-linolenic acid (ALA)
alpha-lipoic acid
alcoholism
Alzheimer's disease (AD)
amygdala
anxiety
arachidonic acid (ARA)
bipolar disorders
chronic fatigue syndrome (CFS)

dementia
depression
dopamine
Diagnostic and Statistical Manual of Mental Disorders (DSM-5)
docosahexaenoic acid (DHA)
eicosapentaenoic acid (EPA)
enteric nervous system (ENS)
epinephrine
fibromyalgia syndrome (FMS)
glutamate
leaky gut (intestinal hyperpermeability)

major depressive disorder (MDD)
mild cognitive impairment (MCI)
MIND diet
neurotransmission
norepinephrine
schizophrenia
schizoaffective disorder
serotonin
serotonin syndrome
synaptic plasticity
vascular dementia

Most illnesses reflect widespread disorders in many parts of the body and are a mix of physical and psychological factors. For example, heart attacks are more common in those with higher levels of hostility (Varghese et al, 2016; Izawa et al, 2011), schizophrenia and autism have been associated with food sensitivities (Jackson et al, 2012; Teitelbaum et al, 2011), and bipolar disorder may be linked to disruption in energy metabolism (Nierenberg et al, 2013). Unfortunately, conditions may be labeled as psychological from a mindset that views the condition as "less real" than other illnesses. This is especially common until a biologic marker or laboratory test is available for an illness. For example, multiple sclerosis was previously called "hysterical paralysis," thought to be caused by an oedipal complex, and lupus was once considered to be a neurosis until tests for these conditions were developed. Chronic fatigue syndrome (CFS) and fibromyalgia (FMS), once thought to be psychosomatic, are now accepted as legitimate physiologic conditions.

As this shift occurs, the artificial and unhealthy boundary between mental and physical illnesses is fading, being replaced with a more accurate reality that treatment in general is most effective when it treats the whole person, recognizing that physiologic imbalances are important to consider in many mental health disorders. The psychological consequences of suboptimal nutritional intake may occur before the physical signs. These include irregular eating habits and unhealthy food choices and can be assessed through careful dietary intake analysis, a nutrition-focused physical examination and biochemical assessment.

The brain weighs approximately 3 lb (1.4 kg). Nerve cells (neurons) gather and transmit electrochemical signals via axons and dendrites. Neurons are the gray matter of the brain; dendrites and axons are the white matter. The cerebrum is the largest part of the brain divided into two halves, which are divided into four lobes, in each hemisphere: (1) the frontal lobes involved with speech, thought, learning, emotion, and movement; (2) the parietal lobes, which process sensory information such as touch, temperature, and pain; (3) the occipital lobes, dealing with vision; and (4) the temporal lobes, which are involved with hearing and memory. The central nervous system consists of the brain and the spinal cord, which connect to the peripheral nervous system, and extends throughout the body (Fig. 40.1).

The brain is approximately 80% fat. The fatty acid composition of neuronal cell membrane phospholipids reflects their intake in the diet. The degree of a fatty acid's unsaturation determines its three-dimensional structure and thus membrane fluidity and function. The ratio between omega-3 and omega-6 polyunsaturated fatty acids (PUFAs) influences various aspects of serotoninergic and catecholaminergic neurotransmission. Beyond their role in brain structure, essential fatty acids (EFAs) are involved in the synthesis and functions of neurotransmitters and in the molecules of the immune system. Nutrition can impact multiple functions in most parts of the brain (Box 40.1).

Nerve cells communicate through the release of molecules of neurotransmitters from the transmitting (releasing) end of one nerve cell, through the synapse between them, to the receiving end (receptors) of

---

Portions of this chapter were written by Jacob Teitelbaum, MD; Alan Weiss, MD; Geri Brewster, RDN, MPH, CDN; and Ruth Leyse-Wallace, PhD.

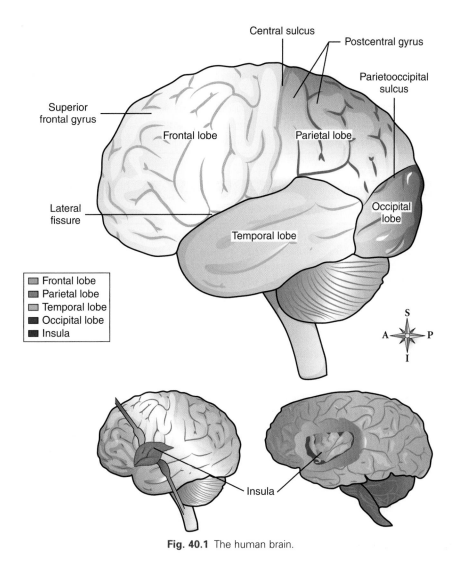

Fig. 40.1 The human brain.

BOX 40.1 How Nutrients Affect Mental Health

Nutrients can affect mental health through a variety of actions:
1. Support the normal development of the brain and central nervous system.
2. Serve as precursors and cofactors for neurotransmitter production.
3. Provide an energy source for the brain.
4. Influence genetic transcription.
5. Support mood and sense of well-being.

Reference: Leyse-Wallace R: *Nutrition and mental health*, Boca Raton, Fla, 2013, Taylor and Francis Inc., CRC Press.

---

a nearby neuron. There are numerous neurotransmitters, including serotonin, acetylcholine, dopamine, norepinephrine, epinephrine, and glutamate.

One of the most important contributions of nutrition to mental health is maintaining the structure and function of the neurons and neurotransmitters in the nervous system. The production of neurotransmitters requires adequate amounts of nutrients. Among these nutrients are amino acids (tryptophan, tyrosine, and glutamine), minerals (zinc, copper, iron, iodine, selenium, magnesium), and B vitamins (B_1, B_2, B_3, B_6, B_{12}, folate). Suboptimal intake of any of these nutrients can impair the production of neurotransmitters and lead to a deterioration of mental health (Table 40.1)

THE ENTERIC NERVOUS SYSTEM

Due to its extensive network of neurons, the gut is often called the enteric nervous system (ENS) or the second brain, which functions autonomously. The ENS contains about 100 million neurons—fewer than the brain, but more than the spinal cord. Acetylcholine, serotonin, and norepinephrine are major neurotransmitters in the ENS. Neural activity in the gut is triggered by receptors that respond to mechanical, thermal, osmotic, and chemical stimuli. Bidirectional information continually passes between the gut and CNS, therefore neurologic and gastrointestinal conditions may have gut and brain components (Sharkey and Savidge, 2014).

The gastrointestinal tract is colonized by more than 10 trillion bacteria, more than there are cells in the body. These bacteria and their byproducts influence brain function and behavior. Gastrointestinal infections with unhealthy microbiota can influence brain function by causing increased intestinal wall permeability, also called leaky gut (intestinal hyperpermeability), which is discussed further in

TABLE 40.1 Neurotransmitters: Precursors and Urinary Metabolites

Neurotransmitter	Precursors	Required Cofactors	Urinary Metabolite
Norepinephrine	Phenylalanine and tyrosine	Copper, *S*-adenosyl-*L*-methionine (SAMe), vitamin C	Vanilmandelate (VMA)
Norepinephrine to epinephrine	Phenylalanine and tyrosine	Copper, SAMe, vitamin C	Vanilmandelate (VMA)
Dopamine	Phenylalanine and tyrosine	Tetrahydrobiopterin (BH$_4$), vitamin B$_6$	Homovanillate (HVA)
Serotonin	Tryptophan	Tetrahydrobiopterin (BH$_4$), vitamin B$_6$	5-Hydroxyindoleacetate (5-HIAA)

✳ NEW DIRECTIONS

Brain-Derived Neurotrophic Factor (BDNF)

Brain-derived neurotrophic factor, also known as *BDNF*, is a protein found in the brain and the peripheral nerves. It plays a role in the growth, differentiation, and maintenance of nerve cells. In the brain, BDNF binds to receptors in the synapses between neurons, increasing voltage and improving signal strength. The synapses can change and adapt over time in response to experience, a characteristic called synaptic plasticity. The BDNF protein helps regulate synaptic plasticity, which is important for learning and memory.

Inside the cells, BDNF activates genes that increase production of more BDNF and other important proteins, as well as serotonin, the neurotransmitter vital for learning and self-esteem. Low levels of BDNF have been associated with depression and even suicide.

The BDNF protein is found in regions of the brain that control eating, drinking, and body weight and likely contributes to the management of these functions.

Certain common genetic variations (polymorphisms; see Chapter 5) in the BDNF gene have been associated with an increased risk of developing psychiatric disorders such as bipolar disorder, schizophrenia, anxiety, and eating disorders.

A particular polymorphism in the *BDNF* gene alters the amino acid sequence in the protein, replacing valine with methionine at position 66 (written as Val66Met or V66M), which impairs the protein's ability to function. Many studies report an association between the Val66Met polymorphism and psychiatric disorders; however, some studies have not supported these findings. It is still unclear how changes in the *BDNF* gene are related to these disorders.

Emerging evidence suggests that moderate aerobic exercise can enhance BDNF expression, which supports the association between exercise and improvements in cognitive function and memory (Wang and Holsinger, 2018).

Chapters 25 and 27. Intestinal wall permeability can result from a host of bowel infections and medications and is associated with many illnesses such as Crohn's disease, celiac disease, multiple sclerosis, and irritable bowel syndrome. See Chapter 27 for more information on these conditions.

BLOOD GLUCOSE REGULATION

Fluctuations in blood glucose can amplify aberrant moods and behavior (Young and Benton, 2014). Rapid and abrupt increases in blood glucose can trigger rapid and excessive release of insulin. This is often followed by a rapid drop in blood glucose as insulin drives the glucose into the cells. The body compensates by raising levels of the compounds epinephrine and cortisol, both of which can trigger marked emotional changes and erratic behavior. The effects of insulin persist well beyond the presence of sugar in the gastrointestinal tract. The natural response is to consume more sugar as it provides immediate relief of the symptoms of low blood glucose; this is the beginning of emotional swings as blood glucose goes up and down.

The habit of eating carbohydrate-rich foods during stress may be physiologically rewarding, as it may raise the level of serotonin in the brain, causing a soothing effect (Wurtman and Wurtman, 2018). With the average American consuming about 100 lb of sugar yearly (U.S. Department of Agriculture, Agricultural Research Service, 2018), this is becoming a major health problem. On the other hand, adequate carbohydrate intake—45% to 65% of total calories, optimally from whole grains and fiber-rich vegetables and fruits—is important for maintaining healthy blood glucose levels, which may protect against mood disturbance and support feelings of well-being (Breymeyer et al, 2016).

Reducing refined carbohydrates and sugar intake can decrease these blood glucose fluctuations considerably. Consuming adequate protein and healthy fats can also contribute to stabilization of

blood sugar levels, often with dramatic clinical and emotional improvement from balancing these three macronutrients (Owen and Corfe, 2017).

THE ROLE OF NUTRIENTS IN MENTAL FUNCTION

Omega-3 Fatty Acids

Omega-3 PUFAs are the preferred fatty acids in the brain and nervous system. From conception through maturity, the essential omega-3 fatty acids eicosapentaenoic acid (EPA) and docosahexaenoic acid (DHA) make unique and irreplaceable contributions to overall brain and nervous system functioning. Clinical research has shown effective and promising roles for EPA and DHA in various psychiatric conditions (Box 40.2) (see *Focus On:* Abbreviations for Fatty Acids).

◎ FOCUS ON

Abbreviations for Fatty Acids

ALA	Alpha (α) linolenic acid
ARA	Arachidonic acid
CLA	Conjugated linoleic acid
DGLA	Dihomo-gamma (γ)-linolenic acid
DHA	Docosahexaenoic acid
EFA	Essential fatty acid
EPA	Eicosapentaenoic acid
GLA	Gamma-linolenic acid
HUFA	Highly unsaturated fatty acid
LA	Linoleic acid
LCFA	Long-chain fatty acids
MUFA	Monounsaturated fatty acids
PUFA	Polyunsaturated fatty acids

BOX 40.2 Some Conditions for Which EPA and DHA May Have Benefit

Alzheimer's disease, dementia, and cognitive function
Age-related macular degeneration
Anxiety
Attention-deficit/hyperactivity disorder (ADHD)
Bipolar disorder
Depression
Postpartum depression
Rheumatoid arthritis
Schizophrenia
Suicidal ideation

DHA, Docosahexanoic acid; *EPA*, eicosapentaenoic acid.
Reference: Office of Dietary Supplements, National Institutes of Health. *Omega-3 Fatty Acids* (website). https://ods.od.nih.gov/factsheets/Omega3FattyAcids-Consumer/.

Alpha-linolenic acid (ALA), a plant-based source of omega-3 fat with 8 carbons and 3 double bonds (18:3), is found in the oil of some seeds and nuts (e.g., flax, chia, sunflower, soybean, and walnuts). Eicosapentaenoic acid (EPA) is a 20-carbon omega-3 fatty acid with 5 double bonds (20:5), and docosahexaenoic acid (DHA) is a 22-carbon fatty acid with 6 double bonds (22:6). EPA and DHA occur naturally in fatty fish and seafood.

ALA serves as a precursor for EPA and DHA, but the conversion of ALA to EPA is approximately 5% to 10%, and conversion of ALA to DHA is even lower (<3%). Health status, other nutritional factors, and genetic variations, particularly in the *FADS1* gene, may influence the conversion rate. Studies have suggested possible differences in conversion rates between vegetarians and carnivores (Welch et al, 2010). Most nutrition and mental health experts do not recommend reliance on ALA as a source of EPA or DHA.

Arachidonic acid (ARA), a 20-carbon omega-6 fatty acid with 4 double bonds (20:4), serves as a precursor to the eicosanoids prostaglandins, thromboxanes, and leukotrienes, which are involved with inflammation, vasoconstriction, and a multitude of metabolic regulations, and also influence mood (see Chapter 7).

Although specific mechanisms remain unclear, clinical research has shown the importance of sufficient EPA intake for general mental health, and particularly as an adjunctive treatment for depression (Grosso et al, 2016). In general, EPA works better when ingested with DHA. They occur together naturally in deep sea fish and seafood. Higher intakes of fish are associated with a decreased risk of depression, particularly in women (Yang et al, 2018). DHA is preferred and selectively stored in brain and nerve cells, and DHA makes up much of the mass of brain tissue. It is required for normal brain growth, development, and maturation and is involved with neurotransmission (brain cells communicating with each other), lipid messaging, genetic expression, and cell membrane synthesis. DHA also provides vital structural contributions; DHA is concentrated in the phospholipids of brain cell membranes.

Oily fish such as salmon, sardines, and tuna are high in EPA and DHA, with the freshest fish having the highest levels. Some canned tuna also has significant amounts and may be more practical for those who cannot get fresh fish. Omega-3 levels of canned albacore tuna are higher than "chunk light" canned tuna, and the tuna should be water and not oil packed, because otherwise the omega-3 oils, which are fat soluble, will be lost when the oil is poured off (see Appendix 26).

During Pregnancy and Lactation

Experts recommend that pregnant women consume at least 200 to 300 mg DHA during pregnancy for optimal development of the infant nervous system. The role of DHA and EPA in pregnancy and lactation is discussed in Chapter 14. Up to 10% of pregnant women may experience depression, and there is considerable interest in finding effective alternatives to prescription medication. Several pilot trials using EPA and DHA from fish oil have been conducted in depressed pregnant women and women with postpartum depression. One dose-ranging study reported measurable improvements in women who consumed as little as 500 mg of combined EPA and DHA.

Research on DHA and EPA intakes by pregnant women and the impact on child cognition has been conflicting. A study that followed more than 9000 pregnant women and their children for 8 years reported lower intelligence quotient and social development in the children of those women who consumed fewer than 12 ounces of fish a week while pregnant. In other words, the children of the women who ate fish two or more times a week during their pregnancy fared better emotionally and mentally (Hibbeln and Davis, 2009). However, a study with the Maastricht Essential Fatty Acid Birth (MEFAB) cohort, with 292 mother-child pairs, showed that there was no association between maternal fatty acid status during pregnancy and child cognition (Brouwer-Brolsma et al, 2017). DHA supplements—as an alternative to DHA from food sources—can be costly and often do not provide the same benefit (Gould et al, 2017). Some concern has been raised about high mercury levels in fish during pregnancy (see Chapter 14). Pregnant women can opt for fish lower in mercury, such as salmon, tuna (canned, light), cod, and catfish. Mercury-free omega-3 fatty acid supplements are also available.

During Childhood

Depression among children is increasing. At the same time, the few studies measuring consumption of EPA and DHA in children report very low average intakes.

Some clinical trials using EPA and DHA supplements from fish oil in children with attention-deficit disorder (ADD) or attention-deficit/hyperactivity disorder (ADHD) have reported benefit, but not all. The difference in findings may be due to many variables, including study design, dose, age of supplementation, the background diet, genetics, and teacher or family dynamics (Gillies et al, 2012). However, it has been shown that children with ADD, ADHD, behavior problems, or who are overweight tend to have lower levels of EPA and DHA in their blood (Milte et al, 2015; Antalis et al, 2006) (see Chapter 43 for further discussion of ADD and ADHD).

During Adulthood

According to the World Health Organization (WHO) major depression is a leading cause of disability around the world (WHO, 2018). The intake of seafood has been shown to be inversely related to the incidence of depression in populations around the world. Increases in homicide occurrence have been associated with less seafood consumption. In active-duty military men, risk of suicide death was 62% greater with lower DHA status (Lewis et al, 2011). When EPA, DHA, and multivitamins were given to prison inmates, antisocial behavior, including violence, fell significantly compared with those on placebo. In another study, teens who had previously attempted suicide made fewer suicide attempts when given EPA and DHA (Hallahan et al, 2007).

With much of the brain composed of the fatty acids found in fish oil (DHA), it is not surprising that fish oil has been shown to be helpful in many conditions. These include depression and schizophrenia

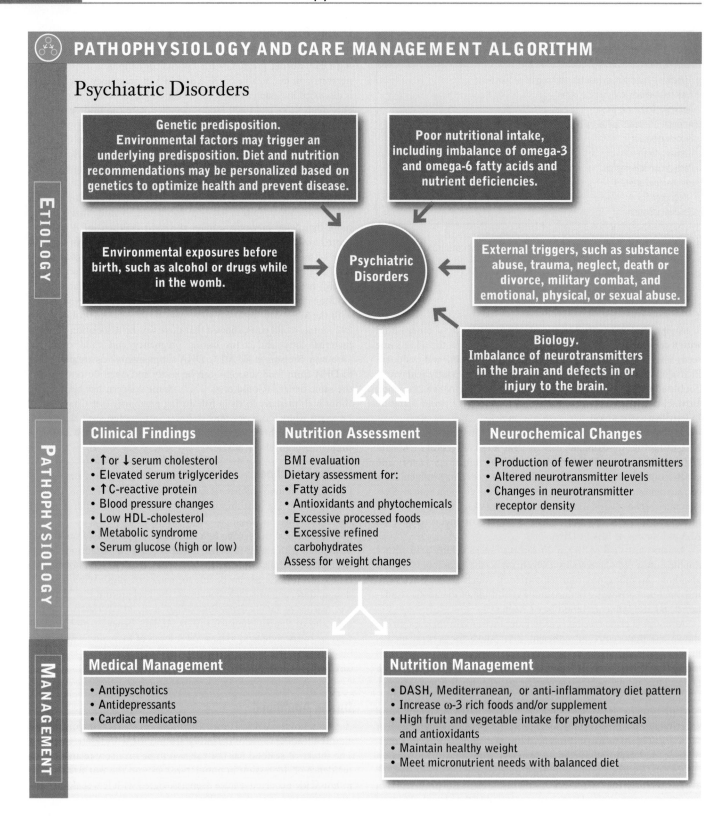

PATHOPHYSIOLOGY AND CARE MANAGEMENT ALGORITHM

Psychiatric Disorders

ETIOLOGY

Genetic predisposition. Environmental factors may trigger an underlying predisposition. Diet and nutrition recommendations may be personalized based on genetics to optimize health and prevent disease.

Poor nutritional intake, including imbalance of omega-3 and omega-6 fatty acids and nutrient deficiencies.

Environmental exposures before birth, such as alcohol or drugs while in the womb.

Psychiatric Disorders

External triggers, such as substance abuse, trauma, neglect, death or divorce, military combat, and emotional, physical, or sexual abuse.

Biology. Imbalance of neurotransmitters in the brain and defects in or injury to the brain.

PATHOPHYSIOLOGY

Clinical Findings

- ↑ or ↓ serum cholesterol
- Elevated serum triglycerides
- ↑ C-reactive protein
- Blood pressure changes
- Low HDL-cholesterol
- Metabolic syndrome
- Serum glucose (high or low)

Nutrition Assessment

BMI evaluation
Dietary assessment for:
- Fatty acids
- Antioxidants and phytochemicals
- Excessive processed foods
- Excessive refined carbohydrates
Assess for weight changes

Neurochemical Changes

- Production of fewer neurotransmitters
- Altered neurotransmitter levels
- Changes in neurotransmitter receptor density

MANAGEMENT

Medical Management

- Antipyschotics
- Antidepressants
- Cardiac medications

Nutrition Management

- DASH, Mediterranean, or anti-inflammatory diet pattern
- Increase ω-3 rich foods and/or supplement
- High fruit and vegetable intake for phytochemicals and antioxidants
- Maintain healthy weight
- Meet micronutrient needs with balanced diet

---

unresponsive to drug treatment alone. EPA was also found to be beneficial in treating the depression associated with bipolar illness (manic depressive illness) (Sarris et al, 2012).

During Adulthood

Research suggests that individuals who consume more fish and seafood during their lifetime have better cognitive function later in life.

Higher blood levels of DHA have been associated with better cognitive function in middle adulthood. Omega-3 fatty acids may have substantial benefits in reducing the risk of cognitive decline in older people (Molfino et al, 2014).

Consumption of a Mediterranean-type diet has also been associated with a decreased rate of cognitive decline with age. It is not clear which aspect of this whole diet approach is responsible for this effect, although it is possible that it is not a single nutrient but the combined effects of the overall diet that produces this benefit. The Mediterranean diet is high in antioxidants and nutrients such as choline and phosphatidylcholine, known to be important for brain function.

Long-chain omega-3 PUFAs, along with other nutrients, have the potential to prevent and reduce comorbidities in older adults. They reduce inflammation, blood lipids, platelet aggregation, and blood pressure. Different mechanisms contribute to these effects, including supporting cell membrane function and composition, eicosanoid production, and gene expression.

The position of the Academy of Nutrition and Dietetics (AND) includes a recommendation for children and adults to eat fish at least twice a week, aiming for intake of 8 ounces or more. The latest recommendation of the International Society for the Study of Fatty Acids and Lipids, released in 2004, is consumption of a daily minimum of 500 mg combined of EPA and DHA. With caveats inherent for ecologic, nutrient disappearance analyses, a healthy dietary allowance for omega-3 fatty acids for current U.S. diets was estimated at 3.5 g/day for a 2000-kcal diet. Higher intakes may be especially helpful in neurologic and psychiatric disorders because of the key roles these omega-3 PUFAs play in the brain.

Omega-3 Supplements

For those who do not eat optimal amounts of omega-3 fats, supplements can be useful. In nature 1000 mg of fish oil contains approximately 180 mg EPA and 120 mg DHA; the remainder is other oils and fatty acids. Therapeutic amounts of EPA and DHA start with around 400 mg of each. Supplement companies sell concentrates of varying dosages, so it is important to read the label. It is also important to make sure the label indicates that the fat is free of heavy metals such as mercury and contaminants such as organophosphates.

Vitamins

Vitamins are critical for energy production as well as many other reactions, and deficiencies can cause serious cognitive and mood problems. Insufficient vitamin intake is defined as intake of an amount below the reference daily vitamin intake amounts, but vitamin deficiency means development of clinically relevant, measurable disorders or characteristic deficiency symptoms due to insufficient intake. Nonetheless, any person with insufficient vitamin intake is also at risk for development of a subclinical functional vitamin deficiency (see Chapter 5).

Mild nutritional deficiencies from poor diet can cause behavioral and cognitive dysfunction, as can increased needs from altered metabolism resulting from genetic mutations (see Chapter 6). Obtaining the levels of micronutrients shown in studies to change brain function often requires a pharmacologic, rather than a dietary reference intake (DRI) level of supplementation, and cannot be reasonably achieved by diet alone. Described below are the function of selected vitamins and minerals involved in psychiatric conditions.

Studies have identified genetic mutations that alter the production and function of serotonin, dopamine, and other neurotransmitters. For example, the methylenetetrahydrofolate reductase (MTHFR) test can reveal alleles (C > T and A > C substitutions) that influence folate metabolism and can lead to a decrease in the production of serotonin and dopamine, as well as an increase in homocysteine levels resulting from an impaired metabolic pathway. People with these genetic single nucleotide polymorphisms (SNPs) (see Chapter 6) with active illness may require folate supplementation in a methylated (5-methyltetrahydrofolate [MTHF]) form. Elevated methylmalonic acid levels suggest

the need for B_{12} supplementation, especially in the presence of elevated serum homocysteine levels (see Appendix 31 for food sources of folate and vitamin B_{12}).

Thiamin (Vitamin B$_1$)

Thiamin diphosphate (TDP), the most bioactive form of thiamin, is an essential coenzyme in glucose metabolism and the biosynthesis of neurotransmitters, including acetylcholine, γ-aminobutyrate, glutamate, aspartate, and serotonin. Norepinephrine, serotonin, and glutamate, as well as their receptors, are potential targets for antidepressant therapies. The degradation rate of TDP, bound to its dependent enzymes, is directly proportional to the available amount of its main substrate, carbohydrate. Body stores of B_1 fall rapidly during fasting. Low TDP concentrations and impaired thiamin-dependent enzymatic activities have been detected in the brains of patients with Alzheimer's disease (AD), Parkinson's dementia (PD), and other neurodegenerative diseases (Zhang et al, 2013).

Wernicke encephalopathy (WE) is a potentially reversible, yet serious neurologic manifestation caused by vitamin B_1 (thiamin) deficiency. It is commonly associated with heavy alcohol consumption but is also reported with the excessive vomiting of hyperemesis gravidarum and vomiting after bariatric surgery. Most patients present with the triad of ocular signs (nystagmus), ataxia, and confusion (see Chapter 28).

Guidelines by the European Federation of Neurological Societies (EFNS) recommend that patients with alcoholism or the conditions mentioned above receive thiamin, 200 mg tid, administered intravenously (IV), before starting any carbohydrate or glucose intake, and that, if directed by a physician, it be continued until there is no further improvement in signs and symptoms. For nonalcoholic patients with thiamin deficiency, an IV dose of thiamin, 100 to 200 mg once daily, may be sufficient (Galvin et al, 2010).

Learning disorders and behavioral problems in young children (sometimes to the point of hospitalization) improved with a high-dose thiamin supplement (Fattal et al, 2011). People with AD were shown to have lower serum thiamin levels than those with other types of dementia (Lu'o'ng and Nguyen, 2011). It has been suggested that the measurement of blood thiamin metabolites may be used as an inexpensive and noninvasive diagnostic tool for distinguishing AD from vascular and frontotemporal dementia (Pan et al, 2015). Some medications may interact with thiamin.

Riboflavin (Vitamin B$_2$)

Biochemical signs of riboflavin depletion appear within a few days of dietary deprivation. Poor riboflavin status interferes with iron absorption and contributes to the etiology of anemia when iron intakes are low. Riboflavin is involved in determining circulating concentrations of homocysteine and may exert some of its effects by reducing the metabolism of other B vitamins, notably folate and vitamin B_6, which are of particular interest in psychiatric disorders. In those with frequent migraines, supplementing with 400 mg of riboflavin a day decreased migraine frequency by 50% to 69% after 6 weeks of use (Markley, 2012).

Niacin (Vitamin B$_3$)

Niacin is a key component of the molecule NADH, which is important for production of the neurotransmitter dopamine. Nicotinamide, the amide form of niacin, plays an important role in neuronal development and in protecting neurons from traumatic injury, stroke, and ischemia (Fricker et al, 2018). One of the signs of pellagra, the niacin-deficiency disease, is dementia. Pellagra can be a cause of delirium during alcohol withdrawal (Oldham and Ivkovic, 2012). Acute pellagra resembles sunburn in its first stages. Psychiatric manifestations are fairly common but are easily overlooked due to their nonspecific nature. Examples include irritability, poor concentration, anxiety, fatigue, restlessness, apathy, and depression.

Vitamin B$_{12}$

The symptoms of vitamin B$_{12}$ deficiency may include agitation, irritability, confusion, disorientation, amnesia, impaired concentration and attention, and insomnia. Mental symptoms may also include stupor, apathy, negativism, memory and judgment disorders or even psychoses, depression, and dementia (Gröber et al, 2013). Catatonia is also described as a psychiatric form of vitamin B$_{12}$ deficiency. Psychiatric disorders that may be diagnosed in patients having B$_{12}$ deficiency include depression, bipolar disorder, panic disorder, psychosis, phobias, and dementia.

A vitamin B$_{12}$ deficiency may express itself in a wide variety of neurologic manifestations such as paresthesias, coordination disorders, reduced nerve conduction velocity, and progressive brain atrophy in the elderly. Cobalamin contributes to hematopoiesis, myelin synthesis, and synthesis of epithelial tissue.

Seventy-five to ninety percent of persons with a clinically relevant B$_{12}$ deficiency have neurologic disorders, and in about 25% of cases these are the only clinical manifestations of the B$_{12}$ deficiency. Levels less than 200 ng/L are sure signs of a B$_{12}$ deficiency, but a functional B$_{12}$ deficiency may also be present at levels under 450 ng/L.

Moderately elevated concentrations of homocysteine ($>10\,\mu mol/L$) have been associated with an increased risk of dementia, notably AD, in many cross-sectional and prospective studies. Raised plasma concentrations of homocysteine are associated with regional and whole-brain atrophy, not only in AD but also in healthy elderly people. Determination of methylmalonic acid and homocysteine are particularly recommended in cases of diagnostically unclarified B$_{12}$ deficiency.

Possible nutrient-drug interactions occur with antibiotics, anticonvulsants, colchicine, metformin, and N$_2$O. Proton pump inhibitors reduce gastric acid secretion and thus the intestinal release of vitamin B$_{12}$ from foods (see Appendix 13).

Hydroxycobalamin, methylcobalamin, and cyanocobalamin are suitable for treatment. The lowest dose of oral cyanocobalamin required to normalize mild vitamin B$_{12}$ deficiency is more than 200 times the recommended dietary allowance of approximately 3 mcg daily (i.e., >500 mcg per day). For deficiency resulting from absorption disorders, doses of 500 to 2000 mcg/day are required.

In a randomized and double-blind interventional study (VITACOG study) involving 168 older adults with mild cognitive impairment (age >70 years), oral supplementation of vitamin B$_{12}$, folate, and vitamin B$_6$ over a period of 24 months slowed the progression of brain atrophy and reduction of cognitive performance by 53.3% (Gröber et al, 2013).

In a study of people being treated for depression, participants with higher levels of vitamin B$_{12}$ tended to get a greater benefit from antidepressants (Moore et al, 2012).

Folate

Folate deficiency is associated with depression, cognitive decline, and dementia. The NHANES 2010 data examined relations between folate and vitamin B$_{12}$ status biomarkers for mental as well as physical conditions. These conditions included lead and neurobehavioral test performance, anemia and cognitive function, hypothyroidism, and gene-nutrient interactions.

Folate deficiency has been identified as a risk factor for schizophrenia through epidemiologic, biochemical, and gene association studies. Folate plus vitamin B$_{12}$ supplementation can improve negative symptoms of schizophrenia. Negative symptoms imply the lack of something, such as social contacts, initiative, energy, motivation, or display of emotion, but treatment response is influenced by genetic variation in folate absorption. These findings support a personalized medicine approach for the treatment of negative symptoms (Roffman et al, 2013).

Folate deficiency may be the result of decreased intake, or increased needs caused by common genetic defects (see MTHFR discussion above). Consequences of inadequate intake are compounded when there is an increased folate requirement, such as during pregnancy, lactation, premature birth, and chronic hemolytic anemias, for example sickle cell anemia and thalassemias (see Chapter 31). Conditions associated with increased cell turnover such as leukemias, aggressive lymphomas, and tumors associated with a high proliferative rate can also cause increased folate demand.

Folate may help cognitive function by decreasing homocysteine levels, improving vascular health, and attenuating antioxidant responses thus inflammatory status (Enderami et al, 2018). However, research is not conclusive. An observational study that included 2900 healthy seniors with high blood levels of homocysteine showed that neither supplementation of folic acid nor vitamin B$_{12}$ improved cognitive performance (van der Zwaluw et al, 2014).

In addition, low folate is associated with AD, with higher folate levels associated with 50% reduction in the risk of developing AD (Luchsinger et al, 2007; Chen et al, 2015). Not all studies have shown a protective effect, however, and one study showed a U-shaped curve, with very high folate levels associated with higher homocysteine levels and a greater risk for developing AD (Faux et al, 2011).

Total homocysteine (tHcy), a nonspecific indicator of inadequate folate status, accumulates with folate inadequacy but is relatively stable across normal folate ranges (Yetley and Johnson, 2011). Folate biomarkers (serum, plasma, and red blood cell folate) increase in response to folate in a dose-response manner (Duffy et al, 2014).

Vitamin D

Vitamin D affects hundreds of genes in the human body and is recognized as an important nutrient for brain health as well as for bone and skeletal health. Clinical research has associated vitamin D deficiency with the presence of mood disorders, all cause dementia including AD, as well as increased risk for major and minor depression in older adults (Littlejohns et al, 2014; Stewart and Hirani, 2010). Supplementing with vitamin D, however, has shown mixed results (Bertone-Johnson et al, 2012; Kjærgaard et al, 2012).

Vitamin D has a crucial role in proliferation, differentiation, neurotrophism, neuroprotection, neurotransmission, and neuroplasticity of cells. Vitamin D exerts its biologic function not only by influencing cellular processes directly, but also by influencing gene expression. The brain has vitamin D receptors, which help provide protection against, and even aid in reversal of, neurocognitive decline. In a study that combined vitamin D with the AD medication memantine, the combination therapy was associated with improvement compared with memantine or vitamin D alone (Annweiler et al, 2012).

Serum levels of vitamin D are most often tested by assessing circulating levels of 25(OH)D, which is the combined product of skin synthesis from sun exposure and dietary sources (see Chapter 5 and Appendix 38). Currently, no "official" agreement has been reached regarding blood levels of 25(OH)D that indicate deficiency, insufficiency, and sufficiency of vitamin D, especially related to brain health. For example, serum levels of 25(OH)D may be low despite a person having an adequate diet or sufficient sun exposure, because of conversion to other forms such as 1,25(OH)D. Many practitioners favor 25(OH)D serum levels of at least 30 ng/mL or 75 nmol/L, although for depression levels of 60 to 80 ng/mL may be beneficial.

The best sources of vitamin D are (1) exposure of the skin to sunlight (the amount of time necessary for an individual to produce adequate vitamin D is dependent on skin type and ultraviolet [UV] index), (2) foods such as oily fish and egg yolks, and (3) vitamin D–fortified foods, such as cow's milk, soy milk, other fortified milks, and fortified cereals. The recommended advice regarding sun exposure is to "avoid sunburn—not sunshine" (see Appendix 38).

Minerals

Iron

Iron deficiency results in poor brain myelination and impaired monoamine metabolism. Glutamate and γ-aminobutyric acid homeostasis is modified by changes in brain iron status. Such changes not only produce deficits in memory, learning capacity, and motor skills but also result in emotional and psychological problems (Kim and Wessling-Resnick, 2014).

Iron deficiency is associated with apathy, depression, and fatigue. Iron deficiency anemia in children is associated with a significantly increased risk of psychiatric disorders, including mood disorders, autism spectrum disorder, ADHD, and developmental disorders (Chen et al, 2013) (see Chapters 31 and 43). At 10 years of age, children given iron supplements from 6 months to 12 months of age smiled and laughed more and needed less prompting to complete a social stress task. However, there were no differences in behaviors such as anxiety, depression, or social problems. Benefits in affect and response to reward may improve performance at school and work, mental health, and personal relationships (Lozoff et al, 2014). Anemia is a late sign of iron deficiency, and therefore a normal blood count in no way precludes its presence.

Iron plays a critical role in dopaminergic signaling. Atypical antipsychotic medications, increasingly used in children and adolescents, modulate brain dopamine. In a study of 115 children who had taken risperidone (an antipsychotic medication commonly used for schizophrenia) for 2.5 ± 1.7 years, 45% had iron depletion and 14% had iron deficiency. Iron status was inversely associated with weight gain during risperidone treatment. It was also inversely associated with the antipsychotic prolactin concentration, which was nearly 50% higher in the iron-deficient group (Calarge and Ziegler, 2013). Nutrition assessment should include evaluation of iron status. Prolactinemia is a challenging side effect of risperidone therapy, especially in males, that may be improved when iron status is normalized.

Selenium

The essential trace mineral selenium is a constituent of selenoproteins, which have important structural and functional roles. Known as antioxidants, they act as a catalyst for the production of active thyroid hormone and are needed for the proper functioning of the immune system. Deficiency has been linked to adverse mood states and depression (Conner et al, 2015; Rayman, 2000). One study found that low dietary selenium intake was associated with an approximate tripling of the likelihood for developing de novo major depression disorder (MDD) (Pasco et al, 2012).

Selenium is available in multivitamin/multimineral supplements and as a stand-alone supplement, often in the forms of selenomethionine or selenium-enriched yeast (grown in a high-selenium medium). An optimal dose for supplementation is ∼ 55 mcg per day for adults, which is equivalent to the recommended dietary allowance (RDA) (Akbaraly et al, 2010). Selenium poisoning from very large intakes is a concern (Nuttall, 2006) (see Appendix 45 on selenium).

Zinc

Zinc imbalance can result not only from insufficient dietary intake but also from impaired activity of zinc transport proteins and zinc-dependent regulation of metabolic pathways. It is known that some neurodegenerative processes are connected with altered zinc homeostasis, and it may influence the state of PD, AD, depression, ADHD, aging-related loss of cognitive function, and possibly psychotic symptoms (Petrilli et al, 2017; Tyszka-Czochara et al, 2014; Grabrucker et al, 2011). Zinc may play a role in regulating the production of dopamine in the brain. Mechanisms of action by which zinc reduces depressive symptoms include (1) decreasing dopamine reuptake (by binding to the dopamine receptor), (2) increasing the conversion of the thyroid hormone T4 to T3, and (3) promoting excitatory neurotransmitter function.

A study of older adults in Australia using a food-frequency questionnaire found those with the highest zinc intake had a 30% to 50% reduction of odds of developing depression. They also reported no association between the zinc-to-iron ratio and developing depression (Vashum et al, 2014). Children with ADHD had lower blood levels of zinc, ferritin, and magnesium than children without ADHD, but they had normal copper levels (Mahmoud et al, 2011).

Amino Acids

In addition to being the building blocks for the key neurotransmitters serotonin (from tryptophan), dopamine, and norepinephrine (both from tyrosine), amino acids are also critical precursors for the antioxidants glutathione (made from glutamine, glycine, and N-acetyl cysteine [NAC]). Amino acid sufficiency can be measured either through plasma or urinary amino acids or by urinary organic acid testing, which measures byproducts of the particular neurotransmitter pathways (see Table 40.1). As more of the neurotransmitters are found in the gut than in the brain, these tests may be helpful but are not absolute indicators of brain neurotransmitter levels or adequacy. Amino acid levels can be low due to inadequate protein intake.

The role of serotonin and dopamine in depression is widely known and it is targeted by many medications, but the role of antioxidants gets less attention, despite its importance. For example, NAC has been shown to be helpful in a wide array of psychiatric conditions, including addiction, compulsive disorders, schizophrenia, and bipolar disorder (Dean et al, 2011). Antioxidant-rich foods, such as dark leafy greens, yellow and orange vegetables, berries, and nuts, can also be incorporated in the diet.

Phytochemicals

New research suggests that plant-based foods rich in bioactive phytochemicals are important to normal brain function and mental health. Promising phytochemicals include three subclasses of flavonoids: flavanols, anthocyanins, and flavanones. These phytochemicals have antioxidant activity, but their more important contributions may be in protecting and preserving brain cell structure and metabolism through a complex cascade of cellular mechanisms, including signaling, transcription, phosphorylation, and gene expression (Spencer, 2010). Foods such as berries, citrus fruits, green tea, and some spices contain phytochemicals, as well as essential vitamins and minerals. Curcumin, derived from turmeric, may be especially neuroprotective, being associated with lower risks of PD and AD.

There is evidence that numerous other plant-based molecules have nutritional and possibly pharmacologic effects in the brain, and the mechanisms are sometimes unknown. These molecules appear to affect brain health through antioxidant, antiinflammatory, and nutrigenomic influences. Other mechanisms are also plausible. Examples of these foods include onion, ginger, turmeric, oregano, sage, rosemary, and garlic. In a study on sulforaphane treatment of autism spectrum disorder (ASD) by Singh et al (2014), participants receiving sulforaphane, a broccoli seed extract, had improvement in social interaction, abnormal behavior, and verbal communication. Sulforaphane, which showed negligible toxicity, was selected because it upregulates genes that protect aerobic cells against oxidative stress, inflammation, and DNA damage, all of which are prominent and possibly mechanistic characteristics of ASD (see Chapter 43). It is plausible that benefits could also be obtained by including more cruciferous vegetables, like broccoli, Brussels sprouts, and cabbage, in the diet (Panjwani et al, 2018).

Nutritional Supplements

People experiencing cognitive and mood dysfunction or psychosis often have difficulty maintaining a healthy diet despite guidance (Davison and Kaplan, 2011). When optimal nutrient levels are not obtained through the diet, a multivitamin may be a reasonable solution.

There are hundreds of psychiatric disorders, which fall into general categories as shown in Table 40.2.

TABLE 40.2 Medical Nutrition Therapy (MNT) for Psychiatric Disorders

A psychiatric diagnosis is based on symptoms observed or reported. A psychoanalytic diagnosis involves the etiology and meaning of symptoms. *The Diagnostic and Statistical Manual of Mental Disorders,* fifth edition (DSM-5), is used by both groups of mental health professionals.

There are hundreds of psychiatric disorders, which fall into the 13 categories below.

MNT therapy for psychiatric disorders requires a nutritional assessment, which takes into account the following:

1. Increase or decrease in appetite
2. Increase or decrease in activity level and therefore calorie requirements
3. Use of medications which cause dry mouth, thirst, constipation, and fluctuations in weight
4. Decrease in ability to concentrate, understand, and follow directions
5. Altered nutritional needs due to use of alcohol, drugs, or tobacco
6. Possible decrease in ability for self-care such as adequate income, shopping, meal preparation
7. History of comorbid conditions that may have resulted in suboptimal or deficient nutritional intake
8. Use of food or nutrition supplements as the "magic answer" in therapy

Psychiatric Disorder	Description	Examples	Nutrition Strategies
Adjustment disorders	A group of symptoms, such as stress, feeling sad or hopeless, and physical symptoms that can occur after a stressful life event. Difficulty coping can result in a stronger reaction than expected for the type of event that occurred.	Sadness, hopelessness, worry, anxiety, excessive crying.	Small, concrete steps and goals. Assess physical symptoms and changes (fatigue, diarrhea, activity level, etc.)
Anxiety disorders	Worry and fear are constant and overwhelming and can be crippling. Anxiety can cause such distress that it interferes with a person's ability to lead a normal life.	Includes generalized anxiety disorder, panic disorder, obsessive-compulsive disorder, social anxiety disorder, post-traumatic stress disorder (PTSD), and specific phobias.	Reassurance and verbal reward for successes. Gradual changes. Use healthy comfort foods. Support blood sugar stability.
Associative disorders	Escape from reality in ways that are involuntary and unhealthy; experience of disconnection and lack of continuity between thoughts, memories, surroundings, actions, and identity.	Symptoms include amnesia and not remembering previous alternate identities.	Support healthy food choices that provide balanced nutrition. Emphasize colorful foods and including all food groups. Omit foods with negative associations.
Eating disorders	A group of serious conditions in which preoccupation with food and weight results in focus on little else. Eating disorders can cause serious physical problems and can even be life-threatening (see Chapter 22).	Includes anorexia nervosa, bulimia, and binge-eating disorders.	Support good food choices already in place. Enlist individual in goal-setting. Encourage use of multivitamin/mineral supplement. Include moderate activity level and social eating.

TABLE 40.2 Medical Nutrition Therapy (MNT) for Psychiatric Disorders—cont'd

Psychiatric Disorder	Description	Examples	Nutrition Strategies
Impulse control disorders (ICDs)	Repetitive or compulsive engagement in a specific behavior (e.g., gambling, hair-pulling) despite adverse consequences, diminished control over the problematic behavior, and tension, or urge state before engagement in the behavior.	Includes pathologic gambling, kleptomania, pyromania, and intermittent explosive disorder. Criteria for other ICDs (compulsive shopping, problematic Internet use, compulsive sexual behavior, and compulsive skin picking) are currently under consideration.	Steer away from overfocus on a single goal. Encourage variety in food choices. Moderate a regular schedule of meals and snacks.
Mood disorders	A general emotional state or mood that is distorted or inconsistent with the circumstances.	Includes: **Major depressive disorder**—prolonged and persistent periods of extreme sadness **Bipolar I and II disorders**—also called manic depression or bipolar affective disorders **Seasonal affective disorder (SAD)**—a form of depression associated with fewer hours of daylight **Cyclothymic disorder**—emotional ups and downs; less extreme than bipolar disorder **Premenstrual dysphoric disorder**—mood changes and irritability that occur during a woman's premenstrual phase and go away with the onset of menses **Persistent depressive disorder (dysthymia)**—a long-term (chronic) form of depression **Disruptive mood dysregulation disorder**—chronic, severe, and persistent irritability in children, often includes frequent temper outbursts that are inconsistent with the child's developmental age	Inquire about history of weight changes. Ensure adequate folate, B_{12}, and omega-3 fatty acid intake. Encourage regular, simple meals and snacks that help maintain healthy blood sugar levels. Detailed planning. Social eating if possible. Bipolar: Assess for consistent fluid and sodium intake. Include plan for social activity and exercise.
Personality disorders	A class of mental disorders characterized by long-term rigid patterns of thought and behavior that deviate markedly from the expectations of the culture. They can cause serious problems and impairment of function.	Includes: behavioral pattern that causes significant distress or impairment in personal, social, or occupational situations. Similar situations do not affect most people's daily functioning to the same degree.	Flexible/variety of food and beverage choices (provide options to give the patient freedom to choose). Flexible eating times.
Psychotic disorders	Serious illnesses that affect the mind and alter a person's ability to think clearly, make good judgments, respond emotionally, communicate effectively, understand reality, and behave appropriately.	Includes: **Schizophrenia**—symptoms such as hallucinations and difficulty staying in touch with reality. Often unable to meet the ordinary demands of daily life. **Schizoaffective disorder**—symptoms of schizophrenia and a mood disorder.	Social eating. Simple meals. Give shopping guidelines and healthy snack ideas. Assess for potential metabolic syndrome. Assess for excess supplement use or water intake.
Sexual dysfunction	Inability to fully enjoy sexual intercourse; disorders that interfere with a full sexual response cycle rarely threaten physical health, but can take a heavy psychological toll, bringing on depression, anxiety, and debilitating feelings of inadequacy.		Support adequate nutrition for healthy physical function. Mediterranean diet may be supportive for vascular function.

Continued

TABLE 40.2	Medical Nutrition Therapy (MNT) for Psychiatric Disorders—cont'd		
Psychiatric Disorder	**Description**	**Examples**	**Nutrition Strategies**
Sexual disorders	Disorders involving sexual functioning, desire, or performance, must cause marked distress or interpersonal difficulty to rate as disorder.	Diagnosis made only when the situation persists, caused at least in part by psychological factors; could occur occasionally or be caused by a temporary factor such as fatigue, sickness, alcohol, or drugs.	Healthy balanced diet to support physical function.
Sleep disorders	Disorders involving changes in sleeping patterns or habits. Signs and symptoms include excessive daytime sleepiness, irregular breathing or increased movement during sleep, difficulty sleeping, and abnormal sleep behaviors.	Includes insomnia, sleep apnea, restless leg syndrome, and narcolepsy.	Food record with times of eating to increase awareness and presence of night eating syndrome. Meet iron requirements.
Somatoform disorders	A group of disorders characterized by thoughts, feelings, or behaviors related to somatic (physical) symptoms, and are excessive for any medical disorder that may be present.	May accompany anxiety disorders and mood disorders, which commonly produce physical symptoms. Somatic symptoms improve with successful treatment of the anxiety or mood disorder.	Review physical symptoms and changes in frequency and severity (abdominal pain, diarrhea, constipation). Eating for comfort.
Substance disorders	Distinct, independent, co-occurring mental disorders, in that all or most of the psychiatric symptoms are the direct result of substance use.	Symptoms of **substance-induced disorders** go from mild anxiety and depression (the most common across all substances) to full-blown manic and other psychotic reactions (much less common). **Psychotic symptoms** can be caused by heavy and long-term amphetamine abuse. **Dementia** (problems with memory, concentration, and problem solving) may result from using substances directly toxic to the brain, which commonly include alcohol, inhalants like gasoline, and amphetamines.	Calculate calories from alcohol, mg of caffeine intake; % of calories from sugar and sweets to increase client awareness and track progress. Moderate goals. Gradual changes. Encourage use of vitamin/mineral supplements (and thiamin in particular for alcoholism). Assess history of irregular food intake and weight changes.

ADDICTION AND SUBSTANCE ABUSE

Addiction is defined as the persistent compulsive use of a substance known by the user to be physically, psychologically, or socially harmful. Addiction to alcohol, or alcoholism, and other substances results in compulsive and relapsing behavior. Addiction may be accompanied by depression or anxiety.

Successful treatment requires attention to the contribution of nutrition in the perpetuation of and recovery from addiction. Addictions may result in poor appetite, craving for sugar and sweets, constipation, and lack of motivation to prepare meals. Poor nutritional status may result from primary malnutrition from insufficient food or nutrient intake, or secondary malnutrition due to alteration in absorption, digestion, metabolism, or excretion of nutrients.

Addiction involves numerous neurotransmitters. The master pleasure molecule, which links and involves most forms of addiction, is dopamine. Its production is triggered by use of heroin, amphetamines, marijuana, alcohol, nicotine, cocaine, and caffeine or the activities of gambling or sex. Compulsive eating behavior may be linked to the same reward system. Other neurotransmitters demonstrated to be involved in addiction include serotonin and glutamate. Nutritional derangements associated with addiction may be severe and can perpetuate addiction, or intensify addiction-related health problems, and make recovery a more difficult process.

Screening for Alcoholism

A moderate intake is defined as no more than two drinks a day for men or one drink a day for women (Centers for Disease Control and Prevention [CDC], 2014). Individuals with intakes larger than this should be assessed using a validated screening tool for alcoholism. One such tool is the Alcohol Use Disorders Identification Test (AUDIT) developed by the WHO and available at their website.

The CAGE questionnaire was commonly used as a screening and evaluation tool for alcoholism (Box 40.3) but has been largely replaced by the AUDIT screening instrument due to its improved sensitivity and specificity. The AUDIT tool is a simple way to screen and identify people at risk of alcohol problems (Box 40.4).

Pathophysiology

In some research on alcohol consumption, light drinking has been shown to be good for the heart and circulatory system and protective against type 2 diabetes and gallstones. However, no level of alcohol consumption has been shown to improve health and reduce all-cause mortality (Burton et al, 2018), thus the only way to minimize health loss is with zero consumption. Heavy drinking is a major cause of preventable death in most countries; it is implicated in about half of fatal traffic accidents in the United States. Heavy drinking can damage the liver and heart, harm an unborn child, increase the chances of developing breast and some other cancers, contribute to depression and violence, and interfere with relationships. When alcohol begins to create problems, and especially when one denies these issues or cannot change the course of them, alcohol addiction must be considered.

Nutrient deficiencies can exacerbate these negative consequences of chronic alcohol consumption:

1. Deficiency of vitamin B_1 can trigger confusion and psychosis (called Wernicke encephalopathy; see Chapter 28)
2. Magnesium deficiency may aggravate withdrawal symptoms such as delirium tremens (DTs) and cardiac arrhythmias. Red blood cell (RBC) magnesium levels are more useful in assessment than serum magnesium levels, which may remain normal even with severe magnesium deficiency. Because magnesium deficiency is so common in alcoholics, deficiency should be presumed to be present.
3. Malnutrition, malabsorption, gastritis, and chronic diarrhea (see Chapters 26 and 27)
4. Hepatitis and cirrhosis (see Chapter 28)
5. Cardiomyopathy (see Chapter 32)
6. Bone marrow disorders
7. Neuropathy, which is also associated with B_{12} deficiency, and dementias

---

BOX 40.3 CAGE Questionnaire for Assessing Alcohol Use

Have you ever felt you should **C**ut down on your drinking?
Have people **A**nnoyed you by criticizing your drinking?
Have you ever felt bad or **G**uilty about your drinking?
Have you ever had a drink first thing in the morning to steady your nerves or to get rid of a hangover (**E**ye opener)?

Item responses on the CAGE are scored 0 or 1, with a higher score as an indication of alcohol problems. A total score of 2 or greater is considered clinically significant.
Ewing JA: Detecting alcoholism. The CAGE questionnaire, *JAMA* 252:1905, 1984.

BOX 40.4 Alcohol Use Disorders Identification Test (AUDIT) Instrument

1. How often do you have a drink containing alcohol?
   (1) Never (skip to questions 9 and10)
   (2) Monthly or less
   (3) 2 to 4 times a month
   (4) 2 to 3 times a week
   (5) 4 or more times a week
2. How many drinks containing alcohol do you have on a typical day when you are drinking?
   (1) 1 or 2
   (2) 3 or 4
   (3) 5 or 6
   (4) 7, 8, or 9
   (5) 10 or more
3. How often do you have six or more drinks on one occasion?
   (1) Never
   (2) Less than monthly
   (3) Monthly
   (4) Weekly
   (5) Daily or almost daily
4. How often during the last year have you found that you were not able to stop drinking once you had started?
   (1) Never
   (2) Less than monthly
   (3) Monthly
   (4) Weekly
   (5) Daily or almost daily
5. How often during the last year have you failed to do what was normally expected from you because of drinking?
   (1) Never
   (2) Less than monthly
   (3) Monthly
   (4) Weekly
   (5) Daily or almost daily

6. How often during the last year have you been unable to remember what happened the night before because you had been drinking?
   (1) Never
   (2) Less than monthly
   (3) Monthly
   (4) Weekly
   (5) Daily or almost daily
7. How often during the last year have you needed an alcoholic drink first thing in the morning to get yourself going after a night of heavy drinking?
   (1) Never
   (2) Less than monthly
   (3) Monthly
   (4) Weekly
   (5) Daily or almost daily
8. How often during the last year have you had a feeling of guilt or remorse after drinking?
   (1) Never
   (2) Less than monthly
   (3) Monthly
   (4) Weekly
   (5) Daily or almost daily
9. Have you or someone else been injured as a result of your drinking?
   (1) No
   (2) Yes, but not in the last year
   (3) Yes, during the last year
10. Has a relative, friend, doctor, or another health professional expressed concern about your drinking or suggested you cut down?
   (1) No
   (2) Yes, but not in the last year
   (3) Yes, during the last year

Add up the points associated with answers. A total score of 8 or more indicates harmful drinking behavior.

Medical Management

The science of treating addictions has evolved considerably. Treatment has progressed from viewing addiction as a character flaw or sign of weakness to thinking of addiction as a chronic brain disorder that results from genetic and environmental inputs.

Any patient or client with active substance abuse issues may be presumed to have nutritional deficiencies. It may be useful to do nutritional testing, especially to document the more dangerous conditions such as thiamin deficiency (see Chapter 5). However, in an acute setting it is critical and may even be lifesaving to presume that B vitamin and magnesium deficiencies are present and treat them rather than wait for laboratory results.

Medical Nutrition Therapy

Medical nutritional therapy for addictions should be individualized, taking into account the current nutritional status of the patient. Some may be homeless and clearly malnourished, whereas others may have less visible deficiencies. Special attention must be given to B vitamins, magnesium, and amino acid deficiencies (see Chapter 5). When possible, the best approach is to evaluate each patient for deficiencies through blood work and then replete as needed or assume poor nutritional status and provide a broad multivitamin/mineral supplement and a diet containing high-quality protein and fats. When gastritis or other intestinal problems are evident, these must be treated to allow for adequate digestion and absorption of nutrients.

Providing adequate levels of amino acids, B vitamins, minerals, and omega-3 fatty acids generally stabilizes function in a patient dealing with addiction of any kind. As seen with many psychiatric disorders, magnesium and NAC are also very helpful in addiction recovery (Bondi et al, 2014; McClure et al, 2014).

Finally, educating addicts about brain function and nutrition enhances their ability to participate successfully in a recovery program, and empowers them to make healthy choices while also understanding the mechanism of addiction (Box 40.5).

ANXIETY

Anxiety disorders are the most common mental illness in the United States (National Institute of Mental Health [NIMH], 2017). According to the CDC, the prevalence rates for anxiety disorder in developed countries range from 13.6% to 28.8% of the population and are higher in developed nations than in developing nations. The underlying etiology of anxiety is not well understood. Different forms of anxiety include generalized anxiety disorder (GAD), panic disorder, obsessive compulsive disorder (OCD), posttraumatic stress disorder (PTSD), and social anxiety disorder (see Table 40.2). Common to all these disorders are heightened and poorly controlled emotional, somatic, and neurologic symptoms triggered by a specific type of circumstance or situation, such as an adverse childhood experience (ACE), death or divorce, substance abuse, military combat, and emotional, physical, or sexual abuse or, in the case of GAD, not related to any specific trigger.

Etiology

At one level, anxiety expressed as a heightened awareness of one's surroundings and of potential danger can be seen as an evolutionary advantage in terms of dealing with threats. However, when this mechanism becomes pervasive and debilitating, it moves into the realm of pathology.

There is a clear genetic component to anxiety. The stress of an ACE can also constitute a significant etiologic factor for anxiety that may impact the individual into and throughout adulthood. It is felt that the anxiety and panic response becomes "hard-wired" at an early age that create hormonal and brain patterns that become entrenched.

Pathophysiology

The structure in the brain thought to generate anxiety is the amygdala (the threat center), which processes fear-related stimuli and then signals other parts of the brain (especially the locus ceruleus) to fire and release norepinephrine; corticotropin-releasing factor (CRF), which ultimately stimulates elevated cortisol levels; and other excitatory components of the sympathetic nervous system. Glutamate is being recognized as playing an increasing role in anxiety disorders (as well as in depression) and is a target for pharmacologic and nonpharmacologic treatment (European College of Neuropsychopharmacology, 2013).

Difficult life circumstances that provoke stress can exacerbate underlying anxiety disorders and may be helpful to address with counseling. These can include marital and relationship stress, job stress, grief, and physiologic stressors such as sleep disorders, menopause, thyroid disease, and food allergies. Hormonal imbalances, including high or low thyroid, low progesterone, and high or low testosterone levels, can also trigger anxiety. Anxiety can be a presenting complaint of perimenopause and of high or low cortisol levels, reflecting adrenal gland dysfunction.

Anxiety provokes physical and emotional symptoms, including rapid heart rate, shallow breathing, diaphoresis, hypervigilance, and sleep disorders. It can be difficult at first to diagnose anxiety because patients present with multiple somatic complaints, and only after somatic pathology is ruled out can a diagnosis of anxiety disorder be established.

Medical Management

The primary pharmacologic therapy for anxiety disorders includes benzodiazepines, selective serotonin reuptake inhibitors (SSRIs), and norepinephrine reuptake inhibitors. Medications used primarily for other conditions can be useful in the treatment of anxiety, such as gabapentin, buspirone, and antipsychotic medications. Each of these can be effective but not for everyone. Each of these treatments carries the potential for side effects.

BOX 40.5 Summary of Medical Nutrition Therapy for Substance Abuse

If warranted by history, assess for high-risk alcohol consumption.

Assess appetite, GI function including nausea, and potential changes in food consumption.

Assess oral health, missing teeth, and chewing ability.

Start multivitamin-mineral supplement; recommend use for 6 months.

Recommend supplement of omega-3 fatty acids: 800 to 1000 mg/day.

Recommend biochemical assessment of thiamin, iron, folic acid, magnesium, selenium.

Recommend 25% to 30% of calories in diet from high quality protein.

Nutritionally adequate diet (moderate intake of up to 300-450 mg caffeine, moderate use of desserts to mediate withdrawal, moderate fiber and adequate fluid intake, inclusion of dairy foods).

Recommend nutrition education group as early as possible during withdrawal.

Reference: Weiss, D: *Nutrition interventions in addiction recovery: the role of the dietitian in substance abuse treatment.* Webinar, September 25, 2013.

Medical Nutritional Therapy

Nutritional therapies that target the underlying metabolic causes of anxiety can be effective. Blood sugar imbalance or being hungry can trigger anxiety and should be suspected if anxiety symptoms are worse in the late morning or afternoon (i.e., after several hours without food). Eating smaller, balanced meals and maintaining routine mealtimes is recommended.

Nutritional deficiencies may be present, especially of vitamin D (Armstrong et al, 2007), B vitamins, and magnesium. Magnesium deficiency can cause anxiety, and anxiety also can cause increased magnesium losses. In hospitalized patients, parenteral magnesium (e.g., 2 g IV over 1 hour, then 1 g per hour for 1 to 3 days) significantly decreased severe anxiety and agitation in agitated psychiatric inpatients. A multivitamin with 100 mg magnesium and high-dose B vitamins was shown to decrease anxiety in a placebo-controlled study. Treatment with B vitamins has also been shown to improve anxiety whether or not deficiency was present (Gaby, 2011). Box 40.6 presents medical nutrition therapy (MNT) and herbal support for anxiety management.

A recent study that included 445 healthy females showed that higher intake of fermented foods that contain probiotics such as yogurt, kefir, pickles, and other lactofermented vegetables may be protective against social anxiety symptoms and neuroticism (Hilimire et al, 2015). Participants were asked to think about their food intake over the past 30 days and indicate how many of certain fermented foods they consumed. "High" and "low" consumption groups were calculated as one standard deviation below and above the mean (9.91 ± 24.51). High consumption of fruits and vegetables as well as exercise frequency were also negatively correlated with social anxiety.

Dietary intake that supports the synthesis of neurotransmitters may also help alleviate anxiety. For example, deficiencies in L-tryptophan, L-phenylalanine, or L-tyrosine, the important building blocks of serotonin, are associated with anxiety (Alramadhan et al, 2012).

Integrative therapies such as meditation, mindfulness, and yoga may also be helpful.

BIPOLAR DISORDER

This is also called bipolar affective disorder and was previously called manic depressive disorder. "Mood Disorders" in the *DSM-IV* has been replaced with separate sections for depressive disorders and bipolar disorders. Bipolar disorder is placed between the psychotic disorders and the depressive disorders in the Diagnostic and Statistical Manual of Mental Disorders (DSM-5), "in recognition of its place as a bridge between the two diagnostic classes in terms of symptomatology, family history and genetics" (Parker, 2014). The criteria for the major psychotic disorders and mood disorders are largely unchanged in the DSM-5.

Bipolar disorder is a disorder in which people experience episodes of an elevated or agitated mood known as mania alternating with episodes of depression. The NIMH reports the 12-month prevalence of bipolar disorder in the U.S. adult population is approximately 2.8% and the lifetime prevalence is about 4.4%. The average age of onset is 25 years (NIMH, 2017). There is a genetic component, but other factors, including hormones, neurotransmitter abnormalities, and stress, are likely to be factors in triggering this illness.

BOX 40.6   Medical Nutrition Therapy for Management of Anxiety

- Assess for vitamin D, magnesium, and B vitamin, and essential fatty acid status (see Chapter 5).
  Eliminating caffeine for 3 to 4 weeks is recommended to see if anxiety decreases. Warn about withdrawal symptoms for 7 to 10 days, including headaches. Cutting intake in half every 4 to 7 days may avoid this. Switching from coffee to green tea can also be helpful as it has less caffeine and contains theanine, a calming amino acid. Anxiety may be triggered by low doses of caffeine (the amounts in decaffeinated coffee); a switch to caffeine-free teas may be necessary.
- Ensure regular meals with protein and low glycemic carbohydrates to promote stable blood sugar.
- Consider adding in a multivitamin (MVI) if dietary intake does not meet the dietary reference intake (DRI) for folate, B_{12}, zinc, magnesium, and vitamin D.

Integrative Therapies for Anxiety

- **GABA:** Deficiency of the neurotransmitter gamma-amino butyric acid (GABA) is associated with anxiety, with GABA being a primary counterbalance for excitatory neurotransmitters (Möhler, 2012).
- **Inositol:** Inositol can be helpful in treating anxiety and panic disorders and is very safe. In high doses it may be valuable in controlling several other mental health disorders, including panic disorder, obsessive compulsive disorder, agoraphobia, and depression.
- **Kava:** Kava has a long history of use for treatment of anxiety at does of 120-280 mg Kavalactones. Safe for short term use (4-8 weeks). Caution in those with liver disease (Sarris, 2018).
- **Lavender:** The smell of lavender is calming, so keeping a vase full of lavender flowers (even dried) around or using a lavender oil spray can be helpful.

In addition, taking a lavender capsule can be calming and reduce the need for tranquilizers (Woelk and Schläfke, 2010).
- **Magnolia:** Magnolia bark has a long history of use in traditional Chinese formulas that relieve both anxiety and depression without the feeling of sedation (Talbott et al, 2013).
- **Passionflower extract:** Doses of 100 to 500 mg 1 to 4 times per day can be helpful (Movafegh et al, 2008).
- **Theanine:** Theanine is derived from green tea. Doses of 200 mg 1 to 2 times per day are helpful (Unno et al, 2013). L-theanine is involved in the formation of the calming neurotransmitter GABA and also stimulates the release of serotonin and dopamine.

Sources

- Möhler H: The GABA system in anxiety and depression and its therapeutic potential, *Neuropharm* 62:1, 2012.
- Sarris J: Herbal medicines in the treatment of psychiatric disorders: 10-year updated review, *Phytother Res*, 32(7):1147-62, 2018.
- Talbott SM, et al: Effect of Magnolia officinalis and Phellodendron amurense (Relora) on cortisol and psychological mood state in moderately stressed subjects, *J Int Soc Sports Nutr* 10:37, 2013.
- Unno K, et al: Anti-stress effect of theanine on students during pharmacy practice: positive correlation among salivary α-amylase activity, trait anxiety and subjective stress, *Pharmacol Biochem Behav* 111:128, 2013.
- Woelk H, Schläfke S: A multi-center, double-blind, randomised study of the Lavender oil preparation Silexan in comparison to Lorazepam for generalized anxiety disorder, *Phytomedicine* 17:94, 2010.

Pathophysiology

Symptoms occur with different levels of severity. At milder levels of mania, known as hypomania, individuals appear energetic, excitable, and may be highly productive. As mania becomes more severe, individuals begin to behave erratically and impulsively, and may have great difficulty with sleep. Behavior may include alcohol abuse, sexual indiscretion, and excessive spending. Eating disorders are a potential comorbidity. The manic phase may result in difficulty in planning and preparing food.

During the depressed phase, 25% to 50% of patients attempt suicide. At the most severe level, individuals can experience psychosis. Bipolar disorder has recently been subdivided into bipolar I (involving cycles of severe mood episodes from mania to depression) and bipolar II (in which milder episodes of mania are mixed with bouts of severe depression) (see Table 40.2). Some individuals experience a mixed state in which features of mania and depression are present at the same time. Manic and depressive episodes last from a few days to several months.

Medical Management

A number of medications are used with varying degrees of success. Medical treatment of bipolar disease is complex and requires frequent monitoring by skilled clinicians. Lithium, a classic treatment, is considered benign when used as lithium orotate at low doses (e.g., 5 mg a day), but when used at high doses as lithium carbonate can cause marked toxicity, including hypothyroidism, renal toxicity, and tremor. Lithium carbonate has a narrow therapeutic index; there is not a large difference between a toxic and therapeutic dose, and blood levels must be closely observed. Other medications used to treat bipolar disorder are mood stabilizers, benzodiazepines, and antipsychotic medications.

The presence of MTHFR reductase genetic mutations should be determined. Some genetic mutations associated with a higher risk of bipolar disorder respond to nutritional treatments of methyl folate (5-MTHF) and methylated B_{12}.

Medical Nutritional Therapy

Lithium and sodium are similar in chemical binding; therefore a stable, moderate, intake of salt (sodium) is necessary to help stabilize lithium levels. Providing dietary guidance based on the Dietary Approaches to Stop Hypertension (DASH) diet may be helpful (see Appendix 17).

Many people starting a course of lithium experience significant dose-dependent weight gain, often resulting in noncompliance with medication. Other side effects that may affect nutritional status include increased thirst, nausea, vomiting, and diarrhea. The usual daily intake of lithium from the diet is 0.65 to 3.1 mg/day (Kapusta et al, 2011).

New information relates bipolar disorder to mitochondrial dysfunction, which leads the possibility of treating bipolar disease with mitochondrial modulators such as coenzyme Q_{10}, NAC, acetyl-L-carnitine (ALCAR), S-adenosyl-L-methionine (SAMe), alpha-lipoic acid, creatine monohydrate, and melatonin (Forester et al, 2015; Nierenberg et al, 2013). This suggests disruption of brain energy metabolism and its relationship to mood disorders and psychiatric disease.

Adequate intake of omega-3 fatty acid may also be important in treatment of bipolar disorder and can be obtained in the diet from deep sea fish or a supplement (Saunders et al, 2016).

Iron excess is also associated with an increased risk of bipolar disorder, so screening of serum ferritin level is warranted to ensure that it is within normal range (Serata et al, 2012). Evaluation in general for mineral and trace element deficiencies is warranted.

As with other mood and psychiatric disorders, the presence of celiac disease or gluten sensitivity should be considered (Dickerson et al, 2011). In nonceliac gluten sensitivity (NCGS), serum and intestinal signs may be absent, but clinical symptoms are reported, and clear within a few days of starting a gluten-free diet. Emerging scientific literature contains several reports linking gluten sensitivity states with neuropsychiatric manifestations including autism, schizophrenia, and ataxia (Genuis and Lobo, 2014).

DEMENTIA AND ALZHEIMER'S DISEASE

Mild cognitive impairment (MCI) is an intermediate stage between the expected cognitive decline of normal aging and the more serious decline of dementia. It can involve problems with memory, language, thinking, and judgment that are greater than normal age-related changes.

Dementia represents a serious loss of cognitive ability characterized by memory loss. It may be stable and nonprogressive, as may occur after brain injuries, or it may be progressive, resulting in long-term decline due to damage or disease in the body. Two of the most common causes are Alzheimer's disease (AD) and vascular disease (called multiinfarct dementia). Other less frequent causes are PD and Lewy body dementia.

Three and a half million Americans have vascular dementia caused by poor circulation to the brain and multiple ministrokes that are also called transient ischemic attacks (TIAs). It is the second leading cause of dementia in Western countries. This syndrome can result from (1) atherosclerotic vascular disease, (2) an embolism usually from the heart due to vascular or arrhythmic disease, (3) poorly controlled hypertension, or (4) an increased tendency to clotting for reasons either inherited or acquired. Recognition of vascular dementia with AD is often delayed until the syndrome is far into its course. Vascular dementia should be considered if the progression of the cognitive dysfunction has progressed in discrete steps, each representing another ministroke.

AD affects an estimated 5.8 million Americans (Alzheimer's Association, 2019). AD is the sixth leading cause of death in the United States and prevalence is increasing at a faster rate than other chronic diseases. For example, whereas deaths from heart disease decreased by 8.9% between 2000 and 2017, deaths from AD increased by 145% (Fig. 40.2). Data from the Framingham Heart Study showed the lifetime risk for AD is about 1 in 10 for men and 1 in 5 for women. See Fig. 40.3 for details. Late-onset AD or LOAD accounts for the large majority of AD cases whereas early-onset, occurring in people ages 30 to 60 years, represents less than 5%. Like other chronic diseases, AD develops as a result of multiple factors. AD appears to be more prevalent in Western countries.

The most proven risk factor for AD is advanced age. Other nonmodifiable risk factors that are associated with higher risk include a positive family history of AD, the presence of the APOE-e4 allele and other genetic risk variants, female gender, and Down's syndrome. Modifiable risk factors include cardiovascular disease risk factors such as hypertension, diabetes, obesity during midlife, and smoking; high amounts of alcohol use; traumatic brain injury; and low educational level. Recent research also links the oxidative stress of air pollution to AD risk (Chen et al, 2017).

Currently AD is incurable. As drug trials for treatment of AD have proven mostly unsuccessful, researchers are turning their focus to prevention as a promising strategy for combating this disease. The pathophysiological changes in the brain associated with AD begin 20 or more years before symptoms appear, providing opportunity for

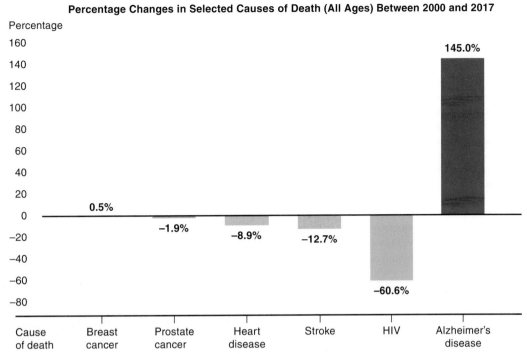

Fig. 40.2 Percentage change in causes of death (all ages) 2000 to 2017. Adapted from Alzheimer's Association, Factors and Figures Report.

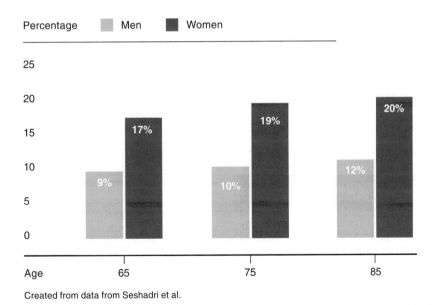

Created from data from Seshadri et al.

Fig. 40.3 Estimated lifetime risk for Alzheimer's by age and sex, from the Framingham Study. Adapted from Seshadri, et al: Lifetime risk of dementia and Alzheimer's disease: the impact of mortality on risk estimates in the Framingham Study. *Neurology* 49(6), 1997. https://n.neurology.org/content/49/6/1498

lifestyle modification for slowing the progression of and/or preventing AD. Factors that may be protective against AD include physical activity, social engagement, and cognitive training. The role of diet and nutrition in AD prevention and treatment is an active and promising area of research.

Pathophysiology

AD is associated with loss of neurons, characterized by microscopic changes in the brain that include deposition of amyloid plaques, tau proteins, and neurofibrillary tangles. The only definitive test for diagnosing AD is a brain biopsy, which, appropriately, is not done. For evaluating dementia the American Academy of Neurology recommends structural neuroimaging, which may include computed tomography (CT) or magnetic resonance imaging (MRI), and screening for depression, vitamin B_{12} deficiency, and hypothyroidism. A recent study demonstrated potential use of a blood test for 10 lipids (eight phosphatidylcholines and two acetyl-L-carnitines) as the best combination lipid blood test panel. A sample of peripheral blood predicted with more than 90% accuracy the development of either amnestic MCI or AD within a 2- or 3-year time frame (Mapstone et al, 2014).

Medical Management

Only half of people with dementia seen by physicians in general practice receive even the basic workup discussed earlier. In only 35% is the correct cause of the dementia determined, and these workups are generally conducted in higher level (secondary care) hospital settings.

A study of autopsies showed that in half the people who had been diagnosed with AD, AD was not seen on their brain biopsy. Rather, they had other causes of dementia that were missed (White, 2011). Although problematic, this also suggests that by looking for and treating nutritional and other issues, function may be improved—sometimes markedly.

Even small changes in brain function can make the difference between being able to care for oneself versus not recognizing one's children. People with dementia can have marked day-to-day fluctuations in cognition. Several types of treatment, including nutritional support and attention to adequate hydration, may significantly improve cognitive function.

It is critical that the practitioner always consider the possible presence of a treatable condition when evaluating a patient for dementia. Examples of treatable and even reversible causes of cognitive decline and memory loss include hormonal imbalances, brain tumors, infections, nutritional deficiencies (e.g., folate and vitamin B_{12}), and the side effects of numerous medications.

It is also important to distinguish between normal fluctuations in mental function and dementia. AD is not when one keeps forgetting where one left the keys, it is when one forgets how to use the keys. Hospitalization can result in poor sleep, loss of routine and familiar surroundings, loss of freedom to make choices, treatment with strong psychoactive medications, and poor diet (e.g., being kept repeatedly nothing by mouth [NPO] for tests, or dietary restrictions from acute illness). This can trigger disorientation that can be confused with dementia. Getting the person into familiar surroundings as quickly as possible, off psychoactive medications, and eating a nutritious diet are important keys to treatment. Other factors may also optimize cognitive function (Box 40.7).

BOX 40.7 Optimizing Cognition in DEMENTIA

Drugs: Wean the person off drugs that are not essential. Being on 10-15 drugs (polypharmacy) is not uncommon in the elderly and can result in abnormal behavior. Anticholinergic medications are especially problematic.

Emotional: Rule out depression and encourage adequate sleep. Nutritional support with favorite foods and comfort foods. Often sweets are preferred.

Metabolic: Levels of hormones should be corrected when possible. Making sure that the person is getting at least the 150 mcg recommended dietary allowance (RDA) of iodine a day is important for maintaining optimal thyroid function (Carcaillon, 2013; Tan et al, 2008) (see Chapter 30).

Ears and eyes: Hearing and vision loss can mimic dementia.

Nutrition: Optimize nutritional intake.

Tumors and other brain lesions: A magnetic resonance imaging (MRI) or computed tomography (CT) scan is appropriate if one is diagnosed with dementia.

Infections: Silent urine and sinus infections can impair mental function.

Anemia, diabetes, and other overt medical problems should be assessed for and treated.

Carcaillon L, et al: Low testosterone and the risk of dementia in elderly men: impact of age and education, *Alzheimers Dement* 10(Suppl 5): S306, 2014; Tan ZS, et al: Thyroid function and the risk of Alzheimer disease: the Framingham study, *Arch Intern Med* 168:1514, 2008.

The medical management of vascular dementia involves decreasing or eliminating further vascular insults to the brain. Treatment may include using aspirin, cholesterol, and blood pressure–lowering agents, and medically managing heart disease when present.

The medical therapies available for AD do not cure nor reverse the disease, though they may help reduce the severity of symptoms and/or slow progression of AD. Therapies are currently limited to (1) acetylcholinesterase inhibitors such as donepezil (Aricept) and rivastigmine tartrate (Exelon), aimed at maintaining levels of acetylcholine in the brain, and (2) memantine (Namenda), an N-methyl-D-aspartate (NMDA) receptor antagonist aimed at reducing glutamate activity, which is excitatory and destructive of brain tissue. Some benefit can be gained from combining these two classes of drugs. Although these medications are generally well tolerated and can modestly slow progression, they often do little to improve symptoms day to day.

Medically managing diabetes and insulin resistance is critical to delaying progression of dementia of any type. Hyper- and hypoglycemia, as well as unchecked insulin resistance, can cause damage to brain structures (Northam and Cameron, 2013) (see *New Directions:* Insulin Resistance in AD and the SNIFF Study [Schiöth et al, 2012]).

✳ NEW DIRECTIONS

Insulin Resistance in AD and the SNIFF Study

Severe insulin resistance in some areas of the brain is present in AD. Brain tissue is one of the few tissues outside of the pancreas that produces insulin, and glucose is the fuel brain cells commonly use. If insulin resistance is present, glucose cannot enter brain cells and the cells essentially starve and cannot function, unless they switch to using ketones for fuel. This suggests that treatment of insulin resistance and metabolic syndrome may be useful in the prevention of or slowing the progression of AD (Willette et al, 2015).

This makes exercise, avoiding excess sugar and saturated fats, and increasing fiber intake especially important. Even just 4 weeks of cutting back on sugar and saturated fats was associated with increased insulin sensitivity and decreased amyloid (Hanson et al, 2013). Intranasal insulin at 10 or 20 IU two times/day is currently being tested in an Alzheimer's randomized controlled trial (the Study of Nasal Insulin to Fight Forgetfulness [SNIFF] study) (Claxton et al, 2015; Morris et al, 2014).

Increasing the level of ketones in the blood and brain may also be considered. The brain can use ketones as fuel, and the metabolism of ketones does not require insulin (Paoli et al, 2014). The role of ketones and ketogenic agents in prevention and management of AD continues to be researched (Sharma et al, 2014; see Appendix 19).

The "4 As" of AD—amnesia, aphasia, apraxia, and agnosia—point to the sequential changes in brain function, behavior, and performance that impair the individual and ultimately can make adequate nutritional intake difficult to maintain (Box 40.8). Specific techniques that take into account the brain deficits must be implemented to improve the ability to eat and enjoy food. An occupational therapist can offer assistance in a dining needs assessment.

Medical Nutritional Therapy

Recent evidence has emerged supporting the connection between dietary intake and cognitive health, particularly in regard to the aging population. A healthier diet during middle-age years (adequate amounts of B vitamins, antioxidants, PUFAs, and phytonutrients [Valls-Pedret et al, 2012]) has been associated with better cognitive function later in life. The MIND Diet or Mediterranean-DASH intervention for neurodegenerative delay has been found to substantially

BOX 40.8   The 4 As of Alzheimer's Dementia

Amnesia: The inability to use or retain memory, including short-term and long-term memory.

The person may constantly repeat questions such as "Where am I?" and "Who are you?" and "When are we going to eat?" or accuse the caregiver of stealing or being an imposter. This type of behavior can continue for hours at a time. This occurs due to damage to the frontal lobes and the hippocampus. This is usually the first area of change noticed by others. At this level of amnesia, the person with dementia does not look ill, so the confusion and inability to remember can appear to be purposeful and is often interpreted as just "annoying" behavior.

NUTRITIONAL IMPACT: May forget to eat, or not trust the caretaker involved in meal preparation or service.

Aphasia: The inability to use or understand language.

The loss of the ability to speak and write is called *expressive aphasia*. An individual may forget words he or she has learned and will provide a lengthy description of an item because he or she cannot find the right word. The individual may call family members by the wrong names. With *receptive aphasia*, an individual may be unable to understand spoken or written words or may read and not understand a word of what is read. Sometimes an individual pretends to understand and even nods in agreement; this is to cover up aphasia. Although individuals may not understand words and grammar, they may still understand nonverbal behavior (i.e., smiling).

NUTRITIONAL IMPACT: May not articulate wants, needs, or requests when it comes to eating.

Apraxia: The inability to use or coordinate purposeful muscle movement or coordination.

In the early stages the person may reach for an item and miss it, have difficulty catching a ball, or clapping hands. The floor may appear to be moving to this person and balance becomes affected, increasing the risk for falls and injury. In time, this loss of ability to move affects the activities of daily living (sleeping, ambulating, toileting, grooming, hygiene, dressing, and eating). In the end stage, the person is not able to properly chew or swallow food, increasing the risk of choking or aspiration. This is linked to damage to parietal lobes (pain, touch, temperature and pressure, sensory perception) and the cortex (skilled movement) and the occipital lobes.

NUTRITIONAL IMPACT: Physically unable to eat, chew, or swallow.

Agnosia: The inability to recognize people or use common objects.

The person may become lost in a familiar place because he or she doesn't recognize the items that alert us to our surroundings. He or she may confuse a fork with a spoon, a toothbrush with a hairbrush, or toothpaste with denture cream. Eventually the ability to recognize objects is lost completely. The person may also confuse a son with a husband or a father or an uncle, or a daughter may be confused with a mother or an aunt or a grandmother. This process is associated with increased damage to the frontal lobes, the occipital lobes (visual association, distance and depth perception), and the temporal lobes.

NUTRITIONAL IMPACT: May not be able to use normal eating utensils or may even forget how to feed himself or herself.

Reference: *Alzheimer's Foundation of America: About Alzheimer's* (website). http://www.alzfdn.org/AboutAlzheimers/symptoms.html, 2014.

slow cognitive decline with aging (Morris et al, 2015; see Appendices 17 and 23.

Three parameters of cognition (delayed recall, learning ability, and memory) were significantly associated with Hb A1c levels in the range of 4.3% to 6.5%, illustrating the effect of even moderate blood glucose levels (American Academy of Neurology, 2015; Kerti et al, 2013).

The metabolic consequences of a high fructose intake and a deficiency of omega-3 fatty acids on cognitive abilities was associated with insulin action, signaling mediators, and lower cognitive scores. Insulin is a vasodilator and its function is blunted in insulin-resistant individuals, which decreases cerebral circulation (Agrawal and Gomez-Pinilla, 2012; Barrett et al, 2009). Insulin resistance, the impairment of the insulin receptor signaling cascade in the hippocampus, may be accompanied by decreasing regional blood flow and reduced memory. Vasoprotective effects that include improved cerebral blood flow have been shown to be associated with a whole food–based diet (Presley et al, 2011).

Research has demonstrated that dietary factors can influence risk for AD due to their effects on vascular function, neuronal function, and synaptic plasticity, which is the ability of synapses to strengthen or weaken over time. Key nutrients that are being investigated for their involvement in AD pathogenesis and brain health overall include the B-vitamins folate, B_{12}, and B_6; choline; folate; iron; potassium; vitamins A, E, and D; omega-3 fatty acids, saturated fat; and cholesterol. Flavanols, polyphenols, caffeine/coffee, and curcumin are also being examined for their roles. Several of these are discussed below.

Historically, folate has been considered an important nutrient for the prevention and treatment of AD. A long-term study using data from the Baltimore Longitudinal Study of Aging, which was begun in 1958 and included more than 1400 participants, found that the participants who had intakes at or above the 400 mcg RDA for folate had a 55% reduction in the risk of developing AD (Corrada et al, 2005).

Most people who reached that level did so by taking folate supplements, which suggests that many people do not get the recommended amounts of folate in their diets. In another study adding folate at 1 mg a day to the anticholinesterase medications used in AD resulted in improved functional status (Connelly et al, 2008). Overall, multivitamins were shown to result in improvement in immediate free recall memory (Grima et al, 2012). A multivitamin, preferably with higher than RDA doses of vitamin B_1 and 400 to 1000 mcg/day of folate, is recommended. More recent studies have focused on folate's role in decreasing inflammation as the key factor in treating AD (Chen et al, 2016).

High folate levels in the presence of low vitamin B_{12} status worsens the enzymatic functions of vitamin B_{12}, which can lead to hyperhomocysteinemia and elevated methylmalonic acid (MMA), and both are associated with cognitive impairment and decline. In a study of 10,413 older individuals (age >/= 60 years) in the 1999–2002 NHANES, it was shown that levels of cognitive impairment increased by 4.7-fold in people with high folate levels (>32.6 nmol/L) and low vitamin B_{12} (<19.3 nmol/L) (Selhub et al, 2007).

Inadequate levels of vitamin B_{12} can affect the risk for cognitive decline, AD, and dementia. This problem is exacerbated by the fact that approximately 10% to 15% of elderly individuals are B_{12} deficient (<200 pmol/L) with reduced ability to absorb vitamin B_{12}. An analysis of 549 individuals from the Framingham Heart Study cohort showed plasma B_{12} levels between 187 and 256.8 pmol/L was predictive of cognitive decline (Morris et al, 2012). B_{12} deficiency is known to damage the myelin sheaths that cover cranial, spinal, and peripheral nerves, which may be correlated with atrophy of gray matter brain regions especially vulnerable to AD pathogenesis. A recent study showed that supplementation of 0.8 mg/day folate, 0.5 mg/day vitamin B_{12}, and 20 mg/day vitamin B_6 over two years significantly slowed brain atrophy in these regions in individuals with MCI and raised levels of plasma tHcy at baseline when compared to those without the supplementation regimen (Douaud et al, 2013).

Vitamin E is vital for maintaining the integrity of cell membranes. Deficiency leads to poor transmission of nerve impulses and nerve damage. Deterioration of neuronal membranes is central to AD. Adequate vitamin E may help slow progression of AD, but only when needs are met through the diet, not supplements (Morris et al, 2002). Most vitamin E supplements are synthetic alpha tocopherols, which not only increase risk of vitamin E deficiency, but do not help AD. The high levels of alpha tocopherol (more than 100 IU/day) can induce a relative deficiency of the other tocopherols. In addition, high dose vitamin E has a pro-oxidative effect, which is linked to increased mortality and incidents of heart failure. Therefore, supplementation with vitamin E, especially at doses more than 100 IU is not recommended, unless a natural mixed tocopherol is used (Usoro and Mousa, 2010).

Iron accumulation in the brain, after tau tangles and the accumulation of beta amyloid plaques, is the third hallmark of AD. Given that at any given moment the brain is using about 20% of the body's entire supply of oxygen (and up to 50% when "thinking hard") iron becomes critical for brain health. It is also released in the breakdown and repair process of myelin sheaths. In this sense, the more myelin sheath breakdown, the greater the accumulation of iron. Iron is also involved in several of the molecular steps leading to the protein deposits, beta-amyloid plaques, and tau characteristic of AD. It has been shown that brain regions most affected by AD have higher levels of ferritin, the storage form of iron in the body. Excessive levels of iron in the brain can promote free radical damage, lipid peroxidation, and cellular death. Iron levels in brain gray matter regions increase with age and are higher in people with age-related neurodegenerative disorders.

The link between iron and AD has been corroborated by nutritional genomic research examining polymorphisms of genes that participate in iron metabolism, transportation, and storage. For example, a risk variant in the transferrin (TF) gene, which leads to defective binding of iron during transport, leads to higher levels of iron and is also a genetic determinant of AD (Wang and Holsinger, 2018) while risk variants in the HFE gene, which lead to hemochromatosis, can increase risk for AD and an earlier age of onset of AD (Lehmann et al, 2006). About 15% of people carry the TF risk variant, which is associated with a 10% to 20% increased risk of AD.

Though iron is implicated in AD neuropathology, the effect of dietary intake of iron within recommended ranges and risk of AD is not clear (Cherbuin et al, 2014). In some regions of the world where consumption of red meat, the richest source of heme iron, in the diet is less, lower incidence of AD is reported. This area of study requires further investigation. Recommendations stand to limit consumption of excessive iron in the diet. If taking a multivitamin, choose one without iron.

Whereas high intakes of saturated fat and cholesterol in the diet are associated with higher risk of cardiovascular disease, the links to AD are not as clear, which may be due, in part, to the individual's APOE genotype. In a meta-analysis of 12 observational studies it was shown that in 4 of the 12 studies, saturated fat increased AD risk while one study showed an inverse relationship (Barnard et al, 2014).

Interestingly, though high cholesterol levels in the periphery increase risk for heart disease and may be associated with AD, cholesterol levels in the brains of AD patients are reduced. Cholesterol balance in the brain is a key parameter for controlling beta amyloid plaque production and clearance. Increasing levels of cholesterol and LDL are generally associated with increased risk of AD though this association is only seen in non-APOE-e4 carriers (Hall et al, 2006). An individual's APOE genotype may have significant influence on dietary recommendations of these nutrients for AD risk reduction.

APOE is a major cholesterol carrier in the brain, mediating lipid transport from one tissue to one cell type or another (and in the brain, primarily neurons). There are three isoforms of APOE: e2, e3, and e4. E2, which is relatively rare, may provide protection against AD; e3, which is most common, presents a neutral risk; e4, which is present in 10% to 15% of the population, increases risk of AD. The isoform type affects the following differently: amyloid plaque aggregation and clearance in the brain, lipid transport, glucose metabolism, neuronal signaling, neuroinflammation, and mitochondrial function. The e4 isoform is less efficient in beta amyloid plaque clearance; thereby its presence can exacerbate the neurotoxicity triggered by plaque accumulation among other deleterious effects.

Each person carries two isoforms of APOE. Those who inherit one copy of e4 have a three-fold higher risk of developing AD, and those with two copies have an 8- to 12-fold higher risk in comparison to those who do not carry a copy of e4. Efforts are being made to understand if dietary modification of cholesterol or saturated fat can modulate the effect of APOE-e4 in the brain and thus risk of AD (Hanson et al, 2013). More research is warranted in this area.

There is growing evidence in the literature that the microbiome composition, species, identity and combinations, density, and distribution of these bacteria may influence how well we age (Mohajeri et al, 2018). As innate immunity predominates over time certain bacteria proliferate, triggering an inflammatory response such as from tumor necrosis factor-alpha (TNF-α). Adequate intake of dietary fiber, fermented foods, and plant-based foods to support a healthy microbiome should be encouraged.

The integrity of the blood-brain barrier (BBB) becomes more difficult to maintain as the bacterial load and sustained TNF-α response occurs. In conditions such as AD, genetic polymorphisms that favor jawbone decay result in increased periodontal pocket depth. This provides the perfect environment for oral anaerobes most closely associated with AD. These conditions in combination with predisposing genetic polymorphisms may increase the propensity for bacteria or endotoxins to gain access to the brain, triggering neuropathology and altering brain function (Shoemark and Allen, 2015). Thus good oral hygiene is important for general wellness of this population.

Advanced glycation end products (AGEs) are implicated in the initiation and progression of Alzheimer-type dementia (Cai et al, 2014). AGEs, also known as glycotoxins, are a diverse group of highly oxidant compounds created through a nonenzymatic reaction between reducing sugars and free amino groups of proteins, lipids, or nucleic acids. The formation of AGEs is a part of normal metabolism, but excessively high levels of AGEs in tissues and the circulation can become pathogenic. AGEs promote oxidative stress and inflammation by binding with cell surface receptors or cross-linking with body proteins, altering their structure and function. In addition to AGEs that form within the body, AGEs also exist in foods. AGEs in foods are formed during dry cooking of food, particularly baking, roasting, and frying. The fat in meat, with beef having generally the most, tends to be richest in AGEs of all foods. AGEs are absorbed and contribute significantly to the body's AGE pool (Uribarri et al, 2010).

Low levels of the omega-3 EFA DHA are present in those with dementia. Increasing omega-3 fat or fish oil intake (from deep sea fish or a supplement if necessary) is more likely to be helpful in those with mild cognitive defects than in those with severe AD (Freund et al, 2014).

AD is 70% less common in India than in the United States, and this is thought to be due to a diet high in turmeric, the source of the bioactive compound curcumin, which is the spice that makes Indian curries yellow (Rigacci and Stefani, 2015). Research has shown that curcumin may combat the buildup of beta amyloid plaques involved in AD

BOX 40.9 Medical Nutrition Therapy for Alzheimer's Disease

A Mediterranean-style diet like that used in the MIND study may slow cognitive decline. A multivitamin supplement containing at least 400 mcg of folate, 1000 IU of vitamin D, and 500 mcg of B_{12}. If the serum vitamin B_{12} level is under 300 pg/mL or serum homocysteine or methylmalonic acid are elevated, a trial of vitamin B_{12} injections is reasonable.

Iron deficiency may be present despite technically normal ferritin (a key laboratory measure for iron) levels. Especially if anemia, cognitive dysfunction, or restless leg syndrome are present, it is reasonable to keep the ferritin level at least 60 mcg/L (ng/mL). Using the standard ferritin cutoffs of 12 and 20 mcg/L (ng/mL) (in females and males respectively) to diagnose iron deficiency is ill advised, as ferritin levels can be higher than this in as many as 92% of people with severe iron deficiency based on bone marrow biopsy.

---

pathogenesis (Reddy et al, 2018). A shortcoming of supplementing curcumin is that it is poorly absorbed. Piperine, however, which is the major active component of black pepper, can increase the bioavailability of curcumin by 2000%. The supplement Meriva is a formulation of both compounds thus providing curcumin in a highly absorbable form. Combining curcumin and vitamin D was also associated with increased amyloid clearance by macrophages (Masoumi et al, 2009; Box 40.9). Curcumin may be generally neuroprotective, also showing benefit in Parkinson's disease (PD) (Pan et al, 2012).

Several prospective studies have shown that intake of specific foods and food groups may influence risk for cognitive decline and AD. In the MIND diet, greater intakes of dark leafy greens, other vegetables, berries, and nuts and seeds rich in monounsaturated and polyunsaturated fatty acids have been shown to be protective in AD and are emphasized whereas red meats, cheeses, and fried foods are limited.

MNT for Advanced Dementia

Advanced dementia almost always results in a decline food intake. Forgetting how to eat and lack of hunger queues can create a challenge for adequate nutrition. It is not uncommon for patients with advanced dementia to develop very different food preferences than what they had earlier in life. As brain function deteriorates, swallowing ability can also be affected, and some people, due to dysphagia, require a texture modified diet (see Chapter 39 and Appendix 20). Providing assistance during meals can become necessary. See Chapter 19 on caring for older adults.

DEPRESSION

Major depressive disorder (MDD) is a common and costly disorder affecting about 6.7% or 16 million Americans. It is usually associated with severe and persistent symptoms, leading to social role impairment and increased mortality, making it the leading cause of disability worldwide (Fig. 40.4) (WHO, 2018). Though rigorously studied, still little is understood of the condition and no definitive cause has been identified. In addition, about one third of people do not respond adequately to available treatments. As is the case for most cognitive disorders, depression affects more women than men. The percent of those who suffer from depression also varies by ethnicity (Fig. 40.5).

There are multiple factors contributing to the development of depression, including genetics, nutrition, environmental stressors, hormonal disruption especially in the hypothalamic-pituitary-adrenal (HPA) axis, and alterations in neurotransmitter biology and function (the monoamine deficiency theory). In addition, people with certain genetic predispositions may be more susceptible to depression following chronic stress (Sutton et al, 2018).

In efforts to better understand the genetic etiology of MDD and develop treatments in particular for the one third of drug nonresponders, a meta-analysis was conducted in 2018 based on the DNA of 135,000 people with reported depression and 350,000 healthy people. The analysis uncovered 44 genetic risk factors linked to MDD (Wray et al, 2018). Though most were associated with targets of current antidepressant medications, this study marked a critical first step for understanding the genetic architecture of depression and possible avenues for treatment. A higher body mass index (BMI) was also linked to MDD.

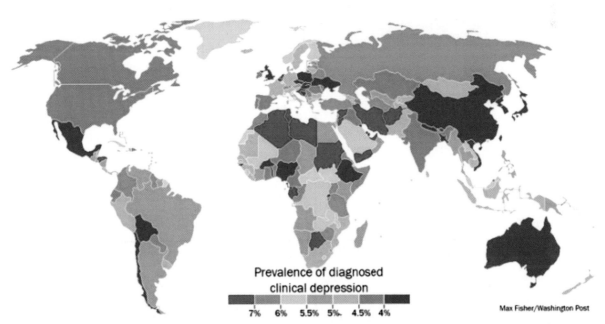

Prevalence of diagnosed clinical depression

7% 6% 5.5% 5%. 4.5% 4%

Max Fisher/Washington Post

Fig. 40.4 Prevalence of diagnosed clinical depression by country. Source: https://www.washingtonpost.com/news/worldviews/wp/2013/11/07/a-stunning-map-of-depression-rates-around-the-world

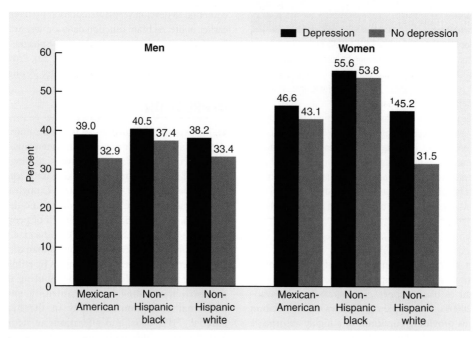

¹Significantly different from no depression.
NOTES: Estimates were age-adjusted by the direct method to the 2000 U.S. census population using the age groups 20–39, 40–59, and 60 and over. Depression is defined as moderate to severe depressive symptoms. Access data table for Figure 3 or https://www.cdc.gov/nchs/data/databriefs/db167_table.pdf#3
SOURCE: CDC/NCHS, National Health and Nutrition Examination Survey, 2005–2010.

Fig. 40.5 Age-adjusted percentage of adults aged 20 and over who were obese, by sex, race/ethnicity, and depression status. United States 2005–2010. Source: https://www.cdc.gov/nchs/products/databriefs/db167.htm

This range of factors and the relative contribution of each to the development of depression in an individual is likely an important reason for the variability of individual response to specific therapies. Thus viewing depression as a heterogeneous condition is useful and demands that the health care provider consider each patient's individuality (see Table 40.2 and Box 40.10).

BOX 40.10 Diagnostic Criteria for Major Depression

- Depressed mood or a loss of interest or pleasure in daily activities for more than 2 weeks.
- Mood representing a change from the person's baseline.
- Impaired function: social, occupational, educational.
- Specific symptoms, at least five of these nine, present nearly every day:
  1. Depressed mood or irritable most of the day, nearly every day, as indicated by subjective report (e.g., feels sad or empty) or observation made by others (e.g., appears tearful)
  2. Decreased interest or pleasure in most activities, most of each day
  3. Significant weight change (5%), or change in appetite
  4. Change in sleep: insomnia or hypersomnia
  5. Change in activity: psychomotor agitation or retardation
  6. Fatigue or loss of energy
  7. Guilt/worthlessness: feelings of worthlessness or excessive or inappropriate guilt
  8. Concentration: diminished ability to think or concentrate, or more indecisiveness
  9. Suicidality: Thoughts of death or suicide, or has suicide plan

American Psychiatric Association (APA): *Diagnostic and Statistical Manual of Mental Disorders*, ed 5, Arlington, VA, 2013, American Psychiatric Association.

Pathophysiology

The monoamine deficiency theory of depression suggests that a deficiency of the monoamines serotonin, dopamine, and norepinephrine, or altered monoamine receptor function in the central nervous system, is the main pathophysiologic factor in depression. This theory has provided a target for the most common pharmacologic methods of treating depression.

In addition to the dietary decrease in fish oils and omega-3 fatty acids already discussed, other factors contribute to depression, including nutritional and hormonal deficiencies. In depression not responsive to antidepressants, a good response is seen using the T3 thyroid hormone despite normal thyroid tests. No significant improvement was seen with T4, the thyroid hormone most often used (Posternak et al, 2008). T3 has also been shown to be helpful in resistant bipolar depression (Kelly and Lieberman, 2009). Testosterone deficiency in men causes depression. Symptoms suggestive of depression can arise in the perimenopausal state, and appropriate therapy including bioidentical hormone therapy can be a useful in addressing this (Joffe, 2011).

As discussed earlier, epidemiologic research has identified associations between lower seafood consumption and increased rates of depression around the world. Dozens of clinical studies using EPA and DHA omega-3 supplements for depression have been conducted, and results are mixed but generally positive (Grosso et al, 2016).

Medical Management

Standard treatment of MDD includes pharmacotherapy as outlined in Box 40.11. Current pharmacologic therapy of depression is inconsistently effective (Garland, 2004). It has been nearly three decades since a new drug has been identified for treatment of MDD. Recent research,

- Selective serotonin reuptake inhibitors (SSRIs), such as fluoxetine, paroxetine, and sertraline among others
- Serotonin norepinephrine reuptake inhibitors, such as duloxetine and venlafaxine
- Norepinephrine-dopamine reuptake inhibitor-bupropion
- Ketamine
- **Older therapies including monoamine oxidase inhibitors and tricyclic antidepressants can be useful but are generally second-line therapies**

receptor), (2) increasing the conversion of T4 to T3, and (3) promoting excitatory neurotransmitter function.

Nutritional approaches to augmenting serotonin and serotonin receptor response include the use of St. John's Wort, tryptophan, 5-hydroxytryptophan (5-HTP), and vitamin D. SAMe can be an effective additive therapy to treat major depressive disorders. It is important to coordinate care with a medical doctor or psychiatrist before recommending these supplements. Caution must be used in treating depression with St. John's Wort, tryptophan, and 5-HTP in patients being treated with serotonergic drugs, such as SSRIs, serotonin-norepinephrine reuptake inhibitors (SNRIs), or tramadol to avoid triggering serotonin syndrome (see *Focus On:* Serotonin Syndrome). St. John's Wort also has a high risk of drug nutrient interactions (see Chapter 11).

however, has found that ketamine may ease symptoms for 60% to 70% of those who are resistant to the treatments currently available (Ionescu and Papakostas, 2017). Clinical trials are underway to investigate two drugs with similar molecular mechanisms of ketamine.

Although a variable moderate percentage of depressed patients receive some benefit from pharmacologic therapy, a majority will not achieve full remission (see *New Directions: Can Genes Help Determine Psychopharmacologic Therapy?*)

✳ NEW DIRECTIONS

Can Genes Help Determine Psychopharmacologic Therapy?

Saliva-based genetic tests for genetic and biological markers can indicate the potential response to different psychiatric drugs. Analysis by a psychopharmacologist can help clinicians more quickly find effective treatment for patients with a range of psychiatric conditions, including depression, bipolar disorder, schizophrenia, anxiety disorders, obsessive compulsive disorders (OCD), and attention-deficit/hyperactivity disorders (ADHD).

◎ FOCUS ON

Serotonin Syndrome

If brain serotonin levels go too high, the result is serotonin syndrome. Serotonin syndrome encompasses a wide range of clinical findings.

- Mild symptoms may consist of increased heart rate, anxiety, sweating, dilated pupils, tremor or twitching, and hyperresponsive reflexes.
- Symptoms of moderate elevation include hyperactive bowel sounds, high blood pressure, and fever.
- Severe symptoms include increases in heart rate and blood pressure that may lead to shock.
- Most often, excess serotonin occurs from combining serotonin raising medications (typically selective serotonin reuptake inhibitors [SSRIs]). It may also come from adding 5-hydroxytryptophan (5-HTP), tryptophan, or herbs (e.g., St. John's Wort, Panax, ginseng, nutmeg, or yohimbe) to high doses of medications which raise serotonin. Treatment is to cut back or stop these adjunctive treatments. Abruptly stopping antidepressants can cause severe withdrawal, so, except in severe situations, dosing is usually lowered rather than stopped completely (Undurraga and Baldessarini, 2012).

Medical Nutritional Therapy

Though it has proved difficult to fundamentally link one specific or a series of nutritional deficiencies or one dietary pattern to MDD, there is somewhat a chicken and egg problem that is presented when using observational research to examine the relationship between nutrition and MDD (and other psychiatric disorders). Is it the disease that leads one to eat less healthfully or does an unhealthy diet potentiate the disease?

A Mediterranean diet–like eating pattern has also been examined in relation to MDD. Studies have shown that diets rich in fruits, vegetables, olive oil, fish, whole grains, low-fat dairy, and antioxidants and low in animal foods may protect against the development of depressive symptoms later in life and decrease risk of MDD (Pagliai et al, 2018; Ylilauri et al, 2017).

Clinical trials examining specific dietary components have shed light on the role of nutrition in MDD risk and development.

Curcumin appears to be a promising treatment for depression due to its antiinflammatory effects (Ng et al, 2017). Effectiveness of common curcumin is decreased because of poor absorption; supplements that provide curcumin with piperine enhance bioavailability.

Low serum zinc levels have been consistently shown in depressed individuals versus healthy controls (Swardfager et al, 2013) and predispose people to treatment-resistance in depression. Repletion of zinc levels may augment otherwise ineffective therapies (Ranjbar et al, 2014). Mechanisms of action by zinc in reducing depressive symptoms include (1) decreasing dopamine reuptake (by binding to the dopamine

Although many clinicians are trained to think that the only presentation of serotonin syndrome is a febrile rigid state requiring emergency medical care, in milder forms patients are simply agitated and have muscle spasms. There is no way to diagnose this other than by clinical suspicion and altering the therapy to reduce serotonin levels and note if symptoms resolve.

In those with vitamin B_{12} or folate deficiency and especially coexisting with an MTHFR methylation mutation or elevated homocysteine levels, optimizing B_{12} and folate levels may help improve depression (Bhatia and Singh, 2015). It can be helpful to evaluate patients with longstanding mood disorders, especially those with a family history of mood disorders, for a genetic methylation mutation of either COMT (catechol-O-methyl transferase) or MTHFR (see Chapter 6). These mutations are involved in inactivation of catecholamine neurotransmitters and are implicated in schizophrenia, OCD, ADHD, and depression as well as vascular disease, thrombotic stroke, homocystinuria, and homocysteinemia.

FATIGUE, CHRONIC FATIGUE SYNDROME (CFS), AND FIBROMYALGIA SYNDROME (FMS)

Although research has shown that fatigue, chronic fatigue syndrome (CFS), and fibromyalgia syndrome (FMS) are physical conditions, discussion of them is included here because cognitive dysfunction (often called "brain fog") is a frequent symptom, and CFS and FMS are often poorly understood. Disorders such as CFS and FMS have a confusing array of diverse symptoms. Some experts believe that CFS and fibromyalgia are variations of the same process; they are discussed here as a single condition (CFS/FMS). Overt fibromyalgia affects approximately 2% of the population (Wolfe et al, 2013), and another approximately 2% have a milder intermediate form.

Women are affected twice as often as men. CFS/FMS can be caused by, and have overlapping symptoms with, autoimmune disorders such as systemic lupus erythematosus (SLE) or hypothyroidism. Viral pathogens, immune dysregulation, central nervous system dysfunction, musculoskeletal disorders, mitochondrial dysfunction, nutrient deficiencies, and other systemic abnormalities and allergies have been proposed as contributing factors in CSF/FMS.

Pathophysiology

Research suggests mitochondrial and hypothalamic dysfunction are common denominators in the syndromes of CFS/FMS (Cordero et al, 2010). Dysfunction of hormonal, sleep, and autonomic control (all centered in the hypothalamus), and energy production can explain the large number of symptoms and why most patients have a similar set of complaints.

Because the hypothalamus controls sleep, the hormonal and autonomic systems, and temperature regulation, it has very high energy

---

BOX 40.12   Effects of Insufficient, High-Quality Sleep

Alteration in moods: irritability, anger, greater risk for depression
Lessened ability to cope with stress
Decreased ability to learn
Decreased memory
Poor insight
Impaired judgment
Increased pain
Immune dysfunction

Source: http://www.webmd.com/sleep-disorders/excessive-sleepiness-10/emotions-cognitive

---

needs for its size, so it malfunctions early in a shortage of energy. In addition, inadequate energy stores in a muscle results in muscle shortening (think of writer's cramp) and pain, which is further accentuated by the loss of deep sleep (Box 40.12). The paradox of severe fatigue combined with insomnia, lasting more than 6 months, indicates the likelihood of a CFS-related process. If a patient also has widespread pain, fibromyalgia is probably present as well (see *Focus On: Fibromyalgia Diagnostic Criteria*).

◎ **FOCUS ON**

Fibromyalgia Diagnostic Criteria

- Widespread pain index (WPI) ≥7 and symptom severity (SS) scale score ≥5, or WPI 3 to 6 and SS scale score ≥9.
- Symptoms have been present at a similar level for at least 3 months.
- The patient does not have a disorder that would otherwise explain the pain.

WPI (Widespread Pain Index)

Check each area below that you've had pain in over the last week. Score 1 point for each you check and enter the total score in the blank space provided.

- Shoulder girdle, left
- Shoulder girdle, right
- Upper arm, left
- Upper arm, right
- Lower arm, left
- Lower arm, right

- Hip (buttock, trochanter), left
- Hip (buttock, trochanter), right
- Upper leg, left
- Upper leg, right
- Lower leg, left
- Lower leg, right

- Jaw, left
- Jaw, right
- Chest
- Abdomen
- Upper back
- Lower back
- Neck

_____ **Total WPI** (score 1 point for each item checked above)

SS (Symptom Severity)

a. Rate each of the three symptoms below according to the severity you've experienced over the past week using the scale shown.

  0 = No problem
  1 = Slight or mild problems, generally intermittent

2 = Moderate, considerable problems, often present and/or at a moderate level
3 = Severe: pervasive, continuous, life-disturbing problems
  _____ Fatigue
  _____ Waking unrefreshed
  _____ Cognitive symptoms ("brain fog")

b. Rate each symptom below that you've experienced during the previous 6 months. Score 1 point for each you check.

  0 = No problem
  1 = Slight or mild problems, generally intermittent
  2 = Moderate, considerable problems, often present and/or at a moderate level
  3 = Severe: pervasive, continuous, life-disturbing problems
  _____ Fatigue
  _____ Waking unrefreshed
  _____ Cognitive symptoms ("brain fog")

c. Check each symptom below that you've experienced during the previous 6 months. Score 1 point for each you check.

- Headaches
- Pain or cramps in lower abdomen
- Depression

_____ **Total SS** (add the scores you entered in step a plus 1 point for each symptom you checked in step b)

Wolf F, Clauw DJ, Fitzcharles MA, et al: The American College of Rheumatology Preliminary Diagnostic Criteria for Fibromyalgia and Measurement of Symptom Severity, *Arthritis Care & Research*, (62)5, 600-610, 2010.

Diagnosis is based on the combination of chronic widespread pain and a symptom severity score based on the amount of fatigue, sleep disturbances, cognitive dysfunction, and other somatic symptoms. The diagnosis of fibromyalgia often overlaps with other chronic pain syndromes, including irritable bowel syndrome, temporomandibular disorders, and idiopathic low back pain. In CFS, chronic fatigue is the major symptom. It lasts 6 months or longer and is accompanied by

hypotension, sore throat, multiple joint pains, headaches, postexertional fatigue, muscle pain, and impaired concentration.

Medical Management

Standard medical therapy is aimed at addressing symptomatology but does not address the underlying metabolic, nutritional, and hormonal derangements. Medications such as low-dose Neurontin, Ambien,

Flexeril, or Desyrel are used to initiate and deepen sleep. Neurontin can also be helpful in reducing pain and restless leg syndrome. Three medications are approved by the Food and Drug Administration (FDA) for treatment of fibromyalgia: duloxetine (Cymbalta), milnacipran (Savella), and the anticonvulsant pregabalin (Lyrica). These can be helpful in some patients suffering from FMS but can have significant side effects.

There are no FDA-approved medications for CFS, and clinicians generally attempt to improve sleep quality in these patients and may attempt a trial of stimulants such as modafinil or amphetamines to improve daytime function. Although there is still much to learn, effective treatment is now available for the majority of these patients. Restoring adequate energy production through nutritional, hormonal, and sleep support, and eliminating the stresses that overuse energy (e.g., infections, situational stresses) restores function in the hypothalamic "circuit breaker" and also allows muscles to release, thus allowing pain to resolve. Massage therapy is an effective non-pharmacological treatment for muscle pain. A placebo-controlled study showed that with these measures, 91% of patients improve, with an average 90% improvement in quality of life, and the majority of patients no longer qualified as having FMS by the end of 3 months (p < 0.0001 vs. placebo) (Teitelbaum, 2012a).

The acronym SHINE, based on the integrated protocol used in the study, is a helpful way to structure treatment recommendations (Box 40.13).

Disordered Sleep

A common element of CFS/FMS is a sleep disorder. Many patients sleep solidly for only 3 to 5 hours a night with multiple awakenings. Even more problematic is the loss of deep stage three and four restorative sleep. Besides the standard medications for sleep improvement, natural sleep remedies can also be very helpful (Box 40.14).

BOX 40.13 SHINE Protocol for Treating Chronic Fatigue and Fibromyalgia

Sleep support
Hormonal support
Infection treatment
Nutritional support
Exercise as able

Teitelbaum JE: Effective treatment of chronic fatigue syndrome, *Integr Med* 10:44, 2012.

BOX 40.14 Natural Sleep Remedies and Recommended Dosages

1. Herbal: Use singly or in combination, once a day at HS (see Chapter 12 for possible interactions).
   Valerian (200-800 mg/day)
   Passionflower (90-360 mg)
   L-Theanine (50-200 mg)
   Hops (30-120 mg)
   Lemon Balm Extract (20-80 mg)
2. Melatonin: 0.5-5 mg at bedtime (0.5 mg is usually optimal for sleep, but higher doses may also decrease nighttime acid reflux).
3. Two to three spritzes or sprays of lavender on the pillow at bedtime helps sleep. Lavender is also available in capsule form.

Source: Teitelbaum JE: Effective treatment of chronic fatigue syndrome, *Integrative Medicine* 10:44, 2012.

Other sleep disturbances must be ruled out. Sleep apnea is suspected if the patient snores, is overweight, is hypertensive, and has a shirt collar size more than 17 inches. Restless leg syndrome (RLS), more accurately called periodic limb movement disorder of sleep (PLMD), is also fairly common in CFS/FMS.

Thyroid function should also be evaluated (see Chapter 30).

Immune Dysfunction and Infections

Immune dysfunction is an integral part of CFS/FMS. Dozens of infections have been implicated in CFS/FMS, including viral, parasitic, and antibiotic-sensitive infections. Most of these infections are known as opportunistic infections, which means they will not survive in the presence of a healthy immune system. Many of them resolve on their own as the immune system recovers with the SHINE protocol (see Box 40.13).

General Pain Relief

Pain often resolves within 3 months of simply treating with the SHINE protocol (Teitelbaum, 2007). Nonsteroidal antiinflammatory drugs (NSAIDs) have been shown to be ineffective in fibromyalgia pain and can contribute to bleeding ulcers, and increased risk of heart attacks and strokes (Bhala et al, 2013; Trelle et al, 2010). Chronic use of acetaminophen depletes glutathione, a key antioxidant. The glutathione depletion from acetaminophen may be prevented by supplementing with NAC (500 to 1000 mg/day) (Woodhead et al, 2012).

Medical Nutritional Therapy

It is recommended that B_{12}, iron, total iron-binding capacity (TIBC), and ferritin levels be assessed, keeping in mind that elevated serum B_{12} may be a sign of an MTHFR mutation and inadequate utilization of B_{12}. Measurement of erythrocyte magnesium and zinc may be helpful, although the laboratory tests are not reliable indicators of nutritional status. Due to a probably low-nutrient-density diet and possible increased nutrient needs, other possible nutrient deficiencies are likely. A multivitamin may be warranted if nutritional needs are not met through diet alone.

These patients often need to increase salt and water intake, especially in the presence of low blood pressure or orthostatic dizziness. Salt restriction is generally ill advised in these patients because of the adrenal dysfunction and orthostatic intolerance. Gluten avoidance may be helpful in a subset as well (Isasi et al, 2014; see Chapter 28).

SCHIZOPHRENIA

Schizophrenia is a severe mental disorder that presents as psychosis, often with paranoia and delusions. Diagnosis requires at least one of the symptoms to be delusions, hallucinations, or disorganized speech. A diagnosis of schizoaffective disorder requires that a person meet all of the criteria for schizophrenia and all of the criteria for an episode of bipolar disorder or depression, with the exception of impaired function (Parker, 2014).

Pathophysiology

The origins and causes of schizophrenia are not completely understood. Ultimately it may be understood as a heterogeneous disorder generated by a combination of biochemical, genetic, structural, nutritional, and environmental factors, including infections and toxins (Altamura et al, 2013). Heritability estimates for schizophrenia are about 80% (Gejman et al, 2010). Symptoms commonly begin to appear in males during their late teens and early 20s and appear in females in their 20s or early 30s.

Medical Management

Pharmaceutical therapy revolves around the use of a combination of dopamine-blocking antipsychotic medications, antidepressants, and tranquilizers. Atypical antipsychotics, the newer, second-generation medications, are generally preferred because they pose a lower risk of serious side effects than do conventional medications.

Conventional, or typical, first-generation antipsychotic medications have frequent and potentially significant neurologic side effects, including the possibility of developing a movement disorder (tardive dyskinesia) that may or may not be reversible. Other treatments include psychosocial interventions such as the following:

- Individual therapy
- Social skills training
- Family therapy
- Vocational rehabilitation and supported employment.

Side effects of antipsychotics may include dry mouth, constipation, and increased appetite. Some antipsychotics should not be used with grapefruit and some other citrus fruits (see Chapter 8). Use of alcohol is contraindicated.

Medical Nutritional Therapy

People with severe mental illnesses (SMI) are more likely than other groups to be overweight, to smoke, and to have hyperglycemia and diabetes, hypertension, and dyslipidemia. Metabolic syndrome and other cardiovascular risk factors, as well as a reduced life expectancy, are common in people with schizophrenia (Vidović et al, 2013).

Schizophrenia appears to be associated with altered metabolism. A CT study showed that with equal total body fat and equal subcutaneous fat, there was three times the amount of visceral fat stored by schizophrenic patients. Reduced energy needs have been found in this population. The energy needs of these patients may be overestimated by the commonly used energy expenditure equations. The antipsychotic medications used are implicated in this decreased energy requirement. Weight gain after the start of antipsychotic medications is a common reason for patients to discontinue medication. Weight gains of 25 to 60 lb over the course of several years have been reported. Many patients are willing, able, and successful with weight management programs when they are offered. The most frequently used interventions included regular visits with a dietitian, a self-directed diet, and a stated treatment goal of weight loss. Behavioral group treatment has been shown successful in preventing weight gain and achieving weight loss.

Dietary factors that affect schizophrenia and depression are similar to those that predict illnesses such as coronary heart disease and diabetes. Low levels of membrane and erythrocyte EFAs have been observed, but do not appear to be related to dietary intake, but rather related to phospholipid metabolism. Supplements have been shown effective in raising the levels of EFAs in cell membranes and erythrocytes. A high intake of fish oil is also associated with a better prognosis, with the EPA fraction being more helpful than the DHA (Marano et al, 2013).

Evaluating for the presence of MTHFR mutations may also contribute to treatment (Zhang et al, 2013a). MTHFR and COMT polymorphisms may increase the predilection for schizophrenia, although the exact mechanism is currently unclear (Roffman et al, 2013). MTHFR defects and elevated plasma homocysteine

---

> ### BOX 40.15 Medical Nutrition Therapy for Schizophrenia
>
> Caution against use of grapefruit and/or grapefruit juice (can alter medication blood levels) and use of alcohol.
>
> Assessment of blood levels for immunoglobulin A (IgA) and IgG transglutaminase antibodies to screen for celiac disease or gluten sensitivity even in the absence of gastrointestinal symptoms.
>
> A gluten-free trial is critical if these are positive, and reasonable even if the tests are negative.
>
> Recommend regular meal pattern and trial of a low glycemic, dairy free Mediterranean diet
>
> Monitor weight: a 7% weight gain should trigger assessment for metabolic syndrome.
>
> Refer to a behavioral weight management program as needed. In addition to nutrition-related material, program should include education regarding smoking, exercise, and alcohol consumption.
>
> Assess diet for quality of fat intake; recommend optimal intake of essential fatty acids eicosapentaenoic acid (EPA) and docosahexaenoic acid (DHA) to replenish or maintain cell membrane and erythrocyte fatty acid status.
>
> Relevant vitamin status includes genetic polymorphism of methylenetetrahydrofolate reductase (MTHFR) and adequacy of folate intake.

---

concentration have been suggested as risk factors for schizophrenia, but the results of epidemiologic studies have been inconsistent (Nishi et al, 2014).

The role of gluten and casein in schizophrenia has been suspected for more than 40 years, with an early blinded, controlled study showing that patients with schizophrenia on a gluten- and casein-free diet were released from the hospital significantly earlier (Niebuhr et al, 2011). Studies of individuals in the Clinical Antipsychotic Trials of Intervention Effectiveness (CATIE) show that 5.5% of those with schizophrenia have a high level of antitransglutaminase (antitTG) antibodies, a measure of gluten intolerance, compared with 1.1% of the healthy control sample (Jackson et al, 2012). Twenty-three percent of those with schizophrenia (age-adjusted) had antigliadin antibodies (AGA) compared with 3.1% in the comparison sample (Cascella et al, 2011). It is strongly recommended that those with schizophrenia have blood levels checked for immunoglobulin A (IgA) and IgG transglutaminase antibodies to screen for celiac disease or gluten sensitivity even in the absence of gastrointestinal symptoms (Jackson et al, 2012a). AGA levels, although not as specific, are also recommended for adequate assessment. A gluten-free trial is critical if these are positive, and reasonable even if the tests are negative (see Chapter 27).

A meta-analysis aimed to determine the prevalence and extent of nutritional deficits in first-episode psychosis in schizophrenia reviewed 28 studies on 6 vitamins and 10 minerals. They concluded that deficits in vitamin D and folate previously observed in long-term schizophrenia appear to exist from illness onset and are associated with worse symptomology. No further conclusions could be made except that more and better studies are needed (Firth et al, 2017).

Schizophrenic patients who smoke have been found to have lower erythrocyte DHA and EPA compared with nonsmokers. Smoking status must be taken into account when studying EFAs in this population (Box 40.15).

CLINICAL CASE STUDY

Adele is a 52-year-old African American woman with a strong family history of Alzheimer's Disease (AD). She recently had genetic testing done and tested positive for APOE-4 genotype. She is on a statin drug for high LDL cholesterol and metformin for a new diagnosis of impaired fasting glucose. She is 5'7" and weighs 180 lbs and says her weight has been increasing slowly over the years. Because she has high cholesterol she tells you she does not eat eggs or butter and tries to eat only lean meats. She does not like fish or seafood and her main source of vegetables is salad which she tries to have most nights with dinner. Adele reports a strong craving for sweets and has a caramel latte on most days as there is a coffee stand in her office building where she works. She is trying to make the transition to whole grain breads and pasta but it is difficult because "no one in the house likes it that much". Because she is trying to lose weight she often skips lunch but then ends up overeating in the evening. She wants to exercise but hasn't in a while due to time limitations with work and family obligations. In addition to being concerned about her cholesterol and blood sugar she is now concerned about her recent test results and wants to discuss preventative measures for AD. After reading an article in the news, she wonders if she should be taking turmeric?

Nutrition Diagnostic Statements

- Undesirable food choices (NB 1.7) related to knowledge deficit about dietary factors that reduce risk of AD as evidenced by regular intake of high glycemic foods, low vegetable intake, elevated LDL cholesterol, and impaired fasting glucose.
- Physical inactivity (NB 2.1) related to busy lifestyle and time limitations as evidenced by report of no regular exercise, steady weight gain, and impaired fasting glucose.
- Excessive energy intake (NI-1.3) related to irregular meal patterns, compensatory overeating and preference for high glycemic foods as evidenced by steady weight gain and a BMI of 28.2.

Nutrition Care Questions

1. What diet changes can you discuss with Adele that are associated with decreasing risk of AD? Are these consistent with what she should be doing for her high cholesterol and high blood sugar?
2. Are there any dietary supplements that may be helpful for Adele?
3. How does exercise fit into the advice you would give her?

USEFUL WEBSITES

Alzheimer's Association
Center for Disease Control and Prevention
National Center for Complementary and Integrative Health
National Center for PTSD
National Center on Sleep Disorders Research
National Institute on Aging
National Institute of Mental Health

REFERENCES

Agrawal R, Gomez-Pinilla F: 'Metabolic syndrome' in the brain: deficiency in omega-3 fatty acid exacerbates dysfunctions in insulin receptor signalling and cognition, *J Physiol* 590:2485–2499, 2012.

Akbaraly TN, Arnaud J, Rayman MP, et al: Plasma selenium and risk of dysglycemia in an elderly French population: results from the prospective Epidemiology of Vascular Ageing Study, *Nutr Metab* 7:21, 2010.

Alramadhan E, Hanna MS, Goldstein TA, et al: Dietary and botanical anxiolytics, *Med Sci Monit* 18:RA40–RA48, 2012.

Altamura AC, Pozzoli S, Fiorentini A, et al: Neurodevelopment and inflammatory patterns in schizophrenia in relation to pathophysiology, *Prog Neuropsychopharmacol Biol Psychiatry* 42:63–70, 2013.

Alzheimer's Association. (2019). *Alzheimer's disease facts and figures.* [Ebook]. Chicago. Available at: https://www.alz.org/media/documents/alzheimers-facts-and-figures-2019-r.pdf.

American Academy of Neurology: *Press release: lower blood sugars may be good for the brain,* 2015. Available at: https://www.aan.com/PressRoom/home/PressRelease/1216.

American College of Rheumatology: *2010 The American College of Rheumatology Preliminary Diagnostic Criteria for Fibromyalgia and Measurement of Symptom Severity.* Avaliable at: https://www.rheumatology.org/Portals/0/Files/2010_Preliminary_Diagnostic_Criteria.pdf.

American Psychiatric Association: *Diagnostic and statistical manual of mental disorders,* ed 5, Arlington, VA, 2013, American Psychiatric Association.

Annweiler C, Herrmann FR, Fantino B, et al: Effectiveness of the combination of memantine plus vitamin D on cognition in patients with Alzheimer disease: a pre-post pilot study, *Cogn Behav Neurol* 25:121–127, 2012.

Antalis CJ, Stevens LJ, Campbell M, et al: Omega-3 fatty acid status in attention-deficit/hyperactivity disorder, *Prostaglandins Leukot Essent Fatty Acids* 75:299–308, 2006.

Armstrong DJ, Meenagh GK, Bickle I, et al: Vitamin D deficiency is associated with anxiety and depression in fibromyalgia, *Clin Rheumatol* 26:551–554, 2007.

Barnard ND, Bunner AE, Agarwal U, et al: Saturated and trans fats and dementia: a systematic review, *Neurobiol Aging* 35(Suppl 2):S65–S73, 2014.

Barrett EJ, Eggleston EM, Inyard AC, et al: The vascular actions of insulin control its delivery to muscle and regulate the rate-limiting step in skeletal muscle insulin action, *Diabetologia* 52:752–764, 2009.

Bertone-Johnson ER, Powers SI, Spangler L, et al: Vitamin D supplementation and depression in the women's health initiative calcium and vitamin D trial, *Am J Epidemiol* 176:1–13, 2012.

Bhala N, Emberson J, Merhi A, et al: Vascular and upper gastrointestinal effects of non-steroidal anti-inflammatory drugs: meta-analyses of individual participant data from randomised trials, *Lancet* 382:769–779, 2013.

Bhatia P, Singh N: Homocysteine excess: delineating the possible mechanism of neurotoxicity and depression, *Fundam Clin Pharmacol* 29(6):522–528, 2015.

Bondi CO, Taha AY, Tock JL, et al: Adolescent behavior and dopamine availability are uniquely sensitive to dietary omega-3 fatty acid deficiency, *Biol Psychiatry* 75:38–46, 2014.

Breymeyer KL, Lampe JW, McGregor BA, et al: Subjective mood and energy levels of healthy weight and overweight/obese healthy adults on high-and low-glycemic load experimental diets, *Appetite* 107:253–259, 2016.

Brouwer-Brolsma EM, van de Rest O, Godschalk R, et al: Associations between maternal long-chain polyunsaturated fatty acid concentrations and child cognition at 7 years of age: The MEFAB birth cohort, *Prostaglandins Leukot Essent Fatty Acids* 126:92–97, 2017.

Burton, et al: No level of alcohol consumption improves health, *Lancet,* 392(10152):987–88, 2018.

Cai W, Uribarri J, Zhu L, et al: Oral glycotoxins are a modifiable cause of dementia and the metabolic syndrome in mice and humans, *Proc Natl Acad Sci U S A* 111:4940–4945, 2014.

Calarge CA, Ziegler EE: Iron deficiency in pediatric patients in long-term risperidone treatment, *J Child Adolesc Psychopharmacol* 23:101–109, 2013.

Cascella NG, Kryszak D, Bhatti B, et al: Prevalence of celiac disease and gluten sensitivity in the United States clinical antipsychotic trials of intervention effectiveness study population, *Schizophr Bull* 37:94–100, 2011.

Centers for Disease Control and Prevention: *Alcohol & public health, frequently asked questions,* 2014. Available at: http://www.cdc.gov/alcohol/faqs.htm.

Centers for Disease Control and Prevention: National Center for Health Statistics (NCHS). National Health and Nutrition Examination Survey Data. Hyattsville, MD: U.S. Department of Health and Human Services, Centers for Disease Control and Prevention, 2017. Available at: https://www.cdc.gov/nchs/data/factsheets/factsheet_nhanes.htm.

Chang CY, Ke DS, Chen JY: Essential fatty acids and human brain, *Acta Neurol Taiwan* 18:231–241, 2009.

Chen H, Kwong JC, Copes R, et al: Living near major roads and the incidence of dementia, Parkinson's disease, and multiple sclerosis: a population-based cohort study, *Lancet* 389(10070):718–726, 2017.

Chen H, Liu S, Ji L, et al: Associations between Alzheimer's disease and blood homocysteine, vitamin B12, and folate: a case-control study, *Curr Alzheimer Res* 12(1):88–94, 2015.

Chen H, Liu S, Ji L, et al: Folic acid supplementation mitigates Alzheimer's Disease by reducing inflammation: a randomized controlled trial. *Mediators Inflamm* 2016;5912146, 2016. doi:10.1155/2016/5912146.

Chen H, Su TP, Chen YS, et al: Association between psychiatric disorders and iron deficiency anemia among children and adolescents: a nationwide population-based study, *BMC Psychiatry* 13:161, 2013.

Cherbuin N, Kumar R, Sachdev PS, et al: Dietary mineral intake and risk of mild cognitive impairment: The PATH through life project, *Front Aging Neurosci* 6:4, 2014.

Claxton A, Baker LD, Hanson A, et al: Long-acting intranasal insulin detemir improves cognition for adults with mild cognitive impairment or early-stage Alzheimer's disease dementia, *J Alzheimers Dis* 44:897–906, 2015.

Connelly PJ, Prentice NP, Cousland G, et al: A randomized double-blind placebo-controlled trial of folic acid supplementation of cholinesterase inhibitors in Alzheimer's disease, *Int J Geriatr Psychiatry* 23:155–160, 2008.

Conner TS, Richardson AC, Miller JC: Optimal serum selenium concentrations are associated with lower depressive symptoms and negative mood among young adults, *J Nutr* 145(1):59–65, 2015.

Cordero MD, de Miguel M, Carmona-López I, et al: Oxidative stress and mitochondrial dysfunction in fibromyalgia, *Neuro Endocrinol Lett* 31:169–173, 2010.

Corrada MM, Kawas CH, Hallfrisch J, et al: Reduced risk of Alzheimer's disease with high folate intake: the Baltimore Longitudinal Study of Aging, *Alzheimers Dement* 1:11–18, 2005.

Davison KM, Kaplan BJ: Vitamin and mineral intakes in adults with mood disorders: comparisons to nutrition standards and associations with sociodemographic and clinical variables, *J Am Coll Nutr* 30:547–558, 2011.

Dean O, Giorlando F, Berk M: N-acetylcysteine in psychiatry: current therapeutic evidence and potential mechanisms of action, *J Psychiatry Neurosci* 36:78–86, 2011.

Dickerson F, Stallings C, Origoni A, et al: Markers of gluten sensitivity and celiac disease in bipolar disorder, *Bipolar Disord* 13:52–58, 2011.

Douaud G, Refsum H, de Jager CA, et al: Preventing Alzheimer's disease-related gray matter atrophy by B-vitamin treatment, *Proc Natl Acad Sci U S A* 110(23):9523–9528, 2013.

Duffy ME, Hoey L, Hughes CF, et al: Biomarker responses to folic acid intervention in healthy adults: a meta-analysis of randomized controlled trials, *Am J Clin Nutr* 99:96–106, 2014.

Enderami A, Zarghami M, Darvishi-Khezri H: The effects and potential mechanisms of folic acid on cognitive function: a comprehensive review, *Neurol Sci* 39(10):1667–1675, 2018.

European College of Neuropsychopharmacology: *Glutamatergic agents show promise for mood, anxiety disorders*, 2013. Available at: www.sciencedaily.com/releases/2013/10/131006142321.htm.

Fattal I, Friedmann N, Fattal-Valevski A: The crucial role of thiamine in the development of syntax and lexical retrieval: a study of infantile thiamine deficiency, *Brain* 134(Pt 6):1720–1739, 2011.

Faux NG, Ellis KA, Porter L, et al: Homocysteine, vitamin B12, and folic acid levels in Alzheimer's disease, mild cognitive impairment, and healthy elderly: baseline characteristics in subjects of the Australian Imaging Biomarker Lifestyle study, *J Alzheimers Dis* 27:909–922, 2011.

Firth J, Carney R, Stubbs B, et al: Nutritional deficiencies and clinical correlates in first-episode psychosis: a systematic review and meta-analysis, *Schizophr Bull* 44(6):1275–1292, 2017.

Forester BP, Harper DG, Georgakas J, et al: Antidepressant effects of open label treatment with Coenzyme Q10 in Geriatric Bipolar Depression, *J Clin Psychopharmacol* 35(3):338–340, 2015.

Freund LY, Vedin I, Cederholm T, et al: Transfer of omega-3 fatty acids across the blood-brain barrier after dietary supplementation with a docosahaenoic acid-rich omega-3 fatty acid preparation in patients with Alzheimer's disease: the OmegAD study, *J Intern Med* 275:428–436, 2014.

Fricker RA, Green EL, Jenkins SI, et al: The influence of nicotinamide on health and disease in the central nervous system, *Int J Tryptophan Res* 11:1178646918776658, 2018.

Gaby AR: *Nutritional medicine*, Concord, NH, 2011, Fritz Perlberg Publishing.

Galvin R, Bråthen G, Ivashynka A, et al: EFNS guidelines for diagnosis, therapy and prevention of Wernicke encephalopathy, *Eur J Neurol* 17:1408–1418, 2010.

Garland EJ: Facing the evidence: antidepressant treatment in children and adolescents, *CMAJ* 170:489–491, 2004.

Gejman P, Sanders AR, Duan J, et al: The role of genetics in the etiology of schizophrenia, *Psychiatr Clin North Am* 33(1):35–66, 2010.

Genuis SJ, Lobo RA: Gluten sensitivity presenting as a neuropsychiatric disorder, *Gastroenterol Res Pract* 2014:293206, 2014. doi:10.1155/2014/293206.

Gillies D, Sinn JKH, Lad SS, et al: Polyunsaturated fatty acids (PUFA) for attention deficit hyperactivity disorder (ADHD) in children and adolescents, *Cochrane Database Syst Rev* (7):CD007986, 2012.

Gould J, Treyvaud K, Yelland L, et al: Seven-year follow-up of children born to women in a randomized trial of prenatal DHA supplementation, *JAMA*, 317(11):1173-1175, 2017.

Grabrucker AM, Rowan M, Garner CC: Brain-delivery of zinc-ions as potential treatment for neurological diseases: mini review, *Drug Deliv Lett* 1(1):13–23, 2011.

Grima NA, Pase MP, Macpherson H, et al: The effects of multivitamins on cognitive performance: a systematic review and meta-analysis, *J Alzheimers Dis* 29:561–569, 2012.

Gröber U, Kisters K, Schmidt J: Neuroenhancement with vitamin B12—underestimated neurological significance, *Nutrients* 5:5031–5045, 2013.

Grosso G, Micek A, Marventano S, et al: Dietary n-3 PUFA, fish consumption and depression: A systematic review and meta-analysis of observational studies, *J Affect Disord* 205:269–281, 2016.

Hall K, Murrell J, Ogunniyi A, et al: Cholesterol, APOE genotype, and Alzheimer disease, *Neurology* 66(2):223–227, 2006.

Hallahan B, Hibbeln JR, Davis JM, et al: Omega-3 fatty acid supplementation in patients with recurrent self-harm. Single-centre double-blind randomized controlled trial, *Br J Psychiatry* 190:118–122, 2007.

Hanson AJ, Bayer-Carter JL, Green PS, et al: Effect of apolipoprotein E genotype and diet on apolipoprotein E lipidation and amyloid peptides: randomized clinical trial, *JAMA Neurol* 70:972–980, 2013.

Hibbeln JR, Davis JM: Considerations regarding neuropsychiatric nutritional requirements for intakes of omega-3 highly unsaturated fatty acids, *Prostaglandins Leukot Essent Fatty Acids* 81:179–186, 2009.

Hilimire MR, DeVylder JE, Forestell CA: Fermented foods, neuroticism, and social anxiety: An interaction model, *Psychiatry Res* 228(2):203–208, 2015.

Ionescu DF, Papakostas GI: Experimental medication treatment approaches for depression, *Transl Psychiatry* 7:e1068, 2017.

Isasi C, Colmenero I, Casco F, et al: Fibromyalgia and non-celiac gluten sensitivity: a description with remission of fibromyalgia, *Rheumatol Int* 34:1607–1612, 2014.

Izawa S, Eto Y, Yamada KC, et al: Cynical hostility, anger expression style, and acute myocardial infarction in middle-aged Japanese men, *Behav Med* 37:81–86, 2011.

Jackson J, Eaton W, Cascella N, et al: A gluten-free diet in people with schizophrenia and anti- tissue transglutaminase or anti-gliadin antibodies, *Schizophr Res* 140:262–263, 2012.

Jackson JR, Eaton WW, Cascella NG, et al: Neurologic and psychiatric manifestations of celiac disease and gluten sensitivity, *Psychiatr Q* 83:91–102, 2012a.

Joffe RT: Hormone treatment of depression, *Dialogues Clin Neurosci* 13:127–138, 2011.

Kapusta ND, Mossaheb N, Etzersdorfer E, et al: Lithium in drinking water and suicide mortality, *Br J Psychiatry* 198:346–350, 2011.

Kelly T, Lieberman DZ: The use of triiodothyronine as an augmentation agent in treatment-resistant bipolar II and bipolar disorder NOS, *J Affect Disord* 116:222–226, 2009.

Kerti L, Witte AV, Winkler A, et al: Higher glucose levels associated with lower memory and reduced hippocampal microstructure, *Neurology* 81:1746–1752, 2013.

Kim J, Wessling-Resnick M: Iron and mechanisms of emotional behavior, *J Nutr Biochem* 25:1101–1107, 2014.

Kjærgaard M, Waterloo K, Wang CE, et al: Effect of vitamin D supplement on depression scores in people with low levels of serum 25-hydroxyvitamin D: nested case-control study and randomised clinical trial, *Br J Psychiatry* 201:360–368, 2012.

Lehmann DJ, Worwood M, Ellis R, et al: Iron genes, iron load and risk of Alzheimer's disease, *J Med Genet* 43(10):e52, 2006.

Lewis MD, Hibbeln JR, Johnson JE, et al: Suicide deaths of active-duty US military and omega-3 fatty-acid status: a case-control comparison, *J Clin Psychiatry*, 721(12):1585–90, 2011.

Littlejohns TJ, Henley WE, Lang IA, et al: Vitamin D and the risk of dementia and Alzheimer disease, *Neurology* 2;83(10):920–928, 2014.

Lozoff B, Castillo M, Clark KM, et al: Iron supplementation in infancy contributes to more adaptive behavior at 10 years of age, *J Nutr* 144:838–845, 2014.

Luchsinger JA, Tanx MX, Miller J, et al: Relation of higher folate intake to lower risk of Alzheimer disease in the elderly, *Arch Neurol* 64:86–92, 2007.

Lu'o'ng Kv, Nguyen LT: Role of thiamine in Alzheimer's disease, *Am J Alzheimers Dis Other Demen* 26:588–598, 2011.

Mahmoud MM, El-Mazary AA, Maher RM, et al: Zinc, ferritin, magnesium and copper in a group of Egyptian children with attention deficit hyperactivity disorder, *Ital J Pediatr* 37:60, 2011.

Mapstone M, Cheema AK, Fiandaca MS, et al: Plasma phospholipids identify antecedent memory impairment in older adults, *Nat Med* 20:415–418, 2014.

Marano G, Traversi G, Nannarelli C, et al: Omega-3 fatty acids and schizophrenia: evidences and recommendations, *Clin Ter* 164:e529–e537, 2013.

Markley HG: CoEnzyme Q10 and riboflavin: the mitochondrial connection, *Headache* 52(Suppl 2):81–87, 2012.

Masoumi A, Goldenson B, Ghirmai S, et al: 1alpha,25-dihydroxyvitamin D3 interacts with curcuminoids to stimulate amyloid-beta clearance by macrophages of Alzheimer's disease patients, *J Alzheimers Dis* 17:703–717, 2009.

McClure EA, Gipson CD, Malcolm RJ, et al: Potential role of N-acetylcysteine in the management of substance use disorders, *CNS Drugs* 28:95–106, 2014.

Milte CM, Parletta N, Buckley JD, et al: Increased erythrocyte eicosapentaenoic acid and docosahexaenoic acid are associated with improved attention and behavior in children with ADHD in a randomized controlled three-way crossover trial, *J Atten Disord* 19(11):954–964, 2015.

Mohajeri MH, La Fata G, Steinert RE, et al: Relationship between the gut microbiome and brain function, *Nutr Rev* 76(7):481–496, 2018.

Möhler H: The GABA system in anxiety and depression and its therapeutic potential. *Neuropharmacology* 62(1):42–53, 2012.

Molfino A, Gioia G, Rossi Fanelli F, et al: The role for dietary omega-3 fatty acids supplementation in older adults, *Nutrients* 6:4058–4073, 2014.

Moore E, Mander A, Ames D, et al: Cognitive impairment and vitamin B12: a review, *Int Psychogeriatr* 24:541–556, 2012.

Morris JK, Vidoni ED, Honea RA, et al: Impaired glycemia inceases disease progression in mild cognitive impairment, *Neurobiol Aging* 35:585–589, 2014.

Morris MC, Evans DA, Bienias JL, et al: Dietary intake of antioxidant nutrients and the risk of incident Alzheimer disease in a biracial community study, *JAMA* 287(24):3230–3237, 2002.

Morris MC, Selhub J, Jacques PF: Vitamin B-12 and folate status in relation to decline in scores on the mini-mental state examination in the framingham heart study, *J Am Geriatr Soc* 60(8):1457–1464, 2012.

Morris MC, Tangney CC, Wang Y, et al: MIND diet slows cognitive decline with aging, *Alzheimers Dement* 11:1015–1022, 2015.

National Institute of Mental Health: *Bipolar disorder*, 2017. Available at: https://www.nimh.nih.gov/health/topics/bipolar-disorder/index.shtml.

Ng QX, Koh SSH, Chan HW, et al: Clinical use of curcumin in depression: a meta-analysis, *J Am Med Dir Assoc* 18(6):503–508, 2017.

Niebuhr DW, Li Y, Cowan DN, et al: Association between bovine casein antibody and new onset schizophrenia among US military personnel, *Schizophr Res* 128:51–55, 2011.

Nierenberg AA, Kansky C, Brennan BP, et al: Mitochondrial modulators for bipolar disorder: a pathophysiologically informed paradigm for new drug development, *Aust N Z J Psychiatry* 47:26–42, 2013.

Nishi A, Numata S, Tajima A, et al: Meta-analyses of blood homocysteine levels for gender and genetic association studies of the MTHFR C677T polymorphism in schizophrenia, *Schizophr Bull* 40:1154–1163, 2014.

Northam EA, Cameron FJ: Understanding the diabetic brain: new technologies but old challenges, *Diabetes* 62:341–342, 2013.

Nuttall KL: Evaluating selenium poisoning, *Ann Clin Lab Sci* 36:409–420, 2006.

Oldham MA, Ivkovic A: Pellagrous encephalopathy presenting as alcohol withdrawal delirium: a case series and literature review, *Addict Sci Clin Pract* 7:12, 2012.

Owen L, Corfe B: The role of diet and nutrition on mental health and wellbeing. *Proc Nutr Soc* 76(4):425–426, 2017.

Pagliai G, Sofi F, Vannetti F, et al: Mediterranean Diet, Food Consumption and Risk of Late-Life Depression: The Mugello Study, *J Nutr Health Aging* 22(5):569–574, 2018.

Pan J, Li H, Ma JF, et al: Curcumin inhibition of JNKs prevents dopaminergic neuronal loss in a mouse model of Parkinson's disease through suppressing mitochondria dysfunction, *Transl Neurodegener* 1:16, 2012.

Pan X, Fei G, Lu J, et al: Measurement of blood thiamine metabolites for Alzheimer's Disease Diagnosis. *EBioMedicine* 26(3):155–162, 2015.

Panjwani AA, Liu H, Fahey JW, et al: Crucifers and related vegetables and supplements for neurologic disorders: what is the evidence? *Curr Opin Clin Nutr Metab Care* 21(6):451–457, 2018.

Paoli A, Bianco A, Damiani E, et al: Ketogenic diet in neuromuscular and neurodegenerative diseases, *Biomed Res Int* 2014:474296, 2014. doi:10.1155/2014/474296.

Parker GF: DSM-5 and psychotic mood disorders, *J Am Acad Psychiatry Law* 42:182–190, 2014.

Pasco JA, Jacka FN, Williams LJ, et al: Dietary selenium and major depression: a nested case-control study, *Complement Ther Med* 20:119–123, 2012.

Petrilli MA, Kranz TM, Kleinhaus K, et al: The emerging role for zinc in depression and psychosis. *Front Pharmacol* 8:414, 2017.

Posternak M, Novak S, Stern R, et al: A pilot effectiveness study: placebo-controlled trial of adjunctive L-triiodothyronine (T3) used to accelerate and potentiate the antidepressant response, Int J Neuropsychopharmacol 11:15–25, 2008.

Presley TD, Morgan AR, Bechtold E, et al: Acute effect of a high nitrate diet on brain perfusion in older adults, *Nitric Oxide* 24:34–42, 2011.

Ranjbar E, Shams J, Sabetkasaei M, et al: Effects of zinc supplementation on efficacy of antidepressant therapy, inflammatory cytokines, and brain-derived neurotrophic factor in patients with major depression, *Nutr Neurosci* 17:65–71, 2014.

Rayman MP: The importance of selenium to human health, *Lancet* 356:233–241, 2000.

Reddy PH, Manczak M, Yin X, et al: Protective Effects of Indian Spice Curcumin Against Amyloid Beta in Alzheimer's Disease, *J Alzheimers Dis* 61(3):843–866, 2018.

Rigacci S, Stefani M: Nutraceuticals and amyloid neurodegenerative diseases: a focus on natural phenols, *Expert Rev Neurother* 15:41–52, 2015.

Roffman JL, Lamberti JS, Achtyes E, et al: Randomized multicenter investigation of folate plus vitamin B12 supplementation in schizophrenia, *JAMA Psychiatry* 70:481–489, 2013.

Sarris J, Mischoulon D, Schweitzer I: Omega-3 for bipolar disorder: meta-analyses of use in mania and biopolar depression. *J Clin Psychiatry*, 73(1):81–86, 2012.

Saunders EF, Ramsden CE, Sherazy MS, et al: Omega-3 and Omega-6 polyunsaturated fatty acids in bipolar disorder: a review of biomarker and treatment studies, *J Clin Psychiatry* 77(10):e1301–e1308, 2016.

Schiöth HB, Craft S, Brooks SJ, et al: Brain insulin signaling and Alzheimer's disease: current evidence and future directions, *Mol Neurobiol* 46:4–10, 2012.

Selhub J, Morris MS, Jacques P: In vitamin B12 deficiency, higher serum folate is associated with increased total homocysteine and methylmalonic acid concentrations, *PNAS* 104(50):19995–20000, 2007.

Serata D, Del Casale A, Rapinesi C, et al: Hemochromatosis-induced bipolar disorder: a case report, *Gen Hosp Psychiatry* 34:101.el-3, 2012.

Seshadri S, Wolf PA, Beiser A, et al: Lifetime risk of dementia and Alzheimer's disease: the impact of mortality on risk estimates in the Framingham Study, *Neurology* 49(6):1498–1504, 1997.

Sharkey KA, Savidge TC: Role of enteric neurotransmission in host defense and protection of the gastrointestinal tract, *Auton Neurosci* 181:94–106, 2014.

Sharma A, Bemis M, Desilets AR: Role of medium chain triglycerides (Axona (R)) in the treatment of mild to moderate Alzheimer's Disease, *Am J Alzheimers Dis Other Demen* 29:409–414, 2014.

Shoemark DK, Allen SJ: The microbiome and disease: reviewing the links between the oral microbiome, aging and Alzheimer's disease, *J Alzheimers Dis* 43:725–738, 2015.

Singh K, Connors SL, Macklin EA, et al: Sulforaphane treatment of autism spectrum disorder (ASD), *Proc Natl Acad Sci U S A* 111:15550–15555, 2014.

Spencer JP: The impact of fruit flavonoids on memory and cognition, *Br J Nutr* 104(Suppl 3):S40–S47, 2010.

Stewart R, Hirani V: Relationship between vitamin D levels and depressive symptoms in older residents from a national survey population, *Psychosom Med* 72:608–612, 2010.

Sutton LP, Orlandi C, Song C, et al: Orphan receptor GPR158 controls stress-induced depression, *Elife* 8:7, 2018.

Swardfager W, Herrmann N, Mazereeuw G, et al: Zinc in depression: a meta-analysis, *Biol Psychiatry* 74(12):872–878, 2013.

Teitelbaum JE: Effective treatment of chronic fatigue syndrome, *Integr Med* 10:44, 2012a.

Teitelbaum JE, Nambudripad DS, Tyson Y, et al: Improving communication skills in children with allergy-related Autism using Nambudripad's allergy elimination techniques: a pilot study, *Integr Med* 10:36–43, 2011.

Tyszka-Czochara M, Grzywacz A, Gdula-Argasińska J, et al: The role of zinc in the pathogenesis and treatment of central nervous system (CNS) diseases. Implications of zinc homeostasis for proper CNS function, *Acta Pol Pharm* 71:369–377, 2014.

Undurraga J, Baldessarini RJ: Randomized, placebo-controlled trials of antidepressants for acute major depression: thirty-year meta-analytic review, *Neuropsychopharmacology* 37:851–864, 2012.

Uribarri J, Woodruff S, Goodman S, et al: Advanced glycation end products in foods and a practical guide to their reduction in the diet, *J Am Diet Assoc* 110:911–916.e12, 2010.

U.S. Department of Agriculture, Agricultural Research Service: Nutrient Intakes per 1000 kcal from Food and Beverages: Mean Energy and Mean Nutrient Amounts per 1000 kcal Consumed per Individual, by Gender and Age, What We Eat in America, *NHANES*, 2015-2016, 2018. Available at: https://www.ars.usda.gov/northeast-area/beltsville-md-bhnrc/beltsville-human-nutrition-research-center/food-surveys-research-group/docs/wweia-data-tables/.

Usoro OB, Mousa SA: Vitamin E forms in Alzheimer's disease: a review of controversial and clinical experiences, *Crit Rev Food Sci Nutr* 50:414–419, 2010.

Valls-Pedret C, Lamuela-Raventós RM, Medina-Remón A, et al: Polyphenol-rich foods in the Mediterranean diet are associated with better cognitive function in elderly subjects at high cardiovascular risk, *J Alzheimers Dis* 29:773–782, 2012.

Varghese T, Hayek SS, Shekiladze N, et al: Psychosocial risk factors related to ischemic heart disease in women, *Curr Pharm Des* 22(25):3853–3870, 2016.

van der Zwaluw NL, Dhonukshe-Rutten RA, van Wijngaarden JP, et al: Results of 2-year vitamin B treatment on cognitive performance: secondary data from an RCT, *Neurology* 83(23):2158–2166, 2014.

Vashum KP, McEvoy M, Milton AH, et al: Dietary zinc is associated with a lower incidence of depression: findings from two Australian cohorts, *J Affect Disord* 166:249–257, 2014.

Vidović B, Dorđević B, Milovanović S, et al: Selenium, zinc, and copper plasma levels in patients with schizophrenia: relationship with metabolic risk factors, *Biol Trace Elem Res* 156:22–28, 2013.

Wang R, Holsinger RMD: Exercise-induced brain-derived neurotrophic factor expression: therapeutic implications for Alzheimer's dementia, *Ageing Res Rev* 48:109–121, 2018.

Welch AA, Shakya-Shrestha S, Lentjes MA et al: Dietary intake and status of n-3 polyunsaturated fatty acids in a population of fish-eating and non-fish-eating meat-eaters, vegetarians, and vegans and the precursor-product-precursor ratio of α-linolenic acid to long–chain n-3 polyunsaturated fatty acids: results from the EPIC-Norfolk cohort, *Am J Clin Nutr* 92:1040–1051, 2010.

White L: *Alzheimer's disease may be easily misdiagnosed*, Honolulu, Hawaii, 2011, American Academy of Neurology- Contemporary and Clinical Issues and Case Studies Plenary Session Annual Meeting.

Willette AA, Johnson SC, Birdsill AC, et al: Insulin resistance predicts brain amyloid deposition in late middle-aged adults, *Alzheimers Dement* 11:504–510.e1, 2015.

Wolf F, Clauw DJ, Fitzcharles MA, et al: The American College of Rheumatology Preliminary Diagnostic Criteria for Fibromyalgia and Measurement of Symptom Severity, *Arthritis Care & Research*, (62)5, 600–610, 2010.

Wolfe F, Clauw DJ, Fitzcharles MA, et al: Fibromyalgia criteria and severity scales for clinical and epidemiological studies: a modification of the ACR Preliminary Diagnostic Criteria for Fibromyalgia, *J Rheumatol* 38:1113–1122, 2011.

Wolfe F, Brähler E, Hinz A, et al: Fibromyalgia prevalence, somatic symptom reporting, and the dimensionality of polysymptomatic distress: results from a survey of the general population, *Arthritis Care Res (Hoboken)* 65:777–785, 2013.

World Health Organization: *Depression*, 2018. Available at: http://www.who.int/mental_health/management/depression/en/.

Woodhead JL, Howell BA, Yang Y, et al: An analysis of N-acetylcysteine treatment for acetaminophen overdose using a systems model of drug-induced liver injury, *J Pharmacol Exp Ther* 342:529–540, 2012.

Wray N, Ripke S, Mattheisen M, et al: Genome-wide association analyses identify 44 risk variants and refine the genetic architecture of major depression, *Nat Genet* 50:668–681, 2018.

Wurtman J, Wurtman R: The trajectory from mood to obesity, *Curr Obes Rep* 7(1):1–5, 2018.

Yang Y, Kim Y, Je Y: Fish consumption and risk of depression: epidemiological evidence from prospective studies, *Asia Pac Psychiatry*, 10:e12335, 2018.

Yetley EA, Johnson CL: Folate and vitamin B-12 biomarkers in NHANES: history of their measurement and use, *Am J Clin Nutr* 94:322S–331S, 2011.

Ylilauri MP, Voutilainen S, Lönnroos E, et al: Association of dietary cholesterol and egg intakes with the risk of incident dementia or Alzheimer disease: the Kuopio Ischaemic Heart Disease Risk Factor Study, *Am J Clin Nutr* 105(2):476–484, 2017.

Young H, Benton D: The nature of the control of blood glucose in those with poorer glucose tolerance influences mood and cognition, *Metab Brain Dis* 29:721–728, 2014.

Zhang G, Ding H, Chen H, et al: Thiamine nutritional status and depressive symptoms are inversely associated among older Chinese adults, *J Nutr* 143:53–58, 2013.

Zhang Y, Yan H, Tian L, et al: Association of MTHFR C677T polymorphism with schizophrenia and its effect on episodic memory and gray matter density in patients, *Behav Brain Res* 243:146–152, 2013a.

PART VI

Pediatric Specialties

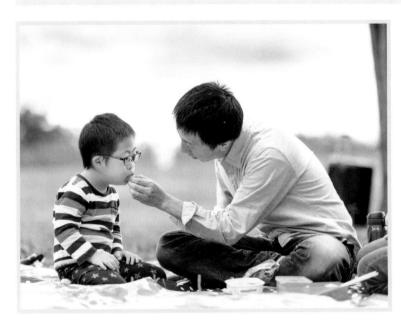

The unique, special role of nutrition in the pediatric population cannot be underestimated. Pediatricians, nurses, and dietitian nutritionists all recognize that unusual feeding problems or disorders can negatively influence growth and health, especially in the very young. This section addresses the specific pediatric conditions affecting the nutritional intake and growth velocity of infants and children. In some cases, adolescents are mentioned if relevant, but most of this section considers younger patients.

Whether in neonatal units, hospital pediatric units, out-patient clinics, long-term care units, or in-home care, children coping with genetic or acquired disorders need appropriate nutrition support in order to grow and thrive. More than ever, nutrition care in this specialty arena requires an understanding of the biochemical, physiologic, social, and economic challenges that our youngest patients face.

41

Medical Nutrition Therapy for Low-Birthweight Infants

Diane M. Anderson, PhD, RDN, FADA

KEY TERMS

apnea of prematurity	human milk fortifiers	oral care with colostrum
appropriate for gestational age (AGA)	infancy	osteopenia of prematurity
bronchopulmonary dysplasia (BPD)	infant mortality rate	perinatal period
carnitine	intrauterine growth restriction (IUGR)	postterm infant
extrauterine growth restriction (EUGR)	kangaroo care	premature (preterm) infant
extremely low birthweight (ELBW)	large for gestational age (LGA)	respiratory distress syndrome (RDS)
gastric gavage	low birthweight (LBW)	small for gestational age (SGA)
gestational age	necrotizing enterocolitis (NEC)	surfactant
glucose load	neonatal period	term infant
hemolytic anemia	neutral thermal environment	very low birthweight (VLBW)

The management of low birthweight (LBW) infants requiring intensive care is continually improving. With new technologies, enhanced understanding of pathophysiologic conditions of the perinatal period (from 20 weeks of gestation to 28 days after birth), current nutrition management principles, and regionalization of perinatal care, the mortality rate during infancy—the period from birth to 1 year of age—has decreased in the United States. In particular, the development and use of surfactant—a mixture of lipoproteins secreted by alveolar cells into the alveoli and respiratory air passages that contributes to the elastic properties of pulmonary tissue—have increased the survival of preterm infants, as has the use of antepartum corticosteroids. Most premature infants have the potential for long and productive lives (Wilson-Costello and Payne, 2015).

Nutrition can be provided to LBW infants in many ways, each of which has certain benefits and limitations. The infant's size, age, and clinical condition dictate the nutrition requirements and the way they can be met. Because of the complexities involved in the neonatal intensive care setting, a team that includes a registered dietitian nutritionist trained in neonatal nutrition should make the decisions necessary to facilitate optimal nutrition (Ehrenkranz, 2014). Neonatal nutritionists monitor compliance with standardized feeding guidelines; ensure that early, intense nutritional support is initiated; facilitate the smooth transition from parenteral to enteral nutrition; and monitor growth and individualized nutrition support to maintain steady infant growth. In regionalized perinatal care systems, the neonatal nutritionist also may consult with health care providers in community hospitals and public health settings.

INFANT MORTALITY AND STATISTICS

In 2016 the infant mortality rate in the United States decreased to 5.87 infant deaths per 1000 live births (Xu et al, 2018). More than 65% of these deaths occur in the neonatal period, with the leading causes being birth defects, prematurity, and LBW. The preterm birth rate was 9.85%, and the incidence of LBW was 8.17% (Martin et al, 2018). The incidence of premature and LBW infants has increased from 2014, which is due to the increased births of late premature infants (Martin et al, 2017). Late premature infants are infants born at 34 to 36 weeks' gestation (Martin and Osterman, 2018). Late premature infants may be near the size of the term infant but will have medical and clinical problems like all premature infants (Williams and Pugh, 2018).

PHYSIOLOGIC DEVELOPMENT

Gestational Age and Size

At birth, an infant who weighs less than 2500 g (5½ lb) is classified as having a low birthweight (LBW); an infant weighing less than 1500 g (3⅓ lb) has a very low birthweight (VLBW); and an infant weighing less than 1000 g (2¼ lb) has an extremely low birthweight (ELBW). LBW may be attributable to a shortened period of gestation, prematurity, or a restricted intrauterine growth rate, which makes the infant small for gestational age (SGA).

The term infant is born between the 37th and 42nd weeks of gestation. A premature (preterm) infant is born before 37 weeks of gestation, whereas a postterm infant is born after 42 weeks of gestation.

Antenatally, an estimate of the infant's gestational age is based on the date of the mother's last menstrual period, clinical parameters of uterine fundal height, the presence of quickening (the first movements of the fetus that can be felt by the mother), fetal heart tones, or ultrasound evaluations. After birth, gestational age is determined by clinical assessment. Clinical parameters fall into two groups: (1) a series of neurologic signs, which depend primarily on postures and tone and

(2) a series of external characteristics that reflect the physical maturity of the infant. The New Ballard Score examination is a frequently used clinical assessment tool (Ballard et al, 1991). An accurate assessment of gestational age is important for establishing nutritional goals for individual infants and differentiating the premature infant from the term SGA infant.

An infant who is small for gestational age (SGA) has a birth weight that is lower than the 10th percentile of the standard weight for that gestational age. An SGA infant whose intrauterine weight gain is poor, but whose linear and head growth are between the 10th and 90th percentiles on the intrauterine growth grid, has experienced asymmetric intrauterine growth restriction (IUGR). An SGA infant whose length and occipital frontal circumference are also below the 10th percentile of the standards has symmetric IUGR. Symmetric IUGR, which usually reflects early and prolonged intrauterine deficit, is apparently more detrimental to later growth and development. Some infants can be SGA because they are genetically small, and these infants usually do well.

An infant whose size is appropriate for gestational age (AGA) has a birth weight between the 10th and 90th percentiles on the intrauterine growth chart. The obstetrician diagnoses IUGR when the fetal growth rate decreases. Serial ultrasound measurements document this reduction in fetal anthropometric measurements, which may be caused by maternal, placental, or fetal abnormalities. The future growth and development of infants who have had IUGR is diverse, depending on the specific cause of the IUGR and treatment. Some infants who suffered from IUGR are SGA, but many may plot as AGA infants at birth. Decreased fetal growth does not always result in an infant who is SGA.

An infant whose birth weight is above the 90th percentile on the intrauterine growth chart is large for gestational age (LGA). Box 41.1 summarizes the weight classifications. Fig. 41.1 shows the classification of neonates based on maturity and intrauterine growth.

Characteristics of Immaturity

The premature or LBW infant has not had the chance to develop fully in utero and is physiologically different from the term infant (Fig. 41.2). Because of this, LBW infants have various clinical problems in the early neonatal period, depending on their intrauterine environment, degree of prematurity, birth-related trauma, and function of immature or stressed organ systems. Certain problems occur with such frequency that they are considered typical of prematurity (Table 41.1). Premature infants are at high risk for poor nutrition status because of poor nutrient stores, physiologic immaturity, illness (which may interfere with nutritional management and needs), and the nutrient demands required for growth.

Most fetal nutrient stores are deposited during the last 3 months of gestation; therefore the premature infant begins life in a compromised

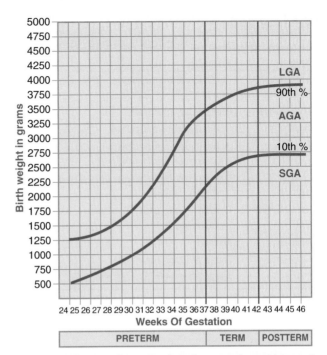

Fig. 41.1 Classification of neonates based on maturity and intrauterine growth (small for gestational age [SGA], appropriate for gestational age [AGA], or large for gestational age [LGA]). (From Battaglia FC, Lubchenco LO: A practical classification of newborn infants by weight and gestational age, *J Pediatr* 71:159, 1967.)

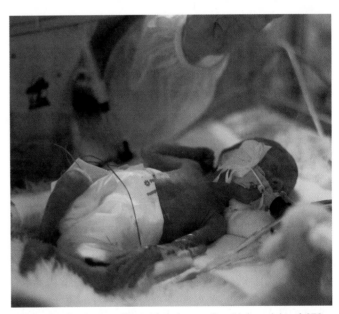

Fig. 41.2 A.R., born at 27 weeks of gestation; birth weight of 870 g (1 lb, 14 oz).

BOX 41.1 Classification of Birthweight and Intrauterine Growth

Low birthweight <2500 g
Very low birthweight <1500 g
Extremely low birthweight <1000 g
Small for gestational age = Birthweight <10th percentile of standard for gestational age
Appropriate for gestational age = Birthweight between the 10th and 90th percentile of standard for gestational age
Large for gestational age = Birthweight >90th percentile of standard for gestational age

nutritional state. Because metabolic (i.e., energy) stores are limited, nutrition support in the form of parenteral nutrition (PN), enteral nutrition (EN), or both should be initiated as soon as possible. In the preterm infant weighing 1000 g, fat constitutes only 1% of total body weight; by contrast the term infant (3500 g) has a fat percentage of approximately 16%. For example, a 1000-g AGA premature infant has a glycogen and fat reserve equivalent to approximately 110 kcal/kg of body weight. With basal metabolic needs of approximately

TABLE 41.1 Common Problems Among Premature Infants

System	Problem
Respiratory	Respiratory distress syndrome, chronic lung disease (bronchopulmonary dysplasia)
Cardiovascular	Patent ductus arteriosus
Renal	Fluid and electrolyte imbalance
Neurologic	Intraventricular hemorrhage, periventricular leukomalacia (cerebral necrosis)
Metabolic	Hypoglycemia, hyperglycemia, hypocalcemia, metabolic acidosis
Gastrointestinal	Hyperbilirubinemia, feeding intolerance, necrotizing enterocolitis
Hematologic	Anemia
Immunologic	Sepsis, pneumonia, meningitis
Other	Apnea, bradycardia, cyanosis, osteopenia

From Eichenwald EC et al, editors: *Cloherty and Stark's Manual of neonatal care*, ed 8, Philadelphia, 2017, Wolters Kluwer.

TABLE 41.2 Expected Survival Time of Starved (H_2O Only) and Semistarved ($D_{10}W$) Infants

	ESTIMATED SURVIVAL TIME (Days)	
Birth Weight (g)	H_2O	$D_{10}W$
1000	4	11
2000	12	30
3500	32	80

Data from Heird WC, et al: Intravenous alimentation in pediatric patients, *J Pediatr* 80:351, 1972.
$D_{10}W$, Dextrose 10% in water; H_2O, water.

50 kcal/kg/day, it is obvious that this infant will rapidly run out of fat and carbohydrate fuel unless adequate nutrition support is established. The depletion time is even shorter for preterm infants weighing less than 1000 g at birth. Nutrient reserves also are depleted most quickly by tiny infants who have IUGR as a result of their decreased nutrient stores.

Theoretic estimates of survival time of starved and semistarved infants are shown in Table 41.2. These estimates assume depletion of all glycogen and fat and approximately one third of body protein tissue at a rate of 50 kcal/kg/day. The effects of fluids such as intravenously provided water (which has no exogenous calories) and 10% dextrose solution ($D_{10}W$) are shown. Currently, PN fluids are started on the day of birth to provide energy and protein for the VLBW infant. Early protein intake promotes positive nitrogen balance, normal plasma amino acid levels, and glucose tolerance.

The small premature infant is particularly vulnerable to undernutrition. Malnutrition in premature infants may increase the risk of infection, prolong chronic illness, and adversely affect brain growth and function. Premature infants fed premature infant formula or human milk demonstrate better growth and development than premature infants fed standard infant formula. Milk from the infant's own mother fed the first month of life has been linked to improved growth and development. Premature infants fed their own mother's milk have

improved neurodevelopment at 30 months of age and higher intelligence test scores at 8 years of age and have brains larger and more developed at 15 years of age (American Academy of Pediatrics [AAP], 2012; Isaacs et al, 2010).

NUTRITION REQUIREMENTS: PARENTERAL FEEDING

Many critically ill preterm infants have difficulty progressing to full enteral feedings in the first several days or even weeks of life. The infant's small stomach capacity, immature gastrointestinal tract, and illness make the progression to full enteral feedings difficult (see *Pathophysiology and Care Management Algorithm:* Nutrition Support of Premature Infants). PN becomes essential for nutrition support, either as a supplement to enteral feedings or as the total source of nutrition. Chapter 12 offers a complete discussion of PN; only aspects related to feeding of the preterm infant are presented here.

Fluid

Because fluid needs vary widely for preterm infants, fluid balance must be monitored. Inadequate intake can lead to dehydration, electrolyte imbalances, and hypotension; excessive intake can lead to edema, congestive heart failure, and possible opening of the ductus arteriosus. Additional neonatal clinical complications reported with high fluid intakes include necrotizing enterocolitis (NEC), and bronchopulmonary dysplasia (BPD) (see Chapter 33).

The premature infant has a greater percentage of body water (especially extracellular water) than the term infant (see Chapter 3). The amount of extracellular water should decrease in all infants during the first few days of life. This reduction is accompanied by a normal loss of 10% to 15% of body weight and improved renal function. Failure of this transition in fluid dynamics and lack of diuresis may complicate the course of preterm infants with respiratory disease.

Water requirements are estimated by the sum of the predicted losses from the lungs and skin, urine, and stool, and the water needed for growth. A major route of water loss in preterm infants is evaporation through the skin and respiratory tract. This insensible water loss is highest in the smallest and least mature infants because of their larger body surface area relative to body weight, increased permeability of the skin epidermis to water, and greater skin blood flow relative to metabolic rate. Insensible water loss is increased by radiant warmers and phototherapy lights and decreased by humidified incubators, heat shields, and thermal blankets. Insensible water loss can vary from 50 to 100 mL/kg/day on the first day of life and increase up to 150 mL/kg/day, depending on the infant's size, gestational age, day of life, and environment. The use of humidified incubators can decrease insensible water losses and thereby reduce fluid requirements.

Excretion of urine, the other major route of water loss, varies from 1 to 3 mL/kg/hr (Doherty, 2017). This loss depends on the fluid volume and solute load presented to the kidneys. The infant's ability to concentrate urine increases with maturity. Stool water loss is generally 5 to 10 mL/kg/day, and 10 to 15 mL/kg/day is suggested as optimal for growth (Dell, 2015).

Because of the many variables affecting neonatal fluid losses, fluid needs must be determined on an individual basis. Usually fluid is administered at a rate of 60 to 100 mL/kg/day the first day of life to meet insensible losses and urine output. Fluid needs then are evaluated by assessing fluid intake and comparing it with the clinical parameters of urine output volume and serum electrolyte, creatinine, and urea nitrogen levels. Assessments of weight, blood pressure, peripheral perfusion, skin turgor, and mucous membrane moisture are performed daily. Daily fluid administration generally increases by 10 to 20 mL/kg/day.

PATHOPHYSIOLOGY AND CARE MANAGEMENT ALGORITHM

Nutrition Support of Premature Infants

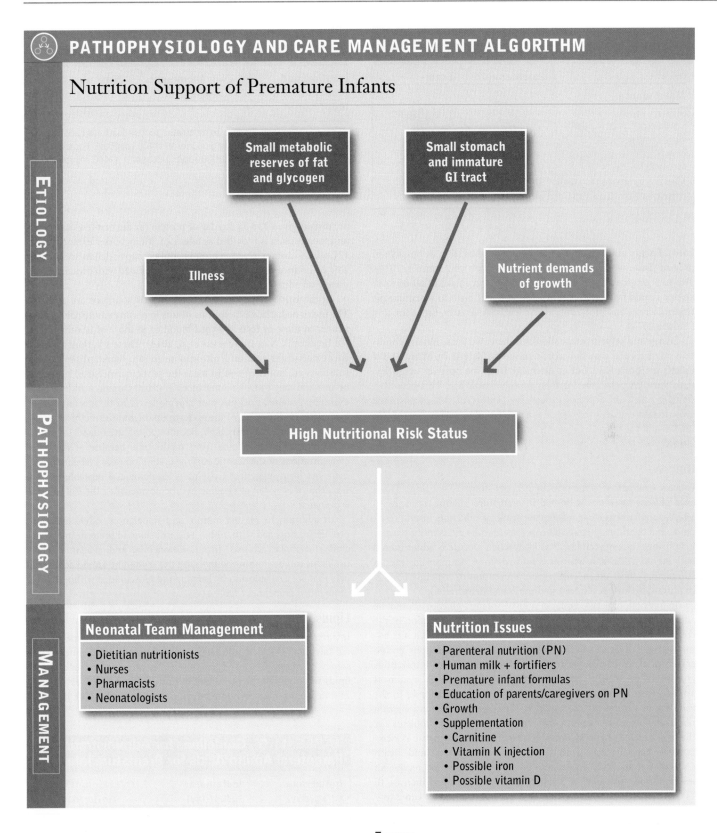

ETIOLOGY

Small metabolic reserves of fat and glycogen

Small stomach and immature GI tract

Illness

Nutrient demands of growth

PATHOPHYSIOLOGY

High Nutritional Risk Status

MANAGEMENT

Neonatal Team Management

- Dietitian nutritionists
- Nurses
- Pharmacists
- Neonatologists

Nutrition Issues

- Parenteral nutrition (PN)
- Human milk + fortifiers
- Premature infant formulas
- Education of parents/caregivers on PN
- Growth
- Supplementation
  - Carnitine
  - Vitamin K injection
  - Possible iron
  - Possible vitamin D

By the end of the first week of life, preterm infants may receive fluids at a rate of 140 to 160 mL/kg/day. Fluid restriction may be necessary in preterm infants with patent ductus arteriosus (an opening between the pulmonary artery and the aorta), congestive heart failure, renal failure, or cerebral edema. However, more fluids are needed by preterm infants who are placed under phototherapy lights or a radiant warmer or when the environmental or body temperature is elevated.

Energy

The energy needs of preterm infants fed parenterally are less than those of enterally fed infants because absorption loss does not occur when nutritional intake bypasses the intestinal tract. Enterally fed preterm infants usually require 110 to 130 kcal/kg/day to grow, whereas parenterally fed premature neonates can grow well if they receive 90 to 100 kcal/kg/day (AAP, 2019; Embleton and Simmer,

TABLE 41.3 Comparison of Parenteral and Enteral Energy Needs of Premature Infants

	Parenteral	Enteral
Maintenance		
Gradually increase intake to meet energy needs by the end of the first week	30-50 kcal/kg/day	50 kcal/kg/day
Growth		
Meet energy needs as soon as the infant's condition is stable	90-100 kcal/kg/day	110-130 kcal/kg/day

TABLE 41.4 Guidelines for Glucose Load in Premature Infants

Initial Load (mg/kg/min)*	Daily Increments (mg/kg/min)	Maximum Load (mg/kg/min)
5-7	1-2	11-12

*Use the following formula to calculate glucose load: (% Glucose × mL/kg/day) × (1000 mg/g glucose) ÷ (1440 min/day). For example, (0.10 × 150 mL/kg/day) × (1000 mg/g glucose) ÷ (1440 min/day) = 10.4 mg/kg/min.

2014). Energy and protein should be provided as soon as possible to prevent tissue catabolism (AAP, 2019; Embleton and Simmer, 2014). Two to 3 g/kg/day of protein with a total energy intake of 60-80 kcal/kg/day should be started within a few hours of birth to maximize nitrogen balance and blood amino acid levels (AAP, 2019; Embleton and Simmer, 2014).

Energy and protein intake should be increased as the infant's condition stabilizes and growth becomes the goal (Table 41.3). Many VLBW infants are born AGA but at discharge from the hospital weigh less than the 10th percentile for their postmenstrual age. This new SGA status is called extrauterine growth restriction (EUGR) or postnatal growth failure. EUGR may occur as a result of poor energy and protein intakes and the decreased growth associated with illness (Griffin et al, 2016).

Glucose

Glucose or dextrose is the principal energy source (3.4 kcal/g). However, glucose tolerance is limited in premature infants, especially in VLBW infants, because of inadequate insulin production, insulin resistance, and continued hepatic glucose release while intravenous glucose is infusing. Hyperglycemia is less likely when glucose is administered with amino acids than when it is infused alone. Amino acids exert a stimulatory effect on insulin release. Prevention of hyperglycemia is important because it can lead to diuresis and dehydration.

To prevent hyperglycemia in VLBW infants, glucose should be administered in small amounts. The glucose load is a function of the concentration of the dextrose infusion and the rate at which it is administered (Table 41.4). The administration of intravenous amino acids stimulates insulin production and the tolerance of intravenous glucose (Hay, 2018). The administration of exogenous insulin is avoided with premature infants (AAP, 2019). Insulin adheres to the intravenous tubing, which results in blood glucose fluctuations as a result of nonsteady insulin concentrations. Additional problems for the infant include hypoglycemia, decreased linear growth, the association of hypoglycemia with poor neurodevelopment, and death (Alsweiler et al, 2012). In general, preterm infants should receive an initial glucose load of 5 to 7 mg/kg/min, with a gradual increase to 11 to 12 mg/kg/min. The glucose load can be advanced by 1 to 2 mg/kg/min/day. Hypoglycemia is not as common a problem as hyperglycemia, but it may occur if the glucose infusion is decreased abruptly or interrupted.

Amino Acids

Protein guidelines range from 3.0 to 4.0 g/kg/day (AAP, 2019). Protein in excess of these parenteral requirements should not be administered because additional protein offers no apparent sdvantage, and increases the risk of metabolic problems (Hay, 2018). In practice preterm infants

are usually given 2 to 3 g/kg/day of protein for the first few days of life, and then protein is provided as tolerated. Many nurseries stock starter PN, which is water, glucose, protein, and perhaps calcium and is available 24 hours a day. Infants then can be provided with protein immediately on admission to the nursery.

In the United States several pediatric PN solutions are available. The use of pediatric PN solutions results in plasma amino acid profiles similar to those of fetal and cord blood or to those of healthy infants fed breastmilk (van Goudoever et al, 2014). These solutions promote adequate weight gain and nitrogen retention. Standard amino acid solutions are not designed to meet the particular needs of immature infants and may provoke imbalances in plasma amino acid levels. For example, cysteine, tyrosine, and taurine levels in these solutions are low relative to the needs of the preterm infant, but the methionine and glycine levels are relatively high. Because premature infants do not effectively synthesize cysteine from methionine because of decreased concentrations of the hepatic enzyme cystathionase, a cysteine supplement has been suggested. Cysteine is insoluble and unstable in solution; thus it is added as cysteine hydrochloride when the PN solution is prepared.

In addition to plasma amino acid imbalances, other metabolic problems associated with amino acid infusions in preterm infants include metabolic acidosis, hyperammonemia, and azotemia. These problems can be minimized by using the crystalline amino acid products that are available and by keeping the protein load within the recommended guidelines (Table 41.5).

Lipids

Intravenous fat emulsions are used for two reasons: (1) to meet essential fatty acid (EFA) requirements and (2) to provide a concentrated source of energy. EFA needs can be met by providing 0.5 g/kg/day of lipids when giving the Intralipid® emulsion. Biochemical evidence of EFA deficiency has been noted during the first week of life in VLBW

TABLE 41.5 Guidelines for Administration of Parenteral Amino Acids for Premature Infants

Initial Rate (g/kg/day)*	Increments (g/kg/day)	Maximum Rate (g/kg/day)
2-3	Advance to meet needs	4

Data from American Academy of Pediatrics, Committee on Nutrition: Nutritional needs of preterm infants. In Kleinman RE, Greer FR, editors: *Pediatric nutrition*, ed 8, Itasca, IL, 2019, American Academy of Pediatrics.
*Use the following formula to calculate protein load: % Protein × mL/kg/day = Protein g/kg/day.
For example: 2% amino acid parenteral solution provided at 150 mL/kg/day *is* 0.02 × 150 mL/kg/day = 3 g/kg/day.

TABLE 41.6 Guidelines for Administration of Parenteral Lipids for Premature Infants

Initial Rate (g/kg/day)*	Increments (g/kg/day)	Maximum Rate (g/kg/day)
2-3	1	3

Data from American Academy of Pediatrics, Committee on Nutrition: Nutritional needs of preterm infants. In Kleinman RE, Greer FR, editors: *Pediatric nutrition*, ed 8, Itasca, IL, 2019, American Academy of Pediatrics.

*Use the following formula to calculate lipid load: % Lipid × mL/kg/day = Lipid g/kg/day. For example, 0.20 × 15 mL/kg = 3 g/kg/day.

infants fed parenterally without fat. The clinical consequences of EFA deficiency may include coagulation abnormalities, abnormal pulmonary surfactant, and adverse effects on lung metabolism.

Lipids can be initiated at 2 to 3 g/kg/day and should be provided over 24 hours (AAP, 2019). Lipids can be advanced by 1 to 2 g/kg/day until a rate of 3 g/kg/day is reached (Table 41.6). Plasma triglycerides should be monitored because elevated triglyceride levels may develop in infants with a decreased ability to hydrolyze triglycerides. These infants usually have lower gestational age, lower birthweight, SGA status, infection, surgical stress, or liver disease. Monitoring of serum triglyceride levels is indicated, and a rate of less than 3 g/kg/day of fat may be required to keep serum triglyceride levels under 200 to 250 mg/dL (AAP, 2019). Once the infant is medically stable and additional energy is needed for growth, lipid loads can be increased slowly. Intralipids can be given to the infant with hyperbilirubinemia. At the present recommendation of 3 g/kg/day, given over 24 hours, the displacement of bilirubin from albumin-binding sites does not occur (AAP, 2014).

The total lipid load is usually 25% to 40% of nonprotein calories (AAP, 2019). (The lipid emulsions currently in use are described in Chapter 12.) In preterm infants 20% Intralipid® solutions providing 2 kcal/mL are recommended because plasma triglyceride, cholesterol, and phospholipid levels are generally lower with these than with the 10% emulsions. The 10% emulsions contain more of the phospholipid emulsifier per gram of lipid and this emulsifier decreases the breakdown of triglycerides.

Intralipid® intravenous fat emulsions are made from soybean oil and contain omega-6 fatty acids, linoleic acid, and arachidonic acid (ARA). These EFAs increase the production of inflammatory mediators and increase the infant's inflammatory state (Premkumar et al, 2014) (see Chapter 7). Omegaven® is a fish-oil base intravenous fat emulsion and contains omega-3 fatty acids: eicosapentaenoic acid (EPA) and docosahexaenoic acid (DHA) and vitamin E. These omega-3 fatty acids are antiinflammatory and the antioxidant properties of vitamin E may be helpful in the treatment of PN-associated liver disease (PNALD) (Premkumar et al, 2014). PNALD can occur with infants who have been on PN for at least 14 days and may be due to a component of the PN and/or the lack of enteral feedings. Infection and prematurity are also risk factors for liver disease. The disease presents with elevated conjugated bilirubin. If not treated, severe liver disease can occur. Intralipid® also contains phytosterols which will decrease bile acid synthesis and flow, which can contribute to the development of PNALD. This fish-oil product is produced in Europe and has recently been approved to treat pediatric patients with PNALD by the Food and Drug Administration (FDA) for patients in the United States. The treatment dose is 1 g/kg/day of the Omegaven® product.

Clinical experience with the fish-oil base intravenous fat is positive with resolution of PNALD in most premature infants (Premkumar et al, 2014). Investigations are needed to determine whether this product can be used to prevent PNALD, which presents with an elevated conjugated bilirubin. Another European fat emulsion, SMOFLipid® (soy oil, medium-chain triglyceride, olive oil, and fish oil), has become available in the United States and has just been approved for adult use by the FDA. SMOFLipid is used off label with the pediatric population. This blend of fat oils may also offer antiinflammatory properties (Vanek et al, 2012). Research must be completed on this product to determine whether it can prevent or treat PNALD and how infants grow on SMOFLipid® (Hojsak et al, 2016). EFA deficiency has been reported with 1 g/kg/day dosing with SMOFLipid, so 2 to 3 g/kg/day should be used with this product (Memon et al, 2019).

Carnitine is frequently added to PN solutions for premature infants. Carnitine facilitates the mechanism by which fatty acids are transported across the mitochondrial membrane, allowing their oxidation to provide energy. Because intravenous lipid does not contain carnitine and premature infants have limited ability to produce carnitine, carnitine supplementation may be helpful for preterm infants who are receiving only PN for 2 to 3 weeks (Hay et al, 2014) The recommended carnitine dose is up to 10 mg/kg/day (AAP, 2019).

Electrolytes

After the first few days of life, sodium, potassium, and chloride are added to parenteral solutions to compensate for the loss of extracellular fluid. To prevent hyperkalemia and cardiac arrhythmia, potassium should be withheld until renal flow is demonstrated. In general, the preterm infant has the same electrolyte requirements as the term infant, but actual requirements vary, depending on factors such as renal function, state of hydration, and the use of diuretics (Table 41.7). Very immature infants may have a limited ability to conserve sodium and thus may require increased amounts of sodium to maintain a normal serum sodium concentration. Serum electrolyte levels should be monitored periodically.

Minerals

Calcium and phosphorus are important components of the PN solution. Premature infants who receive PN with low calcium and phosphorus concentrations are at risk for developing osteopenia of prematurity. This poor bone mineralization is most likely to develop in VLBW infants who receive PN for prolonged periods. Calcium and phosphorus status should be monitored using serum calcium, phosphorus, and alkaline phosphatase activity levels (see Appendix 12). Alkaline phosphatase activity levels in premature infants are greater than the levels seen with adults. It is common to see levels up to 600 IU/L, which may reflect rapid bone growth (Abrams, 2017). When alkaline phosphatase activity levels of 800 IU/L or more persist, knee or wrist radiographs should be examined for rickets (Abrams, 2017).

TABLE 41.7 Guidelines for Administration of Parenteral Electrolytes for Premature Infants

Electrolyte	Amount (mEq/kg/day)
Sodium	2-4
Chloride	2-4
Potassium	1.5-2

Data from American Academy of Pediatrics, Committee on Nutrition: Nutritional needs of preterm infants. In Kleinman RE, Greer FR, editors: *Pediatric nutrition*, ed 8, Itasca, IL, 2019, American Academy of Pediatrics.

TABLE 41.8 Guidelines for Administration of Parenteral Minerals for Premature Infants

Minerals	Amount (mg/kg/day)*
Calcium	60-80
Phosphorus	39-67
Magnesium	4.3-7.2

From American Academy of Pediatrics, Committee on Nutrition: Nutritional needs of preterm infants. In Kleinman RE, Greer FR, editors: *Pediatric nutrition*, ed 8, Itasca, IL, 2019, American Academy of Pediatrics.

*These recommendations assume an average fluid intake of 120 to 150 mL/kg/day with 2.5 g of amino acids per 100 mL. The amino acid concentration prevents the precipitation of these minerals.

TABLE 41.9 Guidelines for Administration of Parenteral Trace Elements for Premature Infants

Trace Elements	Amount (mcg/kg/day)
Zinc	400
Copper	20*
Manganese	1*
Selenium	2.0[†]
Chromium	0.0006[†]
Iodine	1

From Vanek VW: Review of trace mineral requirements for preterm infants: what are the current recommendations for clinical practice? *NCP* 30(5):720, 2015; Vanck VW, et al: ASPEN position paper: recommendations for changes in commercially available parenteral multivitamin and multi-trace element products. *NCP* 27(4):440, 2013.
*Reduced or not provided for infants with obstructive jaundice. Copper may have to be provided based on the infant's blood copper levels.
[†]Reduced or not provided for infants with renal dysfunction.

Elevation in alkaline phosphatase activity also may be seen with liver disease. Serum phosphorous may be low with rickets (Abrams, 2017).

Preterm infants have higher calcium and phosphorus needs than term infants. However, it is difficult to add enough calcium and phosphorus to parenteral solutions to meet these higher requirements without causing precipitation of the minerals. Calcium and phosphorus should be provided simultaneously in PN solutions. Alternate-day infusions are not recommended because abnormal serum mineral levels and decreased mineral retention develop.

Current recommendations for parenteral administration of additional calcium, phosphorus, and magnesium are presented in Table 41.8. The intakes are expressed at a volume intake of 120 to 150 mL/kg/day, with 2.5 g/100 mL of amino acids or protein. Lower fluid volumes or lower protein concentrations may cause the minerals to precipitate out of solution. The addition of cysteine hydrochloride increases the acidity of the fluid, which inhibits precipitation of calcium and phosphorus.

Trace Elements

Zinc should be given to all preterm infants receiving PN. If enteral feedings cannot be started by 2 weeks of age, additional trace elements should be added. However, the amount of copper or manganese should be reduced or omitted for infants with obstructive jaundice, and the amounts of selenium and chromium should be reduced or omitted in infants with renal dysfunction. Copper can be concentrated in the liver with cholestasis, and it is recommended to determine copper status by plasma copper levels or plasma ceruloplasmin levels (AAP, 2019; Domellof, 2014). Parenteral iron is not routinely provided because infants often receive blood transfusions soon after birth, and enteral feedings, which provide a source of iron, often can be initiated. If necessary, the dosage for parenteral iron is approximately 10% of the enteral dosage; guidelines range from 0.2 to 0.25 mg/kg/day (Domellöf, 2014). Table 41.9 provides guidelines for trace minerals.

Vitamins

Shortly after birth all newborn infants receive an intramuscular (IM) injection of 0.3 to 1 mg of vitamin K to prevent hemorrhagic disease of the newborn from vitamin K deficiency. Stores of vitamin K are low in newborn infants, and there is little intestinal bacterial production of vitamin K until bacterial colonization takes place. Because initial dietary intake of vitamin K is limited, neonates are at nutritional risk if they do not receive this IM supplement.

Only intravenous multivitamin preparations currently approved and designed for use in infants should be given to provide the appropriate vitamin intake and prevent toxicity from additives used in adult multivitamin injections. The AAP recommends 40% of the multivitamin for infusion (MVI)-pediatric 5-mL vial per kilogram of weight (AAP, 2019). The maximum dose of 5 mL is given to an infant with a weight of 2.5 kg (Table 41.10).

Respiratory distress syndrome (RDS) is a disease that occurs in premature infants shortly after birth because these infants are deficient in the lung substance surfactant. Surfactant is responsible for keeping the lung elastic while breathing; thus surfactant supplements are given to the infant to prevent RDS or to lessen the illness. Lipids and proteins are components of surfactant, and phospholipids are the major lipid. Choline is required for phospholipid synthesis, but choline supplementation does not increase the production of phospholipids (van Aerde and Narvey, 2006). Choline is a conditionally essential nutrient because the infant can synthesize choline (see Chapter 14 for a discussion of requirement for choline in pregnancy). Choline is added to premature infant formulas at the level contained in human milk. Human milk can be a good source of choline for the infant. The milk choline levels will reflect the mother's intake of choline (Zeisel et al, 2018). The upper level is extrapolated from the adult safe level of intake (Klein, 2002).

TABLE 41.10 Guidelines for Administration of Parenteral Vitamins for Premature Infants

	Preterm
Percentage of one 5-mL vial of MVI-Pediatric/INFUVITE*	40%/kg

MVI, Multivitamin for infusion.
Maximum volume intake is 5 mL/day, which is achieved at 2.5 kg body weight.
*MVI-Pediatric/INFUVITE (5 mL) contains the following vitamins: 80 mg of ascorbic acid, 2300 USP units of vitamin A, 400 USP units of vitamin D, 1.2 mg of thiamin, 1.4 mg of riboflavin, 1 mg of vitamin B$_6$, 17 mg of niacin, 5 mg of pantothenic acid, 7 USP units of vitamin E, 20 mcg of biotin, 140 mcg of folic acid, 1 mcg of vitamin B$_{12}$, and 200 mcg of vitamin K.
Data from American Academy of Pediatrics, Committee on Nutrition: Nutritional needs of preterm infants. In Kleinman RE, Greer FR, editors: *Pediatric nutrition*, ed 8, Itasac, IL, 2019, American Academy of Pediatrics.

Bronchopulmonary dysplasia (BPD) is a chronic lung disease that commonly develops in the premature infant as a result of RDS and the mechanical ventilation and oxygen used to treat it. Because of the role of vitamin A in facilitating tissue repair, and because of reports of preterm infants having low vitamin A stores, large supplemental doses of vitamin A have been suggested for the prevention of BPD. One report suggests that providing ELBW premature infants with IM injections of vitamin A at 5000 units/day three times per week during the first month of life decreases the incidence of BPD (Araki et al, 2018). Physicians may or may not use this supplementation. The decision will be based on the incidence of BPD in their nursery, the lack of proven additional benefits, the acceptability of using IM injections, and the availability of parenteral vitamin A (Darlow et al, 2016). See Chapter 33 for a discussion of BPD.

Apnea of prematurity is when the infant stops breathing for 20 seconds or longer. Apnea can be due to the infant's immature response to breathing. Bradycardia, slowness of the heart rate, and poor blood oxygenation may be associated with apnea. Caffeine can be given daily to prevent apnea of prematurity. Caffeine stimulates the infant to breathe by increasing the brain's sensitivity to carbon dioxide, stimulating the central respiratory drive, and improving skeletal muscle contraction of the diaphragm. Apnea also can be caused by a lack of oxygen, cold or hot environmental temperatures, medications, or illness. The cause of apnea must be determined to provide the correct treatment to the premature infant.

Oral sucrose is given to infants for pain management during procedures such as blood draws by heel stick or venipuncture. The taste of sucrose may release endorphins, but how sucrose aids in pain management is not clear.

TRANSITION FROM PARENTERAL TO ENTERAL FEEDING

It is beneficial to begin enteral feedings for preterm infants as early as possible because the feedings stimulate gastrointestinal enzymatic development and activity, promote bile flow, increase villous growth in the small intestine, and promote mature gastrointestinal motility. These initial enteral feedings also can decrease the incidence of cholestatic jaundice and the duration of physiologic jaundice and can improve subsequent feeding tolerance in preterm infants. At times small, initial feedings are used only to prime the gut and are not intended to optimize enteral nutrient intake until the infant demonstrates feeding tolerance or is clinically stable.

When making the transition from parenteral to enteral feeding, clinicians should maintain parenteral feeding until enteral feeding is well established to maintain adequate net intake of fluid and nutrients. In VLBW infants it may take 7 to 14 days to provide full enteral feeding, and it may take longer for infants with feeding intolerances or illness. The smallest, sickest infants usually receive increments of only 10 to 20 mL/kg/day. Larger, more stable preterm infants may tolerate increments of 20 to 30 mL/kg/day (see Chapter 12 for a more detailed discussion of transitional feeding).

NUTRITION REQUIREMENTS: ENTERAL FEEDING

Enteral alimentation is preferred for preterm infants because it is more physiologic than parenteral alimentation and is nutritionally superior. Initiating a tiny amount of an appropriate breastmilk feeding whenever possible is beneficial (Maffei and Schanler, 2017). However, determining when and how to provide enteral feedings is often difficult and involves consideration of the degree of prematurity, history of

TABLE 41.11 Factors to Consider Before Initiating or Increasing the Volume of Enteral Feedings

Category	Factors
Perinatal	Cardiorespiratory depression
Respiratory	Stability of ventilation, blood gases, apnea, bradycardia, cyanosis
Medical	Vital signs (heart rate, respiratory rate, blood pressure, temperature), lethargy
Gastrointestinal	Anomalies (gastroschisis, omphalocele), patency, gastrointestinal tract function (bowel sounds present, passage of stool), abdominal distension, risk of necrotizing enterocolitis
Infection	Sepsis or suspect sepsis

Data from Adamkin DH, et al: Nutrition and selected disorders of the gastrointestinal tract. In Fanaroff AA, Fanaroff JM, editors: *Klaus and Fanaroff's Care of the high-risk newborn*, Philadelphia, 2013, Elsevier Saunders.

perinatal insults, current medical condition, function of the gastrointestinal tract, respiratory status, and several other individual concerns (Table 41.11).

Preterm infants should be fed enough to promote growth similar to that of a fetus at the same gestational age, but not so much that nutrient toxicity develops. Although the exact nutrient requirements are unknown for preterm infants, several useful guidelines exist. In general the requirements of premature infants are higher than those of term infants because the preterm infant has smaller nutrient stores, decreased digestion and absorption capabilities, and a rapid growth rate. Stress, illness, and certain therapies for illness may further influence nutrient requirements. It is also important to remember that, in general, enteral nutrient requirements are different from parenteral requirements.

Energy

The energy requirements of premature infants vary with individual biologic and environmental factors. It is estimated that an intake of 50 kcal/kg/day is required to meet maintenance energy needs, compared with 110 to 130 kcal/kg/day for growth (Table 41.12). However, energy needs may be increased by stress, illness, and rapid growth. Likewise, energy needs may be decreased if the infant is placed in a neutral thermal environment (the environmental temperature at which an infant expends the least amount of energy to maintain body temperature). It is important to consider the infant's rate of growth in relation to average energy intakes. Some premature infants may need greater than 130 kcal/kg/day to sustain an appropriate rate of growth. Infants with BPD often require such increased amounts. To provide such a large number of calories to infants with a limited ability to tolerate large fluid volumes, it may be necessary to concentrate the feedings to a level of more than 24 kcal/oz (Box 41.2).

Protein

The amount and quality of protein must be considered when establishing protein requirements for the preterm infant. Amino acids should be provided at a level that meets demands without inducing amino acid or protein toxicity.

A reference fetus model has been used to determine the amount of protein that has to be ingested to match the quantity of protein deposited into newly formed fetal tissue (Ziegler, 2014). To achieve these

TABLE 41.12 Estimation of Energy Requirements of the Low Birthweight Infant

Activity	Average Estimation (kcal/kg/day)
Energy expended	40-60
Resting metabolic rate	40-50[*]
Activity	0-5[*]
Thermoregulation	0-5[*]
Synthesis	15[†]
Energy stored	20-30[†]
Energy excreted	15
Energy intake	90-120

Modified from American Academy of Pediatrics, Committee on Nutrition: Nutritional needs of preterm infants. In Kleinman RE, Greer FR, editors: *Pediatric nutrition,* ed 8, Itasca, IL, 2019, American Academy of Pediatrics; Committee on Nutrition of the Preterm Infant, European Society of Paediatric Gastroenterology, Hepatology and Nutrition (ESPGHAN): *Nutrition and feeding of preterm infants,* Oxford, 1987, Blackwell Scientific.
[*]Energy for maintenance.
[†]Energy cost of growth.

BOX 41.2 Recipes for Preparing 90 mL (3 oz) of Concentrated Premature Infant Formula

Kcal/oz RTF[*] Formula	Ratio 24/30 kcal oz RTF Formula	Volume (mL) RTF[*] Premature 24	Volume RTF[*] (mL) Premature 30
24	1/0	90	0
26	2/1	60	30
27	1/1	45	45
28	1/2	30	60
30	0/1	0	90

RTF, Ready-to-feed formula.
[*]RTF (at 24 and 30 kcal/oz).
Example: Recipe for making a 26 kcal/oz formula:
Goal = 90 mL (3 oz) of formula
2 parts of 24 kcal/oz formula + 1 part of 30 kcal/oz formula = 3 parts of formula
90 mL ÷ 3 parts = 30 mL per part
30 mL × 2 parts = 60 mL of RTF Premature 24 kcal/oz formula +
30 mL × 1 part = 30 mL of Premature 30 kcal/oz = 90 mL (3 parts) of 26 kcal/oz formula

fetal accretion rates, additional protein must be supplied to compensate for intestinal losses and obligatory losses in the urine and skin. Based on this method for determining protein needs, the advisable protein intake is 3.5 to 4.5 g/kg/day. This amount of protein is well tolerated. For the ELBW infant, up to 4.5 g/kg/day of protein has been recommended for milk feedings (Agostoni et al, 2010; Koletzko et al, 2014).

The quality or type of protein is an important consideration because premature infants have different amino acid needs than term infants because of immature hepatic enzyme pathways. The amino acid composition of whey protein, which differs from that of casein, is more appropriate for premature infants. The essential amino acid cysteine is more highly concentrated in whey protein, and premature

infants do not synthesize cysteine well. In addition, the amino acids phenylalanine and tyrosine are lower, and the preterm infant has difficulty oxidizing them. Furthermore, metabolic acidosis decreases with consumption of whey-predominant formulas. Because of the advantages of whey protein for premature infants, breastmilk or formulas containing predominately whey proteins should be chosen whenever possible.

Taurine is a sulfonic amino acid that may be important for preterm infants. Human milk is a rich source of taurine, and taurine is added to most infant formulas. Term and preterm infants develop low plasma and urine concentrations of taurine without a dietary supply. The premature infant may have difficulty with synthesizing taurine from cysteine. Although no overt disease has been reported in infants fed low taurine formulas, low taurine may affect the development of vision and hearing (Klein, 2002).

Energy must be provided at sufficient levels to allow protein to be used for growth and not merely for energy expenditure. A range of 2.5 to 3.6 g of protein per 100 kcal is recommended. Inadequate protein intake is growth limiting, whereas excessive intake causes elevated plasma amino acid levels, azotemia, and acidosis.

Lipids

The growing preterm infant needs an adequate intake of well-absorbed dietary fat to help meet the high energy needs of growth, provide EFAs, and facilitate absorption of other important nutrients such as the fat-soluble vitamins and calcium. However, neonates in general, and premature and SGA infants in particular, digest and absorb lipids inefficiently.

Fat should constitute 40% to 50% of total calories. Furthermore, a diet that is high in fat and low in protein may yield more fat deposition than is desirable for the growing preterm infant. To meet EFA needs, linoleic acid should compose 3% of the total calories, and alpha-linolenic acid should be added in small amounts (AAP, 2019). Additional longer-chain fatty acids—ARA and DHA—are present in human milk and are added to infant formulas for term and premature infants to meet federal guidelines.

The premature infant has a greater need than the term infant for ARA and DHA supplementation. These fatty acids accumulate in fatty tissue and the brain during the last 3 months of gestation; thus the premature infant has decreased stores. Premature infants fed formulas supplemented with ARA and DHA frequently demonstrate greater gain in weight and length and higher psychomotor development scores than premature infants not receiving the fatty acid supplementation (Lapillonne and Moltu, 2016). The DHA and ARA content of human milk is variable, and the premature infant may require supplements of ARA and DHA. However, research is needed to document supplementation use for the premature infants provided human milk (AAP, 2019).

Preterm infants have low levels of pancreatic lipase and bile salts, and this decreases their ability to digest and absorb fat. Lipases are needed for triglyceride breakdown, and bile salts solubilize fat for ease of digestion and absorption. Because medium-chain triglycerides (MCTs) do not require pancreatic lipase and bile acids for digestion and absorption, they have been added to the fat mixture in premature infant formulas. Human milk and vegetable oils contain the EFA linoleic acid, but MCT oil does not. Premature infant formulas must contain vegetable oil and MCT oil to provide the essential long-chain fatty acids.

The composition of dietary fat also plays a role in the digestion and absorption of lipid. In general, infants absorb vegetable oils more efficiently than saturated animal fats, although one exception is the saturated fat in human milk. Infants digest and absorb human milk fat better than the saturated fat in cow's milk or the vegetable oil in standard infant formulas. Human milk contains two lipases that facilitate fat digestion and has a special fatty acid composition that aids absorption.

Carbohydrates

Carbohydrates are an important source of energy, and the enzymes for endogenous production of glucose from carbohydrate and protein are present in preterm infants. Approximately 40% of the total calories in human milk and standard infant formulas are derived from carbohydrates. Too little carbohydrate may lead to hypoglycemia, whereas too much may provoke osmotic diuresis or loose stools. The recommended range for carbohydrate intake is 40% to 50% of total calories.

Lactose, a disaccharide composed of glucose and galactose, is the predominant carbohydrate in almost all mammalian milks and may be important to the neonate for glucose homeostasis, perhaps because galactose can be used for either glucose production or glycogen storage. Generally galactose is used for glycogen formation first, and then it becomes available for glucose production as blood glucose levels decrease. Because infants born before 28 to 34 weeks of gestation have low lactase activity, the premature infant's ability to digest lactose may be marginal. In practice, malabsorption is not a clinical problem because lactose is hydrolyzed in the intestine or fermented in the colon and absorbed. Sucrose is another disaccharide that is found in commercial infant formula products. Because sucrase activity early in the third trimester is at 70% of newborn levels, sucrose is well tolerated by most premature infants. Sucrase and lactase are sensitive to changes in the intestinal milieu. Infants who have diarrhea, are undergoing antibiotic therapy, or are undernourished may develop temporary intolerances to lactose and sucrose.

Glucose polymers are common carbohydrates in the preterm infant's diet. These polymers, consisting mainly of chains of five to nine glucose units linked together, are used to achieve the isoosmolality of certain specialized formulas. Glucosidase enzymes for digesting glucose polymers are active in small preterm infants.

Minerals and Vitamins

Premature infants require greater amounts of vitamins and minerals than term infants because they have poor body stores, are physiologically immature, are frequently ill, and will grow rapidly. Formulas and human milk fortifiers that are developed especially for preterm infants contain higher vitamin and mineral concentrations to meet the needs of the infant, obviating the need for additional supplementation in most cases (Table 41.13). One major exception is infants receiving human milk with a fortifier that does not contain iron. An iron supplement of 2 mg/kg/day should be sufficient to meet their needs (AAP, 2019). The other exception is the use of donor human milk fortifier, which requires the addition of a multiple vitamin and an iron supplement.

Calcium and Phosphorus

Calcium and phosphorus are just two of many nutrients that growing premature infants require for optimal bone mineralization. Intake guidelines have been established at levels that promote the bone mineralization rate that occurs in the fetus. An intake of 150 to 220 mg/kg/day of calcium and 75 to 140 mg/kg/day of phosphorus is recommended (Abrams, AAP, 2013). Two thirds of the calcium and phosphorus body content of the term neonate is accumulated through active transport mechanisms during the last trimester of pregnancy. Infants who are born prematurely are deprived of this important intrauterine mineral deposition. With poor mineral stores and low dietary intake, preterm infants can develop osteopenia of prematurity, a disease characterized

TABLE 41.13 Recommendations for Enteral Administration of Vitamins for the Premature Infant

Vitamin	Amount (kg/day)
Vitamin A	1332-3663 IU
Vitamin D	200-400 IU*
Vitamin E	2.2-11 IU
Vitamin K	4.4-28 mcg
Ascorbic acid	20-55 mg
Thiamin	140-300 mcg
Riboflavin	200-400 mcg
Pyridoxine	50-300 mcg
Niacin	1-5.5 mg
Pantothenate	0.5-2.1 mg
Biotin	1.7-16.5 mcg
Folate	35-100 mcg
Vitamin B$_{12}$	0.1-0.8 mcg

Data from Koletzko B, et al: Recommended nutrient intake levels for stable, fully enterally fed very low birth weight infants. In Koletzko B et al, editors: *Nutritional care of preterm infants: scientific basis and practical guidelines.* World Rev Nutr Diet, 110:297, Germany, 2014, S. Karger AG.
*Maximum of 400 IU/day. American Academy of Pediatrics, Committee on Nutrition: Nutritional needs of preterm infants. In Kleinman RE, Greer FR, editors: *Pediatric nutrition,* ed 8, Itasca, IL, 2019, 2014, American Academy of Pediatrics.

by demineralization of growing bones and documented by radiologic evidence of "washed-out" or thin bones. Very immature babies are particularly susceptible to osteopenia and may develop bone fractures or florid rickets with a prolonged dietary deficiency. Osteopenia of prematurity is most likely to develop in preterm infants who are (1) fed infant formula that is not specifically formulated for preterm infants, (2) fed human milk that is not supplemented with calcium and phosphorus, or (3) receiving long-term PN without enteral feedings.

Vitamin D

Human milk with human milk fortifier or infant formula for preterm infants provides adequate vitamin D when infants consume the entire calorie intake suggested. The current recommendations for intake range from 200 to 400 IU/day for preterm infants (Abrams, AAP, 2013).

Vitamin E

Preterm infants require more vitamin E than term infants because of their limited tissue stores, decreased absorption of fat-soluble vitamins, and rapid growth. Vitamin E protects biologic membranes against oxidative lipid breakdown. Because iron is a biologic oxidant, a diet high in either iron or polyunsaturated fatty acids (PUFAs) increases the risk of vitamin E deficiency. The PUFAs are incorporated into the red blood cell membranes and are more susceptible to oxidative damage than when saturated fatty acids compose the membranes.

A premature infant with vitamin E deficiency may experience hemolytic anemia (oxidative destruction of red blood cells). However, this anemia is uncommon today because of improvements in human milk fortifiers and infant formula composition. The human milk fortifiers and premature infant formulas now contain appropriate vitamin E/PUFA ratios for preventing hemolytic anemia.

Because the dietary requirement for vitamin E depends on the PUFA content of the diet, the recommended intake of vitamin E is expressed commonly as a ratio of vitamin E to PUFA. The recommendation for vitamin E is 0.7 IU (0.5 mg of d-alpha-tocopherol) per 100 kcal, and at least 1 IU of vitamin E per gram of linoleic acid.

Pharmacologic dosing of vitamin E (50–100 mg/kg/day) has not proven to be helpful in preventing BPD or retinopathy of prematurity by reducing the toxic effects of oxygen. Furthermore, high doses of vitamin E have been associated with intraventricular hemorrhage, sepsis, NEC, liver and renal failure, and death.

Iron

Preterm infants are at risk for iron deficiency anemia because of the reduced iron stores associated with early birth. At birth most of the available iron is in the circulating hemoglobin. Thus frequent blood sampling further depletes the amount of iron available for erythropoiesis. Transfusions of red blood cells often are needed to treat the early physiologic anemia of prematurity. Recombinant erythropoietin (EPO) therapy has been used to prevent anemia. Iron supplementation is indicated to facilitate red blood cell production, and a dosage of 6 mg/kg/day of enteral iron has been used (AAP, 2014). This therapy has not consistently prevented anemia and the need for blood transfusions and EPO therapy is not recommended (AAP, 2019).

In general the recommendation for iron intake is 2 to 3 mg/kg/day (AAP, 2019). Infants fed human milk should be given ferrous sulfate drops beginning at 2 weeks of age (AAP, 2019). Formulas fortified with iron usually contain sufficient iron to provide 2 mg iron/kg/day (AAP, 2019).

Folic Acid

Premature infants seem to have higher folic acid needs than infants born at term. Although serum folate levels are high at birth, they decrease dramatically, probably as a result of high folic acid use by the premature infant for deoxyribonucleic acid (DNA) and tissue synthesis needed for rapid growth.

A mild form of folic acid deficiency causing low serum folate concentrations and hypersegmentation of neutrophils is not unusual in premature infants. Megaloblastic anemia is much less common. A daily folic acid intake of 25 to 50 mcg/kg effectively maintains normal serum folate concentrations. Fortified human milk and formulas for premature infants meet these guidelines when full enteral feedings are established.

Sodium

Preterm infants, especially those with VLBW, are susceptible to hyponatremia during the neonatal period. These infants may have excessive urinary sodium losses because of renal immaturity and an inability to conserve adequate sodium. Furthermore, their sodium needs are high because of their rapid growth rate.

Daily sodium intakes of 2 to 3 mEq/kg meet the needs of most premature infants, but 4 to 5 mEq/kg or more may be required by some infants to prevent hyponatremia (Dell, 2015). Routine sodium supplementation of fortified human milk and infant formulas is not necessary. However, it is important to consider the possibility of hyponatremia and monitor infants by assessing serum sodium until the blood level is normal. Milk can be supplemented with sodium if repletion is necessary.

FEEDING METHODS

Decisions about breastfeeding, bottle feeding, or tube feeding depend on the gestational age and the clinical condition of the preterm infant. The goal is to feed the infant via the most physiologic method possible and supply nutrients for growth without creating clinical complications.

Oral Care with Colostrum

The mother's colostrum can be used as oral care for her infant as soon as it is available. Drops of colostrum are placed inside the infant's mouth to aid in the prevention of infection. Colostrum is a rich source of proteins, minerals, and immunologic factors which may protect the infant from illness (Gephart and Weller, 2014; AAP, 2019; American College of Obstetricians and Gynecologists [ACOG], 2014). Oral care with colostrum can be initiated before feedings are started.

Gastric Gavage

Gastric gavage by the oral route often is chosen for infants who are unable to suck because of immaturity or problems with the central nervous system. Infants less than 32 to 34 weeks of gestational age, regardless of birthweight, have poorly coordinated sucking, swallowing, and breathing abilities because of their developmental immaturity. Consequently they have difficulty with nipple feeding.

With the oral gastric gavage method, a soft feeding tube is inserted through the infant's mouth and into the stomach. The major risks of this technique include aspiration and gastric distention. Because of weak or absent cough reflexes and poorly developed respiratory muscles, the tiny infant may not be able to dislodge milk from the upper airway, which can cause reflex bradycardia or airway obstruction. However, electronic monitoring of vital functions and proper positioning of the infant during feeding minimize the risk of aspiration from regurgitation of stomach contents. Tiny, immature infants whose small gastric capacity and slow intestinal motility can impede the tolerance of large-volume bolus feeds may need bolus feedings provided with a pump for a 30- to 60-minute infusion to aid in feeding tolerance.

Occasionally, elimination of the distention and vagal bradycardia requires the use of an indwelling tube for continuous gastric gavage feedings rather than intermittent administration of boluses. Continuous feedings may lead to loss of milk fat, calcium, and phosphorus, which deposit in the feeding tubing so that the infant does not receive the total amount of nutrition provided. Bolus feedings provided with the use of the pump infusion can decrease nutrient loss and promote better weight gain (Rogers et al, 2010; Senterre, 2014).

Nasal gastric gavage is sometimes better tolerated than oral tube feeding. However, because neonates must breathe through the nose, this technique may compromise the nasal airway in preterm infants and cause an associated deterioration in respiratory function. This method is helpful for infants who are learning to nipple feed. An infant with a nasal gastric tube can still form a tight seal on the bottle nipple, but it can be difficult if an oral feeding tube is in place during feedings (see Chapter 12).

Transpyloric Feeding

Transpyloric tube feeding is indicated for infants who are at risk for aspirating milk into the lungs or who have slow gastric emptying. The goal of this method is to circumvent the often slow gastric emptying of the immature infant by passing the feeding tube through the stomach and pylorus and placing its tip within the duodenum or jejunum. Infants with severe gastrointestinal reflux do well with this method, which prevents aspiration of feedings into the lungs. This method also is used for infants whose respiratory function is compromised and who are at risk for milk aspiration. The possible disadvantages of transpyloric feedings include decreased fat absorption, diarrhea, dumping syndrome, alterations of the intestinal microflora, intestinal perforation, and bilious fluid in the stomach. In addition, the placement of transpyloric tubes also requires considerable expertise and radiographic confirmation of the catheter tip location. Although associated with many possible complications, transpyloric feedings are used when gastric feeding is not successful.

Nipple Feeding

Nipple feeding may be attempted with infants whose gestational age is greater than 32 weeks and whose ability to feed from a nipple is indicated by evidence of an established sucking reflex and sucking motion. Before this time they are unable to coordinate sucking, swallowing, and breathing. Because sucking requires effort by the infant, any stress from other causes such as hypothermia or hypoxemia diminishes the sucking ability. Therefore nipple feeding should be initiated only when the infant is under minimum stress and is sufficiently mature and strong to sustain the sucking effort. Initial oral feedings may be limited to one to three times per day to prevent undue fatigue or too much energy expenditure, either of which can slow the infant's rate of weight gain. Before oral feedings begin, a standardized oral stimulation program can help infants successfully nipple feed more quickly (Fucile et al, 2011).

Breastfeeding

When the mother of a premature infant chooses to breastfeed, nursing at the breast should begin as soon as the infant is ready. Before this time the mother must express her milk so that it can be tube-fed to her infant. These mothers need emotional and educational support for successful lactation. Studies report that premature breastfed infants have better sucking, swallowing, and breathing coordination and fewer breathing disruptions than bottle-fed infants (Abrams and Hurst, 2018). Kangaroo care—allowing the mother to maintain skin-to-skin contact while holding her infant—facilitates her lactation. In addition, this type of contact promotes continuation of breastfeeding and enhances the mother's confidence in caring for her high-risk infant. The latter benefit also may apply to fathers who engage in kangaroo care with their infants (Kassity-Krich and Jones, 2014).

Feeding infants with cups instead of bottles to supplement breastfeeding has been suggested for preterm infants based on the rationale that it may prevent infant "nipple confusion" (i.e., confusion between nursing at the breast and from a bottle). Complications such as milk aspiration and low volume intakes have to be monitored. Cup feeding has been associated with successful breastfeeding at discharge, but increased length of stay in the hospital for the premature infant (AAP, ACOG, 2014).

Tolerance of Feedings

All preterm babies receiving EN should be monitored for signs of feeding intolerance. Vomiting of feedings usually signals the infant's inability to retain the provided amount of milk. When not associated with other signs of a systemic illness, vomiting may indicate that feeding volumes were increased too quickly or are excessive for the infant's size and maturity. Simply reducing the feeding volume may resolve the problem. If not, or if the infant has signs of a systemic illness, feedings may have to be interrupted until the infant's condition has stabilized.

Abdominal distention may be caused by excessive feeding, organic obstruction, excessive swallowing of air, resuscitation, sepsis (i.e., systemic infection), or NEC. Observing infants for abdominal distention should be a routine practice for nurses. Abdominal distention often indicates the need to interrupt feeding until its cause is determined and resolved.

Gastric residuals, measured by aspiration of the stomach contents, may be determined routinely before each bolus gavage feeding and intermittently in all continuous drip feedings. Whether a residual amount is significant depends partly on its volume in relation to the total volume of the feeding. For example, a residual volume of more than 50% of a bolus feeding or equal to the continuous infusion rate may be a sign of feeding intolerance. However, when interpreting the significance of a gastric residual measurement, clinicians must consider other concurrent signs of feeding intolerance and the previous pattern of residual volumes established for a particular infant.

Residuals are frequently present before feedings are initiated and as small volume feedings are started. As long as no signs of illness are present, feedings should not be withheld.

Bile-stained emesis or residuals frequently may be due to overdistention of the stomach with reflux of bile from the intestine, or to a feeding tube that has slipped into the intestine, or it may indicate that the infant has an intestinal blockage and needs additional evaluation (Hair, 2018). Bloody or bilious gastric residuals are more alarming than those that seem to be undigested milk.

The frequency and consistency of bowel movements should be monitored constantly when feeding preterm infants. Simple inspections can detect the presence of gross blood. All feeding methods for preterm infants have associated complications. Unless close attention is paid to symptoms that indicate poor feeding tolerance, serious complications may ensue. Certain diseases can be recognized by recognizing signs of feeding intolerance. For example, necrotizing enterocolitis (NEC) is a serious and potentially fatal inflammatory disease of the intestines associated with symptoms such as abdominal distention and tenderness, abnormal gastric residuals, and grossly bloody stools.

SELECTION OF ENTERAL FEEDING

During the initial feeding period, premature infants often require additional time to adjust to EN and may experience concurrent stress, weight loss, and diuresis. The primary goal of enteral feeding during this initial period is to establish tolerance to the milk. Infants seem to need a period of adjustment to be able to assimilate a large volume and concentration of nutrients. Thus parenteral fluids may be necessary until infants can tolerate adequate amounts of feedings by mouth.

After the initial period of adjustment, the goal of enteral feeding changes from establishing milk tolerance to providing complete nutrition support for growth and rapid organ development. All essential nutrients should be provided in quantities that support sustained growth. The following feeding choices are appropriate: (1) human milk supplemented with human milk fortifier and iron and vitamins as indicated by fortifier used, (2) iron-fortified premature infant formula for infants who weigh less than 2 kg, or (3) iron-fortified standard infant formula for infants who weigh more than 2 kg.

Premature infants who are discharged from the hospital can be given a transitional formula. Additional vitamin D may be indicated to provide 400 IU per day (Abrams, AAP, 2013). Breast-fed infants may be provided with two to three bottles of transitional formula daily to meet needs. The breastfed premature infant also should receive 2 to 3 mg/kg/day of iron for the first 6 to 12 months and a multiple vitamin for the first year of life (AAP, 2019). Premature infants discharged home on standard formula should receive a multivitamin until the infant reaches 3 kg in weight and then only vitamin D may be needed to provide 400 IU per day (AAP, 2019). Blood ferritin levels can be measured to access the infant's iron status and the need for iron supplements (AAP, 2019).

Human Milk

Human milk is the ideal food for healthy term infants and premature infants. Although human milk requires nutrient supplementation to meet the needs of premature infants, its benefits for the infant are numerous. During the first month of lactation, the composition of milk from mothers of premature infants differs from that of mothers who have given birth to term infants; the protein and sodium concentrations of breastmilk are higher in mothers with preterm infants (Klein, 2002). When premature infants are fed their own mother's milk, they grow more rapidly than infants fed banked, mature breastmilk (Brownell et al, 2018).

In addition to its nutrient concentration, human milk offers nutritional benefits because of its unique mix of amino acids and long-chain fatty acids. The zinc and iron in human milk are more readily absorbed, and fat is more easily digested because of the presence of lipases. Moreover, human milk contains factors that are not present in formulas. These components include (1) macrophages and T and B lymphocytes; (2) antimicrobial factors such as secretory immunoglobulin A, lactoferrin, and others; (3) hormones; (4) enzymes; and (5) growth factors. It has been reported that human milk compared with premature infant formula fed to preterm infants reduces the incidence of NEC and sepsis, improves neurodevelopment, facilitates a more rapid advancement of enteral feedings, and leads to an earlier discharge (AAP, ACOG, 2014). The use of the mother's own milk for her infant supplemented with liquid donor human milk fortifier and donor human milk is linked to decreased incidence of NEC (Sullivan et al, 2010). The use of donor milk and liquid donor human milk fortifier compared with premature infant formula decreases the incidence of NEC treated by surgery and decreases the days of PN (Cristofalo et al, 2013).

However, one well-documented problem is associated with feeding human milk to preterm infants. Whether it is preterm, term, or mature, human milk does not meet the calcium and phosphorus needs for normal bone mineralization in premature infants. Therefore calcium and phosphorus supplements are recommended for rapidly growing preterm infants who are fed predominantly human milk. Currently three human milk fortifiers are available: powder bovine milk base, liquid bovine milk base, and liquid donor human milk base. The bovine products contain calcium and phosphorus, as well as protein, carbohydrates, fat, vitamins, and minerals, and are designed to be added to expressed breastmilk fed to premature infants (Table 41.14). Vitamin supplements are not needed. One bovine fortifier is iron fortified and the other requires the addition of iron. The human-milk base product is made from donor human milk that has been pasteurized, concentrated, and supplemented with calcium, phosphorous, zinc, and electrolytes. A multivitamin and an iron supplement are needed with the use of the human-milk base fortifier. The human-milk base fortifier comes as additives to make the milk 24, 26, 28, or 30 kcal/oz milk. The higher concentrations are used for infants who are volume restricted or not growing on lower caloric-dense milk (Hair et al, 2013). The calories and protein are higher with the increased concentrations, but the concentrations of calcium, phosphorous, and zinc remain the same with the donor human milk fortifier. Often the infant needs more energy and protein, but not increased mineral intake. A donor human milk cream supplement is available that is pasteurized human milk fat and can be added to human milk.

Providing human milk to a premature infant can be a very positive experience for the mother, one that promotes involvement and interaction. Because many preterm infants are neither strong enough nor mature enough to nurse at their mother's breast in the early neonatal period, their mothers usually express their milk for several days (and occasionally for several weeks) before nursing can be established. The proper technique of expression, storage, and transport of milk should be reviewed with the mother (see Table 14.18 in Chapter 14). Many summaries of the special considerations for nursing a preterm infant have been published (AAP, ACOG, 2014).

Donor Human Milk

Pasteurized donor human milk (DM) is recommended for the premature infant when the mother's own milk (MOM) is not available or is contraindicated (AAP, 2017; see *Focus On: What Is a Human Milk Bank?*). Neonatal intensive care units (NICUs) that use donor milk may have guidelines to ensure that the infants most at risk for NEC receive donor milk. For example, an infant with a birthweight less than 1500 g and a gestational age less than 34 weeks would qualify to receive donor milk. The risk for NEC is highest at 32 weeks' gestation (Yee et al, 2012). At 34 weeks, the infant can transfer to a discharge diet of mom's milk and supplementation with transitional formula if needed. Donor milk would not be used after discharge to home.

◎ FOCUS ON

What Is a Human Milk Bank?

Human milk banks are nonprofit and for-profit establishments around the globe that work to pasteurize milk safely from healthy donor mothers and make it available to infants who need it most (Haiden and Ziegler, 2016). Donors are screened carefully for infection and infection risk, medication and supplement use, nonsmoker status, and limited alcohol use. The donating mother's physician and her baby's physician must approve her donation status.

For high-risk infants who are premature, immune compromised, or unable to breastfeed because of human immunodeficiency virus (HIV)-positive mothers, donor breastmilk is a life-saving resource when the mother's own milk, the best choice, is not available (Arslanoglu et al, 2013). In developing countries mothers who are HIV-positive are encouraged to breastfeed and provide their infants the medication therapy for HIV (AAP, ACOG, 2014). The risk of death by infection is very high for the infant when proper water supplies and sanitation are not available. Because of its optimal nutrition profile and unique immunologic properties, no other source of nourishment compares when providing these vulnerable infants with the nutrition needed to get a healthy start in life. This precious commodity has saved lives and improved infant morbidity so greatly that the World Health Organization (WHO) has asked that all nations advocate for breastfeeding and the safe use of donor milk through human milk banking for low birthweight infants (WHO, 2011).

Hospitals with milk-banking systems are usually nonprofit, and each has its own guidelines around distributing the milk so that it remains as a safe and altruistic option for all who need it. Recent research also has shown that unpasteurized sources of human milk can be purchased over the Internet and have a high probability for microbial contamination and the contamination with cow milk products (Keim et al, 2013; Keim et al, 2015). Occasionally, mothers of healthy babies may seek out peer-to-peer sharing to avoid the cost, inconvenience, and depletion of resources for vulnerable babies who need pasteurized donor milk the most. If a mother expresses interest in these options, she should receive education on the risks for her infant of possible exposure to infection, medications, and illegal drugs with unscreened and unpasteurized human milk to discourage direct milk sharing (AAP, 2017).

Effective human milk banks protect, promote, and support breastfeeding at every level and are cradled by governmental support (PATH, 2017). The Human Milk Banking Association of North America (HMBANA) is the premier resource for information on the startup and management of this precious commodity in every community as a means to improve global health (HMBANA, 2018). For more information, see https://www.hmbana.org/. The European Milk Bank Association (EMBA) is a nonprofit organization that provides guidelines for milk banking and encourages international cooperation between milk banks of the countries of Europe (EMBA, 2018). Globally, more than 40 countries have systems developed to provide donor milk (PATH, 2017).

TABLE 41.14 Comparison of the Nutritional Content of Human Milk and Formulas

	Human Milk	Human Milk + Powder Bovine–Based Fortifier*	Human Milk + Liquid Bovine–Based Fortifier†	Human Milk + Liquid Donor Human Milk–Based Fortifier‡	Standard Formula§	Transitional Formula¶	Premature Formula**
Caloric density (kcal/oz)	20	24	24	26	20	22	20, 24, 30
Protein whey/casein ratio	70:30	Whey predominates	Whey predominates or casein hydrolysate	Whey predominates	48:52, 60:40, 100:0	50:50, 80:20	50:50, 60:40, 80:20
Protein (g/L)	9	19	24-26	24	14-15	21	20, 22, & 24, 27, 29 & 30, 33
Carbohydrate	Lactose	Lactose, corn syrup solids	Lactose, maltodextrin	Lactose	Lactose or lactose and corn maltodextrin	Lactose and corn syrup solids or maltodextrin	Lactose and corn syrup solids or maltodextrin
Carbohydrate (g/L)	80	95	76-92	84	72-77	75-77	70-73, 81-88, 78-109
Fat	Human fat	Human fat, MCT oil	Human fat, MCT oil, vegetable oil, DHA, ARA	Human fat	Vegetable oil, DHA, ARA	Vegetable oil, MCT oil, DHA, ARA	Vegetable oil, MCT oil, DHA, ARA
Fat (g/L)	35	38	36-48	52	34-38	39-41	34-37, 41.44, 51-67
Calcium (mg/L)	230	1362	1158-1192	1221	449-530	780-890	1120-1217, 1340-1461, 1670-1826
Phosphorus (mg/L)	130	778	633-675	640	255-290	460-490	610-676, 730-812, 910-1014
Vitamin D (units/L)	10	1177	1175-1575	400	402-507	521-560	1014-2000, 1217-2400. 1522-3000
Vitamin E (units/L)	6	37	38-52	10.2	10-14	27-30	27, 43, 33-51, 41.64
Folic acid (mcg/L)	110	331	325-350	158	101-108	186-193	250-270, 300-320, 375-410
Sodium (mEq/L)	8	14	13-17	23	7-8	11-12	13-20, 15-25, 19-31

ARA, Arachidonic acid; *DHA*, docosahexaenoic acid; *MCT*, medium-chain triglyceride.

*Based on the composition of term human milk fortified with powder Similac Human Milk Fortifiers at four packets per 100 mL.

†Based on the composition of term human milk fortified with Enfamil Human Milk Fortifier Acidified Liquid or Similac Human Milk Fortifier Hydrolyzed Protein Concentrated Liquid at
1 vial/packet + 25 mL milk.

‡Based on the composition of term human milk fortified with Prolact +6.

§Based on the composition of Enfamil Premium, Similac Advance, and Gerber Good Start Gentle formulas.

¶Based on the composition of Enfamil EnfaCare and Similac NeoSure formulas.

**Based on the composition of Enfamil Premature and Similac Special Care formulas.

Data from American Academy of Pediatrics, Committee on Nutrition: Appendix A. Composition of human milk. In Kleinman RE, Greer FR, editors: *Pediatric nutrition*, ed 8, Itasca, IL, 2019, American Academy of Pediatrics.

The use of donor milk has been linked with earlier initiation of feedings, less formula use, and no change in the percentage of MOM use. DM frequently is used with the initiation of feedings before the mother's milk can be expressed. Neonatologists were concerned that the use of DM would lead to mothers not providing milk for their infant, but there was no change in mothers providing milk for their own infants (Marinelli et al, 2014).

Premature Infant Formulas

Formula preparations have been developed to meet the unique nutritional and physiologic needs of growing preterm infants. The quantity and quality of nutrients in these products promote growth at intrauterine rates. These formulas, which have caloric densities of 20, 24, and 30 kcal/oz, are available only in a ready-to-feed form. These premature formulas differ in many respects from standard cow's milk–based formulas (see Table 41.14). The types of carbohydrate, protein, and fat differ to facilitate digestion and absorption of nutrients. These formulas also have higher concentrations of protein, minerals, and vitamins.

Transitional Infant Formulas

Formulas containing 22 kcal/oz have been designed as transition formulas for the premature infant. Their nutrient content is less than that of the nutrient-dense premature infant formulas and more than that of the standard infant formula (see Table 41.14). These formulas can be introduced when the infant reaches a weight of 2000 g, and they can be used throughout the first year of life. Not all premature infants need these formulas to grow appropriately. It is not clear which premature infants need this specialized formula because studies have not always demonstrated improved growth with the use of transitional formula (Young et al, 2016). Gain of weight, length, and head circumference for age and weight for length should be monitored on the World Health Organization growth curves (Lapillonne, 2014). Transitional formulas are available in powder form and in ready-to-feed form.

Formula Adjustments

Occasionally it may be necessary to increase the energy content of the formulas fed to small infants. This may be appropriate when the infant is not growing quickly enough and already is consuming as much as possible during feedings.

Concentration

One approach to providing hypercaloric formula is to prepare the formula with less water, thus concentrating all its nutrients, including energy. Concentrated infant formulas with energy contents of 24 kcal/oz are available to hospitals as ready-to-feed nursettes. However, when using these concentrated formulas, clinicians must consider the infant's fluid intake and losses in relation to the renal solute load of the concentrated feeding to ensure that a positive water balance is maintained. This method of increasing formula density often is preferred because the nutrient balance remains the same; infants who need more energy also need additional nutrients. As mentioned, the transitional formulas are available in ready-to-feed and powder form and can be concentrated from 24 to 30 kcal/oz. However, this formula is still inadequate for infants who need additional calcium (e.g., infants with osteopenia).

A ready-to-feed 30 kcal/oz premature infant formula is available. It meets the nutritional needs for premature infants who must be fluid restricted because of illness. This 30 kcal/oz formula can be diluted with premature infant formula (24 kcal/oz) to make 26, 27, or 28 kcal/oz milks (see Box 41.2). These milks are sterile and are the preferred source of providing concentrated milks to premature infants in the NICU. Infant formula powder is not sterile and is not to be used with high-risk infants when a nutritionally adequate liquid, sterile product is available (Steele and Collins, Pediatric Nutrition Dietetic Practice Group, 2019).

Caloric Supplements

Another approach to increasing the energy content of a formula involves the use of caloric supplements such as vegetable oil, MCT oil, or glucose polymers. These supplements increase the caloric density of the formula without markedly altering solute load or osmolality. However, they do alter the relative distribution of total calories derived from protein, carbohydrate, and fat. Because even small amounts of oil or carbohydrate dilute the percentage of calories derived from protein, adding these supplements to human milk or standard (20 kcal/oz) formulas is not advised. Caloric supplements should be used only

when a formula already meets all nutrient requirements other than energy or when the renal solute load is a concern.

When a high-energy formula is needed, glucose polymers can be added to a base that has a concentration of 24 kcal/oz or greater (either full-strength premature formula or a concentrated standard formula), with a maximum of 50% of total calories from fat and a minimum of 10% of total calories from protein. Vegetable oil should be added to a feeding at the time or given as an oral medication. Vegetable oil added to a day's supply of formula that is chilled will separate out from the milk and cling to the milk storage container and will not be in the feeding to the infant.

NUTRITION ASSESSMENT AND GROWTH

Dietary Intake

Dietary intake must be evaluated to ensure that the nutrition provided meets the infant's needs. Parenteral fluids and milk feedings are advanced as tolerated, and the nutrient intakes must be reviewed to ensure that they are within the guidelines for premature infants and that the infant is thriving on the nutrition provided. Appropriate growth and growth charts are reviewed in the following paragraphs.

Laboratory Indices

Laboratory assessments usually involve measuring the following parameters: (1) fluid and electrolyte balance, (2) PN or EN tolerance, (3) bone mineralization status, and (4) hematologic status (Table 41.15). Hemoglobin and hematocrit are monitored as

TABLE 41.15 Monitoring of the Feeding of the Premature Infant		
Monitor	**Parenteral Nutrition**	**Enteral Nutrition**
Fluid and electrolyte balance	Fluid intake	Fluid intake
	Urine output	Urine output
	Daily weights	Daily weights
	Serum sodium, potassium, and chloride	
	Serum creatinine	
	BUN	
Glucose homeostasis	Serum glucose	Not routine
Fat tolerance	Serum triglycerides	Not indicated
Protein nutriture: BUN	Not helpful	Low levels with human milk–fed infants may indicate need for more protein
Osteopenia	Serum calcium	
	Serum phosphorous	Serum phosphorous
	Serum alkaline phosphatase activity	Serum alkaline phosphatase activity
Parenteral nutrition toxicity	Cholestasis: conjugated bilirubin	Not indicated
	Liver function: ALT	

ALT, Alanine aminotransferase; *BUN,* blood urea nitrogen.

medically indicated. The early decrease in hematocrit reflects the physiologic drop in hemoglobin after birth and blood drawings for laboratory assessments. Early low hemoglobin levels are treated with blood transfusions if needed. Dietary supplementation does not change this early physiologic drop in hemoglobin.

Growth Rates and Growth Charts

All neonates typically lose some weight after birth. Preterm infants are born with more extracellular water than term infants and thus tend to lose more weight than term infants. However, the postnatal weight loss should not be excessive. Preterm infants who lose more than 15% of their birth weight may become dehydrated from the inadequate fluid intake or experience tissue wasting from poor energy intake. An infant's birth weight should be regained by the second or third week of life. The smallest and sickest infants take the longest time to regain their birth weights.

Intrauterine growth curves have been developed using birth weight, birth length, and birth head circumference data of infants born at several successive weeks of gestation. The intrauterine growth curves are the standard of growth recommended for premature infants. During the first week of life premature infants fall away from their birth weight percentile, which reflects the normal postnatal weight loss of newborn infants. After an infant's condition stabilizes and the infant begins consuming all needed nutrients, the infant may be able to grow at a rate that parallels these curves. An intrauterine weight gain of 15 to 20 g/kg/day can be achieved (Fenton et al, 2018).

Although weight is an important anthropometric parameter, measurements of length and head circumference also can be helpful. Premature infants should grow between 0.7 to 1 cm per week in body length and head circumference. A growth curve based on gender can be used to evaluate the adequacy of growth in all three areas (Figs. 41.3 and 41.4). This chart has a built-in correction factor for prematurity; the infant's growth can be followed from 22 to 50 weeks of gestation and it represents cross-sectional data from Canada, Australia, Germany, Italy, Scotland, and the United States (Fenton and Kim, 2013). The intrauterine curves are smooth into the World Health Organization Charts.

Additional intrauterine growth charts based on the birthweight, birth length, and head circumferences of infants born in the United States have been developed (Olsen et al, 2010). Separate charts for male and female infants are available and infants can be plotted from 23 to 41 weeks' gestation.

The 2006 World Health Organization Growth Charts designed for children from birth to 2 years of age also should be used for preterm infants once they reach 40 weeks' gestation, as long as the age is adjusted (see *Focus On: Long-Term Outcome for Premature Infants*). For example, an infant born at 28 weeks of gestation is 12 weeks premature (40 weeks of term gestation minus 28 weeks of birth gestational age). Four months after birth, the growth parameters of a premature infant born at 28 weeks of gestation can be compared with those of a 1-month-old infant born at term (Box 41.3). When using growth grids, age should be adjusted for prematurity until at least 2½ to 3 years of corrected age. In Fig. 41.5 A.R.'s pattern of growth is shown through 18 years of age. These charts are based on term, healthy infants who were breastfed the first year of life (Grummer-Strawn et al, 2010). By using this chart, the infant's growth can be compared with the term infant to assess catch-up growth.

Commonly used problem, etiology, and signs and symptoms (PES) statements for infants are provided in Box 41.4. Assessment of nutrient intakes and infant growth are reviewed.

FOCUS ON

Long-Term Outcome for Premature Infants

As the survival of premature infants continues to improve, their physical growth, cognitive development, health, and quality of life are being evaluated and investigated. Previously it was believed that, if premature infants experienced catch-up growth, it would occur only during the first few years of life. However, catch-up growth for weight and length can continue throughout childhood. Head circumference catch-up growth is limited to 6 to 12 months corrected age (Hack, 2013). Brain development occurs during the first year of life. As adults, extremely low birthweight (ELBW) infants tend to be shorter and weigh the same as infants born at term (Roberts et al, 2013a). The parents of the premature infants are often shorter than the parents of term infants, and this could contribute to the infant's adult height.

Growth in the neonatal intensive care unit (NICU) for ELBW infants is linked to growth and development at 18 to 22 months corrected age (Ehrenkranz, 2014). Infants with weight gains greater than 18 g/kg/day or head circumference growth of 0.9 cm/week had better neurodevelopment and physical growth than infants with slower growth.

Premature infants and very low birthweight infants often develop adult-onset type 2 diabetes. Premature infants have decreased glucose regulation compared with infants born at term. Higher fasting insulin levels, impaired glucose tolerance, and increased insulin resistance may occur (Kajantie and Hovi, 2014). Premature infants or very low birthweight infants have been reported to have higher blood pressures than infants born at term and normal weight (Lapillonne and Griffin, 2013).

More research is needed. What is the optimal rate of growth for premature infants in the NICU and postdischarge to maximize cognitive/developmental outcomes and decrease risk of adult cardiovascular and metabolic diseases (Lapillonne and Griffin, 2013)? How fast should the premature infant grow? What should the body composition be? When should catch-up growth occur?

Tools have been developed and validated that assess how adults report their health status and quality of life. The evaluations may be conducted by interviews or completion of written questionnaires (Saigal, 2014). As adults, premature and very low birthweight infants rate their quality of life to be similar to adults who were born at term. Roberts and colleagues (2013b) reported on 194 ELBW infants and 148 term infants who completed written evaluations at 18 years. Both groups were the same in their reported quality of life, health status, and self-esteem. Quality of life did not differ for the adults with the smallest birth weight or youngest gestational age. Premature infants not completing the evaluation at 18 years were more likely to have a neurosensory disability at 8 years of age, such as cystic periventricular leukomalacia, blindness, cerebral palsy, and a lower intelligence quotient.

Therefore not only are more premature infants surviving, but they also are growing into adults who are enjoying and living productive lives (Hack, 2013; Saigal, 2013). The medical and nutrition care in the hospital nursery continues to progress, which improves outcome in the nursery and sets the stage for later development.

DISCHARGE CARE

Establishment of successful feeding is a pivotal factor determining whether a preterm infant can be discharged from the hospital nursery. Preterm infants must be able to (1) tolerate their feedings and usually obtain all of their feedings from the breast or bottle, (2) grow adequately on a modified-demand feeding schedule (usually every 3–4 hours during the day for bottle-fed infants or every 2–3 hours for breastfed infants), and (3) maintain their body temperature without the help of an incubator. Medically stable premature infants who have delayed feeding development can go home on gavage feedings for a

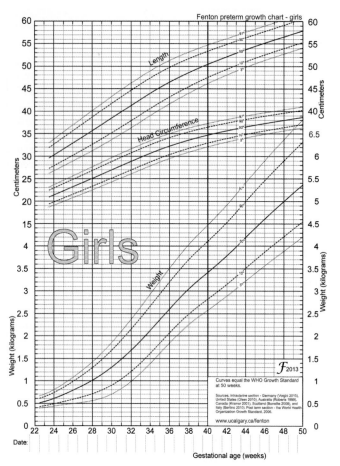

Fig. 41.3 Example of a growth record of weight, length, and head circumference for female infants from 22 to 50 weeks of gestation. This chart has a built-in correction factor for prematurity. https://www.ucalgary.ca/fenton. (From Fenton TR and Kim JH: A systematic review and meta-analysis to revise the Fenton growth chart for preterm infants, *BMC Pediatr* 13:59, 2013.)

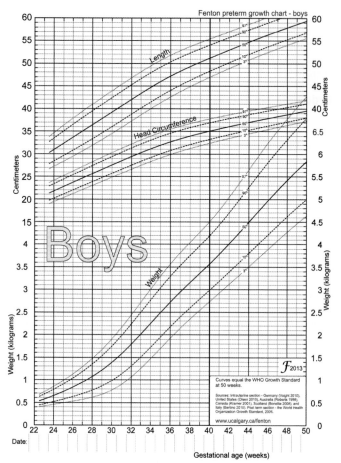

Fig. 41.4 Example of a growth record of weight, length, and head circumference for male infants from 22 to 50 weeks of gestation. This chart has a built-in correction factor for prematurity. https://www.ucalgary.ca/fenton. (From Fenton TR, Kim JH: A systematic review and meta-analysis to revise the Fenton growth chart for preterm infants, *BMC Pediatr* 13:59, 2013.

short period. In addition, it is important that any ongoing chronic illnesses, including nutrition problems, be manageable at home.

Most important, the parents must be ready to care for their infant. In hospitals that allow parents to visit their infants in the nursery 24 hours a day, staff can help parents develop their caregiving skills and learn to care for their infant at home. Often, parents are permitted to "room in" with their infant (i.e., stay with the infant all day and night) before discharge, which helps build confidence in their ability to care for a high-risk infant (Fig. 41.6).

Many preterm infants who are discharged from the hospital weigh less than 5½ lb. Although these infants must meet certain discharge criteria before they can go home, the stress of a new environment may lead to setbacks. Small preterm infants should be followed very closely during the first month after discharge, and parents should be given as much information and support as possible. Within the first week of discharge, a home visit by a nurse, dietitian, or both and a visit to the pediatrician can be extremely educational, and they can provide opportunity for early intervention for developing problems.

Factors that affect the feeding skills and behavior of preterm infants are particularly important after the infants have been discharged. Physical

---

BOX 41.3   Steps for Adjusting Age for Prematurity on Growth Charts

Calculate the number of weeks the infant was premature:
- 40 weeks (term) − Weeks of birth gestational age = Number of weeks premature
- The resulting number of weeks is the correction factor.

Calculate the adjusted age for prematurity:
- Chronologic age − Correction factor = Adjusted age for prematurity

For example:
- 40 weeks − 28 weeks of gestation = 12 weeks premature
- Therefore 12 weeks (3 months) is the correction factor.
- 4 months (chronologic age) − 3 months (correction factor) = 1 month adjusted age

---

factors such as a variable heart rate, a rapid respiratory rate, and tremulousness are examples of physiologic events that interfere with feeding. In addition, infants weighing less than 5½ lb have poor muscle tone. Although muscle tone gradually improves as an infant becomes larger and more mature, it can deteriorate quickly in infants who are

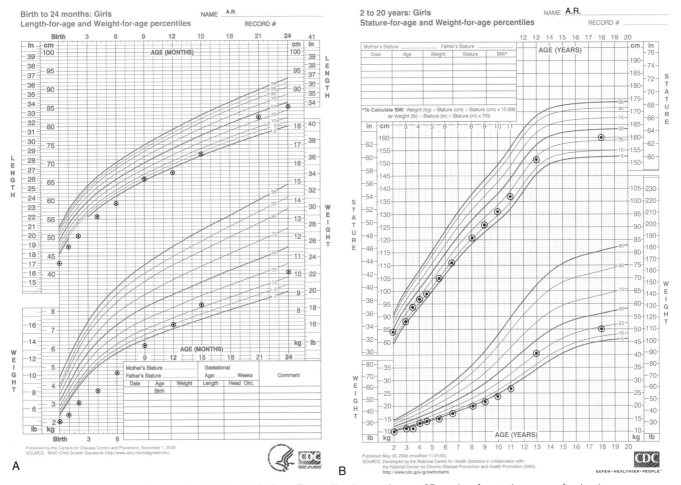

Fig. 41.5 A, Graphs showing how A.R. (from Fig. 41.2), who was born at 27 weeks of gestation, grew after leaving the neonatal unit 1 day before her due date at a weight of 4 ½ lb. Heights and weights until age of 24 months are plotted on the grid at "corrected age" points. A.R. experienced catch-up growth during the first 12 months. **B,** A.R.'s growth pattern from the age of 2 to 18 years. During the first 10 years she grew at the 5th percentile for weight and the 10th percentile for height. She followed her channel of growth but did not experience catch-up growth. However, between the ages of 10 and 13 she began to change growth channels and moved to the 25th percentile for weight and the 25th percentile for height (catch-up growth). At 18 years she crossed the 25th percentile for height and fell slightly below the 25th percentile for weight.

BOX 41.4 Problem, Etiology, and Signs and Symptoms (PES) Statements Commonly Used for Infants

- Increased nutrient (multinutrient) needs (NI-5.1) related to increased metabolic demand from prematurity as evidenced by weight gain less than 15 g/kg/day despite intake meeting estimated needs
- Growth rate below expected (NC-3.5) related to nutrient provision not meeting estimated needs as evidenced by weight gain less than 20 g/day
- No nutrition diagnosis at this time (NO-1.1) related to meeting estimated nutrition needs as evidenced by weight gain/growth appropriate overall

Data taken from commonly used PES statements used by Neonatal Dietitians at Texas Children's Hospital, Houston, Texas, December, 2018.

---

tired or weak. Feeding is often difficult for infants who have limited muscle flexion and strength and poor head and neck control, which are needed to maintain a good feeding posture. Positioning these infants in a manner that supports normal body flexion and ensures proper alignment of the head and neck during feedings is helpful. Premature infants may also need their chin and cheeks supported while bottle feeding.

Small infants tend to sleep more than larger and term infants. It is much easier for preterm infants to feed effectively if they are fully awake. To awaken a preterm infant, the caregiver should provide one type of gentle stimulation for a few minutes and then change to a different type, repeating this pattern until the infant is fully awake. Lightly swaddling of the infant and then placing him or her in a semi-upright position also may help.

The feeding environment should be as quiet as possible. Preterm infants are easily distracted and have difficulty focusing on feeding when noises or movements interrupt their attention. They also tire quickly and are easily overstimulated. When they are overstimulated, they may show only subtle signs of distress. It is important to teach parents of premature infants to recognize the subtle cues that indicate the need for rest or comfort and to respond to them appropriately.

The premature infant may be able to breastfeed all feedings to meet nutritional needs. Infants with a birthweight less than 1500 g may need formula supplementation of human milk to meet their nutritional needs for adequate growth. Two to three feedings of the transitional formula can be provided, and the mother can

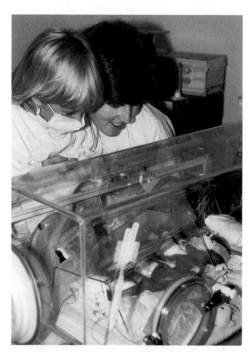

Fig. 41.6 Family in the nursery with their premature infant.

breastfeed the other feedings or provide expressed human milk in bottles. Transitional formula is available as a liquid ready-to-feed formula. The use of powder formula as a supplement can be avoided. Infant formula powders are not sterile and have been linked with *Cronobacter sakazakii* infections. The use of two or three bottles of ready-to-feed formula provides more protein and minerals than provided when human milk is fortified with infant formula powder (AAP, 2014). A multivitamin and iron supplementation should be provided to meet the infant's vitamin D and increased iron demands.

After discharge, most preterm infants need approximately 180 mL/kg/day (2¾ oz/lb/day) of breastmilk or standard infant formula containing 20 kcal/oz. This amount of milk provides 120 kcal/kg/day (55 kcal/lb/day). Alternatively, transitional formula with a concentration of 22 kcal/oz can be provided at a rate of 160 mL/kg/day (or 2.5 oz/lb/day). The best way to determine whether these amounts are adequate for individual infants is to compare their intake with their growth progress over time. Some infants may need a formula that provides 24 kcal/oz. As mentioned previously, powdered transitional formula can be readily altered to a concentration of 24 kcal/oz.

It is important to evaluate needs based on the three growth parameters: weight, length, and head circumference. Patterns of growth should be assessed to determine whether (1) individual growth rate curves at least parallel reference curves, (2) growth curves are shifting inappropriately across growth percentiles, (3) weight is appropriate for length, and (4) growth is proportionate in all three areas.

NEURODEVELOPMENTAL OUTCOME

It is possible to meet the metabolic and nutritional needs of premature infants sufficiently to sustain life and promote growth and development. In fact, more tiny premature infants are surviving than

ever before because of adequate nutrition support and the recent advances in neonatal intensive care technology. There is concern that the ELBW infant is often smaller at discharge than the infant of the same postmenstrual age who was not born prematurely. One report suggests that providing appropriate protein intake during week 1 of life to ELBW infants leads to improved growth of weight, length, and head circumference at 36 weeks' gestation, and improved head circumference in male infants at 18 months' corrected age (Poindexter, 2014). Improved neurodevelopment and growth at 18 months has been reported with ELBW infants who gained more weight and had greater head circumference growth during their stay in the nursery (Ehrenkranz, 2014). The developmental outcome scores for ELBW infants have been higher as the intakes of MOM increase (Lechner and Vohr, 2017). Supplements of donor milk and premature infant formula result in similar developmental outcomes (O'Connor et al, 2016). Research on the neurodevelopment of premature infants who receive fortified donor human milk is needed (Arslanoglu et al, 2013).

Family-centered care where the parents can stay and care for their infants increases the parents' knowledge and skills to care for their infant and the potential for their infant's growth and development (Klaus et al, 2013; Ballard, 2015). A multidisciplinary support is needed to meet the needs for the infant and parents. Complementary therapies have been suggested for improved growth and development of the premature infant. Individual studies have suggested benefits for infant massage and for music therapy (Klaus et al, 2013; Anderson and Patel, 2018). More research is needed to document long-term effect of these therapies.

The increased survival rate of ELBW infants has increased concerns about their short- and long-term neurodevelopmental outcomes. Many questions have been raised about the quality of life awaiting infants who receive neonatal intensive care. As a rule, VLBW infants should be referred to a follow-up clinic to evaluate their development and growth and begin early interventions (Wilson-Costello and Payne, 2015). The survival of ELBW infants has increased, with an increase in the number of children who are developmentally normal who attend school and live independent lives as adults (Wilson-Costello and Payne, 2015). Many of these premature infants reach adulthood with no evidence of any disability (Fig. 41.7).

Complementary and Integrative Approaches

Integrative approaches are frequently used with premature infants to facilitate optimal neurodevelopment. The premature infant develops in a NICU environment that differs from the in utero environment of the fetus during critical brain development. Exposure to sound, light, touch, movement, smell, and taste are different, and it is unclear what exposures are best for premature infants and for infants who are ill (Pineda et al, 2017). Examples of therapies include infant massage, music therapy, kangaroo care, and language exposure (Galicia-Connolly et al, 2012; Pineda et al, 2017). In addition nutrient stores are lower in infants born prematurely, so infant formulas have been supplemented with nutrients that are part of brain development. The addition of long-chain fatty acids and DHA have been helpful (Lapillonne, 2014). Together, parents and caretakers need to identify therapies that work for each infant (Pineda et al, 2017).

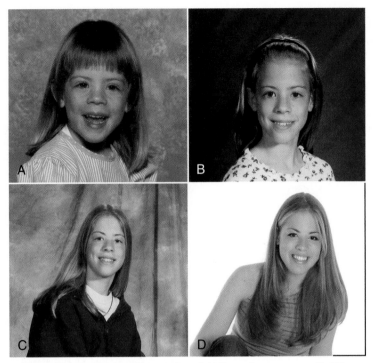

Fig. 41.7 The premature infant A.R. (see Figs. 41.2 and 41.6) as she grows up. **A,** 3½ years. **B,** 10 years. **C,** 14 years. **D,** 18 years. (D, Courtesy Yuen Lui Studio, Seattle, Wash.)

CLINICAL CASE STUDY 1

Heather, a white infant born at 26 weeks of gestation, was admitted to the neonatal intensive care unit. Her birth weight was 850 g (appropriate for gestational age). Heather had respiratory distress syndrome and had to receive a tube for mechanical ventilation. During the first few hours of her life, she was given surfactant, and her ventilator settings were lowered. She was also placed in a humidified incubator and given 100 mL/kg/day of starter parenteral nutrition (dextrose 10% in water with amino acids) intravenously.

On the second day after her birth, she had gained 20 g, and her serum sodium concentration and urine volume output were low. She was diagnosed with excessive fluid intake. Her blood pressure was low and the drug dopamine was provided to increase her urine output.

On the fourth day after birth, her body weight had decreased 50 g—6% of her birth weight—and her serum electrolyte levels were normal. The protein concentration of her parenteral fluids was increased, as was the volume of intravenous fat being provided.

By the fifth day, Heather was clinically stable. She began receiving feedings of milk from her mother—1.0 mL every 3 hours (10 mL/kg of her birth weight)—via bolus oral gastric tube. The feedings were tolerated well. She then began receiving a larger volume of her mother's breastmilk daily and less parenteral fluids.

On day eleven, full enteral feedings were established, and after extubation Heather was successfully breathing on her own.

Nutrition Diagnostic Statement, Day 2
- Excessive fluid intake (NI-3.2) related to intravenous fluids administered as evidenced by gain of 20 g and low serum sodium level.

Nutrition Diagnostic Statement, Day 11
- Inadequate intake (NI-5.11.1) of protein and minerals related to increased needs due to prematurity as evidenced by unfortified human milk not meeting established nutritional needs of premature infants.

Nutrition Care Questions
1. On the second day after birth, should Heather's intravenous fluid volume have been (1) increased because she needed more calories, (2) decreased because she was overhydrated, or (3) changed to enteral feedings because she was clinically stable?
2. How should the intravenous fat that was given to Heather have been administered?
3. The breastmilk from Heather's mother may have inadequate amounts of which nutrients? What do you recommend to resolve this?

CLINICAL CASE STUDY 2

Baby Le was born at 29 weeks of gestation, and his birthweight was 1400 g. He is now 1 week old or 30 weeks' postmenstrual age and weighs 1375 g. He is receiving parenteral nutrition at 130 mL/kg/day that contains 12.5% dextrose and 3.5% amino acids and a 20% intravenous fat emulsion at 15 mL/kg per day. The registered dietitian nutritionist (RDN) assesses the nutrient intake, and calculations are given in the following table. The patient's intakes are compared with the parenteral guidelines of the American Academy of Pediatrics (AAP, 2019) for premature infants.

Nutrient	Nutrient (kg/day)	Guidelines (kg/day)
Kilocalories kcal/kg/day	103	90-100
Glucose mg/kg/min	11.3	11-12
Protein g/kg	4.6	3-4
Fat g/kg	3	1-3

Nutrition Diagnostic Statement

- Excessive protein intake (NI-5.6.2) related to excessive provision in parenteral nutrition as evidenced by protein intake greater than recommendation of 4.0 g of protein per kilogram established by the AAP in 2019.

Nutrition Care Questions

1. The RDN chooses the nutrition diagnosis and writes the problem, etiology, and signs and symptoms statement. Interventions include decreasing the amino acid concentration to 3%, which will provide 4.0 g of protein per kilogram per day.
2. In how many days would you monitor and evaluate baby Le's nutrition status?
3. What guidance is needed for the staff to evaluate him for signs of dehydration?

USEFUL WEBSITES

American Academy of Pediatrics
Fenton Growth Chart
Human Milk Banking Association of North America
March of Dimes
National Center for Education in Maternal and Child Health
Olsen Growth Chart
World Health Organization Growth Curves

REFERENCES

Abrams SA: Osteopenia (metabolic bone disease) of prematurity. In Eichenwald EC, et al, editors: *Cloherty and Starks's Manual of neonatal care,* Philadelphia, PA, 2017, Wolters Kluwer, p 853.

Abrams SA, American Academy of Pediatrics, Committee on Nutrition: Calcium and vitamin D requirements of enterally fed preterm infants, *Pediatrics* 131:e1676–e1683, 2013.

Abrams SA, Hurst NM: Breastfeeding the preterm infant. In Garcia-Prats JA, Hoppin AG, editors: *UpToDate.* 2018. Available at: www.uptodate.com.

Adamkin DH, Radmatcher PG, Lewis S: Nutrition and selected disorders of the gastrointestinal tract. In Fanaroff AA, Fanaroff JM, editors: *Klaus and Fanaroff's care of the high-risk newborn,* Philadelphia, PA, 2013, Elsevier Saunders.

Agostoni C, Buonocore G, Carnielli VP, et al: Enteral nutrient supply for preterm infants: commentary from the European Society for Paediatric Gastroenterology, Heapatology, and Nutrition Committee on Nutrition, *J Pediatr Gastroenterol Nutr* 50:85–91, 2010.

Alsweiler JM, Harding JE, Bloomfield FH: Tight glycemic control with insulin in hyperglycemic preterm babies: A randomized controlled trial, *Pediatrics* 129;639–647, 2012.

American Academy of Pediatrics, American College of Obstetricians and Gynecologists: Lactation support technology. In Schanler RJ et al, editors: *Breastfeeding handbook for physicians,* ed 2, Evanston, Ill, 2014, American Academy of Pediatrics.

American Academy of Pediatrics (AAP), Committee on Nutrition: Nutritional needs of the preterm infant. In Kleinman RE, Greer FR, editors: *Pediatric nutrition handbook,* ed 7, Elk Grove, Ill, 2014, American Academy of Pediatrics.

American Academy of Pediatrics, Committee on Nutrition: Nutritional needs of the preterm infant. In Kleinman RE, Greer FR, editors: *Pediatric nutrition,* ed 8, Itasca, IL, 2019, American Academy of Pediatrics.

American Academy of Pediatrics, Committee on Nutrition, AAP Section on Breastfeeding, AAP Committee on Fetus and the Newborn: Donor human milk for the high-risk infant: preparation, safety, and usage options in the United States, *Pediatrics* 139(1):e20163440, 2017.

American Academy of Pediatrics, Section of Breastfeeding: Breastfeeding and the use of human milk, *Pediatrics* 129:e827, 2012.

Anderson DE, Patel AD: Infants born preterm, stress, and neurodevelopment in the neonatal intensive care unit: might music have an impact? *Dev Med Child Neurol* 60(3):256–266, 2018.

Araki S, Kato S, Namba F, et al: Vitamin A to prevent bronchopulmonary dysplasia in extremely low birth weight infants: a systematic review and meta-analysis, *PLoS One* 29:e0207730, 2018.

Arslanoglu S, Corpeleijn W, Moro G, et al: Donor human milk for preterm infants: current evidence and research directions, *J Pediatr Gastroenterol Nutr* 57:535–542, 2013.

Ballard JL, Khoury JC, Wedig K, et al: New Ballard score, expanded to include extremely premature infants, *J Pediatr* 119:417–423, 1991.

Ballard AR: Attachment challenges with premature or sick infants. In Martin RJ, et al, editors: *Fanaroff and Martin's Neonatal-perinatal medicine diseases of the fetus and infant,* ed 10, Philadelphia, PA, 2015, Elsevier/Saunders.

Brownell EA, Matson AP, Smith KC, et al: Dose-response relationship between donor human milk, mother's own milk, preterm formula, and neonatal growth outcomes, *JPGN* 67:90–96, 2018.

Cristofalo EA, Schanler RJ, Blanco CL, et al: Randomized trial of exclusive human milk versus preterm formula diets in extremely premature infants, *J Pediatr* 163:1592-1595.e1, 2013.

Darlow BA, Graham PJ, Rojas-Reyes MX: Vitamin A supplementation to prevent mortality and short- and long-term morbidity in very low birthweight infants, *Cochrane Datab Syst Rev* (8):CD000501, 2016. doi:10.1002/14651858.CD000501.pub4.

Dell KM: Fluid, electrolyte, and acid-base homeostasis. In Martin RJ, Fanaroff AA, Walsh MC, et al, editors: *Fanaroff and Martin's Neonatal-perinatal medicine diseases of the fetus and infant,* ed 10, Philadelphia, PA, 2015, Elsevier/Saunders.

Doherty EG: Fluid and electrolyte management. In Eichenwald EC, Ann RS, Martin CR, et al, editors: *Cloherty and Starks's manual of neonatal care,* Philadelphia, PA, 2017, Wolters Kluwer, p 296.

Domellöf M: Nutritional care of premature infants: microminerals. In Koletzko B, Poindexter B, Uauy R, et al, editors: *Nutritional care of preterm infants: scientific basis and practical guidelines* (World Rev Nutr Diet, Vol. 110), Germany, 2014, S. Karger AG.

Ehrenkranz RA: Nutrition, growth and clinical outcomes. In Koletzko B, Poindexter B, Uauy R, et al, editors: *Nutritional care of preterm infants: scientific basis and practical guidelines* (World Rev Nutr Diet, Vol. 110), Germany, 2014, S. Karger AG.

Eichenwald EC, Stark AR, Martin CR, et al, editors: *Cloherty and Stark's manual of neonatal care,* ed 8, Philadelphia, PA, 2017, Wolters Kluwer.

Embleton ND, Simmer K: Practice of parenteral nutrition in VLBW and ELBW infants. In Koletzko B, Poindexter B, Uauy R, editors: *Nutritional care of preterm infants: Scientific basis and practical guidelines.* World Rev Nutr Diet (Vol 110), Basel, 2014, Karger, pp 177.

European Milk Bank Association: Human milk banking information provided on European resources, 2018. Available at: https://europeanmilkbanking.com.

Fenton TR, Kim JH: A systematic review and meta-analysis to revise the Fenton growth chart for preterm infants, *BMC Pediatrics* 13:59, 2013.

Fenton TR, Anderson D, Groh-Wargo S, et al: At attempt to standardize the calculation of growth velocity of preterm infants-evaluation of practical bedside methods, *J Pediatr* 196:77–83, 2018.

Fucile S, Gisel EG, McFarland DH, et al: Oral and non-oral sensorimotor interventions enhance oral feeding performance in preterm infants, *Dev Med Child Neurology* 53:829–835, 2011.

Galicia-Connolly E, Shamseer L, Vohra S: Complementary, holistic, and integrative medicine: Therapies for neurodevelopment in preterm infants, *Pediatrics Rev* 33;276–278, 2012.

Gephart SM, Weller M: Colostrum as oral immune therapy to promote neonatal health, *Adv Neonatal Care* 14(1):44–51, 2014.

Griffin IJ, Tancredi DJ, Bertino E, et al: Postnatal growth failure in very low birthweight infants born between 2005 and 2012, *Arch Dis Child Fetal Neonatal Ed* 101:F50–F55, 2016.

Grummer-Strawn LM, Reinold C, Krebs NF, et al: Centers for Disease Control and Prevention, Use of World Health Organization and CDC growth charts for children aged 0-59 months in United States, *MMWR* 59 (RR-9):1–15, 2010. (Erratum in *MMWR Recomm Rep* 59(36):1184, 2010.)

Hack M: The outcome of neonatal intensive care. In Fanaroff AA, Fanaroff JM, editors: *Klaus and Fanaroff's care of the high-risk newborn*, Philadelphia, PA, 2013, Elsevier Saunders.

Haiden J, Ziegler EE: Human milk banking, *Ann Nutr Metab* 69(suppl 2):8–15, 2016.

Hair AB, Hawthorne KM, Chetta KE, et al: Human milk feeding supports adequate growth in infants ≤ 1250 grams birth weight, *BMC Res Notes* 6:459, 2013.

Hair AB: Approach to enteral nutrition in the premature infant. In Abrams SA, Hoppin AG, editors: *UpToDate*, Wolters Kluwer Health. 2018. Available at: www.uptodate.com.

Hay WW, Brown LD, Denne SC: Energy requirements, protein-energy metabolism and balance, and carbohydrates in preterm infants. In Koletzko B, Poindexter B, Uauy R, et al, editors: *Nutritional care of preterm infants: scientific basis and practical guidelines (World Rev Nutr Diet, Vol. 110)*, Germany, 2014, S. Karger AG.

Hay WW: Nutritional support strategies for the preterm infant in the neonatal intensive care unit, *Pediatr Gastroenterol Hepatol Nutr* 21:234–247, 2018.

Heird WC, Driscoll JM, Schullinger JN, et al: Intravenous alimentation in pediatric patients, *J Pediatr* 80:351–372, 1972.

Hojsak I, Colomb V, Bronsky J, et al, ESPGHAN Committee on Nutrition Position Paper: Intravenous lipid emulsions and risk of hepatotoxicity in infants and children: a systematic review and meta-analysis, *JPEN* 62:776–792, 2016.

Human Milk Banking Association of North America: Human milk banking information provided on United States and Canada resources, 2018. Available at: https://www.hmbana.org/.

Isaacs EB, Fischl BR, Quinn BT, et al: Impact of breast milk on intelligence quotient, brain size, and white matter development, *Pediatr Res* 67:357–362, 2010.

Kajantie E, Hovi P: Is very preterm birth a risk factor for adult cardiometabolic disease? *Semin Fetal Neonatal Med* 19:112–117, 2014.

Kassity-Krich NA, Jones JJ: Complementary and integrative therapies. In Kenner C, Lott JW, editors: *Comprehensive neonatal nursing care*, New York, NY, 2014, Springer Publishing.

Keim SA, Hogan JS, McNamara KA, et al: Microbial contamination of human milk purchased via the internet, *Pediatrics* 132:e1227–e1235, 2013.

Keim AS, Kulkarni MM, McNamara K, et al: Cow's milk contamination of human milk purchased via the internet, *Pediatrics* 135:e1157–e1162, 2015.

Klaus MH, Kennell JH, Fanaroff JM: Care of the parents. In Fanaroff AA, Fanaroff JM, editors: *Klaus and Fanaroff's care of the high-risk newborn*, Philadelphia, PA, 2013, Elsevier Saunders.

Klein CJ: Nutrient requirements for preterm infant formula, *J Nutr* 132 (6 Suppl 1):1395S–1577S, 2002.

Koletzko B, Poindexter B, Uauy R: Recommended nutrient intake levels for stable, fully enterally fed very low birth weight infants. In Koletzko B, Poindexter B, Uauy R, editors: *Nutritional care of preterm infants: scientific basis and practical guidelines* (World Rev Nutr Diet, 110:297), Germany, 2014, S. Karger AG.

Lapillonne A: Feeding the preterm infant after discharge. In Koletzko B, Poindexter B, Uauy R, editors: *Nutritional care of preterm infants: Scientific basis and practical guidelines*, World Rev Nutr Diet. Basel, Karger, 2014, vol 110, 264.

Lapillonne A, Moltu SJ: Experimental studies as well as recent clinical trials show that providing larger amounts of DHA than currently and routinely provided is associated with better neurological outcomes at 18 months to 2 years, *Ann Nutr Metab* 69(Suppl 1):35–44, 2016.

Lapillonne A, Griffin IJ: Feeding preterm infants today for later metabolic and cardiovascular outcomes, *J Pediatr* 162(Suppl 3):S7–S16, 2013.

Lechner BE, Vohr BR: Neurodevelopmental outcomes of preterm infants fed human milk, *Clin Perinatol* 44(1):69–83, 2017.

Maffei D, Schanler RJ: Human milk is the feeding strategy to prevent necrotizing enterocolitis! *Semin Perinatol* 41:36–40, 2017.

Marinelli KA, Lussier MM, Brownell E, et al: The effect of a donor milk policy on the diet of very low birth weight infants, *J Hum Lact* 30:310–316, 2014.

Martin JA, Hamilton BE, Osterman MJK: Births in the United States 2016. *NCHS Data Brief*, no 287. Hyattsville, MD, 2017, National Center for Health Statistics.

Martin JA, Hamilton BE, Osterman MJK, et al: Births: final data for 2016. *Natl Vital Stat Rep* 67(1):1–55, 2018.

Martin JA, Osterman MJK: Describing the increase in preterm births in the United States, 2014-2016. *NCHS Data Brief*, no 312. Hyattaville, MD, 2018, National Center for Health Statistics.

Memon N, Hussein K, Hegyi T, et al: Essential fatty acid deficiency with SMOFlipid reduction in an infant with intestinal failure-associated liver disease, *JPEN* in press 43(3):438–441, 2019. doi:10.1002/jpen.1432.

O'Connor DL, Gibbins S, Kiss A, et al: Effect of supplemental donor human milk compared with preterm formula on neurodevelopment of very low-birth-weight infants at 18 months a randomized clinical trial, *JAMA* 316(18):1897–1905, 2016.

Olsen IE, Groveman SA, Lawson ML, et al: New intrauterine growth curves based on United States data, *Pediatrics* 125:e214–e224, 2010.

PATH: *Policy brief: ensuring equitable access to human milk for all infants: a comprehensive approach to essential newborn care*, Seattle: PATH, 2017, Global Breastfeeding Collective.

Pineda R, Guth R, Herring A, et al: Enhancing sensory experiences for very preterm infants in the NICU: an integrative review, *J Perinatol* 37:323–332, 2017.

Poindexter B: Approaches to growth faltering. In Koletzko B, Poindexter B, Uauy R, et al, editors: *Nutritional care of preterm infants: scientific basis and practical guidelines(World Rev Nutr Diet, Vol. 110)*, Germany, 2014, S. Karger AG.

Premkumar MH, Carter BA, Hawthorne KM, et al: Fish oil-based lipid emulsions in the treatment of parenteral nutrition-associated liver disease: An ongoing positive experience, *Adv Nutr* 5:65–70, 2014.

Roberts G, Cheong J, Opie G, et al: Growth of extremely preterm survivors from birth to 18 years of age compared with term controls, *Pediatrics* 131:e439–e445, 2013a.

Roberts G, Burnett AC, Lee KJ, et al: Quality of life at age 18 after extremely preterm birth in the post-surfactant era, *J Pediatr* 163:1008-1013.e1, 2013b.

Rogers SP, Hicks PD, Hamzo M, et al: Continuous feedings of fortified human milk lead to nutrient losses of fat, calcium and phosphorous, *Nutrients* 2:230–240, 2010.

Saigal S: Quality of life of former premature infants during adolescence and beyond, *Early Hum Dev* 89:209–213, 2013.

Saigal S: Functional outcomes of very premature infants into adulthood, *Semin Fetal Neonatal Med*, 19:125–130, 2014.

Senterre T: Practice of enteral nutrition in very low birth weight and extremely low birth weight infants. In Koletzko B, Poindexter B, Uauy R, et al, editors: *Nutritional care of preterm infants: scientific basis and practical guidelines (World Rev Nutr Diet, Vol. 110)*, Germany, 2014, S. Karger AG.

Steele C, Collins EA, Pediatric Nutrition Dietetic Practice Group, editors: *Infant and pediatric feedings: guidelines for preparation of human milk and formula in health care facilities*, 3rd ed, Chicago, 2019, Academy of Nutrition and Dietetics.

Sullivan S, Schanler RJ, Kim JH, et al: An exclusively human milk-based diet is associated with a lower rate of necrotizing enterocolitis than a diet of human milk and bovine milk-based products, *J Pediatr* 156:562-567.e1, 2010.

van Aerde JE, Narvey M: Acute respiratory failure. In Thureen PJ, Hay WW, editors: *Neonatal nutrition and metabolism*, ed 2, Cambridge, 2006, Cambridge University Press.

van Goudoever JB, Vlaardingerbroek H, van den Akker CH, et al: Amino acids and proteins. In Koletzko B, Poindexter B, Uauy R, et al, editors: *Nutritional care of preterm infants: scientific basis and practical guidelines(World Rev Nutr Diet, Vol. 110)*, Germany, 2014, S. Karger AG.

Vanek VW: Review of trace mineral requirements for preterm infants: what are the current recommendations for clinical practice? *Nutr Clin Pract* 30(5):720–721, 2015.

Vanck VW, Borum P, Buchman A, et al: ASPEN position paper: recommendations for changes in commercially available parenteral multivitamin and multi-trace element products, *Nutr Clin Pract* 27(4):440–491, 2013.

Vanek VW, Seidner DL, Allen P, et al: A.S.P.E.N. position paper: Clinical role for alternative intravenous fat emulsions, *Nutr Clin Pract* 27: 150–192, 2012.

Williams JE, Pugh Y: The late preterm: a population at risk, *Crit Care Nurs Clin North Am* 30(4):431–443, 2018.

Wilson-Costello DE, Payne A: Early childhood neurodevelopmental outcomes of high-risk neonates. In Martin RJ, Fanaroff AA, Walsh M, editors: *Fanaroff and Martin's neonatal-perinatal medicine: diseases of the fetus and infant*, 10th ed, Philadelphia, PA, 2015, Elsevier/Saunders.

World Health Organization: *Guidelines on optimal feeding of low birth-weight infants in low-and middle-income countries*, 2011. Available at: www.who.int/maternal_child_adolescent/documents/9789241548366.pdf.

Xu J, Murphy SL, Kochanek KD, et al: Deaths: final data for 2016. *Natl Vital Stat Rep* 67(5):1–76, 2018.

Yee WH, Soraisham AS, Shah VS, et al: Incidence and timing of presentation of necrotizing enterocolitis in preterm infants, *Pediatrics* 129:e298–e304, 2012.

Young L, Embleton ND, McGuire W: Nutrient-enriched formula versus standard term formula for preterm infants following hospital discharge, *Cochrane Database Syst Rev* 12:CD004696, 2016. doi:10.1002/14651858. CD004696.pub5.

Zeisel SH, Klatt KC, Caudill MA: Choline, *Adv Nutr* 8:58–60, 2018.

Ziegler EE: Human milk and human milk fortifiers. In Koletzko B, Poindexter B, Uauy R, et al, editors: *Nutritional Care of Preterm Infants: Scientific basis and practical guidelines(World Rev Nutr Diet, Vol. 110)*, Germany, 2014, S. Karger AG.

42

Medical Nutrition Therapy for Genetic Metabolic Disorders

Beth N. Ogata, MS, RDN, CD, CSP
Cristine M. Trahms, MS, RDN, FADA

KEY TERMS

argininosuccinic aciduria (ASA)
autosomal-recessive
branched-chain ketoaciduria
carbamyl-phosphate synthetase (CPS) deficiency
citrullinemia
fatty acid oxidation disorders
galactokinase deficiency
galactosemia
galactose-1-phosphate uridyltransferase (GALT) deficiency

genetic metabolic disorders
gluconeogenesis
glycogen storage diseases (GSDs)
glycogenolysis
hereditary fructose intolerance (HFI)
ketone utilization disorder
L-carnitine
long-chain 3-hydroxyacyl-CoA dehydrogenase (LCHAD) deficiency
maple syrup urine disease (MSUD)

medium-chain acyl-CoA dehydrogenase (MCAD) deficiency
methylmalonic acidemia
ornithine transcarbamylase (OTC) deficiency
phenylketonuria (PKU)
propionic acidemia
urea cycle disorders (UCDs)

Genetic metabolic disorders are inherited traits that result in the absence or reduced activity of a specific enzyme or cofactor necessary for optimal metabolism. Most genetic metabolic disorders are inherited as autosomal-recessive traits; autosomal means that the gene is located on a chromosome other than the X or Y chromosomes (see Chapter 6). The treatment for many metabolic disorders is medical nutrition therapy (MNT), with intervention specific to the disorder. The goals of MNT are to maintain biochemical equilibrium for the affected pathway, provide adequate nutrients to support typical growth and development, and support social and emotional development. Nutrition interventions are designed to circumvent the missing or inactive enzyme by (1) restricting the amount of substrate available, (2) supplementing the amount of product, (3) supplementing the enzymatic cofactor, or (4) combining any or all of these approaches. The primary conditions commonly found in the United States are discussed here, and Table 42.1 outlines other disorders by the enzymatic defects, distinctive clinical and biochemical features, and current approaches to dietary therapy.

In some instances, when treatment is initiated early in the newborn period and meticulously continued for a lifetime, the affected individual can be cognitively and physically normal. For other conditions, cognitive and physical damage can occur despite early and meticulous treatment. Biochemical disorders range from variations in enzyme activity that are benign, to severe manifestations that are incompatible with life. For many, significant questions related to diagnosis and treatment remain.

NEWBORN SCREENING

Most inherited metabolic disorders are associated with severe clinical illness that often appears soon after birth. Intellectual disability and severe neurologic involvement may be immediately apparent. Diagnosis of a specific disorder may be difficult, and appropriate treatment measures may be uncertain. Prenatal diagnosis is available for many metabolic disorders, but it usually requires the identification of a family at risk, which can be done only after the birth of an affected child. Effective newborn screening programs, as well as advanced diagnostic techniques and treatment modalities, have improved the outcome for many of these infants.

Infants suspected of having a metabolic disorder should be afforded access to care offered by centers with expertise in treating these disorders. Infants who are febrile for no apparent reason, lethargic, vomiting, in respiratory distress, or having seizures should be evaluated for an undiagnosed metabolic disorder. The initial assessment should include blood gas measurements, electrolyte values, glucose and ammonia tests, and a urine test for ketones.

Advances in newborn screening technology offer opportunities for earlier diagnosis, prevention of neurologic crisis, and improved intellectual and physical outcomes. When tandem mass spectrometry techniques are used in newborn screening laboratories, infants with a broader range of metabolic disorders can be detected, and the disorder can be identified earlier (see *Focus On:* Newborn Screening (NBS) and Fig. 42.1).

DISORDERS OF AMINO ACID METABOLISM

Nutrition therapy for amino acid disorders most commonly consists of substrate restriction, which involves limiting one or more essential amino acids to the minimum requirement while providing adequate energy and nutrients to promote typical growth and development (e.g., restricting phenylalanine [Phe] in phenylketonuria [PKU]). An inadequate intake of an essential amino acid is often as detrimental as

TABLE 42.1 Selected Genetic Metabolic Disorders That Respond to Dietary Treatment

Disorder	Affected Enzyme	Prevalence	Clinical and Biochemical Features	Medical Nutrition Therapy	Adjunct Treatment
Urea Cycle Disorders					
Carbamyl-phosphate synthetase deficiency	Carbamyl-phosphate synthetase	1:1,300,000 (1:35,000 for all UCDs)	Vomiting, seizures, sometimes coma → death Survivors usually have ID ↑ plasma ammonia and glutamine	Food: low protein Formula: without non-essential amino acids	L-carnitine, phenylbutyrate,* L-citrulline, L-arginine Hemodialysis or peritoneal dialysis during acute episodes
Ornithine transcarbamylase deficiency	Ornithine transcarbamylase (X-linked)	1:56,500 (1:35,000 for all UCDs)	Vomiting, seizures, coma → death as a newborn ↑ plasma ammonia, glutamine, glutamic acid, and alanine	Food: low protein Formula: without non-essential amino acids	L-carnitine, phenylbutyrate,* L-citrulline, L-arginine
Citrullinemia	Argininosuccinate synthetase	1:250,000 (1:35,000 for all UCDs)	*Neonatal:* vomiting, seizures, coma → death *Infantile:* vomiting, seizures, progressive developmental delay ↑ plasma citrulline and ammonia, alanine	Food: low protein Formula: without non-essential amino acids	L-carnitine, phenylbutyrate,* L-arginine
Argininosuccinic aciduria	Argininosuccinate lyase	1:218,750 (1:35,000 for all UCDs)	*Neonatal:* hypotonia, seizures Subacute: vomiting, FTT, progressive developmental delay ↑ plasma argininosuccinic acid, citrulline, and ammonia	Food: low protein Formula: lower protein SF (without nonessential amino acids)	L-carnitine, phenylbutyrate*
Argininemia	Arginase	1:950,000 (1:35,000 for all UCDs)	Periodic vomiting, seizures, coma Progressive spastic diplegia, developmental delay ↑ arginine and ammonia related to protein intake	Food: low protein Formula: lower protein SF (without non-essential amino acids)	L-carnitine, phenylbutyrate*
Organic Acidemias					
Methylmalonic acidemia	Methylmalonyl-CoA mutase or similar	1:80,000	Metabolic acidosis, vomiting, seizures, coma, often death ↑ organic urine acid and plasma ammonia levels	Food: low protein Formula: lower protein SF (without isoleucine, methionine, threonine, valine)	L-carnitine, vitamin B_{12} IV fluids, bicarbonate during acute episodes
Propionic acidemia	Propionyl-CoA carboxylase or similar	1:105,000 – 1:130,000	Metabolic acidosis, ↑ plasma ammonia and propionic acid, ↑ urine methylcitric acid	Food: low protein Formula: lower protein SF (without isoleucine, methionine, threonine, valine)	L-carnitine, biotin IV fluids, bicarbonate during acute episodes
Isovaleric acidemia	Isovaleryl-CoA dehydrogenase	1:80,000	Poor feeding, lethargy, seizures, metabolic ketoacidosis, hyperammonemia	Food: low protein Formula: SF (without leucine)	L-carnitine, L-glycine
Ketone utilization disorder	2-methylacetoacetyl-CoA-thiolase or similar	Unknown	Vomiting, dehydration, metabolic ketoacidosis	Food: low protein Formula: SF (without isoleucine) Avoid fasting, high complex carbohydrates	L-carnitine, Bicitra

TABLE 42.1 Selected Genetic Metabolic Disorders That Respond to Dietary Treatment—cont'd

Disorder	Affected Enzyme	Prevalence	Clinical and Biochemical Features	Medical Nutrition Therapy	Adjunct Treatment
Biotinidase deficiency	Biotinidase or similar	1:61,067 (both profound and partial)	In *infants*, seizures, hypotonia, rash, stridor, apnea; in *older children*, also see alopecia, ataxia, developmental delay, hearing loss		Supplemental oral biotin
Carbohydrate Disorders					
Galactosemia	Galactose-1-phosphate uridyltransferase	1:48,000	Vomiting, hepatomegaly, FTT, cataracts, ID, often early sepsis ↑ urine and blood galactose	Eliminate lactose, low galactose, use soy protein isolate formula	
Hereditary fructose intolerance	Fructose-1-phosphate aldolase	1:20,000	Vomiting; hepatomegaly; hypoglycemia, FTT, renal tubular defects after fructose introduction ↑ blood and urine fructose after fructose feeding	No sucrose, fructose	
Fructose 1,6-diphosphatase deficiency	Fructose 1,6-diphosphatase	Unknown	Hypoglycemia, hepatomegaly, hypotonia, metabolic acidosis upon fructose introduction No ↑ blood/urine fructose	No sucrose, fructose	
Glycogen storage disease, type Ia	Glucose-6-phosphatase	1:100,000	Profound hypoglycemia, hepatomegaly	Low lactose, fructose, sucrose; low fat; high complex carbohydrate; avoid fasting	Raw cornstarch, iron supplements
Amino Acid Disorders					
Hyperphenylalaninemias					
Phenylketonuria	Phenylalanine hydroxylase	1:15,000		Food: low protein Formula: SF (without Phe, supplemented with tyrosine)	
Mild phenylketonuria	Phenylalanine hydroxylase	1:24,000	↑ blood Phe	Food: low protein Formula: SF (without Phe, supplemented with tyrosine)	
Dihydropteridine reductase deficiency	Dihydropteridine reductase	Rare	↑ blood Phe, irritability, developmental delay, seizures	Food: low protein Formula: SF (without Phe, supplemented with tyrosine)	Biopterin, 5-hydroxytryptophan, L-dopa, folinic acid
Biopterin synthase defect	Biopterin synthase	Rare	Mild ↑ blood Phe, irritability, developmental delay, seizures	None	L-dopa, tetrahydrobiopterin, 5-hydroxytryptophan
Tyrosinemia, type I	Fumarylacetoacetate hydrolase	<1:100,000 to 1:120,000	Vomiting, acidosis, diarrhea, FTT, hepatomegaly, rickets ↑ blood and urine tyrosine, methionine; ↑ urine parahydroxy derivatives of tyrosine; liver cancer	Food: low protein Formula: SF (without tyrosine, Phe, methionine)	Nitisinone[†]
Maple Syrup Urine Disease (MSUD)					
MSUD	Branched-chain ketoacid decarboxylase complex (<2% activity)	1:185,000	Seizures, acidosis Plasma leucine, isoleucine, valine 10× normal	Food: low protein Formula: SF (without leucine, isoleucine, valine)	Thiamin[‡]

Continued

TABLE 42.1 Selected Genetic Metabolic Disorders That Respond to Dietary Treatment—cont'd

Disorder	Affected Enzyme	Prevalence	Clinical and Biochemical Features	Medical Nutrition Therapy	Adjunct Treatment
Intermittent MSUD	Branched-chain ketoacid decarboxylase complex ($<20\%$ activity between episodes)	Rare	Intermittent symptoms Plasma leucine, isoleucine, valine $10\times$ normal during illness	Food: low protein Formula: SF (without leucine, isoleucine, valine)	
Homocystinuria	Cystathionine synthase or similar	1:200,000	Detached retinas; thromboembolic and cardiac disease; mild to moderate ID; bony abnormalities; fair hair and skin; ↑ methionine, homocysteine	Food: low protein Formula: SF (without methionine, supplemented with L-cystine)	Betaine, folate, vitamin B_{12}, vitamin B_6[‡] if folate levels are normal
Fatty Acid Oxidation Disorders					
Long chain acyl-CoA dehydrogenase deficiency	Long-chain acyl-CoA dehydrogenase	Rare	Vomiting, lethargy, hypoglycemia	Low fat, low long-chain fatty acids; avoid fasting	MCT oil, L-carnitine[§]
Long-chain 3-hydroxy-acyl-CoA dehydrogenase deficiency	Long-chain 3-hydroxy-acyl-CoA dehydrogenase	Rare	Vomiting, lethargy, hypoglycemia	Low fat, low long-chain fatty acids; avoid fasting	MCT oil, L-carnitine[§]
Medium-chain acyl-CoA dehydrogenase deficiency	Medium-chain acyl-CoA dehydrogenase	1:13,000 to 1:19,000	Vomiting, lethargy, hypoglycemia	Low fat, low medium-chain fatty acids, avoid fasting	L-carnitine[§]
Short-chain acyl-CoA dehydrogenase deficiency	Short-chain acyl-CoA dehydrogenase	1:35,000	Vomiting, lethargy, hypoglycemia	Low fat, low short-chain fatty acids, avoid fasting	L-carnitine[§]
Very-long-chain acyl-CoA dehydrogenase deficiency	Very-long-chain acyl-CoA dehydrogenase	1:30,000 to 1:100,000	Vomiting, lethargy, hypoglycemia	Low fat, low long-chain fatty acids, avoid fasting	L-carnitine,[§] MCT oil

*Phenylbutyrate is a chemical administered to enhance waste ammonia excretion; other compounds producing the same effect are also used.
†*Nitisinone*, formerly *NTBC*, 2-(2-nitro-4-trifluoromethyl-benzoyl-1,3-cyclohexanedione), commercially available as Orfadin and Nityr.
‡Patient may or may not respond to the compound.
§Use depends on clinic.

CoA, Coenzyme A; *FTT*, failure to thrive; *ID*, intellectual disability; *IV*, intravenous; *MCT*, medium-chain triglyceride; *MSUD*, maple syrup urine disease; *Phe*, phenylalanine; *SF*, specialized formulas are available for medical nutrition therapy for this disorder; *UCD*, urea cycle disorder.

◎ **FOCUS ON**

Newborn Screening (NBS)

Since the 1960s, states across the United States have adopted mandatory newborn screening (NBS) as law (Waisbren, 2006). These programs were developed as a result of the efficacy of the Guthrie bacterial inhibition assay, in which dried blood spots were used to identify phenylketonuria (PKU). This simple, sensitive, and inexpensive screening test became the basis for population-based screening systems for newborns. Hemoglobinopathies, endocrine disorders, metabolic disorders, and some infectious diseases can be identified effectively with the use of dried blood spots.

Tandem mass spectrometry was first used in the 1990s and is now used across the United States. This technology makes it possible to identify multiple disorders from a single dried blood spot. The number of disorders screened for varies by state, and expanded screening also is offered by private, for-profit companies. Follow-up programs also vary; some states have single, organized programs, whereas follow-up in other states is less centralized. Conditions successfully screened for by early NBS programs include congenital hypothyroidism, PKU, congenital adrenal hyperplasia, galactosemia, sickle cell disease, and maple syrup urine disease (Brosco et al, 2006).

The Maternal and Child Health Bureau (MCHB) of the U.S. Health Resources and Services Administration commissioned a report from the American College of Medical Genetics (ACMG). This expert panel identified 29 conditions for which

newborn screening should be mandated and 25 secondary conditions that may be detected incidentally (Watson, 2006). The ACMG developed a series of ACTion (ACT) sheets and confirmatory algorithms for disorders that are identified by NBS screening. The ACT sheets describe the steps health professionals should follow in communicating with the family and determining follow-up (ACMG, 2001).

Other groups, including the World Health Organization, March of Dimes, and Massachusetts Newborn Screening Advisory Committee, also have issued recommendations.

Providers who may be involved in the care and follow-up of families identified by NBS should have a good understanding of their state's system, as well as the confounding factors that may affect results. Communication among families, primary health care providers, and tertiary clinics is critical to timely identification and treatment. Follow-up, including referral to the appropriate specialists, is important for any family who receives positive NBS results. NBS fact sheets from the Committee on Genetics of the American Academy of Pediatrics describe (1) newborn screening; (2) follow-up of abnormal screening results to facilitate timely diagnostic testing and management; (3) diagnostic testing; (4) disease management, which requires coordination with the medical home and genetic counseling; and (5) continuous evaluation and improvement of the NBS system (Kaye et al, 2006).

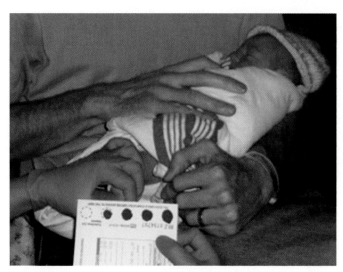

Fig. 42.1 Blood spots are collected from a newborn for newborn screening. (Courtesy Kelly McKean.)

excess. Supplementation of the product of the specific enzymatic reaction usually is required in nutrition therapy for amino acid disorders; for example, tyrosine (Tyr) is supplemented in formulas for treatment of PKU.

Requirements for individual amino acids are difficult to determine because typical growth and development can be achieved over a wide range of intake. The data of Holt and Snyderman (1967) often are used as the basis for prescribing amino acid intakes (Table 42.2). Careful and frequent monitoring is required to ensure the adequacy of the nutritional prescription. Although

nitrogen studies are the most precise, weight gain in infants is a sensitive and easily monitored index of well-being and nutritional adequacy.

PHENYLKETONURIA

Etiology

Phenylketonuria (PKU) is the most common of the hyperphenylalaninemias. In this disorder Phe is not metabolized to Tyr because of a deficiency or inactivity of phenylalanine hydroxylase (PAH) as shown in Fig. 42.2. Of the amino acid disorders, PKU provides a reasonable model for detailed discussion because it (1) occurs relatively frequently and most neonates are screened for it; (2) has a successful MNT treatment; and (3) has a predictable course, with available documentation of "natural" and "intervention" history (see *Focus On:* Timeline of Events in the Diagnosis and Treatment of Phenylketonuria).

Nutritional treatment involves restricting the substrate (Phe) and supplementing the product (Tyr) (see *Pathophysiology and Care Management Algorithm:* Phenylketonuria). Most affected infants exhibit PAH deficiency; the remainder (less than 3%) have defects in associated pathways. Low-Phe nutrition therapy does not prevent the neurologic deterioration present in the disorders of these other associated pathways.

Medical Treatment

All states have newborn screening programs for PKU and other metabolic disorders. Diagnostic criteria for PKU include an elevated blood concentration of Phe and an elevated (i.e., greater than 3) Phe:Tyr ratio. The diagnostic process also should include evaluation for hyperphenylalaninemia that results from the deficiency of

TABLE 42.2 Approximate Daily Requirements for Selected Dietary Components and Amino Acids in Infancy and Childhood

Dietary Component or Amino Acid	AGE AND REQUIREMENT		Dietary Component or Amino Acid	AGE AND REQUIREMENT	
	Birth to 12 mo (mg/kg)	1-10 yr (mg/day)		Birth to 12 mo (mg/kg)	1-10 yr (mg/day)
Phenylalanine	1-5 mo: 47-90	200-500*	Cyst(e)ine§	15-50	400-800
	6-12 mo: 25-47		Lysine	90-120	1200-1600
Histidine	16-34		Threonine	45-87	800-1000
Tyrosine†	1-5 mo: 60-80	25-85 (mg/kg)	Tryptophan	13-22	60-120
	6-12 mo: 40-60		Energy	1-5 mo: 108 kcal/kg	70-102 kcal/kg
Leucine	76-150	1000		6-12 mo: 98 kcal/kg	
Isoleucine	1-5 mo: 79-110	1000	Water	100 mL/kg	1000 mL
	6-12 mo: 50-75		Carbohydrate	kcal × 0.5 ÷ 4 = g/day	kcal × 0.5 ÷ 4 = g/day
Valine	1-5 mo: 65-105	400-600	Total protein	1-5 mo: 2.2 g/kg	16-18
	6-12 mo: 50-80			6-12 mo: 1.6 g/kg	
Methionine‡	20-45	400-800	Fat	kcal × 0.35 ÷ 9 = g/day	kcal × 0.35 ÷ 9 = g/day

Compiled from amino acid data of Holt and Snyderman. Information on amino acid requirements of infants and children at different ages is limited; the figures given here are in excess of minimum requirements. Consequently, this table should be used only as a guide and should not be regarded as an authoritative statement to which individual patients must conform.
*More phenylalanine (>800 mg) is required in the absence of tyrosine.
†Total phenylalanine plus tyrosine should be considered in the prescription because most phenylalanine is converted to tyrosine.
‡More methionine is required in the absence of cyst(e)ine.
§More cyst(e)ine is required in presence of a blocked *trans*-sulfuration outflow pathway for methionine metabolism.
Modified from American Academy of Pediatrics, Committee on Nutrition: Special diets for infants with inborn errors of metabolism, *Pediatrics* 57:783, 1976.

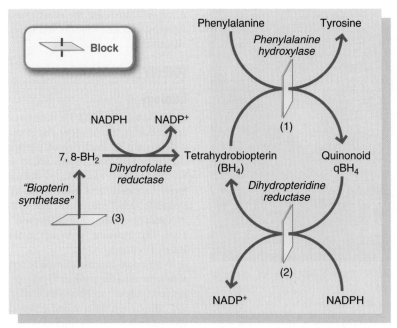

Fig. 42.2 Hyperphenylalaninemias. **1,** Phenylalanine hydroxylase deficiency; **2,** Dihydropteridine reductase deficiency; **3,** Biopterin synthetase deficiency. *NADPH,* Nicotinamide-adenine dinucleotide phosphate (reduced form); *NADP+,* nicotinamide-adenine dinucleotide phosphate (oxidized form).

⊙ FOCUS ON

Timeline of Events in the Diagnosis and Treatment of Phenylketonuria

1934: A. Folling identifies phenylpyruvic acid in the urine of mentally retarded siblings.

1950s: G. Jervis demonstrates a deficiency of phenylalanine oxidation in the liver tissue of an affected patient. H. Bickel demonstrates that dietary phenylalanine restrictions lower the blood concentration of phenylalanine.

1960s: R. Guthrie develops a bacterial inhibition assay for measuring blood phenylalanine levels.

Mid-1960s: Semisynthetic formulas restricted in phenylalanine content become commercially available.

1965-1970: States adopt newborn screening programs to detect phenylketonuria (PKU).

1967-1980: Collaborative Study of Children Treated for Phenylketonuria is conducted. Data from this study form the basis for treatment protocols for PKU clinics in the United States.

Late-1970s: Detrimental effects of maternal PKU are recognized as a significant public health problem.

1980s: Lifelong restriction of phenylalanine intake becomes the standard of care in PKU clinics in the United States.

1983: The Maternal PKU Collaborative Study begins to study the effects of treatment on the pregnancy outcome of women with phenylketonuria.

1987: Techniques for carrier detection and prenatal diagnosis of PKU are developed.

Late-1980s: The gene for phenylalanine hydroxylase deficiency (MIM No. 261600) is located on chromosome 12q22-q24.1. DNA mutation analysis is accomplished with peripheral leukocytes.

1990s: Phenylalanine level of 2-6 mg/dL (120-360 μmol/L), lower than the previous level of less than 10 mg/dL (600 μmol/L), becomes the new standard of care for treatment of PKU.

2000s: Tetrahydrobiopterin-responsive forms of PKU are recognized, especially those with mild mutations.

2007: Sapropterin dihydrochloride (Kuvan), the commercial form of tetrahydrobiopterin receives FDA approval.

2010: Research into alternative and adjunct therapies such as the use of large neutral amino acids, enzyme substitution, and somatic gene therapy continues.

2014: Clinical trials for enzyme replacement therapy using pegylated phenylalanine ammonia lyase (PEG-PAL) injections are underway.

2018: Enzyme replacement therapy (pegvaliase-pqpz injection) receives FDA approval to lower blood Phe levels in adults who have uncontrolled Phe levels on current treatment.

Data from Maternal Child Health Bureau: Newborn screening: toward a uniform screening panel and system, *Genet Med* 8(Suppl 1):1S, 2006; Saugstad LF: From genetics to epigenetics, *Nutr Health* 18:285, 2006; Mitchell JJ, Scriver CR: Phenylalanine hydroxylase deficiency. In Pagon RA et al, editors: GeneReviews [Internet]. Seattle, 1993–2000, University of Washington, Seattle [updated January 5, 2017].

---

enzymes other than PAH, including defects in tetrahydrobiopterin (BH₄) synthesis or regeneration (Vockley et al, 2014). An effective newborn screening program and access to an organized follow-up program are critical to early identification and treatment of infants with PKU.

The advantage of rigorous nutrition therapy has been demonstrated by measurements of intellectual function. Individuals who do not receive diet therapy have severe intellectual disability, whereas individuals who are on therapy from the early neonatal period have normal intellectual function (McPheeters et al, 2012). Outcome,

PATHOPHYSIOLOGY AND CARE MANAGEMENT ALGORITHM

Phenylketonuria

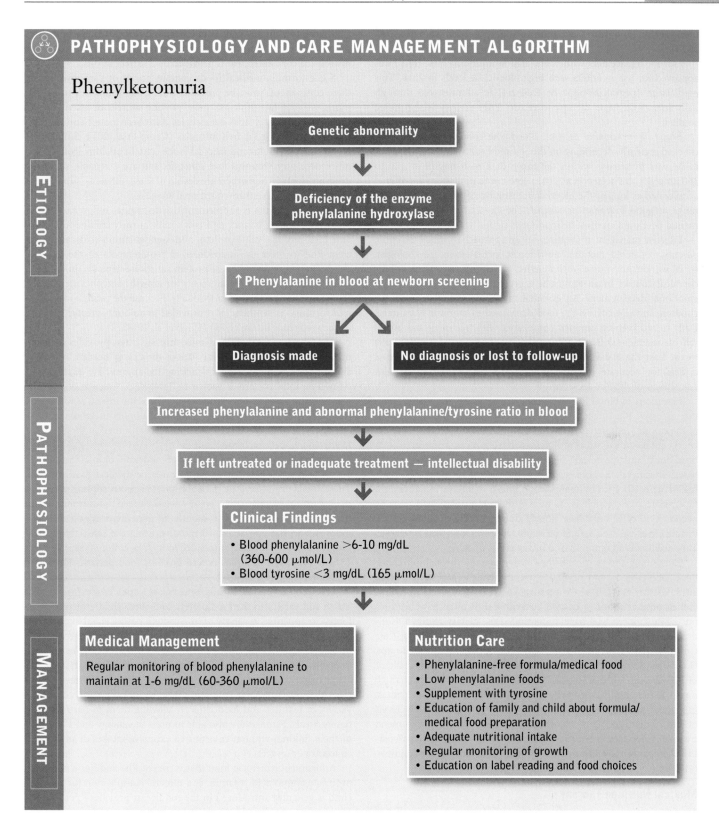

ETIOLOGY

Genetic abnormality

↓

Deficiency of the enzyme phenylalanine hydroxylase

↓

↑ Phenylalanine in blood at newborn screening

Diagnosis made / No diagnosis or lost to follow-up

PATHOPHYSIOLOGY

Increased phenylalanine and abnormal phenylalanine/tyrosine ratio in blood

↓

If left untreated or inadequate treatment — intellectual disability

↓

Clinical Findings

- Blood phenylalanine >6-10 mg/dL (360-600 μmol/L)
- Blood tyrosine <3 mg/dL (165 μmol/L)

MANAGEMENT

Medical Management

Regular monitoring of blood phenylalanine to maintain at 1-6 mg/dL (60-360 μmol/L)

Nutrition Care

- Phenylalanine-free formula/medical food
- Low phenylalanine foods
- Supplement with tyrosine
- Education of family and child about formula/ medical food preparation
- Adequate nutritional intake
- Regular monitoring of growth
- Education on label reading and food choices

measured as intellectual function, depends on the age of the infant at diagnosis and start of nutrition therapy, as well as the individual's biochemical control over time.

BH$_4$ has been studied to evaluate its effectiveness as an alternative treatment to severe dietary Phe restriction, since BH$_4$ is a cofactor needed for proper activity of the enzyme. Treatment with sapropterin (a synthetic form of BH$_4$) is used as an adjunct therapy for some, especially with milder mutations (Longo et al, 2015). Those individuals who respond have what is called BH$_4$-responsive PKU. However, even for BH$_4$-responsive individuals, ongoing intervention and nutrition monitoring is needed (Singh et al, 2010).

Enzyme replacement with phenylalanine ammonia lyase (PAL) was approved for use in adults with high blood Phe levels in 2018. This medication (pegvaliase-pqpz or Palynziq) is administered through daily injections. Gene therapy to restore PAH activity is also being studied.

Blood phenylalanine control. Blood Phe concentration must be checked regularly, depending on the age and health status of the child, to be sure it remains within the range of 2 to 6 mg/dL or 120 to 360 µmol/L (McPheeters et al, 2012). Phe-containing foods are offered as tolerated as long as the blood concentration of Phe remains in the range of good biochemical control. The child's rate of growth and mental development must be monitored carefully.

Effective management requires a team approach in which the child, parents, registered dietitian nutritionist, pediatrician, psychologist, social worker, and nurse work together to achieve and maintain biochemical control in an atmosphere promoting normal mental and emotional development. An essential management tool for parents, children, and clinicians is the food diary used to monitor Phe intake. Daily record keeping supports compliance with treatment and builds self-management skills. An accurate record of food and formula intake for at least the 3 days before a laboratory specimen is obtained is critical for accurate interpretation of the results and subsequent adjustment of the Phe prescription.

Elevations in blood Phe concentration generally are caused by either excessive Phe intake or tissue catabolism. Intake of Phe in excess of the amount required for growth accumulates in the blood. Deficient energy intake or the stress of illness or infection can result in protein breakdown and the release of amino acids, including Phe, into the blood. In general, the anorexia of illness limits energy intake. Preventing tissue catabolism by maintaining intake of the formula/medical food as much as possible is essential. Although it occasionally may be necessary to offer only clear liquids during an illness, the Phe-free formula/medical food should be reintroduced as soon as it is feasible. Tube-feeding is an option if oral intake is not possible.

Continuing the restricted-Phe dietary therapy throughout childhood, adolescence, and beyond is recommended (McPheeters et al, 2012; Vockley et al, 2014). Progressively decreasing IQs, learning difficulties, poor attention span, and behavioral difficulties have been reported in children who have discontinued the dietary regimen. Children who maintain well-controlled blood Phe levels demonstrate comparatively higher intellectual achievement than those who do not. Good dietary control of blood Phe concentrations is the best predictor of IQ, whereas "off-diet" blood Phe concentrations of greater than 20 mg/dL (1200 µmol/L) are the best predictors of IQ loss. Subtle deficits in higher-level cognitive function may persist even at blood Phe levels of 6 to 10 mg/dL (360 to 600 µmol/L). Thus most clinics recommend treatment blood levels of 2 to 6 mg/dL (120 to 360 µmol/L). Restricted-Phe therapy should be continued for life to maintain normal cognitive function.

Medical Nutrition Therapy

Nutrition management guidelines for PKU have been published (Singh et al, 2014).

Formula. For PKU, dietary therapy is planned around the use of a formula/medical food with Phe removed from the protein. Formulas or medical foods provide a major portion of the daily protein and energy needs for affected infants, children, and adults. In general, the protein source in the formula/medical food is L-amino acids, with the critical amino acid (i.e., Phe) omitted. Glycomacropeptide (GMP), a whey protein with very little Phe, is used in a few medical foods as an

alternative to L-amino acids (van Calcar and Ney, 2012). Carbohydrate sources are corn syrup solids, modified tapioca starch, sucrose, and hydrolyzed cornstarch. Fat is provided by a variety of oils.

Some formula/medical foods contain no fat or carbohydrate, so these components must be provided from other sources. If using formulas without fat, clinicians must provide sources of essential fatty acids. Essential fatty acid deficiencies have been noted among individuals consuming fat-free formulas (Camp et al, 2014; Singh et al, 2014). Most formulas and medical foods contain calcium, iron, and all other necessary vitamins and minerals and are a reliable source of these nutrients. When others are devoid of these nutrients, supplementation is needed to ensure nutritional adequacy.

Phe-free formula is supplemented with regular infant formula or breastmilk during infancy and cow's milk in early childhood to provide high-biologic value protein, nonessential amino acids, and sufficient Phe to meet the individualized requirements of the growing child. The optimal amount of protein substitute depends on the individual's age (and thus requirements for growth) and enzyme activity; thus it must be prescribed individually. Because the protein in specialized formulas is synthetic, it is provided in amounts greater than the dietary reference intake (DRI) (Singh et al, 2014).

The Phe-free formula and milk mixture often provides approximately 90% of the protein and 80% of the energy needed by infants and toddlers. A method for calculating the appropriate quantities of a low-Phe food pattern is shown in Table 42.3. Calculations should provide adequate but not excessive energy for the infant, as well as appropriate fluid to maintain hydration. To support metabolic control effectively, formula/medical foods must be consumed in three or four nearly equal portions throughout the day.

Low-phenylalanine foods. Foods of moderate- or low-Phe content are used as a supplement to the formula or medical food mixture. These foods are offered at the appropriate ages to support developmental readiness and to meet energy needs. Pureed foods from a spoon may be introduced at 5 to 6 months of age, finger foods at 7 to 8 months, and the cup at 8 to 9 months, using the same timing and progression of texture recommended for typical children (see Chapters 15 and 16). Table 42.4 lists typical low-Phe food patterns for young children.

Low-protein pastas, breads, and baked goods made from wheat starch add variety to the food pattern and allow children to eat some foods "to appetite." A variety of low-protein pastas, rice, baked goods, egg replacers, and other foods are available. Wheat starch and a variety of low-protein baking mixes for breads, cakes, and cookies are also available. Table 42.5 compares low-protein and regular food items.

In many cases parents create recipes or adapt family favorites to meet the needs of their children. These recipes offer the children a variety of textures and food choices, allowing them to participate in family meals. Families are also able to meet the energy and Phe needs of their children without resorting to excessive intakes of sugars and concentrated sweets.

A formula or medical food that is free of Phe and has a more appropriate amino acid, vitamin, and mineral composition for an older child is generally introduced in the toddler or preschool period. The criteria for introduction of these "next-step" formulas are that the child accept the food pattern and formula well and reliably consume a wide variety of foods from the low-Phe food list. Successful management with consistently low blood Phe levels is based on habit (i.e., the formula/medical food is offered and consumed without negotiation or threat). Children respond favorably to the regularity of the time of ingestion of the formula/medical food and the familiarity of its taste and presentation. Table 42.6 compares a restricted Phe food pattern with a typical food pattern for a child of the same age.

TABLE 42.3 Guidelines for Low-Phenylalanine Food Pattern Calculations

Step 1: Calculate the child's needs for phenylalanine, protein, and energy (kcal).

Phenylalanine

7.7 kg × 40* mg phenylalanine = 308 mg Phe/kg/day

Protein

7.7 kg × 2.5-3† g pro = 19-25 g pro/kg/day

Energy

7.7 kg × 100‡ kcal = 770 kcal/kg/day

Step 2: Estimate the amount of phenylalanine, protein, and energy to be obtained from foods other than the formula mixture.

	APPROXIMATE NEEDS		
	Phenylalanine (mg/day)	Protein (g/day)	Energy (kcal/day)
Foods	30	1-2	100
Formula	~288	18-24	670
Total	*318*	*19-25*	*770*

Step 3: Confirm that a reasonable food pattern is provided with the estimated phenylalanine from food guideline. A sample food pattern:

	Phenylalanine (mg)	Protein (g)	Energy (kcal)
Green beans, strained, 2 Tbsp	15	0.4	8
Banana, mashed, 2 Tbsp	10	0.3	28
Carrots, strained, 2 Tbsp	6	0.2	7
Total	*31*	*0.9*	*43*

Step 4: Determine the amount of standard infant formula to be included in the formula. This information is determined from the infant's estimated phenylalanine needs.

Step 5: Determine the amount of phenylalanine-free formula required per day. This information is determined from the infant's estimated protein and energy needs.

Step 6: Determine the amount of water to mix with the formula. The consistency of the formula will vary according to the infant's age and fluid requirements. For example, for the infant described in the case study, add water to make a total volume of 32 oz.

Step 7: Determine the amounts of phenylalanine, protein, and energy provided by formulas and foods.

	Phenylalanine (mg/day)	Protein (g/day)	Energy (kcal/day)
Phenex-1 powder (70 g)	0	10.5	325
Enfamil powder (70 g)	294	7.4	350
Food	30	1-2	100
Total	*324*	*18.9-19.9*	*775*

Step 8: Determine the actual amounts of phenylalanine, protein, and energy per kilogram body weight.

Phenylalanine

324 ÷ 7.7 kg = 42 mg Phe/kg/day

Protein

19.4 ÷ 7.7 kg = 2.5 g pro/kg/day

Energy

774 ÷ 7.7 kg = 101 kcal/kg/day

*A phenylalanine intake of 40 mg/kg/day is chosen as a moderate intake level. The prescription for phenylalanine must be adapted to individual needs as judged by growth and blood levels.

†Although these intakes are higher than the recommended dietary allowance, they are the intakes found by the Collaborative Study to promote normal growth with consumption of protein hydrolysate-based formula.

‡Total energy intake must be adjusted to meet individual needs, and an excess must be avoided.

Acosta PB: Recommendations for protein and energy intakes by patients with phenylketonuria, *Eur J Pediatr* 155(Suppl 1):S121, 1996; Singh RH, et al: Recommendations for the nutrition management of phenylalanine hydroxylase deficiency, *Genet Med* 16:121, 2014.

TABLE 42.4 Typical Menus for a 3-Year-Old with Phenylketonuria

Tolerance: 300 mg phenylalanine/day		Tolerance: 400 mg phenylalanine/day	
Formula/medical food for 24 hours: 120 g Phe-free-2, 100 g 2% milk, water to 24 oz		Formula/medical food for 24 hours: 120 g Phe-free-2, 100 g 2% milk, water to 24 oz	
This formula mixture provides 30 g protein, 460 kcal, 170 mg phenylalanine.		This formula mixture provides 30 g protein, 460 kcal, 170 mg phenylalanine.	
Menu for 100 mg Phenylalanine from Food	**Phenylalanine (mg)**	**Menu for 200 mg Phenylalanine from Food**	**Phenylalanine (mg)**
Breakfast		**Breakfast**	
Formula mixture, 6 oz		Formula mixture, 6 oz	
Kix cereal, ¼ cup	22	Rice Krispies, 20 g (¼ cup)	25
Peaches, canned, 60 g (¼ cup)	9	Nondairy creamer, 2 Tbsp	9
Lunch		**Lunch**	
Formula mixture, 6 oz		Formula mixture, 6 oz	
Low-protein bread, ½ slice	6	Vegetable soup, ½ cup	82
Jelly, 1 tsp	0	Grapes, 50 g (10)	9
Carrots, cooked, 40 g (¼ cup)	14	Low-protein crackers, 5	3
Apricots, canned, 25 g (½ cup)	32	Low-protein cookie, 2	8
Snack		**Snack**	
Apple slice, peeled, ½ cup	3	Rice cakes, 6 g (2 mini)	25
Goldfish crackers, 10	18	Jelly, 1 tsp	0
Formula mixture, 6 oz		Formula mixture, 6 oz	
Dinner		**Dinner**	
Formula mixture, 6 oz		Formula mixture, 6 oz	
Low-protein pasta, ½ C, cooked	5	Potato, diced, 50 g (5 Tbsp)	39
Tomato sauce, 2 Tbsp	12	Dairy-free margarine, 1 tsp	0
Green beans, cooked, 17 g (2 Tbsp)	9	Zucchini, sauteed, ¼ cup (45 g)	10
Total phenylalanine from food	*130 mg*	*Total phenylalanine from food*	*210*

Education about therapy management. The energy needs and amino acid requirements of children with PKU do not differ appreciably from those of children in general. With proper management, typical growth can be expected (Fig. 42.3). However, parents may tend to offer excessive energy as sweets because they feel their child is being

TABLE 42.5 Comparison of Protein and Energy Content of Foods Used in Low-Protein Diets

Food Item	Energy (kcal)	Protein (g)
Pasta, ½ cup, cooked		
Low-protein	107	0.15
Regular	72	2.4
Bread, 1 slice		
Low-protein	135	0.2
Regular	74	2.4
Cereal, ½ cup, cooked		
Low-protein	45	0.0
Regular	80	1.0
Egg, 1		
Low-protein egg replacer	30	0.0
Regular	67	5.6

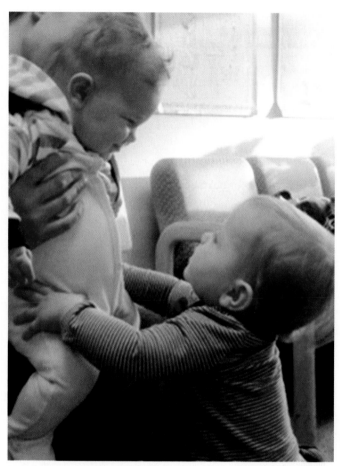

Fig. 42.3 Two young children, both with phenylketonuria, who were identified by a newborn screening program and started on treatment by 7 days of age, demonstrate typical growth and development. (Courtesy Beth Ogata, Seattle.)

deprived of food experiences. Health care providers should support families in recognizing that children with PKU are healthy children who must make careful food choices for themselves, not chronically ill children who require food indulgences.

Appropriate clinical interaction with family members provides them with the information and skills to differentiate between food behaviors that are typical for the age and developmental level of the child and those related specifically to PKU. To avoid power struggles and conflicts over food, it is advisable to involve the child in choosing appropriate foods at an early age. Children who are 2 to 3 years old can master the concept of appropriate choices when foods are categorized as "yes foods" and "no foods." The concept of an appropriate quantity of a food can be introduced to a 3- or 4-year-old child in terms of "how

TABLE 42.6 Comparison of Menus Appropriate for Children With and Without Phenylketonuria

Meal	Menu for PKU	Phenylalanine (mg)	Regular menu	Phenylalanine (mg)
Breakfast	Phenylalanine-free formula	0	Milk	450
	Puffed rice cereal	19	Puffed rice cereal	19
	Orange juice	11	Orange juice	11
Lunch	Jelly sandwich with low-protein bread	18	Peanut butter and jelly sandwich with regular bread	625
	Banana	49	Banana	49
	Carrot and celery sticks	12	Carrot and celery sticks	12
	Low-protein chocolate chip cookies	4	Chocolate chip cookies	60
	Juice	0	Juice	0
Snack	Phenylalanine-free formula	0	Milk	450
	Orange	16	Orange	16
	Potato chips (small bag)	44	Potato chips	44
Dinner	Phenylalanine-free formula	0	Milk	450
	Salad	10	Salad	10
	Low-protein spaghetti with tomato sauce	8	Spaghetti with tomato sauce and meatballs	240 600
	Sorbet	10	Ice cream	120
	Estimated intake	201		3156

PKU, Phenylketonuria.

TABLE 42.7   Tasks Expected of Children with Phenylketonuria by Age Level

Age (yr)	School Level	Task
2-3	Preschool	Distinguishing between "yes" and "no" foods
3-4	Preschool	Counting: how many?
4-5	Preschool	Measuring: how much?
5-6	Kindergarten	Preparing own formula; using scale
6-7	Grade 1-2	Writing basic notes in food diary
7-8	Grade 2	Making some decisions on after-school snack
8-9	Grade 3	Preparing breakfast
9-10	Grade 4	Packing lunches
10-14	Middle school	Managing food choices with increasing independence
14-18	High school	Independently managing phenylketonuria

TABLE 42.8   Frequency of Abnormalities in Children Born to Mothers with Phenylketonuria

Complication (% of Offspring)	MATERNAL PHENYLALANINE LEVELS (mg/dL)				Non-PKU Mother
	20	16-19	11-15	3-10	
Mental retardation	92	73	22	21	5.0
Microcephaly	73	68	35	24	4.8
Congenital heart disease	12	15	6	0	0.8
Low birth weight	40	52	56	13	9.6

Modified from Lenke RR, Levy HL: Maternal phenylketonuria and hyper-phenylalaninemia: an international survey of the outcome of untreated and treated pregnancies, *N Engl J Med* 303:1202, 1980. *PKU*, Phenylketonuria.

many" by counting crackers or raisins and then in terms of "how much" by weighing or measuring foods such as cereal or fruit. The child then moves to more complex tasks (e.g., formula and food preparation) and planning of meals (e.g., breakfast or a packed lunch). Responsibility for planning a full day's menu by calculating the quantity of Phe in portions of food and compiling the daily total is the ultimate goal. These age-related tasks are shown in Table 42.7.

Psychosocial development. The necessity of carefully controlling food intake may prompt parents to overprotect their children and perhaps to restrict their social activities. The children, in turn, may react negatively to their parents and to their nutrition therapy. The ability of the family to respond to the stresses of PKU, as reflected by adaptability and cohesion scores, is demonstrated by improved blood Phe concentrations and the positive coping behaviors of older children with PKU. Thus continuing nutrition therapy beyond early childhood requires that children become knowledgeable about and responsible for managing their own food choices. The health care team becomes responsible for working with families and children to provide strategies that enable children and adolescents to participate in social and school activities, interact with peers, and progress through the typical developmental stages with self-confidence and self-esteem.

Children require parental and professional support as they assume responsibility for their food management. Self-management of food choices is a strategy to prevent the child using dietary noncompliance as a wedge against parental restrictions. Normal intellectual development is a laudable goal of management of PKU, but to be entirely successful children with PKU concomitantly need to develop self-assurance and a strong self-image. This can be achieved in part by fostering self-management, problem-solving skills, independence, and a typical lifestyle.

Maternal PKU

A pregnant woman with elevated blood Phe concentrations endangers her fetus because of the active transport of amino acids across the placenta. The fetus is exposed to approximately twice the Phe level contained in normal maternal blood. Babies whose mothers have elevated blood Phe concentrations have an increased occurrence of cardiac defects, restricted growth, microcephaly, and intellectual disability, as presented in Table 42.8. The fetus appears to be at risk of damage even with minor elevations in maternal blood Phe levels, and the higher the level, the more severe the effect. Strict control of maternal Phe levels before

conception and throughout pregnancy offers the best opportunity for normal fetal development (Koch et al, 2010; Martino et al, 2013).

Nutrition management for pregnant women with hyperphenylalaninemia is complex. The changing physiology of pregnancy and fluctuating nutritional needs are difficult to monitor with the precision required to maintain appropriately low blood-Phe concentrations. Even with meticulous attention to Phe intake, blood concentrations, and the nutrient requirements of pregnancy, a woman cannot be ensured a normal infant (Lee et al, 2005). The risks of abnormal development of the fetus, even with therapeutic dietary management and maintenance of blood Phe concentrations at 1 to 5 mg/dL (60-300 μmol/L), are an important consideration for young women with PKU considering pregnancy (Waisbren and Azen, 2003).

Nutritional management during pregnancy is challenging, even for women who have consistently followed a low-Phe dietary regimen since infancy. Women who have discontinued Phe dietary treatment find that reinstituting medical food consumption and limiting food choices can be difficult and overwhelming. Inadequate maternal nourishment (i.e., inadequate intakes of total protein, fat, and energy) may contribute to poor fetal development and should be prevented. Adherence to nutrition therapy during pregnancy for even the well-motivated woman requires family and professional support, as well as frequent monitoring of biochemical and nutritional aspects of pregnancy and PKU.

Adults Living with Phenylketonuria

Many adults with PKU have had the benefits of early diagnosis and treatment and are less likely to be affected by neurologic damage. However, among those who have had some degree of intellectual disability, hyperactivity and self-abuse are often major concerns. Not all patients respond to late initiation of treatment with improved behavioral or intellectual function. For the difficult-to-manage older patient, a trial of a low-Phe food pattern is recommended. If successful, continued Phe restriction therapy may facilitate behavioral management.

Reinstituting a Phe-restricted food pattern is difficult after the eating pattern has been liberalized. However, the current recommendation of most clinics is effective management of blood Phe concentration throughout a lifetime. This recommendation is based on reports of declining intellectual capabilities and changes in the brain after prolonged, significant elevation of Phe concentrations (Camp et al, 2014). The efficacy of continued treatment throughout adulthood has been documented by reports of improved intellectual performance and problem-solving abilities when blood Phe levels are kept low. Dietary management of PKU throughout the life span is similar to that of other chronic disorders, and prudent MNT results in a normal quality of life.

Maple Syrup Urine Disease

Maple syrup urine disease (MSUD), or branched-chain ketoaciduria, results from a defect in enzymatic activity, specifically the branched-chain alpha-ketoacid dehydrogenase complex. It is an autosomal-recessive disorder. Infants appear normal at birth, but by 4 or 5 days of age they demonstrate poor feeding, vomiting, lethargy, and periodic hypertonia. A characteristic sweet, malty odor from the urine and perspiration can be noted toward the end of the first week of life.

Pathophysiology

The decarboxylation defect of MSUD prevents metabolism of the branched-chain amino acids (BCAAs) leucine, isoleucine, and valine (Fig. 42.4). Leucine tends to be more problematic than the others. The precise mechanism for the complete decarboxylase reaction and the resultant neurologic damage is not known. Neither is the reason why leucine metabolism is significantly more abnormal than that of the other two BCAAs (Strauss et al, 2013).

Medical Treatment

Failure to treat this condition leads to acidosis, neurologic deterioration, seizures, and coma, proceeding eventually to death. Management of acute disease often requires peritoneal dialysis and hydration (see Chapter 34).

Depending on the severity of the enzyme defect, early intervention and meticulous biochemical control can provide a more hopeful prognosis for infants and children with MSUD. Reasonable growth and intellectual development in the normal-to-low-normal range have been described. Diagnosis before 7 days of age and long-term metabolic control are critical factors in long-term normalization of intellectual development. Maintenance of plasma leucine concentrations in infants and preschool children should be as close to physiologically normal as possible. Concentrations greater than 10 mg/dL (760 µmol/L) often are associated with alpha-ketoacidemia and neurologic symptoms.

Because the liver is the central site of metabolic control for amino acids and other compounds that cause acute degeneration of the brain during illness, therapeutic liver transplantation is sometimes an option in MSUD. Liver transplantation can prevent decompensation and crises associated with elevated leucine levels, but it does not reverse existing neurologic damage (Díaz et al, 2014; Oishi et al, 2016).

Medical Nutrition Therapy

Nutrition therapy requires very careful monitoring of blood concentrations of leucine, isoleucine, and valine as well as growth and general nutritional adequacy. Several formulas specifically designed for the treatment of this disorder are available to provide a reasonable amino acid and vitamin mixture. These generally are supplemented with a small quantity of standard infant formula or cow's

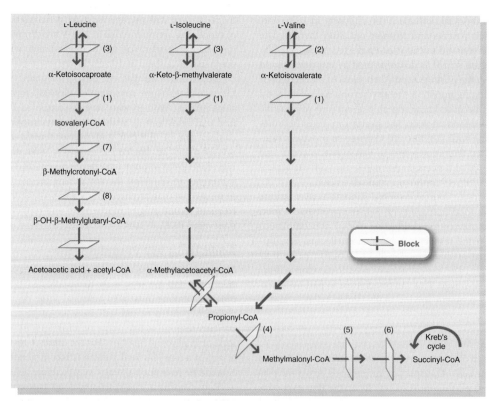

Fig. 42.4 Organic acidemias and maple syrup urine disease (MSUD). **1,** Branched-chain ketoacid decarboxylase (MSUD); **2,** Valine aminotransferase; **3,** Leucine-isoleucine aminotransferase; **4,** Propionyl-CoA carboxylase (propionic acidemia); **5,** Methylmalonyl-CoA racemase (methylmalonic aciduria); **6,** Methylmalonyl-CoA mutase (methylmalonic aciduria); **7,** Isovaleryl-CoA dehydrogenase (isovaleric acidemia); **8,** Beta-methylcrotonyl-CoA carboxylase (biotin-responsive multiple carboxylase deficiency). *CoA,* Coenzyme A.

milk to provide the BCAAs needed to support growth and development. Some infants and children may require additional supplementation with L-valine or L-isoleucine to maintain biochemical balance.

BCAAs may be introduced gradually into the diet when plasma leucine concentrations are decreased sufficiently (Frazier et al, 2014). Clinical relapse is related most often to the degree of elevation of leucine concentrations, and these relapses often are related to infection. Acute infections represent life-threatening medical emergencies in this group of children. If the plasma leucine concentration increases rapidly during illness, BCAAs should be removed from the diet immediately and intravenous therapy can be started.

DISORDERS OF ORGANIC ACID METABOLISM

The organic acid disorders are a group of disorders characterized by the accumulation in the blood of nonamino acid organic acids. Usually most of the organic acids are excreted efficiently in the urine. Diagnosis is based on excretion of compounds not normally present or the presence of abnormally high amounts of other compounds in the urine. The clinical course can vary but is generally marked by vomiting, lethargy, hypotonia, dehydration, seizures, and coma. Survivors often have permanent neurologic damage.

Pathophysiology

Propionic acidemia is a defect of propionyl–coenzyme A (CoA) carboxylase in the pathway of propionyl-CoA to methylmalonyl-CoA, as illustrated in Fig. 42.4. Metabolic acidosis with a marked anion gap and hyperammonemia is characteristic, and long-chain ketonuria also may be present.

At least five separate enzyme deficiencies have been identified that result in methylmalonic acidemia or aciduria. The defect of methylmalonyl-CoA mutase apoenzyme is the most frequently identified. In methylmalonic acidemia, the clinical features are similar to those of propionic acidemia. Acidosis is common, and diagnosis is confirmed by the presence of large amounts of methylmalonic acid in blood and urine. Other findings include hypoglycemia, ketonuria, and elevation of plasma ammonia and lactate levels.

Ketone utilization disorders (mitochondrial 2-methylacetoacetyl-CoA thiolase deficiency or similar enzyme defect) are disorders of isoleucine and ketone body metabolism. Affected individuals are usually older infants or toddlers who present with ketoacidosis, vomiting, and lethargy with secondary dehydration and sometimes coma. This event often is preceded by febrile illness or fasting.

Medical Treatment

Some patients with propionic acidemia may respond to pharmacologic doses of biotin. Long-term outcome in propionic acidemia is variable; hypotonia and cognitive delay may result even in children who are diagnosed early and who receive rigorous treatment. Liver damage and cardiomyopathy are possible sequelae. Liver transplantation may limit intellectual disability and cardiac changes (Sutton et al, 2012).

Individuals with methylmalonic acidemia may respond to pharmacologic doses of vitamin B_{12}. Responsiveness should be determined as part of the diagnostic process (Manoli et al, 2016). Progressive renal insufficiency is often a long-term outcome. Developmental delay is often caused by early and/or prolonged hyperammonemia.

For ketone utilization disorders, the treatment is dietary protein restriction (usually 1.5 g/kg of body weight per day); supplementation with L-carnitine, a carrier of fatty acids across the mitochondrial membranes; avoidance of fasting by providing small, frequent meals

that consist primarily of complex carbohydrates; and the use of Bicitra (sodium citrate-citric acid) to treat ketoacidosis.

Medical Nutrition Therapy

The goals of managing acute episodes of propionic acidemia and methylmalonic acidemia are to achieve and maintain normal nutrient intake and biochemical balance. Maintenance of energy and fluid intake is important to prevent tissue catabolism and dehydration. Intravenous fluids correct electrolyte imbalances, and abnormal metabolites are removed through urinary excretion, promoted by a high fluid intake. Relapses of metabolic acidosis may result from excessive protein intake, infection, constipation, or unidentified factors. Treatment for these episodes must be rapid because coma and death can occur quickly. Parents become skilled at identifying early signs of illness (Southeast Regional Genetics Network [SRGN], 2017).

Restricted protein intake is an essential component of the treatment of organic acid disorders. A daily protein intake of 1 to 1.5 g/kg of body weight is often an effective treatment modality for infants who have a mild form of the disorder. This can be supplied by diluting standard infant formula to decrease the protein content and adding a protein-free formula to meet other nutrient needs. Specialized formulas that limit threonine and isoleucine and omit methionine and valine are used, as clinically indicated, to support an adequate protein intake and growth.

Requirements for the limited amino acids may vary widely. Growth rate, state of health, residual enzyme activity, and overall protein and energy intakes must be monitored carefully and correlated with plasma amino acid levels. Adequate hydration is critical to maintain metabolic equilibrium. Food refusal and lack of appetite may complicate nutrition therapy, which compromises medical management.

DISORDERS OF UREA CYCLE METABOLISM

All urea cycle disorders (UCDs) result in an accumulation of ammonia in the blood. The clinical signs of elevated ammonia are vomiting and lethargy, which may progress to seizures, coma, and ultimately death. In infants the adverse effects of elevated ammonia levels are rapid and devastating. In older children symptoms of elevated ammonia may be preceded by hyperactivity and irritability. Neurologic damage may result from frequent and severe episodes of hyperammonemia. The severity and variation of the clinical courses of some urea cycle defects may be related to the degree of residual enzyme activity. The common urea cycle defects are discussed in a progression that proceeds around the urea cycle, as shown in Fig. 42.5.

Pathophysiology

Ornithine transcarbamylase (OTC) deficiency is an X-linked disorder marked by blockage in the conversion of ornithine and carbamyl phosphate to citrulline. OTC deficiency is identified by hyperammonemia and increased urinary orotic acid, with normal levels of citrulline, argininosuccinic acid, and arginine. Severe OTC deficiency is usually lethal in males. Heterozygous females with various degrees of enzyme activity may not demonstrate symptoms until they are induced by stress, as from an infection, or a significant increase in protein intake.

Citrullinemia is the result of a deficiency of argininosuccinic acid synthetase in the metabolism of citrulline to argininosuccinic acid. Citrullinemia is identified by markedly elevated citrulline levels in the urine and blood. Symptoms may be present in the neonatal period, or they may develop gradually in early infancy. Poor feeding and recurrent vomiting occur which, without immediate treatment, progress to seizures, neurologic abnormalities, and coma.

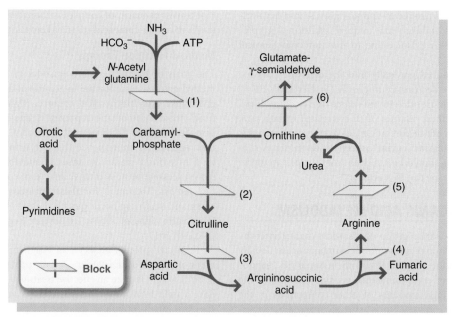

Fig. 42.5 Urea cycle disorders. **1,** Carbamyl-phosphate synthetase deficiency; **2,** Ornithine carbamyl transferase deficiency; **3,** Argininosuccinic acid synthetase (citrullinemia); **4,** Argininosuccinic acid lyase (argininosuccinic aciduria); **5,** Arginase deficiency (argininemia); **6,** Adenosine triphosphate.

Argininosuccinic aciduria (ASA) results from deficiency of argininosuccinate lyase, which is involved in the metabolism of argininosuccinic acid to arginine. ASA is identified by the presence of argininosuccinic acid in urine and blood. L-arginine must be supplemented to provide an alternative pathway for waste nitrogen excretion.

Carbamyl-phosphate synthetase (CPS) deficiency is the result of deficient activity of CPS. The onset is usually in the early neonatal period, with vomiting, irritability, marked hyperammonemia, respiratory distress, altered muscle tone, lethargy, and often coma. Specific laboratory findings usually include low plasma levels of citrulline and arginine and normal orotic acid levels in urine.

Medical Treatment

Acute episodes of illness are managed by discontinuing protein intake and administering intravenous fluids and glucose to correct dehydration and provide energy. If hyperammonemia is severe, peritoneal dialysis, hemodialysis, or exchange transfusion may be required. Intravenous sodium benzoate or other alternative pathway compounds have been beneficial in reducing the hyperammonemia.

Neurologic outcome and intellectual development in individuals with UCDs vary, with a range from normal IQ and motor function to severe intellectual disability and cerebral palsy. Although information on long-term follow-up is limited, the use of alternative pathways for waste nitrogen excretion and a protein-restricted food pattern may improve the outcome.

Medical Nutrition Therapy

Nutritional management of patients who have UCDs is a challenging task. The aim of therapy for the UCDs is to prevent or decrease hyperammonemia and the detrimental neurologic consequences associated with it. Treatment is similar for all of the disorders. For mildly affected infants a standard infant formula can be diluted to provide protein at 1 to 1.5 g/kg body weight per day. The energy, vitamin, and mineral concentrations can be brought up to recommended intake levels with the addition of a protein-free formula that contains these nutrients. However, for most individuals, specialized formulas are needed to adjust protein composition in an effort to limit ammonia production.

The amount of protein tolerated is affected by variables such as the specific enzyme defect, age-related growth rate, health status, level of physical activity, amount of free amino acids administered, energy needs, residual enzyme function, and the use of nitrogen-scavenging medications. Recommendations must take family lifestyle and the individual's eating behaviors into consideration. Long-term therapy consists of restricting dietary protein to 1 to 2 g/kg/day, depending on individual tolerance. For most infants and children with these disorders, L-arginine supplements are required to prevent arginine deficiency and assist in waste nitrogen excretion. L-arginine is supplemented based on individual needs, except in the case of arginase deficiency (Brusilow and Horwich, 2010). Phenylbutyrate or other compounds that enhance alternative metabolic pathways usually are required to normalize ammonia levels.

Protein-Restricted Diets

Infants and children with urea cycle defects or organic acidemias generally require restricted-protein intakes and specialized formulas. The amount of protein prescribed is based on the individual's tolerance or residual enzyme activity, age, and projected growth rate. The highest protein level tolerated should be given to ensure adequate growth and a margin of nutritional safety. The steps for effective planning of a low-protein food pattern are shown in Box 42.1.

In general, low-protein or restricted-protein food patterns can be formulated from readily available, lower-protein infant, toddler, and table foods. Special low-protein foods (see Table 42.5) can be used to provide energy, texture, and variety in the food pattern without appreciably increasing the protein load. The prescribed protein level can be met by adding a protein-free or specialized formula product to standard infant formula. Supplementing carbohydrate and fat makes up the resultant energy deficit.

Specialty formulas are available when needed. The appropriate choice depends on the level of protein restriction, age, and condition of the child. The usual recommendations for energy density and vitamin and mineral composition are generally appropriate to support growth for the infant or child. Osmolarity of the formula and the individual's ability to tolerate hyperosmolar solutions must be considered.

BOX 42.1 Steps in Designing a Low-Protein Eating Plan

1. Determine the protein tolerance of the individual based on (1) diagnosis, (2) age, and (3) growth. Consider the metabolic stability and total protein intake required for the infant's or child's weight.
2. Calculate the protein and energy needs of the individual based on age, activity, and weight.
3. Provide at least 70% of total protein as high-biologic value protein from formula for infants, and from milk or dairy foods for older children. Use a specialized formula if the infant or child cannot tolerate the entire protein intake from intact protein.
4. Provide energy and nutrient sources to meet basic needs.
5. Add water to meet fluid requirements and maintain appropriate concentration of formula mixture.
6. For the older infant and child, provide foods to meet food variety, texture, and energy needs.
7. Provide adequate intake of calcium, iron, zinc, and all other vitamins and minerals for age.

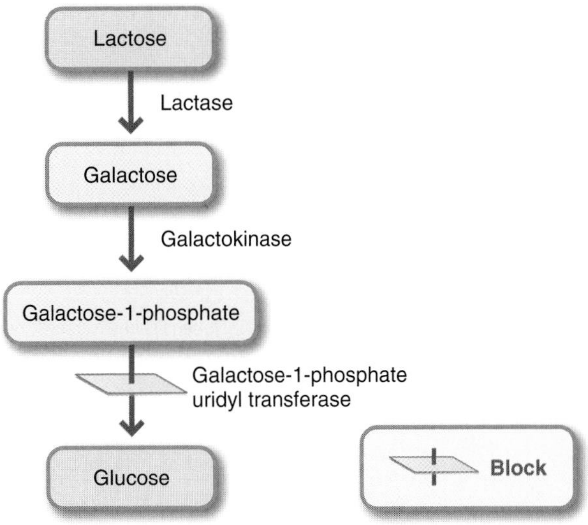

Fig. 42.6 Schematic diagram of the metabolism of galactose in galactosemia.

DISORDERS OF CARBOHYDRATE METABOLISM

Disorders of carbohydrate metabolism vary in presentation, clinical course, and outcome. Galactosemia may present in the early newborn period as life-threatening seizures and sepsis. Hereditary fructose intolerance may present during midinfancy when solids that contain offending ingredients are introduced. Glycogen storage diseases (GSDs) may present at the time when feedings are spaced and subsequent hypoglycemia appears. All of these disorders require early and aggressive nutritional therapy.

Hereditary Fructose Intolerance

Hereditary fructose intolerance (HFI) results from a deficiency of the liver enzyme aldolase B. The disorder typically presents in infancy and toddlerhood, when dietary sources of sucrose and fructose are introduced. Initial symptoms include nausea, bloating, and vomiting. Untreated, liver and kidney damage can occur, along with growth restriction.

Medical Nutrition Therapy

Current management for HFI is restriction of dietary sources of fructose (including disaccharides composed of fructose) and some sugar alcohols, such as sorbitol. HFI (incidence of about 1 in 20,000 to 30,000 in Europe) is different than the more common fructose malabsorption, in which individuals experience gastrointestinal symptoms after ingesting large amounts of fructose (Baker et al, 2015) (see Chapter 27).

Galactosemia

Galactosemia, an elevated level of plasma galactose-1-phosphate combined with galactosuria, is found in two autosomal-recessive metabolic disorders: galactokinase deficiency and galactose-1-phosphate uridyltransferase (GALT) deficiency, which is also called "classic galactosemia." Illness generally occurs within the first 2 weeks of life. Symptoms are vomiting, diarrhea, lethargy, failure to thrive, jaundice, hepatomegaly, and cataracts. Infants with galactosemia may be hypoglycemic and susceptible to infection from gram-negative organisms. If the condition is not treated, death frequently ensues secondarily to septicemia.

Pathophysiology

Galactosemia results from a disturbance in the conversion of galactose to glucose because of the absence or inactivity of one of the enzymes shown in Fig. 42.6. The enzyme deficiency causes an accumulation of galactose, or galactose and galactose-1-phosphate, in body tissues. In addition, expanded newborn screening programs have identified many newborns with Duarte galactosemia. These infants have one allele for galactosemia and one for Duarte galactosemia and are often said to have "D/G galactosemia." The Duarte allele produces approximately 5% to 20% of the GALT enzyme. Little is known about the natural history of D/G galactosemia; apparently infants and children develop normally without medical complications.

Medical Treatment

When diagnosis and therapy are delayed, intellectual disability can result (Berry, 2017). With early diagnosis and treatment, physical and motor development should proceed normally. However, intellectual achievement may be depressed. Patients often have IQs of 85 to 100, visual-perceptual and speech difficulties, and problems with executive function (Doyle et al, 2010; Kaufman et al, 1995). Ovarian failure affects approximately 75% to 95% of women with galactosemia (Forges et al, 2006).

Medical Nutrition Therapy

Galactosemia is treated with lifelong galactose restriction (van Calcar et al, 2014). Although galactose is required for the production of galactolipids and cerebrosides, it can be produced by an alternative pathway if galactose is omitted from the diet. Galactose restriction mandates strict avoidance of all milk and milk products and lactose-containing foods because lactose is hydrolyzed into galactose and glucose. Effective galactose restriction requires careful reading of food product labels. Milk is added to many products, and lactose often appears in the coating of the tablet form of medications. Infants with galactosemia are fed soy-based formula (see Chapter 25). Some fruits and vegetables contain significant amounts of galactose. Table 42.9 presents a low-galactose food pattern.

Medical opinions differ about the intensity and duration of treatment for Duarte galactosemia (Berry, 2017). Many centers eliminate galactose from the diets of these children for the first year of life; other centers do not.

Glycogen Storage Diseases

Glycogen storage diseases (GSDs) reflect an inability to metabolize glycogen to glucose. There are a number of possible enzyme defects along the pathway. The most common of the GSDs are types I and III. Their symptoms are poor physical growth, hypoglycemia, hepatomegaly, and abnormal biochemical parameters, especially for cholesterol

TABLE 42.9   Food Lists for Low-Galactose Food Pattern

Allowable Foods	Galactose-Containing Foods to Be Avoided[*]
Milk and Milk Substitutes	
Similac Soy Isomil	All forms of animal milk
Enfamil Prosobee	Imitation or filled milk
Gerber Good Start Soy	Cream, butter, some margarines
	Cottage cheese, cream cheese
	Hard cheeses
	Yogurt
	Ice cream, ice milk, sherbet
	Breastmilk
Fruits	
All fresh, frozen, canned, or dried fruits except those processed with unsafe ingredients[†]	
Vegetables	
All fresh, frozen, canned, or dried vegetables except those processed with unsafe ingredients,[†] seasoned with butter or margarine, breaded, or creamed	
Meat, Poultry, Fish, Eggs, Nuts	
Plain beef, lamb, veal, pork, ham, fish, turkey, chicken, game, fowl, Kosher frankfurters, eggs, nut butters, nuts	
Breads and Cereals	
Cooked and dry cereals, bread or crackers without milk or unsafe ingredients,[†] macaroni, spaghetti, noodles, rice, tortillas	
Fats	
All vegetable oils; all shortening, lard, margarines, and salad dressings except those made with unsafe ingredients[†]; mayonnaise; olives	

[*]Lactose is often used as a pharmaceutical bulking agent, filler, or excipient; thus tablets, tinctures, and vitamin and mineral mixtures should be evaluated carefully for galactose content. The *Physician's Desk Reference* now lists active and inactive ingredients in medications, as well as manufacturers' telephone numbers.

[†]Unsafe ingredients include milk, buttermilk, cream, lactose, galactose, casein, caseinate, whey, dry milk solids, or curds. Labels should be checked regularly and carefully because formulations of products change often (see Chapter 25).

and triglycerides. Advances in the treatment of GSDs may improve the quality of life for affected children (Weinstein et al, 2018).

Pathophysiology

GSD type Ia is a defect in the enzyme glucose-1-6-phosphatase, which impairs the formation of new glucose (**gluconeogenesis**) and the breakdown of glycogen from storage (**glycogenolysis**). The affected person is unable to metabolize glycogen stored in the liver. Severe hypoglycemia can result and cause irreparable neurologic damage.

Amylo-1, 6-glucosidase deficiency (GSD III or debrancher enzyme deficiency) prevents glycogen breakdown beyond branch points. This disorder is similar to GSD Ia in that glycogenolysis is inefficient but gluconeogenesis is amplified to help maintain glucose production. The symptoms of GSD III are usually less severe and range from hepatomegaly to severe hypoglycemia.

Medical Treatment

The outcome of treatment has been good. The hazard of severe hypoglycemic episodes is diminished, physical growth is improved, and liver size is decreased. The risk of progressive renal dysfunction is not entirely eliminated by current treatment, but liver transplantation for some types of GSD (e.g., type Ib) is sometimes an option. Treatment guidelines include various kinds of carbohydrates at various doses during the day and night (Kishnani et al, 2014). Individual tolerance, body weight, state of health, ambient temperature, and physical activity are important considerations when designing the specific pattern of carbohydrate administration. The goal for all of the protocols remains the same: normalization of blood glucose levels.

Medical Nutrition Therapy

The rationale for intervention is to maintain plasma glucose in a normal range and prevent hypoglycemia by providing a constant supply of exogenous glucose. Administration of raw cornstarch (e.g., a slurry of cornstarch mixed with cold water) at regular intervals and a high–complex carbohydrate, low-fat dietary pattern are advocated to prevent hypoglycemia. Some infants and children do very well with oral cornstarch administration, whereas others require glucose polymers administered via continuous-drip gastric feedings to prevent hypoglycemic episodes during the night. The dose of cornstarch should be individualized; doses of 1.6 to 2.5 g/kg at 4- to 6-hour intervals are generally effective for young children with GSD I (Kishnani et al, 2014). A modified (extended-release) cornstarch product (Glycosade) is also used to manage GSD, typically used at night with older children and adults (Weinstein et al, 2018). Iron supplementation is required to maintain adequate hematologic status because cornstarch interferes with iron absorption.

DISORDERS OF FATTY ACID OXIDATION

Laboratory advancements have enabled identification of fatty acid oxidation disorders such as medium-chain acyl-CoA dehydrogenase (MCAD) deficiency and long-chain 3-hydroxyacyl-CoA dehydrogenase (LCHAD) deficiency (Fig. 42.7). Children who are not identified by newborn screening usually present during periods of fasting or illness with symptoms of variable severity, including failure to thrive, episodic vomiting, and hypotonia.

Pathophysiology

Children with MCAD deficiency who present clinically typically have hypoglycemia without urine ketones, lethargy, seizures, and coma. Children with LCHAD deficiency become hypoglycemic and demonstrate abnormal liver function, reduced or absent ketones in the urine, and often secondary carnitine deficiency. They also may have hepatomegaly and acute liver disease. Hypoglycemia can progress quickly and be fatal (Matern and Rinaldo, 2015). Both disorders are included in the newborn screening panels in all U.S. states.

Medical Nutrition Therapy

The concept underlying effective treatment for fatty acid oxidation disorders is straightforward: avoidance of fasting. This is accomplished

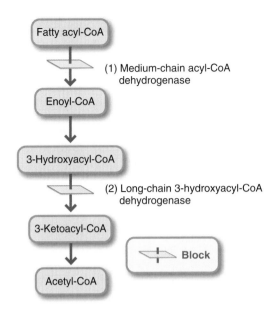

Fig. 42.7 Mitochondrial fatty acid oxidation disorders: **1,** Medium-chain acyl-Coenzyme A dehydrogenase deficiency, the most common fatty acid oxidation disorder. **2,** Long-chain 3-hydroxyacyl-CoA dehydrogenase deficiency.

by the regularly spaced intake of foods that provide an adequate energy intake and are high in carbohydrates. A low-fat diet is advocated because fats are not effectively metabolized. Consumption of not more than 30% of energy as fat has been recommended; some individuals require more restriction. Supplementation with L-carnitine, a substance that functions as a carrier of fatty acids across the mitochondrial membranes, is recommended by some clinics.

Children often do very well with three meals and three snacks offered at regular intervals. Most children may require additional carbohydrate before bed, based on individual ability to maintain blood glucose levels throughout the night (Matern and Rinaldo, 2015). Depending on the disorder, supplementation with specific fatty acids (e.g., medium-chain fats for disorders that involve blocks of long-chain metabolism) may be indicated.

ROLE OF THE NUTRITIONIST IN GENETIC METABOLIC DISORDERS

The role of the pediatric nutrition specialist in the treatment of metabolic disorders is a complex one that requires expertise in MNT for the specific disorder. Preparation and competency requires access to detailed information about the disorders and treatment modalities. A family-centered approach, knowledge of feeding-skill development, and understanding of behavior modification techniques, as well as the support and counsel of a team of health care providers involved in the care of the patient, are also required. Nutrition intervention is often a lifelong consideration. Specific objectives of nutrition care are shown in Box 42.2.

BOX 42.2 Intervention Objectives for the Nutritionist Involved in the Treatment of Genetic Metabolic Disorders

In the clinic the registered dietitian nutritionist (RDN) has a major role in ongoing therapy and planning for each child. These responsibilities include gathering of objective food intake data from the family, assessing the adequacy of the child's intake, and working with the family to incorporate appropriate ways to monitor the restricted food intake pattern. The child with a metabolic disorder often presents with a wide range of concerns, which may include unstable biochemical markers, failure to gain weight, excessive weight gain, difficulty adhering to the diet, and behaviors that cause an adverse feeding situation. Thus managing a child with a metabolic disorder requires input from the entire health care team. The nutritionist uses skills and knowledge of foods as sources of nutrients, parent-child relationships, growth, development, and interviewing to obtain the necessary information for assessing and planning for the child with a genetic metabolic disorder.

I. The RDN functions as an effective interdisciplinary team member by doing the following:
   A. Becoming familiar with the background and current status of the child by reviewing the medical record
   B. Recognizing and accepting the responsibility as the nutritionist by doing the following:
      1. Identifying appropriate intake of nutrients for growth, activity, and biochemical balance
      2. Identifying developmental stages of feeding behavior
      3. Understanding the concept of food as a support of developmental progress
      4. Identifying behavior as it affects nutrient intake
   C. Understanding, respecting, and using the expertise of the team disciplines in providing care for the child
II. The RDN provides adequate and supportive patient services by doing the following:
   A. Establishing a positive, cooperative working relationship with the parent, child, and other family members

   B. Interviewing the family about dietary intake and the feeding situation in a nonjudgmental manner
   C. Assessing the parent-child relationship as it relates to dietary management and control of the disorder
   D. Developing a plan for appropriate dietary management based on growth, biochemical levels, nutrient needs, developmental progress, and nutrition diagnosis, such as:
      Excessive protein intake
      Altered nutrition-related laboratory values
      Intake of inappropriate amino acids
      Inadequate vitamin intake
      Inadequate mineral intake
      Food medication interaction
      Food- and nutrition-related knowledge deficit
      Limited adherence to nutrition-related recommendations
   E. Developing a plan that includes appropriate foods and recognizes the family's skills in food preparation, as well as family routines
   F. Working with the family to establish a method to deal effectively with negative feeding behaviors, if necessary
   G. Contacting the family after receiving laboratory results and calculating food records to make necessary and appropriate changes in diet prescription
III. Supporting families in their efforts at effective dietary and behavior management
IV. The RDN develops a professional knowledge base by doing the following:
   A. Being familiar with the current literature on the treatment of metabolic disorders
   B. Understanding the genetic basis of metabolic disorders
V. The RDN works with team members to understand the long-term patient care and create a written care plan for the patient.

CLINICAL CASE STUDY

Adelaide was born weighing 6 lb, 7 oz and her 1-day newborn screening test result for phenylalanine (Phe) was 3.7 mg/dL (222 μmol/L). She was breastfed with no supplemental formula. A repeat sample was requested to further document the Phe concentration in her blood. The result from this sample, collected on day 4 of life, was 6.2 mg/dL (372 μmol/L). To confirm the diagnosis for this child, which was considered to be "presumptive positive," a quantitative sample was obtained, and Phe and tyrosine levels were both measured. On day of life 9 the serum Phe concentration was 16.6 mg/dL (1328 μmol/L), and the tyrosine level was 1.1 mg/dL (60.5 μmol/L); the Phe to tyrosine ratio was 22.0:1. Blood and urine were collected for biopterin screening; results were later found to be normal.

To provide adequate protein and energy intake and at the same time decrease the serum Phe concentration, a Phe-free formula was introduced at standard dilution without a Phe supplement. Within 24 hours Adelaide's serum Phe concentration had decreased to 8.3 mg/dL (498 μmol/L) while she was being provided an intake of 12 to 14 oz of the Phe-free formula. Breastfeedings were reintroduced; she was offered 3 breastfeedings and Phe-free formula ad lib. Within 48 hours the level was 6.6 mg/dL (396 μmol/L), with an intake of 4 oz of the formula.

Adelaide's Phe concentrations were measured every 4 days, and the levels were 3.6 mg/dL (216 μmol/L) and 2.2 mg/dL (132 μmol/L). In subsequent weeks growth and serum Phe concentrations continued to be monitored carefully, and energy and Phe intakes were adjusted as necessary to maintain blood Phe concentrations between 2 and 6 mg/dL (120 to 360 μmol/L) and to maintain growth in appropriate channels.

By age 2 months, Adelaide's intake had increased to approximately 12 oz formula along with 3 breastfeedings daily (alternating breastmilk and formula feedings), and her feeding pattern was fairly consistent. Blood Phe was measured at 8.7 mg/dL (522 μmol/L), which is outside the desired range. Her Phe-free formula was increased to 14 oz/day to effectively decrease the amount of Phe provided by breastmilk.

Nutrition Diagnostic Statement

- Altered nutrition-related laboratory values (phenylalanine) (NC-2.2) related to phenylketonuria and dietary Phe intake, as evidenced by blood Phe outside desired range.

Nutrition Care Questions

1. What is the expected energy requirement for Adelaide?
2. What are the baseline expectations for intake for a 6-lb, 7-oz neonate? If breastmilk is expected to provide about half of this amount, how much Phe-free formula would you use to provide protein and energy intakes at recommended levels?
3. What are the growth expectations for Adelaide?
4. What steps would you take if Adelaide's plasma Phe concentration exceeded 6 mg/dL (360 μmol/L) on subsequent measurements?

USEFUL WEBSITES

American College of Medical Genetics (ACMG)
Gene Reviews from the National Library of Medicine
Genetic Metabolic Dietitians International (GMDI)
Genetics Home Reference from the National Institutes of Health
MedlinePlus: Metabolic Disorders
National Newborn Screening and Genetics Resource Center
National PKU Alliance
National PKU News

REFERENCES

American College of Medical Genetics: *ACMG ACT sheets and confirmatory algorithms* [Internet], Bethesda, MD, 2001, American College of Medical Genetics.

American College of Medical Genetics Newborn Screening Expert Group: Newborn screening: toward a uniform screening panel and system, *Genet Med* 8(Suppl 1):1S–252S, 2006.

Baker P, Ayres L, Gaughan S, et al: Hereditary fructose intolerance. In Adam MP, Ardinger HH, Pagon RA, et al., editors: *GeneReviews®* [Internet], Seattle, WA, 2015, University of Washington, Seattle.

Berry GT: Classic galactosemia and clinical variant galactosemia. In Adam MP, Ardinger HH, Pagon RA, et al., editors: *GeneReviews®* [Internet], Seattle, WA, 2017, University of Washington, Seattle.

Brosco JP, Seider MI, Dunn AC: Universal newborn screening and adverse medical outcomes: a historical note, *Ment Retard Dev Disabil Res Rev* 12(4):262–269, 2006.

Brusilow SW, Horwich AL: Urea cycle enzymes. In Valle D, Antonarakis S, Ballabio A, et al., editors: *The online metabolic and molecular bases of inherited disease*, New York, NY, 2010, McGraw-Hill.

Camp KM, Parisi MA, Acosta PB, et al: Phenylketonuria Scientific Review Conference: state of the science and future research needs, *Mol Genet Metab* 112(2):87–122, 2014.

Díaz VM, Camarena C, de la Vega Á, et al: Liver transplantation for classical maple syrup urine disease: long-term follow-up, *J Pediatr Gastroenterol Nutr* 59(5):636–639, 2014.

Doyle CM, Channon S, Orlowska D, Lee PJ: The neuropsychological profile of galactosaemia, *J Inherit Metab Dis* 33(5):603–609, 2010.

Forges T, Monnier-Barbarino P, Leheup B, et al: Pathophysiology of impaired ovarian function in galactosaemia, *Hum Reprod Update* 12(5):573–584, 2006.

Frazier DM, Allgeier C, Homer C, et al: Nutrition management guideline for maple syrup urine disease: an evidence- and consensus-based approach, *Mol Genet Metab* 112(3):210–217, 2014.

Holt, LE, Snyderman S: The amino acid requirements of children. In Nyhan WL, editor: *Amino acid metabolism and genetic variation*, New York, NY, 1967, McGraw-Hill.

Kaufman FR, Horton EJ, Gott P, et al: Abnormal somatosensory evoked potentials in patients with classic galactosemia: correlation with neurologic outcome, *J Child Neurol* 10(1):32–36, 1995.

Kaye CI, Accurso F, La Franchi S, et al: Newborn screening fact sheets, *Pediatrics* 118(3):e934–e963, 2006.

Kishnani PS, Austin SL, Abdenur JE, et al: Diagnosis and management of glycogen storage disease type I: a practice guideline of the American College of Medical Genetics and Genomics, *Genet Med* 16(11):e1, 2014.

Koch R, Trefz F, Waisbren S: Psychosocial issues and outcomes in maternal PKU, *Mol Genet Metab* 99(Suppl 1):S68–S74, 2010.

Lee PJ, Ridout D, Walter JH, et al: Maternal phenylketonuria: report from the United Kingdom Registry 1978-97, *Arch Dis Child* 90(2):143–146, 2005.

Longo N, Arnold GL, Pridjian G, et al: Long-term safety and efficacy of sapropterin: the PKUDOS registry experience, *Mol Genet Metab* 114(4):557–563, 2015.

Manoli I, Sloan JL, Venditti CP: Isolated methylmalonic acidemia. In Adam MP, Ardinger HH, Pagon RA, et al., editors: *GeneReviews®* [Internet], Seattle, WA, 2016, University of Washington, Seattle.

Martino T, Koerner C, Yenokyan G, et al: Maternal hyperphenylalaninemia: rapid achievement of metabolic control predicts overall control throughout pregnancy, *Mol Genet Metab* 109(1):3–8, 2013.

Matern D, Rinaldo D: *Medium-chain acyl-coenzyme a dehydrogenase deficiency*. In Pagon R, Adam M, Ardinger H, et al., editors: *GeneReviews®* [Internet], Seattle, WA, 2015, University of Washington, Seattle.

Maternal Child Health Bureau (MCHB): Newborn screening: toward a uniform screening panel and system, *Genet Med* 8(Suppl 1):1S, 2006.

McPheeters ML, Lindegren ML, Sathe N, et al. AHRQ future research needs papers. In *Adjuvant treatment for phenylketonuria: future research needs:*

identification of future research needs from comparative effectiveness review No. 56, Rockville, MD, 2012, Agency for Healthcare Research and Quality.

Oishi K, Arnon R, Wasserstein MP, et al: Liver transplantation for pediatric inherited metabolic disorders: Considerations for indications, complications, and perioperative management, *Pediatr Transplant* 20(6):756–769, 2016.

Singh RH, Quirk ME, Douglas TD, et al: BH(4) therapy impacts the nutrition status and intake in children with phenylketonuria: 2-year follow-up, *J Inherit Metab Dis* 33(6):689–695, 2010.

Singh RH, Rohr F, Frazier D, et al: Recommendations for the nutrition management of phenylalanine hydroxylase deficiency, *Genet Med* 16(2):121–131, 2014.

Southeast Regional Genetics Network, GMDI: *Management guidelines portal*, 2017; Available at: southeastgenetics.org/ngp.

Strauss KA, Puffenberger EG, Morton DH. Maple syrup urine disease. In *GeneReviews®* [Internet], January 30, 2006 [Updated May 9, 2013]. Available at: http://www.ncbi.nlm.nih.gov/books/NBK1319/.

van Calcar SC, Bernstein LE, Rohr FJ, et al: A re-evaluation of life-long severe galactose restriction for the nutrition management of classic galactosemia, *Mol Genet Metab* 112(3):191–197, 2014.

van Calcar SC, Ney DM: Food products made with glycomacropeptide, a low-phenylalanine whey protein, provide a new alternative to amino Acid-based medical foods for nutrition management of phenylketonuria, *J Acad Nutr Diet* 112(8):1201–1210, 2012.

Vockley J, Andersson HC, Antshel KM, et al: Phenylalanine hydroxylase deficiency: diagnosis and management guideline, *Genet Med* 16(2):188–200, 2014.

Waisbren SE: Newborn screening for metabolic disorders, *JAMA* 296(8):993–995, 2006.

Waisbren SE, Azen C: Cognitive and behavioral development in maternal phenylketonuria offspring, *Pediatrics* 112(6 Pt 2):1544–1547, 2003.

Watson MS, Lloyd-Puryear MA, Mann MY, et al: Main Report, *Genet Med* 8:12–252, 2006

Weinstein DA, Steuerwald U, De Souza CFM, et al: Inborn errors of metabolism with hypoglycemia: glycogen storage diseases and inherited disorders of gluconeogenesis, *Pediatr Clin North Am* 65(2):247–265, 2018.

Medical Nutrition Therapy for Intellectual and Developmental Disabilities

Kim Nowak-Cooperman, MS, RDN, CD
Patricia Novak, MPH, RDN
Cam Lanier, RDN, CD
Christine Avgeris, RDN, CD

KEY TERMS

alcohol-related birth defects (ARBD)
alcohol-related neurodevelopmental disorders (ARND)
Arnold Chiari malformation of the brain
Asperger's syndrome
attention-deficit/hyperactivity disorder (ADHD)
autism spectrum disorders (ASD)
cerebral palsy (CP)

cleft lip and/or cleft palate (CL/CP)
developmental disability
Down syndrome (DS)
fetal alcohol spectrum disorders (FASD)
hypotonia
individualized education plan (IEP)
individualized family plan
intellectual disability
midfacial hypoplasia

mosaicism
myelomeningocele (MM)
nondisjunction
oral-motor problems
pervasive developmental disorder (PDD)
Prader-Willi syndrome (PWS)
spina bifida
translocation

Individuals with developmental disabilities were generally housed in institutions for the first half of the 20th century. Little attention was paid to their education, or medical or nutritional care. In 1963 the Developmental Disabilities Assistance and Bill of Rights Act was passed. Through this Act federal funds supported the development and operation of state councils, protection and advocacy systems, university centers, and projects of national significance. This Act provided the structure to assist people with developmental disabilities to pursue meaningful and productive lives. The institutions that housed these individuals gradually were closed or reduced in size. By 1975 these individuals were cared for at home, in schools, or in small residential facilities. In 1975 Public Law (P.L.) 94-142 was passed, opening public schools to children with developmental disabilities. In 1985 P.L. 99-487 (102-119 in 1992), the Early Intervention Act, was passed, bringing services to children from birth to school age. In 2004 the Individuals with Disabilities Education Act (IDEA) reauthorized this legislation.

A developmental disability is defined as a severe chronic disability that is attributable to an intellectual or physical impairment or combination of intellectual and physical impairments. It is manifested before the person reaches age 22; is likely to continue indefinitely; results in substantial functional limitations in three or more areas of major life activity (self-care, receptive and expressive language, learning, mobility, self-direction, capacity for independent living, and economic self-sufficiency); and reflects the person's need for a combination of generic or specialized interdisciplinary care, treatments, or other services that are lifelong or of extended duration and individually planned and co-ordinated. Developmental disabilities affect individuals of all ages and are not a disease state. Intellectual disability replaced the term *mental retardation* in the 11th edition of the *Definition Manual of the American Association on Intellectual and Developmental Disabilities* (AAIDD, 2013).

Intellectual disability is the most common developmental disability, characterized by significantly below-average intellectual functioning along with related limitations in areas such as communication, self-care, functional academics, home living, self-direction, health and safety, leisure, or work and social skills. An estimated 1% to 3% of the population have this diagnosis.

Developmental disabilities have been traced to many causes: chromosomal aberrations, congenital anomalies, specific syndromes, neuromuscular dysfunction, neurologic disorders, prematurity, cerebral palsy (CP), untreated inborn errors of metabolism, toxins in the environment, and nutrient deficiencies. The Centers for Disease Control and Prevention (CDC) reported in 2018 that one in seven or 15% of American children have a developmental disability.

MEDICAL NUTRITION THERAPY

Medical nutrition therapy (MNT) services vary depending on the individual and much has been learned about the role of nutrition in the prevention of disabilities and interventions. The role of the registered dietitian nutritionist (RDN) is essential. Because there is an abundance of information that parents and caretakers use from support groups and websites that are untested scientifically, RDNs often are providing evidence-based counseling to provide support and counteract misinformation.

Numerous nutrition problems have been identified in the individual with developmental disabilities. Growth restriction, obesity, failure to thrive, feeding problems, metabolic disorders, gastrointestinal disorders, drug-nutrient interactions, constipation, and cardiac and renal problems may be present. Other health problems exist, depending on the disorder. Table 43.1 lists the most common developmental disabilities and their associated nutrition problems.

TABLE 43.1 Common Nutrition-Related Issues in Individuals with Intellectual and Developmental Disabilities and Children and Youth with Special Health Care Needs with Suggested Nutrition Diagnosis Terms

Syndrome or Developmental Disability	Nutrition Diagnosis	Etiology and/or Signs and Symptoms
Autism Spectrum Disorders (ASD) ASD is a group of developmental disabilities that are characterized by delayed speech and language development, ritualistic or repetitive behaviors, and impairments in social interactions. Individuals may also have delays in feeding skills and the ability to self-feed.	Inadequate energy intake	Limited food choices Medication side effects affecting appetite
	Limited food acceptance	Sensory processing issues Avoidance of foods/food groups
	Inadequate intake of calcium/vitamin D/iron/other nutrient(s)	Limited food choices; avoidance of foods/food groups Following a special diet, such as a gluten free, casein free diet may place child at risk for nutrient deficiencies, including calcium and fiber if food acceptance is already low.
	Underweight	Inadequate energy intake BMI <5th percentile for children aged 2-20 yr Medication side effects affecting appetite Limited food choices secondary to behaviors
	Overweight/obesity	BMI >85th percentile for children aged 2-20 yr Use of food for behavioral interventions Estimated excessive energy intake Medication side effects affecting appetite Low physical activity level Limited food choices that are excessive in calories
Cerebral Palsy (CP) A nonprogressive disorder of muscle control or coordination that affects different parts of the body. This results from an injury to the brain during fetal, perinatal, or early childhood development. The severity is variable. Intellectual disability is often present.	Increased energy expenditure	Unintended weight loss
	Excessive energy intake	Increased body adiposity Reduced energy expenditure secondary to treatment with medication to reduce muscle tone Hypotonia Weight gain greater than expected Changes in mobility status Enteral nutrition provides more calories than measured/estimated energy expenditure
	Inadequate oral intake	Unintended weight loss Inability to self-feed due to lack of coordination Poor dentition, presence of cavities, and/or abscesses Gastroesophageal reflux disease Oral-motor dysfunction/dysphagia Medications affecting appetite Malnutrition and failure to thrive
	Inadequate fluid and fiber intake	Constipation Inability to independently consume fluid and food Dysphagia Altered thirst sensation, inability to communicate thirst
	Swallowing difficulty	Abnormal swallow study showing aspiration and/or oral/pharyngeal dysphagia Coughing, choking, prolonged chewing, pocketing of food, regurgitating, and facial expression changes during eating Reduced food intake Unintended weight loss Prolonged feeding times, lack of interest in food, food avoidance, mealtime resistance
	Altered GI function	Constipation Gastroesophageal reflux disorder, delayed gastric emptying Medication side effects
	Food–medication interactions	Constipation related to antispasticity medications Increased risk of osteopenia/osteoporosis related to antiseizure and antigastroesophageal reflux disease medications Risk of B_{12} deficiency related to antigastroesophageal reflux disease medications

Continued

TABLE 43.1 Common Nutrition-Related Issues in Individuals with Intellectual and Developmental Disabilities and Children and Youth with Special Health Care Needs with Suggested Nutrition Diagnosis Terms—cont'd

Syndrome or Developmental Disability	Nutrition Diagnosis	Etiology and/or Signs and Symptoms
	Underweight	BMI <5th percentile/age in children aged 2-20 yr Reduced muscle mass, muscle wasting Inadequate energy intake to promote weight gain compared with estimated or measured needs Hypertonia, dystonia
	Overweight	BMI >85th percentile/age for children aged 2-20 yr Excessive energy intake Low physical activity level Hypotonia
Drug exposed and fetal alcohol spectrum disorders Physical, behavioral, mental, or learning disabilities that occur when a fetus is exposed to drugs and/or alcohol during development. Growth may also be affected.	Food–medication interaction	Side effects of medications affecting appetite
	Overweight/obesity	BMI >85th percentile for children aged 2-20 yr Estimated excessive energy intake Sedentary activity level
	Self-monitoring deficit	Altered self-regulation Overweight/obesity Underweight
Down syndrome A genetic disorder that results from an extra chromosome 21, resulting in developmental problems such as congenital heart disease, cognitive delay, short stature, gastrointestinal problems, and decreased muscle tone.	Inadequate oral intake	Dementia Swallowing difficulty Unintended weight loss
	Breastfeeding difficulty	Feeding difficulty with weak suck Poor weight gain
	Altered GI function	Constipation (related to hypotonia, low activity, and/or low fiber intake) Celiac disease
	Overweight/obesity	Increased body adiposity Estimated excessive energy intake Reduced energy needs related to hypotonia BMI >85th percentile for children aged 2-20 yr
Genetic or inherited metabolic disorders Genetic conditions that result in a deficiency or defective enzyme in a metabolic pathway. Some of these, such as phenylketonuria, can result in significant lifetime intellectual and developmental disabilities. Others can cause death if not properly treated.	Imbalance of nutrients Impaired nutrient utilization Altered nutrition-related laboratory values	Food and nutrition knowledge deficit of dietary changes related to new diagnosis Nutrient restriction due to metabolic disorder
	Unintended weight loss	Poor appetite due to metabolic disorder Inadequate energy intake Lack of adequate insurance coverage for low protein foods/special metabolic formulas, limited access to formula Food and nutrition knowledge deficit of dietary changes related to new diagnosis
	Unintended weight gain	Excessive energy intake
Orofacial cleft A birth defect that occurs when the lip and/or the roof of the mouth does not form or close properly, resulting in a cleft lip and/or cleft palate.	Swallowing difficulty	Abnormal swallow study showing aspiration and/or oral/pharyngeal dysphagia Inadequate oral intake Frequent respiratory infections/pneumonias Coughing/choking with foods/liquids Cleft lip/cleft palate
	Breastfeeding difficulty	Inability to form proper latch Inadequate oral intake
	Underweight	Inadequate energy intake Increased energy expenditure

TABLE 43.1 Common Nutrition-Related Issues in Individuals with Intellectual and Developmental Disabilities and Children and Youth with Special Health Care Needs with Suggested Nutrition Diagnosis Terms—cont'd

Syndrome or Developmental Disability	Nutrition Diagnosis	Etiology and/or Signs and Symptoms
Prader-Willi syndrome A genetic disorder resulting from a deletion in chromosome 15. Hypotonia in infancy can result in failure to thrive before onset of hyperphagia. Common medical issues include obesity as a result of hyperphagia, short stature, and varying levels of intellectual abilities.	Breastfeeding difficulty Inadequate oral intake	Feeding difficulty with weak suck Poor weight gain
	Excessive energy intake Overweight/obesity	Increased body adiposity BMI >85th percentile for children aged 2-20 yr Reduced energy needs Self-monitoring deficit
	Limited adherence to nutrition-related recommendations	Inability to limit or refuse foods offered Lack of social support for implementing changes
	Undesirable food choices	Intake inconsistent with diet quality guidelines Unable to independently select foods consistent with food quality and energy controlled guidelines
	Intake of unsafe food	Food obsession Hyperphagia Eating serves a purpose other than nourishment Pica
Spina bifida (myelomeningocele) A neural tube defect resulting from incomplete closure of the spine during early pregnancy. This results in nerve damage, including neurogenic bowel/bladder and paralysis. Other common medical issues include Arnold Chiari II malformation, hydrocephalus, growth hormone deficiency, and learning differences.	Increased protein needs	Chronic, nonhealing wounds
	Swallowing difficulty	Abnormal swallow study showing aspiration and/or oral/pharyngeal dysphagia Frequent respiratory infections/pneumonias Coughing/choking with foods/liquids Presence of Arnold Chiari II malformation of the brain
	Altered GI function	Low fluid and fiber intake Neurogenic bowel Constipation
	Overweight/obesity Unintended weight gain	Increased body adiposity BMI >85th percentile for children aged 2-20 yr Estimated excessive energy intake Self-monitoring deficit Limited mobility Reduced energy needs related to altered body composition, short stature

ASD, Autism spectrum disorder; *BMI*, body mass index; *GI*, gastrointestinal.
Adapted from Figure 1 of 2010 Academy position on developmental disabilities and special health care needs and references 24 and 26.

The Academy of Nutrition and Dietetics confirms that nutrition services provided by RDNs are essential components of comprehensive care for infants and children with special health care needs and adults with intellectual and developmental disabilities. Nutrition services should be provided throughout the life cycle in a manner that is interdisciplinary, family centered, community based, and culturally competent. Poor nutrition-related health habits, limited access to services, and long-term use of multiple medications are considered health risk factors in this population. Timely and cost-effective nutrition interventions promote health maintenance, reduce risk, and reduce the cost of comorbidities and complications (Ptomey and Wittenbrook, 2015).

Nutrition Assessment

Anthropometric Measures

Anthropometric measures are altered when an individual is unable to stand, suffers from contractures or scoliosis, or has other gross motor problems. Measuring body weight may require special equipment such as chair, sling, or bucket scales. Wheelchair scales are used in some clinics but require that the wheelchair weight be known and checked at each clinic visit. Height or length measurements are very challenging to obtain accurately and may be estimated using a recumbent board. Other measures of height include arm span, knee-to-ankle height, or sitting height (Fig. 43.1 and see Appendix 6).

Although growth charts for children with various syndromes do exist, most clinicians recommend using the general CDC charts (see Appendix 3) because the information in the specialized charts is often based on small numbers, mixed populations, and old data (CDC, 2014). For the infant with a developmental disability, the World Health Organization (WHO) growth charts are recommended from birth to 24 months.

Other measures that can be used to explore weight issues include arm circumference, triceps skinfold measures, and body mass index (BMI). BMI is a part of the CDC growth charts and can also be found in Appendix 3. Using the BMI for age can be controversial. For example, BMI is limited for identifying overweight in children with developmental disabilities who are overly fat because of decreased muscle mass and short stature. Also, BMI may not be accurate if height measurement is not accurate. Height age may also be used to assess BMI if an individual plots far below expected height for age.

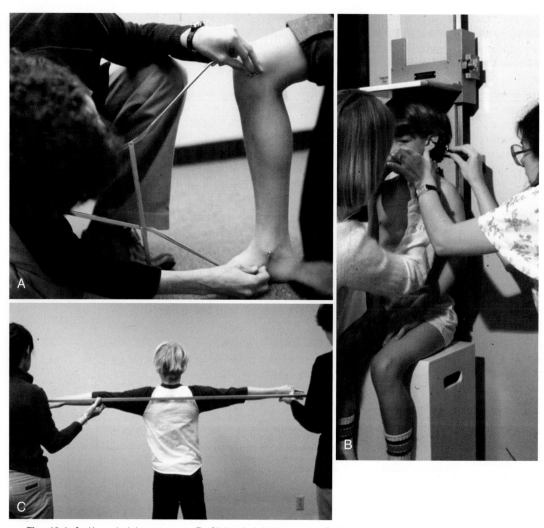

Fig. 43.1 A, Knee height measure. **B,** Sitting height measure. **C,** Arm span measure. (Courtesy Cristine M. Trahms, 2002.)

Biochemical Measures

Laboratory assessment for the child and adult with developmental disabilities is generally the same as that discussed in Chapter 5 and Appendix 13. Additional tests may be indicated for the individual with epilepsy or seizures who is receiving an anticonvulsant medication such as phenytoin, divalproex sodium, topiramate, or carbamazepine. Use of these medications can lead to low blood levels of folate, carnitine, ascorbic acid, vitamin D, alkaline phosphatase, phosphorus, and pyridoxine.

Assessment of thyroid status is part of the protocol for children with Down syndrome (DS), and a glucose tolerance test is recommended for evaluation of the child with Prader-Willi syndrome (PWS). As appropriate, genetic testing may be encouraged for affected individuals and their biological family members to identify any potential risks to the individual and to future pregnancies.

Dietary Intake and Feeding Problems

Dietary information should be obtained for the child with a developmental disability through a diet history or a food frequency questionnaire (see Chapter 4). However, obtaining an accurate recall is difficult as written diaries are difficult to obtain when the child has multiple caretakers or when they are in day care or school. When working with an adult with developmental disabilities, it is often difficult to obtain accurate information unless the individual has supervision, such as in special residential housing. Use of pictures and food models are helpful in obtaining an estimate of the individual's intake (see Box 4.5 Apps for Tracking Intake and Physical Activity in Chapter 4).

Many children and adults with developmental disabilities display feeding problems that seriously impair their ability to eat an adequate diet. Feeding problems are defined as the inability or refusal to eat and/or drink certain foods and liquids because of neuromotor dysfunction, obstructive lesions such as strictures, and behavioral or psychosocial factors. Other causes of feeding problems in this population include oral-motor difficulties, dysphagia, positioning problems, conflict in parent-child relationships, sensory issues, and tactile resistance from previous intubation (Heiss et al, 2010). The nutritional consequences of feeding problems include inadequate or excessive weight gain, poor growth in length, lowered immunity, anemia, vitamin and mineral deficiencies, dental caries, and psychosocial problems. Feeding problems should be assessed with an understanding of the anatomy, physiology, and normal development of feeding (see Chapters 15 through 17 and Chapter 39).

Estimates are that feeding problems are found in 40% to 70% of children with special health care needs and 80% of children with developmental delays. Feeding problems are often classified as oral motor, gross motor, behavioral, or sensory yet feeding problems are usually multifactorial in origin and treatment. Oral-motor problems

BOX 43.1 Oral-Motor Problems

Problem	Description
Tonic bite reflex	Strong jaw closure when teeth and gums are stimulated
Tongue thrust	Forceful and often repetitive protrusion of an often bunched or thick tongue in response to oral stimulation
Jaw thrust	Forceful opening of the jaw to the maximum extent during eating, drinking, attempting to speak, or general excitement
Tongue retraction	Pulling back the tongue within the oral cavity at the presentation of food, spoon, or cup
Lip retraction	Pulling back the lips in a very tight smile-like pattern at the approach of the spoon or cup toward the face
Sensory defensiveness	A strong adverse reaction to sensory input (touch, sound, light)

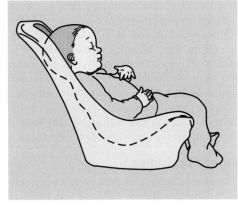

Fig. 43.2 Proper feeding position for the infant. (From Cloud H: *Team approach to pediatric feeding problems*, Chicago, 1987, American Dietetic Association. © American Dietetic Association. Reprinted with permission.)

include difficulty with suckling, sucking, swallowing, and chewing. They also include sensory motor integration and problems with self-feeding and are described as exaggerations of normal neuromotor mechanisms that disrupt the rhythm and organization of oral-motor function and interfere with the feeding process (Box 43.1).

Children with developmental disabilities such as DS, CP, or cleft lip and/or cleft palate (CL/CP) often have oral-motor feeding problems that may be related to the cleft, muscle tone, and inability to accept complex texture. The oral-motor problem also can be related to developmental level, which may be delayed.

Positioning a child for feeding relates to their motor development, head control, trunk stability, and ability to have hips and legs at a right angle (Figs. 43.2 and 43.3). This is frequently a problem for individuals with CP, spina bifida, and DS. Without proper positioning, oral-motor problems are difficult to correct.

The ability to self-feed may be delayed or absent in the child with developmental disabilities and requires intervention and training by a feeding specialist. A feeding evaluation is best completed with actual observation by a team composed of a speech therapist, a dentist, a physical therapist, an occupational therapist, and an RDN. Frequently, adaptive feeding equipment is needed such as special bottles, nipples, cups, utensils, and so on.

Behavioral issues may result from oral-motor or sensory problems, medical problems, certain medications, and the amount of emphasis placed on feeding. Issues such as control of the feeding process along with lack of autonomy in the child may create negative behavior. Environmental factors also influence the eating behavior of the child (see Chapter 16). Examples include where the child is fed, distractibility, serving sizes, delayed weaning, and frequency of feeding. The feeding relationship concept is important and is further discussed in Chapter 16.

Nutrition Diagnosis

Once the nutrition assessment has been completed, problems should be identified related to growth. Excessive or inadequate weight gain velocity; inadequate or excessive dietary intake; excessive or inadequate fluid intake; altered gastrointestinal problems such as constipation, gastroesophageal reflux, vomiting, and diarrhea; intake of foods that are unsafe because of contamination or food allergies; food-medication interactions; chewing and swallowing difficulties; and problems with self-feeding may be issues. The nutrition diagnoses should be listed and priorities established, using a family-centered or client-centered approach.

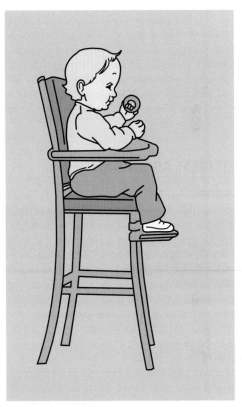

Fig. 43.3 Good feeding position for a child ages 6 to 24 months, showing hip flexion, trunk in midline, and head in midline. Good foot support with a stool should continue throughout childhood. (From Cloud H: *Team approach to pediatric feeding problems*, Chicago, 1987, American Dietetic Association. © American Dietetic Association. Reprinted with permission.)

Interventions

Once the nutrition diagnoses are identified and prioritized, short- and long-term goals should be created. Consideration must be given to the motivational level and readiness of the parent or client, their cultural background, and how the therapy can be community based and family centered. This means that consideration must be given to where the client will be served so that it becomes a part of the individualized education plan (IEP) or the individualized family plan.

Intervention plans should include all aspects of an individual's treatment program to avoid issuing an isolated set of instructions relevant to only one treatment goal. In some cases MNT may not be the family's first priority in the care of the child or adult, making it important for the RDN to recognize the family's needs and goals (see Chapter 13). Even when the family is ready for an intervention, such as weight management for a child with spina bifida, many factors require consideration. The parent or caregiver's educational level and income, language barriers, access to safe and appropriate food, and family coping strategies always should be identified (see Chapter 13).

Monitoring and Evaluation

Once MNT has been initiated, the need for follow-up evaluation and monitoring by either the RDN or another health care professional is important. Giving information in writing, ideally followed by a phone call, gives the chance to repeat some of the discussion and to answer any questions not asked during the initial session. Clarification of suggestions often is needed when monitoring nutrition changes that affect growth and development; a follow-up visit also may be needed.

A case manager may be involved who communicates with the adult with the disability, and a family resource coordinator may be available to assist families of children with disabilities. The RDN may need to assist in finding appropriate resources to pay for supplemental nutrition products, tube feedings, and special food products as a part of the follow-up process. Community and agency resources are identified and discussed, such as the Special Supplemental Nutrition Program for Women, Infants, and Children (WIC) and other government and nongovernment assistance programs.

CHROMOSOMAL ABNORMALITIES

Down Syndrome

Down syndrome (DS) is a chromosomal aberration of chromosome 21 (trisomy 21). It has an incidence of 1 in 600 to 800 live births and results from the presence of an extra chromosome in each cell of the body. This anomaly causes the physical and developmental features of short stature; congenital heart disease; intellectual disability; decreased muscle tone; hyperflexibility of joints; speckling of the iris (Brushfield spots); upward slant of the eyes; epicanthal folds; small oral cavity; short, broad hands with the single palmar crease; and a wide gap between the first and second toes (Bull and Committee on Genetics, 2011; Fig. 43.4).

Pathophysiology

Normally every cell of the human body except for the gametes (sperm or ova) contains 46 chromosomes, which are arranged in pairs (see Chapter 6). With DS there is one extra chromosome for a total of 47. This anomaly can occur by one of these three processes: nondysjunction, translocation, and mosaicism. In nondisjunction, chromosome 21 fails to separate before conception and the abnormal gamete joins with a normal gamete at conception to form a fertilized egg with three of chromosome 21. This also may occur during the first cell division after conception. This type of DS is usually sporadic and has a recurrence rate of 0.5% to 1%. In translocation, the extra chromosome is attached to another chromosome (usually 14, 15, or 22). Approximately half the time, this type of DS is inherited from a parent who is a carrier; it has a much higher risk of recurrence in a subsequent pregnancy. In mosaicism the abnormal separation of chromosome 21 occurs sometime after conception. All future divisions of the affected cell result in cells with an extra chromosome. Therefore the child has some cells with the normal number of chromosomes and other cells with an extra chromosome. Frequently the child with this type of DS lacks some of the more distinctive features of the syndrome (Bull and

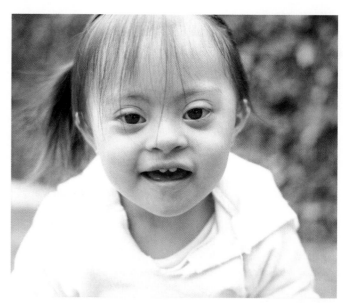

Fig. 43.4 Child with Down syndrome. From www.istockphoto.com

TABLE 43.2 Medical Problems Common in Down Syndrome

Condition	%
Hearing problems	75
Vision problems	60
Cataracts	15
Refractive errors	50
Obstructive sleep apnea	50-75
Otitis media	50-70
Congenital heart disease	40-50
Hypodontia and delayed dental eruption	23
Gastrointestinal atresia	12
Thyroid disease	4-18
Anemia	3
Iron deficiency	10
Transient myeloproliferative disorder	10
Leukemia	1
Celiac disease	5
Atlantoaxial instability	1-2
Autism spectrum disorder	1
Hirschsprung's disease	<1

From Bull MJ, Committee on Genetics: Health supervision for children with Down syndrome, *Pediatrics* 128:393–406, 2011.

Committee on Genetics, 2011) (see *Pathophysiology and Care Management Algorithm:* Down Syndrome).

Medical Treatment

The National Down Syndrome Congress has published a listing of the health concerns for individuals with DS; many have nutrition implications (Table 43.2). The American Academy of Pediatrics (AAP) has published health supervision guidelines for children and young adults up to age 21 (Bull and Committee on Genetics, 2011).

PATHOPHYSIOLOGY AND CARE MANAGEMENT ALGORITHM

Down Syndrome

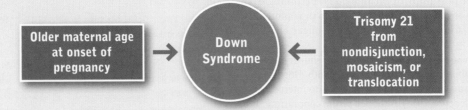

ETIOLOGY

Older maternal age at onset of pregnancy → Down Syndrome ← Trisomy 21 from nondisjunction, mosaicism, or translocation

PATHOPHYSIOLOGY

Clinical Findings

- Hypotonia
- Hyperflexibility/mobility of the joints
- Hip subluxation or dislocation
- Scoliosis
- Foot deformity
- Microbrachycephaly
- Short neck
- Depressed nasal bridge and small nose
- Upward-slanting eyes
- Abnormally shaped ears

- Enlarged, protruding tongue
- Single simian crease in center of the palm
- Excessive space between large and second toe
- Mental retardation
- Speech and motor delay
- Cardiac anomalies
- GI atresia or stenosis
- Hearing loss
- Hypothyroidism
- Dental problems
- Cataracts

MANAGEMENT

Nutrition Assessment

- Feeding problems
- Nutritional intake
- Fluid intake
- BMI compared with Down syndrome standards
- Weight changes
- Dysphagia
- Hemoglobin concentration

Medical Management

- Monitor for leukemia
- Management of infections
- Management of respiratory problems
- Signs of Alzheimer's disease later
- Annual monitoring of hypothyroidism

Nutrition Care

- Assess for feeding challenges
- Provide supportive feeding environment
- Use of adaptive feeding utensils
- Monitor weight changes
- Monitor for signs of nutrient deficiencies

Medical Nutrition Therapy

Anthropometric measures. Height, weight, head circumference, triceps skinfold, and arm circumference are obtained for the child with DS with the usual measurements (see Chapter 5). BMI can be taken but may be higher than normal because of short stature. Muscle tone is low and gross motor ability is often delayed, leading to the possibility of the individual becoming overweight. Monitoring should be frequent, and growth is plotted on the CDC charts or the WHO charts for the younger child (see Appendix 3).

Biochemical measures. Numerous studies have shown biochemical and metabolic abnormalities in individuals with DS; however, many have involved small samples and were difficult to interpret (Bull and Committee on Genetics, 2011). Although serum concentrations of albumin have been found to be low, the guidelines from the Down Syndrome Medical Congress do not list serum albumin assessment as routine. Increased glucose levels have been reported, with an increased incidence of diabetes mellitus.

Current guidelines for the treatment of infants and children with DS include evaluation of thyroid function at birth and thereafter annually. A number of studies have looked at zinc, copper, and selenium as possible deficiencies but concluded that they do not usually exist in children with DS as long as food access and appetite are good (Lima et al, 2010).

Dietary intake. During infancy the food intake of the infant with DS may differ from that of the typically developing infant. Although human breastmilk is recommended, many infants with DS are formula fed. Infant illnesses, admission to the neonatal unit, frustration, depression, perceived milk insufficiency, and difficulty in suckling by the infant are some of the reasons why formula feeding is used.

Progression to solid food has been found to be delayed in children with DS, mostly as a result of delays of oral-motor development. Introduction of solid food may not be offered at 6 months if the infant has poor head control or is not yet sitting. Low tone and sucking problems also delay weaning from the breast or bottle to the cup. IEPs include feeding and feeding progression instruction and practice.

An important part of evaluating dietary intake is determining energy and fluid needs, because children with DS have a high prevalence of obesity. Studies have indicated that the resting energy expenditure (REE) of the child with DS is lower than for children without DS—and may be as much as 10% to 15% lower than the dietary reference intake (DRI) for energy (Medlen, 2006). For the child older than age 5, calculations for energy requirements may have to be based on height rather than weight (Table 43.3 and see Chapter 2).

Feeding skills. Feeding skills are delayed in the infant and child with DS. Some parents find it difficult to initiate oral-motor skills such as suckling and sucking. The infant with DS often has difficulty in coordinating sucking, swallowing, and breathing, which are the foundations for early feeding. When the infant has a congenital heart defect, which occurs in 40% to 60% of DS infants, sucking is weakened, and fatigue interferes with the feeding process. Gastrointestinal anomalies are found in 8% to 12% of infants with DS, and these infants often require nasogastric or gastrostomy feedings.

Other physical factors that make feeding difficult in the first years of life include a midfacial hypoplasia (a craniofacial deformity common in cleft palate), a small oral cavity, a small mandible, delayed or abnormal dentition, misaligned teeth, nasal congestion, facial hypotonia, and small hands and short fingers. Weaning and self-feeding are usually late compared with the typically developing infant and frequently do not emerge until 15 to 18 months of age. The DS infant strives for independence and autonomy approximately 6 months later than the child without DS.

TABLE 43.3 Estimated Caloric Needs for Special Conditions

Condition	kcal/centimeter of height	Comments
Developmentally normal child	Average 16	
Prader-Willi syndrome	Maintain growth: 10-11 Promote weight loss: 8.5	For all children and adolescents
Cerebral palsy Mild Severe, limited mobility	 14 11	 For children ages 5-11 yr For children ages 5-11 yr
Down syndrome	Girls: 14.3 Boys: 16.1	For children ages 5-11 yr
Motor dysfunction Nonambulatory Ambulatory	 7-11 14	 For children ages 5-12 yr For children ages 5-12 yr
Spina bifida	Maintain weight: 9-11 Promote weight loss: 7	For all children older than 8 years of age and minimally active

Modified from Weston S, Murray P: Alternative methods of estimating daily energy requirements based on health condition. In Devore J, Shotton A, editors: *Pocket guide to children with special health care and nutritional needs*, Chicago, 2012, Academy of Nutrition and Dietetics.

Intervention Strategies

Overweight. Children with DS (and all children who have low muscle tone) are at increased risk for becoming overweight because of lower than typical energy expenditure. Weight management includes assessing the feeding developmental level of the child, their physical capability related to gross motor skills and physical activity levels, and environmental challenges. Environmental recommendations are the same as those for all children and include following a regular eating schedule that includes three meals and two to three snacks at regular times with the child sitting either in a high chair or at the table. Planned snacks should be nutrient dense, avoiding foods with excessive amounts of fat and sugar. Soft drinks should be discouraged and physical activity encouraged. It may be helpful to design a calorie-controlled eating plan based on kilocalories per centimeter of height as shown in Table 43.3 (Murray and Ryan-Krause, 2010).

Counseling in which the parent or caregiver helps determine a realistic plan that emphasizes appetite awareness and self-regulation may focus on serving sizes, healthy food choices, and food preparation and decreasing the number of times meals are purchased in fast-food restaurants. If the child or adolescent is school age, a prescription for a special meal at school can be obtained by using the school food service prescription (to be discussed later in the chapter). Prevention of overweight and promotion of an active lifestyle are the goals. Recent studies involving adolescents and young adults have addressed the success of exercise and healthy lifestyles for obese participants with DS. Successful programs include parent training in behavioral intervention and nutrition and activity education over multiple sessions (Curtin et al, 2013).

Eating skills. Parents may wrongly expect more typical eating development for the child with DS. An example of this is the unnecessary delay of weaning to a cup or progression of food textures because of inadequate effort or education. Behavioral problems related to feeding may develop based on what happens between the parent and child at mealtime. An intervention program with a feeding team can guide the parent in working with the child toward attainable feeding skills related to the developmental level.

Constipation. This is a frequent problem for the child with DS because of overall low tone that is exacerbated by a lack of fiber and fluid in the diet. Treatment should involve providing adequate fiber and fluid, with water consumption emphasized. Fiber content of the diet for children after age 3 is 5 to 6 g per year of age per day. For adults the recommendation is for 25 to 30 g of dietary fiber daily (see Chapter 27).

Prader-Willi Syndrome

Prader-Willi syndrome (PWS) was first described in 1956 by Prader, Willi, and Lambert. It is a genetic condition caused by the absence of chromosomal material. PWS occurs with a frequency of 1 in 10,000 to 1 in 25,000 live births. Characteristics of the syndrome include developmental delays, poor muscle tone, short stature, small hands and feet, incomplete sexual development, and unique facial features. Insatiable appetite leading to obesity is the classic feature of PWS; however, in infancy the problem of hypotonia (low muscle tone) interferes with feeding and leads to failure to thrive (Miller et al, 2011; Fig. 43.5). Developmental delays (affecting 50% of the population), learning disabilities, and intellectual disabilities (affecting 10%) are associated with PWS.

The genetic basis of PWS is complex. Individuals with PWS have a portion of genetic material deleted from chromosome 15 received from the father. Of the cases of PWS, 70% are caused from the paternal deletion, occurring in a specific region on the q arm of the chromosome. PWS also can develop if a child receives both chromosome 15s from the mother. This is seen in approximately 25% of the cases of PWS and is called maternal uniparental disomy. Early detection of PWS is now possible because of the use of DNA methylation analysis, which correctly diagnoses 99% of the cases (Miller et al, 2011). This is an important development in the early identification and subsequent treatment of these children to prevent obesity and growth restriction, and it is used to identify the infant born with features and characteristics described previously.

Pathophysiology

Metabolic abnormalities. Short stature in the individual with PWS has been attributed to growth hormone deficiency. In addition to decreased growth hormone release, children have low serum insulin-like growth factor (IGF)-1, low IGF-binding protein-1, and low insulin compared with developmentally typical obese children. Growth hormone (GH) therapy was approved by the Food and Drug Administration (FDA) in 2000, and in one 5-year study in Japan 37 patients from age 3 to 21 years experienced significant increase in height gain velocity when given GH (Obata et al, 2003). A more recent study found that GH therapy of infants and toddlers for 12 months significantly improved body composition and mobility skill acquisition (Carrel et al, 2010).

In addition to the GH deficiency, individuals have a deficiency in the hypothalamic-pituitary-gonadal axis, causing delayed and incomplete sexual development. Finally there is a decreased insulin response to a glucose load in children with PWS compared with age-matched non-PWS obese children (Haqq et al, 2011).

Appetite and obesity. Appetite control and obesity are common problems for individuals with PWS. After the initial period of failure to thrive, children begin to gain excessively between the ages of 1 and 4, and appetite slowly becomes excessive. Based on longitudinal study, Miller et al describe this gradual and complex progression in terms of seven nutritional phases based on levels of appetite, metabolic changes, and growth. In fact, some adults with PWS may progress to the last phase, with no insatiable appetite, and the person is able to feel full (Miller et al, 2011).

This uncontrollable appetite, a classic feature of PWS, when combined with overeating, a low basal metabolic rate, and decreased activity, leads to the characteristic obesity. The cause of the uncontrollable appetite is suspected to involve the hypothalamus and altered levels of satiety hormones and peptides such as ghrelin (Scerif et al, 2011).

Body composition is an important consideration in the evaluation of individuals with PWS. They have decreased lean body mass and increased body fat, even in infancy (Reus et al, 2011). Body fat generally is deposited in the thighs, buttocks, and abdominal area. The lowered energy expenditure is found in young children, adolescents, and adults with PWS, with one study showing adolescents with PWS having a total energy expenditure (TEE) 53% of that of typically developing adolescents who have a larger body size (McCune and Driscoll, 2005). The low muscle tone contributes greatly to the lack of interest in physical activity.

Nutrition Assessment

Anthropometric measures. Height measurements tend to be lower in PWS infants and young children, with the rate of height gain tapering off between the ages of 1 and 4. The usual measurements of length or height, weight, and head circumference should be taken and plotted on the CDC growth curves. Other clinically relevant measurements include arm circumference and triceps skinfold. BMI may be distorted for the individual with PWS because of the short stature; however, plotting the BMI over time is useful in determining unusual changes (see Appendix 3). It is important that anthropometric measures be taken frequently and reported to the parents or caregiver.

Biochemical measures. Biochemical studies are generally the same for the PWS individual, with the exception of either fasting blood glucose tests or glucose tolerance tests. These are added because of the risk for diabetes mellitus, possibly related to the decreased insulin response and obesity that usually accompany PWS.

Dietary intake. Dietary information varies for individuals with PWS depending on their age. In infancy the dietary information should be obtained with a careful dietary history and analyzed for energy and nutrient intake. Infants are commonly difficult to feed because of their hypotonia, poor suck, and delayed motor skills. Generally their feeding development is slower than in the typically developing infant, and transitioning to food at 4 to 6 months of age may be

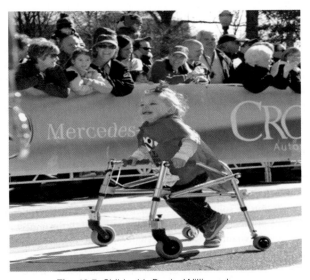

Fig. 43.5 Child with Prader-Willi syndrome.

difficult. Many infants with PWS have gastroesophageal reflux, requiring medication or thickening of their formula. Some infants may require nasogastric or G-tube feeds initially. A video fluoroscopic swallow study (VFSS) may be recommended to rule out dysphagia and aspiration. VFSS is an x-ray done using barium and the speech, or the occupational therapist determines whether there is any aspiration on various liquids. Feeding therapy is also beneficial. Our clinic has been requesting VFSS on infants and we have been finding silent aspiration. We have been proactive in including speech and occupational therapy as part of the assessment (Salehi et al, 2017).

During the toddler years, weight gain may increase rapidly as dietary intake increases. This requires careful assessment of portion sizes, frequency of feeding, and types of foods served. Although some parents may report that the child with PWS does not eat more than other children in the family, they have to be educated that the energy needs of the child are lower because of the reduced lean muscle mass and slow development of motor skills and activity. As the child gets older, interest in food increases; and, starting around ages 5 through 12, the child may be hungry all the time and display difficult behaviors such as tantrums, stubbornness, and food stealing. Information gathered during the dietary interview should include asking about feeding routine and management. The phrase "No doubt, no hope (no chance), no disappointment" has been used. With routines there is no doubt the child is fed, and no chance of getting extra foods leading to no disappointment. Determination of energy needs for the infant with PWS is the same as for a developmentally typical infant. However, when entering the toddler years, children with PWS will need fewer calories to maintain weight gain along the growth curve. This will apply in adulthood when fewer calories are needed to maintain weight. Energy needs have been calculated according to centimeters of height from 2 years and older (Miller et al, 2013) It has been recommended that the macronutrient intake of the diet be 25% protein, 45% carbohydrate, and 30% fat and at least 20 grams of fiber. A reduced energy intake and well-balanced diet improves weight control in children with PWS (Miller et al, 2013) (see Table 43.3).

Feeding skills. The infant with PWS often presents with weak oral skills and poor sucking skills in the first year of life. As the child matures, feeding skills are not a problem, but they may be delayed. Chewing and swallowing problems usually are not seen, although they may be associated with the low muscle tone. Behavioral feeding issues are associated with an insatiable appetite and not being provided with food. This can bring about tantrums.

Intervention Strategies

Intervention for PWS should occur at each developmental stage: infancy, toddler, preschool age, school age, and adult.

Infancy. Providing adequate nutrition as established by the AAP related to breastfeeding or formula feeding is recommended. Because feeding may be difficult related to sucking, concentrating the formula or breastmilk may be necessary to promote adequate weight gain. Feeding intervention will assist in improving the sucking problems caused by hypotonia. As the infant matures, a concentrated formula is not necessary, and solid foods can be added when head control and trunk stability are achieved, usually at approximately ages 4 to 6 months.

Toddler and preschool age. Most children begin to gain excessive weight between 1 and 4 years of age. Beginning a structured dietary plan for the child and the family is important so that the toddler learns that meals are provided at specified times and a pattern of grazing doesn't develop. Encourage parents and caregivers to provide balanced meals including protein, vegetables, whole grains, and fruits and limited amounts of sweets. Early intervention during the preschool years is very important in working with feeding issues and intake regulation as children grow older. Monitoring weight, height, and nutrient intake monthly will help identify early signs of weight acceleration so that dietary patterns and meal composition can be assessed and modified as needed. Regular physical activity is an important part of the IEP, and physical therapy services can be made available if necessary.

School age. For the school-age child, collaboration with the school food service program becomes important. Energy needs should be calculated per centimeter of height (see Table 43.3) and are generally 50% to 75% of the energy needs of typically developing children. This may require using a prescription for special meals through the school food service program.

At home environmental controls may be required, with cupboards and even kitchens being locked, because the child and adolescent have limited satiety and will search for food away from mealtime. Some parents report that GH therapy for their child helps, but it doesn't seem to change the child's lack of satiety. Appetite-suppressing medications have been used but are largely unsuccessful.

Adulthood. Prevention of obesity is truly the key for successful treatment of PWS; however, many adults who are not identified early become very obese. Weight management programs providing a very low 6 to 8 kcal per centimeter of height may be required. If a lower calorie diet is being recommended, patients will likely benefit from vitamin-mineral and essential fatty acid (EFA) supplements if micronutrient needs cannot be met through the diet. Many dietary treatments have been tried such as the ketogenic diet (see Appendix 19) and the protein-sparing modified-fast diets. However, with any approach strict supervision is usually required, and great emphasis must be placed on physical activity. A behavior management approach also has been recommended to implement the dietary management and physical activity plans. In many states there are group homes for adults with PWS, in which supervised independent living is possible and meals can be very structured and exercise programs implemented.

MNT of children and adults with PWS requires follow-up with many health care providers and schools. Fortunately parents of the individual with PWS now have access to a number of support groups and organizations dedicated to education, research, and establishing treatment programs.

NEUROLOGIC DISORDERS

Spina Bifida

Spina bifida is a neural tube defect that presents in a number of ways: meningocele, myelomeningocele (MM), and spina bifida occulta. MM is the most common derangement in the formation of the spinal cord and generally occurs between 26 to 30 days of gestation, with the date of occurrence affecting the location of the lesion. The lesion may occur in the thoracic, lumbar, or sacral area and influences the amount of paralysis. The higher the lesion, the greater is the paralysis. Manifestations range from weakness in the lower extremities to complete paralysis and loss of sensation. Other manifestations include incontinence and hydrocephalus (fluid accumulation in the brain). The incidence of spina bifida is about 2.7 to 3.8 per 10,000 live births in the United States per year, with Hispanics having the highest incidence (Canfield et al, 2014).

Prevention of spina bifida is now possible. In the 1980s, studies reported a positive effect from supplementation of mothers with folic acid plus multivitamins (Smithells et al, 1983). This reduced the risk of a second pregnancy with spina bifida as an outcome. As a result of numerous studies showing folic acid supplementation before conception to be effective, the national recommendation is 400 mcg/day for all women of childbearing age, and 4 mg for women who have had previous affected pregnancies (Committee on Genetics AAP, 1999). Through its Public Health Program, the WHO advocates globally for folic acid supplementation. Folic acid has been added to many flours and other cereal and grain products in the food supply since 1996. The CDC has reported that mandatory folic acid fortification of cereal and grain products has helped about 1300 babies to be born without neural tube defects (NTD) every year (CDC, 2015b). These public health measures have resulted in increased folate blood levels in U.S. women of childbearing age and a decrease of 20% in the national rate of spina bifida (Das et al, 2013; see Chapter 14).

Pathophysiology

The spinal lesion may be open and is typically repaired surgically shortly after birth, usually within 24 hours, to prevent infection. Although the spinal opening can be repaired surgically, the nerve damage is permanent, resulting in the varying degrees of paralysis of the lower limbs. In addition to physical and mobility issues, most individuals have some form of learning disability.

The spinal lesion affects many systems of the body and can result in weakness in the lower extremities, paralysis, and nonambulation; poor skin condition resulting in pressure injuries (see Chapter 19); loss of sensation with bowel and bladder incontinence; hydrocephalus; urinary tract infections; constipation; and obesity. Seizures also occur in approximately 20% of children with MM and may require medication. If medication fails, a ketogenic diet can be tried in some cases (see Appendix 19). Chronic medication is frequently required for prevention and treatment of urinary tract infections and for bladder control. The resultant nutrition problems include obesity, feeding problems, constipation, and drug-nutrient interactions. According to the Spina Bifida Association, children with spina bifida have an increased risk of developing an allergy to latex because of repeated exposers to latex products. The risk is decreasing with the use of latex-free products. Children who are allergic to latex may also develop an allergy to certain foods that cross react with latex such as banana, avocado, chestnut, kiwi, apple, carrot, celery, papaya, tomato, and melon. The Spina Bifida Association recommends that these foods should not be avoided unless there is an established reaction.

Nutrition Assessment

Anthropometric measures. Infants and children with spina bifida are usually shorter than typically developing children because of reduced length and atrophy of the lower extremities, although other problems such as hydrocephalus, scoliosis, renal disease, and malnutrition may contribute. The level of the lesions also can affect the length and height of the individual.

Obtaining accurate length and height measures can be difficult, especially as the child grows older. An alternate measure for determining height, the arm span/height ratio, is used and modified, depending on leg muscle mass. Arm span can be used directly as a height measure (arm span × 1) if there is no leg muscle mass loss, as in a sacral lesion. Arm span × 0.95 can be used to determine height if there is partial leg muscle loss, and arm span × 0.90 is used for a height measurement when there is complete leg muscle loss, such as with a thoracic spinal lesion (Kreutzer and Wittenbrook, 2013; see Fig. 43.1 and Appendix 6).

Weight measures can be obtained for the child unable to stand by using chair, sling, bucket, or wheelchair scales. To monitor weight accurately, it should be obtained in a consistent manner, with the person in light clothing or, if under age 2 years, undressed and wheelchairs weighed at each visit. Triceps skinfold measures can also be used, along with subscapular measures and abdominal and thorax measures, to determine the amount of body fat. They may be used as adjuncts to stature and weight measurements.

Head circumference should be measured in infants and toddlers up to age 3. A high percentage of children with spina bifida have head shunts as a result of their hydrocephalus. Unusual changes in the size of the head may indicate a problem with the shunt.

Biochemical measures. Useful biochemical tests in the health monitoring of individuals with spina bifida include iron status tests, measurements of vitamin D, and other tests related to the nutritional consequences of medications needed for seizures and urinary tract infection control (see Chapter 5 and Appendix 13).

Dietary intake. Many children with spina bifida eat a limited variety of foods, and they are frequently described as "picky eaters" by the parents. When doing a dietary history, it is important to ask about the variety of foods, particularly of high-fiber foods. The school-age child may be prone to skipping breakfast because early morning preparations for school require more time than for the nonaffected child.

Energy needs are lower for the child with spina bifida (see Table 43.3), and calorie requirements must be determined carefully to prevent the obesity to which many are prone. Ekvall and Cerniglia (2005) found that for MM children 8 years or older, the caloric need is 7 cal/cm of height for weight loss and 9 to 11 cal/cm of height to maintain weight. They also found that it is important to evaluate how the mother or caretaker perceives food for the child because it represents sympathy and love for many parents.

It is important to evaluate fluid intake because so many children are prone to having urinary tract infections as a result of daily catheterization. They may be drinking inadequate amounts of water and excessive amounts of soft drinks or tea that contain caffeine, which is a mild diuretic. Cranberry juice can be offered as it may help to prevent urinary tract infections, but calorie intake must be taken into consideration. Physical activity needs to be evaluated and may be found to be very limited, particularly when the child is nonambulatory. Ambulatory individuals with a shunt may be restricted from contact sports but can be involved in walking and running.

Feeding skills need to be evaluated, along with oral-motor function in particular. Many children with spina bifida are born with **Arnold Chiari malformation of the brain**, which affects the brainstem and swallowing (see Chapter 39 and Appendix 20 for dietary recommendations for dysphagia). Difficulty in swallowing may contribute to the child avoiding certain foods. Because of this there may be delays in weaning from the breast or bottle to the cup, but there should be no delays in gaining self-feeding skills.

Clinical evaluation. Evaluation should include looking for pressure injuries and signs of dehydration, along with asking about the amount and type of foods and fluids consumed. Constipation may be caused by the neurogenic bowel (fecal incontinence due to lack of normal bowel function) combined with a diet low in fiber and fluids.

Intervention Strategies

Many children with spina bifida are overweight. The Spina Bifida Association reports that after age 6, 50% of children are overweight and in adolescence and adulthood over 50% are obese (Spina Bifida Association, 2017). This may occur when ambulation is a problem leading to decreased energy needs. Refusal to accept a wide variety of foods is also common. Frequent feeding may be due to an oral-motor or a behavioral problem. Counseling includes introducing foods around age 6 months, limiting the intake of high-sucrose infant jar foods, and supporting the child to accept a wide variety of flavors and textures.

In addition to the generally known health consequences of obesity, specific concerns for individuals who have Spina Bifida include further limits of mobility and increased pressure on skin, increasing the already high risk of skin breakdown. Increased social isolation and decreased self-worth are also consequences (Spina Bifida Association, 2017).

Obesity prevention includes addressing the problems of limited physical activity, increasing fluids and fiber, and estimating the appropriate amount of calories. For school aged children it may be useful to provide a prescription for a low-calorie breakfast and lunch, with weight management listed as a part of the IEP. Enrollment in a group weight management program has been used successfully along with encouraging physical activity. The ideal program uses a team approach with involvement of the individual, the family, RDN, nurse, occupational therapist, physical therapist, educator, and psychologist (see Chapter 20).

In many clinics the child or adult with spina bifida is seen on a semiannual or annual basis. This frequent follow-up is necessary and should include monitoring of growth, particularly weight; food and fluid intake; and medication use. School programs and IEPs are excellent follow-up tools; however, the school often lacks appropriate scales for weighing a nonambulatory student. In this situation the parent should be encouraged to bring the child to the clinic for weight checks or, if distance is a problem, find a long-term care facility that will permit use of its scales. Follow-up by phone contact or email can be done for evaluating dietary intake and fluid management.

Cerebral Palsy

Cerebral palsy (CP) is a group of disorders of motor control or coordination resulting from injury to the brain during its early development. Among the causative agents of CP are prematurity; blood-type incompatibility; placental insufficiency; maternal infection that includes German measles; other viral diseases; neonatal jaundice; anoxia at birth; and other bacterial infections of the mother, fetus, or infant that affect the central nervous system.

The problem in CP lies in the inability of the brain to control the muscles, even though the muscles themselves and the nerves connecting them to the spinal cord are normal. The extent and location of the brain injury determine the type and distribution of CP. The incidence of CP varies with different studies, but the most commonly used rate is 1.5 to 4 in 1000 live births. The prevalence of premature births has contributed to maintenance of this figure despite electronic fetal monitoring (Fig. 43.6).

Pathophysiology

There are various types of CP, which are classified according to the neurologic signs involving muscle tone and abnormal motor patterns and postures. The diagnosis of CP is generally made between 9 to 12 months of age and as late as 2 years with some types (Box 43.2). The severity of CP is classified by levels of self-sufficiency in activities of daily living (ADLs). There are five categories of gross motor function, with category one being the least affected and five the most affected (Box 43.3).

> **BOX 43.2** **Different Types of Cerebral Palsy**
>
> **Spastic cerebral palsy (CP):** Spasticity implies increased muscle tone. This type accounts for 70% to 80% of cases. Muscles continually contract, making limbs stiff, rigid, and resistant to flexing or relaxing. Reflexes can be exaggerated, while movements tend to be jerky and awkward. Often, the arms and legs are affected. The tongue, mouth, and pharynx can be affected as well, impairing speech, eating, breathing, and swallowing.
>
> **Non-spastic CP:** Ataxic CP affects coordinated movements. Balance and posture are involved. Walking gait is often very wide and sometimes irregular. Control of eye movements and depth perception can be impaired. Often, fine motor skills requiring coordination of the eyes and hands, such as writing, are difficult. Does not produce involuntary movements, but instead indicates impaired balance and coordination.
>
> **Dyskinetic:** Dyskinetic CP is separated further into two different groups; athetoid and dystonic.
>
> Athetoid CP includes cases with involuntary movement, especially in the arms, legs, and hands.
>
> Dystonia/Dystonic CP encompasses cases that affect the trunk muscles more than the limbs and results in fixed, twisted posture.
>
> Because non-spastic CP is predominantly associated with involuntary movements, some may classify CP by the specific movement dysfunction, such as:
>
> Athetosis—slow, writhing movements that are often repetitive, sinuous, and rhythmic
>
> Chorea—irregular movements that are not repetitive or rhythmic, and tend to be more jerky and shaky
>
> Choreoathetoid—a combination of chorea and athetosis; movements are irregular, but twisting and curving
>
> Dystonia—involuntary movements accompanied by an abnormal, sustained posture
>
> **Mixed CP:** A child's impairments can fall into both categories, spastic and non-spastic, referred to as mixed CP. The most common form of mixed CP involves some limbs affected by spasticity and others by athetosis.

Data from MYCHILD: Types of Cerebral Palsy (website): http://www.cerebralpalsy.org/types-of-cerebral-palsy/.

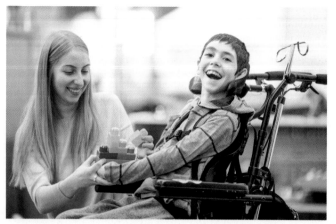

Fig. 43.6 Child with cerebral palsy. From www.istockphoto.com

---

> **BOX 43.3** **Gross Motor Function Classification System (GMFCS)**
>
> The 5-level GMFCS is used in clinical and research settings.
> 1. Walks without limitations
> 2. Walks with limitations
> 3. Walks using a hand-held mobility device
> 4. Self-mobility with limitations, may use powered mobility
> 5. Transported in a manual wheelchair
>   - fed orally without a feeding tube
>   - fed with a feeding tube

Reference: Palisano R, Rosenbaum P, Walter S, et al. Development and reliability of a system to classify gross motor function in children with cerebral palsy. *Cev Med Child Neurol* 1997; 39(4):214-223.

Poor nutrition status and growth failure, often related to feeding problems, are common in children with CP. Meeting energy and nutrient needs is particularly difficult in children and adults with more severe forms of CP such as spastic quadriplegia and athetoid CP, which is typically classified as Gross Motor Function Classification System (GMFCS) 4-5.

For example, bone mineral density of children and adolescents with moderate to severe CP is reduced in those with gross motor function and feeding difficulties (Andrew and Sullivan, 2010).

Other health problems include constipation exacerbated by inactivity, abnormal muscle coordination, and lack of fiber and fluids. Dental problems occur and often are related to malocclusion, dental irregularities, and fractured teeth. Lengthy and prolonged bottle-feedings of milk and juice promote the decay of the primary upper front teeth and molars (see Chapter 24). Hearing problems and especially visual impairments, intellectual disability, respiratory problems, and seizures affect nutrition status. Seizures are controlled with anticonvulsants, and a number of drug-nutrient interaction problems occur (see Appendix 13).

Nutrition Assessment

Anthropometric measures. This is an important area of assessment because of growth failure in the more severely involved child or adult with CP. Children with CP are often shorter, and, depending on the level of severity, some children with CP may have to be measured for length using alternative measuring techniques such as recumbent length boards or standing boards as they grow older (see Appendix 5). However, some of the measuring devices are inappropriate for the child with contractures and inability to be stretched out full length. Arm span can be used when the individual's arms are stretchable, as well as upper arm and lower leg length. Stevenson (1995) has recommended lower leg length or knee height as a possible measure for determining height for children and adults with lower-leg CP (see Fig. 43.1). The CDC recommends using the CDC/WHO curves designed for nonaffected children, plotting sequentially for indications of malnutrition rather than using the disease-specific curves.

Weight measures should be collected over time. Scales may require modifications, with positioning devices for the individual with CP who has developed scoliosis, contractures, and spasticity. Working with a physical therapist to find a positioning device that can be placed in a chair scale or using a bucket scale often works well. Mid–upper arm circumference and triceps skinfold measures are recommended reliable ways to screen for fat stores in children with CP. Head circumference should be measured regularly from birth to 36 months and plotted on the CDC growth charts (see Appendix 3).

Biochemical measures. Although no specific laboratory tests are indicated for the child with CP, a complete blood count, including hemoglobin, hematocrit, and ferritin, should be done when food intake is limited and malnutrition is a possibility. Because bone fractures are a significant problem for many children and adults with spastic quadriplegia, bone mineral density may require evaluating. Medications for seizures may be given; many have nutrition interaction problems (see Appendix 13). Evaluation of vitamin D, carnitine, and vitamin K levels may be useful.

Dietary intake. Oral-motor difficulties can result in limiting the intake of food and fluid, making it difficult for caretakers to meet nutritional needs. The energy needs of the individual with CP vary according to the type of CP. Studies show that the REE and TEE are lower in those with spastic quadriplegic CP than in developmentally typical controls (see Table 43.3).

Intervention Strategies

A high percentage of children with CP have feeding problems that are largely the result of oral-motor, positioning, and behavioral factors. As infants they may have difficulty swallowing and after infancy, coordinating chewing and swallowing, so the normal progression to solid foods is later than usual. Oral-motor problems may be permanent requiring lifelong modifications such as modified textures of foods and fluids to assure swallowing safety and the need for tube feeding for part or all of nutrition and hydration needs. All this may lead to inadequate intake and growth limitations. For those infants and children with IEPs, the team of RDN, speech therapist, occupational therapist, and physical therapist should evaluate the problem and work together in planning therapy to maximize skill development.

Gastroesophageal reflux frequently is seen in these infants and toddlers. Tube feeding may be required if swallowing studies reveal aspiration. Alternative techniques in feeding should be considered, which could include modifying food textures, thickening all beverages, or placing a gastrostomy tube (Mahant et al, 2011). RDNs should evaluate gastrostomy feedings for caloric and nutritional value and volume required for hydration as well as including oral solids and liquids into the tube feeding formula if possible.

Typical problems identified in the evaluation are altered growth, inadequate energy or fluid intakes, drug-nutrient interactions, constipation, and feeding problems. Working out an intervention plan is most successful when it involves the parent as part of the team, addresses cultural issues, and recognizes the importance of the feeding problem. Children with CP have complex problems that require routine follow-up with the family and appropriate agencies, schools, and institutions in the community. State agencies often provide tube-feeding formulas and special wheelchairs and equipment to assist with feeding problems. These agencies vary from state to state.

Autism

Autism spectrum disorders (ASD) were originally described in the 1940s as a behavioral disorder. It is now understood to be a pervasive and systemic syndrome with neurologic, immunologic, gastrointestinal, and endocrine involvement. There is no test to diagnose ASD at this time, rather ASD is diagnosed by the presence of impaired reciprocal social interaction; impaired communication skills with restricted, repetitive, stereotypical interests and behaviors as specified by the *Diagnostic and Statistical Manual of Mental Disorders*, fifth edition (DSM-5) (American Psychiatric Association, 2013).

Before 2013, **pervasive developmental delay (PDD)** and **Asperger's syndrome** were considered to be related but separate disorders (American Psychiatric Association, 2013). Now these disorders are included as part of the diagnosis of ASD as defined by the DSM-5. Rett's syndrome is also a related developmental disorder but is not part of the ASD diagnosis as it is significantly different in causation, is progressive, and is almost exclusively found in girls (Leonard et al, 2013). The CDC estimates 1 in 59 children were identified with ASD in 2014, an increase of 15% from 2012. ASD is four times more common in boys than girls. Most children are diagnosed at 4 years of age, yet it can be reliably diagnosed earlier. Since early diagnosis is essential for best outcomes, the AAP recommends screening all children for autism at the 18- and 24-month well child visits.

Pathophysiology

The etiology of ASD is as complex as the individuals with the disorder. Many theories have been proposed in both the scientific literature and popular press, with some unsubstantiated claims causing harm, such as the discredited link between vaccines and ASD leading to a worldwide resurgence of measles. It is estimated that specific genes or gene mutations account for 10% to 25% of ASD cases, with interaction between genetics and environment assumed to be the primary cause (Ornoy et al, 2016). Various causal theories are listed in Table 43.4.

TABLE 43.4 ASD: Proposed Causes, Contributors, and Associated Disorders

Causes of ASD	Disorders Associated with ASD
Genetics 　Presence of specific gene 　Gene mutation 　Gene deletion	Prematurity, small for gestational age (SGA)
Prenatal Environmental Exposure 　Pesticides 　Air pollution, particularly particulates 　Phthalates, BPA, solvent, flame retardant 　Medication: valproic acid, Misoprostol, 　Thalidomide 　Virus: Rubella, CMV	Birth defects: present in 11% of children with ASD compared with 6.4% of typically developing children
Parental characteristics 　Older age of mother or father 　Maternal autoimmune disorder 　Parental mental health diagnosis 　Obesity	Genetic syndromes: 10% of all children with ASD have a genetic syndrome such as Down Syndrome, fragile X, tuberous sclerosis, neurofibrosis, Angelman's syndrome
Prenatal vitamin deficiency; folate	Psychiatric diagnosis: ADHD, anxiety disorders, depression
Birth spacing: conceived less than 18 months or more than 60 months	IDD: 30% with IDD, additional 23% borderline IQ Sleep disorders: present in 2/3 of individuals with ASD, 80% with presence of IDD and ASD Gastrointestinal disorders prevalence studies vary from 7% up to 90%, constipation and diarrhea primary disorders Allergies; primarily food allergies Seizure disorders with prevalence increasing with age Autoimmune disorders

ADHD, Attention-deficit/hyperactivity disorder; *ASD*, autism spectrum disorder; *BPA*, bisphenol-A; *CMV*, cytomegalovirus; *IDD*, intellectual and developmental disabilities.
Ornoy et al, 2016; Chaidez et al, 2014; Garcia et al, 2017; Campbell et al, 2014; Marshall et al, 2014.

ASD frequently occurs with other developmental or medical diagnoses; these are described in Table 43.4. Children with ASD are more likely to have gastrointestinal (GI) disorders than typically developing children, with up to 90% of children with ASD having some type of GI issue. Compared with children with developmental disabilities, constipation, bloating, or diarrhea are three times more common (Chaidez et al, 2014). GI problems are often expressed atypically as poor sleep, anxiety, aggression, or social withdrawal, resulting in lower quality of life (Garcia et al, 2017). Reasons for GI problems include alterations in the gut microbiome (lack of diversity and characteristic microbiota), carbohydrate intolerance, and limited diets (Chaidez et al, 2014). Children with ASD frequently have restricted diets due to higher rates of food allergies, parent-imposed restricted diet, feeding problems, or selective "picky" eating (Marshall et al, 2014).

Overall, children with ASD who consume adequate nutrition grow well although there is a subgroup of children who demonstrate a general overgrowth pattern with macrocephaly (Campbell et al, 2014).

Nutrition Assessment

Anthropometric measures. Height and weight are determined using standard equipment and growth charts. Head circumference should be monitored up to 36 months, or longer if abnormal growth has been noted (Campbell et al, 2014). Weight gain and growth may be decreased with use of stimulant medicine, and excessive weight gain can occur with psychoactive medications such as risperidone (Ptomey and Wittenbrook, 2015; Richardson et al, 2017).

Biochemical measures. There is no standard pattern of tests other than regular newborn screening and blood work for health monitoring. If pica is noted or restrictive diets followed, pertinent nutrition blood work should be ordered. Since autoimmune disorders and allergies are more common, appropriate testing should be done when suspected (Ly et al, 2017). When psychotropic medicines are used blood lipids, hemoglobin A1C, and liver enzymes should be followed due to risk of metabolic syndrome.

Dietary intake. Dietary assessment is important due to limited diets and frequent constipation (see Chapter 4). Up to 89% of children with ASD exhibit some form of eating issue compared with 25% of typically developing children (Marshall et al, 2014). Limited dietary intake coupled with rigid, monotonous eating patterns place children with ASD at risk for both nutrient deficiencies and excesses (Marshall et al, 2014; Stewart et al, 2015). Idiosyncratic dietary patterns such as avoiding a certain color of food, eating specific foods in specific locations, or avoiding certain food textures are common. One multicenter study found that up to 40% of children with ASD had probable nutrient deficiencies (Stewart et al, 2015). Fruits and vegetables are commonly low in the diet while processed carbohydrates are high (Garcia et al, 2017). When variety is low and only a few foods are regularly consumed, the diet can be unbalanced with high levels of sodium, poor quality fat choices, and low fiber, especially if fortified foods or highly processed foods are consumed in large amounts. Pica or mouthing/chewing nonfood items can be a concern in ASD and cause significant health problems including hepatitis, parasitic disease, lead toxicity, and anemia. Including a feeding assessment along with a diet assessment (see Chapter 4) is helpful in determining whether feeding skills are age appropriate or if sensory processing is interfering with eating—both issues associated with ASD (Ptomey and Wittenbrook, 2015). Since social interaction is impaired, children often do not understand or display typical feeding cues and the feeding relationship may be challenged. Rigid eating habits, poor sense of hunger/satiety, textural aversions, and limited access to physical activity has resulted in a higher rate of obesity in ASD, especially among adolescents (Marshall et al, 2014).

Medical Nutrition Therapy

No one therapy or treatment modality works for all individuals with ASD (Marshall et al, 2014). Most children with ASD participate in a variety of interventions to address rigid or stereotypic behavior, sensory processing, and communication. These can include behavior intervention, structured educational approaches, medication, speech therapy, and occupational therapy. Interdisciplinary feeding therapy is warranted to address selective eating secondary to rigidity, motor planning, or sensory processing. Food rewards are commonly used in behavioral treatment, and alternatives should be explored as food rewards promote eating when not hungry, associate eating with reward, and are linked to emotional eating and obesity.

MNT is an effective complement to other treatments. Addressing selective eating habits can be challenging, and expanding the child's food repertoire takes time due to the rigidity inherent in the disorder. Treatment strategies need to respect the child's and parents' anxiety around mealtime as it can be great due to the child's rigidity, motor skills and sensory preferences, and parents' stress (Marshall et al, 2014). Common techniques include operant behavioral, systematic sensory desensitization, and food chaining (Marshall et al, 2014; Ptomey and Wittenbrook, 2015). Obesity, allergies, intolerances, and GI complaints are all common in children with ASD yet often go untreated (Chaidez et al, 2014; Garcia et al, 2017; Ly et al, 2017). Obesity treatment can be especially challenging due to dietary rigidity, hypersensitivity to sensory characteristics of food, and limited access to physical activity. Specialized diets are often trialed in children with ASD both due to medical concerns (GI complaints, seizures, allergies) as well as media reports (Garcia et al, 2017).

The most popular diet has been the gluten free (GF)–casein free (CF) diet. The majority of studies have not found measurable benefit, but parents often cite subtle improvements (Sathe et al, 2017). It has been theorized that the GF/CF diet or somewhat related Specific Carbohydrate Diet may be helpful in a small group of children as the diet is not treating the ASD per se but addressing undiagnosed immune or GI disorders, which are common in ASD (Garcia et al, 2017). Studies have documented the potential for nutritional deficits with the use of restrictive diets, specifically poor bone status with casein restriction, yet the risk can be minimized with dietitian supervision (Ly et al, 2017; Stewart et al, 2015). Tables 43.5 and 43.6 describe nutritional treatments commonly used in ASD. Care should be taken when beginning a diet trial as once a food is removed from a child's diet, it may be difficult to reintroduce that food if the child is a selective eater. Conversely if special products need to be used, such as GF alternatives, acceptance must be assured before starting the diet trial to assure dietary adequacy. Length of the trial and outcome measures should be clearly identified and the trial continued or ended based on measured effectiveness. When instituting a diet plan, the overarching consideration is to assure a health-promoting, developmentally appropriate diet that allows for social inclusion at home and in the community.

When MNT is used, care providers and the child, when possible, are key contributors to the process, identifying priorities, preferences, and potential challenges (Garcia et al, 2017). Collaborating with occupational therapists, speech and language pathologists, and others on that child's team is critical for success especially if a child is a highly selective eater. As a result of years of rigid and monotonous diets, use of food rewards, psychotropic drug use, and limited physical activity, rates of diet-related disorders such as hypertension, obesity, and diabetes are 40% to 50% higher in adults with ASD compared with the general population (Garcia et al, 2017; Marshall et al, 2014). Nutritional guidance throughout the life course is essential, directed not only toward the caregiver but also toward the adolescent with ASD especially as they achieve independence (Garcia et al, 2017).

Attention-Deficit/Hyperactivity Disorder

Attention-deficit/hyperactivity disorder (ADHD) is a neurobehavioral problem beginning in childhood and often extending into adulthood. Between 9.5% and 11% of children in the United States have been diagnosed with ADHD (CDC, 2018). Nearly two thirds of children with ADHD have another behavioral diagnosis. Diagnosis is based on the presence of specific behaviors noted in different settings: home, school, and community (Wolraich, 2019). According to the DSM-5 criteria for diagnosis, the child must consistently show signs of inattention, hyperactivity, and impulsivity inappropriate for age that

TABLE 43.5	Proposed Dietary Interventions in Neurobehavioral Disorders	
Dietary Interventions	**Associated Disorders**	**Guidance for Use**
Additive/food dye free diet Removal of synthetic food dyes: Blue 1&2, Citrus Red 2, Green 3, Red 40, Yellow 5&6, sodium benzoate	May reduce hyperactive and attentional issues in ADHD, ASD, and typically developing children with sensitivities (Garcia et al, 2017; Lange et al, 2017; Ly et al, 2017)	Requires instruction in label reading, may increase cost of some food products
Elimination diets Elimination of common allergens, usually milk, egg, wheat, soy, peanuts, tree nuts, fish/shellfish May also exclude other foods limiting diet to a handful of hypoallergenic foods	Food allergies Eosinophilic esophagitis ADHD ASD	Used temporarily for identification of problematic foods Requires detailed logs of intake and behavior to detect patterns Foods introduced systematically Removal of food for prolonged time can lead to rebound allergy response in sensitive children and can lead to food refusal in ASD. When foods are reintroduced, identify foods that the whole family can eat to encourage social inclusion. Requires instruction in label reading, may increase constipation especially if highly processed grains are used
FODMAPs diet SCD Elimination of classes of carbohydrate to address low levels of digestive enzymes or alterations in microbiome	Gastrointestinal concerns such as Crohn's disease, ulcerative colitis, carbohydrate intolerance, ASD with gastrointestinal symptoms	Requires detailed education for both consumer and RDN, both diets include staggered restriction/introduction which is helpful for identifying target foods and minimizes risk, specifically with SCD. SCD can lead to nutrient deficits for young children with limited diets. SCD may limit variety of textures which may influence progression of textures in feeding therapy
Gluten free (GF) and Casein free (CF) diets Eliminate casein-containing foods (milk from cow, goat, sheep, etc.) and/or gluten containing foods (wheat, rye, barley)	Celiac disease (GF), commonly used with DS, ASD, and ADHD Cerebral folate deficiency (CF) Food allergies	Identify foods that whole family can eat to encourage social inclusion, requires instruction in label reading, may increase constipation especially if highly processed GF grains are used. Ensure calcium adequacy with CF diet.

ADHD, Attention-deficit/hyperactivity disorder; *ASD,* autism spectrum disorder; *CF,* casein free; *DS,* Down syndrome; *FODMAPs,* fermentable oligosaccharides, disaccharides, monosaccharides, and polyols); *GF,* gluten free; *SCD,* Specific Carbohydrate Diet.
References: Sathe et al, 2017; Ly et al, 2017; Ptomey and Wittenbrook, 2015; Mastrangelo, 2018; Garcia et al, 2017.

TABLE 43.6   Examples of Effects of Nutrient Supplementation in Neurobehavioral Disabilities

Omega-3 fatty acid supplementation	ASD: Little evidence supports the effectiveness of omega-3 supplementation to improve core or associated ASD symptoms (Sathe et al, 2017) ADHD: Modest support for decreased lability, increased attention, and decreased oppositional behavior with GLA and EPA supplementation (Lange et al, 2017) FAS: Possible benefit pre- and postnatally (Murawski et al, 2015)
Digestive enzymes	ASD: Evidence is inadequate to assess the effects of short-term digestive enzyme supplements (Sathe et al, 2017)
Vitamin B$_6$	ALDH7A1 deficiency, Pyridox(am)ine 5'-phosphate oxidase deficiency Hyperprolinemia type II: reduced seizure activity (Mastrangelo, 2018) ASD: Evidence inadequate to support improvements in function, used individually, in various forms or with magnesium (Garcia et al, 2017)
Folic acid, Folacin	Cerebral folate deficiency: Possible reduced seizure activity, improved motor function (Mastrangelo, 2018) Mitochondrial disorders: often included
B$_{12}$ sublingual or injection	ASD: Few significant group communication or behavioral benefits (Sathe et al, 2017)
Multivitamin supplement: riboflavin, ALA, coenzyme Q$_{10}$; often with folinic acid and L-carnitine added when warranted	Mitochondrial disorders: Standard treatment to improve muscle function (Parikh et al, 2015) ASD: May warrant trial for children with ASD if mitochondrial disorder is suspected
Magnesium	ASD: No evidence to support use (Garcia et al, 2017) ADHD: Evidence inadequate to support use (Lange et al, 2017)
Probiotics	ASD: No evidence to support use for ASD, but moderate evidence to support use in treating gastrointestinal issues such as constipation (Garcia et al, 2017) Other disorders: May help to relieve constipation

ADHD, Attention-deficit/hyperactivity disorder; *ASD,* autism spectrum disorders; *EPA,* eicosapentaenoic acid; *FAS,* fetal alcohol syndrome; *GLA,* gamma-linolenic acid.

interfere with daily functioning and are not attributed to other diagnoses. Based on symptoms noted, three types are differentiated: (1) predominately inattentive type, (2) predominately hyperactive-impulse type, and (3) combined presentation. Presentation may change over time as the demands on the child increase. The causes of ADHD are not well understood, but genetic factors play a role. Additionally, other potential causes or risk factors include (Lange et al, 2017):

- Alcohol, drug, or tobacco use during pregnancy
- Premature delivery or low birth weight
- Environment, exposure at a young age; lead, pesticides, institutional care
- Brain injury

Television, parenting styles, sugar, and/or family dysfunction do not cause ADHD although they can exacerbate symptoms.

Nutrition Assessment

Anthropometric measures. Measurements of height and weight should be taken and recorded on a regular basis. Medications used in treatment may cause anorexia resulting in inadequate energy intake and slowing of growth, especially with long-term use (Richardson et al, 2017).

Biochemical measures. Follow recommendations for well child care with increased frequency if child is not gaining weight or has limited intake.

Dietary intake. A detailed dietary history should be obtained (see Chapter 4) especially in children who are exhibiting limited dietary intake. Evaluate the mealtime environment to identify ways to reduce distractions through changing seating or limiting electronics.

Medical Nutrition Therapy

Standard treatment includes behavioral therapy (47% of children) and/or stimulant medication (62% of children). Stimulants tend to reduce appetite and weight gain, especially in the first year of use (Richardson et al,

2017). This contributes to a small but statistically significant lower adult height with long-term treatment with potential negative effects on bone mineralization (Richardson et al, 2017). Since the ability to feel hunger has been reduced, the child cannot be expected to appropriately modulate their own intake. Treatment should consider how to maximize interest in eating, first by adjusting medication timing or dosing when possible (i.e., eating breakfast before medication) (Richardson et al, 2017). When weight gain is a concern, care providers often resort to forcing, bribing, or offering higher fat/sugar foods to encourage intake. These practices rarely are successful and may contribute to the higher rates of obesity seen in adolescents and adults with ADHD. Encourage weight gain by offering calorically dense foods before medication dosing or when effect is waning; small and short frequent meals; and limiting visual/auditory distractions at meals (TV, tablets). In severe cases, a child may need extra support in school meal settings due to the amount of stimulation.

Restricted diets for ADHD have been promoted since the early 1970s starting with the Feingold diet. Despite mixed evidence of success, many families chose to follow this diet, which eliminates naturally occurring salicylates and artificial food dyes (FD&C numbered dyes) and additives (Ly et al, 2017). Recent research suggests that dietary manipulation may be beneficial in a subset of children, specifically the use of Restricted Elimination Diets (RED) and elimination of artificial food dyes (Lange et al, 2017).

Studies on RED and food dyes suggest that there are children with ADHD who have greater sensitivity to food additives and may also have atypical allergic responses (Ly et al, 2017). While there are higher rates of food allergies seen in ADHD, positive response to elimination of a food did not correlate with results of allergy testing, suggesting a non-immunoglobulin E (IgE) response (Ly et al, 2017). Table 43.5 details dietary interventions commonly used.

Supplemental omega-3 fatty acids have also shown mixed results in children with both normal and low blood levels. Meta-analysis has suggested that there is a modest benefit for some children, dependent on age or "critical period," presence of comorbidities, and length of time of use (Lange et al, 2017). Gamma-linolenic acid (GLA) and eicosapentaenoic acid (EPA) appear to be the most effective of the EFAs trialed (Lange et al, 2017). Studies with strict inclusion criteria indicate that there is a subgroup of children who do respond positively to supplementation with slightly improved emotional ability, increased attention, and decreased oppositional behavior (Lange et al, 2017). Typical "Western" diets are low in omega-3 fats and have been linked to ADHD, raising the question if supplementation alone is beneficial or if changing the diet to improve variety of fat intake, and reduce food additive intake, would have the same benefit as supplementation (Ly et al, 2017). Table 43.6 details use of nutritional supplements.

While research on diet and ADHD remains inconclusive and there is significant individual variation in response, reducing intake of processed foods, increasing intake of omega-3 fatty acids, and assuring appropriate weight gain and growth should be part of MNT for ADHD.

Cleft Lip and Palate

Cleft lip and/or cleft palate (CL/CP), also known as orofacial clefts, are some of the most commonly occurring birth defects, with an incidence of 1 in 500 to 700 births worldwide (Shkoukani et al, 2013). There is a wide variation of incidence by ethnic origin and geographic location, with the highest and lowest incidence respectively in Japan and in South Africa. Cleft lip is a condition that creates an opening of the upper lip. It can range from a slight notch to complete separation in one or both sides of the lips and extending upward. If it occurs on one side of the lip, it is called a unilateral cleft lip; if it occurs on both sides, it is called a bilateral cleft lip. The cleft palate occurs when the roof of the mouth has not joined completely; it can be either unilateral or bilateral. Cleft palate can range from just an opening at the back of the soft palate or separation of the roof of the mouth with both soft and hard palate involved. CL/CP result from incomplete merging and fusion of embryonic processes during formation of the face. There is also a condition called submucous cleft palate in which there is incomplete fusion of the muscular layers of the soft palate with fusion of the overlying mucosa (Figs. 43.7 and 43.8).

Lip and palate development occur between 5 and 12 weeks of gestation. Lip development begins first, usually at 5 weeks of gestation, followed by the development of the maxilla prominences and the primary palate. Fusion of the hard palate is completed by 10 weeks of gestation and the soft palate by 12 weeks. Cleft lip, but not cleft palate, can sometimes be identified in-utero with fetal ultrasound. CL/CP have multiple causes: genetic, environmental, and idiopathic. It is estimated that 20% of orofacial clefts are associated with underlying syndromes (syndromic clefts) such as 22q11.2-related disorders, Treacher Collins syndrome, and Stickler syndrome. Syndromic clefts are more likely to be genetic.

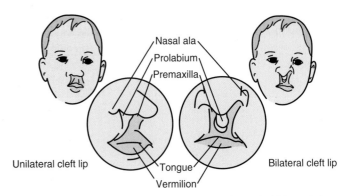

Fig. 43.8 Cleft lip. (From American Cleft Palate-Craniofacial Association, ACPA Family Services. http://acpa-cpf.org/families).

Pierre Robin sequence (RS) is often referred to as a syndrome but it is actually a set of abnormalities affecting the head and face consisting of a small lower jaw (micrognathia), a tongue that is placed further back than normal (glossoptosis), and breathing problems. A horseshoe-shaped cleft palate may or may not be present. Genetic counseling can now identify high-risk families for syndromic and nonsyndromic clefts (Leslie et al, 2013). Environmental causes include teratogens such as maternal smoking, alcohol use, and use of antiepileptic mediations.

Nutrition Assessment

Nutrition assessment for CL/CP includes the usual anthropometric measures for all infants and children. Biochemical measures are also those used with nonaffected children, and dietary intake information depends on the feeding problems that exist. Other problems include dental abnormalities and missing teeth, speech difficulties, and increased incidence of middle ear infections. Some infants (i.e., those with RS) may have increased difficulty breathing. The feeding evaluation is a major part of the assessment and is best accomplished with a team approach, including the parents. Because the major nutrition problem in CL/CP is feeding and providing adequate intake, growth can be jeopardized and must be assessed regularly.

Medical Nutrition Therapy

Treatment for CL/CP includes surgical treatment and nonsurgical treatment. The goal of surgical treatment is to repair the defect for good cosmetic and functional results. Nonsurgical treatment addresses how to feed the infant until the cleft is repaired and how to optimize growth and nutrition and promote successful surgical treatment (Lanier and Wolf, 2017) (Table 43.7).

TABLE 43.7 Feeding and Nutrition Goals for Children with Orofacial Clefts

- Effective feeding method with expected number of feedings and length of feeding in normal range of time
- Expected weight gain and growth for age, taking into account any related syndrome
- Feeding development typical for age (introduction of complementary foods at 6 months, introduction of cup drinking at 6 months)
- Maximized healing and minimized weight loss postsurgeries
- Healthy nutrition and oral health habits appropriate for age, including principles of Ellyn Satter's Division of Responsibility of Eating
- For tube-fed infants and children, feeding plan that promotes oral intake, if appropriate

Adapted from: Lanier, C and Wolf, L. Children with cleft lip and/or palate: Feeding and nutrition. *Nutrition Focus for Children with Special Health Care Needs.* Nov/Dec 2017;32:6.

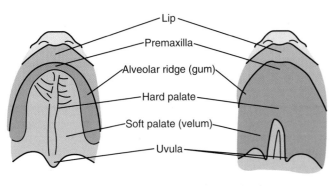

Fig. 43.7 Cleft palate. (From American Cleft Palate-Craniofacial Association, ACPA Family Services. http://acpa-cpf.org/families).

TABLE 43.8 *Surgical, Feeding, and Nutrition Management of Cleft Lip and Palate

Age	Surgical Management	Feeding Modality	Nutrition Management
3-6 months	Lip repair	Cleft lip only: breastfeeding or bottle feeding with wide-based nipple. Cleft palate: Specialty bottle. Upright position helps keep milk out of nasopharynx. Side lying position if tongue-based obstruction (Pierre Robin). Burp often secondary to increased air swallowing. After lip repair: Resume typical feeding modality soon after lip repair.	Breastmilk or standard infant formula. 400 IU vitamin D for babies receiving breastmilk. Introduction of complimentary foods at 6 months or when baby is showing readiness. Progression of textures typical for age. After lip repair: Resume breastmilk or formula
9-15 months	Palate repair (syndromic clefts at late end) Ear tubes for otitis media	See above. Introduction of cup typical for age. Cup must not contain valve. Wean from bottle to cup typical for age (~age 1) or after palate repair After palate repair: For 2-4 weeks, bottle feeding with specialty bottle and/or may use open cup or unvalved cup without hard or long spouts; nothing hard (no utensils or straws or fingers/hands) in mouth.	Wean to whole milk typical for age (age 1) but may wait until after palate is repaired. Toddler diet typical for age. Ensure meeting calcium and vitamin D requirement. After palate repair: For 2-4 weeks, soft, no chew diet.
2-5 years	Velopharyngeal insufficiency (VPI) surgery ("speech surgery") Nose and lip revision considered	After VPI surgery: Nothing hard (no utensils or straws) in mouth for 4-6 weeks.	Preschool diet typical for age. After VPI surgery: Soft, no chew diet for 4-6 weeks.
6-11 years	Bone graft of alveolar cleft after primary dentition complete and closure of oro-nasal fistulae Orthodontic interventions and teeth extractions as needed	After bone grafting: Nothing hard (no utensils or straws) in mouth for 4-6 weeks.	Diet typical for age. After bone grafting: Soft, no chew diet for 4-6 weeks.
12-21 years	Nose revision (rhinoplasty) if needed Jaw surgery in some cases (Orthognathics) Orthodontic bridges and implants	After jaw surgery: Straws are ok.	Diet typical for age. After jaw surgery: Soft, no chew diet for 6-8 weeks; may need blenderized liquid diet.

*Timing of surgeries, feeding modalities, and nutrition interventions may vary between craniofacial centers.
Adapted from Bernstein M and McMahon-Jones K. *Nutrition Across Life Stages.* 2017: Jones & Bartlett Learning, Burlington, MA. www.jblearning.com.

Surgical repair of the cleft lip generally is performed at 3 to 6 months of age, and cleft palate repair at 9 to 15 months. Other operations performed before the child starts school may include ear tubes for otitis media (usually performed at the same time as the palate repair), velopharyngeal insufficiency (VPI) surgery, and minor improvements to the lip or nose. Surgical interventions in later years include alveolar bone graft and, if needed, orthognathic (jaw) surgery (Table 43.8).

Breastfeeding is difficult for these infants because of problems with sucking, although those infants with just the cleft lip may be successful. It is generally recommended that the mother who wishes to breastfeed express her milk and give it to her baby from a specialized bottle and nipple. The use of an appropriate hospital-grade breast pump is recommended for milk expression. Parents and caregivers must be educated in the positioning of the child for feeding, nipple selection, bottle selection, feeding technique, and monitoring of intake (American Cleft Palate-Craniofacial Association, 2018).

Energy needs are generally the same as for a nonaffected infant. The exceptions to this are if the feeding process is too difficult (either adequate volumes are not achieved and/or energy needs are increased with the work of feeding) and if the infant has increased difficulty breathing (which results in increased energy demand). Strategies for solving these problems vary and include adjustment of the feeding modality (appropriate bottles and nipples) and feeding technique/infant

positioning, and/or using more concentrated formula or breastmilk (Table 43.9 and see Chapter 41). Enteral support (tube feeding) is rarely needed, and this may be only for a short while.

Effective feeding requires that the infant be able to form a vacuum inside the mouth and form a seal around the nipple with the lips. This is achieved through the proper bottle, nipple, and position for feeding. Acceptable nipples and bottles include the Mead Johnson Cleft Palate Nurser, the Medela Special Needs Feeder, the Pigeon Bottle and Nipple, and the Dr. Brown's Specialty Feeding System (Dr. Brown's bottle with one-way feeding valve) (Table 43.10). Babies with CL/CP have unique feeding challenges; thus, it is extremely important that an infant-feeding therapist or nurse experienced in feeding infants with clefts evaluate various types of equipment and carefully educate the parent in their use. Positioning in an upright position, choosing the appropriate bottle and nipple, and directing the liquid flow to the side or back of the mouth are strategies for optimal feeding. Babies with clefts swallow more air when feeding and should be given ample opportunities for frequent burping in an upright position.

Introduction of solid foods for the CL/CP infant can follow the usual protocol at 6 months of age or when the baby is showing readiness to feed (i.e., good head control and trunk stability and showing interest in food). Care that the food is presented slowly is important, allowing the infant to control each bite while gradually learning how to direct the

TABLE 43.9 Increasing Calories Through Concentration of Formulas and Addition of Oils and Carbohydrates

Using 20 cal/oz Formula Caloric Density Required Per Ounce

Per Ounce	Measures of Powder	Water Added
20 calories	1 scoop	2 fl oz
22 calories	2 scoops	3.5 fl oz
24 calories	3 scoops	5 fl oz
27 calories	3 scoops	4.25 fl oz

Using 22 cal/oz Formula

22 cal	1 scoop	2 fl oz
24 cal	3 scoops	5.5 fl oz
27 cal	5 scoops	8 fl oz

Adding Oil or Carbohydrates

Product	kcal	Source
Corn oil or safflower oil	9/g or 8.3/mL	Corn or safflower oil
Microlipid	4.5/mL	Safflower oil
MCT oil	8.3/g or 7.6/mL	Fractionated coconut oil
Karo syrup	1 Tbsp = 58 kcal	Polysaccharides
Polycose liquid	2/mL or 60/fl oz	Glucose polymers
Polycose powder	3.8/g; 8/tsp; 23/Tbsp	Glucose polymers
Moducal powder	30/Tbsp	Glucose polymers

food around the cleft. After the repair and healing of the cleft palate, feeding along the developmental pathway should progress slowly but normally (see Chapter 15 and Table 43.9).

FETAL ALCOHOL SYNDROME

Fetal alcohol spectrum disorder (FASD) is a lifelong consequence of maternal alcohol consumption leading to growth retardation, facial malformations, and central nervous system impairment. Since identified in 1973 by Drs. Kenneth Jones and David Smith at the University of Washington School of Medicine, FASD has been documented throughout the world with prevalence ranging from 2.4% to 20.8%; in high-risk populations such as Russian orphanages, rates have been estimated as high as 40% to 68% (Hoyme et al, 2016).

Alcohol consumption during pregnancy interferes with normal fetal growth and development of all body systems and organs. Maternal nutritional status, use of multiple drugs, genetic susceptibility, and alcohol use pattern can influence the severity of the disorder (Murawski et al, 2015). Diagnosis of fetal alcohol syndrome (FAS) requires that the following criteria are fully met: (1) pre- or postnatal growth deficiency, (2) FAS facial features, (3) abnormal brain structures and/or microcephaly, and (4) neurobehavioral impairment, with developmental or cognitive impairment depending on age. The three facial features include smooth filtrum (the groove between the upper lip and the nose), thin upper lip, and small palpebral (between the upper and lower eyelid) fissures. Partial fetal alcohol syndrome (PFAS) is diagnosed when two of the criteria are met with known alcohol exposure, or three of the four criteria when exposure is not documented. Alcohol-related neurodevelopmental disorders (ARND) and alcohol-related birth defects (ARBD) are additional diagnoses used to identify children without facial manifestations or

TABLE 43.10 Specialty Bottles

Specialty Bottle	How It Works	How to Pay and Where to Find
Mead Johnson Cleft Palate Nurser (Squeeze Bottle)	Milk is squeezed into the infant's mouth; flow is controlled by the person feeding.	Some insurance will cover Available through home care companies May be available at no cost from craniofacial centers Available to purchase on the Internet
Medela Special Needs Feeder (Haberman Bottle)	The nipple has a large chamber with a one-way valve. Milk flows into the nipple chamber but cannot flow back into the bottle. Milk is extracted either by squeezing the nipple (by person feeding) or clamping down on the nipple (the baby controls the flow). The nipple has different sized cuts allowing for fast or slow flow.	Some insurance will cover Available through home care companies May be available at no cost from craniofacial centers Available to purchase on the Internet
Pigeon Cleft Palate Nurser	The nipple has a one-way valve and the rubber on one side of the nipple is very thin. Milk flows into the nipple and the baby can extract by clamping down on nipple: the flow is controlled by the baby.	Some insurance will cover Available through home care companies May be available at no cost from craniofacial centers Available to purchase on the Internet
*Dr. Brown's Specialty Feeding System (Dr. Brown's bottle with one-way feeding valve) Nipple options include ultra preemie, preemie, and #1-4.	Same feeding mechanism as Pigeon Nurser.	Not covered by insurance Bottles and/or valves may be available at no cost from craniofacial centers Available to purchase on the Internet

*The valve fits in the nipple of any Dr. Brown bottle.
Adapted from: Lanier, C and Wolf, L. Children with cleft lip and/or palate: Feeding and nutrition. *Nutrition Focus for Children with Special Health Care Needs.* Nov/Dec 2017;32:6.

poor growth but with alcohol-associated psychological or medical problems (Hoyme et al, 2016). Children with ARND may have intellectual disabilities and problems with behavior and learning, particularly with math, memory, attention, judgment, and poor impulse control. Children with ARBD may have problems with the heart, kidney, bones, or hearing. Due to the clinical complexity, a multidisciplinary team should make the diagnosis (Hoyme et al, 2016).

Nutrition Assessment

Anthropometric measures are very important in the assessment of the FASD child due to characteristic growth deficiency. Prenatal growth restriction of the infant often persists postnatally despite a high caloric intake. Growth should be evaluated frequently and plotted on the CDC and WHO growth curves (Hoyme et al, 2016). Feeding problems are associated with FAS, including oral-motor problems expressing as poor suck in infancy and delayed feeding progression in toddlers. Poor growth and feeding issues often result in the diagnosis of failure to thrive (Amos-Kroohs et al, 2016). Impulse control, food hoarding, and hyperphagia are common in older children (Amos-Kroohs et al, 2016; Ptomey and Wittenbrook, 2015).

Medical Nutrition Therapy

Use of MNT with FASD emphasizes prevention of secondary disability beginning with prenatal vitamin-mineral supplementation when alcohol consumption is suspected as this may reduce disability both by addressing maternal nutritional deficits and mitigating teratogenic effects of alcohol (Murawski et al, 2015; Popova et al, 2016). While breastfeeding generally is encouraged, excessive alcohol use is a contraindication. Considering the array of potential nutritional concerns, MNT for the child with FASD is focused on the specific nutrition problem that exists for that child. Motor impairment, ADHD, developmental delay, seizure disorders, communication challenges, hyperphagia, and sensory impairments (visual/hearing) are common comorbidities that can put nutrition at risk (Amos-Kroohs et al, 2016; Popova et al, 2016). Short stature, sensory processing issues, and impulsivity increase the risk of overweight or obesity in the older child and adolescent. In addition, parental substance abuse, past or present, may impact the parent-child feeding relationship, requiring supportive intervention with referral to social services as needed (Amos-Kroohs et al, 2016).

Overall, caloric and nutrient needs do not differ from an unaffected child, although poor fetal nutrition or feeding problems may increase the risk of deficiencies (Popova et al, 2016). Vitamin, mineral, omega fatty acid, and choline supplementation may be warranted to maximize brain development and address prenatal deficits (Murawski et al, 2015). It can be difficult to determine caloric need in the young child when growth restriction is present. Increasing calories potentially can support improved growth but may also lead to excessive weight gain without increasing the rate of growth. Comparing serial measurements of weight to linear gains is necessary to individualize calorie recommendations. Strategies for increasing calorically dense foods may be required for those who have difficulty gaining weight. Food texture may need adaptation if oral-motor impairments are present.

FASD is the leading preventable developmental disability in the world today. Education regarding FASD should occur in all women of child-bearing age as there is no safe time or amount of alcohol during pregnancy (Murawski et al, 2015).

Complementary and Integrative Medicine (CIM) in Intellectual and Developmental Disabilities (IDD)/ASD

Current standard treatments for IDD/ASD include therapies (occupational, physical, speech/language), medication, and MNT. Often, standard interventions are time consuming, are expensive, or have negative side effects (Lindly et al, 2018). These treatments may reduce disease progression and improve function, but they may not provide significant reduction of the child's overall disability. In hoping for greater improvements, caregivers and health professionals seek out CIM to maximize development and quality of life. Over the past 50 years, a variety of studies have been initiated to assess if dietary manipulation or nutritional supplementation can treat or even cure developmental diagnoses. With the exception of the ketogenic diet for seizures and dietary management of metabolic disorders/inborn errors of metabolism, research on supplementation or dietary manipulation has found minimal or transitory improvements in developmental, behavioral, or functional measures (Lewanda et al, 2018; Mastrangelo, 2018; Sathe et al, 2017). As indicated in Chapter 11, research in CIM can be difficult to interpret in pediatrics and even more so in children with IDD/ASD, a very heterogeneous group likely to take multiple medications, participate in multiple therapies, and require frequent medical intervention—all of which will confound research results (Sathe et al, 2017). Studies may have bias, small sample size, multiple agents trialed in one study, lack of long-term follow-up, and flawed assessment of both nutritional adequacy and behavioral/functional change (Garcia et al, 2017; Lewanda et al, 2018; Brizee, 2019; Sathe et al, 2017). Harm is often underassessed, and the long-term effects of supplementation and dietary restriction are unknown (Garcia et al, 2017; Stewart et al, 2015). Despite the lack of clear recommendations, media, consumer groups, and supplement-industry sponsored conferences promote nutritional supplements and special diets in this population. This has resulted in greater use of CIM in this population compared with typically developing children (Lindly et al, 2018; Stewart et al, 2015).

Dietitians and caregivers are challenged with determining whether the potential for benefit from a diet or supplement outweighs the potential risk. Negative side effects include direct effects such as a nutrient deficit or excess and also indirect effects such as the financial and time costs. This can be considerable with use of multiple supplements, need for special dietary products, and payment for practitioners, many of whom are not covered by insurance (Lewanda et al, 2018; Lindly et al, 2018; Stewart et al, 2015). There is also the risk that, considering time and finances, unproven interventions will replace established, evidenced-based treatments (Lindly et al, 2018).

While various CIM methods, including herbs, yoga, and massage, are accessed in this population, the primary CIM modalities used are nutritional supplementation and dietary manipulation; see Chapter 11 for discussion of a wider range of CIM (Lindly et al, 2018).

Nutritional Supplements

Nutritional supplementation has shown benefits in rare metabolic disorders and mitochondrial disorders, but evidence that supplementation improves function in most developmental disorders is lacking (Lewanda et al, 2018; Mastrangelo, 2018; Parikh et al, 2015; Sathe et al, 2017). Other than in those examples, supplementation has been studied without clear or replicated success (supplements studied include B vitamins—B_6, B_{12}, folic acid, biotin, and riboflavin—vitamin E, l-carnitine, magnesium, zinc, and iron) (Garcia et al, 2017; Lewanda et al, 2018). While there often are changes in biochemical indices, significant parallel changes in behavior or function have not been found or replicated (Sathe et al, 2017). Meta-analyses and review articles caution on making supplement conclusions or recommendations due to flawed research methodology. Although research methods are improving, evidence remains insufficient to recommend use of nutritional supplementation (Garcia et al, 2017; Lewanda et al, 2018; Ly et al, 2017; Sathe et al, 2017).

Omega fatty acids and probiotics both have moderate evidence for improvements in mood and attention yet are not necessarily specific to IDD/ASD. It is unclear if this is a direct result of the supplement or of rectifying unbalanced dietary fats (Lange et al, 2017; Ly et al, 2017). Probiotics are thought to improve GI dysbiosis, immune function, and inflammation in ASD and potentially may have more global benefit for ASD and other disabilities (Chaidez et al, 2014; Garcia et al, 2017). This is an emerging area of research; use of probiotics has limited harm but may be contraindicated in children with immune suppression, and it may initially cause bloating and gas (Garcia et al, 2017).

Although data is tenuous, individuals with IDD use supplements twice as frequently as the general population, with use highest when children are young (Lindly et al, 2018). A study of children enrolled in the Autism Treatment Network revealed that more than 50% of children with ASD used nutritional supplements compared with 32% of typically developing children (Stewart et al, 2015). This same study found that supplementation did not address actual areas of deficit and led to excessive nutrient intake. This emphasizes the importance of RDN-supervised supplement use; initiating discussion when clients request use, addressing deficits indicated by poor diet or blood testing, and minimizing harm through attention to dosage, especially when fortified foods are consumed or contraindications exist such as calcium supplementation in William's Syndrome (Ptomey and Wittenbrook, 2015; Stewart et al, 2015). Table 43.6 summarizes use of supplementation. See Chapter 11 for more information about the safe recommendation of dietary supplements.

Special Diets

In 1954 the discovery that restriction of dietary phenylalanine in the diet of a child with phenylketonuria (PKU) prevented intellectual disability created hope that diet could treat or even cure development disabilities. Dietary treatments have been proven effective for some inborn errors of metabolism and for minimizing seizures, but have not yet shown similar success in treating other disabilities (Mastrangelo, 2018; Ptomey and Wittenbrook, 2015). Although there is a lack of empirical evidence, parents report that they chose CIM because they were unhappy with traditional interventions and felt more comfortable and in control using food rather than medication as treatment (Lindly et al, 2018; Ly et al, 2017). Studies of the most popular diets—ketogenic diet, GF diet, CF diet, and Specific Carbohydrate Diet (SCD)—have not found significant behavioral or functional change (other than the noted seizure control), yet caregivers chose to continue the diet after the study ended. It is suggested that parental perceptions of change may be influenced by desire for change, emotional investment in the treatment, and misinterpretation or attribution of any improvement to dietary change (Garcia et al, 2017; Lindly et al, 2018). Conversely, the subtle improvements noted may not be variables being measured, and therefore parents see benefit when researchers do not. For example, parents may see improved bowel movements or sleep, which are not assessed. Use of a special diet may be addressing underlying anemia, GI discomfort, or allergy, reducing discomfort and irritability (Garcia et al, 2017; Ly et al, 2017).

A nutrition assessment may reveal reasons to trial a diet such as a history of or current allergy, reflux, or constipation. The use of special diets is not without nutritional risk, but this can be minimized with RDN supervision. In addition to the risk of nutrient deficits, especially when entire food groups are eliminated or severely restricted, prescribed diets with very limited variety can exacerbate existing conditions like constipation through dependence on highly processed foods. Children with special needs are often socially isolated and restricted diets can further isolate the child by making eating with others challenging. Table 43.5 describes diets frequently used in this population.

Choosing CIM Treatments

Children with neurodevelopmental disorders are at greater risk of harm from both conventional and CIM intervention. Drug-nutrient interactions, GI problems, or altered immune status may make negative response more likely while concurrently making use of CIM attractive for resolving outstanding issues. The RDN can facilitate effective use of CIM by helping parents and other health care providers better understand the applicability and veracity of research (Brizee, 2019; Garcia et al, 2017; Ptomey and Wittenbrook, 2015).

Products that are promoted or advertised as follows should be avoided:
- Personal anecdotes, celebrity endorsement, or industry backed research are the only evidence for effectiveness.
- Claims of effectiveness are grandiose, universal, and apply to many different disorders; the magnitude of improvement is great, and the product is claimed as a cure.
- Reported benefits are general, vague, and unmeasurable.
- Exclusive to this company with a "special" formulation that is a propriety blend; company will not provide ingredients when asked (often necessary for safety concerns).
- Advertised as "opposed by the medical establishment."
- Expensive or costly for what is offered, requires extensive testing that is only available through a partner site, or special promotions that require prepayment; unable to use insurance.
- Clay baths, enemas, and chelation therapy are promoted to remove toxic chemicals to cure or treat various conditions. These procedures can be harmful and have resulted in death. The FDA has issued a warning against use of chelation therapies and highlights the risk of lead exposure in clay baths.

While there is risk for harm, this can be minimized with nutritional monitoring. In some cases the exploration of integrative therapies has led to successful treatment and a better understanding of brain, immune, and GI function in children with neurodevelopmental concerns. Each child should be assessed individually to determine whether any dietary or CIM therapy is appropriate.

COMMUNITY RESOURCES

For many types of nutrition problems and MNT, the school system is an excellent resource through the school lunch and school breakfast programs. Children and adolescents may receive modified meals at school. Child and adult care food programs must provide meals at no extra cost for children and adolescents with special needs and developmental disabilities. School food service is required to offer special meals at no additional cost to children whose disabilities restrict their diets as defined in the U.S. Department of Agriculture's nondiscrimination regulations.

The term "child with a disability" under Part B of IDEA refers to a child evaluated in accordance with IDEA as having one of the 13 recognized disability categories: (1) autism; (2) deaf-blindness; (3) deafness; (4) mental retardation; (5) orthopedic impairments; (6) other health impairments caused by chronic or acute health problems such as asthma, nephritis, diabetes, sickle cell anemia, a heart condition, epilepsy, rheumatic fever, hemophilia, leukemia, lead poisoning, or tuberculosis; (7) emotional disturbances; (8) specific learning disabilities; (9) speech or language impairment; (10) traumatic brain injury; (11) visual impairment; (12) multiple disabilities; and (13) developmental delays. Attention deficit disorder may fall under one of the 13 categories.

When a referral is made to the school system for a special meal related to a developmental disability, it must be accompanied by a medical statement for a child with special dietary needs. The request requires an identification of the medical or other special dietary condition, the food or foods to be omitted, and the food or choice of foods to be substituted. The statement requires the signature of the physician or recognized medical authority. The school food service may make food substitutions for individual children who do not have a disability but who are medically certified as having a special medical or dietary need. An example is the child with severe allergies or an inborn error of metabolism. The availability of school food service for children with developmental disabilities is an important resource in the long-term implementation of MNT.

CLINICAL CASE STUDY

Child with Down Syndrome

Nutrition Assessment
Client History
Colin is a 21-month-old boy with Down syndrome. He was born prematurely (30 weeks of gestation) and was started on nasogastric tube feeding at 10 days of age because of his poor weight gain and severe gastroesophageal reflux. The poor weight gain was caused by a weak suck, although swallowing was not a problem. After hospital discharge he was first seen by a nutritionist in an early intervention program at 4 months of age when it was noted that he had a gastrostomy tube placed at age 2 months.

Food/Nutrition-Related History
Colin received tube feeding instructions while hospitalized for his g-tube placement. He participated in early intervention oral-motor therapy. He was seen every 3 to 6 months for nutrition assessment and adjustment of g-tube formula to meet nutritional needs.

At 16 months Colin was tube fed PediaSure and just started eating table foods. His usual intake was 1 jar of baby food per day along with the tube-feeding formula.

Anthropometric Measurements
At 4 months of age Colin was 22.5 in long (< 5th percentile) and weighed 10 lb 7 oz (< 5th percentile). Weight/length was 10th to 25th percentile.
At 21 months, height was 28 in (< 5th percentile) weight was 18.5 lb (< 5th percentile)
Weight/length was 25th to 50th percentile.

Physical Findings
Colin is crawling but not yet walking, and he has very limited self-feeding skills. Now at age 21 months, his mother's highest priority is to stop the tube feeding and have Colin continue to grow well. She is concerned about his rate of weight gain. She also is concerned that constipation has become a problem requiring use of the medication lactulose. He also has respiratory problems and extreme hypotonia.

Feeding problems identified:
History of weak suck and swallow
Hyperactive gag reflex
Refusal or inability to drink formula from a bottle or cup
Poor appetite for oral foods
Not self-feeding

Nutrition Diagnostic Statements
- Self-feeding difficulty (NB-2.6) related to developmental delays and feeding difficulty as evidenced by poor weight gain and below 5% wt/age.
- Inadequate oral intake (NI-2.1) of food and fluids related to feeding difficulty as evidenced by need of supplement to meet nutritional needs by g-tube.

Nutrition Intervention
1. Tube-fed toddler with daily caloric requirement estimated at 670 (estimated energy requirement [EER] = ~80 cal/kg).
2. Work with occupational therapist (OT) to determine chewing and swallowing challenges and to support development of safe eating and drinking.
3. Introduction of oral foods and fluids as recommended by OT before gastrostomy feedings.
4. Reduction of tube feedings to support transition to oral eating and to meet estimated needs.

Nutrition Care Questions
1. What would be your approach in working with this mother and the other team members?
2. What do you think would be Colin's nutritional needs, starting with energy?
3. How many ounces of a 30 cal/oz tube-feeding formula would you recommend for Colin to promote weight gain?
4. What steps should be taken to increase Colin's oral intake and decrease the tube feeding?
5. What would you recommend for management of his constipation?

CLINICAL CASE STUDY

Adolescent with ASD and Obesity

Nutrition Assessment
History
Alex, a 16-year-old boy with ASD, was admitted to a residential facility after being removed from his special education class. Alex has age-appropriate receptive language but expresses himself usually using phrases from superhero TV shows and movies. Three months before referral, he began a trial of risperidone to address increasing irritability and aggression both at home and at school. Medical evaluation identified sleep apnea, elevated liver enzymes, hypertriglyceridemia, and impaired fasting blood glucose. The contributing factor to the medical problems is his severe obesity.

Food/Nutrition-Related History
Alex's birth weight was 7 lb 8 oz, his birth length was 19 in, and he was full term. He had typical feeding development until 2 years of age when he gradually started refusing previously accepted foods. Gradually, his intake was reduced to primarily crunchy foods including chicken nuggets, fish sticks, French fries, green apples, celery, most crackers, any type of Cheerios, chips, bacon, and beef jerky. Portions are large. His parents have tried to introduce more fruits and have had some success with other crunchy green vegetables such as green peppers or raw broccoli and freeze-dried fruits. Alex drinks milk, usually 24 to 30 ounces a day, and soda is provided as a reward. If he is denied food, he tends to throw a tantrum and family members often relent.

Alex has been overweight since 2 years of age, when his weight for age was between the 85th and 90th percentiles. When he began middle school, his rate of weight gain increased, with his body mass index (BMI) at the 95th percentile. Since starting high school, his rate of weight gain has continued to increase, which his

mother attributes to the role of food in the classroom as part of living skills training and for rewards. Since starting the risperidone, he has gained an additional 15 lbs in 3 months.

Alex enjoys physical activity when it can be related to superheroes. He enjoys watching and playing soccer but has limited opportunity.

Anthropometric Measurements:
Weight 210 lb (95.4 kg) > 97th percentile
Height: 66 in (167.6 cm) - 25th to 50th percentile
BMI index: 34 kg/m², 120% to 130% of the 95th percentile, classified as severe obesity

Biochemical Data
Total cholesterol: 210 mg/dL (high)
High-density lipoprotein (HDL) cholesterol: 29 mg/dL (low)
Triglycerides: 580 mg/dL (very high)
Glucose: 120 mg/dL (high)
Hemoglobin A1C: 6.1% (high)
Liver enzymes: AST 74 U/L, ALT 124 U/L (high)

Nutrition-Focused Physical Findings
Excessive appetite
Poor hygiene
Sedentary with excessive screen time
Constipation (2 to 3 bowel movements [BMs] per week)

CLINICAL CASE STUDY—cont'd

Adolescent with ASD and Obesity

Nutrition Diagnostic Statements

- Obesity, pediatric (NC-3.3.2) related to excessive food and beverage intake, large portion sizes, and high calorie food choices, as evidenced by BMI of 34.
- Altered nutrition related laboratory value (NC-2.2) related to obesity and risperidone use as evidenced by elevated cholesterol and triglycerides and hemoglobin A1C of 6.1%.
- Altered nutrition-related laboratory value (NC-2.2) related to obesity and excessive soda intake as evidenced by elevated liver enzymes ALT and AST.
- Altered gastrointestinal (GI) function (NC-1.4) related to low activity level and insufficient fiber and fluid intake as evidenced by report of only 2 to 3 BMs per week.

Intervention Goals

1. Work with family and school to decrease portion sizes, especially of highly processed foods
2. Increase fiber and fluid intake
3. Reduce sugary beverages due to elevated triglycerides, A1C, and liver enzymes
4. Increase access to physical activity

Nutrition Care Questions

1. When asked to limit food at school, teachers report that reward tokens to purchase snacks at the student store are part of the living skills curriculum. What would be your response?
2. What tools can you offer Alex and his family to help manage portion size and increase fruit/vegetable intake?
3. What resources are available to help Alex increase his physical activity?
4. What suggestions can you make to help Alex's parents respond to his demands for food?

USEFUL WEBSITES

American Cleft Palate Craniofacial Association

Association of Maternal and Child Health: Programs Children and Youth with Special Healthcare Needs

Centers for Disease Control and Prevention Birth Defects Research

March of Dimes

National Autism Association

National Center for Education in Maternal and Child Health

National Dissemination Center for Children with Disabilities

National Folic Acid Campaign

National Human Genome Research Institute Atlas of Human Malformation Syndromes in Diverse Populations

NIH National Institute of Mental Health (ASD)

REFERENCES

American Academy of Pediatrics Subcommittee on Attention-Deficit/Hyperactivity Disorder, Steering Committee on Quality Improvement and Management. ADHD: Clinical Practice Guideline for the Diagnosis, Evaluation and Treatment of Attention-Deficit/Hyperactivity Disorder in Children and Adolescents, *Pediatrics* 128:1007–1022, 2011.

American Association on Intellectual and Developmental Disabilities: *Definitions*, 2013. Available at: http://www.aaidd.org/content_100.cfm?navID=21.

American Cleft Palate-Craniofacial Association: *ACPA family services.* Available at: http://acpa-cpf.org.

American Psychiatric Association. Diagnostic and statistical manual of mental disorders. 5th ed. Arlington, VA: American Psychiatric Association; 2013

Amos-Krooks RM, Fink BA, Smith CJ, et al: Abnormal eating behaviors are common in children with fetal alcohol spectrum disorder, *J Pediatr* 169:194-200.e1, 2016.

Andrew MJ, Sullivan PB: Growth in cerebral palsy, *Nutr Clin Pract* 25: 357–361, 2010.

Brizee LS: Supplements for Children with Special Health Care Needs. *Nutrition Focus for Children with Special Health Care Needs* 34:1–12, 2019.

Bull MJ, Committee on Genetics: Health supervision for children with Down syndrome, *Pediatrics* 128:393–406, 2011.

Campbell DJ, Chang J, Chawarska K: Early generalized overgrowth in autism spectrum disorder: prevalence rates, gender effects, and clinical outcomes, *J Am Acad Child Adolesc Psychiatry* 53(10):1063-1073.e5, 2014.

Canfield MA, Mai CT, Wang Y, et al: The association between race/ethnicity and major birth defects in the United States, 1999-2007, *Am J Public Health* 104:e14–e23, 2014.

Carrel AL, Myers SE, Whitman BY, et al: Long-term growth hormone therapy changes the natural history of body composition and motor function in children with prader-willi syndrome, *J Clin Endocrinol Metab* 95: 1131–1136, 2010.

Centers for Disease Control and Prevention: Updated estimates of neural tube defects prevented by mandatory folic acid fortification-United States, 1995-2011, *MMWR Morb Mortal Wkly Rep* 64(1):1–5, 2015b.

Centers for Disease Control and Prevention: *Key findings: updated national birth prevalence estimates for selected birth defects in the United States, 2004-2006,* 2014. Available at: http://www.cdc.gov/ncbddd/birthdefects/features/birthdefects-keyfindings.html.

Chaidez V, Hansen RL, Hertz-Picciotto I: Gastrointestinal problems in children with autism, developmental delays or typical development, *J Autism Dev Disord* 44(5):1117-1127, 2014.

Committee on Genetics AAP: Folic acid for the prevention of neural tube defects, *Pediatrics* 104(2):325–327, 1999.

Curtin C, Bandini LG, Must A, et al: Parent support improves weight loss in adolescents and young adults with Down syndrome, *J Pediatr* 163: 1402-1408.e1, 2013.

Das JK, Salam RA, Kumar R, et al: Micronutrient fortification of food and its impact on woman and child health: a systematic review, *Syst Rev* 2:67, 2013.

Ekvall SW, Cerniglia F: Myelomeningocele. In Ekvall SW, Ekvall VK, editors: *Pediatric nutrition in developmental disabilities and chronic disorders*, ed 2, New York, 2005, Oxford University Press, 97–104.

Garcia MJ, McPherson P, Patel SY, et al: Diet and supplementation targeted for autism spectrum disorder. In Matson JL, editor: *Handbook of Treatments for Autism Spectrum Disorder*, Cham, Switzerland, 2017, Springer, pp 397–425.

Haqq AM, Muehlbauer MJ, Newgard CB, et al: The metabolic phenotype of Prader-Willi syndrome in childhood: heightened insulin sensitivity relative to body mass index, *J Clin Endocrinol Metab* 96:E225–E232, 2011.

Heiss CJ, Goldberg L, Dzarnoski M: Registered dietitians and speech-language pathologists: an important partnership in dysphagia management, *J Am Diet Assoc* 110:1290, 2010.

Hoyme HE, Kalberg WO, Elliott AJ, et al: Updated clinical guidelines for diagnosing fetal alcohol spectrum disorders, *Pediatrics* 138(2):e20154256, 2016.

Jones KL, Smith DW, Ulleland CN, et al: Pattern of malformation in offspring of chronic alcoholic mothers, *Lancet* 1:1267–1271, 1973.

Kreutzer C, Wittenbrook W: Nutrition issues in children with myelomeningocele (Spina Bifida). In *Nutrition Focus for Children with Special Health Care Needs* 28(5), Seattle, WA, 2013, University of Washington.

Lange KW, Hauser J, Lange KM, et al: The role of nutritional supplements in the treatment of ADHD: what the evidence says, *Curr Psychiatry Rep* 19(2):8, 2017.

Lanier C, Wolf L: Children with cleft lip and/or palate: feeding and nutrition, *Nutrition Focus for Children with Special Health Care Needs* 32:6, 2017.

Leonard H, Ravikumara M, Baikie G, et al: Assessment and management of nutrition and growth in Rett syndrome, *J Pediatr Gastroenterol Nutr* 57(4):451–460; 2013.

Leslie EJ, Marazita ML: Genetics of cleft lip and palate, *Am J Med Genet C Semin Med Genet* 163C:246–248, 2013.

Lewanda AF, Gallegos MF, Summar M: Patterns of dietary supplement use in children with down syndrome, *J Pediatr* 201:100-105.e30, 2018.

Lima AS, Cardoso BR, Cozzolino SF: Nutritional status of zinc in children with Down Syndrome, *Biol Trace Elem Res* 133:20–28, 2010.

Lindly O, Thorburn S, Zuckerman K: Use and nondisclosure of complementary health approaches among US children with developmental disabilities, *J Dev Behav Pediatr* 39(3):217–227, 2018.

Ly V, Bottelier M, Hoekstra PJ, et al. Elimination diets' efficacy and mechanisms in attention deficit hyperactivity disorder and autism spectrum disorder, *Eur Child Adolesc Psychiatry* 26:1067–1079, 2017.

Mahant S, Jovcevska V, Cohen E: Decision-making around gastrostomy-feeding in children with neurologic disabilities, *Pediatrics* 127: e1471–e1481, 2011.

Marshall J, Hill RJ, Ziviani J, et al: Features of feeding difficulty in children with autism spectrum disorder, *Int J Speech Lang Pathol* 16(2):151–158, 2014.

Mastrangelo M: Actual insights into treatable inborn errors of metabolism causing epilepsy, *J Pediatr Neurosci* 13(1):13–23, 2018.

McCune H, Driscoll D: Prader-Willi syndrome. In Ekvall SW, Ekvall VK, editors: *Pediatric nutrition in chronic disease and developmental disorders*, ed 2, New York, NY, 2005, Oxford University Press.

Medlen JG: *The down syndrome nutrition handbook: a guide to promoting healthy lifestyles*, ed 2, Portland, OR, 2006, Phronesis Publishing.

Miller JL, Lynn CH, Driscoll DC, et al: Nutritional phases in Prader-Willi syndrome, *Am J Med Genet A* 155A:1040–1049, 2011.

Miller JL, Lynn CH, Shuster J, et al: A reduced-energy intake, well-balanced diet improves weight control in children with Prader-Willi Syndrome, *J Hum Nutr Diet* 26(1):2–9, 2013.

Murawski NJ, Moore EM, Thomas JD, et al: Advances in diagnosis and treatment of Fetal Alcohol Spectrum Disorders: from animal models to human studies, *Alcohol Res* 37(1):97–108, 2015.

Murray J, Ryan-Krause P: Obesity in children with Down syndrome: background and recommendations for management, *Pediatr Nurs* 36: 314–319, 2010.

Obata K, Sakazume S, Yoshino A, et al: Effects of 5 years growth hormone treatment in patients with Prader-Willi syndrome, *J Pediatr Endocrinol Metab* 16:155–162, 2003.

Ornoy A, Weinstein-Fudim L, Ergaz Z: Genetic syndromes, maternal diseases and antenatal factors associated with autism spectrum disorders (ASD), *Front Neurosci* 10:316, 2016.

Parikh S, Goldstein A, Koenig MK, et al: Diagnosis and management of mitochondrial disease: a consensus statement from the Mitochondrial Medicine Society, *Genet Med* 17(9):689–701, 2015.

Popova S, Lange S, Shield K, et al: Comorbidity of fetal alcohol spectrum disorder: a systematic review and meta-analysis, *Lancet* 387(10022): 978–987, 2016.

Ptomey LT, Wittenbrook W: Position of the Academy of Nutrition and Dietetics: nutrition services for individuals with intellectual and developmental disabilities and special health care needs, *J Acad Nutr Diet* 115(4):593–608, 2015.

Reus L, Zwarts M, van Vlimmeren LA, et al: Motor problems in Prader-Willi syndrome: a systematic review on body composition and neuromuscular functioning, *Neurosci Biobehav Rev* 35:956–969, 2011.

Richardson E, Seibert T, Uli NK: Growth perturbations from stimulant medications and inhaled corticosteroids. *Transl Pediatr* 6(4):237–247, 2017.

Salehi P, Stafford HJ, Glass RP, et al: Silent aspiration in Infants with Prader-Willi syndrome identified by VFSS. *Medicine (Baltimore)* 96(50):e9256, 2017.

Sathe N, Andrews JC, McPheeters ML, et al: Nutritional and dietary interventions for autism spectrum disorder: a systematic review, *Pediatrics* 139(6):e20170346, 2017.

Scerif M, Goldstone AP, Korbonits M: Ghrelin in obesity and endocrine diseases, *Mol Cell Endocrinol* 340:15–25, 2011.

Shkoukani MA, Chen M, Vong A: Cleft lip—a comprehensive review, *Front Pediatr* 1:53, 2013.

Smithells RW, Nevin NC, Seller MJ, et al: Further experience of vitamin supplementation for prevention of neural tube defect recurrences, *Lancet* 1:1027–1031, 1983.

Spina Bifida Association: *Obesity among persons with Spina Bifida*, 2017. Available at: www.spinabifidaassociation.org.

Stevenson RD: Use of segmental measures to estimate stature in children with cerebral palsy, *Arch Pediatr Adolesc Med* 149:658–662, 1995.

Stewart PA, Hyman SL, Schmidt BL, et al: Dietary supplementation in children with autism spectrum disorders: common, insufficient, and excessive, *J Acad Nutr Diet* 115(8):1237–1248, 2015.

Wolraich ML, Hagan JF, Allan C, et. al: Clinical practice guideline for the diagnosis, evaluation, and treatment of attention-deficit/hyperactivity disorder in children and adolescents, *Pediatrics* 144(4), 2019.

Milliequivalents and Milligrams of Electrolytes

To Convert Milligrams to Milliequivalents: Divide milligrams by atomic weight and then multiply by the valence.

$$\text{Example}: \frac{\text{Milligrams}}{\text{Atomic weight}} \times \text{Valence} = \text{Milliequivalents}$$

Mineral Element	Chemical Symbol	Atomic Weight (mg)	Valence
Calcium	Ca	40	2
Chlorine	Cl	35	1
Magnesium	Mg	24	2
Phosphorus	P	31	2
Potassium	K	39	1
Sodium	Na	23	1
Sulfate	SO_4	96	2
Sulfur	S	32	

To Convert Specific Weight of Sodium to Sodium Chloride: Multiply by 2.54.

Example: 1000 mg Sodium
1000 × 2.54 = 2540 mg Sodium chloride (2.5 g)

To Convert Specific Weight of Sodium Chloride to Sodium: Multiply by 0.393.

Example: 2.5 g Sodium chloride
2.5 × 0.393 = 1000 mg sodium

Milligrams	Sodium in Milliequivalents (mEq)	Grams of Sodium Chloride
500	21.8	1.3
1000	43.5	2.5
1500	75.3	3.8
2000	87.0	5.0

Modified from Merck Manual: *Ready Reference Guide.* http://www.merckmanuals.com/professional/print/appendixes/ap1/ap1a.html. Accessed March 22, 2011; Nelson JK, Moxness KE, Jensen MD, et al: *Mayo Clinic diet manual,* ed 7, St. Louis, 1994, Mosby.

Equivalents, Conversions,* and Portion (Scoop) Sizes

LIQUID MEASURE—VOLUME EQUIVALENTS

1 tsp = $^1/_3$ Tbsp = 5 mL or cc
1 Tbsp = 3 tsp = 15 mL or cc
2 Tbsp = 1 fluid oz = $^1/_8$ cup = 30 mL or cc
2 Tbsp + 2 tsp = $^1/_6$ cup = 40 mL or cc
4 Tbsp = ¼ cup = 2 fluid oz = 60 mL or cc
5 Tbsp + 1 tsp = $^1/_3$ cup = 80 mL or cc
6 Tbsp = 3 fluid oz = $^3/_8$ cup = 90 mL or cc
8 Tbsp = ½ cup = 120 mL or cc
10 Tbsp + 2 tsp = $^2/_3$ cup = 160 mL or cc
12 Tbsp = ¾ cup = 180 mL or cc
48 tsp = 16 Tbsp = 1 cup (8 fluid ounces) = ½ pint = 240 mL or cc
2 cups = 1 pint (16 fluid oz) = 0.4732 L
4 cups = 2 pints = 1 quart (32 fluid oz) = 0.9462 L
1.06 quarts = 34 fluid oz = 1000 mL or cc
4 quarts = 1 gallon = 3785 mL or cc

DRY MEASURE

1 quart = 2 pints = 1.101 L
Dry-measure pints and quarts are approximately $^1/_6$ larger than liquid-measure pints and quarts.

WEIGHTS	
English (Avoirdupois Weight**)	Metric
1 oz	Approx 30 g
1 lb (16 oz)	454 g
2.2 lb	1 kg

**A system of weights based on a pound of 16 ounces commonly used in English-speaking countries.

SCOOP SIZES

It is important to use the proper scoop size when portioning out foods to serve to patients.

Number	Approximate Liquid Volume
6	$^2/_3$ cup (5 fluid oz)
8	$^1/_2$ cup (4 fluid oz)
10	$^3/_8$ cup ($3^1/_4$ fluid oz)
12	$^1/_3$ cup ($2^2/_3$ fluid oz)
16	¼ cup (2 fluid oz)
20	$3^1/_5$ Tbsp ($1^3/_5$ fluid oz)
24	$2^3/_3$ Tbsp ($1^1/_3$ fluid oz)
30	$2^1/_5$ Tbsp (1 fluid oz)
40	$1^3/_5$ Tbsp (0.8 fluid oz)
60	1 Tbsp (0.5 fluid oz)

Metric Conversion Factors		
Multiply	By	To Get
Fluid ounces	29.57	Grams
Ounces (dry)	28.35	Grams
Grams	0.0353	Ounces
Grams	0.0022	Pounds
Kilograms	2.21	Pounds
Pounds	453.6	Grams
Pounds	0.4536	Kilograms
Quarts	0.946	Liters
Quarts (dry)	67.2	Cubic inches
Quarts (liquid)	57.7	Cubic inches
Liters	1.0567	Quarts
Gallons	3.785	Cubic centimeters
Gallons	3.785	Liters

From North Carolina Dietetic Association: *Nutrition care manual*, Raleigh, NC, 2011, The Association.

*Note: In the U.S. measuring systems, the same word may have two meanings. For example, an ounce may mean $^1/_{16}$ of a pound and $^1/_{16}$ of a pint, but the former is strictly a weight measure and the latter is a volume measure. Except in the case of water, milk, or other liquids of the same density, a fluid ounce and an ounce of weight are two completely different quantities. These measures are not to be used interchangeably.

Growth Charts

Birth to 24 months: Boys
Length-for-age and Weight-for-age percentiles

NAME _____

RECORD # _____

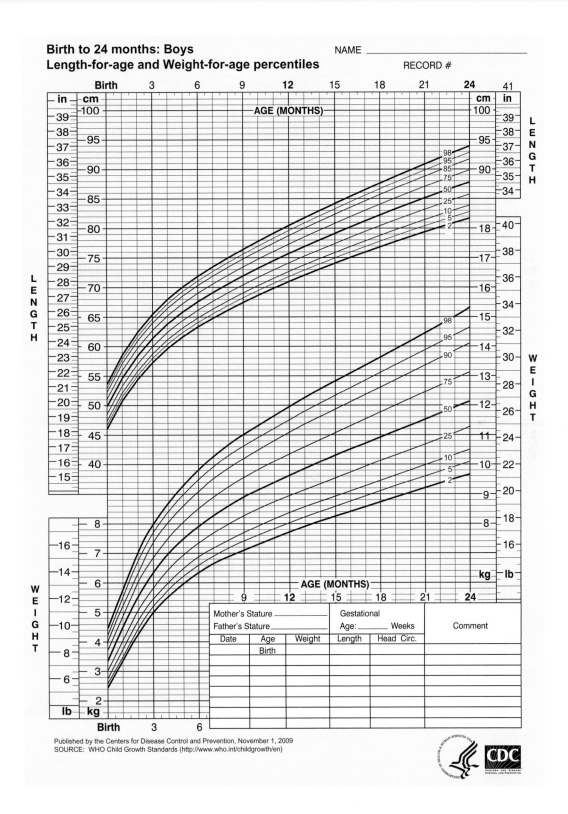

Published by the Centers for Disease Control and Prevention, November 1, 2009
SOURCE: WHO Child Growth Standards (http://www.who.int/childgrowth/en)

Birth to 24 months: Boys
Head circumference-for-age and
Weight-for-length percentiles

NAME _____

RECORD # _____

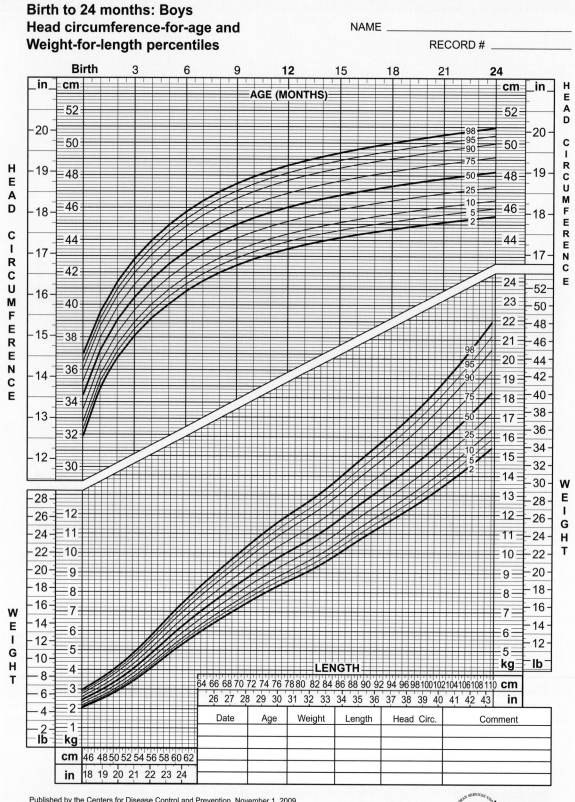

Published by the Centers for Disease Control and Prevention, November 1, 2009
SOURCE: WHO Child Growth Standards (http://www.who.int/childgrowth/en)

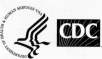

2 to 20 Years: Boys
Stature-for-Age and
Weight-for-Age Percentiles

NAME _____

RECORD # _____

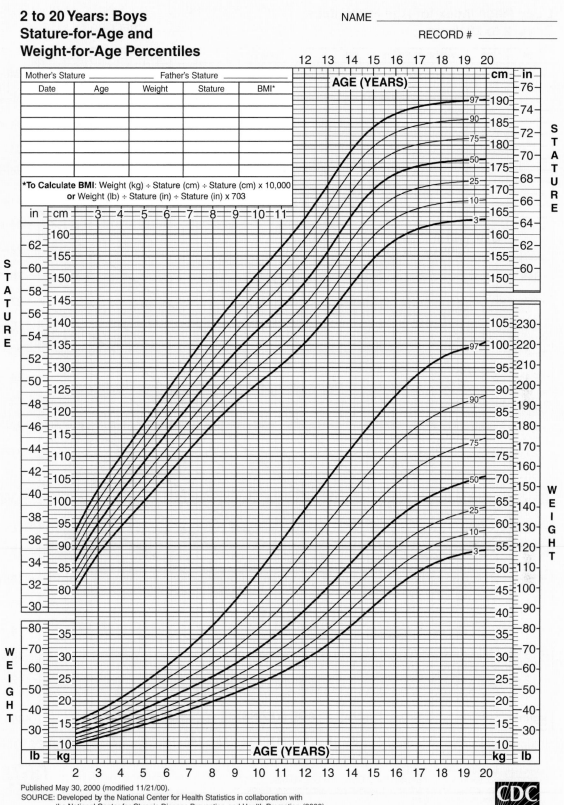

Mother's Stature _____	Father's Stature _____			
Date	Age	Weight	Stature	BMI*

*To Calculate BMI: Weight (kg) ÷ Stature (cm) ÷ Stature (cm) x 10,000
or Weight (lb) ÷ Stature (in) ÷ Stature (in) x 703

Published May 30, 2000 (modified 11/21/00).
SOURCE: Developed by the National Center for Health Statistics in collaboration with
the National Center for Chronic Disease Prevention and Health Promotion (2000).
http://www.cdc.gov/growthcharts

SAFER•HEALTHIER•PEOPLE

Body Mass Index-for-Age Percentiles: Boys, 2 to 20 Years

NAME _____

RECORD # _____

Date	Age	Weight	Stature	BMI*	Comments

*To Calculate BMI: Weight (kg) ÷ Stature (cm) ÷ Stature (cm) x 10,000
or Weight (lb) ÷ Stature (in) ÷ Stature (in) x 703

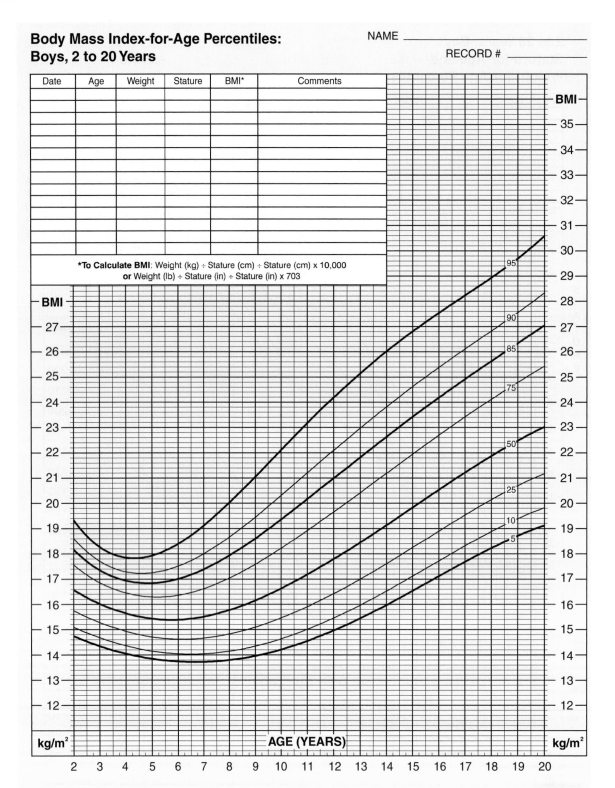

AGE (YEARS)

kg/m²

Published May 30, 2000 (modified 10/16/00).
SOURCE: Developed by the National Center for Health Statistics in collaboration with
the National Center for Chronic Disease Prevention and Health Promotion (2000).
http://www.cdc.gov/growthcharts

SAFER•HEALTHIER•PEOPLE

Birth to 24 months: Girls
Length-for-age and Weight-for-age percentiles

NAME _____

RECORD # _____

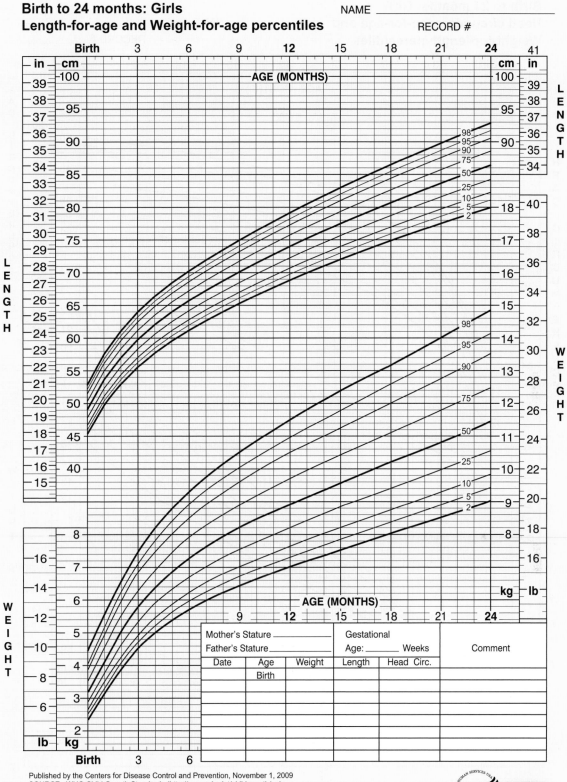

Published by the Centers for Disease Control and Prevention, November 1, 2009
SOURCE: WHO Child Growth Standards (http://www.who.int/childgrowth/en)

Birth to 24 months: Girls
Head circumference-for-age and
Weight-for-length percentiles

NAME _____

RECORD # _____

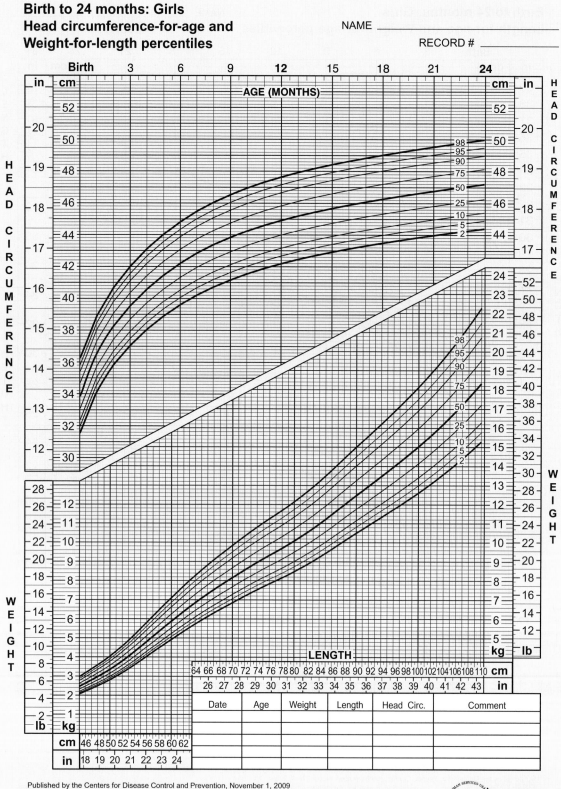

Published by the Centers for Disease Control and Prevention, November 1, 2009
SOURCE: WHO Child Growth Standards (http://www.who.int/childgrowth/en)

2 to 20 Years:
Girls Stature-for-Age and
Weight-for-Age Percentiles

NAME _____

RECORD # _____

Mother's Stature _____		Father's Stature _____		
Date	Age	Weight	Stature	BMI*

*To Calculate BMI: Weight (kg) ÷ Stature (cm) ÷ Stature (cm) x 10,000
or Weight (lb) ÷ Stature (in) ÷ Stature (in) x 703

AGE (YEARS)

12 13 14 15 16 17 18 19 20

STATURE

STATURE

WEIGHT

WEIGHT

AGE (YEARS)

2 3 4 5 6 7 8 9 10 11 12 13 14 15 16 17 18 19 20

Published May 30, 2000 (modified 11/21/00).
SOURCE: Developed by the National Center for Health Statistics in collaboration with
the National Center for Chronic Disease Prevention and Health Promotion (2000).
http://www.cdc.gov/growthcharts

CDC
SAFER·HEALTHIER·PEOPLE

Body Mass Index-for-Age
Percentiles: Girls, 2 to 20 Years

NAME _____

RECORD # _____

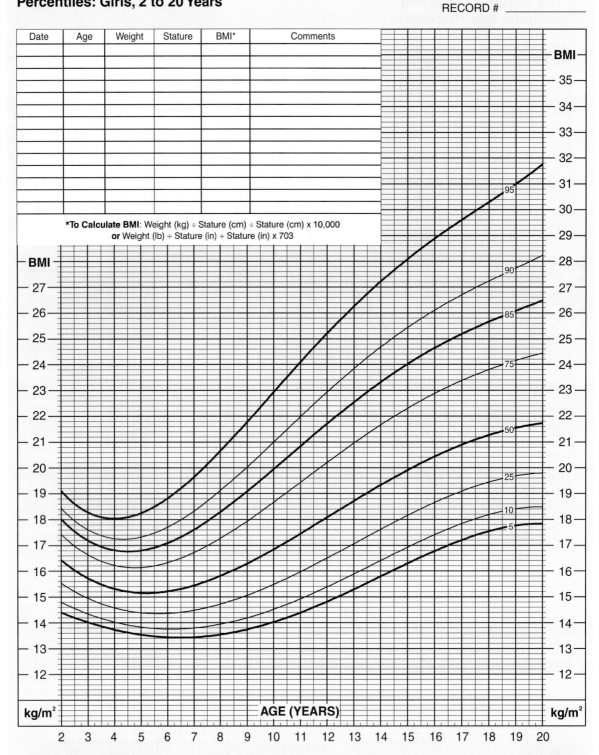

Date	Age	Weight	Stature	BMI*	Comments

*To Calculate BMI: Weight (kg) ÷ Stature (cm) ÷ Stature (cm) x 10,000
or Weight (lb) ÷ Stature (in) ÷ Stature (in) x 703

AGE (YEARS)

Published May 30, 2000 (modified 10/16/00).
SOURCE: Developed by the National Center for Health Statistics in collaboration with
the National Center for Chronic Disease Prevention and Health Promotion (2000).
http://www.cdc.gov/growthcharts

SAFER•HEALTHIER•PEOPLE

PRENATAL WEIGHT GAIN (UNDERWEIGHT)

PRENATAL WEIGHT GAIN (NORMAL WEIGHT)

PRENATAL WEIGHT GAIN (OVERWEIGHT)

PRENATAL WEIGHT GAIN (OBESE)

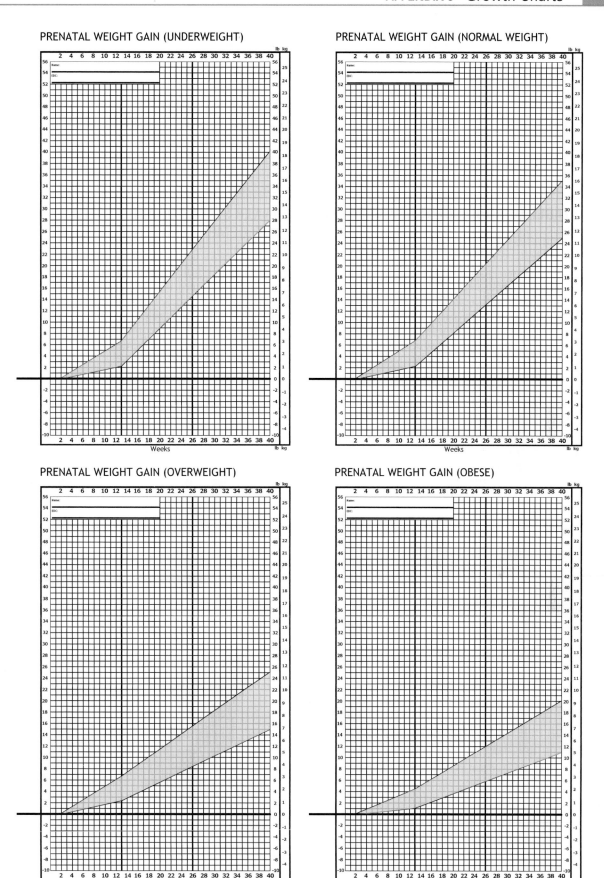

Tanner Stages of Adolescent Development for Girls and Boys

TANNER STAGES OF ADOLESCENT DEVELOPMENT FOR GIRLS

Chronologic age is not always the best way to assess adolescent growth because of individual variations in beginning and completing the growth sequence. A more useful way of describing pubertal development, and thus the varying needs for nutrients throughout adolescence, is to divide growth into stages of breast and pubic hair development in girls. These are termed the *Tanner Stages of Adolescent Development.* Nutritional requirements vary, depending on the stage of development.

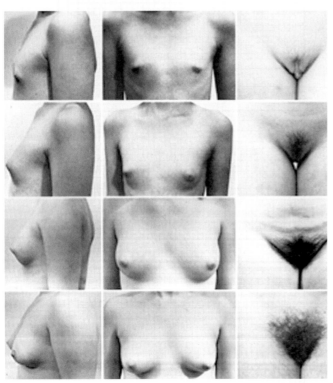

From Mahan LK, Rees JM: *Nutrition in adolescence*, St. Louis, 1984, Mosby.

TANNER STAGES OF ADOLESCENT DEVELOPMENT FOR BOYS

Chronologic age is not always the best way to assess adolescent growth because of individual variations in beginning and completing the growth sequence. A more useful way of describing pubertal development, and thus the varying needs for nutrients throughout adolescence, is to divide growth into stages pubic hair and penis and testicle development in boys. These are termed the *Tanner Stages of Adolescent Development.* Nutritional requirements vary, depending on the stage of development.

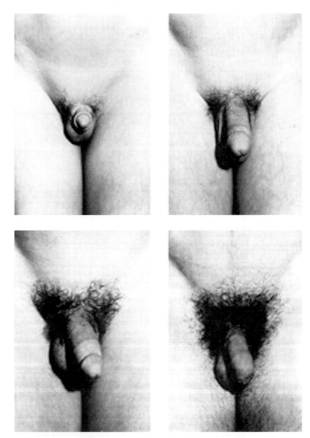

From Mahan LK, Rees JM: *Nutrition in adolescence*, St. Louis, 1984, Mosby.

Direct Methods for Measuring Height and Weight and Indirect Methods for Measuring Height

DIRECT METHODS FOR MEASURING HEIGHT AND WEIGHT

Height

1. Height should be measured without shoes.
2. The individual's feet should be together, with the heels against the wall or measuring board.
3. The individual should stand erect, neither slumped nor stretching, looking straight ahead, without tipping the head up or down. The top of the ear and outer corner of the eye should be in a line parallel to the floor (the "Frankfort plane").
4. A horizontal bar, a rectangular block of wood, or the top of the statiometer should be lowered to rest flat on the top of the head.
5. Height should be read to the nearest ¼ inch or 0.5 cm.

Weight

1. Scale accuracy must be determined. Frequent calibration is required.
2. Use a beam balance scale, not a spring scale, whenever possible.
3. Weigh the subject in light clothing without shoes.
4. Record weight to the nearest ½ lb or 0.2 kg for adults and ¼ lb or 0.1 kg for infants. Measurements above the 90th percentile or below the 10th percentile warrant further evaluation.

INDIRECT METHODS FOR MEASURING HEIGHT

Measuring Arm Span

Steps:

1. The arms are extended straight out to the sides at a 90-degree angle from the body.
2. The distance from the longest fingertip of one hand to the longest finger of the other hand is measured.

Adult Recumbent

Steps:

1. Stand on right side of the body.
2. Align body so that the lower extremities, trunk, shoulders, and head are straight.

3. Place a mark at the top of the sheet in line with the crown of the head and one at the bottom of the sheet in line with the base of the heels.
4. Measure length between marks with measuring tape.

Knee Height

Knee height measurement is highly correlated with upright height. It is useful in those who cannot stand and in those who may have curvatures of the spine.

Steps:

1. Use the left leg for measurements.
2. Bend the left knee and the left ankle to 90-degree angles. A triangle may be used if available.
3. Using knee height calipers, open the caliper and place the fixed part under the heel. Place the sliding blade down against the thigh (approximately 2 inches behind the patella).
4. Measure from the heel to the anterior surface of the thigh, using a cloth measuring tape.

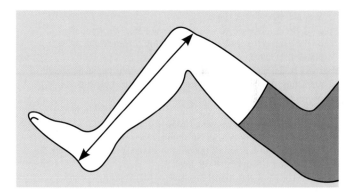

1. Obtain the measurement and convert it to centimeters by multiplying by 2.54.
2. Formulas to use to calculate estimated height from knee height:

Men (height in centimeters) 64.19 (0.04 Age) + (2.02 × Knee height in centimeters)

Women (height in centimeters) 84.8 (0.24 Age) + (1.83 × Knee height in centimeters)

Using Population-Specific Formula, Calculate Height From Standard Formula:

Population and Gender Group	Equation: Stature (cm) =
Non-Hispanic white men (U.S.) [SEE = 3.74 cm]	78.31 + (1.94 × knee height) − (0.14 × age)
Non-Hispanic black men (U.S.) [SEE = 3.80 cm]	79.69 + (1.85 × knee height) − (0.14 × age)
Mexican American men (U.S.) [SEE = 3.68 cm]	82.77 + (1.83 × knee height) − (0.16 × age)
Non-Hispanic white women (U.S.) [SEE = 3.98 cm]	82.21 + (1.85 × knee height) − (0.21 × age)
Non-Hispanic black women (U.S.) [SEE = 3.82 cm]	89.58 + (1.61 × knee height) − (0.17 × age)
Mexican American women (U.S.) [SEE = 3.77 cm]	84.25 + (1.82 × knee height) − (0.26 × age)
Taiwanese men [SEE = 3.86 cm]	85.10 + (1.73 × knee height) − (0.11 × age)
Taiwanese women [SEE = 3.79 cm]	91.45 + (1.53 × knee height) − (0.16 × age)
Elderly Italian men [SEE = 4.3 cm]	94.87 + (1.58 × knee height) − (0.23 × age) + 4.8
Elderly Italian women [SEE = 4.3 cm]	94.87 + (1.58 × knee height) − (0.23 × age)
French men [SEE = 3.8 cm]	74.7 + (2.07 × knee height) − (-0.21 × age)
French women [SEE = 3.5 cm]	67.00 + (2.2 × knee height) − (0.25 × age)
Mexican men [SEE = 3.31 cm]	52.6 + (2.17 × knee height)
Mexican women [SEE = 2.99 cm]	73.70 + (1.99 × knee height) − (0.23 × age)
Filipino men	96.50 + (1.38 × knee height) − (0.08 × age)
Filipino women	89.63 + (1.53 × knee height) − (0.17 × age)
Malaysian men [SEE = 3.51 cm]	(1.924 × knee height) + 69.38
Malaysian women [SEE = 3.40]	(2.225 × knee height) + 50.25

SEE = Standard error of estimate

REFERENCES

Guigoz Y, Vellas B, Garry PJ: Assessing the nutritional status of the elderly: The Mini Nutritional Assessment as part of the geriatric evaluation, *Nutr Rev* 54:S59–S65, 1996.

Fallon C, Bruce I, Eustace A, et al: Nutritional status of community dwelling subjects attending a memory clinic, *J Nutr Health Aging* 6(Suppl):21, 2002.

Kagansky N, Berner Y, Koren-Morag N, et al: Poor nutritional habits are predictors of poor outcome in very old hospitalized patients, *Am J Clin Nutr* 82:784–791, 2005.

Vellas B, Villars H, Abellan G, et al: Overview of the MNA®–Its history and challenges, *J Nutr Health Aging* 10:456–463, 2006.

Guigoz Y, Vellas J, Garry P: Mini Nutritional Assessment: a practical assessment tool for grading the nutritional state of elderly patients, *Facts Res Gerontol* 4(Suppl 2):15–59, 1994.

Guigoz Y: The Mini-Nutritional Assessment (MNA®) review of the literature—what does it tell us? *J Nutr Health Aging* 10:466–485, 2006.

Murphy MC, Brooks CN, New SA, et al: The use of the Mini-Nutritional Assessment (MNA) tool in elderly orthopaedic patients, *Eur J Clin Nutr* 54:555–562, 2000.

Kaiser MJ, Bauer JM, Ramsch C, et al: Validation of the Mini Nutritional Assessment Short-Form (MNA®-SF): a practical tool for identification of nutritional status, *J Nutr Health Aging* 13:782–788, 2009.

Hickson M, Frost G: A comparison of three methods for estimating height in the acutely ill elderly population, *J Hum Nutr Diet* 16: 13–20, 2003.

Kwok T, Whitelaw MN: The use of armspan in nutritional assessment of the elderly, *J Am Geriatr Soc* 39:492–496, 1991.

Chumlea WC, Guo SS, Wholihan K, et al: Stature prediction equations for elderly non-Hispanic white, non-Hispanic black, and Mexican-American persons developed from NHANES III data, *J Am Diet Assoc* 98:137–142, 1998.

Cheng HS, See LC, Shieh YH: Estimating stature from knee height for adults in Taiwan, *Chang Gung Med J* 24:547–556, 2001.

Donini LM, de Felice MR, De Bernardini L, et al: Prediction of stature in the Italian elderly, *J Nutr Health Aging* 4:72–76, 2000.

Guo SS, Wu X, Vellas B, et al: Prediction of stature in the French elderly, *Age & Nutr* 5:169–173, 1994.

Mendoza-Nv√∫nez VM, Sánchez-Rodríguez MA, Cervantes-Sandoval A, et al: Equations for predicting height for elderly Mexican-Americans are not applicable for elderly Mexicans, *Am J Hum Biol* 14:351–355, 2002.

Tanchoco CC, Duante CA, Lopez ES: Arm span and knee height as proxy indicators for height, *J Nutritionist Dietitians Assoc Philipp* 15:84–90, 2001.

Shahar S, Pooy NS: Predictive equations for estimation of stature in Malaysian elderly people, *Asia Pac J Clin Nutr* 12(1):80–84, 2003.

Lefton J, Malone A: Anthropometric assessment. In Charney P, Malone A, editors: *ADA pocket guide to nutrition assessment*, ed 2, Chicago, IL, 2009, American Dietetic Association, pp 160–161.

Osterkamp LK: Current perspective on assessment of human body proportions of relevance to amputees, *J Am Diet Assoc* 95:215–218, 1995.

Determination of Frame Size

Method 1: Height is recorded without shoes. Wrist circumference is measured just distal to the styloid process at the wrist crease on the right arm, using a tape measure. The following formula is used (From Grant JP: *Handbook of total parenteral nutrition*, Philadelphia, PA, 1980, Saunders):

$$r = \frac{\text{Height (cm)}}{\text{Wrist circumstance (cm)}}$$

Frame size can be determined as follows:

Males	Females
r >10.4 small	r >11.0 small
r = 9.6–10.4 medium	r = 10.1–11.0 medium
r <9.6 large	r <10.1 large

Method 2: The patient's right arm is extended forward perpendicular to the body, with the arm bent so the angle at the elbow forms 90 degrees with the fingers pointing up and the palm turned away from the body. The greatest breadth across the elbow joint is measured with a sliding caliper along the axis of the upper arm on the two prominent bones on either side of the elbow. This is recorded as the elbow breadth. The following tables give the elbow breadth measurements for medium-framed men and women of various heights (from Metropolitan Life Insurance Co., 1983). Measurements lower than those listed indicate a small frame size; higher measurements indicate a large frame size.

MEN		WOMEN	
Height in 1″ Heels	Elbow Breadth (inches)	Height in 1″ Heels	Elbow Breadth (inches)
5′2″–5′3″	2½–2⅞	4′10″–4′11″	2¼–2½
5′4″–5′7″	2⅝–2⅞	5′0″–5′3″	2¼–2½
5′8″–5′11″	2¾–3	5′4″–5′7″	2³⁄₈–2⁵⁄₈
6′0″–6′3″	2¾–3⅛	5′8″–5′11″	2³⁄₈–2⁵⁄₈
6′4″	2⅞–3¼	6′0″	

Adjustment of Desirable Body Weight for Amputees

The percentages listed here are estimates because body proportions vary in individuals. Use of these percentages provides an approximation of desirable body weight, which is more accurate than a comparison with the standards for adults without amputations. Ideal body weight (IBW) must be adjusted downward to compensate for missing limbs or paralysis. It is estimated that 5% to 10% should be subtracted from IBW for a paraplegic and from 10% to 15% subtracted for a tetraplegic (quadriplegic).

Adjustment of Ideal Body Weight for Amputees

Body Segment	Average % of Total Weight
Lower arm and hand	2.3
Trunk without extremities	50.0
Entire arm	5.0
Hand	0.7
Entire lower leg	16.0
Below knee including foot	5.9
Lower leg without foot	4.4
Foot	1.5

Lefton J, Malone A: Anthropometric assessment. In Charney P, Malone A, editors: *ADA pocket guide to nutrition assessment*, ed 2, Chicago, IL, 2009, American Dietetic Association, p 160.

$$\text{Estimated IBW} = \frac{100 - \% \text{ amputation}}{100} \times \text{IBW for original height}$$

To use this information, determine the patient's approximate height before the amputation. Span measurement is a rough estimate of height at maturity and is calculated as follows: With the upper extremities, including the hands, fully extended and parallel to the ground, measure the distance between the tip of one middle finger and the tip of the other middle finger. Use this height or actual measurement to calculate the desirable body weight for the normal body size, then adjust the figures according to the type of amputation performed.

Example: To determine the desirable body weight for a 5'10" male with a below-the-knee amputation:

1. Calculate desirable body weight for a 5'10" male:	166 lb
2. Subtract weight of amputated limb (6%) = 166 × 0.06:	− 9.96 (approx. 10 lb)
3. Desirable weight of a 5'10" male with a below-knee amputation:	156 lb

From North Carolina Dietetic Association: *Nutrition care manual*, Raleigh, NC, 2011, The Association.

Body Mass Index Table

BMI	NORMAL WEIGHT						OVERWEIGHT					OBESE					
	19	20	21	22	23	24	25	26	27	28	29	30	31	32	33	34	35
Height							Weight (in pounds)										
4'10" (58")	91	96	100	105	110	115	119	124	129	134	138	143	148	153	158	162	167
4'11" (59")	94	99	104	109	114	119	124	128	133	138	143	148	153	158	163	168	173
5' (60")	97	102	107	112	118	123	128	133	138	143	148	153	158	163	168	174	179
5'1" (61")	100	106	111	116	122	127	132	137	143	148	153	158	164	169	174	180	185
5'2" (62")	104	109	115	120	126	131	136	142	147	153	158	164	169	175	180	186	191
5'3" (63")	107	113	118	124	130	135	141	146	152	158	163	169	175	180	186	191	197
5'4" (64")	110	116	122	128	134	140	145	151	157	163	169	174	180	186	192	197	204
5'5" (65")	114	120	126	132	138	144	150	156	162	168	174	180	186	192	198	204	210
5'6" (66")	118	124	130	136	142	148	155	161	167	173	179	186	192	198	204	210	216
5'7" (67")	121	127	134	140	146	153	159	166	172	178	185	191	198	204	211	217	223
5'8" (68")	125	131	138	144	151	158	164	171	177	184	190	197	203	210	216	223	230
5'9" (69")	128	135	142	149	155	162	169	176	182	189	196	203	209	216	223	230	236
5'10" (70")	132	139	146	153	160	167	174	181	188	195	202	209	216	222	229	236	243
5'11" (71")	136	143	150	157	165	172	179	186	193	200	208	215	222	229	236	243	250
6' (72")	140	147	154	162	169	177	184	191	199	206	213	221	228	235	242	250	258
6'1" (73")	144	151	159	166	174	182	189	197	204	212	219	227	235	242	250	257	265
6'2" (74")	148	155	163	171	179	186	194	202	210	218	225	233	241	249	256	264	272
6'3" (75")	152	160	168	176	184	192	200	208	216	224	232	240	248	256	264	272	279

Data from National Institutes of Health and National Heart, Lung, and Blood Institute: *Evidence report of clinical guidelines on the identification, evaluation, and treatment of overweight and obesity in adults*, Bethesda, MD, 1998, NIH/NHLBI. For a BMI of greater than 35, please go to http://www.nhlbi.nih.gov/health/educational/lose_wt/BMI/bmi_tbl2.htm.

Percentage of Body Fat Based on Four Skinfold Measurements*

Sum of Skinfolds (mm)	MALES (AGE IN YEARS)				FEMALES (AGE IN YEARS)			
	17-29	30-39	40-49	50+	16-29	30-39	40-49	50+
15	4.8	—	—	—	10.5	—	—	—
20	8.1	12.2	12.2	12.6	14.1	17.0	19.8	21.4
25	10.5	14.2	15.0	15.6	16.8	19.4	22.2	24.0
30	12.9	16.2	17.7	18.6	19.5	21.8	24.5	26.6
35	14.7	17.7	19.6	20.8	21.5	23.7	26.4	28.5
40	16.4	19.2	21.4	22.9	23.4	25.5	28.2	30.3
45	17.7	20.4	23.0	24.7	25.0	26.9	29.6	31.9
50	19.0	21.5	24.6	26.5	26.5	28.2	31.0	33.4
55	20.1	22.5	25.9	27.9	27.8	29.4	32.1	34.6
60	21.2	23.5	27.1	29.2	29.1	30.6	33.2	35.7
65	22.2	24.3	28.2	30.4	30.2	31.6	34.1	36.7
70	23.1	25.1	29.3	31.6	31.2	32.5	35.0	37.7
75	24.0	25.9	30.3	32.7	32.2	33.4	35.9	38.7
80	24.8	26.6	31.2	33.8	33.1	34.3	36.7	39.6
85	25.5	27.2	32.1	34.8	34.0	35.1	37.5	40.4
90	26.2	27.8	33.0	35.8	34.8	35.8	38.3	41.2
95	26.9	28.4	33.7	36.6	35.6	36.5	39.0	41.9
100	27.6	29.0	34.4	37.4	36.4	37.2	39.7	42.6
105	28.2	29.6	35.1	38.2	37.1	37.9	40.4	43.3
110	28.8	30.1	35.8	39.0	37.8	38.6	41.0	43.9
115	29.4	30.6	36.4	39.7	38.4	39.1	41.5	44.5
120	30.0	31.1	37.0	40.4	39.0	39.6	42.0	45.1
125	30.5	31.5	37.6	41.1	39.6	40.1	42.5	45.7
130	31.0	31.9	38.2	41.8	40.2	40.6	43.0	46.2
135	31.5	32.3	38.7	42.4	40.8	41.1	43.5	46.7
140	32.0	32.7	39.2	43.0	41.3	41.6	44.0	47.2
145	32.5	33.1	39.7	43.6	41.8	42.1	44.5	47.7
150	32.9	33.5	40.2	44.1	42.3	42.6	45.0	48.2
155	33.3	33.9	40.7	44.6	42.8	43.1	45.4	48.7
160	33.7	34.3	41.2	45.1	43.3	43.6	45.8	49.2
165	34.1	34.6	41.6	45.6	43.7	44.0	46.2	49.6
170	34.5	34.8	42.0	46.1	44.1	44.4	46.6	50.0
175	34.9	—	—	—	—	44.8	47.0	50.4
180	35.3	—	—	—	—	45.2	47.4	50.8
185	35.6	—	—	—	—	45.6	47.8	51.2
190	35.9	—	—	—	—	45.9	48.2	51.6
195	—	—	—	—	—	46.2	48.5	52.0
200	—	—	—	—	—	46.5	48.8	52.4
205	—	—	—	—	—	—	49.1	52.7
210	—	—	—	—	—	—	49.4	53.0

From Durnin JV, Womersley J: Body fat assessed from total body density and its estimation from skinfold thickness: measurements on 481 men and women aged from 16 to 72 years, *Br J Nutr* 32:77–97, 1974.

*Measurements made on the right side of the body, using biceps, triceps, subscapular, and suprailiac skinfolds.

Physical Activity and Calories Expended per Hour

Activity	Type	(110 lb)	(130 lb)	(150 lb)	(170 lb)	(190 lb)	(210 lb)	(230 lb)	(250 lb)
		BODY WEIGHT							
Aerobics class	Water	210	248	286	325	364	401	439	477
Aerobics class	Low impact	263	310	358	406	455	501	549	596
Aerobics class	High impact	368	434	501	568	637	702	768	835
Aerobics class	Step with 6- to 8-inch step	446	527	609	690	774	852	933	1014
Aerobics class	Step with 10- to 12-inch step	525	621	716	812	910	1003	1097	1193
Backpack	General	368	434	501	568	637	702	768	835
Badminton	Singles and doubles	236	279	322	365	410	451	494	537
Badminton	Competitive	368	434	501	568	637	702	768	835
Baseball	Throw, catch	131	155	179	203	228	251	274	298
Baseball	Fast or slow pitch	263	310	358	406	455	501	549	596
Basketball	Shooting baskets	236	279	322	365	410	451	494	537
Basketball	Wheelchair	341	403	465	528	592	652	713	775
Basketball	Game	420	496	573	649	728	802	878	954
Bike	10-11.9 mph, slow	315	372	430	487	546	602	658	716
Bike	12-13.9 mph, moderate	420	496	573	649	728	802	878	954
Bike	14-15.9 mph, fast	525	621	716	812	910	1003	1097	1193
Bike	16-19.9 mph, very fast	630	745	859	974	1092	1203	1317	1431
Bike	>20 mph, racing	840	993	1146	1299	1457	1604	1756	1908
Bike	50 watts, stationary, very light	158	133	215	243	273	301	329	358
Bike	100 watts, stationary, light	289	341	394	446	501	552	603	656
Bike	150 watts, stationary, moderate	368	434	501	568	637	702	768	835
Bike	200 watts, stationary, vigorous	551	652	752	852	956	1053	1152	1252
Bike	250 watts, stationary, very vigorous	656	776	895	1015	1138	1253	1372	1491
Bike	BMX or mountain	446	527	609	690	774	852	933	1014
Boxing	Punching bag	315	372	430	487	546	602	658	716
Boxing	Sparring	473	558	644	730	819	902	988	1074
Calisthenics	Back exercises	184	217	251	284	319	351	384	417
Calisthenics	Pull-ups, jumping jacks	420	496	573	649	728	802	878	954
Calisthenics	Push-ups or sit-ups	420	496	573	649	728	802	878	954
Circuit training	General	420	496	573	649	728	802	878	954
Football	Flag or touch	420	496	573	649	728	802	878	954
Football	Competitive	473	558	644	730	819	902	988	1074
Frisbee	General	158	133	215	243	273	301	329	358
Frisbee	Ultimate	420	496	573	649	728	802	878	954
Golf	Power cart	184	217	251	284	319	351	384	417
Golf	Pull clubs	226	267	308	349	391	431	472	513
Golf	Carry clubs	236	279	322	365	410	451	494	537
Handball	General	630	745	859	974	1092	1203	1317	1431

Continued

Activity	Type	BODY WEIGHT							
		(110 lb)	(130 lb)	(150 lb)	(170 lb)	(190 lb)	(210 lb)	(230 lb)	(250 lb)
Hike	General	315	372	460	487	546	602	658	716
Hockey	Ice, field hockey	420	496	573	649	728	802	878	954
Jog	General	368	434	501	568	637	702	768	835
Jog	Jog-walk combination	315	372	430	487	546	602	658	716
Jump rope	Slow	420	496	573	649	728	802	878	954
Jump rope	Moderate	525	621	716	812	910	1003	1097	1193
Jump rope	Fast	630	745	859	974	1092	1203	1317	1431
Kayak	General	263	310	358	406	455	501	549	596
Martial arts	General	525	621	716	812	910	1003	1097	1193
Racquetball	Casual	368	434	501	568	637	702	768	835
Racquetball	Competition	525	621	716	812	910	1003	1097	1193
Rafting	Whitewater	263	310	358	406	455	501	549	596
Rock climb	General	420	496	573	649	728	802	878	954
Rugby	General	525	621	716	812	910	1003	1097	1193
Run	5 mph, 12 min/mile	420	496	573	649	728	802	878	954
Run	5.2 mph, 11.5 min/mile	473	558	644	730	819	902	988	1074
Run	6 mph, 10 min/mile	525	621	716	812	910	1003	1097	1193
Run	6.7 mph, 9 min/mile	578	683	788	893	1001	1103	1207	1312
Run	7 mph, 8.5 min/mile	604	714	824	933	1047	1153	1262	1372
Run	7.5 mph, 8 min/mile	656	776	895	1015	1138	1253	1372	1491
Run	8 mph, 7.5 min/mile	709	838	967	1096	1229	1354	1481	1610
Run	8.6 mph, 7 min/mile	735	869	1003	1136	1274	1404	1536	1670
Run	9 mph, 6.5 min/mile	788	931	1074	1217	1366	1504	1646	1789
Run	10 mph, 6 min/mile	840	993	1146	1299	1457	1604	1756	1908
Run	10.9 mph, 5.5 min/mile	945	1117	1289	1461	1639	1805	1975	2147
Run	Cross country	473	558	644	730	819	902	988	1074
Skate, ice	General	368	434	501	568	637	702	768	835
Skate, inline	Inline, general	656	776	895	1015	1138	1253	1372	1491
Skateboard	General	263	310	358	406	455	501	549	596
Ski, downhill	Light	263	310	358	406	455	501	549	596
Ski, downhill	Moderate	315	372	430	487	546	602	658	716
Ski, downhill	Vigorous, race	420	496	573	649	728	802	878	954
Ski machine	General	368	434	501	568	637	702	768	835
Ski, cross-country	2.5 mph, slow	368	434	501	568	637	702	768	835
Ski, cross-country	4-4.9 mph, moderate	420	496	573	649	728	802	878	954
Ski, cross-country	5-7.9 mph, brisk	473	558	644	730	819	902	988	1074
Snowboard	General	394	465	537	609	683	752	823	895
Snowshoe	General	420	496	573	649	728	802	878	954
Soccer	Casual	368	434	501	568	637	702	768	835
Soccer	Competitive	525	621	716	812	910	1003	1097	1193
Softball	General	263	310	358	406	455	501	549	596
Stair stepper	General	473	558	644	730	819	902	988	1074
Stationary rower	50 watts, light	184	217	251	284	319	351	384	417
Stationary rower	100 watts, moderate	368	434	501	568	637	702	768	835
Stationary rower	150 watts, vigorous	446	527	609	690	774	852	933	1014
Stationary rower	200 watts, very vigorous	630	745	859	974	1092	1203	1317	1431
Stretch, yoga	General, Hatha	131	155	179	203	228	251	274	298
Swim	Lake, ocean, or river	315	372	430	487	546	602	658	716
Swim	Laps freestyle, slow or moderate	368	434	501	568	637	702	768	835

Activity	Type	BODY WEIGHT							
		(110 lb)	(130 lb)	(150 lb)	(170 lb)	(190 lb)	(210 lb)	(230 lb)	(250 lb)
Swim	Laps freestyle, fast	525	621	716	812	910	1003	1097	1193
Swim	Backstroke	368	434	501	568	637	702	768	835
Swim	Sidestroke	420	496	573	649	728	802	878	954
Swim	Breaststroke	525	621	716	812	910	1003	1097	1193
Swim	Butterfly	578	683	788	893	1001	1103	1207	1312
Tennis	Doubles	315	372	430	487	546	602	658	716
Tennis	Singles	420	496	573	649	728	802	878	954
Treadmill, run	6 mph, 10 min/mile, 0% incline	525	621	716	812	910	1003	1097	1193
Treadmill, run	6 mph, 10 min/mile, 2% incline	578	683	788	893	1001	1103	1207	1312
Treadmill, run	6 mph, 10 min/mile, 4% incline	620	732	845	958	1074	1183	1295	1408
Treadmill, run	6 mph, 10 min/mile, 6% incline	667	788	909	1031	1156	1273	1394	1515
Treadmill, run	7 mph, 8.5 min/mile, 0% incline	604	714	824	933	1047	1153	1262	1372
Treadmill, run	7 mph, 8.5 min/mile, 2% incline	667	788	909	1031	1156	1273	1394	1515
Treadmill, run	7 mph, 8.5 min/mile, 4% incline	719	850	981	1112	1247	1374	1503	1634
Treadmill, run	7 mph, 8.5 min/mile, 6% incline	767	906	1046	1185	1329	1464	1602	1741
Treadmill, run	8 mph, 7.5 min/mile, 0% incline	709	838	967	1096	1229	1354	1481	1610
Treadmill, run	8 mph, 7.5 min/mile, 2% incline	756	894	1031	1169	1311	1444	1580	1718
Treadmill, run	8 mph, 7.5 min/mile, 4% incline	814	962	1110	1258	1411	1554	1701	1849
Treadmill, run	8 mph, 7.5 min/mile, 6% incline	872	1030	1189	1347	1511	1665	1821	1980
Treadmill, run	3 mph, 20 min/mile, 0% incline	173	205	236	268	300	331	362	394
Treadmill, run	3 mph, 20 min/mile, 2% incline	194	230	265	300	337	371	406	441
Treadmill, run	3 mph, 20 min/mile, 4% incline	215	254	293	333	373	411	450	489
Treadmill, run	3 mph, 20 min/mile, 6% incline	236	279	322	365	410	451	494	537
Treadmill, run	4 mph, 15 min/mile, 0% incline	263	310	358	406	455	501	549	596
Treadmill, run	4 mph, 15 min/mile, 2% incline	294	348	401	455	510	562	614	668
Treadmill, run	4 mph, 15 min/mile, 4% incline	326	385	444	503	564	622	680	740
Treadmill, run	4 mph, 15 min/mile, 6% incline	352	416	480	544	610	672	735	799
Tread water	Moderate	210	248	286	325	364	401	439	477
Tread water	Vigorous	525	621	716	812	910	1003	1097	1193
Volleyball	Noncompetitive	158	133	215	243	273	301	329	358
Volleyball	Competitive	420	496	573	649	728	802	878	954
Walk	<2 mph	105	124	143	162	182	201	219	239
Walk	2 mph, 30 min/mile	131	155	179	203	228	251	274	298
Walk	2.5 mph, 24 min/mile	158	133	215	243	273	301	329	358
Walk	3 mph, 20 min/mile	173	205	236	268	300	331	362	394
Walk	3.5 mph, 17 min/mile	200	236	272	308	346	381	417	453
Walk	4 mph, 15 min/mile	263	310	358	406	455	501	549	596
Walk	4.5 mph, 13 min/mile	331	391	451	511	574	632	691	751
Walk	Race walking	341	403	465	528	592	652	713	775
Water polo	General	525	621	716	812	910	1003	1097	1193
Weight training	Free, nautilus, light/moderate	158	133	215	243	273	301	329	358
Weight training	Free, nautilus, vigorous	315	372	430	487	546	602	658	716
Wind surf	Casual	158	133	215	243	273	301	329	358

Copyright 2001 HealtheTech Inc., Golden, Colo.
NOTE: This chart is not intended to be a comprehensive list for all nutritional or metabolic deficiencies or nonnutrition examples.
From Hammond K: Physical Assessment: A Nutritional Perspective, *Nurs Clin North Am* 32(4):779–790, 1997.

11 APPENDIX

Nutrition-Focused Physical Assessment

PART 1 Parameters Useful in the Assessment of General Nutritional Status and the Presence of Malnutrition

Examination Areas	Tips	Severe Malnutrition	Mild-Moderate Malnutrition	Well Nourished
Subcutaneous Fat Loss				
Orbital Region – Surrounding the Eye	View patient when standing directly in front of them, gently touch above cheekbone, below the lower eyelid, and the supraorbital area above the eye below the eyebrow	Hollow look, depressions, dark circles, loose skin, no evidence of fat pads below the lower eyelid or below the eyebrow	Slightly dark circles, somewhat hollow look	Slightly bulged fat pads. Fluid retention may mask loss
Upper Arm Region – Triceps/Biceps	Arm bent, roll skin between fingers, do not include muscle in pinch	Very little space between folds, fingers touch	Some depth pinch but not ample	Ample fat tissue obvious between folds of skin
Thoracic and Lumbar Region – Ribs, Lower Back, Midaxillary Line	Have patient press hands hard against a solid object	Depression between the ribs very apparent. Iliac crest very prominent	Ribs apparent, depressions between them less pronounced. Iliac crest somewhat prominent	Chest is full, ribs do not show. Slight to no protrusion of the iliac crest
Muscle Loss				
Temple Region – Temporalis Muscle	View patient when standing directly in front of them; ask patient to turn head side to side; gently palpate the temple region	Hollowing, scooping, depression	Slight depression	Can see/feel well-defined muscle
Jaw Region – Masseter Muscle	View patient when standing directly in front of him or her; ask patient to clench teeth and move jaw from side to side. Palpate the masseter muscle while the jaw is in motion	Patient is unable to clench teeth or move jaw from side to side. Note: this may be due to a medication condition unrelated to malnutrition	Patient demonstrates moderate ability to clench teeth	Patient demonstrates strong ability to clench teeth
Clavicle Bone Region – Pectoralis Major, Deltoid, Trapezius Muscles	Look for prominent bone. Make sure patient is not hunched forward	Protruding, prominent bone	Visible in male, some protrusion in female	Not visible in male, visible but not prominent in female
Clavicle and Acromion Bone Region – Deltoid Muscle	Patient arms at side; observe shape	Shoulder to arm joint looks square. Bones prominent. Acromion protrusion very prominent	Acromion process may slightly protrude	Rounded, curves at arm/shoulder/neck
Scapular Bone Region – Trapezius, Supraspinatus, Infraspinatus Muscles	Ask patient to extend hands straight out, push against solid object	Prominent, visible bones, depressions between ribs/scapula or shoulder/spine	Mild depression or bone may show slightly	Bones not prominent, no significant depressions
Dorsal Hand – Interosseous Muscle	Look at thumb side of hand; look at pads of thumb when tip of forefinger touching tip of thumb	Depressed area between thumb and forefinger	Slightly depressed	Muscle bulges, could be flat in some well-nourished people

PART 1 Parameters Useful in the Assessment of General Nutritional Status and the Presence of Malnutrition—cont'd

Examination Areas	Tips	Severe Malnutrition	Mild-Moderate Malnutrition	Well Nourished
Lower Body Less Sensitive to Change				
Patellar Region – Quadriceps Muscles	Ask patient to sit with leg propped up, bent at knee	Bones prominent, little sign of muscle around knee	Kneecap less prominent, more rounded	Muscles protrude, bones not prominent
Anterior Thigh Region – Quadriceps Muscles	Ask patient to sit, prop leg up on low furniture. Palpate quads to differentiate amount of muscle tissue from fat tissue	Depression/line on thigh, obviously thin	Mild depression on inner thigh	Well rounded, well developed
Posterior Calf Region- Gastrocnemius Muscle	Palpate the calf muscle to determine amount of tissue	Thin, minimal to no muscle definition; may feel stringy	Not well developed	Well-developed bulb of muscle
Edema				
Rule out other causes of edema, patient at dry weight	View and palpate ankles and hands for evidence of edema	Deep to very deep pitting, depression lasts a short to moderate time (31-60 sec) extremity looks swollen (3-4+)	Mild to moderate pitting, slight swelling of the extremity, indentation subsides quickly (0-30 sec)	No sign of fluid accumulation

Notes:
1. Introduce yourself to the patient/family
2. Provide rationale for examination request
3. Ask the patient for permission to examine him or her
4. Wash/dry hands thoroughly; wear gloves
5. Use standard precautions to prevent disease transmission

References:
1. McCann L: Subjective global assessment as it pertains to the nutritional status of dialysis patients, *Dial Transplant* 25(4):190–202, 1996.
2. Council on Renal Nutrition of the National Kidney Foundation: *Pocket guide to nutrition assessment of the patient with chronic kidney disease*, ed 3, (McCann L, editor), 2005. Available at: http://www.scribd.com/doc/6991983/Pocket-Guide-to-Nut-Crd. Accessed May 30, 2012.
3. Secker DJ, JeeJeebhoy KN: How to perform subjective global nutritional assessment in children, *J Acad Nutr Diet* 112:424–431, 2012.

This table was developed by Jane White, PhD, RDN, FADA, LDN, Louise Merriman, MS, RDN, CDN, Terese Scollard, MBA, RDN, and the Cleveland Clinic Center for Human Nutrition. Content was approved by the Adult Malnutrition Education and Outreach Committee, a joint effort of the Academy of Nutrition and Dietetics and the American Society of Parenteral and Enteral Nutrition.

©2013 Academy of Nutrition and Dietetics. Malnutrition Coding in Biesemeier, C. Ed. Nutrition Care Manual, October 2013 release.

PART 2 Clinical Characteristics That the Clinician Can Obtain and Document to Support a Diagnosis of Malnutrition (Academy/ASPEN)

Clinical Characteristic	MALNUTRITION IN THE CONTEXT OF SOCIAL OR ENVIRONMENTAL CIRCUMSTANCES		MALNUTRITION IN THE CONTEXT OF CHRONIC ILLNESS		MALNUTRITION IN THE CONTEXT OF ACUTE ILLNESS OR INJURY	
	Nonsevere (Moderate) Malnutrition	Severe Malnutrition	Nonsevere (Moderate) Malnutrition	Severe Malnutrition	Nonsevere (Moderate) Malnutrition	Severe Malnutrition
Energy intake[1] Malnutrition is the result of inadequate food and nutrient intake or assimilation; thus recent intake compared with estimated requirements is a primary criterion defining malnutrition. The clinician may obtain or review the food and nutrition history, estimate optimum energy needs, compare them with estimates of energy consumed, and report inadequate intake as a percentage of estimated energy requirements over time.	<75% of estimated energy requirement for >7 days	≤50% of estimated energy requirement for ≥5 days	<75% of estimated energy requirement for ≥1 month	≤75% of estimated energy requirement for ≥1 month	<75% of estimated energy requirement for ≥3 months	≤50% of estimated energy requirement for ≥1 month

Continued

PART 2   Clinical Characteristics That the Clinician Can Obtain and Document to Support a Diagnosis of Malnutrition (Academy/ASPEN)—cont'd

Clinical Characteristic	MALNUTRITION IN THE CONTEXT OF SOCIAL OR ENVIRONMENTAL CIRCUMSTANCES				MALNUTRITION IN THE CONTEXT OF CHRONIC ILLNESS				MALNUTRITION IN THE CONTEXT OF ACUTE ILLNESS OR INJURY			
	Nonsevere (Moderate) Malnutrition		Severe Malnutrition		Nonsevere (Moderate) Malnutrition		Severe Malnutrition		Nonsevere (Moderate) Malnutrition		Severe Malnutrition	
Interpretation of weight loss[2-5] The clinician may evaluate weight in light of other clinical findings, including the presence of under- or overhydration. The clinician may assess weight change over time reported as a percentage of weight lost from baseline.	% 1–2 5 7.5	Time 1 wk 1 mo 3 mo	% >2 >5 >7.5	Time 1 wk 1 mo 3 mo	% 5 7.5 10 20	Time 1 mo 3 mo 6 mo 1 y	% >5 >7.5 >10 >20	Time 1 mo 3 mo 6 mo 1 y	% 5 7.5 10 20	Time 1 mo 3 mo 6 mo 1 y	% >5 >7.5 >10 >20	Time 1 mo 3 mo 6 mo 1 y
Physical Findings[5,6] Malnutrition typically results in changes to the physical examination. The clinician may perform a physical examination and document any one of the physical examination findings below as an indicator of malnutrition.												
Body fat Loss of subcutaneous fat (e.g., orbital, triceps, fat overlying the ribs)	Mild		Moderate		Mild		Severe		Mild		Severe	
Muscle mass Muscle loss (e.g., wasting of the temples [temporalis muscle], clavicles [pectoralis and deltoids], shoulders [deltoids], interosseous muscles, scapula [latissimus dorsi, trapezius, deltoids], thigh [quadriceps], and calf [gastrocnemius])	Mild		Moderate		Mild		Severe		Mild		Severe	
Fluid accumulation The clinician may evaluate generalized or localized fluid accumulation evident on examination (extremities or ascites). Weight loss is often masked by generalized fluid retention (edema), and weight gain may be observed.	Mild		Moderate to severe		Mild		Severe		Mild		Severe	
Reduced grip strength[7] Consult normative standards supplied by the manufacturer of the measurement device	NA		Measurably reduced		NA		Measurably reduced		NA		Measurably reduced	

A minimum of two of the six characteristics above is recommended for diagnosis of either severe or nonsevere malnutrition. *NA*, Not applicable.

Notes:
Height and weight should be measured rather than estimated to determine body mass index (BMI).
Usual weight should be obtained to determine the percentage and to interpret the significance of weight loss.
Basic indicators of nutrition status such as body weight, weight change, and appetite may substantively improve with refeeding in the absence of inflammation. Refeeding and/or nutrition support may stabilize but not significantly improve nutrition parameters in the presence of inflammation. The National Center for Health Statistics defines *chronic* as a disease/condition lasting 3 months or longer.[8]
Serum proteins such as serum albumin and prealbumin are not included as defining characteristics of malnutrition because recent evidence analysis shows that serum levels of these proteins do not change in response to changes in nutrient intake.[9-12]

References

1. Kondrup J: Can food intake in hospitals be improved? *Clin Nutr* 20:153–160, 2001.
2. Blackburn GL, Bistrian BR, Maini BS, et al: Nutritional and metabolic assessment of the hospitalized patient, *JPEN J Parenter Enteral Nutr* 1:11–22, 1977.
3. Klein S, Kinney J, Jeejeebhoy K, et al: Nutrition support in clinical practice: review of published data and recommendations for future research directions. National Institutes of Health, American Society for Parenteral and Enteral Nutrition, and American Society for Clinical Nutrition, *JPEN J Parenter Enteral Nutr* 21:133–156, 1977.
4. Rosenbaum K, Wang J, Pierson RN, et al: Time-dependent variation in weight and body composition in healthy adults, *JPEN J Parenter Enteral Nutr* 24:52–55, 2000.
5. Keys A: Caloric undernutrition and starvation, with notes on protein deficiency, *J Am Med Assoc* 138:500–511, 1948.
6. Sacks GS, Dearman K, Replogle WH, et al: Use of subjective global assessment to identify nutrition-associated complications and death in geriatric long-term care facility residents, *J Am Coll Nutr* 19:570–577, 2000.
7. Norman K, Stobäus N, Gonzalez MC, et al: Hand grip strength: outcome predictor and marker of nutritional status, *Clin Nutr* 30:135–142, 2011.
8. Hagan JC: Acute and chronic diseases. In Mulner RM, editor: *Encyclopedia of health services research* (vol 1), Thousand Oaks, CA, 2009, Sage, p 25.
9. American Dietetic Association Evidence Analysis Library: *Does serum prealbumin correlate with weight loss in four models of prolonged protein-energy restriction: anorexia nervosa, non-malabsorptive gastric partitioning bariatric surgery, calorie-restricted diets or starvation.* Available at: http://www.adaevidencelibrary.com/conclusion.cfm?conclusion_statement_id5251313&highlight5prealbumin& home5. Accessed August 1, 2011.
10. American Dietetic Association Evidence Analysis Library: *Does serum prealbumin correlate with nitrogen balance?* Available at: http://www.adaevidencelibrary.com/conclusion.cfm?conclusion_statement_id5251315&highlight5prealbumin&home51. Accessed August 1, 2011.
11. American Dietetic Association Evidence Analysis Library: *Does serum albumin correlate with weight loss in four models of prolonged protein-energy restriction: anorexia nervosa, non-malabsorptive gastric partitioning bariatric surgery, calorie-restricted diets or starvation.* Available at: http://www.adaevidencelibrary.com/conclusion.cfm?conclusion_statement_id5 251263&highlight5albumin&home5. Accessed August 1, 2011.
12. American Dietetic Association Evidence Analysis Library: *Does serum albumin correlate with nitrogen balance?* Available at: http://www.adaevidencelibrary.com/conclusion.cfm?conclusion_statement_id5251265&highlight5albumin&home51. Accessed August 1, 2011.

This table was developed by Annalynn Skipper PhD, RDN, FADA. The content was developed by an Academy workgroup composed of Jane White, PhD, RDN, FADA, LDN, Chair; Maree Ferguson, MBA, PhD, RDN; Sherri Jones, MS, MBA, RDN, LDN; Ainsley Malone, MS, RDN, LD, CNSD; Louise Merriman, MS, RDN, CDN; Terese Scollard, MBA, RDN; Annalynn Skipper, PhD, RDN, FADA; and Academy staff member Pam Michael, MBA, RDN. Content was approved by an ASPEN committee consisting of Gordon L. Jensen, MD, PhD, Co-Chair; Ainsley Malone, MS, RDN, CNSD, Co-Chair; Rose Ann Dimaria, PhD, RN, CNSN; Christine M. Framson, RDN, PHD, CSND; Nilesh Mehta, MD, DCH; Steve Plogsted, PharmD, RPh, BCNSP; Annalynn Skipper, PhD, RDN, FADA; Jennifer Wooley, MS, RDN, CNSD; Jay Mirtallo, RPh, BCNSP, Board Liaison; and ASPEN staff member Peggi Guenter, PhD, RN. Subsequently, it was approved by the ASPEN Board of Directors. The information in the table is current as of February 1, 2012. Changes are anticipated as new research becomes available. Adapted from Skipper A. Malnutrition coding. In: Skipper A, editor: *Nutrition care manual*, Chicago, IL, 2012, Academy of Nutrition and Dietetics. FROM: White JV, et al: Consensus statement: Academy of Nutrition and Dietetics and American Society for Parenteral and Enteral Nutrition: Characteristics recommended for the identification and documentation of adult malnutrition (undernutrition), *JPEN* 36:275, 2012.

PART 3 Nutrition-Focused Physical Examination

System	Normal Findings	Abnormal Findings	Possible Nutrition and Metabolic Etiologies	Nonnutritional Etiologies
Body Habitus – See Part 1. General Survey	Weight for height appropriate, well-nourished, alert, and cooperative with good stamina	Loss of weight, muscle mass and fat stores, skeletal muscle wasting (hands, face, quadriceps, and deltoids), subcutaneous fat loss (face, triceps, thighs, waist) or overall weight loss, sarcopenia (loss of lean body mass in older adults). See Part 1 Growth retardation in children Inappropriate rates of height and weight gain in children and adolescents	Suboptimal energy and protein intakes Nonsevere malnutrition Severe malnutrition	Endocrine disorders, osteogenic disorders, menopausal disorders secondary to estrogen depletion Sarcopenia related to decreased physical activity, increased cytokine (interleukin-6) and decreased levels of growth hormone and insulin-like growth factor
Skin	Healthy color, soft, moist turgor with instant recoil, smooth appearance	Excess fat stores	Excess energy intake	Diabetes, steroids
		Poor or delayed wound healing, pressure ulcers	Protein deficiency Vitamin C deficiency Zinc deficiency	Poor vascular perfusion
		Dry with fine lines and shedding, scaly (xerosis)	Essential fat deficiency Vitamin A deficiency	Environmental or hygiene factors
		Spine-like plaques around hair follicles on buttocks, thighs, or knees (follicular hyperkeratosis)	Vitamin A deficiency Essential fat deficiency	

Continued

PART 3 Nutrition-Focused Physical Examination—cont'd

System	Normal Findings	Abnormal Findings	Possible Nutrition and Metabolic Etiologies	Nonnutritional Etiologies
		Pellagrous dermatitis (hyperpigmentation of skin exposed to sunlight)	Niacin deficiency Tryptophan deficiency	Thermal, sun, or chemical burns; Addison's disease
		Pallor	Iron deficiency Folic acid deficiency Vitamin B$_{12}$ deficiency	Skin pigmentation disorders, hemorrhage, low volume, low perfusion state
		Generalized dermatitis	Zinc deficiency Essential fatty acid deficiency	Atopic dermatitis, contact dermatitis, allergic or medication rash, psoriasis, connective tissue disease
		Yellow pigmentation	Carotene excess Vitamin B$_{12}$ deficiency	Jaundice
		Poor skin turgor	Fluid loss	Aging process
		Petechiae, ecchymoses	Vitamin K deficiency Vitamin C deficiency	Aspirin overdose, liver disease, or trauma
Nails	Smooth, translucent, slightly curved nail surface and firmly attached to nail bed; nail beds with brisk capillary refill	Spoon-shaped (koilonychia)	Iron deficiency Nonsevere malnutrition Severe malnutrition	COPD, heart disease, aortic stenosis, diabetes, lupus, chemotherapy
		Dull, lackluster	Protein deficiency Iron deficiency	Chemical effects
		Pale, mottled, poor blanching	Vitamin A deficiency Vitamin C deficiency	Infection, chemical effects
		Ridging, transverse-more than one extremity	Protein deficiency	Beau's lines, grooves caused by trauma, coronary occlusion, skin disease, transient illness
Scalp	Pink, no lesions, tenderness; fontanels without softening, bulging	Softening or craniotabes	Vitamin D deficiency	
		Open anterior fontanel (usually closes by <18 months of age)	Vitamin D deficiency	Hydrocephalus
Hair	Natural shine, consistency in color and quantity, fine to coarse texture	Lack of shine and luster, thin, sparse	Protein deficiency Zinc deficiency Biotin deficiency Linoleic acid deficiency	Hypothyroidism, chemotherapy, psoriasis, color treatment
		Easily pluckable	Protein deficiency Biotin deficiency	Hypothyroidism, chemotherapy, psoriasis, color treatment
		Alternating bands of light and dark hair in young children (flag sign)	Protein deficiency	Chemically processed or bleached hair
		"Corkscrew" hair	Copper deficiency Vitamin C deficiency	Menkes disease Chemical alteration
		Premature whitening	Selenium deficiency Vitamin B$_{12}$ deficiency	Graves' disease, medications
Face	Skin warm, smooth, dry, soft, moist with instant recoil	Diffuse depigmentation, swollen	Protein deficiency	Steroids and other medications
		Pallor	Iron deficiency Folic acid deficiency Vitamin B$_{12}$ deficiency	Low-perfusion, low-volume states
		Moon face	Protein deficiency	Cushing's disease, steroids

PART 3 Nutrition-Focused Physical Examination—cont'd

System	Normal Findings	Abnormal Findings	Possible Nutrition and Metabolic Etiologies	Nonnutritional Etiologies
		Bilateral temporal wasting. See Part 1	Protein deficiency Energy deficit	Neuromuscular disorders
		Undifferentiated mucocutaneous border	Riboflavin deficiency	
Eyes	Evenly distributed brows, lids, lashes; conjunctiva pink without discharge; sclerae without spots; cornea clear; skin without cracks or lesions	Pale conjunctiva	Iron deficiency Folate deficiency Vitamin B_{12} deficiency	Low output states
		Night blindness	Vitamin A deficiency	
		Dry, grayish, yellow or white foamy spots on whites of eyes (Bitot's spots)	Vitamin A deficiency	Pterygium, Gaucher's disease
		Dull, milky, or opaque cornea (corneal xerosis)	Vitamin A deficiency	
		Dull, dry, rough appearance to whites of eyes and inner lids (conjunctival xerosis)	Vitamin A deficiency	Chemical, environmental
		Softening of cornea (keratomalacia)	Vitamin A deficiency	
		Cracked and reddened corners of eyes (angular palpebritis)	Riboflavin deficiency Niacin deficiency	Infection, foreign objects
Nose	Uniform shape, septum slightly to left of mid-line, nares patent bi-laterally, mucosa pink and moist, able to identify aromas	Scaly, greasy, with gray or yellowish material around nares (nasolabial seborrhea)	Riboflavin deficiency Niacin deficiency Pyridoxine deficiency	
		Inflammation, redness of sinus tract, discharge, obstruction or polyps	Irritation of skin membranes	Need to reconsider if placing nasoenteric feeding tube; evaluate for nonfood allergies
Oral Cavity				
Lips, mouth	Pink, symmetric, smooth intact	Angular stomatitis (bilateral cracks, redness of lips)	Riboflavin deficiency Niacin deficiency Pyridoxine deficiency Dehydration	Poor-fitting dentures, herpes, syphilis, HIV, environmental exposure
		Cheilosis (vertical cracks of lips or fissuring)	Riboflavin deficiency Niacin deficiency Dehydration	HIV (Kaposi's sarcoma), environmental exposure
		Chapped or peeling	Dehydration	Environmental exposure
		General inflammation	Protein, energy, folic acid	Xerostomia
Tongue	Pink, moist, midline, symmetric with rough texture	Magenta (purplish-red color), inflammation of the tongue (glossitis)	Riboflavin deficiency, B_6 deficiency Niacin deficiency Folate deficiency Vitamin B_{12} deficiency Riboflavin deficiency Iron deficiency	Crohn's Disease, uremia, Infectious disease state, antibiotics, malignancy, Irritants (excess tobacco, alcohol, spices), generalized skin disorder
		Smooth, slick, loss of papillae (atrophic filiform papillae)	Folate deficiency Niacin deficiency Riboflavin deficiency Iron deficiency Vitamin B_{12} deficiency Nonsevere malnutrition Severe malnutrition	

Continued

PART 3   Nutrition-Focused Physical Examination—cont'd

System	Normal Findings	Abnormal Findings	Possible Nutrition and Metabolic Etiologies	Nonnutritional Etiologies
		Distorted taste (dysgeusia)	Zinc deficiency	Cancer therapy, medications, advanced age, trauma, syphilis, xerostomia, poor-fitting dentures, poor hygiene
		Decreased taste (hypogeusia)	Zinc deficiency Vitamin A deficiency	Cancer therapy, advanced age, medications, xerostomia
Gums	Pink, moist without sponginess	Spongy, bleeding, receding	Vitamin C deficiency Riboflavin deficiency	Dilantin and other medication, poor hygiene, lymphoma, polycythemia, thrombocytopenia
		Red, swollen interdental gingival hypertrophy	Vitamin C deficiency Folic acid deficiency, vitamin B_{12} deficiency	Dilantin, poor oral hygiene, lymphoma, vitamin A toxicity
Teeth	Repaired, no loose teeth; color may be various shades of white	Missing, poor repair, caries, loose teeth	Excess sugar intake	Trauma, syphilis, aging, poor dental hygiene
		White or brownish patches (mottled)	Excess fluoride	Enamel hypoplasia, erosion
Cranial nerves	Intact	Abnormal	Feeding route	
Gag reflex	Intact	Absent	Route of feeding	
Jaw	Proper alignment, movement from side to side	Improper alignment and movement	Ability to chew properly	
Parotid gland	Located anterior to earlobe, no enlargement	Bilateral enlargement	Nonsevere malnutrition Severe malnutrition	Bulimia, cysts, tumors, hyperparathyroidism
Neck nodules	Trachea midline, freely movable without enlargement or nodules	Enlarged thyroid	Iodine deficiency	Cancer, allergy, cold infection
Cardiopulmonary				
Chest, lungs	Anterior and posterior thorax; adequate muscle and fat stores, respirations even and unlabored, symmetric rise and fall of chest during inspiration and expiration, lung sounds clear	Somatic muscle- and fat-wasting; labored respirations; breath sounds such as crackles, rhonchi, and wheezing: evaluate for fluid status vs. tenacious secretions that may labor breathing and increase energy expenditure; also consider increased rate and depth, decreased rate and depth	Nonsevere malnutrition Severe malnutrition Metabolic acidosis Metabolic alkalosis	Respiratory disease (e.g., COPD)
Heart	Rhythm regular and rate within normal range; S_1 and S_2 heart sounds	Irregular rhythm	Potassium deficiency or excess Calcium deficiency Magnesium deficiency or excess Phosphorus deficiency	Cardiopulmonary disease states, stress
		Enlarged heart	Thiamin deficiency associated with anemia and beriberi	
		Pitting edema	Retention of sodium chloride, which causes the body to retain water Edema-associated disease of heart, liver, kidneys Fluid leaking into the interstitial tissue spaces	
Vascular access devices intact	No swelling, redness, drainage	Purulent drainage, swelling, excessive redness	Nutrition effects if device has to be removed	

PART 3   Nutrition-Focused Physical Examination—cont'd

System	Normal Findings	Abnormal Findings	Possible Nutrition and Metabolic Etiologies	Nonnutritional Etiologies
Abdomen	Soft, nondistended, symmetric, bilateral without masses, umbilicus in midline, no ascites, bowel sounds present and normoactive; tympanic on percussion; feeding device intact without redness, swelling	Generalized symmetric distention	Obesity	Enlarged organs, fluid, or gas, ileus from other disease
		Protruding, everted umbilicus; tight glistening appearance (ascites)	Effects on protein, fluid, sodium concerns of feeding	
		Scaphoid appearance	Nonsevere malnutrition Severe malnutrition	
		Increased bowel sounds	Nutrition effects in gastroenteritis (normal if hunger pains)	
		High-pitched tinkling	Nutrition effects if intestinal fluid and air present, indicating early obstruction	
		Decreased bowel sounds	Nutrition effects if peritonitis or paralytic ileus present	
Kidney, ureter, bladder	Urine golden yellow (ranges from pale yellow to deep gold), clear without cloudiness, adequate output	Decreased output, extremely dark, concentrated	Dehydration	
Musculoskeletal	Full range of motion without joint swelling or pain, adequate muscle strength	Inability to flex, extend, and rotate neck adequately	Interference with ability to feed or make hand-to-mouth contact	
		Decreased range of motion, swelling, impaired joint mobility of upper extremities; muscle wasting on arms, legs; skin folding on buttocks	Nonsevere malnutrition Severe malnutrition	
		Swollen, painful joints	Vitamin C deficiency Vitamin D deficiency	Connective tissue disease
		Bone tenderness	Vitamin A deficiency	
		Enlargement of epiphyses at wrist, ankle, or knees	Vitamins D deficiency Vitamin C deficiency	Trauma, deformity, or congenital cause
		Bowed legs	Vitamin D deficiency Calcium deficiency	
		Beading of ribs	Vitamin D deficiency Calcium deficiency	Renal rickets, malabsorption
		Pain in calves, thighs	Thiamin deficiency	Deep vein thrombosis, other neuropathy, or other
Neurologic	Alert, oriented, hand-to-mouth coordination; no weakness or tremors	Decreased or absent mental alertness; inadequate or absent hand-to-mouth coordination	Interference with the ability to eat or make hand-to-mouth contact	
		Psychomotor changes, cognitive and sensory deficits, memory loss, confusion, peripheral neuropathy	Nonsevere malnutrition Severe malnutrition Thiamin deficiency Pyridoxine deficiency Vitamin B_{12} deficiency	Trauma, neurologic disease, brain injury, brain tumor, chemotherapy

Continued

PART 3   Nutrition-Focused Physical Examination—cont'd

System	Normal Findings	Abnormal Findings	Possible Nutrition and Metabolic Etiologies	Nonnutritional Etiologies
		Dementia	Thiamin deficiency Niacin deficiency Vitamin B_{12} deficiency	Trauma, neurologic disease, vascular disease, brain injury, brain tumor, chemotherapy
		Tetany	Calcium deficiency Magnesium deficiency	
		Paresthesias or numbness in stocking-glove distribution	Vitamin B_{12} deficiency Thiamin deficiency	Diabetic neuropathy
	Cranial nerves intact: primary nutritionally focused ones include trigeminal, facial, glossopharyngeal, vagus, and hypoglossal			
	Reflexes (biceps, brachioradialis patella, and Achilles common in examination), functioning within normal range of 2^{++}	Hyperactive reflexes	Hypocalcemia	Tetany, upper motor neuron disease
	Hypoactive reflexes	Hypokalemia		Associated with metabolic diseases such as diabetes mellitus and hypothyroidism
		Hypoactive Achilles, patellar reflex	Thiamin deficiency Vitamin B_{12} deficiency	Neurologic disorder

COPD, Chronic obstructive pulmonary disease; *HIV,* human immunodeficiency virus.
From Litchford, MD: *Nutrition-focused physical assessment: making clinical connections.* Greensboro, NC, 2012, CASE Software & Books.
Hammond K: Physical assessment: a nutritional perspective. *Nurse Clin North Am* 32(4):779, 1997. Modified 2010.
Matarese LE, Gottschlich M, editors: *Contemporary nutrition support practice,* Philadelphia, PA, 2003, Saunders Company.
Porter RS, Kaplan JL, editors: *Nutrition disorders, Merck Manual online.* Available at: https://www.merckmanuals.com/professional/nutritional-disorders/undernutrition/overview-of-undernutrition. Accessed February 4, 2019.
This chart is not meant to be a comprehensive list for all nutritional or metabolic deficiencies or nonnutrition examples.

PEDIATRIC MALNUTRITION

Abnormal anthropometric measurements are often the first sign of pediatric malnutrition. Using the Nutrition Care Process, the registered dietitian nutritionist (RDN) uses clinical reasoning skills to determine the etiology of the abnormal pattern of growth (e.g., related to acute or chronic illness and the degree of inflammation present). Illness-related conditions contributing to pediatric malnutrition include starvation, malabsorption, increased rate of metabolism, altered nutrient utilization, and increased nutrient losses. Data gathered in the assessment step will be compared with the diagnostic criteria. There are two categories of diagnostic criteria. The first set of criteria use only one data point. These criteria are anthropometric measurements compared with a growth standard. A growth standard reflects optimal growth or potential growth for children at different ages. Growth standards are defined in terms of percentiles or Z-scores. Percentiles are a percentage of observations that fall above or below the value of the variable. For example, if a child's height is at the 25th percentile, this means that out of 100 normal children of the same gender and age, 75 will be taller than this child and 25 will be shorter.

The characteristics of pediatric malnutrition use Z-scores because these data points are calculated based on the distribution of the reference population including both the means and standard deviation. The advantage of using Z-scores is that the Z-scores are comparable across age and gender and these scores quantify growth status of children whose anthropometric measurements fall outside of the percentile ranges. The criteria include Z-scores for weight to height, BMI, length or height, and midupper arm circumference.

The second set of diagnostic criteria is used when two or more data points are available. The criteria include weight gain velocity, weight loss, deceleration of weight to length or weight to height, Z-score, and inadequate energy and protein intake. For more information, refer to the consensus statement of the Academy of Nutrition and Dietetics/American Society for Parenteral and Enteral Nutrition: Indicators recommended for the identification and documentation of pediatric malnutrition, *J Acad Nutr Diet* 114:1988–2000, 2014.

Laboratory Values for Nutritional Assessment and Monitoring

I. PRINCIPLES OF NUTRITIONAL LABORATORY TESTING

A. Purpose

Laboratory-based testing is used to estimate nutrient availability in biologic fluids and tissues. It is critical for assessment of both nutrient insufficiencies and frank deficiencies. Laboratory data are the only objective data used in nutrition assessment that are "controlled"—that is, the validity of the method of the measurement is checked each time a specimen is assayed by also assaying a sample with a known value. The known sample is called a *control,* and if the value obtained for the sample is outside the range of normal analytic variability, both the specimen and control are measured again.

The nutrition professional can use laboratory test results to support subjective data and clinical findings to determine a personalized nutritional assessment leading to more targeted interventions and successful outcomes. The laboratory values provide objective data useful in regular monitoring and can be used to assess progress and manage side effects such as inflammation, aberrant lipid and glucose metabolism, and immune status.

B. Specimen Types

Ideally the specimen to be tested reflects a high percentage of total body content of the nutrient to be assessed. However, often the best specimen is not readily available. The most common specimens for analysis are the following:

Whole blood—Must be collected with an anticoagulant if entire content of the blood is to be evaluated. The two common anticoagulants for whole blood analyses are ethylenediaminetetraacetic acid, a calcium chelator used in hematologic analyses, and heparin (maintains the blood in its most natural state).

Blood cells—Separated from uncoagulated whole blood for measurement of cellular analyte content: Red blood cells (indicate a 120-day window into intracellular and membrane composition), various blood components like white blood cells, protein-bound molecules, and others.

Plasma—The uncoagulated fluid that bathes the formed elements (blood cells).

Serum—The fluid that remains after whole blood or plasma has coagulated. Coagulation proteins and related substances are missing or significantly reduced.

Urine—Contains a concentrate of excreted metabolites and potential toxins.

Feces—Important in identifying various gastrointestinal functional parameters including inflammatory markers, microbiology, mycology, parasitology, digestive markers, and nutritional analyses when nutrients are not absorbed and therefore are present in fecal material.

Saliva—Laboratory analysis to identify endocrine, inflammatory, infectious, immunologic, some nutrients, and other parameters with buccal cell or whole saliva samples.

Genomic—Expanding beyond the historical metabolic macro- and micronutrient testing, genomic polymerase chain reaction (PCR) assays are emerging genomic clinical indicators for nutrigenetic and nutrigenomic influences on the metabolism of an individual (see Chapter 6).

Expired Air—Concentration of expired gases is a noninvasive and useful estimate of bacterial metabolism. Emerging measurements of expired nitric oxide and ketosis may be useful in estimating inflammatory or ketotic status in selected medical conditions.

Hair—An easy-to-collect tissue; most commonly measuring minerals; usually a poor indicator of actual body levels.

Other tissues—Fat biopsies have been used to estimate vitamin D stores in research studies.

C. Interpretation of Laboratory Data

As with all data, nutrition data may be quantitative (e.g., how much, how often, how fast), semiquantitative (e.g., many, most, few, a lot, usually, majority, several), or qualitative (e.g., color, shape, species). The advantage of quantitative data is that they are less ambiguous or more objective than other types of observations. Although objective laboratory data are extremely important resources in nutrition assessment, one should be extremely cautious about using a single isolated laboratory test value to make an assessment. An isolated value is often misleading, especially when used without the context of an individual's lifestyle habits; clinical status; dietary, medical, and genomic histories; and test results if available. Besides the importance of identifying frank deficiencies or excesses of nutrients, the best data are obtained from analysis of changes in laboratory values and overt clinical physical signs (e.g., compromised skin conditions). It is especially important to monitor laboratory values when contemplating nutritional interventions that involve potentially unsafe levels beyond upper limits (UL), such as fat-soluble vitamins or a mineral like selenium.

When monitoring patients for changes in nutrition test values, one must consider how much change is necessary to give confidence that a difference is significant. The change required for statistical significance has been called the *critical difference.* It is calculated from measurement of the variances calculated from repeated measurements of an analyte: (1) specimens that have been obtained, at several different times, from each of several healthy persons (intrasubject variation), and (2) separate samples from a large specimen pool (analytic variation).

In practice, assessments are not based on the measurement of a single analyte at one point in time except in the case of severe deficiencies or dangerous excesses. Changes in laboratory tests may have biologic significance (e.g., patient's condition is improving) long before statistical significance is achieved. The changes in laboratory data may precede changes in other nutritional indices, but generally, although not always, the data available should point to the same conclusion.

D. Reference Ranges

To determine whether a particular laboratory value is abnormal, particularly when serial data are not available, the value is generally compared with a diagnostic reference range. The reference range is constructed from a large number of test values (20 to >1000). The average value and the standard deviation for these data are determined, and the reference range is calculated from the mean 62 standard deviations. If the sample group is representative of the reference population, the reference range will include values that reflect those found in approximately 95% of the reference population. Approximately 2.5% of this normal population will have values greater than the upper end of the reference range, and 2.5% will have values less than the lower end. This means that one normal individual in 20 would have a value below or above the reference range.

Reference ranges can be made for different populations. For example, reference ranges based on gender, age, ethnicity, and so forth can be developed. In practice, the differences between populations are often ignored because the importance of small differences in a nutrient analyte is not usually significant. However, in the event of borderline values, the possible influence of differences between the patient's population and the reference population may need to be considered.

Reference ranges are often determined by obtaining blood from personnel working in or near the clinical laboratory. This population is often skewed toward younger persons, has limited ethnic diversity, and is overrepresented by women.

As the science of nutrition continues to rapidly evolve due to technological and scientific advances including genomic tests results for individuals, changes in laboratory values can be interpreted as indicating metabolic trends and genotypic influences, even within the reference range of a test. The nutritionist's skill in perceiving nutrient insufficiencies or imbalances related to nutritional influences can provide a more targeted assessment resulting in improved outcomes from therapy.

E. Units

Many types of units are used in reporting nutrient-dependent laboratory values. Two basic systems of units are in common use: the conventional system and the Système Internationale d'Unités (SI) system. The conventional system sometimes lacks convention; thus different laboratories adopt different units to report the same analyte. For example, the conventional report of an ionized calcium value could be 2.3 mEq/L, 46 mg/L, or 4.6 mg/dL. However, in the SI system only 1.15 mmol/L is allowed.

F. Nature of Nutritional Testing and Types of Tests

Typically laboratory tests are static assays (i.e., the concentration of an analyte is measured in a biologic fluid [e.g., a fasting blood specimen] at a point in time). Assessment of nutrient status made by this approach is often inaccurate or distorted. Some nutrients can be assessed by tests that are based on measurements that reflect the endogenous availability of a nutrient to a measurable biologic function (e.g., biochemical, tissue, or organ). Most often, functional assessment of nutrient status may be done by measurement of a biochemical marker (i.e., a normal or abnormal metabolite) of function. The results of this type of testing can be reliably considered to reflect the adequacy of a nutrient pool or possible individual genomic nutrient requirements.

CLINICAL INSIGHT

Bioelectrical Impedance Analysis (BIA) and Bioimpedance Spectroscopy (BIS)—A Functional Test for Nutritional Status

Nutrition assessment is taking on a new level of specificity with the explosion of technology and discoveries of the pathophysiology of disease and functions of the human body. These breakthroughs assist in molecular-level identification of nutrition status. Bioelectrical impedance analysis (BIA) and bioimpedance spectroscopy (BIS) have a credible history of use in research, but recently have found an increasing use as a clinical tool in nutrition assessment.

BIA estimates body composition and cellular activity by measuring the bulk electrical impedance of the body. The testing procedure involves application of conductors (electrodes) to a person's hand and foot and sending a small alternating electric current through the body (see figure on next page). The different electrical conductive properties of various body tissues (adipose, muscular, and skeletal) and hydration affect the impedance measurement. An algorithm derived from statistical analysis of BIA measurements is used to calculate the various parameters that can be measured by this technique.

Normal hydration is critical for results to be valid, with these guidelines before testing:

1. Drink water (16-24 oz during the 4 hours before test)
2. No alcohol for 12 hours before test
3. No food or caffeine drinks for 4 hours before test
4. No moderate to intense exercise for 12 hours before test

Contraindications to BIA testing are pregnancy or the presence of implants like pacemakers or defibrillators. Follow-up monitoring of BIA testing should attempt to be near the same time of day.

There are commercially available BIA devices that measure only body fat % and weight. But professional BIA or BIS instruments are available that provide reliable, more comprehensive full body data, and automatically calculate total body water, intracellular and extracellular water, fat-free mass, percent body fat, phase angle, capacitance, and body cell mass. They are very useful in tracking changes in an individual's progress over time. Research in the past decade has shown promise for the BIA phase angle as a prognostic indicator of some cancers (Norman et al, 2010) and other chronic conditions (Maddocks et al, 2014).

The multiple parameters measured in a BIA or BIS test provide three categories of data:

1. *Anthropometry:* BMI (body mass index), BMR (basal metabolic rate), body fat percentage, and lean body mass percentage. These measurements are used with weight management, monitoring of wasting syndromes, and acute care formulation of dietary prescriptions. Weight, height, age, gender, and date must be entered to obtain these results.
2. *Cellular metabolism:* Phase angle, which measures cell membrane fluidity, is a prognostic marker of mortality, capacitance (electrical resistance of the cell

CLINICAL INSIGHT—cont'd

Bioelectrical Impedance Analysis (BIA) and Bioimpedance Spectroscopy (BIS)—A Functional Test for Nutritional Status

membrane), and body cell mass (the number or amount of metabolically active cells). Using these three measurements provides an easy-to-use, noninvasive, and reproducible technique to evaluate changes in body composition and nutritional status. Phase angle (BIA) detects changes in tissue electrical properties, and it is hypothesized as a marker of malnutrition for investigating various diseases in the clinical setting. Lower phase angles suggest cell death or decreased cell integrity, while higher phase angles suggest large quantities of intact cell membranes (Selberg and Selberg, 2002).

3. *Hydration:* Total body water (in pounds and as a percentage), intracellular water (in pounds and as a percentage), and extracellular water (in pounds and as a percentage).

Every professional practicing nutrition therapy can now consider adding a reasonably priced BIA or BIS instrument to their nutritional assessment toolbox to assist in the management of a client or patient. The four companies from which professional BIA or BIS instruments can currently be obtained are: https://www.impedimed.com

https://www.inbody.com
https://www.biodynamics.com
https://www.rjlsystems.com

These companies also provide informative education on the technology and operation of their bioimpedance or bioimpedance spectroscopy instruments.

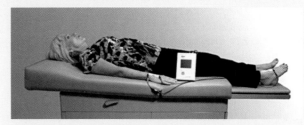

Image reproduced with permission of ImpediMed Limited.

Bauer JM, Kaiser MJ, Anthony P, et al: The Mini Nutritional Assessment—its history, today's practice, and future perspectives, *Nutr Clin Pract* 23:388–396, 2008.

Davis MP, Yavuzsen T, Khoshknabi D, et al: Bioelectrical impedance phase angle changes during hydration and prognosis in advanced cancer, *Am J Hosp Palliat Care* 26(3):180–187, 2009.

Ellis KJ, Bell SJ, Chertow GM, et al: Bioelectrical impedance methods in clinical research: a follow-up to the NIH Technology Assessment Conference, *Nutrition* 12(11-12): 874–880, 1999.

Gupta D, Lis CG, Dahlk SL, et al: The relationship between bioelectrical impedance phase angle and subjective global assessment in advanced colorectal cancer, *Nutr J* 7:19, 2008.

Gupta D, Lammersfeld CA, Vashi PG, et al: Bioelectrical impedance phase angle as a prognostic indicator in breast cancer, *BMC Cancer* 8:249, 2008.

Hengstermann S, Fischer A, Steinhagen-Thiessen E, et al: Nutrition status and pressure ulcer: what we need for nutrition screening, *JPEN J Parenter Enteral Nutr* 31:288–294, 2007.

Jaffrin MY, Morel H: Body fluid volumes measurements by impedance: a review of bioimpedance spectroscopy (BIS) and bioimpedance analysis (BIA) methods, *Med Eng Phys* 30:1257–1269, 2008.

Khalil SF, Mohktar MS, Ibrahim F: The theory and fundamentals of bioimpedance analysis in clinical status monitoring and diagnosis of diseases, *Sensors (Basel)* 14:10895–10928, 2014.

Kyle UG, Bosaeus I, De Lorenzo AD: Bioelectrical impedance analysis-part II: utilization in clinical practice, Clin Nutr 23:1430–1453, 2004.

Methods of body composition tutorials (interactive). Dept. of Nutrition and Food Sciences, University of Vermont. Available at: http://nutrition.uvm.edu/bodycomp/. Accessed May 19, 2011.

Maddocks M, Kon SS, Jones SE, et al: Bioelectrical impedance phase angle relates to function, disease severity and prognosis in stable chronic obstructive pulmonary disease, *Clin Nutr* 34:1245–1250, 2015. doi:10.1016/j.clnu.2014.12.020.

Norman K, Stobäus N, Zocher D, et al: Cutoff percentiles of bioelectrical phase angle predict functionality, quality of life, and mortality in patients with cancer, *Am J Clin Nutr* 92:612–619, 2010.

Selberg O, Selberg D: Norms and correlates of bioimpedance phase angle in healthy human subjects, hospitalized patients, and patients with liver cirrhosis, *Eur J Appl Physiol* 86:509–516, 2002.

Van Loan MD, et al: Use of bioimpedance spectroscopy (BIS) to determine extracellular fluid (ECF), intracellular fluid (ICF), total body water (TBW), and fat free mass (FFM). In Ellis K, editor: *Human body composition: in vivo measurement and studies,* New York, NY, 1993, Plenum Publishing Co., pp 67–70.

Varan HD, Bolayir B, Kara O, et al: Phase angle assessment by bioelectrical impedance analysis and its predictive value for malnutrition risk in hospitalized geriatric patients, *Aging Clin Exp Res* 28:1121–1126, 2016.

II. Clinical Chemistry

A. Protein Markers

Test	Principles	Interpretation	Reference Range	Limitations and Implications
nPCR	nPCR is determined by measuring the intradialytic appearance of urea in body fluids plus any urea lost in the urine in patients with residual renal function. $nPCR = 0.22 + (0.036 \times$ *intradialytic rise in BUN x $\times$ 24)/(intradialytic interval). (also called protein nitrogen appearance (PNA) rate (g/day) $= 13 + 7.31$ UNA (mmol/day) [UNA (mmol/day) $=$ Vd (mL) x Cd (mmol/L) $+$ Vu (mL) $+$ Cu (mmol/L)]	Useful in assessing DPI in patients who are in a steady state on hemodialysis, as a means toward determining adequate nutrition status.	0.81-1.02 g UN/kg per day	nPCR considered superior to sAlb for monitoring nutrition protein status due to sAlb influence by processes other than nutrition status.[2] During hemodialysis, the PCR can also reflect inadequate dialysis.
(U : Cr)	U : Cr concentration in fasting, first-void urine used to compare amino acid catabolism (BUN) with muscle mass (creatinine).	Urine concentration (mg/dL) U : Cr $=$ Urine area (mg/dL) $\div$ Urine creatinine (mg/dL). The U : Cr is used in comparing other markers like microalbumin, albumin, GFR ratios.	**Risk** Low Medium High	**Ratio** >12.0 6.0-12.0 <6.0
UUN	The protein pool (visceral and somatic) N is catabolized to urea; urine urea represents ~80% of N catabolized; requires accurate estimate of protein intake; thus usually used only for PN or tube-feeding patients.	UUN is compared with the actual N intake. Nitrogen Balance $=$ Nitrogen intake (Protein g/day$\div$6.25) $-$ Nitrogen Losses (UUN (g)$+$ 4)[a]	$-$ = Catabolism 0 = Catabolism $+$ = Anabolism (3-6 g/24 hr = optimal use range)	24-hour urine collection must be quantitative (complete); UUN not appropriate in renal insufficiency; does not account for wound leakage, cell losses, or diarrhea; inaccurate in metabolically stressed patients.
TUN	Some N is excreted as nonurea N (e.g., ammonia and creatinine); 24-hour TUN reflects total protein catabolism, accounting for all sources of urinary N; as for UUN, it requires accurate protein intake. Used primarily to accurately follow the protein catabolic response during disease and response to nutritional support.	TUN is compared with the actual N intake; Nitrogen balance $=$ Nitrogen intake (Protein g/day$\div$6.25) $-$ Nitrogen losses (TUN (g)$+$ 2)[b]	$-$ = Catabolism 0 = Catabolism $+$ = Anabolism (3-6 g/24 hr = optimal use range)	Urine 24-hour collection must be quantitative (complete); TUN not appropriate in renal insufficiency; not done in many institutions; does not account for wound leakage, cell losses, or diarrhea.
UKM	Formulas used to estimate nPCR (normalized protein catabolic rate) from changes in BUN concentration in patients with impaired renal function.	Urinary urea (KrU) and BUN levels (urea generation rate—UG) are used to determine nPCR; 1- to 3-day diet intake compared with nPCR. Urea kinetic Modeling (Kt/V$_{urea}$ and nPCR)	In protein balance, nPRC = protein intake (g/kg/day)	Urea lost in dialysis must be accounted for in calculating urea nitrogen appearance. Dietary protein intake is hard to estimate.

B. Inflammatory Markers

Test	Principles	Interpretation	Reference Range	Limitations and Implications
ALB	Easily and quickly measured colorimetrically; large body pool (3-5 g/kg body weight), ~60% is outside the plasma in the extravascular pool; long half-life of 3 weeks.	Decreased levels can occur following acute and chronic inflammatory states; often associated with other deficiencies (i.e., zinc, iron, and vitamin A) reflecting that ALB transports many small molecules.	3.5-5 g/dL (35-50 g/L)	Stable half-life ~3 weeks. A negative phase reactant, impacted by inflammatory stress, (protein losing conditions and hemodilution). Hepatic proteins are indicators of morbidity and mortality.
GLOB	Large body pool (3-5 g/kg body weight), ~35% is outside the plasma in the extravascular pool; long half-life averages 23 days but varies with particular globulins.	GLOB proteins include enzymes and carriers that transport proteins including antibodies that primarily assist in immune function and fight infection.	2.3-3.4 g/dL (23-34 g/L)	Significance confounded by acute stress reaction, infection, inflammatory conditions.

A/G Ratio	Calculated from ALB and GLOB values by direct measurement of TP and ALB.	It represents the relative amounts of ALB and GLOB.	A/G ratio 1:1 - normal <1:1 - disease state	ALB levels fall and globulin levels rise with inflammatory stress.
Tf or TFN	The iron-bound GLOB protein that responds to the need for iron. Can be calculated from TIBC and serum iron; half-life ~9 days.	Tf increased with low iron stores and prevents build-up of highly toxic excess unbound iron in circulation. In iron overload states Tf levels decrease. Because B_6 is required for iron to bind to Hgb, B6 deficiency promotes ↑ Tf from the ↑ circulating iron that binds to Tf; smaller extra-vascular pool than ALB.	Adult male: 215-365 mg/dL (2.15-3.65 g/L) Adult female: 250-380 mg/dL (2.50-3.80 g/L) Newborn: 130-275 mg/dL (1.3-2.75 g/L) Child: 203-360 mg/dL (2.03-3.6 g/L) Pregnancy and estrogen HRT associated with ↑ Tf.	Lead can biologically mimic and displace iron, thus releasing Fe into circulation and ↑ Tf. Tf is a negative acute phase reactant diminished in chronic illness and hypoproteinemia.
Tf-sat	Tf-sat (%) = Serum iron level ÷ TIBC × 100%	Tf-sat decreases to <15% in Fe deficiency; useful in diagnosis of iron toxicity or Fe overload (hemochromatosis). See Chapter 31.	M: 20%-50% F: 15%-50% Chronic illness: normal Tf-sat%. Late pregnancy: low Tf-sat%.	Increased Tf-sat when low vitamin B_6 as in aplastic anemia.
PAB/(TTR)	Transports T_4 and acts as a carrier for retinol-binding protein; PAB also called thyroxin-binding protein; half-life 2 days.	Measure of inflammatory status. Zinc deficiency reduces PAB levels.	15-36 mg/dL or 150-360 mg/L (15-36 mg/dL female, 21-43 mg/dL male) Malnutrition: <8 mg/dL (<0.8g/L or <80 mg/L)	Sensitive to acute zinc deficiency and acute stress reaction. PAB values do not reflect protein status but are a prognostic index for mortality and morbidity.[4]
RBP	Transport retinol; because of low molecular weight, RBP is filtered by glomerulus and catabolized by the kidney tubule; half-life = 12 hours	Measure of inflammatory status.	2.6-7.6 mg/dL (1.43-2.86 mmol/L)	Sensitive to stress response; vitamin A and zinc deficiencies, and hemodilution; increased in chronic renal disease.
hs-CRP	A nonspecific acute phase reactant; short half-life 5-7 hr; CRP responds to inflammation in 6-10 hours. (also called CRP-ultra sensitivity and CRP-cardio)	A sensitive marker of bacterial disease and systemic inflammation; associated with periodontitis, trauma, cardiovascular disease, neoplastic proliferation, and bacterial infections.	Low Risk for CVD = Less than 1.0 mg/L Intermediate Risk for CVD = 2.9 mg/L High Risk for CVD = Greater than 3.0 mg/L Seek inflammatory cause if >10 mg/L	Useful metabolic indicator for adults.[9] Acute-phase reactant; relates mostly to bacterial infection, central adiposity, trauma, and neoplastic activity.
Fibrinogen	Acute-phase reactant protein essential to blood-clotting mechanism/coagulation system.	Decreased fibrinogen related to prolonged PT and PTT; produced in liver; rises sharply during tissue inflammation or necrosis; association with CHD, stroke, myocardial infarction, and peripheral arterial disease.	200-400 mg/dL If <100 mg/dL, increased risk of bleeding. Should be monitored in conjunction with blood platelet levels involved with coagulation status.	Good test and retest reliability, and covariance is stable over time; diets rich in omega-3/6 fatty acids reduce fibrinogen blood levels.

C. Metabolic Indicators

IGF-1 or Somatome-din C	The peptide mediator of growth hormone activity produced by the liver; half-life of a few hours; much less sensitive to stress response than other proteins.	Low in chronic undernutrition; increases rapidly during nutrition repletion; TSAT, PAB, and RBP are not affected. Elevated levels associated with elevated GH in acromegaly and neoplastic activity.	Adult: 42-110 ng/mL Children age 0-19: can vary with age, gender and Tanner Stages (Appendices 17 & 18) used for references per age.	Reduced levels seen in hypopituitarism, hypothyroidism, liver disease, and with estrogen use. Growing evidence of elevated IGF-1 as a prognostic biomarker of neoplastic activity.[5,6]
Hgb A1C	Glycosylated hemoglobin; dependent on blood glucose level over life span of RBC (120 days); the more glucose the Hgb is exposed to, the greater the % Hgb A1C.	Assessment of the mean glycemic blood level and of chronic diabetic control detecting for the previous 2-3 months.[7]	Nondiabetic adult/child: 4%-5.9% Controlled DM: 4%-7% Fair DM control: 7%-8% Poor DM control: >8%	Hgb A1C measurement is a simple, rapid, and objective procedure. Home testing available.

Continued

Insulin, fasting	Pancreatic hormone signaling cell membrane insulin receptors to initiate glucose transport into cell; test fasting 7 hours, or 1 or 2 hours postprandial; usually ordered with blood glucose test.	Elevated levels associated with hyperinsulinemia related to metabolic syndrome; diagnosis of insulin producing neoplasms; excess insulin associated with inflammatory conditions.	Adult values: Fasting 6-27 µ IU/mL 1 or 2 hours PP: see laboratory reference	Good to test and retest reliability, and covariance is stable over time.[8] Insulin antibodies may invalidate the test.

D. Immune Dysregulation Tests
Allergies/Sensitivity

Immunoglobulins (IgA, IgG, IgE, IgM,)	Serologic antibody screening tests; testing of Immunoglobulins; Total IgE ELISA; RAST (radioallergosorbent-blood IgE); Bloodspot: IgG Provocative specific antigen skin prick: (IgE related skin response) used to diagnose allergy and identify the allergen.	Used to determine immunodeficiency states; measurement of +IgE = allergic disorders; (see Table 27-3) +IgG = delayed immunologic sensitivity or intolerance response (see Table 27-3). IgA = largest % Ig primarily made in GI lymphoid tissue and marker of immune strength and response.	Total IgA: Adults = 85-463 mg/dL Children = 1-350 mg/dL Total IgG: <2.0 mcg/mL Total IgE = <10 IU/mL RAST IgE = <1 IU/mL low allergic risk Total IgM: Adults = 48-271 mg/dL Children = 17-200 mg/dL Total IgD = <15.3 mg/dL	NSAIDS, glucocorticoids, vitamin C, bioflavonoids can suppress the immunologic response and promote a false negative. IgA used as a biomarker reference of adequate immune response to enable measurement of IgG, IgE, IgM, IgD.

Innate Immune Factors

TLC	Calculated from the percentage of lymphocytes reported in the hemogram and the WBC count. Units = cells/µl or cells/mm³	Decreased in protein-energy malnutrition and immunocompromised state.	Normal: >2700 Moderate depletion: 900-1800 Severe depletion: <900	
Delayed Cutaneous Hypersensitivity	Anergy for antigens, such as mumps and *Candida*; occurs in malnutrition; antigens intradermal injection; redness (erythema) and hardness (induration) read 1, 2, or 3 days later.	Response affected by protein-energy status and vitamin A, iron, zinc, and vitamin B_6 deficiencies.	*Induration* 1+: <5 mm 2+: 6-10 mm 3+: 11-20 mm 4+: >20 mm Erythema present or absent	Usefulness in acute care limited by drugs, effect of aging and disease (metabolic, malignant, and infectious diseases); difficult to administer and interpret results; semiquantitative.
Cytokines	Serum or joint fluid proteins tested from venous blood. They include lymphocytes (T & B cells), monocytes, leukocytes (interleukins), eosinophils, interferon, and growth factors. (See Chapter 7.)	A group of immune reactant proteins that have many functions even from one cell to another. They respond to the environmental influences to communicate and orchestrate the immune response to protect from cancer, infection, and inflammation.	Cytokine examples: Interleukins: IL-1, IL-6, IL-8, IL-10, TNF-α, TH-1, TH-2 (per laboratory references)	

Adaptive Immune Factors

Eosinophils (Eosinophil leukocyte)	Blood: BAL fluid CSF specimen to rule out eosinophilic meningitis.	Blood: Wide range of clinical conditions reflect nonspecific eosinophilia; elevated related to possible allergies, asthma, sensitivities, or cancers; particularly elevated eosinophils are found with intestinal parasites; noninfectious conditions.	Blood: 1% to 3% 50-500/mm³ BAL negative for infection CSF <10 mm³	Because of the nonspecific nature of blood eosinophilia, it can require further clinical investigation to determine the causal agent.

Food Intolerance/Sensitivity Panels

ALCAT	Measurement of leukocyte cellular reactivity in whole blood, measures levels of mediators by blood cells presented with food or chemical antigens; measures relative changes in cell size.	Food and chemical non-IgE sensitivity (intolerance) testing for up to 350 foods plus gliadin/gluten, casein/whey, and *Candida albicans*; food additives, molds, environmental chemicals, pharmacoactive agents, and other suspected items upon request.	350 Foods: Acceptable Foods Normal = no response Mild intolerance Moderate intolerance Severe intolerance Candida/gluten-gliadin/casein-whey, chemicals/molds: No reaction mild, moderate, or severe reaction.	NSAIDS, glucocorticoids, vitamin C, bioflavonoids can suppress the immunologic response and promote a false negative. IgA used as a biomarker reference of adequate immune response.
MRT (immunologic food reaction test)	Untreated whole blood assay; sample is divided into 150 aliquots plus control samples and incubated with a precise dilution of pure extract of a specific food or food additive[c] (see Chapter 25).	Non IgE-mediated reactions; measurement of blood components; blood specimen checked against the specific signs of cell-mediated reactivity to the antigen challenged (imminent or actual mediator release).	Normal = no response Mild, moderate, or severe reactions are delineated.	NSAIDS, glucocorticoids, vitamin C, bioflavonoids can suppress the immunologic response and promote a false negative. IgA used as a biomarker of adequate immune response.
Celiac Panel/ Gluten Sensitivity Panel	1. Immunologic and genomic for celiac or gluten sensitivity– related genes.	Measurements to identify a possible genetic or immunologic disease of the small bowel in response to exposure to gluten or gliadin molecules in diet. Continued long-term exposure to gluten or gliadin molecules leads to nutrient deficiencies and insufficiencies.	See celiac tests 2-10.	Any of the celiac tests 2-10 should be compared with baseline IgA serum levels and presence of immune suppressive medications to rule out IgA deficiency, which can skew test results to false negative because of compromised or suppressed immune response. Undiagnosed celiac is associated with increased incidence of all chronic diseases and shortened life span.[10,11,12]
	2. EMA	High specificity for celiac disease; may obviate need for small bowel biopsy for diagnosis; become negative on gluten-free diet.	EMA negative	Sensitivity/Specificity 90+%/95%
	3. tTG-IgA, tTG-IgG	Autoantigen of celiac disease, tTG is indicative of villous atrophy secondary to gluten exposure causing damage to GI small intestine villi. tTG negative test results indicate gluten-free diet compliance; marker of restoration of GI villi tight junctions and small bowel villi integrity.	tTG-IgA negative tTG-IgG negative	Sensitivity/specificity 98%/95% in adults; 96%/99% in children. Best age to begin measuring tTG is age 2-3 years.[13]
	4. AGA IgA, AGA IgG)	Positive results are evidence of immune response to the gliadin proteins in gluten-containing foods.	AGA IgA negative AGA IgG negative	Lowest sensitivity among celiac panel (70%-85%) and specificity (70%-90%) for celiac. Also useful for nonceliac gluten sensitivity.
	5. DGP	DGP antibodies improves[14] diagnostic accuracy for diagnosis of CD when tested with tTG; proteins present in the submucosa of affected person's bond to deamidated peptides to form molecular complexes that stimulate the immune system.	DGP negative	Specificity varied between 97.3% and 99.3%. Sensitivity of IgG anti-DGP significantly better than that of IgG anti-tTG (p < 0.05). Specificity was significantly better than IgA and IgG AGA.[15]

Continued

6. Celiac genetic HLA haplotype HLA-DQ2 HLA-DQ8 Cellular assay/MLC to test HLA class II types	HLA-DQ2 and HLA-DQ8 positive indicates a low positive predictive value but a very high negative predictive value for celiac disease. Higher prevalence of CD in patients with type 1 DM or autoimmune thyroid disease (2%-4%) than in general population.	Genotype: HLA DQ2 negative HLA DQ8 negative	More than 97% of individuals with celiac disease share the two HLA markers DQ2 and DQ8, which have high sensitivity and poor specificity. One of the markers can increase possible nonceliac gluten sensitivity (e.g., type 1 DM DQA1*0501:DQB1*0201 haplotype).[14,15,16]
7. Wheat/gluten proteome reactivity & autoimmunity	Functional medicine serum laboratory tests to broaden the view of celiac and gluten sensitivity by assessing antibody production against an array of protein, enzyme, and peptide antigens; includes *glutens, lectins, opioids,* and the enzyme *glutamic decarboxylase* (GAD65) IgG, IgA. Available from https://www .cyrexlabs.com.	ELISA Index Wheat IgG 0.30-1.30 mcg/mL IgA 0.40-2.40 mg/dL Agglutinin IgG 0.30-1.50 mcg/mL IgA 0.90-1.90 mg/dL Alpha Gliadin 17 MER IgG 0.30-1.50 mcg/mL IgA 0.60-2.00 mg/dL Alpha Gliadin 33 MER IgG 0.30-1.40 mcg/mL IgA 0.60-1.80 mg/dL Gamma Gliadin 15 MER Omega Gliadin IgG 0.50-1.60 mcg/mL IgA 0.60-1.80 mg/dL Glutenin IgG 0.20-1.50 mcg/mL IgA 0.50-1.70 mg/dL Gluteomorphin IgG 0.30-1.50 mcg/mL IgA 0.60-1.80 mg/dL Prodynorphin IgG 0.40-1.70 mcg/mL IgA 0.60-1.80 mg/dL GAD65 IgG 0.40-1.30 mcg/mL IgA 0.80-1.50 mg/dL	Enhances clinical sensitivity and specificity in detection of celiac and gluten sensitivity reactions.
8. Gluten-associated cross-reactive foods and foods sensitivity IgG + IgA combined Cow's milk Alpha-casein & beta-casein Casomorphin Milk butyrophilin American cheese Chocolate (Others available)	Functional medicine serum laboratory tests to assess IgG and IgA immune antibody reactions to known cross-reactive food antigens, with the most common being casein. Other foods included are sesame, hemp, rye, barley, wheat, buckwheat, sorghum, millet, spelt, amaranth, quinoa, yeast, tapioca, oats, coffee, corn, rice, potato.	ELISA Index: IgG & IgA combined 0.20 mcg/mL /0.40 mg/ dL -1.80 mcg/mL/ 2.00 mg/dL	Assists further dietary evaluation for celiac or gluten sensitive individuals that are nonresponsive to a gluten-free diet; can relate to gut dysbiosis and continued GI inflammation. Available from https://www.cyrex-labs.com.

III. Tests of Carbohydrate Absorption

Lactose Intolerance

Hydrogen Breath Test for Lactose (HBT-lactose)	Lactose loading (2 g/kg) in lactase deficiency allows bacterial metabolism of lactose with production of H_2 gas. Breath analyzed for H_2 by gas chromatography.	Breath H_2 measured fasting and 0.5 and 2 hours after dosing with lactose; a significant increase is associated with malabsorption.	Normal increase: <50 parts/million (i.e., <50 ppm) Lactose intolerance: 50 ppm or greater	Bacterial overgrowth can cause false-positive results; consumption of soluble fiber or legumes and smoking are associated with H_2 production; false-negative results caused by antibiotics.

Lactose Tolerance Test	Lactose loading (50 g) followed by blood sampling at 5, 10, 30, 60, 90, and 120 min after dose; glucose produced from lactose is assayed.	Lactase deficiency associated with <20 mg/dL increase in serum glucose.	Normal serum glucose Lactose increase >20 mg/dL	Test is not specific (many false positives) or sensitive (many false negatives).
Fructose Intolerance				
Hydrogen Breath Test-Fructose (HBT-fructose)	An assessment for the change in the level of hydrogen and/or methane gas is diagnostic for fructose malabsorption.	HBT-fructose can be used to diagnose a mutation in the aldolase B gene. If hereditary fructose intolerance, may result in GI symptoms and hypoglycemia.	Normal increase <20 parts/million (<20 ppm) Positive HBT-fructose >20 parts per million (>20 ppm)	Positive test results indicate probable benefit of a fructose-restricted diet; research supports use in abdominal pain, IBS, gout.
Fructose Sensitivity	Blood lymphocyte specimen grown with a mitogen to measure growth by incorporating tritiated radioactive thymidine into the DNA of the cells. A functional test of fructose metabolism.	Functional intracellular metabolic test of possible genetic errors compromising fructose metabolism like fructose-6-phosphate.	>34% patient's growth response test media measured by DNA synthesis compared with optimal growth observed in 100% media (valid for male and female of 12 years or older)	Rule out fructose sensitivity in hypoglycemia of unknown etiology, overweight, obesity.
IV. Tests of Lipid Status				
Lipids				
CHOL, Total Serum or Plasma	CHOL is enzymatically released from cholesterol esters; fasting test.	Total CHOL correlated with risk for cardiovascular diseases.	AHA/ACC/NHLBI 2014 Guidelines do not have target levels for CHOL. Generally <200 mg/dL is desirable (see Chapter 32).	CHOL measurements have considerable within subject variability. May partly result from variability in specimen collection or handling.
HDL-c	LDL-c (and VLDL-c) are precipitated from the serum before measurement of residual HDL-c particle size; direct measurement of HDL-c is now done in some laboratories.	HDL-c is called "good cholesterol" to indicate that it is protective against atherosclerotic vascular development.	Generally levels should be above 40 mg/dL. The higher the better.	Some precipitation methods cause underestimation of HDL; HDL can be divided into classes: HDL_1, HDL_2, and HDL_3; elevated HDL_3 correlates with risk of CVD.
LDL-c	LDL-c is estimated by the Friedewald formula, LDL-c = total CHOL − HDL-c − TG/5, or by new direct assays. Available lipid particle size testing examples: https://www.privateMDLab.com (VAP Lipid Profile) https://www.BerkeleyHeartLab.com	LDL-c is called "bad cholesterol" to indicate that it is a positive risk factor for CVD. See NCEP guidelines in Chapter 32. LPP size: Pattern B (small, dense LDL-c) is associated with increased risk of CHD and is responsive to diet. Pattern A (larger, buoyant LDL) is not associated with risk. LPP are not recommended in new ATP4.	Generally, below 130 mg/dL is considered desirable.	Calculation only valid when TG concentration is <400 mg/dL, cannot be determined in nonfasting serum or plasma. Direct assay methods preferred.
TGs	Lipases release glycerol and fatty acids from TGs.	The association of TGs and CHD has been shown. Elevated TG increases blood viscosity.	<150 mg/dL normal >500 mg/dL high	Fasting specimen is essential; sugar concentrated foods and alcohol ingestion can increase TG level; some anticoagulants may affect TG level; carnitine-dependent fatty acids synthesis.
Fat Malabsorption				
Fecal Fat Screening	Microscopic inspection of fat-stained (Sudan stain) specimens for the presence of lipid droplets.	Trained observers are able to identify excessive fat in ~80% of persons with fat malabsorption.	Qualitative results	Patient must be consuming sufficient fat for analysis to reveal malabsorption. Semiquantitative.

Continued

PT	Fat malabsorption decreases absorption of fat-soluble vitamins A, E, D, K, beta-carotene; low vitamin K levels impair coagulation, causing a prolonged PT (also can be called international normalized ratio [INR]).	A prolonged PT is a relatively sensitive but nonspecific indicator of the fat-soluble vitamin K from fat malabsorption.	10-15 sec INR: 0.8-1.1 Possible critical value: >20 sec INR: >5.5	Tests affected by oral anticoagulants and other drugs, reduced platelet count, acquired and hereditary bleeding diseases, and liver disease PT.
Quantitative Fecal Fat Determination	Patient must consume 100 g fat/day (4-8 oz whole milk/day, and 2 Tbsp vegetable oil/meal/day) for 2 days before collection.	Quantitative 72-hour stool collection required for accurate assessment; average daily discharge used for interpretation.	Normal: <5 g fat/24 hr Malabsorption: >10 g/24 hr	Failure to adhere to the diet invalidates the results.
Vitamin A, D, E, K	See V. Tests of Micronutrient Status.			
Fatty Acid Analysis	Whole blood or RBC levels of ALA (C18:3n3) and LA (C18:2n6) reflect essential fatty acid status; also, complex relationships regarding fatty acid analysis are related to neurologic and inflammatory diseases, cell membrane dysfunction and genetic disorders.[17,18]	RBC fatty acid shown to be associated with fatty acid tissue composition. Plasma fatty acid levels are associated with dietary fat or supplement intake or fat digestion and absorption.	AA/EPA = 1.5-3.0 = Normal AA/EPA = High Risk >15 Omega-3 (EP+DHA) Index Risk: Index <2.2 High Index 2.2-3.2 Moderate Index >3.2 Low Omega-6/Omega-3 Ratio 5.7-21 EPA/AA Ratio </= 0.2 AA 520-1490 nmol/mL 5.2-12.9% EPA 14-100 nmol/mL 0.2-1.5% DHA 30-250 nmol/mL 0.2-3.9% GLA 16-150 nmol/mL Omega-6:omega-3 optimal between 1:1 and 4:1.	Is not specific for risk of atherosclerotic disease; inflammation influences this fatty acid test. Likely causes are minor injuries, trauma, and bacterial infections, periodontal/cavitations, orodental disease,[19] *Chlamydia pneumoniae*,[20] dietary fats, and central adiposity.[21]

V. Tests of Micronutrient Status
A. Vitamins

Thiamin (B$_1$)[c]	Thiamin status is usually assessed by measuring the amount of TPP needed to fully activate the RBC enzyme transketolase.	The TPP needed to fully activate transketolase is inversely related to B$_1$ status; percent stimulation by TTP.	Normal: 70-200 nmol/L (for individuals not taking (B$_1$) Stimulation >20% (index >1.2) indicates deficiency	Amount (and activity) of enzyme affected by drugs, iron, folate, or vitamin B$_{12}$ status, malignant or GI diseases, and diabetes.
Riboflavin (B$_2$)	Riboflavin status is assessed by measuring the amount of FAD needed to fully activate RBC enzyme GR.	The FAD needed to fully activate GR is inversely related to B$_2$ status; percent stimulation.	% Stimulation >40% (index >1.4) indicates deficiency	Amount or activity of enzyme may change with age, iron status, liver disease, and glucose-6-phosphate dehydrogenase deficiency.
Niacin (B$_3$)	Urinary excretion of N^1 - NMN is decreased; <0.8 mg/day (<5.8 μmol/day) suggests a niacin deficiency.	Blood: Liquid Chromatography/Tandem Mass Spectrometry (LC/MS/MS). Niacin (nicotinic acid) is a water-soluble vitamin that is also referred to as vitamin B$_3$.	Nicotinic acid: 0.0-5.0 ng/mL Nicotinamide: 5.2-72.1 ng/mL	Niacin (nicotinic acid) is a water-soluble vitamin that is also referred to as vitamin B$_3$. Nicotinamide (nicotinic acid amide) is the derivative of niacin.

Pyridoxine (B₆)ᵉ PLP (pyridoxal-5-phosphate) compounds	1. RBC enzymes, ALT (SGPT) or AST (SGOT),ᵉ are assayed for the presence of PLP as the enzyme's cofactor.	1. Difference between enzyme activities before and after addition of PLP is inversely related to B₆ status.	1. % ALT stimulation of >25% or AST activity of >50% in deficiency.	1. Disease and drugs that affect the liver and heart, and pregnancy confound interpretation.
	2. Plasma PLP can be directly measured by HPLC with fluorescence detection.	2. PLP is major transport form of B₆; therefore serum levels reflect body stores.	2. Normal: 0.50-3.0 mcg/dL (20-120 nmol/L) Male: 5.3-46.7 μg/L Female: 2.0-32.8 μg/L	2. Deficiency may be seen clinically before plasma PLP levels decrease.
	3. Trp load test, measures excretion of the PLP-dependent metabolite XA. 24-hour urine collection required.	3. Functional test indicating marginal vitamin B₆ status when the levels of urinary XA decrease significantly following the ingestion of 3-5 g of L-Trp.	3. Marginal status: Level of urinary XA decreases <50 mg/24 hr	3. Steroid drugs and estrogen enzyme activity and some drugs cause analytic errors. Trp load test most sensitive and responsive to functional adequacy of B₆.
Folateᵍ	1. Because of ↓ DNA synthesis, large RBCs are produced. See Chapter 31.	1. Deficiency leads to increase in MCV and macrocytic RBCs.	1. Normal: MCV 80-100 fL	1. Not sensitive or specific for folate. Possible involvement with B₆, B₁₂, SAMe, and other cofactors in the methionine pathway.
	2. Shape of neutrophil nucleus affected by folate deficiency.	2. Increased neutrophil lobe count seen in folate deficiency.	2. Normal: < or equal 4 lobes per neutrophil	2. Lobe count sensitive but not specific.
	3. Blood folate levels can be directly measured by radioimmunoassay.	3. Both RBC and serum folate are indicators of body stores.	3. 2-10 mcg/L serum; 140-960 ng/L RBC (3.2-22 nmol/L)	3. Plasma from nonfasting subjects may reflect recent intake; RBC folate is not measured accurately.
	4. Functional folate status assayed by FIGLU in 24-hour urine or after oral histidine loading.	4. After 2-15 g loading dose, 10-50 mg of FIGLU should be excreted in 8 hours.	4. Normal: <7.4 mg/24 hours (<42.6 mmol/24 hr) without loading	4. FIGLU affected by vitamin B₁₂, drugs, liver disease, cancer, tuberculosis, and pregnancy.
	5. SNPs MTHFR 677C, MTHFR 1298C	5. SNPs of compromised methylation (transfer of methyl groups in metabolism) potential in use and conversion of folate or folic acid intracellularly. See Chapter 6.	MTHF 677C/1298C Normal = Wild type −/−	Other SNPs are known that affect methylation metabolism: COMT, CYP1B1, and other cytochrome enzymes. See Chapter 6.
Cobalamin (B₁₂)	1. Because of low B₁₂ resulting in decreased DNA synthesis, large RBCs are produced.	1. Deficiency leads to increase in MCV.	1. Normal: MCV 80-100 fL	1. Not sensitive or specific for B₁₂.
	2 Shape of neutrophil nucleus is affected by B₁₂ deficiency.	2. Increased neutrophil lobe count in B₁₂ deficiency.	2. Normal: < or equal 4 lobes per neutrophil	2. Lobe count sensitive but not specific.
	3. B₁₂ can be directly measured by radioimmunoassay.	3. Levels <150 ng/L indicate deficiency (age affects level).	3. 160-950 pg/mL (118-701 pmol/L)	3. Marginal deficiency not correlated with level.
	4. MMA excretion reflects a functional test of B₁₂ availability for BCAA metabolism.	4. MMA excretion >300 mg/24 hr in B₁₂ deficiency. Sensitive test without being overly specific.	4. Normal excretion: 5 mg/24 hr (42 mmol/24 hr) Serum MMA - 0.08-0.56 mmol/L (Normal < 105 ng/mL)	4. Specific for B₁₂ but requires normal BCAA levels; available at most laboratories.
	5. Schilling test for intrinsic factor and B₁₂ absorption assesses radiolabeled B₁₂ absorption as reflected by urinary excretion.	5. Abnormal B₁₂ absorption indicated by excretion <3% of B₁₂ radioactivity per 24 hours.	5. Normal excretion: ~8% of radioactivity per 24 hours	5. Test must be repeated with oral administration of IF to differentiate IF deficiency and malabsorption. Rarely used because of necessity of radioactive B₁₂.
	6. Homocysteine (Hcy)	Hcy level is an independent risk factor for CVD, venous thrombotic disease, and other diseases; folic acid and vitamins B₁₂ and B₆ reduce plasma Hcy levels. Total Hcy (oxidized + reduced forms) is an intermediate amino acid in methionine metabolism.	Normal: 4-14 mmol/L Suggested optimal levels: 4-7 mmol/L	Cardiovascular event risk is increased even at slightly elevated levels. Hcy has a strong association with degenerative neurologic conditions like Parkinson's disease and dementias. Hcy suggests poor methylating capacity of client with need for increased intake of folic acid, B₆, B₁₂, and SAMe.

Continued

Ascorbic Acid (vitamin C)	Plasma or leukocyte vitamin C measured by (1) chromatography; (2) by ascorbate oxidase; (3) spectrophotometrically by reaction with 2,4-dinitrophenylhydrazine.	Leukocyte C is less affected by recent intake, but plasma levels in fasting person parallel leukocyte levels; plasma preferred for acutely ill patients because leukocyte level is affected by infection,[22] some drugs, and hyperglycemia.	Normal: 0-11 months: Not established 1-12 years: 0.2-2.3 mg/dL 13+ years: 0.2-2.0 mg/dL (30-80 mmol/L) Adult: 0.2-1.5 mg/dL (12-90 mmol/L) Leukocyte vitamin C: 20-50 mcg/10^8	Blood samples must be carefully prepared for assay to prevent vitamin C breakdown. Oxalate, glucose, and proteins interfere with some assays; recent intake can mask deficiency.
Retinols (vitamin A)	Serum retinol and retinol esters; functional tests (e.g., dark adaptation) only detect severe deficiency; age and sex are important determining factors for normal retinol levels.	Retinol levels <20 mcg/dL (<0.7 mmol/L) indicate severe deficiency; specific levels are being determined for placental/newborn deficiency serum levels.	Normal: 20-100 mcg/dL (0.7-3.5 mmol/L) Suboptimum (NHANES II/ Gibson): Age 3-11 y: < 0.35 mmol/L Age 12-17 y <0.70 mmol/L Age 18-74 y 0.70-1.05 mmol/L Pregnancy 0.79-1.91 mmol/L Upper Limit: 3.5 mmol\L	Exposure of serum to bright light or oxygen destroys vitamin A; low RBP level is associated with low vitamin A, zinc, and iron (see protein-energy section). Vitamin A's gene transcription is on the nuclear RXR;[22] the vitamin D receptor forms a heterodimer, requiring balance between vitamins A and D for optimum function.
Carotenoids (CARO)	CARO, fat-soluble pigments in plant foods, poorly absorbed in fat malabsorption; light sensitive; transport specimen in amber transport tube; quantitative spectrophotometry testing.	A CARO level of less than 50 mg/dL is seen in ~85% of patients with fat malabsorption.	50-200 mcg/dL (0.74-3.72 mmol/L)	Decreased CARO levels or low spectrophotometry score are also seen in those with low vegetable and fruit diets (e.g., in PN or tube feeding), liver failure, celiac disease, cystic fibrosis, human immunodeficiency virus, and some lipoprotein disorders.
Tocopherols (vitamin E)	Serum alpha- and beta-gamma tocopherols serve different antioxidant functions. Growing evidence that beta and gamma tocopherols may be more important than alpha-tocopherol for human vitamin E nutrition.	Lower values found in infants. Interpretation requires monitoring lipid levels; if hyperlipidemia calculate plasma alpha-tocopherol: cholesterol mmol/L ratio <2.2 or alpha-tocopherol <5 mg/L indicates risk of vitamin E deficiency.[23]	Normal: alpha-tocopherol 5.7-20 mg/L beta-gamma tocopherol 4.3 or less mg/L	Plasma level depends on recent intake and level of lipids, especially TGs, in blood. Smoking and BMI also negatively affect tocopherol levels.
Cholecalciferol (D_3) and (D_2) ergocalciferol	1. Alkaline phosphatase activity reflects level of bone activity and indirectly vitamin D status (see further discussion of ALP in Liver Enzymes section).		1. Adult: 25-100 U/L Child 1-12 yr: <350 U/L	1. Not specific, but a sensitive indicator; serum Ca and PO_4 should also be evaluated. Zinc and B_{12} are rate-limiting cofactors for production of alkaline phosphatase, therefore low levels of < 40 U/L suggest possible zinc or B_{12} or intrinsic factor insufficiencies.
	2. Cholecalciferol (D_3 25-OH-D) and ergocalciferol (D_2 25-OH-D).	2. <20 ng/mL (<50 nmol/L) indicates deficiency; >200 ng/mL (500 nmol/L) indicates hypervitaminosis D.	2. 30-100 ng/mL (75-250 nmol/L)	2. Best indicator of status (liver stores), but marginal levels are hard to interpret.[24] Increased BMI and body fat % may reduce serum D_3 25-OH-D.
	3. Calcitriol (1,25[OH]$_2$$D_3$)	3. Used to show that vitamin D metabolism is occurring normally; active vitamin D to signal nuclear RXR receptor.	3. 2.5-4.5 ng/dL (60-108 pmol/L) (little seasonal change)	3. Poor indicator of status because of tight control of synthesis independent of body stores.

25-hydroxyvitamin D (25-OH-D)/ Calcifediol/ Calcidiol	Prohormone vitamin D malabsorption can lead to secondary malabsorption of calcium. Vitamin D supplementation can lead to increased absorption of calcium and phosphorus; supplementation contraindicated for individuals with kidney or gall stones, sarcoidosis, tuberculosis, lymphoma, or when hypercalcemic with vitamin D supplementation.	Vitamin D insufficiency is defined as the lowest threshold value for plasma 25-OH-D that prevents secondary hyperparathyroidism, bone turnover, bone mineral loss, or seasonal variations in plasma PTH.	25-OH-D: 30-100 ng/mL (85-160 nmol/L) Deficiency: <20 ng/mL (<50 nmol/L (laboratory references vary per individual laboratory)	Available at all laboratories. If elevated serum calcium, further evaluation recommended by testing vitamin 1,25 D-OH, PTH, ionized or free calcium, vitamin A retinol, and osteocalcin (as a vitamin K2 marker) before supplementation.
Phylloquinone (K_1) and Menaquinone (K_2) Menadione (K_3)	Normal coagulation factor synthesis requires K_1; PT assesses coagulation status. K_2 primarily involved with calcium metabolism, including bone health.	In K_1 deficiency, PT increases with increasing production of abnormal coagulation factors.[h] K_1 vegetable plant source; drug-nutrient interaction with blood thinners. K_2 animal and bacterial fermented sources. K_3 synthetic form of Vitamin K; vitamin precursor to Vitamin K_2 known as a provitamin.	K_1: 0.13-1.19 ng/mL (0.29-2.64 nmol/L K_2: (not commercially available—see K_2 marker, Osteocalcin, below)	The level of vitamin K available for vitamin K–dependent bone proteins may not be reflected by the PT; test references vary significantly with method.
OC/ucOC (K_2 marker)	Serum noncollagenous protein specific for bone and dentin formation and turnover. Functional marker of vitamin K_2, a rate-limiting cofactor of formation of osteocalcin. One of the osteocalcin fragments, undercarboxylated osteocalcin, is most sensitive K_2 marker and associated with risk of fracture.	Can be used as a marker of metabolic trend, suggesting low or high vitamin K_2; useful in assessing need for a vitamin K_2-rich diet or K_2 supplementation to optimize formation of intracellular bone osteocalcin. K_2 inhibits soft tissue calcification. OC and ucOC are considered more sensitive markers of bone activity than alkaline phosphatase during corticosteroid therapy.	OC: 11-50 ng/mL ucOC: Normal <1.65 ng/mL High >1.65 ng/mL NOTE: Elevated levels associated with low 25-OH-D levels	Vitamin K_2 is not as involved with coagulation as K_1. Vitamin K_2 is important in calcium metabolism and therefore calcium and vitamin D status. There is a synthetic vitamin K_3, usually administered IV that has similar actions as K_2, and is being used as adjunctive to integrative cancer therapy.

B. Minerals

Electrolytes

Sodium (Na^+) Potassium (K^+) Chloride (Cl^-) Bicarbonate or total CO_2	Serum electrolytes, including bicarbonate, are usually measured together by ion-specific electrodes in autoanalyzers; sometimes Na and K are measured by flame emission spectrophotometry.[i]	Elevated serum Na seen in water loss; decreased serum Na and K occurs in diarrhea and with poor dietary intake or cellular uptake. Decreased chloride levels are seen with cation and osmotic changes in the body. Bicarbonate levels reflect acid-base balance.	Na: 135-145 mEq/L (135-145 mmol/L) K: 3.5-5 mEq/L (3.5-5 mmol/L) Cl: 100-110 mEq/L (100-110 mmol/L) Bicarb or total CO_2: 21-30 mEq/L (21-30 mmol/L)	Electrolytes change rapidly in response to changes in physiology (e.g., hormonal stimulus, renal and other organ dysfunction, acid-base balance changes, and drug action). Serum electrolytes are minimally affected by diet.

Major Minerals

Calcium (Ca^{2+})	1. Total serum Ca^{2+} (bound and unbound)	Usually slightly more than half of the serum Ca^{2+} is bound to ALB or complexed with other molecules; the remaining Ca^{2+} is called *ionized Ca (ICA)*; ICA is available physiologically. Elevated IgE and mast cell release increases intracellular calcium ion levels and negatively distributes ICA.	1. 8.6-10 mg/dL (2.15-2.5 mmol/L)	Calcium status is related to many factors, including vitamin D, vitamin K_2, phosphate, parathyroid function, renal function; medications (thiazide diuretics, lithium), vitamin A toxicity, presence of malignancy.

Continued

	2. Ionized (free) Ca^{2+}	Interpretation of ionized calcium levels requires consideration of other related markers: osteocalcin, vitamin D25-OH-D and D1,25-OH-D, and serum retinol (vitamin A).	2. 4.64-5.28 mg/dL (1.16-1.32 mmol/L)	Ionized calcium depends on vitamin K_2 to enter the bone matrix and to prevent calcification of soft tissue. If phosphate <3.0 mg/dL, check intake of phosphate-binding medications.
Phosphate (H_2PO_4, (Phosphorus)	Phosphorus in body as phosphate form; test measures inorganic phosphate. Most phosphate is part of organic compounds; small part is inorganic.	Abnormal P level is most closely associated with disturbed intake, distribution, or renal function.	1. 7-4.5 mg/dL (0.87-1.45 mmol/L) (higher in children)	Reported as phosphorus (P), not phosphate; hemolyzed blood cannot be used because of high RBC phosphate levels.
Magnesium (Mg^{2+})	1. Total serum Mg^{2+} measured after reaction to form chromogenic or fluorescent complexes.	Neuromuscular function. Hyperirritability, tetany, convulsion, and electrocardiographic changes occur when levels of total serum Mg^{2+} fall to <1 mEq/L.	1. 1.3-2.5 mEq/L (0.65-1.25 mmol/L)	Usually 45% of the serum Mg^{2+} is complexed with other molecules; the remaining Mg^{2+} is called ionized magnesium. Serum levels remain constant until body stores are nearly depleted.
	2. Ionized (free) Mg^{2+}		2. 0.7-1.2 mEq/L (0.35-0.60 mmol/L)	
Trace Minerals				
Iron CBC[k] and RBC indices	1. HCT = % RBC in whole blood 2. Hgb = blood hemoglobin concentration 3. MCV = mean RBC volume = mean corpuscular volume	A CBC with RBC indices is one of the first set of tests that a patient receives; although CBC data are not specific for nutrition status, their universal and repeated presence in the patient's record makes them very important.	1. Females: 35%-47% (0.35-0.47)[l] Males: 42%-52% (0.42-0.52) 2. Females: 12-15 g/dL (7.45-9.31 mmol/L) Males: 14-17 g/dL (8.44-10.6 mmol/L) 3. 82-99 mm³ (82-99 fL)	These tests are affected only when iron stores are essentially depleted. HCT and Hgb are sensitive to hydration status; low MCV also occurs in thalassemias and lead poisoning as well as with iron and copper deficiencies; high MCV suggests macrocytic RBCs and possible inadequate folate, vitamins B_6, or B_{12}.
Serum Iron (Fe)	Serum Fe^{3+} reduced to Fe^{2+} and then complexed with chromogen.	Slightly higher in males than in premenopausal females; reflects recent Fe intake.	F: 40-150 mcg/dL (7.2-26.9 mmol/L) M: 50-160 mg/dL (8.9-28.7 mmol/L)	Very insensitive index of total Fe stores; extremely variable (day-to-day and diurnal).
TIBC	TIBC determined by saturating serum transferrin with Fe and then remeasuring serum Fe.	Reflects transferrin concentration.	250-400 mcg/dL (45-71 mmol/L)	TIBC does not increase until Fe stores are essentially completely depleted. TIBC decreases with increased Fe stores; used to rule out excess iron intake or hemochromatosis. See Chapter 31.
Tf or TFN	The iron-bound globulin protein that responds to the need for iron; half-life ~9 days (see Chapter 5)	(see Section I:A. Protein Status: Tf)	Females: 250-380 mg/dL (2.15-3.80 g/L) Males: 215-365 mg/dL (2.15-3.65 g/L) Newborn: 130-275 mg/dL Child: 203-360 mg/dL	Transferrin is low when Fe stores essentially depleted. Transferrin is low with low vitamin B_6 and low Tf-sat in aplastic anemia.
Tf-sat or TSAT	Tf-sat (%) = Serum iron level ÷ TIBC x 100%	(see Section I:A. Protein Status: Tf-sat)	Females: 15%-50% Males: 20%-50% Chronic illness - normal Tf-sat%. Late pregnancy low Tf-sat%.	
RDW	Measurement of variation in RBC diameter (anisocytosis); reported to be helpful in distinguishing Fe deficiency from anemia associated with chronic inflammation.	Very sensitive indicator of Fe status; normal RDW reportedly rules out anemia caused by chronic inflammatory diseases.[m] Thalassemia (low MCV, normal RDW) differentiated from iron-deficiency (low MCV, high RDW).	Normal value: 11.0-14.5% Microscopic electronic interpretation required.	Specificity of RDW for Fe deficiency is relatively low; interpretation confounded by RBC transfusion; measurement usually not reported.

Ferritin	The primary intracellular Fe storage protein; stored mostly in liver; serum levels parallel iron stores.	Best biochemical index of uncomplicated iron deficiency or overload (iron toxicity) and excess storage. Rule out hemochromatosis or pancreatitis if Ferritin >1000 ng/dL (>1000 mcg/L).	Iron overload: >400 ng/mL (mcg/L) With anemia of chronic disease: <100 ng/mL (<100 mcg/L) F: 10-150 ng/mL (10-150 mcg/L) M: 12-300 ng/mL (12-300 mcg/L) Females with anemia of chronic disease: <20 ng/mL (<20 mcg/L) 6 mo-15 yr: 7-142 ng/mL (7-142 mcg/L) <1 mo-5 mo: 50-200 ng/mL (50-200 mcg/L) Newborn: 25-200 ng/mL (25-200 mcg/L)	A positive acute phase reactant that increases during metabolic response to injury, even when Fe stores are adequate; not useful in anemia of chronic and inflammation diseases.
Zinc (Zn)[n]	Serum levels measured by atomic absorption spectrophotometry.	Serum levels affected by diet and the inflammatory response. Zn deficiency associated with many diseases and trauma.	0.7-1.2 mg/L (11-18 mmol/L)	Serum levels detect frank—but not marginal—deficiency; blood must be collected in Zn-free tubes.
Copper (Cu)	1. Serum levels measured by flame emission atomic AS or ICP/MS.	1. Cu deficiency is associated with neutropenia, anemia, and scurvy-like bone disease and megadoses of Zn (excess Zn suppresses Cu blood and tissue levels).	Adult: 85-150 mcg/dL (13.4-23.6 μmol/L)	1. Serum levels detect frank but not marginal deficiency; use of oral contraceptives lowers serum Cu.
	2. Ceruloplasmin is the major Cu-bound containing plasma protein; measured by immunoassay (e.g., nephelometry).	2. Ceruloplasmin is required for conversion of Fe^{3+} to Fe^{2+} during cellular Fe uptake. Anemia and/or neutropenia can result from low ceruloplasmin. Ceruloplasmin is useful biomarker to follow TM copper chelation for Wilson's Disease (ATP7B gene mutation) and cancer antiangiogenesis copper chelation therapy.[25]	27-50 mg/dL (1.5-2.8 mmol/L)	2. Ceruloplasmin not a useful marker of Cu status, but can be used to assess changes in status after supplementation; useful to calculate free Cu index with serum Cu and serum Zn as potential cancer biomarker.
Selenium (Se)	1. Serum Se test 2. Whole blood levels better reflect long-term status.	Margin between deficiency and toxicity is narrower for Se than any other trace component of the antioxidant enzyme element; important in glutathione peroxidase.	1. 80-320 mcg/L (1-4 mmol/L) 2. 60-340 mcg/L (0.75-4.3 mmol/L)	Cutoff points for deficiency or toxicity are not well established.
Iodine (I)	Urinary excretion is best indicator of I status, either mcg/24 hr or mcg/g creatinine; thyroid hormone level related to I status. Urine test can use 50 mg I/KI challenge.	Excretion should be 24-hour urine >70 mcg/g creatinine. It can be beneficial to test thyroid hormone and antibodies (TSH, T_3-free, T_4-free, thyroid peroxidase, and thyroglobulin antibodies) for improved interpretation. I important for other metabolic functions.	No urinary I reference range; T_4 reference range: F: 5-12 mcg/dL (64-154 mmol/L) M: 4-12 mcg/dL (51-154 mmol/L)	Thyroid hormone levels are affected by many factors besides iodine status. Other halogen elements (Br^+, Fl^+, Cl^+) are known antagonists to iodine metabolism; when completing the iodine urine testing, some laboratories will also test for bromine, fluorine, and chlorine.

Continued

Creatinine (Cr)	Urinary excretion usually tested by atomic absorption spectrophotometry.	Excretion should be 0.63-2.50 g/24 hr; deficiency reported in patients on long-term PN; decreased levels in diabetes mellitus.	10-200 ng/dL (1.9-38 nmol/L)	Test not available in most clinical laboratories; special handling required to prevent specimen contamination during collection.

VI. Blood Gases and Hydration Status

pH	$pH = -\log[H^+]$; H^+ depends mainly on the CO_2 from respiration: $CO_2 + H_2O \rightleftarrows H_2CO_3 \rightleftarrows HCO_3 + H^+$ Measured by ion-selective electrodes (like those found in common pH meters).	Acidosis: pH <7.35 Alkalosis: pH >7.45 pH compatible with life: 6.80-7.80	Whole blood: Arterial pH: 7.35-7.45 Venous pH: 7.32-7.42	Blood must not be exposed to air before or during measurement.
Po$_2$ and O$_2$ saturation (SaO$_2$)	Whole blood O_2 measured by oxygen electrode. P_{O_2} = "pressure" contributed by O_2 to the total "pressure" of all the gases dissolved in blood. O_2 Content (CaO$_2$) = O_2/g SaO$_2$ x Hgb (g/dL) x 1.34 mL + PaO$_2$ x (.003 mL O_2/mm Hg/dL) $PaO_2 = Fio_2(PB-47) - 1.2(Paco_2)$	Affected by alveolar gas exchange, ventilation-perfusion inequalities, and generalized alveolar hypoventilation.	Arterial blood: PaO$_2$: 83-108 mm Hg <40 mm Hg = critical value (gravely dangerous) O_2 saturation: 0.95-0.98 (95%-98%) Elderly = 95% Newborn = 40%-90%	Blood must not be exposed to air before or during measurement.
Pco$_2$	Measured by ion-selective electrode; "pressure" contributed by CO_2 to the total "pressure" of all the gases dissolved in blood.	Increased in respiratory acidosis (increased CO_2 in inspired air or decreased in alveolar ventilation) and decreased in respiratory alkalosis (e.g., in hyperventilation from anxiety, mechanical ventilator, or closed head injury [damaged respiratory center]).	Whole blood: Arterial F: 32-45 mm Hg M: 35-48 mm Hg Venous 6-7 mm Hg higher	Blood must not be exposed to air before or during measurement.
Bicarbonate (HCO$_3^-$) and total CO$_2$ (tCO$_2$)	For whole blood (HCO$_3^-$) is calculated from the equation given in pH section.	Increased in compensated respiratory acidosis and in metabolic acidosis; decreased in metabolic acidosis and in compensated respiratory alkalosis.	Whole blood, arterial: 21-28 mEq/L (21-28 mmol/L)	Blood must not be exposed to air before or during measurement.
Osmolality (Osmol), serum	Osmol depends on the amount of particles (solutes) dissolved in a solution; measurement based on relationship between solute concentration and freezing point; serum osmol assesses hydration status and solute load.	Serum Osmol increases in dehydration, diabetic coma, diabetic ketoacidosis; also estimated from the formula: mOsmol/L = 2 (Na$^+$) + (Glucose mg/dL)/18 + (BUN mg/dL)/2.8	282-300 mOsm/kg H$_2$O (1 Osmol = 1 mol of solute particles; 1 kg serum/L)	Freezing point depression gives a more accurate estimate of osmol than the calculated value (e.g., in ketoacidosis).
Urinalysis: Sp.Gr.	Specimen midstream clean-catch if infection suspected, or regular collection. Dip Stick or laboratory testing for Sp.Gr.	One of a multiple of tests on a urine specimen. Sp.Gr. is a measure of concentration of particles and electrolytes in the urine.	Adult: 1.005-1.030 Sp.Gr. Newborn: 1.001-1.020 Sp.Gr.	Appearance can also give subjective indication of fluid concentration; darker color = higher concentration.

VII. Tests of Antioxidant Status and Oxidative Stress

Water-Soluble Compounds	See Vitamin C above.			
Lipid-Soluble Compounds: see Vitamin E, Carotenoids, and Coenzyme Q$_{10}$	The carotenoids: lutein, xanthine zeaxanthin, alpha- and beta-carotene, and lycopene; carotenoids and coenzyme Q$_{10}$ (ubiquinone-10) are measured chromatographically.	Reference ranges for these compounds vary greatly, depending on the method used for their assay.	See reference for carotenoid range under fat malabsorption.	Tests for carotenoids and coenzyme Q are not yet available for routine clinical use.

Total Antioxidant Capacity (e.g., ORAC, TEAC, FRAP)	ORAC: Oxygen radical absorbance capacity TEAC: Trolox-equivalent antioxidant capacity FRAP: Ferric-reducing ability of plasma.	These assays reflect the presence of all of plasma or serum antioxidants, including vitamins C and E, carotenoids, coenzyme $Q_{1}0$, glutathione, uric acid, bilirubin, superoxide dismutase, catalase, glutathione peroxidase, and ALB.		These assays are now commercially available but are currently performed only in specialized laboratories. Testing botanicals also available.
Oxidative Stress Markers:	Free radical oxidation products of lipids.	8-Isoprostane (also called 8-epiprostaglandin F_{2a}) increases in plasma or urine of patients with lung disease, hypercholesterolemia, or diabetes mellitus. 8HDG represents whole-body cytosolic and nuclear free radical activity, including status of DNA. Lipid peroxides is a marker of membrane oxidative damage by reactive oxygen species (ROS) to PUFAs of cell membranes.	Examples: *o*-tyrosine nitro-tyrosine 8-isoprostane 4-hydroxynonenal malondialdehyde Lipid Peroxides 8-hydroxy-2- deoxyguanosine (8-OHDG) (refer to Laboratory references)	8-Isoprostane assays are now commercially available. Markers of oxidative stress are currently assayed only in specialized laboratories.

VIII. Tests for Monitoring Nutrition Support

CRP (see section V. hs-CRP)	CRP is an acute-phase protein used to assess inflammatory status.	Large increases in CRP are associated with development of a catabolic state during the stress response; CRP levels begin to fall when the anabolic phase is entered.	CRP <10 mg/L	Serial values rather than a single value must be used to specify the stage of the stress response.
Chemistry Panel with Phosphate and Mg^{2+}	Panel includes electrolytes, glucose, creatinine, BUN, and total CO_2 (bicarbonate); see earlier discussion for additional test information.	Used to monitor carbohydrate tolerance, hydration status, and major organ system function.	See earlier discussion on phosphate and magnesium.	Very frequently ordered test panel.
Osmolality	(See discussion in VII. Blood Gases and Hydration Status.)			
Protein-Energy Balance	(See earlier discussion on PAB, RBP, Tf, ALB, nPCR, nitrogen balance, UUN, and TUN.)			
Minerals: Zn, Cu, Se, Cr	(See earlier discussion of serum zinc, serum copper, ceruloplasmin, and lymphocyte micronutrient testing.)			
Vitamins C, D, and A	(See earlier discussion of vitamins C, D, and A) Because vitamins C, 25-OH-D, and A are important in immune function and wound healing, they should be assessed regularly.	Note regarding TPN nutritional monitoring: Vitamin C levels can ↓ sharply in response to stress. Vitamin D and A nuclear receptors share the same connection with the RXR receptor, which have synergistic function and should be monitored congruently.[27,28]		Note regarding TPN nutritional monitoring. Systematic, regular monitoring protocol should be followed. 25-OH- D is produced in the liver and can be suppressed with hepatic stress conditions.[29]
Vitamin K_1 & K_2 status	(TPN only) (see earlier discussion); contribution of the gut flora to vitamin K status is absent during TPN, and basic TPN formulas are devoid of it.			Important to differentiate between vitamin K_1 and K_2.

Continued

IX. Liver Function Tests

BILI T/D (Direct and Indirect)	Total serum bilirubin represents both conjugated or direct bilirubin, and unconjugated or indirect bilirubin. Elevated levels suggest medical problem.	Conjugated bilirubin levels are elevated with cancer of pancreas or liver and bile duct obstruction; unconjugated bilirubin level elevated with hepatitis and jaundice anemias	Total bilirubin: 0.3-1 mg/dL (5.1-17 mmol/L) Direct bilirubin: 0.1-0.3 mg/dL; (1.7-5.1 mmol/L) Indirect bilirubin: 0.2-0.8 mg/dL (3.4-12 mmol/L)	Many medications are associated with elevated bilirubin levels.
ALT	Enzyme found primarily in the liver (also called serum glutamic pyruvic transaminase [SGPT]).	Injury to the liver results in elevated levels of ALT. Depressed in malnutrition.	4-36 U/L Infant: 2 x adult levels	Many medications and alcohol intake are associated with elevated ALT levels. ALT levels are often compared with AST for differential diagnosis.
GGT	Biliary excretory enzyme involved in transfer of amino acids across cell membranes.	Used to evaluate progression of liver disease and screening for alcoholism.	F: 4-25 U/L M: 12-38 U/L	Many medications are associated with elevated GGT levels.
ALP	Enzyme found primarily in the bone, liver, and biliary tract; increased in an alkaline environment.	Elevated levels noted in liver and bone disorders.	30-120 U/L	Nonspecific test; other tests need to confirm diagnosis. Many medications are associated with elevated ALP levels.
AST	Enzyme primarily found in the heart, liver, and skeletal muscle cells (also called serum glutamic oxaloacetic transaminase [SGOT]).	Diagnostic tool when coronary occlusive heart disease or hepatocellular disease is suspected.	0-35 U/L	Many medications are associated with elevated AST levels. AST levels are often compared with ALT for differential diagnosis.
A1AT	A1AT is a serine protease inhibitor secreted primarily by hepatocytes. Most common genetic A1AT variants are ZZ, SS, MZ, SZ. Measured by serum electrophoresis.	Decreased or absent Alpha-1-band in serum electrophoresis; A1AT is an acute-phase reactant associated with emphysema, COPD, and cirrhosis of the liver; A1AT elevated with states of inflammation, infection, or malignancy.	85-213 mg/dL (0.85-2.13 g/L) Homozygous + + variants: severe disease early in life. 80 known variants of A1AT gene: heterozygous ZZ and SS gene variants: majority have hepatic or pulmonary symptoms MZ and SZ milder gene variants: rarely have symptoms.[o,p]	There are 100 known variants of the A1AT gene.[o,p] If a person is not diagnosed with a severe form as a child, an individual may not be identified until an adult with end-stage lung and liver disease.

X. Thyroid Function Tests

Thyroxine Total T_4, and free T_4	Measures the total amount of T_4 in the blood; free T_4 is the active form. See Chapter 30.	T_4 increased in hyperthyroidism; T_4 decreased in hypothyroidism and malnutrition.	T_4, Total F: 5-12 mcg/dL; (64-154 nmol/L) M: 4-12 mcg/dL (51-154 nmol/L) Free T_4 = 0.7-1.9 ng/dL (10-23 pmol/L)	Tests are ordered to distinguish between euthyroidism, or hyperthyroidism and hypothyroidism. Can be related to iodine deficiencies.
Triiodothyronine T_3, Total and Free T_3	Measures the total amount of T_3 in the blood; free T_3 active form. See Chapter 30.	Hyperthyroidism-usually elevated; hypothyroidism-usually decreased and can show low function of thyroid peroxidase enzyme when T_4 normal or high, and T_3 low (poor conversion).	Total T_3 20-50 yr: 70-205 ng/dL (1.2-3.4 nmol/L) >50 yr: 40-180 ng/dL (0.6-2.8 nmol/L) Free T_3: 230-619 pg/mL	Tests are ordered to distinguish between euthyroidism, or hyperthyroidism and hypothyroidism. If low T_3 levels, consider insufficient nutrient cofactors (selenium, vitamin E) for thyroid peroxidase enzyme conversion of T_4 to T_3.

TSH	Used to monitor exogenous thyroid replacement or thyroid suppression; also used as a screening test for thyroid function. See Chapter 30.	Decreased TSH in hyperthyroidism; elevated TSH in hypothyroidism	0.5-5 mIU/L AACE Standards: Target TSH: 0.3-3.0 µIU/mL[o]	Tests are ordered to distinguish between euthyroidism, hyperthyroidism, and hypothyroidism. If depressed, use caution with iodine intake. If elevated, consider assessing nutrient cofactors: iodine, selenium, and vitamins E and A.
anti-TG	Anti-TG blood test used as a marker for autoimmune thyroiditis and related diseases.[30] High prevalence of thyroid autoantibodies in celiac and rheumatoid arthritis patients	Anti-TG autoantibodies bind to thyroglobulin and affect thyroid hormone synthesis, storage and release. Recommend investigation of gluten intolerance if elevated anti-TG.	Titer <4 IU/mL Anti-TG often tested in conjunction with anti-TPO test.	Resulting disordered thyroid function seen most with common related conditions: Hashimoto's thyroiditis and autoimmune hypothyroid.
Anti-TPO or TPO-AB	Anti-TPO blood test used in the diagnosis of thyroid diseases, such as Hashimoto's thyroiditis or chronic lymphocytic thyroiditis (in children). High prevalence of thyroid autoantibodies in celiac and rheumatoid arthritis patients.	Thyroid microsomal antibodies act on section of the microsome in the thyroid cell and initiate inflammatory and cytotoxic effects on the thyroid follicle. Recommend investigation of gluten intolerance if elevated anti-TPO.	TPO-AB <9 IU/mL Anti-TPO often tested in conjunction with Anti-TG test.	Most sensitive assay for antimicrosomal antibody. Nutritional considerations are vitamin E and selenium co-factors for production of TPO enzyme.

XI. Tests for Metabolic Disease

Amino Acidurias	Dietary treatment is the major therapy for many of these genetic diseases: phenylketonuria, cystinuria, maple syrup urine disease, tyrosinemia, homocystinuria, Hartnup disease. See Chapter 42. Urine or plasma amino acid testing.	Monitoring amino acid level in urine or serum is necessary to assess adequacy of treatment.	Examples: Phe: 2-6 g/L (120-360 mmol/L) Phe (during pregnancy): 2-6 mg/dL (120-360 mmol/L) Cys: 2-22 g/L (10-90 mmol/L) Val: 17-37 g/L (145-315 mmol/L) Tyr: 4-16 g/L (20-90 mmol/L)	There are several methods used to measure (e.g., phenylalanine); these usually do not have exactly equivalent reference ranges.
Organic Acids Panel	Urine organic acids panel; home collection of 10 mL sample of nocturnal and first morning urine, frozen and then shipped to laboratory.[q]	Sensitive, broad range test that evaluates comprehensive functional markers for metabolic nutrient pathway functions that can suggest early markers for risk of disease or metabolic imbalances.	(See particular laboratory references)	Excellent for overview of metabolic function and noninvasive pediatric testing.

Diabetes Mellitus (See Chapter 29)

Prediabetes Diagnosis	FBG	Prediabetes, blood glucose levels are higher than normal but not high enough for a diagnosis of diabetes.	Nondiabetic FBG = <99 mg/dL Impaired fasting glucose: 100-125 mg/dL	American Diabetes Association recommends testing for prediabetes in adults without symptoms who are overweight or obese, and who have one or more additional risk factors for diabetes.
Diabetes Diagnosis	1. Serum or whole blood glucose: after fasting 8-16 hours or on a random blood sample.	1. Two or more FBG levels >126 mg/dL are diagnostic; random level >200 mg/dL followed by fasting level >126 mg/dL are diagnostic. Fasting levels of 110 to 126 mg/dL indicate IGT.		1. Elevated glucose levels normally appear with physiologic stress; whole blood gives slightly lower values.

Continued

	2. Glucose tolerance test (GTT); 75 g glucose (100 g during pregnancy) given after fasting; serum glucose measured by before and five times during the next 3 hours after oral dosing. Glucose measured by automated chemistry procedure.	2. Serum levels FBG >200 mg/dL at 2-hour point is diagnostic; 2-hour level <140 and all 0- to 2-hour levels <200 are normal; 140-199 at 2 hours indicates IGT. Gestational diabetes: fasting >105; 1-hour GTT >190; 2-hour GTT >165; and 3-hour GTT >145 mg/dL.	2. Serum: Fasting: <110 mg/dL (<6.1 mmol/L) 30 min: <200 mg/dL (<11.1 mmol/L) 1 hour: <200 mg/dL (<11.1 mmol/L) 2 hours: <140 mg/dL (<7.8 mmol/L) 3 hours: 70-115 mg/dL (<6.4 mmol/L) 4 hours: 70-115 mg/dL (<6.4 mmol/L) Urine: glucose negative	2. Often used for confirmation; ambulatory patient only; bed rest or stress impairs GTT; inadequate carbohydrate consumption before test invalidates results.
Diabetes Monitoring	1. Blood glucose—monitoring requires that the patient monitor blood glucose level. 2. Serum fructosamine—assesses medium-term glucose control by measured glycated serum proteins; currently testing available in the laboratory and home tests. 3. Serum glycated hemoglobin or HgbA1C—assesses longer-term glucose control. 4. Porphyrin urine or whole blood testing for dioxin,[32] a toxin with significant association with promoting diabetes.	1. Tight diabetes control requires frequent monitoring of glucose levels. 2. Allows assessment of average glucose levels for previous 2-3 weeks. 3. Allows assessment of average glucose levels for previous 2-3 months and verification of patient's serum glucose log.	1. 70-99 mg/dL (3.9-5.5 mmol/L) 2. Normal levels: 1%-2% of total protein Ranges vary according to method used. 3. Normal levels: Nondiabetic: 4%-5.9% Good diabetic control: 4%-7% Fair diabetic control: 6%-8% Poor diabetic control: >8%; Mean blood sugar 205 mg/dL or greater is associated with increased risk of side effects	A combination of glucose monitoring (by patient) and laboratory measurement of glycated proteins are needed to effectively monitor glucose control; fructosamine must be interpreted in light of plasma protein half-lives, and HgbA1C must be interpreted in light of RBC half-life. Department of Defense study (July 2005) 47% percent increase in diabetes among veterans with the highest levels of dioxin.[32]

A1AT, Alpha 1 antitrypsin; *AA,* arachidonic acid; *AACE,* American Association of Clinical Endocrinologists; *A/C ratio,* albumin/globulin ratio; *AGA,* antigliadian antibodies; *AHA/ACC/NHLBI,* American Heart Association/American College of Cardiology/National Heart, Lung, and Blood Institute; *ALA,* alpha linolenic acid; *ALB,* albumin; *ALCAT,* Antigen Leucocyte Cellular Antibody Test; *ALP,* alkaline phosphatase; *ALT,* alanine amino transferase; *Anti-TG,* antithyroglobulin antibody; *Anti-TPO,* antithyroid peroxidase antibody; *AS,* absorption spectrophotometry; *AST,* aspartate aminotransferase; *BAL,* bronchoalveolar lavage; *BCAA,* branched-chain amino acid; *BILI T/D,* Bilirubin Total/Direct: *BMI,* body mass index; *BUN,* blood urea nitrogen; *CAPD,* continuous ambulatory peritoneal dialysis; *CARO,* carotene, serum total; *CBC,* complete blood count; *CD,* cardiac disease; *CHD,* coronary heart disease; *CHOL,* cholesterol; *COPD,* chronic obstructive pulmonary disease; *Cr,* chromium; *CRP,* C-reactive protein; *CSF,* cerebrospinal fluid; *CVD,* cardiovascular disease; *DGLA,* dihomo-gamma-linolenic acid; *DGP,* deamidated gliadin peptide antibody; *DHA,* docosahexaenoic acid; *DM,* diabetes mellitus; *DNA,* deoxyribonucleic acid; *DPI,* dietary protein intake; *DRI,* dietary reference intake; *DRT,* diet readiness test; *EDTA,* ethylenediaminetetraacetic acid; *EFA,* essential fatty acid; *ELISA,* enzyme-linked immunosorbent assay; *EMA,* endomysium antibody; *EPA,* eicosapentaenoic acid; *FAD,* flavin adenine dinucleotide; *FIGLU,* formiminoglutamic acid; *FBG,* fasting blood glucose; *FBS,* fasting blood sugar; *FPG,* fasting plasma glucose; *FRAP,* ferric-reducing ability of plasma; *GH,* growth hormone; *GI,* gastrointestinal; *GLA,* Gamma-linolenic acid *GLOB,* globulin; *GOT,* glutamic-oxalacetic transaminase; *GPT,* glutamic-pyruvate transaminase; *GR,* glutathione reductase; *GTT, glucose tolerance test*; *GU,* urea generation rate; *HBT-lactose,* hydrogen breath test-lactose; *HBT-fructose,* hydrogen breath test-fructose; *HCT,* hematocrit; *Hcy,* homocysteine; *Hgb,* hemoglobin; *HDL,* high-density lipoproteins; *HLA,* human leukocyte antigen; *HPLC,* high performance liquid chromatography; *HRT,* hormone replacement therapy *hs-CRP,* high-sensitivity C-reactive protein; *I,* iodine; *ICA,* ionized calcium; *ICP-MS,* inductively coupled plasma/mass spectrometry; *IF,* intrinsic factor; *Ig,* immunoglobulin; *IGF,* insulin-like growth factor; *IGT,* impaired glucose tolerance; *IV,* intravenously; *KrU,* residual renal urea clearance; *Kt/Vurea,* urea kinetics(kinetic dialyzer) x time(min)/volume urea(mL); *LA,* linoleic acid; *LDL,* low-density lipoprotein; *LPP,* lipoprotein particle; *MCV,* mean corpuscular volume; *MLC,* mixed lymphocyte culture; *MMA,* methylmalonic acid; *MRT,* Mediator Release Test; *N,* nitrogen; *NCEP,* National Cholesterol Education Program; *NMN,* methylnicotinamide; *NSAID,* nonsteroidal antiinflammatory drug; *nPCR,* normalized protein catabolic rate; *OC,* osteocalcin; *ORAC,* oxygen radical absorbance capacity; *PAB,* prealbumin; *PCR,* protein catabolic rate; *PEM,* protein-energy malnutrition; *PLP,* pyridoxal phosphate; *PN,* parenteral nutrition; *PNA,* protein equivalent of nitrogen appearance; *PP,* post prandial; *PT,* prothrombin time; *PTH,* parathyroid hormone; *PTT,* partial thromboplastin time; *PUFA,* polyunsaturated fatty acid; *RBC,* red blood cell; *RBP,* retinol-binding protein; *RDW,* RBC distribution width; *ROS,* reaction oxygen species; *RXR,* retinoid X receptor; *sALB,* serum albumin *SAMe,* s-adenosylmethionine; *SNP,* single nucleotide polymorphism; *SP.GR.,* Specific Gravity;

T3, triiodothyronine; *T4,* thyroxine; *T1DM,* type 1 diabetes mellitus; *TEAC,* trolox-equivalent antioxidant capacity; *Tf,* transferrin; *Tf-sat,* transferrin saturation; *TG,* triglyceride; *TIBC,* total iron-binding capacity; *TLC,* total lymphocyte count; *TM,* tetrathiomolybdate; *TP,* total protein; *TPN,* total parenteral nutrition; *TPP,* thiamin pyrophosphate; *Trp,* tryptophan; *TTR,* transthyretin; *TSAT,* transferrin saturation; *tTG,* tissue transglutaminase; *TUN,* total urinary nitrogen; *U: Cr,* urea/creatinine ratio; *ucOC,* undercarboxylated osteocalcin; *UKM,* urea kinetic modeling; *UUN,* urea urinary nitrogen; *VLDL,* very-low-density lipoprotein; *WBC,* white blood cell; *XA,* xanthurenic acid.

[a]Factor = 5.95 for TPN; reflects severity of metabolic stress.

[b]Factor = 5.95 for TPN; reflects severity of metabolic stress; TUN gives the most accurate estimation of total protein catabolism.

[c]Red blood cells are separated from plasma by centrifugation and washed with saline; after hemolyzing the cells, the intracellular material is analyzed for vitamin availability.

[d]No biochemical tests have been developed to assess B_3 status; the fraction of whole blood niacin as nicotinamide adenine dinucleotide (NAD) is a potentially useful test (see Powers HJ: Current knowledge concerning optimum nutritional status of riboflavin, niacin, and pyridoxine, *Proc Nutr Soc* 58:435, 1999).

[e]ALT and GPT are the same enzyme; AST and GOT are the same enzyme.

[f]PLP is a rate-limiting coenzyme in the transamination of amino acids (ALT and AST). PLP found primarily in liver and muscles.

[g]Microbiologic growth assays, the deoxyuridine suppression test, and recently developed research tests for folate and vitamin B_{12} are not generally offered in the contemporary clinical laboratory.

[h]More sensitive procedures for measurement of vitamin K include serum chromatography and determination of the serum level of vitamin K–dependent bone protein called osteocalcin. Deficiency significantly increases the amount of abnormal forms of this protein. These tests are not yet widely available.

[i]These substances are measured by similar techniques when the concentration in urine or other body fluids is determined.

[j]These tests are combined with serum glucose, creatinine, and BUN on a test battery or panel. This set of tests is among the first and most frequently administered laboratory tests.

[k]The CBC includes the red cell count, the red cell indices, Hgb concentration, HCT, MCV, mean cell hemoglobin (MCH), mean cell hemoglobin concentration (MCHC), and white cell and platelet counts. Only HCT, Hgb, and MCV are discussed here (see Savage RA: The red cell indices: yesterday, today, and tomorrow, *Clin Lab Med* 13:773–785, 1993).

[l]Ranges are for adult men and premenopausal women. Pregnant women, infants, and children have different reference ranges.

[m]See van Zeben D, Bieger R, van Wermeskerken RK, et al: Evaluation of microcytosis using serum ferritin and red blood cell distribution width, *Eur J Haematol* 44:106-109, 1990.

[n]Taste acuity tests can be used to supplement laboratory methods (see, e.g., Gibson RS, Vanderkooy PD, MacDonald AC, et al: A growth-limiting, mild zinc-deficiency syndrome in some Southern Ontario boys with low height percentiles, *Am J Clin Nutr* 49:1266–1273, 1989).

[o]AACE supports target TSH level between 0.3 and 3.0 mIU/mL to reduce the incidence of risks associated with subclinical hypothyroidism. AACE Task Force Thyroid Guidelines, *Endocr Pract* 8:466, 2002.

[p]More recent awareness of the highly undiagnosed common disease of A1AT is improving education of health care providers regarding this condition. Köhnlein T, Welte T: Alpha-1 antitrypsin deficiency: pathogenesis, clinical presentation, diagnosis, and treatment, *Am J Med* 121:3–9, 2008.

[q]organic acid functional markers for metabolic effects of micronutrient inadequacies, toxic exposure, neuroendocrine activity and intestinal bacterial overgrowth. Lord R, Bralley J: Organics in urine: assessment of gut dysbiosis, nutrient deficiencies and toxemia, *Nutr Pers* 20:25–31, 1997.

References

1. Parrish CR, series editor: Serum proteins as markers of nutrition: what are we treating? Nutrition Issues in Gastroenterology, series 43, *Pract Gastroenterol* October 2006.
2. Juarez-Congelosi M, Orellana P, Goldstein SL: Normalized protein catabolic rate versus serum albumin as a nutrition status marker in pediatric patients receiving hemodialysis, *J Ren Nutr* 17(4):269–274, 2007.
3. Harty JC, Boulton H, Curwell J, et al: The normalized protein catabolic rate is a flawed marker of nutrition in CAPD patients, *Kidney Int* 45:103–109, 1994.
4. Beck FK, Rosenthal TC: Prealbumin: a marker for nutritional evaluation, *Am Fam Physician* 65:1575–1578, 2002.
5. Wu X, Yu H, Amos CI, et al: Joint effect of insulin-like growth factors and mutagen sensitivity in lung cancer risk, *J Natl Cancer Inst* 92:737–743, 2000.
6. Rowlands MA, Gunnell D, Harris R, et al: Circulating insulin-like growth factor peptides and prostate cancer risk: a systematic review and meta-analysis, *Int J Cancer* 124:2416–2429, 2009.
7. Gonen B, Rubenstein A, Rochman H, et al: Haemoglobin A1: An indicator of the metabolic control of diabetic patients, *Lancet* 2(8041):734–737, 1977.
8. Riese H, Vrijkotte TGM, Meijer P, et al: Covariance of metabolic and hemostatic risk indicators in men and women, *Fibrinolysis Proteolysis* 15(1):9–20, 2001.
9. Bo S, Durazzo M, Guidi S, et al: Dietary magnesium and fiber intakes and inflammatory and metabolic indicators in middle-aged subjects from a population-based cohort, *Am J Clin Nutr* 84:1062–1069, 2006.
10. Douglas D: *MedScape Today News. Improved Diagnosis Does Not Change Celiac Mortality, Reuters Health Information,* February 1, 2011.
11. Grainge MJ, West J, Card TR, et al: Causes of death in people with celiac disease spanning the pre- and post-serology era: a population-based cohort study from Derby, UK, *Am J Gastroenterol* 106:933–939, 2011.
12. Lewis NR, Holmes GK: Risk of morbidity in contemporary celiac disease, *Expert Rev Gastroenterol Hepatol* 4:767–780, 2010.
13. Donaldson MR, Book LS, Leiferman KM, et al: Strongly positive tissue transglutaminase antibodies are associated with Marsh 3 histopathology in adult and pediatric celiac disease, *J Clin Gastroenterol* 42:256–260, 2008.
14. Vermeersch P, Richter T, Hauer AC, et al: Use of likelihood ratios improves clinical interpretation of IgG and IgA anti-DGP antibody testing for celiac disease in adults and children, *Clin Biochem* 44:248–250, 2011.
15. Vermeersch P, Geboes K, Mariën G, et al: Diagnostic performance of IgG anti-deamidated gliadin peptide antibody assays is comparable to IgA anti-tTG in celiac disease, *Clin Chim Acta* 411:931–935, 2010.
16. Sharifi N, Khoshbaten M, Aliasgarzade A, et al: Celiac disease in patients with type-1 diabetes mellitus screened by tissue transglutaminase antibodies in northwest of Iran, *Int J Diabetes Dev Ctries* 28:95–99, 2008.
17. Lampasona V, Bonfanti R, Bazzigaluppi E, et al: Antibodies to tissue transglutaminase C in type I diabetes, *Diabetologia* 42:1195–1198, 1999.

18. Holopainen P, Mustalahti K, Uimari P, et al: Candidate gene regions and genetic heterogeneity in gluten sensitivity, *Gut* 48:696–701, 2001.
19. Feingold KR, Moser A, Patzek SM, et al: Infection decreases fatty acid oxidation and nuclear hormone receptors in the diaphragm, *J Lipid Res* 50:2055–2063, 2009.
20. Lord RS, Bralley JA, editors: *Laboratory evaluations for integrative and functional medicine,* ed 2, Duluth, GA, 2008, MetaMetrix Institute.
21. Sypniewska G: *Pro-inflammatory and prothrombotic factors and metabolic syndrome,* Department of Laboratory Medicine, Collegium Medicum, Nicolae Copernicus University, Bydgoszcz, Poland, 2007.
22. Ng KY, Ma MT, Leung KK, et al: Vitamin D and vitamin A receptor expression and the proliferative effects of ligand activation of these receptors on the development of pancreatic progenitor cells derived from human fetal pancreas, *Stem Cell Rev Rep* 7:53–63, 2011.
23. Aslam A, Misbah SA, Talbot K, et al: Vitamin E deficiency induced neurological disease in common variable immunodeficiency: two cases and a review of the literature of vitamin E deficiency, *Clin Immunol* 112(1):24–29, 2004.
24. Kim K, Valentine RJ, Shin Y, et al: Associations of visceral adiposity and exercise participation with C-reactive protein, insulin resistance, and endothelial dysfunction in Korean healthy adults, *Metabolism* 57:1181–1189, 2008.
25. Finney L, Vogt S, Fukai T, et al: Copper and angiogenesis: unravelling a relationship key to cancer progression, *Clin Exp Pharmacol Physiol* 36:88–94, 2009.
26. Charney P, Malone AM: *Pocket guide to nutrition assessment,* ed 3, Chicago, IL, 2016, American Dietetic Association.
27. Snellman G, Melhus H, Gedeborg R, et al: Determining vitamin D status: a comparison between commercially available assays, *PLoS One* 5(7):e11555, 2010.
28. Katz K, Brar PC, Parekh N, et al: Suspected nonalcoholic fatty liver disease is not associated with vitamin D status in adolescents after adjustment for obesity, *J Obes* 2010:496829, 2010. Published online February 2011.
29. Ahmed A: *The role of 11b-hydroxysteroid dehydrogenase type 1 and hepatic glucocorticoid metabolism in the metabolic syndrome,* Doctoral thesis to College of Medical and Dental Scienc es, University of Birmingham, 2010.
30. Yu VC, Delsert C, Andersen B, et al: RXR beta: a coregulator that enhances binding of retinoic acid, thyroid hormone, and vitamin D receptors to their cognate response elements, *Cell* 67:1251–1266, 1991.
31. Longnecker MP, Michalek JE: Serum dioxin level in relation to diabetes mellitus among Air Force veterans with background levels of exposure, *Epidemiology* 11:44–48, 2000.
32. Longnecker MP, Michalek, JE: Serum dioxin levels in relation to diabetes mellitus among Air Force veterans with background levels of exposure. *Epidemol* 11:44-48, 2000.

Appendix created by Mary Demarest Litchford, PhD, RDN, LDN and Diana Noland, MPH, RDN, CCN, IFMCP, LD.

Nutritional Implications of Selected Drugs

Pharmacology is the study of drugs and their interactions in the body. An interaction between a drug, nutrient, or food can alter the effectiveness of a drug as it moves from its site of administration into the blood and to the target tissues. This is called a *drug-nutrient interaction* (DNI) when there are specific changes to the pharmacokinetics (absorption, distribution, metabolism, or excretion) of a drug caused by foods and nutrients. A drug may also cause a nutrient depletion—either by disrupting absorption or increasing the excretion of one or more nutrients. Older adults and those who take multiple medications (polypharmacy) are at the greatest risk. Additionally, those who take medications along with dietary supplements may also be at increased risk for a DNI.

Many medications also cause side effects such as gastrointestinal (GI) distress, blood sugar imbalance, appetite changes, weight gain or loss, or organ toxicity. They can also affect taste, smell, and hydration status. It is important to evaluate every drug and dietary supplement a client is taking in order to assess for potential DNIs and/or side effects. In many cases these can be minimized or avoided if the diet is modified. Examples include avoidance of certain foods (such as grapefruit with many drugs), limiting certain nutrients (such as tyramine

with monoamine oxidase [MAO] antidepressants and calcium with levothyroxine), or altering the timing of foods (taking drugs either with or without food).

Some drugs have added ingredients, known as *excipients*, that may cause a DNI or side effect, so all drug ingredients should be evaluated when a patient has symptoms. Examples of potentially interactive excipients include alcohol, caffeine, lactose, sorbitol, aspartame, tyramine, and sulfites. Lastly, some drugs contain nutritionally significant ingredients including minerals (calcium, magnesium, or sodium), sugars, and fats that may contribute to a patient's overall nutrient status.

Useful resources for further exploration include:

Food and Drug Administration Center for Drug Evaluation and Research

The Natural Medicines Database (subscription database)

National Institutes of Health (NIH) Clinical Center: Medications

Medscape Drug Interaction Checker

WebMD Drug Interaction Checker

The following is a list of common drugs and their nutritional implications.

Drug	Drug Effect	Nutritional Implications and Cautions
Selected Antiinfective Drugs		
Antibacterial Agents		
Penicillins	Short-term use: diarrhea	Use caution with low potassium diets or in patients with renal failure.
• amoxicillin (Amoxil)	Long-term use: oral candidiasis, diarrhea, epigastric distress, *Clostridium difficile.*	Augmentin: take with food to ↓ GI distress. Replace fluids & electrolytes for diarrhea. Probiotic is advised.
• amoxicillin/clavulanic acid (Augmentin)	Pen VK 250 mg tab contains 0.73 mEq of potassium.	
• Penicillin VK (Pen VK)	Pen VK 500 mg tab contains 1.44 mEq potassium.	
• Piperacillin/Tazobactam (Zosyn)	Pen VK Suspension 125 mg/5 mg = 0.42 mEq potassium.	
	Pen VK Suspension 250 mg/5 mL = 0.85 mEq potassium.	
	Zosyn 2.25 g = 125 mg Na.	
	Zosyn 3.375 g = 192 mg Na.	
	Zosyn 4.5 g = 256 mg Na.	
Macrolides	May cause GI distress (are promotility agents, erythromycin >> clarithromycin >> azithromycin), anorexia, stomatitis, dysgeusia, or diarrhea.	Take with food to ↓ GI distress. Eat frequent, small, appealing meals to counteract anorexia. Use mouth rinses, fresh mint, or lemon water for dysgeusia. Replace fluids & electrolytes for diarrhea. Avoid alcohol. Avoid grapefruit with erythromycin. Probiotic is advised.
• azithromycin (Zithromax)	May increase sedative effect of alcohol. Grapefruit may increase erythromycin levels leading to cardiac conduction abnormalities.	
• clarithromycin (Biaxin)	May cause *Clostridium difficile.*	
• erythromycin (Ery-Tab)		

Continued

Drug	Drug Effect	Nutritional Implications and Cautions
Sulfonamide Combination • sulfamethoxazole/ trimethoprim (Bactrim)	May interfere with folate metabolism, especially with long-term use. May cause stomatitis, anorexia, nausea and vomiting, severe allergic reactions. May inhibit aldehyde dehydrogenase or the elimination of acetaldehyde resulting in disulfiram-type reaction. May increase potassium levels (generally at high doses) and hypoglycemia (more common in the elderly). May cause *Clostridium difficile*.	Take with food and 8 oz fluid to ↓ nausea, vomiting, and anorexia. Replace fluids & electrolytes for diarrhea. Supplement folic acid as needed. Discontinue and consult physician at first sign of allergic reaction. Avoid alcohol. Use with caution in patients with potassium supplements or in renal failure. May potentiate hypoglycemia in diabetic patients. Probiotic is advised.
Cephalosporins **First Generation** • cephalexin (Keflex) • cefazolin (Ancef)	May cause stomatitis, sore mouth and tongue, and may interfere with eating. May cause diarrhea and *Clostridium difficile*.	Replace fluids & electrolytes for diarrhea. Eat moist, soft, low-salt foods and cold foods such as ice chips, sherbet, and yogurt for stomatitis and sore mouth. Probiotic is advised.
Second Generation • cefprozil (Cefzil) • cefuroxime (Ceftin) **Third Generation** • ceftriaxone (Rocephin) • Ceftazidime (Fortaz) • cefdinir (Omnicef) • cefpodoxime (Vantin) **Fourth Generation** • cefepime (Maxipime)	Food ↑ bioavailability of tablets and suspension (cefuroxime). Antacids (H_2 blockers and PPIs), may ↓ bioavailability, avoid combination. Some cefuroxime products contain phenylalanine.	Take with a meal for optimal bioavailability. Take separately from H_2 blockers or proton pump inhibitors or avoid combination (cefuroxime). Probiotic may be advised. Take cefpodoxime with food.
Fluoroquinolones • ciprofloxacin (Cipro) • levofloxacin (Levaquin) • moxifloxacin (Avelox)	Drug will bind to magnesium, calcium, zinc, and iron, forming an insoluble, unabsorbable complex. May cause *Clostridium difficile*. Cipro: Inhibits metabolism of caffeine and can therefore ↑ CNS stimulation. Drug may rarely precipitate in renal tubules.	Limit caffeine intake with ciprofloxacin. Take 2 hours before or 6 hours after antacids, Mg, Ca, Fe, Zn supplements, or multivitamin with minerals. Replace fluids electrolytes for diarrhea. Hold tube feeds 1-2 hours before and 1-2 hours after drug. Probiotic is advised. Take drug with 8 oz of fluid and maintain adequate hydration.
Antimicrobial Agents **Oxazolidinone** • linezolid (Zyvox)	Drug exhibits mild MAO inhibition. May cause taste change, oral candidiasis, and *Clostridium difficile*.	Avoid significant amounts (>100 mg) of high tyramine/pressor foods. See chart in 18th ed. of *Food Medication Interactions*. Eat small, frequent, appealing meals if tastes change. Replace fluids & electrolytes for diarrhea. Probiotic is advised.
Tetracyclines • tetracycline (Sumycin) • doxycycline (Vibramycin)	Often used to treat Lyme disease; may cause anorexia. Binds to Mg, Ca, Zn, and Fe, forming an insoluble unabsorbable complex. May ↓ bacterial production of vitamin K in GI tract. Long-term use may cause B vitamin deficiencies. Combining with vitamin A may ↑ risk of benign intracranial hypertension. May cause *Clostridium difficile*.	Take supplements separately by 3 hours. Eat frequent, small, appealing meals to ↓ anorexia. Avoid excessive vitamin A while taking drug. Long-term use may warrant vitamins K and B supplementation. Probiotic is advised. Replace fluids & electrolytes for diarrhea. Tetracycline: Take drug 1 hour before or 2 hours after food or milk. Both can cause pill esophagitis, take with a full glass of water to ensure passage of pills into stomach.
Antiprotozoal/Antibacterial • metronidazole (Flagyl)	May cause anorexia, GI distress, stomatitis, and metallic taste in mouth. May cause disulfiram-like reaction when ingested with alcohol. Often used to treat *Clostridium difficile*.	Take with food to ↓ GI distress. Eat small, frequent, appealing meals to decrease anorexia. Avoid all alcohol during use and for 3 days after discontinuation. Probiotic is advised.
• clindamycin (Cleocin)	May cause weight loss, increased thirst, esophagitis, nausea, vomiting, cramps, flatulence, bloating, or diarrhea. May cause severe *Clostridium difficile*.	Take oral forms with food or 8 oz water to decrease esophageal irritation. Replace fluids & electrolytes for diarrhea. Probiotic is advised.
Nitrofuran • nitrofurantoin (Macrobid)	Peripheral neuropathy, muscle weakness, and wasting may occur with preexisting anemia, vitamin B deficiency, or electrolyte abnormalities. May cause *Clostridium difficile*.	Drug should be taken with food to maximize absorption, protein, and vitamin B complex. Avoid in G-6-PD deficiency because of increased risk of hemolytic anemia. Replace fluids & electrolytes for diarrhea. Probiotic is advised.
Antituberculars • isoniazid (Nydrazid)	Drug may cause pyridoxine (vitamin B_6) and niacin (vitamin B_3) deficiency resulting in peripheral neuropathy and pellagra. Drug has MAO inhibitor–like activity.	Avoid in malnourished individuals and others at ↑ risk for peripheral neuropathy. Supplement with 25-50 mg of pyridoxine and possibly B-complex if skin changes occur. Avoid foods high in tyramine (e.g., aged cheeses).

Drug	Drug Effect	Nutritional Implications and Cautions
• rifampin (Rifadin) • rifabutin	Drug may increase metabolism of vitamin D. Rare cases of osteomalacia have been reported. Food decreases absorption by 30%. Rifabutin is a less potent enzyme inducer than rifampin with less effects on vitamin D metabolism.	May need vitamin D supplement with long-term use. Take on an empty stomach.
• ethambutol (Myambutol) • pyrazinamide (Rifater)	Drug may ↓ the excretion of uric acid, leading to hyperuricemia and gout. Myambutol: may g copper and zinc.	Maintain adequate hydration and purine-restricted diet. Myambutol: ↑ foods high in Cu and Zn; daily multivitamin with long term use.
Antifungal Agents • amphotericin B (Fungizone)	Drug may cause anorexia and weight loss. Drug causes loss of potassium, magnesium, and calcium. Nephrotoxic	Eat frequent, small, appealing meals high in magnesium, potassium, and calcium. May require PO/IV supplementation. Ensure adequate IV hydration pre and post infusion to reduce renal injury.
• ketoconazole (Nizoral) • fluconazole (Diflucan) • posaconazole (Noxafil) • voriconazole (Vfend)	Drug does not dissolve at pH >5 (Ketoconazole)	Take with food to ↑ absorption. Take with acidic liquid (e.g., orange juice), especially individuals with achlorhydria or those on H_2 blockers or PPIs (for ketoconazole only). Posaconazole tablets (delayed release): Take with a full meal, preferably high-fat (>50g). Suspension: Give during or within 20 minutes following a full meal, liquid nutritional supplement, or an acidic carbonated beverage (e.g., ginger ale). Food decreases voriconazole absorption. Oral voriconazole should be taken 1 hour before or 2 hours after a meal.
• terbinafine (Lamisil)	Drug may cause taste changes or loss, dyspepsia, abdominal pain, diarrhea, weight loss, and headaches. May result in increased adverse effects of caffeine (headache, agitation, insomnia, diuresis).	Avoid taking with acidic foods such as applesauce or fruit-based foods. Limit alcohol and caffeine.
Selected Antiviral Agents • valganciclovir (Valcyte)	Cytomegalovirus antiviral agent. Suppresses bone marrow, renally eliminated.	Must take with a high-fat meal to maximize absorption.
Selected Antithrombotic/Hematologic Drugs ***Anticoagulant Agents*** **Vitamin K Antagonist** • warfarin (Coumadin)	Prevents the conversion of oxidized vitamin K to the active form. Produces systemic anticoagulation. May inhibit mineralization of newly formed bone.	Consistent intake of vitamin K-containing foods and supplements is required, not complete avoidance in order to achieve desired state of anticoagulation. Monitor bone mineral density in individuals on long-term therapy. Data are conflicting on whether consumption of cranberry and pomegranate juice/fruit with warfarin causes increased INR and bleeding episodes. However, it may be prudent to advise patients to avoid drinking large quantities of cranberry juice with warfarin. When concurrent consumption does occur, frequent monitoring for INR changes and for signs or symptoms of bleeding is recommended. The quantity of green and black tea consumed and the method of production affect the amount of vitamin K in the tea. Use caution when enteral nutrition is used in patients receiving warfarin, as there have been reports of development of warfarin resistance in patients receiving concurrent enteral feeding, even when using low vitamin K-containing products. Celery may potentiate the effect of anticoagulants. Apigenin, a constituent of celery, may inhibit thromboxane A_2 formation leading to reduced platelet aggregation (Teng et al, 1988). Celery contains coumarin derivatives, which may produce additional anticoagulant effects. Avoid high doses of fish oil, vitamin E, and herbal products with antiplatelet or anticoagulant effects.

Continued

Drug	Drug Effect	Nutritional Implications and Cautions
Direct Thrombin Inhibitor • dabigatran (Pradaxa)	Drug may cause dyspepsia, abdominal pain, GERD, esophagitis, erosive gastritis, diarrhea, gastric hemorrhage, or GI ulcer. Alcohol may potentiate the effect, increasing the risk of bleeding.	Avoid alcohol and supplements, SJW can ↓ drug effectiveness. Avoid grapefruit, can increase dabigatran concentrations. Chewing can ↓ bioavailability by 75%. Take with food if GI distress occurs.
Factor Xa Inhibitors • rivaroxaban (Xarelto) • apixaban (Eliquis) • edoxaban (Savaysa) • betrixaban (Bevyxxa)	Drug may cause abdominal pain, oropharyngeal pain, toothaches, dyspepsia, and anemia. Excess alcohol can ↑ bleeding risk.	Avoid high doses of fish oil, vitamin E, and herbal products with antiplatelet or anticoagulant effects. Avoid SJW as it can lead to decreased effectiveness. Avoid grapefruit/related citrus (limes, pomelo, Seville oranges) as they can increase risk of bleeding. Minimize alcohol intake.
Antiplatelet Agents **Platelet Aggregation Inhibitors** • aspirin/salicylate (Bayer)	Drug may cause GI irritation and bleeding. Drug may ↓ uptake of vitamin C and ↑ urinary loss.	Incorporate foods high in vitamin C and folate. Monitor electrolytes and hemoglobin to determine need for potassium or iron supplements. Avoid alcohol consumption.
• clopidogrel (Plavix) • prasugrel (Effient) • ticagrelor (Brilinta)	Drug may cause dyspepsia, nausea and vomiting, abdominal pain, GI bleeding/hemorrhage, diarrhea, and constipation.	Food ↑ bioavailability. Take with food if GI distress occurs. Avoid grapefruit/related citrus (limes, pomelo, Seville oranges). Replace fluids & electrolytes for diarrhea.
Selected Antihyperglycemic Drugs ***Insulin Sensitizing Agents*** **Biguanide** • metformin (Glucophage)	Drug may ↓ absorption of vitamin B_{12} and folic acid. May cause lactic acidosis. Drug does not cause hypoglycemia.	Follow American Diabetes Association dietary guidelines. ↑ Foods high in vitamin B_{12} and folate; supplement if necessary. Avoid alcohol to ↓ risk of lactic acidosis.
Thiazolidinedione (TZD) • rosiglitazone (Avandia) • pioglitazone (Actos)	Drugs may lead to ↑ weight and insulin sensitivity, and ↓ gluconeogenesis. Avandia may ↑ total cholesterol, LDL, triglycerides, and ↓ HDL. Actos may g total cholesterol, LDL, triglycerides, and ↑ HDL. Rarely, drugs may cause hypoglycemia.	Black box warning: These agents cause or exacerbate congestive heart failure. Follow American Diabetes Association dietary guidelines. Reduce calorie intake if weight loss is the goal. Avoid SJW. Monitor blood lipid levels closely and encourage antiinflammatory diet to manage undesirable fluctuations.
Insulin Stimulating Agents **Sulfonylureas** • glipizide (Glucotrol) • glyburide (DiaBeta) • glimepiride (Amaryl)	Drug may cause ↑ or ↓ in appetite, weight gain, dyspepsia, nausea, diarrhea, or constipation. Drugs may lead to hypoglycemia. Food can decrease absorption. May enhance the effect of alcohol.	Follow American Diabetes Association dietary guidelines and encourage regular exercise. Time food intake according to pharmaceutical recommendations. Avoid alcohol. Take 30 minutes before meal to avoid erratic absorption.
Meglitinides • repaglinide (Prandin)	Drug stimulates the release of insulin and may lead to weight gain. May also cause nausea, vomiting, diarrhea, or constipation. Drug may cause hypoglycemia if meal not ingested.	Follow American Diabetes Association dietary guidelines and encourage exercise. Reduce calories if weight loss is the goal. Take 30 minutes before meal ingestion, dose should be skipped for that meal if not eating. Limit alcohol intake.
Enzyme Inhibitor Agents **Alpha-Glucosidase Inhibitors** • miglitol (Glyset) • acarbose (Precose)	Drugs may delay the absorption of dietary disaccharides and complex carbohydrates. May also cause abdominal pain, diarrhea, and gas. Glyset: May reduce iron absorption. Drugs do not cause hypoglycemia.	Follow American Diabetes Association dietary guidelines. Avoid digestive enzymes and limit alcohol. Precose: Monitor liver enzymes (AST, ALT) quarterly during the first year. Glyset: Monitor iron levels and supplement as needed.
Dipeptidyl Peptidase-4 (DPP-4) Inhibitors (Gliptins) • sitagliptin (Januvia) • saxagliptin (Onglyza) • linagliptin (Tradjenta) • Alogliptin (Nesina)	Drugs may lead to weight gain, abdominal pain, constipation, diarrhea, gastroenteritis, nausea, vomiting, and rarely, pancreatitis. Drug may cause hypoglycemia.	Follow American Diabetes Association dietary guidelines. ↓ Calories if weight loss is the goal. Onglyza: Avoid grapefruit/related citrus (limes, pomelo, Seville oranges). Onglyza/Tradjenta: Avoid SJW. Januvia: reports of pancreatitis Nesina: reports of hepatotoxicity

Drug	Drug Effect	Nutritional Implications and Cautions
Glucose Reabsorption Inhibitor Agents		
SGLT-2 Inhibitors (Gliflozins) • canagliflozin (Invokana) • dapagliflozin (Farxiga) • empagliflozin (Jardiance) • ertugliflozin (Steglatro)	Drugs ↓ reabsorption of glucose and ↑ urinary glucose excretion. Drugs may lead to weight loss, polydipsia, ↑ LDL, hypovolemia, and dehydration. Drugs may cause hypoglycemia.	Follow American Diabetes Association dietary guidelines. Reduce calorie intake if weight loss is the goal. Monitor LDL and encourage appropriate fat intake. Invokana: Avoid SJW.
Selected Steroidal/Hormonal Drugs		
Corticosteroids • prednisone (Deltasone) • methylprednisolone (Medrol) • dexamethasone (Decadron)	Drug induces protein catabolism, resulting in muscle wasting, atrophy of bone protein matrix, and delayed wound healing. Drug ↓ intestinal absorption of calcium; ↑ urinary loss of calcium, potassium, zinc, vitamin C, and nitrogen; causes sodium retention.	Maintain diet high in Ca, vitamin D, protein, K^+, Zn, and vitamin C, and low in sodium. Ca and vitamin D supplements recommended to prevent osteoporosis with long-term use of drug.
Bisphosphonates • alendronate (Fosamax) • ibandronate (Boniva) • risedronate (Actonel) • zoledronic acid (Reclast)	Drug may induce mild ↓ in serum calcium. Long-term use may cause zinc deficiency.	Pair with diet high in Ca or use Ca/vitamin D supplement. Monitor for signs of zinc deficiency. Drug must be taken 30 minutes to 1 hour before first intake of day with plain water only. Can cause pill-esophagitis; remain upright for 30 minutes after ingesting. Take zinc supplements 2 hours away from drug.
Female Hormones • estrogen (Premarin) • Oral contraceptives	Drug may ↓ absorption and tissue uptake of vitamin C but may ↑ absorption of vitamin A. May inhibit folate conjugate and decrease serum folic acid. Drug may ↓ serum vitamin B_6, B_{12}, riboflavin, magnesium, zinc.	Maintain diet with adequate Mg, folate, vitamin B_6 and B_{12}, riboflavin, and zinc. Calcium and vitamin D supplements may be advised with estrogen as hormone replacement for postmenopausal women.
Thyroid Hormones • levothyroxine (Synthroid) • liothyronine (Cytomel)	Drug may cause appetite changes, weight loss, and nausea/diarrhea. Iron, calcium or magnesium may ↓ absorption of drug. Soy, walnuts, cottonseed oil, or high-fiber foods may also ↓ absorption.	Take Fe, Ca, or Mg supplements away from drug by ≥4 hours; take drug 2-3 hours before soy. Eat walnuts, cottonseed oil, or high-fiber foods away from medication. Use caution with grapefruit/related citrus (limes, pomelo, Seville oranges). Enteral nutrition may reduce bioavailability leading to hypothyroidism. Take on an empty stomach 30 minutes before a meal or 3-4 hours after last meal of the day.
Selected Cardiovascular Drugs		
Cardiac Glycoside Agent • digoxin (Lanoxin)	Drug may ↑ urinary loss of magnesium and ↓ serum levels of potassium.	Monitor potassium and magnesium levels and use caution with calcium supplements and antacids. Take on an empty stomach and avoid consuming high amounts of bran as this may decrease digoxin absorption.
Beta Blocking Agents • metoprolol (Lopressor, Toprol XL) • atenolol (Tenormin) • bisoprolol (Blocadren) • nadolol (Corgard) • propranolol (Inderal)	Do not stop taking abruptly unless under the close monitoring of the physician, can lead to rebound hypertension and cardiac ischemia. Drugs may mask signs of or prolong hypoglycemia. Drug may ↓ insulin release in response to hyperglycemia.	Monitoring of blood glucose levels for hypoglycemia or hyperglycemia may be recommended upon initiation of drugs. Take with food.
• carvedilol (Coreg)	Drug may cause weight gain, nausea, vomiting, and diarrhea. May mask symptoms of diabetic hyperglycemia.	Avoid natural licorice and encourage low sodium diet; ↓ calories if weight loss is the goal. Patients with diabetes should monitor glucose regularly. Take with food to prevent orthostatic hypotension.

Continued

Drug	Drug Effect	Nutritional Implications and Cautions
ACE Inhibitor Agents • enalapril (Vasotec) • lisinopril (Zestril) • benazepril (Lotensin) • ramipril (Altace)	Drugs may ↑ serum potassium. Drugs may cause abdominal pain, constipation, or diarrhea.	Caution with high-potassium diet or supplements. Avoid salt substitutes. Ensure adequate fluid intake. Avoid natural licorice. Limit alcohol.
Angiotensin II Receptor Antagonists losartan (Cozaar) valsartan (Diovan) irbesartan (Avapro) telmisartan (Micardis)	Drugs may ↑ serum potassium.	Caution with high-potassium diet or supplements. Ensure adequate hydration. Avoid natural licorice and salt substitutes. Cozaar: Avoid grapefruit/related citrus (limes, pomelo, Seville oranges).
Calcium Channel Blocking Agents amlodipine (Norvasc)	Drug may cause dysphagia, nausea, cramps, and edema.	If GI distress occurs, take with food. Avoid natural licorice. Reduce sodium intake. Grapefruit can modestly increase amlodipine levels; use caution with combination or avoid altogether.
• diltiazem (Cardizem)	Drug may cause anorexia, dry mouth, dyspepsia, nausea, vomiting, constipation, and diarrhea.	Avoid natural licorice. Strict adherence to a low-sodium diet may ↓ antihypertensive effect. Grapefruit can increase diltiazem levels; avoid grapefruit.
Alpha Adrenergic Agonist • clonidine (Catapres)	Drug commonly causes dizziness, drowsiness, and sedation.	Avoid alcohol and alcohol products. Drug ↑ sensitivity to alcohol, which may ↑ sedation caused by drug alone.
Peripheral Vasodilator • hydralazine (Apresoline)	Drug interferes with pyridoxine (vitamin B_6) metabolism and may result in pyridoxine deficiency. Food and enteral nutrition decrease bioavailability.	Maintain a diet high in pyridoxine. Supplementation may be necessary. Enteral nutrition should be stopped prior to administration or take on an empty stomach.
Antiarrhythmic Agent • amiodarone (Pacerone)	Drug may cause anorexia, nausea, vomiting, taste changes, or increases in liver enzymes or thyroid hormones.	Avoid grapefruit/related citrus (limes, pomelo, Seville oranges) and SJW. Monitor hepatic and thyroid function. Contains 3 mg of inorganic iodide per 100 mg of amiodarone.
Selected Antihyperlipidemic Drugs **HMG Co-A Reductase Inhibitors** • atorvastatin (Lipitor) • simvastatin (Zocor) • pravastatin (Pravachol) • rosuvastatin (Crestor)	Drug may cause significant reduction in CoQ_{10}. Drug lowers LDL cholesterol, raises HDL cholesterol.	Supplementation with CoQ_{10} has not been shown to ↓ statin myopathy but may still be advisable for repletion of the nutrient. Encourage antiinflammatory diet for optimal drug effect. Lipitor/Zocor: Avoid grapefruit/related citrus (limes, pomelo, Seville oranges). Concurrent use of red yeast rice may increase risk of side effects.
Fibric Acid Derivative • gemfibrozil (Lopid) • fenofibrate (Tricor)	Drug decreases serum triglycerides. Lopid: Taste changes may occur.	Encourage antiinflammatory diet for optimal drug effect. Avoid alcohol. Lopid: Small meals are recommended.
Bile Acid Sequestrant • cholestyramine (Questran)	Drug binds fat-soluble vitamins (A, E, D, K), β-carotene, calcium, magnesium, iron, zinc, and folic acid.	Take fat-soluble vitamins in water-miscible form or take vitamin supplement at least 1 hour before first dose of drug daily. Maintain diet high in folate, Mg, Ca, Fe, Zn or supplement as needed. Monitor serum nutrient levels for long-term use.
Nicotinic Acid • niacin (Niaspan)	High dose may elevate blood glucose and uric acid.	Low-purine diet as recommended. Monitor blood glucose with diabetes.

Drug	Drug Effect	Nutritional Implications and Cautions
Selected Diuretic Drugs		
Loop Diuretics		
• furosemide (Lasix) • bumetanide (Bumex)	Drug ↑ urinary excretion of sodium, potassium, magnesium, and calcium. Long-term use can lead to ↑ urinary zinc excretion.	Maintain diet high in zinc, potassium, magnesium, and calcium. Avoid natural licorice, which may counteract diuretic effect of drug. Monitor electrolytes; supplement as needed.
Thiazide Diuretic		
• hydrochlorothiazide (Hydrodiuril) • chlorothiazide (Diuril) • chlorthalidone (Hygroton) • metolazone (Zaroxyln)	Drug ↑ urinary excretion of sodium, potassium, magnesium and ↑ renal resorption of calcium. Long-term use can lead to ↑ urinary zinc excretion.	Maintain diet high in zinc, potassium, and magnesium. Avoid natural licorice, which may counteract diuretic effect of drug. Monitor electrolytes and supplement as needed. Use caution with Ca supplements.
Potassium-Sparing Diuretics		
• triamterene (Dyrenium) • spironolactone (Aldactone)	Drug ↑ renal resorption of potassium. Long-term use can lead to ↑ urinary zinc excretion.	Avoid salt substitutes. Use caution with potassium supplements. Avoid excessive potassium intake in diet. Monitor for signs of zinc deficiency.
Selected Analgesic Drugs		
Non-Narcotic Analgesics		
• acetaminophen (Tylenol)	Drug may cause hepatotoxicity at high dose. Chronic alcohol ingestion ↑ risk of hepatotoxicity.	Maximum safe adult dose is ≤3 g/day. Avoid alcohol or limit to ≤2 drinks/day.
Non-Steroidal Antiinflammatory Drugs (NSAIDs)		
• ibuprofen (Motrin) • naproxen (Naprosyn) • meloxicam (Mobic) • ketorolac (Toradol)	Standard warning with NSAIDs: GI: ↑ risk of serious GI events (bleeding, ulceration, perforation of stomach and intestines) can occur at any time during use without warning. Elderly taking corticosteroids, antiplatelets, or anticoagulants are at greater risk. Renal: ↑ Risk of kidney injury. Cardiovascular: ↑ risk of serious cardiovascular thrombotic events, myocardial infarction, and stroke.	Take drug with food or milk to decrease risk of GI toxicity. Avoid use in the elderly or in individuals with severe cardiovascular disease or renal disease. For chronic ongoing use, consider adding PPI to decrease risk of gastric ulceration.
COX-2 Inhibitor		
• celecoxib (Celebrex)	Drug may cause GI distress, weight gain, taste changes, dyspepsia, nausea, abdominal pain, diarrhea, and flatulence. Rare sudden, serious GI bleeding and colitis can occur.	If GI distress occurs, take with food and limit caffeine. High-fat meals can delay concentration, but ↑ absorption. Similar cardiovascular warnings as for NSAIDS.
Narcotic Analgesic Agents (Opioids)		
• morphine (MS Contin) • codeine/apap (Tylenol #3) • hydrocodone/apap (Norco) • oxycodone (OxyContin) • hydromorphone (Dilaudid) • fentanyl (Duragesic) • methadone (Dolophine)	Narcotics can be highly addictive and may cause severe dose-related sedation, respiratory depression, dry mouth, and constipation. Drugs cause slowing of digestion.	Monitor respiratory function and bowel function (not with paralytic ileus). Do not crush or chew sustained-release. OxyContin/Fentanyl/Methadone: Caution with grapefruit/related citrus (limes, pomelo, Seville oranges); do not take with SJW. Methadone causes QT prolongation; monitor ECG, Mg, and K and replete as necessary. Do not take with alcohol or other CNS depressants.
Synthetic Opioid Analgesic		
• tramadol (Ultram)	Drug may cause anorexia, dry mouth, dyspepsia, nausea/vomiting, abdominal pain, constipation, diarrhea, or gas.	Avoid alcohol. Use caution with SJW. Some products contain phenylalanine. Do not combine with alcohol.

Continued

Drug	Drug Effect	Nutritional Implications and Cautions
Selected Antidepressant Drugs		
Selective Serotonin Reuptake Inhibitors (SSRIs)		
• sertraline (Zoloft) • citalopram (Celexa) • escitalopram (Lexapro) • fluoxetine (Prozac) • paroxetine (Paxil)	Drugs may ↑ weight, appetite, dry mouth, or anorexia. Many drug interactions with herbs and supplements may ↑ toxicity. Prozac: May cause weight loss; may g absorption of leucine. SSRI have antiplatelet effects increasing the risk for intestinal bleeding.	Avoid tryptophan, SJW. Additive effects may produce adverse effects or serotonin syndrome. Monitor weight trends as appropriate. Avoid alcohol. Black box warning: Antidepressants increased the risk compared with placebo of suicidal thinking and behavior (suicidality) in children, adolescents, and young adults (<24 year oldr) in short-term studies of MDD and other psychiatric disorders. Avoid taking with herbal products that have antiplatelet effects. Many drug interactions through CYP450 system, check interactions with all herbs and supplements.
Serotonin Antagonist/Reuptake Inhibitor (SARI) & Serotonin-Norepinephrine Reuptake Inhibitors (SNRIs)		
• trazodone (Desyrel) - SARI • venlafaxine (Effexor XR) - SNRI • desvenlafaxine (Pristiq) – SNRI • duloxetine (Cymbalta) • milnacipran (Savella)	Some herbal and natural products may ↑ toxicity. SNRI have antiplatelet effects increasing the risk for intestinal bleeding.	Alcohol may increase the sedative and psychomotor impairment as well as increase the risk of hepatotoxicity with duloxetine and milnacipran. Avoid tryptophan and SJW. Additive effects may produce adverse effects or serotonin syndrome. Avoid herbs that have antiplatelet effects. Many drug interactions through CYP450 system, check interactions with all herbs and supplements.
Tricyclic Antidepressants (TCAs)		
• amitriptyline (Elavil) • nortriptyline (Pamelor) • doxepin (Silenor) • imipramine (Tofranil)	Drug may cause ↑ appetite (especially for carbohydrates/sweets) and weight gain. Causes dry mouth and constipation. High fiber may ↓ drug absorption.	Monitor caloric intake. Maintain consistent amount of fiber in diet. Avoid alcohol (increased sedation).
Noradrenergic/Specific Serotonic Antidepressants (NaSSA)		
• mirtazapine (Remeron)	Some herbal and natural products may ↑ toxicity. Drug can also be used as an appetite stimulant and may cause significant ↑ in appetite/weight gain. Dry mouth and constipation are common.	Avoid tryptophan and SJW. Additive effects may produce adverse effects or serotonin syndrome. Avoid combining with alcohol and cannabis. Some products contain phenylalanine.
Norepinephrine/Dopamine Reuptake Inhibitor (NDRI)		
• bupropion (Wellbutrin SR, XL)	Drug may cause anorexia, weight loss or gain, ↑ appetite, dry mouth, stomatitis, taste changes, dysphagia, pharyngitis, nausea/vomiting, dyspepsia, or GI distress. Lowers seizure threshold.	Minimize or avoid alcohol (lowers seizure threshold). Take with food to decrease GI irritation. Avoid mixing with SJW.
Monoamine Oxidase Inhibitors (MAOIs)		
• phenelzine (Nardil)	Drug may cause ↑ appetite (especially for carbohydrates and sweets) and weight gain. Risk for severe reaction with dietary tyramine.	Avoid foods high in tyramine, dopamine, tyrosine, phenylalanine, tryptophan, and caffeine during drug use and for 2 weeks after discontinuation to prevent hypertensive crisis. Monitor caloric intake to avoid weight gain.
Mood Stabilizers		
• lithium (Lithobid)	Sodium intake affects drug levels. May cause dry mouth, dehydration, and thirst, reflective of ↑ drug toxicity. Drug may cause GI irritation. Drug can cause nephrotoxicity.	Drink 2 to 3 L of fluid daily to avoid dehydration. Maintain consistent dietary sodium intake. Take with food to ↓ GI irritation. Limit caffeine.

Drug	Drug Effect	Nutritional Implications and Cautions
Selected Antipsychotic & Antianxiety/Hypnotic Drugs		
Typical Antipsychotic Agent		
• haloperidol (Haldol)	May cause ↑ appetite, weight gain or loss, constipation, or dry mouth. Risk for tardive dyskinesia.	Monitor weight and calorie count. Tardive dyskinesia may interfere with biting, chewing, and swallowing. Avoid alcohol.
Atypical Antipsychotic Agents	• Drugs may cause ↑ appetite and weight gain. May also cause ↑ blood sugar, Hgb A1C, or lipids/triglycerides, xerostomia, constipation.	• Monitor weight, fasting blood sugar, Hgb A1C, and lipids/triglycerides.
• aripiprazole (Abilify)		• Do not use in elderly dementia patients; increased risk of cerebrovascular events and greater mortality.
• clozapine (Clozaril)		
• olanzapine (Zyprexa)		
• paliperidone (Invega)		
• quetiapine (Seroquel)		
• risperidone (Risperdal)		
• ziprasidone (Geodon)		
Antianxiety/Hypnotic Agents	Drugs may cause significant sedation. Benzodiazepine drugs are highly addictive.	Avoid concurrent ingestion of alcohol, which will produce CNS depression. Limit or avoid caffeine, which may decrease the therapeutic effect of the drug. Use caution with drugs and herbal and natural products that cause CNS stimulation or sedation that can result in profound respiratory sedation, coma, and death. Avoid using in patients >65 years old.
• lorazepam (Ativan)		
• alprazolam (Xanax)		
• clonazepam (Klonopin)		
• diazepam (Valium)		
• temazepam (Restoril)		
• zolpidem (Ambien)		
Selected Anticonvulsant Drugs		
Carboxamides	Drug may ↓ biotin, folic acid, and vitamin D levels. Long-term therapy (>6 months) may cause loss of bone mineral density. May cause clinically significant hyponatremia.	Maintain diet high in folate and vitamin D. Calcium and vitamin D supplements may be necessary for long-term therapy. Use caution with grapefruit/related citrus (limes, pomelo, Seville oranges). Star fruit or pomegranate may ↑ drug levels and lead to toxicity. Avoid alcohol.
• carbamazepine (Tegretol)		
Hydantoin	Drug may ↓ serum folic acid, calcium, vitamin D, biotin, and thiamine. Drug can cause gingival enlargement, altered taste, dysphagia, nausea, vomiting, and constipation. Alcohol intake decreases drug levels, increases seizure potential, and increases CNS depression. Ca and Mg may ↓ absorption.	May be paired with daily folic acid supplement; monitor levels. Consider Ca, vitamin D and B vitamin supplements with long-term use. Ca, Mg, or antacids should be taken 2 hours away from drug. Holding tube feeds 2 hours before & 2 hours after oral drug is recommended. If continuous tube feeds, switch to IV or may require doubling of the oral phenytoin dose. Avoid alcohol and SJW.
• phenytoin (Dilantin)		
Barbiturate	Drug may induce rapid metabolism of vitamin D, leading to vitamin D and calcium deficiencies. May also ↑ the metabolism of vitamin K and ↓ serum folic acid and vitamin B$_{12}$. Alcohol increases CNS depression and could lead to respiratory depression.	Encourage ↑ dietary intake of Ca, vitamin D, and folate. Consider Ca, vitamin D, folic acid, and vitamin B$_{12}$ supplementation with long-term use. Avoid alcohol.
• phenobarbital (Luminal)		
Valproic Acid Derivatives	Causes competitive inhibition of intestinal SLC22A transport protein, leading to malabsorption of dietary carnitine.	Can cause symptomatic carnitine deficiency in susceptible patients. Supplement as necessary.
• divalproex, valproic acid (Depakote)		
Gamma-Amino Butyric Acid (GABA) Analogs	Drugs used for neuropathy, hot flashes, migraines, and as mood stabilizers. Mg can interfere with drug efficacy by ↓ absorption. Can cause ↑ weight and appetite, nausea, gingivitis, constipation, xerostomia, vomiting, and diarrhea.	Gabapentin: Take Mg supplements separately by 2 hours. Pregabalin: Administer with meals. Avoid alcohol to prevent additive CNS depression.
• gabapentin (Neurontin)		
• pregabalin (Lyrica)		

Continued

Drug	Drug Effect	Nutritional Implications and Cautions
Fructose Derivative • topiramate (Topamax) • lamotrigine (Lamictal)	May cause weight loss, anorexia, dry mouth, gingivitis, taste changes, GERD, nausea, dyspepsia, constipation, or diarrhea.	Topiramate: Encourage adequate fluid intake to ↓ risk of kidney stones. Replace fluids & electrolytes for diarrhea. Avoid alcohol.
Selected Anti-Dementia Drugs **Cholinesterase Inhibitors** • donepezil (Aricept) • rivastigmine (Exelon)	Drug is highly cholinergic; may cause weight loss, diarrhea, nausea/vomiting, ↑ gastric acid, and GI bleeding.	Take with food to prevent GI irritation. Monitor food intake and weight trends.
NMDA Receptor Antagonist • memantine (Namenda)	Drug is cleared from the body almost exclusively by renal excretion. Urine pH >8 decreases renal excretion by 80%.	Avoid diet that alkalinizes the urine (predominantly milk products, citrus fruit) to avoid drug toxicity.
Selected Gastrointestinal Drugs **H_2 Receptor Antagonist** • ranitidine (Zantac) • famotidine (Pepcid)	Drug may reduce the absorption of vitamin B_{12} and iron.	Monitor iron studies, vitamin B_{12} level on long-term therapy. Supplement as needed.
Proton Pump Inhibitors • omeprazole (Prilosec) • lansoprazole (Prevacid) • esomeprazole (Nexium) • pantoprazole (Protonix) • dexlansoprazole (Dexilant)	Long-term ↓ acid secretion may inhibit the absorption of iron and vitamin B_{12}; ↓ calcium absorption may lead to osteoporosis. Low Mg may occur. Inhibition of acid secretion may also ↑ the risk of *Clostridium difficile*. Some studies have also shown correlation between PPI therapy, SIBO, and IBS.	Monitor iron studies, vitamin B_{12}, magnesium levels, and bone density with long-term use; supplement as needed. Consider alternatives in those with a diagnosis of SIBO and/or IBS. Prilosec: Avoid SJW and ginkgo. Hold tube feeds 1 hour before and 1 hour after drug.
Prokinetic Agent • metoclopramide (Reglan)	Drug ↑ gastric emptying; may change insulin requirements in persons with diabetes; may ↑ CNS depressant effects of alcohol. Drug may cause tardive dyskinesia with extended use.	Monitor blood glucose in persons with diabetes carefully when drug is initiated. Avoid alcohol. Tardive dyskinesia may interfere with biting, chewing, swallowing.
Selected Antineoplastic Drugs **Folate Antagonist** • methotrexate (Trexall)	Drug inhibits dihydrofolate reductase; decreased formation of active folate. Drug may cause GI irritation or injury (stomatitis, gingivitis, GI hemorrhage, intestinal perforation), diarrhea, nausea/vomiting, anorexia. All antineoplastic drugs are cytotoxic; potential to damage intestinal mucosa. Drug also used as an antirheumatic.	Maintain diet high in folate and vitamin B_{12}. Daily folic acid supplement may be recommended with antirheumatic doses but is not advised with antineoplastic. Leucovorin rescue may be necessary with antineoplastic doses. Alcohol may increase the risk of hepatotoxicity; avoid alcohol.
Alkylating Agent • cyclophosphamide (Cytoxan)	Drug metabolite causes bladder irritation, acute hemorrhagic cystitis. All antineoplastic drugs are cytotoxic; potential to damage intestinal mucosa. Decreases appetite.	Maintain high fluid intake (2-3 L daily) to induce frequent voiding.
Epidermal Growth Factor Inhibitor • erlotinib (Tarceva)	Drug may cause anorexia, weight loss, stomatitis, nausea, vomiting, diarrhea. Rarely, GI bleeding can occur.	Avoid SJW and grapefruit/related citrus (limes, pomelo, Seville oranges). Hold tube feeds 2 hour before and 1 hour after drug.

Drug	Drug Effect	Nutritional Implications and Cautions
Selected Anti-Parkinson's Drugs		
Dopamine Precursor		
• carbidopa/levodopa (Sinemet)	Carbidopa protects levodopa against pyridoxine-enhanced peripheral decarboxylation to dopamine. Can cause xerostomia.	Pyridoxine supplements >10-25 mg daily may ↑ carbidopa requirements and ↑ adverse effects of levodopa. High protein diet (>2 g/kg) can decrease the efficacy of L-dopa.
Dopamine Agonist		
• bromocriptine (Parlodel)	Drug may cause GI irritation, nausea, vomiting, and GI bleeding.	Take with food to prevent GI irritation. Take at bedtime to ↓ nausea.
MAO-B Inhibitor		
• selegiline (Eldepryl)	Drug selectively inhibits MAO-B at 10 mg or less per day. Drug loses selectivity at higher doses.	Avoid high-tyramine foods at doses >10 mg/day. May precipitate hypertension.
COMT Inhibitor		
• entacapone (Comtan)	Drug chelates iron, which for some patients may ↓ serum iron and make the drug less effective.	Monitor iron levels. Take iron supplement as needed 2-3 hours away from drug. Avoid alcohol.
Selected Attention-Deficit/Hyperactivity Disorder (ADHD) Treatment Drugs		
CNS Stimulants		
• methylphenidate (Ritalin, Concerta) • dextroamphetamine & amphetamine (Adderall)	Drugs may cause anorexia, weight loss, and ↓ growth in children. Dry mouth, metallic taste, and GI upset can occur. May be habit forming.	Monitor children's weight/growth; ensure adequate calories. Limit caffeine & alcohol. Ritalin/Concerta: Avoid SJW. Adderall: High-dose vitamin C and acidifying foods may ↓ absorption and ↑ excretion.
Selected Immunosuppressants		
• tacrolimus (Prograf, Envarsus XR) • cyclosporine (Neoral, Sandimmune)	Inhibits calcineurin to suppress T-lymphocyte activation. Can cause kidney injury, hyperglycemia, hyperkalemia, hypomagnesemia, hyperlipidemia. Also anorexia, constipation, diarrhea. CYP 3A4 substrate.	Monitor potassium; may need low K diet. Monitor Mg and replete as needed. Check fasting blood sugar and lipids at regular intervals. Avoid grapefruit and other herbs that can inhibit 3A4. For Envarsus XR, must avoid alcohol.
• mycophenolate (Cellcept, Myfortic)	Inhibits inosine monophosphate dehydrogenase, preventing de novo guanosine nucleotide synthesis thereby inhibiting T and B cells. Causes nausea, diarrhea, constipation, vomiting, anorexia, and dyspepsia.	Take with food to decrease GI upset. Avoid taking Ca/mg containing antacids within 2 hrs.
• sirolimus (Rapamune)	mTOR inhibitor that halts cell-cycle progression. Antiproliferative. Causes hypercholesterolemia, increased blood sugars, stomatitis, diarrhea, and constipation. Impairs wound healing.	Avoid grapefruit. Check lipids and blood sugars at regular intervals.

ACE, Angiotensin-converting enzyme; *ALT*, alanine amino transferase; *AST*, aspartate aminotransferase; *CNS*, central nervous system; *Co-A*, coenzyme A; *COMT*, catechol-o-methyl transferase; *ECG*, electrocardiogram; *G-6-PD*, glucose-6-phosphate dehydrogenase; *GI*, gastrointestinal; *GERD*, gastroesophageal reflux disease; *HDL*, high-density lipoprotein; *Hgb A1C*, hemoglobin A1c; *HMG*, 3-hydroxy-3-methyl-glutaryl; *IBS*, irritable bowel syndrome; *INR*, international normalized ratio; *LDL*, low-density lipoprotein; *MAO*, monoamine oxidase; *MDD*, major depressive disorder; *mTOR*, mammalian target of rapamycin; *NMDA*, N-methyl-D-aspartate; *NSAID*, nonsteroidal antiinflammatory drug; *PPI*, proton pump inhibitors; *PKU*, phenylketonuria; *↓↑* increase/decrease; *SIBO*, small intestine bacterial overgrowth; *SJW*, St. John's Wort.

REFERENCES

Bailey DG, Dresser G, Arnold JM: Grapefruit-medication interactions: forbidden fruit or avoidable consequences? *CMAJ* 185:309–316, 2013. doi:10.1503/cmaj.120951.

Banach M, Serban C, Sahebkar A, et al: Effects of coenzyme Q10 on statin-induced myopathy: a meta-analysis of randomized controlled trials, *Mayo Clin Proc* 90(1):24–34, 2015.

Crowe JP: *Krause's Food and the Nutrition Care Process*, ed 13, Nutritional Implications of Selected Drugs, Appendix 31. 2012, pp 1100–1106.

Drugs.com web site: *Drug interactions checker*. Available at: https://www.drugs.com/drug_interactions.html. Accessed June, 2015.

Facts and Comparisons. eFacts [online], 2018. Available at Wolter Kluwer Health, Inc. Accessed Dec 18, 2018.

Higdon J: *Linus Pauling Institute Micronutrient Information Center: Zinc*, Updated June 11, 2015. Available at: http://lpi.oregonstate.edu/mic/minerals/zinc#drug-interactions. Accessed June 19, 2015.

Micromedex IBM Corporation [online], 2018. Truven Health Analytics. Accessed Dec 18, 2018.

Nieminen TH, Hagelberg NM, Saari TI, et al: Grapefruit juice enhances the exposure to oral oxycodone, *Basic Clin Pharmacol Toxicol* 107:782–788, 2010.

Novartis Pharmaceuticals: *Product information: Comtan (entacapone)*, East Hanover, NJ, July 2014, Novartis pharmaceuticals. Available at: https://www.pharma.us.novartis.com/product/pi/pdf/comtan.pdf. Accessed June 22, 2015.

Pattani R, Palda VA, Hwang SW, et al: Probiotics for the prevention of antibiotic-associated diarrhea and Clostridium difficile infection among hospitalized patients: systematic review and meta-analysis, *Open Med* 7(2):e56–e67, 2013.

PL Detail-Document, Potential Drug Interactions with Grapefruit. *Pharmacist's Letter/Prescriber's Letter*, January 2013.

Pronsky ZM, Elbe D, Ayoob K: *Food medication interactions*. Birchrunville, PA, 2015, Food-Medication Interactions.

Teng CM, Lee LG, Ko SN, et al. Inhibition of platelet aggregation by apigenin from Apium graveolens. *Asia Pac J Pharmacol*. 1985;3:85.

Appendix created by Glenn Kuz, BSP, PharmD.

Portions of this appendix previously written by Doris Dudley Wales BA, BS, RPh and DeeAnna Wales VanReken, MS, RDN, CD.

Nutritional Facts on Fluid and Hydration

Adequate hydration is essential for life. Body water is necessary to regulate body temperature, transport nutrients, moisten body tissues, compose body fluids, and make waste products soluble for excretion. As the most plentiful substance in the human body, water is also the most plentiful nutrient in the diet. The amount of water recommended for an individual varies with age, activity, medical condition, and physical condition. The water in juice, tea, milk, decaffeinated coffee, and carbonated beverages contributes the majority of water in the diet. Solid foods also contribute water to the diet but usually are not counted in the amount of water provided per day.

Water deficiency, or dehydration, is characterized by dark urine; decreased skin turgor; dry mouth, lips, and mucous membranes; headache; a coated, wrinkled tongue; dry or sunken eyes; weight loss; a lowered body temperature; and increased serum sodium, albumin, blood urea nitrogen (BUN), and creatinine values. Dehydration may be caused by inadequate intake in relation to fluid requirements or excessive fluid losses caused by fever, increased urine output (often related to diuretic therapy), diarrhea, draining wounds, ostomy output, fistulas, environmental temperature, or vomiting. Concentrated or high-protein tube feeding formulas may increase the water requirement.

Thirst is often the first noticeable sign of the need for more water. However, athletes or workers exercising or working physically in hot climates may be significantly dehydrated before they realize they are thirsty. In these situations they should be drinking at regular intervals; they may not be able to rely on thirst to determine their need to drink.

Water excess or overhydration may be the result of inadequate output or excessive intake. Overhydration is characterized by increased blood pressure; decreased pulse rate; edema; and decreased serum sodium, potassium, albumin, BUN, and creatinine values. Fluid restrictions may be necessary for certain medical conditions such as kidney or cardiac disease. For those on fluid restrictions, the fluid needs should be calculated on an individual basis. The usual diet provides approximately 1080 mL (36 oz), a little more than a quart of fluid per day.

Approximate Fluid Content of Common Foods

Food	Fluid Ounces	Household Measure	Metric Measure
Juice	2	¼ cup	60 mL
	3	⅓ cup	90 mL
	4	½ cup	120 mL
	8	1 cup	240 mL
Coffee, tea, decaffeinated coffee	6	⅔ cup	180 mL
Gelatin	4	½ cup	120 mL
Ice cream, sherbet	3	⅓ cup	90 mL
Soup	6	⅔ cup	180 mL
Liquid coffee creamer	1	2 Tbsp	30 mL

©2003, State of California Department of Developmental Services, revised 2004.

Estimating Daily Fluid Requirements for Healthy Individuals

Children	Body Weight	Daily Fluid Requirement
Infants		140 to 150 mL/kg
Children		
Method 1		50 to 60 mL/kg
Method 2	3 to 10 kg of body weight	100 mL/kg
	11 to 20 kg of body weight	1000 mL + 50 mL/kg >10
	More than 20 kg	1500 mL + 20 mL/kg >20

Continued

Estimating Daily Fluid Requirements for Healthy Individuals—cont'd

Children	Body Weight	Daily Fluid Requirement
Adults*		
Method 1	30 to 35 mL per weight in kilograms	
Method 2	1 mL fluid per calorie consumed	
Method 3	First 10 kg of body weight	100 mL/kg
	Second 10 kg of body weight	+50 mL/kg
	Remaining kg of body weight (age <50)	+20 mL/kg
	Remaining kg of body weight (age >50)	+15 mL/kg
Method 4	Age in years	
	16-30 (active)	40 mL/kg
	20-55	35 mL/kg
	55-75	30 mL/kg
	>75	25 mL/kg

*The 1 mL of fluid per calorie method should be used with caution because it will underestimate the fluid needs of those with low-calorie needs. Persons who are significantly obese may best be evaluated by Method 3 because it adjusts for high body weight.

From the California Diet Manual, ©2003, State of California Department of Developmental Services, revised 2004, 2010.

Note: 3 oz is approximately ⅓ cup; 6 oz is approximately ⅔ cup.

Enteral (Tube Feeding) Formulas for Adults Marketed in the United States

This table is meant to be a general reference for types of enteral products marketed in the U.S. It does not reflect precise values for specific formulas as products and formulations are subject to change.

Consult Abbott Nutrition, https://www.abbottnutrition.com/, Nestlé Nutrition, https://www.nestle-nutrition.com, and Functional Formularies (whole foods–based formula), https://www.functional-formularies.com, or Kate Farms (whole foods-based formula), https://www.katefarms.com for current, detailed information.

See *Blenderized Tube Feedings, Suggested Guidelines to Clinicians and Blenderized Feeding Options, The Sky's the Limit* by Carol Rees Parrish, M.S., R.D.N (editor) at the University of Virginia (https://med.virginia.edu/ginutrition/wp-content/uploads/sites/199/2014/06/Parrish-Dec-14.pdf and https://med.virginia.edu/ginutrition/wp-content/uploads/sites/199/2018/06/June-18-Blenderized-EN.pdf) for safety tips, use suggestions, and recipes that may be used to create home blenderized feedings.

Enteral Formulas	kcal/ mL	Protein (g/L)	CHO (g/L)	Fat (g/L)	mOsm/kg water	Water (mL/L)	Notes
Whole foods–based (commercial)	1.06	48	132	40	340	854	Contains chicken, peas, carrots, tomatoes, cranberry juice with added vitamins/minerals. Some formulas are plant based (vegetarian) and contain protein from legumes, nut butter, and quinoa.
Polymeric, standard	1-1.5	44-68	144-216	35-65	300-650	760-1260	Suitable for most patients; higher caloric density products provide less volume; some contain fiber
Polymeric, high-protein	1-1.2	53-63	130-160	26-39	340-490	818-839	Higher protein content relative to energy; some contain fiber
Polymeric, low-electrolyte	1.8-2	35-81	161-290	83-100	600-960	700-736	Volume restricted; lower concentrations of some vitamins/minerals
Polymeric, modified carbohydrate	1-1.5	40-83	96-100	48-75	280-875	859-854	Proprietary carbohydrate blends; some with pureed fruits and vegetables and without sugar alcohols; some with fiber
Polymeric, reduced carbohydrate	1.5	63-68	100-106	93-95	330-785	535-785	Lower carbohydrate with MCT oil; marketed as possible option to reduce diet-induced carbon dioxide production
Peptide-based	1-1.5	40-94	78-188	39-64	345-610	759-848	Di- and tripeptides from whey or casein; MCT oil; some with MCT combined with fish oil; some with fructooligosaccharides; varying protein to energy ratios
Critical care (polymeric or free amino acid options)	1-1.5	50-78	134-176	28-94	460-630	759-868	Various formulations marketed as support for the immune system and healing; some with omega-3 fatty acids, fiber, and/or free amino acids
Modular Additives	**kcal**	**Protein (g)**	**CHO (g)**	**Fat (g)**			
Liquid protein & carbohydrate/30 mL	100	10	14 (glycerin)	0			Hydrolyzed collagen fortified with tryptophan
Powdered protein/7 g	25	6	0	0			Whey protein
Fat & carbohydrate blend/10 g	49	0	7.3	2.2			Cornstarch, vegetable oil, MCT oil

CHO, Carbohydrates; *MCT,* medium-chain triglyceride.

Sample Stepwise Method to Calculate a Parenteral Nutrition (PN) Formula

1. Determine total calories needed (see energy equations in Chapter 2)
2. Determine total protein need: Recommendations—Range of 1 to 2 g protein/kg or provide 20% of total calories as protein
3. Determine total fat needs: Recommendations—1 g/kg/day or 20% to 30% of total calories
4. Balance kcals with carbohydrate (dextrose)

PN FORMULA

Ex: Female, Ht: 65 in (165 cm), Wt: 145 lb (65.9 kg), Age: 43

Recommended Energy Intake: 1800 calories (kcals)/day with 1.4 g protein/kg (moderate stress)

Macronutrients:

1. Protein (amino acids) = 90 g
   (Using a 10% amino acid solution—100 g amino acids/liter)
   EX: 20% of 1800 kcal = 360 kcal from protein divided by 4 kcal/g
      = 90 g protein = 900 mL
2. Fat (lipid emulsion) = ~45 g
   (Using 20% lipid emulsion that provides 2 kcal/mL)
   Ex: 25% of 1800 kcal = 450 kcal = 225 mL
3. Balance of kcals as carbohydrate = 990 kcal = 291 g
   (Using 70% dextrose = 700 g/1000mL 3.4 kcal/g = 2380 kcal/1000 mL)
   Ex: 990 kcal needed × 2380 kcal/1000mL = 415 mL

Macronutrients:

10% amino acids	= 900 mL
20% lipid	= 225 mL
70% dextrose	= 415 mL
Total	= 1540 mL

4. Micronutrients:
   add multivitamin infusion (MVI) + trace elements = 12 to 15 mL
      = 1555 mL
5. Electrolytes/additives: (~100 mL) = 100 mL = 1665 mL
   (to balance—based on current laboratories*)
6. Total nutritional fluids: 1665 mL
7. Fluids needs 2000 mL/day = add 335 mL sterile water to equal = 2000 mL/day

---

*Laboratories that are significantly below normal due to disease fluctuations may need to be treated outside the PN solution.

Dietary Approaches to Stop Hypertension (DASH) Diet

The DASH diet is an eating pattern that reduces high blood pressure. It is not the traditional low-salt diet. DASH uses foods high in the minerals calcium, potassium, and magnesium, which, when combined, help lower blood pressure. It is also low in fat and high in fiber, an eating style recommended for everyone.

The Healthy Eating Pattern is the template for the DASH eating pattern, with inclusion of ½ to 1 serving of nuts, seeds, and legumes daily; limited fats and oils; and use of nonfat or low-fat milk. The eating pattern is reduced in saturated fat, total fat, cholesterol, and sweet and sugar-containing beverages and provides abundant servings of fruits and vegetables.

Although the DASH eating plan is naturally lower in salt because of the emphasis on fruits and vegetables, all adults should still make an effort to reduce packaged and processed foods and high-sodium snacks (such as salted chips, pretzels, and crackers) and use less or no salt at the table.

DASH can be an excellent way to lose weight. Because weight loss can help lower blood pressure, it is often suggested. In addition to following DASH, try adding in daily physical activity such as walking or other exercise. You may want to check with your doctor first.

THE DASH DIET

Food Group	1600 kcal Servings/Day	2000 kcal Servings/Day	2600 kcal Servings/Day	3100 kcal Servings/Day
Grains (whole grains)	6	7-8	10-11	12-13
Vegetables	3-4	4-5	5-6	6
Fruits and juices	4	4-5	5-6	6
Milk, nonfat or low-fat	2-3	2-3	3	3-4
Meats, poultry, and fish	1-2	2 or less	6	2-3
Nuts, seeds, and legumes	3/week	½-1	1	1
Fats and oils	2	2-3	3	4
Sweets	0	5/week	Less than 2	2

DIETARY GUIDELINES

Food Group	Servings/Day	Serving Sizes	Examples	Significance of Each Food Group
Grains	6-13	1 slice bread ½ cup (1 oz) dry cereal* ½ cup cooked rice, pasta, or cereal and fiber	Whole-wheat bread, English muffin, pita bread, bagel, cereals, grits, oatmeal, crackers, unsalted pretzels, and popcorn	Major sources of energy
Vegetables	3-6	1 cup raw, leafy vegetable ½ cup cooked vegetable 6 oz vegetable juice	Tomatoes, potatoes, carrots, peas, kale, squash, broccoli, turnip greens, collards, spinach, artichokes, beans, sweet potatoes	Rich sources of potassium, magnesium, antioxidants, and fiber
Fruits	4-6	6 oz fruit juice 1 medium fruit ¼ cup dried fruit ½ cup fresh, frozen, or canned fruit	Apricots, bananas, dates, grapes, oranges and juice, tangerines, strawberries, mangoes, melons, peaches, pineapples, prunes, raisins, grapefruit and juice	Important sources of energy, potassium, magnesium, and fiber
Low-fat dairy	2-4	8 oz milk, 1 cup yogurt, or 1.5 oz cheese	Fat-free or 1% milk, fat-free or low-fat buttermilk, yogurt, or cheese	Major sources of calcium, vitamin D, and protein
Meat, poultry, fish	1-3	3 oz cooked meats, poultry, or fish 1 egg white†	Select only lean meats; trim away visible fats, broil, roast, boil, instead of frying; remove skin from poultry	Rich sources of protein, zinc, and magnesium

Continued

DIETARY GUIDELINES

Food Group	Servings/Day	Serving Sizes	Examples	Significance of Each Food Group
Nuts, seeds, legumes	3/wk–1/day	1.5 oz ($^1/_2$ cup) nuts, $^1/_2$ oz or 2 Tbsp seeds, $^1/_2$ cup cooked legumes	Almonds, filberts, mixed nuts, walnuts, sunflower seeds, kidney beans, lentils	Rich sources of energy, magnesium, protein, monounsaturated fats, and fiber
Fat	2-4	1 tsp soft margarine, vegetable oil, 1 Tbsp low-fat mayonnaise or salad dressing, or 2 Tbsp light salad dressing‡	Soft margarine, low fat mayonnaise, vegetable oil, light salad dressing	The DASH study had 27% of calories as fat, including fat in or added to foods. Sweets should be low in fat

National Institutes of Health, National Heart, Lung, and Blood Institute: *Your guide to lowering your blood pressure with DASH,* 2006, U.S. Department of Health and Human Services, NIH Publication No. 06-4082.

*Serving sizes vary between ½ cup and 1¼ cup, depending on cereal type. Check the product's Nutrition Facts label.

†Because eggs are high in cholesterol, limit egg yolk intake to no more than four per week; two egg whites have the same protein content as 1 oz of meat.

‡Fat content changes serving amount for fats and oils. For example, 1 Tbsp of regular salad dressing equals one serving; 1 Tbsp of a low-fat dressing equals one-half serving; 1 Tbsp of a fat-free dressing equals zero servings.

SAMPLE MENU

Breakfast	Lunch	Dinner
1 cup calcium-fortified orange juice	3-oz boneless skinless chicken breast	1 cup spaghetti with vegetarian/low-sodium tomato sauce
$^3/_4$ cup Raisin Bran	2 slices reduced-fat cheese	
1 cup skim milk	2 large leaves lettuce	3 Tbsp Parmesan cheese
Mini whole-wheat bagel	2 slices tomato	$^1/_2$ cup green beans
1 ½ tsp soft margarine	1 Tbsp light mayonnaise	1 cup spinach, raw
1 cup coffee	2 slices whole wheat bread	$^1/_2$ cup mushrooms, raw
2 tsp sugar	1 medium apple	2 Tbsp croutons
	$^1/_2$ cup raw carrot sticks	2 Tbsp low-fat Italian dressing
	1 cup iced tea	1 slice Italian bread
		$^1/_2$ cup frozen yogurt

Midmorning Snack	Midafternoon Snack	
1 cup apple juice	1 large banana	
2 oz walnuts		

Nutritional Analysis:

	Calories: 1980	Sodium: 2377 mg
	Protein: 78 g	Potassium: 4129 mg
	Fat: 56 g	Fiber: 32 g
	Saturated fat: 13 g	Magnesium: 517 g
	Carbohydrates: 314 g	

Exchange Lists and Carbohydrate Counting for Meal Planning

HOW THE EXCHANGE LIST WORKS WITH MEAL PLANNING

There are three main groups of foods in this exchange list. They are based on the three major nutrients: carbohydrates, protein (meat and meat substitutes), and fat. Each food list contains foods grouped together because they have similar nutrient content and serving sizes. Each serving of a food has about the same amount of carbohydrate, protein, fat, and calories as the other foods on the same list. Carbohydrate counting is used more often than the full exchange list, although the full exchange list can be useful for overall dietary balance and calorie counts.

- Foods on the **Carbohydrates** list, **Fruits** list, **Milk** list, and **Sweets, Desserts, and Other Carbohydrates** list are similar because they contain 12 to 15 grams of carbohydrate per serving.
- Foods on the **Fat** list and **Meat and Meat Substitutes** list usually do not have carbohydrate (except for the plant-based meat substitutes such as beans and lentils).

- Foods on the Starchy Vegetables list (part of the **Carbohydrates** list and including foods such as potatoes, corn, and peas) contain 15 grams of carbohydrate per serving.
- Foods on the **Nonstarchy Vegetables** list (such as green beans, tomatoes, and carrots) contain 5 grams of carbohydrate per serving.
- Some foods have so little carbohydrate and calories that they are considered "free," if eaten in small amounts. You can find these foods on the **Free Foods** list.
- Foods that have different amounts of carbohydrates and calories are listed as **Combination Foods** (such as lasagna) or **Fast Foods**.

Foods are listed with their serving sizes, which are usually measured after cooking. When you begin, measuring the size of each serving will help you learn to "eyeball" correct serving sizes. The following chart shows the amount of nutrients in one serving from each list:

Food List	Carbohydrate (grams)	Protein (grams)	Fat (grams)	Calories
Carbohydrates				
Carbohydrates: breads, cereals and grains, starchy vegetables, crackers and snacks, and beans, peas, and lentils	15	0-3	0-1	80
Fruits	15	—	—	60
Milk				
Fat-free, low-fat, 1%	12	8	0-3	100
Reduced fat, 2%	12	8	5	120
Whole	12	8	8	160
Sweets, desserts, and other carbohydrates	15	Varies	Varies	Varies
Nonstarchy Vegetables	5	2	—	25
Meat and Meat Substitutes				
Lean	—	7	0-3	45
Medium-fat	—	7	4-7	75
High-fat	—	7	8+	100
Plant-based proteins	Varies	7	Varies	Varies
Fats	—	—	5	45
Alcohol	Varies	—	—	100

CARBOHYDRATES

Cereals, grains, pasta, breads, crackers, snacks, starchy vegetables, and cooked beans, peas, and lentils are carbohydrates. In general, one carbohydrate is:
- $1/2$ cup of cooked cereal, grain, or starchy vegetable
- $1/2$ cup of cooked rice or pasta

- 1 oz of a bread product, such as 1 slice of bread
- $3/4$ oz to 1 oz of most snack foods (some snack foods may also have extra fat)

Nutrition Tips

1. A choice on the **Carbohydrates** list has 15 grams of carbohydrate, 0 to 3 grams of protein, 0 to 1 grams of fat, and 80 calories.

2. For maximum health benefits, eat three or more servings of whole grains each day. A serving of whole grain is about $1/2$ cup of cooked cereal or grain, 1 slice of whole-grain bread, or 1 cup of whole-grain cold breakfast cereal.

Selection Tips

1. Choose low-fat carbohydrates as often as you can.
2. Starchy vegetables, baked goods, and grains prepared with fat count as one carbohydrate and one fat.

3. For many starchy foods (bagels, muffins, dinner rolls, buns), a general rule of thumb is 1 oz equals one serving. Always check the size you eat. Because of their large size, some foods have a lot more carbohydrate (and calories) than you might think. For example, a large bagel may weigh 4 oz and equal four carbohydrate servings.
4. For specific information, read the Nutrition Facts panel on the food label.

Carbohydrates

Food	Serving Size	Food	Serving Size
Bread		Kasha	$1/2$ cup
Bagel, large (about 4 oz)	$1/4$ (1 oz)	Millet, cooked	$1/3$ cup
Biscuit, $2^1/2$ inches across†	1	Muesli	$1/4$ cup
Bread		Pasta, cooked	$1/3$ cup
Reduced-calorie*	2 slices (1½ oz)	Polenta, cooked	$1/3$ cup
White, whole-grain, pumpernickel, rye, unfrosted raisin	1 slice (1 oz)	Quinoa, cooked	$1/3$ cup
Chapati, small, 6 inches across	1	Rice, white or brown, cooked	$1/3$ cup
Cornbread, 1 ¾ inch cube†	1 (1½ oz)	Tabbouleh (tabouli), prepared	$1/2$ cup
English muffin	½	Wheat berries	$1/3$ cup
Hot dog bun or hamburger bun	$1/2$ (1 oz)	Wheat germ, dry	3 Tbsp
Naan, 8 inches by 2 inches	$1/4$	Wild rice, cooked	$1/2$ cup
Pancake, 4 inches across, $1/4$ inch thick	1		
Pita, 6 inches across	½	**Starchy Vegetables**	
Roll, plain, small	1 (1 oz)	Cassava	$1/3$ cup
Stuffing, bread†	$1/3$ cup	Corn	$1/2$ cup
Taco shell, 5 inches across†	2	On cob, large	$1/2$ cob (5 oz)
Tortilla, corn, 6 inches across	1	Hominy, canned*	$3/4$ cup
Tortilla, flour, 6 inches across	1	Hummus	$1/3$ cup
Tortilla, flour, 10 inches across	$1/3$ tortilla	Mixed vegetables with corn, peas, or pasta*	1 cup
Waffle, 4-inch square or 4 inches across†	1	Parsnips*	$1/2$ cup
		Peas, green*	$1/2$ cup
Cereals and Grains		Plantain, ripe	$1/3$ cup
Barley, cooked	$1/3$ cup		
Bran, dry		*Potato*	
Oat*	$1/4$ cup	Baked with skin	$1/4$ large (3 oz)
Wheat*	$1/2$ cup	Boiled, all kinds	$1/2$ cup or $1/2$ medium (3 oz)
Bulgur (cooked)*	$1/2$ cup	French fried (oven-baked)	1 cup (2 oz)
		Mashed, with milk and fat†	$1/2$ cup
Cereals		Pumpkin, canned, no sugar added*	1 cup
Bran*	$1/2$ cup	Spaghetti/pasta sauce	$1/2$ cup
Cooked (grits, oats, oatmeal)	$1/2$ cup	Squash, winter (acorn, butternut, delicata)*	1 cup
Puffed	$1^1/2$ cup	Succotash*	$1/2$ cup
Shredded wheat, plain	$1/2$ cup	Yam, sweet potato, plain	$1/2$ cup
Sugar-coated	$1/2$ cup		
Unsweetened, ready-to-eat	$3/4$ cup	**Crackers and Snacks**	
Couscous	$1/3$ cup	*Crackers*	
		Animal crackers	8
Granola		Graham cracker, $2^1/2$-inch square	3
Low-fat	$1/4$ cup	Matzo	$3/4$ oz
Regular†	$1/4$ cup	Melba toast, about 2-inch by 4-inch piece	4 pieces
Granola bar	1	Oyster crackers	20
		Round-butter type†	6

Carbohydrates—cont'd

Food	Serving Size		Food	Serving Size
Rye crisps	4		**Chips**	
Saltine-type	6		Fat-free or baked (tortilla, potato), baked pita chips	15-20 ($^3/_4$ oz)
Sandwich-style, cheese or peanut butter filling[†]	3		Regular (tortilla, potato)[†]	9-13 ($^3/_4$ oz)
Whole-wheat regular[†]	2-5 ($^3/_4$ oz)		**Beans, Peas, and Lentils**	
Whole-wheat lower fat or crispbreads[*]	2-5 ($^3/_4$ oz)		***The Choices on this List Count as One Carbohydrate + One Lean Meat.***	
Popcorn (Microwave Popped)			Baked beans[*]	$^1/_3$ cup
With butter[†*]	3 cups		Beans, cooked (black, garbanzo, kidney, lima, navy, pinto, white)[*]	$^1/_2$ cup
No fat added[*]	3 cups		Lentils, cooked (brown, green, red, yellow)[*]	$^1/_2$ cup
Lower fat[*]	3 cups		Peas, cooked (black-eyed, split)[*]	$^1/_2$ cup
Pretzels	$^3/_4$ oz		Refried beans, canned[‡*]	$^1/_2$ cup
Rice cakes, 4 inches across	2			

[*]More than 3 grams of dietary fiber per serving.
[†]Extra fat or prepared with added fat. (Count as one carbohydrate + one fat.)
[‡]480 milligrams or more of sodium per serving.

FRUIT

Fresh, frozen, canned, and dried fruits and fruit juices are on this list. In general, 1 fruit choice is:

- $^1/_2$ cup of canned or fresh fruit or unsweetened fruit juice
- 1 small fresh fruit (4 oz)
- 2 tablespoons of dried fruit

Nutrition Tips

1. A choice on the **Fruits** list has 15 grams of carbohydrate, 0 grams of protein, 0 grams of fat, and 60 calories.
2. Fresh, frozen, and dried fruits are good sources of fiber. Fruit juices contain very little fiber. Choose fruits instead of juices whenever possible.
3. Citrus fruits, berries, and melons are good sources of vitamin C.

Selection Tips

1. Use a food scale to weigh fresh fruits. Practice builds portion skills.
2. The weight listed includes skin, core, seeds, and rind.
3. Read the Nutrition Facts on the food label. If one serving has more than 15 g of carbohydrate, you may need to adjust the size of the serving.
4. Portion sizes for canned fruits are for the fruit and a small amount of juice (1 to 2 tablespoons).
5. Food labels for fruits may contain the words *no sugar added* or *unsweetened*. This means that no sucrose (table sugar) has been added; it *does not* mean the food contains no sugar.
6. Fruit canned in *extra light syrup* has the same amount of carbohydrate per serving as the *no sugar added* or *the juice pack*. All canned fruits on the **Fruits** list are based on one of these three types of pack. Avoid fruit canned in heavy syrup.

Fruit

Food	Serving Size		Food	Serving Size
Apple			Dates	3
Unpeeled, small	1 (4 oz)		Dried fruits (blueberries, cherries, cranberries, mixed fruit, raisins)	2 Tbsp
Dried	4 rings			
Applesauce, unsweetened	$^1/_2$ cup		**Figs**	
			Dried	$1^1/_2$
Apricots			Fresh[*]	$1^1/_2$ large or 2 medium ($3^1/_2$ oz)
Canned	$^1/_2$ cup		Fruit cocktail	$^1/_2$ cup
Dried	8 halves			
Fresh[*]	4 whole ($5^1/_2$ oz)		**Grapefruit**	
Banana, extra small	1 (4 oz)		Large	$^1/_2$ (11 oz)
Banana, regular	1		Sections, canned	$^3/_4$ cup
Blackberries[*]	$^3/_4$ cup		Grapes, small	17 (3 oz)
Blueberries	$^3/_4$ cup		Guava[*]	$^1/_2$
Cantaloupe, small	$^1/_3$ melon or 1 cup cubed (11 oz)		Honeydew melon	1 slice or 1 cup cubed (10 oz)
			Kiwi[*]	1 ($3^1/_2$ oz)
Cherries			Kumquats[*]	5 ($3^1/_2$ oz)
Sweet, canned	$^1/_2$ cup		Mandarin oranges, canned	3/4 cup
Sweet fresh	12 (3 oz)		Mango, small	$^1/_2$ fruit ($5^1/_2$ oz) or $^1/_2$ cup

Continued

Fruit—cont'd

Food	Serving Size
Nectarine, small	1 (5 oz)
Orange, small*	1 (6½ oz)
Papaya	½ fruit or 1 cup cubed (8 oz)
Peaches	
Canned	½ cup
Fresh, medium	1 (6 oz)
Pears	
Canned	½ cup
Fresh, large	½ (4 oz)
Persimmon, medium	2
Pineapple	
Canned	½ cup
Fresh	¾ cup
Plums	
Canned	½ cup

Food	Serving Size
Dried (prunes)	3
Fresh, small	2 (5 oz)
Pomegranate*	½
Raspberries*	1 cup
Strawberries*	1¼ cup whole berries
Tangerines, small*	2 (8 oz)
Watermelon	1 slice or 1¼ cups cubes (6½ oz)
Fruit Juice	
Apple juice/cider	½ cup
Fruit juice blends, 100% juice, unsweetened	⅓ cup
Grape juice	⅓ cup
Grapefruit juice	½ cup
Orange juice	½ cup
Pineapple juice	½ cup
Prune juice	⅓ cup

*More than 3 grams of dietary fiber per serving.

MILK

Different types of milk and nondairy beverages are on this list. However, two types of milk products are found in other lists:

- Cheeses are on the **Meat and Meat Substitutes** list (because they are rich in protein).
- Cream and other dairy fats are on the **Fats** list.

Milks and yogurts are grouped in three categories (fat-free/low-fat, reduced-fat, or whole) based on the amount of fat they have. The following chart shows you what one milk choice contains:

Milk

	Carbohydrate (grams)	Protein (grams)	Fat (grams)	Calories
Fat-free (skim), low-fat (1%)	12	8	0-3	100
Reduced-fat (2%)	12	8	5	120
Whole	12	8	8	160

Nutrition Tips

1. Milk and yogurt are good sources of calcium and protein.
2. The higher the fat content of milk and yogurt, the more saturated fat and cholesterol it has.
3. Children over the age of 2 and adults should choose lower-fat varieties such as skim, 1%, or 2% milks or yogurts.

Selection Tips

1. 1 cup equals 8 fluid oz or ½ pint.
2. If you choose 2%, or whole-milk foods, be aware of the extra fat.

Milk and Yogurts

Food	Serving Size	Count As
Fat-free (skim) or low-fat (1%)		
Milk, buttermilk, acidophilus milk, Lactaid	1 cup	1 fat-free milk
Evaporated milk	½ cup	1 fat-free milk
Chocolate milk	1 cup	1 fat-free milk + 1 carbohydrate
Eggnog	⅓ cup	1 carbohydrate
Yogurt, plain or Greek	⅔ cup (6 oz)	1 fat-free milk
Yogurt with fruit or juice	⅔ cup (6 oz)	1 fat-free milk + 1 carbohydrate
Yogurt, low carbohydrate (less than 6 grams carbohydrate per choice)	⅔ cup (6 oz)	½ fat-free milk
Reduced-fat (2%)		
Milk, acidophilus milk, kefir, Lactaid	1 cup	1 reduced-fat milk
Chocolate milk	1 cup	1 reduced-fat milk + 1 carbohydrate
Eggnog	⅓ cup	1 carbohydrate + 1 fat
Yogurt, plain or Greek	⅔ cup (6 oz)	1 reduced-fat milk
Yogurt with fruit or juice	⅔ cup (6 oz)	1 reduced-fat milk + 1 carbohydrate

Milk and Yogurts—cont'd

Food	Serving Size	Count As
Whole		
Milk, buttermilk, goat's milk	1 cup	1 whole milk
Evaporated milk	½ cup	1 whole milk
Chocolate milk	1 cup	1 whole milk + 1 carbohydrate
Eggnog	½ cup	1 carbohydrate + 2 fats
Yogurt, plain or Greek	8 oz	1 whole milk
Yogurt with fruit or juice	⅔ cup (6 oz)	1 whole milk + 1 carbohydrate
Non-Dairy Beverages		
Almond milk		
Original	1 cup	½ carbohydrate + ½ fat
Flavored	1 cup	1 carbohydrate + ½ fat
Cashew milk		
Original	1 cup	½ carbohydrate + 1 fat
Flavored	1 cup	1 carbohydrate + 1 fat
Hemp milk		
Original	1 cup	1 carbohydrate + 1 fat
Flavored	1 cup	2 carbohydrates + 1 fat
Rice milk		
Original	1 cup	2 carbohydrates + 1 fat
Flavored	1 cup	2 carbohydrates + 1 fat
Soymilk		
Original	1 cup	½ carbohydrate + 1 fat
Flavored	1 cup	1 carbohydrate + 1 fat

SWEETS, DESSERTS, AND OTHER CARBOHYDRATES

You can substitute food choices from this list for other carbohydrate-containing foods (such as those found on the **Carbohydrates**, **Fruit**, or **Milk** lists) in your meal plan, even though these foods have added sugars or fat.

Common Measurements

Dry:
3 tsp = 1 Tbsp
4 oz = ½ cup
8 oz = 1 cup

Liquid:
4 Tbsp = ¼ cup
8 oz = ½ pint

Nutrition Tips

1. A serving from this list has 15 grams of carbohydrate, variable grams of protein, variable grams of fat, and variable calories.
2. The foods on this list do not have as many vitamins, minerals, and fiber as the choices on the **Carbohydrates**, **Fruits**, or **Milk** lists. When choosing sweets, desserts, and other carbohydrate foods, you should also eat foods from other food lists to balance out your meals.
3. Many of these foods do not equal a single choice. Some will also count as one or more fat choices.
4. If you are trying to lose weight, choose foods from this list less often.
5. The serving sizes for these foods are small because of their fat content.

Selection Tips

1. Read the Nutrition Facts on the food label to find the serving size and nutrient information.
2. Many sugar-free, fat-free, or reduced-fat products are made with ingredients that contain carbohydrates. These types of food usually have the same amount of carbohydrates as the regular foods they are replacing. Talk with your registered dietitian nutritionist (RDN) and find out how to fit these foods into your meal plan.

Sweets, Desserts, and Other Carbohydrates

Food	Serving Size	Count As	Food	Serving Size	Count As
Beverages, Soda, and Energy/Sports Drinks			**Brownies, Cake, Cookies, Gelatin, Pie, and Pudding**		
Cranberry juice cocktail	½ cup	1 carbohydrate	Brownie, small, unfrosted	1¼-inch square, ⅞-inch high (about 1 oz)	1 carbohydrate + 1 fat
Energy drink	1 can (8.3 oz)	2 carbohydrates			
Fruit juice or lemonade	1 cup (8 oz)	2 carbohydrates	**Cake**		
Hot Chocolate			Angel food, unfrosted	1/12 of cake (about 2 oz)	2 carbohydrates
Regular	1 envelope added to 8 oz water	1 carbohydrate + 1 fat	Frosted	2-inch square (about 2 oz)	2 carbohydrates + 1 fat
Sugar-free or light	1 envelope added to 8 oz water	1 carbohydrate	Unfrosted	2-inch square (about 2 oz)	1 carbohydrate + 1 fat
Soft drink (soda), regular	1 can (12 oz)	2½ carbohydrates			
Sports drink	1 cup (8 oz)	1 carbohydrate			

Continued

Sweets, Desserts, and Other Carbohydrates—cont'd

Food	Serving Size	Count As
Cookies		
Chocolate chip	2 cookies (2¼ inches across)	1 carbohydrate + 2 fats
Gingersnap	3 cookies	1 carbohydrate
Sandwich, with cream filling	2 small (about ⅔ oz)	1 carbohydrate + 1 fat
Sugar-free	3 small or 1 large (¾-1 oz)	1 carbohydrate + 1-2 fats
Vanilla wafer	5 cookies	1 carbohydrate + 1 fat
Cupcake, frosted	1 small (about 1¾ oz)	2 carbohydrates + 1-1½ fats
Fruit cobbler	1/2 cup (3½ oz)	3 carbohydrates + 1 fat
Pie		
Commercially prepared fruit, 2 crusts	⅙ of 8-inch pie	3 carbohydrates + 2 fats
Pumpkin or custard	⅓ of 8-inch pie	1½ carbohydrates + 1½ fats
Pudding		
Regular (made with reduced-fat milk)	½ cup	2 carbohydrates
Sugar-free or sugar- and fat-free (made with fat-free milk)	½ cup	1 carbohydrate
Candy, Spreads, Sweets, Sweeteners, Syrups, and Toppings		
Candy bar, chocolate/peanut	2 "fun size" bars (1 oz)	1½ carbohydrates + 1½ fats
Candy, hard	3 pieces	1 carbohydrate
Chocolate "kisses"	5 pieces	1 carbohydrate + 1 fat
Coffee Creamer		
Dry, flavored	4 tsp	½ carbohydrate + ½ fat
Liquid, flavored	2 Tbsp	1 carbohydrate
Fruit snacks, chewy (pureed fruit concentrate)	1 roll (¾ oz)	1 carbohydrate
Fruit spreads, 100% fruit	1½ Tbsp	1 carbohydrate
Honey	1 Tbsp	1 carbohydrate
Jam or jelly, regular	1 Tbsp	1 carbohydrate
Sugar	1 Tbsp	1 carbohydrate
Syrup		
Chocolate	2 Tbsp	2 carbohydrates
Light (pancake type)	2 Tbsp	1 carbohydrate
Maple	1 Tbsp	1 carbohydrate
Condiments and Sauces		
Barbecue sauce	3 Tbsp	1 carbohydrate

Food	Serving Size	Count As
Cranberry sauce, jellied	¼ cup	1½ carbohydrates
Gravy, mushroom, canned[‡]	½ cup	½ carbohydrate + ½ fat
Salad dressing, fat-free, low fat, cream-based	3 Tbsp	1 carbohydrate
Sweet and sour sauce	3 Tbsp	1 carbohydrate
Donuts, Muffins, Pastries, and Sweet Breads		
Banana nut bread	1-inch slice (1 oz)	2 carbohydrates + 1 fat
Donuts		
Cake, plain	1 medium (1½ oz)	1½ carbohydrates + 2 fats
Glazed	3¾ inches across (2 oz)	2 carbohydrates + 2 fats
Muffin (4 oz)	¼ muffin (1 oz)	1 carbohydrate + ½ fat
Sweet roll or Danish	1 (2½ oz)	2½ carbohydrates + 2 fats
Frozen Bars, Frozen Desserts, Frozen Yogurt, and Ice Cream		
Frozen pops	1	½ carbohydrate
Fruit juice bars, frozen, 100% juice	1 bar (3 oz)	1 carbohydrate
Ice Cream		
Fat-free	½ cup	1½ carbohydrates
Light	½ cup	1 carbohydrate + 1 fat
No sugar added	½ cup	1 carbohydrate + 1 fat
Regular	½ cup	1 carbohydrate + 2 fats
Sherbet, sorbet	½ cup	2 carbohydrates
Yogurt, Frozen		
Fat-free	⅓ cup	1 carbohydrate
Regular	½ cup	1 carbohydrate + 0-1 fat
Granola Bars, Meal Replacement Bars/Shakes, and Trail Mix		
Granola or snack bar, regular or low-fat	1 bar (1 oz)	1½ carbohydrates
Meal replacement bar	1 bar (1⅓ oz)	1½ carbohydrates + 0-1 fat
Meal replacement bar	1 bar (2 oz)	2 carbohydrates + 1 fat
Meal replacement shake, reduced calorie	1 can (10-11 oz)	1½ carbohydrates + 0-1 fat
Trail Mix		
Candy/nut-based	1 oz	1 carbohydrate + 2 fats
Dried fruit-based	1 oz	1 carbohydrate + 1 fat

[‡]480 mg or more of sodium per serving.

NONSTARCHY VEGETABLES

Vegetable choices include vegetables in this **Nonstarchy Vegetables** list and the Starchy Vegetables list found within the **Carbohydrates** list. Vegetables with small amounts of carbohydrate and calories are on the **Nonstarchy Vegetables** list. Vegetables contain important nutrients. Try to eat at least two to three nonstarchy vegetable choices each day (as well as choices from the Starchy Vegetables list). In general, one nonstarchy vegetable choice is:

- $1/2$ cup of cooked vegetables or vegetable juice
- 1 cup of raw vegetables

If you eat 3 cups or more of raw vegetables or $1^1/2$ cups of cooked vegetables in a meal, count them as one carbohydrate choice.

Nutrition Tips

1. A choice on this list ($1/2$ cup cooked or 1 cup raw) equals 5 grams of carbohydrate, 2 grams of protein, 0 grams of fat, and 25 calories.
2. Fresh and frozen vegetables have less added salt than canned vegetables. Drain and rinse canned vegetables to remove some salt.

3. Choose dark green and dark yellow vegetables each day. Spinach, broccoli, romaine, carrots, chilies, squash, and peppers are great choices.
4. Brussels sprouts, broccoli, cauliflower, greens, peppers, spinach, and tomatoes are good sources of vitamin C.
5. Eat vegetables from the cruciferous family several times each week. Cruciferous vegetables include bok choy, broccoli, Brussels sprouts, cabbage, cauliflower, collards, kale, kohlrabi, radishes, rutabaga, turnip, and watercress.

Selection Tips

1. Canned vegetables and juices are also available without added salt.
2. A 1-cup portion of broccoli is a portion about the size of a regular light bulb.
3. Starchy vegetables such as corn, peas, winter squash, and potatoes that have more calories and carbohydrates are on the Starchy Vegetables section in the **Carbohydrates** list.
4. The tomato sauce referred to in this list is different from spaghetti/pasta sauce, which is on the Starchy Vegetables list.

Nonstarchy Vegetables

Amaranth or Chinese spinach	Chayote*	Peppers (all varieties)*
Artichoke	Coleslaw, packaged, no dressing	Radishes (breakfast, daikon, watermelon)
Artichoke hearts	Cucumber	Rutabaga
Asparagus	Eggplant	Sauerkraut‡
Baby corn	Gourds (bitter, bottle, luffa, bitter melon)	Spinach
Bamboo shoots	Green onions or scallions	Sprouts (alfalfa, broccoli, clover, mung bean, radish, soybean)
Beans (green, wax, Italian)	Greens (dandelion, collard, kale, mustard, turnip)	Squash (summer, crookneck, zucchini)
Bean sprouts	Hearts of palm	
Beets	Jicama	Sugar pea snaps
Borscht‡	Kohlrabi	Swiss chard*
Broccoli	Leeks	Tomato, fresh or canned
Brussels sprouts*	Mixed vegetables (without corn, peas, or pasta)	Tomato sauce‡
Cabbage (purple, green, bok choy, Chinese)	Mushrooms, all kinds, fresh	Tomato/vegetable juice‡
Carrots*	Okra	Turnips
Cauliflower	Onions (green, pearl, red, shallots, sweet, white, yellow)	Water chestnuts
Celery	Pea pods	Watercress
		Yard-long beans

*More than 3 grams of dietary fiber per serving.
‡480 milligrams or more of sodium per serving.

MEAT AND MEAT SUBSTITUTES

Meat and meat substitutes are rich in protein. Foods from this list are divided into four groups based on the amount of fat they contain. These groups are lean meat, medium-fat meat, high-fat meat, and plant-based proteins. The following chart shows you what one choice includes:

Meat and Meat Substitutes

	Carbohydrate (grams)	Protein (grams)	Fat (grams)	Calories
Lean meat	—	7	0-3	45
Medium-fat meat	—	7	4-7	75
High-fat meat	—	7	8+	100
Plant-based protein	Varies	7	Varies	Varies

Nutrition Tips

1. Read labels to find foods low in fat and cholesterol. Try for 3 grams of fat or less per serving.
2. Read labels to find "hidden" carbohydrate. For example, hot dogs actually contain a lot of carbohydrate. Most hot dogs are also high in fat but are often sold in lower-fat versions.

3. Whenever possible, choose lean meats.
   a. Select grades of meat that are the leanest.
   b. Choice grades have a moderate amount of fat.
   c. Prime cuts of meat have the highest amount of fat.
4. Fish such as herring, mackerel, salmon, sardines, halibut, trout, and tuna are rich in omega-3 fats, which may help reduce risk for heart disease. Choose fish (not commercially fried fish fillets) two or more times each week.
5. Bake, roast, broil, grill, poach, steam, or boil instead of frying.

Selection Tips

1. Trim off visible fat or skin.
2. Roast, broil, or grill meat on a rack so that the fat will drain off during cooking.
3. Use a nonstick spray and a nonstick pan to brown or fry foods.
4. Some processed meats, seafood, and soy products contain carbohydrates. Read the food label to see if the amount of carbohydrates in the serving size you plan to eat is 12 to 15 grams. If so, count it as one carbohydrate choice and one or more meat choice.
5. Meat or fish that is breaded with cornmeal, flour, or dried breadcrumbs contain carbohydrates. Count 3 Tbsp of one of these dry grains as 15 grams of carbohydrate.

Lean Meats and Meat Substitutes

Food	Amount
Beef: Select or Choice grades trimmed of fat: ground round, roast (chuck, rib, rump), round, sirloin, steak (cubed, flank, porterhouse, T-bone), tenderloin	1 oz
Beef jerky‡	1 oz
Cheeses with 3 grams of fat or less per oz	1 oz
Cottage cheese	1/4 cup
Egg substitutes, plain	1/4 cup
Egg whites	2
Fish, fresh, frozen, or canned, plain: catfish, cod, flounder, haddock, halibut, orange roughy, salmon, tilapia, trout, tuna	1 oz
Fish, smoked: herring or salmon (lox)‡	1 oz
Game: buffalo, ostrich, rabbit, venison	1 oz
Hot dog with 3 grams of fat or less per oz‡ (8 dogs per 14 oz package) *(Note: May be high in carbohydrate)*	1
Lamb: chop, leg, or roast	1 oz
Organ meats: heart, kidney, liver *(Note: May be high in cholesterol)*	1 oz
Oysters, fresh or frozen	6 medium
Pork, Lean	
Canadian bacon‡	1 oz
Rib or loin chop/roast, ham, tenderloin	1 oz
Poultry, without skin: Cornish hen, chicken, domestic duck or goose (well-drained of fat), turkey	1 oz
Processed sandwich meats with 3 grams of fat or less per oz: chipped beef, deli thin-sliced meats, turkey ham, turkey kielbasa, turkey pastrami	1 oz
Salmon, canned	1 oz
Sardines, canned	2 medium
Sausage with 3 grams of fat or less per oz‡	1 oz
Shellfish: clams, crab, imitation shellfish, lobster, scallops, shrimp	1 oz
Veal, loin chop, roast	1 oz
Medium-Fat Meat and Meat Substitutes	
Beef: corned beef, ground beef, meatloaf, prime grades trimmed of fat (prime rib), short ribs, tongue	1 oz
Cheeses with 4-7 grams of fat per oz: feta, mozzarella, pasteurized processed cheese spread, reduced-fat cheeses, string	1 oz
Egg *(Note: High in cholesterol, so limit to 3 per week)*	1
Fish, any fried product	1 oz
Lamb: ground, rib roast	1 oz
Pork: cutlet, shoulder roast	1 oz
Poultry: chicken with skin; dove, pheasant, wild duck, or goose; fried chicken; ground turkey	1 oz
Ricotta cheese	2 oz or 1/4 cup
Sausage with 4-7 grams of fat per oz‡	1 oz
Veal, cutlet (no breading)	1 oz

‡480 milligrams or more of sodium per serving.

The following foods are high in saturated fat, cholesterol, and calories and may raise blood cholesterol levels if eaten on a regular basis. Try to eat three or fewer servings from this group per week.

High-Fat Meat and Meat Substitutes

Food	Amount
Bacon	
Pork‡	2 slices (16 slices per lb or 1 oz each, before cooking)
Turkey‡	3 slices (1/2 oz each before cooking)
Cheese, regular: American, bleu, brie, cheddar, hard goat, Monterey jack, queso, and Swiss	1 oz
Hot dog: beef, pork, or combination (10 per lb-sized package)‡†	1
Hot dog: turkey or chicken (10 per lb-sized package)‡	1
Pork: ground, sausage, spareribs	1 oz
Processed sandwich meats with 8 grams of fat or more per oz: bologna, pastrami, hard salami	1 oz
Sausage with 8 grams fat or more per oz: bratwurst, chorizo, Italian, knockwurst, Polish, smoked, summer‡†	1 oz

†Extra fat or prepared with added fat. (Add an additional fat choice to this food.)
‡480 milligrams or more of sodium per serving.

Because carbohydrate content varies among plant-based proteins, you should read the food label.

Plant-Based Proteins

Food	Amount	Count As
"Bacon" strips, soy-based	3 strips	1 medium-fat meat
Baked beans*	1/3 cup	1 carbohydrate + 1 lean meat
Beans, cooked: black, garbanzo, kidney, lima, navy, pinto, white*	1/2 cup	1 carbohydrate + 1 lean meat
"Beef" or "sausage" crumbles, soy-based*	2 oz	1/2 carbohydrate + 1 lean meat
"Chicken" nuggets, soy-based	2 nuggets (1 1/2 oz)	1/2 carbohydrate + 1 medium-fat meat
Edamame*	1/2 cup	1/2 carbohydrate + 1 lean meat
Falafel (spiced chickpea and wheat patties)	3 patties (about 2 inches across)	1 carbohydrate + 1 high-fat meat

Plant-Based Proteins—cont'd

Food	Amount	Count As
Hot dog, soy-based	1 (1½ oz)	½ carbohydrate + 1 lean meat
Hummus*	⅓ cup	1 carbohydrate + 1 high-fat meat
Lentils, brown, green, or yellow*	½ cup	1 carbohydrate + 1 lean meat
Meatless burger, soy-based*	3 oz	½ carbohydrate + 2 lean meats
Meatless burger, vegetable- and starch-based*	1 patty (about 2½ oz)	1 carbohydrate + 2 lean meats
Nut spreads: almond butter, cashew butter, peanut butter, soy nut butter	1 Tbsp	1 high-fat meat
Peas, cooked: black-eyed and split peas*	½ cup	1 carbohydrate + 1 lean meat
Refried beans, canned‡*	½ cup	1 carbohydrate + 1 lean meat
"Sausage" patties, soy-based	1 (1½ oz)	1 medium-fat meat
Soy nuts, unsalted	¾ oz	½ carbohydrate + 1 medium-fat meat
Tempeh	¼ cup	1 medium-fat meat
Tofu	4 oz (½ oz)	1 medium-fat meat
Tofu, light	4 oz (½ oz)	1 lean meat

*More than 3 grams of dietary fiber per serving.
‡480 milligrams or more of sodium per serving.

FATS

Fats are divided into three groups, based on the main type of fat they contain:

- **Unsaturated fats** (omega-3, monounsaturated, and polyunsaturated) are primarily vegetable and are liquid at room temperature. These fats have good health benefits.
  - **Omega-3 fats** are a type of polyunsaturated fat and can help lower triglyceride levels and the risk of heart disease.
  - **Monounsaturated fats** also help lower cholesterol levels and may help raise high-density lipoprotein (HDL) (good) cholesterol levels.
  - **Polyunsaturated fats** can help lower cholesterol levels.
- **Saturated fats** have been linked with heart disease. They can raise low-density lipoprotein (LDL) (bad) cholesterol levels and should be eaten in small amounts. Saturated fats are solid at room temperature.
- **Trans fats** are made in a process that changes vegetable oils into semisolid fats. These fats can raise blood cholesterol levels and should be eaten in small amounts. Partially hydrogenated and hydrogenated fats are types of man-made trans fats and should be avoided. Trans fats are also found naturally occurring in some animal products such as meat, cheese, butter, and dairy products.

Nutrition Tips

1. A choice on the **Fats** list contains 5 grams of fat and 45 calories.
2. All fats are high in calories. Limit serving sizes for good nutrition and health.

3. Limit the amount of fried foods you eat.
4. Nuts and seeds are good sources of unsaturated fats if eaten in moderation. They have small amounts of fiber, protein, and magnesium.
5. Good sources of omega-3 fatty acids include:
   a. Fish such as albacore tuna, halibut, herring, mackerel, salmon, sardines, and trout.
   b. Flaxseeds, chia seeds, and English walnuts.
   c. Oils such as canola, soybean, flaxseed, and walnut.

Selection Tips

1. Read the Nutrition Facts on food labels for serving sizes. One fat choice is based on a serving size that has 5 grams of fat.
2. The food label also lists total fat grams, saturated fat, and trans fat grams per serving. When most of the calories come from saturated fat, the food is part of the Saturated Fats list.
3. When selecting fats, consider replacing saturated fats with monounsaturated fats and omega-3 fats.

Fats and oils have mixtures of unsaturated (polyunsaturated and monounsaturated) and saturated fats. Foods on the Fats list are grouped together based on the major type of fat they contain. In general, one fat choice equals:

- 1 teaspoon of vegetable oil or butter
- 1 tablespoon of regular salad dressing

Fats

Food	Serving Size
Monounsaturated Fats	
Avocado, medium	2 Tbsp (1 oz)
Nut butters: almond butter, cashew butter, peanut butter (smooth or crunchy)	1½ tsp
Nuts	
Almonds	6 nuts
Brazil	2 nuts
Cashews	6 nuts
Filberts (hazelnuts)	5 nuts
Macadamia	3 nuts
Mixed (50% peanuts)	6 nuts
Peanuts	10 nuts
Pecans	4 halves
Pistachios	16 nuts
Oil: canola, olive, peanut	1 tsp
Olives	
Black (ripe)	8 large
Green, stuffed	10 large
Polyunsaturated Fats	
Mayonnaise	
Reduced-fat	1 Tbsp
Regular	1 tsp
Mayonnaise-Style Salad Dressing	
Reduced-fat	1 Tbsp
Regular	2 tsp
Non-Dairy Spread, stick or tub	1 tsp

Continued

Fats—cont'd

Food	Serving Size
Nuts	
Walnuts, English	4 halves
Pignolia (pine nuts)	1 Tbsp
Oil: canola, corn, cottonseed, flaxseed, grape seed, safflower, soybean, sunflower	1 tsp
Salad Dressing	
Reduced-fat (Note: May be high in carbohydrate)‡	2 Tbsp
Regular‡	1 Tbsp
Seeds	
Chia, flaxseed (whole), pumpkin, sunflower, sesame	1 Tbsp
Tahini or sesame paste	2 tsp
Saturated Fats	
Bacon, cooked, regular, or turkey	1 slice
Butter	
Stick	1 tsp
Whipped	2 tsp
Butter Blend made with Oil	
Reduced-fat or light	1 Tbsp
Regular	1½ tsp
Coconut, sweetened, shredded	2 Tbsp
Coconut Milk	
Light	⅓ cup
Regular	1½ Tbsp
Cream	
Half and half	2 Tbsp
Heavy	1 Tbsp
Light	1½ Tbsp
Whipped	2 Tbsp
Whipped, pressurized	¼ cup
Cream Cheese	
Reduced-fat	1½ Tbsp (¾ oz)
Regular	1 Tbsp (½ oz)
Lard	1 tsp
Oil: coconut, palm, palm kernel	1 tsp
Salt pork	¼ oz
Shortening, solid	1 tsp
Sour Cream	
Reduced-fat or light	3 Tbsp
Regular	2 Tbsp

‡480 milligrams or more of sodium per serving.

FREE FOODS

A "free" food is any food or drink choice that has less than 20 calories and 5 grams or less of carbohydrate per serving.

Selection Tips

1. Most foods on this list should be limited to three servings (as listed here) per day. Spread out the servings throughout the day. If you eat all three servings at once, it could raise your blood glucose level.
2. Food and drink choices listed here without a serving size can be eaten whenever you like.

Free Foods

Food	Serving Size
Low Carbohydrate Foods	
Cabbage, raw	½ cup
Candy, hard (sugar-free)	1 piece
Carrots, cauliflower, or green beans, cooked	¼ cup
Cranberries, sweetened with sugar substitute	½ cup
Cucumber, sliced	½ cup
Gum, sugar free	1 stick
Jam or jelly, light or no sugar added	2 tsp
Rhubarb, sweetened with sugar substitute	½ cup
Salad greens	1 cup raw
Sugar substitutes (artificial sweeteners)	
Syrup, sugar-free	2 Tbsp
Modified Fat Foods with Carbohydrate	
Cream cheese, fat-free	1 Tbsp (½ oz)
Creamers	
Nondairy, liquid	1 Tbsp
Nondairy, powdered	2 tsp
Mayonnaise	
Fat-free	1 Tbsp
Reduced-fat	1 tsp
Mayonnaise-Style Salad Dressing	
Fat-free	1 Tbsp
Reduced-fat	1 tsp
Salad Dressing	
Fat-free or low-fat	1 Tbsp
Fat-free, Italian	2 Tbsp
Sour cream, fat-free or reduced-fat	1 Tbsp
Whipped Topping	
Light or fat-free	2 Tbsp
Regular	1 Tbsp
Condiments	
Barbecue sauce	2 tsp
Honey mustard	1 Tbsp
Horseradish	1 tsp
Ketchup	1 Tbsp
Lemon juice	1 Tbsp
Miso	1½ tsp
Mustard	1 Tbsp
Parmesan cheese, freshly grated	1 Tbsp
Pickle relish	1 Tbsp
Salsa	¼ cup

Free Foods—cont'd

Food	Serving Size
Soy sauce, light or regular‡	1 Tbsp
Sweet and sour sauce	2 tsp
Sweet chili sauce	2 tsp
Taco sauce	1 Tbsp
Vinegar	1 Tbsp
Pickles	
Dill‡	1½ medium
Sweet, bread and butter	2 slices
Sweet, gherkin	¾ oz

‡480 milligrams or more of sodium per serving.

Drinks/Mixes

Any food on this list—without a serving size listed—can be consumed in any moderate amount:

- Bouillon, broth, consommé‡
- Bouillon or broth, low-sodium
- Carbonated or mineral water
- Club soda
- Cocoa powder, unsweetened (1 Tbsp)
- Coffee, unsweetened or with sugar substitute
- Diet soft drinks, sugar-free
- Drink mixes, sugar-free
- Tea, unsweetened or with sugar substitute
- Tonic water, diet
- Water
- Water, flavored, carbohydrate free

Seasonings

Any food on this list can be consumed in any moderate amount:

- Flavoring extracts (e.g., vanilla, almond, peppermint)
- Garlic
- Herbs, fresh or dried
- Nonstick cooking spray
- Pimento
- Spices
- Hot pepper sauce
- Wine, used in cooking
- Worcestershire sauce

COMBINATION FOODS

Many of the foods you eat are mixed together in various combinations, such as casseroles. These "combination" foods do not fit into any one choice list. This is a list of choices for some typical combination foods. This list will help you fit these foods into your meal plan. Ask your RDN for nutrient information about other combination foods you would like to eat, including your own recipes.

Combination Foods

Food	Serving Size	Count As
Entrees		
Casserole type (tuna noodle, lasagna, spaghetti with meatballs, chili with beans, macaroni and cheese)‡	1 cup (8 oz)	2 carbohydrates + 2 medium-fat meats

Combination Foods—cont'd

Food	Serving Size	Count As
Stews (beef/other meats and vegetables)‡	1 cup (8 oz)	1 carbohydrate + 1 medium-fat meat + 0-3 fats
Tuna salad or chicken salad	½ cup (3½ oz)	½ carbohydrate + 2 lean meats + 1 fat
Frozen Meals/Entrees		
Burrito (beef and bean)‡*	1 (5 oz)	3 carbohydrates + 1 lean meat + 2 fats
Entree or meal with more than 340 calories‡	Generally 14-17 oz	3 carbohydrates + 3 medium-fat meats + 3 fats
Entree or meal with less than 340 calories‡	About 8-11 oz	2-3 carbohydrates + 1-2 lean meats
Pizza		
Cheese/vegetarian, thin crust‡	¼ of a 12 inch (4½-5 oz)	2 carbohydrates + 2 medium-fat meats
Meat topping, thin crust‡	¼ of a 12 inch (5 oz)	2 carbohydrates + 2 medium-fat meats + 1½ fats
Pocket sandwich‡	1 (4½ oz)	3 carbohydrates + 1 lean meat + 1-2 fats
Pot pie‡	1 (7 oz)	2½ carbohydrates + 1 medium-fat meat + 3 fats
Salads (Deli-Style)		
Coleslaw	½ cup	1 carbohydrate + 1½ fats
Macaroni/pasta salad	½ cup	2 carbohydrates + 3 fats
Potato salad‡	½ cup	1½-2 carbohydrates + 1-2 fats
Soups		
Asian noodle (pho, ramen)‡	1 cup	2 carbohydrates + 2 fats
Bean, lentil, or split pea‡	1 cup	1 carbohydrate + 1 lean meat
Chowder (made with milk)‡	1 cup (8 oz)	1 carbohydrate + 1 lean meat + 1½ fats
Instant‡	6 oz prepared	1 carbohydrate
With beans or lentils‡	8 oz prepared	2½ carbohydrates + 1 lean meat
Miso soup‡	1 cup	½ carbohydrate + 1 fat
Rice (congee)	1 cup	1 carbohydrate
Tomato (made with water)‡	1 cup (8 oz)	1 carbohydrate
Vegetable beef, chicken noodle, or other broth-type‡	1 cup (8 oz)	1 carbohydrate

*More than 3 grams of dietary fiber per serving.
‡600 milligrams or more of sodium per serving (for combination food main dishes/meals).

FAST FOOD

The choices in the **Fast Food** list are not specific fast food meals or items but are estimates based on popular foods. You can get specific nutrition information for almost every fast food or restaurant chain. Ask the restaurant or check its website for nutrition information about your favorite fast foods.

Fast Food

Food	Serving Size	Count As
Asian		
Beef/chicken/shrimp with vegetables in sauce‡	1 cup (about 5 oz)	1 carbohydrate + 1 lean meat + 1 fat
Egg roll, meat‡	1 (about 3 oz)	1 carbohydrate + 1 lean meat + 1 fat
Fried rice, vegetarian	¹/₂ cup	1 ¹/₂ carbohydrates + 1 ¹/₂ fats
Meat and sweet sauce (orange chicken)‡	1 cup	3 carbohydrates + 3 medium-fat meats + 2 fats
Noodles and vegetables in sauce (chow mein, lo mein)‡*	1 cup	1 carbohydrate + 1 medium-fat meat + 1 ¹/₂ fats
Soup, hot and sour	1 cup	½ carbohydrate + ½ fat
Breakfast Sandwiches		
Egg, cheese, meat, English muffin‡	1 sandwich	2 carbohydrates + 2 medium-fat meats
Sausage biscuit sandwich‡	1 sandwich	2 carbohydrates + 2 high-fat meats + 3¹/₂ fats
Main Dishes/Entrees		
Burrito		
Bean and cheese‡*	1 (about 8 oz)	3 1/2 carbohydrates + 1 medium-fat meats + 1 fats
Beef and beans‡*	1 (about 8 oz)	3 carbohydrates + 3 medium-fat meats + 3 fats
Chicken breast, breaded and fried‡	1 (about 5 oz)	1 carbohydrate + 4 medium-fat meats
Chicken drumstick, breaded and fried	1 (about 2 oz)	2 medium-fat meats
Chicken nuggets‡	6 (about 3¹/₂ oz)	1 carbohydrate + 2 medium-fat meats + 1 fat
Chicken thigh, breaded and fried‡	1 (about 4 oz)	¹/₂ carbohydrate + 3 medium-fat meats + 1¹/₂ fats
Chicken wings, hot‡	6 (5 oz)	5 medium-fat meats + 1¹/₂ fats
Spaghetti with meatballs	1 cup	2 carbohydrates + 2 medium-fat meats
Taco, hard or soft shell (meat and cheese)	1 small	1 carbohydrate + 1 medium-fat meat + 1¹/₂ fats
Taco salad with chicken and tortilla bowl	16 oz	3¹/₂ carbohydrates + 4 medium-fat meat + 3 fats
Pizza		
Cheese, pepperoni, regular crust‡	¹/₈ of a 14 inch (about 4 oz)	2¹/₂ carbohydrates + 1 medium-fat meat + 1¹/₂ fats

Food	Serving Size	Count As
Cheese/vegetarian, thin crust‡	¹/₄ of a 12 inch (about 6 oz)	2¹/₂ carbohydrates + 2 medium-fat meats + 1¹/₂ fats
Sandwiches		
Chicken sandwich, grilled‡	1	3 carbohydrates + 4 lean meats
Chicken sandwich, crispy‡	1	3¹/₂ carbohydrates + 3 medium-fat meats + 1 fat
Fish sandwich with tartar sauce	1	2¹/₂ carbohydrates + 2 medium-fat meats + 2 fats
Hamburger		
Large with cheese‡	1	2¹/₂ carbohydrates + 4 medium-fat meats + 1 fat
Regular	1	2 carbohydrates + 1 medium-fat meat + 1 fat
Soy (meatless)	1	¹/₂ carbohydrate + 2 lean meats
Veggie and grain	1	1 carbohydrate + 2 lean meats
Hot dog with bun‡	1	1 carbohydrate + 1 high-fat meat + 1 fat
Submarine Sandwiches		
Less than 6 grams fat‡	6-inch sub	3 carbohydrates + 2 lean meats
Regular‡	6-inch sub	3 ¹/₂ carbohydrates + 2 medium-fat meats + 1 fat
Salads		
Salad, main dish (grilled chicken type, no dressing or croutons)‡*	Salad	1 carbohydrate + 4 lean meats
Salad, side, no dressing or cheese	Small (about 5 oz)	1 vegetable
Sides/Appetizers		
Falafel patties	3	1 carbohydrate + 1 high-fat meat
French fries, restaurant style†	Small	3 carbohydrates + 3 fats
	Medium	4 carbohydrates + 4 fats
	Large	5 carbohydrates + 6 fats
Hummus	¹/₃ cup	1 carbohydrate + 1 medium-fat meat

Fast Food—cont'd

Food	Serving Size	Count As
Nachos with cheese‡	Small (about 4¹/₂ oz)	2¹/₃ carbohydrates + 4 fats
Onion rings‡	1 serving (about 3 oz)	2¹/₂ carbohydrates + 3 fats
Refried beans‡*	½ cup	1 carbohydrate + 1 lean meat

Food	Serving Size	Count As
Desserts		
Milkshake, any flavor	12 oz	6 carbohydrates + 2 fats
Soft-serve ice cream cone	1 small	2¹/₂ carbohydrates + 1 fat

*More than 3 grams of dietary fiber per serving.
†Extra fat or prepared with extra fat.
‡600 milligrams or more of sodium per serving (for fast food main dishes/meals).

ALCOHOL

Nutrition Tips

1. In general, one alcohol choice (¹/₂ oz absolute alcohol) has about 100 calories.

Selection Tips

1. If you choose to drink alcohol, you should limit it to one drink or fewer per day for women, and two drinks or fewer per day for men.

2. To reduce your risk of low blood glucose (hypoglycemia), especially if you take insulin or a diabetes pill that increases insulin, always drink alcohol with food.

3. While alcohol, by itself, does not directly affect blood glucose, be aware of the carbohydrate (for example, in mixed drinks, beer, and wine) that may raise your blood glucose.

4. Check with your RDN if you would like to fit alcohol into your meal plan.

Alcohol

Alcoholic Beverage	Serving Size	Count As
Beer		
Light (4.2%)	12 fl oz	1 alcohol equivalent + ¹/₂ carbohydrate
Regular (4.9%)	12 fl oz	1 alcohol equivalent + 1 carbohydrate
Distilled spirits: vodka, rum, gin, whiskey 80 or 86 proof	1¹/₂ fl oz	1 alcohol equivalent
Liqueur, coffee (53 proof)	1 fl oz	1 alcohol equivalent + 1 carbohydrate
Sake	1 fl oz	¹/₂ alcohol equivalent
Wine		
Dessert (sherry)	3¹/₂ fl oz	1 alcohol equivalent + 1 carbohydrate
Dry, red or white (10%)	5 fl oz	1 alcohol equivalent

Adapted from: *Choose your foods: food lists for diabetes,* American Diabetes Association and Academy of Nutrition and Dietetics, 2014.
USDA Food Composition Database: United States Department of Agriculture: Agricultural Research Service.
Food Exchange Lists: Diabetes Teaching Center at the University of California, San Francisco, 2018.

ESTIMATED EXCHANGE RECOMMENDATIONS BASED ON CALORIE LEVEL

Omnivore or Vegetarian Diet

Calorie Level	Vegetables	Fruit	Breads, Cereals & Starchy Vegetables	Legumes	Fats	Milk	Meat, Fish, Cheese & Eggs
1500	5	2 - 3	6	1	5	1	2
2000	5	2 - 3	13	2	7	1	2
2500	8	2 - 3	17	2	8	1	3
3000	10	3	20	2	10	1	3

Vegan Diet

Calorie Level	Vegetables	Fruit	Breads, Cereals & Starchy Vegetables	Legumes	Fats
1500	5	2	9	2 - 3	4
2000	5 - 6	2	11	5	8
2500	8	3	17	5	8
3000	10	4	17	6	10

19 APPENDIX

The Ketogenic Diet

The ketogenic diet is a high-fat diet that is low in carbohydrate, adequate in protein, and mimics fasting.[1,2] Under the condition of reduced carbohydrate and increased fat intake, fats are converted into ketone bodies in the liver, resulting in a state of ketosis. Ketone bodies are then utilized as the main energy source by the brain and other organs, instead of the usual energy source, glucose.[1]

A ketogenic diet is an evidence-based and effective treatment primarily for epilepsy that has been utilized and researched for nearly 100 years. Dating back to biblical times, fasting has been noted to treat epilepsy.[1] In the early 1920s, Dr. Russell Wilde at the Mayo Clinic suggested that a high-fat and low-carbohydrate diet can mimic fasting and produce ketosis.[1,2] The diet was developed and utilized for the treatment of epilepsy, but the use of the diet decreased with the introduction of additional antiseizure medications in 1930s.[2] The diet gained increased popularity again in 1990s. The increase in its popularity has been attributed to the efforts of Jim Abraham's family, who, in 1994, founded the Charlie Foundation. The Charlie Foundation is a not-for-profit organization established in the United States to educate the public on the use of ketogenic diets for the treatment of epilepsy after the founder's son, Charlie Abrahams, became seizure-free on the diet. Since then, numerous studies have been published on the use of the ketogenic diet. In 2017, the American College of Nutrition awarded the Charlie Foundation with the Humanitarian Award for being "an organization that has worked selflessly and effectively in the broader field of nutrition to benefit humanity."[3]

Less restrictive variations of ketogenic diet have been developed, including modified Atkins diet (MAD), low glycemic index treatment (LGIT), and medium chain triglyceride (MCT) oil diet (see Tables 1 and 2). The diet type is chosen by the medical team based on individual diet needs, preferences, medical history, and age of each patient.[4] Overall, more than 50% of patients with epilepsy will develop greater than 50% seizure reduction and some will become seizure-free on a ketogenic type diet.[2]

A classic ketogenic diet is the strictest type of a ketogenic diet. Patients are usually young children and are admitted to the hospital for the diet initiation. All meal ingredients are weighed on a gram scale with 0.1 gram accuracy. The diet ratio is calculated for every meal and snack (see Table 3). There is commonly 3 to 4 parts of fat for every 1 part of the sum of protein and net carbohydrates (net carbohydrates = total carbohydrates minus fiber).[1] For example, if a meal contains 40 grams fat, 7 grams protein, and 3 grams net carbohydrates, it has 4:1 ratio, because 40:(7 + 3) = 40:10 = 4:1. A 2016 review of randomized controlled studies showed that with a 4:1 ratio classic ketogenic diet, up to 55% patients became seizure-free and up to 85% had a reduction in seizures.[5] Although 4:1 and 3:1 ratios are the most commonly used, lower diet ratios that accommodate more carbohydrates and contain less fat are used as well and are called a modified ketogenic diet. Lower-ratio diet may provide higher compliance and less side effects; however, diet efficacy can be reduced. The KetoDietCalculator™ (https://www.KetoDietCalculator.org) is a free online program that is used to calculate meal plans.

The MCT oil diet incorporates MCT oil, which is absorbed faster and results in a higher level of ketosis, allowing for more carbohydrates in the diet. The MCT oil diet and classic ketogenic diet have shown to have similar effectiveness and tolerability.[6]

MAD and LGIT utilize household measurements or estimate portion sizes instead of using a gram scale and calculate total amount of net carbohydrate allowance per day instead of calculating a diet ratio for every meal and snack[1] (see Tables 4 and 5). These diets are usually initiated in a home setting.[1,4] These less restrictive forms of ketogenic diet produce less side effects and may be easier to follow, thus increasing compliance.[2] The diet is considered a better fit for older children and adults.[7] However, the MAD and LGIT appear to be slightly less effective than the classic ketogenic diet.[2]

The diet is contraindicated for some individuals, especially those with carnitine or fatty acid oxidation disorders, failure to thrive, eating disorders, history of kidney stones, gastrointestinal (GI) disorders, major organ dysfunction, and dyslipidemia among others (see Table 6).[2,4] The exact mechanism of the diet action is unknown, but its effectiveness is due to a combination of several factors, including decreased inflammation and changes in blood glucose levels and neurotransmitters.[2] Emerging research suggests that changes in the microbiota may also play a role.[8]

The multidisciplinary team approach, with a neurologist, a nurse, and a dietitian trained in ketogenic diets, is key to the successful diet initiation and maintenance.[2] Pharmacists and social workers also play an important role in supporting the patient and the family on the diet and assuring compliance.[2,4] Many potential side effects of the diet can be prevented by appropriate diet initiation, laboratory monitoring, and nutrient supplementation (see Tables 7, 8).[2,4]

Although the diet has been originally used for the treatment of epilepsy, it has since been studied and utilized in a variety of other conditions, including cancer, Alzheimer's disease, Parkinson's disease, weight loss, traumatic brain injury, mitochondrial disorders, autism, diabetes, migraines, bipolar disorder, multiple sclerosis, and amyotrophic lateral sclerosis[3] with varying levels of success. The utilization of ketogenic diets in the treatment of cancer, especially brain tumors, is promising but requires additional research.[9,10] For example, the use of a ketogenic diet in the treatment of gliomas is considered experimental but generally safe according to the available research.[9] There is a need for more research to help better understand the safety, tolerability, effectiveness, and appropriate administration of ketogenic diets for cancer[9,10] and other disorders.

TABLE 1 Example of Approximate Macronutrient Composition of Available Ketogenic Diet Therapies*

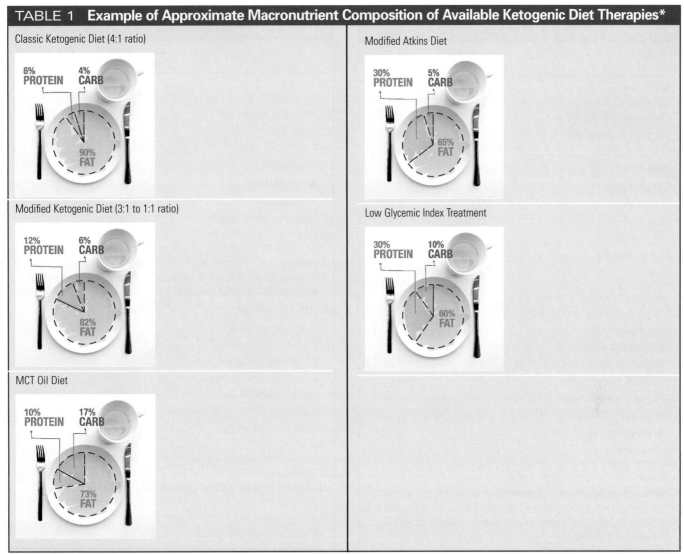

Classic Ketogenic Diet (4:1 ratio)
6% PROTEIN   4% CARB   90% FAT

Modified Ketogenic Diet (3:1 to 1:1 ratio)
12% PROTEIN   6% CARB   82% FAT

MCT Oil Diet
10% PROTEIN   17% CARB   73% FAT

Modified Atkins Diet
30% PROTEIN   5% CARB   65% FAT

Low Glycemic Index Treatment
30% PROTEIN   10% CARB   60% FAT

*Note: Ratio and specific macronutrient composition can vary on each type of ketogenic diet. The above images serve as a visual comparison of diet compositions. Images obtained from The Charlie Foundation for Ketogenic Therapies www.CharlieFoundation.org website.

TABLE 2 Comparison of Macronutrient Composition and Initiation Requirements Between Various Ketogenic Diets and the 2015–2020 Dietary Guidelines for Americans[a]

Diet	Fat	Carbohydrate	Protein	Hospital Admission
	←	range (%)	→	
2015-2020 Dietary Guidelines for Americans	20-35	45-65	10-35	No
Ketogenic diet ratio[b]				
4:1	90	2-4	6-8	Yes
3:1	85-90	2-5	8-12	Varies
2:1	80-85	5-10	10-15	Varies
Modified Atkins diet (1:1 ratio[b])	60-65	5-10	25-35	No
Low glycemic index treatment (1:1 ratio[b])	60-70	20-30	10-20	No
Medium-chain triglyceride diet (1:1 ratio[b])	60-70	20-30	10	Yes

[a]Based on data from the Charlie Foundation for Ketogenic Therapies and U.S. Department of Health and Human Services.
[b]Ratio refers to grams of (fat) : (net carbohydrates + protein).
Note: Kossoff 2018 guidelines do not recommend hospital admission for most, though individual cases may vary.
(From Roehl K, Sewak SL: Practice paper of the Academy of Nutrition and Dietetics: classic and modified ketogenic diets for treatment of epilepsy, J Acad Nutr Diet 117(8):1279–1292, 2017.)

TABLE 3 Sample Menu for the Classic Ketogenic Diet, 3:1 Ratio[a]

	Grams Net Carbohydrate	Fat (in Grams)
Breakfast		
Egg Scramble (To prepare: Melt butter in frying pan; scramble all items together on medium heat.)		
71 g raw egg mixed well	0.51	6.75
17 g heavy cream	0.51	6.12
28 g butter	0.02	22.71
29 g feta cheese	1.2	6.17
21 g spinach	0.3	0.08
10 g mushrooms, chopped	0.23	0.02
10 g olive oil	0	22.71
Breakfast Subtotal:	2.76	64.56
Lunch		
Cobb Salad (To prepare: Toss all salad ingredients together in a bowl, top with olive oil and red wine vinegar.)		
72 g mixed greens	0.9	0.22
18 g avocado, sliced	0.33	2.77
68 g hard-boiled egg, chopped	0.76	7.21
14 g finely chopped bacon	0.42	6.3
15 g hard cheese shredded	0.27	4.55
31 g olive oil	0	31
15 g red wine vinegar	0	0
Lunch Subtotal:	2.68	52.05
Dinner		
Chicken and Zucchini "Pasta" (To prepare: Slice zucchini thinly into "noodles" and sauté in olive oil. Mix half the pesto into the zucchini and spread the other half on top of chicken. Basil Pesto recipe available at https://www.ketodietcalculator.org.)		
39 g baked chicken breast	0	1.4
80 g sliced or spiraled zucchini	1.69	0.26
28 g olive oil	0	28
32 g basil pesto	0.62	16.7
Dinner Subtotal:	2.76	46.36
Snacks		
Celery & Cream Cheese		
10 g stalk of celery, sliced	0.14	0
30 g full-fat cream cheese	1.1	10.3
Snacks Subtotal:	1.24	0
Daily Total:	9.44	173.27

[a]Approximate daily total: 1700 kcal; (173.27 g fat): (9.44 g net carbohydrate + 45 g protein) = 3:1 diet ratio.
Nutrition information obtained from: https://www.ketodietcalculator.org.
(Roehl K, Sewak SL: Practice paper of the Academy of Nutrition and Dietetics: classic and modified ketogenic diets for treatment of epilepsy, J Acad Nutr Diet 117(8):1279 -1292, 2017.)

TABLE 4 Sample Menu for the Modified Atkins Diet[a]

	Grams Net Carbohydrate	Fat (in Servings[b])
Breakfast		
Egg Scramble (To prepare: Melt butter in frying pan; scramble all items together on medium heat.)		
2 large eggs	1	1
2 Tbsp heavy cream	½	1
1 Tbsp butter	0	1
¼ cup feta cheese	2	½
½ cup spinach	½	0
½ cup mushrooms, chopped	1	0
Breakfast Subtotal:	5	3½
Lunch		
Cobb Salad (To prepare: Toss all salad ingredients together in a bowl, top with olive oil and red wine vinegar.)		
1½ cups mixed greens	½	0
½ cup avocado, sliced	2	1
1 hard-boiled egg, sliced	1	½
1 Tbsp finely chopped bacon	0	½
¼ cup blue cheese or cheddar cheese, shredded	1	1
2 Tbsp olive oil	0	2
1 Tbsp red wine vinegar	0	0
Lunch Subtotal:	4½	5
Dinner		
Chicken and Zucchini "Pasta" (To prepare: Slice zucchini thinly into "noodles" and sauté in olive oil. Mix half the pesto into the zucchini and spread the other half on top of chicken.)		
1 medium baked chicken breast	0	0
1 cup sliced or spiraled zucchini	2½	0
1 Tbsp olive oil	0	1
2 Tbsp pesto	1	1
Dinner Subtotal:	3½	2
Snacks		
Celery & Cream Cheese		
1 stalk of celery, sliced	1	1
2 Tbsp full-fat cream cheese	2	0
½ cup sugar-free gelatin	½	0
Snacks Subtotal:	3½	1
Daily Total:	16½	11½

[a]Approximate daily total: 1700 kcal, 16½ g net carbohydrate, 75 g protein, 150 g fat (11½ servings).
[b]1 serving = 14 g of fat.
(Roehl K, Sewak SL: Practice paper of the Academy of Nutrition and Dietetics: classic and modified ketogenic diets for treatment of epilepsy, J Acad Nutr Diet 117(8):1279 -1292, 2017.)

TABLE 5 Sample Menu for Low Glycemic Index Treatment[a]

	Grams Net Carbohydrate	Fat (in Servings[b])		Grams Net Carbohydrate	Fat (in Servings[b])
Breakfast			**Dinner**		
Egg Scramble (To prepare: Melt butter in frying pan; scramble all items together on medium heat.)			Chicken and Zucchini "Pasta" (To prepare: Slice zucchini thinly into "noodles" and sauté in olive oil. Mix half the pesto into the zucchini and spread the other half on top of chicken.)		
2 large eggs	1	1	1 medium baked chicken breast	0	0
1 Tbsp heavy cream	½	½	1 cup sliced or spiraled zucchini	2½	0
1 Tbsp butter	0	1	1 Tbsp olive oil	0	1
¼ cup feta cheese	2	½	2 Tbsp pesto	1	1
½ cup spinach	½	0	Dinner Subtotal:	3½	2
½ cup mushrooms, chopped	1	0			
1 medium grapefruit	18	0	**Snacks**		
Breakfast Subtotal:	23	3	*Celery & Cream Cheese*		
			3 small stalks of celery, sliced	½	0
Lunch			2 Tbsp full-fat cream cheese	1	1
Cobb Salad (To prepare: Toss all salad ingredients together in a bowl; top with olive oil and red wine vinegar.)			*Yogurt & Strawberries*		
1½ cups mixed greens	½	0	8 oz plain/unsweetened Greek yogurt (4% milkfat)	8	1
½ cup avocado, sliced	1	½	½ cup strawberry halves (mix into yogurt)	5	0
1 hard-boiled egg, sliced	½	½	Snacks Subtotal:	14½	2
1 Tbsp finely chopped bacon	0	½	Daily Total:	44	10½
¼ cup blue cheese or cheddar cheese, shredded	1	1			
1 Tbsp olive oil	0	1			
1 Tbsp red wine vinegar	0	0			
Lunch Subtotal:	3	3½			

[a]Approximate daily total: 1700 kcal, 44 g net carbohydrate, 75 g protein, 140 g fat (10½ servings).
[b]1 serving = 14 g of fat.
(Roehl K, Sewak SL: Practice paper of the Academy of Nutrition and Dietetics: classic and modified ketogenic diets for treatment of epilepsy, J Acad Nutr Diet 117(8):1279 -1292, 2017.)

TABLE 6 Contraindications for the Use of Ketogenic Diet, Absolute and Relative, With Suggested Workups for Relative Concerns

Contraindication/Concern	Action
Absolute	Do not initiate ketogenic diet
Carnitine deficiency (primary)	
Carnitine palmitoyltransferase (CPT) I or II deficiency	
Carnitine translocase deficiency	
Beta-oxidation defects	
• Medium-chain acyl dehydrogenase deficiency (MCAD)	
• Long-chain acyl dehydrogenase deficiency (LCAD)	
• Short-chain acyl dehydrogenase deficiency (SCAD)	
• Long-chain 3-hydroxyacyl-CoA deficiency	
• Medium-chain 3-hydroxyacyl-CoA deficiency	
Pyruvate carboxylase deficiency	
Porphyria	
Surgical focus identified by neuroimaging and video-electroencephalography (EEG) monitoring	
Propofol concurrent use (risk of propofol infusion syndrome may be higher)	• Consult with physician
Relative Contraindications	• Obtain gastrointestinal consult
• Inability to maintain adequate nutrition or hydration	• Obtain swallow evaluation
• Failure to thrive	• Consider need for gastronomy tube placement
• Dysphagia	• Increase fat/kcal before initiation
• Gastrointestinal issues (chronic diarrhea, vomiting, reflux)	• Trial of 4:1 ketogenic formula

TABLE 6   Contraindications for the Use of Ketogenic Diet, Absolute and Relative, With Suggested Workups for Relative Concerns

Contraindication/Concern	Action
• Not able to meet fluid goals • Extreme picky eating/limited food acceptance	• Provide recipes/foods to trial • Behavioral feeding consult
Concerning medical history • Extreme dyslipidemia • Cardiomyopathy • Renal disease/renal calculi • Liver disease • Baseline metabolic acidosis	• Obtain cardiology, nephrology, or hepatology consult for clearance • Adjust fluid minimums • Add citrate, consider bicitrate to alkalize urine, avoid drugs such as topiramate and zonisamide • Taper off contraindicated medications if possible, increase fluid minimums, consider beginning with lower diet ratio
Social constraints • Access to food and kitchen • Caregiver noncompliance • Multiple caregivers/unstable home environment	• Connect family with social worker to discuss access to services, for example (but not limited to) durable medical equipment; Special Supplemental Program for Women, Infants, and Children; respite care; in home supportive services; formula company's assistance programs • Registered dietitian nutritionist can discuss meal and food options that may be feasible for family

Table created by Maggie Moon, MS, RDN, combined data from: Roehl K, Sewak SL: Practice paper of the Academy of Nutrition and Dietetics: classic and modified ketogenic diets for treatment of epilepsy, J Acad Nutr Diet 117(8):1279 -1292, 2017; and Kossoff EH, Zupec-Kania BA, Auvin S, et al: Optimal clinical management of children receiving dietary therapies for epilepsy: updated recommendations of the International Ketogenic Diet Study Group, Epilepsia Open 3(2):175 -192, 2018. doi:10.1002/epi4.12225.

TABLE 7   Dietary Supplements for Orally Fed Patients on Ketogenic Diet

Recommended supplements:*
• Multivitamin with minerals and trace minerals, especially selenium
• Calcium with vitamin D (meeting daily recommended dietary allowance [RDA] requirements)

Optional supplements to consider based on specific patient needs:
• Vitamin D (above RDA)
• Oral citrates
• Laxatives (Miralax, mineral oil, glycerin suppository)
• Additional selenium, magnesium, zinc, phosphorus, iron, copper
• Carnitine
• Probiotic
• Eicosapentaenoic acid/docosahexaenoic acid
• Medium chain triglyceride oil
• Table salt/light salt
• Digestive enzymes

*All supplements should be provided as carbohydrate-free when possible.

Table created by Maggie Moon, MS, RDN, combined data from: Roehl K, Sewak SL: Practice paper of the Academy of Nutrition and Dietetics: classic and modified ketogenic diets for treatment of epilepsy, J Acad Nutr Diet 117(8):1279 -1292, 2017; and Kossoff EH, Zupec-Kania BA, Auvin S, et al: Optimal clinical management of children receiving dietary therapies for epilepsy: updated recommendations of the International Ketogenic Diet Study Group, Epilepsia Open 3(2):175 -192, 2018. doi:10.1002/epi4.12225.

Medical, social, and nutrition history should be taken into account when determining whether a patient is an appropriate candidate for a ketogenic diet. It is important to take a comprehensive look at the patient's family history, genetics (including increased cardiovascular risk), and lifestyle and to communicate any potential risks and benefits of following any restrictive diet, such as a ketogenic diet.

Suggested Organizations for Additional Information:
Charlie Foundation https://www.charliefoundation.org
Matthew's Friends https://www.matthewsfriends.org
International League Against Epilepsy https://www.ilae.org
Keto Hope Foundation https://www.ketohope.org

TABLE 8 Laboratory Values Taken at Ketogenic Diet Therapy Follow-up Visits

Standard laboratory assessment recommendations throughout various states of ketogenic diet therapy. Protocols may vary by institution, individual patient, and diet type. Based on data from the Charlie Foundation for Ketogenic Therapies.[3]

Laboratory values	Prediet baseline	Daily during admission	1 and 3 mo post diet initiation	Every 3 mo until stable	Every 6 to 12 mo
Urine organic acids	X				
Plasma amino acids	X				
Complete metabolic panel	X	X	X	X	X
Complete blood count with platelets	X	X	X	X	X
Liver profile	X		X	X	X
Ionized calcium	X		X	X	X
Magnesium	X		X	X	X
Phosphate	X		X	X	X
Prealbumin	X		X	X	X
Lipid panel (fasting)	X		X	X	X
Vitamin D$_3$	X			X	X
Free and total carnitine	X		X	X	X
β-hydroxybutyrate	X	X	X	X	X
Selenium	X			X	X
Zinc	X		X	X	X
Urinalysis	X		X	X	X
Urine calcium	X		X	X	X
Urine creatinine	X		X	X	X
Vitamins A, E, and B$_{12}$				X	X
Copper				X	X
Folate/ferritin				X	X

(Roehl K, Sewak SL: Practice paper of the Academy of Nutrition and Dietetics: classic and modified ketogenic diets for treatment of epilepsy, J Acad Nutr Diet 117(8):1279 -1292, 2017.)

REFERENCES

1. Kossoff EH, Turner Z, Doerrer S, et al: *The ketogenic and modified Atkins diets: treatments for epilepsy and other disorders*, 6 ed, New York, NY, 2016, Demos Health.
2. Roehl K, Sewak SL: Practice paper of the Academy of Nutrition and Dietetics: classic and modified ketogenic diets for treatment of epilepsy, *J Acad Nutr Diet* 117(8):1279–1292, 2017.
3. Charlie Foundation for Ketogenic Therapies. 2018. Available at: https://www.charliefoundation.org. Accessed January 21, 2019.
4. Kossoff EH, Zupec-Kania BA, Auvin S, et al: Optimal clinical management of children receiving dietary therapies for epilepsy: updated recommendations of the International Ketogenic Diet Study Group, *Epilepsia Open* 3(2):175–192, 2018. doi:10.1002/epi4.12225.
5. Martin K, Jackson CF, Levy RG, et al: Ketogenic diet and other dietary treatments for epilepsy, *Cochrane Database Syst Rev* 9(2):CD001903, 2016. doi:10.1002/14651858.CD001903.pub3.
6. Neal EG, Chaffe H, Schwartz RH, et al: The ketogenic diet for the treatment of childhood epilepsy: a randomised controlled trial, *Lancet Neurol* 7(6):500–506, 2008. doi:10.1016/S1474-4422(08)70092-9.
7. Cervenka MC, Kossoff EH: Dietary treatment of intractable epilepsy, *Continuum (Minneap Minn)* 19(3 Epilepsy):756–766, 2013. doi:10.1212/01.CON.0000431396.23852.56.
8. Zhang Y, Zhou S, Zhou Y, et al: Altered gut microbiome composition in children with refractory epilepsy after ketogenic diet, *Epilepsy Res* 145: 163–168, 2018. doi:10.1016/j.eplepsyres.2018.06.015.
9. Noorlag L, De Vos FY, Kok A, et al: Treatment of malignant gliomas with ketogenic or caloric restricted diets: a systematic review of preclinical and early clinical studies, *Clin Nutr* 38(5):1986–1994, 2019. doi:10.1016/j.clnu.2018.10.024.
10. Sremanakova J, Sowerbutts AM, Burden S: A systematic review of the use of ketogenic diets in adult patients with cancer, *J Hum Nutr Diet* 31(6):793–802, 2018. doi:10.1111/jhn.12587.

Appendix created by Lisa I. Shkoda, RDN, CSO, CSP, CNSC, FAND.

The International Dysphagia Diet Standardisation Initiative (IDDSI)

INTRODUCTION AND BACKGROUND

The clinical disorder of swallowing, known as dysphagia, is addressed by multiple professionals at different phases of diagnosis, treatment, and management. The clinical management must be approached as an interdisciplinary venture in that a primary mechanism is through diet texture modification (Lam et al, 2017). The communication between speech-language pathologists (SLPs) and nutrition professionals supports the identification of food preferences, the modifications to food to support safe oropharyngeal transit, and the active consideration of an individual's quality of life.

How does the existing classification system under the National Dysphagia Diet (NDD) fit in this framework?

A universal language for the various diet textures had been attempted under the National Dysphagia Diet (NDD) initiative in 2002. At that time the American Dietetic Association, now the Academy of Nutrition and Dietetics (AND), through the National Dysphagia Diet Task Force (NDDTF), described terminology related to dysphagia, texture, and viscosity of common food and liquid modifications, and created an implementation strategy using the NDD for hospitals.

Though a task force composed of dietetic professionals and SLPs existed, the resulting framework was not peer-reviewed by the American Speech-Language-Hearing Association (ASHA). Though widely used, the framework was not considered an evidenced-based standard for SLPs (NDDTF, 2002). Resulting research addressed concerns of fidelity within implementation and consistency across settings. However, the framework also made apparent that multiple key components were absent in the medical language used to diagnose and manage dysphagia. Therefore the resulting widespread use of the NDD system was adopted in practice by SLPs. Important recommendations that resulted from the NDDTF were as follows:

- a need for scientific foundations of diet texture modification;
- a need for consistency in food preparation;
- consideration of texture modifications for both liquids and solids;
- prescriptive integration for the diagnosis, treatment, and management of dysphagia;
- standardization of practice;
- application within health care facilities and in the transition home; and
- and continuity among all settings.

The diet classifications were established using an exemplary food item within each category with the understanding that the diet descriptions needed to have flexibility to address all possible foods (NDDTF, 2002). However, one limitation of the framework immediately recognized was the inability to specifically categorize all foods (McCullough et al, 2003). Further, the NDD did not provide testing methods to determine classification with certainty.

Food textures were characterized on levels with anchor foods to aid in characterization:

- Level 1, or dysphagia puree;
- Level 2, or dysphagia mechanically altered;
- Level 3, or dysphagia advanced; and
- Regular, or all foods allowed.

In a similar manner, specifications for viscosity of fluids were outlined as follows:

- Thin liquids, described as 1 to 50 centipoise
- Nectar-like, described as 51 to 350 centipoise
- Honey-like, described as 351 to 1750 centipoise
- Spoon-thick, described as >1750 centipoise

Initial intentions included correlation of a standardized severity scale, such as the Dysphagia Outcome and Severity Scale (DOSS), to aid in classification. The idea behind this was to support an evidence-based decision component for the use of a particular diet texture (McCullough et al, 2003). However, ASHA never supported the use of a scale to determine a specific texture modification as this would diminish the role of clinical judgment and expertise of SLPs in assessing the swallow mechanism (McCullough et al, 2003). Therefore the standard of practice remained a combination of testing methods paired with clinical judgment.

Emergence of a New International Dysphagia Diet Standardisation Initiative (IDDSI)

Within the use of the NDD, dysphagia management professionals expressed concerns relating to characterizations of foods not found on the exemplary list or not matching closely enough with the exemplary item (Lam et al, 2017). Continued challenges persisted in managing the difficulties with the consistency of preparation to attain a specified level and subsequent quality control assessments. Managing external factors on foods when textures are modified, and availability of commercially produced modified diets in maintaining described textures, were also of concern (Cichero, 2014). Finally, despite attempts at a consistent language, the terminology of the NDD still seemed to vary across and within settings, which created uncertainty (Lam et al, 2017).

Rather than modify the existing framework by overlaying standardized components, a team of diverse professionals reviewed existing research, professional concerns related to implementation and use, and patient reports of use and confusion to create a new framework (Cichero, 2014). Professionals represented included dietitians, SLPs, food scientists, physicians, occupational therapists, engineers, and nurses (IDDSI, 2018). The initial goal was directed toward patient safety and better treatment of dysphagia by tracking outcomes (Cichero et al, 2013). This goal expanded to include a system across the life span, cultural terms and uses, detailed definitions, accessible and inexpensive testing, input of professionals involved in food preparation, and publication-level standardization of use (Cichero et al, 2017).

The resulting framework addressed gaps in research related to inconsistent descriptions and uses for diet texture modifications. Steele et al (2015) noted combining "nectar-thick" and "slightly thicker than thin" to encapsulate research for swallowing impaired individuals who required modification to their liquid. Even more so, solids were sometimes minimally categorized as "soft," "hard," or "puree," a significant reduction from even the NDD framework recommendations (Steele et al, 2015). As such, research attempting to understand the therapeutic and physiologic benefits of modified diets were unable to address basic questions related to consistency across multiple settings, carryover of findings into new settings, and actual consistency of foods tested (Steele et al, 2015). What resulted was better insight into patient safety and professional oversight for diet texture modification, and consequently, an entirely new framework.

DEVELOPMENT

In 2013, the committee members created the International Dysphagia Diet Standardisation Initiative (IDDSI) to address the need for a standardized global terminology (IDDSI, 2017). Within their research and experimentation methods, the committee defined eight distinctive groups across liquids and solids, as well as the intersection of liquids and solids. The continuum is identified by number, description, and color coding to support users across language differences, global cuisines, education level, and food service industry familiarity (IDDSI, 2017). See Figure 1.

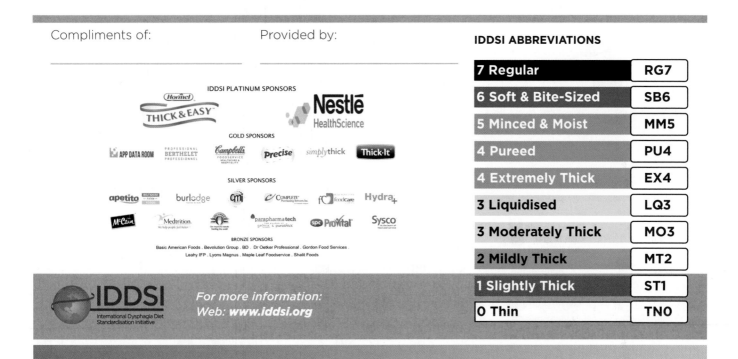

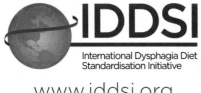

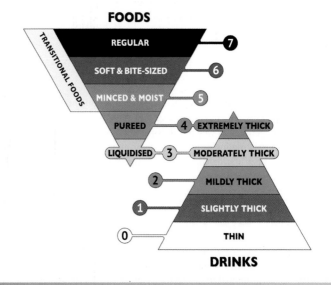

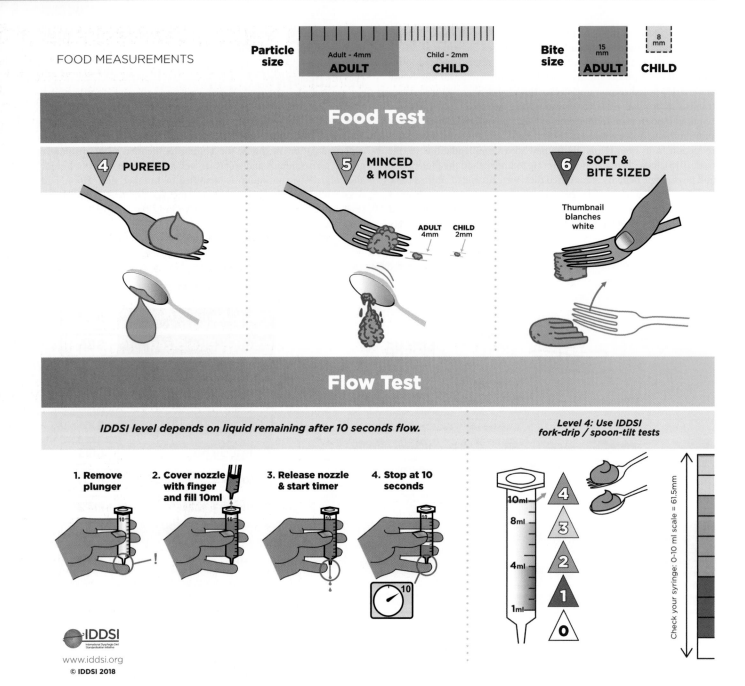

Another inclusion element is that the dysphagia continuum is now across all age groups. The framework incorporates aspects of pediatric dysphagia management as well as adults with considerations for food preparation and testing inside and outside of medical facilities. Unlike prior attempts at a standardized system, the IDDSI committee expanded considerations for cultural foods (Cichero et al, 2017). This consideration allowed for the development of different testing methods and a departure from terminology that would only be understood by professionals within the medical or food service industry (Cichero et al, 2017).

As such, the resulting labels are defined in multiple ways to support users of varied training and education in food preparation. Each level is defined by its number, 0 to 7. The direction of the triangle identifies the food as a solid or a liquid with the presence of two triangles for textures which are present in both areas (IDDSI, 2017). Information is available to support clinical decision making for the use of a particular texture. However, no texture is mandated for a particular clinical presentation. The key component for each diet texture is the testing method available to accurately identify the uncertain food item within a category description (IDDSI, 2017). The ability to test any food item and classify it within the framework allows for the IDDSI framework to be implemented consistently in any setting. Simple training for family members allows for transition to the home setting with carryover of the recommended diet texture.

FRAMEWORK

One of the unique components of the IDDSI framework is the ease of testing available. This component allows for the framework to apply to any potential food without relying on exemplar foods as the standard.

The tests used are the Flow Test, Fork Drip Test, Fork Pressure Test, Spoon Tilt Test, Chopstick Test, and the Finger Test.

- The Flow Test involves using a 10 mL syringe where fluid is filled to the 10 mL line and then allowed to flow for 10 seconds. The remaining amount of fluid defines the consistency.
- The Fork Drip Test requires a standard fork. Food is scooped onto the fork, and classification is based on how it drips, if at all, through the tines.
- The Fork Pressure Test involves using a standard fork which typically has a 4 mm space between each tine. This spacing serves as a measurement for adults as "bite-sized." Using the tines on the food and a thumb pressed on the solid portion of the fork, the pressure required to blanch the fingernail is comparable to the lingual pressure required within a swallow. The way the food changes, or not, determines the food texture level.
- The Spoon Tilt Test involves a standard spoon used to scoop food in a small mound. The spoon can then be tipped slightly. The manner of which the food falls off the spoon and its ability to maintain shape on the plate, or not, define the consistency.
- The Chopstick Test is similar to the Finger Test where the food is picked up and squeezed between the chopsticks. The ability to hold shape, or not, defines the consistency.

The first three levels describe liquids only. Within the framework these triangles are right-side up and identify these consistencies as only liquids. These levels are best tested and differentiated with a 10 mL syringe (i.e., the Flow Test). The three levels are differentiated by how much fluid is left in the syringe after 10 seconds.

- 0 – Thin: no residue
- 1 – Slightly Thick: will leave 1 to 4 mL in the syringe
- 2 – Mildly Thick: will leave 4 to 8 mL in the syringe

The expectations for thin, level 0, is for the liquid to flow "like water" (IDDSI, 2017). As such, a thin liquid can pass through a teat, a nipple, a cup, or a straw without difficulty. The expectation for slightly thick, level 1, is for the liquid to be a little thicker than water (IDDSI, 2017). The thickness described is commercially found in "anti-regurgitation infant formula" (IDDSI, 2017). This level requires a little more effort to pass through a straw, syringe, teat, or nipple than a level 0 would require. A level 2, or mildly thick, liquid should easily flow off a spoon, but sipping from a standard straw would require effort given the slower flow (IDDSI, 2017). IDDSI (2017) recommends this level if tongue control is slightly reduced, or if the individual is unable to manage faster flowing fluids as would be found in a level 0.

The next two levels, 3 and 4, comprise the overlap of liquids and solids; these levels maintain two triangles, one right-side up and one upside-down on the framework (see Figure 1). As such, the availability of testing options increases if the item being tested is meeting a liquids requirement verses a solids texture. Available methods for testing include the Flow Test, the Fork Drip Test, the Spoon Tilt Test, the Chopstick Test, and the Finger Test.

- 3 – Liquidized/Moderately Thick:
  - Flow Test: >8 mL will remain in the syringe.
  - Fork Drip Test: Dollops through the prongs, fork does not leave a pattern on the surface, and food will spread out on the plate.
  - Spoon Tilt Test: Will not stick to the spoon when poured from the spoon.
  - Chopstick Test: Not suitable.
  - Finger Test: Not suitable.
- 4 – Pureed/Extremely Thick:
  - Flow Test: Not suitable.
  - Fork Drip Test: Fork tines will leave a clear pattern on the surface; no lumps in the food; food will sit in a mound on the plate; food may seep between tines, but it will not drip continuously.

- Spoon Tilt Test: Food will hold a shape on the spoon, and it will hold together and fall off the spoon all at once. It may spread out a little bit on a plate.
- Chopstick Test: Not suitable.
- Finger Test: Difficult, but able to hold a small sample between fingers. When rubbing fingers together, no noticeable residue will remain.

Levels 3 and 4 integrate foods and liquids that share properties. A level 3 liquid could be drunk from a cup or sipped through a straw with effort. A level 3 cannot hold shape, so serving on a plate or eating with a fork would not be appropriate. No chewing or oral processing is required for this food (IDDSI, 2017). IDDSI (2017) recommends this texture for individuals with pain on swallow or the need for extra time for oral control. A level 4 is differentiated in that it can be eaten with a fork, and it will hold its shape on a plate. A key component for a level 4 is that it must be cohesive but not sticky. IDDSI differentiates between cohesion and adhesion when identifying foods in level 4. Consider a scoop of chocolate pudding versus a scoop of peanut butter. Both are cohesive (i.e., stick together), but peanut butter is adhesive as well, so it will leave significant residue on the spoon whereas pudding will leave minimal residue. IDDSI (2017) recommends a level 4 when tongue control is significantly reduced; the texture requires no chewing or biting.

The remaining three levels, 5 through 7, define solids. As such, the triangle is upside-down on the framework for these levels. The availability of testing options includes the Fork Pressure Test, Fork Drip Test, Spoon Tilt Test, Chopstick test, and Finger Test. The Flow Test is not appropriate for this level.

- 5 – Minced and Moist:
  - Fork Pressure Test: Food will easily separate when pressed; little pressure (i.e., nail blanching not required) will mash food out of its presented shape.
  - Fork Drip Test: Food will sit in a pile on the fork without falling through the tines.
  - Spoon Tilt Test: When the spoon is tilted, food should easily fall off. It may spread slightly on a plate.
  - Chopstick Test: When chopsticks are pressed together, food can be scooped or held in position.
  - Finger Test: When placed between the fingers, the food can be held in place. The food will leave the fingers wet.
- 6 – Soft and Bite-Sized:
  - Fork Pressure Test: A fork can be used to cut the food. When using pressure and the thumbnail blanches, the sample will change shape and is unable to return to prior shape.
  - Spoon Pressure Test: A spoon can be used to cut the food. When using pressure and the thumbnail blanches, the sample will change shape and not return to the prior shape.
  - Chopstick Test: Can break the food into smaller pieces.
  - Finger Test: With pressure between the thumb and index finger to blanch the nail, the food will change shape and be unable to return to its prior shape.
- 7 – Regular:
  - There are no tests for this level as all foods are acceptable.

Levels 5 and 6 create differentiation from prior systems in the specificity of food size. For a level 5, adult-sized food is to be within 4 mm lump sizes, or the space between the tines of a fork (IDDSI, 2017). For pediatric populations, this is 2 mm (IDDSI, 2017). Minimal oral processing in terms of chewing is required for this level, with the tongue being necessary to support bolus transit. For a level 6, the adult-sized piece is 1.5 cm, or a standard fork's width (IDDSI, 2017). For pediatric populations, this size is reduced to 8 mm (IDDSI, 2017). A level 6 mandates the need for chewing and enough lingual control for bolus movement and transit. Level 7 is meant to include foods that are naturally hard or soft, may include chewy, sticky, crunchy, combined textures, variable sizes (i.e., seeds), and layers of complexity (i.e., pith inside skin) (IDDSI, 2017). Foods considered to be regular have no tests because there are no exclusions or exceptions.

Another unique aspect of the IDDSI framework is in the consideration of "transitional food" (IDDSI, 2017). These foods are defined as items that change from one texture to another when moisture or changes in temperature are presented to the food item. As such, minimal chewing may support modifying the bolus, but often the lingual pressure is sufficient. Tests may be applied after the modification (i.e., moisture or temperature change). The results would be as follows:

- Fork Pressure Test: With a "bite-size" portion, the fork pressure for blanching the thumbnail should result in the sample changing shape, or it has melted into a different shape.
- Chopstick Test: With a "bite-size" portion, the food will break apart with the pressure from squeezing the chopsticks together.
- Finger Test: With a "bite-size" portion, the food will break apart with the pressure from squeezing the fingers together.

Implementation and Utilization: Where and How Is the IDDSI Being Utilized?

While this is continually changing, IDDSI.org tracks policy related to implementation. As such, Australia, Canada, and the United States have scheduled adoption of the IDDSI framework as the standard by May 1, 2019 (IDDSI, 2018; AND, n.d.). Discussions for implementation are in process in Belgium, Brazil, China, Denmark, France, Germany, Ireland, Israel, Japan, the Netherlands, New Zealand, Norway, Poland, Slovenia, Sweden, South Africa, Thailand, and Turkey (IDDSI, 2018). The United Kingdom has an adoption date of April 2019 (IDDSI, 2018). The United States has endorsed the need for creating an implementation process. This commitment has been led by joint work of the Academy and the ASHA.

Challenges: How Do We Understand Patient Choice Within This Framework? How Do We Implement to Fidelity? How Do We Address Exceptions?

Many challenges that arise result from applying the IDDSI framework to individuals who do not have dysphagia. Though common practice to qualify a diet texture in the absence of dysphagia, the IDDSI framework was not created to capture diet modifications for purposes outside of dysphagia management and risk reduction (Cichero et al, 2013). Therefore the diet textures do not address elements of nutritional adequacy or quantity measurements in the context of thickened fluids (Cichero et al, 2013). Further, as was a concern for the NDD, the IDDSI is not meant to be prescriptive in coordination with a standardized swallow function test to determine a particular diet texture (Cichero et al, 2013). The levels are defined in a particular manner with specific testing results that aid in classification. Once the presence of dysphagia is established, clinical expertise and judgment identify appropriate textures based on physiologic presentations. As such, there are no exceptions if the IDDSI framework is implemented correctly (IDDSI, 2018).

Patient choice remains an integral element of dysphagia management. Discussing with the patient and family the risks associated with a diet texture outside of the recommended levels is meant to be a professional discussion between a provider and a patient.

Training food service providers in the different levels and how to test them will aid in increasing staff knowledge and understanding of the IDDSI framework (Garcia et al, 2018). A continued challenge in medical settings is the consistency of implementation for diet texture modifications. This challenge involves training food service staff so they understand how to prepare foods in levels 5 and 6, how to cut into bite-size to attain a level 6, how to mix fluids to attain a level 2 or 3, and

how to use sauces within the different levels. Furthermore, in institutional food service, holding times in warmers and steam tables can affect the food texture and must be taken into consideration. These challenges have carried over from prior systems, such as the NDD, and remain a challenge of implementation under the IDDSI (Garcia et al, 2018). The role of testing supports accuracy of diet texture modifications (Garcia et al, 2018).

WEBSITES RECOMMENDED FOR ADDITIONAL RESEARCH

International Dysphagia Diet Standardisation Initiative
https://www.iddsi.org
Academy of Nutrition and Dietetics
http://www.eatright.org
https://www.eatrightpro.org/practice/practice-resources/post-acute-care-management/international-dysphagia-diet-standardization-initiative
https://www.eatrightpro.org/media/press-releases/positions-and-issues/academy-and-asha-support-new-global-standardization-of-diets-for-swallowing-disorders
American Speech-Language Hearing Association
http://www.asha.org
https://blog.asha.org/2018/05/17/iddsi-implementation-hows-it-going/
https://blog.asha.org/2017/11/07/iddsi-next-steps-tools-tips-for-smooth-implementation/

REFERENCES

Academy of Nutrition and Dietetics (AND): Available at https://www.eatright-pro.org/search-results?keyword=IDDSI, n.d.

Cichero JA: Standardization of dysphagia diet terminology across the lifespan: an international perspective, *SIG 13 Perspectives on Swal and Swal Dis (Dysphagia)* 23:166–172, 2014. doi:10.1044/sasd23.4.166.

Cichero JA, Lam P, Steele CM, et al: Development of international terminology and definitions for texture-modified foods and thickened fluids used in dysphagia management: the IDDSI framework, *Dysphagia* 32:293–314, 2017. doi:10.1007/s00455-016-9758-y.

Cichero JA, Steele C, Duivestein J, et al: The need for international terminology and definitions for texture-modified foods and thickened liquids used in dysphagia management: foundations of a global initiative, *Curr Phys Med Rehabil Rep* 1:280–291, 2013. doi:10.1007/s40141-013-0024-z.

International Dysphagia Diet Standardisation Initiative. 2018. Available at: http://iddsi.org.

International Dysphagia Diet Standardisation Initiative: *Complete IDDSI framework detailed definitions*, 2017. Available at: http://iddsi.org/Documents/IDDSIFramework-CompleteFramework.pdf .

Garcia JM, Chambers IV E, Russell EG, et al: Modifying food textures: practices and beliefs of staff involved in nutrition care, *Am J Speech Lang Pathol*, 27(4):1458–1473, 2018. doi:10.1044/2018_AJSLP-18-0021.

Lam P, Stanschus S, Zaman R, et al: The international dysphagia diet standardisation initiative (IDDSI) framework: the Kempen pilot, *BJNN/Stroke Assoc Suppl* S18–S26, 2017.

McCullough G, Pelletier C, Steele C: National dysphagia diet: What to swallow? *ASHA Lead* 8:16–27, 2003. doi:10.1044/leader.FTR3.08202003.16.

National Dysphagia Diet Task Force: *National dysphagia diet: standardization for optimal care*, Chicago, IL, 2002, Academy of Nutrition & Dietetics.

Steele CM, Namasivayam-MacDonald AM, Guida BT, et al: Creation and initial validation of the international dysphagia diet standardisation initiative functional diet scale, *Arch Phys Med Rehabil* 99:934–944, 2018.

Steele CM, Alsanei WA, Ayanikalath S, et al: The influence of food texture and liquid consistency modification on swallowing physiology and function: a systematic review, *Dysphagia* 30:2–26, 2015. doi:10.1007/s00455-014-9578-x.

Appendix created by Ashley Contreras-France, MA, MS, CCC-SLP.

Renal Diet for Dialysis

Your diet depends on your kidney function. Most of the information here relates to people on dialysis. What is right for others is not always right for you. As your kidney function changes, your diet may change as well. This guide will help you do two things: plan nutritious meals you enjoy and keep your body working at its best. Your renal dietitian will work with you to make any changes needed to your usual meal plan, but this will provide helpful guidelines.

1. Increase Protein

   You will need to eat a high-protein diet. Your protein needs are based on your weight. Most people need at least 6 to 8 oz of protein per day.

2. Limit Potassium

   Most foods contain some potassium, but fruits and vegetables are the easiest to control. Limit high potassium foods to 1 serving from the high, 2 from the medium and 2-3 from the low list per day (see list on following page).

   Do not use salt substitute or "lite" salt because they are made with potassium.

3. Limit Salt

   Limit the salt you eat. Don't add salt during cooking or at the table. Avoid high-salt foods such as frozen meals; canned or dried foods; "fast foods"; and salted meats such as ham, sausage, and luncheon meats. Use salt-free spices or spice mixes such as Mrs. Dash instead of salt to add flavor to your food.

4. Limit Phosphorus

   Use only one serving of milk or dairy food per day. A serving is usually ½ to 1 cup. Take phosphate binders such as Tums, PhosLo, Renagel, or Fosrenol with your meals as prescribed by your doctor.

5. Fluid

   A safe amount of fluid to drink is different for everyone. It depends on how much urine you are making. Try not to drink more than 3 cups (24 oz) of fluid each day plus the amount equal to your urine output. If you are limiting your salt intake, you should not feel thirsty.

   Fluids include all beverages and foods that are liquid at room temperature such as Jell-O, ice cream, popcicles, ice, and soup.

6. Poor Appetite and Weight Loss

   It is common to have a poor appetite if you are new to dialysis. If your appetite has been poor, try eating small frequent meals and extra snacks. Try adding high-calorie fats such as butter, non-hydrogenated margarine, and oils; sauces and gravies; and sour cream, cream cheese, or whipped cream for extra calories. Adding rice, pasta, bread, and rolls to meals also adds calories. Talk to your dietitian about adding a high calorie nutritional supplement.

PROTEIN

When on dialysis, you need to eat a high-protein diet. This is because you lose protein during each dialysis treatment. To stay healthy, you need to eat enough protein for your daily needs and also make up for the amount lost during dialysis. Meat, fish, poultry, eggs, and other animal foods provide most of the protein in your diet, although some vegetarian foods are acceptable options too (see list below). Your body uses protein to build and repair muscles, skin, blood, and other tissues.

ALBUMIN

Albumin is a protein found in blood. Each month a laboratory test measures your albumin. It is a good way to know how healthy you are. Your albumin level should be more than 3.4 mg/dL. To maintain a healthy albumin level, make sure to eat enough protein. Find your weight on the chart below to identify the number of servings you need each day.

PROTEIN SERVINGS FOR YOU

If you weigh:	You need:
40 kg	4-5 servings
50 kg	5-6 servings
60 kg	6-7 servings
70 kg	7-8 servings
80 kg	8-9 servings
90 kg	9-10 servings
Your weight: _____ kg	
You need: _____ protein servings each day	

ONE SERVING OF PROTEIN

1 egg
1 oz cooked meat, fish, poultry
¼ cup cooked or canned fish, seafood
½ cup tofu
1 cup milk
1 oz cheese
¼ cup cottage cheese
¾ cup pudding or custard
2 Tbsp peanut butter
1 scoop protein powder
½ protein bar

COMMON SERVING SIZES

Most people eat protein foods in portions larger than one serving. Here are some examples:
Average hamburger patty (3 oz) = 3 protein servings
Small beefsteak (3 in × 4 in) = 4 protein servings
Half chicken breast (3 oz) = 3 protein servings
Chicken drumstick or thigh (2 oz) = 2 protein servings
Average pork chop (3 oz) = 3 protein servings
Fish fillet (3 in × 3 in) = 3 protein servings

ESTIMATING SERVING SIZES

Here are some other easy ways to estimate protein serving sizes:
- Your whole thumb is about the size of 1 oz.
- Three stacked dice are about the size of 1 oz.
- A deck of cards is about the size of 3 oz.
- The palm of your hand is about the size of 3 to 4 oz.
- Your clenched fist is about the size of 1 cup.

TIPS FOR EATING MORE PROTEIN

Some people on dialysis dislike the taste of protein. Some people find cooking smells unpleasant. Still others are not able to eat enough protein each day.
The following tips will be helpful:
- Use gravy, sauces, seasonings, or spices to improve or hide flavors.
- Prepare meals ahead of time or stay away from kitchen smells if they spoil your appetite.
- Eat cooked protein foods cold. Try cold fried chicken, a roast beef sandwich, or shrimp salad.
- Add cut-up meats or beans to soups or salads.
- Use more eggs. Try hardboiled eggs, egg salad sandwiches, custards, or quiches. Stir beaten eggs into casseroles and soups.
- Try other protein foods such as angel food cake, peanut butter, or bean salads.
- Eat a protein bar. Your nutritionist can help you choose one.
- Use a protein powder. Your nutritionist can help you choose one and give you ideas for using it.

NUTRITIONAL SUPPLEMENTS

Nutritional supplements provide extra calories and protein. In general, use one can of supplement as a snack each day. Add one extra can for each meal you miss.

Not all nutritional supplements are safe for dialysis patients. Check with your nutritionist before using any supplement. Some of the supplements that are used by people on dialysis are listed below.

MALNUTRITION

If you are not eating enough high-protein foods, your albumin level will drop below the recommended level.

If your albumin level is low, the cells in your body cannot hold fluid well. This leads to swelling (edema) and low blood pressure during dialysis. Low albumin increases your risk of death. Patients with albumin levels above four have the lowest death rate.

It is also important to eat enough calories. Your nutritionist can help you make sure you are getting plenty of protein and calories.

EXERCISE

Try to be active in some way each day (e.g., walk, swim, garden, stretch). Using your muscles helps keep them strong. Protein that is stored in your muscles helps support your albumin level.

POTASSIUM FOR PEOPLE ON HEMODIALYSIS

- Most foods have some potassium, but fruits and vegetables are the easiest form to control in your diet. The following list groups vegetables and fruits by the amount of potassium in one serving.
- Remember, there are no foods that you cannot eat on your diet. What is important is the amount of foods you eat and how often you eat them. Keep this list handy for shopping or eating out.
- If there are fruits and vegetables you enjoy that are not on the list, ask your nutritionist about them.

MOST PEOPLE ON HEMODIALYSIS MAY HAVE

- One serving per day from the high-potassium group
- Two servings per day from the medium-potassium group
- Two to three servings per day from the low-potassium group
This is approximately 2000 to 3000 mg of potassium per day with the other foods you eat. Check the serving size for each food, listed in parentheses next to the item.

SOAKING VEGETABLES AND BEANS

Soaking works well for high-potassium foods such as potatoes, parsnips, sweet potatoes, winter squash, and beans. The procedure for soaking follows.
1. Peel vegetables and slice thinly (1/8 inch). Rinse well. Place them in a bowl of warm water, using four times more water than vegetable. For example, soak 1 cup of sliced vegetables in 4 cups of water. Soak at least 1 hour. Drain and rinse again.
2. Vegetables that have been soaked this way can then be fried, mashed, scalloped, put in soups or stews, or served fresh. If you are boiling the food, use four times more water than food and cook as usual.
3. Dried beans should be cooked and then chopped and soaked, using the preceding directions. Canned beans can simply be chopped, rinsed, and soaked.

	Low-Potassium Foods 5-150 mg	Medium-Potassium Foods 150-250 mg	High-Potassium Foods 250-500 mg
		Food Category	
Fruits	Applesauce (½ cup)	Apple (1 medium), cherries (8-10)	Apricots (3)
	Blackberries (½ cup)	Fruit cocktail (½ cup)	Avocados (¼)
	Blueberries (1 cup)	Grapes (10-15)	Banana (1 medium)
	Grapefruit (½ cup)	Mango (½ medium)	Dates (5)
	Pears, canned (½ cup)	Melons: cantaloupe, honeydew (½ cup),	Figs (3)
	Pineapple (½ cup)	papaya (½ cup)	Kiwi (1)
	Plums, canned (½ cup)	Peaches, canned (½ cup)	Nectarine (1 medium)
	Raspberries (½ cup)	Pear, fresh (1 medium)	Orange (1 medium)
	Rhubarb, cooked (½ cup)	Plums (2)	Peach, fresh (1 medium)
	Strawberries (½ cup)	Watermelon (1 cup)	Prunes (5)
	Tangerine (1)		Raisins and dried fruit (¼ cup)
Vegetables	Asparagus (4 spears)	Broccoli (½ cup)	Artichoke (1 medium)
	Bean sprouts (½ cup)	Brussels sprouts (4-6)	Beans: lima, kidney, navy, pinto (½ cup)
	Cabbage (½ cup)	Beets (½ cup)	Greens: beet, collard, mustard, spinach, turnip (½ cup)
	Cauliflower (½ cup)	Carrots (½ cup)	Lentils, split peas, chickpeas, black-eyed peas (½ cup)
	Corn (½ cup)	Celery (½ cup)	Nuts: all kinds (½ cup)
	Cucumber (½)	Eggplant (½ cup)	Parsnips (½ cup)
	Green and wax beans (½ cup)	Mixed vegetables (½ cup)	Potatoes (½ cup or 1 small)
	Lettuce (1 cup)	Mushrooms (½ cup)	Pumpkin (½ cup)
	Okra (3 pods)	Peanut butter (2 Tbsp)	Spinach (½ cup)
	Onions (½ cup)	Pepper, green (1)	Tomato (1 medium)
	Peas (½ cup)	Potato chips (10)	Tomato sauce, tomato salsa (¼ cup)
	Radishes (5)	Soaked potatoes (½ cup)	Winter squash (½ cup)
	Rutabagas (½ cup)		Yams, sweet potatoes (½ cup)
	Summer squash (½ cup)		
	Turnips (½ cup)		
	Water chestnuts (4)		
Juices	Apple juice (½ cup)	Apricot nectar (½ cup)	Pomegranate juice (½ cup)
	Cranberry juices (1 cup)	Grape juice, canned (½ cup)	Prune juice (½ cup)
	Grape juice, frozen (1 cup)	Grapefruit juice (½ cup)	Tomato juice (½ cup)
	Tang, Hi-C and other fruit drinks (1 cup),	Pineapple juice (½ cup)	V-8 juice (½ cup)
	Kool-Aid (1 cup)		
	Lemonade and limeade (1 cup)		
	Peach or pear nectar (½ cup)		

OTHER HIGH-POTASSIUM FOODS

- Milk is high in potassium. Limit milk to 1 cup per day unless you are told to do otherwise.
- Supplements such as Ensure Plus also contain a lot of potassium. Always speak to your nutritionist before using supplements.
- Most salt substitutes and "lite" salt products are made with potassium. Do not use these products. If you are unsure, ask your nutritionist.

SHAKING THE SALT HABIT

Salt, or sodium chloride, is found in convenience and preserved foods. Foods that do not spoil easily are usually high in sodium. The more sodium you eat, the thirstier you will be. The following list of foods is grouped by sodium levels.

Following a low-sodium diet can be challenging. This list of sodium levels of foods is meant to help you learn what foods and how much of them you can enjoy.

Remember, there are no foods that you cannot eat on your diet. What is important is the amount of foods you eat and how often you eat them. Keep this list handy for shopping or dining.

MOST PEOPLE ON DIALYSIS MAY HAVE

- 1 serving per day from the high group
- 3 servings per day from the medium group
- As many servings as desired from the low group*
    *Your daily sodium should not exceed 2000 mg of sodium per day.
Check the serving size for each and the sodium content.

RINSING CANNED FOODS TO LOWER SODIUM (CANNED VEGETABLES, CHUNK OR FLAKED FISH OR SHELLFISH, POULTRY, OR MEATS)

1. Empty can into colander or sieve.
2. Drain brine and discard.
3. Break up chunks into flakes or smaller pieces.
4. Rinse under running water for 1 min.
5. Drain food until most moisture is gone.

	Low-Sodium Foods 1-150 mg	Medium-Sodium Foods 150-250 mg	High-Sodium Foods 250-700 mg
		Food Category	
Breads and cereals	Breads, white, whole grain Cakes, cookies, crepes, doughnuts Cereals: cooked, granola, puffed rice, puffed wheat, Shredded Wheat, Sugar Pops, Sugar Smacks, Sugar Crisps Crackers: graham, low salt, melba toast Macaroni, noodles, spaghetti, rice Corn tortillas	Biscuits, rolls, muffins: homemade (1) Pancakes (1) "Ready-to-eat" cereals (¾ cup) Saltine crackers (6) Sweet roll (1)	All Bran (¼ cup) Instant mixes: noodles, potatoes, rice (½ cup) Instant mixes: biscuits, breads, muffins, rolls (1 serving) Flour tortillas Waffles (1)
Condiments	Butter, margarine, oil Horseradish, mustard, spices, herbs, sugar, syrup, Tabasco, vinegar, Worcestershire	Bacon (2 slices) Catsup, steak sauce (1 Tbsp) Commercial salad dressing (1 Tbsp) Gravy (2 Tbsp) Low-sodium soy sauce (2 tsp) Mayonnaise (2 Tbsp) Pickle relish (2 Tbsp) Sweet pickles (2 small)	Salt (¼ tsp)
Dairy products	Cheeses: cream, Monterey, mozzarella, ricotta, low-salt types Cream: half-and-half, sour, whipping Custard, ice cream, sherbet Milk: all kinds, yogurt Nondairy creamer	Cheeses (1-oz slice) Cottage cheese (½ cup) Pudding (¾ cup)	Buttermilk (1 cup) Processed cheeses and cheese spreads (1 slice or 2 Tbsp)
Main dishes	All unprocessed meats, fish, poultry Eggs Peanut butter Tuna: low-sodium or rinsed		Broth (½ cup) Canned fish, meat (¼ cup) Canned soups (½ cup) Hot dog (1) Luncheon meat (1 slice) Canned entrees (e.g., pork and beans, spaghetti, stew) (1 cup) Sausage (1 oz)
Fruits and vegetables	All fresh or frozen vegetables All fruits and juices Canned tomatoes, tomato paste Canned vegetables: low-sodium or rinsed	Vegetables (½ cup) Juices: tomato, vegetable (½ cup)	Canned tomato sauce or puree (¼ cup) Frozen vegetables with special sauce (½ cup) Sauerkraut (¼ cup)
Beverages and snacks	Beer, wine, coffee, tea Candy: all kinds Fruit drinks, Popsicles, soda pop, Kool-Aid, Tang Low-salt products: without potassium substitutes Unsalted nuts, unsalted popcorn	Potato and corn chips (1 cup) Snack crackers (5-10)	Commercial dips (¼ cup) Dill pickle chips (3 slices) Olives (5) Salted nuts (½ cup)

PHOSPHORUS

Low-Phosphorus Diet

When phosphorus is high for too long, bones become brittle and weak. You may have joint and bone pain. Extra phosphorus may go into your soft tissue, causing hard or soft lumps. Also, you may have severe itching.

The good news is that with diet, binders, and good dialysis, you can keep your phosphorus level under control.

Phosphorus is a mineral found in most foods. Dialysis does not remove it easily. Your phosphorus level depends on the foods you eat and your medications. Keeping your phosphorus at a safe level will help keep your bones healthy.

Each month your phosphorus level will be measured. High phosphorus is a common problem for people on dialysis. A good phosphorus level in your blood is between 3 and 6 g/dL.

High-Phosphorus Foods

Phosphorus is found in most foods you eat, especially protein foods. The foods that are highest in phosphorus are milk and things made from milk (dairy foods).

By limiting these foods you can cut down on the phosphorus you are eating. Most people on dialysis can have one serving daily from this list of dairy foods. The serving size is also noted.

You can also eat part of a serving of different foods to add up to one serving.

Milk (1 cup)
Cheese (2 oz)
Cottage cheese (2/3 cup)
Yogurt (1 cup)
Ice cream (1½ cup)
Frozen yogurt (1½ cup)
Milkshake (1 cup)
Hot chocolate (1 cup)
Pudding or custard (1 cup)

Other High-Phosphorus Foods

When your phosphorus level is high, you may need to limit these foods to once a week.
Bran cereals (1 oz)
Dried beans or peas (½ cup cooked)
Chili (½ cup)
Nuts (½ cup)
Frozen waffles (1)

Phosphorus and Potassium

High-phosphorus foods are often high in potassium as well. This is another reason to limit dairy foods and other high-phosphorus foods.

Phosphate Binders

Phosphate binders are pills you take when you eat. Binders help keep phosphorus in your food from going into your blood.

Your doctor will decide which binder is best for you and how many you should take each time you eat.

It is important to take all your binders planned for each day.

You can take your binders just before you start a meal, during the meal, or right after eating.

If you forget to take them or skip a meal, it may be difficult to get your full binder dose. Ask your doctor what to do if this happens.

It may take some hard work to remember to take binders each time you eat. Try these ideas:
- Each morning take out the number of binders you need that day. Put them in a small container to carry with you. It should be empty at the end of the day.

- Carry a spare container of binders for when you travel or eat out.
- Take your binders with high-protein snacks such as sandwiches or dairy foods.
- Binders may cause constipation. Talk with your nutritionist about ideas to help with bowel movements.
- There are many types of binders. If you don't like the kind you are taking, talk with your doctor, pharmacist, or nutritionist about other kinds.

Lower Phosphorus Ideas

Following are some lower phosphorus choices you can make in the place of milk and other creamy dairy products. Check those you will try.
- Use nondairy creamer such as Mocha Mix, Coffee Rich, or rice or soy milk on cereal, for creamy sauces or soups, and in shakes.
- Try soy cheese or soy yogurt. They are available in a variety of flavors.
- Use cream cheese in the place of regular cheese or cottage cheese.
- Use sour cream or imitation sour cream on fruits or to replace yogurt in dips.
- Try a nondairy frozen ice cream made from soy, rice, or nondairy creamer such as Mocha Mix.
- Enjoy sorbet or sherbet instead of ice cream.

High Phosphorus Levels

Following are some reasons for a high phosphorus level. Check the ones that you think may apply to you:
- Eating too many high-phosphorus foods
- Forgetting to take your binders
- Not taking all the phosphate binders ordered for you
- Not taking your phosphate binders at the right times

Even if you follow your diet and take your binders, your phosphorus level may be high. When calcium and phosphorus are out of balance, your parathyroid gland becomes overactive. High levels of parathyroid hormone damage your bones. Your doctor can test for this problem and recommend treatment.

Appendix created by Katy G. Wilkens, MS, RDN.
Northwest Kidney Centers, Seattle, Washington
NOTE: Some foods are very high in sodium and should be used only once a week. These include East Asian foods; corned beef, ham, and pastrami; fast foods (e.g., commercial hamburgers, pizza, tacos); pickles; soy sauce; and TV dinners and frozen entrees.

The Antiinflammatory Diet

DIETARY APPROACHES TO REDUCE INFLAMMATION

Inflammation is thought to underlie most chronic health conditions including metabolic syndrome, type 2 diabetes, cancer, cardiovascular disease, arthritis, autoimmune diseases, atopic conditions, inflammatory bowel disease, and cognitive decline. Various nutrients, foods, and dietary patterns have been shown to reduce inflammatory markers as well as subjective and objective measures of inflammation.

Multiple iterations of an antiinflammatory diet exist: Dietary Approaches to Stop Hypertension (DASH), Mediterranean, Mediterranean-DASH Intervention for Neurodegenerative Delay (MIND), vegetarian, food allergy elimination, calorie restriction, intermittent fasting, and low histamine. In most cases, overall dietary and lifestyle habits are more important to consider rather than any single change. Which diet is right for any individual often depends on trial and error (Casas et al, 2016; Kaluza et al, 2019).

The Dietary Inflammatory Index (DII) has been developed and validated as a tool to evaluate the overall inflammatory potential of the diet based on evaluation of over 6500 peer-reviewed research articles. The DII consists of 45 foods, spices, nutrients, and bioactive compounds in relation to six inflammatory biomarkers: IL-1β, IL-4, IL-6, IL-10, TNF-α, and C-reactive protein (Garcia-Arellano et al, 2015; Shivappa et al, 2014). In recent studies, dietary patterns with a higher DII have been associated with an increased risk of cancer, asthma, cardiovascular disease, low bone density, depression, and metabolic syndrome (Bergmans and Malecki, 2017; Fowler and Akinyemiju, 2017; Neufcourt et al, 2015; Shivappa et al, 2016).

Dietary components with the most antiinflammatory effects are included as negative numbers in the Overall Inflammatory Effect Score as shown in the table below.

Food Parameters in the Dietary Inflammatory Index and Overall Inflammatory Effect Score

Food Parameter	Overall Inflammatory Effect Score	Food Parameter	Overall Inflammatory Effect Score
Alcohol (g)	−0-278	Riboflavin (mg)	−0-068
Vitamin B$_{12}$ (μg)	0-106	Saffron (g)	−0-140
Vitamin B$_6$ (mg)	−0-365	Saturated fat (g)	0-373
β-Carotene (μg)	−0-584	Se (μg)	−0-191
Caffeine (g)	−0-110	Thiamin (mg)	−0-098
Carbohydrate (g)	0-097	Trans fat (g)	0-229
Cholesterol (mg)	0-110	Turmeric (mg)	−0-785
Energy (kcal)	0-180	Vitamin A (RE)	−0-401
Eugenol (mg)	−0-140	Vitamin C (mg)	−0-424
Total fat (g)	0-298	Vitamin D (μg)	−0-446
Fiber (g)	−0-663	Vitamin E (mg)	−0-419
Folic acid (μg)	−0-190	Zn (mg)	−0-313
Garlic (g)	−0-412	Green/black tea (g)	−0-536
Ginger (g)	−0-453	Flavan-3-ol (mg)	−0-415
Fe (mg)	0-032	Flavones (mg)	−0-616
Mg (mg)	−0-484	Flavonols (mg)	−0-467
MUFA (g)	−0-009	Flavonones (mg)	−0-250
Niacin (mg)	−0-246	Anthocyanidins (mg)	−0-131
n-3 Fatty acids (g)	−0-436	Isoflavones (mg)	−0-593
n-6 Fatty acids (g)	−0-159	Pepper (g)	−0-131
Onion (g)	−0-301	Thyme/oregano (mg)	−0-102
Protein (g)	0-021	Rosemary (mg)	−0-013
PUFA (g)	−0-337		

MUFA, Monounsaturated fatty acid; PUFA, polyunsaturated fatty acid; RE, Retinol equivalents.
Adapted from Shivappa N, Steck SE, Hurley TG, et al: Designing and developing a literature-derived, population-based dietary inflammatory index, Public Health Nutr 17:1689–1696, 2014.

The following recommendations reflect an effort to consolidate similarities among the various antiinflammatory diets.

CONSUME AN ABUNDANCE OF FRUITS, VEGETABLES, HERBS, AND SPICES

Colorful fruits and vegetables contain a myriad of antiinflammatory phytochemicals and fiber and are thought to be the cornerstone of an antiinflammatory diet due to their ability to down-regulate markers such as C-reactive protein (CRP), Nuclear Factor-kappa Beta (NFkB), histamine, and other inflammatory cytokines in vivo and in vitro.

Most plant-based foods contain antiinflammatory properties, but the following fruits and vegetables appear to be the most antiinflammatory based on their mention in research: cruciferous vegetables, onions, berries, purple grapes, cherries, citrus fruits, tomatoes, and pomegranates. Antiinflammatory herbs and spices include: green and black tea, turmeric, garlic, ginger, rosemary, oregano, fenugreek, caraway, anise, cocoa, mint, clove, coriander, cinnamon, nutmeg, red chili powder, lemongrass, fennel, saffron, black pepper, parsley, sage, dill, bay leaf, and basil (Aggarwal and Shishodia, 2004; Galland, 2010; Habauzit and Morand, 2012; Jiang et al, 2014; Jungbauer and Medjakovic, 2012; Panahi et al, 2016).

ENCOURAGE A LOW GLYCEMIC DIET PATTERN

Excessive amounts of refined carbohydrates and sugars may be proinflammatory. Regular consumption of these high glycemic foods can increase blood glucose and insulin levels, which, when chronically elevated, can trigger an inflammatory response. Choosing low glycemic foods has been shown to reduce post-prandial glucose and insulin levels and modestly lower concentrations of insulin-like growth factor (IGF) and improve the inflammatory and adipokine (inflammatory proteins secreted by adipose tissue) profiles (Neuhouser et al, 2012; Runchey et al, 2012). It is important to look at the glycemic load of a food versus the glycemic index because the glycemic load is a better indicator of the actual portion of food. See Appendix 28. For example, beets have a high glycemic index: 64, but a low glycemic load: 5.

High Glycemic Foods	Low Glycemic Foods
Cookies, cakes, pastries,* chips, white flour breads, crackers, tortillas, pasta, white rice	Whole and unprocessed grains, (like oats, brown rice, quinoa, whole wheat) high-fiber or whole grain pastas
Fruit juice and dried fruits	Fresh fruit
White (russet potatoes) mashed or baked without the skin	Sweet potatoes, pumpkin, squashes, beans and lentils, nuts and seeds
Sugar-sweetened sodas and other beverages	Most vegetables**

*cookies, cakes etc., can be made using low glycemic ingredients like oats and nuts, which can reduce their glycemic load.
**Consuming large amounts of certain juiced vegetables like carrots or beets will produce a higher glycemic load.

INCLUDE NUTS AND SEEDS OR NUT AND SEED BUTTERS EVERY DAY

Nuts and seeds not only provide antiinflammatory and valuable phenolic compounds, but they provide a beneficial ratio of polyunsaturated fats (omega-6 and omega-3) that helps to support a healthy inflammatory response in the body. Consume a variety of nuts in order to gain the spectrum of nutrients that each has to offer. Especially beneficial are pumpkin seeds, sunflower seeds, almonds, cashews, Brazil nuts, flaxseed, sesame seeds, and walnuts.

ADJUST THE QUALITY AND QUANTITY OF DIETARY FAT AND OILS

Increase:
Unsaturated fats high in omega-3 fatty acids (alpha-linolenic acid), which are antiinflammatory. Best sources include coldwater fish, flax, chia and hemp seeds, and walnuts. Flaxseed, walnut and expeller pressed canola oils are excellent plant sources of omega-3 fatty acids but should not be heated. Choose brands that use low-heat processing for best quality.
Monounsaturated fats:
Use extra virgin olive oil as the main ingredient for sauces, salad dressings, and marinades. It can also be used for low-heat sautéing.
Avocados can replace cheese or mayonnaise on sandwiches, and can be added to dips, smoothies, and salads.

Decrease:
Red meats contain arachidonic acid and saturated fats, which can increase inflammation if eaten in excess, especially in those with a higher body mass index (BMI) (Chai et al, 2017).
Processed foods and oils are high in omega-6 fatty acids (linoleic acid) such as soybean, corn, safflower, and sunflower oils. Omega-6 fatty acids can increase proinflammatory markers in the body if eaten in excess. Many of these oils are common in highly processed foods. Deep fried foods or oils heated (and reheated) to high temperatures may result in oxidation and trans fat formation causing a pro-inflammatory effect.

Avoid:
Hydrogenated fats and trans fats that are found in many baked and prepackaged foods and are in hydrogenated vegetable shortening and many margarines. Trans fat consumption has been shown to increase markers of systemic inflammation and is particularly associated with coronary artery disease. Trans fats were banned in processed foods in the United States in July 2015, and manufacturers had 3 years to completely remove it.

SUPPORT A HEALTHY MICROBIOME

Preliminary studies suggest that consumptions of fermented foods (probiotics) and plant fibers (prebiotics) may help reduce inflammation by supporting a healthy microbiome in the gut (Hiippala et al, 2018). Fermented and cultured foods are an excellent source of probiotic bacteria. Sources include miso, sauerkraut, yogurt, kefir, kimchi, tempeh, and kombucha (a fermented beverage). Prebiotic foods feed the good bacteria and are also important for gut health. Inulin and fructooligosaccharides are examples of prebiotics and can be found in bananas, asparagus, maple syrup, onions, garlic, chicory, artichoke, and many other plant foods.

ELIMINATE FOODS THAT CAUSE SYMPTOMS OF ALLERGY AND INTOLERANCE

Adverse reactions to food can induce the production of a variety of inflammatory mediators including immunoglobulins, cytokines, and histamine. Reactions can be either immediate or delayed, and their intensity may depend on dose and individual tolerance. Risk may depend on timing and composition of food exposure in early life, diet quality, and gastrointestinal microflora balance.

AVOID CHEMICALS

Many industrial chemicals and pesticides can irritate or disrupt the immune system and cause inflammation. Choose organic or low pesticide foods and "green" personal care and cleaning products to reduce exposure. Many canned foods contain bisphenol A in their linings. Bisphenol A (BPA), which is also found in many plastic bottles and food containers, is an endocrine disrupter, impairs the action of insulin in the body, and upregulates inflammatory pathways (Valentino et al, 2013). Seek out "BPA-Free" cans and use glass containers and bottles as often as possible. Refer online to the Environmental Working Group for more information.

DRINK ALCOHOL IN MODERATION

Alcohol can have the effect of both increasing and decreasing markers of inflammation, depending on the individual person and the amount consumed. High intake, especially for prolonged periods, can increase inflammatory cytokines (Miller et al, 2011). In the PREDIMED trial, moderate alcohol consumption was associated with improved lipid profiles, blood pressure, endothelial function, and reduced reactive oxygen species (ROS) and was associated with about a one drink equivalent (10 g) per day. Red wine is the most commonly featured as antiinflammatory.

CALORIE RESTRICTION AND INTERMITTANT FASTING

Modification of dietary patterns including calorie restriction (CR) and intermittent fasting (IF) have been studied for their effect on inflammation, longevity, and metabolic health. CR involves a reduction of calories by 20% to 40% while maintaining a consistent meal pattern. In multiple animal models, CR has led to significant lengthening of lifespan and reduction of inflammatory markers (González, 2012). In humans, CR has shown improvements in metabolic health, but the effect on longevity is still under investigation. Studies have demonstrated a similar metabolic and antiinflammatory benefits with the use of IF. Although several methods exist, the most common application of IF includes a 13-hour overnight fast (also called prolonged nightly fasting) and alternate-day fasting where participants alternate fasting with ad libitum eating (Patterson and Sears, 2017). Both of these interventions should be employed with care to ensure they are used appropriately. While most of the research is positive, there is theoretically a potential for harm in certain populations, especially those with disordered eating or in those with critical illness.

REDUCE STRESS AND IMPROVE SLEEP

High stress levels and lack of adequate sleep are both associated with inflammation. Elevated circulating cortisol levels found under conditions of psychological stress are associated with elevated inflammatory cytokines. Sustained sleep deprivation has also been associated with an inflammatory state and an elevation of CRP, TNF-α, interleukin (IL)-1β, IL-2, IL-4, and monocyte chemo-attractant protein-1 (MCP-1) (Axelsson et al, 2013; Richardson and Churilla, 2017). Intentionally practicing stress reduction techniques such as meditation has been shown to reduce the inflammatory response in human experimental models (Kox et al, 2014).

EXAMPLE OF AN ANTIINFLAMMATORY 1-DAY DIET BASED ON THE DASH, MIND, AND MEDITERRANEAN MEAL PATTERNS

Breakfast: Vegetable frittata with onions, garlic, basil, spinach, artichoke hearts, and tomato. Baked sweet potato wedges. Herbal tea.

Lunch: Lentil vegetable soup and a green salad with arugula, purple cabbage, red onion, cucumber, carrot, walnuts, and a mustard vinaigrette. Whole grain bread or crackers. Green tea with lemon.

Snack: Greek yogurt with berries.

Dinner: Lemon dill baked fish over brown rice with garlic sautéed kale and a glass of red wine.

Dessert: Dark chocolate and cherries.

REFERENCES

Aggarwal BB, Shishodia S: Suppression of the nuclear factor-kappa-B activation pathway by spice-derived phytochemicals: reasoning for seasoning, *Ann N Y Acad Sci* 1030:434–441, 2004.

Axelsson J, Rehman JU, Akerstedt T, et al: Effects of sustained sleep restriction on mitogen-stimulated cytokines, chemokines and T helper 1/T helper 2 balance in humans, *PLoS One* 8(12):e82291, 2013.

Bahna SL, Burkhardt JG: The dilemma of allergy to food additives, *Allergy Asthma Proc* 39(1):3–8, 2018.

Bergmans RS, Malecki KM: The association of dietary inflammatory potential with depression and mental well-being among U.S. adults, *Prev Med* 99:313–319, 2017.

Casas R, Sacanella E, Urpí-Sardà M, et al: Long-term immunomodulatory effects of a mediterranean diet in adults at high risk of cardiovascular disease in the PREvención con DIeta MEDiterránea (PREDIMED) randomized controlled trial, *J Nutr* 146(9):1684–1693, 2016.

Chai W, Morimoto Y, Cooney RV, et al: Dietary red and processed meat intake and markers of adiposity and inflammation: the multiethnic cohort study, *J Am Coll Nutr* 36(5):378–385, 2017.

Fowler ME, Akinyemiju TF: Meta-analysis of the association between dietary inflammatory index (DII) and cancer outcomes, *Int J Cancer* 141(11):2215–2227, 2017.

Galland L: Diet and Inflammation, *Nutr Clin Pract* 25:634–640, 2010.

Garcia-Arellano A, Ramallal R, Ruiz-Canela M, et al: Dietary inflammatory index and incidence of cardiovascular disease in the PREDIMED study, *Nutrients* 7(6):4124–4138, 2015.

González O, Tobia C, Ebersole J, et al: Caloric restriction and chronic inflammatory diseases, *Oral Dis* 18(1):16–31, 2012.

Habauzit V, Morand C: Evidence for a protective effect of polyphenols-containing foods on cardiovascular health: an update for clinicians, *Ther Adv Chronic Dis* 3(2):87–106, 2012.

Hiippala K, Jouhten H, Ronkainen A, et al: The potential of gut commensals in reinforcing intestinal barrier function and alleviating inflammation, *Nutrients* 10(8):E988, 2018.

Jiang Y, Wu SH, Shu XO, et al: Cruciferous vegetable intake is inversely correlated with circulating levels of proinflammatory markers in women, *J Acad Nutr Diet* 114(5):700-708.e2, 2014.

Jungbauer A, Medjakovic S: Anti-inflammatory properties of culinary herbs and spices that ameliorate the effects of metabolic syndrome, *Maturitas* 71:227–239, 2012.

Kaluza J, Håkansson N, Harris HR, et al: Influence of anti-inflammatory diet and smoking on mortality and survival in men and women: two prospective cohort studies, *J Intern Med* 285(1):75–91, 2019. doi:10.1111/joim.12823.

Kox M, van Eijk LT, Zwaag J, et al: Voluntary activation of the sympathetic nervous system and attenuation of the innate immune response in humans, *Proc Natl Acad Sci U S A* 111(20): 7379–7384, 2014.

Miller AM, Horiguchi N, Jeong WI, et al: Molecular mechanisms of alcoholic liver disease: innate immunity and cytokines, *Alcohol Clin Exp Res* 35(5):787–793, 2011.

Neufcourt L, Assmann KE, Fezeu LK, et al: Prospective association between the dietary inflammatory index and metabolic syndrome: findings from the SU.VI.MAX study, *Nutr Metab Cardiovasc Dis* 25(11):988–996, 2015.

Neuhouser ML, Schwarz Y, Wang C, et al: A low-glycemic load diet reduces serum C-reactive protein and modestly increases adiponectin in overweight and obese adults, *J Nutr* 142(2):369–374, 2012.

Panahi Y, Hosseini MS, Khalili N, et al: Effects of curcumin on serum cytokine concentrations in subjects with metabolic syndrome: a post-hoc analysis of a randomized controlled trial, *Biomed Pharmacother* 82:578–582, 2016.

Patterson RE, Sears DD: Metabolic effects of intermittent fasting, *Annu Rev Nutr* 37:371–393, 2017.

Richardson MR, Churilla JR: Sleep duration and C-reactive protein in US Adults, *South Med J* 110(4):314–317, 2017.

Runchey SS, Pollak MN, Valsta LM, et al: Glycemic load effect on fasting and post-prandial serum glucose, insulin, IGF-1 and IGFBP-3 in a randomized, controlled feeding study, *Eur J Clin Nutr* 66(10):1146–1152, 2012.

Shivappa N, Hébert JR, Karamati M, et al: Increased inflammatory potential of diet is associated with bone mineral density among postmenopausal women in Iran, *Eur J Nutr* 55(2):561–568, 2016.

Shivappa N, Steck SE, Hurley TG, et al. Designing and developing a literature-derived, population-based dietary inflammatory index, *Public Health Nutr* 17(8):1689–1696, 2014.

Valentino R, D'Esposito V, Passaretti F, et al: Bisphenol-A impairs insulin action and up-regulates inflammatory pathways in human subcutaneous adipocytes and 3T3-L1 cells, *PLoS One* 8(12):e82099, 2013. doi:10.1371/journal.pone.0082099.

Widmer RJ, Flammer AJ, Lerman LO, et al: The Mediterranean diet, its components, and cardiovascular disease, *Am J Med* 128(3):229–238, 2015.

Appendix created by Mary Purdy, PhD and Kelly Morrow, MS, RDN, FAND.

The Mediterranean Diet

SIGNIFICANCE

The Mediterranean diet emulates both the traditional diet and lifestyle of countries bordering the Mediterranean Sea. It is known as one of the healthiest dietary patterns in the world, specifically for its prevention of various chronic diseases. The diet places emphasis on the consumption of fruits, vegetables, nuts, seeds, whole grains, legumes, fish, lean meats, red wine (in moderation), and olive oil, and minimizes consumption of red meat and sugar. Additionally, the diet prioritizes daily physical activity, as well as getting adequate sleep, spending time with friends and family, and living a low-stress lifestyle. While the diet is specific to the Mediterranean region, its principles can easily be adapted to incorporate foods and recipes characteristic of other global cuisines.

One of the greatest risk factors for developing chronic diseases is inflammation. Eating a Mediterranean diet pattern has been demonstrated to reduce the following inflammatory markers: C-reactive protein (CRP), IL-1β, IL-4, IL-5, IL-6, IL-7, IL-18, TNF-α, TGFβ, COX-2, fibrinogen, and homocysteine. Notable antiinflammatory components of the Mediterranean diet include polyphenols, omega-3 fatty acids, fiber, and various phytochemicals including anthocyanin and lycopene (Donovan et al, 2017). Significant associations have also been demonstrated between consuming a Mediterranean diet and physical function, mental function, health-related quality of life for men and women, and life satisfaction for women (Zaragoza-Martí et al, 2018). Additionally, by choosing to include olive oil, vegetables, legumes, fish, nuts, and wine in food patterns, dependence on polypharmacy significantly decreases. Specifically, a high adherence to the Mediterranean diet is inversely associated with overall number of medications used for controlling health conditions (Vicinanza et al, 2018).

Common Health Conditions Managed With the Mediterranean Diet

- *Cardiovascular disease*
- *Cancer*
- *Diabetes*
- *Reproductive Health*
- *Brain Health*

Foods and Lifestyle Factors Emphasized

- *Fruits and vegetables:* Incorporating a colorful variety of fruits and vegetables into the diet ensures adequate consumption of many vitamins, minerals, and phytonutrients. Snack on vegetables in the morning and include them on half of the plate at lunch and dinner. Enjoy fruits and vegetables both in their cooked and raw forms.
  - Fruits to include: Apples, apricots, bananas, blackberries, blueberries, cantaloupe, cherries, clementines, cranberries, dates, figs, goji berries, grapefruit, grapes, lemons, limes, mango, marionberries, melons, nectarines, oranges, papaya, peaches, pears, persimmons, pineapples, plums, pomegranates, prunes, raspberries, star fruit, strawberries, tangerines, watermelon
  - Vegetables to include: Artichokes, arugula, asparagus, avocados, bean sprouts, beets, bell peppers, bok choy, broccoli, broccolini, Brussels sprouts, cabbage, carrots, cauliflower, celeriac, celery, chicory, collards, cucumbers, daikon, dandelion greens, eggplant, fennel, jicama, kale, leeks, lettuce, mushrooms, mustard greens, nettles, okra, olives, onions, peas, peppers, purslane, radicchio, radishes, scallions, shallots, spinach, tomatoes, watercress, zucchini
- *Nuts and seeds:* Nuts and seeds are both rich sources of essential fats, protein, fiber, and vitamins and minerals, including calcium, magnesium, B vitamins, and vitamin E. Nuts and seeds are healthiest when consumed in their raw, natural form or in butters made without hydrogenated oils. Choose them for a snack or to accompany a favorite meal.
  - Nuts to include: Almonds, cashews, hazelnuts, peanuts, pecans, pine nuts, pistachios, walnuts
  - Seeds to include: Chia, flax, hemp, pumpkin, sesame, sunflower
- *Whole grains and starches:* Unlike refined grains, whole grains consist of complex carbohydrates and are richer sources of fiber, essential fats, B vitamins, antioxidants, and phytonutrients. They provide lasting energy throughout the day, balance blood sugar, and regulate appetite.
  - Whole grains and starches to include: Amaranth, barley, brown rice, buckwheat, bulgur, corn, couscous, durum, farro, millet, oats, polenta, potatoes, pumpkin, quinoa, rice, rutabaga, rye, spelt, sweet potatoes, squash (acorn, buttercup, butternut, carnival, delicata, kabocha, spaghetti), turnips, wheat berries, whole wheat bread
- *Legumes:* This plant-based protein is a great meat alternative, for it is also rich in fiber, vitamins, minerals, antioxidants, and phytonutrients that help fight inflammation.
  - Legumes to include: Beans (adzuki, black, black eyed, cannellini, fava, garbanzo, green, kidney, pinto, red), edamame, lentils (black, brown, French, green, red, yellow), split peas
- *Lean animal protein:* When following a Mediterranean eating pattern, meat is eaten as an accent on the plate and not the main dish. Smaller portions of less than 3 oz are usually consumed, which is equivalent to the size of a deck of cards. Alternative protein sources include eggs, fish, and seafood. It is recommended to consume fish and seafood at least two times per week.
  - Lean animal protein to include: Chicken, turkey
  - Eggs to include: Chicken, duck, quail
  - Fish to include: Cod, flounder, salmon, sardines, sea bass, tilapia, tuna, yellowtail
  - Seafood to include: Clams, crab, lobster, mussels, oysters, shrimp
- *Healthy fats:* The Mediterranean diet emphasizes the consumption of fats at every meal and snack. Nuts and seeds can be added to any dish, as they are rich in both healthy fats and protein. Choose oils high in omega-3, monounsaturated, and polyunsaturated fatty acids to dress salads, and incorporate avocado and olives into meals. Dairy products usually only accompany main dishes in small portions or are eaten in fermented forms such as kefir and yogurt.

- Healthy fats to include: Avocado, cheese, coconut, milk, nuts (see above), oils (avocado, coconut, flaxseed, grapeseed, hemp seed, olive, safflower, sunflower seed, sesame, walnut), olives (kalamata, niçoise, picholine), seeds (see above), yogurt
- *Herbs and spices:* Cooking with these seasonings not only enhances the flavor of food but also increases its nutrient content by contributing vitamins, minerals, and antioxidants and protective phytonutrients.
  - Herbs to include: Basil, bay leaf, cilantro, lavender, mint, parsley, rosemary, sage, tarragon, thyme
  - Spices to include: Anise, chili peppers, cinnamon, clove, cumin, fennel, garlic, ginger, marjoram, oregano, pepper, turmeric, za'atar
- *Beverages to include:* Herbal tea, water, coffee, and a small glass of red wine, which contains beneficial antioxidants and phytonutrients.

EXAMPLES OF A 1-DAY MEAL PLAN BASED ON THE MEDITERRANEAN DIET

Breakfast: Shakshuka with baked eggs, onions, garlic, tomatoes, crumbled feta served with cooked quinoa or whole wheat bread. Season with paprika and cumin. Black coffee, tea, or water.

Lunch: Veggie wrap with whole wheat tortilla, spinach, cucumber, shredded carrots, hummus, avocado. Eat with a piece of fruit. Water or tea.

Snack: Hardboiled egg with grapes and mixed nuts.

Dinner: Paella with shrimp, brown rice, bell pepper, stewed tomatoes, onion, garlic, extra virgin olive oil. Season with saffron. Water, tea, or one small glass of red wine.

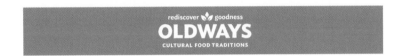

Mediterranean Diet Pyramid

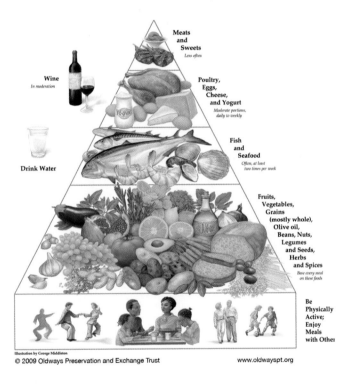

Illustration by George Middleton
© 2009 Oldways Preservation and Exchange Trust   www.oldwayspt.org

INFORMATION FOR FURTHER READING

Old Ways Foundation

REFERENCES

Donovan MG, Selmin OI, Doetschman TC, et al: Mediterranean diet: prevention of colorectal cancer, *Front Nutr* 4:59, 2017.

Huang CH, Hou YC, Yeh CL, et al: A soybean and fish oil mixture with different n-6/n-3 PUFA ratios modulates the inflammatory reaction in mice with dextran sulfate sodium-induced acute colitis, *Clin Nutr* 34:1018–1024, 2015.

Maraki MI, Yannakoulia M, Stamelou M, et al: Mediterranean diet adherence is related to reduced probability of prodromal Parkinson's disease, *Mov Disord* 34(1):48–57, 2019.

Vicinanza R, Troisi G, Cangemi R, et al: Aging and adherence to the Mediterranean diet: relationship with cardiometabolic disorders and polypharmacy, *J Nutr Health Aging* 22(1):73–81, 2018.

Zaragoza-Martí A, Ferrer-Cascales R, Hurtado-Sánchez JA, et al: Relationship between adherence to the Mediterranean diet and health-related quality of life and life satisfaction among older adults, *J Nutr Health Aging* 22(1):89–96, 2018.

Appendix created by Kelly Morrow, MS, RDN, FAND.

Nutritional Facts on Alcoholic Beverages

According to the 2015 National Survey on Drug Use and Health, 86% of U.S. adults 18 and older report drinking alcohol at some time in their life; 26% report binge drinking in the past month, and 7% report excessive drinking in the past month. An estimated 15 million adults in the United States have alcohol use disorder according to the National Institute on Alcohol Abuse and Alcoholism (National Institutes of Health [NIH], 2019). Recent studies have disputed the overall health benefits of drinking alcohol, although some research demonstrates a small positive effect of moderate drinking on cardiovascular risk and mortality (Centers for Disease Control [CDC], 2019). A growing body of evidence suggests that regular alcohol intake, especially if excessive, is associated with liver disease, hypertension and left ventricular function, multiple forms of cancer (breast, mouth, esophagus, larynx, throat), as well as motor vehicle accidents, violence, and sexual assault (CDC, 2019).

The 2015–2020 Dietary Guidelines for Americans (DGA) recommend moderate drinking for those who do drink alcohol and do not recommend that individuals start drinking for any potential health benefit if they do not drink already. The DGA guidelines recommend the following:

- Alcoholic beverages should not be consumed by some individuals, including those who cannot control their alcohol intake, women of childbearing age who may become pregnant, pregnant and lactating women, children and adolescents, individuals taking medications that can interact with alcohol, and those with specific medical conditions.
- Those who choose to drink alcoholic beverages should do so sensibly and in moderation—defined as the consumption of up to one drink per day for women and up to two drinks per day for men.
- Combining alcohol and caffeine is not recommended. This can lead to excessive drinking because caffeine can mask the effects of alcohol.
- Alcoholic beverages should be avoided by individuals engaging in activities that require attention, skill, or coordination, such as driving or operating machinery.

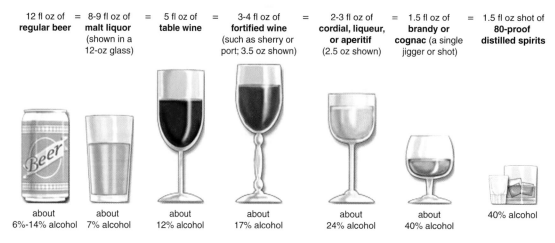

| 12 fl oz of **regular beer** | = | 8-9 fl oz of **malt liquor** (shown in a 12-oz glass) | = | 5 fl oz of **table wine** | = | 3-4 fl oz of **fortified wine** (such as sherry or port; 3.5 oz shown) | = | 2-3 fl oz of **cordial, liqueur, or aperitif** (2.5 oz shown) | = | 1.5 fl oz of **brandy or cognac** (a single jigger or shot) | = | 1.5 fl oz shot of **80-proof distilled spirits** |

about 6%-14% alcohol — about 7% alcohol — about 12% alcohol — about 17% alcohol — about 24% alcohol — about 40% alcohol — 40% alcohol

Each beverage portrayed above represents one U.S. standard drink (also known as an alcoholic drink-equivalent). The percent of pure alcohol, expressed here as alcohol by volume (alc/vol), varies within and across beverage types.

ALCOHOL AND CALORIE CONTENT IN SELECTED ALCOHOLIC BEVERAGES

This table is a guide to estimate the alcohol percentage and calories from various alcoholic beverages. A sample serving volume and the calories in that drink are shown for beer, wine, and distilled spirits.

Higher alcohol content (higher percent alcohol or higher proof) and mixing alcohol with other beverages such as sweetened soft drinks, fruit juice, or cream increase the amount of calories in the beverage. Alcoholic beverages supply calories but provide few essential nutrients apart from small amounts of B vitamins in some beer (USDA, 2019; Cronometer, 2019).

One standard drink equivalent contains ~14 grams of alcohol. This equates to roughly 12 ounces of regular beer (6%–14% alcohol), 5 ounces of wine (12% alcohol), and 1.5 ounces of distilled spirits (hard alcohol 40% alcohol).

Image: National Institutes of Health, National Institute on Alcohol Abuse and Alcoholism: *Rethinking drinking.* Available at: https://www.rethinking drinking.niaaa.nih.gov/How-much-is-too-much/What-counts-as-a-drink/Whats-A-Standard-Drink.aspx. Accessed February 4, 2019.

Beverage	Serving (oz)	Alcohol (%)	Calories (Approximate)
Beer and Cider			
Regular	12	5%	120-150
Microbrew/Craft beer	12	6%-14%	160-250
Gluten Free Beer	12	4%-5%	120-200
Light beer	12	4%-5%	100
Nonalcoholic beer	12	Trace	100-130
Hard Cider	12	3.4%-8.5%	140-200
Hard Lemonade	11.2	5%	220
Distilled Spirits (gin, vodka, rum, brandy, whisky, scotch)			
80 Proof	1.5	40%	90-100
100 Proof	1.5	50%	105-120
Wine			
White	4	10%-12%	80-100
Zinfandel and Shiraz	4	14%-16%	115-120
Red	4	12%-15%	85-100
Rose	4	11.5%-13.5%	85-110
Wine cooler	12	4%-6%	200
Champagne	4	12%	100
Sweet wine	4	12%	130
Sherry, port, muscatel	2	17%-21%	75-90
Sake	4	17%-21%	150
Cordials, liqueurs	2-3	24%	160
Mixed Drinks			
Bloody Mary	8	18%-20%	160
Daiquiri	6	18%-20%	350
Manhattan	4	25%-30%	220
Martini	4	30%	225
Drink Mixes			
Mineral water	Any	0	0
Club soda	Any	0	0
Diet soda	Any	0	0
Tomato juice	4	0	25
Bloody Mary mix	4	0	25
Orange juice	4	0	60
Grapefruit juice	4	0	60
Pineapple juice	4	0	60
Miscellaneous			
Kombucha	12	Less than 0.5% (unless sold as an alcoholic beverage then up to 2.5%)	Varies 40-100

American Addiction Centers (AAC): *Alcohol by volume: beer, wine, & liquor.* Available at: https://www.alcohol.org/statistics-information/abv/. Accessed February 4, 2019

Centers for Disease Control (CDC): *Fact Sheets: Moderate drinking.* Available at: https://www.cdc.gov/alcohol/fact-sheets/moderate-drinking.htm. Accessed February 3, 2019.

Cronometer. Available at: https://cronometer.com/. Accessed February 5, 2019

National Institutes of Health (NIH), National Institute on Alcohol Abuse and Alcoholism: *What is a standard drink?* Available at: https://www.niaaa.nih.gov/alcohol-health/overview-alcohol-consumption/what-standard-drink. Accessed February 3, 2019.

USDA: *Nutrient database standard release.* Available at: https://ndb.nal.usda.gov/ndb/search/list. Accessed. February 3, 2019.

The caloric contribution from alcohol of an alcoholic beverage can be estimated by multiplying the number of ounces by the proof and then again by the factor 0.8. For beers and wines, kilocalories from alcohol can be estimated by multiplying ounces by percentage of alcohol (by volume) and then by the factor 1.6.

Nutritional Facts on Caffeine-Containing Products

Caffeine is similar in structure to adenosine, a chemical found in the brain that slows down its activity. Because the two compete, the more caffeine is consumed, the less adenosine is available, up to a point. Caffeine temporarily heightens concentration and wards off fatigue. Within 30 to 60 minutes of drinking a cup of coffee, caffeine reaches peak concentrations in the bloodstream and takes 4 to 6 hours for its effects to wear off. The average American adult consumes about 200 mg of caffeine a day, and many may consume twice that level. It is generally safe to consume no more than the equivalent amount of caffeine in 1 to 2 cups of coffee daily during pregnancy or lactation. Individuals with heart disease and hypertension may benefit from a reduction in caffeine consumption. To reduce caffeine and its stimulant effects, monitor intake from foods and beverages listed below.

Selected Food and Beverage Sources of Caffeine

Caffeine-Containing Products	Serving (mg)
Coffee	
Starbucks coffee (in store), 16 oz	330
Starbucks coffee (at home), 16 oz	260
Brewed, drip method, 6 oz	103
Brewed, percolator method, 6 oz	75
Instant, 1 rounded tsp	57
Flavored, regular and sugar-free, 6 oz	26-75
Espresso, 1 oz	40
Café Latte, short (8 oz) or tall (12 oz) (Starbucks)	35
Decaffeinated, 6 oz	2
Tea	
Black or green tea, 16 oz	60-100
3-minute brew, 12 oz	72
Lipton, Arizona, or Snapple tea, 16 oz	30-60
Instant, 1 rounded tsp in 8 oz of water	25-35
Tea, green brewed, 8 oz	30
Tea, bottles (12 oz) or from instant mix, 8 oz	14
Decaffeinated, 5-minute brew, 6-oz cup	1
Carbonated Beverages	
7-Eleven Big Gulp cola, 64 oz	190
Mountain Dew MDX or Vault, 12 oz	120
Diet Pepsi Max, 20 oz	70
Mountain Dew, 12 oz, regular or diet	54
Mellow Yellow, 12 oz, regular or diet	52
Regular or diet cola, cherry colas, Dr. Pepper, Mr. Pibb, 12 oz	35-50
Decaffeinated drinks, 12 oz	Trace

Caffeine-Containing Products	Serving (mg)
Cocoa and Chocolate	
Chocolate, baking, unsweetened, 1 oz	58
Chocolate, sweet, semisweet, dark, milk, 1 oz	8-20
Milk chocolate bar, 1.5 oz	10
Chocolate milk, 8 oz	8
Cocoa beverage, 6-oz cup	4
Chocolate-flavored syrup, 1 oz	5
Chocolate pudding, ½ cup	4-8
Energy Drinks	
Rockstar (16 oz)	160
Red Bull (8.3 oz)	80
Full Throttle (16 oz)	160
Monster (16)	160
Jolt (8 oz)	80
Miscellaneous	
NoDoz, Maximum Strength (1), or Vivarin (1)	200
Pit Bull Energy Bar, 2 oz	165
Excedrin (2)	130
NoDoz, Regular Strength (1)	100
Water, caffeinated (Edge 2 O), (8 oz)	70
Anacin (2)	65
Bud Extra Beer, 10 oz	55
Propel Invigorating water	50
Bai Antioxidant Infusion (16 oz)	70
Crystal Light Energy (1 packet)	60
Starbucks Refresher (12 ounces)	50

Center for Science in the Public Interest: *Caffeine Chart*. Available at: https://cspinet.org/eating-healthy/ingredients-of-concern/caffeine-chart. Accessed February 2, 2019.

USDA Agricultural Research Service: *National nutrient database for standard reference*. Available at: http://ndb.nal.usda.gov/ndb/search. Accessed February 1, 2019.

Nutritional Facts on Essential (Omega) Fatty Acids

Essential fatty acids (EFAs) are fatty acids that are required in the human diet. They must be obtained from food because human cells have no biochemical pathways capable of producing them internally. There are two closely related families of EFAs: **omega-3 (Ω-3 or ω-3)** and **omega-6 (Ω-6 or ω-6)**. Only one substance in each of these families is truly essential, because, for example, the body can convert one ω-3 to another ω-3 but cannot create ω-3 endogenously.

In the body essential fatty acids serve multiple functions. In each of these the balance between dietary ω-3 and ω-6 strongly affects function. They are modified to make the eicosanoids (affecting inflammation and many other cellular functions); the endogenous cannabinoids (affecting mood, behavior, and inflammation); the lipoxins from ω-6 EFAs and resolvins from ω-3 (in the presence of aspirin, down-regulating inflammation); the isofurans, isoprostanes, hepoxilins, epoxyeicosatrienoic acids, and neuroprotectin D; and the lipid rafts (affecting cellular signaling). They also act on deoxyribonucleic acid (activating or inhibiting transcription factors for nuclear factor–κ-B [NFκB], a proinflammatory cytokine).

Between 1930 and 1950, arachidonic and linolenic acids were termed *essential* because each was more or less able to meet the growth requirements of rats given fat-free diets. Further research has shown that human metabolism requires both fatty acids. To some extent any ω-3 and any ω-6 can relieve the worst symptoms of fatty acid deficiency. However, in many people the ability to convert the ω-3 α-linolenic acid (ALA) to the ω-3 eicosapentaenoic (EPA) and docosahexaenoic acid (DHA) is only 5% efficient. Therefore it is important to incorporate the EPA and DHA directly into the diet, usually as fish or a fish oil supplement. Particular fatty acids such as DHA are needed at critical life stages (e.g., infancy and lactation) and in some disease states.

The essential fatty acids are:
- ALA (18:3)-ω-3
- Linoleic acid (18:2)- ω-6

These two fatty acids cannot be synthesized by humans because humans lack the desaturase enzymes required for their production. They form the starting point for the creation of longer and more desaturated fatty acids, which are also referred to as long-chain polyunsaturates:

Ω-3 FATTY ACIDS:

- EPA (20:5) eicosapentanoic acid
- DHA (22:6) docosahexanoic acid
- ALA (18:) alpha-linolenic acid

Ω-6 FATTY ACIDS:

- Gamma-linolenic acid (GLA) (18:3)
- Dihomo-γ-linolenic acid (DGLA) (20:3)
- Arachidonic acid (AA) (20:4)

Ω-9 Fatty acids are not essential in humans, because humans possess all the enzymes required for their synthesis.

ADEQUATE INTAKES FOR Ω-3 FATTY ACIDS FOR CHILDREN AND ADULTS				ADEQUATE INTAKES FOR Ω-6 FATTY ACIDS FOR CHILDREN AND ADULTS			
Age (years)	Males and Females (g/day)	Pregnancy (g/day)	Lactation (g/day)	Age (years)	Males and Females (g/day)	Pregnancy (g/day)	Lactation (g/day)
1-3	0.7	N/A	N/A	1-3	7	N/A	N/A
4-8	0.9	N/A	N/A	4-8	10	N/A	N/A
9-13	1.2 for boys, 1 for girls	N/A	N/A	9-13	12 for boys, 10 for girls	N/A	N/A
14-18	1.6 for boys, 1.1 for girls	1.4	1.3	14-18	16 for boys, 11 for girls	13	13
19+	1.6 for men, 1.1 for women	1.4	1.3	19+	17 for men, 12 for women	13	13

N/A, Not applicable.

DIETARY SOURCES

Some of the food sources of ω-3 and ω-6 fatty acids are fish and shellfish, flaxseed (linseed), soya oil, canola (rapeseed) oil, hemp oil, chia seeds, pumpkin seeds, sunflower seeds, leafy vegetables, and walnuts.

EFAs play a part in many metabolic processes, and there is evidence to suggest that low levels of EFAs or the wrong balance of types among the EFAs may be a factor in a number of illnesses.

Plant sources of ω-3s do not contain EPA and DHA. This is thought to be the reason that absorption of EFAs is much greater from animal rather than plant sources.

EFA content of vegetable sources varies with cultivation conditions. Animal sources vary widely, both with the animal's feed and that the EFA makeup varies markedly with fats from different body parts.

OMEGA-3 FATTY ACIDS

There is some evidence that suggests that ω-3s may:
- Help lower elevated triglyceride levels. High triglyceride levels can contribute to coronary heart disease.
- Reduce the blood's tendency to clot, which may relate to the clotting that occurs with the initial atherosclerotic plaque.
- Reduce the inflammation involved in conditions such as rheumatoid arthritis.
- Improve symptoms of depression and other mental health disorders in some individuals.

Dietary sources of ω-3 fatty acids include fish oil and certain plant and nut oils. Fish oil contains both DHA and EPA, whereas some nuts (English walnuts) and vegetable oils (canola, soybean, flaxseed and linseed, olive) contain only the ω-3 ALA.

There is evidence from multiple large-scale population (epidemiologic) studies and randomized controlled trials that intake of recommended amounts of DHA and EPA in the form of fish or fish oil supplements lowers triglycerides and raises HDL cholesterol. However, high doses may have harmful effects such as an increased risk of bleeding. Some species of fish carry a higher risk of environmental contamination such as with methyl mercury. Refer to the U.S. Environmental Protection Agency for more information about safely consuming fish: https://www.epa.gov/fish-tech.

Common Food Sources of Omega-3 Fats

Omega-3 Fat	Food Source
ALA	Ground flaxseed and walnuts and soybeans
	Flaxseed (ground), walnut, soybean and canola oils, and nonhydrogenated canola and soy margarines
DHA and EPA	Mackerel, salmon, herring, trout and sardines, and other fish and shellfish
	Marine algae supplements

Fish or Other Food Source	Omega-3 Content in a 4-oz Serving
English walnuts	6.8 g
Chinook salmon	3.6 g
Sockeye salmon	2.3 g
Mackerel	1.8-2.6 g
Herring	1.2-2.7 g
Rainbow trout	1.0 g
Wheat germ and oat germ	0.7-1.4 g
Halibut	0.5-1.3 g
White tuna	0.97 g
Light tuna	0.35 g
Whiting	0.9 g
Spinach	0.9 g
Flounder	0.6 g
King crab	0.6 g
Shrimp	0.5 g
Tofu	0.4 g (less in "lite" tofu)
Clam	0.32 g
Cod	0.3 g
Scallop	0.23 g

Supplements*	
Cod liver oil	800-100 mg/tsp
Fish oil	1200-1800 mg/tsp
Omega-3 fatty acid concentrate	~250 mg/capsule

Enhancing Intake of Omega-3 Fats

- Eat fish at least two times each week.
- Include canned fish in your diet (examples: salmon, sardines, light tuna). Try sardines on toast.
- Add ground flaxseed to foods such as hot or cold cereal or yogurt (flaxseed must be ground for the fatty acids to be fully available for absorption).
- Add walnuts to salads, cereals, baking (examples, muffins, cookies, breads), and pancakes or have on their own as a snack.
- Have fresh or frozen soybeans (edamame) as a vegetable at meals or as a snack.
- Use soybean oil or canola oil in salad dressings and recipes.
- Use nonhydrogenated margarine made from canola or soybean as a spread or in baking.
- Cook with ω-3 eggs. Enjoy scrambled, hardboiled, poached, or over easy.
- Use other ω-3 fortified products such as milk, yogurt, nutritional beverages, bars, cereal, bread, and pasta.
- Substitute ¼ cup ground flaxseed for ¼ cup flour in bread, pizza dough, muffin, cookie, or meatloaf recipes.
- Replace 1 egg with 1 Tbsp ground flaxseed blended with 3 Tbsp water in recipes.

*Exact omega-3 content varies per manufacturer. Check label.
EPA, Eicosapentaenoic; *DHA*, docosahexaenoic acid.
National Institutes of Health Office of Dietary Supplements Fact Sheets for Health Professionals: Omega-3 Fatty Acids. Updated October 17, 2019. https://ods.od.nih.gov/factsheets/Omega3FattyAcids-HealthProfessional/ Accessed December 30, 2019; U.S. Department of Agriculture Food Data Central. https://fdc.nal.usda.gov Accessed February 4, 2019.

Nutritional Facts on a High-Fiber Diet

This diet is a modification of the regular diet. The purpose of this diet is to decrease transit time through the intestine, promote more frequent bowel movements, and promote softer stools. A high fiber diet may be prescribed as a treatment for diverticulosis, irritable bowel syndrome, hemorrhoids, or constipation. A high-fiber diet is also prescribed for weight loss, cardiovascular disease, and diabetes. It includes all the foods on a regular diet, with emphasis on the proper planning and selection of foods to increase the daily intake of fiber. Fluid intake should be also increased. The Academy of Nutrition and Dietetics recommends that the average adult have a daily fiber intake of 20 to 35 g from a variety of sources. For children, the child's age plus 5 g of fiber is recommended daily. In cases of severe constipation, more fiber is recommended. Following the guidelines for the Mediterranean diet will provide a high fiber diet.

Dietary Reference Intakes for Fiber for Children and Adults

Age (years)	Males and Females (g/day)	Pregnancy (g/day)	Lactation (g/day)
1-3	19	N/A	N/A
4-8	25	N/A	N/A
9-13	31 for boys, 26 for girls	N/A	N/A
14-18	38 for boys, 26 for girls	28	29
19+	38 for men, 25 for women	28	29

N/A, Not applicable.

Although numerous over-the-counter fiber supplements are available, food sources provide many nutrients and are the preferred method of increasing dietary fiber. Adequate liquid consumption (at least eight 8-oz glasses per day) is recommended. Fiber should be added to the diet slowly because of possible cramps, bloating, and diarrhea with a sudden fiber increase. Maximum therapeutic benefits of fiber are obtained after several months of compliance. There are two components of dietary fiber, each providing health benefits: insoluble and soluble.

Types of Dietary Fiber

Type of Fiber	Components of Cells	Food Sources	Health Benefits
Soluble fibers	Gums, mucilages, pectin, certain hemicelluloses	Vegetables, fruits, barley; legumes, oats, and oat-bran	Decrease total blood cholesterol. Guard against diabetes. Prevent constipation. May help manage irritable bowel syndrome. May protect against colon cancer and gallstones.
Insoluble fibers	Cellulose, lignin, some hemicelluloses	Whole-wheat products, wheat and corn bran, and many vegetables (including cauliflower, green beans, potatoes, and skins of root vegetables)	May prevent diverticular disease. Prevents constipation. May delay glucose absorption (probably insignificant). May increase satiety and therefore assist with weight loss. Lower cholesterol. May protect against colon cancer.

GUIDELINES FOR HIGH-FIBER DIET

1. Increase consumption of whole-grain breads, cereals, flours, and other whole-grain productions to 6 to 11 servings daily.
2. Increase consumption of vegetables, legumes and fruits, nuts, and edible seeds to 5 to 8 servings daily.
3. Consume high-fiber cereals, granolas, and legumes as needed to bring fiber intake to 25 g or more daily.
4. Increase consumption of fluids to at least 2 L (or approximately 2 qt) daily.
5. For a high-fiber diet of approximately 24 g of dietary fiber: use 12 or more servings of the foods from the groups below (each food contains approximately 2 g of dietary fiber). For example, ½ cup of baked beans (8 Tbsp) would count as 4 servings.

EACH OF THESE FOODS IN THIS AMOUNT CONTAINS 2 G OF DIETARY FIBER

Apple, 1 small	Strawberries, ½ cup
Orange, 1 small	Pear, ½ small
Banana, 1 small	Cherries, 10 large
Peach, 1 medium	Plums, 2 small
Whole-wheat bread, 1 slice	Oatmeal, dry, 3 Tbsp
All Bran, 1 Tbsp	Shredded wheat, ½ biscuit
Rye bread, 1 slice	Wheat bran, 1 tsp
Corn flakes, ⅔ cup	Grape-nuts, 3 Tbsp
Cracked wheat bread, 1 slice	Puffed wheat, 1½ cup
Broccoli, ½ stalk	Potato, 2-in diameter
Lettuce, raw, 2 cups	Celery, 1 cup
Brussels sprouts, 4	Tomato, raw, 1 medium
Green beans, ½ cup	Corn on the cob, 2 in
Carrots, ⅔ cup	Baked beans, canned, 2 Tbsp

SELECTED FOOD SOURCES OF FIBER

Food	Grams per Serving	% Daily Value*
Navy beans, cooked, ½ cup	9.5	38
Bran ready-to-eat cereal (100%), ½ cup	8.8	35
Kidney beans, canned, ½ cup	8.2	33
Split peas, cooked, ½ cup	8.1	32
Lentils, cooked, ½ cup	7.8	31
Black beans, cooked, ½ cup	7.5	30
Pinto beans, cooked, ½ cup	7.7	31
Lima beans, cooked, ½ cup	6.6	26
Artichoke, globe, cooked, 1 each	6.5	26
White beans, canned, ½ cup	6.3	25
Chickpeas, cooked, ½ cup	6.2	24
Great northern beans, cooked, ½ cup	6.2	24
Cowpeas, cooked, ½ cup	5.6	22
Soybeans, mature, cooked, ½ cup	5.2	21
Bran ready-to-eat cereals, various, 1 oz	2.6-5.0	10-20
Crackers, rye wafers, plain, 2 wafers	5.0	20
Sweet potato, baked, with peel, 1 medium (146 g)	4.8	19
Asian pear, raw, 1 small	4.4	18
Green peas, cooked, ½ cup	4.4	18
Whole-wheat English muffin, 1 each	4.4	18
Pear, raw, 1 small	4.3	17

SELECTED FOOD SOURCES OF FIBER

Food	Grams per Serving	% Daily Value*
Bulgur, cooked, ½ cup	4.1	16
Mixed vegetables, cooked, ½ cup	4.0	16
Raspberries, raw, ½ cup	4.0	16
Sweet potato, boiled, no peel, 1 medium (156 g)	3.9	15.5
Blackberries, raw, ½ cup	3.8	15
Potato, baked, with skin, 1 medium	3.8	15
Soybeans, green, cooked, ½ cup	3.8	15
Stewed prunes, ½ cup	3.8	15
Figs, dried, ¼ cup	3.7	14.5
Dates, ¼ cup	3.6	14
Oat bran, raw, ¼ cup	3.6	14
Pumpkin, canned, ½ cup	3.6	14
Spinach, frozen, cooked, ½ cup	3.5	14
Shredded wheat ready-to-eat cereals, various, ≈1 oz	2.8-3.4	11-13
Almonds, 1 oz	3.3	13
Apple with skin, raw, 1 medium	3.3	13
Brussels sprouts, frozen, cooked, ½ cup	3.2	13
Whole-wheat spaghetti, cooked, ½ cup	3.1	12
Banana, 1 medium	3.1	12
Orange, raw, 1 medium	3.1	12
Oat bran muffin, 1 small	3.0	12
Guava, 1 medium	3.0	12
Pearled barley, cooked, ½ cup	3.0	12
Sauerkraut, canned, solids, and liquids, ½ cup	3.0	12
Tomato paste, ¼ cup	2.9	11.5
Winter squash, cooked, ½ cup	2.9	11.5
Broccoli, cooked, ½ cup	2.8	11
Parsnips, cooked, chopped, ½ cup	2.8	11
Turnip greens, cooked, ½ cup	2.5	10
Collards, cooked, ½ cup	2.7	11
Okra, frozen, cooked, ½ cup	2.6	10
Peas, edible-podded, cooked, ½ cup	2.5	10

*Daily values (DVs) are reference numbers based on the recommended dietary allowance. They were developed to help consumers determine whether a food contains a lot or a little of a specific nutrient. The DV for fiber is 25 g. The percent DV (%DV) listed on the Nutrition Facts panel of food labels states the percentage of the DV provided in one serving. %DVs are based on a 2000-calorie diet.

Food sources of dietary fiber ranked by grams of dietary fiber per standard amount. (All are ≥10% of adequate intake for adult women, which is 25 g/day.)

Glycemic Index (GI) and Glycemic Load (GL) of Selected Foods[*]

The glycemic index (GI) is a measure of the predicted rise in blood glucose of a variety of carbohydrate foods on a scale of 1–100 as compared to pure glucose, which has a value of 100. The GI ranking is as follows: high GI >70; moderate GI 56–69; and low GI <55 (University of Sydney, 2019). Foods with a high GI cause a rapid rise in blood glucose, whereas lower GI foods cause blood glucose to rise more slowly which could be helpful in managing conditions such as diabetes, cardiovascular disease, and obesity (Augustin et al, 2015).

The glycemic load (GL) takes this measurement one step further and looks at the predicted rise in blood glucose in a typical portion of carbohydrate food using this equation: GI × grams carbohydrate in a typical portion of food ÷ 100. The ranking is as follows: high GL ≥20; medium GL 11–19; and low GL ≤10 (Monro and Shaw, 2008).

Additional factors that affect the GI and the GL include portion eaten, whether it was eaten on an empty stomach or not, and overall macronutrient and fiber content of the meal. Pairing a high GI food with some fat and protein will lead to a slower rise in blood glucose.

	GI	GL
Breakfast Cereals		
Kashi Seven Whole Grains	65	16
Kellogg's All-Bran	30	4
Kellogg's Cocoa Puffs	77	20
Kellogg's Corn Flakes	92	24
Kellogg's MiniWheats	58	12
Kellogg's Nutrigrain	66	10
Old-fashioned oatmeal	42	9
Kellogg's Rice Krispies	82	22
Kellogg's Special K	69	14
Kellogg's Raisin Bran	61	12
Grains and Pastas		
Buckwheat	54	16
Bulgur	48	12
Quinoa	53	13
Rice		
Basmati	58	22
Brown	50	16
Instant	87	36
Uncle Ben's	39	14
Converted, white	4	
Noodles—instant	7	19
Pasta		
Egg fettuccine (avg)	40	18
Spaghetti (avg)	38	18
Vermicelli	35	16
Whole wheat	50	1
Bread		
Bagel	72	25
Croissant[†]	67	17
Crumpet	69	13

	GI	GL
"Grainy" breads (avg)	49	6
Pita bread	57	10
Pumpernickel (avg)	50	6
Rye bread (avg)	58	8
White bread (avg)	70	10
Whole-wheat bread (avg)	77	9
Crackers and Crispbread		
Kavli	71	12
Puffed crisp bread	81	15
Ryvita	69	11
Water cracker	78	14
Cookies		
Oatmeal	55	12
Milk Arrowroot	69	12
Shortbread (commercial)[†]	64	10
Cake		
Chocolate, frosted, Betty Crocker	38	20
Oat bran muffin	69	24
Sponge cake	46	17
Waffles	76	10
Vegetables		
Beets, canned	64	5
Carrots (avg)	47	3
Parsnip	97	12
Peas (green, avg)	48	3
Potato		
Baked (avg)	85	26
Boiled	88	16
French fries	75	22
Microwaved	82	27

	GI	GL		GI	GL
Pumpkin	75	3	Ice cream		
Sweet corn	60	11	Regular (avg)	61	8
Sweet potato (avg)	61	17	Low-fat	50	3
Rutabaga	72	7	Yogurt, low-fat	33	10
Yam (avg)	37	13			
			Beverages		
Legumes			Apple juice	40	12
Baked beans (avg)	48	7	Coca Cola	63	16
Broad beans	79	9	Lemonade	66	13
Butter beans	31	6	Fanta	68	23
Chickpeas (avg)	28	8	Orange juice (avg)	52	12
Cannellini beans (avg)	38	12			
Kidney beans (avg)	28	7	**Snack Foods**		
Lentils (avg)	29	5	Tortilla chips[†] (avg)	63	17
Soy beans (avg)	18	1	Fish sticks	38	7
			Peanuts[†] (avg)	14	1
Fruit			Popcorn	72	8
Apple (avg)	38	6	Potato chips[†]	57	10
Apricot (dried)	31	9			
Banana (avg)	51	13	**Convenience Foods**		
Cherries	22	3	Macaroni and cheese	64	32
Grapefruit	25	3	Soup		
Grapes (avg)	46	8	Lentil	44	9
Kiwi fruit (avg)	53	6	Split-pea	60	16
Mango	51	8	Tomato	38	6
Orange (avg)	48	5	Sushi (avg)	52	19
Papaya	59	10	Pizza, cheese	60	16
Peach (avg)					
Canned (natural juice)	38	4	**Sweets**		
Fresh (avg)	42	5	Chocolate[†]	44	13
Pear (avg)	38	4	Jelly beans (avg)	78	22
Pineapple	59	7	Life Savers	70	21
Plum	39	5	Mars Bar	68	27
Raisins	64	28	Kudo whole-grain chocolate-chip bar	62	20
Cantaloupe	65	4			
Watermelon	72	4	**Sugars**		
			Honey (avg)	55	10
Dairy Foods			Fructose (avg)	19	2
Milk			Glucose[*]	100	10
Full-fat	27	3	Lactose (avg)	46	5
Skim	32	4	Sucrose (avg)	68	7
Chocolate-flavored	42	13			
Condensed	61	33	**Sports Bars**		
Custard	43	7	Clif bar (cookies and cream)	101	3
			PowerBar (chocolate)	83	35
			Zone Perfect (chocolate)	44	8

[*]The numbers above are compared to pure glucose with a value of 100.
[†]These foods are high in saturated fat.
Atkinson FS, Foster-Powell K, Brand-Miller JC: International tables of glycemic index and glycemic load values: 2008, *Diabetes Care* 31(12): 2281–2283, 2008.

REFERENCES

Augustin LS, Kendall CW, Jenkins DJ, et al: Glycemic index, glycemic load and glycemic response: An International Scientific Consensus Summit from the International Carbohydrate Quality Consortium (ICQC), *Nutr Metab Cardiovasc Dis* 25(9):795–815, 2015.

Monro JA, Shaw M: Glycemic impact, glycemic glucose equivalents, glycemic index, and glycemic load: definitions, distinctions, and implications, *Am J Clin Nutr* 87(1):237S–243S, 2008.
The University of Sydney: *About Glycemic Index: measuring the GI*. Updated November 26, 2019. Available at: http://www.glycemicindex.com/about.php. Accessed December 31, 2019.

Nutritional Facts on a High-Protein Diet

A diet high in protein is recommended most often for increased needs for healing. A diet of 1.2 g/kg to 1.5 g/kg is recommended for healing by the National Pressure Injury Advisory Panel. It is now recommended for people on dialysis and for those with some types of liver disease. Diets as high as 2.0 g/kg have been recommended after major trauma. High-protein diets of 1.6g/kg are recommended for athletes who are building muscle. Historically, a high-protein diet has been defined as one with at least 100 g of protein per day. This has been replaced by recommendations based on weight. How to accurately determine protein needs in an obese person remains debatable. A high-protein diet of 1.75 g/kg of ideal body weight (IBW) is sometimes beneficial for treating those with obesity.

BEST FOOD SOURCES OF PROTEIN

1 cup = 240 mL; 1 ounce = 28 grams
Meat: most types of meat provide 7 g per ounce
Fish and shellfish: 7 g per ounce
Eggs: 6 to 7 g per egg, depends on the egg size
Cow's milk: 8 g per cup
Goat's milk: 9 g per cup
Soy milk: 7 to 8 g per cup
Nonfat milk powder: 8 grams per 3 Tbsp. (24g)
Plain yogurt: 6 to 7 g per ½ cup
Greek yogurt: 11 to 15 g per ½ cup
Cheese: 7 g per ¼ cup of cottage cheese OR 1 ounce hard cheese.

Peanut butter or nut butter: 8 g per 2 Tbsp. (34g)
Tofu: 4.6 g per ounce
Lentils: 10 g per ½ cup, cooked
Chickpeas: 8 g per ½ cup, cooked
Quinoa: 4 g per ½ cup, cooked
Teff: 5 g per ½ cup, cooked
Chia seeds: 5 g per ounce
Hemp seeds: 9 grams per 3 Tbsp. (30g)

PROTEIN SUPPLEMENTS

Nonfat dry milk (NFDM) may be added to cooked foods to increase protein intake. However when it is added, carbohydrate is also added as the sugar lactose. NFDM can be added to regular milk to create more concentrated milk. Protein powders are a popular way to increase the protein content of the diet, either by adding it to foods or by using it in smoothies or shakes. Whey-based supplements are the most common because they are water-soluble and provide complete protein. Soy-based supplements are also popular, especially for those avoiding animal products. For other vegetable protein sources, see Appendix 30. There are now hundreds of products available, most with other added nutrients.

It is important to note that almond milk, hemp milk, oat milk, and coconut milk in their fluid forms are relatively low in protein. If used for high-nutrition impact drinks, an added source of powdered protein may be necessary to meet nutrition goals.

Nutritional Facts on Vegetarian Eating

A well-planned vegetarian diet can meet nutritional needs and can be a healthy way to meet the dietary guidelines. Vegetarian diets are chosen for nutritional, religious, ecologic, or personal reasons. It is the position of the Academy of Nutrition and Dietetics (AND) that "appropriately planned vegetarian diets are healthful, nutritionally adequate and provide health benefits in the prevention and treatment of certain diseases" (Melina et al, 2016).

The Academy's practice guideline contains recommendations, based on scientific evidence, designed to assist in the appropriate nutrition care for vegetarians. The guideline includes recommendations for children, adolescents, adults, and women who are pregnant or lactating, providing more than 30 nutrition recommendations related to vegetarian nutrition, including:

- Macronutrients, including protein
- Micronutrients, including vitamin B_{12}
- Knowledge, beliefs, and motivations
- Diet diversity
- Nutrition counseling
- Treatment of hyperlipidemia, obesity, type 2 diabetes
- Adherence to a vegetarian diet

Vegetarian adaptations of the U.S. Department of Agriculture (USDA) food patterns were included in the 2010 *Dietary Guidelines for Americans,* with sample vegetarian food patterns that allow for additional flexibility in food group choices. However, those adaptations did not modify the underlying structure of the patterns but substituted the same amounts of plant foods for animal foods in each food group. In contrast, the current Healthy Vegetarian Pattern in the 2015 U.S. Dietary Guidelines includes changes in food group composition and amounts, based on assessing the food choices of vegetarians. The Healthy Vegetarian Pattern is similar in meeting nutrient standards to the Healthy U.S.-Style Pattern, but somewhat higher in calcium and fiber and lower in vitamin D due to differences in the foods included.

Vegetarian diets are usually classified into one of the following three types:

1. Lacto-ovo-vegetarian is a modification of the diet that eliminates all dietary sources of animal protein except dairy products and eggs. This is the most common type of vegetarian diet and is the easiest of the vegetarian diets to prepare.
2. Lacto-vegetarian is a modification of the diet that eliminates all dietary sources of animal protein except dairy products. This requires that baked products be made without eggs and the elimination of egg noodles.
3. Strict vegetarian (vegan diet) is a modification of the diet that eliminates all dietary sources of animal protein.

Adequacy: The more restrictive the diet, the more challenging it is to ensure adequacy. Lacto-ovo and lacto-vegetarian diets require the same planning as any other diet. The vegan diet is a little more difficult but can be adequate with some planning. The Power Plate is a tool developed by Physicians Committee for Responsible Medicine to assist in planning a nutritionally complete vegan diet and can be accessed at PCRM.org.

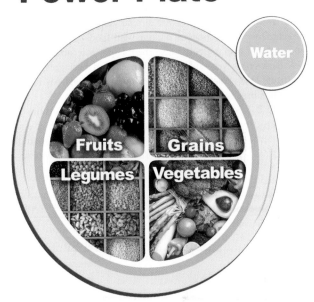

The **Sustainable Power Plate**

SustainablePowerPlate.org

NUTRIENTS TO CONSIDER WHEN PLANNING A VEGETARIAN MENU

Protein

Foods that provide approximately 7 grams of protein per serving:

¼ cup cottage cheese	½ cup legumes, cooked
1 cup cow's milk, goat's milk or soymilk	¼ cup soybeans
	¾ cup of almonds
1 oz cheese	¼ cup tofu (soy cheese)
$1/3$ cup mixed nuts	¾ cup yogurt
1 egg	¼ cup plain, Greek style yogurt
2 Tbsp peanut butter	1 cup of quinoa

Foods that contain the essential amino acids are considered complete proteins. However, foods that are incomplete proteins can be combined to make a complete protein. These are known as complementary proteins. They do not have to be eaten together at the same meal. The most common combination of complementary proteins is beans (legumes) combined with rice or corn.

Calcium: All vegetarians, especially young women, should ensure adequate calcium intake for development and maintenance of strong bones. In place of dairy products, choose abundant amounts of dark, leafy greens (e.g., kale, mustard and turnip greens, collards); bok choy; broccoli; legumes; tofu processed with calcium; dried figs; sesame seeds; and calcium-fortified cereals and juices can be incorporated into the diet. The following foods provide approximately the same amount of calcium as 1 cup of cow's milk (approximately 300 mg).

1 cup calcium-fortified orange juice, soy milk, nut milk, grain, or hemp milk	2-3 cups cooked dried beans
¼ cup sesame seeds or 2 Tbsp. sesame butter (Tahini)	1 cup almonds
	1.5 oz chia seeds
1 cup collards or kale, cooked	¾ cup blanched nettles
	3 ounces (100g) extra firm tofu made with calcium

Iron: Iron deficiency rates are similar between vegetarians and nonvegetarians. When consumed along with foods rich in vitamin C, plant sources of iron are better absorbed. High-iron foods include legumes, dark-green vegetables (i.e., spinach and beet greens), dried fruits, prune juice, blackstrap molasses, pumpkin seeds, soy nuts, and iron-fortified breads and cereals.

Vitamin B₁₂: Found only in animal foods, vitamin B_{12} is not a nutrient of great concern for vegetarians who regularly consume eggs or dairy products (lacto-ovo-vegetarians). However, vegans should include vitamin B_{12}–fortified foods such as fortified soymilk and commercial breakfast cereals, or a B_{12} supplement in their diets. Vitamin B_{12} is also found in some brands of Brewer's yeast (check the label).

Vitamin D: In the United States, the primary source of vitamin D is dairy products, most of which are fortified with vitamin D. However, cheese and yogurt do not have to be made from vitamin D–fortified milk and thus are not reliable sources of vitamin D. The other main source results from sunlight exposure, causing vitamin D to be synthesized in the skin. See Appendix 38. If dairy products are not consumed and direct sunlight exposure is limited, supplementation is warranted. Foods containing vitamin D include fortified cow's milk, soy milk, rice milk, or nut milk. Supplementation (at least 1000 IU/day) is needed for individuals who do not consume milk products or who spend little time in the sun.

Zinc: Because zinc is found in higher amounts in animal foods, the vegetarian diet may be limited. The following foods can be included in the diet to increase zinc intake:

Wheat germ
Tofu
Nuts including cashews and almonds
Seeds including sunflower, flax, pumpkin (pepitas), and chia seeds
Dried beans
Breakfast cereals, fortified

To follow the Dietary Guidelines for Americans Healthy Vegetarian Eating Pattern, identifying an appropriate calorie level is the first step (see table below). Then choose a variety of foods in each group and subgroup over time in recommended amounts, and limit choices that are not in nutrient-dense forms so that the overall calorie limit is not exceeded.

Calorie Level of Pattern	1000	1200	1400	1600	1800	2000
Food Group	Daily Amount of Food From Each Group (vegetable and protein foods subgroup amounts are per week)					
Vegetables	1 c-eq	1½ c-eq	1½ c-eq	2 c-eq	2½ c-eq	2½ c-eq
Dark-green vegetables (c-eq/wk)	½	1	1	1½	1½	1½
Red and orange vegetables (c-eq/wk)	2½	3	3	4	5½	5½
Legumes (beans and peas) (c-eq/wk)	½	½	½	1	1½	1½
Starchy vegetables (c-eq/wk)	2	3½	3½	4	5	5
Other vegetables (c-eq/wk)	1½	2½	2½	3½	4	4
Fruits	1 c-eq	1 c-eq	1½ c-eq	1½ c-eq	1½ c-eq	2 c-eq
Grains	3 oz-eq	4 oz-eq	5 oz-eq	5½ oz-eq	6½ oz-eq	6½ oz-eq
Whole grains (oz-eq/day)	1½	2	2½	3	3½	3½
Refined grains (oz-eq/day)	1½	2	2½	2½	3	3
Dairy	2 c-eq	2.5 c-eq	2.5 c-eq	3 c-eq	3 c-eq	3 c-eq
Protein Foods	1 oz-eq	1½ oz-eq	2 oz-eq	2½ oz-eq	3 oz-eq	3½ oz-eq
Eggs (oz-eq/wk)	2	3	3	3	3	3
Legumes (beans and peas) (oz-eq/wk)	1	2	4	4	6	6
Soy products (oz-eq/wk)	2	3	4	6	6	8
Nuts and seeds (oz-eq/wk)	2	2	3	5	6	7
Oils	15 g	17 g	17 g	22 g	24 g	27 g
Limit on Calories for Other Uses, calories (% of calories)	190 (19%)	170 (14%)	190 (14%)	180 (11%)	190 (11%)	290 (15%)

U.S. Dietary Guidelines 2015-2020 Appendix 5. USDA Food Patterns: Healthy Vegetarian Eating Pattern. https://health.gov/dietaryguidelines/2015/guidelines/appendix-5/. Accessed February 7, 2019.

SPECIAL NOTES

Pregnancy and Lactation: Well-planned vegan and lacto-ovo-vegetarian eating patterns adequately provide for the nutritional needs of pregnant and lactating women. Folate supplements are recommended for all pregnant women, including vegetarians. Vegans must ensure daily intake of 2 mcg of vitamin B_{12} daily during pregnancy and 2.6 mcg during lactation, whether through supplements or fortified foods. Women with limited sun exposure should include vitamin D–fortified foods and possibly a vitamin D supplement. Caution should be used with vitamin D supplementation because excess vitamin D can cause fetal abnormalities.

Infants, Children, and Adolescents: According to the Academy, well-planned vegan and lacto-ovo-vegetarian eating patterns adequately provide for the nutritional needs of infants, children, and adolescents. Because of the high bulk of low-fat vegetarian eating patterns, it may be difficult for children and adolescents to consume enough food to provide for their energy needs. Frequent meals and snacks with nutrient-dense foods can help meet energy and nutrient needs. If sun exposure is limited, vitamin D–fortified foods or supplements should be used. For vegan children, a reliable source of vitamin B_{12} should be included in their diets. To provide for growth, calcium, iron, and zinc intakes deserve special attention. It is recommended that parents of vegetarian infants and youth consult a registered dietitian nutritionist (RDN) with expertise in the vegetarian eating pattern.

Meal Pattern: Lacto-Vegetarian

Breakfast	Lunch	Dinner	Snack
½ cup orange juice	Vegetarian chili	Quinoa patties	½ peanut butter sandwich and 8 oz milk
Whole grain cereal and milk	Corn bread	Brown rice	
Berry yogurt parfait	Green salad	Fresh spinach served with lemon and butter if desired	
	Fresh fruit	Banana pudding made with coconut milk	

Meal Pattern: Lacto-Ovo-Vegetarian

Breakfast	Lunch	Dinner	Snack
Fresh fruit	Egg salad sandwich on whole wheat bread with lettuce	Black bean burritos with cheese, avocado, and salsa	Apple and cheese
½ cup oatmeal served with Greek yogurt	Cup of tomato soup	Lettuce salad	
1 cup (8 oz) milk	Carrot sticks	Peanut butter cookie and 8 oz milk	
	Fresh fruit		

Meal Pattern: Vegan

Breakfast	Lunch	Dinner	Snack
½ cup orange juice (calcium fortified)	Bean burritos served with guacamole and salsa	Tofu-vegetable stir-fry (include bok choy and spinach for calcium) Top with cashews	½ peanut butter sandwich or ½ cup of edamame
3 whole grain pancakes topped with walnuts, applesauce, and cinnamon	Green salad with oil and vinegar salad dressing	Brown rice	
1 cup fortified soy milk or soy yogurt	1 fresh apple	Cardamom-flavored chia pudding made with soymilk	
	1 cup fortified soymilk	Beverage of choice	

Reference: AND Evidence Analysis Library, Vegetarian Nutrition Guideline, 2011.

REFERENCE

Melina V, Craig W, Levin S: Academy of Nutrition and Dietetics Position Paper: Vegetarian Diets, *J Acad Nutr Diet* 116(12):1970–1980, 2016.

Nutritional Facts on Folic Acid, Vitamin B$_6$, and Vitamin B$_{12}$

FOLATE

Folate is a water-soluble B vitamin that occurs naturally in food. Folic acid is the synthetic form of folate that is found in supplements and is added to fortified foods. Folate, formerly known as folacin, is the generic term to refer to both folate and folic acid. Folate functions as an enzyme in single carbon transfers and is involved in the production and maintenance of new cells, which is especially important during periods of rapid cell division and growth such as infancy, adolescence, and pregnancy. Folate is needed to make deoxyribonucleic acid (DNA) and ribonucleic acid, the building blocks of cells. Both adults and children need folate to make normal red blood cells and prevent anemia. Folate is also essential for the conversion of homocysteine to methionine in the synthesis of s-adenosyl-methionine, and important methyl donor.

A genetic mutation of a folate-metabolizing enzyme (5,10-methylenetetrahydrofolate reductase [MTHFR]) results in the inability to convert dietary folate or folic acid into the active form, 5-methyltetrahydrofolate (5-MTHFA). The result is folate deficiency unless folate is consumed in the methylated form as methyltetrahydrofolic acid (MTHFA).

Recommended Intakes

Intake recommendations for folate and other nutrients are provided in the dietary reference intakes (DRIs) developed by the Food and Nutrition Board (FNB), Institute of Medicine (IOM) of the National Academies (formerly National Academy of Sciences). DRI is the general term for a set of reference values used for planning and assessing nutrient intakes of healthy people.

The table lists the current RDAs for folate as micrograms (mcg) of dietary folate equivalents (DFEs). The FNB developed DFEs to reflect the higher bioavailability of folic acid than that of food folate. At least 85% of supplemental folic acid is estimated to be bioavailable when taken with food, whereas only about 50% of folate naturally present in food is bioavailable. Based on these values, the FNB defined DFE as follows:

- 1 mcg DFE = 1 mcg food folate
- 1 mcg DFE = 0.6 mcg folic acid from fortified foods or dietary supplements consumed with foods
- 1 mcg DFE = 0.5 mcg folic acid from dietary supplements taken on an empty stomach

For infants from birth to 12 months of age, AIs were established that are equivalent to the mean intake of folate in healthy, breastfed infants in the United States. For a list of tolerable upper intake levels (UL), see the DRI table on the inside cover of this book.

Recommended Dietary Allowances (RDAs) for Folate

Age	Male	Female	Pregnant	Lactating
Birth to 6 months*	65 mcg DFE*	65 mcg DFE*	N/A	N/A
7-12 months*	80 mcg DFE*	80 mcg DFE*	N/A	N/A
1-3 years	150 mcg DFE	150 mcg DFE	N/A	N/A
4-8 years	200 mcg DFE	200 mcg DFE	N/A	N/A
9-13 years	300 mcg DFE	300 mcg DFE	N/A	N/A
14-18 years	400 mcg DFE	400 mcg DFE	600 mcg DFE	500 mcg DFE
19+ years	400 mcg DFE	400 mcg DFE	600 mcg DFE	500 mcg DFE

N/A, Not applicable.

*Adequate intake (AI)

Tolerable upper intake level (UL): 0-12 mos not determined; 1-3y 300 mcg/d; 4-8y 400 mcg/d; 9-13y 600 mcg/d; 14-18y (also for pregnancy and lactation) 800 mcg/d; 19+ (also for pregnancy and lactation) 1000 mcg/d.

Selected Food Sources of Folate and Folic Acid

Food	mcg DFE per Serving	Percent DV*	Food	mcg DFE per Serving	Percent DV*
Beef liver, braised, 3 ounces	215	54	Peanuts, dry roasted, 1 ounce	41	10
Spinach, boiled, ½ cup	131	33	Wheat germ, 2 tablespoons	40	10
Black-eyed peas (cowpeas), boiled, ½ cup	105	26	Tomato juice, canned, ¾ cup	36	9
Breakfast cereals, fortified with 25% of the DV†	100	25	Crab, Dungeness, 3 ounces	36	9
Rice, white, medium-grain, cooked, ½ cup†	90	23	Orange juice, ¾ cup	35	9
Asparagus, boiled, 4 spears	89	22	Turnip greens, frozen, boiled, ½ cup	32	8
Spaghetti, cooked, enriched, ½ cup†	83	21	Orange, fresh, 1 small	29	7
Brussels sprouts, frozen, boiled, ½ cup	78	20	Papaya, raw, cubed, ½ cup	27	7
Lettuce, romaine, shredded, 1 cup	64	16	Banana, 1 medium	24	6
Avocado, raw, sliced, ½ cup	59	15	Yeast, baker's, ¼ teaspoon	23	6
Spinach, raw, 1 cup	58	15	Egg, whole, hard-boiled, 1 large	22	6
Broccoli, chopped, frozen, cooked, ½ cup	52	13	Vegetarian baked beans, canned, ½ cup	15	4
Mustard greens, chopped, frozen, boiled, ½ cup	52	13	Cantaloupe, raw, 1 wedge	14	4
Green peas, frozen, boiled, ½ cup	47	12	Fish, halibut, cooked, 3 ounces	12	3
Kidney beans, canned, ½ cup	46	12	Milk, 1% fat, 1 cup	12	3
Bread, white, 1 slice†	43	11	Ground beef, 85% lean, cooked, 3 ounces	7	2
			Chicken breast, roasted, ½ breast	3	1

*DV = Daily value. The Food and Drug Administration (FDA) developed DVs to help consumers compare the nutrient contents of products within the context of a total diet. The DV for folate is 400 mcg for adults and children aged 4 and older. However, the FDA does not require food labels to list folate content unless a food has been fortified with this nutrient. Foods providing 20% or more of the DV are considered to be high sources of a nutrient.

†Fortified with folic acid as part of the folate fortification program.

VITAMIN B₆

Vitamin B₆ is a water-soluble vitamin that exists in three major chemical forms: pyridoxine, pyridoxal, and pyridoxamine and their respective esters. Pyridoxal 5' phosphate (PLP) and pyridoxamine 5' phosphate (PMP) are the active coenzyme forms of vitamin B₆. Vitamin B₆ is naturally present in many foods, is added to others, and also exists as a dietary supplement.

Vitamin B₆ performs a wide variety of functions in the body. It is needed for more than 100 enzymes involved in protein metabolism and is essential for red blood cell metabolism. The nervous and immune systems need vitamin B₆ to function efficiently, and it is also needed for the conversion of tryptophan (an amino acid) to niacin. A vitamin B₆ deficiency can result in a form of anemia that is similar to iron deficiency anemia.

Through its involvement in protein metabolism and cellular growth, vitamin B₆ is important to the immune system. It helps maintain the health of lymphoid organs (thymus, spleen, and lymph nodes) that make white blood cells. It is also important for maintaining normal blood glucose levels.

Recommended Intakes

Intake recommendations for vitamin B₆ and other nutrients are provided in the DRIs developed by the FNB of the IOM of the National Academies.

Recommended Dietary Allowances for Vitamin B₆ for Children and Adults

Age (years)	Males (mg/day)	Females (mg/day)	Pregnancy (mg/day)	Lactation (mg/day)
0-6 mo	0.1*	0.1*	N/A	N/A
7-12 mo	0.3*	0.3*	N/A	N/A
1-3	0.5	0.5	N/A	N/A
4-8	0.6	0.6	N/A	N/A
9-13	1.0	1.0	N/A	N/A
14-18	1.3	1.2	1.9	2.0
19-50	1.3	1.3	1.9	2.0
51+	1.7	1.5	N/A	N/A

N/A, Not applicable.

*Adequate intake (AI). AI for vitamin B₆ is equivalent to the mean intake of vitamin B₆ in healthy, breastfed infants.

Tolerable upper intake level (UL): 0-12 mos not determined; 1-3y 30 mg/d; 4-8y 40 mg/d; 9-13y 60 mg/d; 14-18y (also for pregnancy and lactation) 80 mg/d; 19+ (also for pregnancy and lactation) 100 mg/d.

Substantial proportions of the naturally occurring pyridoxine in fruits, vegetables, and grains exist in glycosylated forms that exhibit reduced bioavailability.

Selected Food Sources of Vitamin B₆

Food	Milligrams (mg) per Serving	Percent DV*
Chickpeas, canned, 1 cup	1.1	55
Beef liver, pan fried, 3 ounces	0.9	45
Tuna, yellowfin, fresh, cooked, 3 ounces	0.9	45
Salmon, sockeye, cooked, 3 ounces	0.6	30
Chicken breast, roasted, 3 ounces	0.5	25
Breakfast cereals, fortified with 25% of the DV for vitamin B₆	0.5	25
Potatoes, boiled, 1 cup	0.4	20
Turkey, meat only, roasted, 3 ounces	0.4	20
Banana, 1 medium	0.4	20
Marinara (spaghetti) sauce, ready to serve, 1 cup	0.4	20
Ground beef, patty, 85% lean, broiled, 3 ounces	0.3	15
Waffles, plain, ready to heat, toasted, 1 waffle	0.3	15
Bulgur, cooked, 1 cup	0.2	10
Cottage cheese, 1% low-fat, 1 cup	0.2	10
Squash, winter, baked, ½ cup	0.2	10
Rice, white, long-grain, enriched, cooked, 1 cup	0.1	5
Nuts, mixed, dry-roasted, 1 ounce	0.1	5
Raisins, seedless, ½ cup	0.1	5
Onions, chopped, ½ cup	0.1	5
Spinach, frozen, chopped, boiled, ½ cup	0.1	5
Tofu, raw, firm, prepared with calcium sulfate, ½ cup	0.1	5
Watermelon, raw, 1 cup	0.1	5

*DV = Daily value. DVs were developed by the Food and Drug Administration (FDA) to help consumers compare the nutrient contents of products within the context of a total diet. The DV for vitamin B₆ is 2 mg for adults and children age 4 and older. However, the FDA does not require food labels to list vitamin B₆ content unless a food has been fortified with this nutrient. Foods providing 20% or more of the DV are considered to be high sources of a nutrient.

VITAMIN B₁₂

Vitamin B_{12} is a member of the vitamin B complex. It contains cobalt; thus it is also known as *cobalamin*. Methylcobalamin and 5-deoxyadenosylcobalamin are the active forms of vitamin B_{12}. Like folate, vitamin B_{12} is involved in the conversion of homocysteine to methionine.

Vitamin B_{12} is necessary for the synthesis of red blood cells, the maintenance of the nervous system, DNA synthesis, and growth.

Deficiency can cause anemia. Vitamin B_{12} neuropathy, involving the degeneration of nerve fibers and irreversible neurologic damage, can also occur.

Proper vitamin B_{12} absorption requires the presence of hydrochloric acid (HCL) and gastric protease, which cause its release from the protein it is bound to in food, allowing it to be absorbed. B_{12} then combines with intrinsic factor (IF), secreted by the stomach's parietal cells, and travels down the gastrointestinal (GI) tract where it is absorbed as the B_{12}-IF complex in the distal ileum. Because HCL production tends to diminish with age, B_{12} supplementation where the B_{12} is already separated from the protein molecule and is in its free form can be useful in treating or preventing a deficiency. Total body store of B_{12} is 2 to 5 mg in adults. Approximately 80% of this is stored in the liver.

Along with folate and vitamin B_6, vitamin B_{12} is helpful in lowering the level of the amino acid homocysteine in the blood. It has been hypothesized that at high levels homocysteine might damage coronary arteries or make it easier for blood-clotting cells to clump together and form a clot. This could increase risks for a heart attack or stroke.

The table below lists the current RDAs for vitamin B_{12} in micrograms (mcg). For infants aged 0 to 12 months, there are AIs that are equivalent to the mean intake of vitamin B_{12} in healthy, breastfed infants.

Recommended Dietary Allowances for Vitamin B₁₂ for Children and Adults

Age (years)	Males and Females (mcg/day)	Pregnancy (mcg/day)	Lactation (mcg/day)
0-6 mo	0.4*	N/A	N/A
7-12 mo	0.5*	N/A	N/A
1-3	0.9	N/A	N/A
4-8	1.2	N/A	N/A
9-13	1.8	N/A	N/A
14 +	2.4	2.6	2.8

N/A, Not applicable.
*Adequate intake (AI)
Tolerable upper intake level (UL) not established for B₁₂.

Vitamin B_{12} is found primarily in animal foods such as fish, meat, poultry, eggs, and dairy products. However, it is also synthesized by bacteria, and there has been considerable research into proposed plant sources of vitamin B_{12}. Fermented soy products, seaweeds, and algae (spirulina) have all been suggested as containing significant B_{12}. However, the present consensus is that any B_{12} present in plant foods is likely to be unavailable to humans; thus these foods should not be relied on as safe sources. Vegans need B_{12} from fortified foods or as a supplement. Fortified breakfast cereals are a readily available source of vitamin B_{12} with high bioavailability for vegans. Some nutritional yeast products also contain vitamin B_{12}. Fortified foods vary in formulation, so it is important to read product labels.

Many vegan foods are supplemented with B_{12}.

Selected Food Sources of Vitamin B$_{12}$

Food	Micrograms (mcg) per Serving	Percent DV*
Clams, cooked, 3 ounces	84.1	1,402
Liver, beef, cooked, 3 ounces	70.7	1,178
Breakfast cereals, fortified with 100% of the DV for vitamin B$_{12}$, 1 serving	6.0	100
Trout, rainbow, wild, cooked, 3 ounces	5.4	90
Salmon, sockeye, cooked, 3 ounces	4.8	80
Trout, rainbow, farmed, cooked, 3 ounces	3.5	58
Tuna fish, light, canned in water, 3 ounces	2.5	42
Cheeseburger, double patty and bun, 1 sandwich	2.1	35
Haddock, cooked, 3 ounces	1.8	30
Breakfast cereals, fortified with 25% of the DV for vitamin B$_{12}$, 1 serving	1.5	25
Beef, top sirloin, broiled, 3 ounces	1.4	23
Milk, low-fat, 1 cup	1.2	18
Yogurt, fruit, low-fat, 8 ounces	1.1	18
Cheese, Swiss, 1 ounce	0.9	15
Beef taco, 1 soft taco	0.9	15
Ham, cured, roasted, 3 ounces	0.6	10
Egg, whole, hard boiled, 1 large	0.6	10
Chicken, breast meat, roasted, 3 ounces	0.3	5

*DV = Daily value. DVs were developed by the Food and Drug Administration (FDA) to help consumers determine the level of various nutrients in a standard serving of food in relation to their approximate requirement for it. The DV for adults and children aged 4 and older is 6.0 mcg. The %DV listed on the Nutrition Facts label states the percentage of the DV provided per serving. However, the FDA does not require food labels to list vitamin B$_{12}$ content unless a food has been fortified with this nutrient. Foods providing 20% or more of the DV are considered to be high sources of a nutrient, but foods providing lower percentages of the DV also contribute to a healthful diet.

REFERENCES

Institute of Medicine: *Food and Nutrition Board: dietary reference intakes for Thiamin, Riboflavin, Niacin, Vitamin B$_6$, Folate, Vitamin B$_{12}$, Pantothenic Acid, Biotin, and Choline,* Washington, DC, 1998, National Academies Press.

U.S. Department of Agriculture: *Food data central,* Released April 1, 2019. Available at: https://fdc.nal.usda.gov. Accessed December 30, 2019.

Nutritional Facts on Choline

Choline is an essential nutrient synthesized in the liver but must be consumed through diet to adequately meet human needs. It is found in many foods but is most concentrated in meat, poultry, fish, and eggs. Choline supports the structural integrity of cells as a precursor to two essential membrane phospholipids, phosphatidylcholine and sphingomyelin. It also supports the synthesis of ceramide and diacylglycerol, which are important in cell signaling as intracellular messengers. Choline has a role in stimulating the synthesis of catecholamine neurotransmitters and is a precursor for acetylcholine, which is needed for muscle control, memory, mood, circadian rhythm, and other neurologic functions.

Additionally, phosphatidylcholine is needed for the formation and secretion of very-low-density lipoprotein (VLDL) from the liver; therefore a choline deficiency can lead to nonalcoholic fatty liver disease (NAFLD) and nonalcoholic steatohepatitis (NASH).

Choline acts as a methyl donor, modulating gene expression as well as many metabolic steps, including homocysteine metabolism. Homocysteine accumulation is associated with elevated risk of cardiovascular disease (CVD). Betaine, a metabolite of choline, serves as the methyl donor for up to 60% of the methylation needed to convert homocysteine back to methionine. Yet research suggests high choline intake coupled with certain intestinal microbiota may also increase risk for CVD. Choline and phosphatidylcholine can be converted to trimethylamine (TMA) by the microbiota, which is converted to trimethylamine-N-oxide (TMAO) in the liver. Elevated TMAO has been linked with increased CVD risk, but more research is needed to elucidate the relationship between choline, microbiota composition, and CVD risk (Bu and Wang, 2018).

GROUPS WITH INCREASED CHOLINE NEEDS

Most pregnant women consume less than the AI of choline, and it is rarely included in prenatal supplements. Higher choline intake may be especially important for pregnant women with impaired methylation status resulting from low folic acid or vitamin B_{12} intake or a single nucleotide polymorphism (SNP) for methylenetetrahydrofolate dehydrogenase.

Other SNPs can also raise the risk for choline deficiency, such as one for the enzyme phosphatidylethanolamine N-methyltransferase (PEMT). PEMT governs de novo choline synthesis. When impaired, individuals are more susceptible to a choline deficiency and resulting organ dysfunction. Estrogen induces PEMT, therefore this SNP is of greatest concern for postmenopausal women. Other SNPs that correlate with race can modify choline requirements. Those of European descent are more likely to have four SNPs that elevate risk for organ dysfunction when consuming a low-choline diet.

Another group at risk of developing choline-insufficiency-induced organ damage are adult and pediatric patients receiving long-term total parenteral nutrition (TPN). Currently, routine TPN formulations lack choline.

Finally, because choline is a methyl donor nutrient with critical roles in neuronal functions, cognitive processes, and DNA methylation, it may be particularly important for developing children as well as older adults facing neurologic decline and diseases such as Alzheimer's disease.

EXCESSIVE CHOLINE INTAKE

Excessive choline intake is characterized by fishy body odor, vomiting, extreme sweating and salivation, hypotension, and liver toxicity.

Dietary Reference Intakes: Adequate Intakes (AIs) for Choline for Children and Adults

Age (years)	Male (mg/day)	Female (mg/day)	Pregnancy (mg/day)	Lactation (mg/day)
Birth-6 mo	125	125		
7-12 mo	150	150		
1-3	200	200		
4-8	250	250		
9-13	375	375		
14-18	550	400	450	550
19+	550	425	450	550

Tolerable upper intake level (UL): 0-12 mos not determined; 1-3y 1 g/d; 4-8y 1 g/d; 9-13y 2 g/d; 14-18y (also for pregnancy and lactation) 3 g/d; 19+ (also for pregnancy and lactation) 3.5 g/d.

Food Sources of Choline

Food	Milligrams (mg) per Serving	% Daily Value*	Food	Milligrams (mg) per Serving	% Daily Value*
Beef kidney, 3 oz	436	79	Cod, Atlantic, cooked, 3 oz	71	13
Pork chitterlings, 3 oz	400	73	Chicken, light meat, 3 oz	71	13
Beef liver, 3 oz	362	65	Pork loin, 3 oz	65	11
Beef liver, pan fried, 3 oz	356	65	Brussels sprouts, boiled, 1 cup	63	11
Chicken liver, 3 oz	277	50	Broccoli, boiled, 1 cup	63	11
Wheat germ, toasted, 1 cup	202	37	Mushrooms, shiitake, cooked, ½ cup	58	11
Beef heart, 3 oz	195	35	Potato, red, baked, with skin, 1 large	57	10
Peas, green, split, raw, ½ cup	154	28			
Egg, hard boiled	147	27	Cauliflower, boiled, 1 cup	48	8
Egg yolk, 1 large	140	25	Beans, kidney, canned, ½ cup	45	8
Shrimp, 3 oz	115	21	Milk, (whole or skim), 1 cup	35	6
Oysters, 3 oz	110	20	Quinoa, cooked, ½ cup	22	4
Soybeans, roasted, ½ cup	107	19	Peanut butter, smooth, 2 tablespoons	20	4
Chickpeas, raw, ½ cup	99	18			
Beef, trim cut, cooked, 3 oz	97	18	Cheese, cheddar, 1.5 oz	7	1.3
Chicken, dark meat, 3 oz	84	15	Cheese, mozzarella, 1.5 oz	7	1.3
Salmon, pink, canned, 3 oz	73	13	Egg white, 1 large	0.04	0.007
Chicken breast, roasted, 3 oz	72	13			

*DV 5 Daily value. DVs were developed by the Food and Drug Administration (FDA) to help consumers determine the level of various nutrients in a standard serving of food in relation to their approximate requirement for it. The DV for adults and children aged 4 and older is 6.0 mcg. The %DV listed on the Nutrition Facts label states the percentage of the DV provided per serving. However, the FDA does not require food labels to list vitamin B12 content unless a food has been fortified with this nutrient. Foods providing 20% or more of the DV are considered to be high sources of a nutrient, but foods providing lower percentages of the DV also contribute to a healthful diet.

Drug Nutrient Interaction: Methotrexate

Methotrexate inhibits methyl group donation from folate derivatives. Therefore patients taking methotrexate may need more choline to compensate (akin to folate deficiency).

REFERENCES

Institute of Medicine: *Food and nutrition board: dietary reference intakes for Thiamin, Riboflavin, Niacin, Vitamin B₆, Folate, Vitamin B₁₂, Pantothenic Acid, Biotin, and Choline,* Washington DC, 1998, National Academies.

Oregon State University: *Linus Pauling Institute Micronutrient Information Center: Choline* (website), January 2015. Available at: https://lpi.oregonstate.edu/mic/other-nutrients/choline#reference82. Accessed September 24, 2018.

U.S. Department of Agriculture: *Food Data Central,* Released April 1, 2019. Available at: https://fdc.nal.usda.gov. Accessed December 30, 2019.

Nutritional Facts on Biotin

Biotin is an essential nutrient that is naturally present in some foods and available as a dietary supplement. Biotin is a water-soluble B vitamin and functions as a cofactor for five carboxylase enzymes needed for important steps in the metabolism of amino acids, glucose, and fatty acids. Biotin is also used in histone modification, gene regulation, and cell signaling. While some biotin found in foods is in the free form, most biotin is bound to protein. Once released and processed by enzymes in the gastrointestinal tract, free biotin is absorbed in the small intestine and predominantly stored in the liver.

There is not currently sufficient data available to derive an estimated average requirement and recommended dietary allowance for biotin, resulting in only an established adequate intake (AI) for biotin. The Food and Nutrition Board has determined the AI for all age groups by taking the amount of biotin in human breastmilk consumed by infants and extrapolating AI to the other groups using body weight.

Daily Reference Intakes: Adequate Intakes (AIs) for Biotin for Children and Adults

Age	Males and Females	Pregnancy	Lactation
0-6 months	5 mcg	N/A	N/A
7-12 months	6 mcg	N/A	N/A
1-3 years	8 mcg	N/A	N/A
4-8 years	12 mcg	N/A	N/A
9-13 years	20 mcg	N/A	N/A
14-18 years	25 mcg	30 mcg	35 mcg
19+ years	30 mcg	30 mcg	35 mcg

N/A, Not applicable.
Tolerable upper intake level (UL) has not been established for biotin.

Biotin is found in appreciable amounts in organ meats, egg, fish, and meat, but is also found in seeds, nuts, and some vegetables. Raw egg whites contain a glycoprotein, avidin, that inhibits biotin's absorption in the gastrointestinal tract. Individuals consuming large amounts of raw egg whites may be at risk for biotin deficiency. Cooking egg whites denatures the avidin, preventing this interference. In healthy individuals eating a normal mixed diet, biotin deficiency is rare. There are currently no upper limits set for biotin due to lack of evidence of toxicity at high exposures. However, high levels of biotin supplementation may interfere with clinical tests, such as producing falsely normal or abnormal results on thyroid function tests.

Selected Food Sources of Biotin*

Food	Biotin (mcg)
Beef liver, cooked, 3 ounces	30.8
Egg, whole, cooked	10.0
Salmon, pink, canned in water, 3 ounces	5.0
Pork chop, cooked, 3 ounces	3.8
Hamburger patty, cooked, 3 ounces	3.8
Sunflower seeds, roasted, ¼ cup	2.6
Sweet potato, cooked, ½ cup	2.4
Almonds, roasted, ¼ cup	1.5
Tuna, canned in water, 3 ounces	0.6
Spinach, boiled, ½ cup	0.5
Broccoli, fresh, ½ cup	0.4
Cheddar cheese, mild, 1 ounce	0.4
Milk, 2%, 1 cup	0.3
Plain yogurt, 1 cup	0.2
Oatmeal, 1 cup	0.2
Banana, ½ cup	0.2
Whole-wheat bread, 1 slice	0.0
Apple, ½ cup	0.0

*Biotin does not currently have a daily value (DV) but will have a DV of 30 mcg for adults and children age 4+ on updated Nutrition and Supplement Facts labels starting in January 2020.

REFERENCES

Institute of Medicine: *Food and nutrition board: dietary reference intakes for thiamin, Riboflavin, Niacin, Vitamin B₆, Folate, Vitamin B₁₂, Pantothenic Acid, Biotin, and Choline,* Washington DC, 1998, National Academies.

U.S. Department of Agriculture: *Food data central,* Released April 1, 2019. Available at: https://fdc.nal.usda.gov. Accessed December 30, 2019.

Nutritional Facts on Vitamin A and Carotenoids

Vitamin A includes a group of compounds that affect vision, bone growth, reproduction, cell division, immunity, and healthy surface linings of the respiratory tract and mucous membranes. There are two categories of vitamin A, depending on whether the food source is an animal or a plant. Vitamin A found in animal foods is called *preformed vitamin A* and is absorbed as retinol. Sources include liver, whole milk, and some fortified food products. In the body retinol can be made into retinal and retinoic acid (other active forms of vitamin A).

Plant sources of vitamin A provide the provitamin A, called *carotenoids.* They can be made into retinol in the body and then into the other active forms of vitamin A. In the United States, approximately 26% to 34% of vitamin A consumed is in the form of provitamin A carotenoids. Common provitamin A carotenoids, which give plants their color, are β-carotene, α-carotene, and β-cryptoxanthin. Among these, β-carotene is most efficiently made into retinol. The darker the color of a fruit or vegetable, the greater is its carotenoid content.

Vitamin A deficiency rarely occurs in the United States. Vitamin A deficiency is more common in developing countries, where access to sufficient animal and beta-carotene containing plant sources is limited. Vitamin A deficiency is a leading cause of preventable blindness in children. Children with measles or diarrhea can significantly benefit from increased vitamin A. Fat malabsorption can result in diarrhea and prevent normal absorption of vitamin A; this may result in vitamin A deficiency in celiac disease, Crohn's disease, and pancreatic disorders. The best absorbed form of vitamin A is in the oil form such as in cod liver oil.

Excess intake of retinol (preformed vitamin A) can be toxic to the liver and can lead to birth defects. The tolerable upper limit (UL) for adults is 3000 RAE/10,000 IU. This does not apply to intake of vitamin A derived from carrotenoids.

All dietary sources of vitamin A are converted to retinol. Intake recommendations for vitamin A in foods are expressed as micrograms of retinol activity equivalents (RAEs) as a way to standardize the variation in bioactivities of retinol and provitamin A carotenoids, and account for the differences based on source. International units (IU) are a helpful guideline, but conversion rates also vary based on source:

- 1 IU retinol = 0.3 mcg RAE
- 1 IU beta-carotene from dietary supplements = 0.15 mcg RAE
- 1 IU beta-carotene from food = 0.05 mcg RAE
- 1 IU alpha-carotene or beta-cryptoxanthin = 0.025 mcg RAE

Recommended Daily Allowances

Age (years)	Males and Females (mcg RAEs/IU/day)	Pregnancy (mcg RAEs/IU/day)	Lactation (mcg RAEs/IU/day)
0-6 mo	400*/1333	N/A	N/A
0-7 mo	500*/1666	N/A	N/A
1-3	300/1000	N/A	N/A
4-8	400/1333	N/A	N/A
9-13	600/2000	N/A	N/A
14-18	900/3000 for boys 700/2333 for girls	750/2500	1200/4000
19+	900/3000 for men 700/2333 for women	770/2566	1300/4333

N/A, Not applicable; *RAE,* retinol activity equivalent.
*Adequate intakes

Tolerable upper intake level (UL): 0-12 mos 600 mcg/ 2000 IU/d; 1-3y 600 mcg/2000 IU/d; 4-8y 900 mcg/ 3000 IU/d; 9-13y 1700 mcg/ 5666 IU/d; 14-18y (also for pregnancy and lactation) 2800 mcg/ 9333/d; 19+ (also for pregnancy and lactation) 3000 mcg/ 10000 IU/d.

FOOD SOURCES OF VITAMIN A

Selected Animal Sources of Vitamin A

Food	Vitamin A (IU)	% Daily Value
Liver, beef, cooked, 3 oz	27,185	545
Liver, chicken, cooked, 3 oz	12,325	245
Cod Liver Oil, 1Tbs	4080	13,600
Milk, fortified skim, 1 cup	500	10
Cheese, cheddar, 1 oz	284	6
Milk, fortified whole (3.25% fat), 1 cup	249	5
Egg, whole, large	266	5.6
Egg substitute, ¼ cup	226	5
Egg yolk, large	216	4.5

Selected Plant Sources of Vitamin A (from β-Carotene)

Food	Vitamin A (IU)	% Daily Value*	Food	Vitamin A (IU)	% Daily Value*
Sweet potato, 1 medium	28,058	561	Papaya, cubes, 1 cup	1532	30
Carrot juice, canned, ½ cup	22,567	450	Mango, sliced, 1 cup	1262	25
Carrots, boiled, slices, ½ cup	13,418	270	Oatmeal, instant, fortified, plain, prepared with water, 1 cup	1252	25
Spinach, frozen, boiled, ½ cup	11,458	230			
Kale, frozen, boiled, ½ cup	9558	190	Peas, frozen, boiled, ½ cup	1050	20
Carrots, 1 raw (7½ in)	8666	175	Tomato juice, canned, 6 oz	819	15
Vegetable soup, canned, chunky, ready-to-serve, 1 cup	5820	115	Peaches, canned, juice pack, halves or slices, ½ cup	473	10
Cantaloupe, cubes, 1 cup	5411	110	Peach, 1 medium	319	6
Spinach, raw, 1 cup	2813	55	Pepper, sweet, red, raw, 1 ring (3 inches diameter by ¼ inch thick)	313	6
Apricots with skin, juice pack, ½ cup	2063	40			
Apricot nectar, canned, ½ cup	1651	35			

*Daily values (DVs) are reference numbers based on the RDA. They were developed to help consumers determine whether a food contains a lot or a little of a nutrient. The DV for vitamin A is 5000 IU. Most food labels do not list vitamin A content. The %DV column in this table indicates the percentage of the DV provided in one serving. A food providing 5% or less of the DV is a low source, whereas a food that provides 10% to 19% of the DV is a good source. A food that provides 20% or more of the DV is high in that nutrient. It is important to remember that foods that provide lower percentages of the DV also contribute to a healthful diet.

Carotenoids in Fruits and Vegetables (mole %)

	Neoxanthins and Violaxanthins	Lutein and Zeaxanthin	Lutein	Zeaxanthin	Cryptoxanthins	Lycopenes	α-Carotene	β-Carotene
Egg yolk	8	89	54	35	4	0	0	0
Maize (corn)	9	86	60	26	5	0	0	0
Kiwi	38	54	54	0	0	0	0	8
Red seedless grapes	23	53	43	10	4	5	3	16
Zucchini squash	19	52	47	5	24	0	0	5
Pumpkin	30	49	49	0	0	0	0	21
Spinach	14	47	47	0	19	4	0	16
Orange pepper	4	45	8	37	22	0	8	21
Yellow squash	19	44	44	0	0	0	28	9
Cucumber	16	42	38	4	38	0	0	4
Pea	33	41	41	0	21	0	0	5
Green pepper	29	39	36	3	20	0	0	12
Red grape	27	37	33	4	29	0	1	6
Butternut squash	24	37	37	0	34	0	5	0
Orange juice	28	35	15	20	25	0	3	8
Honeydew	18	35	17	18	0	0	0	48
Celery (stalks, leaves)	12	34	32	2	40	1	13	0
Green grapes	10	31	25	6	52	0	0	7
Brussels sprouts	20	29	27	2	39	0	0	11
Scallions	32	29	27	2	35	4	0	0
Green beans	27	25	22	3	42	0	1	5
Orange	36	22	7	15	12	11	8	11
Broccoli	3	22	22	0	49	0	0	27

Carotenoids in Fruits and Vegetables (mole %)—cont'd

	Neoxanthins and Violaxanthins	Lutein and Zeaxanthin	Lutein	Zeaxanthin	Cryptoxanthins	Lycopenes	α-Carotene	β-Carotene
Apple (red delicious)	22	20	19	1	23	13	5	17
Mango	52	18	2	16	4	6	0	20
Green lettuce	33	15	15	0	36	0	16	0
Tomato juice	0	13	11	2	2	57	12	16
Peach	20	13	5	8	8	0	10	50
Yellow pepper	86	12	12	0	1	0	1	0
Nectarine	18	11	6	5	23	0	0	48
Red pepper	56	7	7	0	2	8	24	3
Tomato (fruit)	0	6	6	0	0	82	0	12
Carrots	0	2	2	0	0	0	43	55
Cantaloupe	9	1	1	0	0	3	0	87
Dried apricots	2	1	1	0	9	0	0	87
Green kidney beans	72	0	0	0	28	0	0	0

Table from Sommerburg O, Keunen JE, Bird AC, et al: Fruits and vegetables that are sources for lutein and zeaxanthin: the macular pigment in human eyes, *Br J Ophthalmol* 82:907–910, 1998.

The contents of the major carotenoids are given in mole %. The amounts of the carotenoids were shown in seven major groups, as (1) neoxanthins and violaxanthins (neoxanthin, violaxanthin, and their related isomers, lutein 5, 6 epoxide), (2) lutein, (3) zeaxanthin, (4) cryptoxanthins (α-cryptoxanthin, β-cryptoxanthins, and related isomers), (5) lycopenes (lycopene and related isomers), (6) alpha-carotenes, and (7) β-carotene (all *trans* β-carotene and *cis* isomers). Lutein and zeaxanthin are given combined and as single amounts. The data are sorted by the combined amount of lutein and zeaxanthin.

REFERENCES

Institute of Medicine: *Food and nutrition board: dietary reference intakes for Vitamin A, Vitamin K, Arsenic, Boron, Chromium, Copper, Iodine, Iron, Manganese, Molybdenum, Nickel, Silicon, Vanadium, and Zinc*, Washington DC, 2001, National Academies Press.

Oregon State University: *Linus Pauling Institute Micronutrient Information Center: Vitamin A* (website), Updated March, 2015. Available at: https://lpi.oregonstate.edu/mic/vitamins/vitamin-A Accessed December 30, 2019.

U.S. Department of Agriculture: *Food data central*, Released April 1, 2019. Available at: https://fdc.nal.usda.gov. Accessed December 30, 2019.

Nutritional Facts on Vitamin C

Vitamin C is a nutrient naturally present in foods (mainly fruits and vegetables) and is also known by the chemical name of its principal form, L-ascorbic acid or, simply, ascorbic acid. Unlike most animals, humans are unable to synthesize vitamin C. Vitamin C is principally known as a water-soluble antioxidant, preventing the damaging effects of free radicals, and it regenerates other antioxidants in the body including vitamin E or alpha-tocopherol.

Vitamin C is required for the biosynthesis of collagen, L-carnitine, and certain neurotransmitters; it is also involved in protein metabolism. Collagen is an essential component of connective tissue, which plays a vital role in wound healing, and it plays an important role in immune function. It also improves the absorption of nonheme iron, the form of iron present in plant-based foods. Vitamin C prevents scurvy, characterized by fatigue or lassitude, widespread connective tissue weakness, and capillary fragility.

The recommended dietary allowances (RDAs) for vitamin C are based on its known physiologic and antioxidant functions in white blood cells and are much higher than the amount required for protection from deficiency. For infants from birth to 12 months, the Food and Nutrition Board (FNB) established an adequate intake (AI) for vitamin C that is equivalent to the mean intake of vitamin C in healthy, breastfed infants.

Fruits and vegetables are the best sources of vitamin C, especially citrus fruits, red and green peppers, kiwi fruit, and tomatoes and tomato juice. Other good food sources include broccoli, strawberries, Brussels sprouts, and cantaloupe. Some fortified breakfast cereals are also good sources of vitamin C.

The vitamin C content of food can be lessened by prolonged storage and by cooking because ascorbic acid is water soluble and is destroyed by heat. Steaming or microwaving vegetables rather than boiling them may reduce cooking losses. Fortunately, many of the best food sources of vitamin C, such as fruits and vegetables, are usually consumed raw.

Recommended Dietary Allowances (RDAs) for Vitamin C for Children and Adults

Age (years)	Males and Females (mg/day)	Pregnancy (mg/day)	Lactation (mg/day)
0-6 mo	40	N/A	N/A
7-12 mo	50	N/A	N/A
1-3	15	N/A	N/A
4-8	25	N/A	N/A
9-13	45	N/A	N/A
14-18	75 for boys, 65 for girls	80	115
19+	90 for men, 75 for women	85	120
Smokers	Individuals who smoke require 35 mg/day more vitamin C than nonsmokers.		

N/A, Not applicable.
Tolerable upper intake level (UL): 0-12 mos not determined; 1-3y 400 mg/d; 4-8y 650 mg/d; 9-13y 1200 mg/d; 14-18y (also for pregnancy and lactation) 1800 mg/d; 19+ (also for pregnancy and lactation) 2000 mg/d.

Selected Food Sources of Vitamin C

Food	Milligrams (mg) per Serving	Percent (%) DV*
Red pepper, sweet, raw, ½ cup	95	158
Orange juice, ¾ cup	93	155
Orange, 1 medium	70	117
Grapefruit juice, ¾ cup	70	117
Kiwifruit, 1 medium	64	107
Green pepper, sweet, raw, ½ cup	60	100
Broccoli, cooked, ½ cup	51	85
Strawberries, fresh, sliced, ½ cup	49	82
Brussels sprouts, cooked, ½ cup	48	80
Grapefruit, ½ medium	39	65
Broccoli, raw, ½ cup	39	65
Tomato juice, ¾ cup	33	55
Cantaloupe, ½ cup	29	48
Cabbage, cooked, ½ cup	28	47
Cauliflower, raw, ½ cup	26	43
Potato, baked, 1 medium	17	28
Tomato, raw, 1 medium	17	28
Spinach, cooked, ½ cup	9	15
Green peas, frozen, cooked, ½ cup	8	13

*DV = Daily value. DVs were developed by the Food and Drug Administration (FDA) to help consumers compare the nutrient contents of products within the context of a total diet. The DV for vitamin C is 60 mg for adults and children aged 4 and older. The FDA requires all food labels to list the percent DV for vitamin C. Foods providing 20% or more of the DV are considered to be high sources of a nutrient.

Dietary Supplements

Supplements typically contain vitamin C in the form of ascorbic acid, which has equivalent bioavailability to that of naturally occurring ascorbic acid in foods, such as orange juice and broccoli. Other forms of vitamin C supplements include sodium ascorbate; calcium ascorbate; other mineral ascorbates; ascorbic acid with bioflavonoids; and combination products, such as Ester-C, which contains calcium ascorbate, dehydroascorbate, calcium threonate, xylonate, and lyxonate. It is not established whether Ester-C is more bioavailable or effective than ascorbic acid in improving vitamin C status.

REFERENCES

Institute of Medicine, Food and Nutrition Board: *Dietary reference intakes for Vitamin C, Vitamin E, Selenium, and Carotenoids*, Washington, DC, 2000, National Academies Press.

U.S. Department of Agriculture: *Food data central*, Released April 1, 2019. Available at: https://fdc.nal.usda.gov. Accessed December 30, 2019.

Nutritional Facts on Vitamin E

Vitamin E is a naturally occurring fat-soluble vitamin that exists in eight different forms: alpha-, beta-, gamma-, and delta-tocopherol, and alpha-, beta-, gamma-, and delta-tocotrienol that have varying levels of biological activity. Alpha- (or α-) tocopherol appears to be the most active form and is the only form that is recognized to meet human requirements. Serum concentrations of alpha-tocopherol depend on the liver, which takes up the nutrient after absorption of all the forms from the small intestine. The liver then preferentially secretes only alpha-tocopherol and metabolizes and excretes the other vitamin E forms. As a result, blood and cellular concentrations of other forms of vitamin E are lower than those of alpha-tocopherol and thus have been less studied.

Vitamin E has powerful antioxidant activities, which protect cells from the damaging effects of free radicals. Free radicals combine with oxygen and form reactive oxygen species (ROS) that damage cells. Free radicals are produced endogenously when the body metabolizes food to energy. Exogenous sources come from exposure to cigarette smoke, air pollution, and ultraviolet radiation from the sun. ROS are part of signaling mechanisms among cells, and antioxidant vitamin E protects the cells against free radical damage. Scientists are investigating whether, by limiting free-radical production and possibly through other mechanisms, vitamin E might help prevent or delay the chronic diseases associated with free radicals. Besides functioning as an antioxidant, vitamin E is also involved in immune function and, as shown primarily by in vitro studies of cells, cell signaling, regulation of gene expression, and other metabolic processes.

Vitamin E in supplements is usually sold as α-tocopherol acetate, a form of α-tocopherol that protects its ability to function as an antioxidant. The synthetic form is labeled dl, whereas the natural form is labeled d. The synthetic form is only half as active as the natural form. It is important to include foods high in vitamin E on a daily basis to get enough vitamin E from foods alone. Vegetable oils, nuts, green leafy vegetables, and fortified cereals are common food sources of vitamin E.

Vitamin E content of food is stated as milligrams of α-tocopherol, milligrams of α-tocopherol equivalents (mg α-TE), or as international units (IUs) on supplement labels. 1 unit = 0.67 α-TE in the d form and approximately ½ of that in the dl or synthetic form. The vitamin E content of foods and dietary supplements is listed on labels in IUs, a measure of biological activity rather than quantity. Naturally sourced vitamin E is called d-alpha-tocopherol; the synthetically produced form is dl-alpha-tocopherol. Conversion rules are as follows:

- To convert from mg to IU: 1 mg of alpha-tocopherol is equivalent to 1.49 IU of the natural form or 2.22 IU of the synthetic form.
- To convert from IU to mg: 1 IU of alpha-tocopherol is equivalent to 0.67 mg of the natural form or 0.45 mg of the synthetic form.

Numerous foods provide vitamin E. Nuts, seeds, and vegetable oils are among the best sources of alpha-tocopherol, and significant amounts are available in green leafy vegetables and fortified cereals (see the table below). Most vitamin E in American diets is in the form of gamma-tocopherol from soybean, canola, corn, and other vegetable oils and food products.

Recommended Dietary Allowances (RDAs) for Vitamin E of α-Tocopherol Equivalents (TE) for Children and Adults

Age	Males and Females (mg/day)	Pregnancy (mg/day)	Lactation (mg/day)
0-6 mo	4 mg (6 IU)*	N/A	N/A
7-12 mo	6 mg (7.5 IU)*	N/A	N/A
1-3 years	6 (9 IU)	N/A	N/A
4-8 years	7 (10.4 IU)	N/A	N/A
9-13 years	11 (16.4 IU)	N/A	N/A
14-18 years	15 (22.4 IU)	15 (22.4 IU)	19 (28.4 IU)
19+ years	15 (22.4 IU)	15 (22.4 IU)	19 (28.4 IU)

N/A, Not applicable.
*Adequate intake (AI)
Tolerable upper intake level (UL): 0-12 mos not determined; 1-3y 200 mg/d; 4-8y 300 mg/d; 9-13y 600 mg/d; 14-18y (also for pregnancy and lactation) 800 mg/d; 19-50 (also for pregnancy and lactation) 1000 mg/d.

Selected Food Sources of Vitamin E (α-Tocopherol)

Food	Milligrams (mg) per Serving	Percent DV*
Wheat germ oil, 1 tablespoon	20.3	100
Sunflower seeds, dry roasted, 1 ounce	7.4	37
Almonds, dry roasted, 1 ounce	6.8	34
Sunflower oil, 1 tablespoon	5.6	28
Safflower oil, 1 tablespoon	4.6	25
Hazelnuts, dry roasted, 1 ounce	4.3	22
Peanut butter, 2 tablespoons	2.9	15
Peanuts, dry roasted, 1 ounce	2.2	11
Corn oil, 1 tablespoon	1.9	10
Spinach, boiled, ½ cup	1.9	10
Broccoli, chopped, boiled, ½ cup	1.2	6
Soybean oil, 1 tablespoon	1.1	6
Kiwifruit, 1 medium	1.1	6
Mango, sliced, ½ cup	0.7	4
Tomato, raw, 1 medium	0.7	4
Spinach, raw, 1 cup	0.6	3

*DV = Daily value. DVs were developed by the Food and Drug Administration (FDA) to help consumers compare the nutrient content of different foods within the context of a total diet. The DV for vitamin E is 30 IU (approximately 20 mg of natural alpha-tocopherol) for adults and children age 4 and older. However, the FDA does not require food labels to list vitamin E content unless a food has been fortified with this nutrient. Foods providing 20% or more of the DV are considered to be high sources of a nutrient, but foods providing lower percentages of the DV also contribute to a healthful diet.

REFERENCES

Institute of Medicine: *Food and nutrition board: dietary reference intakes for Vitamin C, Vitamin E, Selenium, and Carotenoids,* Washington DC, 2000, National Academies Press.

Oregon State University: *Linus Pauling Institute Micronutrient Information Center: Vitamin E* (website). Updated May, 2015. Available at: https://lpi.oregonstate.edu/mic/vitamins/vitamin-E. Accessed December 30, 2019.

U.S. Department of Agriculture: *Food data central*, Released April 1, 2019. Available at: https://fdc.nal.usda.gov. Accessed December 30, 2019.

Nutritional Facts on Vitamin K

Vitamin K refers to a family of compounds with a common chemical structure. These compounds include phylloquinone (vitamin K_1) and a series of menaquinones known as vitamin K_2. They are further designated as MK-4 through MK-13 depending on the length of their individual side chains. Vitamin K is fat soluble and is naturally present in some foods, is produced by the bacteria naturally present in the gastrointestinal tract, and is available as a dietary supplement. Vitamin K_1, the main dietary form of vitamin K, is present mainly in green leafy vegetables. Menaquinones, primarily of bacterial origin, are found in some animal-based foods and in fermented foods. Natto, a Japanese fermented soy food, is an excellent source of vitamin K_2. Menaquinones are also produced by the naturally occurring bacteria in the gut. However, MK-4 is unique in that it is produced from phylloquinone by a conversion process that does not involve bacteria.

Vitamin K functions as a coenzyme for vitamin K-dependent carboxylase, an enzyme required for the synthesis of proteins involved in hemostasis (blood clotting) and bone metabolism, and other diverse physiologic functions. Prothrombin (clotting factor II) is a vitamin K–dependent protein in plasma that is directly involved in blood clotting.

Matrix Gla-protein is another vitamin K–dependent protein present in vascular smooth muscle, bone, and cartilage. Matrix Gla-protein is the focus of considerable scientific research because it might help reduce abnormal calcification. Osteocalcin is another vitamin K–dependent protein, and it is present in bone and may be involved in bone mineralization or turnover.

Antibiotics may interfere with this normal production. Circumstances that may lead to vitamin K deficiency include liver disease, serious burns, health problems that can prevent the absorption of vitamin K (such as gallbladder or biliary disease, which may alter the absorption of fat), cystic fibrosis, celiac disease, Crohn's disease, and chronic antibiotic therapy. Excess vitamin E can inhibit vitamin K activity and precipitate signs of deficiency. The classic sign of a vitamin K deficiency is a prolonged prothrombin time, which increases the risk of spontaneous hemorrhage. Because vitamin K is stored in the liver, clinical deficiencies are rare.

Vitamin K is needed to make clotting factors that help the blood to clot and prevent bleeding. The amount of vitamin K in food may affect drug therapy, such as that from warfarin or other anticoagulants. Warfarin (Coumadin) and some anticoagulants used primarily in Europe antagonize the activity of vitamin K and, in turn, prothrombin. For this reason, individuals who are taking these anticoagulants need to maintain consistent vitamin K intakes. When taking these medications, it is necessary to eat a normal, balanced diet, maintaining a consistent amount of vitamin K and avoiding large changes in vitamin K intake.

In general, leafy green vegetables and certain legumes and vegetable oils contain high amounts of vitamin K. Foods that contain a significant amount of vitamin K include beef liver, green tea, turnip greens, broccoli, kale, spinach, cabbage, asparagus, and dark-green lettuce. Chlorophyll, which is water soluble, is the substance in plants that gives them their green color and provides vitamin K; thus chlorophyll supplements need to be considered when assessing vitamin K intake. Foods that appear to contain low amounts of vitamin K include roots, bulbs, tubers, the fleshy portion of fruits, fruit juices and other beverages, and cereal grains and their milled products.

Dietary Reference Intakes: Adequate Intakes (AIs) for Vitamin K for Children and Adults			
Age (years)	Males and Females (mcg/day)	Pregnancy (mcg/day)	Lactation (mcg/day)
Birth-6 mo	2	N/A	N/A
7-12 mo	2.5	N/A	N/A
1-3	30	N/A	N/A
4-8	55	N/A	N/A
9-13	60	N/A	N/A
14-18	75	75	75
19+	120 for men; 90 for women	90	90

N/A, Not applicable.
Tolerable upper intake level not determined.

Selected Food Sources of Vitamin K (Phylloquinone, Except as Indicated)

Food	Micrograms (mcg) per Serving	Percent DV*	Food	Micrograms (mcg) per Serving	Percent DV*
Natto, 3 ounces (as MK-7)	850	1062	Grapes, ½ cup	11	14
Collards, frozen, boiled, ½ cup	530	662	Vegetable juice cocktail, ¾ cup	10	13
Turnip greens, frozen, boiled ½ cup	426	532	Canola oil, 1 tablespoon	10	13
Spinach, raw, 1 cup	145	181	Cashews, dry roasted, 1 ounce	10	13
Kale, raw, 1 cup	113	141	Carrots, raw, 1 medium	8	10
Broccoli, chopped, boiled, ½ cup	110	138	Olive oil, 1 tablespoon	8	10
Soybeans, roasted, ½ cup	43	54	Ground beef, broiled, 3 ounces (as MK-4)	6	8
Carrot juice, ¾ cup	28	34	Figs, dried, ¾ cup	6	8
Soybean oil, 1 tablespoon	25	31	Chicken liver, braised, 3 ounces (as MK-4)	6	8
Edamame, frozen, prepared, ½ cup	21	26	Ham, roasted or pan-broiled, 3 ounces (as MK-4)	4	5
Pumpkin, canned, ½ cup	20	25	Cheddar cheese, 1½ ounces (as MK-4)	4	5
Pomegranate juice, ¾ cup	19	24	Mixed nuts, dry roasted, 1 ounce	4	5
Okra, raw, ½ cup	16	20	Egg, hard boiled, 1 large (as MK-4)	4	5
Salad dressing, Caesar, 1 tablespoon	15	19	Mozzarella cheese, 1½ ounces (as MK-4)	2	3
Pine nuts, dried, 1 ounce	15	19	Milk, 2%, 1 cup (as MK-4)	1	1
Blueberries, raw, ½ cup	14	18	Salmon, sockeye, cooked, 3 ounces (as MK-4)	0.3	0
Iceberg lettuce, raw, 1 cup	14	18	Shrimp, cooked, 3 ounces (as MK-4)	0.3	0
Chicken, breast, rotisserie, 3 ounces (as MK-4)	13	17			

*DV = Daily value. DVs were developed by the Food and Drug Administration (FDA) to help consumers compare the nutrient contents of products within the context of a total diet. The DV for vitamin K is 80 mcg for adults and children age 4 and older. However, the FDA does not require food labels to list vitamin K content unless a food has been fortified with this nutrient. Foods providing 20% or more of the DV are considered to be high sources of a nutrient.

REFERENCES

Institute of Medicine: *Food and nutrition board: dietary reference intakes for Vitamin A, Vitamin K, Arsenic, Boron, Chromium, Copper, Iodine, Iron, Manganese, Molybdenum, Nickel, Silicon, Vanadium, and Zinc*, Washington DC, 2001, National Academies Press.

Oregon State University: *Linus Pauling Institute Micronutrient Information Center: Vitamin K* (website), Updated July, 2014. Available at: https://lpi.oregonstate.edu/mic/vitamins/vitamin-K. Accessed December 30, 2019.

U.S. Department of Agriculture: *Food data central*, Released April 1, 2019. Available at: https://fdc.nal.usda.gov. Accessed December 30, 2019.

Nutritional Facts on Vitamin D

Vitamin D is a fat-soluble vitamin that is naturally present in very few foods, is added to some foods, is available as a nutritional supplement, and is made when ultraviolet light, specifically UVB rays from the sun, strike the skin and stimulate its synthesis. Both the vitamin D that is absorbed from food and supplements, and the vitamin D that is made by the skin, is biologically inert. It must be hydroxylated twice in the body—first into 25(OH)D (calcidiol) by the liver, and again into 1,25(OH)D_2 (calcitriol) by the kidney.

Vitamin D is needed for the absorption of calcium from the small intestine and for the functioning of calcium in the body. Vitamin D also acts like a hormone and has many functions unrelated to its co-functions with calcium absorption and bone growth and remodeling. Besides being in bone, receptors for vitamin D have been identified in the gastrointestinal tract, brain, breast, nerve, and many other tissues. Vitamin D maintains adequate serum calcium and phosphate concentrations to prevent hypocalcemic tetany. It also modulates cell growth, neuromuscular and immune function, and reduction of inflammation. Many genes that encode for the regulation of cell proliferation, differentiation, and apoptosis are modulated by vitamin D. Recommended dietary allowances (RDAs) were established for vitamin D in 2011 and are presented in Table 1.

VITAMIN D SYNTHESIZED FROM SUNLIGHT EXPOSURE

Vitamin D made in the skin lasts twice as long in the blood as vitamin D ingested from the diet. The skin not only makes vitamin D upon exposure to UVB rays but also makes other photoproducts that cannot be obtained from food or supplements. It is unknown if any of these products have unique benefits to health, but research continues in this area.

UVB light cannot pass through glass; exposure of the skin to sunlight through glass will not result in vitamin D synthesis. Another deterrent to vitamin D synthesis by the skin is sunscreen. A sunscreen with an SPF 15 reduces skin synthesis of vitamin D by 95%, and an SPF 30 reduces it by 99%.

How much sun exposure is the correct amount to maintain optimal vitamin D levels in the body? A person sunbathing in a bathing suit will have received a dose of between 10,000 and 25,000 IU of vitamin D when he or she has sunbathed long enough to be slightly pink 24 hours later (technically called a minimal erythemal dose or "1 MED.") Exposing 25% of the body (arms and legs) for ¼ to ½ the time it takes to get slightly pink will allow the body to make 2000 to 4000 IU of vitamin D with each exposure.

The amount of time necessary for sunlight exposure to produce adequate vitamin D depends on the person's skin type (pale skin requires less time than dark skin with a lot of the burn-protecting pigment melanin), season of the year (the lower the sun on the horizon in the winter, the greater the time needed), the latitude (within + or − 35 degrees from the equator, the most vitamin D can be produced when skin is exposed to UVB rays), and the time of day (more vitamin D is synthesized by the skin when the sun is directly overhead between 11 AM and 3 PM). A person should be exposed to sunlight two to three times per week from March through October in northern climates to accumulate enough vitamin D to get through the winter with adequate vitamin D. See Holick (2010) for tables of time of sun exposure needed to make adequate amounts of vitamin D. Several apps are also available to determine this—Vitamin D Calculator, Vitamin D Pro, and D-Minder.

VITAMIN D IN FOODS

Vitamin D is measured in international units (IUs). 1 mcg = 40 IU of vitamin D or calciferol. IUs are used on food and supplement labels and both are used in the 2011 RDAs for vitamin D. The vitamin D in foods is measured as calciferol. There are only a few food sources of vitamin calciferol. Fish such as salmon, tuna, and mackerel and fish oils are one of the few natural sources of vitamin D. Beef liver, cheese, and egg yolks contain small amounts of vitamin D_3, a metabolite of vitamin D, which appears to be approximately five times more potent than the parent vitamin (calciferol) in raising serum 25(OH)D concentrations. At the present time, the USDA's Nutrient Database does not include this vitamin D metabolite when reporting the vitamin D content of foods. Actual vitamin D intakes in the U.S. population may be underestimated for this reason.

Mushrooms are the only plant food known to contain vitamin D, and the amount varies widely depending on the type of mushroom and amount of sunlight exposure during growth. Commercially raised

TABLE 1 Recommended Dietary Allowances (RDAs) for Vitamin D

Age	Male	Female	Pregnancy	Lactation
0-12 months*	400 IU (10 mcg)	400 IU (10 mcg)	N/A	N/A
1-13 years	600 IU (15 mcg)	600 IU (15 mcg)	N/A	N/A
14-18 years	600 IU (15 mcg)	600 IU (15 mcg)	600 IU (15 mcg)	600 IU (15 mcg)
19-50 years	600 IU (15 mcg)	600 IU (15 mcg)	600 IU (15 mcg)	600 IU (15 mcg)
51-70 years	600 IU (15 mcg)	600 IU (15 mcg)	N/A	N/A
70 years	800 IU (20 mcg)	800 IU (20 mcg)	N/A	N/A

N/A, Not applicable.

*Adequate intake (AI)

Tolerable upper intake level (UL): 0-6 mos 25 mcg/d; 7-12 mos 38 mcg/d; 1-3y 63 mcg/d; 4-8y 75 mcg/d; 9-13y 100 mcg/d; 14-18y (also for pregnancy and lactation) 100 mcg/d; 19-50 (also for pregnancy and lactation) 100 mcg/d.

TABLE 2 Selected Food Sources of Vitamin D

Food	IUs per Serving*	Percent DV**	Food	IUs per Serving*	Percent DV**
Cod liver oil, 1 tablespoon	1360	340	Milk, nonfat, reduced fat, and whole, vitamin D-fortified, 1 cup	115	29-31
Swordfish, cooked, 3 ounces	566	142	Yogurt, fortified, with 20% of the DV for vitamin D, 6 ounces (some yogurts are more heavily fortified—check label)	80	20
Salmon (sockeye), cooked, 3 ounces	447	112			
Mushrooms, maitake, raw, 3 ounces	943	235			
Mushrooms, portabella, exposed to UV light, raw, 3 ounces	375	94	Margarine, fortified, 1 tablespoon	60	15
Mushrooms, chanterelle, raw, 3 ounces	15	4	Sardines, canned in oil, drained, 2 sardines	46	12
Mushrooms, shiitake, raw, 3 ounces	178	45	Liver, beef, cooked, 3 ounces	42	11
Mushrooms, white, raw, 3 ounces	6	2	Egg, 1 large (vitamin D is found in yolk)	41	10
Tuna fish, canned in water, drained, 3 ounces	100	39	Ready-to-eat cereal, fortified with 10% of the DV for vitamin D, 0.75-1 cup (more heavily fortified cereals might provide more of the DV)	40	10
Orange juice fortified with vitamin D, 1 cup (check product labels, as amount of added vitamin D varies)	137	34			
			Cheese, Swiss, 1 ounce	6	2

DV, Daily value; *UV*, ultraviolet.
*IUs 5 international units.
**DV for vitamin D is 400 IU (10 mcg).

mushrooms are now being grown with controlled UVB exposure so that they synthesize and thus contain much more vitamin D than if grown in the wild. In fact, grown with lots of UVB exposure, four to five button or crimini mushrooms may contain as much as 400 IU of vitamin D.

Good sources of vitamin D are fortified foods and beverages such as milk; fortified soy, rice, and nut beverages; some yogurts and margarine; fortified breakfast cereals, fortified orange juice and other juices; and fortified products (check the labels on these foods). These fortified foods supply most of the calcium in the American diet. Cow's milk in the United States is voluntarily fortified to 100 IU/cup and in Canada is fortified by law to 35 to 40 IU/100 mL (84 to 96 IU/cup). Yogurt, cheese, cottage cheese, quark, and other milk products, unless made with vitamin D fortified milk (which is not required) or are fortified with vitamin D during production, are not good sources of vitamin D. See Table 2 for the vitamin D content of selected foods.

VITAMIN D IN SUPPLEMENTS

In supplements, as well as in fortified foods, vitamin D is available in two forms, D_2 (ergocalciferol) and D_3 (cholecalciferol). Vitamin D_2 is manufactured by the UV irradiation of ergosterol in yeast, and vitamin D_3 is manufactured by the irradiation of 7-dehydrocholesterol from lanolin and the chemical conversion of cholesterol. Both forms

effectively raise serum 25(OH)D levels. Firm conclusions about any different effects of these two forms of vitamin D cannot be drawn at this time. However, it appears that at nutritional doses vitamins D_2 and D_3 are equivalent, but at high doses vitamin D_2 appears to be less potent. https://ods.od.nih.gov/factsheets/VitaminD-HealthProfessional/. It also appears that frequent smaller dosing (daily) rather than much, much larger bolus dosing (weekly or monthly) of vitamin D may be more effective in improving 25(OH)D levels.

REFERENCES

Holick MF: *The Vitamin D Solution*, 2010, Penguin Group, pp 180–188.

Hollis BW, Wagner CL: Clinical review: the role of the parent compound vitamin D with respect to metabolism and function: why clinical dose intervals can affect clinical outcomes, *J Clin Endocrinol Metab* 98: 4619–4628, 2013. doi:10.1210/jc.2013-2653.

Institute of Medicine, Food and Nutrition Board: *Dietary Reference Intakes for Calcium and Vitamin D*, Washington, DC, 2010, National Academies Press.

Taylor CL, Patterson KY, Roseland JM, et al: Including food 25-hydroxyvitamin D in intake estimates may reduce the discrepancy between dietary and serum measures of vitamin D status, *J Nutr* 144:654–659, 2014.

U.S. Department of Agriculture, Agricultural Research Service: *USDA National Nutrient Database for Standard Reference*, Release 24, 2011, Nutrient Data Laboratory Home Page.

Nutritional Facts on Calcium

Calcium, the most abundant mineral in the body, is found in some foods, is added to others, is available as a dietary supplement, and is present in some medications such as antacids. Less than 1% of total body calcium supports critical metabolic functions required for vascular contraction and vasodilation, muscle function, nerve transmission, intracellular signaling, and hormonal secretion. The remaining 99% of the body's calcium supply is stored in the bones and teeth where it supports their structure and function.

Serum calcium is very tightly regulated and does not fluctuate with changes in dietary intakes; the body uses bone tissue as a reservoir for and source of calcium, in order to maintain constant concentrations of calcium in blood, muscle, and intercellular fluids. The website https://ods.od.nih.gov/factsheets/Calcium-HealthProfessional is an excellent resource for additional calcium nutrition information.

Recommended Dietary Allowances (RDAs) for Calcium

Age	Male	Female	Pregnancy	Lactating
0-6 months*	200 mg	200 mg		
7-12 months*	260 mg	260 mg		
1-3 years	700 mg	700 mg		
4-8 years	1000 mg	1000 mg		
9-13 years	1300 mg	1300 mg		
14-18 years	1300 mg	1300 mg	1300 mg	1300 mg
19-50 years	1000 mg	1000 mg	1000 mg	1000 mg
51-70 years	1000 mg	1200 mg		
71+ years	1200 mg	1200 mg		

*Adequate intake (AI)
Tolerable upper intake level (UL): 0-6 mos 1000 mg/d; 7-12 mos 1500 mg/d; 1-3y 2500 mg/d; 4-8y 2500 mg/d; 9-13y 3000 mg/d; 14-18y (also for pregnancy and lactation) 3000 mg/d; 19-50 (also for pregnancy and lactation) 2500 mg/d; 51+ 2000 mg/d.

CALCIUM IN FOODS

There are many dietary sources of calcium, but low-fat milk or yogurt or fortified substitutes are the most efficient and readily available. The lactose in mammalian milks appears to improve the absorption of calcium from milk. Lactose-free milk and soy, nut, rice, and other grain milks fortified with calcium and vitamin D are now available. They are usually fortified to 300 mg calcium per cup, equivalent to the amount of calcium in cow's or goat's milk, but the nutrition label should be checked.

In addition to milk, a variety of foods and calcium-fortified juices contain calcium and can help children, teens, and adults get sufficient levels of calcium in their diets. If it is difficult to get the recommended amounts of calcium from foods alone, a combination of food sources and supplements may be needed.

The absorption of calcium from the gut is increased when there is high body need such as during pregnancy and lactation, growth in infancy, childhood and adolescence, and when there is adequate vitamin D. Absorption is decreased by the presence of phytic acid and oxalic acid containing foods in the gut, alcohol, and caffeine.

Selected Food Sources of Calcium

Food	Milligrams per Serving
Dairy Foods	
Milk, with added calcium, 1 cup	420
Milk, whole, 2%, 1% skim, 1 cup	300
Yogurt, low fat, plain, ¾ cup	300
Cheese, processed slices, 2 slices	265
Yogurt, fruit on the bottom, ¾ cup	250
Processed cheese spread, 3 Tbsp	250
Cheese, hard, 1 oz	240
Milk, evaporated, ¼ cup	165
Cottage cheese, ¾ cup	120
Frozen yogurt, soft serve, ½ cup	100
Ice cream, ½ cup	85
Macaroni and cheese, prepared as per box instructions, ½ cup	80
Beans and Bean Products	
Soy cheese substitutes, 1 oz	0-200
Tofu, firm, made with calcium sulfate, 3½ oz	125
White beans, ½ cup	100
Navy beans, ½ cup	60
Black turtle beans, canned, ½ cup	42
Pinto beans, chickpeas, ½ cup	40
Nuts and Seeds	
Almonds, dry roasted, ¼ cup	95
Whole sesame seeds (black or white), 1 Tbsp	90
Tahini (sesame seed butter), 1 Tbsp	63
Brazil, hazelnuts, ¼ cup	55
Almond butter, 1 Tbsp	43
Meats, Fish, and Poultry	
Sardines, canned, 3½ oz (8 med)	370
Salmon, canned with bones, 3 oz	180
Oysters, canned, ½ cup	60
Shrimp, canned, ½ cup	40
Turnip greens, boiled, ½ cup	99
Okra, frozen, ½ cup	75
Chinese cabbage or bok choy, ½ cup	75

Food	Milligrams per Serving
Kale, raw, chopped, ½ cup	50
Mustard greens, boiled, ½ cup	76
Chinese broccoli (gai lan), ½ cup	44
Broccoli, raw, ½ cup	21
Fruit	
Orange, 1 med	55
Dried figs, 2 med	54
Nondairy Drinks	
Calcium enriched orange juice, 1 cup	300
Fortified rice milk, 1 cup	300
Fortified almond milk, 1 cup	300
Fortified soy milk, 1 cup	300
Regular soy milk, 1 cup	20
Grains	
Amaranth, raw, ½ cup	150
Whole wheat flour, 1 cup	40
Pizza, cheese, 1 small slice (l oz)	120
Macaroni and cheese, boxed mix, prepared as per label, 1 cup	80
Other	
Blackstrap molasses, 1 Tbsp	80
Regular molasses, 1 Tbsp	41
Asian Foods	
Sea cucumber, fresh, 3 oz	285
Shrimp, small, dried, 1 oz	167
Dried fish, smelt, 2 Tbsp	140
Seaweed, dry (hijiki), 10 g	140
Seaweed, dry (agar), 10 g	76
Boiled bone soup, ½ cup	Negligible
Laver, nori, and wakame seaweeds are low in calcium.	
Native Foods	
Oolichan, salted, cooked, 3 oz	210
Fish head soup, 1 cup	150
Native American ice cream (whipped soapberries), ½ cup	130

CALCIUM SUPPLEMENTS

Calcium carbonate is the most common and least expensive calcium supplement. It can be difficult to digest and causes gas and constipation in some people. Calcium carbonate is 40% elemental calcium; 1000 mg will provide 400 mg of calcium. This supplement should be taken with food to aid in absorption. Taking magnesium with it can help prevent constipation.

Calcium citrate is more easily absorbed, easier to digest, and less likely to cause constipation and gas than calcium carbonate. It is a better choice for those with malabsorption diseases and in the elderly. However, it is less concentrated, providing approximately 21% elemental calcium; 1000 mg will provide 210 mg of calcium. It is more expensive than calcium carbonate, and more of it must be taken to get the same amount of calcium, but it is better absorbed. It can be taken with or without food.

Calcium phosphate costs more than calcium carbonate but less than calcium citrate. It is easily absorbed and is less likely to cause constipation and gas.

Calcium lactate and calcium aspartate are both more easily digested but more expensive than calcium carbonate.

As the dose of calcium supplement increases, the percentage absorbed decreases. Because it appears that absorption is highest with dosages of <500 mg at a time, it is best to take calcium supplements in at least two dosages per day.

CALCIUM IN MEDICATIONS

Many over-the-counter antacids such as Tums and Rolaids contain calcium carbonate because of calcium carbonate's ability to neutralize stomach acid. Depending on the product, each chewable pill or soft chew contains 200 to 300 mg of elemental calcium, which can be a significant source of calcium supplementation for the person with normal levels of stomach acid.

REFERENCES

Institute of Medicine: *Food and nutrition board: dietary reference intakes for Calcium and Vitamin D,* Washington DC, 2011, National Academies Press.

Oregon State University: *Calcium,* Linus Pauling Institute, Available at: https://lpi.oregonstate.edu/mic/minerals/calcium. Updated May 2017. Accessed February 1, 2019.

U.S. Department of Agriculture: *Food data central,* Released April 1, 2019. Available at: https://fdc.nal.usda.gov. Accessed December 30, 2019.

Nutritional Facts on Chromium

Chromium is known to enhance the action of insulin; chromium was identified as the active ingredient in the "glucose tolerance factor" many years ago. Chromium also appears to be directly involved in carbohydrate, fat, and protein metabolism, but more research is needed to determine the full range of its roles in the body.

Chromium is widely distributed in the food supply, but most foods provide only small amounts (less than 2 mcg per serving). Meat and whole-grain products, as well as some fruits, vegetables, and spices, are relatively good sources, but Brewer's yeast is by far the most concentrated food source. Foods high in simple sugars (such as sucrose and fructose) are low in chromium. Dietary intakes of chromium cannot be reliably determined because the content of the mineral in foods is substantially affected by agricultural and manufacturing processes and food-composition databases are inadequate. Chromium values in foods are approximate and should only serve as a guide. It appears that chromium picolinate and chromium nicotinate used in supplements are more bioavailable than chromic chloride.

Dietary reference intakes for chromium are adequate intakes (AIs). See table below.

Dietary Reference Intakes (AIs) for Chromium for Children and Adults

Age (years)	Males and Females (mcg/day)	Pregnancy (mcg/day)	Lactation (mcg/day)
0-6 months	0.2		
7-12 months	5.5		
1-3	11	N/A	N/A
4-8	15	N/A	N/A
9-13	25 for boys 21 for girls	N/A	N/A
14-18	35 for men 24 for women	29	44
19+	35 for men 25 for women	30	45
50+	30 for men 29 for women	N/A	N/A

N/A, Not applicable.
Tolerable upper intake level not determined.

Selected Food Sources of Chromium

Food	Micrograms per Serving
Broccoli, ½ cup	11
Grape juice, 1 cup	8
English muffin, whole wheat, 1	4
Potatoes, mashed, 1 cup	3
Garlic, dried, 1 tsp	3
Basil, dried, 1 Tbsp	2
Beef cubes, 3 oz	2
Orange juice, 1 cup	2
Turkey breast, 3 oz	2
Whole wheat bread, 2 slices	2
Red wine, 5 oz	1-13
Apple, unpeeled, 1 med	1
Banana, 1 med	1
Green beans, ½ cup	1

DV = Daily value. DVs were developed by the Food and Drug Administration (FDA) to help consumers compare the nutrient contents of products within the context of a total diet. The DV for chromium is 120 mcg. The percentage DV listed on the label indicates the percentage of the DV provided in one serving. A food providing 5% of the DV or less is a source, whereas a food that provides 10% to 19% of the DV is a good source. A food that provides 20% or more of the DV is high in that nutrient.

REFERENCES

Institute of Medicine: *Food and nutrition board: dietary reference intakes for Vitamin A, Vitamin K, Arsenic, Boron, Chromium, Copper, Iodine, Iron, Manganese, Molybdenum, Nickel, Silicon, Vanadium, and Zinc,* Washington DC, 2001, National Academies Press.

U.S. Department of Agriculture: *Food Data Central,* Released April 1, 2019. Available at: https://fdc.nal.usda.gov. Accessed December 30, 2019.

Nutritional Facts on Iodine

Iodine is an important mineral that is naturally found in some foods and added to others (primarily iodized salt). It is most concentrated in foods from the ocean. More than 70 countries, including the United States and Canada, have salt iodization programs.

Iodine is an essential component of thyroid hormones, thyroxine (T_4) and triiodothyronine (T_3), which help regulate metabolic rate, body temperature, growth, reproduction, blood cell production, muscle function, nerve function, and even gene expression. Iodine appears to have physiologic functions including a role in the immune response and possibly a beneficial effect on mammary dysplasia and fibrocystic breast disease.

The most useful clinical tool for measuring thyroid function and thus iodine sufficiency is to measure thyroid-stimulating hormone (TSH), which is released from the pituitary gland and stimulates thyroid hormone production and release. If the TSH is high, thyroid function should be evaluated further. Selenium-dependent enzymes are also required for the conversion of thyroxine (T_4) to the biologically active thyroid hormone, triiodothyronine (T_3); thus deficiencies of selenium, vitamin A, or iron may also affect iodine status. Another method to assess iodine status is the urinary iodine excretion test.

DEFICIENCY

Iodine deficiency is an important health problem throughout much of the world. Most of the earth's iodine is found in its oceans and soils; thus parts of the world away from the oceans exposed for millions of years longer have iodine-deficient soils, and the foods grown in these soils have low iodine content. Thus large percentages of people eating foods from those iodine-deficient soils, and not able to consume fish, can become iodine deficient unless public health measures are taken. Iodine deficiency can cause developmental and cognitive delay, hypothyroidism, goiter, and varying degrees of other growth and developmental abnormalities. Iodine is now recognized as the most common cause of preventable brain damage in the world, with millions living in iodine-deficient areas.

The major source of dietary iodine in the United States is iodized salt, which has been fortified with iodine. In the United States, assume that any salt in processed foods is iodized unless the product label shows that it is not iodized. In the United States and Canada, iodized salt contains 77 mcg of iodine per gram of salt. Iodine is also added in the diet because it is used in the feed of animals and in many processed or preserved foods as a stabilizer and as a component of red food dyes.

Diets that exclude iodized salt, fish, and seaweed have been found to contain very little iodine. Urinary iodine excretion studies suggest that iodine intakes are declining in the United States, possibly as a result of increased adherence to dietary recommendations to reduce salt intake.

GOITROGENS

Substances that interfere with iodine use or thyroid hormone production are known as goitrogens and occur in some foods. Some species of millet and cruciferous vegetables (e.g., cabbage, broccoli, cauliflower, and Brussels sprouts) contain goitrogens, and the soybean isoflavones genistein and daidzein have also been found to inhibit thyroid hormone synthesis. Most of these goitrogens are not of clinical importance unless they are consumed raw and in large amounts or there is a coexisting iodine or selenium deficiency. Cooking food will decrease the goitrogenic effect.

Recommended Dietary Allowances (RDAs) for Iodine				
Age	Male mcg/day	Female mcg/day	Pregnancy mcg/day	Lactation mcg/day
0-6 months	110*	110*	N/A	N/A
7-12 months	130*	130*	N/A	N/A
1-3 years	90	90	N/A	N/A
4-8 years	90	90	N/A	N/A
9-13 years	120	120	N/A	N/A
14-18 years	150	150	220	290
19+	150	150	220	290

N/A, Not applicable.
*Adequate intake (AI).
Tolerable upper intake level (UL): 0-12 mos not determined; 1-3y 200 mcg/d; 4-8y 300 mcg/d; 9-13y 600 mcg/d; 14-18y (also for pregnancy and lactation) 900 mcg/d; 19+ (also for pregnancy and lactation) 1,100 mcg/d.

The World Health Organization, United Nations Children's Fund, and the International Council for the Control of Iodine Deficiency Disorders recommend a slightly higher iodine intake for pregnant women of 250 mcg per day.

The iodine contents of some common foods containing iodine are given in the table below. As already mentioned, the iodine content of fruits and vegetables depends on the soil in which they were grown; the iodine content of animal foods, outside of those from the ocean, depends on where they were raised and which plants they consumed. Therefore these values are average approximations.

Selected Food Sources of Iodine

Food	Serving	Micrograms (mcg) per Serving	% Daily Value*
Salt (iodized)	1 g	47.5	31.3%
Cod	3 oz	99	66
Shrimp	3 oz	35	23
Fish sticks	2 fish sticks (2 oz)	54	36
Tuna, canned in oil	3 oz (½ can)	17	11
Milk (cow's), reduced fat	1 cup (8 fluid oz)	56	37
Egg, boiled	1 large	24	16
Navy beans, cooked	½ cup	35	23
Potato with peel, baked	1 medium	63	42
Seaweed	1 g, dried	Variable; 16 to 2984; may be greater than 18,000 mcg (18 mg)	11 to 1989

*DVs were developed by the Food and Drug Administration (FDA) to help consumers to compare the nutrient content of products. The DV for iodine is 150 mcg for adults and children 4 years and older. Foods containing 20% or more of the DV are considered to be excellent sources. However, the FDA does not require food labels to list iodine content unless the food has been fortified with iodine.

REFERENCES

Institute of Medicine: *Food and nutrition board: dietary reference intakes for Vitamin A, Vitamin K, Arsenic, Boron, Chromium, Copper, Iodine, Iron, Manganese, Molybdenum, Nickel, Silicon, Vanadium, and Zinc,* Washington DC, 2001, National Academies Press.

U.S. Department of Agriculture: *Food data central,* Released April 1, 2019. Available at: https://fdc.nal.usda.gov. Accessed December 30, 2019.

Nutritional Facts on Iron

Iron is a nutrient found in trace amounts in every cell of the body. Iron is part of hemoglobin in red blood cells and myoglobin in muscles. The role of both of these molecules is to carry oxygen. Iron also makes up part of many proteins and enzymes in the body. Iron deficiency anemia is common in children, adolescent girls, and women of childbearing age. It is usually treated with an iron-rich diet as well as iron supplements. Iron exists in foods in two forms: heme iron and nonheme iron. Vitamin C–containing foods (see Appendix 35) enhance the absorption of nonheme iron and should be consumed at the same time as an iron-rich food or meal. The presence of heme iron in the meal also enhances the absorption of nonheme iron. Substances that decrease the absorption of nonheme iron are as follows:

Oxalic acid, found in raw spinach and chocolate

Phytic acid, found in wheat bran and beans (legumes)

Tannins, found in commercial black or pekoe teas

Polyphenols, found in coffee

Calcium carbonate supplements

Heme iron found in animal foods is absorbed more efficiently than nonheme iron. The richest dietary sources of heme iron are oysters, liver, lean red meat (especially beef), poultry (the dark red meat), tuna, and salmon. Less rich sources are lamb, pork, shellfish, and eggs (especially the yolks).

Nonheme iron is harder for the body to absorb. Sources of nonheme iron are iron-fortified cereals, dried beans, whole grains (wheat, millet, oats, brown rice), legumes (lima beans, soybeans, dried beans and peas, kidney beans), nuts (almonds, Brazil nuts), dried fruits (especially prunes, raisins, apricots), vegetables, and greens (broccoli, spinach, kale, collards, asparagus, dandelion greens). See Table: Selected Food Sources of Iron.

Breastmilk contains a highly bioavailable form of iron that is well absorbed by infants, but the amount is not enough to meet the needs of the infant older than 4 to 6 months, so a food source of iron (usually as infant cereal) should be offered to the older infant.

Recommended Dietary Allowances for Iron for Children and Adults

Age	Male	Female	Pregnancy	Lactation
0-6 months	0.27 mg*	0.27 mg*		
7-12 months	11 mg	11 mg		
1-3 years	7 mg	7 mg		
4-8 years	10 mg	10 mg		
9-13 years	8 mg	8 mg		
14-18 years	11 mg	15 mg	27 mg	10 mg
19-50 years	8 mg	18 mg	27 mg	9 mg
51+ years	8 mg	8 mg		

*Adequate intake (AI)

Tolerable upper intake level (UL): 0-12 mos 40 mg; 1-3y 40 mg/d; 4-8y 119 mg/d; 9-13y 40 mg/d; 14-18y (also for pregnancy and lactation) 45 mg/d; 19+ (also for pregnancy and lactation) 45 mg/d.

Selected Food Sources of Iron

Food	Milligrams Per Serving	% Daily Value*
Clams, canned, drained, 3 oz	2.28	12.67
Fortified ready-to-eat cereals (various), ≈1 oz	1.8-19.2	10-107
Oysters, eastern, wild, cooked, moist heat, 3 oz	8	44
Organ meats (liver, giblets), various, cooked, 3 oz†	5.2-9.9 1.77-33.46	29-55 9.83-185.9
Fortified instant cooked cereals (various), 1 packet	3.40-10.55	18.9-58.6
Soybeans, mature, cooked, ½ cup	4.4	24
White beans, canned, ½ cup	3.9	22
Molasses, 1 Tbsp	3.5	19
Lentils, cooked, ½ cup	3.3	18
Spinach, cooked from fresh, ½ cup	3.2	18
Beef, chuck, blade roast, lean, cooked, 3 oz	3.1	17
Beef, bottom round, lean, 0 in fat, all grades, cooked, 3 oz	2.8	15.5
Kidney beans, cooked, ½ cup	2.6	14
Sardines, canned in oil, drained, 3 oz	2.5	14
Beef, rib, lean, ¼ in. fat, all grades, 3 oz	2.4	13
Chickpeas, cooked, ½ cup	2.4	13
Pumpkin and squash seed kernels, roasted, 1 oz	2.3	12.7
Duck, meat only, roasted, 3 oz	2.3	13
Lamb, shoulder, arm, lean, ¼ in fat, choice, cooked, 3 oz	2.3	13
Prune juice, ¾ cup	2.3	13
Shrimp, canned, 3 oz	1.8	10
Cowpeas, cooked, ½ cup	2.2	12
Ground beef, 15% fat, cooked, 3 oz	2.2	12
Tomato puree, ½ cup	2.2	12
Lima beans, cooked, ½ cup	2.2	12
Soybeans, green, cooked, ½ cup	2.3	13
Navy beans, cooked, ½ cup	2.2	12
Refried beans, ½ cup	2.1	11.5
Beef, top sirloin, lean, 0 in fat, all grades, cooked, 3 oz	2.0	11
Tomato paste, ¼ cup	2.0	11

DV = Daily value.

*DVs were developed by the Food and Drug Administration to help consumers compare the nutrient content of products. The % DV listed on the Nutrition Facts panel of food labels states the percentage of the DV provided in one serving. The DV for iron is 18 mg. Foods containing 20% or more of the DV are considered to be excellent sources of the nutrient.

†High in cholesterol.

TIPS FOR INCREASING IRON INTAKE

The amount of iron the body absorbs varies depending on several factors. For example, the body will absorb more iron from foods when iron stores are low and will absorb less when stores are sufficient. In addition, use these tips to enhance absorption:

- Include heme and nonheme iron at the same meal
- Include a vitamin C rich food in a meal
- Drink coffee or tea between meals rather than with a meal
- Cook acidic foods in cast iron pots, which can increase the iron content of food up to 30 times.

WHAT ABOUT TOO MUCH IRON?

It is unlikely that a healthy person would take iron at toxic (too high) levels. However, children can sometimes develop iron toxicity by eating iron supplements, mistaking them for candy. Symptoms include the following: fatigue, anorexia, dizziness, nausea, vomiting, headache, weight loss, shortness of breath, and grayish color to the skin.

Hemochromatosis is a genetic disorder that affects the regulation of iron absorption. Treatment consists of a low-iron diet, no iron supplements, and phlebotomy (blood removal) on a regular basis.

Excess storage of iron in the body is known as hemosiderosis. The high iron stores come from eating excessive iron supplements or from receiving frequent blood transfusions, not from increased iron intake in the diet.

To reduce the iron from dietary sources, review the list of foods and exclude or severely limit their intake until the iron overload is alleviated. Pay particular attention to sports drinks, energy bars, fortified cereals, and multivitamin mineral supplements that have significant amounts of added iron.

REFERENCES

Institute of Medicine: *Food and nutrition board: dietary reference intakes for Vitamin A, Vitamin K, Arsenic, Boron, Chromium, Copper, Iodine, Iron, Manganese, Molybdenum, Nickel, Silicon, Vanadium, and Zinc,* Washington DC, 2001, National Academies Press.

U.S. Department of Agriculture: *Food data Central,* Released April 1, 2019. Available at: https://fdc.nal.usda.gov. Accessed December 30, 2019.

43 | APPENDIX

Nutritional Facts on Magnesium

The mineral magnesium is important for every organ in the body, particularly the heart, muscles, and kidneys. It also contributes to the composition of teeth and bones. Most important, it is a cofactor in hundreds of enzyme systems, contributing to energy production and deoxyribonucleic acid (DNA) synthesis, and it helps regulate calcium levels, as well as copper, zinc, potassium, vitamin D, and other important nutrients in the body.

DIETARY SOURCES

Rich sources of magnesium include tofu, legumes, whole grains, green leafy vegetables, wheat bran, Brazil nuts, soybean flour, almonds, cashews, blackstrap molasses, pumpkin and squash seeds, pine nuts, and black walnuts. Other good dietary sources of this mineral include peanuts, whole-wheat flour, oat flour, beet greens, spinach, pistachio nuts, shredded wheat, bran cereals, oatmeal, bananas, baked potatoes (with skin), chocolate, and cocoa powder. Many herbs, spices, and seaweeds supply magnesium, such as agar seaweed, coriander, dill weed, celery seed, sage, dried mustard, basil, cocoa powder, fennel seed, savory, cumin seed, tarragon, marjoram, and poppy seed. See Table: Selected Food Sources of Magnesium.

Recommended Dietary Allowance (RDA) for Magnesium for Children and Adults

Age	Males and Females (mg/day)	Females (mg/day)	Pregnancy (mg/day)	Lactation (mg/day)
0-6 months	30	30	N/A	N/A
7-12 months	75	75	N/A	N/A
1-3	80	80	N/A	N/A
4-8	130	130	N/A	N/A
9-13 years	240	240	N/A	N/A
14-18 years	410	360	400	360
19-30 years	400	310	350	310
31-50 years	420	320	360	320
51+ years	420	320	N/A	N/A

N/A, Not applicable.
Tolerable upper intake level (UL): 0-12 mos not determined; 1-3y 65 mg/d; 4-8y 119 mg/d; 9-13y 350 mg/d; 14-18y (also for pregnancy and lactation) 350 mg/d; 19+ (also for pregnancy and lactation) 350 mg/d.

Selected Food Sources of Magnesium

Food	Milligram per Serving	% Daily Value*	Food	Milligram per Serving	% Daily Value*
Pumpkin and squash seed kernels, roasted, 1 oz	156	39	Navy beans, cooked, ½ cup	48	12
Brazil nuts, 1 oz	107	27	Tofu, firm, prepared with nigari,† ½ cup	47	11.7
Bran ready-to-eat cereal (100%), ≈1 oz	103	25.5	Soy milk, not fortified 1 cup	61	15.2
Quinoa, dry, ¼ cup	84	21	Cowpeas, cooked, ½ cup	46	11.5
Mackerel, baked, 3 oz	82	20.5	Hazelnuts, 1 oz	46	11.5
Spinach, canned, ½ cup	81	20	Oat bran muffin, 1 oz	45	11.3
Almonds, 1 oz	78	19.5	Great northern beans, cooked, ½ cup	44	11
Spinach, cooked from fresh, ½ cup	78	19.5	Oat bran, cooked, ½ cup	44	11
Buckwheat flour, ¼ cup	75	19	Buckwheat groats, roasted, cooked, ½ cup	43	10.7
Cashews, dry roasted, 1 oz	74	18.5	Brown rice, cooked, ½ cup	42	10.5
Soybeans, mature, cooked, ½ cup	74	18.5	Okra, cooked from frozen, ½ cup	37	9.2
Pine nuts, dried, 1 oz	71	17.5	Tuna, yellowfin, cooked, 3 oz	36	9
Pollock, walleye, cooked, 3 oz	69	17	Cod, baked, 3 oz	36	9
White beans, canned, ½ cup	67	17	Artichokes (hearts), cooked, ½ cup	35	9
Mixed nuts, oil roasted, with peanuts, 1 oz	65	16.5	Turkey, roasted, white meat, 3 oz	27	6.8
Black beans, cooked, ½ cup	60	15	Halibut, cooked, 3 oz	24	6
Bulgur, dry, ¼ cup	57	14	Veal, cutlet, cooked, 3 oz	24	6
Oat bran, raw, ¼ cup	55	13.5	Haddock, cooked, 3 oz	22.1	5.5
Soybeans, green, cooked, ½ cup	54	13.7	Chicken, cooked, 3 oz	22	6
Lima beans, baby, cooked from frozen, ½ cup	50	12.5	T-bone steak, broiled, lean only, 3 oz	22	5.7
Peanuts, dry roasted, 1 oz	50	12.5	Beef, ground, cooked, extra lean, 17% fat, 3 oz	17	4
Beet greens, cooked, ½ cup	49	12			

DV = Daily value.
*DVs were developed by the Food and Drug Administration to help consumers compare the nutrient content of products. The %DV listed on the Nutrition Facts panel of food labels states the percentage of the DV provided in one serving. The DV for magnesium is 400 mg. Foods containing 20% or more of the DV are considered to be excellent sources of the nutrient.
†Calcium sulfate and magnesium chloride.

REFERENCES

Institute of Medicine: *Food and nutrition board: dietary reference intakes for Calcium, Phosphorus, Vitamin D and Fluoride*, Washington DC, 1997, National Academies Press.

U.S. Department of Agriculture: *Food data central*, Released April 1, 2019. Available at: https://fdc.nal.usda.gov. Accessed December 30, 2019.

Nutritional Facts on Potassium

A potassium-rich diet is useful for cardiac patients who are trying to lower their blood pressure using diet. If diuretics are also used, it is important to know if potassium is retained or depleted by the diuretic, and it should be monitored. Most patients with chronic kidney disease or on renal dialysis may need to restrict potassium in their diets. Because potassium is lost in sweat, athletes need to pay attention to the potassium in their diets.

There is no recommended dietary allowance (RDA) for potassium. Dietary reference intake (DRI) is a general term for a set of reference values used to plan and assess nutrient intakes of healthy people. The DRIs for potassium are stated as adequate intakes (AIs). For breastfed infants, the AI is the mean intake; for older individuals, the AI is believed to cover the needs of all individuals in the group, but there is a lack data to be more specific. AIs are given in the following table.

Dietary Reference Intakes: Adequate Intakes (AIs) for Potassium for Children and Adults

Age	Males and Females (mg/day)	Pregnancy (g/day)	Lactation (g/day)
0-6 months	400	N/A	N/A
7-12 months	860	N/A	N/A
1-3 years	2000	N/A	N/A
4-8 years	2300	N/A	N/A
9-13 years	3000	N/A	N/A
14-18 years	3400	2600	2500
19+ years	3400	2900	2800

N/A, Not applicable.
There is no tolerable upper intake level for healthy people.

Selected Food Sources of Potassium

Food	Milligrams (mg) per Serving	% Daily Value*
Sweet potato, baked, 1 potato (146 g)	694	19.8
Tomato paste, ¼ cup	669	19
Beet greens, cooked, ½ cup	655	18.7
Potato, baked, flesh, 1 potato (156 g)	610	17.4
White beans, canned, ½ cup	595	17
Yogurt, plain, nonfat, 8-oz container	579	16.5
Tomato puree, ½ cup	549	15.7
Clams, canned, 3 oz	534	15.3
Yogurt, plain, low-fat, 8-oz container	531	15.2
Prune or carrot juice, ¾ cup	530	15.1
Soy or lima beans, green, cooked, ½ cup	485	13.9
Halibut or yellowfin tuna, cooked, 3 oz	449	12.8
Winter squash, cooked, ½ cup	448	9.5
Bananas, 1 med	422	12.1
Spinach, cooked, ½ cup	419	12
Peaches, dried, uncooked, ¼ cup	398	11.4
Prunes, stewed, ½ cup	398	11.4
Rockfish, Pacific, cooked, 3 oz	397	11.3

Food	Milligrams (mg) per Serving	% Daily Value*
Tomato juice, ¾ cup	395	11.3
Milk, nonfat, 1 cup	382	10.9
Pork chop, center loin, cooked, 3 oz	382	10.9
Rainbow trout, farmed, cooked, 3 oz	382	10.9
Apricots, dried, uncooked, ¼ cup	378	10.8
Orange juice, ¾ cup	372	10.6
Buttermilk, cultured, low-fat, 1 cup	370	10.5
Cantaloupe, ¼ med	368	10.5
1%-2% milk, 1 cup	366	10.4
Honeydew melon, $\frac{1}{8}$ med	365	10.4
Lentils, cooked, ½ cup	365	10.4
Tomato sauce, ½ cup	364	10.4
Pork loin, rib (roasts), lean, roasted, 3 oz	358	10.2
Plantains, cooked, ½ cup slices	358	10.2
Kidney beans or split peas, cooked, ½ cup	358	10.2
Yogurt, plain, whole milk, 8-oz container	352	10.0
Cod, Pacific, cooked, 3 oz	246	7.0

*Daily values (DVs) are reference numbers based on the recommended dietary allowance. They were developed to help consumers determine whether a food contains a lot or a little of a specific nutrient. The DV for potassium is 3500 mg. The %DV listed on the Nutrition Facts panel of food labels states the percentage of the DV provided in one serving. Percent DVs are based on a 2000-calorie diet.

REFERENCES

National Academies of Medicine: *Food and nutrition board: dietary reference intakes for sodium and potassium,* Washington DC, 2019, National Academies Press.

U.S. Department of Agriculture: *Food data central,* Released April 1, 2019. Available at: https://fdc.nal.usda.gov. Accessed December 30, 2019.

Nutritional Facts on Selenium

Selenium is incorporated into proteins to make selenoproteins, which are important antioxidant enzymes. The antioxidant properties of selenoproteins prevent cellular damage from free radicals. Other selenoproteins help regulate thyroid function and play a role in the immune system. Selenium, as a nutrient that functions as an antioxidant, may be protective against some types of cancer and heart disease.

Plant foods are the major dietary sources of selenium. The content of selenium in food depends on the selenium content of the soil where plants are grown or animals are raised. Soil in Nebraska and the Dakotas has very high levels of selenium. The southeast coastal areas in the United States have very low levels; selenium deficiency is often reported in these regions. Selenium is also found in some meats and seafood. Animals that eat grains or plants that were grown in selenium-rich soil have higher levels of selenium in their muscle. In the United States, meats, bread, and Brazil nuts are common sources of dietary selenium. Most food labels do not list the selenium content of a food; however, if they do, it is listed as a % Daily value (DV).

Dietary Reference Intakes for Selenium for Children and Adults

Age (years)	Males and Females (mcg/day)	Pregnancy (mcg/day)	Lactation (mcg/day)
1-3	20	N/A	N/A
4-8	30	N/A	N/A
9-13	40	N/A	N/A
14-18	55	60	70
19+	55	60	70

N/A, Not applicable.
Tolerable upper intake level (UL): 0-6 mos 45 mcg; 7-12 mos 60 mcg; 1-3y 90 mcg/d; 4-8y 150 mcg/d; 9-13y 280 mcg/d; 14-18y (also for pregnancy and lactation) 400 mcg/d; 19+ (also for pregnancy and lactation) 400 mcg/d.

Selected Food Sources of Selenium

Food	Micrograms per Serving	% DV*	Food	Micrograms per Serving	% DV*
Brazil nuts, dried, unblanched, 1 oz	544	777	Macaroni, elbow, enriched, boiled, 1 cup	37	53
Tuna, yellowfin, cooked, dry heat, 3 oz	92	131	Egg, whole, 1 med	15	21
Ground beef, 25% fat, cooked, oz	18	26	Cottage cheese, 1% fat, 1 cup	20	29
Spaghetti sauce, marinara, 1 cup	4	6	Oatmeal, instant, fortified, cooked, 1 cup	13	19
Corn Flakes, 1 cup	2	3	Milk, 1 %, 1 cup	8	11
Turkey, light meat, roasted, 3 oz	31	44	Lentils, boiled, 1 cup	6	9
Spinach, frozen, boiled, 1 cup	11	16	Bread, whole wheat, 1 slice	13	19
Chicken breast, meat only, roasted, 3 oz	22	31	Rice, brown, long grain, cooked, 1 cup	19	27
Noodles, enriched, boiled, ½ cup	19	27	Cashew nuts, dry roasted, 1 oz	3	4

DV = Daily value.
*DVs were developed by the Food and Drug Administration to help consumers compare the nutrient content of products.
The % DV listed on the Nutrition Facts panel of food labels states the percentage of the DV provided in one serving. The DV for selenium for adults and children aged 4 and over is 70 mcg. Foods containing 20% or more of the DV are considered to be excellent sources of the nutrient.

REFERENCES

Institute of Medicine: *Food and nutrition board: dietary reference intakes for Vitamin C, Vitamin E, Selenium, and Carotenoids,* Washington DC, 2000, National Academies Press.
U.S. Department of Agriculture: *Food data central,* Released April 1, 2019. Available at: https://fdc.nal.usda.gov. Accessed December 30, 2019.

46 APPENDIX

Sodium in Food

The National Academies of Sciences updated the AI's for sodium in March, 2019 and are as follows: 110 mg for infants 6-12 mos; 800 mg for children 1-3; 1000 mg for ages 4-8; 1200 mg for 9-13; and 1500 mg for 14 and older. Both the National Academies and the 2015–2020 U.S. Dietary Guidelines specify an upper limit of 2300 mg/day of sodium for adults. This is approximately a teaspoon of table salt. In the past this level of sodium was considered to be a restriction. Currently, the average American eats almost double the recommended daily amount of sodium, so sodium restrictions continue to be commonly prescribed for patients with heart disease, kidney disease, and liver disease.

The sodium in food is added in processing. Virtually no food is naturally high in sodium (see selected food list below). Food manufacturers have been responding to the call from health professionals and consumers to lower the amount of sodium in processed foods, but processed foods remain the main source of sodium in the U.S. diet.

SPECIAL CONSIDERATIONS

A therapeutic sodium-restricted meal plan should be prescribed in terms of milligrams of sodium desired on a daily basis. The following are the commonly used levels of sodium restrictions:

No added salt (NAS): This is the least restrictive of the sodium-restricted diets. Table salt should not be used, and salt should not be added in cooking. High-sodium foods such as smoked, cured, or dried meats and cheeses; condiments and seasonings; salted snacks; and canned and dried soups and bouillon are restricted. The NAS diet provides no more than 3000 mg of sodium daily. It is desirable to be closer to the 2300 mg of sodium when possible.

2000 mg sodium: This diet may be appropriate for people with some types of liver disease and renal disease. It is no longer recommended for patients with heart failure. This diet *eliminates* processed and prepared foods and beverages that are high in sodium. In addition to limiting all the foods in the NAS diet, baked products must also be limited. Milk and milk products are limited to 16 oz daily. Only salt-free commercially prepared foods should be used.

GUIDELINES FOR SODIUM RESTRICTION

Salt substitutes containing potassium chloride should be recommended only if approved by a physician. Potassium is generally contraindicated for patients with renal disease and for people on potassium sparing diuretics. Salt-free, herb-based seasoning products are readily available in most grocery stores and should be suggested instead.

- Instruct patients/clients on reading the Nutrition Facts food label for sodium content of foods.
- Encourage patients to prepare food at home without adding salt and to limit eating in restaurants.

- Recommend baked products that use sodium-free baking powder, potassium bicarbonate (instead of sodium bicarbonate or baking soda), and salt-free shortening in place of those containing sodium.
- Limit or avoid obviously salted foods such as bouillon, soup and gravy bases, canned soups and stews, bread and rolls with salt toppings, salted crackers, salted nuts or popcorn, potato chips, pretzels, and other salted snack foods. Avoid buying vegetables prepared in sauce.
- Limit or avoid smoked or cured meats, such as bacon, bologna, cold cuts, other processed meats, chipped or corned beef, frankfurters, ham, kosher or kosher-style meats, and canned meat poultry.
- Limit or avoid salted and smoked fish such as cod, herring, and sardines.
- Limit or avoid sauerkraut, olives, pickles, relishes, kimchi, and other vegetables prepared in brine, tomato, and vegetable cocktail juices.
- Limit or avoid seasonings such as celery salt, garlic salt, Worcestershire sauce, fish sauce, and soy sauce. Reduced sodium versions of items like soy sauce can still be very high in sodium.
- Serve cheeses in limited amounts. Swiss cheese and cream cheese are relatively low in sodium.
- Monitor the sodium content of various medications, including over-the-counter brands.

The front of the food package can be used to quickly identify foods that may contain less sodium, but it is important to understand the terminology. For example, look for foods with claims such as:

- **Salt/Sodium-Free** → Less than 5 mg of sodium per serving
- **Very Low Sodium** → 35 mg of sodium or less per serving
- **Low Sodium** → 140 mg of sodium or less per serving
- **Reduced Sodium** → At least 25% less sodium than in the original product
- **Light in Sodium or Lightly Salted** → At least 50% less sodium added than in the regular product
- **No-Salt-Added or Unsalted** → No salt is added during processing, but not necessarily sodium-free. Check the Nutrition Facts label.

Seasoning without salt: Flavorings or seasonings will make food more appetizing. For example:

- Lemon or vinegar is excellent with fish or meat and with many vegetables such as broccoli, asparagus, green beans, or salads.
- Meat may be seasoned with onion, garlic, green pepper, nutmeg, ginger, dry mustard, sage, cumin and marjoram. It may be cooked with fresh mushrooms or unsalted tomato juice. Curries made without salt are a good way to season meats and lentils.
- Cranberry sauce, applesauce, or jellies make appetizing accompaniments to meats and poultry.
- Vegetables can be flavored by the addition of onion, mint, ginger, mace, dill seed, parsley, green pepper, or fresh mushrooms.
- Unsalted cottage cheese can be flavored with minced onion, chopped chives, raw green pepper, grated carrots, chopped parsley, or crushed pineapple.
- A number of salt-free seasonings for use in cooking are available in the spice section of most supermarkets.

Sodium Content of Selected Common Foods

Food	Sodium	Food	Sodium
1 cup of whole or reduced fat milk	107 mg	1 avocado	11 mg
1 slice whole-wheat bread	110-170 mg	1 small potato with skin, baked	12 mg
1 hamburger bun	300-375 mg	1 cup chopped broccoli, raw	30 mg
1 slice American cheese	270-280 mg	½ cup broccoli in cheese sauce (Green Giant)	420 mg
1 slice Swiss cheese (nonprocessed)	50-65 mg	1 cup brown rice, cooked	8 mg
2 oz mozzarella cheese, part skim	350 mg	1 cup white rice, cooked	0 mg
2 oz cream cheese	178 mg	1 cup prepared rice pilaf (Rice-A-Roni)	970 mg
3 oz corned beef (brisket)	900-1100 mg	1 cup pasta, enriched	3-8 mg
3 oz lean ground beef	55-60 mg	1 large egg, raw	71 mg
3 oz chicken, raw broiler without the skin	65 mg	1 large olive, ripe	65 mg
1 slice bacon, pork	185 mgR	1 tbsp olive oil	0 mg
1 cup kidney beans, cooked without salt	2 mg	2 tbsp ranch dressing	270 mg
1 cup canned kidney beans, drained	230-250 mg	2 tbsp balsamic vinegar	8 mg
1 tbsp soy sauce (tamari)	1000 mg	2 tbsp sour cream, cultured	8 mg
1 tbsp reduced-sodium soy sauce	450 mg	12 oz cola, regular	11 mg
1 cup chopped celery, raw	80 mg	1 slice cheese pizza (Domino's)	565 mg
1 cup chopped onion, raw	6 mg	1 slice pepperoni pizza (Pizza Hut)	769 mg
1 tbsp garlic	0 mg	1 Big Mac (McDonald's)	460 mg
1 med banana	1 mg	1 6-in. Subway Club on white bread	720 mg

REFERENCES

National Academies of Medicine: *Food and nutrition board: dietary reference intakes for Sodium and Potassium,* Washington DC, 2019, National Academies Press.

U.S. Department of Agriculture: *Food data central,* Released April 1, 2019. Available at: https://fdc.nal.usda.gov. Accessed December 30, 2019.

Nutritional Facts on Zinc

Zinc is an essential mineral that is found in almost every cell. It stimulates the activity of approximately 100 enzymes, which are substances that promote biochemical reactions in the body. Zinc supports immunity; is needed for wound healing; helps maintain the sense of taste and smell; is needed for deoxyribonucleic acid (DNA) synthesis; and supports normal growth and development during pregnancy, childhood, and adolescence.

Zinc is found in a wide variety of foods. Oysters and Alaskan crab are some of the best food sources of zinc, but red meat and poultry provide the majority of zinc in the American diet. Other good food sources include beans, nuts, certain seafood, whole grains, fortified breakfast cereals, and dairy products.

Because zinc absorption is greater from a diet high in animal protein than a diet rich in plant proteins, vegetarians may become deficient if they are not monitored carefully. Phytates from whole-grain breads, cereals, legumes, and other products can decrease zinc absorption.

Recommended Dietary Allowance (RDA) for Zinc for Children and Adults

Age	Males and Females (mg/day)	Pregnancy (mg/day)	Lactation (mg/day)
0-6 months	2	N/A	N/A
7-12 months	2	N/A	N/A
1-3	3	N/A	N/A
4-8	5	N/A	N/A
9-13	8	N/A	N/A
14-18	11 for boys, 9 for girls	12	13
19+	11 for men, 8 for women	11	12

N/A, Not applicable.

DV = Daily value. The DV for zinc is 15 mg.

Tolerable upper intake level (UL): 0-6 mos 4 mg; 7-12 mos 5 mg; 1-3y 7 mg/d; 4-8y 12 mg/d; 9-13y 23 mg/d; 14-18y (also for pregnancy and lactation) 34 mg/d; 19+ (also for pregnancy and lactation) 40 mg/d.

Selected Food Sources of Zinc

Food	Milligrams (mg) per Serving	% Daily Value*
Oysters, battered and fried, 6 med	16.0	100
RTE breakfast cereal, fortified with 100% of the DV for zinc per serving, ¾ cup serving	15.0	100
Beef shank, lean only, cooked 3 oz	8.9	60
Beef chuck, arm pot roast, lean only, cooked, 3 oz	7.1	47
Beef tenderloin, lean only, cooked, 3 oz	4.8	30
Beef, eye of round, lean only, cooked, 3 oz	4.0	25
RTE breakfast cereal, fortified with 25% of the DV for zinc per serving, ¾ cup	3.8	25
Pork shoulder, lean, cooked, 3 oz	3.5	25
Baked beans, canned, plain or vegetarian, ½ cup	2.9	19
Chicken leg, meat only, roasted, 1 leg	2.7	20
Pork tenderloin, lean only, cooked, 3 oz	2.5	15
Pork loin, sirloin roast, lean only, cooked, 3 oz	2.2	15
Yogurt, plain, low fat, 1 cup	2.2	15
Baked beans, canned, with pork, ½ cup	1.8	10
Cashews, dry roasted without salt, 1 oz	1.6	10
Yogurt, fruit, low fat, 1 cup	1.6	10
Chickpeas, mature seeds, canned, ½ cup	1.5	9
Pecans, dry roasted without salt, 1 oz	1.4	10
Oatmeal, instant, low sodium, 1 packet	1.3	9
Cheese, Swiss, 1 oz	1.2	8
Mixed nuts, dry roasted with peanuts, 1 oz	1.1	8
Walnuts, black, dried, 1 oz	1.0	6
Almonds, dry roasted, without salt, 1 oz	1.0	6
Milk, fluid, any kind, 1 cup	0.9	6
Chicken breast, meat only, roasted, ½ breast with bone and skin removed	0.9	6
Cheese, cheddar, 1 oz	0.9	6
Cheese, mozzarella, part skim, low moisture, 1 oz	0.9	6
Beans, kidney, California red, cooked, ½ cup	0.9	6

RTE, Ready to eat.

*DV = Daily value: developed by the Food and Drug Administration to help consumers compare the nutrient content of products. Foods containing 20% or more of the DV are considered to be excellent sources.

REFERENCES

Institute of Medicine: *Food and nutrition board: dietary reference intakes for Vitamin A, Vitamin K, Arsenic, Boron, Chromium, Copper, Iodine, Iron, Manganese, Molybdenum, Nickel, Silicon, Vanadium, and Zinc,* Washington DC, 2001, National Academies Press.

U.S. Department of Agriculture: *Food data central,* Released April 1, 2019. Available at: https://fdc.nal.usda.gov. Accessed December 30, 2019.

INDEX

A

A/G ratio, 1028t
AAD *see* Antibiotic-associated diarrhea
AASs *see* Androgenic-anabolic steroids
Abdomen
 distention of, 923
 nutrition-focused physical examination of, 1003–1008t
 open, 816
 radiation therapy to, 778t, 779
Abdominal compartment syndrome, 816
Abdominal trauma, 816
Abducens nerve, 849t
ABG (arterial blood gas) values, 38t
Absence seizure (petit mal), 870
Absorption
 of carbohydrates and fiber, 11–12, 11f
 in large intestine, 11–15
 of lipids, 13
 overview of, 3–9
 of proteins, 12–13
 neural mechanisms as, 6t
 regulators of, 4–8
 sites of, 4f, 5f
 in small intestine, 9
 of fats, 14f
 mechanisms of, 9
 structure and, 9
 of vitamins and minerals, 13–15
Academic Consortium for Integrative Medicine and Health, 191
Academy of Nutrition and Dietetics
 fish intake recommendations, 887
 on food insecurity, 175
 Standards of Professional Performance, 143
Acanthosis nigricans, 611
Acarbose (Precose), 1031–1041t
 for type 2 diabetes, 621–622t, 622
Acceptable intake (AI), 52–53
Acceptable macronutrient distribution ranges (AMDRs), 52–53, 167, 174t
Acceptance and commitment therapy (ACT), 228–229
Accreditation, 151
Accumulated damage, and aging, 375t
ACD *see* Anemia of chronic and inflammatory disease
Acesulfame-K, during pregnancy, 278
Acetaldehyde, in alcoholic liver disease, 583, 583b, 584f
Acetaminophen (Tylenol), 1031–1041t
Acetate, in parenteral solutions, 218t
Acetylcholine, 872
 regulation of gastrointestinal activity by, 6t
Acetylcholine receptors (AchRs), 872
Achalasia, 525
Achlorhydria, 378, 533, 537
Achylia gastrica, 537
Acid(s)
 defined, 37
 fixed, 38
 generation of, 38
 organic, 38

Acid-base balance, 37–38, 38t
 guidelines and applications of, 39
 regulation of, 32f, 38
Acid-base disorder(s), 38
 compensation for, 39
 imbalances, 38t
 metabolic acidosis as, 38–39
 metabolic alkalosis as, 39
 respiratory acidosis as, 39
Acid foods, 730b
Acid pocket, 528
Acid reflux, integrative approaches to, 531b
Acidemia, 38–39
Acidosis
 metabolic, 38–39
 anion gap, 39
 nongap, 39
 respiratory, 39
Acinar destruction, 709
Acquired immune deficiency syndrome (AIDS), 787. *see also* Human immunodeficiency virus
 epidemiology and trends in, 788
 global, 788, 789f
 in United States, 788, 789f
 etiology of, 794f
 opportunistic infections in, 790
 oral manifestations of, 490, 490t
Action plan, 235
Active listening, 231b
Active transport, 9
Activities of daily living (ADLs), of older adults, 379
Activity level, unintentional weight loss due to changes in, 416t
Activity-related energy expenditure, 21
Activity thermogenesis (AT), 19, 395–397
 nonexercise, 19, 395–397
Actomyosin, 441
Actos (pioglitazone), for type 2 diabetes, 621–622t
Acupuncture, 188–189t, 190
Acute kidney injury (AKI), 736–737
 causes of, 736t
 medical management of, 736
 medical nutrition therapy for, 736–737, 737t
 energy in, 737
 fluid and sodium in, 737
 potassium in, 737
 protein in, 736–737
 pathophysiology of, 736–737
Acute pancreatitis (AP), 600
Acute-phase proteins, 825
 in metabolic response to stress, 808
Acute-phase reactants, 63t
 negative, 64
 positive, 62–64
Acute renal failure (ARF) *see* Acute kidney injury
Acute respiratory distress syndrome (ARDS), 39, 720–721
 medical management of, 721
 medical nutrition therapy for, 721, 721t
 pathophysiology of, 720–721, 721t
Acute rheumatic fever, 829
ADA *see* American Dietetic Association

Adaptive immune factors, 1028t
Addiction
 definition of, 892
 medical nutritional therapy for, 894, 894b
 neurotransmitters involved in, 892
 nutritional derangements associated, 892
Addison's disease, 645, 652
Adenosine diphosphate (ADP), 441
Adenosine triphosphate (ATP), 9f, 441–442
 mitochondrial production of, 111
 resynthesis of, 441–442
Adenosine triphosphate-creatine phosphate (ATP-CP) system, 441–442
Adequate intake (AI), 167
 for potassium, 1126t
ADH *see* Antidiuretic hormone
ADHD *see* Attention-deficit/hyperactivity disorder
Adherence, to antiretroviral therapy, 791
ADIME (assessment, diagnosis, interventions, monitoring, evaluation) format, 152–153, 152b, 153t
Adipocytes, size and number of, 394
Adipokines
 definition of, 106
 visceral adipose tissue and, 110–111
Adiponectin, 714–715
 in heart failure, 697
 in regulation of body weight, 396–397t, 397b
Adiponectin (ADIPOQ) gene, 398
Adipose tissue
 brown, 394
 composition of, 394
 visceral, 109, 394
 white, 394
Adiposity, 831
Adiposity rebound, 324, 394
Adjustment disorders, 890–892t
ADLs *see* Activities of daily living
Adolescence
 definition of, 341
 diabetes mellitus in, energy balance and weight in, 615
 food habits and eating behaviors of, 348–351
 dieting and body image as, 351
 family meals as, 350, 350b
 fast foods and convenience foods as, 349–350, 349b, 350f
 irregular meals and snacking as, 348–349, 349b
 media and advertising and, 350–351
 growth and development during, 341–343
 linear growth in, 343, 344f
 physiologic anemia of, 347
 psychological changes in, 341–342
 sexual maturation in, 342, 342f, 343t
 hypertension in, 692–693
 late, 350–351
 nutrient requirements in, 344–348, 359b
 for carbohydrates and fiber, 345–346
 for energy, 344, 345t
 for fat, 346
 for minerals and vitamins, 346–348, 346t, 347t

Adolescence *(Continued)*
    calcium as, 346–347
    folate as, 347
    iron as, 347, 347b
    vitamin D as, 347–348
    for protein, 344–345, 345t
  nutrition screening, assessment, and counseling
    for, 351, 352f, 352t
  special topics during, 351–359
    nutritional needs during pregnancy as,
      358–359
    preventing and screening for diabetes as, 358,
      358b
    promoting cardiovascular health as, 355–358,
      356t, 357t
      dietary counseling and weight management
        for, 355–357
      dietary recommendations for, with
        elevated triglyceride or non-high-
        density lipoprotein cholesterol levels,
        357b
      dietary recommendations for elevated
        low-density lipoprotein cholesterol,
        357b
    promoting healthy weight-related attitudes
      and behaviors as, 354
    promoting healthy weight status as, 354,
      355b
    promoting physical activity as, 358
    skin health as, 353–354
    vegetarian dietary patterns as, 351–353, 353t
  supplement use by, 348
  type 2 diabetes in, 358, 358b
  vegetarian diet in, 1097
Adolescent development, Tanner staging of
  in boys, 990, 990f
  in girls, 990, 990f
Adolescent pregnancy, 269, 270b, 358
ADP *see* Adenosine diphosphate
Adrenal dysfunction, and hypothyroidism, 646
Adrenal fatigue, 652–653
Adrenal glands, 652
Adrenal insufficiency, 652–653
  primary, 652
Adrenocorticotropic hormone, in metabolic
  response to stress, 807–808
Adrenoleukodystrophy, 847–848t
  X-linked recessive, 94
Adrenomedullin, in regulation of body weight,
  396–397t
Adrenomyeloleukodystrophy, 865–866
Adrenomyeloneuropathy, 865–866
Adult Family Home (AFH), 386t
Adults
  cancer in, monitoring and evaluation of, 782b
  diabetes mellitus in, energy balance and weight
    in, 615–620
  food security for, 365
  food trends and patterns in, 369
  health disparities in, 367
  lifestyle and health risk factors in, 366–367
  nutrition in, 362, 366b, 371b
    factors affecting, 367–368
    functional foods, 369–370, 370b
    information sources, 364–365
    interventions for, 368
    messages, 362–363, 363f
    supplementation, 369

Adults *(Continued)*
  prevention strategies for, 368
  quality of life in, 365
  recumbent measurement, 991
  wellness in, 365
  work-life balance for, 365
Advance directives, 160, 222
Advanced glycation end products (AGEs), 900
Adverse childhood experience (ACE), 894
Adverse events (AEs), 194
Adverse reactions to food (ARFs), 493, 495f
  assessment of, 514
    immunologic testing for, 515–516
      other tests in, 516
      serum antibody tests in, 516
      skin-prick test in, 515–516, 516f
  defined, 494
  definitions for, 494–497, 497b
  diagnosis of, 514–516
  etiology of, 498
    genetics and epigenetics in, 498
  food allergy
    defined, 494–495
    food protein-induced enterocolitis syndrome
      as, 508–511
    IgE-mediated, 501, 502t
      defined, 501
      food-dependent, exercise-induced
        anaphylaxis as, 501–511
      food-induced anaphylaxis as, 501
      latex-fruit or latex-food syndrome as, 503
      oral allergy syndrome as, 503
    mixed IgE- and non-IgE-mediated, 502t
      eosinophilic esophagitis, 505–507
      eosinophilic gastroenteritis, 507
  food intolerances as, 496–497t, 511–514
    to amines, 513–514
    defined, 495
    to FODMAPs, 511
    to food additives, 513–514
    to histamine, 512
    to lactose, 511
    to microbial contamination and toxins,
      496–497t, 514
    to pharmacologic reactions, 512
    to tyramine, 513
  food sensitivity as, 495–497
  immune system in, 498–501
  interventions for, 516–517
    avoidance of suspect food as, 516
      allergen labeling of foods in, 517b
      hidden allergens in, 517, 517b
    monitoring and evaluation as, 517–518
  medical nutrition therapy for, 493
    elimination diets in, 508t, 516–517
    food and symptom diary in, 514, 515f
    oral food challenge in, 517
  pathophysiology of, 498
    immune system in, 498–501
    sensitization in, 500f
  prevalence of, 497–498
  prevention of, 519–522
    allergen avoidance hypothesis in, 521
    antibiotic use in, 520
    breastfeeding for, 521
    dual allergen hypothesis in, 521
    fatty acids in, 522
    folate in, 522

Adverse reactions to food *(Continued)*
    future directions in, 522
    future innovations in, 522
    genetics and omics in, 522
    immunotherapy in, 522
    infant formula for, 521
    introduction of solids for, 521–522
    microbial exposure hypotheses for, 519–520
    nutritional immunomodulation for, 522
    prebiotics and probiotics in, 521
    route of delivery in, 520
    vitamin D in, 522
Advertising, and food intake
  of adolescents, 350–351
  of children, 330
Adynamic bone disease, 749
Aerobic metabolism, 441
Aerobic pathway, 442, 442f
Aerobic training, for weight loss, 409
Aerophagia, 544
Affirming, 231–232
Affordable Care Act (ACA), 155, 157b
Africa, 163
After-School Snack Program, 134–135t
Age
  dietary reference intakes based on, 174
  gestational *see* Gestational age
  gynecologic, 358
  and resting energy expenditure, 18
Age-related macular degeneration (AMD), 377
Ageusia, due to chemotherapy, 777
Aging, 374f. *see also* Older adults
  and coronary heart disease, 678
  and heart failure, 696b, 698t
  and hypothyroidism, 646
  latent autoimmune diabetes of, 607
  nutrition in, 373
  spectrum of, 374
  theories on, 374–375, 375t
Aging Network, 385
Agnosia, 899b
agouti gene, 89b
Agreeing with a twist, for resistance
  behaviors, 234
AHA *see* American Heart Association
AHD *see* Atherosclerotic cardiovascular disease
AIDS *see* Acquired immune deficiency syndrome
AITDs *see* Autoimmune thyroid disorders
AKI *see* Acute kidney injury
Alanine aminotransferase (ALT), 580–581t
  in chemistry panels, 59–60t
Albright hereditary osteodystrophy, 93
Albumin, 64
  in chemistry panels, 59–60t
  in dialysis patients, 1073
  in end-stage renal disease, 745–747t
  as inflammatory marker, 1028t
  serum, 580–581t
ALCAT *see* Antigen leukocyte cellular antibody
  test
Alcohol
  and bone health, 478
  calories from, 1084–1085, 1085t
  exchange lists for, 1061, 1061t
    nutrition tips, 1061
    selection tips, 1061
  nutritional facts on, 1084, 1084f, 1085t
  withdrawal symptoms from, 893

Alcohol consumption
in carcinogenesis, 759
complications of excessive, 584f
with diabetes mellitus, 618
and exercise and sports, 464
gout caused by, 840
and heart failure, 699
and hypertension, 687t, 689, 692
hypoglycemia due to, 636
metabolic consequences of, 583b
during pregnancy, 278
and resting energy expenditure, 18
in restricted-energy diet, 404
Alcohol-related birth defects (ARBD), 973–974
Alcohol-related neurodevelopmental disorders
(ARND), 973–974
Alcohol Use Disorders Identification Test
(AUDIT), 892, 893b
Alcoholic beverages
energy value of, 25
proof of, 25
Alcoholic cirrhosis, 585
Alcoholic hepatitis, 584f, 585
clinical case study on, 603b
Alcoholic liver disease, 583–585
alcoholic cirrhosis as, 585
alcoholic hepatitis as, 585
hepatic steatosis as, 585
histopathology of, 584f
malnutrition and, 585b
pathogenesis of, 583, 583b, 584f
prevalence of, 583
Alcoholics
folic acid deficiency in, 663
malnutrition in, 585b
Alcoholism
CAGE questionnaire for, 892
definition of, 892
medical management of, 894
pathophysiology of, 892–893
screening for, 892–894, 893b
ALD see Adrenomyeloleukodystrophy
Aldosterone
during exercise and sports, 453
in metabolic response to stress, 808–809
and sodium balance, 35
Alendronate (Fosamax), 1031–1041t
ALF see Assisted Living Facility
Alignment, 231–232
Alkalemia, 39
Alkaline diet
of anticancer dietary plan, 774t
and bone health, 478
Alkaline foods, 730b
Alkaline phosphatase, 1028t
in chemistry panels, 59–60t
serum, 580–581t
Alkalosis
contraction, 39
metabolic, 39
respiratory, 39
Alkylating agents, 775–776t, 1031–1041t
Alleles, 88
Allergen(s), 498
definition of, 497b
hidden, 517
Allergen immunotherapy (AIT), 522
Allergen labeling, of foods, 517, 517b

Allergenic peptides, 12–13
Allergic response, in food allergy, 499–501, 500f
Allergy(ies)
in children, 336–337
to food see Food allergy
Alli see Orlistat
Allium sativum, 198–205b
Allostasis, 105, 106
Almond milk, 1052–1053t
ALP see Alkaline phosphatase
Alpha adrenergic agonist, 1031–1041t
Alpha-glucosidase inhibitors, 1031–1041t
Alpha-linolenic acid, 836b, 885
Alpha-lipoic acid, 198–205b, 896
for diabetes mellitus, 618
as sports supplement, 457–458t
Alpha-gal, 502–503
Alprazolam (Xanax), 1031–1041t
ALS see Amyotrophic lateral sclerosis
ALT see Alanine aminotransferase
Altered neurotransmitter theory, of hepatic
encephalopathy, 588
Alternative medicine, 187
Aluminum, in end-stage renal disease, 745–747t
Alveolar bone, 483f
Alveoli, 706f
Alzheimer's disease, 107–109, 866
"4 As" of, 898, 899b
dementia caused by, 896
folate levels and, 888
folate prevention of, 899
insulin resistance in, 898b
medical management of, 898
medical nutritional therapy for, 898–901, 901b
pathophysiology of, 897–898
risk factor for, 896
vitamin B_{12} levels and, 899
Amaryl (glimepiride), for type 2 diabetes,
621–622t
Ambivalence, 229
AMD see Age-related macular degeneration
Amenorrhea, due to anorexia nervosa, 424
American Cancer Society, 758b, 760t
American Dietetic Association (ADA), 146–147
American Heart Association (AHA), for lifestyle
management, 677b
American Institute for Cancer Research, 131
American Society for Parenteral and Enteral
Nutrition (ASPEN), 810
Americans
Dietary Guidelines for, 132, 176, 176b
nutritional status of, 174–175
Amines, food intolerances due to, 513–514
Amino acid(s)
aromatic, in hepatic encephalopathy, 588
branched-chain
in hepatic encephalopathy, 588
as sports supplements, 457–458t, 462t
description of, 883–884
digestion and absorption of, 12
essential, as sports supplements, 457–458t
in infancy and childhood, 939t
insulin production affected by, 916
mental health and, 889
in parenteral solutions, 217
premature infant requirements for, 916, 916t, 919
in protein synthesis, 83f
as sports supplements, 457–458t

Amino acid metabolism, disorders of, 935–939,
936–938t
maple syrup urine disease as, 936–938t,
946–947, 946f
medical nutrition therapy for, 946–947
medical treatment of, 946
pathophysiology of, 946
phenylketonuria as, 936–938t, 939–947, 939t,
943t, 944f, 944t
adults living with, 945–946
care management algorithm for, 941f
clinical case study on, 952
formula for, 942
low-phenylalanine foods for, 942, 943t
maternal, 945, 945t
medical nutrition therapy for, 942–945
medical treatment of, 939–942
pathophysiology of, 939, 940f, 941f
patient education on, 943–945
psychosocial development with, 945
tasks expected of children with, 945t
timeline of events in, 940b
requirements for individual amino
acids, 939
Amino acidurias, 1028t
γ-aminobutyric acid (GABA), 895b
regulation of gastrointestinal activity by, 6t
Aminopeptidase, in digestion, 6t
Amiodarone (Pacerone), 1031–1041t
Amitriptyline (Elavil), 1031–1041t
Amlodipine (Norvasc), 1031–1041t
Ammonia (NH_3)
in hepatic encephalopathy, 588
in viral hepatitis, 580–581t
Amnesia, 899b
Amoxicillin (Amoxil), 1031–1041t
Amoxicillin/clavulanic acid (Augmentin),
1031–1041t
Amphotericin B (Fungizone), 1031–1041t
Ampulla of Vater, 599
Amputations, desirable body weight adjustments
in patients with, 994
Amygdala, 894
Amylase
pancreatic, in digestion, 8–9
of carbohydrates, 11
in infants, 311
salivary, in digestion, 3, 8
of carbohydrates, 11
in infants, 311
α-Amylase, in digestion, 6t
Amylin, in type 1 diabetes mellitus, 622
Amylin agonists, for type 2 diabetes,
621–622t, 622
Amylo-1, 6-glucosidase deficiency, 950
Amylopectin, 11
Amylophagia, during pregnancy, 270
Amylose, 11
Amyotrophic lateral sclerosis, 847–848t, 868–870
AN see Anorexia nervosa
Anabolic effects, of steroids, 465
Anabolic steroids, as sports supplements, 465
Anaerobic metabolism, 441
Anaerobic pathway, 442
Analgesics, 1031–1041t
for rheumatic disease, 826, 826t
Analyte, 58
in chemistry panels, 59–60t

Anaphylaxis, 495
 food-dependent, exercise-induced, 501–511
 food-induced, 501
Androgen(s), in polycystic ovary syndrome, 649
Androgenic-anabolic steroids (AASs), as sports
  supplements, 461–462t, 464–465
Androgenic effects, of steroids, 465
Android fat distribution, 402
Androstenedione, as sports supplement, 465–467
Anemia(s), 655
 aplastic, 660–661
 B vitamin deficiencies, 66
  folate and vitamin B_{12} in, 66
  methylmalonic acid in, 66
  serum homocysteine in, 66
 of chronic renal disease, 750
 classification of, 65, 655, 656t
 copper deficiency, 666
 defined, 65, 655
 folic-deficiency, 662–664
  clinical findings in, 662–663
  etiology of, 662–663
  medical management of, 664
  medical nutrition therapy for, 664
  methylfolate trap in, 663, 663f
  MTHFR allele in, 663
  pathophysiology of, 663–664, 663b
  stages of, 663, 664f
 hemolytic, 667
  in premature infants, 921
  vitamin E-responsive, 667
 hypochromic, 655, 656t
  microcytic transient, 668
  of protein-energy malnutrition, 666
 iron deficiency, 65–66, 657–660, 657b
  assessment of, 659, 659t
  in athletes, 459
  care management algorithm for, 658f
  clinical findings in, 658f
  diagnosis of, 659, 659t
  hematocrit or packed cell volume and
   hemoglobin in, 65
  laboratory assessment of, 65–66
  medical management of, 659–660
   oral supplementation in, 659–660, 660t
   parenteral iron-dextran in, 660
  medical nutrition therapy for, 660
   bioavailability of dietary iron in, 660
   forms of iron in, 660
   inhibitors in, 660
  pathophysiology of, 657–658, 658f
  serum ferritin in, 65
  serum iron in, 65
  total iron-binding capacity and transferrin
   saturation in, 65–66
 macrocytic, 65, 655, 656t
  from B vitamin deficiencies, 66
 megaloblastic, 661–666
  in vegans, 180
 microcytic, 65, 655, 656t
 nonnutritional, 667–669
 normocytic, 655, 656t
 nutritional, 655
 pernicious, 664–666, 665b, 847–848t, 847t
  assessment of, 666
  clinical findings in, 665–666
  defined, 665
  etiology of, 665

Anemia(s) (Continued)
  medical management of, 666
  medical nutrition therapy for, 666
  pathophysiology of, 665
  stages of, 665
 physiologic, of growth, 347
 of pregnancy, 667
 of protein-energy malnutrition, 666
 sickle cell, 667–668
  clinical case study on, 668–669b
  clinical findings in, 667
  medical management of, 667–668
  medical nutrition therapy for, 668
  pathophysiology of, 667, 667f
 sideroblastic (pyridoxine-responsive), 666–667
 sports, 459, 668
 vitamin B_{12} deficiency, 664–666, 665b
  assessment of, 666
  clinical findings in, 665–666
  etiology of, 665
  medical management of, 666
  medical nutrition therapy for, 666
  stages of, 662f, 665
Anemia of chronic and inflammatory disease
  (ACD), 65, 667
 ferritin in, 63–64
Angelman's syndrome, 90b
Angina, 672
Angiogenesis, 758
Angiography, 674
Angiotensin-converting enzyme (ACE), 739
Angiotensin-converting enzyme (ACE) inhibitors,
  1031–1041t
Angiotensin II, 728
 and water balance, 30
Angiotensin II receptor antagonists, 1031–1041t
Anion(s), 33t
Anion gap, 38–39
Anion gap metabolic acidosis, 39
Ankylosing spondylitis (AS), 842
Anorexia, due to cancer treatment, 770
 pharmacotherapy for, 773
Anorexia athletica (AA), 446–447
Anorexia nervosa, 421
 in adults, 367
 amenorrhea due to, 424
 anthropometric assessment of, 430–431, 430b
 binge eating or purging type of, 421
 biochemical assessment for, 428–429
 clinical characteristics and medical complications
  of, 424–425, 424f
 diagnostic criteria for, 422–423b
 eating behavior in, 428–429, 428b
 energy expenditure in, 429–430
 fluid and electrolyte balance in, 429
 fluid intake with, 427
 lanugo in, 424
 medical nutrition therapy for, 432–434, 432b
 mortality rates for, 421
 nutrition assessment for, 427
 nutrition education for, 437, 437b
 PES statements related to, 155t
 prognosis for, 437
 psychologic management of, 426–427
 refeeding syndrome in, 432–433, 433t
 restricting type of, 427
 treatment approach to, 426
 and vegetarian diet, 427

Anorexia nervosa (Continued)
 vitamin and mineral deficiencies in, 429
 weight gain in
  assessment of, 430–431, 430b
  medical nutrition therapy for, 432–434, 432b
Anosmia, 850
Antacids, for upper GI disorders, 529, 529t
Antecedents, 105
Anthropometric measurements
 for attention-deficit/hyperactivity disorder, 970
 for autism, 968
 for cerebral palsy, 967
 for developmental disabilities, 957
 for Down's syndrome, 962
 for eating disorders, 430–431, 430b
 in nutrition assessment, 957, 958f
 for Prader-Willi syndrome, 963
 in premature infants, 927
 for spina bifida, 965
Anti-dementia drugs, 1031–1041t
Anti-HBe, 580–581t
Anti-HBs, 580–581t
Anti-HCV, 580–581t
Anti-Parkinson's drugs, 1031–1041t
Antiandrogens, nutrition-related effects of,
  775–776t
Antiangiogens, 767
Antianxiety agents, 1031–1041t
Antiarrhythmic agents, 1031–1041t
Antibiotic-associated diarrhea (AAD), 548–550
Antibiotics, and vitamin K production, 1112
Antibodies, in allergic reaction, 498, 500f
Anticariogenic foods, 484
Anticholinesterases, 873
Anticonvulsants
 nutrition status affected by, 870
 nutritional implications of, 1031–1041t
Antidepressants, 888, 901, 1031–1041t
 tricyclic, 1031–1041t
Antidiarrheal medication, for upper
  GI disorders, 529
Antidiuretic hormone (ADH), 30
 in control of water excretion, 727–728
 in metabolic response to stress, 808–809
Antidumping medications, for upper GI
  disorders, 529t
Antifungal agents, 1031–1041t
Antigas medications, for upper GI disorders, 529t
Antigen(s), 498
 inflammation caused by, 109–110
Antigen leukocyte cellular antibody test (ALCAT),
  516, 1028t
Antigen-presenting cells (APCs), in allergic reaction,
  498–499, 500f
Antigenic load, 109–110
Antihyperglycemic drugs insulin sensitizing
  agents, 1031–1041t
Antihyperlipidemic drugs, 1031–1041t
Antiinfective drugs, 1031–1041t
Antiinfective factors, in human milk, 315
Antiinflammatory diet, 828, 828b, 835, 1078
 alcohol, 1080
 avoid chemicals, 1080
 calorie restriction and intermittent fasting, 1080
 dietary approaches to reduce, 1078–1079, 1078t
 example of, 1080
 fat and oils, quality and quantity of, 1079
 food allergy or sensitivity elimination, 1079

Antiinflammatory diet (Continued)
  fruits, vegetables, herbs, and spices, 1079
  healthy microbiome, 1079
  low glycemic diet pattern, 1079, 1079t
  nuts and seeds or nut and seed butters, 1079
  stress and sleep, 1080
Antimetabolites, nutrition-related effects of,
    775–776t
Antimicrobial agents, 1031–1041t
Antineoplastic drugs, 766
  nutrition-related effects of, 775–776t
  nutritional implications of, 1031–1041t
Antinuclear antibodies (ANA), 580–581t, 825, 832
Antioxidant(s)
  burn patient requirements for, 819
  in carcinogenesis, 764
  and coronary heart disease, 682
  for exercise and sports, 456–458
  flavonoids and, 120–121, 120b
  laboratory testing of, 1028t
  for prevention of food allergy, 522
  reactive oxygen species and, 120
  in rheumatoid arthritis patients, 836
  supplements, 192
Antiplatelet agents, 1031–1041t
Antiprotozoals, 1031–1041t
Antipsychotics, nutritional implications of,
    1031–1041t
Antiretroviral therapy (ART), 787
  classes of drugs in, 790–791
  drug resistance to, 791
  food-drug interactions with, 791, 792t
  predictors of adherence to, 791
Antisecretory medications, for upper
    GI disorders, 529t
Antithrombotic/hematologic drugs anticoagulant
    agents, 1031–1041t
Antithymocyte globulin (ATG), after liver
    transplantation, 594t
Antithyroglobulin antibody (anti-TG), 1028t
Antithyroid peroxidase antibody (Anti-TPO),
    1028t
Antithyroidal antibodies, reduction of, 651
α₁-antitrypsin, 580–581t, 1028t
α₁-antitrypsin deficiency, 586
Antitubercular drugs, 1031–1041t
Antitumor antibiotics, nutrition-related effects of,
    775–776t
Antiviral agents, 1031–1041t
Antrum, 7–8
Anxiety, unintentional weight loss due to, 416t
Anxiety disorders, 890–892t, 894–895, 895b
APCs see Antigen-presenting cells
Aphasia, 850, 857, 899b
Apidra (insulin glulisine), 622–623
Apixaban (Eliquis), 1031–1041t
Aplastic anemia, 660–661
Apnea of prematurity, 919
Apolipoprotein(s), in coronary heart disease, 673
Apolipoprotein A-I (APOA1), and vascular
    disease, 100
Apolipoprotein A-IV (APOA4), in regulation of
    body weight, 396–397t
Apolipoprotein B (apoB) phenotype, and
    cardiovascular disease, 69
Apolipoprotein E (apoE) phenotype, and
    cardiovascular disease, 69
Apoptosis, 758

Appetite control, in Prader-Willi syndrome, 963
Appetite enhancers, for unintentional weight loss, 416
Appetite loss, due to HIV infection, 795t
Appetizers, fast foods and, 1061t
Apple, fruits and, 1051–1052t
Appropriate for gestational age, 913, 913b
Apraxia, 850, 899b
Apricots, fruits and, 1051–1052t
Arachidonic acid (ARA), 113–115, 825b, 885
  for infants, 312
ARDS see Acute respiratory distress syndrome
Area Agencies on Aging, 134–135t
Areflexia, 872
ARFs see Adverse reactions to food
Arginase deficiency, 936–938t, 948f
Arginine, 198–205b
  as sports supplement, 457–458t
Argininemia, 936–938t, 948f
Argininosuccinate lyase deficiency, 936–938t, 948
Argininosuccinic acid synthetase deficiency,
    936–938t, 947, 948f
Argininosuccinic aciduria (ASA), 936–938t, 948,
    948f
Aripiprazole (Abilify), 1031–1041t
Arm span measurement, 991
Armour Thyroid (desiccated natural thyroid), for
    hypothyroidism, 646t
Arnold Chiari malformation of brain, 965
Aromatase inhibitors (AIs), nutrition-related
    effects of, 775–776t
Aromatic amino acids (AAAs), in hepatic
    encephalopathy, 588
Arsenic, 54t
ART see Antiretroviral therapy
Arterial blood gas (ABG) values, 38t, 1028t
Arteriovenous fistula, for hemodialysis, 742f
Arthritis
  autoimmune, 823
  definition of, 823
  etiology of, 824
  medical nutrition therapy for, 824t
  microbiota and, 829
  osteoarthritis
    adiposity management in, 831
    chondroitin for, 832
    complementary integrative therapies for, 832
    etiology of, 830f
    exercise for, 831
    glucosamine for, 832
    inflammation in, 824
    joints commonly affected in, 831, 831f
    medical management of, 830f, 831
    medical nutrition therapy for, 824t, 831
    minerals for, 831–832
    pathophysiology of, 829–831, 830f, 831f
    risk factors for, 829
    surgical management of, 831
    vitamins for, 831–832
    weight management for, 831
  prevalence of, 823
  reactive, 829
  rheumatoid see Rheumatoid arthritis
Artificial food dyes, and attention-deficit/
    hyperactivity disorder, 970
Artificial loop graft, for hemodialysis, 742f
Artificial sweeteners
  during pregnancy, 278–279
  in restricted-energy diet, 404–405

ASA see Argininosuccinic aciduria
Ascites, in end-stage liver disease, 587–589
  alcoholic, 585
  medical nutrition therapy for, 588
  paracentesis for, 590–591
  pathophysiology and medical treatment of, 587
Ascorbate, 120–121
Ascorbic acid, 1012t. see also Vitamin C
  for hypertension, 691t
  in parenteral solutions, 218t
  during pregnancy, 261
    with twins, 269t
ASCVD see Atherosclerotic cardiovascular disease
ASDs see Autism spectrum disorders
Ash content, of human vs. cow's milk, 315
Asian, fast foods, 1061t
Aspartame, during pregnancy, 278
Aspartate aminotransferase (AST), 580–581t
  in chemistry panels, 59–60t
  laboratory values for, 1028t
Asperger's syndrome, 967, 968t
Aspiration, 852
  with enteral nutrition, 215
Aspiration pneumonia, 721, 721b, 855–856
Aspirin/salicylate (Bayer), 1031–1041t
Assessment, diagnosis, interventions, monitoring,
    evaluation (ADIME) format, 152–153, 152b,
    153t
Assessment information, sources for, 130
Assessment terminology, 197b
Assisted living, 385
Assisted Living Facility (ALF), 386t
Assisted reproductive technology (ART), 245
Associative disorders, 890–892t
AST see Aspartate aminotransferase
Asthma, 711–712
  allergic (extrinsic), 712
  defined, 711
  medical management of, 712
  medical nutrition therapy for, 712
  nonallergic (intrinsic), 712
  pathophysiology of, 711–712
Asymptomatic HIV infection, 788–790
Atenolol (Tenormin), 1031–1041t
ATG see Antithymocyte globulin
Atheroma, 671–672
Atherosclerosis, 670–673
  anatomy and physiology of, 670–671
  clinical manifestations of, 673f
  description of, 121
  due to genetic hyperlipidemias, 674–683
    familial combined hyperlipidemia as, 674
    familial dysbetalipoproteinemia as, 674
    familial hypercholesterolemia as, 674
    polygenic familial hypercholesterolemia as,
      674
  medical diagnosis of, 674
  medical intervention of, 683
  medical management of, 682–683
  pathophysiology of, 671–673, 671f, 672f,
    673f, 680f
    lipoproteins in, 673
    total cholesterol in, 673
    triglycerides in, 673
  pharmacologic management of, 682–683
  prevention and risk factor management of,
    674–676
    in adults, 676

Atherosclerosis *(Continued)*
  in children, 674–675
    Framingham Heart Study on, 674–675, 675b
    inflammatory markers for, 676, 676b
    lifestyle guidelines in, 676–677, 677b
    nonmodifiable risk factors in, 678–679
    risk factor identification for, 674, 675b
Atherosclerotic cardiovascular disease
    (ASCVD), 670
  in end-stage renal disease, 750
Athletes *see* Exercise and sports performance
Athletic energy deficit (AED), 447
Atopic dermatitis, 498
  skin-prick test with, 516f
Atopic eczema, 501f
Atopic march, 521
Atopy, 497b
Atorvastatin (Lipitor), 1031–1041t
ATP *see* Adenosine triphosphate
Attention-deficit/hyperactivity disorder (ADHD),
    969–971
  anthropometric measures in, 970
  biochemical measures in, 970
  in children, 337
  defined, 969–970
  dietary intake in, 970
  medical nutrition therapy for, 970–971
  nutrition assessment for, 970
  treatment drugs, 1031–1041t
Atypical antipsychotic agents, 1031–1041t
Australia, 167f
Autism, 857, 967–969
  anthropometric measures in, 968
  biochemical measures in, 968
  defined, 967
  dietary intake in, 968
  nutrition assessment for, 968
  nutrition diagnoses with, 955–957t
  pathophysiology of, 967–968
Autism spectrum disorders (ASDs), 967, 968t
  clinical scenario on, 976
Autoantibodies, 825
Autoimmune arthritis, 823
Autoimmune diseases, inflammatory biomarkers
    in, 107–109, 110t
Autoimmune thyroid disorders (AITDs), 641
Autonomic symptoms, of insulin reaction, 633
Autophagy, 105
Autosomal dominant single-gene disorders, 93
Autosomal recessive disorders, 93
Autosomal-recessive traits, 935
Autosomes, 87
Aversions, during pregnancy, 270, 271t
Avoidant/restrictive food intake disorder
    (ARFID), 422–423b, 424
Axons, 849
Ayurveda, 188–189t, 188t
Azathioprine, after liver transplantation, 594t
Azithromycin (Zithromax), 1031–1041t
Azotemia, 728

B

B cells, in allergic reaction, 498–499, 500f
B-complex vitamins
  for exercise and sports, 456
  in inflammation reduction, 120, 120b
B-natriuretic peptide (BNP), in heart failure, 696
B vitamins, for exercise and sports, 456

Baby boomers, 373
"Baby-bottle tooth decay" *see* Early childhood
    caries
Baby-led weaning, 319, 320b
Bacillus cereus, 136–138t
Bacon, meat and meat substitute, 1056–1057t
Bacteria, as intestinal microflora, 10f, 12
Bacterial action, of large intestine, 10–11, 10f
Bacterial overgrowth
  gastritis and, 10
  small intestine, 570–571
    defined, 570
    etiology of, 570–571
    medical nutrition therapy for, 571
    medical treatment of, 571
    pathophysiology of, 571
Bamboo spine, 842
Barbiturate, 1031–1041t
Bariatric surgery, 411, 413t
  gastric bypass, gastroplasty, and gastric banding
    as, 411–413, 412f, 413t
  and kidney stones, 729
  and prediabetes, 616
  pregnancy after, 268
Barrett's esophagus (BE), 528
Basal energy expenditure (BEE), 17–18
Basal metabolic rate (BMR), 17
Basal or background insulin dose, 623
Base, 37
Base-pairing rules, 83f
Basic foods, 730b
Basic metabolic panel (BMP), 59, 59–60t
Basilar skull fractures, 860
Basopenia, 61t
Basophil(s)
  in allergic reaction, 499
  in differential count, 61t
Basophilia, 61t
BAT *see* Brown adipose tissue
Battle's sign, 860
Baxter Clinimix Compounding System, 212f
BCAAs *see* Branched-chain amino acids
Beckwith-Wiedemann's syndrome, 93
BED *see* Binge eating disorder
Bedsores, in older adults, 379, 380t
BEE *see* Basal energy expenditure
Beer, alcohol and, 1061t
Behavior change, 226–227
  defined, 226
Behavior change counseling, 226–227
  assessing readiness for, 232
  clinical scenario on, 236b
  defined, 226
  evaluation of effectiveness of, 235–236
  factors affecting
    communication as, 231b
    counselor, 230b
    cultural competency as, 229–230
    health literacy as, 232
  models for, 227–228, 228t
    health belief model as, 227, 228t
    social cognitive theory as, 227, 228t
    theory of planned behavior as, 227–228, 228t
    transtheoretical (stages of change) model as,
      228, 228t
  new directions on, 235b
  not-ready-to-change sessions in, 232–233
    affirming in, 231–232

Behavior change counseling *(Continued)*
    asking open-ended questions in, 231
    building rapport in, 231
    concern in, 233
    eliciting self-motivational statements in, 232
    ending session in, 233
    intention to change in, 233
    optimism in, 233
    problem recognition in, 232
    reflective listening in, 231
    summarizing in, 232
  ready-to-change sessions in, 235
    action plan in, 235
    setting goals in, 235
  resistance to, 234
    agreeing with a twist for, 234
    double-sided reflection for, 234
    ending session in, 234
    reflecting for, 234
    reframing for, 234
    shifting focus for, 234
  stages of, 228f
  strategies for
    acceptance and commitment therapy as, 228–229
    cognitive behavioral therapy as, 228
    developing discrepancy in, 229
    empathy and rapport in, 230
    motivational interviewing as, 229
    self-efficacy in, 229
  unsure-about-change sessions in, 233–234
Behavior modification, 226
  for obesity, 404
Behavioral-environmental domain, of nutrition
    diagnosis, 127
  for cancer, 770b
Behavioral factors, food allergy and, 514
Benazepril (Lotensin), 1031–1041t
Benign tumor, 766
Benzoic acid, food intolerance due to, 496–497t
Berberine, 618
Beta blocking agents, 1031–1041t
Beta-glucans, 198–205b
Beta-hydroxy-beta-methylbutyrate (HMB), as
    sports supplement, 457–458t
Beta3-adrenoreceptor gene, 398
Betrixaban (Bevyxxa), 1031–1041t
Beverages, 192b
  Mediterranean diet and, 1083
Bezoar, 540
BH$_4$ *see* Tetrahydrobiopterin
BIA *see* Bioelectrical impedance analysis
Bicarbonate (HCO$_3^-$), 38–39, 38t, 1028t
  in chemistry panels, 59–60t
  laboratory values for, 1028t
Bifidobacteria spp., 10
Biguanides, 1031–1041t
  for type 2 diabetes, 620, 621–622t
Bile
  in digestion, 13
  in liver, 579
Bile acid(s)
  in digestion, 8
  recycling of, 9
  serum, 580–581t
Bile acid sequestrants, 1031–1041t
  for coronary heart disease, 682–683
Bile salt(s), 580
  in digestion, 8, 13

Bile salt export pump (BSEP), 595
Biliary cirrhosis
    primary, 582f, 585
    secondary, 596
Bilirubin, 580
    serum
      in chemistry panels, 59–60t
        direct, 580–581t
        indirect, 580–581t
        total, 580–581t
    urine, 62t, 580–581t
Billroth I (gastroduodenostomy), 537–538, 538f
Billroth II (gastrojejunostomy), 537–538, 538f
Binge, 421
Binge eating disorder (BED), 423–424
    diagnostic criteria for, 422–423b
    medical nutrition therapy for, 436
Bioactive compounds, 53, 54t, 191
    in carcinogenesis, 764
Bioactive food components, 86b, 97
Bioactive substances and integrative care, 187
Biochemical assessment, 57–59, 58f
    C-reactive protein in, 62–63
    of chronic disease risk, 68–70
      hemoglobin A1C and diabetes in, 69
      lipid indices of cardiovascular risk in, 68–69, 69b
      oxidative stress in, 68t
        markers of, 68t
    clinical case study on, 77–78b
    creatinine in, 68
    definitions in, 58
    for eating disorders, 428–429
    of fat-soluble vitamins, 66–67
      vitamin A as, 67
      vitamin D as, 67
      vitamin E as, 67
      vitamin K as, 67
    hepatic transport proteins in, 64
      albumin as, 64
      prealbumin (transthyretin) as, 64
      retinol-binding protein as, 64
      transferrin as, 64
    of hydration status, 61–64
      bioelectrical impedance analysis for, 72
    immunocompetence in, 64
    inflammation and, 62
    nitrogen balance in, 68
    of nutritional anemias, 65–66
      from B vitamin deficiencies, 66
        folate and vitamin B_{12} in, 66
        methylmalonic acid in, 66
        serum homocysteine in, 66
      classification of, 65
      iron deficiency, 65–66, 657–660, 657b
        hematocrit or packed cell volume and hemoglobin in, 65
        serum ferritin in, 65
        serum iron in, 65
        total iron-binding capacity and transferrin saturation in, 65–66
    routine medical laboratory tests in, 59–61
      clinical chemistry panels as, 59, 59–60t
      complete blood count as, 59, 61t
      stool testing as, 59–60
      urinalysis as, 61, 62t
    specimen types in, 58–59
Biochemical data, in nutrition assessment, 958

Biochemical individuality, 110
Biochemical measures
    for attention-deficit/hyperactivity disorder, 970
    for autism, 968
    for cerebral palsy, 967
    for developmental disabilities, 958
    for Down's syndrome, 962
    for Prader-Willi syndrome, 963
    for spina bifida, 965
Bioelectrical impedance analysis (BIA), 72, 74f, 796, 1010–1011b
    for anorexia nervosa, 430
Bioenergetics, 441–442
Bioflavonoids, 120
Bioimpedance spectroscopy, 1010–1011b
Bioinformatics, 82b
Biologic response modifiers (BRMs), 826t, 827
Biomarkers, inflammation
    description of, 107–108t, 107–109, 111b, 112
    transferrin, 1028t
Biopterin synthetase deficiency, 936–938t, 940f
Bioterrorism, 140–142
Biotherapy, for cancer, 777
    nutritional impact of, 775–776t
Biotin
    daily reference intakes of, 1104t
    nutritional facts on, 1104, 1104t
    in parenteral solutions, 218t
    sources of, 1104t
Biotinidase deficiency, 936–938t
Biotransformation (detoxification), 96–97
Bipolar disorders, 890–892t, 895–896
Birth control, breastfeeding with, 298–299
Birth defects, risk factors for, 249b
Birthweight, 913b
    low see Low birthweight (LBW) infant
Bisoprolol (Blocadren), 1031–1041t
Bisphenol-A (BPA), 54t
    and infant feeding, 317
    during pregnancy, 279
Bisphenol A (BPA) toxicity, in carcinogenesis, 762, 762b
Bisphosphonates, 479
    for end-stage renal disease, 749t
    nutritional implications of, 1031–1041t
Bitter orange, for weight loss, 408t
Black pepper (Piper nigrum), 194
Blackburn, George L., 393t
Bladder
    neurogenic, 874
    nutrition-focused physical examination, 1003–1008t
Blastocyst, 246–249t
Blind loop syndrome see Small intestine bacterial overgrowth
Blood, in urine, 62t
Blood cells, as specimens, 58, 1009
Blood composition, during pregnancy, 250, 250t, 251t
Blood gases values, 38t
Blood glucose
    fasting, 609
      impaired, 607
    fluctuations in, 884
    postprandial (after a meal), 609
    during pregnancy, 628, 628t
    preprandial (fasting/premeal), 609
    regulation of, 884

Blood glucose (Continued)
    self-monitoring of, 613–614, 625
    target goals for, 614t, 624–625
Blood pressure
    in adolescence, 357t
    categories of, 683t
    with diabetes mellitus, 614, 635t
      monitoring of, 625
    diastolic, 683
    high see Hypertension
    during pregnancy, 250
    systolic, 683
Blood spots, as specimens, 58
Blood urea nitrogen (BUN)
    in chemistry panels, 59–60t
    in end-stage renal disease, 745–747t
Blood urea nitrogen to creatinine (BUN/Cr) ratio, in acute kidney injury, 736
Blood volume, during pregnancy, 250, 250t, 251t
Blue zones, 375b
BMC see Bone mineral content
BMD see Bone mineral density
BMI see Body mass index
BMP see Basic metabolic panel
BMR see Basal metabolic rate
Body composition
    with aging, 375–376
    inflammation and, 110–111
    and resting energy expenditure, 18
Body fat, 394
    malnutrition and, 1001–1002t
    skinfold measurements for percentage determinations, 996, 996t
Body fluids, viscosity of, 112
Body habitus, 1003–1008t
Body image, in adolescence, 341, 351
Body language, 231b
Body mass index (BMI), 70, 71, 76b, 342, 351
    for anorexia nervosa, 421
    body composition phenotypes and, 110–111
    for developmental disabilities, 957
    and obesity, 401
    table of, 995, 995t
Body size, and resting energy expenditure, 18
Body water, 28–33
    distribution of, 28–29
Body weight
    for amputees adjustment, 994t
    in carcinogenesis, 759–760
    components of, 394–395, 394f
    in eating disorders, 430
    and energy adequacy, 17
    maintaining reduced, 414
    regulation of, 395–397
Bolus, 8
Bolus feedings, 212
Bombesin
    in regulation of body weight, 396–397t
    in regulation of gastrointestinal activity by, 5
Bone(s)
    composition of, 471
    cortical, 471, 472f
    defined, 471
    nutrition and, 476–478
      alcohol in, 478
      alkaline diets in, 478
      caffeine in, 478
      dietary fiber in, 478

Bone(s) (Continued)
energy in, 476
isoflavones in, 478
minerals for, 476–477
calcium as, 476–477, 477t
phosphate as, 477
trace minerals as, 477
protein in, 476
sodium in, 478
vegetarian diets in, 478
vitamins for, 477–478
vitamin A as, 477
vitamin D as, 477
vitamin K as, 477–478
osteopenia and osteoporosis of, 473–476
appearance of bone in, 474f
causes and risk factors of, 474–475, 474b
alcohol as, 474
body weight as, 474
cigarette smoking as, 474
ethnicity as, 474
limited weight-bearing exercise as, 474–475
loss of menses as, 475
medications as, 475, 475b
nutrients as, 475
sarcopenia as, 475
clinical scenario on, 479b
definitions, 475
diagnosis and monitoring of, 475
drugs for, 479
integrative approaches for, 479b
prevalence of, 474
prevention of, 478
screening tools for, 476t
treatment of, 478–479
types of, 474, 474b
rebuilding or formation stage of, 473
structure and physiology of, 471–473
trabecular (cancellous, spongy), 471, 472f
ultrasound measurements of, 475
Bone cells, 472, 472t
Bone densitometry, 475
Bone health, 471
in children, 337
Bone loss, due to anorexia nervosa, 424
Bone markers, 475–476
Bone mass, 471
peak, 472
Bone metastases, hypercalcemia due to, 773
Bone mineral content (BMC), 471
Bone mineral density (BMD), 471
in anorexia nervosa, 424
peak, 473f
Bone modeling, 472–473, 473f
Bone remodeling, 473, 473f
Bone resorption, 474
Bone tissue
and calcium homeostasis, 472
types of, 471, 472f
Bone turnover, normal, 473, 473f
Botanical formulations, 192b
Botanicals, 188–189t, 191
and thyroid health, 651
Bottle, weaning from, 320
Botulism, in infancy, 312
Bowman's capsule, 727, 728f

Boys
estimated energy requirement for, 23–24b
head circumference-for-age and weight-for-length percentiles, 982f, 983f, 984f
length-for-age and weight-for-age percentiles, 981f
weight maintenance TEE for, 23–24b
BPA see Bisphenol-A
BPD see Bronchopulmonary dysplasia
Bradycardia, 919
Brain
Arnold Chiari malformation of, 965
with HIV infection, 793t
lobes of, 882, 883f
neurons of, 882
nutrition effects on, 883b
Brain-derived neurotrophic factor, 884b
Brain neurotransmitters, in regulation of body weight, 396–397t
Brainstem
anatomy of, 851f
lesions of, 850
Branched-chain amino acids (BCAAs)
in hepatic encephalopathy, 588
as sports supplements, 457–458t, 462t
Branched-chain ketoacid decarboxylase complex deficiency, 946f
Branched-chain ketoaciduria, 946
intermittent, 936–938t
medical nutrition therapy for, 946–947
medical treatment of, 946
pathophysiology of, 946
Bravewell Collaborative, 191
Bread, carbohydrates and, 1050–1051t
Breakfast, of children, 334
and learning, 334b
Breakfast sandwiches, fast foods and, 1061t
Breast augmentation, breastfeeding with, 297–298
Breast development, 342, 342f
Breastfed infants, iron supplementation for, 314b
Breastfeeding, 286–300, 287f. see also Lactation
benefits of, 287–288, 287b, 314
birth control and, 298–299
breast augmentation and, 297–298
with cleft lip and palate, 972
clinical scenario on, 300
contraindications to, 288–289
exclusive, 314–315
exercise and, 297
health risk not associated with, 288b
of infant, 294
colostrum in, 292
preparation for, 294
initiation of, 293–294
overweight and, 297
postpartum depression and, 298
pregnancy during, 299
of premature infants, 923, 929–930
preservation of, 295–297, 296f
for prevention of food allergies, 521
problems of, 294, 294–295t
recommendations on, 314–315
reduction mammoplasty and, 298
return to work or school and, 299–300
tandem nursing and, 299
ten steps to successful, 288b
tips for, 293b
weaning and, 299

Breastfeeding (Continued)
weaning from, 320
by women with diabetes, 293–294
Breastmilk, 314
antiinfective factors in, 315
composition of, 289, 315
iron from, 1122
transfer of drugs into, 297
type of, 300t
Breath tests, 58–59
Brewer's yeast, 1119
Bristol stool scale, 545, 546f
Bromocriptine (Parlodel), 1031–1041t
Bronchiectasis, 708
Bronchioles, 706f
Bronchogenic carcinomas, 718
Bronchopulmonary dysplasia (BPD), 722–724, 919
medical management of, 722–723
medical nutrition therapy for, 723–724, 723b
in premature infants, 722–723
Brown adipose tissue (BAT), 394
Brownies, sweet, desserts, and other carbohydrates, 1053–1054t
Brush border, 9
Buddhist dietary practices, 181t
Budwig diet, of anticancer dietary plan, 774t
Buffer systems, 38
Bulimia nervosa (BN), 421
binging in, 421
biochemical assessment for, 429
clinical characteristics and medical complications of, 425
cognitive behavioral therapy for, 426, 435
defined, 421
diagnostic criteria for, 422–423b
eating behavior in, 428
energy expenditure in, 429–430
fluid and electrolyte balance in, 429
medical nutrition therapy for, 434–435, 434b
mortality rates for, 421
nutrition assessment for, 427–428, 428b
nutrition counseling for, 435, 435t
nutrition education for, 437, 437b
prognosis for, 437
psychologic management of, 426–427
Russell's sign in, 425, 425f
treatment approach to, 425–426
Bulk herbs, 192b, 198–205b
Bumetanide (Bumex), 1031–1041t
BUN see Blood urea nitrogen
Bupropion (Wellbutrin SR, XL), 1031–1041t
Burns
ancillary measures for, 817
calcium levels after, 819
classification of, 816–819, 817f
electrolyte imbalances and, 819
hypophosphatemia and, 819
medical management of, 817
ancillary measures in, 817
electrolyte repletion, 817
fluid, 817
wound management in, 817
medical nutrition therapy for, 817–819
antioxidants, 819
energy, 818
energy requirements in, 816–817
goals of, 818b

Burns (*Continued*)
methods of nutrition support for, 819
micronutrients, 819
micronutrients and antioxidants in, 819
protein, 818–819
vitamins, 815
pathophysiology of, 816–817
total body surface area, 817
vitamin D deficiency and, 819
zinc deficiency in, 819
Burrito, fast foods and, 1061t
Butter, fats and, 1058–1059t
Butylated hydroxyanisole (BHA), food intolerance due to, 496–497t
Butylated hydroxytoluene (BHT), food intolerance due to, 496–497t
Byetta (exenatide), for type 2 diabetes, 620–622, 621–622t

C
C-peptide, 70
C-reactive protein (CRP), 62–63
and coronary heart disease, 676
high-sensitivity, and cardiovascular disease, 69b
as inflammation marker, 825, 1028t
C-reactive protein-high sensitivity (CRP-hs), 105
Ca *see* Calcium
CABG (coronary artery bypass graft) surgery, 683
Cachexia
cancer, 772
pharmacotherapy for, 773
cardiac, 696
rheumatoid arthritis as cause of, 835
Cadmium, during pregnancy, 279–280
Caffeine
and bone health, 478
and exercise and sports, 464
and heart failure, 699
and infertility, 241–242
nutritional facts on products containing, 1086, 1086t
and resting energy expenditure, 18
CAGE questionnaire, 892, 893b
Cake, sweet, desserts, and other carbohydrates, 1053–1054t
Calciferol *see* Vitamin D
Calcification, metastatic, 749
Calcimimetics, for end-stage renal disease, 749t
Calciphylaxis, 749
Calcitonin, 641–642
and bone remodeling, 479
Calcitriol, 826–827
in calcium homeostasis, 472
Calcium aspartate, 1117
Calcium (Ca), 33–34, 198–205b
absorption of, 34
for adolescence, 346–347
in burn patients, 819
in cancer prevention, 764
for children, 327
and bone health, 337
dietary reference intakes for, 34
electrolyte classification of, 33t
in end-stage renal disease, 745–747t, 748–750
excretion of, 34
for exercise and sports, 459–460
food sources of, 1117t
in foods, 1116–1117

Calcium (*Continued*)
functions of, 33–34
for heart failure, 699
and hypertension, 687t, 688–689, 692
for infants, 313
ionized Ca^{++}, 33
laboratory testing of, 1028t
for lactation, 290
magnesium and, 106, 119
in medications, 1118
nutritional facts on, 1116
for older adults, 383t
in parenteral solutions, 218t
and periodontal disease, 488–489
during pregnancy
requirements for, 262–263, 263t
with twins, 269t
premature infant requirements for, 917–918, 921
recommended dietary allowances for, 1116t
sources of, 34
supplements, 1117–1118
total, in chemistry panels, 59–60t
in vegetarian diet, 1096, 1096t
Calcium carbonate, 1117
Calcium channel blocking agents, 1031–1041t
Calcium citrate, 1117
Calcium homeostasis, 472
Calcium intake, and bone health, 476–477, 477t
Calcium lactate, 1117
Calcium phosphate, 1117
Calcium-phosphorus homeostasis, 728
Calcium stones, 729–731
Calcium supplements
for end-stage renal disease, 749t
and kidney stones, 730
Calculus
dental, 485
renal *see* Kidney stones
Caloric intake, for exercise, 445
Caloric prescription
for anorexia nervosa, 433
for bulimia nervosa, 435
Caloric values, for diabetes, 630, 631t
Calorie(s), 19
in alcoholic beverages, 1084–1085, 1085t
for lactation, 289
physical activity expenditure of, 997, 999t
during pregnancy, 257
exercise and, 257–258
restriction of, 257–258
with twins, 269t
Calorie count, 47–48t, 48
Calorie deficit, for weight loss, 403
Calorie restriction (CR)
for hypothyroidism, 646–647
Calorimetry
direct, 19
indirect, 19–20, 20f
Calvarial skull fractures, 860
CAM *see* Complementary and alternative medicine
Camellia sinensis, 198–205b
Campylobacter jejuni, 136–138t
Canada, dietary guidelines in, 162, 175b
Canagliflozin (Invokana), 1031–1041t
Cancellous bone, 471, 472f

Cancer
antiangiogenic agents for, 767
biotherapy for, 777
nutritional impact of, 774–781
care management algorithm for, 763f
case study on, 783–784b
chemotherapy for, 767
nutritional impact of, 774–776
diarrhea as, 776–777
food-drug interactions as, 777
mucositis as, 777
nausea and vomiting as, 777
oral changes as, 777
classification of, 766
complementary and integrative therapies for
dietary supplements as, 773–774
cost of, 756, 757f
defined, 756
development *see* Carcinogenesis
etiology of, 756
foods for, 764t
hematopoietic cell transplantation for, 781
nutritional impact of, 774–781
with graft-*versus*-host disease, 781
with neutropenia, 768
hormone therapy for, 778
inflammation in, 111b, 120
liquid, 766
managed with Mediterranean diet, 1082
medical diagnosis of, 765–766, 766t
medical nutrition therapy for, 768–773
energy in, 768–769, 769b, 769t
fluid in, 769
general assessment in, 768
micronutrients in, 769–770
protein in, 769
supplement use in, 773–774
medical treatment of, 766–768
cultural considerations, 768
goals of, 768
response to, 767–768
nutrition impact symptoms in, 770
nutrition intervention for
for alterations in energy metabolism, 772
for anorexia and alterations in taste and smell, 771–772
for cancer cachexia, 772
oral nutrition management strategies in, 770–771, 771–772t
for other cancer-related metabolic abnormalities, 773
with pharmacotherapy, 773
nutrition monitoring and evaluation for, 781
nutrition recommendations for, 782–784
nutrition screening and assessment for, 768
nutritional genomics and, 97
palliative care for, 782
pathophysiology of, 758
pediatric, 781–782
PES statements related to, 155t
physical activity with, 765
prevention of, 756, 758b
coffee and tea in, 764
fruits and vegetables in, 765
soy and phytoestrogens in, 765
vegetarian and vegan plant-based diets, 765
vitamin D in, 764
radiation therapy for, 767

Cancer (Continued)
nutritional impact of, 774–781, 778t
to abdomen or pelvis, 779
to head and neck, 779
to thorax, 778–779
total-body, 779
risk for, 760b
selenium and, 1127
solid, 766
staging of, 765–766, 766t
surgery for, 771–772t, 779–781
esophageal, 779
gastric, 779
head and neck, 779
intestinal tract, 781
nutrition-related effects of, 780t
pancreatic, 779
symptoms of, 765–766
unintentional weight loss due to, 416t
Cancer cachexia, 719, 772
pharmacotherapy for, 773
Cancer survivors
integrative therapies used by, 783b
nutrition recommendations for, 782–784
physical activity for, 783b
Cancer vaccines, 777
nutrition-related effects of, 775–776t
Candida albicans, with chemotherapy, 777
Candidate gene approach, 92b
Candidiasis, with HIV infection, 793t
oral, 490
Cannabinoid hyperemesis syndrome, 541b
CAPD see Continuous ambulatory peritoneal dialysis
Capsules, 192b, 196
Carbamazepine (Tegretol), 1031–1041t
Carbamoyl-phosphate synthetase (CPS) deficiency, 936–938t, 948f
Carbidopa/levodopa (Sinemet), 1031–1041t
Carbohydrate(s)
absorption of, laboratory testing of, 1028t
for adolescence, 345–346
and carcinogenesis, 760
digestion and absorption of, 11–12, 11f, 12f
in enteral formulas, 213–214
on exchange list, 1049–1051, 1050–1051t
nutrition tips, 1049–1050
selection tips, 1050–1051
for exercise and sports, 448–451
types of, 450–451
fermentable, in development of dental caries, 483
glycemic index of, 1093t
for infants, 312
for lactation, 290
for older adults, 383t
in parenteral solutions, 217
during pregnancy, 259
with twins, 269t
premature infant requirements for, 921
Carbohydrate counting
for diabetes mellitus, 616, 632, 632f
for hypoglycemia, 637
Carbohydrate intake
for anorexia nervosa, 433
for diabetes mellitus, 616–617
exercise guidelines for, 619–620
during exercise, 450–451, 451f

Carbohydrate intake (Continued)
postworkout and recovery, 451
pretraining fasting, 450, 450b
Carbohydrate metabolism
disorders of, 949–950
galactosemia as, 936–938t, 949
medical nutrition therapy for, 949, 950t
medical treatment of, 949
pathophysiology of, 949
glycogen storage diseases as, 936–938t, 949–950
medical nutrition therapy for, 950
medical treatment of, 950
pathophysiology of, 950
insulin and, 614t
in liver, 579
Carbohydrate requirements
for end-stage liver disease, 592
in infancy and childhood, 939t
Carbohydrate restriction, for hypothyroidism, 646–647
Carbon dioxide (CO$_2$)
electrolyte classification of, 33t
in end-stage renal disease, 745–747t
partial pressure of dissolved, 38
total, 38
Carbonic acid (H$_2$CO$_3$), 38
Carboxypeptidase, in digestion, 6t
of proteins, 12
Carcinogen, 758
Carcinogenesis
alcohol in, 759
antioxidants in, 764
bisphenol A toxicity in, 762
chemical exposures in, 762
defined, 758
energy intake and body weight in, 759–760
epidemiologic studies of, 765
fat in, 761
nutrition and, 758–762
phases of, 758
phytochemicals in, 759t
protein in, 761
smoked, grilled, and preserved foods in, 761
sugar and nonnutritive sweeteners in, 761
Carcinomas, 766
Cardiac cachexia, 696
Cardiac catheterization, 674
Cardiac glycoside agent, 1031–1041t
Cardiac output, during pregnancy, 250
Cardiac remodeling, 694
Cardiac transplantation, 700–702
nutrition support after
immediate, 701, 701t
long-term, 701–702
pretransplant medical nutrition therapy, 701
Cardiomyopathies, 700
Cardiopulmonary system, 1003–1008t
Cardiovascular changes, with aging, 379
Cardiovascular disease (CVD), 346, 670
atherosclerosis and coronary heart disease as, 670–673
anatomy and physiology of, 670–671
clinical manifestations of, 673f
due to genetic hyperlipidemias, 674–683
familial combined hyperlipidemia as, 674
familial dysbetalipoproteinemia as, 674
familial hypercholesterolemia as, 674

Cardiovascular disease (Continued)
polygenic familial hypercholesterolemia as, 674
medical diagnosis of, 674
medical intervention of, 683
medical management of, 682–683
medical nutrition therapy for, 679–682
pathophysiology of, 671–673, 671f, 672f, 673f, 681f
lipoproteins in, 673
total cholesterol in, 673
triglycerides in, 673
pharmacologic management of, 682–683
prevention and risk factor management of, 674–676
in adults, 676
in children, 674–675
Framingham Heart Study on, 674–675, 675b
inflammatory markers for, 676, 676b
lifestyle guidelines in, 676–677, 677b
nonmodifiable risk factors in, 678–679
risk factor identification for, 674, 675b
cardiac transplantation for, 700–702
nutrition support after
immediate, 701, 701t
long-term, 701–702
pretransplant medical nutrition therapy, 701
clinical case study on, 702b
defined, 670
diabetes and, 635
heart failure as, 693–700
adiponectin in, 697
B-natriuretic peptide in, 696
cardiac cachexia in, 696
cardiac remodeling in, 694
case management algorithm for, 695f
classification of, 696t
medical management of, 697
medical nutrition therapy for, 697–700
alcohol in, 699
caffeine in, 699
calcium in, 699
coenzyme Q$_{10}$ in, 700
D-ribose in, 700
energy in, 700
fats in, 700
folate, vitamin B$_6$, and vitamin B$_{12}$ in, 700
L-arginine in, 699–700
magnesium in, 700
meal strategies in, 700
salt restriction in, 698–699, 698t, 699b
thiamin in, 700
vitamin D in, 700
in middle age vs. older adulthood, 698t
pathophysiology of, 694–697, 694f
prevention of, 697
risk factors for, 696b, 697
skeletal muscle changes in, 696t
structure of heart pump and, 693f
symptoms of, 696
hypertension as, 683–693
in children and adolescents, 692–693
defined, 683
essential, 684
manifestations of, 685t
medical management of, 689, 690f
medical nutrition therapy of, 689–692

Cardiovascular disease (Continued)
  in older adults, 693
  pathophysiology of, 685–686, 686f, 695f
  pre-, 683, 683t
  prevalence and incidence of, 684–685, 684f
  primary prevention of, 686–689, 687t
  risk factors and adverse prognosis in, 685b
  secondary, 684
  lipid indices of risk for, 68–69
  managed with Mediterranean diet, 1082
  in older adults, 378
  risk factors for, 674
    identification of, 674, 675b
    major, 675b
    modifiable
      cardiovascular, 675b
      lifestyle, 675b
    nonmodifiable, 678–679
    related conditions as, 675b
  types and incidence of, 670, 671b
Cardiovascular drugs, 1031–1041t
Cardiovascular function, during pregnancy, 250
Caries see Dental caries
Cariogenic foods, 484
Cariogenicity, of food, 483, 484b
  factors affecting, 484–485
    exposure as, 484
    form and consistency as, 484
    nutrient composition as, 484–485
    sequence and frequency of eating as, 485
Cariostatic foods, 484
Carnegie Stages, 246, 246–249t
Carnitine, 917
Carotene, 1028t
β-Carotene
  and coronary heart disease, 682
  deficiency of, with HIV, 802t
Carotenoids
  β-carotene, 1106t
  in fruits and vegetables, 1106–1107t
  nutritional facts on, 1105
  in vitamin A deficiency, 67
Carrier, 88
Cartilage, 472
Carvedilol (Coreg), 1031–1041t
Case management, 156–157
Casein, 906
  in human vs. cow's milk, 315
Casein free diet, for autism, 969t
Casein hydrolysate, infant formulas made from, 316–317
Casein phosphopeptide-amorphous calcium phosphate (CPP-ACP, Recaldent), for remineralization, 484
Cashew milk, 1052–1053t
Cataract, 378
Catch-up growth, 310, 325
Catecholamine(s)
  description of, 807
  in metabolic response to stress, 808
Cation(s), 33t
Cation exchange resin, for end-stage renal disease, 749t
CBC see Complete blood count
CBT see Cognitive behavioral therapy
CCK see Cholecystokinin
CCPD see Continuous cyclic peritoneal dialysis

CCR5 antagonists, medication interactions and common adverse effects of, 791
CD4+ cells, in HIV, 788
CD4 count, in HIV, 790
Cecum, 9
Cefazolin (Ancef), 1031–1041t
Cefdinir (Omnicef), 1031–1041t
Cefepime (Maxipime), 1031–1041t
Cefpodoxime (Vantin), 1031–1041t
Cefprozil (Cefzil), 1031–1041t
Ceftazidime (Fortaz), 1031–1041t
Ceftriaxone (Rocephin), 1031–1041t
Cefuroxime (Ceftin), 1031–1041t
Celecoxib (Celebrex), 1031–1041t
Celery/celeriac, avoidance guidelines for, 508t
Celiac disease, 553–558
  assessment of, 555
  in autism, 857
  care management algorithm for, 557f
  clinical insight on, 555b
  defined, 554
  etiology of, 554, 554b
  gluten-free diet for, 556b
  hidden gluten exposure and cross-contamination with, 558b
  medical nutrition therapy for, 555–558
  pathophysiology of, 554–555, 554f, 557f
  and pregnancy, 276
  refractory, 555
  resources on, 558, 559b
  unintentional weight loss due to, 416t
Celiac panel, 1028t
Cell(s), 83f
  T cells, 841
Cell division, 83f
Cell-mediated reaction, 505
Cell-mediated response, to metabolic stress, 807–809
Cell-signaling molecules, 106
Cellulose, digestion of, 12
Celsus, Aulus Cornelius, 106b
Centenarians, 373, 375b
Centers for Disease Control and Prevention, 131, 760f
  community guide, 129
  food security operations of, 142
  foodborne illness statistics of, 133
  national nutrition monitoring by, 131
Centers for Medicare and Medicaid Services (CMS), 151
Central nervous system (CNS)
  cranial nerves, 849t
  description of, 846–849
  mass lesions, 850
  radiation therapy to, 778t
Central parenteral nutrition (CPN), 216
  description of, 810
  long-term, 217
  short-term, 217, 217f
Cephalexin (Keflex), 1031–1041t
Cephalosporins, 1031–1041t
Cereals
  carbohydrates and, 1050–1051t
  infant, 317
    introduction of, 318
Cerebellum
  anatomy of, 851f
  lesions of, 850

Cerebral palsy, 966–967, 966f
  anthropometric measures in, 967
  ataxic, 966b
  biochemical measures in, 967
  defined, 966
  dietary intake in, 967
  dyskinetic, 966b
    athetoid, 966b
  health concerns with, 967
  intervention strategies for, 967
  mixed, 966b
  nutrition assessment for, 967
  nutrition diagnoses with, 955–957t
  spastic, 966b
  types of, 966b
Certified specialist in oncology nutrition (CSO), 768
Ceruloplasmin, 836
  in copper deficiency anemia, 666
  in liver function, 580–581t
  in metabolic response to stress, 809
CF see Cystic fibrosis
CF-related diabetes, 708–709
CFS see Chronic fatigue syndrome
CGM see Continuous glucose monitoring
Chamomile, 198–205b
CHD see Coronary heart disease
Chelated minerals, 196
Chelation, 14
Chemical exposures, in carcinogenesis, 762
Chemoprevention, of cancer, 762–765
  coffee and tea in, 764
  fruits and vegetables in, 765
  soy and phytoestrogens in, 765
  vitamin D in, 764
Chemotherapy, 767
  drug resistance to, 767–768
  nutritional impact of, 774–776, 775–776t
    diarrhea as, 776–777
    food-drug interactions as, 777
    mucositis as, 777
    nausea and vomiting as, 777
    oral changes as, 777
Cherries, fruits and, 1051–1052t
Chest, nutrition-focused physical examination of, 1003–1008t
CHI see Creatinine-height index
Chi (qi), 188–189t
Child and Adult Care Food Program, 134–135t
Childhood disintegrative disorder, 968t
Children, 324
  breakfast of, 334
    and learning, 334b
  cancer in, 781–782
  chronic kidney disease and end-stage renal disease in, 751
  clinical case study on, 338b
  constipation in, 336, 545
    medical management of, 547
  with developmental disabilities, feeding position for, 959f
  diabetes mellitus in
    energy balance and weight in, 615
    type 1, 627
    type 2, 628
  diarrhea in, 553, 553t
  docosahexaenoic acid intake in, 885–886
  eating disorders in, 423t

Children (Continued)
  eicosapentaenoic acid intake in, 885–886
  estimated energy requirement for, 23–24b
  feeding of
    in group setting, 332, 333f
    preschool, 331–332, 332f
    school-age, 333–334
  fluid intake during exercise and sports for, 455
  food insecurity of, 329–330
  food intake of
    factors influencing, 329–331
      family environment as, 329, 329f
      illness or disease as, 331
      media messages as, 330
      peer influence as, 330
      socioeconomic influences as, 329–330
    patterns of, 328–329
  growth of, 324–325
    assessing, 324–325, 325f, 326f
    catch-up, 310, 325
    patterns of, 324
  HIV in, 803
  hunger in, effect on cognition and behavior, 330b
  hypertension in, 692–693
  nutrient requirements of, 326–328
    for energy, 326, 327b
    for minerals and vitamins, 326–328
      calcium as, 327
      iron as, 327
      vitamin D as, 327
      zinc as, 327
    for protein, 326, 327t
  nutrition education for, 334–335
  nutritional concerns in, 335–337
    allergies as, 336–337
    attention-deficit/hyperactivity disorder as, 337
    dental caries as, 336
    iron deficiency as, 336
    overweight and obesity as, 335–336
    underweight and failure to thrive as, 336
  nutritional concerns in, overweight and obesity as, 398b
  oral health for, 485t
  physical activity in, 25
  portion sizes for, 333t
  prevention of chronic disease in, 337–338
    calcium and bone health in, 337
    cardiovascular health and, 337
    fiber in, 337
    gut microbiome in, 337
    physical activity in, 337–338, 338f
  providing adequate diet for, 328–335, 328t
  school lunch for, 333
  snacks of, 334
  undernutrition in, 336
  vegetarian diet in, 1097
  vitamin-mineral supplements for, 327–328
"Chinese restaurant syndrome," 514
Chiropractic, 188–189t, 190
Chitosan, for weight loss, 408t
Chloride (Cl⁻), 1028t
  in chemistry panels, 59–60t
  electrolyte classification of, 33t
  in parenteral solutions, 218t
Chlorophyll, vitamin K from, 1112–1113
Chlorothiazide (Diuril), 1031–1041t

Chlorthalidone (Hygroton), 1031–1041t
Cholangitis, 599
  sclerosing, 582f, 585
Cholecalciferol (D₃), 1028t
Cholecystectomy, 596
Cholecystitis, 597–599
  acalculous, 596
  acute, 597–598
  calculous, 597
  chronic, 598–599
  defined, 597
  medical nutrition therapy for, 597–599
  pathophysiology of, 597
  surgical management of, 597
Cholecystokinin (CCK)
  in digestion of lipids, 7, 13
  in regulation of body weight, 396–397t
  regulation of gastrointestinal activity by, 7, 7t
Choledocholithiasis, 596
Cholelithiasis, 596
  defined, 596
  medical and surgical management of, 596
  medical nutrition therapy for, 596
  pathophysiology of, 596
Cholestasis
  laboratory tests of, 580–581t
  pathophysiology and medical management of, 596
Cholestatic liver disease, 585
  primary biliary cirrhosis as, 582f, 585
  sclerosing cholangitis as, 582f, 585
Cholesterol
  in adolescence, 354, 357b, 357t
  in adults, 676
  in breastmilk, 290
  and coronary heart disease, 672–673
  with diabetes mellitus, 635t
  digestion of, 13
  in human vs. cow's milk, 315
  laboratory testing of, 1028t
  total
    in chemistry panels, 59–60t
    and coronary heart disease, 673
    laboratory testing of, 1028t
Cholesterol esterase, in digestion, 6t
Cholesterol gallstones, 596
Cholestyramine (Questran), 1031–1041t
Choline, 918
  dietary reference intakes of, 1102t
  food sources of, 1103t
  intake of, 1102–1103
  needs, 1102
  nutritional facts on, 1102, 1102t, 1103t
  during pregnancy, 261
Cholinesterase inhibitors, 1031–1041t
Chondroitin
  for osteoarthritis, 832
  as sports supplement, 457–458t
Chromium, 198–205b
  for diabetes mellitus, 618
  dietary reference intake of, 1119t
  nutritional facts on, 1119
  in parenteral solutions, 219t
  selected food sources of, 1119t
Chromosomal abnormalities, 960–964
  autism spectrum disorders as, clinical scenario on, 976
  Down's syndrome as, 960–964, 960f

Chromosomal abnormalities (Continued)
  anthropometric measures in, 962
  biochemical measures in, 962
  care management algorithm for, 962f
  clinical scenario on, 976
  constipation in, 963
  defined, 960
  dietary intake in, 962, 962t
  eating skills in, 962–963
  feeding skills in, 962
  health concerns with, 962t
  intervention strategies for, 962–963
  medical nutrition therapy for, 962
  medical treatment for, 960, 960t
  overweight in, 962
  pathophysiology of, 960
  Prader-Willi syndrome as, 963, 963f
    anthropometric measures in, 963
    appetite and obesity in, 963
    biochemical measures in, 963
    defined, 962t
    dietary intake in, 963–964
    feeding skills in, 964
    genetics of, 963
    intervention strategies for, 964
    metabolic abnormalities in, 963
    nutrition assessment for, 963–964
    nutrition diagnoses with, 955–957t
    pathophysiology of, 963
Chromosomal level, disease at, 92–93
Chromosomes, 82
Chronic bronchitis, 713
Chronic care model (CCM), 157b
Chronic disease
  allostasis in, 105, 106
  anemia of, 667, 776–777
    ferritin in, 667
  autophagy in, 105
  body composition and, 110–111
  common denominator of, 106–113
  epidemic of, 104–105, 104b
  genesis of, 105
  inflammation and pathophysiology of, 104
  as "lifestyle diseases," 104–105
  long-latency nutrient insufficiencies and, 105
  nutrient-partner principle and, 106, 106b
  nutritional genomics and, 94–101
  pathophysiology concepts in, 105–106
  as "smoldering disease," 107
  systems biology in, 105
  triage theory of, 106
Chronic disease, global health, 367
Chronic disease risk assessment, 68–70
  C-peptide in, 70
  diabetes in, 69–70
  hemoglobin A1C and diabetes in, 69
  lipid indices of cardiovascular risk in, 68–69, 69b
  oxidative stress in, 68t
Chronic fatigue syndrome (CFS), 882, 903–907, 905b
Chronic inflammatory demyelinating polyneuropathy, 871–872
Chronic kidney disease, and potassium, 1126
Chronic kidney disease (CKD), 737–740
  anemia of, 750
  causes of, 738b
  in children, 751

Chronic kidney disease (Continued)
diabetes and, 737
and heart disease, 739b
medical management of, 738–739
medical nutrition therapy for, 739–740
energy in, 739
lipids in, 740
phosphorus in, 740
potassium in, 740
protein in, 739
sodium in, 739–740
vitamins in, 740
pathophysiology of, 737
prevalence of, 738–739
stages of, 738t
Chronic obstructive pulmonary disease (COPD), 713–716
advanced stage of, 716
medical management of, 713–714, 714f
medical nutrition therapy for, 714–716, 715t
energy, 715
fat, 715
macronutrients, 715
protein, 715
vitamins and minerals, 715–716
pathophysiology of, 713, 713f
risk factors for, 713t
Chronic pancreatitis, 600–602
Chronic pulmonary disease, 707–711
cystic fibrosis, 707, 708f
medical management of, 709–711
pathophysiology of, 708–709
bone disease, 709
pancreatic disease, 708–709
pulmonary and sinus disease, 708, 708f
Chylomicrons, in coronary heart disease, 673
Chylothorax, 720
medical management of, 720
medical nutrition therapy for, 720
Chyme, 3
Chymotrypsin, in digestion, 6t
of proteins, 12
Chymotrypsinogen, activated, 6t
Cigarette smoking, reflux and, 530
Cilia, 706
Cinnamon, 198–205b
Ciprofloxacin (Cipro), 1031–1041t
Circadian rhythms, overweight and obesity due to, 400
Cirrhosis
alcoholic, 585
ascites due to, 587–588
in alcoholic liver disease, 585
medical nutrition therapy for, 588
pathophysiology and medical treatment of, 587
biliary
primary, 582f, 585
secondary, 596
clinical manifestations of, 586, 587–589
fat malabsorption due to, 589
medical nutrition therapy for, 589
pathophysiology of, 589
glucose alterations due to, 589
medical nutrition therapy for, 589
pathophysiology of, 589
hepatic encephalopathy due to, 588
medical nutrition therapy for, 588

Cirrhosis (Continued)
pathophysiology and medical treatment of, 588
stages of, 588b
hyponatremia due to, 588
medical nutrition therapy for, 588
pathophysiology of, 588
nutrient requirements with, 592–593
for carbohydrates, 592
for energy, 592
herbal supplement for, 593–594
for lipids, 592
for protein, 592
for vitamins and minerals, 592–593
nutrition assessment for, 589–590
factors that affect interpretation of, 590t
of malnutrition, 590–591, 590f, 591f
route of nutrition, 590–592
subjective global assessment parameters for, 589–590, 590b
osteopenia due to, 589
medical nutrition therapy for, 589
pathophysiology of, 589
portal hypertension due to, 587
in alcoholic liver disease, 585
pathophysiology and medical treatment of, 587
renal insufficiency and hepatorenal syndrome due to, 589
Citalopram (Celexa), 1031–1041t
Citrate intake, and kidney stones, 735
Citrullinemia, 936–938t, 947
CKD see Chronic kidney disease
Cl⁻ see Chloride
Clarithromycin (Biaxin), 1031–1041t
Clear liquid diets, 159
Cleft lip (CL), 971–973, 971f
bilateral, 971
medical nutrition therapy for, 971–973, 972t, 973t
nutrition assessment for, 971
unilateral, 971
Cleft palate, 971–973, 971f
medical nutrition therapy for, 971–973, 972t, 973t
nutrition assessment for, 971
submucous (incomplete), 971
Client's perspective, 230
Climate, and resting energy expenditure, 18
Clindamycin (Cleocin), 1031–1041t
Clinical chemistry panels, 59, 59–60t
Clinical domain, of nutrition diagnosis, for cancer, 770b
Clinical latency, of HIV infection, 788–790
Clonazepam (Klonopin), 1031–1041t
Clonidine (Catapres), 1031–1041t
Clopidogrel (Plavix), 1031–1041t
Closed enteral system, 214
Clostridium botulinum, 136–138t
Clostridium difficile, diarrhea due to, 548–549
probiotics for, 550, 550b
Clostridium perfringens, 136–138t
Clozapine (Clozaril), 1031–1041t
Clubbing, 708, 708f
CMP see Comprehensive metabolic panel
CMS see Centers for Medicare and Medicaid Services
CNS see Central nervous system
CNS stimulants, 1031–1041t
CO₂ see Carbon dioxide

Cobalamin see Vitamin B₁₂
Coconut milk, fats and, 1058–1059t
Codeine/apap (Tylenol), 1031–1041t
Codex Alimentarius Commission (Codex), 195
Coding, 157b
Coding region, 83
Codon, 83–84
Coenzyme Q₁₀ (CoQ₁₀), 120–121, 198–205b
for heart failure, 700
for hypertension, 691t
Coffee see also Caffeine
in cancer prevention, 764
Coffee creamer, sweet, desserts, and other carbohydrates, 1053–1054t
Cognition
in dementia, 898b
parameters of, 899
Cognitive behavioral therapy (CBT), 228
for bulimia nervosa, 426, 435
Cognitive development, and feeding and nutrition of children, 328t
Cognitive dissonance, 230
Cognitive impairment, managed with Mediterranean diet, 1082
Cognitive restructuring, for weight loss, 404
Colchicine, for gout, 838
Colectomy, ileal pouch after
defined, 574
medical treatment of, 574–575
Colipase, 8–9
Colitis
collagenous, 565–566
lymphocytic, 565–566
microscopic, 565–567
ulcerative, 562–564
care management algorithm for, 563f
clinical features of, 562f, 562t
complications of, 562t
etiology of, 561–562
extraintestinal manifestations of, 562t
gross pathology of, 562t
histopathology of, 562t
medical management of, 564
medical nutrition therapy for, 564–565
pathophysiology of, 562–564, 563f
and risk of malignancy, 561
surgical management of, 564
vs. Crohn's disease, 562t
Collagen, in bone remodeling, 473
Collagen fibrils, in bone, 472f
Collagenous colitis, 565–566
Collecting duct, 727, 728f
Colloidal osmotic pressure, 31b
Colon, 9. see also Large intestine
Colon cancer see Colorectal cancer
Colonic salvage, of malabsorbed energy sources and short-chain fatty acids, 11
Colorectal cancer, 568–569
etiology of, 568–569
medical management of, 569
medical nutrition therapy for, 569
pathophysiology of, 569
Colostomy
defined, 572
medical nutrition therapy for, 573–574, 573t
medical treatment of, 572–573
nutritional consequences of, 572, 572f
pathophysiology of, 572

Colostrum, 292, 314
Combination foods, on exchange list, 1049, 1059, 1060–1061t
Combined hyperlipidemia, familial, 674
Commission E Monographs, 191
Commodity Supplemental Food Program (CSFP), 134–135t, 385
Communication
  and behavior change, 231b
  nonverbal, 231b
Community needs assessment, 130, 130b
Community nutrition, 127
  assessment sources, 131b
  description of, 127
  Institute of Medicine report on, 127
  needs assessment for, 129–130
  nutrition professionals in, 128
Comorbidity(ies), 402
Comparative standards, 147
Compensation, for acid-base imbalance and, 39
Complementary and alternative medicine (CAM), 46t, 54–55, 187, 190
  commonly used, 188–189t, 190f
  for osteoarthritis, 832
  for rheumatic diseases, 828–829
  rheumatoid arthritis managed with, 836–837
  use of, 187–191
Complementary strands, 83f
Complete blood count (CBC), 59, 61t
Complete response, to cancer treatment, 768
Complete spinal cord injury, 864
Component resolved diagnostics (CRD), 516
Compounding methods, for parenteral solutions, 219
Comprehensive metabolic panel (CMP), 59, 59–60t
Computerized provider order entry (CPOE), 209
COMT inhibitor, 1031–1041t
Conception, 245–246, 246–249t
Concern, in behavior change, 233
Concrete operational period, and feeding and nutrition of children, 328t
Concussion, 860
Condiments, free foods and, 1059t
"Conditionally essential," term, 115
Confidentiality, 154
Congenital anomalies
  developmental disabilities due to, 954
  obesity and, 244
Congestive heart failure see Heart failure
Conjugated linoleic acids (CLAs), for weight loss, 408t
Conservative treatment, for end-stage renal disease, 752–753
Consistency modifications, 159
Consolidation, in bone modeling, 472
Constipation, 545–548
  in adults, medical management of, 547
  in children, 336, 545
    medical management of, 547
  defined, 545
  with Down syndrome, 963
  with enteral nutrition, 216
  etiology of, 545
  functional, 547b
  medical nutrition therapy for, 547–548, 548b
  in older adults, 378
  pathophysiology of, 545–547, 546b
  during pregnancy, 270
  primary, 545–547

Consumer price index (CPI), 369
Contaminants, in food, 139
  during pregnancy, 279, 280f
Continuing Survey of Food Intake of Individuals, 131
Continuous ambulatory peritoneal dialysis (CAPD), 740, 743f
  advantages of, 742
  complications of, 742
Continuous Care Retirement Community (CCRC), 386t
Continuous cyclic peritoneal dialysis (CCPD), 740
Continuous glucose monitoring (CGM), 625
Continuous infusion
  of enteral formula, 215
  of parenteral solution, 219
Continuous positive airway pressure (CPAP), 719
Continuous renal replacement therapy (CRRT), 736
Continuous venovenous hemodialysis (CVVHD), 736
Continuous venovenous hemofiltration (CVVH), 736
Contraction alkalosis, 39
Contusion, 860
Convenience foods, in adolescence, 349–350, 349b, 350f
Conversions, for food measurements, 980
Cookies, sweet, desserts, and other carbohydrates, 1053–1054t
Coordination of care
  for end-stage renal disease, 752
  nutrition interventions and, 159–160
COPD see Chronic obstructive pulmonary disease
Copper (Cu)
  deficiency of, 666
  deficiency of, during pregnancy, 263
  in end-stage liver disease, 593
  laboratory testing of, 1028t
  in parenteral solutions, 219t
  during pregnancy, 263
  premature infant requirements for, 918
  rheumatoid arthritis levels of, 836
Copper-chelating agents, for Wilson's disease, 586
Copper deficiency anemia, 666
CoQ10 see Coenzyme Q10
Cor pulmonale, 714
Coronal caries, 486
Coronary artery bypass graft (CABG) surgery, 683
Coronary heart disease (CHD), 670–673
  causes of, 738b
  chronic kidney disease and, 739b
  clinical manifestations of, 673f
  due to genetic hyperlipidemias, 674–683
    familial combined hyperlipidemia as, 674
    familial dysbetalipoproteinemia as, 674
    familial hypercholesterolemia as, 674
    polygenic familial hypercholesterolemia as, 674
  medical diagnosis of, 674
  medical intervention of, 683
  medical management of, 682–683
  medical nutrition therapy for, 679–682
    antioxidants in, 682
    dietary cholesterol in, 679
    fiber in, 679–682
    monounsaturated fatty acids in, 679
    omega-3 fatty acids in, 679

Coronary heart disease (Continued)
    polyunsaturated fatty acids in, 679
    saturated fatty acids in, 679
    stanols and sterols in, 682
    trans fatty acids in, 679–680
    weight loss in, 682
  pathophysiology of, 671–673
    lipoproteins in, 673
    total cholesterol in, 673
    triglycerides in, 673
  pharmacologic management of, 682–683
  prevention and risk factor management of, 674–676
    in adults, 676
    in children, 674–675
    Framingham Heart Study on, 674–675, 675b
    inflammatory markers for, 676, 676b
    lifestyle guidelines in, 676–677, 677b
    nonmodifiable risk factors in, 678–679
    risk factor identification for, 674, 675b
Corpus, of stomach, 8
Corrected calcium formula, 33–34
Correction factor, in self-monitoring of blood glucose, 625
Cortical blindness, 850
Cortical bone, 471, 472f
Corticosteroids, 1031–1041t
  for rheumatic diseases, 826t, 827
Corticotropin-releasing factor (CRF)
  description of, 894
  in regulation of body weight, 396–397t
Cortisol, 652, 827
  excess, 651–652
  in metabolic response to stress, 807–808
CORTRAK system, 211f
Counseling, for behavior change, 226
  assessing readiness for, 232
  clinical scenario on, 236b
  defined, 226
  evaluation of effectiveness of, 235–236
  factors affecting
    communication as, 231b
    counselor, 230b
    cultural competency as, 229–230
    health literacy as, 232
  models for, 227–228, 228t
    health belief model as, 227, 228t
    social cognitive theory as, 227, 228t
    theory of planned behavior as, 227–228, 228t
    transtheoretical (stages of change) model as, 228, 228t
  new directions on, 235b
  not-ready-to-change sessions in, 232–233
    affirming in, 231–232
    asking open-ended questions in, 231
    building rapport in, 231
    concern in, 233
    eliciting self-motivational statements in, 232
    ending session in, 233
    intention to change in, 233
    optimism in, 233
    problem recognition in, 232
    reflective listening in, 231
    summarizing in, 232
  ready-to-change sessions in, 235
    action plan in, 235
    setting goals in, 235
  resistance to, 234

Counseling, for behavior change (Continued)
    agreeing with a twist for, 234
    double-sided reflection for, 234
    ending session in, 234
    reflecting for, 234
    reframing for, 234
    shifting focus for, 234
    stages of, 228f
    strategies for
        acceptance and commitment therapy as, 228–229
        cognitive behavioral therapy as, 228
        developing discrepancy in, 229
        empathy and rapport in, 230
        motivational interviewing as, 229
        self-efficacy in, 229
    unsure-about-change sessions in, 233–234
Counterregulatory hormones
    insulin and, 613
    in metabolic response to stress, 807–808
Country mallow, for weight loss, 408t
Cow's milk
    composition of, 315
    human vs., 315
    for infants, 317
Cow's milk protein allergy (CMPA), 501
COX see Cyclooxygenase
COX-1, 825b, 826
COX-2, 825b, 826
COX-2 inhibitor, 1031–1041t
COX-3, 825b
CPN see Central parenteral nutrition
CPP-ACP see Casein phosphopeptide-amorphous calcium phosphate
CPS deficiency see Carbamoyl-phosphate synthetase (CPS) deficiency
Crackers, carbohydrates and, 1050–1051t
Cranberry, 198–205b
Cranial nerves, 849t
    nutrition-focused physical examination, 1003–1008t
Cravings, during pregnancy, 270, 271t
Cream, fats and, 1058–1059t
Cream cheese, fats and, 1058–1059t
Creamers, free foods and, 1059t
Creatine, 198–205b
    as sports supplement, 463
Creatine kinase, 441
Creatine phosphate, 441
Creatinine (Cr), 63t, 68
    in chemistry panels, 59–60t
    in end-stage renal disease, 745–747t
    laboratory testing of, 1028t
    in renal disorders, 728
Creatinine-height index (CHI), 63t, 68
Cretinism, 646, 847t
CRF see Corticotropin-releasing factor
CRISPR, 91b
Critical care
    definition of, 807
    equipment used in, 808f
    glycemic control in, 812–813
    multiple organ dysfunction syndrome, 810
    systemic inflammatory response syndrome, 810, 810b
Critical illness
    due to abdominal trauma and open abdomen, 816

Critical illness (Continued)
    due to burns, 816–819
        medical management of, 817
            ancillary measures in, 817
            fluid and electrolyte repletion in, 817
            wound management in, 817
        medical nutrition therapy for, 817–819
            energy requirements in, 816–817
            methods of, 819
            micronutrients and antioxidants in, 819
        pathophysiology of, 816–817
    ebb phase of, 807, 814f
    enteral nutrition in, 810
    equipment used in, 808f
    feeding strategies in, 815
    flow phase of, 807, 814f
    hypermetabolic response in, 814f
    malnutrition in, 810–816
        medical management of, 814f
        medical nutrition therapy for
            nutrition support therapy in, 812–813
            nutritional requirements in
                formula selection for, 816
                minerals, 815
                protein, 815
                trace elements, 815
                vitamins, 815
        metabolic response to stress in, 807
            hormonal and cell-mediated response in, 807–809
            starvation vs., 809
        neuroendocrine consequences of, 808f
        nutrition management of, 814f
        nutrition requirements of
            energy, 813, 813t
            minerals, 815
            protein, 815
            trace elements, 815
            vitamins, 815
        nutrition support therapy in, 812–813
        obese patients with, 813–814
        surgery for, 819–821
        systemic inflammatory response syndrome, 809–810, 810b
        timing and route of feeding in, 815–816, 815t
Critical pathways, 155–156
Crohn's disease, 562
    care management algorithm for, 563f
    clinical features of, 562f, 562t
    complications of, 562t
    etiology of, 561–562
    extraintestinal manifestations of, 562t
    gross pathology of, 562t
    histopathology of, 562t
    medical management of, 564
    medical nutrition therapy for, 564–565
    pathophysiology of, 562, 563f
    and risk of malignancy, 561
    surgical management of, 564
    vs. ulcerative colitis, 562t
Cross-reactivity, 503
    definition of, 497b
Crosslink/glycosylation theory, of aging, 375t
CRP see C-reactive protein
CRRT see Continuous renal replacement therapy
Cryptosporidiosis, with HIV infection, 793t
Cryptosporidium parvum, 136–138t
Crypts, 3, 5f

CSFP see Commodity Supplemental Food Program
Cu see Copper
Cultural awareness, 230
Cultural competence
    and behavior change, 229–230
    models of, 181–182
    planning diet with, 162, 185b
Cultural context, 181
Culture, dietary planning considerations, 180–185, 181t
Culture change, 381b
Cup, weaning from breast or bottle to, 320
Curcumin, 54t, 120, 852f, 900–901, 903
Cushing's syndrome, 651–652
CVD see Cardiovascular disease
CVVH see Continuous venovenous hemofiltration
CVVHD see Continuous venovenous hemodialysis
Cyanocobalamin, 592t, 888
Cyanosis, 716
Cyclic infusion, of parenteral solution, 220
Cyclooxygenase (COX), 824
Cyclophosphamide (Cytoxan), 1031–1041t
Cyclosporine, 594t, 1031–1041t
Cyclothymic disorder, 890–892t
Cystathionase, 916
Cystathionine synthase deficiency, 936–938t
Cysteine, 920
    in human vs. cow's milk, 315
    in infancy and childhood, 939t
Cysteine stones, 732
Cystic fibrosis (CF), 707, 708f
    care management algorithm for, 710f
    food intolerance due to, 496–497t
    medical management of, 709–711
    medical nutrition therapy for
        energy, 711
        salt, 711
        vitamins and minerals, 711
        zinc, 711
    pathophysiology of, 708–709, 710f
    unintentional weight loss due to, 416t
Cystic fibrosis-related diabetes (CFRD), 708–709
Cystine see Cysteine
Cytochrome P450 enzymes
    definition of, 119
    in inflammation reduction, 119
    single nucleotide polymorphisms, 119
Cytochrome P450 enzymes (CYPs) genes, 96
Cytokines, 106, 809, 832–833, 1028t
    in bone remodeling, 473
    in cancer cachexia, 772
    for cancer therapy, 772, 775–776t
    in food allergy, 499
    in metabolic response to stress, 809
Cytomegalovirus, with HIV infection, 793t
Cytomel (liothyronine), for hypothyroidism, 646t

D

Dabigatran (Pradaxa), 1031–1041t
Daily reference values (DRVs), 177–178, 178t
Daily value (DV), 177, 177t
Dakota, levels of selenium in, 1127
Dapagliflozin (Farxiga), 1031–1041t
DASH see Dietary Approaches to Stop Hypertension
Daughter cells, 83f
Dawn phenomenon, 634

DBPCFC *see* Double-blind, placebo-controlled food challenge
DCCT *see* Diabetes Control and Complications Trial
Debrancher enzyme deficiency, 950
Decarboxylase, 878
Decoctions, 192b
Decubitus ulcer(s), in older adults, 379, 380t
Deep structure culture, 230
Defecation, 9–10
Degenerative arthritis *see* Osteoarthritis
Degenerative joint disease *see* Osteoarthritis
Deglutition, 8
Deglutory dysfunction, 873
Dehydration, 28
  characteristics of, 1043
  defined, 61
  during exercise and sports, 453
    in children, 453
    daily fluid needs and, 454
    electrolyte replacement for, 455–456, 455t
      of potassium, 456
      of sodium, 455–456
    fluid absorption and, 454–455
    fluid balance and, 453–454
    fluid replacement for, 454, 454b
    at high altitudes, 455
    in older athletes, 455
  signs of, 32
7-dehydrocholesterol, 477
Dehydroepiandrosterone (DHEA), 198–205b
  as sports supplement, 465
5-Deiodinase, 642–643
5-Deiodinase inhibitors, 643–644, 644b
Delayed cutaneous hypersensitivity, 1028t
Deletion, 92
Delirium tremens, 893
Delta-6-desaturase, 118
Dementia, 847–848t, 866
  AIDS, 793t
  Alzheimer's disease and, 896–901, 897f
  cognition in, 898b
  ESPEN guidelines on nutrition in, 868t
  homocysteine and, 888
  medical management of, 898
  multiinfarct, 896
  symptoms of, 890–892t
  vascular, 896, 898
Demineralization, of tooth enamel, 482–483, 483f
Dendritic cells (DCs), 499
Dental caries, 482–487
  in children, 336
  decay process in, 485–486
    roles of saliva in, 486
  defined, 482–483
  development of
    by individual foods, 484
      exposure as, 484
      form and consistency as, 484
      nutrient composition as, 484–485
      sequence and frequency of eating as, 485
    oral microbiome and, 483
    substrate and, 483–484, 484b
    susceptible tooth and, 483
  early childhood, 320, 487
    nutrition care and, 487
    pathophysiology and incidence of, 487, 487f
  factors causing, 482–483, 483f

Dental caries (*Continued*)
  lingual, 486
  pathophysiology of, 482–484, 483f
  patterns of, 486
  prevention of, 487–488
    diet for, 487, 488f
    fluoride for, 486–487, 487t
      excess, 487
      food sources of, 486
      mechanism of action of, 486
      supplementation with, 486–487, 487t
      in water, 487t
    guidelines for, 485b
    messages for children on, 485t
  root, 486
Dental erosion, 485–486
Dental health
  for children, 485t
  clinical case study on, 490b
  nutrition for, 482
Dentin, 482, 483f
Dentures, 488
  nutrition care for, 488
Deoxyribonuclease, in digestion, 6t
Deoxyribonucleic acid (DNA), 82
  mitochondrial, 88
  transcription of, 83
Deoxyribonucleic acid (DNA) methylation, 85f, 87b
Deoxyribonucleic acid (DNA) replication, 83f
Department of Homeland Security (DHS), 142
Depot fat, 394
Depression, 901f, 902f
  dopamine's role in, 889
  major depressive disorder, 890–892t, 901, 902b
  managed with Mediterranean diet, 1082
  medical management of, 902–903
  medical nutrition therapy for, 890–892t, 903, 903b
  monoamine deficiency theory of, 902
  in older adults, 379–381
  pathophysiology of, 902
  serotonin's role in, 889
  unintentional weight loss due to, 416t
Dermatitis
  atopic, 498
    skin-prick test with, 515–516, 516f
  herpetiformis, 554
Desensitization, definition of, 497b
Desiccated natural thyroid (Armour Thyroid), for hypothyroidism, 646t
Desserts
  on exchange list, 1049, 1052–1053, 1053–1054t
    nutrition tips, 1053
    selection tips, 1053
  fast foods and, 1061t
Desvenlafaxine (Pristiq), 1031–1041t
Detoxification, in adults, 370
Development *see* Growth and development
Developmental disabilities, 954
  cleft lip and palate as, 971–973, 971f
    medical nutrition therapy for, 971–973, 971t, 972t, 973t
    nutrition assessment for, 971
  clinical scenarios on, 976
  due to chromosomal abnormalities, 960–964
    autism spectrum disorders as, clinical scenario on, 976

Developmental disabilities (*Continued*)
  Down's syndrome as, 960–964, 960f
    anthropometric measures in, 962
    biochemical measures in, 962
    care management algorithm for, 962f
    clinical scenario on, 976
    constipation in, 963
    defined, 960
    dietary intake in, 962, 962t
    eating skills in, 962–963
    feeding skills in, 962
    health concerns with, 962t
    intervention strategies for, 962–963
    medical nutrition therapy for, 962
    medical treatment for, 960, 960t
    nutrition diagnoses with, 959
    overweight in, 962
    pathophysiology of, 960
  Prader-Willi syndrome as, 963, 963f
    anthropometric measures in, 963
    appetite and obesity in, 963
    biochemical measures in, 963
    defined, 963
    dietary intake in, 963–964
    feeding skills in, 964
    genetics of, 963
    intervention strategies for, 964
    metabolic abnormalities in, 963
    nutrition assessment for, 963–964
    nutrition diagnoses with, 955–957t
    pathophysiology of, 963
  due to neurologic disorders, 964–973
    attention-deficit/hyperactivity disorder as, 969–971
      anthropometric measures in, 970
      biochemical measures in, 970
      defined, 969–970
      dietary intake in, 970
      medical nutrition therapy for, 970–971
      nutrition assessment for, 970
    autism as, 967–969
      anthropometric measures in, 968
      biochemical measures in, 968
      defined, 967
      dietary intake in, 968
      nutrition assessment for, 968
      nutrition diagnoses with, 955–957t
      pathophysiology of, 967–968
    cerebral palsy as, 966–967, 966f
      anthropometric measures in, 967
      biochemical measures in, 967
      defined, 966
      dietary intake in, 967
      health concerns with, 967
      intervention strategies for, 967
      nutrition assessment for, 967
      nutrition diagnoses with, 955–957t
      types of, 966b
    spina bifida as, 964–966
      anthropometric measures in, 965
      biochemical measures in, 965
      clinical evaluation of, 965
      defined, 964
      dietary intake in, 965
      health concerns with, 964
      intervention strategies for, 967
      nutrition assessment for, 965

Developmental disabilities (Continued)
　　nutrition diagnoses with, 955–957t
　　prevention of, 964–965
　fetal alcohol syndrome as, 973–975
　　defined, 973
　　diagnosis of, 973–974
　　medical nutrition therapy for, 974
　　nutrition assessment for, 974
　medical nutrition therapy for, 954–960
　nutrition assessment for, 957–959
　　anthropometric measures in, 957
　　biochemical measures in, 958
　　of dietary intake and feeding problems, 958–959
　　　due to oral-motor problems, 958–959
　nutrition diagnoses for, 955–957t, 959
　nutrition interventions for, 959–960
　nutrition monitoring and evaluation for, 960
　position for feeding with, 959f
Developmental inflammatory-related conditions, 122
Developmental landmarks, and addition of semisolid foods, 318, 319t
Developmental origins, of health and disease, 240
Dexamethasone (Decadron), 1031–1041t
Dexfenfluramine, for weight loss, 409
Dexlansoprazole (Dexilant), 1031–1041t
Dexpanthenol, in parenteral solutions, 218t
α-dextrinase, in digestion, 6t
Dextrins, digestion of, 11, 12f
Dextroamphetamine amphetamine (Adderall), 1031–1041t
Dextrose monohydrate, in parenteral solutions, 217
DHA see Docosahexaenoic acid
DHEA see Dehydroepiandrosterone
Diabetes Control and Complications Trial (DCCT), 613
Diabetes insipidus, X-linked recessive nephrogenic, 94
Diabetes mellitus, 606
　categories of glucose intolerance in, 607–611
　and chronic kidney disease, 737
　clinical case study on, 637–638b
　complications of
　　acute, 633–634
　　　hyperglycemia and diabetic ketoacidosis as, 634, 634b
　　　hypoglycemia as, 633–634
　　long-term, 634–636
　　　diabetic kidney disease as, 635
　　　dyslipidemia as, 635
　　　hypertension as, 635
　　　macrovascular diseases as, 635
　　　microvascular diseases as, 635–636
　　　neuropathy as, 635–636
　　　retinopathy as, 635
　and coronary heart disease, 678
　defined, 606
　diagnosis, 1028t
　diagnostic criteria for, 611t, 612
　end-stage renal disease in, 751
　gestational, 270–272, 609–611, 611t
　　blood glucose goals for, 628–629, 628t
　　diagnostic criteria for, 272t, 612
　　incidence and prevalence of, 609
　　and macrosomia, 271, 611
　　management of, 609
　　nutrition intervention for, 628–629

Diabetes mellitus (Continued)
　overweight and obesity and, 270
　screening for, 609
　vs. undiagnosed diabetes, 609
　hemoglobin A1C and, 69
　and hypertension, 685
　immune-mediated, 607
　incidence and prevalence of, 606–607
　latent autoimmune diabetes of aging as, 607
　management of, 613–625
　　medical, 613–614
　　　glycemic control in, 613–614, 614t
　　　insulin in, 622–623, 623t, 624f
　　medical nutrition therapy for, 614–615
　　　alcohol in, 618
　　　carbohydrate intake in, 616–617
　　　dietary fat in, 617–618
　　　fiber in, 617
　　　glycemic index and glycemic load in, 617
　　　goals and desired outcomes of, 615
　　　herbal supplements in, 618–619
　　　micronutrients in, 618–619
　　　nutrition therapy interventions with, 626
　　　protein intake in, 617
　　　sweeteners in, 617
　　medications for, 620–624
　　　glucose-lowering, 620, 621–622t
　　　insulin as, 622–623, 623t, 624f, 1028t
　　monitoring in, 624–625
　　　of A1C, 625
　　　of ketones, lipids, and blood pressure, 625
　　　laboratory testing for, 1028t
　　　self-monitoring of blood glucose for, 613–614, 625
　　physical activity and exercise for
　　　and carbohydrates, 619–620
　　　guidelines for, 619–620
　　　and insulin, 620
　　　potential problems with, 619
　　　precautions with, 620
　　　recommendations for, 620
　　physical activity/exercise for, 619
　　self-management education for, 624
　nutrition care process for, 625–632
　　follow-up encounters in, 632
　　nutrition assessment in, 625–626, 626b
　　nutrition diagnosis in, 612, 626b
　　nutrition education and counseling in, 632, 632f
　　nutrition intervention in, 626–632
　　nutrition monitoring and evaluation in, 632, 633b
　　nutrition prescription in, 629–632, 630f, 631f
　　for specific populations, 626–627, 628t
　in older adults, 629
　oral manifestations of, 489
　PES statements related to, 155t
　pre-, 607
　　defined, 607
　　diagnostic criteria for, 611t
　　incidence and prevalence of, 607
　　management of, 612–613
　　　bariatric surgery for, 616
　　　lifestyle interventions for, 612–613
　　　medical, 613
　　　medical nutrition therapy for, 613
　　　physical activity in, 613
　during pregnancy

Diabetes mellitus (Continued)
　gestational see Diabetes mellitus, gestational
　preexisting, 628
　　nutrition intervention for, 628, 628t
　　vs. gestational, 611
　screening for, 611–612, 612t
　type 1, 607
　　care management algorithm for, 608f
　　genetic predisposition to, 607
　　honeymoon phase of, 607
　　idiopathic, 607
　　immune-mediated, 607
　　incidence and prevalence of, 607
　　nutrition intervention for
　　　with insulin, 627
　　　in youth, 627–628
　　pathophysiology of, 607, 608f
　type 2, 607–609
　　care management algorithm for, 610f
　　exercise guidelines for, 619–620
　　glucose-lowering medications for, 620, 621–622t
　　incidence and prevalence of, 607
　　nutrition intervention for
　　　with glucose-lowering medications, 627
　　　with medical nutrition therapy along, 627
　　　in youth, 628
　　pathophysiology of, 609, 610f
　　progressive, 614
　　risk factors for, 609
　unintentional weight loss due to, 416t
Diabetic ketoacidosis (DKA), 634, 634b
Diabetic nephropathy, 635
Diabetic neuropathy, 635–636
Diabetic retinopathy, 635
Diagnosis terminology, 197b
Diagnostic and Statistical Manual of Mental Disorders, fifth Edition (DSM-5), 422–423b, 895
Diagnostic-related groups (DRGs), 151
Dialysate, 740–742
Dialysis, 740–742
　emergency diets with, 752, 753b
　evaluation of efficiency of, 742
　exercise considerations, 1074
　hemo-, 740, 742f
　　access for, 742f
　　mechanism of action of, 743f
　malnutrition concerns in, 1074
　medical nutrition therapy for, 742, 744f, 745t
　peritoneal, 740, 743f
　renal diet for, 1073
　　albumin, 1073
　　canned foods to lower sodium, 1075–1076, 1076t
　　common serving sizes, 1074
　　estimating serving sizes, 1074
　　nutritional supplements, 1074
　　phosphorus, 1076–1077
　　potassium, 1074
　　proteins, 1073
　　salt habit, 1075
　　vegetables and beans, 1074–1075, 1075t
Diamine oxidase (DAO), 512
Diaphragm, 706f
Diarrhea, 548–553, 551f
　antibiotic-associated, 548–550
　defined, 548

Diarrhea (Continued)
due to cancer or chemotherapy, 776–777
due to Clostridium difficile, 548–549
with enteral nutrition, 216
exudative, 548
with HIV, 548, 795t
in infants and children, 553, 553t
malabsorptive, 548, 549b
medical nutrition therapy for, 552–553, 552t
medical treatment of, 550–552, 550b
osmotic, 548
pathophysiology of, 548, 549b
probiotics for, 550, 550b
secretory, 548
types of, 548, 549b
Diastolic blood pressure (DBP), 683
Diazepam (Valium), 1031–1041t
Diet(s)
adequate and balanced, 162
by adolescence, 351
antiinflammatory, 828, 828b, 835
body fluid viscosity affected by, 112
clear liquid, 159
coronary heart disease and, 677–678
DASH, 364
disease and, relationships between, 179b
elimination, 508t, 516
high-energy, 416–417, 417t
high-fiber, nutritional facts on, 1090, 1090t
high-phosphorus, 1076–1077
high-protein, 1094
ketogenic, 869, 871
low-carbohydrate, high-fat, 407
low-phosphorus, 1076
Mediterranean, 828, 886–887
osteoporosis and, 478
popular, 405t, 406
randomized controlled trial, 400b
regular or general, 159
religion and, 180–181, 181t
restricted-energy, 404–405
vegetarian
in adults, 368
description of, 180
very-low-calorie, 407
very-low-fat, 407
Diet history
for eating disorders, 427
in nutrition assessment, 958–959
in rheumatoid arthritis, 835
Diet-induced thermogenesis (DIT), 18, 429–430
Diet programs, 405–406, 408t
Dietary Approaches to Stop Hypertension
(DASH), 355–357, 364, 677, 1047,
1047–1048t, 1048t
antiinflammatory diet based on, 1080
calcium in, 688–689
for hypertension, 686–688, 690–691
magnesium in, 689
potassium in, 689
sodium in, 688
Dietary fat, 109t, 115–116
Dietary fiber, 548
and bone health, 478
Dietary guidelines, 162–174, 163f, 164f, 166f, 167f,
168f, 169f, 170f, 171f, 172f, 173f
Dietary Guidelines for Americans (DGA), 132,
175, 176, 176b, 368

Dietary Inflammatory Index (DII), 1078
Dietary intake
with attention-deficit/hyperactivity disorder, 970
with autism, 968
with cerebral palsy, 967
data on, 46
with developmental disabilities, 958–959
with Down's syndrome, 962, 962t
with Prader-Willi syndrome, 963–964
with spina bifida, 965
Dietary modifications
in consistency, 159
in hospitalized clients, 158–159
of normal diet, 158
for obesity, 404–405
balanced lower calorie diets as, 407
commercial programs of, 405, 406f
meal replacement programs as, 405
popular diets and practices in, 406, 408t
restricted-energy diets as, 404–405
very low-calorie diets of, 405–406
of regular or general diet, 159
Dietary patterns, 180
Dietary planning
cultural aspects of, 180–185, 181t
national guidelines for, 176
Dietary reference intake (DRIs), 41
Dietary reference intakes (DRIs), 22, 22t, 41, 167, 362
adequate intake, 167
for adolescence, 344, 345t
age groupings, 174
of choline, 1102t
components of, 167–174
definition of, 133
development of, 167
estimated average requirement, 167
for fiber, 1090t
gender grouping, 174
physical activity level and, 24, 24t
during pregnancy, 257
recommended dietary allowances and, 133, 167
reference men and women, 174
for sodium, 35
target population, 174
tolerable upper intake level, 174
Dietary supplement(s)
for cancer, 773–774
for exercise and sports see Ergogenic aids
Dietary supplement facts label, 193f
Dietary Supplement Health and Education Act of
1994 (DSHEA), 193, 193f
Dietary Supplement Label Database, 194–195
Dietary supplementation, 191–193, 205b
assessment of, 196–197b, 196–205
definition of, 191
formulations, 195–196
guidelines for, and botanical products, 198b
popular, and their efficacy, 198–205b
for potentially at-risk populations, 192–193,
193t
quality issues of, 195–196
quantity of ingredients of, 195
recommendation and sale of, 197
regulation, 193–196
resources for clinicians, 197–205
safety of, 194–195
that affect blood clotting, 197b

Dietary supplementation (Continued)
third party certification of, 195
trends in, 191
use of, 195f
Differential count, 59, 61t
Diffuse axonal injury, 860
Diffuse parenchymal lung disease (DPLD),
716–717
medical management of, 717
medical nutrition management for, 717
pathophysiology of, 717
pulmonary diagnostic tests for, 717
Diffusion, 9, 9f
Digestion
of carbohydrates and fiber, 11–12, 11f, 12f
enzymes in, 4, 6t
by infants, 311
of lipids, 13
in mouth, 8
overview of, 3–9
of proteins, 12–13
regulators of, 4–8
sites of, 4f, 5f
in small intestine, 8–9
in stomach, 8
of vitamins and minerals, 13–15
Digestive system, 2–3
anatomy of, 3f
functions of, 3–9
sites of secretion, digestion, and absorption in,
4f, 5f
Digoxin (Lanoxin), 1031–1041t
Dihomo-γ-linolenic acid (DGLA), 825b
Dihydrofolate, 663
Dihydropteridine reductase deficiency, 936–938t, 940f
1,25-Dihydroxy vitamin D_3, in calcium
homeostasis, 472
Diiodotyrosine, 642f
Dilantin see Phenytoin
Diltiazem (Cardizem), 1031–1041t
Dipeptidase, in digestion, 6t
Dipeptides, digestion and absorption of, 12
Dipeptidyl peptidase 4 (DPP-4) inhibitors, for
type 2 diabetes, 621–622t, 622
Direct calorimetry, 19
Direct thrombin inhibitor, 1031–1041t
Disability Adjusted Life Years (DALY), 846
Disaccharides
digestion of, 11, 12f
by infants, 311
Disaster Feeding Program, 134–135t
Disaster planning, 142
Discharge planning, nutrition interventions and,
159–160
Discrepancy, developing, 229
Disease
antecedents of, 105
developmental origins of, 240
diet and, relationships between, 179b
fetal origins of, 240
and food intake of children, 331
inheritance and, 90–94
at chromosomal level, 92–93
at epigenetic level, 94
at mitochondrial level, 93
at molecular level, 93–94
mediators of, 105
triggers of, 105

Disease management, 155–156

Disease-modifying antirheumatic drugs
(DMARDs), 826t, 827, 833

Disease prevention
managed with Mediterranean diet, 1082
for older adults, 374

Disease progression, after cancer treatment,
767–768

Disordered eating, in adolescence, 351, 352–353

Displacement, 860

Disruptive mood dysregulation disorder, 890–892t

Distal convoluted tubule, 728f

Distal intestinal obstruction syndrome (DIOS, 709b

Diuretics, 1031–1041t
for ascites, 587
for hypertension, 689
loop, 1031–1041t

Divalproex, 1031–1041t

Diverticular disease, 568
etiology of, 568
medical and surgical treatment of, 568
medical nutrition therapy for, 568
pathophysiology of, 568

Diverticulitis, 568

Diverticulosis, 378, 568
defined, 568
etiology of, 568
pathophysiology of, 568

DKA see Diabetic ketoacidosis

DLW see Doubly labeled water

DMD see Duchenne muscular dystrophy

DNA see Deoxyribonucleic acid

Docosahexaenoic acid (DHA)
adult intake of, 885–886
childhood intake of, 885–886
conditions treated with, 885b
in dementia patients, 900
description of, 116, 825b, 864
food sources of, 885
for infants, 312
lactation intake of, 885
older adult intake of, 886–887
during pregnancy, 242
with twins, 269t
pregnancy intake of, 885
structure of, 885
supplementation of, 887

Documentation, 151–154
electronic health records and nutrition
informatics for, 153–154
medical record charting as, 152–153
ADIME format for, 152–153, 152b, 153t
PES statements in, 152–153, 155t
POMR for, 152
SOAP note format for, 152, 152t

Dogbane plant, for hypertension, 691t

Dolomite, during pregnancy, 279

Dominant gene, 88

Donepezil (Aricept), 1031–1041t

Donor human milk, 924–925, 924b

Donuts, sweet, desserts, and other carbohydrates,
1053–1054t

Dopamine, 876, 892
in regulation of body weight, 396–397t

Dopamine agonist, 1031–1041t

Dopamine precursor, 1031–1041t

Double-blind, placebo-controlled food challenge
(DBPCFC), 511t, 514

Double-sided reflection, for resistance behaviors, 234

Doubly labeled water (DLW), for measuring
energy expenditure, 21
activity-related, 21

Down's syndrome, 93, 960–964, 960f
anthropometric measures in, 962
biochemical measures in, 962
care management algorithm for, 962f
clinical scenario on, 976
constipation in, 963
defined, 960
dietary intake in, 962, 962t
eating skills in, 962–963
feeding skills in, 962
health concerns with, 962t
intervention strategies for, 962–963
medical nutrition therapy for, 962
medical treatment for, 960, 960t
midfacial hypoplasia in, 962
nutrition diagnoses with, 955–957t
overweight in, 962
pathophysiology of, 960

Doxepin (Silenor), 1031–1041t

Doxycycline (Vibramycin), 1031–1041t

DPP-4 see Dipeptidyl peptidase 4

Dr. Dean Ornish's Program for Reversing Heart
Disease, 407

DRGs see Diagnostic-related groups

DRI(s) see Dietary reference intakes

Dronabinol
for chemotherapy-induced nausea and
vomiting, 416
for unintentional weight loss, 416

Drug(s)
in breastmilk, 297
nutritional implications of, 1031–1041t, 1031
unintentional weight loss due to, 416t

Drug-nutrient interaction (DNI), 194, 1031–1041t

Drug resistance
to antiretroviral therapy drugs, 791
to chemotherapy, 767–768

Dry measure equivalents, 980

Dry mouth, 486, 490
with aging, 378
due to medications, 486, 490b

Dual allergen hypothesis, 521
definition of, 497b

Duchenne muscular dystrophy (DMD), 94

Duloxetine (Cymbalta), 1031–1041t

Dumping syndrome, 539–540
after gastric surgery, 779
clinical case study on, 541–542b
defined, 539
medical management of, 539
medical nutrition therapy for, 539–540, 540b
pathophysiology of, 539

Duodenal resection, nutritional consequences
of, 569

Duodenal ulcers, 536, 536f

Duodenum, digestion in, 8

Duration, of exercise, and energy sources, 443

Dutch famine study, 89b

Dysarthria, 866

Dysbetalipoproteinemia, familial, 674

Dysbiosis, 10
and food allergy, 499–500

Dysgeusia, 376
due to chemotherapy, 777

Dyslipidemia, 672–673
in diabetes mellitus, 635

Dysosmia, 850

Dyspepsia, 532–533
defined, 532
functional, 532–533
medical nutrition therapy for, 532–533
pathophysiology of, 532

Dysphagia, 526, 531
with aging, 378
in amyotrophic lateral sclerosis, 869
definition of, 852–857
diet developments of, 853b
enteral tube nutrition for, 856–857
medical nutrition therapy for, 854–855
National Dysphagia Diet (NDD), 854, 854f
PES statements related to, 155t
in stroke, 858–860
symptoms of, 852
textures of food, 856
unintentional weight loss due to, 416t

Dyspnea
in heart failure, 693–694
in pulmonary disease, 707

Dysthymia, 890–892t

E

EAAs see Essential amino acids

EAL see Evidence Analysis Library

Early childhood caries (ECC), 320, 487, 487f
nutrition care for, 487
pathophysiology and incidence of, 487

East Asian medicine, 188–189t, 188t

Eastern Orthodox dietary practices, 181t

Eat Smart to Play Hard, 337, 338f

Eating, exercise, and body image (EEBI) disorders,
447

Eating behaviors
of adolescence, 348–351
dieting and body image as, 351
family meals as, 350, 350b
fast foods and convenience foods as, 349–
350, 349b, 350f
irregular meals and snacking as, 348–349,
349b
media and advertising and, 350–351
diabetes and, 616
in eating disorders, 428, 428b

Eating disorder(s), 421
in adolescence, 354
anorexia nervosa as, 421, 422–423b
anthropometric assessment of, 430–431,
430b
biochemical assessment for, 428–429
in childhood, 423t
clinical characteristics and medical
complications of, 424–425, 424f
diagnostic criteria for, 422–423b
eating behavior in, 428, 428b
energy expenditure in, 429–430
fluid and electrolyte balance in, 429
medical nutrition therapy for, 430b, 432–434
nutrition assessment for, 427
nutrition education for, 437, 437b
prognosis for, 437
vitamin and mineral deficiencies in, 429
anthropometric assessment for, 430–431,
430b

Eating disorder(s) (Continued)
  binge
    diagnostic criteria for, 423–424
    medical nutrition therapy for, 436
  biochemical assessment for, 428–429
  bulimia nervosa as
    biochemical assessment for, 429
    clinical characteristics and medical
        complications of, 425
    diagnostic criteria for, 421
    eating behavior in, 428, 428b
    fluid and electrolyte balance in, 429
    medical nutrition therapy for, 434–435, 434b
    nutrition assessment for, 427–428, 428b
    nutrition education for, 437, 437b
    prognosis for, 437
  in childhood, 423t
  clinical characteristics and medical
      complications of, 424–425, 424f
  defined, 421
  diagnostic criteria for, 421, 422–423b
  eating behavior in, 428, 428b
  energy expenditure in, 429–430
  fluid and electrolyte balance in, 429
  medical nutrition therapy and counseling for,
      431–437, 431t, 432b, 434b, 435t
  medical nutrition therapy for, 890–892t
  nutrition assessment for, 427–428
  nutrition education for, 437, 437b
  patient monitoring for, 436–437, 436b
  prognosis for, 437
  psychologic management of, 426–427
  treatment approach for, 425–426
  vitamin and mineral deficiencies in, 429
Eating skills, in Down's syndrome, 962–963
Eating Well with Canada's Food Guide, 163–167,
    164f
Eatwell Guide (United Kingdom), 173f
Ebb phase, of stress, 807
EBF see Epithelial barrier function
EBGs see Evidence-based guidelines
EBNPGs see Evidence-based nutrition practice
    guidelines
ECC see Early childhood caries
ECF see Enterocutaneous fistula
Echinacea angustifolia, 198–205b
ECSWL see Extracorporeal shockwave lithotripsy
Eczema, 497b
  skin-prick test with, 516f
Edema, 28, 29b, 29f, 30f, 61–62, 1000–1001t
  in heart failure, 698
  lower extremity, during pregnancy, 250, 273
Edentulism, 488
  nutrition care for, 488
Edoxaban (Savaysa), 1031–1041t
Education tools, culturally specific, 182
EER see Estimated energy requirement
EFAs see Essential fatty acids
EFNEP see Expanded Food and Nutrition
    Education Program
EGD see Esophagogastroduodenoscopy
EGE see Eosinophilic gastroenteritis
Egg, avoidance guidelines for, 508t
EHRs see Electronic health records
Eicosanoid cascade, 116
Eicosanoids, 824
  metabolism of, 116
  in prostaglandin formation, 115–116

Eicosapentaenoic acid (EPA)
  adult intake of, 885–886
  childhood intake of, 885–886
  conditions treated with, 885b
  description of, 116, 825b, 864
  food sources of, 885
  lactation intake of, 885
  older adult intake of, 886–887
  pregnancy intake of, 885
  structure of, 885
  supplementation of, 887
  during twin pregnancy, 269t
El Plato del Bien Corner, 166f
Elastase, in digestion, 6t
Elavil see Amitriptyline
Elderly see Older adults
Electrolyte(s), 33–37, 33t
  calcium as, 33–34, 33t
    absorption and excretion of, 34
    functions of, 33–34
    recommended intakes of, 34
    sources of, 34
  chloride as, 33t
  defined, 33
  in enteral formulas, 218–219
  laboratory testing of, 1028t
  magnesium as, 33t, 35–36
    absorption and excretion of, 36
    dietary reference intakes for, 36
    function of, 35–36
    sources of, 36
  milliequivalents and milligrams of, 979, 979t
  in parenteral solutions, 218–219, 218t, 219t
  phosphorus as, 33t, 36
    absorption and excretion of, 36
    dietary reference intakes for, 36
    functions of, 36
    sources of, 36
  potassium as, 36–37
    absorption and excretion of, 36
    dietary reference intakes for, 37
    functions of, 36
    sources of, 36–37, 37b
  premature infant requirements for, 917, 917t
  sodium as, 33t, 34–35
    absorption and excretion of, 35
    dietary reference intakes for, 35
    functions of, 34–35
    sources of, 35
Electrolyte replacement
  for burns, 817
  for diarrhea, 550
  for exercise and sports, 455–456, 455t
Electrolytically reduced iron, 317
Electronic chart note, 156f
Electronic health records (EHRs), 147, 153–154
Electronic medical record (EMR), 154
Elimination diets, 508t, 516–517
  for autism, 969t
  replacements in, 518–519t
  for rheumatic diseases, 829
Embolic stroke, 857
Emergency diets, for dialysis patients, 752, 753b
Emergency Food and Shelter Program, 134–135t
Emetogenic (nausea-causing) chemotherapy
    agents, 773
Empagliflozin (Jardiance), 1031–1041t
Empathy, 230

Emphysema, 713
EMR see Electronic medical record
Enalapril (Vasotec), 1031–1041t
Enamel, 482, 483f
  demineralization of, 482–483, 483f
  remineralization of, 484
Encephalopathy
  hepatic, 588
    medical nutrition therapy for, 588
    pathophysiology and medical treatment of,
        588
    stages of, 588b
  HIV, 793t
  portal systemic, 588
  Wernicke, 593
End-stage liver disease (ESLD)
  ascites due to, 587f
    medical nutrition therapy for, 588
    pathophysiology and medical treatment of,
        587
  clinical manifestations of, 586, 587f
  fat malabsorption due to, 589
    medical nutrition therapy for, 589
    pathophysiology of, 589
  glucose alterations due to, 589
    medical nutrition therapy for, 589
    pathophysiology of, 589
  hepatic encephalopathy due to, 588
    medical nutrition therapy for, 588
    pathophysiology and medical treatment of,
        588
    stages of, 588b
  hyponatremia due to, 588
    medical nutrition therapy for, 588
    pathophysiology of, 588
  liver resection and transplantation for, 594,
      594t, 595t
  nutrient requirements with, 592–593
    for carbohydrates, 592
    for energy, 592
    herbal supplement for, 593–594
    for lipids, 592
    for protein, 592
    for vitamins and minerals, 592–593
  nutrition assessment for, 589–590
    factors that affect interpretation of, 590t
    of malnutrition, 590–591, 590f, 591f
    route of nutrition, 590–592
    subjective global assessment parameters for,
        589–590
  osteopenia due to, 589
    medical nutrition therapy for, 589
    pathophysiology of, 589
  portal hypertension due to, 587
    in alcoholic liver disease, 585
    medical nutrition therapy for, 587
    pathophysiology and medical treatment of,
        587
  renal insufficiency and hepatorenal syndrome
      due to, 589
End-stage renal disease (ESRD), 740–753
  care management algorithm for, 741f
  in children, 751
  conservative treatment or palliative care for,
      752–753
  coordination of care for, 752
  with diabetes, 751
  dialysis for, 740–741

End-stage renal disease *(Continued)*
  emergency diets with, 752, 753b
  evaluation of efficiency of, 742
  hemo-, 740, 742f
    access for, 742
    mechanism of action of, 743f
    procedure for, 743f
    peritoneal, 740, 743f
  kidney transplantation for, 752
  medical nutrition therapy for, 742, 744f, 745–747t, 745t
    calcium and parathyroid hormone in, 745–747t, 748–750
    energy in, 744–747
    ferritin in, 745–747t
    fluid and sodium balance in, 745–747t, 747–748
    iron and erythropoietin in, 749t, 750
    lipid in, 750
    magnesium in, 745–747t
    phosphorus in, 745–747t, 748, 749t
    potassium in, 745–747t, 748
    protein in, 742–744
    vitamins in, 749t, 750
  medical treatment of, 740–750
  nutrition support in, 750–751
    enteral tube feeding for, 750–751
    intradialytic parenteral nutrition for, 749t, 751
    oral protein supplementation during dialysis, 751
    parenteral nutrition for, 751
  pathophysiology of, 740–741, 741f
  patient counseling for, 752
  patient education for, 752
  treatment in, 744t
Endocrine conditions, and fertility, 244–245
Endocrine specific inflammatory markers, 117t
Endorphins, in regulation of body weight, 396–397t
Endoscopy, 534, 534b
Endothelial cells, 670–671
Energy, 17
  and bone, 476
  burn patient requirements for, 818
  for chronic obstructive pulmonary disease, 715
  critical illness requirements, 813, 813t
  for cystic fibrosis, 711
  defined, 17
  food, calculation of, 25–26
  and heart failure, 700
  premature infant requirements for, 915–916, 916t, 919
  in rheumatoid arthritis, 835
  for tuberculosis, 718
Energy adequacy, body weight and, 17
Energy balance, in diabetes mellitus, 615
Energy continuum, 442, 443f
Energy expenditure, 17
  activity-related
    estimation of, 19–21, 23–24b, 24–25
    in children, 25
    doubly labeled water technique for, 21
    physical activity questionnaire for, 21
    triaxial monitors for, 21
    uniaxial monitors for, 21
    using metabolic equivalents, 24–25
  activity thermogenesis in, 19

Energy expenditure *(Continued)*
  additional considerations in, 19
  basal, 17–18
  components of, 17–21, 18f, 19f
  in eating disorders, 429–430
  measurement of, 19–21
    activity-related, 21
    direct calorimetry for, 19
    doubly labeled water technique for, 21
    indirect calorimetry for, 19–20, 20f
    methods of, 21
    respiratory quotient for, 20–21
  resting, 17–18, 18f, 20t
    defined, 17–18
    estimation of, 21–22
    factors affecting, 18
      age as, 18
      body composition as, 18
      body size as, 18
      climate as, 18
      gender as, 18
      hormonal status as, 18
      other, 18
      temperature as, 18
  thermal effect of food in, 18–19
  total, 17, 19f
    determining, 21–22
    for overweight and obese men, 22
    for overweight and obese women, 22
    weight maintenance, 22
Energy intake
  in carcinogenesis, 759–760
  for chronic kidney disease, 739
  for end-stage renal disease, 744–747
  estimating energy requirements from, 22
  for hypertension, 690
  malnutrition and, 1001–1002t
Energy metabolism, alterations in, due to cancer, 772
Energy needs *see* Energy requirements
Energy production
  adenosine triphosphate in, 441–442
  aerobic pathway of, 442, 442f
  anaerobic or lactic acid pathway of, 442
  energy continuum for, 442, 443f
Energy requirements, 17
  for acute kidney injury, 737
  for adolescence, 344, 345t
  for burn patient, 816–817
  with cancer, 768–769
  for children, 326, 327b, 939t
  defined, 17
  for end-stage liver disease, 592
  estimating, 21–25
    in children, 25
    energy expended in physical activity in, 24–25
      using metabolic equivalents, 24–25
    from energy intake, 22
    equations for estimating resting energy expenditure for, 21–22
    prediction equations for, 22–24
  of exercise, 444–445, 445b
  with HIV, 798
  of infants, 311, 311t, 939t
  for lactation, 289
  for older adults, 383t
  prediction equations for, 22–24

Energy requirements *(Continued)*
  during pregnancy, 257–258
    exercise and, 257–258
    restriction of, 257–258
    with twins, 269t
Energy/sports drinks, sweet, desserts, and other carbohydrates, 1053–1054t
Energy value
  of alcoholic beverages, 25
  of food, 26f
Engaging content, in reading materials, 183
Enhanced Recovery After Surgery (ERAS), 821b, 821f
Entacapone (Comtan), 1031–1041t
Enteral nutrition, 209, 209t
  administration of, 214–215
    via bolus, 214–215
    via continuous drip, 215
    via intermittent drip, 215
  closed enteral system for, 214
  in critically ill patients, 810
  for dysphagia, 856–857
  for end-stage renal disease, 750–751
  formula for, 212–214, 993t, 1045
    carbohydrate in, 213–214
    composition of, 925t
    for critically ill patients, 816
    factors to consider when choosing, 213b
    fluid in, 214
    immune modulating, 816
    lactose free, 212–213
    lipid in, 214
    osmolality of, 212
    polymeric, 212–213
    in premature infants, 925–926
    protein in, 213
    standard, 213
    vitamins, minerals, and electrolytes in, 214
  hang time in, 214
  for inflammatory bowel disease, 564
  long-term, 211–212
    gastrostomy or jejunostomy for, 211–212, 212f
    multiple lumen tube for, 212
    other minimally invasive techniques for, 212
  monitoring and evaluation of, 215–216
    for complications, 215–216, 215b
    for tolerance and nutrient intake goals, 216, 216b
  nutrition care process for, 220b
  open enteral system for, 214
  with pediatric cancer, 782
  postoperative, 820
  for premature infants
    calcium, 921
    carbohydrates, 921
    description of, 919–922
    energy, 919, 920b, 920t
    folic acid, 922
    formula, 925–926
    human milk, 923–924, 925t
    iron, 922
    lipids, 920–921
    minerals, 921–922
    parenteral nutrition transition to, 919
    phosphorus, 921
    protein, 919–920
    selection of, 923–926
    sodium, 922

Enteral nutrition (Continued)
    tolerance of, 923
    transitional infant formulas, 926
    vitamins, 921–922, 921t
    volume of, 919t
  refeeding syndrome with, 220–221
  route selection for, 210f
  short-term, 209–211
    gastric *versus* small-bowel access for, 210
    nasoduodenal or nasojejunal access for, 210–211
    nasogastric access for, 209–210, 211f
  transitional feeding, 221–222
Enteric nervous system, 883–884
Enteritis, chronic radiation, 779
Enterocolitis syndrome, food protein-induced, 508–511
Enterocutaneous fistula (ECF), 571
Enterocytes, 3
Enterohemorrhagic *Escherichia coli* (EHEC), 136–138t
Enterohepatic circulation, 13
Enteroimmunology, 112, 113f
Enterokinase, in digestion, 6t
  of proteins, 12
Enteropathy, HIV-induced, 793t
Enteropeptidase, in digestion, 8–9
Enterostatin, in regulation of body weight, 396–397t
Enterotoxigenic *Escherichia coli* (ETEC), 136–138t
Entrees, combination foods and, 1060–1061t
Environmental factors, and genetics, 83
Enzyme(s), in digestion, 4
Enzyme deficiencies, food intolerances due to, 496–497t
EoE *see* Eosinophilic esophagitis
Eosinopenia, 61t
Eosinophil(s), 61t, 499, 1028t
Eosinophil leukocyte, 1028t
Eosinophilia, 61t
Eosinophilic esophagitis (EoE), 505–507, 528
Eosinophilic gastroenteritis (EGE), 507
Eosinophilic gastrointestinal diseases (EGID), 505–507
EPA *see* Eicosapentaenoic acid
Ephedra, for weight loss, 408t
Epidemiologic studies, of carcinogenesis, 759
Epidermal growth factor inhibitor, 1031–1041t
Epidural hematomas, 860
Epigastric pain, 528
Epigenetic effects, 256–257, 257f
Epigenetic inheritance, 88–90, 89b
Epigenetic marks, 87
Epigenetic modification, of genome, 498
Epigenetic regulation, 85f
Epigenetic silencing, 89b
Epigenetics, 87, 87b, 94
  and cancer, 97
  and obesity, 99–100
  and T2DM, 98
  and vascular disease, 101
Epigenome, 88
Epigenomics, 87, 94
Epilepsy
  characteristics of, 870
  medical management of, 870–871
  medical nutrition therapy for, 847–848t, 871, 871b, 872f
  pathophysiology of, 870

Epinephrine, 882–883
Epithelial barrier function (EBF), 810
Epithelial cells, 3
Epitope(s), in allergic reaction, 498–499
EPO *see* Erythropoietin
EPOC *see* Excess postexercise oxygen consumption
Equivalents, for food measurements, 980
Ergocalciferol, 1028t
Ergogenic aids, 457–458t, 461–463
  defined, 461
  muscle-building supplements as
    amino acids as, 457–458t
    androstenedione as, 465–467
    beta-hydroxy-beta-methylbutyrate, 457–458t
    branched-chain amino acids as, 457–458t, 462t
    creatine as, 463
    dehydroepiandrosterone as, 465
    human growth hormone as, 457–458t, 465
    prohormones as, 465–467
    steroids as, 461–462t, 464–465
Erlotinib (Tarceva), 1031–1041t
Ertugliflozin (Steglatro), 1031–1041t
Eructation, 544
Erythrocyte sedimentation rate, 64
Erythromycin (Ery-Tab), 1031–1041t
Erythropoietin (EPO), 728, 922
  in anemia of chronic kidney disease, 750
  in children, 751
  in end-stage renal disease, 749t, 750
  as sports supplement, 465
Escherichia coli, food intolerance due to, 496–497t
Escherichia coli O157:H7, 136–138t
Escitalopram, 1031–1041t
ESLD *see* End-stage liver disease
Esomeprazole (Nexium), 1031–1041t
Esophageal cancer, surgery for, 779
Esophageal disorders, 525–532
  achalasia as, 525
  anatomy and, 525, 526f
  gastroesophageal reflux and esophagitis as, 526–531
    etiology of, 526
    medical and surgical management of, 529, 529f, 529t
    medical nutrition therapy for, 529–531
    pathophysiology of, 526–528
  odynophagia as, 531–532
  transport in, 3
Esophageal phase, of swallowing, 853f, 854
Esophageal reflux *see* Gastroesophageal reflux disease
Esophageal ulcers, due to HIV infection, 795t
Esophagectomy, 531
  nutrition guidelines after, 532b
Esophagitis, 526
  acute, 528
  eosinophilic, 528
  etiology of, 526
  medical and surgical management of, 529, 529f, 529t
  medical nutrition therapy for, 529–531
  nutrition care guidelines for, 530b
  pathophysiology of, 526–528, 535f
Esophagogastroduodenoscopy (EGD), 526, 534b

Esophagus
  anatomy of, 525, 526f
  Barrett's, 528
  surgery for, 531
    medical nutrition therapy for, 531
ESRD *see* End-stage renal disease
Essential amino acids (EAAs), as sports supplements, 457–458t
Essential fat, 394
Essential fatty acids (EFAs)
  for attention-deficit/hyperactivity disorder, 964
  in brain structure, 882
  with enteral formulas, 214
  inflammation and, 115–116
  nutritional facts on, 1087, 1087t
  for premature infants, 920
Essential oils, 192b
Essiac diet, of anticancer dietary plan, 774t
Ester-C, 1109
Estimated average requirement (EAR), 167
Estimated energy requirement (EER)
  for adolescence, 344, 345t
  for children, 326, 327b
  defined, 22
  metabolic equivalents and, 24–25
  physical activity level and, 24, 24t
  prediction equations for, 23–24b
Estimated glomerular filtration rate (eGFR), 737
Estrogen
  nutritional implications of, 1031–1041t
  and sodium balance, 35
Estrogen agonists, 479
Estrogen receptors (ER), 479
Ethambutol (Myambutol), 1031–1041t
Ethical implications, of genomics, 95b
Etiology, in nutrition diagnosis, 148
Euthyroid sick syndrome, 645
Evidence Analysis Library (EAL), 147
Evidence-based guidelines (EBGs), 151
Evidence-based nutrition practice guidelines (EBNPGs), 151
  for diabetes mellitus, 615
Excess postexercise oxygen consumption (EPOC), 19
Excessive leanness, 415–417
  appetite enhancers in, 416
  assessment of, 415
  cause of, 415
  high-energy diets in, 416–417, 417t
  management of, 415–416, 416t
Exchange lists
  for diabetes mellitus, 615
  for meal planning, 1049
Excipients, 196
Exclusive breastfeeding (EBF), 314–315
Exenatide (Byetta), for type 2 diabetes, 620–622, 621–622t
Exercise and sports performance, 441
  by adolescence, 351
  alcohol and, 464
  bioenergetics of, 441–442
  and breastfeeding, 297
  caffeine and, 464
  clinical case study on, 466–467b
  for diabetes mellitus, 619
    and carbohydrates, 619–620
    guidelines for, 619–620
    and insulin, 620

Exercise and sports performance (Continued)
    potential problems with, 619
    precautions with, 620
    recommendations for, 620
    in dialysis patients, 1074
    duration of, and energy sources, 443
    energy production in
        adenosine triphosphate in, 441–442
        aerobic pathway of, 442, 442f
        anaerobic or lactic acid pathway of, 442
        energy continuum for, 442, 443f
    ergogenic aids for, 457–458t, 461–463
        muscle-building supplements as
            amino acids as, 457–458t
            androstenedione as, 465–467
            beta-hydroxy-beta-methylbutyrate,
                457–458t
            branched-chain amino acids as, 457–458t,
                462t
            creatine as, 463
            human growth hormone as, 457–458t, 465
            prohormones as, 465–467
            steroids as, 461–462t, 464–465
    fluids for, 453–456
        absorption, 454–455
            in children, 455
            in older athletes, 455
        daily needs for, 454
        and electrolyte replacement, 455–456, 455t
            of potassium, 456
            of sodium, 455–456
        and fluid balance, 453–454
        and hydration at high altitudes, 455
        replacement of, 454, 454b
    fuels for contracting muscles in, 442–444
        duration of exercise and, 443
        effect of training on, 443–444
        intensity of exercise and, 443, 443f
        sources of, 442–443
    for hypertension, 687t, 689, 692
    intensity of, and energy sources, 443, 443f
    macronutrients for, 447–448, 448f
        carbohydrates as, 448–451
            during exercise, 450–451, 451f
            postworkout and recovery, 451
            pretraining fasting, 450, 450b
            types of, 450–451
        fat as, 452–453
        protein as, 451–452
            for resistance exercise, 451–452
    nutritional requirements of, 444–445
        energy as, 444–445, 445f
        sports supplements for, 442–444, 448t
    osteoarthritis managed with, 831
    osteoporosis and, 478, 479
    for prediabetes, 615b
    during pregnancy, 257–258
    rheumatoid arthritis managed with, 834
    vitamins and minerals for, 456–459
        antioxidants as, 456–458
        B vitamins as, 456
        calcium as, 459–460
        iron as, 459
        vitamin D as, 458–459, 458b
    for weight loss, 409f
    weight management with, 445–446, 446t
Exercise related transient abdominal pain (ETAP),
    460b

Exons, 83
Exophthalmos, in Graves' disease, 650f
Expanded Food and Nutrition Education
    Program (EFNEP), 231
Expired air specimen, 1009
Expression genome-wide association study
    (eGWAS), 99
Extensively hydrolyzed infant formula, 521
Extracellular electrolytes, 33
Extracellular fluid, 28
Extracorporeal shockwave lithotripsy (ECSWL),
    732
Extracts, 192b
Extrauterine growth restriction, 916
Extremely low birthweight (ELBW), 912, 913b, 930
Eyes, nutrition-focused physical examination of,
    1003–1008t
Eyesight, with aging, 376–378

F

Face, nutrition-focused physical examination of,
    1003–1008t
Facial nerve, 849t
Facilitated diffusion, 9
Factor Xa inhibitor, 1031–1041t
Facultative thermogenesis, 18
FAILSAFE diet, 514
Failure to thrive (FTT)
    in childhood, 336
    in older adults, 381
FALCPA see Food Allergen Labeling and Consumer
    Protection Act
Familial combined hyperlipidemia (FCHL), 674
Familial dysbetalipoproteinemia, 674
Familial hypercholesterolemia (FH), 674
    polygenic, 674
Family-based therapy (FBT), 426
Family environment, and food intake of children,
    329, 329f
Family history, and coronary heart disease, 678
Family meals, during adolescence, 350, 350b
Famotidine (Pepcid), 1031–1041t
Farmers Market Nutrition Program, 134–135t
FAS see Fetal alcohol syndrome
Fast foods
    in adolescence, 349–350, 349b, 350f
    on exchange list, 1049, 1060–1061, 1061t
Fasting, 181, 406
    for hypothyroidism, 646–647
Fasting blood glucose see Fasting plasma glucose
Fasting hypoglycemia, 636–637
    in end-stage liver disease, 589, 589b
Fasting plasma glucose (FPG), 607
Fat(s)
    abdominal, 402
    for adolescence, 346
    body, 394
        skinfold measurements for percentage
            determinations, 996, 996t
    for chronic obstructive pulmonary disease, 715
    depot, 394
    dietary intake of, 109t, 115–116
    in digestion, 920–921
    digestion and absorption of, 13, 14f
        by infants, 311
    essential, 394
    exchange lists for, 1049, 1052, 1052t, 1055–1057,
        1058–1059t

Fat(s) (Continued)
    nutrition tips, 1057
    selection tips, 1057
    malabsorption of, laboratory testing of, 1028t
    in rheumatoid arthritis patients, 835–836
Fat adaptation strategy, 449
Fat deposition, and metabolic syndrome, 402–403
Fat distribution
    android, 402
    gynoid, 402
Fat-free mass (FFM), 18, 394, 394f
Fat-free milk, 1052–1053t
Fat intake
    for anorexia nervosa, 433
    for bulimia nervosa, 433
    in carcinogenesis, 761
    and cardiovascular disease in children, 337
    for diabetes mellitus, 617–618
    for exercise and sports, 452–453
    and heart failure, 700
    with HIV, 801
    and hypertension, 686
    for infants, 312
    and inflammation, 452–453
    for lactation, 289
    for older adults, 380t
    during pregnancy, 258–259
        with twins, 269t
Fat loss, toxins in, 395b
Fat malabsorption, and vitamin A, 1105
Fat malabsorption, in end-stage liver disease, 589
    medical nutrition therapy for, 589
    pathophysiology of, 589
Fat mass, 394
Fat metabolism, insulin and, 614t
Fat-restricted diet, for cholecystitis, 597–598t,
    597–598
Fat-soluble vitamin(s)
    absorption of, 13
    biochemical assessment of, 66–67
    vitamin A as, 67
    vitamin D as, 67
    vitamin E as, 67
    vitamin K as, 67
Fat storage, 394–395
Fatigue
    chronic fatigue syndrome, 882, 903–907, 905b
    mitochondrial dysfunction and, 111
Fatty acid(s)
    abbreviations for, 884b
    analysis of, 1028t
    dietary fat intake assessments, 115–116
    digestion and absorption of, 13
    essential
        for attention-deficit/hyperactivity disorder,
            964
        in brain structure, 882
        with enteral formulas, 214
        inflammation and, 115–116
        nutritional facts on, 1087, 1087t
        for premature infants, 920
    in food allergy, 522
    inflammation and, 836b
    monounsaturated, and coronary heart disease,
        679
    omega-3, 1057
        adult intake of, 885–886
        in cancer prevention, 761

Fatty acid(s) *(Continued)*
  cognition affected by, 899
  and coronary heart disease, 679
  description of, 884–885
  food sources of, 1088, 1088t
  for gastritis and peptic ulcers, 537b
  and hypertension, 687t
  inflammation and, 836b
  and kidney stones, 735–736
  in lactation, 885
  as ligands, 86
  nutritional facts on, 1087, 1087t, 1088, 1088t
  older adult intake of, 886–887
  in pregnancy and lactation, 242
  pregnancy intake of, 885
  supplementation of, 887
  omega-6
    dietary sources of, 1088
    nutritional facts on, 1087, 1087t, 1088t
  polyunsaturated, and coronary heart disease, 679
  in regulation of body weight, 396–397t
  saturated, and coronary heart disease, 679
  short-chain
    colonic salvage of, 11
    production of, 4
  trans, and coronary heart disease, 679–680
Fatty acid oxidation, genetic disorders of,
    936–938t, 950–951, 951f
Fatty liver disease
  alcoholic, 583–585
  nonalcoholic, 402, 582–583
Fatty streaks, in atherosclerotic cardiovascular
    disease, 671, 671f
FCHL *see* Familial combined hyperlipidemia
FDC yellow no. 5, food intolerance due to,
    496–497t
FDEIA *see* Food-dependent, exercise-induced
    anaphylaxis
Fecal elastase, 709b
Fecal fat screening, 1028t
Fecal impaction, 548
Fecal microbiota transplant (FMT), 550
Feces
  composition of, 9–10
  samples of, 58
  specimen of, 1009
Federal Emergency Management Agency
    (FEMA), 142
Feeding
  of children
    in group setting, 332, 333f
    preschool, 331–332, 332f
    school-age, 333–334
  of infants, 318–322
    addition of semisolid foods for, 318–320
    clinical case study on, 322b
    development of feeding skills in, 318, 319f,
        320f
    developmental landmarks and, 319t
    and early childhood caries, 320
    early patterns in, 318
    environment for, 321–322
    forced, 321
    new look at, 321b
    for older infants, 320–322, 320f
    satiety behaviors and, 318t
    serving size in, 321
    weaning from breast or bottle to cup in, 320

Feeding Infants and Toddlers Study, 321b
Feeding position, with developmental
    disabilities, 959f
Feeding problems, with developmental
    disabilities, 958–959
Feeding skills
  in critical illness, 815
  development of, in infants, 318, 319f, 320f
  in Down's syndrome, 962
  in Prader-Willi syndrome, 964
Feeding tube *see* Enteral nutrition
Female athlete triad, 447
Fenfluramine-phentermine (fen-phen), for weight
    loss, 409
Fenofibrate (Tricor), 1031–1041t
Fentanyl (Duragesic), 1031–1041t
Fermentable carbohydrates, in development of
    dental caries, 482, 483f
Fermentable oligo-, di-, and monosaccharides and
    polyols (FODMAPs)
  for autism, 969t
  intolerance of, 496–497t, 511
  in irritable bowel syndrome, 567
Fermentation, in large intestine, 9
Ferric iron, 659–660, 660t
Ferritin
  laboratory testing of, 1028t
  serum, 580–581t, 656
    in end-stage renal disease, 745–747t
    in iron deficiency anemia, 65, 659
Ferroprotein, 661
Ferrous iron, for iron deficiency anemia, 659–660,
    660t
Fertility, 240–245
  diet and, 240–241
  endocrine conditions and, 244–245
  obesity and, 244–245
  toxins and, 241–244, 243–244t
Fertilization, 246–249t
  in vitro, 244
Fetal alcohol syndrome (FAS), 278, 973–975
  clinical features of, 278
  defined, 973
  diagnosis of, 973–974
  medical nutrition therapy for, 974
  nutrition assessment for, 974
Fetal origins of disease, 240
α-fetoprotein, 580–581t
FFM *see* Fat-free mass
Fiber
  for adolescence, 345–346
  dietary reference intake for, 1090t
  digestion and absorption of, 11–12, 11f
  food sources of, 1091t
  insoluble, for diarrhea, 548
  soluble, for diarrhea, 548
  types of, 1090t
Fiber intake
  for children, 337
  and colonic salvage, 11
  for constipation, 548, 548b
  and coronary heart disease, 679–682
  in diabetes mellitus, 617
  for diverticular disease, 568
  during pregnancy, 259
Fibric acid derivative, 1031–1041t
Fibrinogen, 1028t
  and coronary heart disease, 676

Fibromyalgia syndrome, 882, 903–907, 904b, 905b
Figs, fruits and, 1051–1052t
First trimester, 246–249t
Fish
  avoidance guidelines for, 508t
  mercury levels in, 139
Fish oil, 198–205b
  adult intake of, 885–886
  docosahexaenoic acid in, 885
  eicosapentaenoic acid in, 885
  for hypertension, 691t
  metabolism of, 116
Fistula(s), 571–572, 816
  defined, 571
  enterocutaneous, 571
  etiology of, 571, 571b
  for hemodialysis, 740, 742f
  medical nutrition therapy for, 572
  medical treatment of, 571–572
Fixed acids, 38
Flatulence, 544–545
  defined, 545
  medical nutrition therapy for, 545, 545b
  pathophysiology of, 544–545
Flatus, 544
Flavonoids, 54t
  in inflammation reduction, 120–121, 120b
  and thyroid hormone metabolism, 651
Flexitarians, 180
Flow phase, of metabolic response to stress, 814f
Fluconazole (Diflucan), 1031–1041t
Fluid(s)
  in enteral formulas, 214, 219
  nutritional facts on, 1043, 1043–1044t, 1043t
  in parenteral solutions, 219
  premature infant requirements for, 914–915
Fluid absorption, during exercise and sports,
    454–455
  by children, 455
  at high altitudes, 455
  by older athletes, 455
Fluid accumulation, malnutrition and, 1001–1002t
Fluid balance
  for acute kidney injury, 737
  in eating disorders, 429
  in end-stage renal disease, 745–747t, 747–748
  during exercise and sports, 453–454
Fluid intake
  in anorexia nervosa, 427
  for exercise and sports, 453–456
    absorption of, 454–455
      in children, 455
      in older athletes, 455
    daily needs for, 454
    and electrolyte replacement, 455–456, 455t
      of potassium, 456
      of sodium, 455–456
    and fluid balance, 453–454
    and hydration at high altitudes, 455
    replacement of, 454, 454b
  for kidney stones, 733
  during pregnancy, 283
Fluid losses, 31
  during exercise and sports, 453
Fluid management, with cancer, 769
Fluid needs
  during exercise and sports, 454
  with HIV, 790

Fluid overload, 31
    PES statements related to, 155t
Fluid replacement
    for diarrhea, 550
    with exercise and sports, 454, 454b
Fluid resuscitation, for burns, 817
Fluid status, clinical assessment of, 32–33
Fluoridation, of water, 486, 487t
Fluoride
    for caries prevention, 486–487
        excess, 487
        food sources of, 486
        mechanism of action of, 486
        supplementation with, 486–487, 487t
        in water, 487t
    for children, 327
    for infants, 313
    during pregnancy, 263
    in water, 487t
Fluoride supplementation, 486, 487t
Fluoroapatite, 486
Fluoroquinolones, 1031–1041t
Fluorosis, 487
Fluoxetine (Prozac), 1031–1041t
Foam cells, in atherosclerotic cardiovascular
    disease, 671
FODMAPs see Fermentable oligo-, di-, and
    monosaccharides and polyols
Folacins see Folate
Folate, 67–68, 198b. see also Folic acid
    absorption, transport, and storage of, 663
    for adolescence, 347
    Alzheimer's disease and, 888, 899
    assessment of, biochemical, 66
    deficiency of, 888
        in alcoholic liver disease, 592–593
        in alcoholics, 663
        causes of, 663b
        in end-stage liver disease, 592t
        maternal, 259–260
        stages of, 663, 664f
    dietary folate equivalents, 1098
    for exercise and sports, 456
    for heart failure, 700
    intake of, 1098–1099
    laboratory testing of, 1028t
    nutritional facts on, 1098–1099, 1098t, 1099t
    for older adults, 383t
    for prevention of food allergy, 522
    recommended dietary allowances for, 1098t
Folate antagonists, 1031–1041t
Folic acid, 198b. see also Folate
    deficiency of, in premature infants, 922
    nutritional facts on, 1098, 1098t, 1099t
    in parenteral solutions, 218t
    during pregnancy, 259–260
        with twins, 269t
    premature infant requirements for, 922
    recommended dietary allowances for, 1098t
    supplementation of, 888
Folic-deficiency anemia, 662–664
    clinical findings in, 662–663
    etiology of, 662–663
    medical management of, 664
    medical nutrition therapy for, 664
    methylfolate trap in, 663, 663f
    MTHFR allele in, 663
    pathophysiology of, 663–664, 663b
    stages of, 663, 664f

Folinic acid, 827
Follow-up encounters, for diabetes mellitus, 632
Food(s)
    adverse reactions to see Adverse reactions to
        food
    allergen labeling of, 517, 517b
    cariogenicity of, 483, 484b
        factors affecting, 484–485
            exposure as, 484
            form and consistency as, 484
            nutrient composition as, 484–485
            sequence and frequency of eating as, 485
    contamination of, 139
    disaster planning for, 142
    genetic modification/genetic engineering,
        139–140
    glycemic index of, 1092, 1093t
    glycemic load of, 1092, 1093t
    for infants, 317
        home preparation of, 317b
        semisolid, 318–320
        types of, 321
    and nutrient intake data, 174–175
    nutrient labeling and, 176–179
        health claims on, 178–179, 179b
        mandatory, 176–177
        nutrient content claims on, 178, 178b
        nutrition facts label, 177–178, 177t, 178b
        standardized serving sizes, 176f, 177
        tips for reading and understanding, 178b
    organic, and pesticide use, 139, 141–142b
    purine content of, 840b
    safety of, 139–142, 141t
    specific effect of, 18
    sustainability issues, 142–143
    thermic effect of, 18–19
    and water supply, 143
Food additives, reactions to, 496–497t, 512,
    513–514
Food Allergen Labeling and Consumer Protection
    Act (FALCPA), 517, 517b
Food allergen-specific serum IgE testing, 516
Food allergy
    assessment of, 504t, 514
        immunologic testing for, 515–516
            other tests in, 516
            serum antibody tests in, 516
            skin-prick test in, 515–516, 516f
        and behavioral factors, 514
    cell-mediated, food protein-induced
        enterocolitis syndrome as, 508–511
    in children, 336–337
    comparison of allergic reactions in, 502t
    definitions for, 494–495, 497b
    etiology of, 498
        genetics and epigenetics in, 498
    IgE-mediated, 501, 502t
        defined, 501
        food-dependent, exercise-induced
            anaphylaxis as, 501–511
        food-induced anaphylaxis as, 501
        latex-fruit or latex-food syndrome as, 503
        oral allergy syndrome as, 503
    and inflammatory bowel disease, 564
    interventions for
        avoidance of suspect food as, 516
            allergen labeling of foods in, 517b
            hidden allergens in, 517, 517b
            monitoring and evaluation as, 517–518

Food allergy (Continued)
    medical nutrition therapy for, 493
        elimination diets in, 508t, 516–517
        food and symptom diary in, 514, 515f
        oral food challenge in, 517
    mixed IgE- and non-IgE-mediated, 502t
        eosinophilic esophagitis as, 505–507
        eosinophilic gastroenteritis as, 507
    pathophysiology of, 498
        immune system in, 498–501
        sensitization in, 500f
    prevention of, 519–522
        allergen avoidance hypothesis in, 521
        antibiotic use in, 520
        breastfeeding for, 521
        dual allergen hypothesis in, 521
        fatty acids in, 522
        folate in, 522
        future directions in, 522
        future innovations in, 522
        genetics and omics in, 522
        immunotherapy in, 522
        infant formula for, 521
        introduction of solids for, 521–522
        microbial exposure hypotheses for,
            519–520
        nutritional immunomodulation for, 522
        prebiotics and probiotics in, 521
        route of delivery in, 520
        vitamin D in, 522
    strategies for coping with, 520b
Food Allergy and Anaphylaxis Network, 517
Food and Agriculture Organization (FAO), 162
Food and Drug Administration (FDA), dietary
    supplements by, 191, 191b
Food and nutrient administration, 46t, 53–54
Food and nutrient intake, 46–53, 46t, 47–48t
    beverages in, 50f, 51–52
    bioactive dietary components in, 53
    calorie count for, 47–48t, 48
    energy intake in, 50, 51f
    food diary for, 46–48, 47–48t, 47f
    food frequency questionnaire for, 47–48t,
        48, 49f
    food group quantity and balance in, 50–51, 52f
    food quality in, 51
    food record for, 46–48, 47–48t, 47f
    macronutrients in, 52–53
    micronutrients in, 53
    24-hour recall for, 47–48t, 48
Food assistance and nutrition programs, 133,
    134–135t
Food autoimmune or immune reactivity, 495–497,
    497b
Food Balance Wheels, 173f
Food biosecurity, 140
Food challenge
    double-blind, placebo-controlled, 514
    oral, 517
    protocols, 511t
Food defense, 140
Food delivery, nutrition interventions and, 158
    acceptance and psychologic factors as, 159
    consistency modifications as, 159
    diet modifications in hospitalized clients as,
        158–159
    food intake as, 159
    modifications of normal diet as, 158
    regular or general diet in, 159

Food-dependent, exercise-induced anaphylaxis (FDEIA), 501–511
Food deserts, 133, 175, 367
Food diary, 46–48, 47–48t, 47f
  for food allergies, 514, 515f
Food-drug interactions
  with antiretroviral therapy for HIV infection, 791, 792t
  with chemotherapy, 777
  pharmacogenomics and, 84b
Food energy, calculation of, 25–26
Food first, 382b
Food frequency questionnaire (FFQ), 47–48t, 48, 49f
Food guides, 132
Food habits, of adolescence, 348–351
  dieting and body image as, 351
  family meals as, 350, 350b
  fast foods and convenience foods as, 349–350, 349b, 350f
  irregular meals and snacking as, 348–349, 349b
  media and advertising and, 350–351
Food hypersensitivities
  allergic see Food allergy
  nonallergic
    to amines, 513–514
    to FODMAPs, 511
    to food additives, 513–514
    to histamine, 512
    to lactose, 511
    to microbial contamination and toxins, 496–497t, 514
    to pharmacologic reactions, 512
    to tyramine, 513
Food-induced anaphylaxis, 501
Food insecurity, 175, 329–330
Food intake
  of children
    factors influencing, 329–331
      family environment as, 329, 329f
      illness or disease as, 331
      media messages as, 330
      peer influence as, 330–331
      socioeconomic influences as, 329–330
    patterns of, 328–329
  nutrition interventions and, 159
  during pregnancy, 283, 284b, 284t
Food intolerances, 496–497t, 511–514
  to amines, 513–514
  defined, 495, 497b
  to FODMAPs, 511
  to food additives, 513–514
  to gluten, 511–512
  to histamine, 512
  and inflammatory bowel disease, 564
  laboratory testing for, 1028t
  to lactose, 511
  to microbial contamination and toxins, 496–497t, 514
  to pharmacologic reactions, 512
  to tyramine, 513
Food jags, 332
Food lists, for diabetes, 630, 631t
Food-nutrient delivery
  bioactive substance and integrative care, 187
  planning diet with cultural competence, 162, 185b
Food Pagoda, 163–167, 168f
Food Prodigy, 22

Food protein-induced enterocolitis syndrome (FPIES), 508–511
Food protein-induced proctitis or proctocolitis (FPIP), 511
Food record see Food diary
Food safety
  bioterrorism, 140–142
  contamination, 139
  in Dietary Guidelines for Americans, 133
  global, 139b
  public education campaigns for, 139
  resources for, 141t
Food Safety and Inspection Service (FSIS), 142
Food security, 133, 142, 365
Food sensitivity, 495–497, 497b
Food toxicity, 496–497t, 514
Food-water safety, 140–142
Foodborne illness
  bioterrorism uses of, 140–142
  causes of, 133
  government agency information, 139
  hazard analysis critical control points, 139, 140f
  high-risk populations for, 133
  prevalence of, 133
  public education campaigns for, 139
  types of, 136–138t
"Foodies," 364
Forced feeding, of infants, 321
Formal operational period, and feeding and nutrition of children, 328t
Formula(s)
  composition of, 925t
  infant, 316–317, 316t
    preparation of, 317
    for prevention of food allergy, 521
  for phenylketonuria, 942
  premature infant
    adjustments to, 926
    caloric supplements added to, 926
    concentration of, 926
    transitional infant formulas, 926
  selection, for critically ill patients, 816
Formula-fed infants, iron supplementation for, 314b
Fortified foods, 369
FPG see Fasting plasma glucose
FPIES see Food protein-induced enterocolitis syndrome
Fracture risk assessment, 475
Fragile X syndrome, 93
Frailty, in older adults, 381
Frame size, determination of, 993, 993t
Framingham Heart Study, 674–675, 675b
Frazier Free Water Protocol, 856
Free fatty acids, digestion of, 13
Free foods, on exchange list, 1049, 1057–1058, 1059t
  drinks/mixes, 1058–1059
  free snacks, 1058–1059
  seasonings, 1058–1059
  selection tips, 1058–1059
Free radical(s), in exercise and sports, 456–458
Free radical theory, of aging, 375t
Free T_4, 642–643, 644t
French size, of feeding tubes, 209
French Stairs, 169f
Fresh Fruit and Vegetable Program, 333
Friedan's pyramid, 128
Frieden, Thomas, 128, 129f

Friedewald equation, 69
Frontal lobes, 850, 882
Frozen meals, combination foods and, 1060–1061t
Frozen yogurt, sweet, desserts, and other carbohydrates, 1053–1054t
Fructooligosaccharides (FOS), in enteral formulas, 214
Fructose
  absorption of, 11–12, 12f
  intolerance to, 1028t
  transport of, 12
Fructose-1-phosphate aldolase deficiency, 936–938t
Fructose 1,6-diphosphatase deficiency, 936–938t
Fructose derivative, 1031–1041t
Fructose intake
  in diabetes mellitus, 617
  and kidney stones, 735
Fructose intolerance, 496–497t
  hereditary, 93, 936–938t
Fructose malabsorption, 561
  medical nutrition therapy for, 561
  pathophysiology of, 561
Fructose sensitivity, 1028t
Fruit(s)
  in cancer prevention, 765
  and dental caries, 483–484
  on exchange list, 1049, 1051–1052t
    nutrition tips, 1051
    selection tips, 1051
  and hypertension, 686–688, 687t
  Mediterranean diet and, 1082
  strained and junior, 317
Fruit juice, 1051–1052t
FTO gene, 398
  in weight management, 97
FTT see Failure to thrive
Fuels, for muscle contraction, 442–444
  duration of exercise and, 443
  effect of training on, 443–444
  intensity of exercise and, 443, 443f
  sources of, 442–443
Fulminant hepatitis, 586
Fulminant liver disease, 586
Fumarylacetoacetate hydrolase deficiency, 936–938t
Functional foods, 162
  for adults, 369–370, 370b
Functional medicine, 187
Functional nutrition assessment (FNA), 77, 77t
Functionality, of older adults, 381
Fundoplication, for GERD, 529
Fundus, of stomach, 8
Fungal infections, oropharyngeal, 489
Furosemide (Lasix), 1031–1041t
Fusion inhibitors, medication interactions and common adverse effects of, 791

G

G6PD (glucose-6-phosphate dehydrogenase) deficiency
  food intolerance due to, 496–497t
GABA see γ-aminobutyric acid
Gabapentin (Neurontin), 1031–1041t
Gag reflex, 1003–1008t
Galactogogues, 295, 296t
Galactokinase deficiency, 949
Galactose, 921
  absorption of, 12f
  metabolism of, 949f

Galactose-1-phosphate uridyltransferase (GALT) deficiency
GALT, 936–938t, 949
Galactose cotransporter, 11–12
Galactose-1-phosphate uridyltransferase deficiency, 936–938t, 949
Galactose-α-1, 3-galactose anaphylaxis (alpha-gal), 502–503
Galactosemia, 936–938t, 949
    Duarte, 949
    food intolerance due to, 496–497t
    medical nutrition therapy for, 949, 950t
    medical treatment of, 949
    pathophysiology of, 949
Gallbladder
    physiology and functions of, 595, 595f
    during pregnancy, 250
Gallbladder disease, 595–599
    cholangitis as, 599
    cholecystitis as, 597–599
        chronic, 598–599
        medical nutrition therapy for, 597–599
        pathophysiology of, 597
        surgical management of, 597
    cholelithiasis as, 596
        medical and surgical management of, 596
        medical nutrition therapy for, 596
        pathophysiology of, 596
    cholestasis as, 596
    food intolerance due to, 496–497t
Gallstones, 596
    cholesterol, 596
    medical and surgical management of, 596
    medical nutrition therapy for, 596
    pathophysiology of, 596
    pigmented, 596
    risk factors for, 596t
GALT see Gut-associated lymphoid tissue
Gamma-amino butyric acid (GABA) analogs, 1031–1041t
Gamma-linolenic acid (GLA), 111, 113–115, 836–837
Garlic, 198–205b
    for hypertension, 691t
Gas, intestinal, 544–545
    medical nutrition therapy for, 545, 545b
    pathophysiology of, 544–545
Gastrectomy, 537
    total, 537
Gastric banding, 411–413, 412f
Gastric bypass, 411–413, 412f
Gastric carcinoma
    dumping syndrome after, 779
    Helicobacter pylori and, 533
Gastric disorders
    carcinoma as, 537
        medical nutrition therapy for, 537
        pathophysiology of, 537
    dumping syndrome as, 539–540
        medical management of, 539
        medical nutrition therapy for, 539–540, 540b
        pathophysiology of, 539
    dyspepsia as, 532–533
        medical nutrition therapy for, 532–533
        pathophysiology of, 532
    endoscopy for, 534, 534b

Gastric disorders (Continued)
    gastric surgeries for, 537
        medical nutrition therapy after, 538–539
        types of, 537–539, 538f
    gastritis as, 533–534
        due to Helicobacter pylori, 533
        medical treatment of, 534
        non-Helicobacter pylori, 534
    gastroparesis as, 540–542
        medical management of, 540
        medical nutrition therapy for, 540–542
        pathophysiology of, 540
    peptic ulcers as, 534–535
        care management algorithm for, 535f
        emergency symptoms of, 535
        etiology of, 534–535
        gastric vs. duodenal, 536–537, 536f
        medical and surgical management of, 536
        medical nutrition therapy for, 536–537
        pathophysiology of, 535f
Gastric emptying, 7
Gastric feedings, 210–211
Gastric gavage, 922
Gastric juice, digestive enzymes in, 6t, 8
Gastric lipase, 8
    in digestion, 13
Gastric pull-up, 531, 531f
Gastric residual volume, with enteral nutrition, 215–216
Gastric surgeries, 537
    medical nutrition therapy after, 538–539
    nutritional complications of, 539t
    types of, 537–539, 538f
Gastric ulcers, 536, 536f
Gastrin, regulation of gastrointestinal activity by, 7, 7t
Gastrin-releasing polypeptide, regulation of gastrointestinal activity by, 5
Gastritis, 533–534
    acute, 533
    atrophic, 533, 536
    autoimmune, 665
    chronic, 533
    due to Helicobacter pylori, 533
    medical treatment of, 534
    non-Helicobacter pylori, 534
Gastritis, and bacterial overgrowth, 10
Gastroenteritis, eosinophilic, 507
Gastroesophageal reflux disease (GERD), 526
    and Barrett's esophagus, 528
    with cerebral palsy, 967
    defined, 526
    erosive, 526
    esophagogastroduodenoscopy for, 526, 534b
    mechanisms involved in, 526b
    medical and surgical management of, 529, 529f, 529t
    medical nutrition therapy for, 532–533
    nocturnal, 526
    pathophysiology of, 526
    symptoms of, 526, 528t
Gastroesophageal reflux (GER), 526
    nutrition care guidelines for, 530b
Gastrointestinal (GI) activity, regulators of, neural mechanisms as, 4–8
Gastrointestinal (GI) changes, with aging, 378–379

Gastrointestinal (GI) complications, of anorexia nervosa, 424
Gastrointestinal (GI) decompression, multiple lumen tube with, 212
Gastrointestinal (GI) function, during pregnancy, 250
Gastrointestinal (GI) hormones, functions of, 7t
Gastrointestinal (GI) microbiota, 10–11, 10f, 883–884
    human milk and, 315
Gastrointestinal (GI) obstruction, 553
    medical nutrition therapy for, 553
    pathophysiology of, 553
Gastrointestinal (GI) strictures, 553
    medical nutrition therapy for, 553
    pathophysiology of, 553
Gastrointestinal (GI) surgery, PES statements related to, 155t
Gastrointestinal (GI) transit time, 9–10
Gastrointestinal tract (GIT), 2–3
    absorption in, 1
    anatomy of, 2
    assessment of, 112–113
    digestion by, 1
    excretion in, 1
    functions of, 15, 121
    sites of secretion, digestion, and absorption in, 4f, 5f, 15f
Gastrointestinal tract (GIT) disorders see Lower gastrointestinal tract disorders; Upper gastrointestinal tract disorders
Gastrojejunal dual tubes, 212
Gastrojejunostomy, 212
Gastroparesis, 540–542
    defined, 540
    in diabetic neuropathy, 636
    medical management of, 540
    medical nutrition therapy for, 540–542
    pathophysiology of, 540
Gastroplasty, 411–413, 412f
Gastrostomy, 211–212, 212f
GBS see Guillain-Barré syndrome
GBV-C (hepatitis GB-C virus), 583t
GDM see Gestational diabetes mellitus
Gelatin, sweet, desserts, and other carbohydrates, 1053–1054t
Gelatin capsules, 196
Gemfibrozil (Lopid), 1031–1041t
Gender differences
    dietary reference intakes based on, 174
    in resting energy expenditure, 18
Gene, 82
    determining psychopharmacologic therapy, 903b
    food and, 86b
Gene expression, 83–84
    epigenomics and, 87
    regulation of, 84–87
Gene therapy, 91b
Gene variant, 88–89
    and cancer, 97
    and obesity, 99
    and T2DM, 97–98
    and vascular disease, 100–101
General diet, 159
Generally recognized as safe (GRAS), 193–194
Genesis of disease, 105
Genetic code, 87
    variations in, 84f

Genetic diseases, 90
Genetic hyperlipidemias, 674–683
    familial combined hyperlipidemia as, 674
    familial dysbetalipoproteinemia as, 674
    familial hypercholesterolemia as, 674
    polygenic familial hypercholesterolemia as, 674
Genetic information, variations in, 84f
Genetic Information Nondiscrimination Act
    (GINA), 95b
Genetic metabolic disorders, 935
    of amino acid metabolism, 935–939, 936–938t
        maple syrup urine disease as, 936–938t,
            946–947, 946f
            medical nutrition therapy for, 946–947
            medical treatment of, 946
            pathophysiology of, 946
        phenylketonuria as, 936–938t, 939–947, 943t,
            944f, 944t
            adults living with, 945–946
            care management algorithm for, 941f
            clinical case study on, 952
            formula for, 942
            low-phenylalanine foods for, 942, 943t
            maternal, 945, 945t
            medical nutrition therapy for, 942–945
            medical treatment of, 939–942
            pathophysiology of, 941f
            patient education on, 943–945
            psychosocial development with, 945
            tasks expected of children with, 945t
            timeline of events in, 940b
        requirements for individual amino acids,
            939t
    autosomal-recessive, 93, 935
    of carbohydrate metabolism, 949–950
        galactosemia as, 936–938t, 949
            medical nutrition therapy for, 949, 950t
            medical treatment of, 949
            pathophysiology of, 949
        glycogen storage diseases as, 936–938t,
            949–950
            medical nutrition therapy for, 950
            medical treatment of, 950
            pathophysiology of, 950
    clinical case study on, 952
    defined, 935
    of fatty acid oxidation, 936–938t, 950–951
        medical nutrition therapy for, 950–951
        pathophysiology of, 950
    organic acidemias as, 936–938t, 947
        medical nutrition therapy for, 947
        medical treatment of, 947
        pathophysiology of, 947
    role of nutritionist in, 951–952, 951b
    screening for
        newborn, 935–938, 938b
        tandem mass spectrometer for, 939f
    of urea cycle metabolism, 936–938t, 947–948
        medical nutrition therapy for, 948
        medical treatment of, 948
        pathophysiology of, 947–948
Genetic technologies, 84b
Genetic testing, 94–96
Genetic theory, of aging, 375t
Genetic variability, and chronic disease, 96b
Genetic variation, 84b, 90–94
Genetically modified (GM) foods, 139–140,
    761–762

Genetics
    cell division in, 83f
    cells in, 83f
    and coronary heart disease, 678
    defined, 82
    fundamentals of, 82–87, 83f, 84f
    genetic variation in, 84b, 90–94
    and nutrition therapy, 93
    proteins in, 83f
Genitalia, in sexual maturation, 342f, 343t
Genome, 82
Genome editing, 91b
Genome sequencing, 94–95
Genome-wide association studies (GWAS),
    91, 92b
Genomic imprinting, 90
Genomic specimen, 1009
Genomic testing, 122
Genomics, 82, 84b, 765b
    ethical, legal, and social implications of, 95b
    inflammation and, 110
    nutritional, 81
Genotype, 82, 104–105
Geophagia, during pregnancy, 270
GERD see Gastroesophageal reflux disease
Geriatrics, 374
Germline cells, 88
Gerontologists, 374–375
Gerontology, 374
Gerson therapy, of anticancer dietary plan, 774t
Gestational age, 912–913
    appropriate for, 913, 913b, 913f
    large for, 256, 913, 913b, 913f
    small, 913, 913b, 913f
Gestational diabetes mellitus (GDM), 270–272,
    609–611, 611t
    blood glucose goals for, 628–629, 628t
    diagnostic criteria for, 272t
    incidence and prevalence of, 609
    and macrosomia, 271, 611
    management of, 609
    nutrition intervention for, 628–629
    overweight and obesity and, 270
    screening for, 609
    vs. undiagnosed diabetes, 609
Gestational hypertension, 273
GFD see Gluten-free diet
GFR see Gluten-free diet
Ghrelin, 400, 714–715, 719
    in regulation of body weight, 396–397t, 397b
    regulation of gastrointestinal activity by, 5
"Gin-and-tonic" syndrome, 636
GINA see Genetic Information Nondiscrimination
    Act
Gingiva, 482, 483f
Gingival sulcus, 483f, 488
Ginkgo biloba, 198–205b
GIP see Glucose-dependent insulinotropic
    polypeptide
Girls
    estimated energy requirement for, 23–24b
    head circumference-for-age and weight-for-
        length percentiles, 986f, 987f, 988f
    length-for-age and weight-for-age percentiles,
        985f
    weight maintenance TEE for, 23–24b
GIT see Gastrointestinal tract
Glandular secreting cells of Paneth, 5f

Glasgow Coma Scale, 860, 861f
Glaucoma, 378
Glimepiride (Amaryl), 1031–1041t
    for type 2 diabetes, 621–622t
Glinides, for type 2 diabetes, 621–622t, 622
Glipizide (Glucotrol), 1031–1041t
    for type 2 diabetes, 621–622t
Glitazones
    for prediabetes, 620
    for type 2 diabetes, 621–622t
Globulin (GLOB), 1028t
    serum, 580–581t
Glomerular filtration rate (GFR)
    in acute kidney injury, 736
    in chronic kidney disease, 738t
    during pregnancy, 251
Glomerulus, 727, 728f
Glossopharyngeal nerve, 849t
Glucagon
    in hypoglycemia, 636
    in regulation of body weight, 396–397t
Glucagon-like peptide-1 (GLP-1)
    in regulation of body weight, 396–397t
    regulation of gastrointestinal activity by, 5, 7t
Glucagon-like peptide-1 (GLP-1) agonists, for
    type 2 diabetes, 620–622, 621–622t
Glucagon-like peptide-2 (GLP-2), regulation of
    gastrointestinal activity by, 5–7
Glucocorticoids, after liver transplantation, 594t
Gluconeogenesis
    during exercise, 448
    in glycogen storage diseases, 950
Glucophage see Metformin
Glucosamine, 198–205b, 832
    as sports supplement, 457–458t
Glucose
    absorption of, 11, 12f
    blood
        fasting, impaired, 607
        fluctuations in, 884
        postprandial (after a meal), 609
        during pregnancy, 628, 628t
        preprandial (fasting/premeal), 609
        regulation of, 884
        self-monitoring of, 613–614, 625
        target goals for, 614t, 624–625
    capillary plasma
        postprandial, 614t
        preprandial, 614t
    in chemistry panels, 59–60t
    in end-stage renal disease, 745–747t
    premature infant requirements for, 916, 916t
    transport of, 11–12
    in urine, 62t
Glucose-6-phosphatase deficiency, 936–938t
Glucose alterations, in end-stage liver disease, 589
    medical nutrition therapy for, 589
    pathophysiology of, 589
Glucose cotransporter, 11–12
Glucose-dependent insulinotropic polypeptide
    (GIP)
    in regulation of body weight, 396–397t
    regulation of gastrointestinal activity by, 5, 7t
Glucose intolerance
    categories of, 607–611
    in end-stage liver disease, 589
Glucose load, 916

Glucose-lowering medications, for diabetes mellitus, 615
  nutrition therapy interventions with, 627
Glucose monitoring, continuous, 625
Glucose polymers, 921
Glucose reabsorption inhibitor agents, 1031–1041t
Glucose tolerance, impaired, 607
Glucose tolerance factor, 1119
Glucose tolerance test (GTT), 1028t
  for gestational diabetes mellitus, 609
  for pancreatic function, 599t
Glucose transporter 2 (GLUT 2), 11–12, 12f
Glucose transporter type I deficiency syndrome, 871
α-glucosidase inhibitors
  for prediabetes, 613
  for type 2 diabetes, 621–622t, 622
Glucotoxicity, 609
Glucotrol (glipizide), for type 2 diabetes, 621–622t
GLUT 2 (glucose transporter 2), 11–12, 12f
Glutamate, 882–883
Glutamic oxaloacetic transaminase, serum, 580–581t
Glutamic pyruvic transaminase, serum, 580–581t
Glutamine, 198–205b
  for small bowel resections and short-bowel syndrome, 570
γ-glutamyl transpeptidase (GGT), 580–581t
Glutathione, 120–121
Glutathione peroxidase, 648
Glutathione S-transferases (GST) genes, 96
Gluten, 554, 906
  hypothyroidism and, 644b
Gluten exposure, hidden, in celiac disease, 558b
Gluten-free diet (GFD)
  for autism, 969t
  for celiac disease, 556b
Gluten intolerance, 511–512, 554–555
Gluten-sensitive enteropathy, 553–558
  assessment of, 555
  care management algorithm for, 557f
  clinical insight on, 555b
  defined, 554
  etiology of, 554, 554b
  gluten-free diet for, 556b
  hidden gluten exposure and cross-contamination with, 558b
  medical nutrition therapy for, 555–558
  pathophysiology of, 554–555, 554f, 557f
  refractory, 555
  resources on, 558, 559b
Gluten sensitivity, 554–555, 1028t
  symptoms of, 857
Glyburide (DiaBeta), 1031–1041t
Glyburide (Glynase PresTab), for type 2 diabetes, 621–622t
Glycemic control
  for critically ill patient, 812–813
  for diabetes mellitus, 613–614
    recommendations on, 614t
Glycemic index, 1092, 1093t
  and carcinogenesis, 761
  in diabetes mellitus, 617
  for exercise and sports, 450
Glycemic load, 1092, 1093t
  in diabetes mellitus, 617
Glycerites, 192b
Glycogen, during exercise, 442

Glycogen depletion, during exercise, 448
Glycogen loading, for exercise and sports, 449
Glycogen storage diseases (GSDs), 936–938t, 949–950
  medical nutrition therapy for, 950
  medical treatment of, 950
  pathophysiology of, 950
Glycogen supercompensation, for exercise and sports, 449
Glycogenolysis
  during exercise, 448
  in glycogen storage diseases, 950
Glycolysis, 442
Glycosylated hemoglobin see Hemoglobin A1C
Glynase PresTab (glyburide), for type 2 diabetes, 621–622t
Glyset (miglitol), for type 2 diabetes, 621–622t, 622
Goblet cell, 5f
Goiter, in Graves' disease, 650f
Goitrin, 647
Goitrogens, 1120
  and hypothyroidism, 647
Goldenseal (Hydrastis canadensis), 194
Gout
  alcohol consumption as risk factor for, 840
  colchicine for, 838
  definition of, 838
  medical management of, 838–839
  medical nutrition therapy for, 824t, 839–840
  pathophysiology of, 838, 839f
Government, public health role of, 128–129, 129b
Graft, for hemodialysis, 740, 742f
Graft-versus-host disease (GVHD), 781
Grains, carbohydrates and, 1050–1051t
Granola bars, sweet, desserts, and other carbohydrates, 1053–1054t
Granulocytes, in allergic reaction, 499
Grapefruit, fruits and, 1051–1052t
Graves' disease, 649–650, 650f
Gravida, 241
Greek Food Pyramid, 170f
Green tea, 198–205b
  for weight loss, 408t
Greenville gastric bypass, 412f
Grilled foods, in carcinogenesis, 761
Grip strength, malnutrition and, 1001–1002t
Gross motor function classification system (GMFCS), 966b
Growth and development
  during adolescence, 341–343
    linear growth in, 343, 344f
    psychological changes in, 341–342
    sexual maturation in, 342, 342f, 343t
  of children, 324–325
    assessing, 324–325, 325f, 326f
    catch-up, 310, 325
    patterns of, 324–325
  lag-down, 310
  latent or quiescent period of, 324
  physiologic anemia of, 347
  stunted, 325
Growth channels, 310, 324
Growth charts, 324, 325f, 326f, 981
  boys
    head circumference-for-age and weight-for-length percentiles, 982f, 983f, 984f
    length-for-age and weight-for-age percentiles, 981f

Growth charts (Continued)
  for developmental disabilities, 957
  girls
    head circumference-for-age and weight-for-length percentiles, 986f, 987f, 988f
    length-for-age and weight-for-age percentiles, 985f
Growth deficiency, 336
Growth hormone, for Prader-Willi syndrome, 963
Growth spurt, 343, 343t
GSDs see Glycogen storage diseases
GST genes, 96
GTT see Glucose tolerance test
Guar gum, for weight loss, 408t
Guillain-Barré syndrome (GBS), 847–848t, 850, 871–872
Gum(s)
  digestion of, 12
  nutrition-focused physical examination of, 1003–1008t
Gut-associated lymphoid tissue (GALT), 121
  and food allergy, 499–500
Gut-brain axis, 2
Gut ecology, 121
Gut hormones, in regulation of body weight, 396–397t
Gut microbiome
  in children, 337
  human milk and, 315
  in sensitization to food antigens, 499–500
GVHD see Graft-versus-host disease
Gynecologic age, 358
Gynoid fat distribution, 402

H

H₂ blockers, for upper GI disorders, 529, 529t
H₂-receptor antagonist, 1031–1041t
H₂CO₃ see Carbonic acid
Hair
  nutrition-focused physical examination, 1003–1008t
  specimen of, 59, 1009
Haloperidol (Haldol), 1031–1041t
HALS see HIV-associated lipodystrophy syndrome
Hamburger, fast foods and, 1061t
Hang time, in enteral nutrition, 214
Hapten, 497b
Harris-Benedict equations, 21
Hashimoto's thyroiditis, 644
HAV see Hepatitis A virus
Haversian systems, 471, 472f
Hawthorn berry, for hypertension, 691t
Hazard analysis critical control points (HACCP), 139, 140f
HBeAg, 580–581t
HBM see Health belief model
HBsAg, 580–581t
HBV see Hepatitis B virus
HCAs see Heterocyclic amines
HCBS see Home- and community-based services
HCO₃⁻ see Bicarbonate
HCT see Hematopoietic cell transplantation
Hct see Hematocrit
HCV see Hepatitis C virus
HCV-RNA, 580–581t
Hcy see Homocysteine
HD see Hemodialysis
HDL see High-density lipoprotein

HDL-c, 1028t
HDV *see* Hepatitis D virus
Head and neck cancer, 489–490, 531–532
   medical nutrition therapy for, 532
   pathophysiology of, 531–532
   radiation therapy for, 778–779, 778t
   surgery for, 779
Head circumference, 71b, 72
Head Start, 134–135t, 334
Health
   developmental origins of, 240
   social determinants of, 128
Health at Every Size (HAES®), 409
Health belief model (HBM), 227, 228t
Health Canada, 162–163
Health care, influences on, 154–157
Health claims, 193–194
   on food labels, 178–179, 179b
Health continuum, 105
Health disparities, 366b, 367
Health Food Palm, 171f
Health history, 122
Health Impact Pyramid, 128, 129f
Health Insurance Portability and Accountability
    Act (HIPAA), 154
Health literacy, 181, 232
Health policy think tanks, 130b
Health promotion, for older adults, 374
Health-related quality of life (HRQOL), 365
Health risk(s), of obesity, 401
Healthy Children 2020, on breast feeding,
    314–315, 315b
Healthy Eating Index, 175
Healthy fats, Mediterranean diet and, 1082–1083
"Healthy Food in Health Care" pledge, 175b
Healthy People 2020, 128, 130, 132
Hearing loss, with aging, 376, 377
Heart, nutrition-focused physical examination of,
    1003–1008t
Heart disease *see also* Cardiovascular disease
   atherosclerotic, 670–673
   coronary *see* Coronary heart disease
   inflammation in, 121
   selenium and, 1127
Heart failure (HF), 693–700
   adiponectin in, 697
   B-natriuretic peptide in, 696
   cardiac cachexia in, 696
   cardiac remodeling in, 694
   case management algorithm for, 695f
   classification of, 696t
   defined, 693–694
   medical management of, 697
   medical nutrition therapy for, 697–700
     alcohol in, 699
     caffeine in, 699
     calcium in, 699
     coenzyme Q_{10} in, 700
     D-ribose in, 700
     energy in, 700
     fats in, 700
     folate, vitamin B_6, and vitamin B_{12} in, 700
     L-arginine in, 699–700
     magnesium in, 700
     meal strategies in, 700
     salt restriction in, 698–699, 698t, 699b
     thiamin in, 700
     vitamin D in, 700

Heart failure *(Continued)*
   in middle age *vs.* older adulthood, 698t
   pathophysiology of, 694–697, 694f, 695f
   PES statements related to, 155t
   prevention of, 697
   risk factors for, 696b, 697
   skeletal muscle changes in, 696t
   structure of heart pump and, 693f
   symptoms of, 696
Heart pump, structure of, 693f
Heart transplantation, 700–702
   nutrition support after
     immediate, 701, 701t
     long-term, 701–702
   pretransplant medical nutrition therapy, 701
Heartburn, 526
   integrative approaches to, 531b
   during pregnancy, 273
Heartleaf, for weight loss, 408t
Height measurements
   calculation from standard formula, 992t
   direct methods for, 991, 992t
   indirect methods for, 991
Height spurt, 342f
Helicobacter pylori, 533
   gastritis from, 533
   integrative approaches to, 537b
   medical nutrition therapy for, 536
   and pernicious anemia, 665
Hematemesis, 528, 535
Hematocrit (Hct)
   in complete blood count, 61t
   defined, 655
   in iron deficiency anemia, 65
Hematomas
   definition of, 860
   epidural, 860
   subdural, 860
Hematopoietic cell transplantation (HCT), 781
   with neutropenia, 768
   nutritional impact of, 781
     with graft-*versus*-host disease, 781
     with neutropenia, 768
Hematopoietic growth factors, for cancer
    therapy, 777
Heme iron, 660
Hemianopsia, 848–849b, 849f
Hemicellulose, digestion of, 12
Hemiparesis, 848–849b
Hemochromatosis, 586, 661
   assessment of, 661
   clinical findings in, 661
   medical management of, 661
   medical nutrition therapy for, 661
   pathophysiology of, 661
Hemodialysis (HD), 740
   access for, 742f
   continuous venovenous, 736
   mechanism of action of, 743f
   medical nutrition therapy for, 742, 744f, 745t
   simple menu plan for, 744f
Hemodynamic stability
   of critically ill patient, 812
   with parenteral nutrition, 220
Hemofiltration, continuous venovenous, 736
Hemoglobin A1C (HgbA1C)
   in diabetes mellitus, 69
     for diagnosis, 612, 612f, 612t

Hemoglobin A1C *(Continued)*
    for glycemic control, 614t
     monitoring of, 625
   laboratory values for, 1028t
   in prediabetes, 607
Hemoglobin (Hgb)
   defined, 655
   glycosylated *see* Hemoglobin A1C
   in iron deficiency anemia, 64
Hemoglobin (Hgb) concentration
   in complete blood count, 61t
   in iron deficiency anemia, 64
Hemoglobin S disease *see* Sickle cell anemia
Hemogram, 59, 61t
Hemolytic anemia, 667
   in premature infants, 921
   vitamin E-responsive, 667
Hemorrhage
   intracranial, 857
   intraparenchymal, 857
   subarachnoid, 857
Hemorrhoids, during pregnancy, 270
Hemp milk, 1052–1053t
Hepatic disease *see* Liver disease
Hepatic encephalopathy, 588
   medical nutrition therapy for, 588
   pathophysiology and medical treatment of, 588
   stages of, 588b
Hepatic enzymes, laboratory tests of, 580–581t
Hepatic excretion, laboratory tests of, 580–581t
Hepatic failure, 588
Hepatic osteodystrophy, 585
Hepatic steatosis, 584f, 585
Hepatic transport proteins, 64
Hepatitis
   alcoholic, 584f, 585
     clinical case study on, 603b
   chronic, 586
     active, 582f
   fulminant, 586
   viral
     acute, 581–582
     markers for, 580–581t
     types of, 583t
Hepatitis A virus (HAV), 581, 583t
Hepatitis B virus (HBV), 581, 583t
Hepatitis C virus (HCV), 112, 581, 583t
   and HIV coinfection, 791b
Hepatitis D virus (HDV), 581, 583t
Hepatitis E virus (HEV), 581, 583t
Hepatitis G virus (HGV), 583t
Hepatitis GB-C virus (GBV-C), 583t
Hepatobiliary disease *see* Gallbladder disease;
    Liver disease
Hepatobiliary disorders, 579
Hepatocellular carcinoma, 586
Hepatorenal syndrome, 589
Hepatotoxicity, of herbal supplements, 593
Hepcidin, 661
Herb-based seasoning, 1128
Herbal medicine, 191
Herbal supplement(s)
   for adolescents, 348
   for diabetes mellitus, 618–619
   hepatotoxicity of, 593
   for liver disease, 593–594
   Mediterranean diet and, 1083
Hereditary fructose intolerance, 93, 936–938t

Hernia, hiatal, 528, 528f, 528t
Heterocyclic amines (HCAs), in carcinogenesis, 761
Heterozygous individual, 88
HEV *see* Hepatitis E virus
HF *see* Heart failure
Hgb *see* Hemoglobin
HGH *see* Human growth hormone
HGV *see* Hepatitis G virus
HHS *see* Hyperglycemic hyperosmolar state
Hiatal hernia, 528, 528f, 528t
High altitudes, hydration at, during exercise and sports, 455
High-carbohydrate diet, for exercise and sports, 449
High-density lipoprotein(s) (HDLs), in coronary heart disease, 672–673
High-density lipoprotein cholesterol (HDL-C), 1028t
 with diabetes mellitus, 635t
High-energy diets, for unintentional weight loss, 416–417, 417t
High-fiber diet
 for constipation, 548, 548b
 for diverticular disease, 568
 nutritional facts on, 1090, 1090t
  2 G of, 1091, 1091t
  guidelines for, 1090
High-intensity interval training (HIIT), beta-alanine for, 463
High-metabolic-rate organs (HMROs), 18
High-metabolic-rate organs (HRMOs), 18
High-protein diet, 1094
High-protein nutrition support therapy, 813
High-sensitivity C-reactive protein (hs-CRP), 62–63, 105, 1028t
HIIT *see* High-intensity interval training
Hindu dietary practices, 181t
Hip circumference, 73
Hip fracture, 476b
HIPAA *see* Health Insurance Portability and Accountability Act
Histamine
 in allergic reaction, 499
 food intolerance due to, 496–497t, 512
Histamine-N-methyltransferase (HNMT), 512
Histamine-releasing agents, food intolerance due to, 496–497t
Histamine-restricted diet, 512–513b
Histidine (His), in infancy and childhood, 939t
Histone modification, 90
Histones, 82
HIV *see* Human immunodeficiency virus
HIV-associated lipodystrophy syndrome (HALS), 796, 797f
HIV-associated lipohypertrophy and lipoatrophy, 796t, 797f
HIV ribonucleic acid (RNA), 788
HMG-CoA *see* 3-Hydroxy-3-methylglutaryl coenzyme A (HMG-CoA) reductase inhibitors
Holistic medicine, 187, 188t
Holotranscobalamin II (holo TCII), 665
Home- and community-based services (HCBS), 385
 Waivers, 384
Home care, 223, 223b
Home enteral nutrition (HEN), 223

Home parenteral nutrition (HPN), 223
Homeopathy, 188–189t, 188t
Homocysteine
 in B vitamin deficiencies, 66
 and coronary heart disease, 676
 and creatinine, 68
 dementia and, 888
 total, 888
 in vitamin B_{12} deficiency, 666
Homocystinuria, 936–938t
Homozygous individual, 88
Honeymoon phase, of type 1 diabetes mellitus, 607
Hoodia, for weight loss, 408t
Hormonal response, to metabolic stress, 807–809
Hormonal status, and resting energy expenditure, 18
Hormonal therapy, 766
 for cancer, nutritional impact of, 775–776t, 778
Hormone(s)
 counterregulatory, 807–808
 functions of, 5–8
 in regulation of body weight, 397b
Hormone-sensitive lipase (HSL), 395
Hospice
 for cancer, 768
 nutrition for client in, 160
Hospice care, 386–388
Hot chocolate, sweet, desserts, and other carbohydrates, 1053–1054t
House diet, 159
House of Healthy Nutrition, 170f
HPT *see* Hypothalamic-pituitary-thyroid (HPT) axis
HSL *see* Hormone-sensitive lipase
5-HT *see* 5-Hydroxytryptamine
Humalog (insulin lispro), 622–623
Human Genome Project, 82, 82b, 110
Human growth hormone (HGH), as sports supplement, 457–458t, 465
Human immunodeficiency virus (HIV), 787
 acute infection with, 788
 anthropometry and body composition measurements, 796
 antiretroviral therapy for, 787, 790–791
  classes of drugs in, 790–791
  drug resistance to, 791
  food-drug interactions with, 791
  predictors of adherence to, 791
 appetite loss due to, 795t
 asymptomatic infection with, 788–790
 cardiometabolic risk, 796–798
 care management algorithm for, 794f
 CD4 count in, 790
 changing face of, 787–788, 787–788b
 in children, 803
 classification of, 788–790
 clinical latency of, 788–790
 clinical scenario on, 804b
 diarrhea with, 548, 795t
 encephalopathy, 793t
 epidemiology and trends in, 788
  global, 788, 789f
  in United States, 788, 789f
 etiology of, 794f
 and hepatitis C virus coinfection, 791b
 HIV-associated lipodystrophy syndrome in, 796, 797f
 hyperglycemia due to, 795t
 hyperlipidemia due to, 795t

Human immunodeficiency virus *(Continued)*
 illicit drug use and, 791
 integrative and functional nutrition (IFN), 803–804
 long-term nonprogression of, 788–790
 medical management of, 791
 medical nutrition therapy for, 793–801, 799f
  factors to consider in nutrition assessment for, 796t
  gastrointestinal health, 801
  nutrient recommendations in, 798–801
   for energy and fluid, 798
   for fat, 801
   for micronutrients, 801, 802t
   for protein, 798–801
  social and economic factors in, 798
 mouth and esophageal ulcers due to, 795t
 nausea and vomiting due to, 795t
 obesity and, 798
 opportunistic infections with, 790
 oral manifestations of, 490, 490t
 pancreatitis due to, 795t
 pathophysiology of, 788–790, 790b, 794f
 seroconversion in, 788
 sore throat due to, 795t
 symptomatic HIV infection, 790
 taste alterations due to, 795t
 transmission of, 788
 wasting in, 796
 weight loss due to, 795t
 in women, 802–803
  postpartum and other considerations with, 803
  preconception and prenatal considerations with, 803
Human immunodeficiency virus (HIV)-associated lipodystrophy syndrome (HALS), 796, 797f
Human immunodeficiency virus (HIV)-induced enteropathy, 793t
Human milk *see also* Breastmilk
 composition of, 925t
 donor, 924b
 fortifiers for, 921, 923
 for premature infants, 923–924, 925t
Human milk bank, 924b
Hunger, childhood, effect on cognition and behavior, 330b
Hunger-Free Kids Act, 133
Hydantoin, 1031–1041t
Hydralazine (Apresoline), 1031–1041t
Hydration
 for exercise and sports, 454, 454b
  at high altitudes, 455
 importance of, 1043
 nutritional facts on, 1043
Hydration status
 assessment of, 61–64
  bioelectrical impedance analysis for, 72
 laboratory testing of, 1028t
Hydrocephalus, 850
Hydrochloric acid, 1100
Hydrochlorothiazide (Hydrodiuril), 1031–1041t
Hydrocodone/apap (Norco), 1031–1041t
Hydrogen, in alcoholic liver disease, 584f
Hydrogen breath test, 559, 1028t
Hydromorphone (Dilaudid), 1031–1041t
Hydrostatic pressure, 29b

3-Hydroxy-3-methylglutaryl coenzyme A (HMG-CoA) reductase inhibitors, 1031–1041t
  for coronary heart disease, 682–683
25-hydroxy-vitamin D, 477
  biochemical assessment of, 67
Hydroxyapatite
  in bone, 471, 472f
  in bone remodeling, 473
  in tooth development, 482
Hydroxychloroquine, 841
5-Hydroxytryptamine (5-HT), regulation of gastrointestinal activity by, 6t
Hyperandrogenism, in polycystic ovary syndrome, 649
Hypercalciuria, 729–731
  idiopathic, 729
Hypercapnia, 713
Hypercarotenemia, due to anorexia nervosa, 429
Hypercatabolism, 860
Hypercholesterolemia, familial, 674
  polygenic, 674
Hypercoagulation, 112
Hyperemesis gravidarum (HG), 274–276
Hyperglycemia
  in carcinogenesis, 777
  defined, 606
  in diabetes mellitus, 634, 634b
    exercise and, 619
    in older adults, 629
    "rebound," 634
    type 2, 607, 609
  due to HIV infection, 795t
  in metabolic response to stress, 818
  in metabolic stress, 808–809
  in very low birthweight infants, 916
Hyperglycemic hyperosmolar state (HHS), 629
Hyperinsulinemia, 122, 609
Hyperinsulinism, in end-stage liver disease, 589
Hyperlipidemia(s)
  in adolescence, 355, 356t
  due to HIV infection, 795t
  familial combined, 674
  genetic, 674–683
    familial combined hyperlipidemia as, 674
    familial dysbetalipoproteinemia as, 674
    familial hypercholesterolemia as, 674
    polygenic familial hypercholesterolemia as, 674
Hypermetabolic response, 814f. see also Metabolic stress
Hypermetabolism, 860
Hypernatremia, 34–35
Hyperosmia, 850
Hyperoxaluria, 729, 731
Hyperphagia, in regulation of body weight, 395
Hyperphenylalaninemias, 940f
Hyperplasia, 394
Hyperproliferative zone, in bone, 472f
Hypertension
  in adolescence, 355, 356t, 357t
  algorithm for treatment of, 690f
  and coronary heart disease, 683–693
  defined, 683
  in diabetes mellitus, 635
  essential, 684
  gestational, 273
  manifestations of, 685t

Hypertension (Continued)
  medical management of, 689, 690f
  medical nutrition therapy for, 689–692
    alcohol in, 692
    complementary and alternative approaches for, 691t
    DASH diet in, 690–691
    energy intake in, 690
    exercise in, 692
    lipids in, 692
    potassium, calcium, and magnesium in, 692
    salt restriction in, 691–692, 692b
  in older adults, 693
  pathophysiology of, 685–686, 686f
  portal, 587
    in alcoholic liver disease, 585
    medical nutrition therapy for, 587
    pathophysiology and medical treatment of, 587
  pre-, 683, 683t
  pregnancy-induced, 273–274
    overweight and obesity and, 271
  prevalence and incidence of, 684–685, 684f
  primary prevention of, 686–689, 687t
    alcohol consumption in, 687t, 689
    calcium in, 687t, 688–689
    DASH diet for, 687t, 690–691
    dietary patterns for, 686–688
    fats in, 686
    fruits and vegetables in, 686–688, 687t
    magnesium in, 687t, 689
    omega-3 fatty acids in, 687t
    physical activity in, 687t, 689
    potassium in, 687t, 689
    protein in, 686
    sodium in, 687t, 688
    vitamin D, 687t
    weight reduction in, 687t, 688
  risk factors and adverse prognosis in, 685b
  salt-resistant, 688
  salt-sensitive, 688
  secondary, 684
Hyperthyroidism, 649–650
  care management algorithm for, 645f
  due to Graves' disease, 649–650, 650f
  medical management of, 650, 650t
  pathophysiology of, 645f, 650
  symptoms of, 644b
  triggers for, 650
    genetics as, 650
    stress as, 650
  unintentional weight loss due to, 416t
Hypertriglyceridemia, 673
Hypertrophy, 394
Hyperuricemia, 838
Hypervolemia, 31
Hypnotic agents, 1031–1041t
Hypocalcemia, 847t
  in burn patients, 819
Hypocaloric feeding, 813
Hypochromic microcytic transient anemia, 668
Hypocitraturia, 735
Hypogeusia, due to chemotherapy, 777
Hypoglossal nerve, 849t
Hypoglycemia
  defined, 633
  in diabetes mellitus, 633–634
    causes of, 633, 633b
    exercise and, 619

Hypoglycemia (Continued)
    followed by in "rebound" hyperglycemia, 634
    treatment of, 633, 634b
  fasting, 636–637
    in end-stage liver disease, 589, 589b
  lactation, 293–294
  neonatal, gestational diabetes mellitus and, 611
  of nondiabetic origin, 636–638
    defined, 636
    diagnostic criteria for, 637
    management of, 637–638, 637b
    pathophysiology of, 636
    types of, 636–637
  postprandial, in dumping syndrome, 540
  prevention of, 637
  reactive, 636
    idiopathic, 636
    postprandial, 636
  rebound, with parenteral nutrition, 219
Hypohydration, in older athletes, 453
Hypokalemia, in burn patients, 819
Hypolactasia, 559
Hyponatremia, 34, 478, 588
  in burn patients, 819
  medical nutrition therapy for, 588
  pathophysiology of, 588
Hypophagia, in regulation of body weight, 395
Hypophosphatemia, 819
Hypopnea, 719
Hyposmia, 376
Hypothalamic-pituitary-thyroid (HPT) axis, 642, 642f
  managing imbalances of, 650–651, 651b
Hypothalamus, 642
  lesions of, 850
Hypothyroidism, 644–648
  care management algorithm for, 645f
  and celiac disease, 644
  clinical case study on, 653b
  due to Hashimoto's thyroiditis, 644
  and fertility, 244
  gluten and, 644b
  medical management of, 646, 646t
  medical nutrition therapy for, 646–648
    fasting or restrictive diets in, 646–647
    goitrogens and, 647
    iodine in, 647
    iron in, 647
    magnesium in, 648
    selenium in, 647–648
    vitamin D in, 648
  pathophysiology of, 644–646, 645f
  in polycystic ovary syndrome, 649
  and pregnancy, 648
  risk factors for, 644
  subclinical, 644
  symptoms of, 644b
  triggers for, 646
    adrenal dysfunction and oxidative stress as, 646
    aging as, 646
    pregnancy as, 646
Hypotonia, in Prader-Willi syndrome, 963

I

IADLs see Instrumental activities of daily living
Ibandronate (Boniva), 1031–1041t
IBD see Inflammatory bowel disease

IBS *see* Irritable bowel syndrome
Ibuprofen (Motrin), 1031–1041t
IBW *see* Ideal body weight
Ice cream, sweet, desserts, and other carbohydrates, 1053–1054t
IDDSI *see* International Dysphagia Diet Standardisation Initiative
IDEA *see* Individuals with Disabilities Education Act
Ideal body weight (IBW), 994
Ideal body weight (UBW), 71
Identical twins, 87b
Idiopathic hypercalciuria (IH), 729
Idiopathic pulmonary fibrosis (IPF), 716, 717
IDLs *see* Intermediate-density lipoproteins
IDPN *see* Intradialytic parenteral nutrition
IEP *see* Individualized education plan
IFAb *see* Intrinsic factor antibody
IGF-1 *see* Insulin-like growth factor-1
Ileal pouch anal anastomosis, restorative proctocolectomy with, 574–575
  defined, 574
  medical nutrition therapy of, 575
  medical treatment of, 574–575
Ileal resections, nutritional consequences of, 569
Ileocecal valve, 9
Ileostomy, 572–574, 573f
  medical nutrition therapy for, 573–574, 573t
  medical treatment of, 572–573
Ileum, digestion in, 4f, 8
Ileus, 810
Illicit drug use, and HIV infection, 791
Illness, and food intake of children, 331
Imipramine (Tofranil), 1031–1041t
Immaturity, 913–914, 914t
Immune dysregulation tests, 1028t
Immune-mediated diabetes mellitus, 607
Immune system
  in allergic reaction, 498–501
  dysfunction of, 905
  function of, 106
Immune system theory, of aging, 375t
Immunocompetence, 64
Immunoglobulins, 1028t
  in allergic reaction, 498, 499b
Immunoglobulin A (IgA), 499b, 1028t
  secretory, in human milk, 315
Immunoglobulin D (IgD), 499b
Immunoglobulin E (IgE), 499b, 1028t
Immunoglobulin E (IgE)-mediated food allergy, 502t
  defined, 501
  food-dependent, exercise-induced anaphylaxis as, 501–511
  food-induced anaphylaxis as, 501
  latex-fruit or latex-food syndrome as, 503
  oral allergy syndrome as, 503
Immunoglobulin E (IgE) testing, food allergen-specific, 516
Immunoglobulin G (IgG), 499b, 1028t
Immunoglobulin G (IgG) anti-HAV, 580–581t
Immunoglobulin M (IgM), 499b, 1028t
Immunologic testing, for food allergies, 515–516
  other tests in, 516
  serum antibody tests in, 516
  skin-prick test in, 515–516, 516f
Immunosuppressants, 1031–1041t
  after liver transplantation, 594t

Impaired fasting glucose (IFG), 607
Impaired glucose tolerance (IGT), 607
Implantation, 246–249t
Impulse control disorders (ICDs), medical nutrition therapy for, 890–892t
In vitro fertilization (IVF), 244
Inborn errors of metabolism (IEM), 93. *see also* Genetic metabolic disorders
  food intolerances due to, 496–497t
Increased intracranial pressure (ICP), 850
Incretins
  in diabetes mellitus, 620–622
  in regulation of body weight, 396–397t
Independent Living Facility (ILF), 386t
Indigenous food sovereignty movement, 184b
Indigestion, 532
  defined, 532
  medical nutrition therapy for, 532–533
  pathophysiology of, 532
Indinavir stones, 732
Indirect calorimetry (IC), 19–20, 20f
  energy requirements in critical illness determined using, 813
Individualized education plan (IEP), 959
Individualized family plan, 959
Individuals with Disabilities Education Act (IDEA), 975
Infant(s), 310
  botulism in, 312
  diarrhea in, 553, 553t
  estimated energy requirement for, 23–24b
  feeding of, 318–322
    addition of semisolid foods for, 318–320
    clinical case study on, 322b
    development of feeding skills in, 318, 319f, 320f
    with developmental disabilities, 959f
    developmental landmarks and, 319t
    and early childhood caries, 320
    early patterns in, 318
    environment for, 321–322
    forced, 321
    new look at, 321b
    for older infants, 320–322, 320f
    satiety behaviors and, 318t
    serving size, 321
    weaning from breast or bottle to cup in, 320
  food for, 317
    home preparation of, 317b
    types of, 321
  gestational age of, 912–913
  milk for, 314–317
    formulas as, 316–317, 316t
      preparation of, 317
    human, 314–315
      antiinfective factors in, 315
      composition of, 315
      recommendations on, 314–315
    whole cow's, 317
      human *vs.*, 315
  nutrient requirements of, 311–314
    for carbohydrates, 312
    for energy, 311, 311t
    for lipids, 312
    for minerals, 313
      calcium as, 313
      fluoride as, 313
      iron as, 313
      zinc as, 313

Infant(s) *(Continued)*
    for protein, 311–312, 311t
    for vitamins, 313–314
      vitamin B_{12}, 313
      vitamin D as, 313–314
      vitamin K as, 314
    for water, 312–313, 312t
  nutrient requirements of, vitamin K, 918
  physiologic development of, 310–311, 912–914
  premature (preterm) *see* Premature infant(s)
  size of, 912–913
  term, 912
  vegetarian diet in, 1097
  vitamin and mineral supplement for, 314, 314b
Infant cereals, 317
  introduction of, 318
Infant formula(s), 316–317, 316t
  extensively hydrolyzed, 521
  free amino acid-based, 316–317
  partially hydrolyzed, 521
  preparation of, 317
  for prevention of food allergy, 521
Infant Formula Act, 316, 316t
Infant mortality rate, 912
Infections
  inflammation in, 112–113
  opportunistic, 905
  with parenteral nutrition, 220
  signs and symptoms of, 112
  spinal cord injury and, 856
Infertility
  caffeine and, 241–242
  causes of, 240
  diet and, 240–241
  managed with Mediterranean diet, 1082
Inflammaging, 112b
Inflammation, 106–113
  acute-phase proteins in, 825
  antigens as source of, 109–110
  antiinflammatory diet for, 828, 828b, 835
  arachidonic acid in, 113–115
  assessment of, 122
  in autoimmune diseases, 107–109, 110t
  biochemistry of, 825b
  biomarkers of
    C-reactive protein, 825
    description of, 107–108t, 107–109, 111b, 112
    globulin, 1028t
  body composition and, 110–111
  in cancer, 111b, 120
  definition of, 106
  in developmental inflammatory-related conditions, 122
  endocrine specific inflammatory markers, 117t
  energy dysregulation in, 111–112
  fat intake and, 452–453
  fatty acids and, 836b
  functions of, 824
  genomics and, 110
  in heart disease, 107–109
  hypercoagulation secondary to, 112
  in infection, 112–113
  in metabolic syndrome, 109, 122
  microbiome and, 112, 113f
  in neurologic conditions, 110t, 122
  nutrient insufficiencies associated with, 112–113, 115
  nutrient modulators of, 113–118, 115f, 116f

Inflammation (Continued)
  cyclooxygenases, 118
  essential fatty acids, 115–116
  lipoxygenases, 118
  omega-3 alpha-linoleic acid, 115–116
  omega-6 linoleic acid, 115–116
  prostaglandin 1 series, 117
  prostaglandin 2 series, 117
  prostaglandin 3 series, 117–118
  prostaglandins, 113, 114f
  specialized proresolving mediators, 118
  omega-3 fatty acids and, 836b
  in osteoarthritis, 824
  overweight and obesity due to, 401–402
  phytonutrients and, 120
  polyunsaturated fatty acids in, 824
  prolonged, 106–113, 107–108t
    reducing, 122
  reduction of, 118–122, 119f
    B complex vitamins for, 120, 120b
    bioflavonoids in, 120
    clinical insight in, 121–122
    cytochrome P450 enzymes in, 119
    flavonoids in, 120–121, 120b
    foods for, 123b
    lifestyle for, 121, 123b
    magnesium for, 119
    methylation in, 120, 120b, 120f
    minerals in, 119–121
    nutraceuticals for, 123b
    physical activity for, 121
    sleep for, 121
    stress of life in, 121
    toxin load in, 121–122
    vitamin D in, 119
    zinc for, 119
  in rheumatoid arthritis, 824
  role of vagus nerve in, 121
  signs of, 106b
  stress and, 113, 121
  total inflammatory load and, 109, 111f, 122
Inflammatory bowel disease (IBD), 561–569
  care management algorithm for, 563f
  clinical features of, 562f, 562t
  comparison of, 562f, 562t
  complications of, 562t
  etiology of, 561–562
  extraintestinal manifestations of, 562t
  food intolerance due to, 512
  gross pathology of, 562t
  histopathology of, 562t
  medical management of, 564
  medical nutrition therapy for, 564–565
  pathophysiology of, 562–564, 563f
  and risk of malignancy, 561
  surgical management of, 564
  weight loss due to, 561
Inflammatory diseases
  anemia of, 65–66, 667
    ferritin in, 63–64
  nutritional genomics and, 96
Inflammatory markers, 1028t
  for cardiovascular disease, 676, 676b
Inflammatory mediators, 499
Informed negotiation, 230
Infusions, 192b
Ingestion, digestion, and utilization (IDU)
    model, 2

Inheritance
  and disease, 90–94
    at chromosomal level, 92–93
    at mitochondrial level, 93
    at molecular level, 93–94
  epigenetic, 88–90
  mendelian, 87–88
  mitochondrial, 88
  modes of, 87–90
Inherited metabolic disorders see Genetic
    metabolic disorders
Initiation, in carcinogenesis, 758
Innate immune factors, 1028t
Inositol, 895b
Insensible water loss, 31, 914–915
Institute of Medicine (IOM), community
    nutrition report from, 127
Instrumental activities of daily living (IADLs), of
    older adults, 381
Insulin
  actions of carbohydrate, protein, and fat
      metabolism, 614t
  amino acids effect on, 916
  and counterregulatory (stress) hormones,
      613
  defined, 606
  for diabetes mellitus, 622–623
    action times of, 623t
    bolus or mealtime, 623
    exercise guidelines for, 620
    indications for, 622–623
    intermediate-acting, 623, 623t
    long-acting, 623, 623t
    nutrition therapy interventions with, 627
    during pregnancy, 628
    premixed, 623, 623t
    rapid-acting, 622–623, 623t
    regimens for, 623–624, 624f
    regular, 623
    type 2, 621–622t, 622–623
  fasting, 1028t
  in regulation of body weight, 396–397t,
      397b
Insulin aspart (Novolog), 622–623
Insulin deficiency, 607
Insulin detemir (Levemir), 623, 623t
Insulin glargine (Lantus), 623, 623t
Insulin glulisine (Apidra), 622–623
Insulin-like growth factor-1 (IGF-1), 1028t
  in carcinogenesis, 759–760
Insulin lispro (Humalog), 622–623
Insulin pump therapy, 624, 624f
Insulin reaction, 633
Insulin resistance, 609
  in Alzheimer's disease, 898b
  in polycystic ovary syndrome, 649
Insulin secretagogues
  alcohol and, 618
  exercise with, 619
Insulin to carbohydrate ratio, 623–624
Intake domain, of nutrition diagnosis, 770b
  for cancer, 770b
Integrative and functional nutrition (IFN),
    803–804
Integrative medicine, 187, 773
  for cancer, 773–774
  commonly used, 188–189t, 189, 190f
  use of, 187–191

Intellectual disabilities, 954
  clinical scenarios on, 976
  community resources on, 975–976
  defined, 954
  due to chromosomal abnormalities, 960–964
    Down's syndrome as, 960–964, 960f
      anthropometric measures in, 962
      biochemical measures in, 962
      care management algorithm for, 962f
      constipation in, 963
      defined, 954
      dietary intake in, 962, 962t
      eating skills in, 962–963
      feeding skills in, 962
      health concerns with, 962t
      intervention strategies for, 962–963
      medical nutrition therapy for, 962
      medical treatment for, 960, 960t
      nutrition diagnoses with, 955–957t
      overweight in, 962
      pathophysiology of, 960
    fetal alcohol syndrome as, 973–975
      defined, 973
      diagnosis of, 973–974
      medical nutrition therapy for, 974
      nutrition assessment for, 974
    medical nutrition therapy for, 954–960
    nutrition assessment for, 957–959
      anthropometric measures in, 957–959
      biochemical measure in, 958
      of dietary intake and feeding problems,
          958–959
        due to oral-motor problems, 958–959
    nutrition diagnoses for, 955–957t, 959
    nutrition interventions for, 959–960
    nutrition monitoring and evaluation for, 960
    position for feeding with, 959f
    Prader-Willi syndrome as, 963, 963f
      anthropometric measures in, 963
      appetite and obesity in, 963
      biochemical measures in, 963
      defined, 963
      dietary intake in, 963–964
      feeding skills in, 964
      intervention strategies for, 964
      metabolic abnormalities in, 963
      nutrition assessment for, 963–964
      nutrition diagnoses with, 955–957t
      pathophysiology of, 963
Intensity, of exercise, and energy source,
    443, 443f
Intensive care unit (ICU) see Critical illness
Intention, in behavior change, 233
Interleukin(s) (ILs), in allergic reaction, 500f
Interleukin-1 (IL-1)
  in bone remodelling, 473
  injury response regulated by, 809
  in Sjögren syndrome, 837
Interleukin-1beta (IL1β) gene, in inflammatory
    disorders, 96
Interleukin-6 (IL-6), 107–109
  in metabolic response to stress, 809
  in regulation of body weight, 396–397t
Interleukin-6 (IL6) gene, in inflammatory
    disorders, 96
Intermediate-density lipoproteins (IDLs), in
    coronary heart disease, 673
Intermittent drip feeding, 215

Intermittent fasting (IF), of anticancer dietary plan, 774t
International Dietetics and Nutrition Terminology (IDNT), 197b
International Dysphagia Diet Standardisation Initiative (IDDSI), 1068
  background of, 1068–1069
  development of, 1069–1070, 1069f
  emergence of, 1068–1069
  framework of, 1070–1072
    implementation and utilization of, 1072
    patient choice within, 1072
International Dysphagia Diet Standardisation Initiative (IDDSI) Framework, 855t
Interpreters, 230
Interproximal spaces, 484
Interstitial fluid, 28
Intervening sequences, 82
Intervention terminology, 197b
Intestinal brush-border enzyme deficiencies, 559–561
  fructose malabsorption due to, 561
    medical nutrition therapy for, 561
    pathophysiology of, 561
  lactose intolerance due to, 559–561
    etiology, 559–560
    medical nutrition therapy for, 560–561, 560t
    medical treatment of, 559–560
    as norm, 560b
    pathophysiology, 559
Intestinal fistulas, 816
Intestinal gas, 544–545
  medical nutrition therapy for, 545, 545b
  pathophysiology of, 544–545
Intestinal (GI) flora, human milk and, 315
Intestinal hyperpermeability, 883–884
Intestinal ischemia, unintentional weight loss due to, 416t
Intestinal ostomies, nutritional consequences of, 572, 572t
Intestinal permeability, increased, and food allergy, 499–500
Intestinal polyps, and colorectal cancer, 568–569
Intestinal surgery, 569–575
  colostomy as, 572
  fistulas after, 571–572
    etiology of, 571, 571b
    medical nutrition therapy for, 572
    medical treatment of, 571–572
  ileal pouch anal anastomosis, restorative proctocolectomy with, 574–575
    medical nutrition therapy of, 575
    medical treatment of, 574–575
  ileostomy as, 572–574, 573f
    medical nutrition therapy for, 573–574, 573t
    medical treatment of, 572–573
  intestinal ostomies as, 572, 572t
  medical nutrition therapy for, 575
  small bowel resections and short-bowel syndrome, 569
    etiology of, 569
    medical and surgical management of, 570
    medical nutrition therapy for, 570
    pathophysiology of, 569
  small intestine bacterial overgrowth after, 570–571
    etiology of, 570–571
    medical nutrition therapy for, 571
    medical treatment of, 571
    pathophysiology of, 571

Intestinal tract cancers, surgery for, 781
Intraabdominal obesity, and type 2 diabetes mellitus, 609
Intracellular electrolytes, 33
Intracellular fluid, 28
Intracranial hemorrhage, 857
Intracranial pressure, increased, 850, 857
Intradialytic parenteral nutrition (IDPN), 749t, 751
Intraparenchymal hemorrhage, 857
Intraperitoneal nutrition (IPN), for end-stage renal disease, 751
Intrauterine fetal demise (IUFD), overweight and obesity and, 244
Intrauterine growth restriction (IUGR), 252, 913
  after bariatric surgery, 267–268
  causes of, 256b
Intrinsic factor antibody (IFAb), 666
Intrinsic factor (IF), 664–665
Introns, 83
Inverted nipples, breastfeeding with, 294–295t
Iodine
  deficiency of, 1120
  food sources of, 1121t
  for hypothyroidism, 647
  laboratory testing of, 1028t
  lactation, 290
  nutritional facts on, 1120
  during pregnancy, 255t, 263–264
    supplementation of, 263–264
  radioactive, for hyperthyroidism, 650t
  recommended dietary allowances of, 1120t
  recommended intakes of, 1120–1121
Iodized salt, 1120
Ionizing radiation, 767
Irbesartan (Avapro), 1031–1041t
Iron (Fe), 198–205b
  absorption of, inhibitors of, 659–660
  for adolescents, 347
  bioavailability of, 660
  for children, 327
  deficiency of, 657–660, 657b
    in adolescents, 347b
    in children, 313
    in end-stage liver disease, 592t, 593
    with HIV, 802t
    in infants, 313
    pathophysiology and care management algorithm for, 658f
  electrolytically reduced, 317
  in end-stage renal disease, 749t, 750
  for exercise and sports, 459
  ferric, 659–660, 660t
  ferrous, 659–660, 660t
  food sources of, 1122t
  form of, 660
  heme, 660, 1122
  in human vs. cow's milk, 315
  for hypothyroidism, 647
  for infants, 313
  laboratory testing of, 1028t
  in metabolic response to stress, 809
  nonheme, 660, 1122
  nutritional facts on, 1122
  parenteral, in premature infants, 918
  during pregnancy, 264–266
    supplementation of, 264
    with twins, 269t
  premature infant requirements for, 922
  recommended dietary allowance of, 1122t

Iron (Continued)
  recommended intakes of, 1122
  serum
    in iron deficiency anemia, 65
    laboratory testing of, 1028t
  toxic levels of, 1123
  in vegetarian diet, 1096
Iron-binding capacity, total, 656
  in iron deficiency anemia, 65
Iron deficiency anemia, 65–66, 657–660, 657b, 1122
  assessment of, 659, 659t
  in athletes, 459
  care management algorithm for, 658f
  clinical findings in, 658f
  diagnosis of, 659, 659t
  laboratory assessment of
    hematocrit or packed cell volume and hemoglobin in, 65
    serum ferritin in, 65
    serum iron in, 65
    total iron-binding capacity and transferrin saturation in, 65–66
  medical management of, 659–660
    oral supplementation in, 659–660, 660t
    parenteral iron-dextran in, 660
  medical nutrition therapy for, 660
    bioavailability of dietary iron in, 660
    form of iron in, 660
    inhibitors in, 660
  mental health affected by, 889
  pathophysiology of, 657–658, 658f
Iron depletion, 657b, 657f
Iron-dextran, parenteral, for iron deficiency anemia, 660
Iron excess, 657b, 657f, 660
Iron intake
  in adult men, 368
  increased, 1123
Iron overload, 655–656, 657b, 657f, 660–661
Iron-related blood disorders, 655–660, 657b
Iron requirements, in anorexia nervosa, 429
Iron status, 657b, 657f, 889
Iron supplementation, for iron deficiency anemia, 659–660, 660t
Irregular meals, of adolescents, 348–349, 349b
Irritable bowel syndrome (IBS), 566
  defined, 566
  diagnosis of, 566, 566b
  etiology of, 566
  medical management of, 567, 567t
  medical nutrition therapy for, 567
  pathophysiology of, 566–567
  subtypes of, 566t
Ischemia, 672
Isoflavones
  for adults, 370, 765
  as bioactive compound, 85
  and bone health, 478
  in soy-based infant formulas, 316
Isoleucine (Ile)
  in infancy and childhood, 939t
  as sports supplement, 462t
Isomaltase, in digestion, 6t, 11
Isoniazid (Nydrazid), 1031–1041t
Isoprostanes, as biomarker of oxidative stress, 68t
Isothiocyanates, 54t, 162
Isotonic water, 781
Isovaleric acidemia, 936–938t
Isovaleryl-CoA dehydrogenase deficiency, 946f

Isovolemic hyponatremia, 34
IUFD *see* Intrauterine fetal demise
IUGR *see* Intrauterine growth restriction
IVF *see* In vitro fertilization

J

J-pouch, 574, 574f
Januvia (sitagliptin), for type 2 diabetes, 621–622t
Japanese Food Guide Spinning Top, 168f
Jaundice, in acute viral hepatitis, 581–582
Jaw, nutrition-focused physical examination, 1003–1008t
Jejunal resections, nutritional consequences of, 569
Jejunostomy, 211–212
Jejunum, digestion in, 8
Jewish dietary practices, 181t
Joints
    gouty, 839f
    osteoarthritis effects on, 830f
    rheumatoid arthritis effects on, 832, 833f
Joule (J), 19
Juices, childhood consumption of, 332
Junior vegetables and fruits, 317
Juxtaglomerular apparatus, 728, 728f

K

K *see* Potassium
Kangaroo care, 923
Kaposi sarcoma, with HIV infection, 793t
Karyotype, 92–93
Kava Kava, 198–205b
Kayser-Fleischer rings, 586
kcal (kilocalorie), 19
KDOQI panel *see* Kidney Dialysis Outcome Quality Initiative (KDOQI) panel
Ketoacidosis, diabetic, 634, 634b
Ketoconazole (Nizoral), 1031–1041t
Ketogenic diet, 406–407, 774t, 869, 871, 1062, 1063t, 1064t, 1065t, 1066t, 1067t
Ketone(s), 898
    with diabetes, 625
    during fasting, 647
    in urine, 62t
Ketone utilization disorders, 936–938t, 947
Ketorolac (Toradol), 1031–1041t
Ketosis, 871
Kidney(s)
    of infants, 311
    nutrition-focused physical examination of, 1003–1008t
    physiology and function of, 727–728, 728f
Kidney Dialysis Outcome Quality Initiative (KDOQI) panel, 739
Kidney disease *see* Renal disorders
Kidney stones, 728–736
    with bariatric procedures, 729
    baseline information and metabolic evaluation of, 729t
    calcium, 729–731
    case management algorithm for, 734f
    causes and composition of, 729t
    cystine, 732
    medical management of, 732
    medical nutrition therapy for, 732–736, 732t
        animal protein in, 733
        citrate in, 735
        fluid and urine volume in, 733
        fructose in, 735

Kidney stones (*Continued*)
        magnesium in, 735
        omega-3 fatty acids in, 735–736
        oxalate, 733–735
        phosphate in, 735
        potassium in, 735
        sodium in, 735
        vitamins in, 735
    melamine and indinavir, 732
    obesity and, 729
    oxalate, 731, 731b
    pathophysiology of, 728–732, 729t, 734f
    struvite, 732
    uric acid, 729, 731t
Kidney transplantation, 752
Kilocalorie (kcal), 19
Kinetic modeling, for evaluation of dialysis efficiency, 742
Klebsiella, food intolerance due to, 496–497t
Knee height measurement, 958f, 991–992, 992t
    anthropometric measures, 967
Koch pouch, 574
Koilonychia, 658, 659f
Krebs cycle, 442, 442f
Kt/V
    in end-stage renal disease, 745–747t
    for evaluation of dialysis efficiency, 742
Kupffer cells, 580
Kyphosis, 709

L

L-arginine, 699–700
L-ascorbic acid, 1108
L-Carnitine, for ketone utilization disorders, 947
L-Dopa, 877, 877t
Laboratory assessment *see* Biochemical assessment
Laboratory data
    in biochemical assessment, 58
    interpretation of, 59–61
Laboratory testing, 58
    data interpretation of, 1009–1010
    nature of nutritional testing and types of tests, 1010–1030
    nutrition-based, 1009–1030
    principles of, 1009–1030
    purpose of, 1009
    reference ranges, 1010
    specimen types for, 1009
    units, 1010
Lactalbumin, in human *vs.* cow's milk, 315
Lactase, in digestion, 6t, 11
    in infants, 311
Lactase deficiency, 496–497t, 511
Lactate, electrolyte classification of, 33t
Lactation, 240, 286–300, 287f. *see also* Breastfeeding
    docosahexaenoic acid intake in, 885
    estimated energy requirement during, 23–24b
    mercury during, 280–281, 281b
    nutritional requirements of, 289–291, 291b
        for carbohydrates, 290
        for energy, 289
        for lipid, 290
        for protein, 289–290
        for vitamins and minerals, 290–291
    omega-3 fatty acids during, 242, 885
    physiology of, 291–297, 292f
    vegetarian diet in, 1097

Lactation hypoglycemia, 293–294
Lacteal, 5f
Lactic acid pathway, 442
Lactic dehydrogenase, serum, 580–581t
Lactobacillus
    in development of dental caries, 482–483
    for diarrhea, 552
Lactobacillus bifidus, human milk and, 315
Lactoferrin, in human milk, 315
Lactoovovegetarian, 180, 1097t
Lactose
    in common foods, 560t
    description of, 921
    in human *vs.* cow's milk, 315
Lactose free formulas, 212–213
Lactose intolerance, 511, 559–561
    defined, 559
    diagnosis of, 559
    etiology of, 559–560
    intestinal gas and flatulence due to, 545
    medical nutrition therapy for, 560–561, 560t
    medical treatment of, 559–560
    as norm, 560b
    pathophysiology of, 559
    secondary, 559
Lactose tolerance test, 559–560, 1028t
    laboratory testing of, 1028t
Lactovegetarian, 180, 1097t
LADA *see* Latent autoimmune diabetes of aging
Lag-down growth, 310
Lag time, 627
Lamina propria, of small intestine, 9
Lamotrigine (Lamictal), 1031–1041t
Lansoprazole (Prevacid), 1031–1041t
Lantus (insulin glargine), 623, 623t
Lanugo, 424
Laparoscopic sleeve gastrectomy (LSG), 411
Large for gestational age (LGA), 256, 913, 913b, 913f
Large intestine, 4, 9–15
    fermentation in, 9
    microbiota, 10–11, 10f
    salvage of malabsorbed energy sources and short-chain fatty acids in, 11
    structure of, 9
    transport in, 4
Larynx, 706f
Latent autoimmune diabetes of aging (LADA), 607
Latent period, of growth, 324
Latex-food syndrome, 503
Latex-fruit syndrome, 503
Lavender, 895b
LBM *see* Lean body mass
LBW infant *see* Low birthweight (LBW) infant
LCHAD deficiency *see* Long-chain 3-hydroxy-acyl-CoA dehydrogenase (LCHAD) deficiency
LDL *see* Low-density lipoprotein
Lead, 54t
    during pregnancy, 279–280, 280f
"Leaky gut," and food allergy, 499–500
Lean animal protein, Mediterranean diet and, 1082
Lean body mass (LBM), 18, 110–111, 394
Leanness, excessive, 415–417, 416t
    assessment of, 415
    cause of, 415
    management of, 415–416
        appetite enhancers in, 416
        high-energy diets in, 416–417, 417t

Learning, breakfast and, 334b
Learning disorders, 887
Left ventricular hypertrophy (LVH), and heart failure, 697
Leg cramps, during pregnancy, 273
Legal implications, of genetic testing, 95b
Legumes, Mediterranean diet and, 1082
Leptin, 400, 714–715
    in regulation of body weight, 396–397t, 397b
LES see Lower esophageal sphincter
Let-down, 292
Leucine (Leu)
    in infancy and childhood, 939t
    as sports supplement, 462t
Leukemia, 766
Leukocyte esterase, in urine, 62t
Leukotrienes, 116, 824
Levemir (insulin detemir), 623, 623t
Levofloxacin (Levaquin), 1031–1041t
Levothyroxine (Synthroid, Levoxyl), 1031–1041t
    for hypothyroidism, 646t
Lewy bodies, 876
LGA see Large for gestational age
Lifestyle changes
    for diabetes, 628
        in children, 628
    for hypertension, 686, 687t
    for inflammation, 121, 123b
    for obesity, 404
"Lifestyle diseases," 104–105
Lifestyle risk factors, for coronary heart disease, 675b, 676–677
    diet as, 676–677, 677b
    physical inactivity as, 677–678
    stress as, 678
Ligand, 84–85
    omega-3 fatty acids as, 86b
Linear growth, in adolescence, 343, 344f
Linezolid (Zyvox), 1031–1041t
Lingual caries, 486
Linoleic acids
    conjugated
        for weight loss, 408t
        and coronary heart disease, 679–680
    in human vs. cow's milk, 315
    for infants, 312
    omega-3, 115–116
    omega-6, 115–116
Linolenic acid
    alpha-, 115–116, 836b
    gamma-, 836–837
    omega-6 dihomo-γ-, 111, 113–115
α-Linolenic acid, for infants, 312
Liothyronine (Cytomel), 1031–1041t
    for hypothyroidism, 646t
Liotrix (Thyrolar), for hypothyroidism, 646t
Lipase, 6t
    gastric, 6t
    pancreatic, 8–9
Lipid(s)
    digestion and absorption of, 13
    in enteral formulas, 214
    in human vs. cow's milk, 315
    laboratory testing of, 1028t
    for older adults, 383t
    in parenteral solutions, 217–218
    premature infant requirements for, 916–917, 917t, 920–921

Lipid emulsions, 217
    intravenous, 917
Lipid indices, of cardiovascular risk, 68–69
Lipid intake
    and cardiovascular disease in children, 337
    for chronic kidney disease, 740
    with diabetes, 625
    in end-stage renal disease, 750
    and hypertension, 692
    for infants, 312
    for lactation, 290
    during pregnancy, 259
Lipid levels, with diabetes mellitus, 614, 635t
Lipid metabolism, in metabolic response to stress, 808
Lipid requirements
    for end-stage liver disease, 592
    in infancy and childhood, 939t
Lipid-soluble compounds, 1028t
Lipid status test, 1028t
Lipid transfer protein syndrome (LTPS), 503, 505b
Lipoatrophy, 796, 797f
Lipogenesis, 394
Lipoic acid, 120–121
    and thyroid health, 651
Lipolysis, in type 2 diabetes mellitus, 609
Lipoprotein(s) (Lps)
    in coronary heart disease, 673
    high-density, 672–673
    low-density, 672–673
Lipoprotein lipase (LPL), 395
Lipoprotein (Lp) profile, in adults, 676
Lipotoxicity, in type 2 diabetes mellitus, 609
Lipoxygenase (LOX)
    description of, 824
    in inflammation, 118
Lips, nutrition-focused physical examination of, 1003–1008t
Liquid measure equivalents, 980, 980t
Liquid supplements, for anorexia nervosa, 433
Liquids, swallowing of, 855–856
Liraglutide (Victoza), for type 2 diabetes, 620–622, 621–622t
Lisinopril (Zestril), 1031–1041t
Listening
    active, 231b
    reflective, 231, 231f
Listeria monocytogenes, 136–138t
    during pregnancy, 280, 281b
Lithium, 1031–1041t
    for bipolar disorder, 896
Liver
    detoxification in, 370
    functions of, 579–580
    normal appearance of, 582f
    regeneration of, 579
    structure of, 579
Liver disease, 581–586
    alcoholic, 583–585
        alcoholic cirrhosis as, 585
        alcoholic hepatitis as, 585
        hepatic steatosis as, 585
        histopathology of, 584f
        malnutrition and, 585b
        pathogenesis of, 583, 583b, 584f
    cholestatic, 585
        primary biliary cirrhosis as, 582f, 585
        sclerosing cholangitis as, 582f, 585

Liver disease (Continued)
    cirrhosis as
        ascites due to, 587f
            in alcoholic liver disease, 585
            medical nutrition therapy for, 588
            pathophysiology and medical treatment of, 587
        clinical manifestations of, 586, 587f
        fat malabsorption due to, 589
            medical nutrition therapy for, 589
        glucose alterations due to, 589
            medical nutrition therapy for, 589
            pathophysiology of, 589
        hepatic encephalopathy due to
            medical nutrition therapy for, 588
            pathophysiology and medical treatment of, 588
            stages of, 588b
        hyponatremia due to, 588
            medical nutrition therapy for, 588
            pathophysiology of, 588
        nutrient requirements with, 592–593
            for carbohydrates, 592
            for energy, 592
            herbal supplement for, 593–594
            for lipids, 592
            for protein, 592
            for vitamins and minerals, 592–593
        nutrition assessment for, 589–590
            factors that affect interpretation of, 590t
            of malnutrition, 590–591, 590f, 591f
            route of nutrition, 590–592
            subjective global assessment parameters for, 589–590, 590b
        osteopenia due to, 589
            medical nutrition therapy for, 589
            pathophysiology of, 589
        portal hypertension due to, 587
            in alcoholic liver disease, 585
            medical nutrition therapy for, 587
            pathophysiology and medical treatment of, 587
        renal insufficiency and hepatorenal syndrome due to, 589
    end-stage
        ascites due to, 587f
            medical nutrition therapy for, 588
            pathophysiology and medical treatment of, 587
        clinical manifestations of, 586, 587f
        fat malabsorption due to, 589
            medical nutrition therapy for, 589
            pathophysiology of, 589
        glucose alterations due to, 589
            medical nutrition therapy for, 589
            pathophysiology of, 589
        hepatic encephalopathy due to, 588
            medical nutrition therapy for, 588
            pathophysiology and medical treatment of, 588
            stages of, 588b
        hyponatremia due to, 588
            medical nutrition therapy for, 588
            pathophysiology of, 588
        liver resection and transplantation for, 594, 594t, 595t
        nutrient requirements with
            for carbohydrates, 592

Liver disease (Continued)
    for energy, 592
    herbal supplement for, 593–594
    for lipids, 592
    for protein, 592
    for vitamins and minerals, 592–593
    nutrition assessment for, 589–590
      factors that affect interpretation of, 590t
      of malnutrition, 590–591, 590f, 591f
      route of nutrition, 590–592
      subjective global assessment parameters for, 589–590, 590b
    osteopenia due to, 589
      medical nutrition therapy for, 589
      pathophysiology of, 589
    portal hypertension due to, 585, 587
      in alcoholic liver disease, 585
      medical nutrition therapy for, 587
      pathophysiology and medical treatment of, 587
    renal insufficiency and hepatorenal syndrome due to, 589
    hepatitis as
      acute viral, 581–582
      chronic, 586
      chronic active, 582f
      fulminant, 586
    inherited, 585–586
      α_1-antitrypsin deficiency as, 586
      hemochromatosis as, 586, 661
      Wilson's disease as, 586
    markers of specific, 580–581t
    nonalcoholic fatty, 582–583
    other, 586
    polycystic, 582f
Liver failure, 585
Liver function tests, 580–581t, 1028t
Liver resection, 594, 594t, 595t
Liver transplantation, 594, 595t
Liver tumors, 586
Long-chain 3-hydroxy-acyl-CoA dehydrogenase (LCHAD) deficiency, 936–938t, 951f
    pathophysiology of, 950
Long-chain acyl-CoA dehydrogenase deficiency, 936–938t
Long-latency nutrient insufficiencies, 105
Long-term care (LTC), 222–223
Long-term nonprogression, of HIV infection, 788–790
"Long-term services and supports" (LSS), 384
Longevity
    obesity, 401, 402f
Loop diuretics, 1031–1041t
Loop of Henle, 727, 728f
Lorazepam (Ativan), 1031–1041t
Losartan (Cozaar), 1031–1041t
Lou Gehrig disease see Amyotrophic lateral sclerosis
Low birthweight (LBW) infant, 279
Low birthweight (LBW) infants
    classification of, 912, 913b
    incidence of, 912
    management of, 912
    medical nutrition therapy for, 911
Low-carbohydrate foods
    free foods and, 1059t
    high-fat diet, 407

Low-density lipoprotein(s) (LDLs), in coronary heart disease, 672–673
Low-density lipoprotein cholesterol (LDL-C), 635t
    with diabetes mellitus, 614, 635t
Low density lipoprotein (LDL-c), 1028t
Low-fat milk, 1052–1053t
Low-fiber diet, for diarrhea, 552t
Low glycemic index treatment (LGIT), 1062, 1063t, 1065t
Low-phenylalanine foods, for phenylketonuria, 942, 943t
    guidelines for calculations of, 942, 943t
    low-protein foods in, 943t
    menus of, 943–945, 943t
    in young children, 942, 944t
Low-protein diet, for disorders of urea cycle metabolism, 948, 949b
Low-protein foods, for phenylketonuria, 944t
Low-sodium diet
    for heart failure, 699b
    for hypertension, 687t, 692b
Low T3 syndrome, due to eating disorders, 425
Low turnover bone disease, 750
Lower body less sensitive to change, 1000–1001t
Lower esophageal sphincter (LES), 8, 525, 526f
    in GERD, 526
Lower gastrointestinal tract disorders, 544
    clinical case study on, 575b
    common, 544–553
      constipation as, 545–548
        medical management for adults, 547
        medical management for infants and children, 547
        medical nutrition therapy for, 547–548, 548b
        pathophysiology of, 545–547
      diarrhea as, 548–553, 551f
        medical nutrition therapy for, 552–553, 552t
        medical treatment of, 550–552, 550b
        pathophysiology of, 548, 549b
        treatment in infants and children for, 553, 553t
        types, 548, 549b
      gastrointestinal strictures and obstruction as, 553
        medical nutrition therapy for, 553
        pathophysiology of, 553
      intestinal gas and flatulence as, 544–545
        medical nutrition therapy for, 545, 545b
        pathophysiology, 544–545
    diverticular disease as, 568
      etiology of, 568
      medical and surgical treatment of, 568
      medical nutrition therapy for, 568
      pathophysiology of, 568
    inflammatory bowel diseases (Crohn's disease and ulcerative colitis) as, 561–569
      care management algorithm for, 563f
      clinical features of, 562f, 562t
      comparison of, 562f, 562t
      complications of, 562t
      etiology of, 561–562
      extraintestinal manifestations of, 562t
      gross pathology of, 562t
      histopathology of, 562t
      medical management of, 564
      medical nutrition therapy for, 564–565

Lower gastrointestinal tract disorders (Continued)
      pathophysiology of, 562–564, 563f
      and risk of malignancy, 561
      surgical management of, 564
    intestinal brush-border enzyme deficiencies as, 559–561
      frets malabsorption due to
        medical nutrition therapy for, 561
        pathophysiology of, 561
      fructose malabsorption due to, 561
      lactose intolerance due to, 559–561
        etiology of, 559–560
        medical nutrition therapy for, 560–561, 560t
        medical treatment of, 559–560
        as norm, 560b
        pathophysiology of, 559
    intestinal polyps and colorectal cancer as, 568–569
      etiology of, 568–569
      medical management of, 569
      medical nutrition therapy for, 569
      pathophysiology of, 569
    irritable bowel syndrome as, 566
      medical management of, 567, 567t
      medical nutrition therapy for, 567
      pathophysiology of, 566–567
    microscopic colitis as, 565–567
    nutritional consequences of intestinal surgery for, 569–575
      with colostomy, 572
      fistulas as, 571–572
        etiology of, 571, 571b
        medical nutrition therapy for, 572
        medical treatment of, 571–572
      with ileal pouch anal anastomosis, 574–575
        medical nutrition therapy of, 575
        medical treatment of, 574–575
      with ileostomy, 572–574, 573f
        medical nutrition therapy for, 573–574, 573t
        medical treatment of, 572–573
      with intestinal ostomies, 572, 572t
      medical nutrition therapy for, 570
      small bowel resections and short-bowel syndrome as, 569
        etiology of, 569
        medical and surgical management of, 570
        medical nutrition therapy for, 570
        pathophysiology of, 569
      small intestine bacterial overgrowth as, 570–571
        etiology of, 570–571
        medical nutrition therapy for, 571
        medical treatment of, 571
        pathophysiology of, 571
    of small intestine, 553–559
      celiac disease (gluten-sensitive enteropathy) as, 553–558
        assessment of, 555
        care management algorithm for, 557f
        clinical insight on, 555b
        etiology of, 554, 554b
        gluten-free diet for, 556b
        hidden gluten exposure and cross-contamination with, 558b
        medical nutrition therapy for, 555–558
        pathophysiology of, 554–555, 554f, 557f

Lower gastrointestinal tract disorders (*Continued*)
  refractory, 555
    resources on, 558, 559b
  tropical sprue as, 558–559
    medical nutrition therapy for, 559
    medical treatment of, 559
    pathophysiology of, 559
Lower motor neurons, 849
Lower respiratory tract, 706f
Lozenges, 192b
LPL (lipoprotein lipase), 395
Lung(s), 705, 706f
  nutrition-focused physical examination of, 1003–1008t
Lung cancer, 718–719
  medical management of, 719
  medical nutrition therapy for, 719
  pathophysiology of, 718–719
Lung transplantation, 722
  medical nutrition therapy for, 722
Lupin, avoidance guidelines for, 508t
Lupus *see* Systemic lupus erythematosus
Luteinizing hormone-releasing hormone (LHRH)
  antagonist, nutrition-related effects of, 775–776t
LVH *see* Left ventricular hypertrophy
Lymph edema, 29b
Lymphocyte(s)
  in allergic reaction, 498–499
  in differential count, 61t
Lymphocytic colitis, 565–566
Lymphocytopenia, 61t
Lymphocytosis, 61t
Lymphomas, 766
  with HIV infection, 793t
Lysine (Lys), in infancy and childhood, 939t
Lysozymes, in human milk, 315

M

Ma huang, for weight loss, 408t
Macrobiotic diet, of anticancer dietary plan, 774t
Macrocytic anemias, 65, 655, 656t
  from B vitamin deficiencies, 66
Macrolides, 1031–1041t
Macronutrient(s)
  for anorexia nervosa, 433
  for bulimia nervosa, 435
  for chronic obstructive pulmonary disease, 715
  for diabetes, 616, 630, 631t
  distribution ranges for, 174t
  for exercise and sports, 447–448, 448f
Macrophages, in allergic reaction, 498–499
Macrosomia, gestational diabetes mellitus and, 271, 611
Macrovascular diseases, in diabetes mellitus, 635
Macular degeneration, age-related, 377
Magnesium (Mg), 35–36, 198–205b
  absorption, transport, storage, and excretion of, 36
  antiinflammatory effects of, 119
  calcium and, 106, 119
  deficiency of, 847t, 895
    in end-stage liver disease, 592t, 593
  dietary reference intake for, 119
  dietary sources of, 1124–1125
  electrolyte classification of, 33t
  food sources of, 1125t
  function of, 35–36
  for hypothyroidism, 648

Magnesium (*Continued*)
  laboratory testing of, 1028t
  nutritional facts on, 1124
  in parenteral solutions, 218t
  recommended dietary allowance of, 1124t
Magnesium (Mg) intake
  dietary reference, 36
  in end-stage renal disease, 745–747t
  for heart failure, 700
  and hypertension, 687t, 689, 692
  and kidney stones, 735
  during pregnancy, 266
Magnolia, 895b
Major depressive disorder, 890–892t, 901, 902b
Major trauma, PES statements related to, 155t
Malabsorbed energy sources, colonic salvage of, 11
Malabsorption
  after gastric surgery, 779
  in end-stage liver disease, 590–591
  fat, laboratory testing of, 1028t
Malabsorptive diarrhea, 548
Maldigestion, in end-stage liver disease, 590–591
Male(s), sexual maturation of, 342, 342f, 343t
Maleficence, 230b
Malnutrition
  in acute illness and injury, 812b
  in alcoholics, 585b
  definitions, 811f
  diagnosis of, 1001–1002t
  in dialysis patients, 1074
  in end-stage liver disease, 590–591, 590f, 591f
  etiology-based definition of, 810–816
  medical nutrition therapy for, 810–816
  nutrition support for, 812–813
  in older adults, 381–382
  and pregnancy outcome, 256, 256f
  in premature infants, 914
  presence of, 1000–1001t
  protein-energy
    anemia of, 666
    in older adults, 382
  in Sjögren syndrome, 837
Malnutrition Screening Tool (MST), 147
Malondialdehyde, as biomarker of oxidative stress, 68t
Maltase, 6t, 11
Maltose, digestion of, 11
Maltotriose, 12f
Mammary gland development, 291–292
Managed-care organizations (MCOs), 154–155
Manganese
  in end-stage liver disease, 593
  in parenteral solutions, 219t
MAO-B inhibitor, 1031–1041t
MAOIs *see* Monoamine oxidase inhibitors
Maple syrup urine disease (MSUD), 936–938t, 946–947, 946f
  intermittent, 936–938t
  medical nutrition therapy for, 946–947
  medical treatment of, 946
  pathophysiology of, 946
Maresins, 825b
Marfan syndrome, 93
Marinol (dronabinol), for unintentional weight loss, 416
Market research, 130
Mass lesions, 850

Massage therapy, 188–189t
Mast cells, in allergic reaction, 499, 500f
Maternal diet, and food allergy, 521
Maternal inheritance, 88
Maternal uniparental disomy, 963
Matrix Gla-protein, 1112
Maturity onset diabetes of youth (MODY), 611
Maximum oxygen uptake (VO2max), 443, 443f
Mayonnaise
  fats and, 1058–1059t
  free foods and, 1059t
MCAD deficiency *see* Medium-chain acyl-CoA dehydrogenase (MCAD) deficiency
MCH *see* Mean corpuscular hemoglobin
MCHC *see* Mean corpuscular hemoglobin concentration
MCOs *see* Managed-care organizations
MCTs *see* Medium-chain triglyceride
MCV *see* Mean corpuscular volume
MDS *see* Minimum Data Set
Meal planning
  for anorexia nervosa, 434
  exchange lists for, 1049
Meal replacement programs, 405
Meal skipping, by adolescents, 348
Meal strategies, for heart failure, 700
Meals on wheels, 384
Mean corpuscular hemoglobin concentration (MCHC), 61t
Mean corpuscular hemoglobin (MCH), 61t
Mean corpuscular volume (MCV), 61t
Meat(s)
  exchange lists for, 1049, 1049t, 1052, 1055, 1056t
    nutrition tips, 1055
    selection tips, 1055
  strained and junior, 317
Meat-fish-poultry (MFP) factor, 660
Meat substitutes, on exchange list, 1049, 1052, 1055, 1056–1057t
Media messages, and food intake
  of adolescents, 350–351
  of children, 330
Mediator release test (MRT), 516, 1028t
Mediators, 105
Medicaid, 385
Medical history, 122
Medical nutrition therapy (MNT)
  for acute kidney injury, 736–737, 737t
    energy in, 737
    fluid and sodium in, 737
    potassium in, 737
    protein in, 736–737
  for acute respiratory distress syndrome, 721, 721t
  for addiction, 894, 894b
  for adverse reactions of food, 514
    elimination diet in, 508t, 516–517
    food and symptom diary in, 514, 515f
    oral food challenge in, 517
  after gastric surgeries, 538–539
  after ileostomy, 573–574, 573t
  for Alzheimer's disease, 898–901, 901b
  for amyotrophic lateral sclerosis, 869–870
  for anxiety, 895, 895b
  for ascites, 588
  for asthma, 712
  for attention-deficit/hyperactivity disorder, 970–971

Medical nutrition therapy (Continued)
 for autism, 968–969, 969t, 970t
 for bipolar disorder, 896
 for bronchopulmonary dysplasia, 723–724,
  723b
 for burns, 817–819
  energy requirements in, 816–817
  methods of, 819
  micronutrients and antioxidants in, 819
 for cancer
  energy in, 768–769, 769t
  fluid in, 769
  general assessment in, 768
  micronutrients, 769–770
  protein in, 769
  supplement use in, 773–774
 for celiac disease, 555–558
 for cholecystitis, 597–599
 for cholelithiasis, 596
 for chronic fatigue syndrome, 905
 for chronic kidney disease, 739–740
  energy in, 739
  lipids in, 740
  phosphorus in, 740
  potassium in, 740
  protein in, 739
  sodium in, 739–740
  vitamins in, 740
 for chronic obstructive pulmonary disease,
  714–716, 715t
  energy, 715
  fat, 715
  macronutrients, 715
  protein, 715
  vitamins and minerals, 715–716
 for chylothorax, 720
 for cleft lip and palate, 971–973, 971t, 972t, 973t
 for colorectal cancer, 569
 for constipation, 547–548, 548b
 for coronary heart disease, 679–682
  antioxidants in, 682
  dietary cholesterol in, 679
  fiber in, 679–682
  monounsaturated fatty acids in, 679
  nutrition factors that affect LDL cholesterol
   in, 677b
  omega-3 fatty acids in, 679
  polyunsaturated fatty acids in, 679
  stanols and sterols in, 682
  trans fatty acids in, 679–680
  weight loss in, 682
 for critically ill patient
  nutrition requirements in
   formula selection for, 816
  nutrition support therapy in, 812–816
 for cystic fibrosis, 711
  energy, 711
  salt, 711
  vitamins and minerals, 711
  zinc, 711
 for depression, 903
 for developmental disabilities, 954
 for diabetes mellitus, 614–615
  alcohol in, 618
  carbohydrate intake in, 616–617
  dietary fat in, 617–618
  fiber in, 617
  gestational, 628–629

Medical nutrition therapy (Continued)
  glycemic index and glycemic load in, 617
  goals and desired outcomes of, 615
  herbal supplements in, 618–619
  micronutrients in, 618–619
  nutrition therapy interventions with, 627
  protein intake in, 617
  sweeteners in, 617
 for diarrhea, 552–553, 552t
 for diffuse parenchymal lung disease, 717
 for diverticular disease, 568
 for Down's syndrome, 960–964, 960f
 for dumping syndrome, 539–540, 540b
 for dyspepsia, 532–533
 for dysphagia, 854–855
 for eating disorders, 431–437, 431t
 in end-stage liver disease
  for fat malabsorption, 589
  for glucose alterations, 589
  for osteopenia, 589
 for end-stage renal disease, 742, 744f, 745–747t,
  745t
  calcium and parathyroid hormone in,
   745–747t, 748–750
  energy in, 744–747
  ferritin in, 745–747t
  fluid and sodium balance in, 744–747,
   745–747t
  iron and erythropoietin in, 749t, 750
  lipid in, 750
  magnesium in, 745–747t
  phosphorus in, 745–747t, 748, 749t
  potassium in, 745–747t, 748
  protein in, 742–744
  vitamins in, 749t, 750
 for epilepsy, 871, 871b, 872f
 for fetal alcohol syndrome, 974
 for fibromyalgia syndrome, 905
 for fistulas, 572
 for folic-deficiency anemia, 664
 for fructose malabsorption, 561
 for galactosemia, 936–938t, 949
 for gastroesophageal reflux and esophagitis,
  529–531
 for gastrointestinal strictures and obstruction,
  555–558
 for gastroparesis, 540–542
 for glycogen storage diseases, 936–938t,
  949–950
 for head and neck cancer, 532
 for heart failure, 697–700
  alcohol in, 699
  caffeine in, 699
  calcium in, 699
  coenzyme Q_{10} in, 700
  D-ribose in, 700
  energy in, 700
  fats in, 700
  folate, vitamin B_6, and vitamin B_{12} in, 700
  L-arginine in, 699–700
  magnesium in, 700
  meal strategies in, 700
  salt restriction in, 698–699, 698t, 699b
  thiamin in, 700
  vitamin D in, 700
 for hemochromatosis, 661
 for hepatic encephalopathy, 588
 for hepatorenal syndrome, 589

Medical nutrition therapy (Continued)
 for HIV infection, 787
  factors to consider in nutrition assessment
   for, 796t
  gastrointestinal health in, 801
  medical management, 790–791
  nutrient recommendations in, 798–801
   for energy and fluid, 798
   for fat, 801
   for micronutrients, 801, 802t
   for protein, 798–801
  social and economic factors in, 798
 for hypertension, 689–692
  alcohol in, 692
  complementary and alternative approaches
   for, 691t
  DASH diet in, 690–691
  energy intake in, 690
  exercise in, 692
  lipids in, 692
  potassium, calcium and magnesium in, 692
  salt restriction in, 691–692, 692b
 for hyponatremia, 588
 for hypothyroidism, 646–648
  fasting or restrictive diets, 646–647
  goitrogens and, 647
  iodine in, 647
  iron in, 647
  magnesium in, 648
  selenium in, 647–648
  vitamin D in, 648
 for ileal pouch after colectomy, 575
 for inflammatory bowel disease, 564–565
 for intestinal gas and flatulence, 545, 545b
 for iron deficiency anemia, 660
 for irritable bowel syndrome, 567
 for kidney stones, 732–736, 732t
  animal protein in, 733
  citrate in, 735
  fluid and urine volume in, 733
  fructose in, 735
  magnesium in, 735
  omega-3 fatty acids in, 735–736
  oxalate in, 733–735
  phosphate in, 735
  potassium in, 735
  sodium in, 735
  vitamins in, 735
 for lactose intolerance, 560–561, 560t
 for lung cancer, 719
 for lung transplantation, 722
 for malnutrition, 810–816
 for maple syrup urine disease, 936–938t,
  946–947, 946f
 for multiple sclerosis, 874–876, 875–876t
 for myasthenia gravis, 873
  nutrition professionals in, 128
 for obesity hypoventilation syndrome, 719–720
 for organic acidemias, 936–938t, 947
 for osteoarthritis, 824t, 831
 for osteoporosis, 478–479
 for pancreatitis, 600–602
 for Parkinson's disease, 877–878
 for peptic ulcers, 536–537
 for phenylketonuria, 936–938t, 943t, 944f, 944t
  formula in, 942
  low-phenylalanine foods in, 942, 943t
   guidelines for calculations of, 943t

Medical nutrition therapy (Continued)
    low-protein foods in, 944t
    menus of, 943t
    in young children, 942, 944t
  for pleural effusion, 720
  for polycystic ovary syndrome, 649
  for portal hypertension, 587
  for prediabetes, 615b
  pretransplant, 701
  for pulmonary hypertension, 716
  for renal transplantation, 752
  for rheumatoid arthritis, 824t
  for schizophrenia, 906–907, 906b
  for scleroderma, 824t
  for sickle cell anemia, 668
  for Sjögren's syndrome, 824t, 837
  for small bowel resections and short-bowel
    syndromes, 570
  for small intestine bacterial overgrowth, 571
  for stomach carcinoma, 537
  for stroke, 857–860
  for substance abuse, 894b
  for surgery, 819–821
    postoperative, 820–821
    preoperative, 819–820
  for systemic lupus erythematosus, 824t, 841–842
  for temporomandibular disorder, 824t, 838
  for traumatic brain injury, 860–864
  for tropical sprue, 559
  for tuberculosis, 718
    energy, 718
    protein, 718
    vitamins and minerals, 718
  for urea cycle metabolism disorders, 936–938t,
    947–948
  for vitamins B$_{12}$ deficiency anemia, 666
Medical record charting, 152–153
  ADIME format for, 152–153, 152b, 153t
  PES statements in, 152–153, 155t
  POMR for, 152
  SOAP note format for, 152, 152t
Medicare benefits, 384
Medication(s) see Drug(s)
Mediterranean-DASH Intervention for
  Neurodegenerative Delay (MIND) diet, 867t,
  898–899
  antiinflammatory diet based on, 1080
Mediterranean diet, 828, 886–887, 1082
  antiinflammatory diet based on, 1080
  and coronary heart disease, 677, 679, 681f, 682f
  examples of, 1083
  significance of, 1082–1083
    common health conditions managed with,
    1082
    foods and lifestyle factors, 1082–1083
Medium-chain acyl-CoA dehydrogenase (MCAD)
  deficiency, 936–938t, 951f
  pathophysiology of, 950
Medium-chain triglyceride(s) (MCTs), 1062, 1063t
  in enteral formulas, 214
  for inflammatory bowel disease, 565
  for short bowel resections and short-bowel
    syndrome, 570
Megaloblastic anemia(s), 661–666
  folic-deficiency, 662–664
    clinical findings in, 662–663
    etiology of, 662–663
    medical management of, 664

Megaloblastic anemia(s) (Continued)
    medical nutrition therapy for, 664
    methylfolate trap in, 663, 663f
    MTHFR allele in, 663
    pathophysiology of, 663–664, 663b
    stages, 663, 664f
  iron deficiency see Iron deficiency anemia
  pernicious, 664–666, 665b
    assessment of, 666
    clinical finding in, 665–666
    defined, 665
    medical management of, 666
    medical nutrition therapy for, 666
    pathophysiology of, 665
    stages, 665
  in premature infants, 922
  in vegans, 180
Meglitinides, 1031–1041t
  for type 2 diabetes, 621–622t, 622
Meiosis, 87
Melamine stones, 732
Melatonin, 198–205b
Melena, 535
Meloxicam (Mobic), 1031–1041t
Memantine (Namenda), 1031–1041t
Men
  estimated energy requirement for, 23–24b
  health of, nutritional factors affecting, 368
  iron intake by, 368
  obesity in, 368
Menaquinones, 1028t, 1112. see also Vitamin K
Menarche, 342, 342f
Mendel, Gregor, 87–88
Mendelian inheritance, 87–88
Menopause, 368
  and coronary heart disease, 678–679
Menses, 367–368
Mental health
  amino acids and, 889
  eicosapentaenoic acid for, 884
  folate and, 888
  iron deficiency effects on, 889
  minerals that affect, 889–890
  niacin and, 887–888
  nutritional supplements and, 890
  nutrition's role in, 882, 883b
  omega-3 fatty acid for, 884–885, 887
  phytochemicals and, 889–890
  riboflavin and, 887
  selenium deficiency effects on, 889
  thiamin and, 887
  vitamin B$_{12}$ and, 888
  vitamin D and, 888–889
  vitamins for, 887–889
  zinc intake and, 889
Mental illness see Psychiatric disorders
Mercury, 54t
  during pregnancy and lactation, 280–281, 281b
  pregnancy exposure to, 885
  in seafood, 139
Meridians, 188–189t
Messenger RNA (mRNA), 83–84
Metabolic acidosis, 38–39
  anion gap, 39
  nongap, 39
Metabolic alkalosis, 39
Metabolic changes, in starvation, 809f
Metabolic consequences, of injury, 808f

Metabolic disease test, 1028t
Metabolic equivalents (METs), 24, 445
Metabolic measurement cart, 20
Metabolic panel
  basic, 59–60t
  comprehensive, 59–60t
Metabolic rate, in regulation of body weight,
  395–397
Metabolic stress
  cell-mediated response, 807–809
  clinical scenario on, 820–821b, 821b
  description of, 807–808
  due to abdominal trauma and open abdomen,
    816
  due to burns, 816–819
    medical management of, 817
      ancillary measures in, 817
      fluid and electrolyte repletion in, 817
      wound management in, 817
    medical nutrition therapy for, 817–819
      energy requirements in, 816–817
      methods of, 819
      micronutrients and antioxidants, 819
    pathophysiology of, 816–817
  due to surgery, 819–821
    medical nutrition therapy for, 819–821
    postoperative, 820–821
    preoperative, 819–820
  hormonal and cell-mediated response in, 809t
  hormonal response, 807–809
  hyperglycemia during, 808–809
  malnutrition due to, 810–816
  medical nutrition therapy for
    nutrition support therapy in, 812–813
    nutritional requirements in, 813–816
      formula selection for, 816
  pathophysiology and care management
    algorithm for, 814f
  starvation versus, 809, 809f
Metabolic syndrome, 122, 367, 402–403
  in carcinogenesis, 760
  and coronary heart disease, 673, 678
  in diabetes mellitus, 635
  obesity and, 109
Metabolic water, 30
Metabolism
  assessment of, 105
  inborn errors of, 93. see also Genetic metabolic
    disorders
    food intolerances due to, 496–497t
Metabolomics, 84b
Metastasis, 758
Metastatic calcification, 749
Metformin (Glucophage), 1031–1041t
  for prediabetes, 613
  for type 2 diabetes, 620, 621–622t
Methadone (Dolophine), 1031–1041t
Methimazole (Tapazole), for hyperthyroidism, 650t
Methionine (Met), in infancy and childhood, 939t
Methotrexate (Trexall), 1103
  nutritional implications of, 1031–1041t
  for rheumatic diseases, 827
  for rheumatoid arthritis, 833
2-Methylacetoacetyl-CoA-thiolase deficiency,
  936–938t
Methylation
  of DNA, 87b
  in inflammation reduction, 120, 120b, 120f

Methylenetetrahydrofolate reductase, deficiency, 887
Methylenetetrahydrofolate reductase (MTHFR)
    allele, 663
    genetic variation in, 94
Methylfolate trap, 663, 663f
Methylmalonic acid
    in B vitamin deficiencies, 66
    in vitamin B12 assessments, 887
Methylmalonic acidemia, 936–938t, 947
    medical nutrition therapy for, 947
    medical treatment of, 947
    pathophysiology of, 947
Methylmalonyl-CoA mutase deficiency, 946f
Methylmercury exposure and toxicity, 331b
Methylphenidate (Ritalin, Concerta), 1031–1041t
Methylprednisolone (Medrol), 1031–1041t
5-Methyltetrahydrofolate, 903, 1098
5-Methyltetrahydrofolic acid, 663
Metoclopramide (Reglan), 1031–1041t
Metolazone (Zaroxolyn), 1031–1041t
Metoprolol (Lopressor, Toprol XL), 1031–1041t
Metric conversion factors, 980t
Metronidazole (Flagyl), 1031–1041t
MFAs see Monounsaturated fatty acids
Mg see Magnesium
Micelles, 13
Microalbuminuria, 635
Microarray chips, 94–95
Microbial contaminants, food intolerance due to, 496–497t
Microbial exposure hypotheses, for prevention of food allergy, 519–520
Microbiome, 121, 460b
    genes in, 112
    of gut, 99–100
    inflammation and, 112
    oral, in development of dental caries, 483
Microbiota, 548, 549f
    arthritis and, 829
Microcytic anemia, 65, 655, 656t
Micronutrient(s) see also Mineral(s); Vitamin(s)
    for anorexia nervosa, 432b
    for bulimia nervosa, 434b
    for burn patient, 819
    burn patient requirements for, 819
    for diabetes mellitus, 618–619
    with HIV, 801
    laboratory testing of, 1028t
Microorganisms, in food, 8
Microscopic colitis, 565–567
Microvascular diseases, in diabetes mellitus, 635–636
Microvilli, 3
Midarm circumference, 72–73
Midclavicular catheter, 217
Midfacial hypoplasia, in Down's syndrome, 962
Midline catheter, 217
Mifflin-St. Jeor energy equation, 21, 383–384
Miglitol (Glyset), 1031–1041t
    for type 2 diabetes, 621–622t, 622
Migraine headache, 847–848t
Mild cognitive impairment (MCI), 896
Milk
    avoidance guidelines for, 508t
    on exchange list, 1049, 1052–1053t
        nutrition tips, 1052
        selection tips, 1052
    for infants, 314–317

Milk (Continued)
    formulas as, 316–317, 316t
        preparation of, 317
    human, 314–315
        antiinfective factors in, 315
        composition of, 315
        recommendations on, 314–315
        vs. cow's, 315
    whole cow's, 317
Milk production see also Breastfeeding; Lactation
    nutritional requirements for, 289–291, 291b
    physiology of, 291–297, 292f
Milk thistle, 198–205b
    for liver disease, 593–594
Millennium Development Goals, 367
Milliequivalents, of electrolytes, 979, 979t
Milligrams, of electrolytes, 979, 979t
Milliosmoles (mOsm), 31b
Milnacipran (Savella), 1031–1041t
Mineral(s), 196, 198–205b, 1028t
    absorption of, 13–15
    for adolescence, 346–348, 346t, 347t
    and bone, 476–477
    for chronic obstructive pulmonary disease, 715–716
    critical illness requirements, 815
    for cystic fibrosis, 711
    digestion of, 13–15
    in enteral formulas, 214
    in inflammation reduction, 119–121, 836
    interactions among, 13–15
    laboratory testing of, 1028t
    for older adults, 383t
    osteoarthritis managed with, 831–832
    premature infant requirements for, 917–918, 918t, 921–922
    in rheumatoid arthritis patients, 836
    trace see Trace element(s)
    for tuberculosis, 718
Mineral deficiencies
    in alcoholic liver disease, 585b
    in eating disorders, 429
    in end-stage liver disease, 592t, 593
Mineral intake
    for children, 326–328
    for exercise and sports, 456–459
    with HIV, 801
    for infants, 313
    for lactation, 290–291
    during pregnancy, 262–266
        with twins, 269t
Mineral metabolism, in liver, 579
Mineral requirements, for end-stage liver disease, 592–593
Mineral supplements
    for adolescence, 353
    for anorexia nervosa, 433
    for children, 327–328
    for diabetes mellitus, 618
    for end-stage liver disease, 592–593
    for infants, 314, 314b
    during pregnancy, 269t
    with restricted-energy diet, 405
Mini Nutritional Assessment (MNA), 43, 45f
    for older adults, 382
Minimal residue diet, for diarrhea, 552t
Minimum Data Set (MDS), 386, 387f

Mirtazapine (Remeron), 1031–1041t
    for unintentional weight loss, 416
Mistletoe, for hypertension, 691t
Mitochondria
    adenosine triphosphate production by, 111
    in aerobic pathway, 442
    dysfunction of, 111
Mitochondrial antibody, 580–581t
Mitochondrial DNA (mtDNA), 88
Mitochondrial inheritance, 88
Mitochondrial level, disease at, 93
Mitogen, 760
Mitosis, 87
Mitotic inhibitors, nutrition-related effects of, 775–776t
Mixed antibody reactions, 502t
MNA see Mini Nutritional Assessment
MNT see Medical nutrition therapy
Model systems, 82b
Modification of Diet in Renal Disease, 739
Modified Atkins diet (MAD), 1062, 1063t, 1064t
Modular additives, 1045t
Molecular level, disease at, 93–94
Molecular mimicry, 829
Mollusks, avoidance guidelines for, 508t
Monitoring nutrition support test, 1028t
Monoamine oxidase inhibitors (MAOIs)
    nutritional implications of, 1031–1041t
    and tyramine, 513
Monoamine oxidase (MAO), 513
Monoclonal antibodies
    for cancer therapy, 777
    nutrition-related effects of, 775–776t
Monocytes
    in allergic reaction, 498–499
    in differential count, 61t
Monogenic obesity, 99
Monoglycerides, digestion of, 13
Monosaccharides
    absorption of, 11
    digestion into, 11–12
Monosodium glutamate (MSG), adverse reactions to, 496–497t, 513
Monosodium urate (MSU) crystals, 838
Monounsaturated fats, 1057, 1058–1059t
Monounsaturated fatty acids (MFAs), and coronary heart disease, 679
Montgomery glands, 299
Mood disorders, 890–892t
Mood stabilizers, 1031–1041t
Morbid obesity, 404
Mormon dietary practices, 181t
Morphine (MS Contin), 1031–1041t
Mosaicism, 960
mOsm (milliosmoles), 31b
Motilin, regulation of gastrointestinal activity by, 7, 7t
Motivational interviewing (MI), 229
    developing discrepancy in, 229
    expressing empathy in, 229
    self-efficacy, 229
Motor dysfunction, estimated caloric needs with, 962t
Motor strips, 850
Mouth
    digestion in, 8
    nutrition-focused physical examination of, 1003–1008t

Mouth-to-anus transit time, 9–10
Mouth ulcers, due to HIV infection, 795t
Moxifloxacin (Avelox), 1031–1041t
mRNA *see* Messenger RNA
MSG *see* Monosodium glutamate
MSUD *see* Maple syrup urine disease
MTHFR allele, 663
Mucosa-associated lymphoid tissue (MALT), 121, 533
Mucositis, due to chemotherapy, 777
Mulberry, for hypertension, 691t
Multifetal gestations, 268
Multiinfarct dementia, 896
Multiple births, 268–269
Multiple lumen tube, 212
Multiple organ dysfunction syndrome (MODS), 810
Multiple sclerosis, 847–848t, 873–876
Multivitamin, for infants, 918
Multivitamin efficacy, 191–192
Muscle-building supplements
    androstenedione as, 465–467
    branched-chain amino acids as, 462t
    creatine as, 463
    dehydroepiandrosterone as, 465
    erythropoietin as, 465
    human growth hormone as, 465
    steroids as, 461–462t, 464–465
Muscle contraction, fuels for, 442–444
    duration of exercise and, 443
    effect of training on, 443–444
    intensity of exercise and, 443, 443f
    sources of, 442–443
Muscle dysmorphia, 447, 447b
Muscle loss, 1000–1001t
Muscle mass, malnutrition and, 1001–1002t
Musculoskeletal system, 1003–1008t
Mushrooms, as source of vitamin D, 1114–1115
Muslim dietary practices, 181t
Mustard, avoidance guidelines for, 508t
Mutations, 91, 758
    silent, 91
Myasthenia gravis, 847–848t, 850, 872–873
Mycobacterium avium complex, with HIV infection, 793t
Mycophenolate (Cellcept, Myfortic), 1031–1041t
Mycophenolate mofetil, after liver transplantation, 594t
Mycophenolic acid, after liver transplantation, 594t
Myelin, 872
Myelomeningocele (MM), 964
    nutrition diagnoses with, 955–957t
Myelopathy, 856
Myeloperoxidase (MPO), as biomarker of oxidative stress, 68t
Myelosuppression, due to chemotherapy, 775
Myocardial infarction (MI), 670
Myoglobin, in exercise and sports, 459
MyPlate, 132
MyPlate Food Guidance System, 163–167, 163f
MyPlate Tracker, 22
Mypyramid.gov, 132

N

N-acetylcysteine, 198–205b
N-nitroso compounds (NOCs), in carcinogenesis, 761
Na/K-ATPase (sodium-potassium adenosine triphosphatase) pump, 29–30, 33

NAD *see* Nicotinic acid dehydrogenase
Nadolol (Corgard), 1031–1041t
NAFLD *see* Nonalcoholic fatty liver disease
Nails
    as specimens, 59
    spoon-shaped, 658, 659f
Nails, nutrition-focused physical examination, 1003–1008t
Naproxen (Naprosyn), 1031–1041t
Narcotic analgesic agents (opioids), 1031–1041t
Nares, 706f
Nasal cavity, 706f
Nasal gastric gavage, 922
NASH *see* Nonalcoholic steatohepatitis
Nasoduodenal tube (NDT), 210–211
Nasogastric tubes (NGTs), 209, 211b
Nasojejunal tube (NJT), 210–211
Nateglinide (Starlix), for type 2 diabetes, 621–622t, 622
National Center for Complementary and Integrative Health (NCCIH), 190
    common holistic therapies according to, 188t
National Cholesterol Education Program (NCEP), 676
National Dysphagia Diet (NDD), 854, 854f, 1068
National Health and Nutrition Examination Survey (NHANES), 130–131, 174, 397
National Heart, Lung, and Blood Institute (NHLBI), 131, 364
National Nutrient Databank, 131
National nutrition guidelines and goals, 131–133
    Dietary Guidelines for Americans, 132
    dietary reference intakes, 133
    food guides, 132
    Healthy People, 132
    National School Lunch Program, 132–133, 134–135t
    recommended dietary allowances, 133
    Surgeon General's Report on Nutrition and Health, 132
National Nutrition Monitoring and Related Research Act, 131
National nutrition surveys, 130–131
    Continuing Survey of Food Intake of Individuals, 131
    National Health and Nutrition Examination Survey, 130–131
    National Nutrient Databank, 131
    National Nutrition Monitoring and Related Research Act, 131
    What We Eat in America, 131
National provider identifier (NPI), 157b
National School Breakfast Program, 132–133, 134–135t
National School Lunch Program (NSLP), 132–133, 134–135t, 333
Native Americans, diet planning for, 180
Naturopathy, 188–189t, 188t
Nausea and vomiting
    chemotherapy induced, 777
    due to HIV infection, 795t
    in pregnancy, 274–276
    unintentional weight loss due to, 416t
NCEP *see* National Cholesterol Education Program
NCP *see* Nutrition care process
NEAT *see* Nonexercise activity thermogenesis
Nebraska, levels of selenium in, 1127

Neck cancer, 531–532
    medical nutrition therapy for, 532
    pathophysiology of, 531–532
Neck nodules, 1003–1008t
Necrotizing enterocolitis, 923
Needs assessment
    community, 130, 130b
    description of, 129
Negative acute-phase reactants, 64
Neglect, 848–849b, 850
Negotiation, in behavior change, 233
Neonatal period, 913
Neonates *see* Infant(s)
Neoplasm, defined, 758
Nephritic syndrome, chronic interstitial, 740
Nephrogenic diabetes insipidus, X-linked recessive, 94
Nephrolithiasis, 728. *see also* Kidney stones
Nephron, 727, 728f
Nephropathy, diabetic, 635
Nervous system, 846–852
NES *see* Night-eating syndrome
Neural tube defects (NTDs)
    folate and, 259–260, 260t
    maternal nutrition and, 256
    maternal obesity and, 268
Neuroendocrine consequences, of injury, 808f
Neurogenic bladder, 874
Neurogenic bowel, 547, 874–876
Neuroglycopenic symptoms, of insulin reaction, 633
Neurologic changes, with aging, 379
Neurologic disorders
    adrenomyeloleukodystrophy, 865–866
    amyotrophic lateral sclerosis, 847–848t, 868–870
    case study of, 878
    developmental disabilities due to, 964–973
        attention-deficit/hyperactivity disorder as, 969–971
            anthropometric measures in, 970
            biochemical measures in, 970
            defined, 969–970
            dietary intake in, 970
            medical nutrition therapy for, 970–971
            nutrition assessment for, 970
        autism as, 967–969
            anthropometric measures in, 968
            biochemical measures in, 968
            defined, 967
            dietary intake in, 968
            nutrition assessment for, 968
            pathophysiology of, 967–968
        cerebral palsy as, 966–967, 966f
            anthropometric measures in, 967
            biochemical measures in, 967
            defined, 966
            dietary intake in, 967
            health concerns with, 967
            intervention strategies for, 967
            nutrition assessment for, 967
            nutrition diagnoses with, 955–957t
            types of, 966b
        spina bifida as, 964–966
            anthropometric measures in, 965
            biochemical measures in, 965
            clinical evaluation of, 965
            defined, 964
            dietary intake in, 965

Neurologic disorders (Continued)
  health concerns with, 964
  intervention strategies for, 967
  nutrition assessment for, 965
  nutrition diagnoses with, 955–957t
  prevention of, 964–965
  Guillain-Barré syndrome, 847–848t, 850,
    871–872
  impairments with, 851t
  inflammatory biomarkers in, 110t, 122
  issues complicating nutrition therapy in,
    848–849b
  medical nutrition therapy for, 846
  multiple sclerosis, 847–848t, 873–876
  myasthenia gravis, 850, 872–873
  nutrition factors for, 851–852, 852f
  of nutritional origin, 847t, 857
  Parkinson's disease, 847–848t, 876–878
  spine trauma, 864–878
  symptoms of, 849
Neurologic reactions, food intolerances due to,
  496–497t
Neurologic system, nutrition-focused physical
  examination, 1003–1008t
Neuromuscular junction, 872
Neurons, 882
Neuropathy, diabetic, 635–636
Neuropeptide Y, in regulation of body weight,
  396–397t
Neurotensin, regulation of gastrointestinal
  activity by, 6t
Neurotransmission, 885
Neurotransmitter(s)
  in addiction, 892
  regulation of gastrointestinal activity by, 4–8, 6t
  types of, 882–883, 884t
Neurotrauma, 860–864
Neurulation, 246–249t
Neutral foods, 730b
Neutral protamine hagedorn (NPH) insulin, 623,
  623t
Neutral thermal environment, 919
Neutropenia, 61t
  due to chemotherapy, 781
  nutritional precautions with, 768
Neutrophil(s), in differential count, 61t
Neutrophilia, 61t
"Never events," 156–157
New Ballard Score, 912–913
New dietary ingredients (NDIs), 194
"New-to-nature" molecules, 104, 121
Newborn(s) see Infant(s)
Newborn screening, for genetic metabolic
  disorders, 935–938, 938b
NHANES see National Health and Nutrition
  Examination Survey
Niacin, 887–888, 1028t, 1031–1041t
  deficiency of, in end-stage liver disease, 592t
  for end-stage renal disease, 750
Niacinamide, in parenteral solutions, 218t
Nicotinamide (Nam) see Niacin
Nicotine, and resting energy expenditure, 18
Nicotinic acid, 1031t. see also Niacin
Nicotinic acid dehydrogenase (NAD), 442
Night-eating syndrome (NES), 400
Nightshade, 829
Nipple(s), inverted, breastfeeding with, 294–295t
Nipple feeding, 923

Nissen fundoplication, 529, 529f, 530b
Nitrates
  in carcinogenesis, 761
  food intolerance due to, 496–497t
Nitric oxide (NO), 670–671
  regulation of gastrointestinal activity by, 6t
  as sports supplement, 457–458t
Nitrite
  in urine, 62t
Nitrites
  in carcinogenesis, 761
  food intolerance due to, 496–497t
Nitrofuran, 1031–1041t
Nitrofurantoin (Macrobid), 1031–1041t
Nitrogen balance, 68
  for burn patient, 818–819
Nitrogen-containing compounds, 68
Nitrosamides
  in carcinogenesis, 761
Nitrosamines
  in carcinogenesis, 761
Nitrotyrosine (3-NO2-tyr), as biomarker of
  oxidative stress, 68t
NMDA receptor antagonists, 1031–1041t
NO see Nitric oxide
No Added Salt (NAS) diet, 1128
NOCs see N-nitroso compounds
Non-IgE-mediated reactions, 501, 502t, 505
Non-narcotic analgesics, 1031–1041t
Non-steroidal antiinflammatory drugs (NSAIDS),
  1031–1041t
Nonalcoholic fatty liver disease (NAFLD), 402,
  582–583
Nonalcoholic steatohepatitis (NASH), 583
Nonallergic food hypersensitivities
  to amines, 513–514
  to FODMAPs, 511
  to food additives, 513–514
  to histamine, 512
  to lactose, 511
  to microbial contamination and toxins,
    496–497t, 514
  to pharmacologic reactions, 512
  to tyramine, 513
Noncoding RNAs, 86–87
Nondysjunction, 960
Nonexercise activity thermogenesis (NEAT), 19,
  395–397
Nonfat dry milk, 1094
Nonheme iron, 660
Nonnucleoside reverse transcriptase inhibitors
  (NNRTIs), 790
Nonnutritive substances, in foods, during pregnancy
  artificial sweeteners as, 278–279
  bisphenol-A as, 279
  lead and cadmium as, 279–280, 280f
  Listeria monocytogenes as, 280, 281b
  mercury as, 280–281, 281b
  polychlorinated biphenyls as, 280–281, 281b
Nonnutritive sweeteners
  and carcinogenesis, 761
  for diabetes mellitus, 617
  during pregnancy, 278–279
Nonprofit organizations, 130
Nonstarchy vegetable(s), on exchange list, 1049,
  1053–1054
  nutrition tips, 1055
  selection tips, 1055, 1055t

Nonsteroidal antiinflammatory drugs (NSAIDs),
  for rheumatic diseases, 826–827
Nonverbal communication, 231b
Noradrenergic/specific serotonic antidepressants
  (NASSA), 1031–1041t
Norepinephrine, 882–883
  in regulation of body weight, 396–397t
  regulation of gastrointestinal activity by, 6t
Norepinephrine/dopamine reuptake inhibitor
  (NDRI), 1031–1041t
Normalization, 231–232
Normalized protein catabolic rate (nPCR), 1028t
Normocytic anemia, 65, 655, 656t
Normoglycemia, 613
Norovirus, 136–138t
Northyx (methimazole), for hyperthyroidism, 650t
Nortriptyline (Pamelor), 1031–1041t
Nose, nutrition-focused physical examination of,
  1003–1008t
Not-ready-to-change counseling sessions, 232–233
  affirming in, 231–232
  asking open-ended questions in, 231
  building rapport in, 231
  concern in, 233
  eliciting self-motivational statements in, 232
  ending session in, 233
  intention to change in, 233
  optimism in, 233
  problem recognition in, 232
  reflective listening in, 231, 231f
  summarizing in, 232
Novolog (insulin aspart), 622–623
NPH see Neutral protamine hagedorn
NRTIs see Nucleoside and nucleotide reverse
  transcriptase inhibitors
NSAIDs see Nonsteroidal antiinflammatory
  drugs
NSLP see National School Lunch Program
NTDs see Neural tube defects
Nucleosidase, in digestion, 6t
Nucleoside and nucleotide reverse transcriptase
  inhibitors (NRTIs), 790
Nucleotidase(s), in digestion, 6t
Nucleotides, 82
  for small bowel resections and short-bowel
    syndrome, 570
Numeracy skills
  in health and nutrition, 183
  measuring, 183
  tools for, 183–185
Nutraceuticals, 123b
Nutrient content claims, on food labels,
  178, 178b
Nutrient delivery, nutrition interventions and, 158
  acceptance and psychologic factors as, 159
  consistency modifications as, 159
  diet modifications in hospitalized clients as,
    158–159
  food intake as, 159
  modifications of normal diet as, 158
  regular or general diet in, 159
Nutrient insufficiencies
  long-latency, 105
  in prolonged inflammation, 112–113, 115
Nutrient-partner principle, 106, 106b
Nutrient pool, size of, 58, 58f
Nutrient recommendations, during twin
  pregnancy, 269t

Nutrient requirements
  of adolescents, 344–348
  of children, 326–328
    for energy, 326, 327b
    for minerals and vitamins, 326–328
      calcium as, 327
      iron as, 327
      vitamin D as, 327
      zinc as, 327
    for protein, 326, 327t
  of infants, 311–314
Nutrients
  megadoses of, 195
  needs for, 162
Nutrigenetics, 94
Nutrigenomics, 94, 765b
Nutrition
  epigenetic inheritance and, 89b
  influences on, 154–157
Nutrition access, 46t, 55
Nutrition assessment, 43–44, 44f
  in adolescence, 351, 352f, 352t
  for attention-deficit/hyperactivity disorder, 970
  for autism, 968
  biochemical assessment in, 57–59
  for cancer, 768
  for cerebral palsy, 967
  for cleft lip and palate, 971
  clinical case study on, 101b
  for developmental disabilities, 957–959
    anthropometric measures in, 957
    biochemical measures in, 958
    of dietary intake and feeding problems, 958–959
  for diabetes mellitus, 625–626, 626b
  of digestion, absorption, transport, and excretion of nutrients, 2–3
  for eating disorders, 427–428
  for fetal alcohol syndrome, 974
  health history for, 122
  for HIV infection, 796t
    nutrition implications in, 793t
  medical history for, 122
  in nutrition care process, 147, 147t
  nutritional genomics in, 81
  of older adults, 382
  patient's story in, 122
  for Prader-Willi syndrome, 963–964
  in premature infants, 926–927
  for spina bifida, 965
  of water, electrolytes, and acid-base balance, 28
Nutrition behaviors, 46t, 54
Nutrition care, during pregnancy, 284b
Nutrition care indicators, 43–44
Nutrition care process model (NCPM), 146
Nutrition care process (NCP), 41, 43b, 44f, 46t, 94–96, 146–151
  accreditation and surveys for, 151
  application of, 150b
  for diabetes mellitus, 625–632
    follow-up encounters in, 632
    nutrition assessment in, 625–626, 626b
    nutrition diagnosis in, 626, 626b
    nutrition education and counseling in, 632, 632f
    nutrition intervention in, 627
    nutrition monitoring and evaluation in, 632, 633b

Nutrition care process (Continued)
    nutrition prescription in, 629–632, 630f, 631f
    for specific populations, 626–627, 628t
  for enteral and parenteral nutrition, 220b
  evidence-based guidelines in, 151
  monitoring and evaluation of nutrition care in, 149–151
  nutrition assessment and reassessment in, 147, 148f
  nutrition diagnosis in, 147–149, 626, 626b
  nutrition intervention in, 149
  nutrition screening, 147, 147t
  overview of, 146–147
Nutrition care process terminology (NCPT), 147
Nutrition care record, 151–154
  electronic health records and nutrition informatics for, 153–154
  medical record charting as, 152–153
    ADIME format for, 152–153, 152b, 153t
    PES statements in, 152–153, 155t
    POMR for, 152
    SOAP note format for, 152, 152t
Nutrition counseling
  in adolescence, 351, 352f, 352t
  for bulimia nervosa, 435, 435t
  for diabetes mellitus, 632, 632f
  for end-stage renal disease, 752
  nutrition interventions and, 159
Nutrition diagnosis etiology matrix, 148–149
Nutrition diagnosis(es)
  for cancer, 770
    behavioral-environmental domain in, 770b
    clinical domain in, 770b
    intake domain in, 770b
  for critically ill patient, 812
  with developmental disorders, 959
  for diabetes mellitus, 626, 626b
  and intervention, 145
    clinical case study on, 160b
  in nutrition care process, 147–149
Nutrition education
  for adults, 364–365
  for children, 334–335
  for diabetes mellitus, 632, 632f
  for eating disorders, 437
  for end-stage renal disease, 752
  with HIV infection, 800b
  nutrition intervention related to, 159
  for phenylketonuria, 943–945
Nutrition evaluation, 149–151
  for cancer, 781
  for developmental disorders, 960
  for diabetes mellitus, 632, 633b
Nutrition facts label, 177–178, 177t, 178b
Nutrition-focused physical examination (NFPE), 74–78, 1003–1008t
  approach for, 74
  functional medicine in, 76–78, 78f
  functionality in, 75
  malnutrition in adults, 75, 75f, 76t
  malnutrition in children, 75
  physical activity assessment in, 73b, 75
  strength in, 76
  techniques and findings in, 75, 75t
Nutrition impact symptoms, in cancer, 770
Nutrition informatics, 153–154

Nutrition intervention(s), 158–160
  for cancer, 770–773
    for alterations in energy metabolism, 772
    for anorexia and alterations in taste and smell, 771–772
    for cancer cachexia, 772
    oral nutrition management strategies in, 770–771, 771–772t
    for other cancer-related metabolic abnormalities, 773
    with pharmacotherapy, 773
  for cerebral palsy, 967
  coordination of care as, 159–160
  definition of, 149
  for developmental disorders, 959–960
  for diabetes mellitus, 626–632
    for specific populations, 626–627, 628t
  for Down's syndrome, 959–960
  for food and nutrient delivery, 158
    acceptance and psychologic factors as, 159
    consistency modifications as, 159
    diet modifications in hospitalized clients as, 158–159
    food intake as, 159
    modifications of normal diet as, 158
    regular or general diet in, 159
  implementation phase of, 149
  monitoring and evaluation of, 149–151
  in nutrition care process, 149
  nutrition education and counseling as, 159, 632, 632f
  planning phase of, 149
  for Prader-Willi syndrome, 964
  specificity of, 149
  for spina bifida, 967
Nutrition knowledge/beliefs/attitudes, 46t, 54
Nutrition labeling, 176–177, 414b
Nutrition Labeling and Education Act (NLEA), 176
Nutrition monitoring, 149–151
  for cancer, 781
  for developmental disorders, 960
  for diabetes mellitus, 624–625, 632, 633b
  for eating disorders, 436–437, 436b
Nutrition periodization, 448
Nutrition planning, 130
Nutrition policy, 129–130
Nutrition practice, in community, 128–129
Nutrition prescription, 149
  for diabetes mellitus, 629–632, 630f, 631f
Nutrition Program for the Elderly, 134–135t
Nutrition Quality of Life, 55
Nutrition rehabilitation, for eating disorders, 427–431
Nutrition-related history, 44–46
  clinical case study on, 55b
Nutrition screening, 41–43, 44b, 46b
  in adolescence, 351, 352f, 352t
  for cancer, 768
  in nutrition care process, 147, 147t
  for older adults, 382
Nutrition standardized language, 157b
Nutrition status
  of Americans, 174–175
  anticonvulsants effect on, 870
  assessment of, parameters used in, 1000–1001t

Nutrition support, 239
  for burn patient, 819
  in end-stage renal disease, 750–751
  enteral nutrition for, 209–216
    administration of, 214–215
      via bolus, 214–215
      via continuous drip, 215
      via intermittent drip, 215
    closed enteral system for, 214
    formula for
      carbohydrate in, 213–214
      factors to consider when choosing, 213b
      fluid in, 214
      lactose free, 212–213
      lipid in, 214
      osmolality of, 212
      polymeric, 212–213
      protein in, 213
      standard, 213
      vitamins, minerals, and electrolytes, 214
    hang time in, 214
    long-term, 211–212
      gastrostomy or jejunostomy for, 211–212, 212f
      multiple lumen tube for, 212
    monitoring and evaluation of, 215–216
      for complications, 215–216, 215b
      for tolerance and nutrient intake goals, 216, 216b
    nutrition care process for, 220b
    open system for, 214
    other minimally invasive techniques for multiple lumen tube for, 212
    refeeding syndrome with, 220–221
    route selection for, 210f
    short-term, 209–211
      gastric vs. small-bowel access for, 210
      nasoduodenal or nasojejunal access for, 210–211
      nasogastric access for, 209–210, 211f
  ethical issues, 223–224, 224b
  in long-term and home care, 222–224
  for malnutrition, 812–813
  for older adults, 384–385
  parenteral nutrition for, 216–220
    access for, 217
      central, 217
      long-term central, 217
      peripheral, 217
      short-term central, 217, 217f
    administration of, 219–220
      via continuous infusion, 219
      via cyclic infusion, 220
    algorithm for route selection for, 210f
    central
      long-term, 217
      short-term, 217, 217f
    monitoring and evaluation of, 220
      for complications, 220
    nutrition care process for, 220b
    osmolarity of nutrients in, 216, 216t
    parenteral solutions for, 217–219
      carbohydrates in, 217
      compounding methods for, 219
      electrolytes in, 218–219, 218t, 219t
      fluid in, 219
      lipid in, 217–218
      protein in, 217–219

Nutrition support (Continued)
      trace elements, 218–219
      trace elements in, 219t
      vitamins in, 218–219, 218t
    peripheral, 217
    refeeding syndrome with, 220–221
  for premature infants, 915f
  refeeding syndrome with, 220–221
  route selection for, 210f
  sentinel events in, 209
Nutrition therapy see Medical nutrition therapy
Nutrition transition, 104, 184b
Nutritional anemia(s), 655
  B vitamin deficiencies, 66
    folate and vitamin B$_{12}$ in, 66
    methylmalonic acid in, 66
    serum homocysteine in, 66
  classification of, 65
  copper deficiency, 666
  folic-deficiency, 662–664
    clinical findings in, 662–663
    etiology of, 662–663
    medical management of, 664
    medical nutrition therapy for, 664
    methylfolate trap in, 663, 663f
    MTHFR allele in, 663
    pathophysiology of, 663–664, 663b
    stages of, 663, 664f
  iron deficiency see Iron deficiency anemia
  pernicious, 664–666, 665b
    assessment of, 666
    clinical findings in, 665–666
    defined, 665
    medical management of, 666
    medical nutrition therapy for, 666
    pathophysiology of, 665
    stages of, 665
  of protein-energy malnutrition, 65–66, 666
  sideroblastic (pyridoxine-responsive), 666–667
  vitamin E-responsive hemolytic, 667
Nutritional deficiencies, in anxiety disorder patients, 895
Nutritional facts
  on alcohol, 1084, 1084f, 1085t
  on biotin, 1104, 1104t
  on caffeine-containing products, 1086, 1086t
  on choline, 1102, 1102t, 1103t
  on essential fatty acids, 1087, 1087t
  on fluids, 1043
  on folate, 1098–1099, 1098t, 1099t
  on folic acid, 1098, 1098t, 1099t
  on high-fiber diet, 1090, 1090t
  on high-protein diet, 1094
  on hydration, 1043
  on omega-3 fatty acids, 1087, 1087t, 1088, 1088t
  on omega-6 fatty acids, 1087, 1087t
  on vegetarian diets, 1095, 1095f, 1096t, 1097t
  on vitamin B$_6$, 1099–1100, 1099t, 1100t
  on vitamin B$_{12}$, 1100–1101, 1100t, 1101t
Nutritional genomics, 81, 362, 397–398
  and chronic disease, 94–101
Nutritional immunomodulation, for prevention of food allergy, 522
Nutritional needs, of older adults, 382–384
Nutritional requirements
  of critically ill patient, 813–816, 813t
    formula selection for, 816
    minerals, 815

Nutritional requirements (Continued)
    protein, 815
    trace elements, 815
    vitamins, 815
  for end-stage liver disease, 592–593
  of exercise, 444–445
    energy as, 444–445, 445b
    sports supplements for, 442–444, 448t
  during twin pregnancy, 269, 269t
Nutritional status, 41, 42f
Nutritional supplementation
  for children, 327–328
  for infants, 314, 314b
  during pregnancy, 269t, 283–285
  with restricted-energy diet, 405
Nutritional supplementation, in dialysis patients, 1074
Nutriture, 115
Nuts
  fats and, 1058–1059t
  Mediterranean diet and, 1082

O
O$_2$ see Oxygen
OA see Osteoarthritis
OAA (Older Americans Act) Nutrition Program, 384–385
OAS (oral allergy syndrome), 503
Ob gene, 398
Obama, Michelle, 398b
Obese men, TEE for, 23–24b
Obese women, TEE for, 23–24b
Obesity, 397–398
  in adults, 367, 403–415
  in Americans, 174
  assessment of, 415
  breastfeeding with, 297
  in carcinogenesis, 759–760
  causes of
    inadequate physical activity as, 400
    inflammation as, 401–402
    medication usage, 400
    obesogens as, 400
    sleep, stress, and circadian rhythms as, 400
    taste, satiety, and portion sizes as, 400
    viruses and pathogens as, 400–401
  in childhood, 335–336
    and diabetes, 628
  classification of, 401t
  and coronary heart disease, 678, 683b
  defined, 401
  discrimination due to, 403
  and fertility, 244–245
  global prevalence of, 367
  health risks of, 367, 401
  with HIV, 798
  intraabdominal, and type 2 diabetes mellitus, 609
  and kidney stones, 729
  and longevity, 401, 402f
  management of, 403–415
    bariatric surgery in, 411, 413t
      gastric bypass, gastroplasty, and gastric banding as, 411–413, 412f, 413t
    common problems in
      maintaining reduced body weight as, 414
      plateau effect as, 414
      weight cycling as, 414–415

Obesity *(Continued)*
dietary modification in, 404–405
commercial programs of, 405, 406f
intermittent fasting as, 406
meal replacement programs as, 405
popular diets and practices in, 406, 408t
restricted-energy diets as, 404–405
very-low-calorie diets as, 407
very low-calorie diets of, 405–406
goals of, 403
lifestyle modification in, 404
pharmacotherapy in, 409
physical activity in, 407–409, 409f
rate and extent of weight loss in, 403–404
metabolic syndrome and, 109, 402–403
morbid, 404
and neural tube defects, 268
and nutritional genomics, 98–100
in older adults, 381
PES statements related to, 155t
in Prader-Willi syndrome, 963
and pregnancy, 267–268
prevalence of, 397–398, 398f, 399f
sarcopenic, 110–111, 112b, 376
severe, in adolescence, 354
toxins in, 395b
Obesity hypoventilation syndrome (OSH),
719–720
medical management of, 719
medical nutrition therapy for, 719–720
Obesogens, 99, 400
Obligatory thermogenesis, 18
OBRA *see* Omnibus Reconciliation Act
Obstruction, gastrointestinal, 553
medical nutrition therapy for, 553
pathophysiology of, 553
Obstructive sleep apnea (OSA), 719
OC/ucOC (K_2 marker), 1028t
Occipital lobes, 850, 882
Oculomotor nerve, 849t
Odynophagia, 531–532
OGTT *see* Oral glucose tolerance test
25(OH)D, 888–889, 1028t
25-(OH)D₃ (25-hydroxy-vitamin D)
biochemical assessment of, 67
Oil, 109t, 116
OIs *see* Opportunistic infections
Olanzapine (Zyprexa), 1031–1041t
Older adults, 373, 374f
classification of, 373
clinical case study on, 387–388b
community and residential facilities for,
385–388, 387f
demographics of, 373
depression in, 379–381
diabetes in, 629
docosahexaenoic acid intake in, 886–887
eicosapentaenoic acid intake in, 886–887
frailty and failure to thrive as, 381
health promotion and disease prevention
for, 374
heart failure in, 696b, 698t
hypertension in, 693
hypothyroidism in, 647–648
Medicare benefits for, 384
Minimum Data Set (MDS) for, 386, 387f
nutrition needs of, 382–384, 383t
nutrition screening and assessment of, 382

Older adults *(Continued)*
nutrition support services for, 384–385
Commodity Supplemental Food Program
(CSFP) as, 385
Medicaid and nutrition services as, 385
Seniors' Farmers Market Nutrition Program
(SFMNP) as, 385
U.S. Department of Health and Human
Services Older Americans Act (OAA)
Nutrition Program as, 384–385
USDA food assistance programs as, 385
omega-3 fatty acid intake in, 886–887
physical activity for, 376
physiologic changes in, 375–379
in body composition, 375–376
cardiovascular, 379
gastrointestinal, 377b, 378–379
in hearing and eyesight, 376–378, 377b
in immunocompetence, 378
neurologic, 379
oral, 378
renal, 379
in taste and smell, 376
pressure injuries in, 379, 380t
quality of life of, 379–382
functionality in, 381
weight maintenance in, 381–382
and obesity, 381
and underweight and malnutrition,
381–382
study of, 374
theories on aging and, 374–375, 375t
Older Americans Act (OAA) Nutrition Program,
384–385
Older athletes, hydration during exercise and
sports, 455
Oleic acid, and coronary heart disease, 679
Olfactory nerve, 849t
Oligosaccharides, 316
digestion of, 11
Oliguria, 728
Olives, fats and, 1058–1059t
Omega-3 alpha-linoleic acid, 115–116
Omega-3 fatty acids, 1057
adult intake of, 885–886
in cancer prevention, 761
cognition affected by, 899
and coronary heart disease, 679
description of, 884–885
food sources of, 1088, 1088t
for gastritis and peptic ulcers, 537b
and hypertension, 687t
inflammation and, 836b
and kidney stones, 735–736
in lactation, 885
as ligands, 86
nutritional facts on, 1087, 1087t, 1088, 1088t
older adult intake of, 886–887
pregnancy intake of, 885
supplementation of, 887
Omega-6 dihomo-γ-linolenic acid, 111, 113–115
Omega-6 fatty acids
dietary sources of, 1088
nutritional facts on, 1087, 1087t, 1088t
Omega-6 linoleic acid, 115–116
Omeprazole (Prilosec), 1031–1041t
Omnibus Reconciliation act (OBRA), 386
Oncogenes, 758

Oncology, 758
Oncology Toolkit, 770
Oncotic pressure, 29b, 31b
1000 Genomes Project, 92, 92b
Onglyza (saxagliptin), for type 2 diabetes, 621–622t
Oocyte, 246–249t
Open abdomen, 816
Open-ended questions, 231
Open enteral system, 214
Open fractures, 860
Open oral food challenge, 511t
Opioid analgesics, 826
Opportunistic infections (OIs), 905
in AIDS, 790
Optic nerve, 849t
Optimal Macronutrient Intake Trial for Heart
Health (OmniHeart) trial, 688
Optimism, in behavior change, 233
Oral allergy syndrome (OAS), 503
Oral care with colostrum, 922
Oral cavity
digestion in, 3
nutrition-focused physical examination, 1003–1008t
Oral changes
with aging, 378
with chemotherapy, 777
Oral communication tools, 182
Oral contraceptives, 1031–1041t
Oral disorders, 488–489
Oral feeding
enteral to, 222
parenteral to, 222
Oral food challenge, 517
Oral glucose tolerance test (OGTT), for
gestational diabetes mellitus, 609
Oral health
for children, 485t
clinical case study on, 490b
natural products in, 489b
nutrition for, 482
Oral literacy, 182
Oral manifestations, of systemic disease, 489–490
Oral-motor problems, with developmental
disabilities, 958–959, 959b
Oral mucositis, due to chemotherapy, 777
Oral nutrition, with cancer, 770–771
Oral phase, of swallowing, 852–854, 853f
Oral rehydration solution (ORS), 31
for diarrhea, 550, 553t
Oral supplements, 222
nutrition intervention related to, 159
Oral tolerance, 497b, 520b
breakdown of, 499
Order-writing privileges (OWPs), 158
Orexigenic agents, for unintentional weight loss, 416
Organic acid(s), 947, 1028t
Organic acidemias, 936–938t, 946f, 947
medical nutrition therapy for, 947
medical treatment of, 947
pathophysiology of, 947
Organic foods, 139, 141–142b
Organogenesis, 241t
Orlistat (Xenical, Alli)
for prediabetes, 613
for weight loss, 408t, 409, 410t
Ornish Program, 407
Ornithine transcarbamylase (OTC) deficiency,
936–938t, 947

ORS *see* Oral rehydration solution
Orthopnea, in heart failure, 696
OSFED *see* Other specified feeding or eating disorder
Osmolality (Osmol), 30, 31b, 1028t
    of enteral formula, 212
Osmolarity, 29–30, 31b
    of nutrients in parenteral nutrition, 216, 216t
Osmoles, 31b
Osmotic agents, for constipation, 547
Osmotic forces, 31b
Osmotic pressure, 31b
Osteitis fibrosa cystica, 749
Osteoarthritis (OA), 823
    adiposity management in, 831
    chondroitin for, 832
    complementary integrative therapies for, 832
    etiology of, 830f
    exercise for, 831
    glucosamine for, 832
    inflammation in, 824
    joints commonly affected in, 831, 831f
    medical management of, 830f, 831
    medical nutrition therapy for, 824t, 831
    minerals for, 831–832
    pathophysiology of, 829–831, 830f, 831f
    risk factors for, 829
    surgical management of, 831
    vitamins for, 831–832
    weight management for, 831
Osteoblasts, 472, 472t
    in bone remodeling, 473f
Osteocalcin, 67, 477
    as vitamin K–dependent protein, 1112
Osteoclasts, 472, 472t
    in bone remodeling, 473f
Osteocytes, 472
Osteodystrophy
    hepatic, 585
    renal, 749
Osteoid, in bone, 471
Osteomalacia, 471, 749
Osteons, 471, 472f
Osteopenia, 473–476, 712
    in end-stage liver disease, 589
        medical nutrition therapy for, 589
        pathophysiology of, 589
    of prematurity, 917–918, 921, 926t
Osteoporosis, 473–476
    appearance of bone in, 474f
    causes and risk factors of, 474–475, 474b
        alcohol as, 474
        body weight as, 474
        cigarette smoking as, 474
        ethnicity as, 474
        limited weight-bearing exercise as, 474–475
        loss of menses as, 475
        medications as, 475, 475b
        nutrients as, 475
        sarcopenia as, 475
    clinical scenario on, 479b
    definitions, 475
    diagnosis and monitoring of, 475
    drugs for, 479
    due to anorexia nervosa, 424
    integrative approaches for, 479b
    prevalence of, 474
    prevention of, 478

Osteoporosis *(Continued)*
    screening tools for, 476t
    treatment of, 478–479
    types of, 474, 474b
    vitamin B$_{12}$ deficiency and, 666
Osteoradionecrosis, 778
Ostomy, 572
OTC deficiency *see* Ornithine transcarbamylase (OTC) deficiency
Other specified feeding or eating disorder (OSFED), 422–423b, 424
Otorrhea, 860
Overhydration, 61–62, 1043
Overweight, 397–398
    in adolescence, 354
    adults, 367
    assessment of, 415
    breastfeeding with, 297
    causes of
        inadequate physical activity as, 400
        inflammation as, 401–402
        medication usage, 400
        obesogens as, 400
        sleep, stress, and circadian rhythms as, 400
        taste, satiety, and portion sizes as, 400
        viruses and pathogens as, 400–401
    in childhood, 335–336, 398b
    classification of, 401t
    defined, 401
    discrimination due to, 403
    with Down's syndrome, 962, 962t
    health risks of, 401
    and longevity, 401, 402f
    and metabolic syndrome, 402–403
    and pregnancy, 267–268
    prevalence of, 397–398, 398f, 399f
Overweight boys, weight maintenance TEE for, 23–24b
Overweight girls, weight maintenance TEE for, 23–24b
Overweight men, TEE for, 23–24b
Overweight women, TEE for, 23–24b
Owen equations, 21
Oxalate intake, and kidney stones, 733–735
Oxalate stones, 731, 731b
Oxalobacter formigenes, 731
Oxazolidinone, 1031–1041t
Oxidative phosphorylation, 441
Oxidative stress, 68t
    and hypothyroidism, 646
    laboratory testing of, 1028t
    markers of, 68t, 1028t
Oxidized LDL cholesterol (OxLDL), as biomarker of oxidative stress, 68t
Oxycodone (OxyContin), 1031–1041t
Oxygen consumption, excess postexercise, 19
Oxygen metabolism theory, of aging, 375t
Oxygen requirements, during pregnancy, 250
Oxygen saturation, 38t
Oxyntomodulin, regulation of gastrointestinal activity by, 5
Oxytocin, in lactation, 292
Oysters, zinc from, 1130

P

PAB *see* Prealbumin
Pacemaker theory, of aging, 375t
Pagophagia, 657

PAHs *see* Polycyclic aromatic hydrocarbons
Pain relief, 905
PAL *see* Physical activity level
Paliperidone (Invega), 1031–1041t
Palliative care, 160, 386–388
    for cancer, 768, 782
    for end-stage renal disease, 752–753
Palmar grasp, and feeding skills, 318
Pancreas, exocrine, 599
    pancreatitis of, 599–602
        acute, 600
        chronic, 600–602
        clinical manifestations of, 599
        medical nutrition therapy for, 600–602
        pathophysiology and medical management of, 599
        tests of pancreatic function for, 599t
    physiology and functions of, 599
Pancreatic acinus, 709
Pancreatic amylase, in digestion, 8–9
    of carbohydrates, 11
    in infants, 311
Pancreatic cancer, surgery for, 779
Pancreatic disease, food intolerance due to, 496–497t
Pancreatic disorders, 579
Pancreatic duct, 599
Pancreatic enzyme(s), in digestion, 6t, 8–9
Pancreatic enzyme replacement therapy (PERT), 709, 709b
Pancreatic function, tests of, 599t
Pancreatic insufficiency (PI), 708
Pancreatic lipase, 920
    in digestion, 8–9
Pancreatic polypeptide, regulation of gastrointestinal activity by, 5
Pancreatic secretions, exocrine, 599
Pancreatic surgery, 602–603
Pancreaticoduodenectomy, 602
Pancreatitis, 599–602, 708
    acute, 600
    chronic, 600–602
    clinical manifestations of, 599
    defined, 599
    due to HIV infection, 795t
    medical nutrition therapy for, 600–602
    pathophysiology and medical management of, 599
    tests of pancreatic function for, 599t
    unintentional weight loss due to, 416t
Pancytopenia, with hematopoietic cell transplantation, 781
Pandemic control, 127
Pantoprazole (Protonix), 1031–1041t
PAQ *see* Physical activity questionnaire
Paracentesis, in end-stage liver disease, 590–591
Paraplegia, 864
Parasympathetic nervous system, regulation of gastrointestinal activity by, 5
Parathyroid hormone (PTH)
    in calcium homeostasis, 472
    and calcium metabolism, 472
    in end-stage renal disease, 745–747t, 748–750
Parent strands, 83f
Parenteral nutrition (PN), 209t, 216–220
    access for, 217
        central, 216
            long-term, 217
            short-term, 217, 217f
        peripheral, 217

Parenteral nutrition (Continued)
  administration of, 219–220
    via continuous infusion, 219
    via cyclic infusion, 220
  algorithm for route selection for, 210f
  for burn patients, 819
  central, 810
  for end-stage renal disease, 745–747t, 751
  fluid, 914–915
  for inflammatory bowel disease, 564
  method to calculate, 1046
  monitoring and evaluation of, 220, 221t
    for complications, 220, 221b
  nutrition care process for, 220b
  parenteral solutions for, 217–219
    carbohydrates in, 217
    compounding methods for, 219
    electrolytes in, 218–219, 218t, 219t
    fluid in, 219
    lipid in, 217–218
    osmolarity of nutrients in, 216, 216t
    protein in, 217
    trace elements in, 218–219, 219t
    vitamins in, 218–219, 218t
  with pediatric cancer, 782
  peripheral, 217
  for premature infants
    amino acids, 916
    calcium, 917–918
    electrolytes, 917, 917t
    energy, 915–916, 916t
    enteral nutrition transition of, 919
    fluid, 914–915
    glucose, 916, 916t
    lipids, 916–917, 917t
    minerals, 917–918, 918t
    monitoring of, 926t
    phosphorus, 917–918
    protein, 916
    trace elements, 918, 918t
    vitamins, 918–919, 918t
  solutions for
    pediatric, 916
    premature infants, 917
Paresthesia, 872
Parietal cells, 5, 532, 538
Parietal lobes, 882
Parkinson's disease, 847–848t, 876–878
Parotid gland, nutrition-focused physical
  examination, 1003–1008t
Paroxetine (Paxil), 1031–1041t
Partial pressure of dissolved carbon dioxide
  (PCO_2), 38, 38t, 1028t
Partial seizures, 870
Partially hydrolyzed formula (PHF), 521
Partnership for a Healthier America, 398b
Passionflower extract, 895b
Passive diffusion, 9
Pathogens, and overweight and obesity, 400–401
Patient-centered care, 156–157
Patient-centered medical home (PCMH), 156
Patient Protection and Affordable Care Act, 155
Patient Reported Outcome Measure (PROMs), 160
Patient's story, 122
Payment systems, 154–155
PBC see Primary biliary cirrhosis
PBM see Peak bone mass
PCBs see Polychlorinated biphenyls

PCI see Percutaneous coronary intervention
PCMH see Patient-centered medical home
PCO_2 see Partial pressure of dissolved carbon
  dioxide
PCOS see Polycystic ovary syndrome
PDD see Pervasive developmental disorder
Peaches, fruits and, 1051–1052t
Peak bone mass (PBM), 472
Peak height gain velocity, 343
Peanut
  allergy to, 522
  avoidance guidelines for, 508t
Pears, fruits and, 1051–1052t
Pectin(s), digestion of, 12
Pediatric clients see Children
Pediatric undernutrition, 336
Pedigree, 87–88
Peer educator, 231
Peer influence, and food intake of children,
  330–331
PEG see percutaneous endoscopic gastrostomy
Pegloticase, 839
Pellagra, 847t, 887–888
Pelvis, radiation therapy to, 778t, 779
PEM see Protein-energy malnutrition
Penetrance, 88
  reduced, 88
Penicillin VK (Pen VK), 1031–1041t
Penicillins, 1031–1041t
People-centered care (PCC), 156–157
Pepsin, in digestion, 6t, 8
  of proteins, 6t
Peptic ulcers, 534–535
  care management algorithm for, 535f
  defined, 534
  emergency symptoms of, 535
  etiology of, 534–535
  gastric vs. duodenal, 536–537, 536f
  medical and surgical management of, 536
  medical nutrition therapy for, 536–537
  pathophysiology of, 535f
Peptide(s), allergenic, 12–13
Peptide YY_{3-36} (PYY_{3-36})
  in regulation of body weight, 396–397t
  regulation of gastrointestinal activity by, 5
Peptones, digestion of, 12
Percutaneous coronary intervention (PCI), 683
Percutaneous endoscopic gastrostomy (PEG), 211–212
Periconceptual period, 241t
Perimenopause, 368
Perinatal mortality, low birth weight and, 255
Perinatal period, 912
Periodic limb movement disorder of sleep, 905
Periodontal disease, 488–489
  nutrition care for, 488–489
  pathophysiology of, 488
Periodontal ligament, 483f
Periodontitis, 105
Peripheral nervous system (PNS), 846–849
Peripheral neuropathy, 775–776t, 865
Peripheral parenteral nutrition (PPN), 216
Peripherally inserted central catheter (PICC,
  PIC), 217
Peristalsis, 8
Peritoneal dialysis (PD), 740
  continuous
    ambulatory, 740, 743f
    cyclic, 740

Peritoneal dialysis (Continued)
  mechanism of action of, 743f
  medical nutrition therapy for, 742, 744f, 745t
  types of, 742
Pernicious anemia, 664–666, 665b, 847–848t, 847t
  assessment of, 666
  clinical findings in, 665–666
  defined, 665
  etiology of, 665
  medical management of, 666
  medical nutrition therapy for, 666
  pathophysiology of, 665
  stages of, 665
Peroxisome proliferator-activated receptor gamma
  (PPARG), 97
Persistent depressive disorder, 890–892t
Personal health record (PHR), 154
Personality disorders, 890–892t
Pervasive developmental disorder (PDD), 967, 968t
PES statements (problem, etiology, signs and
  symptoms), 41, 43b
Pesticides, 139, 141–142b
PFAS see Pollen-food allergy syndrome
pH
  laboratory testing of, 1028t
  normal arterial blood gas values for, 38t
  regulation of, 38
  urinary, 62t
    diet and, 730b
    and stone formation, 731t
Pharmacogenomics, 84b
  application of, 96b
Pharmacognosy, 188–189t
Pharmacologic reactions, food intolerances due
  to, 496–497t, 512
Pharmacotherapy, for weight loss, 409, 410t
Pharyngeal phase, of swallowing, 853f, 854
Pharynx, 706f
Phe see Phenylalanine
Phe-free formula, 942
Phenelzine (Nardil), 1031–1041t
Phenobarbital (Luminal), 870, 1031–1041t
Phenolic acid, 86b
Phenotype, 88
Phenylalanine hydroxylase deficiency, 939, 940f
Phenylalanine (Phe)
  blood concentrations of, in phenylketonuria, 942
  foods low in, for phenylketonuria, 942
    guidelines for calculations of, 943t
    low-protein foods in, 944t
    menus of, 943t
    in young children, 942, 944t
  in infancy and childhood, 939t
Phenylethylamine, food intolerance due to,
  496–497t
Phenylketonuria (PKU), 93, 936–938t, 939–947,
  943t, 944f, 944t
  adults living with, 945–946
  care management algorithm for, 941f
  clinical case study on, 952
  food intolerance due to, 496–497t
  formula for, 942
  low-phenylalanine foods for, 942, 943t
  maternal, 945, 945t
  medical nutrition therapy for, 942–945
  medical treatment of, 939–942
  mild, 936–938t
  pathophysiology of, 941f

Phenylketonuria *(Continued)*
  patient education on, 943–945
  psychosocial development with, 945
  tasks expected of children with, 945t
  timeline of events in, 940b
Phenytoin (Dilantin), 1031–1041t
PHI *see* Protected health information
Phosphate(s), 1012t. *see also* Phosphorus
  and bone health, 477
  in chemistry panels, 59–60t
  laboratory testing of, 1028t
  in parenteral solutions, 218t
Phosphate binders, 1077
  for chronic kidney disease, 740
  for end-stage renal disease, 748, 748b, 749t
Phosphate intake, and kidney stones, 735
Phospholipids, digestion of, 13
Phosphorus, 36
  absorption, transport, storage, and excretion
    of, 36
  deficiency of, in end-stage liver disease, 592t
  in dialysis patients, 1076–1077
    binders, 1077
    high, 1076–1077
    low, 1076, 1077
    potassium and, 1077
  electrolyte concentration of, 33t
  functions of, 36
  premature infant requirements for, 917–918, 921
  serum, in chemistry panels, 59–60t
  sources of, 36
Phosphorus intake
  for chronic kidney disease, 740
  dietary reference, 36
  in end-stage renal disease, 745–747t, 748, 749t
  during pregnancy, 266
Phosphorus supplements, for end-stage renal
  disease, 749t
Phosphorylase, in digestion, 6t
PHR *see* Personal health record
Phylloquinone, 1012t. *see also* Vitamin K
  food sources of, 1113t
Physical activity, 46t, 55
  in adolescence, 358
  apps for tracking, 50b
  calories expended per hour with, 997, 999t
  with cancer, 765
  in children, 25, 337–338, 338f
  for diabetes mellitus, 619
    and carbohydrates, 619–620
    guidelines for, 619–620
    and insulin, 620
    potential problems with, 619
    precautions with, 620
    recommendations for, 620
  for hypertension, 687t, 689
  inadequate, overweight and obesity due to, 400
  inflammation levels affected by, 121
  for older adults, 376
  for prediabetes, 613
  for weight loss, 407–409, 409f
Physical activity level (PAL)
  change in, 24
  and estimated energy expenditure, 24
  and estimated energy requirements
    for adolescence, 344, 345t
  intensity and effect of various activities on, 25t
  walking equivalent of, 24t

Physical activity questionnaire (PAQ), 21
Physical assessments, 70–74
  anthropometry in, 70
  body composition in, 71–72
    air displacement plethysmogram, 74, 74f
    dual-energy x-ray absorptiometry, 73f, 74
    indirect calorimetry, 74
  body mass index in, 71, 76b
  circumference measurements in, 72
    adults, 73
    children, 72
    waist, 72f, 73
  height and weight in, interpretation of
    adults, 70–71, 70b
    children and teens, 70
  length and height in, 70, 70f
  nutrition-focused, 1000
    parameters used in, 1000–1001t
  skinfold thickness in, subcutaneous fat in, 72
  weight in, 69b, 70
Physical examination, nutrition-focused,
  1003–1008t
Physical findings, malnutrition and, 1001–1002t
Physical function, 46t, 55
Physical inactivity, coronary heart disease and,
  677–678
Physiologic anemia of growth, 347
Physiologic changes, with aging, 375–379
Phytic acid, calcium and, 1116
Phytochemicals, 86b, 162, 191, 370, 889–890
  as carcinogen inhibitors, 759
Phytoestrogens, 368
  in cancer prevention, 765
  in soy-based infant formulas, 316
Phytonutrients, 86b
  definition of, 370
  flavonoids, 120
  inflammation and, 120
Phytosterols, 54t
Piaget's theory of cognitive development, and
  feeding and nutrition of children, 328t
Pica, during pregnancy, 270
Pickles, free foods and, 1059t
Pie, sweet, desserts, and other carbohydrates,
  1053–1054t
Pierre Robin sequence, 971
Pigmented gallstones, 596
PIH *see* Pregnancy-induced hypertension
Pill forms, 192b
Pincer grasp, and feeding skills, 318
Pineapple, fruits and, 1051–1052t
Pioglitazone (Actos), 1031–1041t
  for type 2 diabetes, 621–622t
Piper methysticum, 198–205b
Piperacillin/tazobactam (Zosyn), 1031–1041t
PIs *see* Protease inhibitors
Pituitary gland, 642
  lesions of, 850
Pizza
  combination foods and, 1060–1061t
  fast foods and, 1061t
PKU *see* Phenylketonuria
Placenta, 251–255, 253f
Placental membrane, representation of, 253f
Plant alkaloids, nutrition-related effects of,
  774–775
Plant-based proteins, meat and meat substitute,
  1056–1057t

Plant foods, selenium from, 1127
Plaque
  atherosclerotic
    advanced, 672f
    fibrous, 672f
    mature, 671f
    natural progression of, 672f
    rupture of, 670
    stable, 671f
    and thrombus formation, 672f
    unstable, 671f
  dental, 485
Plasma, 655, 1028t
  specimen of, 1009
Plasma cells, in allergic reaction, 500f
Plasma specimens, 58
Plateau effect, with weight loss, 414
Platelet aggregation inhibitors, 1031–1041t
Plato Saludable de la Familia Colombiana, 166f
Pleural effusion, 720, 720f
  medical management of, 720
  medical nutrition therapy for, 720
Plums, fruits and, 1051–1052t
PNA rate *see* Protein-nitrogen appearance
  (PNA) rate
Pneumocystis jiroveci pneumonia, with HIV
  infection, 793t
Pneumocystis pneumonia (PCP), with HIV
  infection, 793t
Pneumonia, 721–722
  medical management of, 722
  medical nutrition therapy for, 722
  pathophysiology of, 722
  Pneumocystis jiroveci, with HIV infection, 793t
PO_2 and O_2 saturation (SaO_2), 1028t
PO_2 (oxygen partial pressure), 38t
Policy development, 131
Pollen-food allergy syndrome (PFAS), 503, 505b
Polychlorinated biphenyls (PCBs), during
  pregnancy, 280–281, 281b
Polycyclic aromatic hydrocarbons (PAHs), in
  carcinogenesis, 759
Polycystic liver disease, 582f
Polycystic ovary syndrome (PCOS), 648–649, 649t
  defined, 648–649
  and fertility, 240–241
  medical management of, 649
  medical nutrition therapy for, 649
  pathophysiology of, 649
Polycythemia, 666
Polydipsia, 607
Polygenic familial hypercholesterolemia, 674
Polygenic obesity, 99
Polymeric enteric formula, 212–213
Polymorphism, 88–89
  single nucleotide, 88–89
Polymyalgia rheumatica (PMR), 823, 842
Polymyositis (PM), 842
Polyp(s), intestinal, and colorectal cancer, 569
Polypeptides, digestion of, 12
Polypharmacy, 378
Polyunsaturated fats, 1057, 1058–1059t
Polyunsaturated fatty acids (PUFAs), 823
  conversion of, to prostaglandins, 113
  and coronary heart disease, 679
  in inflammation, 824
  vitamin E deficiency and, 921
Polyuria, 607

POMR *see* problem-oriented medical record
Popcorn, carbohydrates and, 1050–1051t
Popular Anticancer Dietary Plan, 774t
Popular diets, 405t, 406
Population-based public health, 127
Portal hypertension
    in alcoholic liver disease, 585
    medical nutrition therapy for, 587
    pathophysiology and medical treatment of, 587
Portal systemic encephalopathy, 588
Portion sizes *see* Serving sizes
Posaconazole (Noxafil), 1031–1041t
Positioning, for feeding, with developmental disabilities, 959f
Positive acute-phase reactants, 62–64
Postgastrectomy syndrome, 779
Postmenopausal women, osteoporosis and, 476b
Postpartum depression, breastfeeding with, 298
Postprandial blood glucose, 609
Postprandial capillary plasma glucose, in diabetes mellitus, 614t
Postprandial hypoglycemia, 636
    in dumping syndrome, 540
Postterm infant, 912
Posttranscriptional processing, 83–84
Posttranslational modification, 83–84
Potassium (K), 36–37
    absorption and excretion of, 36
    in chemistry panels, 59–60t
    in dialysis patients, 1074
        high-, 1075
        phosphorus and, 1077
    dietary reference intakes of, 1126t
    electrolyte classification of, 33t
    functions of, 36
    laboratory testing of, 1028t
    nutritional facts on, 1126
    for older adults, 383t
    in parenteral solutions, 218t
    sources of, 36–37, 37b, 1126t
Potassium bisulfite, food intolerance due to, 496–497t
Potassium chloride, as salt substitute, 1128
Potassium intake
    with acute kidney injury, 737
    for chronic kidney disease, 740
    dietary reference, 37
    in end-stage renal disease, 745–747t, 748
    and hypertension, 687t, 689, 692
    and kidney stones, 735
Potassium metabisulfite, food intolerance due to, 496–497t
Potassium replacement, for exercise and sports, 456
Potassium-sparing diuretics, 1031–1041t
Potassium sulfite, food intolerance due to, 496–497t
Potato, carbohydrates and, 1050–1051t
Pouchitis, 574
PPARG *see* Peroxisome proliferator-activated receptor gamma
PPIs *see* Proton pump inhibitors
PPN *see* Peripheral parenteral nutrition
PPOs *see* Preferred-provider organizations
Prader-Willi syndrome (PWS), 90b, 963, 963f
    anthropometric measures in, 963
    appetite and obesity in, 963
    biochemical measures in, 963

Prader-Willi syndrome *(Continued)*
    dietary intake in, 963–964
    feeding skills in, 964
    genetics of, 963
    hypotonia in, 963
    intervention strategies for, 964
    metabolic abnormalities in, 963
    nutrition assessment for, 963–964
    nutrition diagnoses with, 955–957t
    pathophysiology of, 963
Pramlintide (Symlin), for type 2 diabetes, 621–622t, 622
Prandin (repaglinide), for type 2 diabetes, 621–622t
Prasugrel (Effient), 1031–1041t
Pravastatin (Pravachol), 1031–1041t
Prealbumin (PAB), 64, 1028t
    in end-stage renal disease, 743–744
Prebiotics
    function of, 10
    for inflammatory bowel disease, 567
    for prevention of food allergy, 521
Precautionary allergen labeling (PAL), 517
PRECEDE-PROCEED model, 229
Precision (personalized) health, 81
Preconception, 240–245
Precose *see* Acarbose
Predetermination, and aging, 375t
Prediabetes, 607
    defined, 607
    diagnostic criteria for, 612t
    incidence and prevalence of, 607
    laboratory testing of, 1028t
    management of, 612–613
        bariatric surgery for, 616
        lifestyle interventions for, 612–613
        medical, 613
        medical nutrition therapy for, 613
        physical activity in, 613
Prednisone (Deltasone), 1031–1041t
Preeclampsia, 273, 274b
Preexercise fuel prescription, 450
Preferred-provider organizations (PPOs), 154–155
Preformed vitamin A, 1105
Pregabalin (Lyrica), 1031–1041t
Pregnancy, 250–286
    in adolescence, 358–359
    adolescent, 269, 270b
    after bariatric surgery, 268
    anemia of, 667
    breastfeeding during, 299
    clinical scenario on, 300
    complications of, 269–276
        constipation, hemorrhoids, and diarrhea as, 270
        diabetes mellitus as, 270–272, 272t
        edema and leg cramps as, 273
        heartburn as, 273
        nausea, vomiting, and hyperemesis gravidarum as, 274–276
        pregnancy-induced hypertension as, 273–274
    cravings and aversions during, 270, 271t
    diabetes mellitus during
        gestational *see* Diabetes mellitus, gestational
        preexisting, 270–272
            nutrition intervention for, 628, 628t
            vs. gestational, 611
    docosahexaenoic acid intake in, 885

Pregnancy *(Continued)*
    eicosapentaenoic acid intake in, 885
    epigenetic effects in, 256–257, 257f
    estimated energy requirement during, 23–24b
    food safety during, 276–283, 277b
    guide for eating during, 283–285, 284b
        alcohol in, 278
        fluids in, 283
        nonnutritive substances in foods in
            artificial sweeteners as, 278–279
            bisphenol-A as, 279
            lead and cadmium as, 279–280, 280f
            Listeria monocytogenes as, 280, 281b
            mercury as, 280–281, 281b
            polychlorinated biphenyls as, 280–281, 281b
        recommended food intake in, 283, 284t
    high-risk, 254
    with hypothyroidism, 646
    mercury exposure in, 885
    metabolic responses during, 251, 252t
    multiple birth, 268–269
    nutrition requirements during, 257–266, 258f
        carbohydrates, 259
        energy, 257–258
            exercise and, 257
        fiber, 259
        lipids, 259
        minerals, 262–266
            calcium as, 262–263, 263t
            copper as, 263
            fluoride as, 263
            iodine as, 255t, 263–264
            iron as, 264–266
            magnesium as, 266
            phosphorus as, 266
            sodium as, 266
            zinc as, 266
        protein, 258–259, 259t
        vitamins, 259–262
            choline as, 261
            folic acid as, 259–260
            vitamin A as, 261
            vitamin B₆ as, 260
            vitamin B₁₂ as, 260–261
            vitamin C as, 261
            vitamin D as, 261–262
            vitamin E as, 262
            vitamin K as, 262
    nutritional supplementation during, 269t, 283–285
    obesity and, 267–268
    omega-3 fatty acids during, 242
    phenylketonuria during, 945
    physiologic changes of, 250–255
        in blood volume and composition, 250, 250t, 251t
        in cardiovascular and pulmonary function, 250
        in gastrointestinal function, 250
        in renal function, 251
    pica during, 270
    placenta during, 251–255
    uterine environment during, 251–255
    vegetarian diet in, 1097
    weight gain during, 266–269, 266f, 267t
    weight loss during, 267
Pregnancy-induced hypertension (PIH), 273–274
    overweight and obesity and, 258, 268

Pregnancy outcome, effects of nutritional status on, 255–257
Prehypertension, 683, 683t
Premature infant(s)
  anthropometric measurements in, 927
  body water in, 914
  breastfeeding of, 923
  bronchopulmonary dysplasia in, 722
  case study of, 931b, 932b
  definition of, 912
  dietary intake in, 926
  discharge care for, 927–930, 930f
  enteral nutrition for
    calcium, 921
    carbohydrates, 921
    description of, 919–922
    energy, 919, 920b, 920t
    folic acid, 922
    formula, 925–926
    human milk, 923–924, 925t
    iron, 922
    lipids, 920–921
    minerals, 921–922
    parenteral nutrition transition to, 919
    phosphorus, 921
    protein, 919–920
    selection of, 923–926
    sodium, 922
    tolerance of, 923
    transitional infant formulas, 926
    vitamin D, 921
    vitamin E, 921–922
    vitamins, 921–922, 921t
    volume of, 919t
  extremely low birthweight, 912, 913b, 930
  feeding of
    breastfeeding of, 923, 929–930
    discharge determinations based on, 927–928
    formula, 925–926
    gastric gavage, 922
    monitoring of, 926t
    nipple, 923
    transpyloric, 922
  glucose load in, 916t
  growth charts for, 927, 928b, 928f, 929f
  growth rates for, 927, 928f
  human milk for, 923–924, 925t
  insensible water loss in, 914–915
  laboratory indices in, 926–927
  lipases in, 920
  long-term outcome for, 927b
  malnutrition in, 914
  megaloblastic anemia in, 922
  neurodevelopmental outcome of, 930–932, 931f
  nutrition assessment of, 926–927
  nutrition support of, 915f
  osteopenia of prematurity in, 921, 926t
  pancreatic lipase in, 920
  parental readiness for caring of, 928
  parenteral nutrition for
    amino acids, 916
    calcium, 917–918
    electrolytes, 917, 917t
    energy, 915–916, 916t
    enteral nutrition transition of, 919
    fluid, 914–915
    glucose, 916, 916t
    lipids, 916–917, 917t

Premature infant(s) (Continued)
    minerals, 917–918, 918t
    monitoring of, 926t
    phosphorus, 917–918
    protein, 916
    trace elements, 918, 918t
    vitamins, 918–919, 918t
  PES statements commonly used for, 929b
  problems among, 914t
  weight of, 927
Premeal blood glucose, 616
Premenstrual dysphoric disorder, 890–892t
Premenstrual syndrome (PMS), 367–368
Preoperational period, and feeding and nutrition of children, 328t
Preosteoclastic cells, in bone remodeling, 473
Preprandial blood glucose, 609
Preprandial capillary plasma glucose, in diabetes mellitus, 614t
Presbyopia, 377–378
Preschool children, feeding of, 331–332, 332f
Preserved foods, in carcinogenesis, 761
Pressure injuries, in older adults, 379, 380t
Preterm birth rate, 912
Preterm infant see Premature infant(s)
Prevention
  for older adults, 374
  primary, 374
  secondary, 374
  tertiary, 374
Prevotella copri, 829
Primarily wasted, 325
Primary biliary cirrhosis (PBC), 582f, 585
Primary osteoporosis, 474
Primary prevention, 127, 374
Primitive streak, 246–249t
Print literacy, 183
Pritikin Program, 407
Probiotics, 198–205b
  for diarrhea, 550, 550b
  function of, 10
  for gastritis and peptic ulcers, 537b
  for inflammatory bowel disease, 567
  for irritable bowel syndrome, 567
  for prevention of food allergy, 521
Problem, etiology, signs, and symptoms (PES) statements, 41, 43b, 148–149, 152–153, 155t, 927, 929b
Problem-oriented medical record (POMR), 152
Problem recognition, in behavior change, 232
Problem solving, for weight loss, 404
Proctocolectomy, 574–575
Progesterones, nutrition-related effects of, 775–776t
Program of All-Inclusive Care for the Elderly (PACE), 384
Progression, in carcinogenesis, 758
Prohormones, as sports supplements, 465–467
Prokinetics, 1031–1041t
  for upper GI disorders, 529t
Prolactin, in lactation, 289, 292f
Promoter region, 83
Promotion, in carcinogenesis, 758
Proof, of alcoholic beverages, 25
Propionic acidemia, 936–938t, 947
  medical nutrition therapy for, 947
  medical treatment of, 947
  pathophysiology of, 947
Propionyl-CoA carboxylase deficiency, 936–938t, 946f

Propranolol (Inderal), 1031–1041t
Propylthiouracil (Northyx), for hyperthyroidism, 650t
Prostaglandin 1 series (PGE1), 117
Prostaglandin 2 series (PGE2), 117
Prostaglandin 3 series (PGE3), 117–118
Prostaglandin-endoperoxide synthase (PTGS), 825b
Prostaglandins, 824
  eicosanoids in formation of, 115–116
  functions of, 116
  inflammation and, 113, 114f
  metabolites of, 115–116
Prostanoids, 824
Protease inhibitors (PIs), 790
Protected health information (PHI), 154
Protectins, 825b
"Protective diet," 163
Protein(s)
  for adolescence, 344–345, 345t
  and bone, 476
  burn patient requirements for, 818–819
  for chronic obstructive pulmonary disease, 715
  critical illness requirements, 815
  in dialysis patients, 1073
    one serving, 1074
    servings for you, 1073, 1073t
    tips for eating more, 1074
  digestion and absorption of, 11–12
  electrolyte classification of, 33t
  in enteral formulas, 213
  food sources of, 1094
  high-protein diet, 1094
  in human vs. cow's milk, 315
  L-dopa therapy and, 877t
  markers of, 1028t
  for older adults, 383t
  in parenteral solutions, 217
  premature infant requirements for, 916, 919–920
  in rheumatoid arthritis patients, 835
  serum, in liver function tests, 580–581t
  sources of, 12–13
  supplements, 1094
  synthesis of, 83f
  for tuberculosis, 718
  in urine, 62t
  in vegetarian diet, 1095–1096, 1095t
Protein-calorie deprivation, 847t
Protein carriers, for mineral transport, 15
Protein-energy balance, 1028t
Protein-energy malnutrition (PEM)
  anemia of, 666
  due to anorexia nervosa, 424
  in older adults, 382
Protein intake, 12
  for acute kidney injury, 736–737
  for anorexia nervosa, 433
  for bulimia nervosa, 433
  in carcinogenesis, 761
  for children, 326, 327t
  for chronic kidney disease, 739
  for diabetes mellitus, 617
  with diabetic nephropathy, 635
  in end-stage renal disease, 742–744
  for exercise and sports, 451–452
    for resistance exercise, 451–452
  with HIV, 798–801

Protein intake *(Continued)*
    and hypertension, 686
    for infants, 311–312, 311t
    for lactation, 289–290
    during pregnancy, 258–259, 259t
        with twins, 269t
Protein metabolism
    insulin and, 614t
    in liver, 579
Protein-nitrogen appearance (PNA) rate
    in end-stage renal disease, 745–747t
    for evaluation of dialysis efficiency, 742
Protein requirements
    with cancer, 769
    for end-stage liver disease, 592
    in infancy and childhood, 939t
Protein-restricted diets, for disorders of urea cycle
        metabolism, 948
Proteolytic enzymes, in digestion, 8–9
Proteolytic peptidases, in digestion, 12
Proteomics, 84b
Proteoses, digestion of, 12
Proteus, food intolerance due to, 496–497t
Prothrombin, 1112
Prothrombin time (PT), 580–581t, 1028t
Proton pump inhibitors (PPIs), 888, 1031–1041t
    for upper GI disorders, 529, 529t
Protoporphyrin, in iron deficiency anemia, 659
Proximal convoluted tubule, 727, 728f
Pseudoanemia, 459
Psychiatric disorders
    algorithm for, 886f
    anxiety disorders, 890–892t, 894–895
    bipolar disorders, 890–892t, 895–896
    chronic fatigue syndrome, 882, 903–907
    depression, 888
    etiology of, 886f
    fibromyalgia, 882, 903–907, 904b
    major depressive disorder, 890–892t, 901, 902b
    medical management of, 886f
    medical nutrition therapy in, 882, 890–892t
    pathophysiology of, 886f
    schizophrenia, 888, 890–892t
Psychologic management, of eating disorders,
        426–427
Psychological changes, during adolescence,
        341–342
Psychological reactions, food intolerances due to,
        496–497t
Psychosocial development, with phenylketonuria,
        945
Psychotic disorders, 890–892t
PT *see* Prothrombin time
PTH *see* Parathyroid hormone
Ptyalin, in digestion, 6t
Ptyalism gravidarum, 276
Pubarche, 342, 342f, 343t
Puberty, 341, 342f, 343t
Pubic hair, in sexual maturation, 342, 342f, 343t
Public health
    core functions of, 128
    definition of, 127
    framework for, 128
    funding sources for, 128
    government's role in, 128–129, 129b
    Health Impact Pyramid and, 128, 129f
    population-based, 127
Public health assurance, 133

Pudding, sweet, desserts, and other carbohydrates,
        1053–1054t
PUFAs *see* Polyunsaturated fatty acids
Pulmonary cachexia, 716, 716b
Pulmonary disease, 705, 708f
    acute respiratory distress syndrome as, 720–721
        medical management of, 721
        medical nutrition therapy for, 721, 721t
        pathophysiology of, 720–721, 721t
    asthma as, 711–712
        allergic (extrinsic), 712
        defined, 711
        medical management of, 712
        medical nutrition therapy for, 712
        nonallergic (intrinsic), 712
        pathophysiology of, 711–712
    bronchopulmonary dysplasia as, 722–724
        medical management of, 722–723
        medical nutrition therapy for, 723–724, 723b
        in premature infants, 722–723
    care management algorithm for, 710f
    chronic, 707–711
    chronic obstructive, 713–716
        advanced stage of, 716
        medical management of, 713–714, 714f
        medical nutrition therapy for, 714–716, 715t
        pathophysiology of, 713, 713f
        risk factors for, 713t
    chylothorax as, 720
        medical management of, 720
        medical nutrition therapy for, 720
    clinical case study on, 724b
    cystic fibrosis as, 707, 708f
        care management algorithm for, 710f
        medical management of, 709–711
        medical nutrition therapy in, 711
        pathophysiology of, 708–709, 710f
    diffuse parenchymal lung disease as, 716–717
        medical management of, 717
        medical nutrition management for, 717
        pathophysiology of, 717
        pulmonary diagnostic tests for, 717
    lung cancer as, 718–719
        medical management of, 719
        medical nutrition therapy for, 719
        pathophysiology of, 718–719
    lung transplantation, 722
        medical nutrition therapy for, 722
    malnutrition on, 706
    on nutritional status, 706–707, 707b
    obesity hypoventilation syndrome as, 719–720
        medical management of, 719
        medical nutrition therapy for, 719–720
    pleural effusion as, 720, 720f
        medical management of, 720
        medical nutrition therapy for, 720
    pneumonia as, 721–722
        medical management of, 722
        medical nutrition therapy for, 722
        pathophysiology of, 722
    pulmonary hypertension as, 716
        medical management of, 716
        medical nutrition therapy for, 716
    tuberculosis as, 717–718
        medical management of, 718
        medical nutrition therapy for, 718
        pathophysiology of, 717–718
Pulmonary function, during pregnancy, 250

Pulmonary function tests, 707
Pulmonary hypertension (PH), 716
    medical management of, 716
    medical nutrition therapy for, 716
Pulmonary status, assessment of, 707, 707f
Pulmonary system, 705–707, 706f
Pulp, of tooth, 483f
Pulse oximetry, 707, 707f
Pureed by gastronomy tube, 213b
Purging, 421
Purines, 838
PWS *see* Prader-Willi syndrome
Pyloric sphincter, 8
Pyloroplasty, 538, 538f
Pylorus, 7–8
Pyrazinamide (Rifater), 1031–1041t
Pyridoxamine (PM) *see* Vitamin B$_6$
Pyridoxine, 1012t. *see also* Vitamin B6
Pyridoxine-responsive anemia, 666
Pyruvate dehydrogenase deficiency, 871
PYY$_{3-36}$ *see* Peptide YY$_{3-36}$

Q

Quality management, 155–156
Quality of life, in adults, 365, 366f, 379–382
    functionality in, 381
    weight maintenance in, 381–382
        and obesity, 381
        and underweight and malnutrition, 381–382
Quantitative fecal fat determination, 1028t
Quantitative food patterns, 50
Quercetin, 120
    for hypertension, 691t
Questions, open-ended, 231
Quetelet index (W/H^2), 71
Quetiapine (Seroquel), 1031–1041t
Quick Sequential Organ Failure Assessment
        (qSOFA) Criteria, 810t
Quiescent period, of growth, 324

R

RA *see* Rheumatoid arthritis
Radiation, ionizing, 767
Radiation-induced enteritis, chronic, 779
Radiation therapy, nutritional impact of, 778, 778t
    to abdomen or pelvis, 779
    to head and neck, 779
    to thorax, 778–779
    total-body, 779
Radioactive iodine, for hyperthyroidism, 650t
Raffinose, intestinal gas and flatulence due to, 545
RAI *see* Resident Assessment Instrument
Ramipril (Altace), 1031–1041t
Ranitidine (Zantac), 1031–1041t
Rapport, 230
RAS *see* Renin-angiotensin system
Rate of living theory, of aging, 375t
Raw food diet, of anticancer dietary plan, 774t
Raynaud's syndrome, 840
RBC count *see* Red blood cell (RBC) count
RBC distribution width (RDW), 1028t
RBD *see* Retinol-binding protein
RBP *see* Retinol-binding protein
RDS *see* respiratory distress syndrome
Reactive arthritis, 829
Reactive hypoglycemia
    idiopathic, 636
    postprandial, 636

Reactive oxygen species (ROS), 120, 456
  antioxidant protection against, 120–121
Ready-to-change counseling sessions, 235
  action plan in, 235
  setting goals in, 235
Rebaudinoside A (stevia), during pregnancy, 279
Rebound hypoglycemia, with parenteral nutrition, 219
Recaldent (casein phosphopeptide-amorphous calcium phosphate), for remineralization, 484
Recessive gene, 88
Recombinant human EPO (rHuEPO), 750
Recommended dietary allowances (RDAs), 52–53, 133, 167
  folate, 1098t
  folic acid, 1098t
  vitamin B$_6$, 1099t
  vitamin B$_{12}$, 1100t
Recommended food intake, during pregnancy, 283, 284b, 284t
Recovery apps, 427b
Rectum, 9
Red blood cell (RBC) count, in complete blood count, 61t
Red wine, and coronary heart disease, 682
Red yeast, 198–205b
Reduced calorie sweeteners, for diabetes mellitus, 617
Reduced-fat milk, 1052–1053t
Reduced penetrance, 88
Reduction mammoplasty, breastfeeding with, 298
REE see Resting energy expenditure
Refeeding syndrome, 35b
  in anorexia nervosa, 432–433, 433t
Reference daily intakes (RDIs), 177–178, 177t
Reference SNP (rs) number, 95–96
Reflection, for resistance behaviors, 234
  double-sided, 234
Reflective listening, 231, 231f
Refractory epilepsy, 871
Reframing, for resistance behaviors, 234
Registered dietitian nutritionist, 105
Regular diet, 159
Regulatory B-cells (B-reg cells), 499
Regulatory region, 83
Rehabilitation Hospital, 386t
Relative energy deficit in sports (RED-S), 447
Religion, food and, 180–181, 181t
Remineralization, of dental enamel, 484
Renal dialysis, and potassium, 1126
Renal disorders, 727
  acute kidney injury (acute renal failure) as, 736–737
    causes of, 736t
    medical management of, 736
    medical nutrition therapy for, 736–737, 737t
      energy in, 737
      fluid and sodium in, 737
      potassium in, 737
      protein in, 736–737
    pathophysiology of, 736–737
  chronic kidney disease as, 737–740
    causes of, 738b
    in children, 751
    diabetes and, 737
    and heart disease, 739b
    medical management of, 738–739

Renal disorders (Continued)
    medical nutrition therapy for, 739–740
      energy in, 739
      lipids in, 740
      phosphorus in, 740
      potassium in, 740
      protein in, 739
      sodium in, 739–740
      vitamins in, 740
    pathophysiology of, 737
    prevalence of, 738–739
    stages of, 738t
  clinical case study on, 753b
  education, adherence, and compliance, 736
  end-stage renal disease as, 740–753
    care management algorithm for, 741f
    in children, 751
    conservative treatment or palliative care for, 752–753
    coordination of care for, 752
    with diabetes, 751
    dialysis for, 740–741
      emergency diets with, 752, 753b
      evaluation of efficiency of, 742
      hemo-, 740, 742f
      peritoneal, 740, 743f
    kidney transplantation for, 752
    medical nutrition therapy for, 742, 744f, 745–747t, 745t
      calcium and parathyroid hormone in, 745–747t, 748–750
      energy in, 744–747
      ferritin in, 745–747t
      fluid and sodium balance in, 745–747t, 747–748
      iron and erythropoietin in, 749t, 750
      lipid in, 750
      magnesium in, 745–747t
      phosphorus in, 745–747t, 748, 749t
      potassium in, 745–747t, 748
      protein in, 742–744
      vitamins in, 749t, 750
    medical treatment of, 740–750
    nutrition support in, 750–751
      enteral tube feeding for, 750–751
      intradialytic parenteral nutrition for, 749t, 751
      oral protein supplementation during dialysis, 751
      parenteral nutrition for, 751
    pathophysiology of, 740–741, 741f
    patient counseling for, 752
    patient education for, 752
  kidney stones (nephrolithiasis) as, 728–736
    with bariatric procedures, 729
    baseline information and metabolic evaluation of, 729t
    calcium, 729–731
    case management algorithm for, 734f
    causes and composition of, 729t
    cystine, 732
    medical management of, 732
    medical nutrition therapy for, 732–736, 732t
      animal protein in, 733
      citrate in, 735
      fluid and urine volume in, 733
      fructose in, 735
      magnesium in, 735

Renal disorders (Continued)
      omega-3 fatty acids in, 735–736
      oxalate in, 733–735
      phosphate in, 735
      potassium in, 735
      sodium in, 735
      vitamins in, 735
    melamine and indinavir, 732
    obesity and, 729
    oxalate, 731, 731b
    pathophysiology of, 728–732, 729t, 734f
    struvite, 732
    uric acid, 729, 731t
Renal failure
  acute see Acute kidney injury
  defined, 728
Renal function, 727–728, 728f
  age-related changes in, 379
  impaired, nutrient requirements for, 745t
  during pregnancy, 251
Renal insufficiency, in end-stage liver disease, 589
Renal osteodystrophy, 749
Renal replacement therapy (RRT), for acute kidney injury, 736
Renal solute load, of human vs. cow's milk, 315
Renal tubular acidosis (RTA), 735
Renal tubules, 727, 728f
Renin, 728
Renin-angiotensin mechanism, 728
Renin-angiotensin system (RAS)
  in hypertension, 685, 686f
  and water balance, 30
Repaglinide (Prandin), 1031–1041t
  for type 2 diabetes, 621–622t
Replication, of DNA, 83f
RER see Respiratory exchange ratio
Resident Assessment Instrument (RAI), 386
Residential care communities, 385
Residential housing, types of, 386t
Residue, 548
Resilience, 143
Resistance behaviors, 234
  agreeing with a twist for, 234
  double-sided reflection for, 234
  ending session in, 234
  reflecting for, 234
  reframing for, 234
  shifting focus for, 234
Resistance training
  protein needs for, 451–452
  for weight loss, 409
Resistant starch, 4
Resistin, 714–715
  in regulation of body weight, 396–397t
Resolvins, 118, 715, 825b
Respiratory acidosis, 39
Respiratory alkalosis, 39
Respiratory disease see Pulmonary disease
Respiratory distress syndrome (RDS), 918
  acute, 39
Respiratory exchange ratio (RER), in athletes, 444
Respiratory quotient (RQ), 20–21
Respiratory system see Pulmonary system
Respiratory tract
  lower, 706f
  upper, 706f
Response elements, 83

Resting energy expenditure (REE), 17–18, 18f, 20t
defined, 17–18
in eating disorders, 429–430
in end-stage liver disease, 592
estimation of, 21–22
factors affecting, 18
age as, 18
body composition as, 18
body size as, 18
climate as, 18
gender as, 18
hormonal status as, 18
other, 18
temperature as, 18
Resting metabolic rate (RMR), 17–18, 394. *see also*
Resting energy expenditure
Restless legs syndrome (RLS), 658, 905
Restricted-energy diets, 404–405
Restrictive diet, for hypothyroidism, 646–647
Resveratrol, 852f
for hypertension, 691t
Reticulocytosis, after iron administration, 660
Retinoic acid, 1105
Retinol *see also* Vitamin A
biochemical assessment of, 64
Retinol activity equivalents (RAEs), of
vitamin A, 1105
Retinol-binding protein (RBP), 64, 1028t
Retinols (vitamin A), 1028t
Retinopathy, diabetic, 635
Rett syndrome, 968t
Reverse T₃ (rT₃), 641–642
Rheumatic and musculoskeletal diseases (RMDs)
acute-phase proteins in, 825
antiinflammatory diet for, 828, 828b
autoantibodies in, 825
biochemical assessment of, 825
complementary and integrative health
approaches for, 828–829
description of, 823
elimination diets for, 829
etiology of, 824
inflammation in, 824
medical diagnosis of, 825
medical nutrition therapy for, 823, 842–843b
pathophysiology of, 824
pharmacology for
analgesics, 826, 826t
biologics, 826t, 827
corticosteroids, 826t, 827
disease-modifying antirheumatic drugs,
826t, 827
nonsteroidal antiinflammatory drugs,
826–827
prevalence of, 823
risk factors for, 824
scleroderma, 824t, 840–841
systemic lupus erythematosus, 824t, 841–842
temporomandibular disorder, 824t, 837–838
treatment of, 825
vitamin D deficiency and, 827
Rheumatic fever, 829
Rheumatoid arthritis, 832f
algorithm for, 834f
antiinflammatory diet for, 828, 828b
articular manifestations of, 835
cachexia caused by, 835
diet history in, 835

Rheumatoid arthritis (Continued)
disease-modifying antirheumatic drugs for,
826t, 833
etiology of, 834f
exercise for, 834
extraarticular manifestations of, 835
inflammation in, 824
medical nutrition therapy for, 824t, 834–837
antioxidants, 836
complementary and integrative therapies,
836–837
energy, 835
fat, 835–836
minerals, 836
protein, 835
vitamins, 836
methotrexate for, 833
pathophysiology of, 832–834, 833f, 834f
pharmacologic therapy for, 833
salicylates for, 833
surgery for, 833–834
Rheumatoid factor (RF), 825
Rhinorrhea, 860
Riboflavin
laboratory testing of, 1028t
mental health and, 887
in parenteral solutions, 218t
Ribonuclease, in digestion, 6t
Ribonucleic acid (RNA)
messenger, 83–84
translation of, 83–84
D-ribose, for heart failure, 700
Rice milk, 1052–1053t
Rifabutin, 1031–1041t
Rifampin (Rifadin), 1031–1041t
Risedronate (Actonel), 1031–1041t
Risk assessment, 139
Risk management, 139
Risperidone (Risperdal), 1031–1041t
Rivaroxaban (Xarelto), 1031–1041t
Rivastigmine (Exelon), 1031–1041t
RLS *see* Restless legs syndrome
RNA *see* Ribonucleic acid
Roman Catholic dietary practices, 181t
Rome IV criteria, 532, 541b
for irritable bowel syndrome, 566,
566b, 566t
Room service, 159
Root caries, 486
ROS-induced changes, to gene expression,
as biomarker of oxidative stress, 68t
ROS (reactive oxygen species), 456
Roselle, for hypertension, 691t
Rosiglitazone (Avandia), 1031–1041t
for type 2 diabetes, 621–622t
Rosuvastatin (Crestor), 1031–1041t
Roux-en-Y gastric bypass, 411, 412f
Roux-en-Y procedure, 537–538, 538f
RQ *see* Respiratory quotient
RRT *see* Renal replacement therapy
rT₃ (reverse), 641–642
Russell's sign, 425, 425f

S

S-adenosyl-L-methionine (SAMe), for liver
disease, 593
S-adenosylmethionine (SAM), in B vitamin
deficiencies, 66

S-glutathionylation, as biomarker of oxidative
stress, 68t
S-pouch, 574
Saccharin, during pregnancy, 278
Saccharomyces boulardii, for diarrhea, 550b, 552
Salad dressing
fats and, 1058–1059t
free foods and, 1059t
Salads
combination foods and, 1060–1061t
fast foods and, 1061t
Salicylates, food intolerance due to, 496–497t
Saliva
and dental caries, 486
in digestion, 8
digestive enzymes in, 6t
excessive, during pregnancy, 276
as specimens, 59, 1009
Salivary amylase, in digestion, 3
of carbohydrates, 11
in infants, 311
Salivary glands, in digestion, 8
Salmonella, 136–138t
Salt *see also* Sodium
for cystic fibrosis, 711
dietary reference intakes for, 35
measurement equivalents for, 699b
seasoning without, 1128–1129
Salt-resistant hypertension, 688
Salt restriction
for heart failure, 698–699, 698t, 699b
for hypertension, 687t, 691–692, 692b
Salt-sensitive hypertension, 688
Salt substitutes, 1128
Salve, 192b
SAM *see* S-adenosylmethionine
SAMe *see* S-adenosyl-L-methionine
Sandwiches, fast foods and, 1061t
Sarcoma, Kaposi's, with HIV infection, 793t
Sarcopenia, 375–376
pathophysiology of, 110–111
Sarcopenic obesity, 110–111, 112b
Satiety behaviors
in infants, 318t
and overweight and obesity, 400
sensory-specific, 400
Saturated fats, 1057, 1058–1059t
Saturated fatty acids (SFAs), and coronary heart
disease, 679
Saw palmetto, 198–205b
Saxagliptin (Onglyza), 1031–1041t
for type 2 diabetes, 621–622t
SBP *see* Systolic blood pressure
SBS *see* Short-bowel syndrome
SCA *see* Sickle cell anemia
Scalp, 1003–1008t
SCFAs *see* Short-chain fatty acids
Schizoaffective disorder, 890–892t, 905
Schizophrenia, 888, 890–892t, 905–907
Schmidt syndrome, 645
School, return to, breastfeeding with, 299–300
School-age children, feeding of, 333–334
School Nutrition Dietary Assessment Study, 133
SCI *see* Spinal cord injury
Scintigraphy, 540
Scleroderma, 824t, 840–841
Sclerosing cholangitis, 582f, 585
SCOFF Questionnaire, 427, 427b

Scoop sizes, 980
Screenings, alcoholism, 892–894, 893b
SCT see Social cognitive theory
Scurvy, 105
Seafood, 139
Seasonal affective disorder, 890–892t
Seasoning(s), without salt, 1128–1129
Second trimester, 246–249t
Secondary osteoporosis, 474
Secondary prevention, 127, 374
Secretin, regulation of gastrointestinal activity by, 7, 7t
Secretin stimulation test, for pancreatic function, 599t
Secretion(s)
    sites of, 4f, 5f, 15f
    in small intestine, 3
Secretory immunoglobulin A (sIgA), in human milk, 315
Sedentary death syndrome (SeDS), 376
Sedentary lifestyle, 376
Sedimentation rate, 107–109
Seeds
    fats and, 1058–1059t
    Mediterranean diet and, 1082
Seizures see also Epilepsy
    absence, 870
    tonic-clonic, 870
Selective estrogen receptor modulators (SERMS), 479
Selective estrogen receptor modulators (SERMs)
    nutrition-related effects of, 775–776t
Selective serotonin reuptake inhibitors (SSRIs), 1031–1041t
Selegiline (Eldepryl), 1031–1041t
Selenium-dependent enzymes, 1120
Selenium (Se), 198–205b
    deficiency of, 1127
        mental health affected by, 889
    dietary reference intakes for, 1127t
    food sources of, 1127t
    with HIV, 802t
    for hypothyroidism, 647–648
    laboratory testing of, 1028t
    nutritional facts on, 1127
    supplementation of, description of, 889
Selenium (Se), in parenteral solutions, 219t
Selenoproteins, 889, 1127
Self-efficacy, 229
Self-management, 230b
Self-management education, for diabetes, 624
Self-monitoring
    for behavior change, 235
    for weight loss, 404
Self-monitoring of blood glucose (SMBG), 613–614, 625
Self-motivational statements, 232
Semisolid foods, for infants, 318–320
Semivegetarian, 180
Semivolatile organic compounds (SVOCs), 394
Senescence, 375
Seniors Farmers' Market Nutrition Program (SFMNP), 134–135t, 385
Senna, for weight loss, 408t
Sensible water loss, 31
Sensitivity-related illness, 495–497, 497b
Sensitization, 499–500, 500f

Sensorimotor period, and feeding and nutrition of children, 328t
Sensory-specific satiety, 400
Sentinel events, 151
    in nutrition support, 209
Sepsis, 807. see also Critical illness
    metabolic responses during, 807
Seroconversion, in HIV, 788
Serotonin, 882–883
    in irritable bowel syndrome, 566
    in regulation of body weight, 396–397t
    regulation of gastrointestinal activity by, 396–397t
Serotonin antagonist/reuptake inhibitor, 1031–1041t
Serotonin-norepinephrine reuptake inhibitors (SNRIs), 1031–1041t
Serotonin syndrome, 903, 903b
Sertraline (Zoloft), 1031–1041t
Serum, 655
    specimen of, 1009
Serum antibody tests, for food allergies, 516
Serum antioxidant capacity, as biomarker of oxidative stress, 68t
Serum calcium, 1116
Serum glutamic oxaloacetic transaminase (SGOT), 580–581t
Serum glutamic pyruvic transaminase (SGPT), 580–581t
Serum specimens, 58
Serving sizes
    for children, 332, 333t
    for infants, 321
    and overweight and obesity, 400
Sesame seed, avoidance guidelines for, 508t
Session, ending, in behavior change, 233, 234
Set point theory, 395
Setting goals, 235
Seventh Day Adventist dietary practices, 181t
72-hr stool fat test, for pancreatic function, 599t
Sex, and coronary heart disease, 678
Sex chromosomes, 82
Sex hormones, 1031–1041t
Sex-linked inheritance, 88
Sexual disorders, 890–892t
Sexual dysfunction, 890–892t
Sexual maturity, during adolescence, 342, 342f, 343t
Sexual maturity rating (SMR), 342, 342f
SFAs see Saturated fatty acids
SFMNP see Seniors Farmers' Market Nutrition Program
SGLT-2 inhibitors (Gliflozins), 1031–1041t
SGOT see Serum glutamic oxaloacetic transaminase
SGPT see Serum glutamic pyruvic transaminase
Shellfish, avoidance guidelines for, 508t
Shifting focus, for resistance behaviors, 234
Shigellosis, 136–138t
Shock, 810
Short-bowel syndrome (SBS), 569
    defined, 569
    etiology of, 569
    medical and surgical management of, 570
    medical nutrition therapy for, 570
    pathophysiology of, 569
Short-chain acyl-CoA dehydrogenase deficiency, 936–938t

Short-chain fatty acids (SCFAs), 552
    colonic salvage of, 11
    production of, 4
SIBO see Small intestine bacterial overgrowth
Sickle cell anemia (SCA), 667–668
    clinical case study on, 668–669b
    clinical findings in, 667
    medical management of, 667–668
    medical nutrition therapy for, 668
    pathophysiology of, 667, 667f
Sideroblastic anemia, 666–667
sIgA see Secretory immunoglobulin A
Signal transduction, 85, 86b
Silent mutations, 91
Simple diffusion, 9f
Simvastatin (Zocor), 1031–1041t
Single-blind food challenge, 511t
Single nucleotide polymorphisms (SNPs), 88–89
    cytochrome P450, 119
    testing for, 120
Sirolimus, 1031–1041t
    after liver transplantation, 594t
Sitagliptin (Januvia), 1031–1041t
    for type 2 diabetes, 621–622t
Six-food elimination diet (SFED), 506
Sjögren's syndrome (SS), 823
    definition of, 837
    malnutrition in, 837
    medical management of, 837
    medical nutrition therapy for, 824t, 837
    pathophysiology of, 837
    xerostomia in, 837
Skilled nursing facilities (SNFs), 385, 386t
Skin
    nutrition-focused physical examination, 1003–1008t
Skin-prick test, for food allergies, 515–516, 516f
Skinfold measurements, for body fat percentage determinations, 996, 996t
Skull fractures, 860
SLE see Systemic lupus erythematosus
Sleep
    in inflammation reduction, 121
    insufficient amount of, 121, 904b
    natural remedies for, 905b
Sleep deprivation, overweight and obesity due to, 400
Sleep disorders, 890–892t, 905
Slovenia, Food Pyramid, 172f
Small bowel, with HIV infection, 793t
Small-bowel access, 210
Small bowel resections, nutritional consequences of, 569
    etiology of, 569
    medical and surgical management of, 570
    medical nutrition therapy for, 570
    pathophysiology of, 569
Small for gestational age, 912, 913, 913b, 913f
Small intestine
    absorption in, 9
        of fats, 13
        mechanisms of, 9, 14f
        structure and, 9
    anatomy of, 4f, 9
    digestion in, 8–9
    structure and function of, 9
    transport in, 9

Small intestine bacterial overgrowth (SIBO), 570–571
  defined, 570
  etiology of, 570–571
  medical nutrition therapy for, 571
  medical treatment of, 571
  pathophysiology of, 571
Small intestine diseases, 553–559
  celiac disease (gluten-sensitive enteropathy) as, 553–558
    assessment of, 555
    care management algorithm for, 557f
    clinical insight on, 555b
    defined, 554
    etiology of, 554, 554b
    gluten-free diet for, 556b
    hidden gluten exposure and cross-contamination with, 558b
    medical nutrition therapy for, 555–558
    pathophysiology of, 554–555, 554f, 557f
    refractory, 555
    resources on, 558, 559b
  tropical sprue as, 558–559
    defined, 558
    medical nutrition therapy for, 559
    medical treatment of, 559
    pathophysiology of, 559
Small molecule inhibitors, nutrition-related effects of, 775–776t
SMBG see Self-monitoring of blood glucose
Smell, with aging, 376
SMOFLipid®, 917
Smoked foods, in carcinogenesis, 761
Smoking
  multiple sclerosis and, 873
  reflux and, 530
"Smoldering disease," 107
SMR see Sexual maturity rating
Snacking
  adolescence by, 348–349, 349b
  by children, 334
SNFs see Skilled nursing facilities
SNPs see Single nucleotide polymorphisms
SNS see Sympathetic nervous system
SOAP (subjective, objective, assessment, plan) note format, 152, 152t
Social cognitive theory (SCT), 227, 228t
Social determinants of health, 128
Social-ecological model, 226, 227f
Social epigenomics, 88b
Social implications, of genetic testing, 95b
Social Security, 384
Social services, referral for, PES statements related to, 155t
Socioeconomic influences, and food intake of children, 329–330
SOD (super oxide dismutase) genes, 96–97
Soda, sweet, desserts, and other carbohydrates, 1053–1054t
Sodium (Na)
  absorption and excretion of, 35
  and bone health, 478
  childhood consumption of, 332
  electrolyte classification of, 33t
  food industry and, 692b
  food labeling guide for, 699b
  foods high in, 699b
  functions of, 34–35

Sodium (Continued)
  ionized (Na⁺), in chemistry panels, 59–60t
  laboratory testing of, 1028t
  measurement equivalents for, 699b
  for older adults, 383t
  parenteral solutions, 218t
  premature infant requirements for, 922
  sources of, 35
Sodium benzoate, food intolerance due to, 496–497t
Sodium bicarbonate, as sports supplement, 457–458t
Sodium bisulfite, food intolerance due to, 496–497t
Sodium chloride, 35
Sodium content
  of common foods, 1129t
  of over-the-counter brands, 1128
Sodium-dependent transport, of monosaccharides, 11–12
Sodium intake
  with acute kidney injury, 737
  for chronic kidney disease, 739–740
  dietary reference, 35
  in end-stage renal disease, 745–747t, 747–748
  and hypertension, 687t, 688, 692b
  for kidney stones, 735
  during pregnancy, 266
Sodium metabisulfite, food intolerance due to, 496–497t
Sodium phosphate, as sports supplement, 457–458t
Sodium-potassium adenosine triphosphatase (Na/K-ATPase) pump, 29–30, 33
Sodium replacement, for exercise and sports, 455–456
Sodium-restricted diets, 1128
Sodium restriction
  for acute kidney injury, 737
  guidelines for, 1128–1129
  for heart failure, 698–699, 698t, 699b
  for hypertension, 687t, 691–692, 692b
Sodium sulfite, food intolerance due to, 496–497t
Soft gels, 192b
Solid food, introduction of, and prevention of food allergy, 521–522
Soluble fibers, for diarrhea, 552
Soluble serum transferrin receptors (STfR), 659
Somatic cells, 88
Somatic mutation theory, of aging, 375t
Somatoform disorders, 890–892t
Somatomedin C, 1028t
Somatostatin, regulation of gastrointestinal activity by, 7–8
Somites, 246–249t
Somogyi effect, 634
SOPPs see Standards of Professional Performance
Sore throat, due to HIV infection, 795t
"Soul food," 180
Soups, combination foods and, 1060–1061t
Sour cream, fats and, 1058–1059t
South America, diet planning for, 162–163
South Beach Diet, 407
Soy
  for adults, 370
  avoidance guidelines for, 508t
  and bone health, 478
  in cancer prevention, 765
Soy-based infant formulas, 316
Soy isoflavones, 54t
Soymilk, 1052–1053t
Span measurement, for amputees adjustment, 994

Spastic quadriplegia, 967
Special Milk Program, 134–135t, 333
Special Supplemental Nutrition Program for Women, Infants, and Children (WIC), 128, 134–135t
Specialized intestinal metaplasia, 528
Specialized proresolving mediators (SPMs), 116, 825b
Specific dynamic action, 18
Specific effect of food, 18
Specific gravity
  laboratory values for, 1028t
  of urine, 62t
Specimen(s), types of, 58–59, 1009
Speech-language pathologists (SLP), 852
Spices
  and GI disorders, 537
  Mediterranean diet and, 1083
Spina bifida, 964–966
  anthropometric measures in, 965
  biochemical measures in, 965
  clinical evaluation of, 965
  defined, 964
  dietary intake in, 965
  health concerns with, 964
  intervention strategies for, 967
  nutrition assessment for, 965
  nutrition diagnoses with, 955–957t
  prevention of, 964–965
Spinal accessory nerve, 849t
Spinal cord
  lesions of, 850
  in vertebral canal, 850f
Spinal cord injury (SCI), 850, 866b
Spinal trauma, 865f, 847–848t, 864–878
Spirometry, 707
Spironolactone (Aldactone), 1031–1041t
Spondylarthritides, 842–843
Spoon-shaped nails, 658, 659f
Sports anemia, 459, 668
Sports drinks, electrolyte content of, 455t
Sports injury, fat intake and, 452–453
Sports performance see Exercise and sports performance
Sports supplements, 442–444, 448t
Sprue, tropical, 558–559
  defined, 558
  medical nutrition therapy for, 559
  medical treatment of, 559
  pathophysiology of, 559
St. John's wort, 194, 198–205b
Stable disease, after cancer treatment, 767–768
Staffing, 157
Stages of change model, 228, 228t
Staging, of cancer, 766
Standardized serving sizes, 176f, 177
Standards of care, 151
Standards of Professional Performance (SOPPs), 143, 151
Stanols, and coronary heart disease, 682
Staphylococcus aureus, 136–138t
Starch(es)
  in diabetes mellitus, 617
  digestion of, 11
  Mediterranean diet and, 1082
Starchy vegetables, carbohydrates and, 1050–1051t
Starlix (nateglinide), for type 2 diabetes, 621–622t, 622

Starvation, 809, 809f
  metabolic changes in, 809f
  vs. stress, 809
Statins, for coronary heart disease, 682–683
Statiometer, 70
Status asthmaticus, 712
Steatohepatitis, nonalcoholic, 583
Steatorrhea, 13, 548, 708
  in alcoholic liver disease, 590–591
  in end-stage liver disease, 590–591
Steatosis, hepatic, 584f, 585
Step up two-four-six food elimination diets, 506, 506–507b
Steroids, 1031–1041t
  as sports supplements, 461–462t, 464–465
Sterols, and coronary heart disease, 682
Stevia (Rebaudinoside A), during pregnancy, 279
STfR *see* Soluble serum transferrin receptors
Stimulant laxatives, for constipation, 547
Stimulus control, for weight loss, 404
Stomach
  anatomy and physiology of, 532–540
  carcinoma of, 537
    medical nutrition therapy for, 537
    pathophysiology of, 537
  digestion in, 8
  disorders of *see* Gastric disorders
Stomach capacity, of infants, 310–311
Stomach carcinoma, *Helicobacter pylori* and, 533
Stomatitis, in HIV infection and AIDS, 490
Stool softeners, for constipation, 547
Stool testing, 59–60
Stool weight, 9–10
Storage fat, 394
Strained meats, 317
Strained vegetables and fruits, 317
Streptococcus mutans, in development of dental caries, 483
Streptococcus pyogenes, 136–138t
Streptococcus sanguis, in development of dental caries, 483
Stress
  coronary heart disease and, 678
  ebb phase of, 807, 814f
  and Graves' disease, 650
  inflammation and, 113, 121
  metabolic response to, 807. *see also* Metabolic stress
  overweight and obesity due to, 400
  oxidative, and hypothyroidism, 646
  unintentional weight loss due to, 416t
Stress hormone, insulin and, 613
Stress ulcers, 536
Strictures, gastrointestinal, 553
  medical nutrition therapy for, 553
  pathophysiology of, 553
Stroke
  coronary heart disease and, 670
  definition of, 857
  dysphagia in, 858–860
  medical management of, 857
  medical nutrition therapy for, 857–860
  nutrition guidance for, 858–859t
  nutritional therapy for, 847–848t
  pathophysiology of, 857
  primary prevention of, 857
  thrombotic, 857
Structure function claim, 193–194

Struvite stones, 732
Stunted growth, 325
Subarachnoid hemorrhage (SAH), 857
Subclavian catheter, for hemodialysis, 740, 742f
Subcutaneous fat loss, 1000–1001t
Subdural hematomas, 860
Subjective, objective, assessment, plan (SOAP) note format, 152, 152t
Subluxations, 188–189t
Submarine sandwiches, fast foods and, 1061t
Substance abuse, medical nutritional therapy for, 894b
Substance disorders, 890–892t
Substance P, regulation of gastrointestinal activity by, 6t
Substrate, in development of dental caries, 483–484, 484b
Sucralose, during pregnancy, 278
Sucrase, in digestion, 6t, 11
Sucrose
  and dental caries, 484
  digestion of, 12f
Sucrose intake, in diabetes mellitus, 617
Sugar, and dental caries, 484
Sugar intake, 884
  in diabetes mellitus, 617
Suicide attempt, 896
Sulfamethoxazole/ trimethoprim (Bactrim), 1031–1041t
Sulfates, electrolyte classification of, 33t
Sulfites, food intolerance due to, 496–497t, 513
Sulfonamide combination, 1031–1041t
Sulfonylureas
  nutritional implications of, 1031–1041t
  for type 2 diabetes, 620, 621–622t
Sulforaphane, 890
Sulfur dioxide, food intolerance due to, 496–497t
Summarizing, 232
Summer Food Service Program, 134–135t, 333
Supplemental Nutrition Assistance Program (SNAP), 133, 134–135t, 138b, 365
Surface structure, 230
Surfactant, 706, 706f, 912, 918
Surgeon General's Report on Nutrition and Health, 132
Surgery
  for cancer, 771–772t, 779–781
    esophageal, 779
    gastric, 779
    head and neck, 779
    intestinal tract, 781
    pancreatic, 779
  medical nutrition therapy after, 819–821
  metabolic stress due to, 819–821
    medical nutrition therapy for, 819–821
      postoperative, 820–821
      preoperative, 819–820
  for rheumatoid arthritis, 833–834
Surveys, 151
Surveys, national nutrition, 130–131
  Continuing Survey of Food Intake of Individuals, 131
  National Health and Nutrition Examination Survey, 130–131
  National Nutrient Databank, 131
  National Nutrition Monitoring and Related Research Act, 131
  What We Eat in America, 131

Sustainable Development Goals (SDGs), 128
SVOCs *see* Semivolatile organic compounds
Swallowing
  of liquids, 855–856
  phases of, 852, 853f
Sweat, as specimens, 59
Sweet(s), on exchange list, 1049, 1052–1053, 1053–1054t
  nutrition tips, 1053
  selection tips, 1053
Sweetened beverages, childhood consumption of, 332
Sweeteners
  and carcinogenesis, 761
  in diabetes mellitus, 617
Symlin (pramlintide), for type 2 diabetes, 621–622t, 622
Symmetric intrauterine growth restriction, 913
Sympathetic nervous system (SNS), regulation of gastrointestinal activity by, 5
Synaptic plasticity, 899
Synbiotics, 10
  for diarrhea, 551
Syncope, in heart failure, 696
Syndrome of inappropriate antidiuretic hormone secretion (SIADH), 850
Synthetic opioid analgesic, 1031–1041t
Synthroid (levothyroxine), for hypothyroidism, 646t
Syrup, sweet, desserts, and other carbohydrates, 1053–1054t
Systemic disease, oral manifestations of, 489–490
Systemic inflammatory response syndrome (SIRS), 809–810, 810b
Systemic lupus erythematosus (SLE), 823, 824t, 841–842
Systemic nickel allergy syndrome (SNAS), 503–505
Systemic sclerosis (SSc), 823, 840–841
Systems biology, 105
Systolic blood pressure (SBP), 683

T

T cells, in allergic reaction, 498–499, 500f
T helper (Th) cells
  in allergic reaction, 499, 500f
  in HIV, 788
T-lymphocytes, 119
T-regulatory cells (T-reg cells), 499
T-suppressor cells, 499
T1DM *see* Type 1 diabetes mellitus
T2DM *see* Type 2 diabetes mellitus
T₃ *see* Triiodothyronine
T₄ *see* Thyroxine
Tablets, 192b, 196
Tachypnea, in pulmonary disease, 707
Tacrolimus (Prograf, Envarsus XR), 1031–1041t
Tandem mass spectrometry, 939f
Tanner staging of adolescent development, 342, 342f
  in boys, 990, 990f
  in girls, 990, 990f
Tapazole (methimazole), for hyperthyroidism, 650t
Target blood glucose goals, for diabetes, 613–614, 624–625
Tartrazine, food intolerance due to, 496–497t

Taste
  with aging, 376
  and overweight and obesity, 400
Taste alterations
  due to cancer treatment, 771–772
  due to HIV infection, 795t
Taurine, 920
  in human *vs.* cow's milk, 315
TB *see* Tuberculosis
TBG *see* Thyroid-binding globulin
TBI *see* Traumatic brain injury
TCF7L2 see Transcription factor 7-like 2
TCI *see* Transcobalamin I
TCIII *see* Transcobalamin III
TCO₂ *see* Total carbon dioxide
TDD *see* Total daily dose
Teas, in cancer prevention, 764
TEE *see* Total energy expenditure
Teen pregnancy, 269, 270b
Teenagers *see* Adolescence
Teeth *see* Tooth
Tegretol *see* Carbamazepine
Tela submucosa, 5f
Telehealth, 404
Telmisartan (Micardis), 1031–1041t
Telomere length, 375t
Temazepam (Restoril), 1031–1041t
Temperature, and resting energy
    expenditure, 18
Temporal lobes, 850, 882
Temporomandibular disorder, 824t,
    837–838
Teratogenicity, of alcohol, 278
Terbinafine (Lamisil), 1031–1041t
Term infant, 912
Terminally ill patient, nutrition for, 160
Tertiary prevention, 127, 374
Tetany seizures, 847t
Tetracycline (Sumycin), 1031–1041t
Tetrahydrobiopterin (BH₄), for phenylketonuria,
    939–940
Tetrahydrofolic acid (THFA), in folic-deficiency
    anemia, 663, 663f
Tetraplegia, 864
Tf *see* Transferrin
TGB *see* Thyroglobulin
TGB Ab *see* Thyroglobulin antibodies
Th (T helper) cells
  in allergic reaction, 499
  in HIV, 788
Th1 cells, in allergic reaction, 499
Th2 cells, in allergic reaction, 499, 500f
Thalassemias, 668–669
The Joint Commission (TJC), 151
Theanine, 895b
Thelarche, 342, 342f
Theory of planned behavior (TPB),
    227–228, 228t
Thermic effect of food (TEF), 18–19
Thermogenesis
  activity, 19, 395–397
    nonexercise, 19
  diet-induced, 18
  facultative, 18
  obligatory, 18
Thermoregulation, during exercise and sports, 453
THFA *see* Tetrahydrofolic acid

Thiamin, 67–68
  deficiency of
    in alcoholic liver disease, 585b
    in alcoholics, 894
    in end-stage liver disease, 592–593, 592t
  for heart failure, 700
  laboratory testing of, 1028t
  mental health and, 887
  in parenteral solutions, 218t
Thiamin diphosphate, 887
Thiazide diuretic, 1031–1041t
Thiazolidinediones (TZDs)
  for prediabetes, 613
  for type 2 diabetes, 620, 621–622t
Third party certification, dietary supplementation
    and, 195
"Third space" fluid, 28, 31b
Thirst, 33
Thorax, radiation therapy to, 778–779, 778t
Threonine, in infancy and childhood, 939t
Thrombocytopenia, 775–776
Thromboembolic event, 857
Thrombotic stroke, 857
Thromboxanes, 118, 824
Thrombus, 671–672, 672f
Thrush, with chemotherapy, 777
Thymus gland, 119
Thyroglobulin (TGB), 642f
Thyroglobulin antibodies (TGB Ab), 644–645
Thyroid-binding globulin (TBG), 642–643
Thyroid disorders, 641
  assessment of, 643–644
    laboratory norms in, 643–644, 644b, 644t
  autoimmune, 641
  hyperthyroidism as, 649–650
    care management algorithm for, 645f
    due to Graves' disease, 649–650, 650f
    medical management of, 650, 650t
    pathophysiology of, 645f, 650
    symptoms of, 644b
    triggers for, 650
      genetics as, 650
      stress as, 650
  hypothyroidism as, 644–648
    care management algorithm for, 645f
    and celiac disease, 644
    clinical case study on, 653b
    due to Hashimoto's thyroiditis, 644
    medical management of, 646, 646t
    medical nutrition therapy for, 646–648
      fasting or restrictive diets in, 646–647
      goitrogens and, 647
      iodine in, 647
      iron in, 647
      magnesium in, 648
      selenium in, 647–648
      vitamin D in, 648
    pathophysiology of, 644–646, 645f
    risk factors for, 644
    subclinical, 644
    symptoms of, 644b
    triggers for, 646
      adrenal dysfunction and oxidative stress
        as, 646
      aging as, 646
      pregnancy as, 646
  during pregnancy, management of, 648

Thyroid function, assessment of, 643, 644b, 644t
Thyroid function tests, 1028t
Thyroid gland
  desiccated natural, for hypothyroidism, 646t
  physiology of, 641–643
Thyroid health, promotion of, 651b
Thyroid hormones, 641–642
  flavonoids and, 651
  metabolism of, 643f
  nutritional implications of, 1031–1041t
  in regulation of body weight, 396–397t
  release of, 642
  synthesis of, 642, 642f
Thyroid peroxidase (TPO), 642, 643f
Thyroid peroxidase antibodies (TPO Abs), 644–645
Thyroid-stimulating hormone (TSH), 641–642, 642f
  iodine sufficiency and, 1120
  reference range for, 643, 644t
Thyroid-stimulating immunoglobulin, 650
Thyroiditis, Hashimoto's, 644
Thyrolar (liotrix), for hypothyroidism, 646t
Thyrotropin-releasing hormone (TRH), 642, 643f
Thyroxine (T₄), 641–642, 1028t
  free, 642–643, 644t
  improving conversion to T₃ of, 651
  iodine and, 1120
  metabolism of, 643f
  precursors for formation of, 651
  synthesis of, 642f
  synthetic, for hypothyroidism, 646t
TIBC *see* Total iron-binding capacity
Ticagrelor (Brilinta), 1031–1041t
Tight junctions, in intestinal villus, 810, 811f
Tinctures, 192b
TJC *see* The Joint Commission
TNF-alpha, 107–109
TNM *see* Tumor-node-metastasis
Tobacco, use of, reflux and, 530
Tocopherol(s), 900, 1012t. *see also* Vitamin E
  α-Tocopherol, 1110, 1110t
    food sources of, 1110t
Tocotrienols, 196. *see also* Vitamin E
Tolerable upper intake level (UL), 174
  of DRI value, 53
Tongue, nutrition-focused physical examination
    of, 1003–1008t
Tonic-clonic (grand mal) seizure, 870
Tooth decay *see* Dental caries
Tooth development, nutrition for, 482, 483f
Tooth loss, 488
  nutrition care for, 488
Tooth (teeth)
  anatomy of, 483f
  nutrition-focused physical examination,
    1003–1008t
Tophi, 838
Topiramate (Topamax), 1031–1041t
Topoisomerase inhibitors, nutrition-related effects
    of, 775–776t
Total antioxidant capacity, 1028t
Total-body irradiation (TBI), 779
Total body surface area, 817
Total body water (TBW), 28
Total carbon dioxide (TCO₂), 38, 1028t
  in chemistry panels, 59–60t
Total daily dose (TDD), in self-monitoring of
    blood glucose, 625

Total energy expenditure (TEE), 17, 19f
  determining, 21–22
  for overweight and obese men, 22
  for overweight and obese women, 22
  weight maintenance, 22
Total inflammatory load, 109, 111f, 122
Total iron-binding capacity (TIBC), 65,
    656, 1028t
  in iron deficiency anemia, 65
Total lymphocyte count (TLC), 1028t
Total nutrient admixture, 219
Total protein, in chemistry panels, 59–60t
Total urinary nitrogen (TUN), 1028t
Toxic Substances Control Act, 762
Toxin load, 121–122
Toxins
  and fertility, 241–244, 243–244t
  in obesity development and fat loss, 395b
Toxoplasma, during pregnancy, 283b
TPB *see* Theory of planned behavior
TPO *see* Thyroid peroxidase
TPO Abs *see* Thyroid peroxidase antibodies
Trabecular bone, 471, 472f
Trace element(s), 918, 918t, 1028t
  biochemical assessment of, 67–68
    ascorbic acid, 67
    body composition, 68
    B-vitamins, 67–68
  and bone health, 477
  in parenteral solutions, 218–219, 219t
Trachea, 706f
Trail mix, sweet, desserts, and other carbohydrates,
    1053–1054t
Training *see* Exercise and sports performance
Tramadol (Ultram), 1031–1041t
Trans fats, 1057
Trans fatty acids, 121
  and coronary heart disease, 679–680
Transcobalamin I (TCI), 665
Transcobalamin III (TCIII), 665
Transcription, 83–84
Transcription factor(s), 83
Transcription factor 7-like 2 (*TCF7L2*) gene, in
    diabetes mellitus, 97
Transcriptomics, 84b
Transferrin, 64, 1028t
  as inflammatory marker, 1028t
  in iron deficiency anemia, 659
Transferrin receptors, in iron deficiency
    anemia, 659
Transferrin saturation (Tf-sat), 656, 1028t
Transient ischemic attacks (TIAs), 672, 857
Transit time, 9–10
Transitional feeding, 221–222
Translation, 83–84
Translators, 230b
Translocation, 960
Transport
  in large intestine, 4
  in small intestine, 9, 9f
Transport proteins, 9
Transpyloric feeding, 922
Transtheoretical model (TM), 228, 228t
Transthyretin (TTHY), 64
Trauma *see also* Critical illness
  abdominal, 816
  spinal, 847–848t, 864–878

Traumatic brain injury (TBI)
  definition of, 860
  medical management of, 860
  medical nutrition therapy for, 860–864
  pathophysiology of, 860
  role of dietary compounds in, 862–863t
  stress caused by, 860
Trazodone (Desyrel), 1031–1041t
Tree nut, avoidance guidelines for, 508t
TRH *see* Thyrotropin-releasing hormone
Triage theory, 106
Triamterene (Dyrenium), 1031–1041t
Triaxial monitor, for activity-related energy
    expenditure, 21
Tricyclic antidepressants (TCAs), 1031–1041t
Trigeminal nerve, 849t
Triggers, 105
Triglycerides, 1028t
  and cardiovascular disease, 69b
  in chemistry panels, 59–60t
  and coronary heart disease, 673
  with diabetes mellitus, 635t
  digestion and absorption of, 13
Triiodothyronine (T_3), 641–642, 1028t
  enhancing influence on mitochondrial
    bioenergetics of, 651
  improving conversion of T_4 to, 651
  iodine and, 1120
  metabolism of, 643f
  reverse, 641–642
  structure of, 643f
  synthetic, for hypothyroidism, 646t
Trimethylamine-N-oxide (TMAO), and coronary
    heart disease, 676
Tripeptides, digestion and absorption of, 12
Trismus, 778
Trochlear nerve, 849t
Tropical sprue, 558–559
  defined, 558
  medical nutrition therapy for, 559
  medical treatment of, 559
  pathophysiology of, 559
Trypsin, in digestion, 6t
  of proteins, 12
Trypsinogen, activated, in digestion, 6t
Tryptophan (Trp), 939t
TSH *see* Thyroid-stimulating hormone
TTHY *see* Transthyretin
Tube feedings, 213. *see also* Enteral nutrition
Tuberculosis (TB), 717–718
  medical management of, 718
  medical nutrition therapy for, 718
    energy, 718
    protein, 718
    vitamins and minerals, 718
  pathophysiology of, 717–718
Tumor angiogenesis, 758
Tumor burden, 767–768
Tumor necrosis factor-α (TNF-α), 107–109
  in cancer cachexia, 772
  in regulation of body weight, 396–397t
Tumor necrosis factor alpha (*TNF*) gene, in
    inflammatory disorders, 96
Tumor necrosis factor-β (TNF-β), in cancer
    cachexia, 772
Tumor necrosis factor (TNF), in metabolic
    response to stress, 809

Tumor-node-metastasis (TNM) staging system,
    766, 767f
Tumor suppressor genes, 758
Tumor(s)
  benign, 766
  defined, 758
  liquid, 766
  solid, 766
"Tunneled" catheter, 217
Turmeric, 198–205b, 900–901
24-hour recall, 47–48t, 48
Twins, 268–269, 269f
Type 1 diabetes mellitus (T1DM) *see also* Diabetes
    mellitus
  care management algorithm for, 608f
  genetic predisposition to, 607
  honeymoon phase of, 607
  idiopathic, 607
  immune-mediated, 607
  incidence and prevalence of, 607
  nutrition intervention for
    with insulin, 627
    in youth, 627–628
  pathophysiology of, 607, 608f
Type 2 diabetes mellitus (T2DM) *see also* Diabetes
    mellitus
  care management algorithm for, 610f
  exercise guidelines for, 619–620
  glucose-lowering medications for, 620, 621–622t
  incidence and prevalence of, 607
  nutrition intervention for
    with glucose-lowering medications, 627
    with medical nutrition therapy along, 627
    in youth, 628
  and nutritional genomics, 97–98
  pathophysiology of, 609, 610f
  PES statements related to, 155t
  progressive, 614
  risk factors for, 609
Typical antipsychotic agent, 1031–1041t
Tyramine, food intolerance due to, 496–497t, 513
Tyrosine (Tyr)
  in infancy and childhood, 939t
  and thyroid hormones, 642, 642f
Tyrosinemia, type I, 936–938t
TZDs *see* Thiazolidinediones

U

UC *see* Ulcerative colitis
UKPDS *see* United Kingdom Prospective Diabetes
    Study
Ulcer(s)
  decubitus, in older adults, 379, 380t
  duodenal, 536, 536f
  gastric, 536, 536f
  mouth and esophageal, due to HIV infection,
    795t
  peptic, 534–535
    care management algorithm for, 535f
    defined, 534
    emergency symptoms of, 535
    etiology of, 534–535
    gastric *vs.* duodenal, 536–537, 536f
    medical and surgical management of, 536
    medical nutrition therapy for, 536–537
    pathophysiology of, 535f
  stress, 536

Ulcerative colitis (UC), 562–564
  care management algorithm for, 563f
  clinical features of, 562f, 562t
  complications of, 562t
  etiology of, 561–562
  extraintestinal manifestations of, 562t
  gross pathology of, 562t
  histopathology of, 562t
  medical management of, 564
  medical nutrition therapy for, 564–565
  pathophysiology of, 562–564
  and risk of malignancy, 561
  surgical management of, 564
  vs. Crohn's disease, 562t
Ultrafiltrate, 727
Undernutrition, pediatric, 336
Underweight, 415
  assessment of, 415
  cause of, 415
  in childhood, 336
  defined, 415
  management of, 415–416, 416t
    appetite enhancers in, 416
    high-energy diets in, 416–417, 417t
  in older adults, 381–382
Uniaxial monitors, for activity-related energy
    expenditure, 21
Unintentional weight loss, 415–417
  cause of, 415
  management of, 415–416, 416t
    appetite enhancers in, 416
    high-energy diets in, 416–417, 417t
United Kingdom Prospective Diabetes Study
    (UKPDS), 613
Unsaturated fats, 1057
Unstirred water layer (UWL), 13
Unsure-about-change counseling sessions, 233–234
Upper esophageal sphincter (UES), 525
Upper gastrointestinal tract disorders, 525
  clinical case study on, 541–542b
  of esophagus, 525–532
    achalasia as, 525
    anatomy and, 525, 526f
    gastroesophageal reflux and esophagitis as,
        526–531
      etiology of, 526
      medical and surgical management of, 529,
          529f, 529t
      medical nutrition therapy for, 529–531
      pathophysiology of, 526–528
    odynophagia as, 531–532
  head and neck cancer as, 531–532
    medical nutrition therapy for, 532
    pathophysiology of, 531–532
  of stomach, 532–540
    carcinoma as, 537
      medical nutrition therapy for, 537
      pathophysiology of, 537
    dumping syndrome as, 539–540
      clinical case study on, 541–542b
      medical management of, 539
      medical nutrition therapy for, 539–540, 540b
      pathophysiology of, 539
    dyspepsia as, 532–533
      medical nutrition therapy for, 532–533
      pathophysiology of, 532
    endoscopy for, 534, 534b
    gastric surgeries for, 537

Upper gastrointestinal tract disorders (Continued)
    medical nutrition therapy after, 538–539
    types of, 537–539, 538f
  gastritis as, 533–534
    due to Helicobacter pylori, 533
    medical treatment of, 534
    non-Helicobacter pylori, 534
  gastroparesis as, 540–542
    medical management of, 540
    medical nutrition therapy for, 540–542
    pathophysiology of, 540
  peptic ulcers as, 534–535
    care management algorithm for, 535f
    etiology of, 534–535
    gastric vs. duodenal, 536–537, 536f
    medical and surgical management of, 536
    medical nutrition therapy for, 536–537
    pathophysiology of, 535f
Upper motor neurons, 849
Upper respiratory tract, 706f
Urate transporter 1, 838
Urea, in chemistry panels, 59–60t
Urea cycle metabolism, disorders of, 936–938t,
    947–948, 948f
  medical nutrition therapy for, 948
  medical treatment of, 948
  pathophysiology of, 947–948
Urea kinetic modeling (UKM), 1028t
Urea nitrogen, blood
  in chemistry panels, 59–60t
  in end-stage renal disease, 745–747t
Urea reduction ratio (URR)
  in end-stage renal disease, 745–747t
  for evaluation of dialysis efficiency, 742
Urea urinary nitrogen (UUN), 1028t
Uremia, 740
Ureter, nutrition-focused physical examination,
    1003–1008t
Uric acid stones, 729, 731–732, 731t
Uricostatic drugs, 838
Uricosuric drugs, 838
Urinalysis, 61, 62t
  laboratory values for, 1028t
Urinary pH
  diet and, 730b
  and stone formation, 731t
Urinary tract infections (UTIs), spinal cord injury
    and, 856
Urine
  bilirubin in, 62t
  blood in, 62t
  glucose in, 62t
  ketones in, 62t
  leukocyte esterase in, 62t
  nitrite in, 62t
  pH of, 62t
  protein in, 62t
  specific gravity of, 62t
  specimens, 58, 1009
  urobilinogen in, 62t
  water loss through excretion of, 914
Urine volume, with kidney stones, 733
Urobilinogen, urine, 62t, 580–581t
Urolithiasis see Kidney stones
URR see Urea reduction ratio
U.S. Department of Agriculture (USDA)
  dietary recommendations from, 162–163
  Economic Research Service of, 133

U.S. Department of Agriculture (Continued)
  food assistance programs of, 385
  Food Safety and Inspection Service, 142
U.S. Department of Health and Human Services
    (USDHHS), 130
  dietary recommendations from, 162–163
  Older Americans Act (OAA) Nutrition Program
    of, 384–385
Usual body weight (UBW), 71
Uterine environment, during pregnancy, 251–255
Utilization management, 156
UVB light, and vitamin D synthesis, 1114

V

Vagotomy, 538, 538f
  parietal cell, 538
  truncal, 538
Vagus nerve, 121, 538, 849t
  in metabolic response to stress, 809
  in regulation of body weight, 397b
Valganciclovir (Valcyte), 1031–1041t
Valine (Val)
  in infancy and childhood, 939t
  as sports supplement, 462t
Valproic acid (Depakote), 1031–1041t
Valsartan (Diovan), 1031–1041t
Varices, in portal hypertension, 587
Vascular access devices intact, nutrition-focused
    physical examination, 1003–1008t
Vascular dementia, 896, 898
Vascular disease, nutritional genomics and,
    100–101
Vasodilators, peripheral, 1031–1041t
Vasopressin
  in control of water excretion, 727–728
  and water balance, 30
VAT see Visceral adipose tissue
Vegan diets, 180, 677, 1097t
  of adolescents, 353
  in cancer prevention, 765
Vegetable(s)
  in cancer prevention, 765
  and hypertension, 686–688, 687t
  Mediterranean diet and, 1082
  strained and junior, 317
Vegetarian diets, 180
  of adolescents, 352–353, 352f, 353t
  in adults, 368
  and anorexia nervosa, 427
  and bone health, 478
  nutritional facts on, 1095, 1095f, 1096t, 1097t
  planning, 1095–1096, 1095t, 1096t
Vending machine nutrition labeling, 414b
Venlafaxine (Effexor XR), 1031–1041t
Venous access, for central parenteral nutrition,
    217f
Vertebral canal, spinal cord in, 850f
Very-long-chain acyl-CoA dehydrogenase
    deficiency, 936–938t
Very-long-chain fatty acids, 865
Very low birthweight infants
  description of, 912, 913b
  hyperglycemia in, 916
Very-low-calorie diets (VLCDs), 407
Very-low-density lipoproteins (VLDLs), in
    coronary heart disease, 673
Very-low-fat diets, 407
Vestibulocochlear nerve, 849t

Vibrio vulnificus, 136–138t
Victoza (liraglutide), for type 2 diabetes, 620–622, 621–622t
Villi, 3, 5f, 9
Viral load, in HIV, 788
Viruses, and overweight and obesity, 400–401
Vis medicatrix naturae, 187
Visceral adipose tissue (VAT), 109, 394
Viscous (soluble) fiber, 54t
Visfatin, in regulation of body weight, 396–397t
Vision, poor, with aging, 377–378
Vitamin(s), 196, 198–205b
    for adolescence, 346–348, 346t, 347t
    and bone health, 477–478
    burn patient requirements for, 819
    for children, 326–328
    for chronic kidney disease, 740
    for chronic obstructive pulmonary disease, 715–716
    critical illness requirements, 815
    for cystic fibrosis, 711
    deficiencies of, 887
        in alcoholic liver disease, 585b
        in eating disorders, 429
        in end-stage liver disease, 592t, 593
    digestion and absorption of, 13–15
    for end-stage liver disease, 593
    for end-stage renal disease, 749t, 750
    in enteral formulas, 218–219
    for exercise and sports, 456–459
    fat-soluble, 66–67
        biochemical assessment of, 66–67
        vitamin A as, 67
        vitamin D as, 67
        vitamin E as, 67
        vitamin K as, 67
    with HIV, 801
    in human *vs.* cow's milk, 315
    for infants, 313–314
    insufficient intake of, 887
    and kidney stones, 735
    for lactation, 290–291
    in liver metabolism of, 579
    in mental health, 887–889
    for older adults, 383t
    osteoarthritis managed with, 831–832
    in parenteral solutions, 218–219, 218t
    during pregnancy, 259–262
    premature infant requirements for, 918–919, 918t, 921–922, 921t
    in rheumatoid arthritis patients, 836
    and thyroid health, 651
    for tuberculosis, 718
    with twins, 269t
    water-soluble
        biochemical assessment of, 67–68
        in human *vs.* cow's milk, 315
Vitamin A
    animal sources of, 1105t
    and bone health, 477
    burn patient requirements for, 819
    deficiency of
        in end-stage liver disease, 592t, 593
        with HIV, 802t
    food sources of, 1105–1107
    laboratory testing of, 1028t
    nutritional facts on, 1105
    in parenteral solutions, 218t

Vitamin A *(Continued)*
    plant sources of of, 1106t
    during pregnancy, 261
    recommended dietary allowances for, 1105t
    for rheumatic diseases, 827–828
    vitamin D and, 119
Vitamin B$_1$ *see* Thiamin
Vitamin B$_2$ *see* Riboflavin
Vitamin B$_2$ deficiency, 847t
Vitamin B$_3$ *see* Niacin
Vitamin B$_5$ deficiency, 847t
Vitamin B$_6$, 198–205b, 1099
    deficiency of, 847t
        in end-stage liver disease, 592t
    food sources of, 1100t
    functions of, 1099
    for heart failure, 700
    intake of, 1099–1100
    for kidney stones, 735
    nutritional facts on, 1099–1100, 1099t, 1100t
    in parenteral solutions, 218t
    during pregnancy, 260
    recommended dietary allowances for, 1099t
Vitamin B$_6$-responsive anemia, 666–667
Vitamin B$_7$ *see* Biotin
Vitamin B$_9$ *see* Folate
Vitamin B$_9$ deficiency, 847t
Vitamin B$_{12}$, 67–68, 198–205b
    Alzheimer's disease and, 899
    assessment of, 66
    deficiency of, 664–666
        causes of, 665b
        in end-stage liver disease, 592t
        etiology of, 665
        with HIV, 802t
        mental health affected by, 888
        neurologic disorder associated with, 888
        and osteoporosis, 666
        stages of, 662f
        symptoms of, 888
    for exercise and sports, 456
    food sources of, 1100, 1101t
    for heart failure, 700
    hydrochloric acid effects on metabolism of, 1100
    for infants, 313
    laboratory testing of, 1028t
    nutritional facts on, 1100–1101, 1100t, 1101t
    for older adults, 383t
    in parenteral solutions, 218t
    during pregnancy, 260–261
    recommended dietary allowances for, 1100t
    in vegetarian diet, 1096
Vitamin B$_{12}$ balance, negative, 665
Vitamin C, 198–205b
    burn patient requirements for, 819
    and coronary heart disease, 682
    deficiency of, 105
    dietary supplements with, 1109
    food sources of, 1108t
    for hypertension, 691t
    for kidney stones, 735
    laboratory testing of, 1028t
    nutritional facts on, 1108
    recommended intakes of, 1108t
Vitamin D, 198–205b, 1028t
    for adolescence, 347–348
    antiinflammatory effects of, 119

Vitamin D *(Continued)*
    assessment of, 888–889
    and bone health, 477
    calcium and, 1116
    in calcium homeostasis, 472
    in cancer prevention, 122, 764
    for children, 327
    deficiency of
        in adolescents, 348
        in burn patient, 819
        in end-stage liver disease, 592t, 593
        with HIV, 802t
        in rheumatic diseases, 827
    dietary sources of, 119
    for end-stage renal disease, 749t
    for exercise and sports, 458–459, 458b
    for food allergy prevention, 522
    in foods, 1114–1115, 1115t
    functions of, 888
    for heart failure, 700
    for hypertension, 687t, 691t
    for hypothyroidism, 648
    for infants, 313–314
    in inflammation reduction, 119
    for lactation, 290
    mental health and, 888–889
    nutritional facts on, 1114
    for older adults, 383t
    in parenteral solutions, 218t
    preconceptual, 261–262
    during pregnancy, 261–262
        with twins, 269t
    premature infant requirements for, 921
    production of, 119
    recommended dietary allowances for, 1114t
    sun exposure as source of, 888–889
    from sunlight exposure, 1114
    in supplements, 1115
    and thyroid health, 651
    in vegetarian diet, 1096
    vitamin A and, 119
Vitamin D receptors, description of, 119, 122
Vitamin E, 198–205b, 1028t
    and coronary heart disease, 682
    deficiency of
        in end-stage liver disease, 592t
        with HIV, 802t
    for hypertension, 691t
    nutritional facts on, 1110
    in parenteral solutions, 218t
    during pregnancy, 262
        with twins, 269t
    premature infant requirements for, 921–922
    recommended dietary allowances for, 1110t
Vitamin E-responsive hemolytic anemia, 667
Vitamin K, 1028t
    and bone health, 477–478
    deficiency of, in end-stage liver disease, 592t, 593
    dietary reference intakes of, 1112t
    food sources of, 1113t
    infant requirements for, 918
    for infants, 314
    nutritional facts on, 1112
    in parenteral solutions, 218t
    during pregnancy, 262
Vitamin K antagonist, 1031–1041t

Vitamin supplements
  for anorexia nervosa, 433
  for children, 327–328
  for diabetes mellitus, 618
  for end-stage liver disease, 592–593
  for end-stage renal disease, 750
  for infants, 314, 314b
  during pregnancy, 269t
  with restricted-energy diet, 405
VLCDs *see* Very-low-calorie diets
VLDLs *see* Very-low-density lipoproteins
VO₂max (maximum oxygen uptake), 443
Volume equivalents, 980, 980t
Voluntary activity, in regulation of body weight,
    395–397
Vomiting
  chemotherapy induced, 777
  due to HIV infection, 791
  during pregnancy, 274–276
Voriconazole (Vfend), 1031–1041t

W

W-pouch, 574
Waist circumference, 72f, 73
  and obesity, 401
Waist-to-height ratio, 73, 73t
Waist-to-hip ratio (WHR), 73
  and obesity, 401
Warfarin (Coumadin), 96b, 1031–1041t, 1112
Wasted, primarily, 325
Wasting, with HIV, 796
WAT *see* white adipose tissue
Water, 28
  bioterrorism concerns, 140–142
  body, 28–33
  in common foods, 30t
  contamination of, 139
  disaster planning for, 142
  distribution of, 28–29
  extracellular, 28
  fluoride supplement in, 487t
  and food supply, 143
  functions of, 28
  intracellular, 28
  metabolic, 30
  for older adults, 383t
  safety of, 139–142, 141t
  sustainability issues, 142–143
Water balance, 29–31
Water deficits, in infants, 312–313
Water elimination, 31–32
Water intake, 30–31, 30t, 31t
Water intoxication, 31, 313
Water loss, 31
  insensible, 31
  sensible, 31
Water requirements, 33b
  in infancy and childhood, 312–313, 312t
Water-soluble compounds, 1028t
Water-soluble vitamin(s)
  biochemical assessment of, 67–68
  in human *vs.* cow's milk, 315
WBC count *see* White blood cell (WBC)
    count
Weaning
  from breast or bottle to cup, 320
  breastfeeding and, 299

Wear-and-tear theory, of aging, 375t
Weight(s)
  in carcinogenesis, 759–760
  components of, 394–395, 394f
  conversions for, 980t
  in diabetes mellitus, 615
  in eating disorders, 430
  and energy adequacy, 17
  maintaining reduced, 414
  regulation of, 395–397
Weight cycling, 414–415
Weight discrimination, 403
Weight gain
  in adults, 368
  in anorexia nervosa
    assessment of, 430–431, 430b
    medical nutrition therapy for, 432
  by infants, 310
  during pregnancy, 266–269, 266f, 267t
Weight goals, 403
Weight imbalance
  excessive leanness or unintentional weight loss
      as, 415–417
    assessment of, 415
    cause of, 415
    management of, 415–416, 416t
      appetite enhancers for, 416
      high-energy diets for, 416–417, 417t
  overweight and obesity as *see* Obesity; Overweight
Weight loss
  and coronary heart disease, 682, 683b
  due to HIV infection, 795t
  for hypertension, 687t, 688
  by infants, 310
  interpretation of, 1001–1002t
  for obesity, 394f
    bariatric surgery in, 411, 413t
      gastric bypass, gastroplasty, and gastric
          banding as, 411–413, 412f, 413t
    common problems in
      maintaining reduced body weight as, 414
      plateau effect as, 414
      weight cycling as, 414–415
    dietary modification in, 404–405
      commercial programs of, 405, 406f
      intermittent fasting as, 406
      meal replacement programs as, 405
      popular diets and practices in, 406, 408t
      restricted-energy diets as, 404–405
      very-low-calorie diets as, 407
      very low-calorie diets of, 405–406
    goals of, 403
    lifestyle modification in, 404
    pharmacotherapy in, 409
    physical activity in, 407–409, 409f
    rate and extent of, 403–404
  osteoarthritis managed with, 831–832
  during pregnancy, 267
  rate and extent of, 403–404
  in Sjögren syndrome, 837
  unintentional, 415–417
    assessment of, 415
    cause of, 415
    management of, 415–416, 416t
      appetite enhancers in, 416
      high-energy diets in, 416–417, 417t
Weight loss programs, 404

Weight maintenance, for older adults, 381–382
Weight maintenance TEE, 23–24b
Weight management
  for athletes, 445–446, 446t
  in children, 415
  clinical case study on, 417b
  for excessive leanness or unintentional weight
      loss, 415–417, 416t
    appetite enhancers for, 416
    high-energy diets for, 416–417, 417t
  in nutrition, 391
  for obesity, 403–415
    bariatric surgery in, 411, 413t
      gastric bypass, gastroplasty, and gastric
          banding as, 411–413, 412f, 413t
    common problems in
      maintaining reduced body weight as, 414
      plateau effect as, 414
      weight cycling as, 414–415
    dietary modification in, 404–405
      commercial programs of, 405, 406f
      intermittent fasting as, 406
      meal replacement programs as, 405
      popular diets and practices in, 406, 408t
      restricted-energy diets as, 404–405
      very-low-calorie diets as, 407
      very low-calorie diets of, 405–406
    foundation in nutritional medicine, 392–393
    goals of, 403
    lifestyle modification in, 404
    pharmacotherapy in, 409
    physical activity in, 407–409, 409f
    rate and extent of weight loss in,
        403–404
  regulatory factors involved in, 396–397t
Weight measurements
  with developmental disabilities, 957
  direct methods for, 991
Weir equation, 19–20
Wellness, in adults, 365
Wellness Councils of America (WELCOA), 365
Wernicke encephalopathy, 593, 887
Wernicke-Korsakoff syndrome, 847–848t, 847t, 857
Wet beriberi, 847t
What We Eat in America, 131
Wheal and flare reaction, 515
Wheat, avoidance guidelines for, 508t
Wheel of Five (Netherlands), 169f
Whey proteins, in human *vs.* cow's milk, 315
WHI *see* Women's Health Initiative
Whipped topping, free foods and, 1059t
Whipple procedure, 602
Whipple's triad, 636
White adipose tissue (WAT), 394
White blood cell (WBC) count, 61t
Whole blood specimens, 58
Whole grains, Mediterranean diet and, 1082
Whole milk, 1052–1053t
WHR *see* Waist-to-hip ratio
Wilson's disease, 586, 847t
Wine, alcohol and, 1061t
Wolfram's syndrome, 93
Women
  estimated energy requirement for, 23–24b
  health of, nutritional factors affecting, 367–368
  HIV in, 802–803
    postpartum and other considerations with, 803

Women (Continued)
 preconception and prenatal considerations
   with, 803
 sexual maturation of, 342
 weight gain by, 368
Women's Health Initiative (WHI), 761
Work, return to, breastfeeding with, 299–300
Work-life balance, 365, 366f
Worksheet, for nutrition prescription, for
   diabetes, 630f, 631f
World Health Organization (WHO), obesity
   and, 367
Wound management, for burns, 817
Written communication tools, 183

X

X-inactivation, 90
X-linked dominant disorders, 93
X-linked recessive disorders, 94
Xanthan gum, 856
Xanthomas, in familial hypercholesterolemia,
   674
Xenical *see* Orlistat
Xenical (orlistat)
 for prediabetes, 613
 for weight loss, 408t, 409

Xenobiotics, 121
Xerostomia, 486, 490, 770–771, 775
 with aging, 378
 due to medications, 486, 490b
 in Sjögren syndrome, 837
Xylitol, as anticariogenic food, 484

Y

Y-linked inheritance disorders, 94
Yersinia enterocolitica, 136–138t
Yo-yo effect, 414–415
Youth *see* Children

Z

Zantac (ranitidine), 1031–1041t
Zinc (Zn), 198–205b
 absorption of, 14
 antiinflammatory effects of, 119
 for children, 327
 for cystic fibrosis, 711
 deficiency of, 119, 819, 847t
   in anorexia nervosa, 429
   in end-stage liver disease, 592t
   with HIV, 802t
 depression and, 903
 dietary recommended intakes for, 1130

Zinc (Continued)
 food sources of, 1130t
 for infants, 313
 laboratory testing of, 1028t
 for lactation, 290–291
 mental health and, 889
 nutritional facts on, 1130
 for older adults, 383t
 in parenteral solutions, 219t
 during pregnancy, 266
   with twins, 269t
 recommended dietary allowance for,
   1130t
Zinc supplementation
 for sickle cell anemia, 668
 for Wilson's disease, 586
Ziprasidone (Geodon), 1031–1041t
Zithromax (azithromycin), 1031–1041t
Zn *see* Zinc
Zocor (simvastatin), 1031–1041t
Zoledronic acid (Reclast), 1031–1041t
Zoloft (sertraline), 1031–1041t
Zolpidem (Ambien), 1031–1041t
The Zone, 407
Zyprexa (olanzapine), 1031–1041t
Zyvox (linezolid), 1031–1041t

Dietary Reference Intakes (DRIs): Acceptable Macronutrient Distribution Ranges

Food and Nutrition Board, Institute of Medicine, National Academies

Macronutrient	RANGE (PERCENT OF ENERGY)		
	Children, 1-3 yr	Children, 4-18 yr	Adults
Fat	30-40	25-35	20-35
n-6 polyunsaturated fatty acids[a] (linoleic acid)	5-10	5-10	5-10
n-3 polyunsaturated fatty acids[a] (α-linolenic acid)	0.6-1.2	0.6-1.2	0.6-1.2
Carbohydrate	45-65	45-65	45-65
Protein	5-20	10-30	10-35

Source: *Dietary Reference Intakes for Energy, Carbohydrate, Fiber, Fat, Fatty Acids, Cholesterol, Protein, and Amino Acids* (2002/2005). The report may be accessed via www.nap.edu.
[a]Approximately 10% of the total can come from longer-chain *n*-3 or *n*-6 fatty acids.

Dietary Reference Intakes (DRIs): Acceptable Macronutrient Distribution Ranges

Food and Nutrition Board, Institute of Medicine, National Academies

Macronutrient	Recommendation
Dietary cholesterol	As low as possible while consuming a nutritionally adequate diet
Trans fatty acids	As low as possible while consuming a nutritionally adequate diet
Saturated fatty acids	As low as possible while consuming a nutritionally adequate diet
Added sugars[a]	Limit to no more than 25% of total energy

Source: *Dietary Reference Intakes for Enemy, Carbohydrate, Fiber, Fat, Fatty Acids, Cholesterol, Protein, and Amino Acids* (2002/2005). The report may be accessed via www.nap.edu.
[a]Not a recommended intake. A daily intake of added sugars that individuals should aim for to achieve a healthful diet was not set.

Dietary Reference Intakes (DRIs): Tolerable upper Intake Levels, Vitamins*
Food and Nutrition Board, Institute of Medicine, National Academies

Life Stage Group	Vitamin A (mcg/d)[a]	Vitamin C (mg/d)	Vitamin D (IU/d)	Vitamin E (mg/d)[b,c]	Niacin (mg/d)[c]	Vitamin B_6 (mg/d)	Folate (mcg/d)[c]	Choline (g/d)
Infants								
Birth to 6 mo	600	ND[e]	1000	ND	ND	ND	ND	ND
6 to 12 mo	600	ND	1500	ND	ND	ND	ND	ND
Children								
1-3 yr	600	400	2500	200	10	30	300	1.0
4-8 yr	900	650	3000	300	15	40	400	1.0
Males								
9-13 yr	1700	1200	4000	600	20	60	600	2.0
14-18 yr	2800	1800	4000	800	30	80	800	3.0
19-30 yr	3000	2000	4000	1000	35	100	1000	3.5
31-50 yr	3000	2000	4000	1000	35	100	1000	3.5
51-70 yr	3000	2000	4000	1000	35	100	1000	3.5
>70 yr	3000	2000	4000	1000	35	100	1000	3.5
Females								
9-13 yr	1700	1200	4000	600	20	60	600	2.0
14-18 yr	2800	1800	4000	800	30	80	800	3.0
19-30 yr	3000	2000	4000	1000	35	100	1000	3.5
31-50 yr	3000	2000	4000	1000	35	100	1000	3.5
51-70 yr	3000	2000	4000	1000	35	100	1000	3.5
>70 yr	3,000	2000	4000	1000	35	100	1000	3.5
Pregnancy								
14-18 yr	2800	1800	4000	800	30	80	800	3.0
19-30 yr	3000	2000	4000	1000	35	100	1000	3.5
31-50 yr	3000	2000	4000	1000	35	100	1000	3.5
Lactation								
14-18 yr	2,800	1,800	4000	800	30	80	800	3.0
19-30 yr	3,000	2,000	4000	1000	35	100	1000	3.5
31-50 yr	3,000	2,000	4000	1000	35	100	1000	3.5

NOTE: A Tolerable Upper Intake Level (UL) is the highest level of daily nutrient intake that is likely to pose no risk of adverse health effects to almost all individuals in the general population. Unless otherwise specified, the UL represents total intake from food, water, and supplements. Due to a lack of suitable data, ULs could not be established for vitamin K, thiamin, riboflavin, vitamin B_{12}, pantothenic acid, biotin, and carotenoids. In the absence of a UL, extra caution may be warranted in consuming levels above recommended intakes. Members of the general population should be advised not to routinely exceed the UL. The UL is not meant to apply to individuals who are treated with the nutrient under medical supervision or to individuals with predisposing conditions that modify their sensitivity to the nutrient.

*The tolerable upper intake levels for the following nutrients have not been determined: vitamin K, thiamin, riboflavin, vitamin B_{12}, pantothenic acid, biotin, and the carotenoids. The levels have not been determinable due to lack of data of adverse effects in this age group and concern with regard to lack of ability to handle excess amounts. Source of intake should be from food only to prevent high levels of intake.

[a]As preformed vitamin A only.

[b]As α-tocopherol; applies to any form of supplemental -tocopherol.

[c]The ULs for vitamin E, niacin, and folate apply to synthetic forms obtained from supplements, fortified foods, or a combination of the two.

[d]β-Carotene supplements are advised only to serve as a provitamin A source for individuals at risk of vitamin A deficiency.

SOURCES: *Dietary Reference Intakes for Calcium, Phosphorus, Magnesium, Vitamin D, and Fluoride* (1997); *Dietary Reference Intakes for Thiamin, Riboflavin, Niacin, Vitamin B_6, Folate, Vitamin B_{12}, Pantothenic Acid, Biotin, and Choline* (1998); *Dietary Reference Intakes for Vitamin C, Vitamin E, Selenium, and Carotenoids* (2000); *Dietary Reference Intakes for Vitamin A, Vitamin K, Arsenic, Boron, Chromium, Copper, Iodine, Iron, Manganese, Molybdenum, Nickel, Silicon, Vanadium, and Zinc* (2001); and *Dietary Reference Intakes for Calcium and Vitamin D* (2011). These reports may be accessed via www.nap.edu.